VOLUME 6

3rd Edition

DIAGNOSIS OF BONE AND JOINT DISORDERS

Donald Resnick, M.D.

Professor of Radiology
University of California, San Diego
Chief of Osteoradiology Section
Veterans Administration Medical Center
San Diego, California

With the Editorial Assistance of Catherine F. Fix
With the Technical Assistance of Debra J. Trudell

W.B. SAUNDERS COMPANY
A Division of Harcourt Brace & Company
Philadelphia   London   Toronto   Montreal   Sydney   Tokyo

W.B. SAUNDERS COMPANY
A Division of
Harcourt Brace & Company

The Curtis Center
Independence Square West
Philadelphia, Pennsylvania 19106

Library of Congress Cataloging-in-Publication Data

Resnick, Donald

Diagnosis of bone and joint disorders / Donald Resnick.—3rd ed.

p. cm.

Includes bibliographical references and indexes.

ISBN 0–7216–5066–X (set)

1. Musculoskeletal system—Diseases—Diagnosis.   2. Bones—Diseases—
   Diagnosis.   3. Joints—Diseases—Diagnosis.   4. Diagnostic
   imaging.   I. Title.

[DNLM: 1. Bone Diseases—diagnosis.   2. Joint Diseases—diagnosis.
3. Diagnosis Imaging.   WE 300 R434d 1995]

RC925.7.R47 1995

616.7′1075—dc20

DNLM/DLC   93–48321

Diagnosis of Bone and Joint Disorders, 3rd edition

Volume One	ISBN	0–7216–5067–8
Volume Two	ISBN	0–7216–5068–6
Volume Three	ISBN	0–7216–5069–4
Volume Four	ISBN	0–7216–5070–8
Volume Five	ISBN	0–7216–5071–6
Volume Six	ISBN	0–7216–5072–4
Six Volume Set	ISBN	0–7216–5066–X

Printed in the United States of America.

Last digit is the print number: 9   8   7   6   5   4   3   2   1

CONTENTS

▼

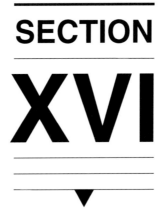

SECTION
XVI

Tumors and Tumor-Like Diseases

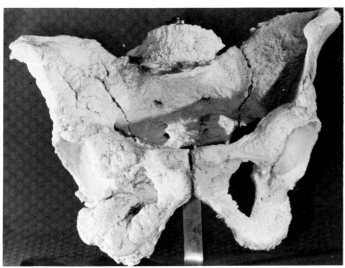

A

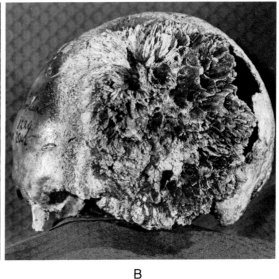

B

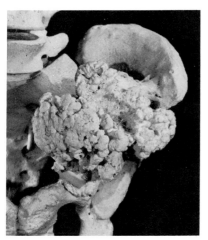

C

A Skeletal metastasis from carcinoma of the prostate: Note diffuse nodular hyperostosis with enlargement of the bones of the pelvis.
B Osteosarcoma: Irregular tumor bone projects outward from the frontoparietal area. It also extends from the inner aspect of the cranial vault.
C Osteosarcoma: A pedunculated lesion arises from the ilium. (From Ortner DJ, Putschar WGJ: Identification of Pathological Conditions in Human Skeletal Remains. Washington, DC, Smithsonian Institution Press, 1981.)

82

Tumors and Tumor-Like Lesions of Bone: Radiographic Principles

Donald Resnick, M.D.

Owing to the great number of tumors and tumor-like lesions of bone, accurate diagnosis of the nature of the process on the basis of its radiographic characteristics or features evident on other imaging studies often is not possible. Data concerning the patient's history, physical examination, and laboratory evaluation must be considered during the interpretation of the radiographs and, in many instances, findings provided by histologic analysis of material derived from closed or open biopsy procedures are required. In no other area of musculoskeletal disease is the cooperation of the orthopedic surgeon, radiologist, and pathologist more important. Any of the three specialists working independently of the others is more likely to err. The "Aunt Minnie" approach to the interpretation of the radiographs, in which a diagnosis is offered immediately because of the similarity of the findings to those remembered from a previous case, relies on an accurate memory and considerable examiner experience and ignores the possibility that Aunt Minnie may have close relatives or other look-alikes and the fact that bone responds to the insult of disease in only a limited number of ways.

Although the radiographic findings may not allow a simple, precise diagnosis in a patient with a tumor or tumor-like lesion, they do provide reliable information regarding its aggressiveness or rate of growth,[1] and this information, coupled with data reflecting the site of the lesion and the age of the patient, allows the formulation of a reasonable diagnosis in most cases. A note of warning in this analysis is required. Although aggressive lesions commonly are malignant and benign tumors commonly are nonaggressive, this is not uniformly true. Rapid osseous expansion, an aggressive characteristic, can occur in nonmalignant conditions such as an aneurysmal bone cyst. Similarly, a rim of bone sclerosis about a lesion is a nonaggressive characteristic that, in rare circumstances, becomes evident in malignant neoplasms. Furthermore, osteomyelitis frequently is associated with poorly demarcated osteolysis and periostitis, findings resembling those of a malignant tumor.

The solitary bone lesion often is a tumor or is tumor-like in nature, although congenital, inflammatory, ischemic, and traumatic disorders of bone also can appear in this fashion. Obviously, the initial step in the radiographic diagnosis of the solitary lesion is deciding if the finding really is present or an artifact of the x-ray technique (is there a lesion?). Subsequent diagnostic steps include an analysis of the behavior of the lesion (is it aggressive or nonaggressive?), a decision regarding the need for pathologic inspection (is a biopsy necessary and, if so, from what site(s)?), and some consideration regarding the likelihood of the proposed pathologic diagnosis (are the histologic findings compatible with those of the radiographs?).

In the pages that follow, it is the answer to the second question—regarding the aggressiveness of the process, on the basis of its appearance on conventional radiographs—that will be emphasized.[2–4] The role of other diagnostic techniques, such as xeroradiography, scintigraphy, CT, and MR imaging, in the evaluation of musculoskeletal neoplasms, has been commented on in earlier chapters and will be illustrated in Chapter 83, in which individual lesions are discussed.

MORPHOLOGY

Morphologic features that aid in the differential diagnosis of osseous tumors and tumor-like lesions include, among others, the pattern of bone destruction, the presence and nature of visible tumor matrix or periosteal response, the pattern of cortical erosion, expansion, or penetration, and the presence and characteristics of an adjacent soft tissue mass. These features have been extremely well summarized by Lodwick and collaborators,[5–7] who applied them to the computer analysis of bone and joint neoplasms. Many of their concepts are included in this discussion.

Pattern of Bone Destruction

The radiograph is not extremely sensitive in the detection of small amounts of bone destruction, especially if the destructive focus is located in cancellous bone.[8] Cortical lesions are detected more readily than those in cancellous bone (Fig. 82–1). In some sites, such as the diaphyses of tubular bones, few trabeculae are present in the medullary canal so that radiographic identification of a lesion is extremely difficult. In fact, the detection of a sharply margin-ated radiolucent area overlying the medullary portion of a tubular bone in a single radiographic projection almost always implies cortical involvement, which readily becomes apparent when a second projection is obtained. In certain sites, such as the ribs and spine, technical factors, including the size or thickness of the body part, and the presence of considerable overlying shadows accentuate the radiograph's insensitivity in delineating small lesions. Still, even with optimal technique, the destruction of all cancellous trabec-ulae may not be detected with routine radiography if the surrounding cortex is not affected.

Three radiographic patterns of bone destruction have been identified: geographic, motheaten, and permeative.[5]

Geographic Bone Destruction (Fig. 82–2). The geographic pattern is the least aggressive pattern of bone destruction, and it generally is indicative of a slow-growing lesion. The margin of the lesion is well defined and easily separated from the surrounding normal bone. This margin may be smooth or irregular, but in either instance, it usually is clearly demarcated, with a short zone of transition from

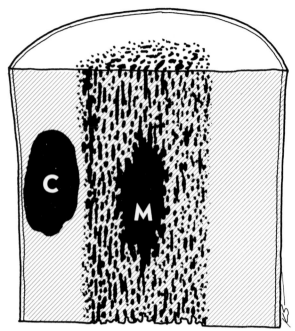

FIGURE 82–1. Cortical versus medullary involvement. A lesion in the medullary bone (M) may be more difficult to recognize than one in the cortical bone (C). In addition, a nonaggressive cortical lesion will produce a sharp interface with the surrounding bone, whereas such a lesion in the medullary bone may not.

normal to abnormal bone. In some instances, a sclerotic margin of variable thickness surrounds the lesion. The thicker and more complete the sclerotic margin, the less aggressive is the process. Benign bone tumors usually demonstrate geographic bone destruction. Malignant diseases (such as plasma cell myeloma and metastasis) and osteomyelitis (particularly granulomatous infections) can demonstrate a similar pattern of bone destruction, however.

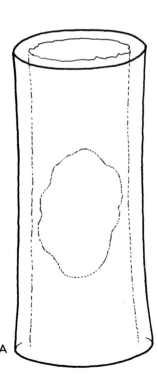

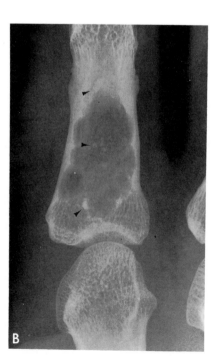

FIGURE 82–2. Geographic bone destruction.
  A This pattern of bone destruction is characterized by well-defined lesional margins and a short zone of transition from normal to abnormal bone.
  B The lesion in the proximal phalanx demonstrates geographic bone destruction, a central location, lobulated margins, and small foci of calcification (arrowheads). (Final diagnosis—enchondroma.)

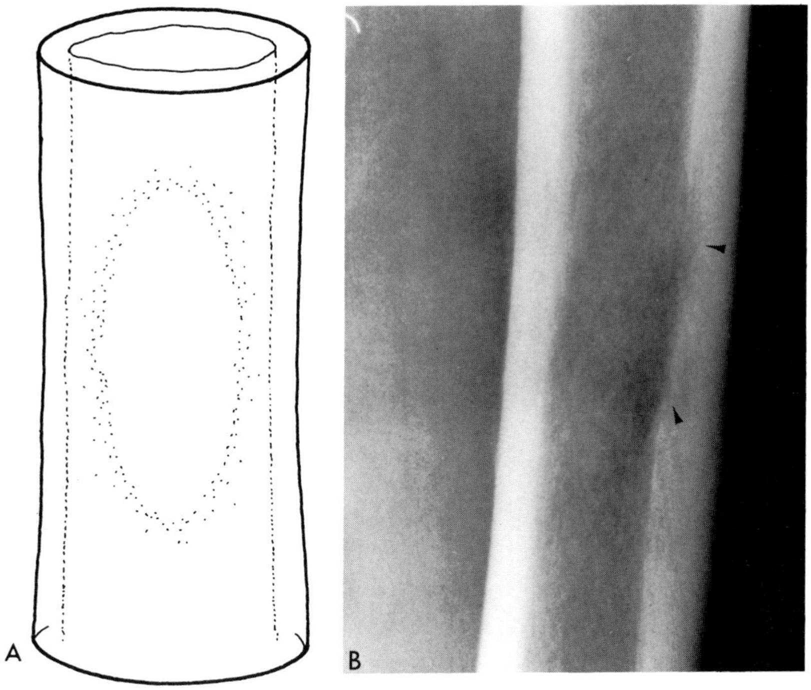

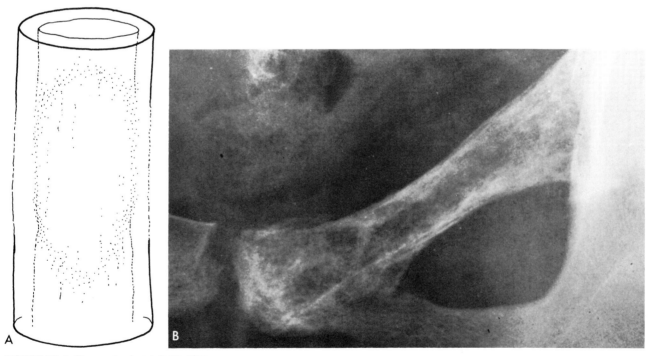

FIGURE 82–3. Motheaten bone destruction.

A This pattern of bone destruction is associated with lesional margins that are less well defined and a longer zone of transition from normal to abnormal bone.

B A lesion with motheaten bone destruction is identified in this femur. Note its poorly defined margins and its erosion of the endosteal margin of the cortex (arrowheads.) (Final diagnosis—histiocytic lymphoma.)

Motheaten Bone Destruction (Fig. 82–3). The motheaten pattern is a more aggressive pattern of bone destruction, characteristic of a lesion that is growing more rapidly than one that demonstrates geographic bone destruction. The motheaten pattern of bone destruction is associated with a less well defined or demarcated lesional margin and with a longer zone of transition from normal to abnormal bone. Malignant bone tumors and osteomyelitis may demonstrate the motheaten pattern of bone destruction. Some benign processes, such as eosinophilic granuloma, may be associated with motheaten bone destruction, however.

Permeative Bone Destruction (Fig. 82–4). The permeative pattern indicates an aggressive bone lesion with rapid growth potential. The lesion is poorly demarcated and not easily separated from the surrounding normal bone. In fact, it may merge imperceptibly with uninvolved osseous seg-

FIGURE 82–4. Permeative bone destruction.

A This pattern of bone destruction is associated with very poorly defined lesional margins and a very long zone of transition from normal to abnormal bone.

B The lesion in the superior pubic ramus reveals permeative bone destruction with cortical erosion, periostitis, and a soft tissue mass. (Final diagnosis—histiocytic lymphoma.)

ments, creating a zone of transition that is very long. Its true size is larger than that evident on the radiographs. Certain malignant bone tumors, such as Ewing's sarcoma, may demonstrate permeative bone destruction. Osteomyelitis and rapidly developing osteoporosis, as in reflex sympathetic dystrophy, may reveal permeative bone destruction, however.

Size, Shape, and Margin of Lesion

Lodwick[5] has indicated that size and shape of the lesion can be useful in differential diagnosis. In general, primary malignant tumors of bone are larger than benign tumors and may be greater than 6 cm in size when first discovered. Although the shape of a lesion is a relatively poor guide to its nature, elongated lesions, in which the greatest lesional diameter is at least 1.5 times the smallest diameter, may be indicative of Ewing's sarcoma, histiocytic lymphoma, chondrosarcoma, and angiosarcoma. Osteomyelitis, including a Brodie's abscess, however, may be elongated.

The growth rate of a lesion is of great importance in assessing the aggressiveness of any skeletal process. Although radiographs obtained at a particular time do provide clues regarding growth rate, more accurate information requires serial examinations, which, when available, generally imply indecision or procrastination on the part of the physician. Benign tumors usually grow more slowly than malignant tumors, or they may show no change in size over a long period of observation; however, exceptions to this rule are encountered. Plasma cell myeloma occasionally is associated with slow growth, and histologically low grade or benign giant cell tumors may enlarge rapidly.

Slowly growing lesions can be associated with reactive sclerosis of the surrounding normal bone. The sclerotic margin can be of variable thickness and may surround the bone lesion partially or completely. A vigorous bony reaction is especially characteristic of cortical osteoid osteomas, and this reaction may obscure the radiolucent nidus of the lesion.

Presence and Nature of Visible Tumor Matrix

Certain tumors produce matrix that calcifies or ossifies.[5, 9] The resulting radiodense areas must be distinguished from calcification that may develop in regions of necrotic or degenerative tissue, from callus formation that may indicate the presence of a pathologic fracture, and from a sclerotic response of non-neoplastic bone to the adjacent tumorous deposit. In the last of these situations, the bone is formed by the host's normal osteoblasts and has the capacity to be remodeled into lamellar bone.[9]

Certain cartilage tumors are associated with matrix calcification (Fig. 82–5). These include chondromas, chondroblastomas, chondrosarcomas, and, less frequently, chondromyxoid fibromas. In most instances, the frequency and extent of pathologically evident calcification are greater than the frequency and extent of radiographically evident calcification. Cartilage matrix calcification frequently is located centrally and may appear as ringlike, flocculent, or flecklike radiodense areas.[12] Similar findings can be apparent within the cartilaginous cap of an osteochondroma. In some instances, ossification occurring as a result of endochondral bone formation may accompany cartilage tumors.[9]

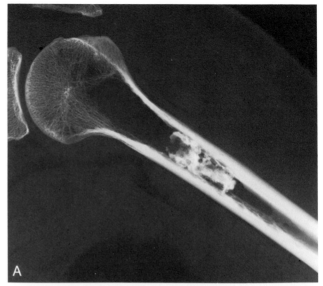

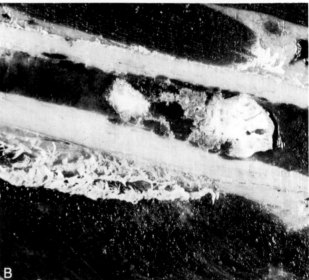

FIGURE 82–5. Matrix calcification. A sectional radiograph and photograph of a coronal section of the humerus reveal a centrally located tumor containing calcification. (Final diagnosis—enchondroma).

Such ossification is more frequent in benign lesions than in malignant lesions and arises through calcification of the pathologic cartilage and its subsequent transformation into bone.[9]

Visible tumor matrix also is associated with neoplastic bone.[5] Primary formation of pathologic bone by neoplastic cells of osteogenic cell origin leads to direct deposition as woven bone and does not develop by endochondral bone formation.[9] Examples of neoplasms producing such tumor matrix are osteosarcomas, parosteal osteosarcomas, ossifying fibromas, osteomas, and osteoblastomas. The resulting radiodense collections are of variable size; they may occupy an entire lesion or a part of a lesion and can be inhomogeneous or homogeneous.

Certain lesions, such as fibrous dysplasia, can be accompanied by a uniform increase in radiodensity, an appearance that is designated the ground-glass pattern. This pattern is associated with obscuration or obliteration of neighboring trabeculae.

Internal or External Trabeculation

Within or around the lesion, trabeculated shadows may be identified on the radiograph. In some instances, these reflect the location of residual trabeculae that have been modified or displaced by the neighboring tumor. In other instances, the trabeculation represents new bone formation evoked as a response to the presence of a nearby neoplasm. Such bony proliferation frequently is located at the interface between the endosteal and periosteal envelopes.[5] The location and appearance of the trabeculation provide information regarding the nature of the neoplasm (Table 82–1). For example, giant cell tumors commonly are associated with delicate or thin trabeculae (Fig. 82–6A), chondromyxoid fibromas and desmoplastic fibromas (Fig. 82–7) can be accompanied by coarse or thick trabeculae, and aneurysmal bone cysts can be characterized by horizontally oriented, delicate trabeculation extending into the surrounding soft tissues. Hemangiomas can stimulate a coarse periosteal response leading to a honeycombed, striated, or radiating appearance (Figs. 82–6B and 82–7), and nonossifying fibromas may reveal lobulated trabeculation (Fig. 82–6C).

Cortical Erosion, Penetration, and Expansion

The bony cortex can serve as an effective barrier to the further lateral growth of certain tumors, whereas in other instances, the neoplasm may penetrate the cortex partially or completely. Nonaggressive medullary lesions may provoke little change in the endosteal surface of the cortex and, in fact, may extend in a path of least resistance within the medullary canal. Other slow-growing lesions, such as enchondromas, can lead to lobulated erosion of the inner margin of the cortex, producing a scalloped endosteal margin, which may be associated with uniform periosteal proliferation or buttressing of the outer cortical surface. If progressive endosteal erosion is associated with periosteal bone deposition, an expanded osseous contour can be created. The rate of bone expansion is variable. Certain tumors expand bone very slowly, and the accompanying periosteal response eventually may produce a surrounding cortical shell of such thickness that further expansion of the cortex is resisted. Other lesions, such as an aneurysmal bone cyst, cause very rapid bone expansion.

Aggressive bone lesions can penetrate the entire thickness of the cortex in one or more places. As the tumor reaches the outer aspect of the cortex, the periosteal membrane may be elevated, leading to a variety of patterns of periosteal new bone formation.

Periosteal Response (Fig. 82–8)

Lodwick[5] has characterized the various patterns of periosteal response to adjacent tumor. A slowly growing tumor

TABLE 82–1. Some Trabeculated Lesions

Lesion	Pattern
Giant cell tumor	Delicate, thin
Chondromyxoid fibroma	Coarse, thick
Desmoplastic fibroma	Coarse, thick
Nonossifying fibroma	Lobulated
Aneurysmal bone cyst	Delicate, horizontally oriented
Hemangioma	Striated, radiating

that is eroding or penetrating the cortex can evoke a periosteal response in which additional layers of new bone are added to the exterior, creating an expanded osseous contour. In these instances, the ultimate thickness of the surrounding cortical bone depends on the extent of endosteal erosion and periosteal proliferation. It can be of diminished or of ''normal'' thickness compared with the original thickness of the cortex, or the new cortex can be thickened in a uniform or nonuniform fashion. If the interface between the normal and expanded cortex is ''filled in'' with bone, a buttressed pattern has evolved. The buttressed pattern is not specific for a particular tumor or tumor-like lesion, although it is encountered regularly in cases of eosinophilic granuloma involving tubular bones. With more rapid tumor growth, the periosteal response may be characterized by delicate layers of new bone. Single or multiple laminated bone formation may be identified. Multiple concentric layers of periosteal new bone produce the onion-peel pattern,[5] which has been interpreted by some investigators to indicate alternating periods of rapid and slow growth,[10] although others regard it as indicating only an acceleration of the normal periosteal bone response.[11] The onion-peel pattern can be identified in some cases of Ewing's sarcoma and osteosarcoma.

At the edges or periphery of a neoplasm or an infective focus, a triangular elevation of the periosteum may be identified, termed Codman's triangle. In these cases, histologic evaluation frequently will confirm that the periosteum has been elevated by adjacent neoplasm, although the subperiosteal area in the region of the Codman's triangle itself is free of tumor.

In some patients with aggressive bone tumors, delicate rays of periosteal bone formation can form, separated by spaces containing blood vessels.[5] In certain neoplasms, such as osteosarcoma, the rays extend away from the bone in a radiating or sunburst pattern, emanating from a single focus in the bone; in other neoplasms, such as Ewing's sarcoma, the rays extend in a direction perpendicular to the underlying bone, creating a hair-on-end periosteal pattern.

Soft Tissue Mass

Soft tissue masses not infrequently are associated with malignant bone neoplasms. In some tumors, such as histiocytic lymphoma, the masses may be quite large at the time of clinical presentation, as other physical signs and symptoms are not marked. In other tumors, considerable pain and tenderness may lead a patient to the hospital quickly, so that the finding of a small mass or even no mass cannot be regarded as a uniformly good prognostic sign. Osteomyelitis also is associated with a soft tissue mass or swelling. Although radiographic characteristics that may separate an inflammatory mass from a neoplastic mass have been identified, these are not extremely reliable and often depend on modification of the imaging technique to optimize soft tissue detail or use of other diagnostic techniques, such as low kV radiography, xeroradiography, CT, or MR imaging. A soft tissue mass related to tumor may reveal displacement of adjacent soft tissue planes, whereas one related to infection may be associated with distortion or obliteration of these planes.

Text continued on page 3623

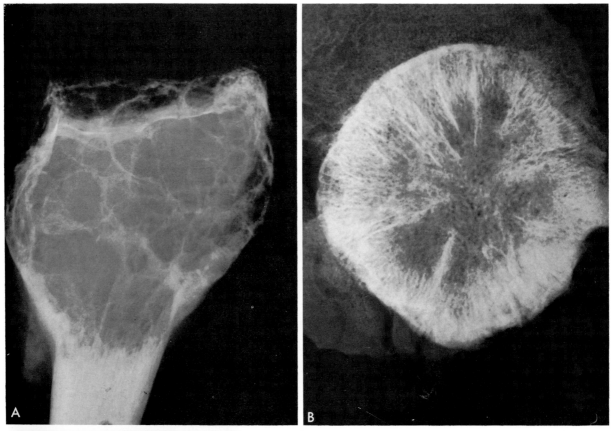

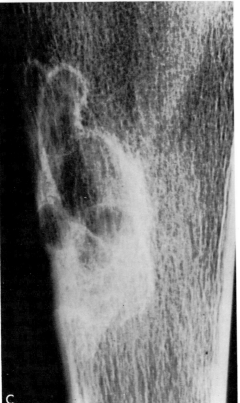

FIGURE 82–6. Trabeculation.

A Giant cell tumor. Note delicate trabeculae that extend through and around this lesion of the distal portion of the radius (specimen radiograph).

B Hemangioma. Observe the radiating pattern of trabeculation associated with this lesion of the cranial vault (specimen radiograph).

C Nonossifying fibroma. A lobulated pattern of trabeculation characterizes this lesion of the proximal portion of the tibia (specimen radiograph).

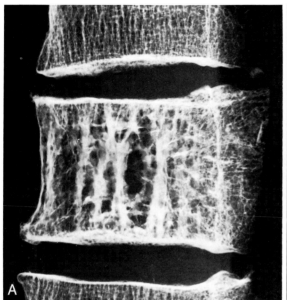
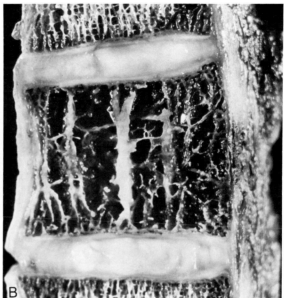

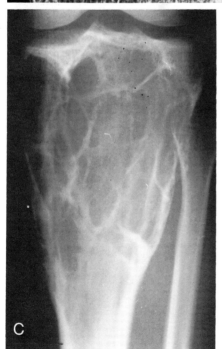

FIGURE 82–7. Trabeculation.

A, B Hemangioma. A specimen radiograph **(A)** and photograph **(B)** show the typical "corduroy" appearance of a vertebral body that contains a hemangioma. Accentuation of the vertical trabecular pattern is present.

C Desmoplastic fibroma. Note the coarse trabeculation that characterizes this lesion.

(**C,** Courtesy of B. Flanagan, M.D., Los Angeles, California.)

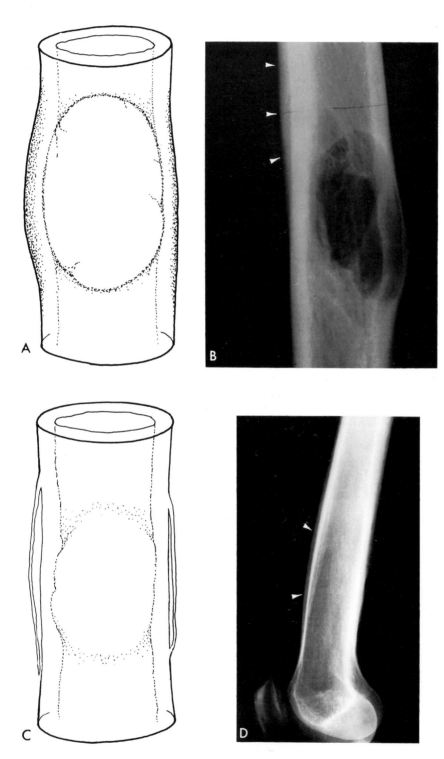

FIGURE 82–8. Periosteal response.

A, B Periosteal buttressing. The diagram **(A)** indicates that periosteal bone formation in response to a lesion may merge with the underlying cortex, producing a buttressed appearance. On the radiograph **(B)**, a thick single layer of periosteal bone (arrowheads) about this femoral lesion still is separated from the underlying cortex. The thickness of the periosteal response would indicate a relatively slow-growing lesion. (Final diagnosis—simple bone cyst.)

C, D Single layer of periosteal bone. The diagram **(C)** demonstrates the appearance of a single thin layer of periosteal bone about a lesion, separated from the underlying bone. The radiograph **(D)** indicates a single layer of periosteal bone on both the anterior and posterior surfaces of the femur. Anteriorly, the periosteal layer is quite thick and still separated from the underlying bone (arrowheads). Posteriorly, the periosteal bone has merged with the femur. (Final diagnosis—hypertrophic osteoarthropathy.)

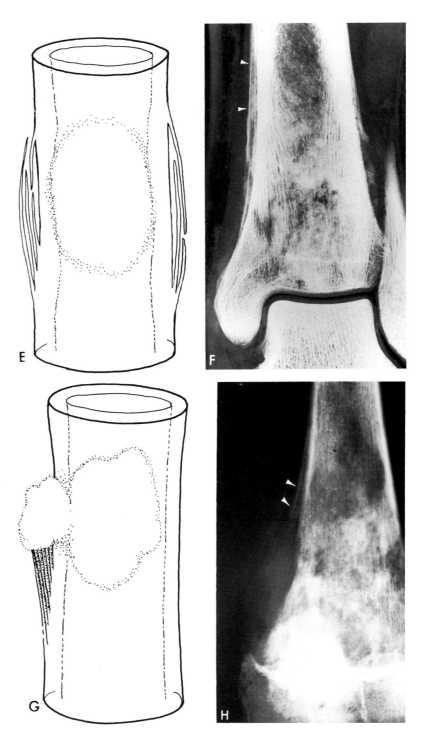

FIGURE 82–8. *Continued*

E, F Multiple layers of periosteal bone: Onion-peel pattern. The diagram **(E)** indicates multiple concentric layers of periosteal bone about the lesion. The specimen radiograph **(F)** shows such a pattern along one side of the distal portion of the tibia (arrowheads). On the other side of the bone, a more complex pattern of periostitis is seen. The medullary lesion contains radiopaque foci. (Final diagnosis—osteosarcoma.)

G, H Codman's triangle. The diagram **(G)** reveals triangular elevation of the periosteum beneath an aggressive lesion that is penetrating the cortex. The specimen radiograph **(H)** shows such a Codman's triangle (arrowheads). Note the medullary and cortical bone destruction, soft tissue mass, and radiodense foci within the lesion. (Final diagnosis—osteosarcoma.)

Illustration continued on following page

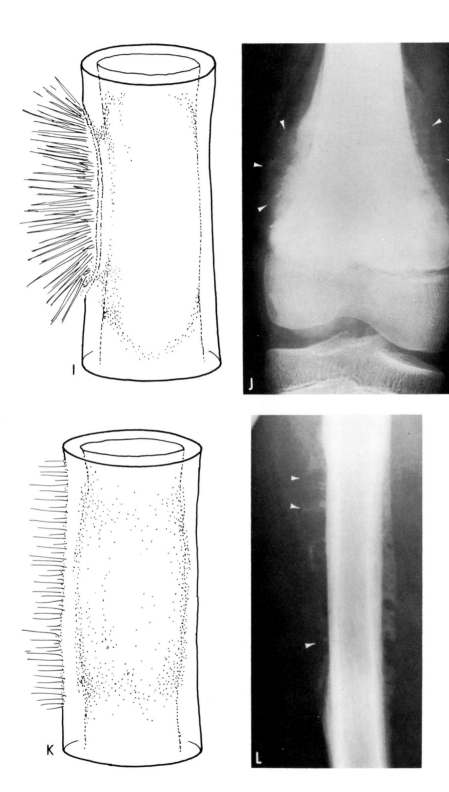

FIGURE 82–8. *Continued*

I, J Radiating spicules of periosteal bone: Sunburst pattern. The diagram **(I)** shows radiating spicules that emanate from a single focus within the bone. The radiograph **(J)** indicates such a sunburst pattern of periosteal bone (arrowheads), which is intermixed with tumor bone formation. Note the radiodense lesion in the medullary bone and the Codman's triangle. (Final diagnosis—osteosarcoma.)

K, L Radiating spicules of periosteal bone: Hair-on-end pattern. The diagram **(K)** demonstrates the parallel horizontal spicules that emanate from the underlying bone. The radiograph **(L)** indicates a femoral lesion characterized by a hair-on-end pattern (arrowheads). The individual striations of periosteal bone have created an inhomogeneous band of radiodensity on the opposite side of the bone. (Final diagnosis—Ewing's sarcoma.)

DISTRIBUTION IN A SINGLE BONE

The distribution of a solitary lesion within a bone provides an important clue to the correct diagnosis. Lodwick's analysis,[5] which is summarized here, is based predominantly on lesions in tubular bones, although in some instances the analysis can be extended to involvement of flat or irregular bones.

Position of Lesion in Transverse Plane
(Figs. 82–9 and 82–10)

The identification of a lesion's center is of fundamental importance in establishing a correct diagnosis. The position of the center of a lesion frequently can be identified as of central, eccentric, cortical, juxtacortical (parosteal or periosteal), or soft tissue location. This analysis is facilitated when the lesion is not of great size, as the center may be more difficult to define when a large lesion is encountered. Furthermore, establishing the position of the center of a lesion is less reliable when a narrow tubular bone, such as the fibula, is the site of involvement, as eccentric lesions in small tubular bones soon appear central in location.

Some lesions characteristically lie on or close to the central axis of the bone (i.e., central lesions) within the medullary canal. These include, among others, enchondromas, fibrous dysplasia, and simple bone cysts. Other lesions arise to one side of the central axis of the bone, still within the medullary canal (i.e., eccentric lesions) or within the cortex (i.e., cortical lesions). It may be difficult to differentiate a lesion arising subcortically from one originating in the cortex. Eccentric lesions include giant cell tumors, mesenchymal sarcomas, such as osteosarcoma, chondrosarcoma, and fibrosarcoma, and chondromyxoid fibromas. Cortical lesions include nonossifying fibromas and osteoid osteomas. Lesions arising adjacent to the outer surface of the cortex are juxtacortical. Juxtacortical lesions can be divided further into those that are derived from the deep layer of the periosteum, separating it from the cortex (i.e., periosteal lesions), and those that are derived from the outer layer of the periosteum, growing in an exophytic pattern (i.e., parosteal lesions).[12] Typical examples of juxtacortical lesions are juxtacortical chondromas, periosteal osteosarcomas, and parosteal osteosarcomas. Soft tissue lesions may be located near the surface of a bone but external to the periosteum (i.e., paraosseous lesions) or at a distance from the bone (i.e., extraosseous lesions). These lesions are discussed in Chapter 95. Complicating the precise classification of some processes are the occurrence of extensive bone reaction beneath parosteal lesions (e.g., parosteal lipoma), the extension of some lesions from the surface of the bone (e.g., osteochondroma), changes in position of the lesion during stages of its development (e.g., juxtacortical myositis ossificans), and the occurrence of lesions that have several components that differ in location (e.g., adamantinoma). Furthermore, some kinds of lesions, such as osteosarcomas, chondrosarcomas, fibrosarcomas, and osteoblastomas, may arise from various locations.[5]

Position of Lesion in Longitudinal Plane

Certain solitary lesions in the tubular bones show a remarkable propensity to develop in specific anatomic locations, such as the epiphysis, metaphysis, and diaphysis.

Examples of lesions that may involve the epiphyses of adults are clear cell chondrosarcoma, metastasis, lipoma (Fig. 82–11A), and intraosseous ganglion. Although originating in the metaphysis, giant cell tumors quickly penetrate the closed growth plate, involving the epiphysis with extension to the subchondral bone adjacent to the joint (Fig. 82–11B). Examples of epiphyseal lesions in children are chondroblastoma (Fig. 82–11C), osteomyelitis, and, less frequently, osteoid osteoma, enchondroma, and eosinophilic granuloma.[13] Transarticular spread of epiphyseal tumors is encountered most consistently with aggressive lesions, such as bone sarcomas, plasma cell myeloma, and skeletal metastasis, and in joints that lack or have limited mobility, such as the sacroiliac and discovertebral joints.[14]

Metaphyseal lesions include nonossifying fibroma, which characteristically develops at a short distance from the growth plate; chondromyxoid fibroma, which abuts on the growth plate; simple bone cyst; osteochondroma; Brodie's abscess; and mesenchymal sarcomas, such as osteosarcoma and chondrosarcoma (Table 81–2).

Aggressive lesions that may develop in a diaphysis include round cell tumors, such as Ewing's sarcoma. Nonaggressive lesions that may appear in the diaphysis of a tubular bone include nonossifying fibromas, simple bone cysts, aneurysmal bone cysts, enchondromas, osteoblastomas, and fibrous dysplasia.

Although these anatomic divisions are not applied as accurately to lesions in flat bones,[5] epiphyseal equivalent areas exist beneath the articular cartilage in the bones of the pelvic and shoulder girdles (Fig. 82–12), such that lesions within these areas commonly are those that show predilection for the epiphyses in the tubular bones. Similar ''epiphyseal'' lesions may develop in the small bones of the wrist and midfoot and in the patella.

LOCATION IN THE SKELETON

Despite an ever-increasing number of reports that indicate variability in the skeletal distribution of most bone tumors, selection of specific sites represents one of the most important diagnostic characteristics of such tumors. Knowledge of typical locations of osseous neoplasms, although perhaps not entirely permitting the selection or the elimination of a particular diagnosis, certainly allows the physician to better gauge diagnostic probabilities in any individual case.

Certain tumors predominate in areas of red, or hematopoietic, marrow, related either to their being derived from cells of the red marrow or to their being transported to such areas by the vasculature of the marrow.[15] The distribution of the hematopoietic marrow is dependent directly on the age of the person and is influenced further by the presence of pathologic conditions that cause reconversion of yellow, or fatty, marrow to red marrow.

The hematopoietic function of the bone marrow is established in utero and, at birth, the marrow is fully responsible for red cell production.[15] Immediately prior to birth and increasingly thereafter, a normal conversion of red to yellow marrow becomes evident, a process that proceeds from distal locations to more proximal ones. By adulthood, red marrow predominates in the axial skeleton (spine, pelvis, ribs, sternum, and skull) and the proximal portions of the shafts of the femora and humeri.[16] The ability of fatty mar-

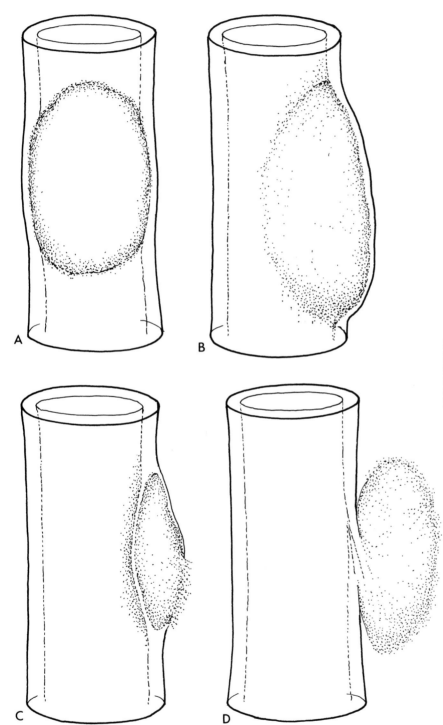

A

B

C

D

FIGURE 82–9. Position of lesion in transverse plane. Lesions may be central **(A)**, eccentric **(B)**, cortical **(C)**, or juxtacortical **(D)**. Identification of the precise position of the lesion requires that radiographs be obtained in more than one projection.

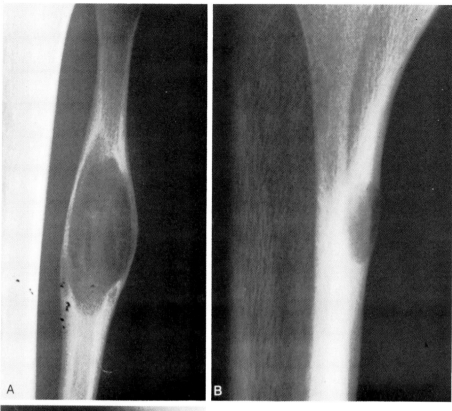

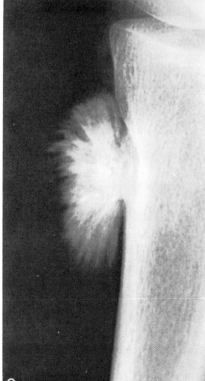

FIGURE 82–10. Position of lesion in transverse plane.
 A Central (simple bone cyst).
 B Cortical (nonossifying fibroma).
 C Juxtacortical (parosteal osteosarcoma).
 (**A,** Courtesy of V. Vint, M.D., San Diego, California; **C,** Courtesy of A. D'Abreu, M.D., Porto Alegre, Brazil.)

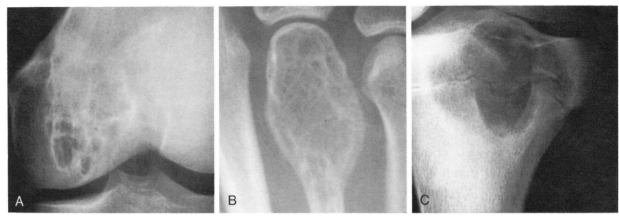

FIGURE 82–11. Position of lesion in longitudinal plane. Lesions involving epiphyses.
A Intraosseous lipoma.
B Giant cell tumor.
C Chondroblastoma.
(**A,** Courtesy of A. G. Bergman, M.D., Stanford, California; **C,** Courtesy of R. Stiles, M.D., Atlanta, Georgia.)

row to convert to hematopoietic red marrow quickly is well established and represents the body's protective response to the stress produced by chronic anemias, myelofibrosis, plasma cell myeloma, and skeletal metastasis, in which the capacity of the normal sites of hematopoiesis is reduced.[15]

Metastatic disease, plasma cell myeloma, Ewing's sarcoma, and histiocytic lymphoma are among the tumors that localize primarily to hematopoietic marrow. The tendency for these neoplasms to involve both the appendicular and the axial skeleton in the young, and predominantly the axial skeleton in the aged, is consistent with the changing distribution of red marrow that takes place with advancing age. The occurrence of such lesions in an atypical site, such as a peripherally located bone in an adult, should arouse suspicion that reconversion of yellow to red marrow has occurred as a response to axial skeletal involvement.[15] As microscopic rests of hematopoietic marrow exist in all bones even during the adult years, exceptions to the expected sites of involvement are encountered.

Many primary osseous neoplasms develop in areas of rapid bone growth, especially the distal portion of the femur and the proximal portions of the tibia and the humerus. Because it has been suggested that a tumor of a given cell type typically arises in a location where the homologous normal cells are most active,[17] the predilection of many bone tumors for the metaphysis and physeal regions of an enlarging tubular bone is not unexpected. Furthermore, the vascular anatomy peculiar to this region, consisting of looped vessels and sinusoidal channels, promotes sluggish blood flow and, with it, metastatic seeding of tumor (and infection).[8, 15] An affinity of cancer cells for vascular endothelium[18] may further accentuate this tendency for metaphyseal localization.

Certain tumors, because of their derivation, predominate in one or more particular areas of the skeleton. A variety of neoplasms related to dentition virtually are confined to the mandible and maxilla. Chordomas, developing from the remnants of the primitive notochord, typically are seen at the cranial and caudal limits of the vertebral column. Epidermoid cysts, apparently occurring because of implantation of cells from superficial tissues, have a definite predilection for the terminal phalanges and calvarium. Neurilemomas occur most commonly in sites containing extensive intraosseous nerves, such as the mandible and the sacrum.

A few other tendencies regarding specific sites of involvement deserve emphasis. Lesions of the vertebrae in adults relate most frequently to skeletal metastasis, plasma cell myeloma, hemangioma, lymphoma, and osteomyelitis. In children, important diagnostic considerations for spinal lesions are eosinophilic granuloma, aneurysmal bone cyst, osteoblastoma, osteoid osteoma, lymphoma, leukemia, and osteomyelitis. In addition to chordomas, other important lesions of the sacrum include plasmacytomas, metastases, giant cell tumors, and a variety of neurogenic cystic lesions.[19] Sternal lesions in adults typically relate to malignant tumors such as metastasis, plasma cell myeloma, lymphoma, and chondrosarcoma. Similarly, clavicular lesions in adults usually are malignant tumors. Metastasis is the dominant cause of rib lesions in adults, although enchon-

TABLE 82–2. Mesenchymal Sarcoma Versus Round Cell Sarcoma*

	Mesenchymal	Round Cell
Examples	Osteosarcoma, chondrosarcoma, fibrosarcoma	Ewing's sarcoma, leukemias
Location in tubular bones	Metaphyseal	Metadiaphyseal
Types of bone destruction	Motheaten pattern	Permeative pattern
Visible tumor matrix	Common (osteosarcoma, chondrosarcoma)	Rare
Periostitis	Sunburst, Codman's triangle	Onion-peel, hair-on-end, Codman's triangle

*Classic features are indicated for each type of sarcoma, although considerable variability can be evident.

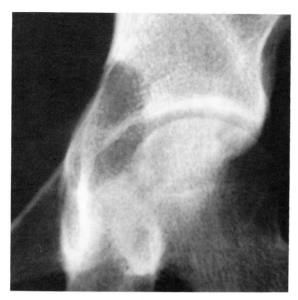

FIGURE 82–12. Lesions in epiphyseal equivalent areas: An osteolytic lesion involves the subchondral bone of the acetabulum (chondroblastoma).

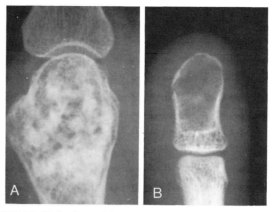

FIGURE 82–13. Lesions of the metacarpal bones and phalanges of the hand.
  A Enchondroma.
  B Inclusion cyst.
  (**A,** Courtesy of S. Kursunoglu-Brahme, M.D., San Diego, California; **B,** Courtesy of G. Greenway, M.D., Dallas, Texas.)

dromas and fibrous dysplasia are other commonly encountered causes of such lesions. Although enchondroma (Fig. 82–13A) and giant cell tumor should be given serious diagnostic consideration in patients with well-defined lesions of the metacarpal bones and phalanges of the hand, sarcoidosis, giant cell reparative granuloma, fibrous dysplasia, and aneurysmal bone cyst also should be considered. With regard to the terminal phalanges, additional diagnostic choices include an inclusion cyst (Fig. 82–13B), glomus tumor, and even metastasis.[20] Patellar lesions generally are benign and include chondroblastoma, giant cell tumor, simple bone cyst, hemangioma, dorsal defect, osteochondritis dissecans, and gout.[21, 22]

SUMMARY

Conventional radiographic techniques remain of fundamental importance in the analysis of bone tumors and tumor-like lesions. The morphologic characteristics of the process, including the pattern of bone destruction, the tumor's size, shape, and margin, the presence and nature of visible tumor matrix, any internal or external trabeculation, the existence of cortical erosion, penetration, and expansion, the type of periosteal response, and the presence of a soft tissue mass, provide important diagnostic information regarding the aggressive or nonaggressive behavior of the lesion. The foregoing data, when combined with information related to the site or distribution of skeletal involvement, allow the formulation of a single diagnostic choice or several choices that are most likely in any patient. The addition of clinical information, including the age of the patient, information derived from other imaging techniques, and, in some cases, histologic data, also is essential and underscores the importance of close cooperation among the radiologist, orthopedic surgeon, and pathologist. In Chapter 83, a discussion of the individual tumors and tumor-like lesions of the skeleton emphasizes how such cooperation can lead to diagnostic success.

References

1. Lodwick GS, Wilson AJ, Farrell C, et al: Estimating the rate of growth in bone lesions: Observer performance and error. Radiology *134:*585, 1980.
2. Lichtenstein L: Bone Tumors. 4th Ed. St Louis, CV Mosby Co, 1972.
3. Huvos AG: Bone Tumors: Diagnosis, Treatment, Prognosis. Philadelphia, WB Saunders Co, 1979.
4. Dahlin DC: Bone Tumors: General Aspects and Data on 6,221 Cases. 3rd Ed. Springfield, Ill, Charles C Thomas, 1978.
5. Lodwick GS: The bones and joints. *In* PJ Hodes (Ed): Atlas of Tumor Radiology. Chicago, Year Book Medical Publishers, 1971.
6. Lodwick GS, Wilson AJ, Farrell C, et al: Determining growth rates of focal lesions of bone from radiographs. Radiology *134:*577, 1980.
7. Lodwick GS: A systematic approach to the roentgen diagnosis of bone tumors. *In* Tumors of Bone and Soft Tissues. Papers, MD Anderson Hospital. Chicago, Year Book Medical Publishers, 1965, p 49.
8. Kricun ME: Radiographic evaluation of solitary bone lesions. Orthop Clin North Am *14:*39, 1983.
9. Puzas JE, Miller MD, Rosier RN: Pathologic bone formation. Clin Orthop *245:*269, 1989.
10. Braunschwig A, Harman PH: Studies in bone sarcoma. III. An experimental and pathological study of role of the periosteum in formation of bone in various primary bone tumors. Surg Gynecol Obstet *60:*30, 1935.
11. Volberg FM Jr, Whalen JP, Krook L, et al: Lamellated periosteal reactions: A radiologic and histologic investigation. AJR *128:*85, 1977.
12. Whalen E: International Skeletal Society: Eighteenth annual refresher course, September 1991. AJR *158:*449, 1992.
13. Gardner DJ, Azouz EM: Solitary lucent epiphyseal lesions in children. Skel Radiol *17:*497, 1988.
14. Abdelwahab IF, Miller TT, Hermann G, et al: Transarticular invasion of joints by tumors: Hypothesis. Skel Radiol *20:*279, 1991.
15. Kricun ME: Red-yellow marrow conversion: Its effect on the location of some solitary bone lesions. Skel Radiol *14:*10, 1985.
16. Piney A: The anatomy of the bone marrow. Br Med J *2:*792, 1922.
17. Johnson LC: A general theory of bone tumors. Bull NY Acad Med *29:*164, 1953.
18. Johnston AD: Pathology of metastatic tumors in bone. Clin Orthop *73:*8, 1970.
19. Willinsky RA, Grossman H, Cooper PW, et al: The radiology of sacral cysts. J Can Assoc Radiol *39:*21, 1988.
20. Jones SN, Stoker DJ: Radiology at your fingertips: Lesions of the terminal phalanx. Clin Radiol *39:*478, 1988.
21. Kransdorf MJ, Moser RP Jr, Vinh TN, et al: Primary tumors of the patella. A review of 42 cases. Skel Radiol *18:*365, 1989.
22. Ehara S, Khurana JS, Kattapuram SV, et al: Osteolytic lesions of the patella. AJR *153:*103, 1989.

83

Tumors and Tumor-Like Lesions of Bone: Imaging and Pathology of Specific Lesions

Donald Resnick, M.D., Michael Kyriakos, M.D., and Guerdon D. Greenway, M.D.

Bone-Forming Tumors
    Benign Tumors
        Osteoma
        Enostosis (Bone Island)
        Osteoid Osteoma
        Osteoblastoma
        Ossifying Fibroma
    Malignant Tumors
        Osteosarcoma
Cartilage-Forming Tumors
    Benign Tumors
        Chondroma
        Chondroblastoma
        Chondromyxoid Fibroma
        Osteochondroma
    Malignant Tumors
        Chondrosarcoma
Tumors Arising from or Forming Fibrous Connective Tissue
    Benign Tumors
        Nonossifying Fibroma
        Periosteal (Juxtacortical) Desmoid
        Desmoplastic Fibroma
    Malignant Tumors
        Fibrosarcoma
Histiocytic or Fibrohistiocytic Tumors
    Benign Tumors
        Fibrous Histiocytoma
    Locally Aggressive Tumors
        Giant Cell Tumor
    Malignant Tumors
        Malignant Fibrous Histiocytoma
Tumors of Fatty Differentiation
    Benign Tumors
        Lipoma
    Malignant Tumors
        Liposarcoma
Tumors of Muscle Differentiation
    Benign Tumors
        Leiomyoma
    Malignant Tumors
        Leiomyosarcoma
        Rhabdomyosarcoma

Tumors of Vascular Differentiation
    Benign Tumors
        Hemangioma
        Cystic Angiomatosis
        Lymphangioma and Lymphangiomatosis
        Glomus Tumor
    Benign or Malignant Tumors
        Hemangiopericytoma
    Malignant Tumors
        Angiosarcoma (Hemangioendothelioma)
Tumors of Neural Differentiation
    Benign Tumors
        Solitary Neurofibroma
        Neurilemoma
    Malignant Tumors
        Neurogenic Sarcoma (Malignant Schwannoma)
Tumors of Notochord Origin
    Locally Aggressive or Malignant Tumors
        Chordoma
        Chondroid Chordoma
Tumors of Hematopoietic Origin
    Malignant Tumors
        Non-Hodgkin's Lymphomas, Hodgkin's Disease,
          Leukemias
Plasma Cell Dyscrasias
    Locally Aggressive or Malignant Tumors
        Plasmacytoma, Multiple Myeloma
Tumors and Tumor-Like Lesions of Miscellaneous or Unknown Origin
    Benign Tumors
        Simple (Solitary or Unicameral) Bone Cyst
        Epidermoid Cyst
        Aneurysmal Bone Cyst
        Intraosseous Ganglion Cyst
    Locally Aggressive or Malignant Tumors
        Adamantinoma (Angioblastoma)
    Malignant Tumors
        Ewing's Sarcoma
Tumors of Dental Origin and Related Lesions
    Locally Aggressive or Malignant Tumors
        Ameloblastoma
Summary

It is with regard to tumors and tumor-like lesions that the interpreter of skeletal radiographs faces his or her greatest diagnostic challenge. The number of specific tumors that affect the skeleton is large and to select one from among this group of neoplasms as most likely on the basis of the roentgenographic findings can sorely test the clinical acumen of even the keenest observer. Furthermore, many of these lesions are rare and are encountered a few times, once, or perhaps not at all during professional careers that span decades, so that the personal experience guiding many physicians in the accurate radiographic interpretation of bone neoplasms frequently is very limited. Although additional imaging methods exist, such as scintigraphy, angiography, CT scanning, and MR, that can be used to provide diagnostic help in many of these cases, the importance of complete and accurate clinical information cannot be overstated. Attempting to interpret the imaging studies in the absence of such clinical data will increase significantly the likelihood of misdiagnosis (Tables 83–1 and 83–2). In particular, knowledge of the age of the patient is fundamental to the correct interpretation of the imaging abnormalities.[1804] The propensity of any specific variety of tumor to affect infants, children, adolescents, young or middle-aged adults, or the elderly represents one of the most characteristic features of many tumors and tumor-like lesions of the skeleton (Table 83–2). Almost equal in diagnostic importance is knowledge of skeletal sites that characteristically are affected by each of these lesions (Table 83–1).

In Chapter 82, the principles fundamental to the interpretation of conventional radiographs in cases of tumor and tumor-like lesions of the skeleton are outlined. Also contained in that chapter is a statement stressing the necessity of close cooperation among orthopedic surgeon, radiologist, and pathologist to ensure optimal diagnosis and treatment. In the present chapter, further emphasis is placed on the requirement of close correlation of imaging and pathologic aberrations (as well as clinical data) in each of the important neoplastic lesions that affect the skeleton.

BONE-FORMING TUMORS

Benign Tumors

Osteoma

Osteomas, which are benign lesions that usually arise from membranous bones and are composed of dense, compact osseous tissue, are discussed in Chapter 93. They are evident in both children and adults, are most prevalent in the skull, nasal sinuses, and mandible, and may be associated with intestinal polyposis, indicative of Gardner's syndrome. The radiographic features, consisting of a mass of dense bone of varying size protruding from the outer surface or, more rarely, the inner surface of a bone, are virtually diagnostic, differing from the abnormalities that accompany other exophytic processes, including osteophytes, enthesophytes, and osteochondromas; enostoses, or bone islands; and disorders (such as hypertrophic osteoarthropathy and tuberous sclerosis) in which periostitis or hyperostosis, or both, is present.

Enostosis (Bone Island)

As indicated in Chapter 93, the common lesions known as enostoses also have been designated focal sclerosis, calcified island in bone, and bone nucleus. They are encountered in all age groups, in both men and women, and typically as an incidental finding on radiographs obtained for unrelated reasons. Enostoses occur most frequently in the bones of the pelvis, the ribs, and the femur.[1–3] Although occurring predominantly in flat and irregular bones, enostoses are observed in tubular bones, more frequently those in the lower extremity, in 45 per cent of cases. When a tubular bone is affected, a solitary lesion and involvement of the epiphysis or metaphysis are most typical.[1] Location in the skull, mandible, maxilla, or sternum is extremely rare. In the spine, enostoses are seen most commonly in the thoracic or lumbar vertebral bodies,[4, 5] producing radiodense foci that simulate those associated with skeletal metastasis. Of diagnostic help in such cases, bone scintigraphy almost uniformly is negative in instances of enostoses, whereas in patients with osteoblastic metastasis, accumulation of the radiopharmaceutical agent is expected.

Enostoses, or bone islands, appear radiographically as single or multiple, ovoid, round, or oblong, intraosseous sclerotic areas with discrete margins and thorny, radiating spicules. Although enostoses generally are small in size and stable, giant bone islands—especially in the pelvis[6]—and those that grow[7, 8] or diminish[3] in size on serial radiographic studies have been described. When sectioned, enostoses are dense, hard, white or yellow-white lesions with a smooth surface.[2, 9] They consist of compact lamellar bone in which haversian systems are present[2, 10] (Fig. 83–1), although woven bone, at times, also may be evident. The bone is uniform, with regular cement lines, and there is no evidence of cartilage to suggest an origin from endochondral ossification.[8] Radiating projections about the lesion connect to surrounding trabeculae.

The general radiographic and pathologic features of enostoses are identical to those of osteopoikilosis (see Chapter 93), with some minor differences in histologic abnormalities between the two conditions noted by some investigators.[11]

Osteoid Osteoma

The term osteoid osteoma was introduced by Jaffe[12] in 1935 to describe a benign osteoblastic tumor with distinctive histologic abnormalities consisting of a central core of vascular osteoid tissue and a peripheral zone of sclerotic bone. Subsequent descriptions of this lesion have been numerous, with in excess of 1000 cases being reported in the literature, firmly establishing the osteoid osteoma as one of the more frequent and characteristic tumors or tumor-like lesions of bone. A focus of intense interest and investigation, osteoid osteoma also has been subject to heated debate regarding, for example, its neoplastic or infectious origin and its precise relationship to a second lesion of bone, the osteoblastoma. Indeed, the term osteoblastoma has been used by some investigators to encompass both of these osseous lesions,[13] whereas others use the designation osteoid osteoma–osteoblastoma complex for this purpose. Regardless of this controversy, osteoid osteoma and osteoblastoma are considered separately in this chapter.

Clinical Abnormalities. Although osteoid osteomas are observed most frequently in patients between the ages of 7 and 25 years, descriptions of this lesion can be found in very young children[14, 15, 1927] as well as in elderly persons.[16, 1924] The ratio of male patients to female patients

TABLE 83–1. Tumors and Tumor-Like Lesions: Typical Sites of Skeletal Localization

Tumor or Tumor-Like Lesion (Number of Cases Evaluated)	Site*								
	Femur	Tibia	Fibula	Foot	Patella	Humerus	Radius	Ulna	Hand, Wrist
Enostosis (371)	25	7	1	5	<1	9	1	<1	9
Osteoid Osteoma (661)	32	24	4	11	<1	7	1	3	9
Osteoblastoma (Conventional) (298)	14	10	4	7	<1	3	1	2	3
Osteoblastoma (Aggressive) (47)	11	13	6	11		2			2
Osteosarcoma (Conventional) (3844)	46	21	3	1	<1	11	<1	<1	<1
Osteosarcoma (Telangiectatic) (191)	54	16	5	<1		14	<1	<1	<1
Osteosarcoma (Periosteal) (69)	44	41	4			7			
Osteosarcoma (Parosteal) (300)	64	11	3	2		15	2	1	<1
Chondroma (Enchondroma) (1028)	11	3	2	7	<1	7	2	<1	57
Chondroma (Periosteal) (130)	25	8	3	5		32	2	2	20
Chondroblastoma (642)	33	18	1	10	2	22	1		2
Chondromyxoid Fibroma (231)	17	38	8	16		1	3	3	2
Osteochondroma (Solitary) (1604)	31	18	4	6	<1	19	1	1	5
Chondrosarcoma (Conventional) (1937)	24	7	2	2	<1	10	1	1	3
Chondrosarcoma (Clear Cell) (64)	64	5				16		2	2
Chondrosarcoma (Mesenchymal) (92)	15	7	1	8		7		1	
Chondrosarcoma (Dedifferentiated) (107)	43	7				17			
Nonossifying Fibroma (833)	38	43	8	1		5	1	<1	1
Desmoplastic Fibroma (121)	12	8	2	2		10	8	2	1
Fibrosarcoma (621)	39	16	3	2		11	1	1	<1
Giant Cell Tumor (1949)	31	27	4	2	<1	6	10	3	4
Fibrous Histiocytoma (Malignant) (271)	44	21	2	2	1	9	1	1	
Lipoma (66)	15	14	20	15		9		2	
Hemangioma (Solitary) (195)	4	3	2	5	1	3	1	1	2
Hemangiopericytoma (48)	10		6	4		15	4	2	2
Hemangioendothelioma (151)	18	23	4	6	1	13	2		2
Neurofibroma (42)		7	5			2			
Neurilemoma (76)	7	4	1	3	3	4		5	8
Chordoma (503)									
Simple Bone Cyst (884)	27	6	5	1		56	1	1	1
Aneurysmal Bone Cyst (465)	14	15	7	8	<1	9	3	4	5
Adamantinoma (189)	3	81	3	1		6	1	4	1
Ewing's Sarcoma (1974)	22	11	9	3		10	2	1	1

*Numbers indicate percentages of the lesions that affect each of the skeletal sites based upon analysis of major reports containing the greatest number of cases. Percentages may not always total 100 per cent because numbers were rounded to nearest whole number.

Table continued on opposite page

TABLE 83–1. Tumors and Tumor-Like Lesions: Typical Sites of Skeletal Localization *Continued*

Tumor or Tumor-Like Lesion (Number of Cases Evaluated)	Site*								
	Scapula	Clavicle	Sternum	Ribs	Vertebrae, Including Sacrum and Coccyx	Innominate Bone	Skull	Face	Mandible, Maxilla
Enostosis (371)	1	<1		12	2	25			
Osteoid Osteoma (661)	1			<1	6	2	<1		<1
Osteoblastoma (Conventional) (298)	1	<1		4	30	2	—4—		11
Osteoblastoma (Aggressive) (47)	4			2	23	13	11		2
Osteosarcoma (Conventional) (3844)	1	<1	<1	1	2	7	1	<1	4
Osteosarcoma (Telangiectatic) (191)	2			2		3	2		<1
Osteosarcoma (Periosteal) (69)				1		1			1
Osteosarcoma (Parosteal) (300)	<1					1			
Chondroma (Enchondroma) (1028)	1	<1	1	5	1	3	<1		
Chondroma (Periosteal) (130)				2	1	2			
Chondroblastoma (642)	2	<1	<1	2	1	4	1		<1
Chondromyxoid Fibroma (231)	1		<1	3	2	6	<1		
Osteochondroma (Solitary) (1604)	4	<1	<1	2	2	5	<1		
Chondrosarcoma (Conventional) (1937)	5	1	2	8	6	24	1	1	2
Chondrosarcoma (Clear Cell) (64)	2			3	3	2	2		2
Chondrosarcoma (Mesenchymal) (92)	2		1	12	11	12	8	1	14
Chondrosarcoma (Dedifferentiated) (107)	8		<1	4	1	22			
Nonossifying Fibroma (833)	<1	<1		1		1	<1		<1
Desmoplastic Fibroma (121)	3	2		2	3	11	1		33
Fibrosarcoma (621)	2	1	<1	1	4	10	1		7
Giant Cell Tumor (1949)	<1	<1	<1	1	7	4	1	<1	<1
Fibrous Histiocytoma (Malignant) (271)	1	1	<1	3	2	9	2		3
Lipoma (66)				8	5		5		9
Hemangioma (Solitary) (195)	2	1		9	25	3	29	2	8
Hemangiopericytoma (48)	2	4	4	8	15	11	2		10
Hemangioendothelioma (151)	3		1	5	10	8	3		2
Neurofibroma (42)					7			2	76
Neurilemoma (76)	1			3	16	1	3		42
Chordoma (503)					75		25		
Simple Bone Cyst (884)	<1	<1		<1		2			
Aneurysmal Bone Cyst (465)	2	3		3	14	9	2	<1	2
Adamantinoma (189)				1		1			
Ewing's Sarcoma (1974)	5	2	<1	8	6	18	1	<1	1

*Numbers indicate percentages of the lesions that affect each of the skeletal sites based upon analysis of major reports containing the greatest number of cases. Percentages may not always total 100 per cent because numbers were rounded to nearest whole number.

TABLE 83–2. Tumors and Tumor-Like Lesions: Typical Ages of Patients

Tumor	Age (Years)
	0 — 10 — 20 — 30 — 40 — 50 — 60 — 70 — 80

Malignant
- Osteosarcoma
- Parosteal osteosarcoma
- Chondrosarcoma
- Fibrosarcoma
- Fibrous histiocytoma
- Malignant giant cell tumor
- Ewing's Sarcoma
- Adamantinoma
- Hemangioendothelioma
- Histiocytic lymphoma
- Chordoma
- Plasma cell myeloma
- Skeletal metastasis

Benign
- Osteoma
- Osteochondroma
- Enchondroma
- Chondroblastoma
- Chondromyxoid fibroma
- Osteoid osteoma
- Osteoblastoma
- Nonossifying fibroma
- Desmoplastic fibroma
- Lipoma
- Hemangioma
- Giant cell tumor
- Neurilemoma
- Simple bone cyst
- Aneurysmal bone cyst

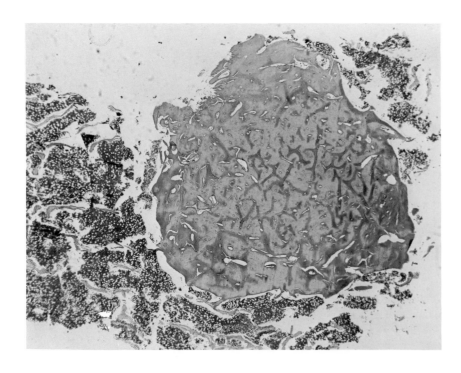

FIGURE 83–1. Enostosis (bone island): Microscopic abnormalities. The lesion is composed of compact lamellar bone and is surrounded by cancellous trabeculae and bone marrow elements. Note that some of the cancellous trabeculae merge with the peripheral portion of the enostosis, accounting for the radiographic appearance of thorny radiations that is characteristic of this lesion. (11×.)

is approximately 3 to 1. With rare exceptions,[17, 1805, 1926] pain is the hallmark of the lesion and, without this symptom, the diagnosis is suspect. The pain typically is more dramatic at night and ameliorated when small doses of salicylates are used; however, these are not invariable clinical characteristics of the lesion and, furthermore, other skeletal processes can be associated with similar abnormalities. Pain usually is described as dull or aching; it initially is mild and inconstant, accounting for a delay of months or, sometimes, years before the patient seeks the aid of a physician. Later the pain increases in severity, becomes more persistent, and may be accompanied by soft tissue swelling and tenderness. The mechanism of pain in osteoid osteomas is not entirely clear, although it has been postulated that local stimulation of sensory nerve endings, owing to changes in vascular pressure perhaps mediated through the production of prostaglandins by the tumor tissue, is a causative factor.[18, 1806, 2431] The identification of unmyelinated nerve fibers in the fibrous zone around the central nidus of the lesion[19] or in the nidus itself[20–22, 1925] lends support to this theory.

Additional clinical manifestations of osteoid osteoma are encountered frequently and depend on the age of the patient and the precise skeletal location of the lesion. In the immature skeleton, significant aberrations in growth, muscle atrophy, and skeletal deformity are recognized complications of osteoid osteomas. Torticollis, spinal stiffness, and scoliosis are among the clinical characteristics of those lesions that develop in the vertebral column, whereas joint tenderness, swelling, synovitis, and limitation of motion may represent the initial clinical manifestations of intra-articular osteoid osteomas (see later discussion). In any location, symptoms and signs of a systemic process generally are lacking; laboratory studies usually are unremarkable.

Skeletal Location. In defining the precise anatomic distribution of osteoid osteoma on the basis of previous descriptions of this lesion, a critical factor relates to the criteria that were used to separate osteoid osteoma and osteoblastoma. This separation has been based primarily on the size of the lesion. Although some investigators have used 1.0 cm as the upper limit of the size of an osteoid osteoma, others have used 1.5 cm for this purpose and still others designate as osteoid osteomas lesions that have been as large as 2.5 cm.[13, 18, 23–27] Although these different criteria cause some variation in the frequency with which individual bones have been designated as sites for either osteoid osteoma or osteoblastoma, osteoid osteoma generally is more common in the long tubular bones, especially those in the lower extremities; approximately 50 to 60 per cent occur in the femur or tibia,[23, 24, 28–30] whereas osteoblastoma is more common in the flat bones and the vertebrae.[29]

In an analysis of the anatomic distribution of 661 cases of osteoid osteoma derived from seven series, each containing 30 or more cases,[23, 25, 30–34] the femur was the bone involved most frequently, followed by the tibia. These two bones together accounted for 57 per cent of the total cases, and the long bones were the site of origin in 71 per cent of cases. The bones in the hands and feet were involved in 20 per cent of cases. In the hands, osteoid osteomas usually were found in a proximal phalanx or a metacarpal bone; osteoid osteoma occurring in a distal phalanx was quite rare. Of the carpal bones, the scaphoid was affected most frequently, whereas in the foot, the talus and the calcaneus

were involved most commonly.[44–56, 1886, 1928] Within long bones, osteoid osteoma usually is located in the diaphysis, but it may extend into the metaphysis.[16, 25] Epiphyseal and intra-articular osteoid osteomas are rare (see later discussion). In the femur, there is predilection for the proximal end of the bone, especially the neck and intertrochanteric region.[13, 25, 34]

Vertebral osteoid osteomas usually arise from the posterior elements with the base of the transverse process, the lamina, and the pedicle being the most common sites; the vertebral body is involved only rarely.[32, 35–43] The lumbar vertebrae are the sites most typically affected followed in order of frequency by the cervical and thoracic vertebrae, with the sacrum or coccyx representing a rare site of involvement.[35, 37, 40–42, 1929, 2380] Additional infrequent sites of localization of osteoid osteomas are the innominate bone,[1930, 1931] skull,[57–59] mandible or maxilla,[60] clavicle,[61, 62] scapula,[1932] ribs,[63, 64, 1933–1935] and radius.[65, 1936]

Radiographic Abnormalities. Conventional radiography represents an effective initial technique in the evaluation of patients in whom an osteoid osteoma is suspected. When present, the classic roentgenographic appearance of a centrally located, oval or round radiolucent area, measuring less than 1 cm in diameter, surrounded by a zone of uniform bone sclerosis is virtually diagnostic of this lesion. Unfortunately, this appearance is not present uniformly, being modified according to the specific bone that is affected as well as the precise site of involvement in that bone. As an example, an osteoid osteoma arising in the vertebral column, in a small bone in the wrist, hand, or foot, or within an articulation reveals unique radiographic characteristics that differ from those associated with an osteoid osteoma in the diaphysis of a long tubular bone. Furthermore, this lesion may occur in the cortex, in the medullary or cancellous bone, or in a subperiosteal location, and the resulting radiographic abnormalities are not identical in these three locations.

Long Tubular Bones. With regard to the long tubular bones, those osteoid osteomas that are *diaphyseal* in location (and some that are metaphyseal in location) typically are observed in the cortex, appearing as a radiolucent lesion, representing the nidus, that is surrounded by bone sclerosis with cortical thickening owing to endosteal and subperiosteal new bone formation (Fig. 83–2). The nidus itself may be uniformly radiolucent or contain variable amounts of calcification. It usually is small (almost always less than 1 cm in diameter) and oval or round in configuration; these characteristics have diagnostic significance, generally allowing differentiation of an osteoid osteoma from a stress fracture (which is accompanied by a linear, radiolucent cortical area) and an osteoblastoma (which commonly is a larger lesion). In rare circumstances, a single osteoid osteoma may contain more than one nidus,[66, 67] or more than one osteoid osteoma, each with its own nidus, may be found in the same bone[13] or neighboring bones[68, 69] (Fig. 83–3).

The degree and extent of the sclerotic reaction about an osteoid osteoma are variable. When exuberant, such sclerosis may resemble the osseous response to a malignant tumor, such as a Ewing's sarcoma; be accompanied by bone formation in an adjacent bone; or completely obscure the nidus itself. As a general rule, the nidus is located in the center of the sclerotic reaction, but its precise delinea-

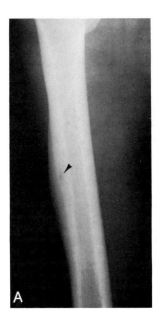

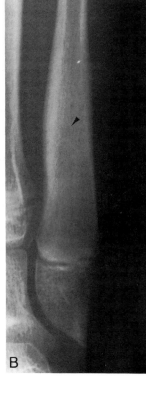

FIGURE 83–2. Osteoid osteoma: Radiographic abnormalities—long tubular bones.

A Femur. Note the radiolucent nidus (arrowhead) with surrounding endosteal and periosteal bone formation in the diaphysis of the femur.

B Fibula. The nidus of the lesion is difficult to see (arrowhead), although the fibula is expanded due to adjacent bone formation.

tion may require additional imaging techniques, such as conventional or computed tomography. Those osteoid osteomas that are subperiosteal in location may evoke more limited osseous proliferation immediately adjacent to or at a distance from the lesion. This situation is encountered most typically in lesions of the neck of the femur, where the nidus may be identified in a subperiosteal (or cortical) location, usually along the medial aspect of the bone. Here

new bone formation may be limited, and accurate diagnosis may be extremely difficult: The slightly thickened cortex in the medial portion of the femoral neck may be overlooked owing to the prominence of the femoral cortex that normally is seen in this region; the combination of a subperiosteal or cortical radiolucent focus and reactive bone formation may be misinterpreted as evidence of an osseous response to stress; or the intracapsular osteoid osteoma may

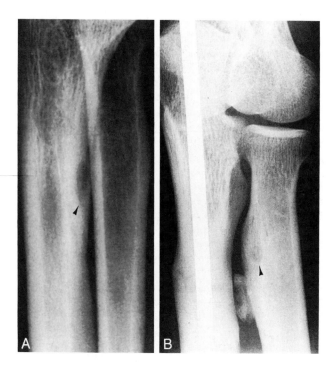

FIGURE 83–3. Osteoid osteoma: Radiographic abnormalities—metachronous lesions. This 27 year old man developed pain in the forearm of 4 months' duration.

A An osteoid osteoma of the ulna (arrowhead) is evident, manifested as a radiolucent nidus and cortical thickening. An en bloc excision of this lesion documented a classic osteoid osteoma.

B Two months later, pain of an identical nature and in a similar location developed, and a radiograph reveals a new lesion in the proximal portion of the radius (arrowhead). The central radiolucent nidus is partially calcified. This lesion, too, was removed with histologic documentation of an osteoid osteoma. The patient subsequently has been asymptomatic for 10 years.

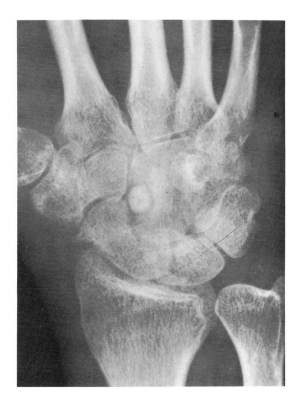

FIGURE 83–4. Osteoid osteoma: Radiographic abnormalities—carpal bones. This osteoid osteoma in the capitate of a 17 year old man is manifested as a partially calcified lesion with osteopenia in all of the carpal bones.

be accompanied by clinical findings that suggest an articular disorder (see later discussion).

Carpus, Tarsus, and Epiphyses. In the carpal or tarsal bones (Fig. 83–4) as well as in the epiphyses of the long tubular bones (Fig. 83–5), an osteoid osteoma usually arises in the medullary spongiosa and, radiographically, appears

as a well-circumscribed lesion that is partially or completely calcified.[1807–1809, 1937–1945] A radiolucent zone may surround the lesion, and extensive reactive sclerosis generally is absent. These features, which are at variance with the classic radiographic abnormalities of a cortical osteoid osteoma, may lead to considerable diagnostic difficulty, es-

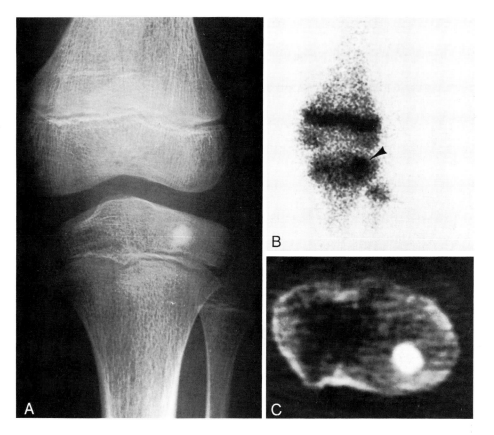

FIGURE 83–5. Osteoid osteoma: Radiographic abnormalities—epiphysis of the long tubular bones.

A The routine radiograph in this 8 year old boy with night pain reveals a well-defined, circular, sclerotic lesion in the proximal epiphysis of the tibia. A knee effusion was not evident on physical examination.

B The bone scan shows increased accumulation of the radiopharmaceutical agent at the site of the lesion (arrowhead).

C A transaxial CT scan reveals the calcified lesion. Surgery and histologic examination confirmed the presence of an osteoid osteoma.

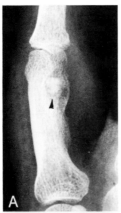

FIGURE 83–6. Osteoid osteoma: Radiographic abnormalities—phalanges. Three lesions of the hand in different patients are shown. The first (A) is present in the proximal phalanx of the fifth finger; the nidus (arrowhead) is partially calcified, and considerable soft tissue swelling is evident. The second (B) is partially calcified and located in a subperiosteal location (arrowhead), and it has led to cortical irregularity and soft tissue swelling. The third (C) appears as a radiodense focus (arrowhead) in a terminal phalanx with adjacent soft tissue swelling. (A, Courtesy of P. Major, M.D., Winnipeg, Manitoba, Canada.)

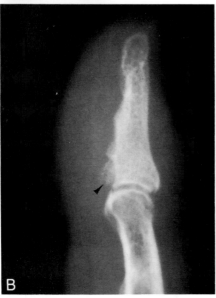

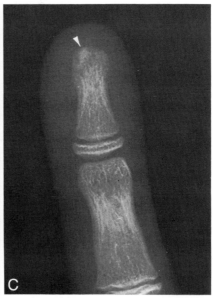

pecially when clinical manifestations are dominated by symptoms and signs of an articular process.[70] In the immature skeleton of children and adolescents, an osteoid osteoma arising in an epiphyseal ossification center can lead to alterations in normal physeal growth and, if not diagnosed and treated at an early stage, may result in significant osseous deformity.[71, 72] A similar complication is well recognized in children with osteoid osteomas arising in the neck of the femur and in other tubular bones.[73, 74]

Small Bones of the Hand and Foot. In the metacarpals, metatarsals, and phalanges (Figs. 83–6 and 83–7), osteoid osteomas have a variable radiographic appearance.[1946, 2432] When located in the cortex, they generally provoke a periosteal response similar to that observed in the diaphysis of the long tubular bones. In subperiosteal sites, they produce scalloping of the adjacent cortical surface; and in the cancellous bone, a partially or totally calcified lesion with or without a radiolucent margin is identified. In any of these

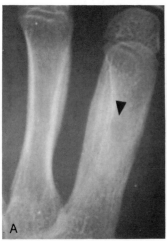

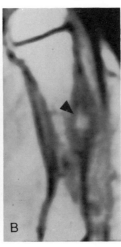

FIGURE 83–7. Osteoid osteoma: Radiographic abnormalities—metacarpal bones. The routine radiograph (A) reveals a subtle radiolucent focus (arrowhead) in the diaphysis of the fifth metacarpal bone with periostitis of this bone as well as the ulnar aspect of the fourth metacarpal bone. A sagittal proton density–weighted (TR/TE, 2000/20) spin echo MR image (B) through the fifth metacarpal bone reveals the nidus (arrowhead), marrow edema, and periosteal reaction. (Courtesy of A. Nemcek, M.D., Chicago, Illinois.)

locations, soft tissue swelling may be prominent, simulating the appearance of infection or arthritis. Painless osteoid osteomas appear to be more frequent in the phalanges than in other sites, however.

Intra-articular Sites. Osteoid osteomas arising in an intra-articular location deserve special emphasis (Figs. 83–8 to 83–11). Clinical manifestations in such cases, which include pain, soft tissue swelling, a joint effusion, and restriction of articular motion, may be attributed falsely to a primary articular disorder. Accurate diagnosis commonly is delayed, sometimes for a period of years, while unnecessary investigations and surgical procedures are performed.[75–77] Persistent hyperemia and a synovial inflammatory response that is characterized as lymphofollicular in type[78–80, 1887] may lead to irreversible cartilaginous and osseous destruction. Osteopenia, uniform narrowing of the interosseous space, and periarticular subperiosteal bone apposition may be encountered,[78] particularly in the hip[81–83, 1951] but also in such locations as the elbow[78, 1810, 1952, 1953, 1956] and ankle.[75, 1954, 1955] Eventually, hypertrophic changes similar to those in osteoarthritis may be seen.[81] Although early diagnosis and effective treatment with surgical removal of the nidus are essential in these cases, such steps do not always prevent subsequent articular deterioration.[81]

Spine. Osteoid osteomas arising in the spine also represent a diagnostic challenge owing to the complex anatomy of the vertebral column, the obscuration of bone by overlying soft tissue shadows during conventional radiography, and atypical and variable clinical findings (Figs. 83–12 and 83–13). Pain, which may be radicular in type, commonly is prominent, especially at night and during spinal motion, and is accompanied in a majority of cases by an abnormality of spinal curvature. Scoliosis, particularly when combined with pain, has repeatedly been emphasized as an important clinical manifestation of a spinal (or a rib) osteoid osteoma,[37, 41, 84, 85] although this combination certainly is not specific and is evident in other vertebral lesions as well, including osteoblastoma, pyogenic infection, aneurysmal bone cyst, and eosinophilic granuloma.[86] Excision of the lesion in an adolescent usually ensures complete resolution of the abnormal spinal curvature, whereas in a child, this favorable response is less predictable.[87] Local tenderness and paraspinal muscle atrophy[88] are additional clinical manifestations; neurologic abnormalities are relatively infrequent.[41] Neck stiffness, pain, and torticollis may accompany an osteoid osteoma in the cervical spine.[39, 42, 1888]

On radiographs, the lesion characteristically is located on the concave aspect of the scoliotic curve, near its apex. Osteosclerosis of a pedicle, lamina, articular process, or, less commonly, a transverse or spinous process[1957] is observed. A radiolucent nidus may be present, but its identification frequently requires conventional or computed tomography.[89–91] Rare radiographic patterns include localization in a vertebral body with or without transdiscal extension,[38]

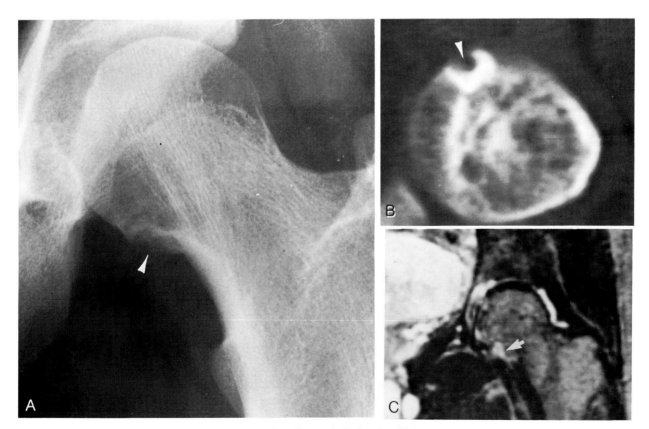

FIGURE 83–8. Osteoid osteoma: Radiographic abnormalities—intra-articular location (hip).

A The routine radiograph reveals subtle osseous irregularity (arrowhead) in the superomedial aspect of the femoral neck.

B A transaxial CT scan shows the subsynovial osteoid osteoma (arrowhead).

(**A, B,** Courtesy of P. VanderStoep, M.D., St. Cloud, Minnesota.)

C In a different patient, a coronal T2-weighted (TR/TE, 1500/70) spin echo MR image reveals an osteoid osteoma (arrow) in the femoral neck and a joint effusion. (**C,** Courtesy of W. Peck, M.D., Orange, California.)

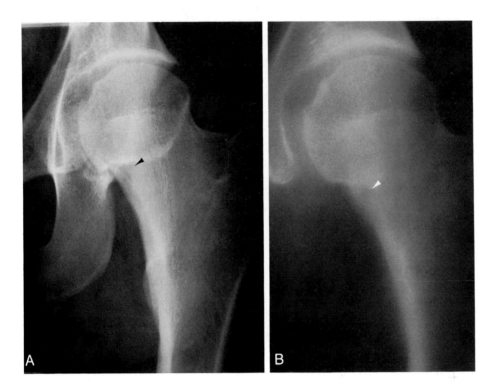

FIGURE 83–9. Osteoid osteoma: Radiographic abnormalities—intra-articular location (hip). An osteoid osteoma with a radiolucent nidus (arrowheads) in the femoral neck has produced extensive adjacent new bone formation, osteophytosis, and mild narrowing of the hip joint.

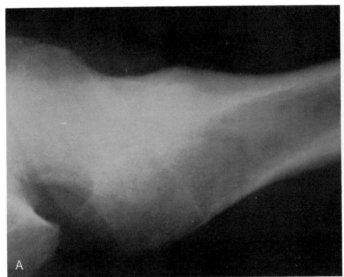
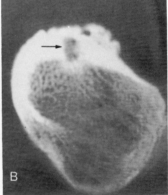

FIGURE 83–10. Osteoid osteoma: Radiographic abnormalities—intra-articular location (hip). A lateral radiograph of the hip **(A)** shows considerable new bone formation involving the anterior aspect of the femoral neck. The nidus is not visible. Transaxial CT **(B)** reveals the radiolucent nidus (arrow) in the anterior aspect of the femoral neck with adjacent bone proliferation. (Courtesy of P. Kindynis, M.D., Geneva, Switzerland.)

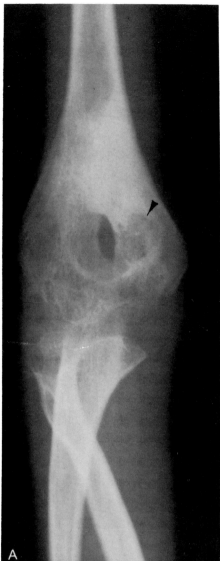

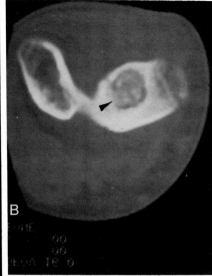

FIGURE 83–11. Osteoid osteoma: Radiographic abnormalities—intra-articular location (elbow). A partially calcified osteoid osteoma (arrowheads) of the distal portion of the humerus in a child is well shown with routine radiography **(A)** and transaxial CT **(B)**. Note soft tissue atrophy, osteopenia, epiphyseal enlargement, and irregularity of subchondral bone. (Courtesy of R. Kerr, M.D., Los Angeles, California.)

multiple lesions in a single or several vertebrae,[1958, 1959] and bone sclerosis at more than one vertebral level as a response to a single lesion.[92]

It should be emphasized that although an osteosclerotic focus in the posterior osseous elements represents an important diagnostic sign of an osteoid osteoma, a similar abnormality may occur in patients with other disorders, including skeletal metastasis and infection, such as tuberculosis, and as a response to a contralateral spondylolysis or hypoplastic neural arch.

Other Skeletal Sites. In other skeletal sites, osteoid osteomas are associated with a variety of radiographic abnormalities. In the innominate bones of the pelvis (Fig. 83–14) and in the scapula, an osteoid osteoma most typically appears as a radiolucent or partially calcified lesion with limited surrounding bone sclerosis. A para-articular location, such as the glenoid or acetabular region, is characteristic. In a rib (Fig. 83–15), the lesion may be accompanied by a profound sclerotic reaction, which can extend to adjacent ribs[1933] and, rarely, by scoliosis.[1811, 1934] Extensive bone sclerosis also can accompany a clavicular osteoid osteoma. Osteoid osteomas in the skull or facial bones are so rare

that characteristic radiographic patterns have not been established.

Other Imaging Techniques. Scintigraphy (Fig. 83–16) has been used in the preoperative and intraoperative evaluation of patients with osteoid osteoma. It is well recognized that preoperatively, with rare exceptions,[93] these lesions avidly accumulate bone-seeking radiopharmaceutical agents during the vascular, blood-pool, and delayed phases of the scintigraphic examination.[94, 95] The resulting abnormalities initially were considered to be relatively nonspecific, being duplicated by a variety of other skeletal processes, but the sensitivity of the technique and its applicability to those osteoid osteomas in sites such as the spine,[96, 97, 1812] in which routine radiography might be inadequate, were not questioned. It was suggested subsequently that supplemental gallium imaging could improve the specificity of the bone scan by documenting disproportionately low accumulation of the radioisotope when compared with the high accumulation of the technetium radiopharmaceutical agent.[95] More recently, a distinctive pattern of abnormality, designated the double-density sign, has been observed in radionuclide bone scans in patients with osteoid osteoma.[98, 1960] This sign

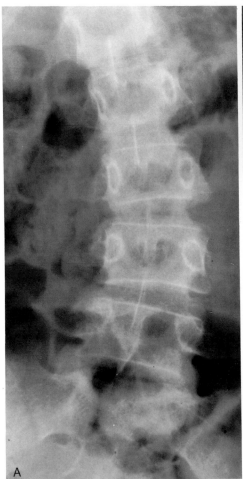

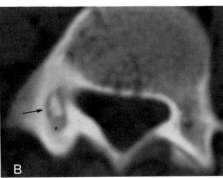

FIGURE 83–12. Osteoid osteoma: Radiographic abnormalities—spine.

A A frontal radiograph of the lumbar spine shows scoliosis but no other significant abnormalities.

B A transaxial CT scan at the level of the fifth lumbar vertebra reveals the partially calcified nidus (arrow) of an osteoid osteoma. (Courtesy of J. Kirkham, M.D., Minneapolis, Minnesota.)

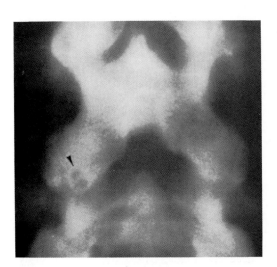

FIGURE 83–13. Osteoid osteoma: Radiographic abnormalities—spine. Note the radiolucent nidus (arrowhead) of an osteoid osteoma in the inferior articular process of a lumbar vertebra. (Courtesy of V. Vint, M.D., San Diego, California.)

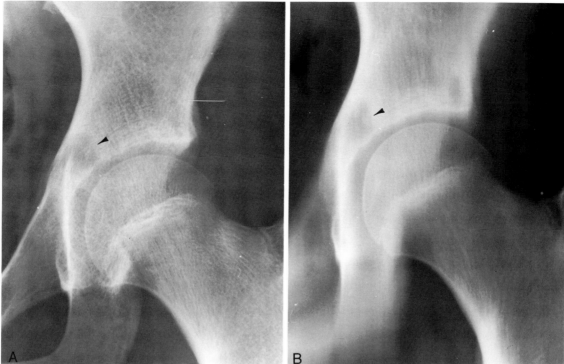

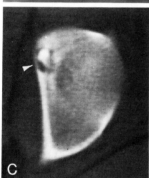

FIGURE 83–14. Osteoid osteoma: Radiographic abnormalities—innominate bones.

A, B Hip pain in this 13 year old boy resulted from an osteoid osteoma (arrowheads) in the acetabular region.

C In a different patient, a transaxial CT scan shows a partially calcified nidus (arrowhead) in the acetabulum.

(**C,** From Gamba JL, et al: Am J Roentgenol *142*:769, 1984. Copyright 1984, American Roentgen Ray Society.)

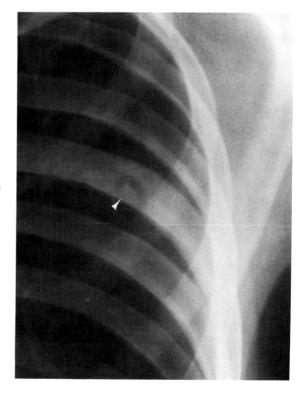

FIGURE 83–15. Osteoid osteoma: Radiographic abnormalities—ribs. In a young child, a partially calcified nidus of an osteoid osteoma (arrowhead) is identified. Note the bone sclerosis and osseous expansion in adjacent ribs. (Courtesy of A. Brower, M.D., Norfolk, Virginia.)

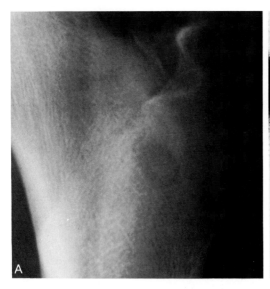
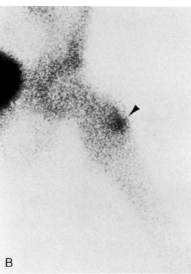

FIGURE 83–16. Osteoid osteoma: Scintigraphic abnormalities. As shown in this classic osteoid osteoma of the proximal portion of the femur in a 15 year old boy, avid accumulation of a bone-seeking radionuclide (arrowhead) corresponds in location to the site of the radiographically evident lesion **(A).** Note that the region of most intense scintigraphic activity is surrounded by a zone of less intense but abnormal activity **(B).**

is characterized by intense scintigraphic activity centrally in the region of the nidus and less intense accumulation of the radionuclide peripherally in the sclerotic bone. This pattern differs from that typically observed in osteomyelitis, in which more uniform radionuclide accumulation is seen, or in an abscess cavity, which may actually reveal decreased radionuclide uptake. Indium-111 chloride radionuclide imaging also may be useful in the differentiation of a cortical osteoid osteoma and a cortical abscess; the former lesion has been reported not to be associated with increased accumulation of the radionuclide whereas the latter lesion has been found to be associated with radionuclide accumulation.[1961]

Intraoperative radionuclide methods also have been used in patients with osteoid osteoma, particularly for precise localization of the nidus.[99–103] As excision of the nidus results in complete cure (see later discussion), its accurate delineation at the time of surgery assumes clinical importance.[1889] Briefly, the scintigraphic technique used for this purpose involves the injection of a bone-seeking radiopharmaceutical agent 2 hours prior to surgery. At the time of surgery, a sterilized sodium iodide scintillation probe is used to identify the osseous area containing the greatest amount of scintigraphic activity,[103, 104] and the biopsy samples can subsequently be placed in a scintillation-well counter until a specimen with peak activity is identified and additional samples obtained from the adjacent bone show a return to normal basal activity.[105] Modifications in this technique as well as other methods (such as preoperative labeling with tetracycline[1813]) also are described,[104, 106, 1962] but all are designed to ensure complete operative removal of the nidus.

Ultrasonography appears to have a limited role in the assessment of osteoid osteomas, although it has been used successfully for the detection of osteoid osteomas in the femoral neck.[2433]

CT scanning (Figs. 83–17 and 83–18) has largely replaced conventional tomography in the imaging evaluation of osteoid osteomas, although neither technique is essential in the majority of cases. In those instances in which the lesion is small or not readily apparent on conventional radiography, CT may be required. The method is most

valuable in defining osteoid osteomas in the spine,[43, 89, 90, 107, 108] osseous pelvis and femoral neck,[109, 110, 2434] and, occasionally, in other sites.[111, 1814, 1815, 1963] The choice of adequate window settings for visualization of cortical bone is essential for accurate computed tomographic documentation of the nidus.[111]

Angiography occasionally has been used to localize an osteoid osteoma revealing a homogeneous accumulation of contrast material, or blush, of variable density in the region of the nidus that appears early in the arterial phase and persists late into the venous phase of the study.[112–115] The procedure, however, generally is not required in the evaluation of such lesions.

Although *MR imaging* has been used in the evaluation of osteoid osteomas,[1964–1970, 2436, 2437] it generally is considered less useful than CT scanning in the detection of the nidus[2435] (Figs. 83–17 and 83–19), and furthermore, MR imaging findings in cases of osteoid osteoma may simulate those of a malignant tumor or osteomyelitis, owing to the presence of marrow and soft tissue edema and even a soft tissue mass. The soft tissue mass consists of reactive, myxomatous tissue whose signal intensity may increase following the intravenous administration of a gadolinium compound.[1969] MR imaging findings of synovitis and joint effusion (Fig. 83–20) may accompany intra-articular osteoid osteomas.[1970] When seen in the MR images, the nidus of an osteoid osteoma reveals variable patterns of signal intensity dependent on the size of the nidus and the amount of calcification or fibrous tissue present. The extent of juxtanidal marrow edema also is variable, appearing as regions of increased signal intensity in T2-weighted spin echo MR images and revealing enhancement of signal intensity following the intravenous administration of a gadolinium compound. The extent of both bone marrow and soft tissue edema may be reduced with the use of therapeutic doses of salicylates or nonsteroidal anti-inflammatory medications.[2435]

Pathologic Abnormalities. An osteoid osteoma is composed of a circumscribed region of active bone formation within a highly vascular stroma. As indicated previously, this nidus may be within the cancellous bone (Fig. 83–21) or the cortex or in a subperiosteal location.[13, 34, 116, 1890] Intracortical osteoid osteoma is most common and, in this posi-

FIGURE 83–17. Osteoid osteoma: CT abnormalities.

A, B Although conventional tomography **(A)** reveals the nidus (arrowhead) of an osteoid osteoma in the tibia, it is far better seen (arrowhead) with transaxial CT **(B).**

C In a different patient, note the partially calcified nidus (arrowhead) of an osteoid osteoma of the tibia that is exquisitely shown with transaxial CT.

(C, Courtesy of C. Dayton, M.D., Eugene, Oregon.)

D, E An osteoid osteoma (arrowheads) of the sixth cervical vertebra is shown by transaxial CT **(D)** and MR imaging **(E).** The partially calcified nidus (arrow) and the sclerotic bone have a low signal intensity in the spin echo MR image in E.

(D, E, Courtesy of J. Tsurada, M.D., San Francisco, California.)

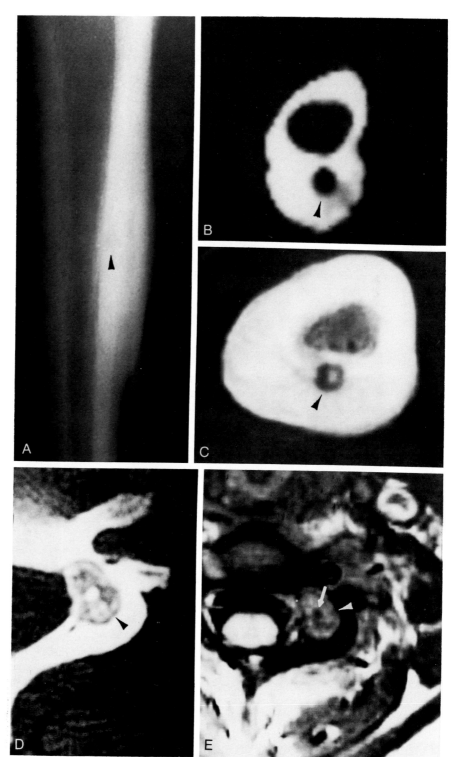

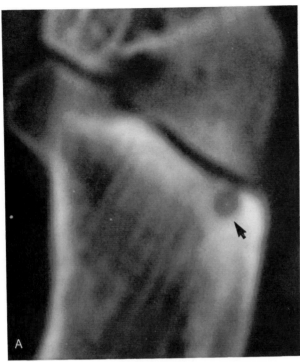

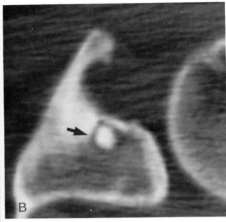

FIGURE 83–18. Osteoid osteoma: CT abnormalities.

A Calcaneus. A coronal CT scan shows the radiolucent nidus (arrow) adjacent to the posterior subtalar joint. (Courtesy of G. In der Maur, M.D., Zwolle, The Netherlands.)

B Scapula. A transaxial CT scan reveals the calcified nidus (arrow) adjacent to the glenoid cavity. (Courtesy of P. Kindynis, M.D., Geneva, Switzerland.)

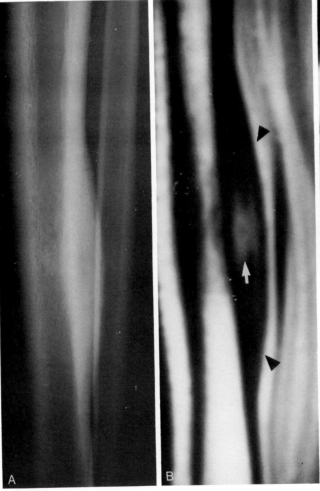

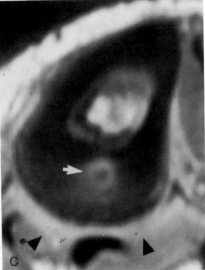

FIGURE 83–19. Osteoid osteoma: MR imaging abnormalities.

A A routine radiograph reveals fusiform cortical thickening in the posterior aspect of the diaphysis of the tibia, although the nidus cannot be identified.

B A sagittal proton density–weighted (TR/TE, 2500/20) spin echo MR image shows the cortical thickening (arrowheads) and a region of intermediate signal intensity (arrow) representing the nidus.

C A transaxial proton density–weighted (TR/TE, 2500/20) spin echo MR image shows the partially calcified nidus (arrow) within the area of cortical thickening. Surrounding soft tissue edema (arrowheads) is seen.

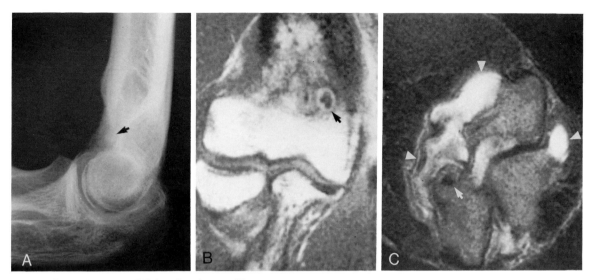

FIGURE 83–20. Osteoid osteoma: MR imaging abnormalities.

A A lateral radiograph of the elbow shows cortical thickening in the distal portion of the humerus and a partially calcified nidus (arrow) of an osteoid osteoma.

B In a coronal T1-weighted (TR/TE, 600/20) spin echo MR image, the partially calcified nidus (arrow) is identified.

C A transaxial T2-weighted (TR/TE, 2500/70) spin echo MR image through the distal portion of the humerus reveals the nidus (arrow) and a large joint effusion (arrowheads). (Courtesy of P. VanderStoep, M.D., St. Cloud, Minnesota.)

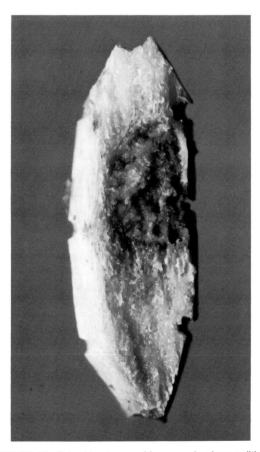

FIGURE 83–21. Osteoid osteoma: Macroscopic abnormalities. An en bloc resection of a lesion in the cancellous bone of the tibia reveals no thickening of the adjacent cortex. The osteoid osteoma is granular in appearance with foci of calcification.

tion, the tumor produces the characteristic gross pathologic appearance of a nidus, usually less than 1 cm in diameter, surrounded by abundant white sclerotic bone.[13, 26, 71] If removed during its active growth phase, when there is still considerable vascularity and bone production, an osteoid osteoma appears as a discrete round or oval lesion marked by its cherry-red or reddish-brown color.[18, 24, 26, 32, 71] It may be quite friable and granular and, if located in the cortex, may easily be displaced from the surrounding sclerotic bone.[18] Depending on its content of calcium and bone, the consistency of the nidus can be soft or hard and gritty.[16, 28, 34, 71]

Microscopically, the nidus of an osteoid osteoma consists of bone in various stages of maturity within a highly vascular connective tissue stroma containing numerous dilated capillaries (Fig. 83–22). Seams of osteoid are found that are lined by plump osteoblasts lacking nuclear pleomorphism or atypia. Some nuclei occasionally may be quite large, hyperchromatic, and associated with numerous mitoses, however.[28, 117] The osteoid undergoes calcification and forms irregular trabeculae of woven or reticular bone. Osteoclasts in the stroma erode and remodel this immature bone. The process of active bone production and resorption eventually yields bone that has a mosaic pattern similar to that seen in Paget's disease.[13, 30, 34, 118, 119] The proportion of this pagetoid bone to that of unmineralized osteoid varies from tumor to tumor. In some, the nidus may consist entirely of osteoid arranged in broad sheets with focal calcification, whereas in others abundant calcification and woven bone may be evident. Usually the center of the tumor is its most highly mineralized portion and, with the production of bone, the nidus, which formerly was radiolucent owing to its content of unmineralized osteoid, may become uniformly sclerotic and appear radiodense on roentgenograms. Toward the periphery of the nidus, the bone may be more

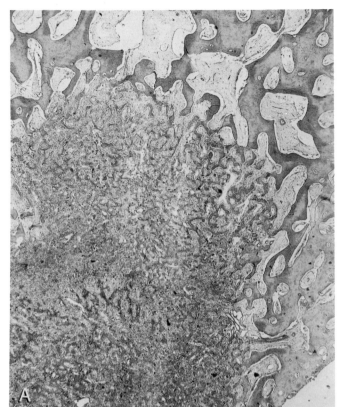

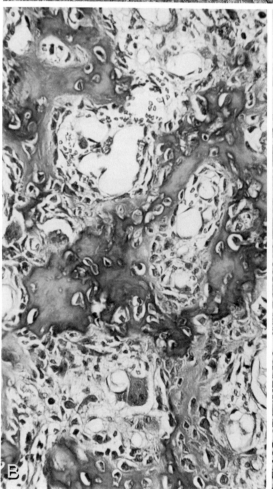

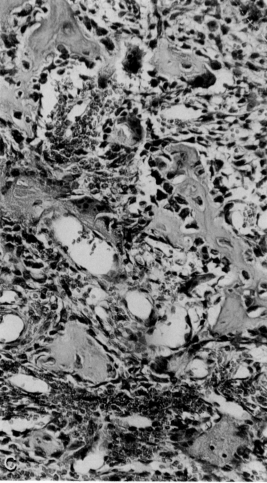

FIGURE 83–22. Osteoid osteoma: Microscopic abnormalities.

A The nidus of an osteoid osteoma shows a central portion composed of abundant trabeculae. The deeper region of the nidus appears darker owing to the presence of more compact bone and calcified osteoid. At the periphery of the lesion, there is a rim of thickened normal bone with which the peripheral trabeculae of the nidus merge. (20×.)

B An area in the center of the nidus shows highly vascular stroma with calcified osteoid, which, in some areas, is rimmed by osteoblasts. A few osteoclast-type giant cells are present. (300×.)

C Another portion of the nidus shows hemorrhagic stroma with trabeculae of osteoid lined by plump active osteoblasts. (300×.)

mature and fuse to form an anastomotic or interlacing network of trabeculae separated by the vascular stroma. Foci of cavernous sinuses similar to those of an aneurysmal bone cyst, at times, may be found in an osteoid osteoma.[29]

In osteoid osteomas located in the spongiosa, the nidus is separated from the adjacent cancellous bone by a thin rim of vascular connective tissue. No marrow elements are found within the nidus of these cancellous lesions.[32] In the cortex, the nidus is encased by bone, which may have two distinct layers. The inner layer consists of remnants of the original cortex that was eroded by the vascular stroma and its osteoclasts, whereas the outer layer consists of compact lamellar bone produced by the periosteum.[120]

Histologically, osteoid osteoma and osteoblastoma are essentially similar, although some investigators believe that osteoblastomas may be more vascular and possess more osteoblasts, wider trabeculae, and less organization than osteoid osteomas. The distinction between the two tumors, however, depends essentially on their size, location, and clinical features. It has been emphasized, however, that this distinction not always is clear, and tumors may be encountered that have features of both lesions.[13] In this regard, in an electron microscopic study of five cases of osteoid osteoma, Steiner[121] found that the tumor osteoblasts were morphologically similar to normal osteoblasts with only minor differences. In two of these cases, the osteoblasts contained atypical mitochondria that had a honeycombed appearance. A case of osteoblastoma also was studied by Steiner,[121] and the osteoblasts of this tumor had a similar cell morphology, including the presence of the atypical mitochondria.

Natural History. As it is well recognized that surgical resection of the entire nidus is a prerequisite for an optimal clinical response, considerable attention has been directed toward methods that document that the nidus has been completely removed before the surgical procedure is terminated.[1971–1973] In addition to intraoperative scintigraphy and tetracycline labeling (see previous discussion), conventional radiography and even tomography[122] of the specimen have been used for this purpose (Fig. 83–23). The importance of this determination relates to the fact that although patients occasionally have been ''cured'' even when no nidus has been found on pathologic inspection of the resected tissue, recurrences are likely when surgical removal of the lesion is incomplete.[23, 29, 32, 123, 124, 1979, 1980] True recurrences following complete resection of the nidus indeed are rare and, in some cases, relate to the presence of more than one nidus in a single osteoid osteoma or a second osteoid osteoma in the same bone or a different bone.[69, 123, 125, 1958, 1959] Failure of surgery to relieve the patient's symptoms and signs also may indicate that the initial diagnosis of an osteoid osteoma was incorrect.[126]

Recently, percutaneous resection of an osteoid osteoma has been suggested as an alternative to open surgery.[1974–1976] The method usually involves drilling the cortical bone under CT guidance and appears to be better suited to removal of osteoid osteomas in the long tubular bones (Fig. 83–24) than in small bones or the spine.[1976] Percutaneously placed electrodes also may be used for the ablation of osteoid osteomas.[1977]

The natural history of those osteoid osteomas that are not removed surgically (or percutaneously) is not clear as a precise diagnosis of the lesion requires verification of typical histologic features. There are several reported instances in which lesions with clinical and radiologic characteristics of an osteoid osteoma have healed spontaneously, with or without the administration of anti-inflammatory medications, over a varying period of time.[18, 127–129, 1978] The benign nature of an osteoid osteoma is not in question, as there have been no reports of malignant transformation or of metastases from the lesion.[16]

Differential Diagnosis. In the majority of cases, the radiographic abnormalities of an osteoid osteoma are sufficiently characteristic to allow accurate diagnosis. In an intracortical location, a lesion containing a radiolucent center (with or without calcification) and a peripheral zone of bone sclerosis is almost certainly an osteoid osteoma despite occasional reports in which an abscess or a bone tumor (i.e., hemangioma, osteosarcoma) has had a similar radiographic appearance. In a subperiosteal or intramedullary location or within an articulation, the roentgenographic diagnosis of an osteoid osteoma is more difficult (see previous discussion) and in certain sites, such as the spine, additional diagnostic methods may be required for precise delineation of the nidus. Even with CT, however, differentiation of an osteoid osteoma from another lesion, such as an abscess, may be difficult.[1814] With MR imaging, diagnostic difficulties may be accentuated.

Osteoblastoma

Osteoblastoma can be further categorized into conventional and aggressive types.

Conventional Osteoblastoma. Benign osteoblastoma is a relatively uncommon primary neoplasm of bone that is composed of a well-vascularized connective tissue stroma in which there occurs active production of osteoid and primitive woven bone. Initially designated as a giant osteoid osteoma[130] and osteogenic fibroma,[131, 132] osteoblastoma obtained its currently accepted name in 1956 with independent descriptions by Jaffe[133] and Lichtenstein.[134] As a precise relationship between this lesion and osteoid osteoma is not clear and, in recent years, an aggressive variety of osteoblastoma has been recognized (see later discussion), the designation of benign osteoblastoma may require some future modification.

Clinical Abnormalities. Although there are reports of osteoblastomas in patients as young as 2 years of age and as old as 70 years,[135, 136] the lesion is observed most frequently in persons under 30 years old, with approximately 70 per cent of cases appearing in the second or third decade of life.[135] Male patients are affected more frequently than female patients, in a ratio of approximately 2 to 1. As in cases of osteoid osteoma, local pain is a common manifestation of osteoblastoma, although generally it is mild. Accentuation of pain at night and its amelioration with salicylates are inconstant clinical features of osteoblastoma. Spinal lesions may be accompanied by muscle spasm, scoliosis, and neurologic manifestations, including paresthesias and weakness.

Skeletal Location. Although osteoblastoma may affect virtually any bone, it is most frequently observed in the flat bones or the vertebrae, as opposed to the distribution of osteoid osteoma, which is predominantly a tumor of the tubular bones.[28–30, 33, 34, 135, 137, 138] Among 298 osteoblastomas found in six published series,[34, 135–139] each with a minimum of 16 cases, the vertebrae were the site of origin in 30 per

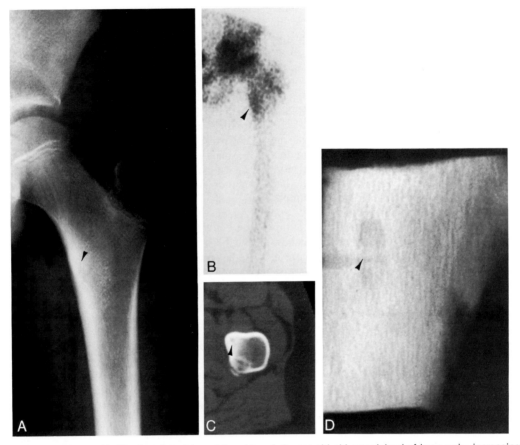

FIGURE 83–23. Osteoid osteoma: Verification of excision of the nidus. A 9 year old girl complained of knee pain, increasing at night and relieved with aspirin, that initially was diagnosed as evidence of Osgood-Schlatter disease.

A–C Preoperatively, routine radiography **(A)**, bone scintigraphy **(B)**, and transaxial CT **(C)** document the presence of a typical osteoid osteoma (arrowheads) in the femoral neck.

D Confirmation that the nidus (arrowhead) was removed surgically is accomplished with specimen radiography.

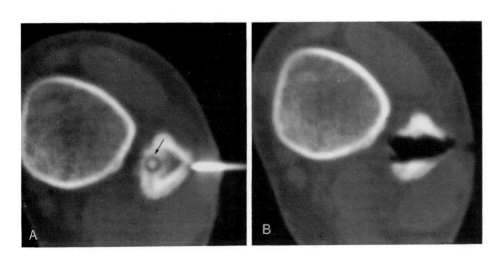

FIGURE 83–24. Osteoid osteoma: Percutaneous resection. Two transaxial CT scans obtained during **(A)** and after **(B)** the percutaneous removal of an osteoid osteoma (arrow) of the fibula are shown. (Courtesy of J. J. Railhac, M.D., Toulouse, France.)

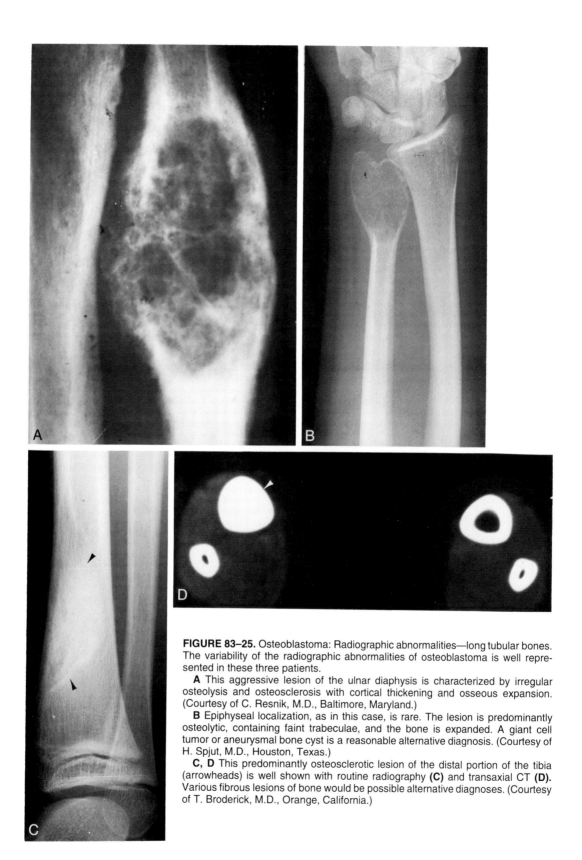

FIGURE 83–25. Osteoblastoma: Radiographic abnormalities—long tubular bones. The variability of the radiographic abnormalities of osteoblastoma is well represented in these three patients.

A This aggressive lesion of the ulnar diaphysis is characterized by irregular osteolysis and osteosclerosis with cortical thickening and osseous expansion. (Courtesy of C. Resnik, M.D., Baltimore, Maryland.)

B Epiphyseal localization, as in this case, is rare. The lesion is predominantly osteolytic, containing faint trabeculae, and the bone is expanded. A giant cell tumor or aneurysmal bone cyst is a reasonable alternative diagnosis. (Courtesy of H. Spjut, M.D., Houston, Texas.)

C, D This predominantly osteosclerotic lesion of the distal portion of the tibia (arrowheads) is well shown with routine radiography **(C)** and transaxial CT **(D).** Various fibrous lesions of bone would be possible alternative diagnoses. (Courtesy of T. Broderick, M.D., Orange, California.)

cent of patients and the long tubular bones were involved in 34 per cent of patients. The bones of the lower extremity were affected in 35 per cent of these patients, and those of the upper extremity in 9 per cent. Fifteen per cent of tumors affected the skull, mandible, or maxilla, 5 per cent of tumors occurred in the innominate bone, and 10 per cent of the osteoblastomas were localized in the bones of the hands and feet. Other reports dealing with a single patient or a few patients confirm these sites of predilection and document the occurrence of osteoblastomas in unusual locations such as the carpal or tarsal bones, sternum, patella, scapula, sacrum, clavicle, orbit, ribs, and paranasal sinuses.[140–161, 1981–1985, 2438, 2439]

With regard to the anatomic location of osteoblastoma versus that of osteoid osteoma, both lesions occur more frequently in the lower extremities than in the upper extremities. Osteoid osteomas are found about twice as commonly in the long tubular bones and the bones of the hands and feet than are osteoblastomas. The latter tumor, however, is far more common in the vertebrae and also occurs more frequently in the skull, mandible, ribs, and innominate bone.

In the long tubular bones, approximately 75 per cent of osteoblastomas are situated in the diaphysis with the remainder in the metaphysis.[28, 30, 33, 135, 1985] Epiphyseal involvement is distinctly unusual[137, 143] except for those osteoblastomas that occur within the short tubular bones of the hands or feet.[33, 137] Although the femur is the long bone most typically affected by osteoblastoma, the proximal portion of this bone rarely is involved.[160] In the spine, the thoracic and lumbar vertebrae are the most frequent sites of involvement.[34, 41, 43] Vertebral osteoblastomas arise mainly in the pedicles, the laminae, and, less commonly, the transverse and spinous processes.[33, 41, 43, 135, 1812] Involvement of the vertebral body is less typical.[1986, 1987]

Rare multicentric foci of osteoblastoma within a single bone have been reported but, owing to the small size of these individual foci, some investigators would consider them to represent multiple nidi of an osteoid osteoma.[33, 34, 41]

Radiographic Abnormalities. The radiographic features of osteoblastoma are varied and, in most instances, nondiagnostic. Osteolysis alone, osteosclerosis alone, or a combination of both osteolysis and osteosclerosis may be observed. Expansion of bone, cortical thinning, and a soft tissue mass may accompany this lesion and, in some cases, suggest a far more ominous neoplasm. When radiographs reveal an expansile, well-circumscribed, partially calcified lesion or one that resembles a large osteoid osteoma, the diagnosis of osteoblastoma should be considered.

In the *long tubular bones,* osteoblastomas may originate in the medullary or cortical bone (Figs. 83–25 to 83–27) or, rarely, in a subperiosteal location[162, 163] (Fig. 83–28). Variable in size and sometimes quite large, these lesions usually are round or oval and predominantly osteolytic, with areas of calcification or ossification, well marginated, and expansile. Bone sclerosis and periostitis may be exuberant, and the latter finding may resemble the periosteal reaction that characterizes malignant neoplasms. Pathologic fractures and multifocal lesions are rare.[135, 1996] Similar radiographic alterations may accompany osteoblastomas in the small bones of the *hands* and *feet* and in the *innominate bone*[135, 137, 152, 164, 1988] (Fig. 83–29). Two radiographic features related to osteoblastomas of the appendicular skeleton should be emphasized: Owing to considerable variability in their appearance, accurate diagnosis often is not possible; in some instances, aggressive characteristics are misinterpreted as evidence of a malignant tumor.

In the *spine,* a well-defined, expansile osteolytic lesion that is partially or extensively calcified or ossified, arising

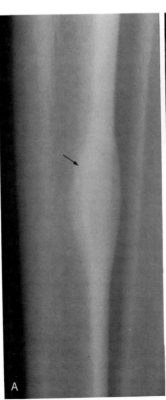
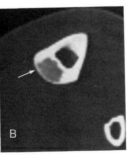

FIGURE 83–26. Osteoblastoma: Radiographic abnormalities—long tubular bones. This 19 year old man complained of leg pain.

A A routine radiograph shows a region of cortical thickening (arrow) containing an elongated radiolucent focus in the posterior aspect of the diaphysis of the tibia.

B Transaxial CT shows the intracortical tumor (arrow). The radiolucent region is larger than a typical osteoid osteoma.

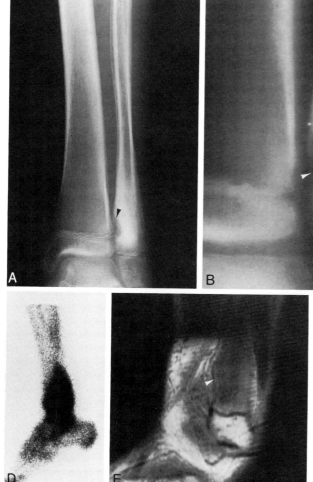
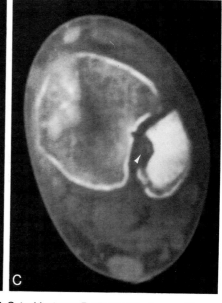

FIGURE 83–27. Osteoblastoma: Radiographic abnormalities—long tubular bones. This 14 year old boy developed progressive pain and swelling in the lateral aspect of the lower portion of the leg over a 3 month period.

A, B Routine radiography **(A)** and conventional tomography **(B)** reveal an osteolytic focus (arrowheads) with considerable sclerosis and periostitis, the latter affecting a long segment of the fibula and the adjacent surface of the tibia.

C A transaxial CT scan at the level of the lesion shows that the area of osteolysis contains a ring-like focus of calcification (arrowhead).

D A bone scan shows considerable accumulation of the radionuclide in the fibula and tibia.

E A sagittal T1-weighted (TR/TE, 500/30) spin echo MR image reveals decreased signal intensity at the site of the fibular lesion (arrowhead). Following curettage, the initial histologic diagnosis was osteoid osteoma; further evaluation confirmed the diagnosis of an osteoblastoma.

from the posterior osseous elements, especially in the thoracic or lumbar segment, should suggest the diagnosis of an osteoblastoma[165, 166] (Figs. 83–30 and 83–31). This appearance is not invariable and, occasionally, a small lesion may be entirely overlooked, destruction of a vertebral body may occur alone or in combination with involvement of the dorsal osseous elements, a nidus may be seen similar to that of an osteoid osteoma, or a large and purely radiolucent osteoblastoma in the posterior arch may resemble an aneurysmal bone cyst (Fig. 83–32). Although not so characteristic as in cases of osteoid osteoma, scoliosis may accompany spinal osteoblastomas[167, 168]; this finding is more typical of thoracic or lumbar lesions, whereas in the cervical spine, where osteoblastomas not uncommonly affect the spinous process, abnormalities of spinal curvature may be absent.[169, 170] Scoliosis also may be associated with osteoblastomas in the *ribs*[158, 159] (Fig. 83–33).

Osteoblastomas are infrequent in the *skull*.[171–173] The precise location is variable, including the temporal, occipital, ethmoid, frontal, and sphenoid bones. A circumscribed oval radiolucent defect, with varying degrees of central calcification, involving both the inner and the outer tables of the skull, is typical. Although the tumor generally is small in size, massive osteoblastomas of the skull have been de-

scribed.[174] Those with features suggesting an aneurysmal bone cyst also may be encountered.[175, 176]

Osteoblastomas are somewhat more frequent in the *mandible* than in the *maxilla*, usually affecting the tooth-bearing regions of the bones with the premolar area being the most typical location.[177, 178] Rarely, the mandibular condyle is affected.[1989] The tumor often begins centrally, consisting of a spherical calcified lesion surrounded by a well-defined radiolucent halo. Displacement of adjacent teeth may be evident, and reactive osteosclerosis is infrequent.

Other Imaging Techniques. As in the case of osteoid osteomas, bone scintigraphy, CT scanning, and MR imaging can be used to assess osteoblastomas. Bone scintigraphy reveals increased accumulation of the radionuclide at the site of the lesion, and CT scanning and MR imaging allow full delineation of the extent of the process. An inflammatory reaction in the bone about the tumor or in the nearby soft tissues may lead to a misleading appearance in MR images that simulates a malignant tumor.[1985, 1995] This inflammatory reaction may include a mass that reveals enhancement of signal intensity following the intravenous administration of a gadolinium compound.[1995]

Pathologic Abnormalities. With regard to *macroscopic pathology,* an osteoblastoma may have a subperiosteal, cor-

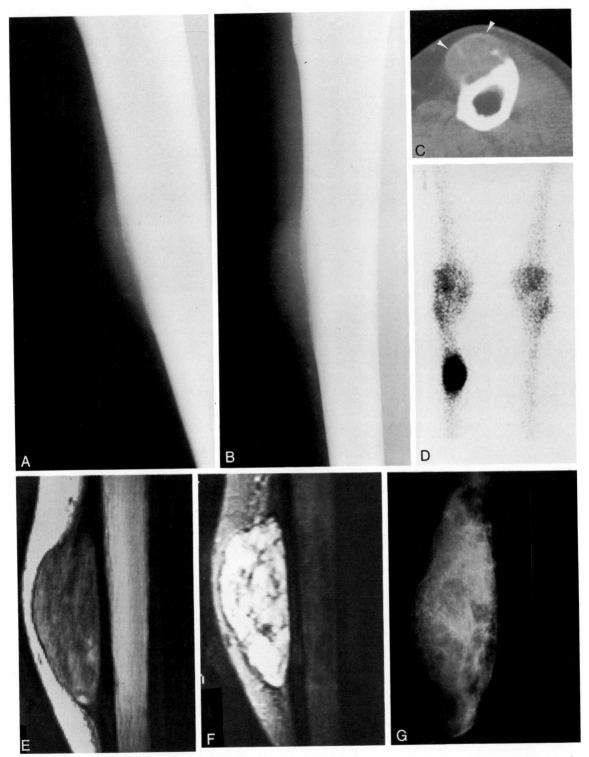

FIGURE 83–28. Osteoblastoma: Radiographic abnormalities—long tubular bones. A 37 year old woman developed a lump on the anterior surface of the tibia over a 2 month period following minor trauma. On physical examination, a 2 × 3 cm mass was palpated.

A, B Radiographs obtained 2 months apart (2 and 4 months following the injury) show an enlarging mass adjacent to the anterior surface of the tibia. The hazy, radiodense lesion contains horizontally oriented trabeculae and is accompanied by excavation of the external cortical surface and periostitis.

C A transaxial CT scan reveals a rim of increased attenuation (arrowheads) at the margin of the lesion and cortical erosion.

D Intense accumulation of the bone-seeking radionuclide is apparent.

E, F Sagittal MR images reveal low signal intensity with T1 weighting **(E)** and high signal intensity with T2 weighting **(F).** The medullary portion of the tibia is uninvolved.

G Radiograph of the lesion following total excision shows its trabecular pattern. Histologic analysis confirmed the presence of a subperiosteal osteoblastoma with some microscopic features of an aneurysmal bone cyst.

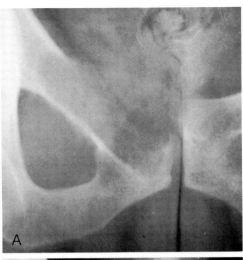

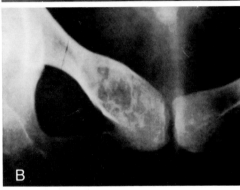

FIGURE 83–29. Osteoblastoma: Radiographic abnormalities—innominate bone. Two examples show the variability of the radiographic features of this tumor.

A An osteolytic, expansile lesion of the parasymphyseal bone is present. (Courtesy of R. S. Howell, M.D., Louisville, Kentucky.)

B Considerable osteosclerosis and calcification are evident in a lesion in a similar location. (Courtesy of P. Feldman, M.D., Toronto, Ontario, Canada.)

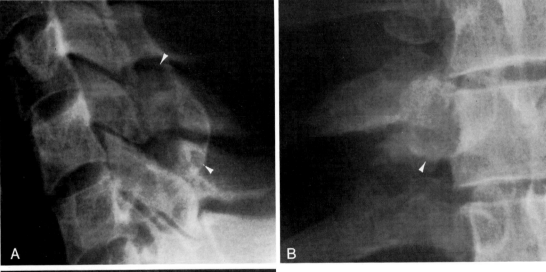

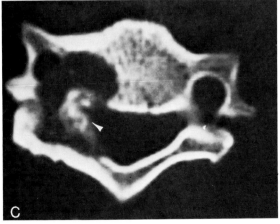

FIGURE 83–30. Osteoblastoma: Radiographic abnormalities—spine. Three different examples are shown. In **A,** an expansile lesion (arrowheads) in the lamina of the fifth cervical vertebra is evident. In **B,** an osteosclerotic lesion (arrowhead) is located primarily in the transverse process of a thoracic vertebra. In **C,** note an osteolytic lesion containing calcification or ossification (arrowhead) affecting the body, transverse and costal elements, and lamina of a cervical vertebra as depicted in a transaxial CT scan. (**B,** Courtesy of V. Vint, M.D., San Diego, California; **C,** courtesy of J. A. Amberg, M.D., San Diego, California.)

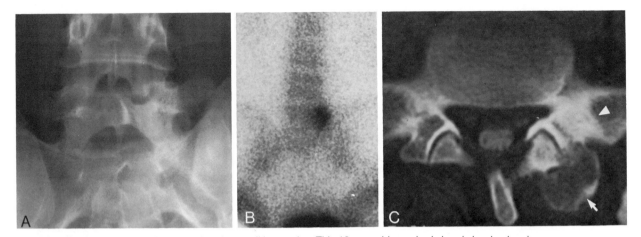

FIGURE 83–31. Osteoblastoma: Radiographic abnormalities—spine. This 18 year old man had chronic low back pain.
  A A routine radiograph shows bone sclerosis involving the posterior elements in the left side of the fifth lumbar vertebra.
  B A bone scan reveals increased uptake of the radiopharmaceutical agent in the left side of the fifth lumbar vertebra.
  C Transaxial CT reveals an expansile lesion (arrow) accompanied by bone sclerosis (arrowhead). (Courtesy of A. Newberg, M.D., Boston, Massachusetts.)

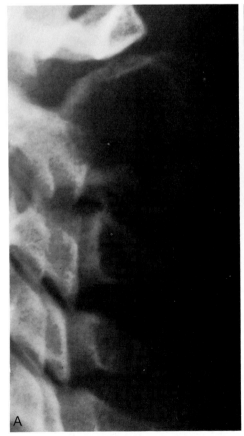

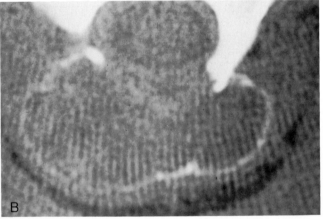

FIGURE 83–32. Osteoblastoma: Radiographic abnormalities—spine. A radiograph **(A)** and a transaxial CT scan **(B)** in a 13 year old girl reveal a large, expansile, osteolytic lesion with an osseous rim involving the spinous process of the axis. It resembles an aneurysmal bone cyst.

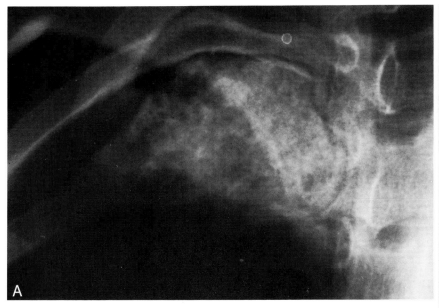

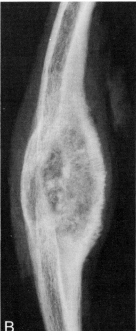

FIGURE 83–33. Osteoblastoma: Radiographic abnormalities—ribs.

A In a 16 year old boy, a large, expansile, heavily calcified lesion involves the posterior portion of the rib, extending to the costovertebral articulations.

B In a second case, an expansile osteolytic lesion containing calcification is evident in this specimen radiograph. Note the extraordinary amount of cortical thickening.

(**B**, Courtesy of W. F. Keller, M.D., Oklahoma City, Oklahoma.)

tical, or medullary location.[28, 135, 137] Although cortical or medullary tumors are most frequent, subperiosteal osteoblastomas are not uncommon in the facial and cranial bones, especially the maxilla, and also occur in the humerus, radius, ribs, femur, and tibia.[13, 33, 34, 144, 154, 161, 162, 1990] Intracortical osteoblastomas are associated with a marked amount of surrounding sclerotic bone (Fig. 83–34A) similar to that found in an osteoid osteoma, but the nidus of an osteoblastoma is larger.[13, 30, 34, 135, 163] Because the periosteum apparently is required for the production of sclerotic bone, osteoblastomas located in the spongiosa lack abundant osteosclerosis.[13, 30, 34, 137]

In the long tubular bones, osteoblastomas vary in size from 2 to 13.5 cm in their maximum dimension and frequently cause a bulge in the osseous contour related to cortical erosion by the tumor.[28, 135] The outer margin of the tumor usually is covered by periosteum as well as by a thin rim of reactive bone, however.[28, 33, 34] In the short tubular bones of the hands and feet, the lesion may produce fusiform osseous expansion. Unlike long bone osteoblastomas, which seldom extend into the soft tissue,[28] vertebral osteoblastomas not infrequently have epidural extension and may even extend into the paraspinal tissue or involve adjacent vertebrae.[41, 1991]

When sectioned, osteoblastomas are fairly well delineated, and a thin rim of limiting bone may be present on the medullary aspect of a tumor of cancellous bone.[28] The neoplasms are hemorrhagic, purple to reddish-brown in color, and have a gritty or granular consistency with occasional softer cystic regions.[28, 30, 33, 130, 135]

Microscopically, the basic pattern of osteoblastoma is similar to that of osteoid osteoma, consisting of a well-vascularized connective tissue stroma in which there is active production of osteoid and primitive woven bone[13, 28, 30, 33, 34, 134, 135, 179] (Fig. 83–34B). There is considerable variation in this pattern, however. In less mature lesions, there is an abundance of connective tissue stroma in which multinucleated osteoclast-type giant cells and small osteoid foci are present, leading in some instances to a lace-like pattern. With maturation of the tumor, there is progressive mineralization of the osteoid, which is converted to trabeculae of coarse woven bone that may fuse to form an anastomosing network. The trabeculae are rimmed by plump, active osteoblasts (Fig. 83–34C). Such osteoblasts, as well as those that may be present as broad sheets in the adjacent stroma, usually lack any significant atypia and possess round to oval regular nuclei and, perhaps, prominent nucleoli. Mitotic activity is infrequent. In some instances, the characteristic osteoblast-rimmed trabeculae of bone may not be found throughout the entire tumor, instead being replaced by large sheets of osteoid with little or no stroma and few osteoblasts.[180] Stromal osteoclasts are present, which frequently are actively involved in remodeling the primitive bone trabeculae. The presence of active bone production and remodeling may create pagetoid bone that has prominent cement lines.[33, 34] The degree of calcification is variable; some lesions are extensively calcified. Although cartilage usually is not considered a part of the histologic spectrum of osteoblastoma, rare examples are reported in which the tumor contained hyaline cartilage or chondroid matrix.[2440]

Although the histologic diagnosis of osteoblastoma generally is not difficult, especially when radiologic and clinical data also are considered, there are occasions in which the microscopic features in this tumor may be more difficult to interpret. The overall pattern of osteoblastoma tends to

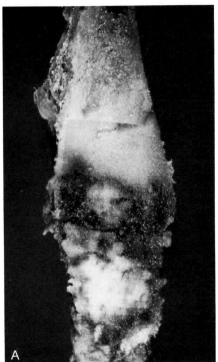

FIGURE 83–34. Osteoblastoma: Macroscopic and microscopic abnormalities.

A This lesion of the ilium is associated with considerable cortical sclerosis. Its cut surface reveals calcified osteoid (white foci) as well as granular vascular regions (dark foci). (Courtesy of B. Perez, M.D., St. Louis, Missouri.)

B A section through the nidus of an osteoblastoma reveals highly vascular stroma with numerous, dilated blood vessels. Abundant osteoid and primitive trabeculae are present, most of which lack any osteoblastic rimming. (150×.)

C In another area of the nidus of the osteoblastoma illustrated in **A**, trabeculae are lined by plump osteoblasts. (150×.)

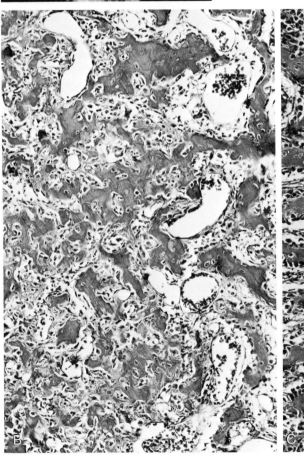

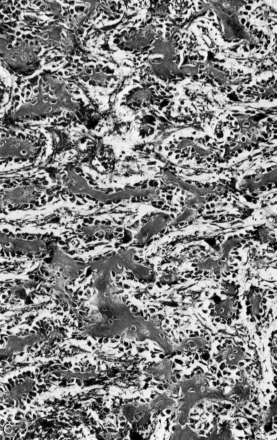

be less well organized than that of osteoid osteoma, with the trabeculae of woven bone in osteoblastoma being larger, wider, more widely separated, and less likely to mature to lamellar bone than the trabeculae of osteoid osteoma.[34, 137, 138, 179] The abundant vascularity characteristic of the osteoblastoma consists mainly of widely dilated capillaries; however, areas of large dilated blood sinusoids similar to those in aneurysmal bone cyst occasionally may be found.[30, 33, 135–137] Some osteoblastomas have large tumor cells with highly bizarre, atypical hyperchromatic nuclei containing prominent nucleoli, or cartilaginous matrix, simulating the findings of osteosarcoma,[28, 30, 135, 181, 1992] and, conversely, there exist cases of osteosarcoma that histologically resemble osteoblastoma. Indeed, with small biopsy specimens, it may be impossible to distinguish between these two tumors.[28, 30, 182] Cases are encountered in which foci of osteosarcoma coexist with areas of osteoblastoma,[135, 183, 2441] and, furthermore, osteoblastomas have recurred with ''transformation'' to osteosarcoma. Whether these phenomena are the result of initial misdiagnosis of an osteosarcoma or a true transformation of an osteoblastoma sometimes is unclear.[182–187, 1870] As true osteoblastomas treated by en bloc excision are claimed not to recur, recurrence of the tumor should alert the pathologist to the possibility that either malignant transformation of an osteoblastoma has occurred or the initial diagnosis of osteoblastoma was in error.[188] Electron microscopy, unfortunately, is of no value in distinguishing the osteoblasts of osteoblastoma from those of osteosarcoma.[189]

Differential Diagnosis. The radiographic abnormalities of osteoblastoma commonly do not allow a precise diagnosis, although those tumors in the posterior osseous elements of the vertebrae (which lead to an expansile, partially calcified area of osteolysis) or in the skull (which produce a sharply marginated radiolucent defect containing central calcification or ossification) may be identified accurately as osteoblastomas. In other sites, this neoplasm has a highly variable radiologic appearance, which may include features suggestive of other diagnoses, including osteoid osteoma, aneurysmal bone cyst, eosinophilic granuloma, enchondroma, fibrous dysplasia, chondromyxoid fibroma, or solitary bone cyst. Furthermore, in cases of aggressive osteoblastomas (see following discussion), the osseous expansion and soft tissue extension that are evident radiographically can simulate the abnormalities associated with osteosarcoma, Ewing's sarcoma, or other malignant tumors.

Aggressive (Malignant) Osteoblastoma. As osteoblastoma had been considered a benign tumor for which conservative excision, when possible, represented the treatment of choice, the identification by Mayer[184] in 1967 of a more aggressive pattern of tumor behavior that led to the patient's death was unexpected. Although typical osteoblastomas had been known to recur in as many as 10 per cent of cases, particularly following incomplete excision,[188, 190, 191, 1816, 1993] the documentation of recurrent osteoblastoma in which the histologic appearance was more aggressive than that of the original tumor, as provided by Mayer[184] and others,[182, 186, 192, 193, 1817, 1818, 1994] served as a warning that osteoblastomas should not be regarded as uniformly benign. Unfortunately, the precise definitions of malignant osteoblastoma and aggressive osteoblastoma still are not clearly established, and the two have been regarded as either identical or different lesions.[183, 194, 195] Further, Bertoni and collaborators[196] recently have reported examples of osteosar-

comas that histologically resembled osteoblastoma and postulated that such tumors were similar to those designated malignant or aggressive osteoblastoma.

In general, the anatomic distribution of aggressive (malignant) osteoblastoma parallels that of conventional osteoblastoma. The vertebrae, tibia, femur, and skull are the most common sites of involvement.[1817, 1818] Other bones, however, may be affected.[2442] In the long tubular bones, metaphyseal location with extension to the epiphysis may be evident. In all sites, the radiologic and macropathologic features of these lesions resemble the findings of typical osteoblastoma but with a greater likelihood of soft tissue involvement[194, 197] (Figs. 83–35 to 83–37).

The histologic characteristics of aggressive osteoblastoma include findings of conventional osteoblastoma as well as those suggestive of malignancy. Descriptions of the histologic features of aggressive osteoblastoma emphasize the presence of highly cellular tumors containing compact areas of osteoblasts that are larger and have more frequent mitoses than the osteoblasts in conventional osteoblastoma. The osteoblasts also may have an epithelial appearance and have been designated epithelioid osteoblasts. Additional characteristics of aggressive osteoblastoma include the presence of numerous multinucleated osteoclast-type giant cells and abundant osteoid and trabeculae of woven bone. Atypical, highly calcified tumor bone is evident that stains intensely with hematoxylin. This spiculated tumor bone is similar to that occurring in conventional osteosarcoma. Also, in aggressive osteoblastoma, large sheets of osteoblasts are evident that are approximately twice the size of conventional osteoblasts and that appear plump, with prominent nucleoli. These cells are round (rather than spindle-shaped, as are the stromal cells of conventional osteosarcoma), and contain hyperchromatic atypical nuclei and abundant, clear to eosinophilic cytoplasm. Such cells are termed epithelioid osteoblasts and are the histologic hallmark of the tumor. Vascular stroma with cellular, fibroblastic regions, variable mitotic activity that may be brisk, lace-like ribbons of osteoid, and irregular trabeculae are further microscopic characteristics of aggressive osteoblastoma.

The major diagnostic problem is differentiating these aggressive or malignant osteoblastomas from osteosarcoma. In general, those investigators who believe that these aggressive osteoblastomas differ from osteosarcoma are of the view that when adequate tissue is examined, the tumors have an overall pattern that is more structured than that of osteosarcoma, with more orderly trabeculae that are lined by plump osteoblasts that lack the bizarre nuclear configurations seen in osteosarcoma. They also lack the atypical mitotic figures, necrosis, and malignant cartilage of osteosarcoma.[194, 198]

It is important to differentiate between aggressive osteoblastomas and conventional osteoblastomas, as the former tumors show a far greater likelihood to recur (approaching 50 per cent of cases). In some instances, aggressive osteoblastomas have led to the patient's death, exhibiting patterns of tumor growth similar to those of low grade osteosarcomas, including metastases.[1818]

Ossifying Fibroma

This fibro-osseous lesion is closely related radiographically and pathologically to fibrous dysplasia. Most ossifying fibromas arise in the facial bones, particularly in the

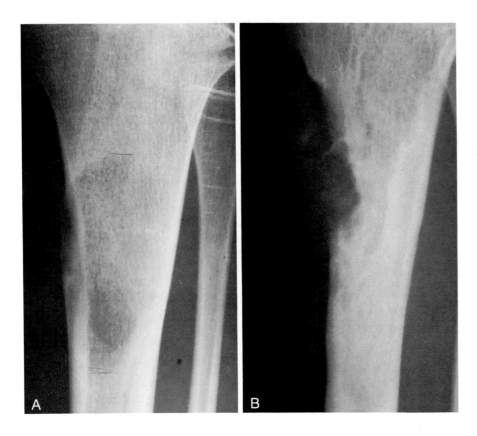

FIGURE 83–35. Aggressive (malignant) osteoblastoma: Radiographic abnormalities.

A The initial radiograph in a 16 year old girl reveals a well-defined, slightly expansile, osteolytic lesion of the tibia. Biopsy confirmed the presence of an osteoblastoma. Following conservative surgery, recurrence of tumor occurred.

B Four years after **A**, following multiple surgical procedures, an aggressive eccentric lesion is evident in the tibia. Note the soft tissue extension of the tumor with extraosseous ossification.

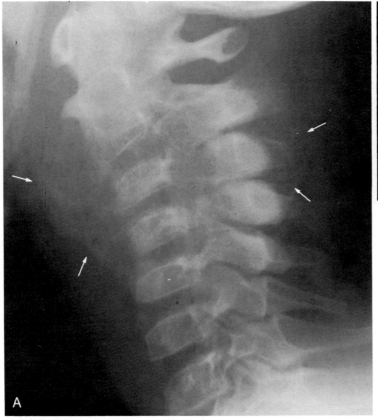

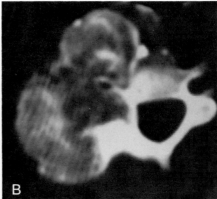

FIGURE 83–36. Aggressive (malignant) osteoblastoma: Radiographic abnormalities.

A A lateral radiograph in this 6 year old boy shows a large expansile lesion (arrows) involving the upper cervical vertebrae.

B Transaxial CT scan at the level of the second cervical vertebra documents the expansile nature of the tumor.

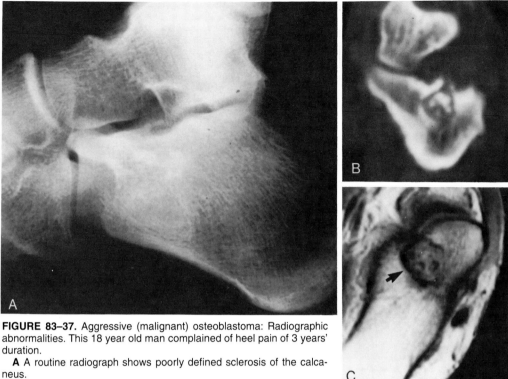

FIGURE 83–37. Aggressive (malignant) osteoblastoma: Radiographic abnormalities. This 18 year old man complained of heel pain of 3 years' duration.

A A routine radiograph shows poorly defined sclerosis of the calcaneus.

B A coronal CT scan reveals a partially calcified lesion in the calcaneus with an appearance similar to that of an osteoid osteoma.

C A transverse proton density–weighted (TR/TE, 2600/20) spin echo MR image shows the tumor (arrow) containing regions of low signal intensity, representing calcification. At surgery, a mass extended into the tarsal sinus.

mandible and maxilla, in the second, third, and fourth decades of life, predominantly in women. A similar tumor can appear in a tubular bone, almost exclusively in the tibia, with an earlier age of onset.

Ossifying Fibroma of Facial Bones. The ossifying fibromas of the jaws are well-circumscribed, slowly growing lesions, which enlarge in an expansile manner.[199] Their similarity to fibrous dysplasia has been emphasized repeatedly, although differentiation of the two conditions is important; ossifying fibromas are well demarcated and amenable to surgical enucleation or curettage, whereas fibrous dysplasia typically lacks clearly demarcated borders.[200] As summarized by Eversole and colleagues,[201] ossifying fibromas elaborate bone, cementum, and spheroidal calcifications, leading to some variation in terminology: When bone predominates, the appellation of ossifying fibroma is most appropriate; when curvilinear trabeculae or spheroidal calcifications are encountered, cementifying fibroma is the assigned term; and when both bone and cemental tissues are observed, cemento-ossifying fibroma is the accepted nomenclature.

In general, a painless expansion of the tooth-bearing portion of the mandible or, less commonly, the maxilla is observed on clinical examination. Radiographically, the lesion typically is 1 to 5 cm in diameter, although larger (and more aggressive) tumors are encountered, especially in children, that have been designated juvenile aggressive or active ossifying fibromas.[201–204] Well-defined unilocular or multilocular areas of osteolysis containing varying degrees of calcification are seen, and cortical thinning and expan-

sion with displacement of adjacent teeth are additional radiographic abnormalities.[199, 201] The ease with which ossifying fibromas can be separated from the surrounding bone at the time of surgery is a feature usually allowing their differentiation from monostotic fibrous dysplasia.[199] Histologic findings include osseous products consisting of woven and lamellar trabeculae, spheroid products with nonpolarizable features or exhibiting Sharpey's fiber-like fringes, and a fasciculated or storiform stroma containing dystrophic calcification.[201]

Ossifying Fibroma of Tubular Bones. Ossifying fibromas of the tubular bones are rare,[205–217] being first reported by Kempson in 1966.[205] In subsequent descriptions, these lesions also have been designated *osteofibrous dysplasia*,[206, 210] although, in all reports, the predominant involvement of the tibia and, to a lesser extent, the fibula has been emphasized. The majority of cases have consisted of lesions isolated to the tibia (Fig. 83–38); additional patterns of distribution have included involvement of the tibia and ipsilateral fibula (Fig. 83–39), of the fibula alone, and of both tibiae and fibulae. Exceptional sites of ossifying fibromas are the ulna, radius, humerus, and metatarsal and phalangeal bones,[206, 207, 1997] although, in some of these instances, histologic verification has been lacking. Diaphyseal localization is typical, especially the middle third of the tibia, although such lesions can extend into the metaphysis. Involvement of the distal diaphyseal segment of the fibula also is characteristic. In the tibia, the lesion usually is located in the anterior aspect of the bone, apparently beginning as an intracortical tumor that subsequently violates the spongiosa. Multiple separate

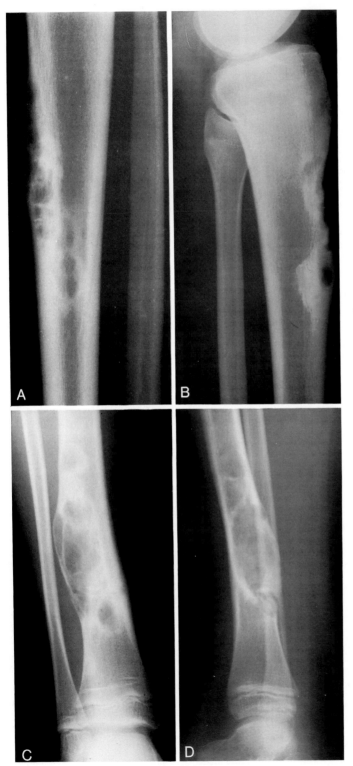

FIGURE 83–38. Ossifying fibroma: Radiographic abnormalities—tibia.

A In a 16 year old girl with progressive pain in the anterior portion of the lower leg, a lateral radiograph reveals a sharply marginated, lobulated, eccentric lesion in the diaphysis, affecting mainly the anterior cortex.

B In a second patient, observe multiple anterior cortical radiolucent areas with bone sclerosis. (**B,** Courtesy of E.G. Hardy, M.D., Adelaide, South Australia.)

C, D Anteroposterior (**C**) and lateral (**D**) radiographs in a child reveal a bubbly, multilocular radiolucent lesion with associated bone sclerosis, osseous expansion and bowing, and a pathologic fracture. The appearance is reminiscent of a nonossifying fibroma.

(**A,** From Goergen TG, et al: Cancer *39*:2067, 1977.)

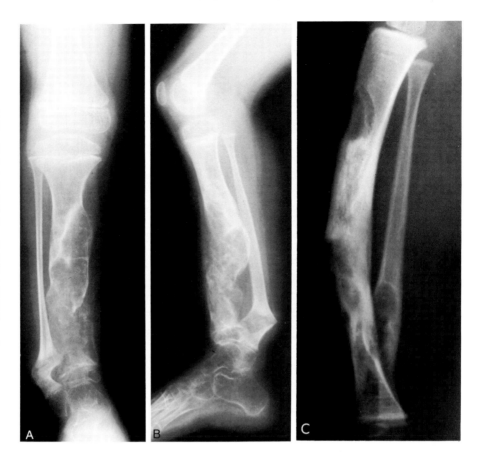

FIGURE 83–39. Ossifying fibroma: Radiographic abnormalities—tibia and fibula.

A, B Anteroposterior **(A)** and lateral **(B)** radiographs in a child show an extensive lesion of the diaphysis and metaphysis of the tibia leading to osseous expansion and a pathologic fracture; note the additional involvement of the distal portion of the fibula with osseous deformity.

C In this 2 year old child note the multiloculated, eccentric cortical lesion of the tibia with an additional lesion of the fibula. Other bones were not affected. Although the biopsy indicated only "fibrous" tissue, the appearance is compatible with osteofibrous dysplasia (see text).

(**C,** Courtesy of J.E.L. Desautels, M.D., Calgary, Alberta, Canada.)

foci within the same bone may occur or, as indicated previously, more than one bone may be involved simultaneously or metachronously.[206, 209, 210]

Ossifying fibromas of the tubular bones generally are seen in the first or second decade of life, in boys or girls with approximately equal frequency, leading to painless enlargement and bowing of the bone.[1998, 1999] Neonates may be affected.[2000, 2001] In the tibia, slight or moderate anterior or anterolateral bowing is the rule. Osseous deformity may be accentuated by pathologic fractures that occur with minor trauma and may be followed by pseudarthrosis. Intracortical osteolysis clearly marginated by a band of sclerosis may be seen as a single confluent region or multiple, elongated, bubble-like areas.[210] A hazy or ground-glass appearance similar to that of fibrous dysplasia commonly is evident. Occasionally, the tumor is entirely osteosclerotic. Although ossifying fibroma of the tubular bones usually is stable or may even regress spontaneously on serial radiographic examinations,[218, 2000] progression of the lesion, especially before puberty, occasionally is observed, and tumor recurrence following curettage or subperiosteal resection is well documented.

At the time of surgery, the cortex of the involved bone is found to be quite thin or even absent focally, but the periosteum is intact over the lesion. The tumor itself varies from 1 to 10 cm in its maximum dimension. On section, the tibial tumors are found to be located eccentrically and to bulge from the cortex into the medullary cavity, but to rarely extend to involve the complete circumference of the bone. In the fibula, however, the entire width of the bone usually is involved. The tumor appears well demarcated from the adjacent uninvolved bone, frequently by a thin band of sclerosis. It is pale white to yellow-white and varies in consistency from rubbery to firm or gritty, depending on the amount of osseous or fibrous tissue that is present.

Histologically, ossifying fibroma consists of a fairly abundant well-vascularized fibrous stroma in which reside trabeculae of new bone.[205, 206, 208, 210] The stroma is composed of well-differentiated fibroblasts that may demonstrate a whorled or storiform pattern (Fig. 83–40). The fibroblasts may be loosely arranged and separated from each other or closely arranged and compact. Multinucleated giant cells may be scattered within the stroma or aggregated focally about areas of stromal hemorrhage or microfracture. The trabeculae are arranged randomly throughout the stroma in no apparent functional pattern, have the coarse appearance of woven bone, and, characteristically, are rimmed by osteoblasts and occasional osteoclasts. Although by ordinary light microscopy, these trabeculae appear immature, some have a peripheral rim of lamellar bone when examined by polarized light. Fully mature spicules of lamellar bone may be found, but they are not frequent. Such spicules usually are evident at the periphery of the lesion where it merges with cortical bone; here, a zonal pattern is created in which the central portion of the lesion consists of immature woven bone and the peripheral portion contains more mature bone.[206, 210, 2443] The trabeculae of ossifying fibroma do not have the irregular C or S shapes that typically are found in fibrous dysplasia.[216] Some ossifying fibromas contain small foci of cartilage, either as part of an area of reparative callus or as an isolated island without any associated evidence of prior trauma.

In an electron microscopic study of a single case, Kempson[205] noted that the osteoblasts of ossifying fibroma had

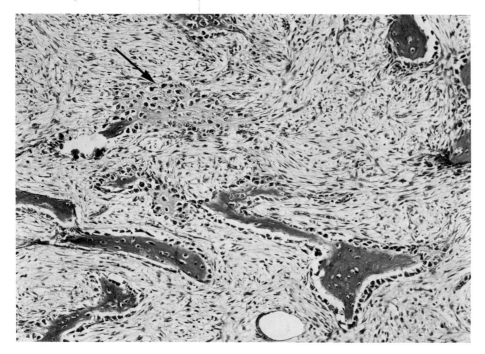

FIGURE 83–40. Ossifying fibroma: Microscopic abnormalities. Observe the loosely arranged, whorled fibroblastic stroma of an ossifying fibroma in which active bone formation is seen. As with fibrous dysplasia, the new bone in the form of osteoid (arrow) arises directly from the stroma; however, unlike the case with fibrous dysplasia, this bone is rimmed by osteoblasts. (150×.)

the same features as osteoblasts in reactive bone. In addition, he found that at sites of active bone formation, the stromal cells had features of both fibroblasts and osteoblasts.

With regard to accurate diagnosis, the radiographic features of ossifying fibromas in the tubular bones most resemble those of fibrous dysplasia. Tibial involvement with predilection for the anterior cortex of the diaphysis, a unilocular or multilocular elongated lesion, osseous bowing and, in some cases, associated abnormalities of the fibula are highly characteristic of ossifying fibroma, although similar alterations may be evident in fibrous dysplasia, leading to considerable diagnostic difficulty. Monostotic fibrous dysplasia commonly affects patients in the second and third decades of life and, in addition to the tibia, frequently involves the rib, femur, facial bones, or skull. Adamantinoma represents a second lesion sharing many radiographic features with ossifying fibroma, including a propensity to affect the middle region of the tibia. Indeed, a relationship between adamantinoma in young persons and ossifying fibroma may exist (see later discussion). Of interest in this regard are reports of tibial lesions with histologic features of adamantinoma and fibrous regions similar but not identical to those of fibrous dysplasia.[208, 217] These problems in precise radiographic diagnosis are accentuated by histologic similarity between ossifying fibroma and other lesions, specifically fibrous dysplasia. The major point of difference between ossifying fibroma and fibrous dysplasia is the lack of osteoblastic rimming on the metaplastic trabeculae in the latter lesion.[205, 207] Although occasional bone spicules in fibrous dysplasia are lined by osteoblasts, this finding is indeed infrequent and usually is accompanied by histologic evidence of previous trauma, including hemosiderin deposition, chronic inflammatory cells, macrophages, or actual callus formation, indicating that the new bone is a reparative phenomenon and not part of the actual tumor.[205] Furthermore, the trabeculae of fibrous dysplasia do not show peripheral maturation to lamellar bone, as is found in ossi-

fying fibroma. Another potential source of diagnostic difficulty is distinguishing histologically between ossifying fibroma and well-differentiated intraosseous osteosarcoma. The trabeculae in this latter tumor lack the zonal arrangement of ossifying fibroma, and the osteocytes, osteoblasts, and stromal cells of well-differentiated osteosarcoma have a degree of nuclear atypia that is not present in the cells of ossifying fibroma.

Malignant Tumors

Osteosarcoma

Osteosarcoma, which also has been designated osteogenic sarcoma, is second in frequency only to plasma cell myeloma as a primary malignant neoplasm of bone. It is characterized histologically by proliferating tumor cells that, in most instances, produce osteoid or immature bone. Infrequently, such cells remain so immature that osteoid or bone is not elaborated, leading to difficulties in tumor classification and to considerable interest in identifying diagnostic methods not dependent on routine microscopy. As an example, one histochemical technique relies for diagnosis on the abundance of alkaline phosphatase in the tumor cells of osteosarcoma,[219, 220] although conspicuous alkaline phosphatase activity may not be detected in those neoplastic foci that contain predominantly fibroblastic or cartilaginous tissue.[221] Additional diagnostic methods employ immunohistology, immunoscintigraphy, or immunofluorescence.[221–224]

Extensive modifications in the classification scheme of osteosarcomas have appeared in recent years. Traditional systems using the designations of conventional and parosteal tumors have been replaced owing to the identification of many clinical, radiologic, and histologic varieties of osteosarcoma, although no single method of classification is accepted uniformly. Available systems employ such features as the precise location of the tumor within the bone (intramedullary or central, intracortical, surface, periosteal, or parosteal); the degree of cellular differentiation (high grade or low grade); the histologic composition (osteoblastic, chondroblastic, fibroblastic, fibrohistiocytic, telangiectactic, small cell, clear cell); the number of foci of involvement (single or multicentric); and the status of the underlying bone (normal or the site of disease such as Paget's disease, of injury as occurs with a vascular insult or following irradiation, or of another neoplasm, such as an osteochondroma, chondroma, or osteoblastoma).

In the following discussion, a summary of some of the recognizable varieties of osteosarcoma is provided. The importance of each of the specific subdivisions of the neoplasm should be judged on the basis of the uniqueness of its clinical, radiologic, histologic, or behavioral characteristics, and with full knowledge that alternative methods of tumor classification exist.

Conventional Osteosarcoma. Conventional osteosarcoma generally is seen in the second and third decades of life,[225–227] although the neoplasm has been identified in patients of all ages, including infants and very young children[228, 229] and the elderly.[230, 1819] Men are affected more frequently than women in a ratio of approximately 2 to 1, and osteosarcomas occurring in more than one member of a single family have been encountered.[231, 232] Clinical manifestations include pain and swelling, restriction of motion, warmth, and pyrexia.[225, 226] Frequently, the patient seeks medical assistance only after a traumatic episode, which may or may not result in a pathologic fracture.[227]

Skeletal Location. The most typical sites of involvement are the tubular bones in the appendicular skeleton (80 per cent of cases), particularly the femur (40 per cent), the tibia (16 per cent), and the humerus (15 per cent); it is the distal portion of the femur and the proximal portions of the tibia and humerus that represent the areas involved most frequently.[30, 33, 34, 180, 225, 233–237, 2002] Fifty to 75 per cent of all cases develop in the osseous structures about the knee. Osteosarcomas are relatively infrequent in the fibula, innominate bone, mandible, maxilla, and spine[234, 238, 239, 1820, 2003, 2004] and are rare in the skull, ribs, scapula, clavicle, sternum, radius, ulna, and small bones of the hands and feet.[240–249, 1821, 1891, 2005–2010] With regard to the long tubular bones, metaphyseal location predominates. Initial involvement of the diaphysis occurs in 2 to 11 per cent of cases and may be accompanied by relatively subtle or innocent osteosclerotic changes.[250–254] Although osteosarcoma may extend into the epiphysis,[255] especially when the physis is closed,[234, 237] a primary epiphyseal origin is quite rare.[256, 257, 2011, 2012] Epiphyseal osteosarcomas predominate in the femoral condyles.[2011]

Radiographic Abnormalities. Although descriptions exist of subtle radiographic abnormalities in the early stages of osteosarcoma,[258] the roentgenographic findings usually are obvious at the time of the initial examination of the patient. The pattern of osseous involvement is variable, depending to large extent on the amount of bone produced by the tumor[235] (Fig. 83–41). A mixed pattern consisting of both osteolysis and osteosclerosis is most typical (Fig. 83–42), with purely osteolytic or osteosclerotic lesions (Figs. 83–43 and 83–44) being encountered less frequently.[259] Osteolysis is especially characteristic of the telangiectatic variety of osteosarcoma (see later discussion). With regard to the tubular bones of the appendicular skeleton, conventional osteosarcoma usually is evident as an ill-defined,

intramedullary, metaphyseal lesion that has extended through the cortex and produced a sizeable soft tissue mass[235, 260] (Fig. 83–45). Periosteal reaction in the form of a Codman's triangle or with a "sunburst" appearance[260, 261] and, rarely, a pathologic fracture[225] are additional radiographic features (Fig. 83–46). Osteosarcomas in the diaphysis of a tubular bone (Fig. 83–47) may reveal osteosclerotic foci and endosteal thickening with the absence of cortical destruction or periostitis.[250, 251] Those arising in an epiphysis usually are osteolytic.

The radiographic features of osteosarcoma in other skeletal sites are similar to those in the tubular bones and include varying degrees of osteolysis and osteosclerosis, cortical violation, periostitis, and a soft tissue mass (Fig. 83–48). Five to 10 per cent of osteosarcomas involve the flat bones, including those of the pelvis, and such involvement may be more frequent in older patients.[1819] Analysis of the rarely occurring spinal osteosarcomas indicates that the vertebral bodies are the preferred site of involvement. When localized in the posterior elements of a vertebra, an osteosarcoma may be misdiagnosed as an osteoblastoma.[1820] Rib lesions may be accompanied by large, extrapleural masses similar to those seen in plasma cell myeloma. In the skull, osteolysis is the predominant radiographic abnormality.[1821]

Other Imaging Techniques. Additional imaging methods that have been used in the evaluation of osteosarcoma include bone scintigraphy,[262–266, 1822, 1823, 2013, 2014] arteriography,[267, 268, 2015] CT,[269–273, 1892, 2016] and MR imaging.[1824, 1893, 1894, 2017–2028] It should be emphasized, however, that the "gold standard" in the specific diagnosis of this tumor remains the conventional radiograph and that these other techniques are more useful in defining the extent of the neoplasm and its relationship to surrounding neurovascular structures (information that is vital to the orthopedic surgeon who is contemplating operative intervention) and in evaluating the response of the tumor to therapy (see later discussion). The radionuclide examination uniformly shows an increased accumulation of the bone-seeking radiopharmaceutical agent within the primary tumor itself and, less uniformly, at sites of skeletal or extraskeletal metastasis. Although this technique provides additional information regarding the anatomic extent of the osseous tumor, an extended pattern of radionuclide accumulation beyond the true margin of the osteosarcoma, perhaps related to marrow hyperemia, medullary reactive bone, and periostitis, is well documented and creates difficulty in accurate interpretation of the scintigraphic findings[262] (Fig. 83–49). Angiography provides identification of the extraosseous component of the tumor and defines the degree of displacement (or invasion) of vessels (Fig. 83–50); its precise role as a diagnostic method allowing differentiation of osteosarcoma from other sarcomas is controversial. CT is useful in assessing the intramedullary and soft tissue extent of the neoplasm, although limitations in the interpretation of the data are recognized. An increase in the attenuation values of the tissue within the medullary canal generally is indicative of tumor extension or "skip" metastases; however, similar findings may relate to nutrient vessels or osseous ridges.[269] Soft tissue involvement in osteosarcoma is better defined with CT when intermuscular fasciae are visible; the presence of edema or hemorrhage in the soft tissues leads to diagnostic difficulties.[269]

Text continued on page 3668

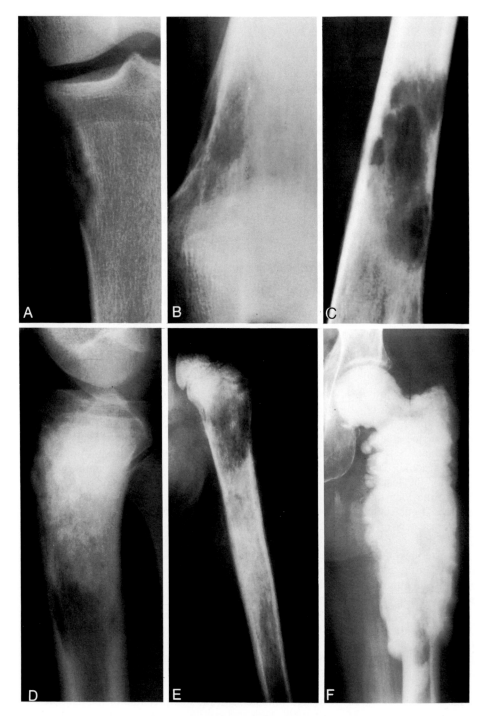

FIGURE 83–41. Conventional osteosarcoma: Radiographic abnormalities—basic patterns of osseous involvement.

A Purely osteolytic pattern (metaphyseal and epiphyseal).

B Purely osteolytic pattern (metaphyseal and diaphyseal).

C Purely osteolytic pattern (diaphyseal).

D Mixed osteolytic and osteosclerotic pattern (metaphyseal and diaphyseal).

E Mixed osteolytic and osteosclerotic pattern (metaphyseal and diaphyseal).

F Purely osteosclerotic pattern (epiphyseal, metaphyseal, and diaphyseal).

(**F,** Courtesy of P. Major, M.D., Winnipeg, Manitoba, Canada.)

FIGURE 83–42. Conventional osteosarcoma: Radiographic abnormalities—mixed osteolytic and osteosclerotic pattern.

A, B This 66 year old man developed left hip and thigh pain that initially was diagnosed as a muscle strain. The routine radiograph **(A)** reveals a large lesion of the metaphyseal region of the proximal portion of the femur with diaphyseal extension. Its major component is osteolytic with adjacent bone sclerosis, and there is disruption of the lateral cortex of the femoral neck. A bone scan **(B)** shows increased accumulation of the radionuclide at the site of the lesion (arrow). The tumor was resected and a Thompson endoprosthesis was inserted. The final histologic diagnosis was a fibroblastic osteosarcoma.

C, D This 51 year old woman developed pain in the right knee over a 6 month period. She had fallen 1 month prior to her current evaluation. On physical examination, soft tissue prominence was palpated on the superolateral aspect of the knee. There was no joint effusion, and neurovascular status was normal. The routine radiograph **(C)** documents the presence of a large lesion involving the metaphysis and diaphysis of the distal portion of the femur with osteolysis and bone production. A pathologic fracture is evident although not well shown on this oblique projection. A bone scan **(D)** reveals increased accumulation of the radionuclide (arrow) at the site of the tumor. Histologic evaluation of this lesion indicated a chondroblastic osteosarcoma.

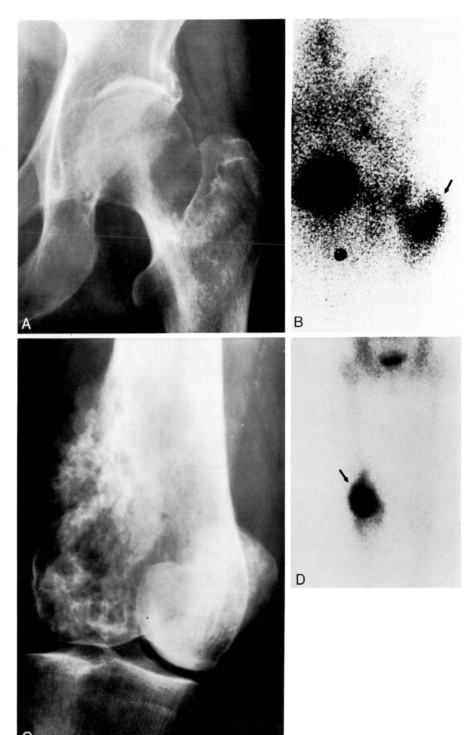

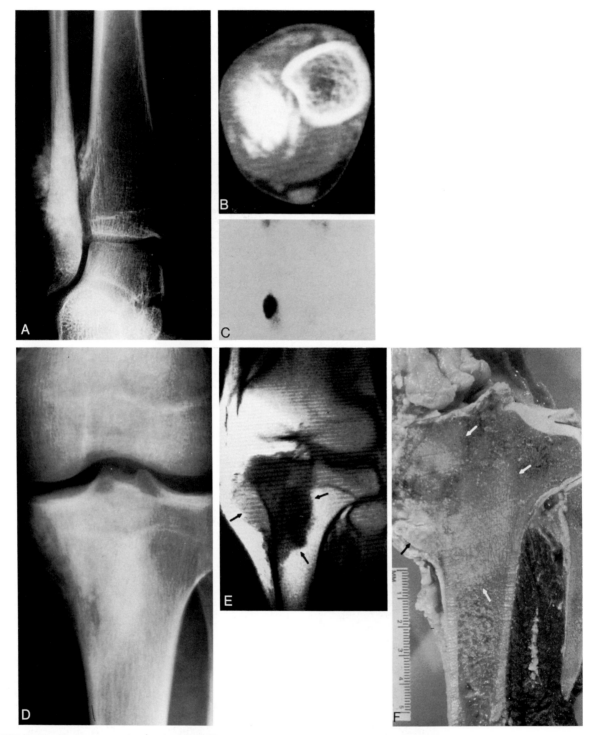

FIGURE 83–43. Conventional osteosarcoma: Radiographic abnormalities—purely osteosclerotic pattern.

A–C Pain and swelling in the ankle of 1 month's duration occurred in a 17 year old man. On physical examination, a 6 × 8 cm mass was palpated in the soft tissues about the lateral aspect of the ankle. The routine radiograph **(A)** shows an osteosclerotic lesion in the diaphysis and metaphysis of the distal portion of the fibula. Note the bone formation within the adjacent soft tissues. A transaxial CT scan **(B)** at the level of the lesion documents the involvement of both the fibula and the soft tissues. A bone scan **(C)** reveals increased accumulation of the radionuclide at the site of the tumor. An osteoblastic osteosarcoma was the final histologic diagnosis.

D–F In an 18 year old man with an unreliable medical history, a conventional radiograph **(D)** shows the purely osteosclerotic lesion in the medial aspect of the metaphysis and epiphysis of the proximal portion of the tibia. In **E,** a coronal T1-weighted (TR/TE, 500/30) spin echo MR image reveals low signal intensity in the intraosseous and extraosseous components of the tumor (arrows). A coronal section of the amputated specimen **(F)** shows the extent of the tumor (arrows) which corresponds to the extent defined in **E.** The final histologic diagnosis was a chondroblastic osteosarcoma.

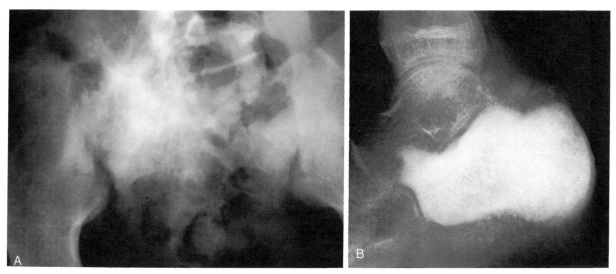

FIGURE 83–44. Conventional osteosarcoma: Radiographic abnormalities—purely osteosclerotic pattern.
A In a 13 year old girl with a 2 month history of foot and leg pain note osteosclerosis involving the sacrum, representing an osteosarcoma. Myelography (not shown) confirmed an extradural lesion in the lower lumbar spine.
B A lateral radiograph reveals osteosclerosis of the entire calcaneus and adjacent soft tissues in a second patient. (**B**, Courtesy of S. Grazelle, M.D., Boston, Massachusetts.)

FIGURE 83–45. Conventional osteosarcoma: Radiographic abnormalities—tubular bones. In a 7 year old boy, a lateral radiograph (**A**) and photograph (**B**) of the amputated specimen reveal the classic metaphyseal location of an osteosarcoma. In this case, epiphyseal extension of the tumor is evident. In **A,** observe osteolysis, osteosclerosis, periostitis and a soft tissue mass. (Courtesy of C. Resnik, M.D., Baltimore, Maryland.)

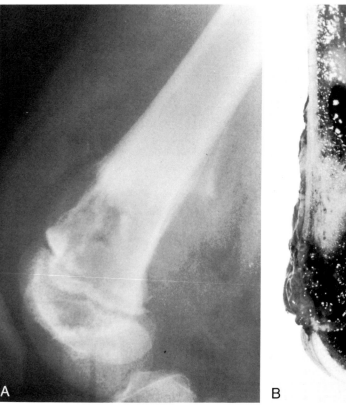
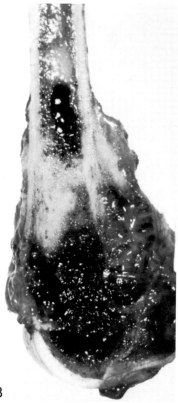

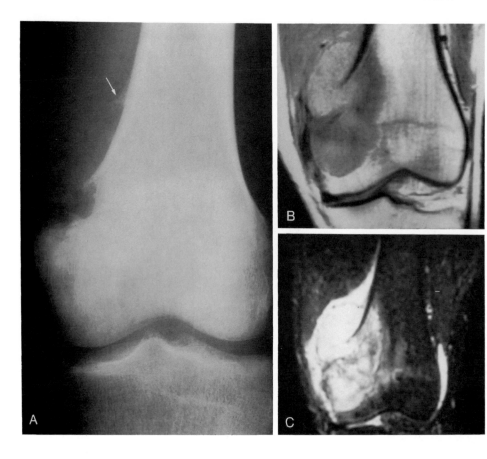

FIGURE 83–46. Conventional osteosarcoma: Radiographic abnormalities—tubular bones. This 17 year old man had a 2 month history of knee pain.

A A routine radiograph reveals an osteolytic lesion involving the medial aspect of the metaphysis of the femur. A Codman's triangle (arrow) is seen.

B A coronal T1-weighted (TR/TE, 700/20) spin echo MR image shows the intraosseous and extraosseous extent of the tumor.

C A coronal T2-weighted (TR/TE, 2500/80) spin echo MR image obtained with chemical presaturation of fat (ChemSat) shows high signal intensity in the tumor, as well as a joint effusion. A total knee arthroplasty was performed.

MR imaging appears to be superior to CT scanning in defining the intraosseous and extraosseous extent of the tumor.[2020, 2025, 2027] The neoplasm typically is of low signal intensity on T1-weighted spin echo MR images and, in such images, can be differentiated from normal fatty marrow (Figs. 83–50 and 83–51). Inhomogeneous or homogeneous high signal intensity within the tumor usually is evident in T2-weighted spin echo MR images (Fig. 83–52). In some instances, differentiation of soft tissue and intraosseous extension of osteosarcoma and peritumoral edema is difficult on the basis of MR imaging.[2508] Enhancement of signal intensity in the tumor is evident following intravenous administration of gadolinium compounds (Fig. 83–53). This may lead to obscuration of the tumor-marrow interface in T1-weighted spin echo MR images that are not combined with fat suppression techniques.[2022] Similarly, contrast-enhanced MR images may lead to diagnostic difficulty with tumor infiltration into perineurovascular fat; such images, however, may be useful in allowing differentiation of intra-articular invasion by tumor and a joint effusion.[2022]

Pathologic Abnormalities. With regard to *macroscopic pathology,* conventional osteosarcomas commonly are large (averaging 8 to 10 cm in maximum dimension), they frequently are observed to invade adjacent soft tissues, and their gross appearance and consistency vary considerably depending on the proportions of cartilage, fibrous tissue, and bone that are present[34, 180] (Fig. 83–54). The tumor may be pink or gray-white and friable with a "fish-flesh" appearance, or gray to blue-gray, owing to the presence of abundant cartilage, with firm, white, fibrous nodular masses.[34, 274] Yellow to yellow-white calcified foci as well as areas of necrosis, hemorrhage, and cystic degeneration commonly are evident. In most osteosarcomas, including the highly

sclerotic ones, the margin of the soft tissue component usually will have highly cellular areas that may be sectioned easily with a scalpel blade, and it is these regions that should be evaluated by frozen section biopsy.[274]

As most osteosarcomas occur in young children and adolescents, the neoplasm usually is noted to abut on an open physeal plate. It had long been considered that an open physis served as a barrier in preventing extension of the tumor into the epiphysis[237]; however, some investigators have indicated that macroscopic or microscopic evidence of transphyseal extension may be quite common, related either to direct invasion through the physeal plate or, less commonly, to tumor extension beneath the perichondrium at the periphery of the plate[255, 275, 276] (Fig. 83–55). Osteosarcomas that involve the epiphysis may extend to the articular cartilage, but generally they do not penetrate the cartilage to enter the joint space.[255, 277] Although osteosarcomas usually do not contain areas of tumor that are separate from the main neoplasm,[180, 278, 279] such "skip" areas have been observed in as many as 25 per cent of cases.[280, 281] These separate foci are found either in the same bone as the main tumor or in an adjacent bone, indicative of transarticular spread.

The *microscopic pathology* of conventional osteosarcoma traditionally has been subdivided into three categories, osteoblastic, chondroblastic, and fibroblastic, depending on the predominant differentiation of tumor cells. Approximately 50 per cent of these tumors produce osteoid in significant amounts to be considered osteoblastic osteosarcomas; 25 per cent of these neoplasms show predominant differentiation toward cartilage and are termed chondroblastic osteosarcomas; and the remaining 25 per cent of osteosarcomas reveal a spindle cell stroma with a herring-

Text continued on page 3676

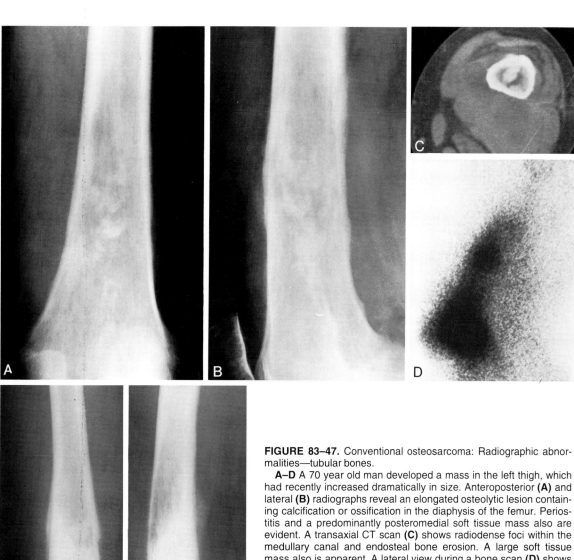

FIGURE 83–47. Conventional osteosarcoma: Radiographic abnormalities—tubular bones.

A–D A 70 year old man developed a mass in the left thigh, which had recently increased dramatically in size. Anteroposterior **(A)** and lateral **(B)** radiographs reveal an elongated osteolytic lesion containing calcification or ossification in the diaphysis of the femur. Periostitis and a predominantly posteromedial soft tissue mass also are evident. A transaxial CT scan **(C)** shows radiodense foci within the medullary canal and endosteal bone erosion. A large soft tissue mass also is apparent. A lateral view during a bone scan **(D)** shows increased accumulation of the radionuclide in the lesion. Needle biopsy of the tumor and subsequent amputation were performed. The final diagnosis was a chondroblastic or fibroblastic osteosarcoma.

E, F In a 13 year old boy with a 2 month history of pain, weight loss, and weakness, an osteosclerotic lesion in the femoral diaphysis is seen. Observe periostitis and soft tissue extension. A biopsy led to the diagnosis of an osteoblastic osteosarcoma.

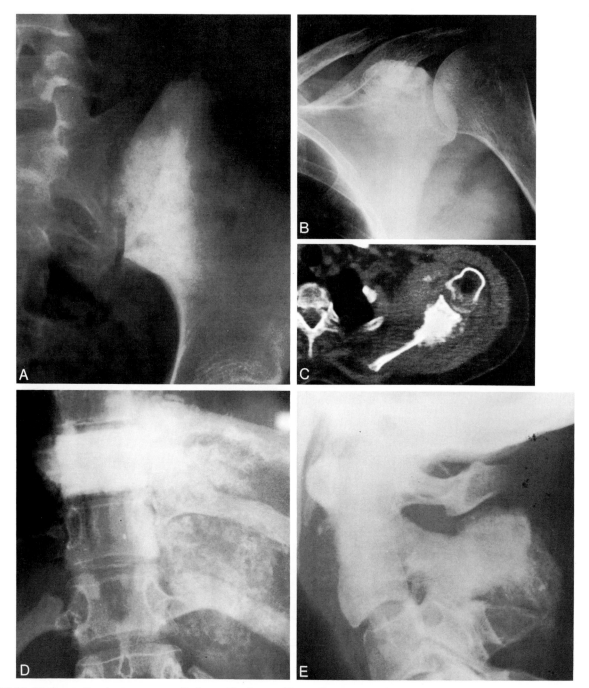

FIGURE 83–48. Conventional osteosarcoma: Radiographic abnormalities—other osseous sites.
A Ilium. An osteosclerotic lesion involves the bone about the sacroiliac joint.
B, C Scapula. Routine radiograph **(B)** and transaxial CT **(C)** document an osteosclerotic lesion of the scapula. In **C,** observe a soft tissue mass.
D Thoracic spine. An extraordinary amount of soft tissue ossification is evident. Note the ivory-like vertebral body.
E Cervical spine. This osteosarcoma, arising in the posterior elements of the axis, is predominantly osteosclerotic. The vertebral body also is affected, and there is a retropharyngeal mass containing calcification or ossification.

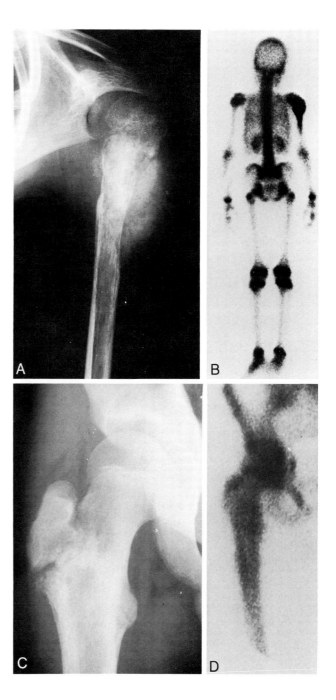

FIGURE 83–49. Conventional osteosarcoma: Scintigraphic abnormalities.

A, B This 7 year old boy developed pain in the left shoulder. The radiograph **(A)** reveals an osteosclerotic lesion in the metaphysis and diaphysis of the humerus. The epiphysis appears uninvolved. Note the soft tissue component of the neoplasm and the erosion of the external surface of the humerus. A bone scan **(B)** reveals an extended pattern of uptake involving the humeral epiphysis and scapula as well as the metaphysis and diaphysis of the humerus. Amputation was required, with subsequent pathologic examination documenting the presence of an osteoblastic osteosarcoma.

C, D In a 12 year old boy with a 1 year history of intermittent right hip pain, a mixed osteolytic and osteosclerotic lesion in the proximal metaphysis of the femur is evident on the conventional radiograph **(C)**. The greater trochanter of the femur also is affected. The bone scan **(D)** reveals uptake of the radiopharmaceutical agent in the metaphysis of the femur as well as in its diaphysis and epiphysis. Inspection of the specimen following hemipelvectomy indicated that the lesion, a fibroblastic osteosarcoma, largely was confined to the metaphysis and trochanteric regions.

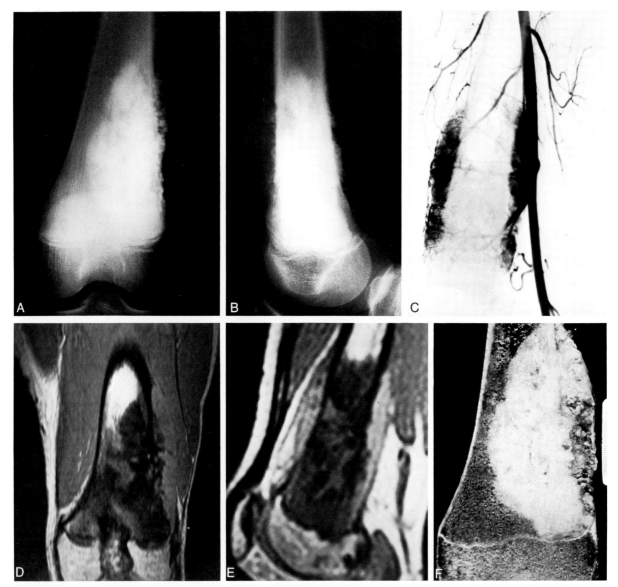

FIGURE 83–50. Conventional osteosarcoma: Angiographic and MR imaging abnormalities. A 15 year old boy noted increasing pain in the thigh of 2 months' duration. Diffuse soft tissue enlargement was apparent on physical examination.

  A, B Anteroposterior **(A)** and lateral **(B)** radiographs show a purely osteosclerotic lesion of the distal metaphysis and diaphysis of the femur. Note the irregular periosteal bone formation.

  C A subtraction lateral image during an angiogram reveals a vascular lesion with new tumor vessels. Arteriovenous shunting also was apparent.

  D, E Coronal **(D)** and sagittal **(E)** T1-weighted spin echo MR images obtained immediately following amputation of the leg exquisitely show the full extent of the tumor, which appears as an area of decreased signal intensity.

  F A photograph of a coronal section of the osteoblastic osteosarcoma reveals the intraosseous and extraosseous components of the tumor. Compare with **A** and **D.**

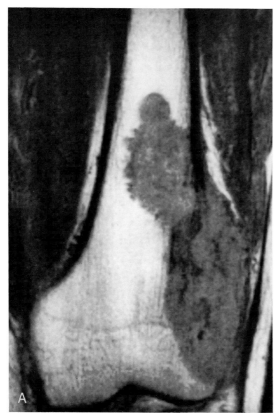

FIGURE 83–51. Conventional osteosarcoma: MR imaging abnormalities.

A Femur. A coronal T1-weighted (TR/TE, 500/30) spin echo MR image reveals the tumor as a region of low signal intensity. (Courtesy of M. Solomon, M.D., Los Gatos, California.)

B, C Tibia. A coronal T1-weighted (TR/TE, 600/15) spin echo MR image **(B)** shows the intraosseous and extraosseous extent of the tumor, which is of low signal intensity. A coronal short tau inversion recovery (STIR) MR image (TR/TE, 5550/60; inversion time, 150 msec) **(C)** reveals inhomogeneous signal intensity in the tumor. Note regions of high signal intensity, representing edema. (Courtesy of C. Wakeley, M.D., Bristol, England.)

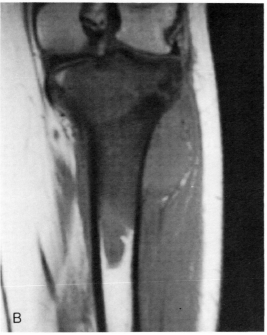

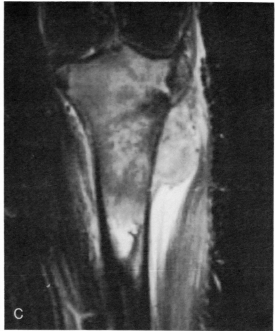

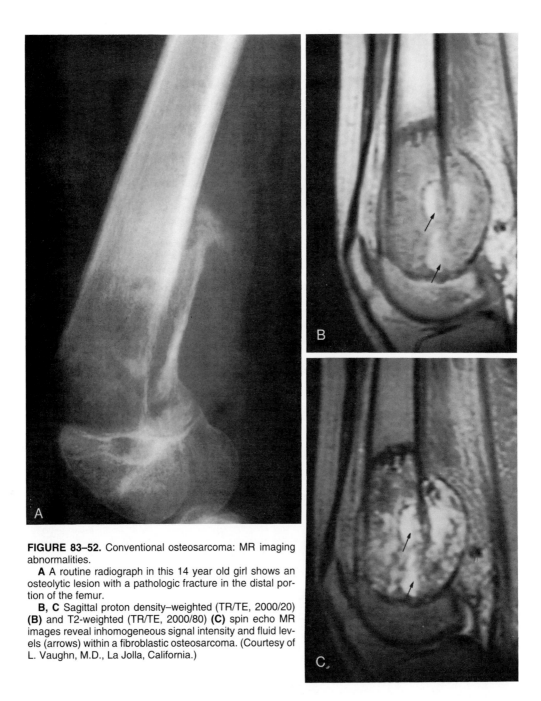

FIGURE 83–52. Conventional osteosarcoma: MR imaging abnormalities.

A A routine radiograph in this 14 year old girl shows an osteolytic lesion with a pathologic fracture in the distal portion of the femur.

B, C Sagittal proton density–weighted (TR/TE, 2000/20) **(B)** and T2-weighted (TR/TE, 2000/80) **(C)** spin echo MR images reveal inhomogeneous signal intensity and fluid levels (arrows) within a fibroblastic osteosarcoma. (Courtesy of L. Vaughn, M.D., La Jolla, California.)

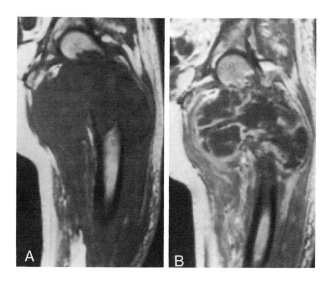

FIGURE 83–53. Conventional osteosarcoma: MR imaging abnormalities. Coronal T1-weighted (TR/TE, 700/15) spin echo MR images obtained before **(A)** and after **(B)** the intravenous injection of a gadolinium-based contrast agent reveal a tumor of low signal intensity in the femur and adjacent soft tissue with inhomogeneous enhancement of signal intensity in **B.** (Courtesy of J. Kramer, M.D., Vienna, Austria.)

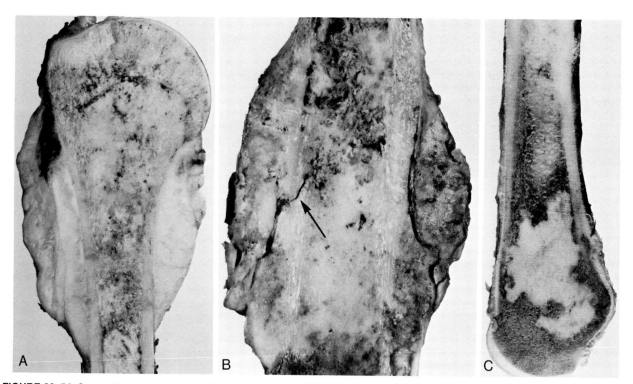

FIGURE 83–54. Conventional osteosarcoma: Macroscopic abnormalities.
 A This tumor involves the entire medullary cavity of the proximal portion of the humerus. Foci of dense calcification (white areas) are scattered throughout the neoplasm. Note the cortical violation and periosteal elevation in the form of Codman's triangles.
 B This osteosarcoma of the femur has led to cortical destruction and extraosseous extension. Observe a pathologic fracture (arrow).
 C A third neoplasm involves the distal portion of the femur. It is white with sharp margins.

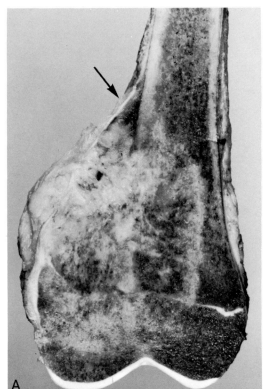
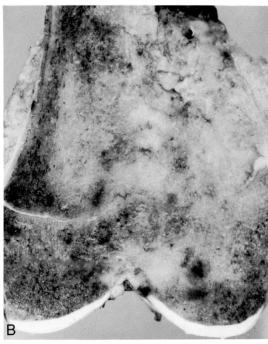

FIGURE 83–55. Conventional osteosarcoma: Macroscopic abnormalities—transphyseal extension.

A An osteosarcoma in the distal portion of the femur has eroded the cortex, producing elevation of the periosteal membrane with a Codman's triangle (arrow). Note transphyseal spread of the neoplasm into the epiphysis.

B A second osteosarcoma has extended from the metaphysis through the growth plate into the epiphysis, with invasion of articular cartilage.

bone pattern similar to that seen in fibrosarcoma and are designated fibroblastic osteosarcomas.[235] The recent identification of additional histologic types, such as chondroblastoma-like osteosarcomas,[2030] chondromyxoid fibroma–like osteosarcomas, osteoblastoma-like osteosarcomas, osteosarcomas with a clear cell component,[2031] and fibrohistiocytic osteosarcomas,[282, 283, 2029] indicates that the traditional classification system is not ideal, although a better method of categorizing these neoplasms currently does not exist, owing to the marked variability of the microscopic features.[180, 274] Even those neoplasms that are classified as osteoblastic may contain focal areas of malignant fibrous, fibrohistiocytic, or cartilaginous tissue (Fig. 83–56A). In general, all conventional osteosarcomas contain pleomorphic stromal elements that are either plump, spindle-shaped fibroblast-like cells or plump, round to oval osteoblasts with irregular, hyperchromatic nuclei (Fig. 83–56), and many contain multinucleated tumor cells with grotesque shapes.[180, 235, 274] At times, the malignant stromal cells may have an epithelioid appearance and occur in large, sheet-like configurations, features that may suggest alternative diagnoses, such as metastatic carcinoma and malignant melanoma or lymphoma.[28] Abnormal mitotic activity and foci of necrosis, hemorrhage, hemosiderin pigment, and even cyst-like vascular spaces similar to those in an aneurysmal bone cyst frequently are evident. The form and shape of the malignant osteoid also are highly variable.[28] Classically, it consists of an eosinophilic hyalin-like material arranged in thin strands among the malignant stromal cells, producing a lace-like pattern. Large, irregular trabeculae not rimmed by osteoblasts may be evident. When in the form of narrow ribbons, the osteoid may be impossible

to distinguish from collagen. Indeed, there is no histologic stain that allows differentiation between collagen and osteoid; however, in undecalcified sections, the presence of calcification in these strands indicates that the material is osteoid. With calcification, the osteoid may be converted to coarse, woven bone or tumor bone that resembles irregular lamellar bone but whose osteocytes are small, irregular, and hyperchromatic.

Osteoblastic osteosarcomas (Fig. 83–56D) produce an abundance of osteoid, woven bone, and irregular tumor bone that frequently are deposited on the remnants of the normal cancellous trabeculae. Chondroblastic osteosarcomas produce lobules or islands of chondroid tissue and cartilage with malignant-appearing cells lying within lacunae.[235] The cells appear similar to those found in high grade chondrosarcomas. Fibroblastic osteosarcomas contain large areas of spindle cells (that are indistinguishable from those in fibrosarcoma) and, in the better differentiated tumors, a herringbone pattern. Fibrohistiocytic osteosarcomas are characterized by an abundance of large, pleomorphic cells with bizarre and prominent nuclei, multinucleated giant cells that have considerable eosinophilic cytoplasm, and phagocytic, histiocytic-type cells; in some instances, these osteosarcomas have a microscopic appearance similar to that of a pleomorphic liposarcoma or rhabdomyosarcoma.

Histologic grading of osteosarcomas, based on the degree of cellular differentiation, has been used by some investigators to separate the tumors into four categories, I to IV, with grade IV being the least differentiated[30]; other investigators use mitotic activity alone or a combination of cellular atypia and mitotic activity to divide the osteosarcomas

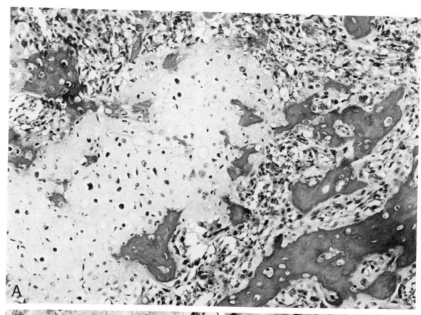

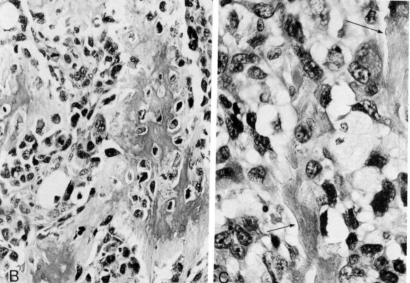

FIGURE 83–56. Conventional osteosarcoma: Microscopic abnormalities.

A Portions of the malignant cartilage in this neoplasm reveal metaplastic bone. The diagnosis of osteosarcoma rests on the identification of the production of tumor bone by the malignant cells in the stroma. (150×.)

B Large masses of osteoid are being produced by the malignant-appearing stroma cells. The osteoid is partially calcified and has formed irregular woven tumor bone. (300×.)

C Strands of osteoid (arrows) are being produced by the anaplastic, plump stromal tumor cells. These strands may be difficult to distinguish from ordinary collagen. (600×.)

D A photomicrograph of this osteoblastic osteosarcoma reveals irregular, thin tumor trabeculae forming a lattice-type network that is continuous with a remnant of a normal bone spicule. (150×.)

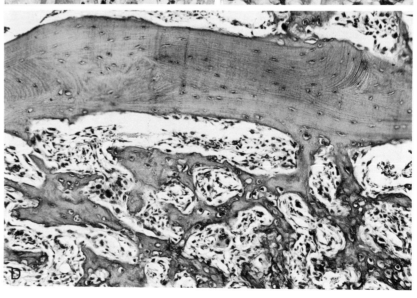

into three grades.[285] As the histology of osteosarcomas may vary greatly from one area to another in the same tumor and the grade of the tumor has not been shown to have prognostic importance, with the exception of the relatively rare, well-differentiated (grade I) intraosseous osteosarcoma (see later discussion), many pathologists do not use any such grading system.

Numerous *electron microscopic studies* of osteosarcoma have been accomplished, disclosing a variety of cell types, including fibroblasts, myofibroblasts, chondroblasts, osteoblasts, multinucleated giant cells, histiocytes, angioblasts, and primitive undifferentiated mesenchymal cells.[286–297] Some osteosarcoma tumor cells have intranuclear bundles of microfilaments or dot-like or tubular structures suggestive of virus particles.[286, 288, 296] The electron microscopic evidence suggests a common multipotent progenitor cell with the ability to differentiate along a variety of pathways, producing the mixture of cells found in osteosarcoma.

Natural History. With regard to the natural history and prognosis of conventional osteosarcomas, the application of new and innovative chemotherapeutic strategies as a supplement to surgery and irradiation has resulted in a dramatic increase in the number of patients who can be expected to survive for 5 years or more. The response of the neoplasm to intense chemotherapy can be evaluated with serial radiographs; a favorable response is characterized by a decrease in the size of the soft tissue mass and an increase in periostitis, medullary sclerosis, and calcification.[298, 299] Angiography[298, 1825] and CT[300, 1892] represent additional imaging methods that allow assessment of the tumor response to such therapy, and that can be supplemented with histologic evaluation of biopsy samples from the osteosarcoma (during chemotherapy and prior to amputation of an affected limb). The demonstration of greater degrees of tumor necrosis during assessment of pathologic specimens is a favorable prognostic sign.[2445, 2446] Local recurrence and distant skeletal metastasis following such amputation lead to osseous alterations that are similar to those of the primary tumor and, in some instances, that must be differentiated from multifocal osteosarcomatosis (see later discussion).[301, 302] Of interest, lymph node, soft tissue, or visceral metastases from osteosarcoma may appear as calcified or ossified lesions on the radiograph,[303–307, 2032] and pulmonary metastatic foci can be associated with a spontaneous pneumothorax (Fig. 83–57).

Although MR imaging has been used to monitor the response of the tumor to chemotherapy, its effectiveness is not entirely clear.[2444] Several different patterns of signal intensity have been observed after preoperative chemotherapy,[2024] although detection of decreased signal intensity in the soft tissue mass (when compared with the signal intensity of the mass prior to chemotherapy) has been associated with a favorable histologic response in some patients.[2019, 2023] A reduction in the extent of peritumoral edema also may be identified following effective chemotherapy. Diagnostic difficulty arises, however, owing to the presence of radiation-induced inflammation that may lead to changes in signal intensity similar to those of residual or recurrent tumor.[2033] Supplementary use of intravenous administration of gadolinium compounds has been recommended as a technique that provides additional information in patients with malignant tumors (such as osteosarcomas). Enhancement of signal intensity is expected in viable tumor tissue, although the fibrous and sclerotic portions of the tumor do not show such enhancement, and granulation tissue and peritumoral edema may reveal increases in signal intensity following administration of the contrast agent.[2021] Dynamic MR imaging studies in which rapid gradient echo imaging is ac-

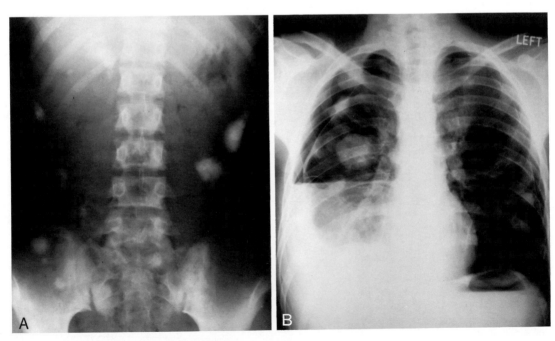

FIGURE 83–57. Conventional osteosarcoma: Natural history.
   A Ossified soft tissue metastases. Ossified metastatic lesions in the soft tissues arose from an osteosarcoma of the humerus in this 14 year old girl. (Courtesy of S. Wootton, M.D., Denver, Colorado.)
   B Pulmonary metastases with hydropneumothorax. Bilateral pneumothoraces with an air-fluid level on the right side are associated with metastases in both lungs resulting from an osteosarcoma of the femur in a 21 year old man. (Courtesy of R. Kerr, M.D., Los Angeles, California.)

complished after the intravenous injection of a gadolinium compound is a further technical modification that has been used to assess tumor viability following chemotherapy.[2023, 2034] Tumor signal intensity is plotted from serial images obtained at 15- to 20-sec intervals, and the slope of the resultant time-intensity curve is calculated.[2021] Steeper slopes (>30 per cent) suggest the presence of viable tumor; more gradual increases in signal intensity are seen in necrotic areas as well as in cystic regions and in cartilaginous and myxomatous tissue.[2021]

A gadolinium-enhanced subtraction MR imaging technique also has been used to assess the chemotherapeutic response of patients with osteosarcoma.[2017] This method relates to subtracting precontrast T1-weighted spin echo MR images from those obtained following the intravenous administration of a gadolinium compound. The more profound the difference in signal intensity in the two images, the more likely the existence of viable tumor.

It appears that the absence of regions of high signal intensity in T2-weighted spin echo MR images is a good prognostic sign in patients with osteosarcoma who have undergone chemotherapy. The significance of such regions in T2-weighted spin echo MR images is not certain, however. When areas of high signal intensity are evident in the T2-weighted spin echo MR images, a role appears to exist for dynamic MR imaging following the intravenous administration of a gadolinium compound. Rapid enhancement of signal intensity with such imaging is most consistent with residual tumor. Nontumorous causes of such enhancement do exist, however (Fig. 83–58).

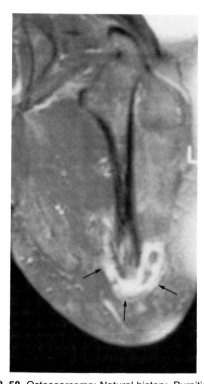

FIGURE 83–58. Osteosarcoma: Natural history. Bursitis developing at an amputation site. In a 20 year old man, an amputation at the midfemoral level was the treatment for an osteosarcoma in the distal portion of the femur. A coronal T1-weighted (TR/TE, 800/20) spin echo MR image obtained with chemical presaturation of fat (ChemSat) following the intravenous administration of a gadolinium compound shows a region of high signal intensity (arrows) about the femoral stump, consistent with bursitis.

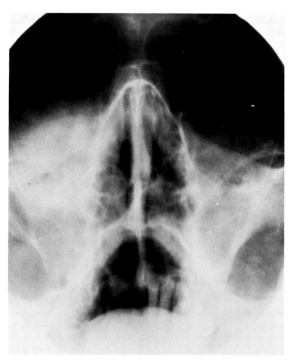

FIGURE 83–59. Gnathic osteosarcoma: Radiographic abnormalities. Observe the osteosclerotic tumor arising in the right maxilla and involving the adjacent maxillary sinus.

Gnathic Osteosarcoma. Osteosarcomas of the mandible or maxilla are considered by some investigators to be tumors that are distinct from conventional osteosarcomas owing to an older age of onset (average age of approximately 30 years) and a decreased tendency for systemic metastases.[235] Tumors arising in the mandible are slightly more frequent than those occurring in the maxilla and predominate in the body of the bone[1895]; maxillary osteosarcomas usually affect the alveolar ridge and antrum[308-318] (Fig. 83–59). Although gnathic osteosarcoma may be purely osteolytic or purely osteosclerotic or demonstrate a mixed pattern of osteolysis and osteosclerosis, the finding of a small, radiodense tumor presents a particular diagnostic challenge. This latter radiographic appearance may be interpreted as evidence of a benign process; however, the frequently associated permeation of the cortex, periostitis, and soft tissue mass containing bone are important in the accurate appraisal of the roentgenograms.

CT findings of gnathic osteosarcomas include tumor calcification, involvement of the cortex, and soft tissue and intramedullary bone extension.[2035] MR imaging reveals similar features, although the detection of matrix calcifications and bone destruction or reaction is better accomplished with CT scanning.[2035]

Descriptions of the histologic features of gnathic osteosarcomas have been conflicting. Some investigators indicate that these lesions commonly are chondroblastic and highly differentiated[235, 308, 317]; others believe that there are no significant differences between the microscopic appearance of these tumors and those of osteosarcomas in extragnathic sites.[311, 312, 319]

Telangiectatic Osteosarcoma. The presence in some osteosarcomas of microscopic features that include large cystic cavities filled with fresh and clotted blood has led to the segregation of a distinct clinicopathologic variety of tumor that has been designated telangiectatic (or hemorrhagic) osteosarcoma.[221, 235, 320–329] Although some authors report that such neoplasms represent as many as 11 per cent of all osteosarcomas,[327] most investigators indicate a lesser frequency.[221] Disagreement also exists regarding the ultimate prognosis of telangiectatic osteosarcoma, with varying opinions indicating rapid progression[320] or an outcome similar to that of ordinary osteosarcoma.[327, 328, 1871]

Telangiectatic osteosarcoma primarily is a tumor of the long tubular bones; the femur is involved most frequently, followed in frequency by the tibia and humerus, a distribution similar to that of conventional osteosarcoma.[2036] In these bones, the metaphysis is the usual site of origin, but the tumor can extend into the epiphysis and subchondral region when the physeal plate is closed. Diaphyseal involvement occurs in approximately 10 per cent of cases. Other bones, such as the sternum[2036] and mandible,[2037] may be involved.

The osteolytic nature of the process is the radiographic hallmark of telangiectatic osteosarcoma (Figs. 83–60 and 83–61). Intralesional sclerosis is infrequent and mild. A large, multilocular or pseudocystic, expansile lesion often lacking periosteal bone production[1826] and possessing, in some instances, a relatively well-defined margin is characteristic.[327] Pathologic fractures (in approximately 25 to 30 per cent of cases) and soft tissue masses also are encountered. MR imaging may show areas of high signal intensity in T1-weighted spin echo images and fluid-fluid levels similar to those seen in an aneurysmal bone cyst.

When sectioned, the tumor is friable and contains cystic spaces filled with blood and areas of soft, necrotic solid tissue with calcific foci (Fig. 83–62). Dense, sclerotic tumor bone typically is lacking. Microscopically, telangiectatic osteosarcoma has features resembling those of an aggressive aneurysmal bone cyst. The dominant histologic pattern is that of large cystic blood spaces (Fig. 83–63A) separated by usually thin fibrous septa, creating a sponge-like appearance.[321] These spaces vary in size but usually are large and may communicate with each other to form anastomosing channels. The spaces are lined not by endothelial cells but by benign multinucleated osteoclast-like giant cells and mononuclear malignant tumor cells[320, 328] (Fig. 83–63B). The neoplasms are quite vascular, with numerous normal, endothelial-lined blood vessels coursing within the fibrous septa, in which also are found mononuclear anaplastic tumor cells that form osteoid seams and trabeculae (Fig. 83–63C). The amount of osteoid formed in these osteosarcomas is scant, requiring careful histologic analysis for identification. In some instances, such osteoid formation is entirely absent.[320, 2447] Electron microscopic data have suggested that this tumor should be considered an osteosarcoma that is characterized by predominance of an angiosarcomatous component.[324]

The radiographic and histologic features of telangiectatic osteosarcoma most resemble those of an aneurysmal bone cyst, giant cell tumor, or angiosarcoma.[322, 324, 326, 327] Differentiation of this lesion from a benign tumor on the basis of its imaging abnormalities alone may be difficult.[1826]

Small Cell Osteosarcoma. In 1979, Sim and associates[330] described 24 osteosarcomas whose component cells were small and resembled those of Ewing's sarcoma, to which they gave the designation of small cell osteosarcoma.

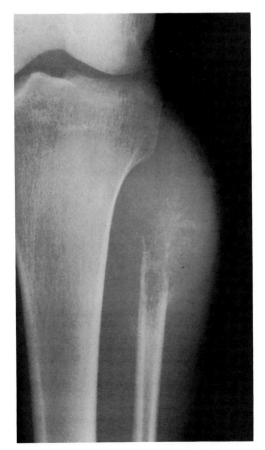

FIGURE 83–60. Telangiectatic osteosarcoma: Radiographic abnormalities. A 19 year old Mexican man reported a 5 month history of pain and swelling below the knee. The radiograph reveals extensive osteolysis in the proximal portion of the fibula. Note complete dissolution of the fibular head and permeative bone destruction distally. A large soft tissue mass is evident. Only minor periostitis is apparent.

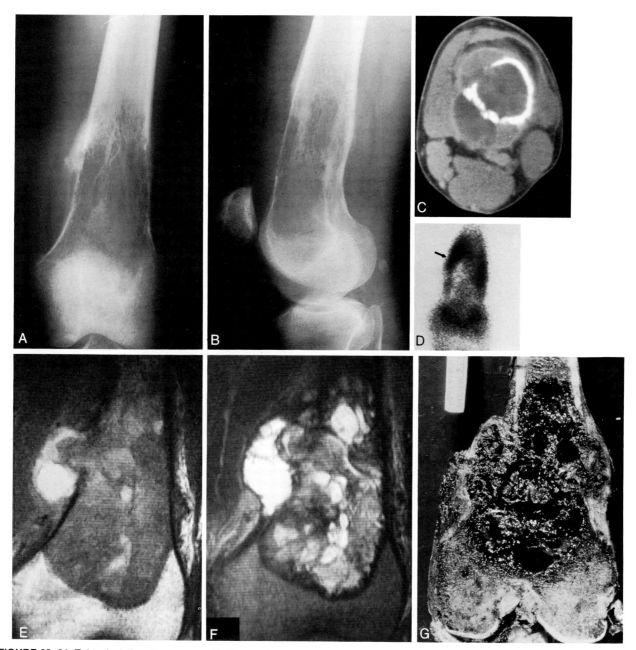

FIGURE 83–61. Telangiectatic osteosarcoma: Radiographic abnormalities. Over a 2 month period, a 19 year old man developed pain and a palpable mass in the anteromedial aspect of the thigh.

A, B Anteroposterior **(A)** and lateral **(B)** radiographs show an osteolytic lesion containing small and large areas of bone destruction in the femur. The cortex is thinned or perforated, and Codman's triangles and a large soft tissue mass are evident.

C A transaxial CT scan reveals the intraosseous and extraosseous components of the lesion and cortical erosion. Note a partial rim of greater attenuation at the periphery of the soft tissue mass.

D On a bone scan, the periphery of the lesion has accumulated the radionuclide (arrow) and its central portion is photopenic.

E, F T1-weighted (TR/TE, 500/30) **(E)** and T2-weighted (TR/TE, 2000/120) **(F)** spin echo coronal MR images vividly demonstrate the extent of the tumor. In **E,** only the soft tissue component of the lesion has a high signal intensity; in **F,** the overall intensity of the tumor has increased. Following a biopsy, which established the diagnosis of telangiectatic osteosarcoma, the patient was treated with intra-arterial infusion of doxorubicin hydrochloride (Adriamycin) and irradiation. He subsequently returned following a pathologic fracture, and amputation of the limb was required.

G A coronal section of the specimen reveals the pathologic fracture and the tumor. Note that this hemorrhagic neoplasm contains cystic spaces and solid tissue.

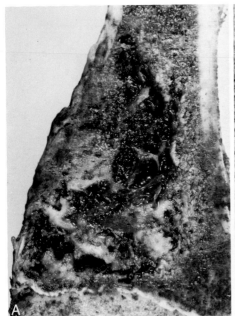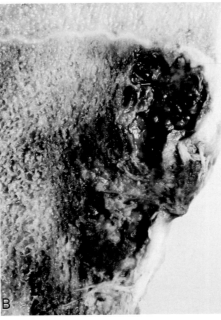

FIGURE 83–62. Telangiectatic osteosarcoma; Macroscopic abnormalities.
A This section of a tumor in the distal portion of the femur reveals solid white islands of tissue separated by cystic blood-filled cavities. The neoplasm extends distally to the physeal plate and through the metaphyseal cortex.
B A second neoplasm in the proximal portion of the tibia has focally violated the cortex. Its medullary border is poorly defined.

On the basis of data from this investigation and a few additional reports,[331, 332, 2038–2041] the neoplasm usually is seen in a male or female patient in the second, third, or fourth decade of life, although small children and even elderly persons may be affected. Pain and swelling of short duration are the typical clinical manifestations. Sites of involvement, in order of decreasing frequency, include the femur, humerus, tibia, and ilium. Uncommon locations of this tumor include the facial bones, fibula, radius, ribs, scapula, skull, sacrum, and small bones in the hand and feet.[2038] Lesions in the tubular bones predominate in the epiphysis and metaphysis. The prognosis of the tumor appears to be poorer than for conventional osteosarcoma, with most reported patients dying within the first year following diagnosis.

Radiographically, a large, predominantly osteolytic lesion involving the medullary and cortical bone is accompanied by periostitis or a soft tissue mass, or both, in approximately 50 per cent of cases.[330] Rarely, an intracortical lesion may be detected.[2040] The presence of a tumor with osteoblastic features extending from the metaphysis into the diaphysis and associated with permeative bone destruction is suggestive but not diagnostic of a small cell osteosarcoma.[2038]

Microscopically, small cell osteosarcoma, as its name implies, is composed of small cells arranged in solid sheets or separated into lobules by dense fibrous septa (Fig. 83–64A). The cells are round to spindle-shaped, with oval nuclei that vary only moderately in size (Fig. 83–64B,C). The chromatin usually is finely and uniformly distributed, nucleoli only rarely are prominent, the cytoplasm is scanty, and the cell borders are either indistinct[330] or distinct.[331] Mitotic figures are found but may not be frequent (Fig. 83–64C). Well-defined cartilage is evident inconsistently, appearing as a myxoid or extracellular stroma in which individual cells reside in lacunae. All small cell osteosarcomas contain variable amounts of intercellular osteoid that usually is in the form of focal, fine, lacelike strands (Fig. 83–64A); however, occasional tumors reveal broad, thick tra-

becular seams in such abundance as to simulate the appearance of sclerotic osteosarcoma.[332]

The histologic features of small cell osteosarcoma must be differentiated from those of other primary, small cell neoplasms of bone, especially Ewing's sarcoma. Typically, the nuclei occupying the tumor cells of Ewing's sarcoma are much more uniform than those of small cell osteosarcoma, but variations exist in these histologic patterns.[330] Although the presence of glycogen within the cytoplasm of tumor cells (as demonstrated by periodic acid–Schiff reaction) is considered by some to be diagnostic of Ewing's sarcoma, staining for glycogen has been positive in some small cell osteosarcomas,[331, 332] and a negative glycogen stain does not, in the view of some investigators,[330] eliminate the diagnosis of Ewing's sarcoma. Furthermore, although the identification of unequivocal osteoid formation by the tumor cells strongly suggests the diagnosis of a small cell osteosarcoma, some investigators would interpret these results as indicative of a Ewing's sarcoma containing rare foci of reactive or metaplastic bone or cartilage.[221]

Intraosseous Low Grade Osteosarcoma. Low grade or well-differentiated osteosarcomas arising within a bone are uncommon compared with the frequency of highly aggressive, intraosseous osteosarcomas. These low grade neoplasms, which appear to represent the intramedullary counterpart of the parosteal variety of tumor (see later discussion), lead to clinical, radiologic, and histologic characteristics that may simulate those of benign neoplasms.

Following the initial report of this tumor by Unni and associates[333] in 1977, other investigators have further confirmed the occurrence of low grade or well-differentiated osteosarcomas arising within a bone.[334–336, 2042, 2043] Such tumors typically affect young or middle-aged adults and are located mainly in the tibia or femur.[334, 337] Indeed, the femur is involved in approximately 50 per cent of cases. Flat and irregular bones, however, also may be affected.[2448] The clinical manifestations may be mild and of relatively long duration. Radiographs usually reveal a relatively large, metaphyseal lesion, which may be purely osteosclerotic or both

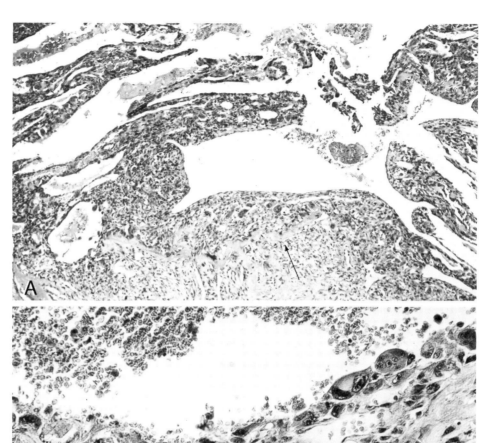

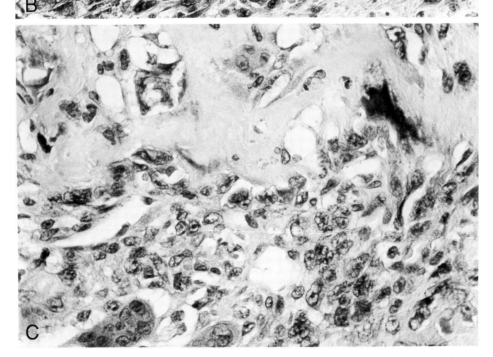

FIGURE 83–63. Telangiectatic osteosarcoma: Microscopic abnormalities.

A Fibrous septa create large and small vascular spaces. A strand of osteoid (arrow) is present in one of these septa. Scattered multinucleated giant cells are evident. (90×.)

B The cystic spaces are lined by anaplastic tumor cells, which also reside in the adjacent stroma. (300×.)

C Note the partially calcified osteoid that is being produced by the malignant stromal cells. A benign osteoclast-type giant cell is seen at the lower left portion of the photomicrograph. (600×.)

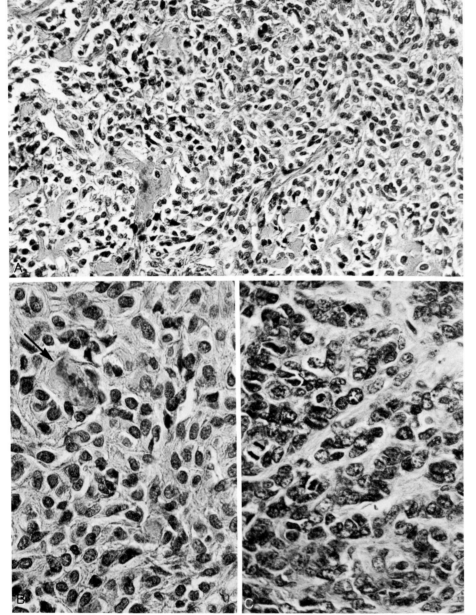

FIGURE 83–64. Small cell osteosarcoma: Microscopic abnormalities.

A Note sheet-like proliferation of fairly uniform, small cells. Foci of osteoid are observed in the form of either thin ribbons or large, clump-like collections. (300×.)

B The nuclei of the tumor cells are uniform in appearance with fine, diffuse chromatin. The cytoplasm is relatively abundant and the cell borders are distinct. A small focus of osteoid (arrow) is present. (600×.)

C The cells in a more anaplastic small cell osteosarcoma show a greater degree of nuclear atypia and hyperchromasia and a lesser amount of cytoplasm. The borders of the cells are indistinct. A mitotic figure is evident at the left side of the photomicrograph. (600×.)

osteolytic and osteosclerotic in appearance (Figs. 83–65 and 83–66). Epiphyseal extension, cortical violation, osseous expansion, and soft tissue extension are features that are encountered inconsistently. Owing to the presence of bone sclerosis, the diagnosis of an osteosarcoma is possible, although the lesion generally lacks the highly aggressive characteristics of a conventional osteosarcoma.[2449] Reports of diagnostic histologic features are misleading as initial interpretations of biopsy material frequently have been incorrect, resulting in alternative diagnoses, including a variety of benign fibrous tumors and tumor-like lesions, particularly fibrous dysplasia. When clinical and radiologic data also are considered, microscopic analysis is more accurate. Well-differentiated intraosseous osteosarcomas are composed of spindle cells arranged in interlacing fascicles separated by collagen fibers (Fig. 83–67). In general, the nuclei are slender to plump, and the nuclear atypia and pleomorphism of conventional osteosarcoma characteristically are lacking. Mitoses are rare or absent entirely. Benign giant cells, arranged in focal clusters or scattered singly throughout the tumor, are evident in more than 50 per cent of cases. Chondroid foci are uncommon and, when present, appear malignant. Within the fibrous stroma are irregular trabeculae. In most cases, this bone appears to arise directly from or is intimately associated with the stromal spindle cells, much in the same manner as the bone produced in fibrous dysplasia. Some trabeculae are lined by osteoblasts and fuse to form a lattice-like network. The amount of osteoid produced by the tumor is variable; in some instances, abundant, broad, irregular trabecular seams are evident, whereas in other cases, minute, lacelike foci of osteoid are difficult to find or distinguish from ordinary collagen. The histologic features of this tumor, at times, may resemble those of parosteal osteosarcoma or desmoid lesions, as well as fibrous dysplasia.

Intraosseous low grade osteosarcoma is associated with a

better prognosis than conventional osteosarcoma,[1827] although inadequate surgery generally is followed by local tumor recurrence,[333] which, in some instances, is characterized by a more anaplastic and high grade histologic pattern.[334, 2048] Rarely, a more aggressive histologic pattern is evident at the time of initial presentation of the tumor.[2044]

Intracortical Osteosarcoma. This tumor appears to represent the rarest form of osteosarcoma, with only a few cases being documented.[338–341, 2045–2047] Its existence as a distinct entity has been challenged by those investigators who would consider it a form of periosteal osteosarcoma or an early manifestation of conventional osteosarcoma.[340] Unlike periosteal osteosarcoma, however, which arises on the surface of the bone and has a spiculated radiologic appearance, intracortical osteosarcoma arises within the confines of the cortex as an osteolytic lesion with surrounding cortical sclerosis and without radiating osseous spicules.[339] Typically affecting young adults (and, in rare instances, affecting children), intracortical osteosarcoma is a diaphyseal lesion of the tibia or femur. A radiolucent focus containing osteoid and surrounded in part by a sclerotic margin usually is seen[339] (Fig. 83–68A,B). Reactive thickening of the adjacent cancellous trabeculae may be evident.[341]

On macroscopic inspection of resected specimens, the cortex in the vicinity of this small tumor is thick and sclerotic, with slight expansion of the bone (Fig. 83–68C). The neoplasm is located within the cortex, without involvement of the medullary cavity. Soft tissue involvement is absent at the time of initial diagnosis. The majority of intracortical osteosarcomas reveal a microscopic pattern identical to that of a conventional osteoblastic osteosarcoma. One example of an intracortical small cell osteosarcoma has been documented.[2040] Examples of this tumor possessing a histologic appearance similar to an osteoid osteoma also can be found,[339] however, a diagnostic problem that is accentuated by the similarity in the radiologic appearance of intracortical osteosarcoma and osteoid osteoma.

Whether there is any prognostic difference between the intracortical and conventional types of osteosarcoma is not yet clear.

Surface High Grade Osteosarcoma. With regard to general nomenclature of surface lesions of bone, periosteal lesions are defined as processes originating from the deep layer of the periosteum; parosteal lesions are defined as those originating from the outer fibrous layer of the periosteum; and subperiosteal lesions are processes that separate the periosteum from the cortex.[2049] The term juxtacortical is flexible and is applied to surface lesions of extracortical origin regardless of their exact anatomic relation to the periosteum; paraosseous lesions are those that originate completely outside the periosteum and are separated from the adjacent cortex and periosteum by a soft tissue cleavage plane.[2049]

According to Dahlin, Unni, and their collaborators,[235, 342, 343] three types of osteosarcoma involve predominantly the surface of a bone: parosteal osteosarcoma, periosteal osteosarcoma, and high grade conventional osteosarcoma. Surface high grade osteosarcomas occur in male or female patients of various ages. Tubular bones, especially the femur, are involved most frequently, and a diaphyseal location is typical.[2050–2052] Histologically, these tumors are identical to conventional osteosarcoma, and it is only their localization to the surface of the bone that represents a

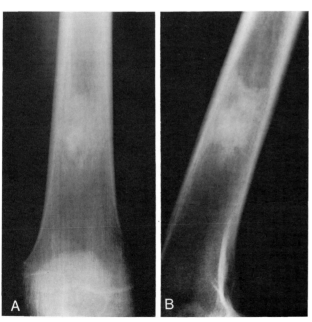

FIGURE 83–65. Intraosseous low grade osteosarcoma: Radiographic abnormalities. Frontal **(A)** and lateral **(B)** radiographs reveal a poorly defined osteosclerotic tumor in the distal portion of the femur. Subtle endosteal erosion is evident.

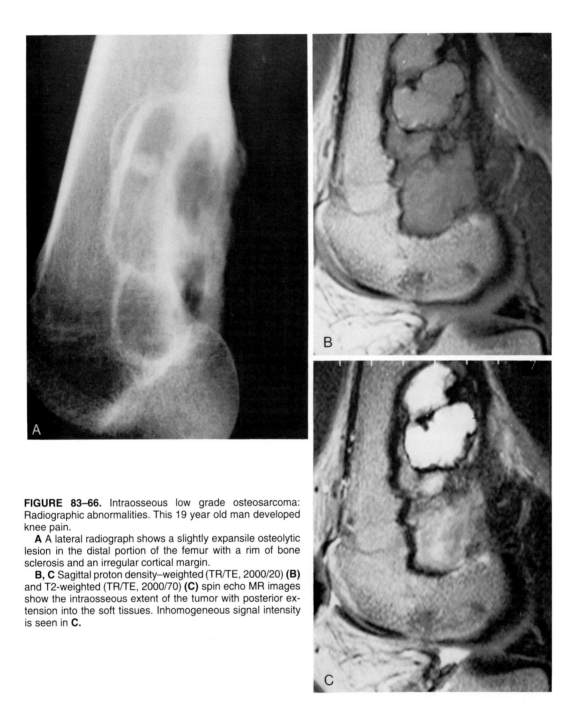

FIGURE 83–66. Intraosseous low grade osteosarcoma: Radiographic abnormalities. This 19 year old man developed knee pain.

A A lateral radiograph shows a slightly expansile osteolytic lesion in the distal portion of the femur with a rim of bone sclerosis and an irregular cortical margin.

B, C Sagittal proton density–weighted (TR/TE, 2000/20) **(B)** and T2-weighted (TR/TE, 2000/70) **(C)** spin echo MR images show the intraosseous extent of the tumor with posterior extension into the soft tissues. Inhomogeneous signal intensity is seen in **C.**

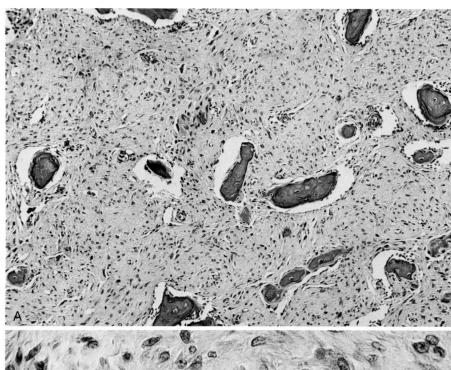

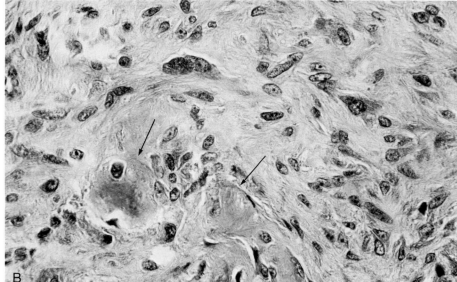

FIGURE 83–67. Intraosseous low grade osteosarcoma: Microscopic abnormalities.

A Note spicules of bone that are irregularly distributed within a bland fibrous stroma. The pattern simulates that of fibrous dysplasia. (150×.)

B At higher magnification, some of the stromal cells contain atypical nuclei and small indistinct strands of osteoid (arrows). (600×.)

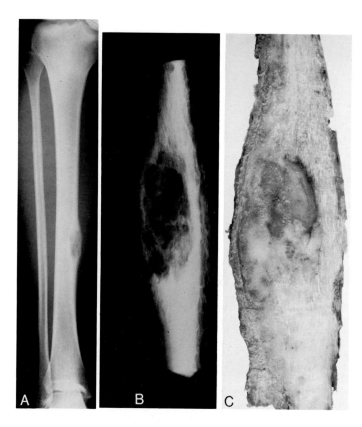

FIGURE 83–68. Intracortical osteosarcoma: Radiographic and macroscopic abnormalities.

A A radiolucent lesion of the diaphyseal cortex of the tibia is accompanied by cortical thickening, slight osseous expansion, and narrowing of the medullary canal.

B, C A radiograph **(B)** and photograph **(C)** of the resected specimen show the cortical location of the predominantly osteolytic process and surrounding sclerotic bone.

(**A,** From Kyriakos M: Cancer 46:2525, 1980.)

differentiating feature. The radiographic appearance of surface high grade osteosarcoma resembles that of periosteal osteosarcoma (see later discussion) and is characterized by a broad-based, partially or completely calcified or ossified lesion arising from the external surface of the cortex (Fig. 83–69). The cortical bone may be destroyed and, infrequently, medullary sclerosis indicative of tumor extension is seen.[342] The prognosis of this type of tumor appears to be identical to that of conventional high grade osteosarcoma and poorer than that of parosteal or periosteal osteosarcoma.

Periosteal Osteosarcoma. Periosteal osteosarcomas, which also arise on the surface of a bone, were first identified as a distinct type of tumor by Unni and collaborators[344] in 1976. Although subsequent reports have confirmed the existence of this tumor,[345–353, 2050, 2053, 2054] its relationship to juxtacortical chondrosarcoma remains unclear (see later discussion).[221] Periosteal osteosarcoma is an infrequent neoplasm; the age range of affected patients is broad, with most reports indicating that the tumor predominates in the second and third decades of life. Involvement of the diaphysis (or, less commonly, the diametaphysis or metaphysis) of a long tubular bone, especially the femur or the tibia, is most typical. The humerus also may be affected, and rare sites of involvement include other long tubular bones, the ilium, the maxilla and mandible, the rib, the calcaneus, and the clavicle. It is significant that when a periosteal osteosarcoma is seen in the distal region of the femur, it usually is located in the anterior, lateral or medial portion of the bone, differing from the posterior femoral involvement that characterizes a parosteal osteosarcoma.

Periosteal osteosarcomas are variable in size, appearing radiographically as a lesion on the surface of the bone. The

tumor is limited to the cortex, which is thickened and irregular externally, and is commonly accompanied by nonhomogeneous, radiating osseous spicules that extend from the superficial region of the cortex into the adjacent soft tissues (Figs. 83–70 and 83–71). It should be emphasized that the medullary cavity, with rare exceptions,[351] is uninvolved.

On gross examination, a soft, lobulated lesion is seen on the surface of the bone[235] (Fig. 83–72). When sectioned, the periphery of the tumor is found to be well rounded and distinctly chondroid in appearance, with glistening gray or gray-white lobules. The more central areas may be hard and gritty owing to the presence of calcification or ossification. Histologically, periosteal osteosarcoma (generally but not universally) is relatively poorly differentiated and predominantly chondroblastic (Fig. 83–73A–C), although osteoblastic or fibroblastic elements may predominate.[347, 351] In a typical case, therefore, it may not be possible on histologic analysis alone to differentiate between the periosteal and conventional varieties of osteosarcoma. At the periphery of the lesion, large lobules of high grade malignant cartilage are identified, and careful evaluation generally will reveal variable amounts of lacelike ribbons of osteoid (Fig. 83–73D).

The prognosis of this tumor definitely is better than that of conventional osteosarcoma, although local recurrences or systemic metastases occur if surgical resection is inadequate.[344]

Parosteal Osteosarcoma. This lesion is the third type of osteosarcoma arising on the surface of a bone. Affected patients generally are adults in the second to fifth decades of life, an age distribution that is significantly different from that of conventional osteosarcoma.[354–360] Symptoms and signs typically are insidious, consisting of pain, swelling,

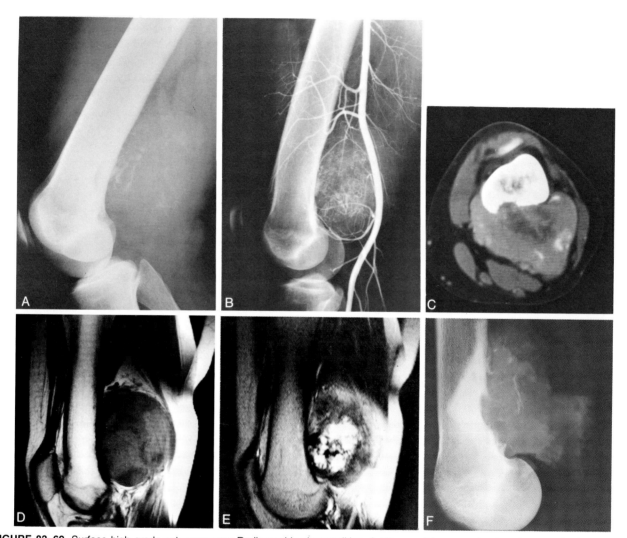

FIGURE 83–69. Surface high grade osteosarcoma: Radiographic abnormalities. A 23 year old woman developed a mass in the posterior aspect of the thigh that increased in size over a 6 month period.

A A lateral radiograph reveals a large soft tissue mass behind the distal portion of the femur. It is partially ossified or calcified, and there is evidence of cortical erosion and sclerosis.

B Angiography demonstrates posterior displacement of the popliteal artery with numerous tumor vessels and a tumor "blush."

C Transaxial CT reveals a soft tissue mass containing both calcification and areas of low attenuation, as well as cortical erosion of the femur.

D, E T1-weighted **(D)** and T2-weighted **(E)** sagittal spin echo MR images show the full extent of the soft tissue mass. It is of uniformly low signal intensity in **D** and contains areas of high signal intensity in **E**. The marrow appears to be uninvolved in these images.

F A lateral radiograph of the amputated femur shows the soft tissue mass and the extent of cortical involvement.

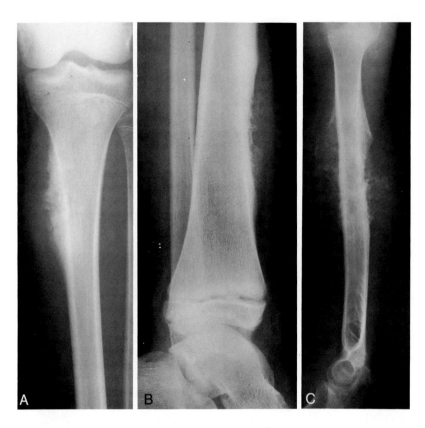

FIGURE 83–70. Periosteal osteosarcoma: Radiographic abnormalities.

A Tibia. Observe the location of the lesion in the medial cortex of the tibia, cortical thickening, and radiating and cloud-like osseous proliferation in the external surface of the bone. The medullary portion is uninvolved.

B Tibia. An anterior lesion has led to external cortical saucerization, irregular bone proliferation, and soft tissue prominence. The spongiosa is unaffected.

C Humerus. A diaphyseal location, exuberant periostitis, including Codman's triangles, osseous proliferation, and soft tissue prominence are observed.

and a palpable mass, and a delay in the patient's consulting a physician accounts for the enormous size of the tumor that often is present at the time of initial clinical evaluation.

Skeletal Location. Parosteal osteosarcomas occur almost exclusively in the long tubular bones; the femur is the predominant site of involvement (approximately 65 per cent of cases), followed in order of frequency by the humerus (15 per cent), tibia (10 per cent), fibula (3 per cent), radius (2 per cent), and ulna (1 per cent). Other bones of the appendicular skeleton and those of the axial skeleton, skull, and face rarely are affected.[361–365, 2055–2058, 2450–2453] Parosteal osteosarcomas are particularly common in the posterior surface of the distal portion of the femur (50 to 70 per cent of femoral tumors) and proximal regions of the tibia (80 per cent of tibial tumors), fibula (90 per cent of fibular tumors), and humerus (90 per cent of humeral tumors). Involvement of the bones about the knee occurs in approximately 70 per cent of all parosteal osteosarcomas. These tumors characteristically arise in the metaphyseal region of a tubular bone[357, 360, 366] and only occasionally affect the epiphysis[367]; a diaphyseal location is distinctly uncommon.[350, 354, 355, 359, 368, 369, 2059, 2060]

Radiographic Abnormalities. The radiographic abnormalities of this tumor are highly characteristic (Figs. 83–74 to 83–76). A large, radiodense, oval or spheroid mass possessing smooth lobulated or irregular margins is evident. Typically it is attached in a sessile fashion to the external cortex, which itself may be thickened, and a thin radiolucent line, or cleavage plane, may separate the remaining portion of the tumor from the underlying bone, although this latter finding is not constant.[2060] With progressive enlargement of the neoplasm, it may grow around the surface of the bone with partial obliteration of the radiolucent plane. Ossification within the tumor proceeds from the base of the lesion to its periphery and may be homogeneous or

contain distinctive radiolucent or cystic areas that are well demonstrated by CT (see later discussion). The pattern of ossification differs from that seen in posttraumatic heterotopic bone formation (myositis ossificans) in which the periphery of the lesion is the first to ossify. Medullary destruction is infrequent, although the bulky nature of the ossifying tumor makes radiographic evaluation of the underlying bone quite difficult.

CT represents an additional imaging method that may be used to evaluate a parosteal osteosarcoma, although the interpretation of the image data is not without difficulty.[370–372] The technique can define the extent of the neoplasm and, in some cases, the presence of medullary involvement[1896, 1897]; however, the differentiation between (1) neoplastic invasion of the medullary cavity and reactive non-neoplastic loss of cancellous bone[371] and (2) tumor bone and thickened adjacent host cortex[370] is not always possible. Of interest is the identification with CT (as well as conventional radiography) of radiolucent regions within the otherwise dense tumor mass that can represent fibrous or cartilaginous tissue, normal fat, entrapped benign soft tissues, or dedifferentiated, high grade areas of parosteal osteosarcoma.[370, 373] The precise location of the radiolucent areas within the tumor provides insight into their specific cause; those intralesional radiolucent shadows that are superficial generally are composed of low grade malignant cartilaginous or fibrous tissue that is mixed with fat and trabeculae, and those that are deeply situated more often correspond to sites of high grade dedifferentiated tissue.[373]

Dedifferentiated parosteal osteosarcoma appears to evolve from a low grade parosteal osteosarcoma and after a long period of time or a history of local recurrence develops an additional high grade mesenchymal component.[2049] This type of dedifferentiation may occur in as many as 20 to 25

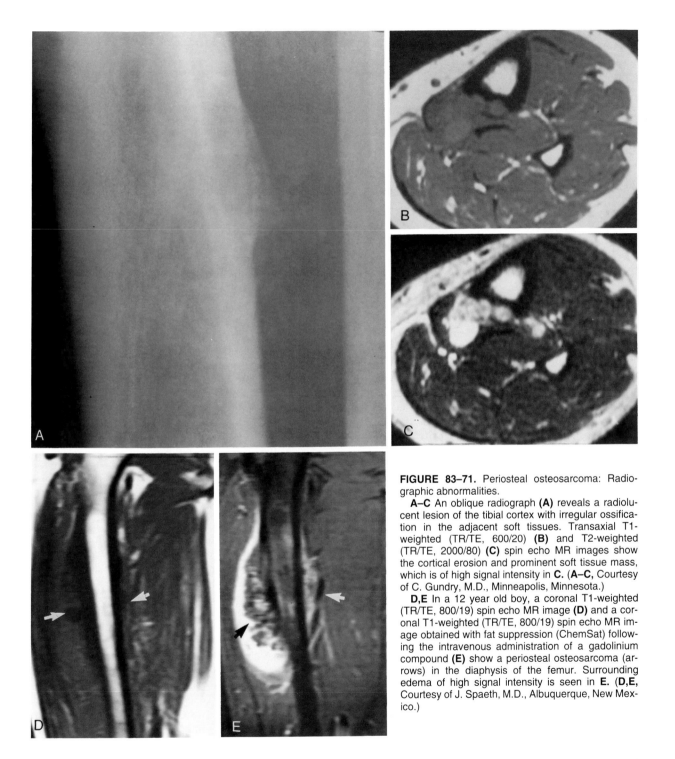

FIGURE 83–71. Periosteal osteosarcoma: Radiographic abnormalities.

A–C An oblique radiograph **(A)** reveals a radiolucent lesion of the tibial cortex with irregular ossification in the adjacent soft tissues. Transaxial T1-weighted (TR/TE, 600/20) **(B)** and T2-weighted (TR/TE, 2000/80) **(C)** spin echo MR images show the cortical erosion and prominent soft tissue mass, which is of high signal intensity in **C.** (**A–C,** Courtesy of C. Gundry, M.D., Minneapolis, Minnesota.)

D,E In a 12 year old boy, a coronal T1-weighted (TR/TE, 800/19) spin echo MR image **(D)** and a coronal T1-weighted (TR/TE, 800/19) spin echo MR image obtained with fat suppression (ChemSat) following the intravenous administration of a gadolinium compound **(E)** show a periosteal osteosarcoma (arrows) in the diaphysis of the femur. Surrounding edema of high signal intensity is seen in **E.** (**D,E,** Courtesy of J. Spaeth, M.D., Albuquerque, New Mexico.)

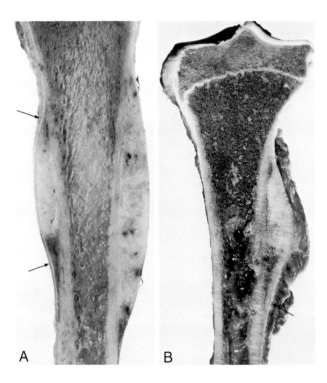

FIGURE 83–72. Periosteal osteosarcoma: Macroscopic abnormalities.
   A Tibia. This diaphyseal lesion rests on the cortex and is covered by a grossly intact periosteum, which is observed as a thin white line (arrows). The medullary cavity is uninvolved.
   B Tibia. In a second example, the tumor resides beneath the periosteal membrane (arrow). The subjacent cortex is invaded.

per cent of all parosteal osteosarcomas. Rarely, a high grade sarcoma develops within a parosteal osteosarcoma that shows no signs of dedifferentiation.[2050] In either situation, routine radiographic findings may be identical to those of a typical parosteal osteosarcoma, although radiolucent regions (as indicated previously), cortical permeation and, in some cases, bizarre enlargement of the lesion may be noted.[2049, 2061–2063] The femur, particularly the posterior aspect of the distal metaphysis, is the usual site of a dedifferentiated parosteal osteosarcoma.

   Pathologic Abnormalities. The *macroscopic pathology* of parosteal osteosarcomas is consistent with their radiographic appearance. These tumors originate from the parosteal soft tissue and form a coarsely lobulated, broad-based mass that bulges from the external surface of the bone (Fig. 83–77). Cortical thickening, the absence of periostitis, and infrequent medullary invasion are additional findings. Intramedullary extension appears to correlate with the length of time the neoplasm has been present and is more frequent when inadequate initial treatment leads to tumor recurrence. Although parosteal osteosarcomas usually appear well delineated, may possess a fibrous capsule, and are easily separated from the parent bone, they may invade the adjacent soft tissues, frequently incorporating skeletal muscle and fat into their peripheral growth zone.[355, 374] The consistency of the tumor varies according to the proportion of fibrous, osseous, and cartilaginous tissue that is present. Any soft or fleshy regions within the neoplasm require careful histologic sampling as they represent the more cellular areas and may contain cells of a higher degree of malignancy than those in the remainder of the tumor.[359]

   With regard to *microscopic pathology,* many of the features of the parosteal osteosarcoma resemble those of intraosseous low grade osteosarcoma. The paucity of histologic abnormalities suggesting malignancy may lead to an initial diagnosis of a benign neoplasm and certainly is re-

flected in the early designation of this tumor as a parosteal osteoma.[375] The basic cellular background of parosteal osteosarcoma consists of a fibrous stroma in which reside irregular osseous spicules and trabeculae (Fig. 83–78A). This stroma may be relatively hypocellular, with abundant collagen, or highly cellular, especially at the periphery of the tumor, with compact cells and little intervening matrix.[357, 358] Such cells may be spindle-shaped and lack any nuclear features of malignancy; however, in some instances, the nuclei are plumper, are more atypical, and create fibrosarcoma-like foci (Fig. 83–78B). Mitotic figures are, as a rule, infrequent. The osseous spicules and trabeculae are irregular in shape and either woven or lamellar in form. Unlike conventional osteosarcoma, in which the tumor bone lacks a rim of osteoblastic cells, the trabeculae of parosteal osteosarcoma may be bordered by a single layer of plump but otherwise bland-appearing osteoblasts. Elsewhere, the tumor appears to arise by metaplastic transformation of the fibrous stroma similar to the bone that is formed in fibrous dysplasia.[28] At the periphery of the tumor can be found abundant cells containing anaplastic features and direct osteoid formation. Also peripherally, connective tissue, fat, and skeletal muscle may become entrapped within the substance of the tumor, as it advances into the soft tissue. Chondroid islands of various size, revealing cellular characteristics of low grade chondrosarcoma, are present in 50 to 80 per cent of cases. These cartilaginous areas, however, are never the dominant feature in parosteal osteosarcoma (as they may be in periosteal osteosarcoma).

   In recurrent parosteal osteosarcomas and, occasionally, even in primary tumors, areas of high grade conventional osteosarcoma may occur in an otherwise histologically typical parosteal tumor.[311, 357, 366, 374, 376, 377] Such dedifferentiated parosteal osteosarcomas resemble the surface high grade variety of osteosarcoma described earlier in this chapter.

   A few examples of parosteal osteosarcomas have been studied by *electron microscopy.*[348, 378, 379] In addition to fi-

Text continued on page 3697

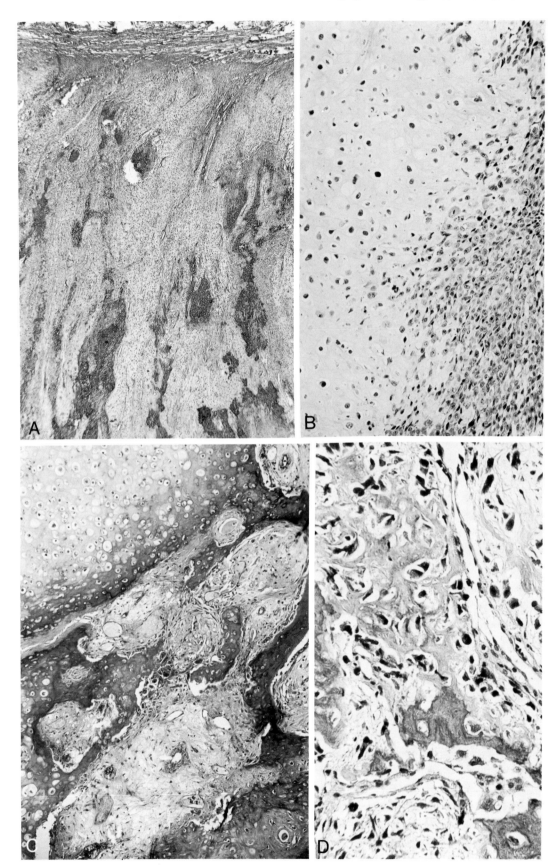

FIGURE 83–73. Periosteal osteosarcoma: Microscopic abnormalities.
  A The periosteum (top of photomicrograph) covers the tumor, which is composed of cartilage with strand-like areas of ossification (dark regions). (25×.)
  B At the periphery of this tumor, low grade malignant cartilage with transition to malignant ovoid and spindle cells is identified. (150×.)
  C Centrally, malignant cartilage (top of photomicrograph) is calcifying and undergoing endochondral ossification. (90×.)
  D In this area, malignant stromal cells are forming osteoid without an intervening cartilage matrix. (300×.)

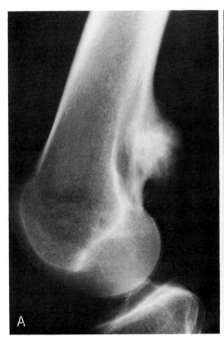 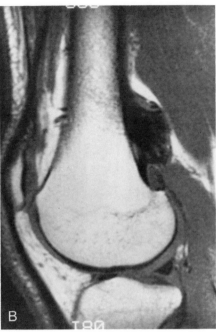

FIGURE 83–74. Parosteal osteosarcoma: Radiographic abnormalities—femur.

A A lateral radiograph shows an irregular ossified lesion involving the posterior aspect of the distal femoral metaphysis.

B In a sagittal T1-weighted (TR/TE, 550/20) spin echo MR image, the tumor is of low signal intensity and the adjacent marrow of the femur is normal.

FIGURE 83–75. Parosteal osteosarcoma: Radiographic abnormalities—femur.

A An exuberant, densely ossified lesion involves the posterior metaphyseal and diaphyseal regions of the femur. It has wrapped itself around the femur, accounting for the radiodense shadows seen anterior to the bone. The lesion is lobulated and irregular in outline, and the underlying cortex is thickened.

B, C Transaxial CT scans at diaphyseal **(B)** and metaphyseal **(C)** levels show the extent of the ossifying process, which involves not only the posterior surface of the bone but also the medial and lateral surfaces. The cortex is thickened and the medullary bone appears to be involved.

(Courtesy of Regional Naval Medical Center, San Diego, California.)

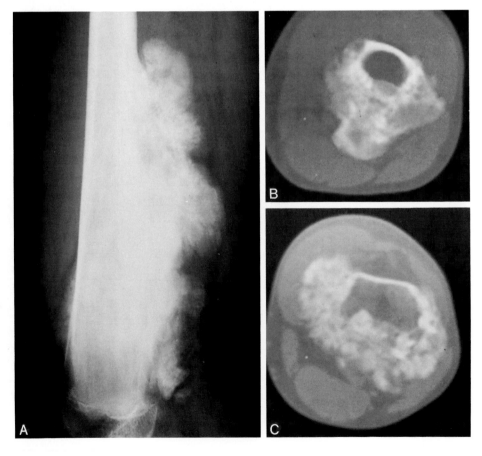

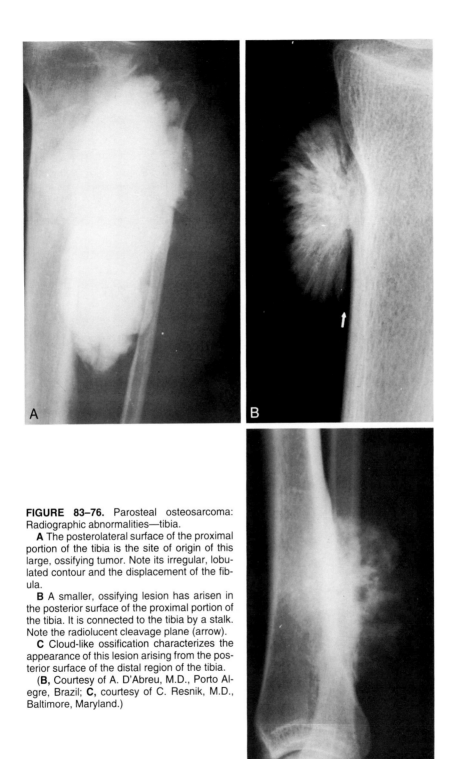

FIGURE 83–76. Parosteal osteosarcoma: Radiographic abnormalities—tibia.

A The posterolateral surface of the proximal portion of the tibia is the site of origin of this large, ossifying tumor. Note its irregular, lobulated contour and the displacement of the fibula.

B A smaller, ossifying lesion has arisen in the posterior surface of the proximal portion of the tibia. It is connected to the tibia by a stalk. Note the radiolucent cleavage plane (arrow).

C Cloud-like ossification characterizes the appearance of this lesion arising from the posterior surface of the distal region of the tibia.

(**B,** Courtesy of A. D'Abreu, M.D., Porto Alegre, Brazil; **C,** courtesy of C. Resnik, M.D., Baltimore, Maryland.)

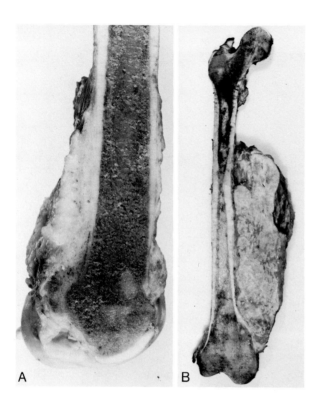

FIGURE 83–77. Parosteal osteosarcoma: Macroscopic abnormalities.
   A This tumor in the posterior aspect of the distal portion of the femur is broad-based, resting on the cortex. The medullary bone is uninvolved.
   B A large neoplasm involves more than one half the length of the femur. Despite its large size, the tumor does not involve the medullary cavity.

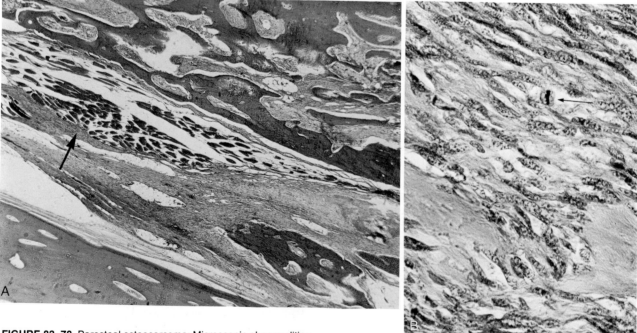

FIGURE 83–78. Parosteal osteosarcoma: Microscopic abnormalities.
   A The normal cortex of the parent bone is located at the lower left portion of this photomicrograph. The tumor consists of lamellar-type bone residing in a fibrous stroma. Skeletal muscle (arrow) is entrapped by the neoplasm. (25×.)
   B The stroma in this neoplasm is highly cellular and composed of spindle-shaped fibroblasts with atypical nuclei and mitotic figures (arrow), creating an appearance resembling that of a fibrosarcoma. (600×.)

broblast-like and osteoblast-like tumor cells, an abundance of myofibroblasts may be present. Hence, the spindle-shaped stromal cells noted by light microscopy represent either osteoblasts, fibroblasts, or myofibroblasts.[379]

Differential Diagnosis. The radiographic and pathologic features of parosteal osteosarcoma must be differentiated from posttraumatic heterotopic bone formation (myositis ossificans) and sessile osteochondroma. A clinical history of trauma followed by the rapid appearance of a soft tissue mass, a lesion that initially ossifies at its periphery and is separated by a thick radiolucent band from the underlying bone, and a zonal pattern of maturation in which the periphery of the lesion consists of lamellar bone and the center consists of proliferating mesenchymal cells represent the distinguishing features of myositis ossificans. An osteochondroma is characterized radiologically by continuity between the cortex and spongiosa of the excrescence and the underlying normal bone; histologically it is characterized by a benign, hyaline cartilage cap, the presence of fat or hematopoietic elements within its deeper portions, and the absence of fibrous stroma with cellular atypia. A periosteal osteosarcoma represents a lesion that usually is small compared with the size of a parosteal osteosarcoma, that is accompanied by a distinctive spiculated periosteal reaction, and that histologically is predominantly chondroblastic. Other tumors that arise from the cortical surface, such as a high grade osteosarcoma, an osteoma, and a chondrosarcoma developing in an osteochondroma, usually can be differentiated from parosteal osteosarcoma when clinical, imaging, and histologic data are analyzed together.

Multicentric Osteosarcoma. Involvement of more than one skeletal site by osteosarcoma in a single person may be related to several different mechanisms: multicentric lesions that arise simultaneously (osteosarcomatosis); multicentric lesions that arise metachronously; or a unicentric lesion in which a second neoplastic focus develops in the same bone or in an adjacent bone owing to transarticular spread (skip metastasis) or that metastasizes to a distant bone (with or without pulmonary metastases).[380] As differentiating among these causes of multiple foci of osteosarcoma is difficult (Fig. 83–79), considerable disagreement and debate exist regarding the accuracy of any classification system.[2454]

Osteosarcomatosis, representing the simultaneous occurrence of multiple skeletal osteosarcomas, is regarded by many investigators as a rare, distinct form of disease that predominates in children.[381, 382] It is the similarity in size and radiologic and histologic appearance of the osseous lesions with the absence of a larger (or dominant) bone tumor that is used to support the contention that multiple primary osteosarcomas, rather than secondary deposits arising from a single osteosarcoma, are present. Certainly, the symmetric, osteosclerotic foci in the metaphyseal regions of tubular bones that are evident in childhood osteosarcomatosis support this interpretation, although the presence of pulmonary metastasis in some of these cases and the known frequency of osseous metastasis in cases of osteosarcoma are features that invite alternative explanations for the findings and promote the introduction of additional classification schemes.[383-385] Separation of such cases into those with pulmonary metastasis and those without such metastasis has failed to disclose any notable clinical or pathologic differences between the two groups.[382] What is agreed on is the uniformly poor prognosis of this form of the disease.[386, 387, 2064-2067]

Multiple, metachronous osteosarcomas have been well documented, typically occurring in adolescents and young adults.[388, 389, 2068] In this situation, one or more new tumors develop after the initial treatment of a primary osteosarcoma. Such metachronous sarcomas may represent late metastases from the original neoplasm or new primary tumors.[388] The lesions are distributed asymmetrically, vary in size, and are not necessarily osteosclerotic. Long-term survival is possible when each of the tumors is treated adequately.

A *unicentric osteosarcoma with subsequent skeletal metastasis* represents a definite cause of multicentric lesions. Osseous dissemination in patients with a primary osteosarcoma appears to occur in 10 to 20 per cent of cases, especially in the setting of recurrence of the primary tumor, predominates in the spine and pelvic bones, and may be more common when the initial lesion is located in a tubular bone.[380] Radiographic surveys of the entire skeleton or scintigraphy, or both, should be used to evaluate all patients with an osteosarcoma to allow identification of those with distant skeletal metastasis (Fig. 83–80). In such cases, pulmonary foci of tumor may or may not be present.

Multicentric osteosarcomas also may occur in persons with *Paget's disease* (see Chapter 54) or the Rothmund-Thomson syndrome (autosomal recessive disorder associated with short stature, dystrophic nails, cutaneous abnormalities, cataracts, skeletal anomalies, and a propensity to develop tumors),[2069] or following *irradiation* or exposure to *radium* (see Chapter 73).

CARTILAGE-FORMING TUMORS

Benign Tumors

Chondroma

A chondroma may arise within a bone (enchondroma) or on the surface of a bone (periosteal chondroma), it may be solitary or multiple (enchondromatosis), and the tumor may be accompanied by soft tissue hemangiomas (Maffucci's syndrome).

Enchondroma. The solitary enchondroma is a tumor that develops in the medullary cavity and is composed of lobules of hyaline cartilage.[390-392] The neoplasm usually is discovered in the third or fourth decade of life and is equally frequent in men and women. Lesions, particularly those in the hand, usually are asymptomatic or associated with painless swelling. The appearance of pain should arouse suspicion of malignant transformation, a complication that, although infrequent, is noted more commonly in the long tubular bones and especially in those bones of the pelvic and shoulder girdles.

Skeletal Location. As a general rule, the bones commonly affected by enchondromas rarely are involved by chondrosarcomas.[28, 30, 34, 393] Approximately 40 to 65 per cent of solitary enchondromas occur in the hands or, much less frequently, the feet.[391, 394-398, 2070] Within the hand, the proximal phalanges are the most common site of involvement (40 to 50 per cent of cases), followed in frequency by the metacarpal bones (15 to 30 per cent of cases) and middle phalanges (20 to 30 per cent of cases); enchondromas are unusual in the terminal phalanges (5 to 15 per cent of cases) and are rare in the carpal bones (less than 2 per cent of cases).[390, 391, 399, 400, 2071] The bones of the thumb are

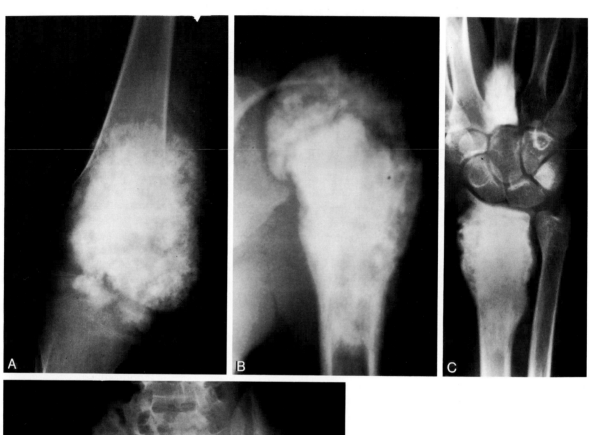

FIGURE 83–79. Multicentric osteosarcoma: Radiographic abnormalities. This 14 year old boy developed pain in his right knee. Skeletal radiographs reveal multiple foci of osteosarcoma involving the femur **(A)**, humerus **(B)**, radius, triquetrum, and metacarpal bone **(C)** and innominate bones **(D)**. It is difficult in these cases to document whether the lesions arose simultaneously or metachronously and whether they represent multiple primary tumors or a single primary neoplasm and multiple metastatic foci.

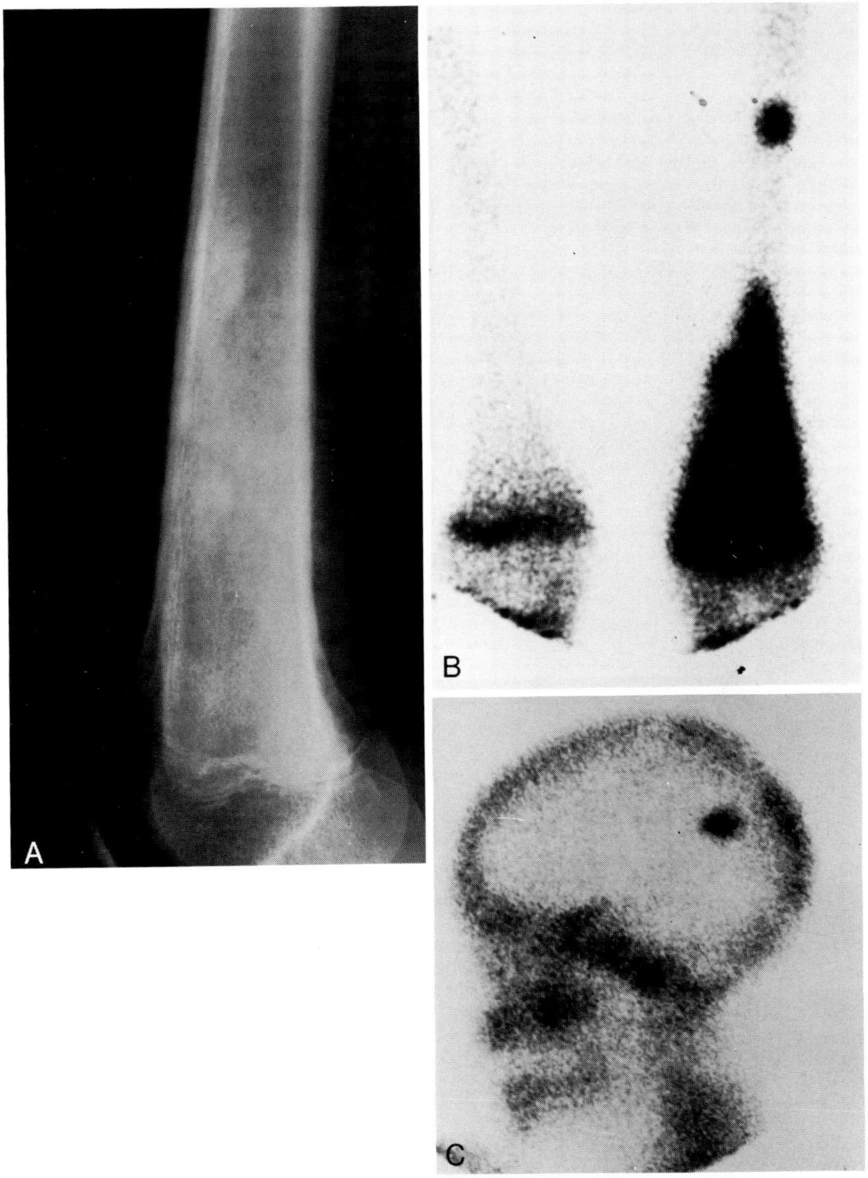

FIGURE 83–80. Unicentric osteosarcoma with skeletal metastasis: Radiographic and scintigraphic abnormalities.

A The primary tumor in the femur is accompanied by multiple, focal radiodense areas in the metaphysis and diaphysis. Periostitis is evident.

B A bone scan shows increased uptake of the radiopharmaceutical agent in the distal portion of the femur and in a separate, more proximal satellite nodule.

C Increased accumulation of the radionuclide also is seen in the skull. This cranial lesion was biopsied, confirming the presence of metastatic osteosarcoma. There was no evidence of pulmonary metastasis.

affected least commonly, whereas those of the fifth finger are involved most frequently. In the foot, which is the site of the tumor in approximately 6 per cent of all enchondromas, a phalanx, a metatarsal bone, or a tarsal bone, in order of decreasing frequency, is affected.

Solitary enchondromas occur in the long tubular bones in approximately 25 per cent of cases and are more frequent in the bones of the upper extremity than in those of the lower extremity. Typical sites of involvement are the humerus, femur, and tibia. The innominate bones, in which chondrosarcomas are relatively frequent, account for fewer than 3 per cent of all enchondromas. Rare areas of skeletal localization are the skull, facial bones, patella, clavicle, sternum, scapula, ulna, and vertebrae.[401–412, 2455] Those tumors in the ribs[413–417] (as well as some enchondromas in the tubular bones[418]) may lead to osseous expansion, designated as enchondroma protuberans,[2072] that simulates the appearance of an osteochondroma, or to massive enlargement of the bone. Enchondromas and osteochondromas rarely can occur simultaneously or in close proximity in a single patient.[2072, 2073]

Enchondromas usually are central tumors that are located in the metaphysis of a long tubular bone (where they may extend into the shaft or epiphysis if the physis is closed) or in the diaphysis of a short tubular bone in the hand or foot. The rare cranial chondromas usually arise in the base of the skull with an origin in the sella turcica, clivus, parasellar area, or posterior fossa at one of the synchondroses; these neoplasms are considered by some investigators to represent chondroid chordomas (see later discussion). In the flat bones, such as those of the pelvis, or in the ribs, it may be impossible to determine whether the tumor began centrally or in a periosteal location.

Radiographic Abnormalities. The radiographic appearance of solitary enchondromas in the hand (Fig. 83–81) or foot (Fig. 83–82) usually is characteristic. A well-defined, medullary lesion with some degree of calcification, a lobulated contour, and endosteal erosion allow precise diagnosis in most cases. Cortical expansion or thickening and pathologic fracture are other potential radiographic characteristics. It should be emphasized that although the presence of calcification is a relatively diagnostic radiographic finding,

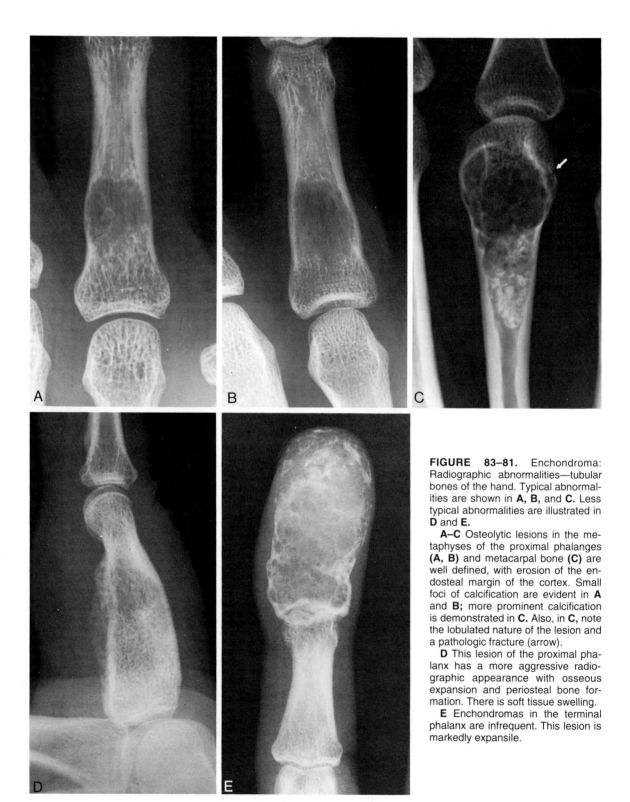

FIGURE 83–81. Enchondroma: Radiographic abnormalities—tubular bones of the hand. Typical abnormalities are shown in **A, B,** and **C.** Less typical abnormalities are illustrated in **D** and **E.**

A–C Osteolytic lesions in the metaphyses of the proximal phalanges **(A, B)** and metacarpal bone **(C)** are well defined, with erosion of the endosteal margin of the cortex. Small foci of calcification are evident in **A** and **B;** more prominent calcification is demonstrated in **C.** Also, in **C,** note the lobulated nature of the lesion and a pathologic fracture (arrow).

D This lesion of the proximal phalanx has a more aggressive radiographic appearance with osseous expansion and periosteal bone formation. There is soft tissue swelling.

E Enchondromas in the terminal phalanx are infrequent. This lesion is markedly expansile.

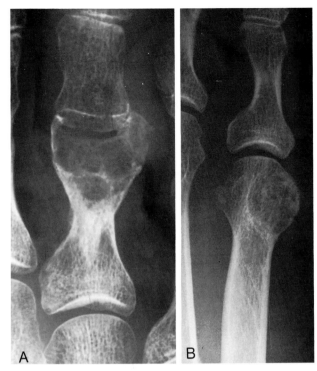

FIGURE 83–82. Enchondroma: Radiographic abnormalities—tubular bones of the foot.

A An expansile, osteolytic lesion of the distal portion of the proximal phalanx is associated with collapse of the articular surface. An unrelated fracture of the base of this phalanx is seen.

B An eccentric lesion in the fifth metatarsal bone contains a sclerotic margin and subtle punctate calcification and has led to osseous expansion.

it is not seen invariably; as enchondromas represent the most common benign tumor of the hand, the identification of a solitary, well-marginated, and lobulated intraosseous lesion in the bones of the hands (with, perhaps, the exception of the distal phalanges) should be considered evidence of an enchondroma until proved otherwise. Elsewhere, enchondromas also possess typical roentgenographic features. In the long tubular bones, a centrally or eccentrically placed medullary, osteolytic tumor of variable size with or without calcification, leading to lobulated erosion of the endosteal margin of the cortex, is most typical (Figs. 83–83 and 83–84). In some cases, channel-like radiolucent areas in the metaphysis are seen (Fig. 83–85), although the finding is more common in Ollier's disease. The radiographic abnormalities accompanying an enchondroma in a flat or irregular bone may not be diagnostic.

MR imaging in cases of enchondroma usually shows a well-circumscribed lesion of low signal intensity in T1-weighted spin echo MR images and of high signal intensity in T2-weighted spin echo MR images (Figs. 83–86 and 83–87). A lobulated configuration is typical. Calcific foci appear as regions of low signal intensity.

Pathologic Abnormalities. With regard to *macroscopic pathology,* fragments of partially calcified, blue-white or blue-gray cartilage that are derived from curettage of the tumor usually are available for examination. Rarely, following en bloc excision, the tumor shows a well-delineated blue to blue-gray translucent surface that has a distinct lobular configuration (Fig. 83–88). White to yellow-white foci of calcium may be found within the lobules. In the

short tubular bones, the cortex may be expanded, scalloped, and thin owing to an eccentric location of the neoplasm. Although most enchondromas are only a few centimeters in size, those in the long tubular bones are often larger, measuring up to 8 cm or more in diameter. It should be noted, however, that the larger a cartilaginous lesion is, the greater is the likelihood that it is a chondrosarcoma.

Microscopically, most enchondromas consist of lobules of hyaline-type cartilage (Fig. 83–89*A*) in which chondrocytes reside in well-formed lacunae.[419] These chondrocytes typically are small, with pale, indistinct cytoplasm and small, round, and hyperchromatic nuclei[420] (Fig. 83–89*B*). A few binucleated cells occasionally may be found residing within a single lacuna (Fig. 83–89*C*), but the occurrence of more than a few of these cells should raise the possibility of chondrosarcoma, especially when the tumor is not located within a bone in the hand or foot. Enchondromas frequently contain calcified regions in which the cells may appear degenerate or necrotic and possess enlarged, irregular, plump nuclei. It is important in the histologic evaluation of cartilaginous lesions to avoid analysis of such calcified areas as the cellular changes may be misinterpreted as evidence of chondrosarcoma.

When sufficient material is available for histologic evaluation, the individual lobules of cartilage frequently are seen to be encased at their periphery by woven or lamellar bone and to be separated from each other by normal marrow elements. The lobules are not confluent, and there is no evidence of infiltration within the intertrabecular marrow spaces.[1872]

The degree of cellularity in enchondromas varies greatly and cannot by itself be used as an indicator of malignancy.[34] Such tumors in the hands and feet, especially in children and adolescents, frequently are hypercellular and may contain cells with enlarged, plump, and atypical nuclei as well as an increased number of binucleated forms.[30, 180] Because of these characteristics, the general histologic criteria that are used for distinguishing a benign chondroma from a chondrosarcoma do not apply when evaluating a cartilaginous tumor in the hands or feet; in these locations, the radiologic findings are of critical importance to accurate diagnosis. The presence of cortical erosion and destruction with extension of the tumor into the soft tissues is an indicator of malignancy that takes precedence over the histologic findings. Mitotic figures are quite rare or totally absent in benign enchondromas[390]; hence, the discovery of more than a rare mitotic figure in a cartilaginous tumor indicates a high probability that it is malignant. Furthermore, the presence of individual chondrocyte necrosis, numerous binucleated cells, occasional mitotic figures, and enlarged plump chondrocytes with prominent visible chromatin and nucleoli and the absence of peripheral bone maturation in the cartilage lobules are all factors favoring a diagnosis of chondrosarcoma. Important also is the occurrence of confluence of the cartilage lobules and invasion of the intertrabecular spaces by the cartilage with entrapment of residual normal trabeculae in cases of chondrosarcoma and the lack of these features in enchondromas.

Studies using *electron microscopy* have shown no essential differences in the morphology of the cells of an enchondroma and those of a well-differentiated chondrosarcoma.[421]

The occurrence of *malignant transformation* of a solitary, benign enchondroma is a matter of great debate. On

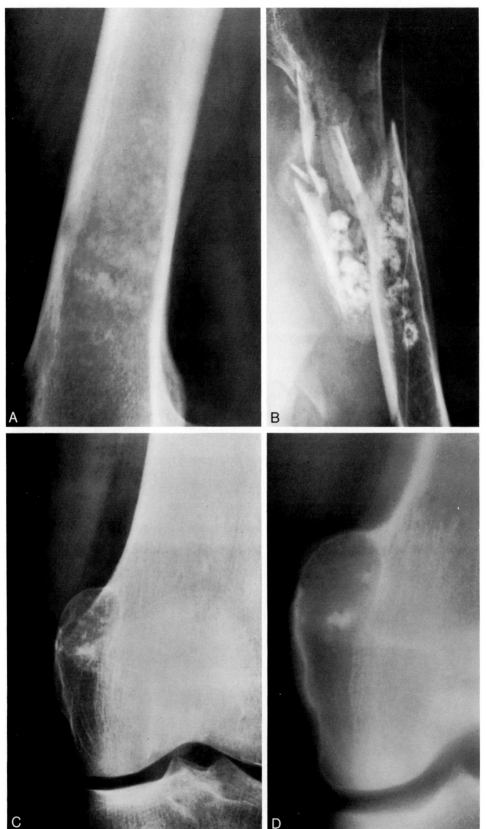

FIGURE 83–83. Enchondroma: Radiographic abnormalities—long tubular bones.

A A lateral radiograph reveals an elongated, calcified medullary lesion in the diaphysis of the femur with endosteal erosion of the cortex.

B A subacute pathologic fracture is evident, related to the presence of a large, heavily calcified enchondroma in the humerus.

C, D A 52 year old woman developed pain and swelling about the knee over a 3 month period. Increased uptake of the bone-seeking radionuclide at the site of the lesion was evident (not shown). Conventional radiography **(C)** and tomography **(D)** document an eccentric, radiolucent metaphyseal and epiphyseal lesion of the femur with osseous expansion and calcification. Presence of an enchondroma was confirmed histologically.

FIGURE 83–84. Enchondroma: Radiographic abnormalities—long tubular bones. This lesion was detected as an incidental finding in a 31 year old man.

A A lateral radiograph shows distinctive small focal calcific collections in the medullary cavity of the tibia.

B A transaxial three-dimensional spoiled gradient recalled acquisition in the steady state (SPGR) MR image (TR/TE, 50/10; flip angle, 60 degrees) obtained with chemical presaturation of fat (ChemSat) reveals the lesion of high signal intensity (arrow) in the tibia. Note foci of low signal intensity representing calcification and mild endosteal erosion. A biopsy was not performed.

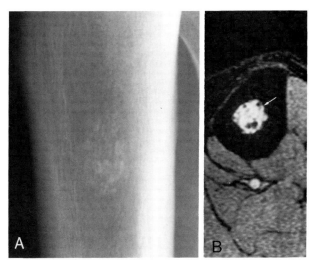

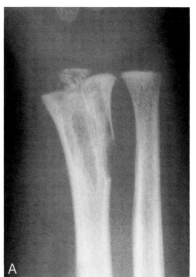

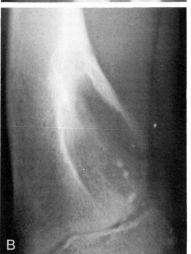

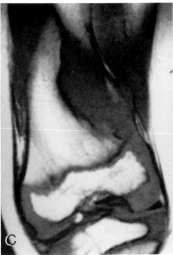

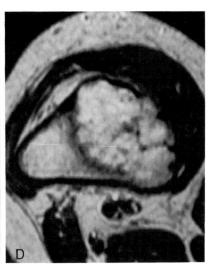

FIGURE 83–85. Enchondroma: Radiographic abnormalities—long tubular bones.

A In this child with a solitary lesion, observe channel-like radiolucent areas extending into the metaphysis of the radius. The appearance is diagnostic of an enchondroma. (Courtesy of E. Bosch, M.D., Santiago, Chile.)

B–D In a second child, a routine radiograph **(B)** shows an elongated lesion containing calcification in the distal femoral metaphysis. The bone is bowed. A coronal T1-weighted (TR/TE, 600/20) spin echo MR image **(C)** shows a well-marginated lesion of low signal intensity. A transaxial T2-weighted (TR/TE, 2000/80) spin echo MR image **(D)** reveals that the lesion is of high signal intensity, is lobulated, and contains septations of low signal intensity. **(B–D,** Courtesy of T. Broderick, M.D., Orange, California.)

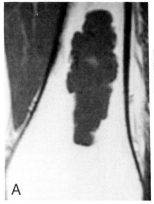
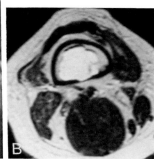

FIGURE 83–86. Enchondroma: MR imaging abnormalities—long tubular bones.

A A coronal T1-weighted (TR/TE, 500/19) spin echo MR image in a 32 year old woman shows a lobulated intramedullary lesion of low signal intensity in the distal portion of the femur.

B A transaxial T2-weighted (TR/TE, 2500/80) spin echo MR image shows that the lesion is of high signal intensity, is lobulated, and erodes the endosteal portion of the cortex posteriorly. (Courtesy of L. Vaughn, M.D., La Jolla, California.)

FIGURE 83–87. Enchondroma: MR imaging abnormalities—long tubular bones. This lesion was discovered as an incidental finding in a 41 year old woman.

A A coronal proton density–weighted (TR/TE, 1500/20) spin echo MR image shows a lobulated lesion of low signal intensity in the proximal humeral metaphysis.

B In a short tau inversion recovery (STIR) MR image (TR/TE, 2200/20; inversion time, 160 msec), the lesion is of high signal intensity with linear regions of low signal intensity.

C A transaxial multiplanar gradient recalled (MPGR) MR image (TR/TE, 650/12; flip angle, 20 degrees) reveals the well-marginated lesion of high signal intensity. Two focal areas of low signal intensity are consistent with calcifications.

D In a transaxial CT image, the calcific collections are well seen.

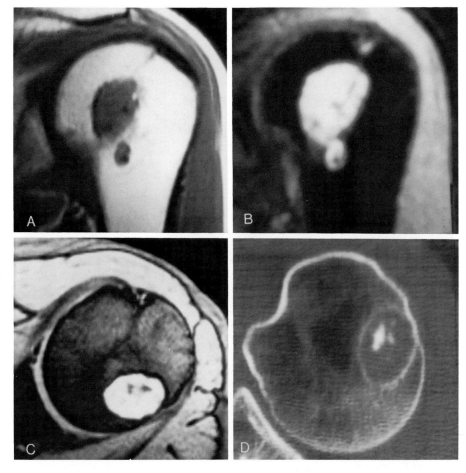

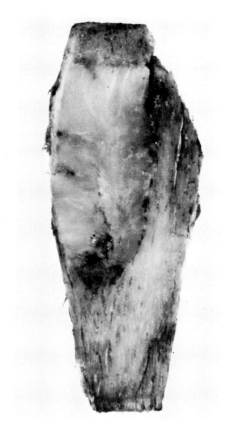

FIGURE 83–88. Enchondroma: Macroscopic abnormalities. A specimen derived from an en bloc excision of a tibial enchondroma shows a homogeneous tumor that is sharply delineated from the cortical bone. The latter is expanded.

the basis of available data, it appears reasonable to suggest that such transformation is exceptional in those enchondromas that are located in the small bones of the hand or foot[422] (Fig. 83–90) and more likely in those enchondromas that are present in the long tubular or flat bones.[1828] Although chondrosarcoma is the expected result following malignant transformation of an enchondroma, additional neoplasms, including malignant fibrous histiocytoma, fibrosarcoma, and osteosarcoma, have been reported in this situation.[423–425] In some instances, a sarcoma may arise adjacent to an enchondroma as an independent event, and these neoplasms may merge subsequently to form a ''collision'' tumor.[1829] An enlarging radiolucent area, pathologic fracture, soft tissue mass, or disappearance of preexisting calcification within the enchondroma are reported radiographic features indicating malignant transformation.

Enchondromatosis (Ollier's Disease). Although enchondromatosis, including Ollier's disease, is discussed in Chapter 90, a few additional comments are appropriate here. Originally described by Ollier in 1899,[426] this disorder is rare and nonhereditary, consisting of multiple, asymmetrically distributed intraosseous cartilaginous foci and subperiosteal deposition of cartilage, either exclusively or predominantly involving one side of the body; the affected bones often are shortened and deformed[427, 1830] (Fig. 83–91). In childhood, the cartilaginous lesions are subject to pathologic fractures, and in adult life they are at risk for malignant transformation.[427] It is the widespread distribution of the cartilaginous lesions that distinguishes Ollier's disease from cases in which several enchondromas are evident, particularly in the bones of the hands and feet.[428] The chondromas in Ollier's disease predominate in the extremities, localizing both to the long tubular bones—particularly the tibia, femur,[1898] and fibula—and, less commonly, to the

metacarpal and metatarsal bones and phalanges. The flat bones, especially those in the pelvis, also are affected.

Clinical manifestations usually appear in the first decade of life and consist of palpable bony masses, asymmetric shortening of the extremities, and osseous deformities related to fractures, a complication that is most frequent in the femur. On radiographs, linear or columnar translucencies in the metaphyses, which may reveal calcification, represent sites of persistent cartilaginous tissue.[429, 2362] In some instances, erosion and proliferation of the bone surface are seen, similar in appearance to the changes associated with juxtacortical chondroma.[2363] Linear radiolucent areas containing calcification also may be evident in the flat bones. Some of the lesions may regress during the years of growth, being replaced by normal bone, and even may disappear completely, although persistent growth disturbances are common.[429, 430] Following cessation of normal growth, the lesions do not increase in size unless malignant transformation has occurred (Fig. 83–92). This complication has been noted in 5 to 30 per cent of cases,[2364] resulting in a chondrosarcoma or, less frequently, a dedifferentiated chondrosarcoma, an osteosarcoma, or a chondroid chordoma.[431, 2365] Rarely, other tumors, including ovarian or brain neoplasms, have been seen in patients with Ollier's disease.[2366–2368] Because the cartilage in cases of Ollier's disease may be more cellular and the chondrocytes may be more atypical than findings in conventional enchondromas, difficulties may be encountered in accurate assessment of the histologic findings in Ollier's disease with regard to the diagnosis of a complicating chondrosarcoma. Helpful in this assessment are the facts that cartilage in Ollier's disease does not show necrotic change, does not destroy trabeculae, is solid rather than myxoid in type, and usually is not as cellular as in a chondrosarcoma.[2364]

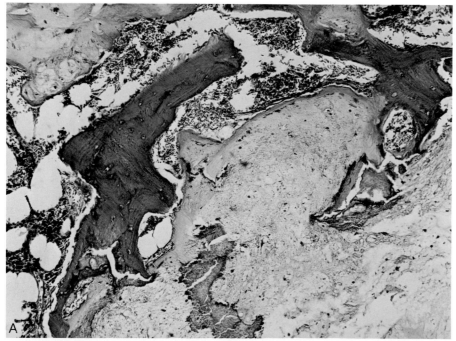

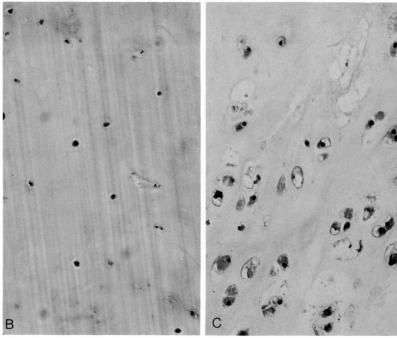

FIGURE 83–89. Enchondroma: Microscopic abnormalities.

A The periphery of this lobule of cartilage is ossified in the form of lamellar bone. (150×.)

B The chondrocytes are well separated and reside in small lacunae. Their nuclei are small and hyperchromatic, and the cells have little or no visible cytoplasm. (150×.)

C In this more cellular enchondroma, larger cells and binucleated cells (arrows) are present. The nuclei still are small and dense. (300×.)

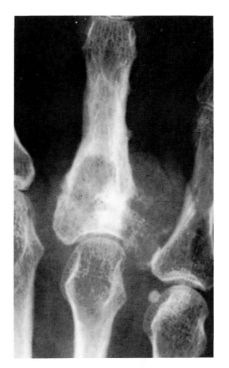

FIGURE 83–90. Enchondroma: Malignant transformation. A chondrosarcoma developing in an enchondroma of the proximal phalanx of the fourth finger is associated with cortical erosion, bone proliferation, and a soft tissue mass.

In recent years, it has become increasingly apparent that several different forms of enchondromatosis exist and that the classification of all such cases as Ollier's disease or Maffucci's syndrome (see following discussion) is no longer appropriate.[433] In some instances, vertebral lesions are prominent,[2369–2372] and in others, soft tissue alterations, such as lipomas and hemangiomas, resemble those of Maffucci's syndrome.[434–436] In fact, skeletal changes combining features of cartilaginous exostoses and enchondromas (metachondromatosis) have been described.[437–439]

Maffucci's Syndrome. Maffucci's syndrome represents a rare, congenital, nonhereditary mesodermal dysplasia manifested by multiple enchondromas and soft tissue hemangiomas. It causes varying degrees of disability, but malignant transformation in the cartilage is the most severe complication, occurring with a frequency of approximately 20 per cent.[441, 2373] Maffucci's syndrome usually is observed in boys and girls in the first decade of life and, not infrequently, the diagnosis is established at birth.[422] Clinical manifestations relate to osseous deformities and soft tissue abnormalities that include cavernous or capillary hemangiomas and, less commonly, lymphangiomas. The soft tissue lesions typically are painless, although mild discomfort as well as increased skin temperature may be noted.[442] Hemangiomas also may occur in the mucous membranes or viscera.

With regard to the skeletal abnormalities, a unilateral distribution is observed in approximately 50 per cent of the cases. Sites of osseous alterations include, most frequently, the metacarpals and phalanges in the hand, which may be the only area of involvement in approximately 5 per cent of patients.[442] Skeletal changes may be limited to one or both upper extremities or one or both lower extremities in some instances, and resulting discrepancies in limb length on the two sides of the body and scoliosis are encountered. The sites of chondromas and soft tissue vascular lesions need not coincide, although, most typically, the distribution of the osseous and soft tissue alterations is similar.[442–444]

Radiographic abnormalities are characteristic, consisting of typical central or eccentric radiolucent lesions containing variable amounts of calcification, and phleboliths within the affected soft tissues[445, 446] (Fig. 83–93). Additionally, radiographs often reveal sequelae of a dysplasia, including limb length discrepancy, a shortened ulna with inferior radioulnar subluxation or dislocation, and tubulation deformities owing to lack of normal bone modeling.[441]

The potential for both bone and soft tissue lesions to undergo sarcomatous transformation in this syndrome has been emphasized, although the risk is greater for the skeletal component.[442] Chondrosarcoma is the dominant malignant tumor encountered,[2374, 2375] although other neoplasms of the musculoskeletal system, such as hemangiosarcoma, lymphangiosarcoma, and fibrosarcoma, are reported in patients with Maffucci's syndrome, and benign and malignant mesenchymal and nonmesenchymal tumors may be evident in other organ systems.[441, 442, 447, 448, 2376] Multiple skeletal lesions in a single patient may, in fact, undergo sarcomatous transformation.[442] Malignant transformation, particularly into a chondrosarcoma, usually is seen in adults after the age of 40 years and in patients with widely distributed osseous lesions.[441] Radiographs may reveal cortical erosion or destruction, disappearance of previously documented calcification in the chondroma, and a soft tissue mass; the presence of osseous expansion and deformity is more difficult to interpret, as such abnormality may accompany the benign lesions of Maffucci's syndrome.[441] Similarly, pathologic fracture is not diagnostic of malignant transformation.

Periosteal (Juxtacortical) Chondroma. Periosteal chondroma, composed of hyaline cartilage, develops adjacent to the cortical surface, beneath the periosteal membrane. It was first described by Lichtenstein and Hall[449] in 1952. Periosteal chondromas are discovered in men more frequently than in women, in a ratio of approximately 2 to 1, and occur in patients of all ages, although they predominate in persons who are less than 30 years of age,[450] with the highest frequency in the second decade of life.[451, 452, 2074]

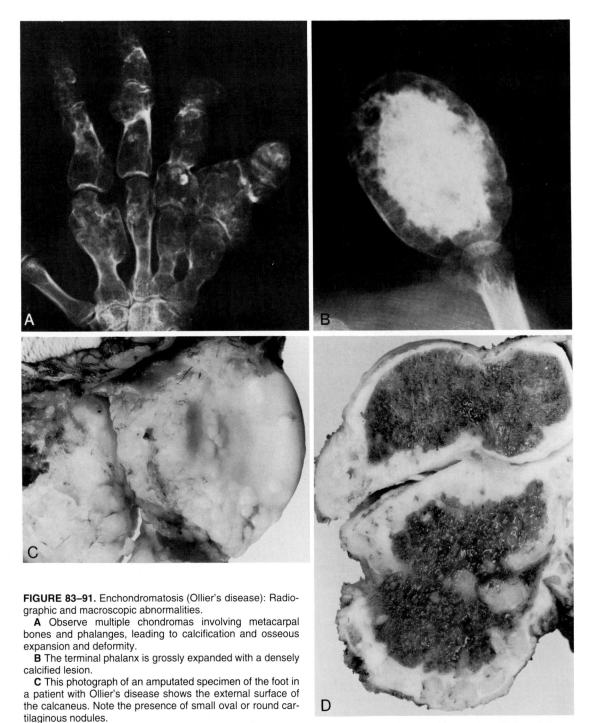

FIGURE 83–91. Enchondromatosis (Ollier's disease): Radiographic and macroscopic abnormalities.

A Observe multiple chondromas involving metacarpal bones and phalanges, leading to calcification and osseous expansion and deformity.

B The terminal phalanx is grossly expanded with a densely calcified lesion.

C This photograph of an amputated specimen of the foot in a patient with Ollier's disease shows the external surface of the calcaneus. Note the presence of small oval or round cartilaginous nodules.

D A section through the calcaneus illustrated in **C** (the talus is at the top of the photograph) reveals multiple nodules in the cartilaginous and osseous portions of the bone.

(**A, B,** Courtesy of C. Pineda, M.D., Mexico City, Mexico.)

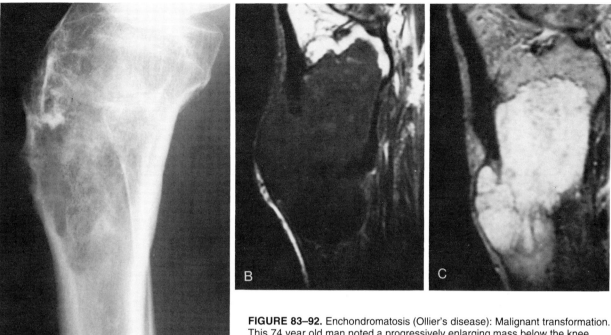

FIGURE 83–92. Enchondromatosis (Ollier's disease): Malignant transformation. This 74 year old man noted a progressively enlarging mass below the knee.

A Routine radiography reveals an osteolytic lesion containing calcification in the proximal portion of the tibia. The anterior tibial cortex is eroded. Additional radiographs confirmed enchondromas in many other tubular bones.

B, C Sagittal T1-weighted (TR/TE, 800/20) **(B)** and T2-weighted (TR/TE, 2000/80) **(C)** spin echo MR images show that the mass penetrates the tibial cortex anteriorly. The findings are compatible with a chondrosarcoma.

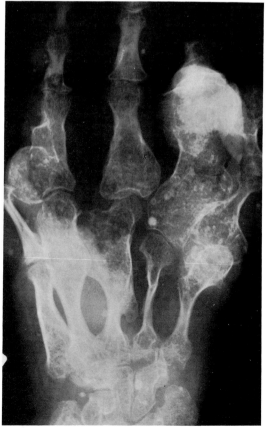

FIGURE 83–93. Maffucci's syndrome: Radiographic abnormalities. This 32 year old woman originally was diagnosed as having Ollier's disease until hemangiomas were discovered on physical examination. This radiograph reveals enchondromas of virtually every bone as well as soft tissue calcifications, or phleboliths.

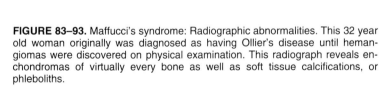

Clinical manifestations are prolonged and include initial local swelling followed by intermittent mild to moderate pain.[450, 451] The long tubular bones, particularly the humerus and the femur, are affected in approximately 70 per cent of cases, and the bones in the hands or, less commonly, the feet are affected in approximately 25 per cent of cases.[450, 451, 453–455] Metaphyseal localization predominates, with typical sites of involvement including the proximal portions of the humerus and the tibia and the proximal and distal portions of the femur. It has been observed that periosteal chondromas frequently are found at the osseous sites of insertion of tendons or ligaments.[456] Rarely, periosteal

chondromas are described that are multiple, involving several sites in one bone or different bones,[445, 456] that are accompanied by solitary or multiple enchondromas,[451, 457] or that occur in flat or irregular bones, such as the clavicle, ribs, scapula, or innominate bone, in the spine, or in other sites.[458, 459, 2074, 2075] Periosteal chondromas occurring in one unusual location, the tibial tubercle, are associated with characteristic radiographic findings.[460]

Radiographically, a soft tissue mass with erosion or saucerization of the adjacent cortex is evident (Figs. 83–94 and 83–95). Medullary sclerosis and periostitis may be seen. Calcification within the lesion is evident in approximately

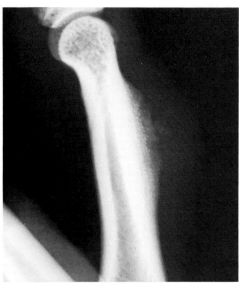

FIGURE 83–94. Periosteal (juxtacortical) chondroma: Radiographic abnormalities.

A A partially calcified lesion on the dorsum of the proximal phalanx has led to considerable periostitis and soft tissue swelling.

B In this lesion, findings include a calcified soft tissue mass, cortical excavation, and periostitis.

C A large calcified lesion adjacent to the tibial tuberosity is associated with osseous erosion.

(**C,** Courtesy of J. Kaye, M.D., New York, New York.)

A

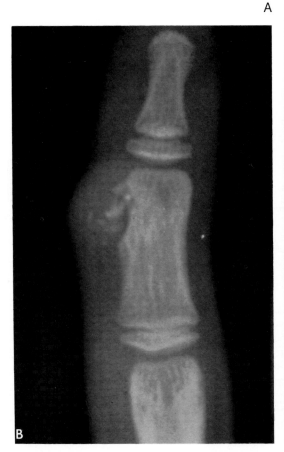

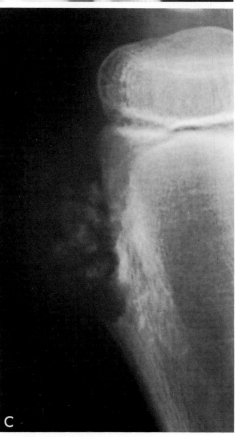

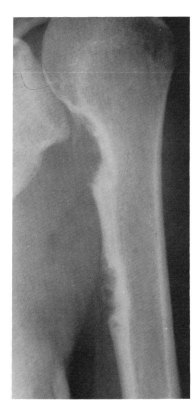

FIGURE 83–95. Periosteal (juxtacortical) chondroma: Radiographic abnormalities. In this example, multiple lesions involve the medial aspect of the humerus. Scalloped erosions and calcification are apparent. (Courtesy of M. Ozonoff, M.D., Hartford, Connecticut.)

50 per cent of cases and may be extensive in some instances.[450, 454, 461–466, 2076] Marked irregularity of an elongated segment of the osseous surface may be misinterpreted as evidence of a malignant tumor, although the scalloped appearance and sclerotic margin of the bone erosions represent important diagnostic clues. In some cases, periosteal chondromas lead to an osseous excrescence simulating an osteochondroma[2077] or a well-defined intracortical radiolucent area.[2078] With MR imaging, these tumors are of high signal intensity in T2-weighted spin echo images (Fig. 83–96).

Gross pathologic examination typically reveals an oval or round tumor of variable size (most do not exceed 4 cm in diameter) that is well circumscribed, located on the surface of a bone, and contained within the periosteum[449–451] (Fig. 83–97*A*). The external surface of the chondroma is either smooth or bosselated (Fig. 83–97*B*). When sectioned, it is firm to rubbery in consistency and consists of lobules of blue to blue-gray glistening cartilage in which yellow-white flecks or streaks of calcification may be seen. The tumor resides within a cuplike or saucer-like crater in the adjacent cortical bone. The proximal and distal ends of the crater frequently show periosteal new bone formation that produces osseous ledges that extend over the tumor cartilage.[450] There is no evidence of invasion of either the soft tissue or the medullary bone.[451]

Microscopically, a periosteal chondroma is composed of lobules of hyaline cartilage that varies in cellularity (Fig. 83–98). Some tumors reveal cellular features typical of an enchondroma, with small, widely separated chondrocytes

that have dense nuclei, whereas others are hypercellular, with large, plump cells that show nuclear atypia and binucleation such that the diagnosis of low grade chondrosarcoma is suggested.[449, 451] The periphery of the tumor frequently contains numerous thin-walled blood vessels and foci of reactive new bone formation. This new bone may form a thin shell about the growing margin of the neoplasm. The base of the lesion may reveal sclerotic new bone that becomes continuous with the cortex. On a purely histologic basis, it is not possible to distinguish a chondroma arising in the soft tissue from one that develops in the periosteum.[467–469]

A periosteal chondroma must be differentiated from a periosteal, or juxtacortical, chondrosarcoma. Unfortunately, this is not always easily accomplished. Although patients with a periosteal chondrosarcoma are somewhat older than those with a periosteal chondroma and the chondrosarcomas tend to be larger, these features do not allow accurate diagnosis in many cases. The histologic abnormalities of these two tumors also may be indistinguishable. If the lesion has an aggressive radiologic pattern with cortical destruction, or if there is evidence of soft tissue invasion on macroscopic or microscopic examination, a diagnosis of chondrosarcoma should be considered.[451]

Chondroblastoma

Chondroblastoma probably was first recognized in 1923 by Ewing,[470] who used the designation calcifying giant cell tumor; subsequently, in 1927, Kolodny identified this neoplasm as a cartilage-containing giant cell tumor,[471] and, in 1931, Codman[472] described a series of patients with what he termed an epiphyseal chondromatous giant cell tumor. In 1942, Jaffe and Lichtenstein[473] introduced the term benign chondroblastoma to emphasize its distinction from giant cell tumor. Although today such neoplasms occasionally are referred to as Codman's tumors, the designation of chondroblastoma is widely accepted. Rarely reported as an extraosseous lesion,[474, 475] chondroblastoma generally is considered to be an uncommon, benign, cartilaginous neoplasm originating in bone.

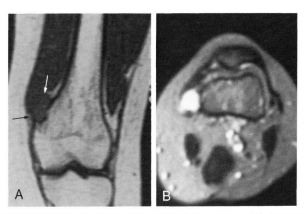

FIGURE 83–96. Periosteal (juxtacortical) chondroma: MR imaging abnormalities.
  A Coronal T1-weighted (TR/TE, 800/25) spin echo MR image reveals the tumor (arrows), of low signal intensity, leading to erosion of the subjacent bone.
  B In a transaxial T2-weighted (TR/TE, 2500/80) spin echo MR image, the tumor is of high signal intensity. (Courtesy of M. Abel, M.D., Stanford, California.)

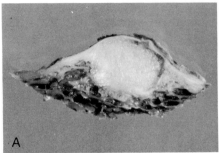

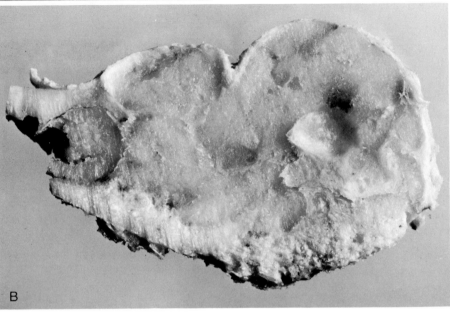

FIGURE 83–97. Periosteal (juxtacortical) chondroma: Macroscopic abnormalities.

A This specimen derived from an en bloc resection of a small periosteal chondroma in the fibula shows that the tumor extends beyond the osseous contour and elevates the adjacent periosteum.

B This tumor in the humerus has a bosselated contour and is covered by an intact periosteal membrane. The surface has a vague, lobular pattern.

Clinical Abnormalities. Chondroblastomas are most frequent in the second and third decades of life, although they have been encountered in patients as young as 3 years and as old as 70 years.[476–480] Approximately 90 per cent of chondroblastomas occur in persons between the ages of 5 and 25 years. Men are affected more commonly than women, in a ratio of approximately 2 to 1. Nonspecific symptoms and signs, including local pain, swelling and tenderness, are evident, varying in duration from several months to many years. As the neoplasms most typically are located in para-articular bone, joint manifestations are not unexpected, may simulate a primary synovial process, and have been accompanied by effusions in as many as 30 per cent of cases.[478]

Skeletal Location. Chondroblastomas generally arise in an epiphysis or apophysis of a long tubular bone. Although metaphyseal extension of an epiphyseal tumor is not uncommon, chondroblastomas originating in the metaphysis or diaphysis of a tubular bone are exceedingly rare.[481–483, 1873, 2079, 2090] The femur (33 per cent of cases), the humerus (20 per cent of cases), and the tibia (18 per cent of cases) are the most frequent sites of involvement. In the humerus or tibia, it is the proximal epiphysis that is affected predominantly (more than 90 per cent of cases); in the femur, proximal and distal epiphyseal involvement occurs with approximately equal frequency. The bones in the lower extremity are affected more commonly than those in the upper extremity. Chondroblastomas in other long tubular bones, such as the ulna, radius, and fibula, are unusual.

Approximately 10 per cent of chondroblastomas arise in the bones of the hands and feet, with particular predilection for the talus and the calcaneus.[484–486, 1831, 1874, 2080] Although infrequent, tumors occurring in the innominate bone reveal a para-acetabular distribution,[2081, 2082] and those occurring in the ribs (and other unusual sites) may predominate in older patients.[477, 487, 2083, 2084] The skull, mandible, and maxilla (including the maxillary sinus) are rare sites of chondroblastomas,[488–490, 2085] as are the vertebrae, scapula, patella, and sternum.[491–493, 2086–2088] In the skull, involvement of the temporal bone is most frequent.[2456] Only one case of multifocal chondroblastomas has been reported in detail, with the tumors occurring in two different bones, one neoplasm appearing several years before the other.[494]

Radiographic Abnormalities. The radiographic features of this neoplasm are highly characteristic,[495–498] consisting of an osteolytic lesion, eccentrically or centrally located in an epiphysis or apophysis, usually less than 5 or 6 cm in size, which is well defined and spheroid or oval in shape (Figs. 83–99 to 83–101). A thin sclerotic rim may separate the tumor from the adjacent normal bone, and the overlying cartilage may be thinned or eroded. Extension of the lesion to subarticular bone (or, rarely, into the joint space) and to the metaphysis is well recognized; metaphyseal involvement occurs in 25 to 50 per cent of cases. Calcific foci within the lesion are documented in approximately 30 to 50 per cent of patients, although the degree of calcification is variable and its identification may require conventional or computed tomography. Rarely, calcification may be exten-

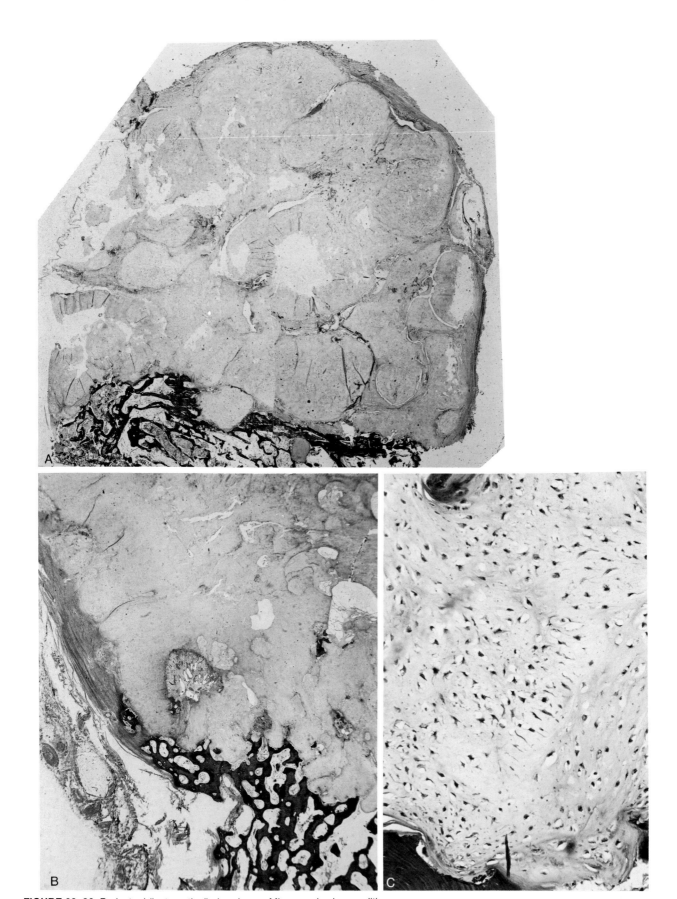

FIGURE 83–98. Periosteal (juxtacortical) chondroma: Microscopic abnormalities.

A A composite photomicrograph shows a periosteal chondroma that is located on the cortical surface (at bottom of photograph) and is covered by the periosteum. The lobular character of the cartilage is evident. A small cartilaginous nodule is extending into the subjacent bone. (5×.)

B The peripheral portion of this tumor is sharply demarcated. The periosteum represents the band of gray tissue to the left of the lesion. Note the scalloped erosion of the bone beneath the tumor. (8×.)

C Increased cellularity of the chondrocytes in these lesions may suggest the presence of a more aggressive process. (150×.)

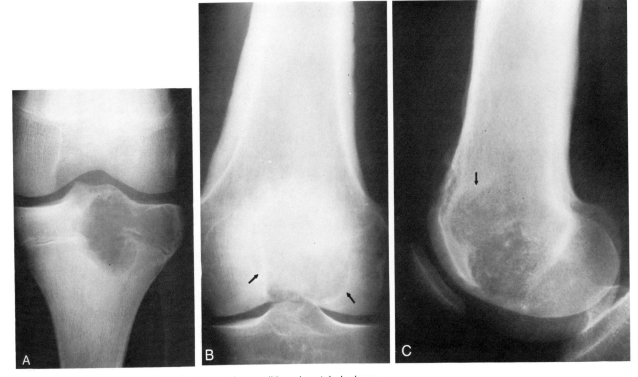

FIGURE 83–99. Chondroblastoma: Radiographic abnormalities—long tubular bones.
  A Tibia. Note the radiolucent lesion involving the metaphysis and epiphysis of the proximal portion of the tibia.
  B, C Frontal **(B)** and lateral **(C)** radiographs of the femur in a 22 year old man show a large epiphyseal and metaphyseal lesion (arrows) that contains foci of calcification. An unusual degree of periostitis is apparent in the metaphysis and diaphysis.

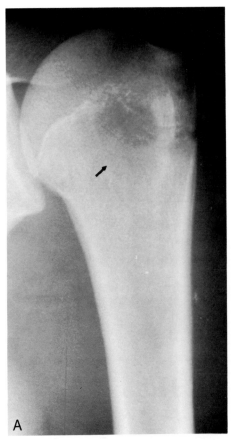

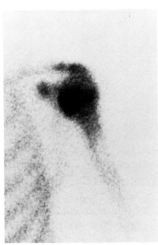

FIGURE 83–100. Chondroblastoma: Radiographic, abnormalities—long tubular bones. This 18 year old man had pain and a decreased range of motion in his shoulder of several weeks' duration.
  A An osteolytic lesion involves the proximal metaphysis of the humerus (arrow). Periostitis in the metaphysis and diaphysis is evident.
  B The bone scan shows increased accumulation of the radionuclide.

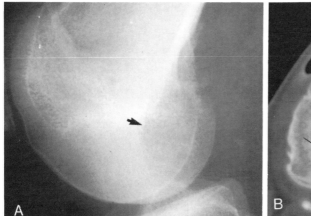
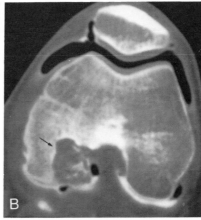

FIGURE 83–101. Chondroblastoma: Radiographic abnormalities—long tubular bones. This 14 year old boy developed knee pain following an injury. Several arthroscopic examinations documented the presence of thickened synovial membrane. The pain continued, however.
  A Routine radiograph shows an osteolytic lesion (arrow) involving the posterior aspect of the medial femoral condyle.
  B Transaxial CT scan performed following the intra-articular injection of air shows the osteolytic lesion containing calcification (arrow). The cortex is eroded. A chondroblastoma was verified at surgery.

sive, producing a radiopaque lesion that may be mistaken for an osteoblastoma.[499] Soft tissue masses and pathologic fractures also are rare.

Periostitis in the adjacent metaphysis or diaphysis is evident in approximately 30 to 50 per cent of cases.[500, 2089] Such periostitis is most frequent in those chondroblastomas that involve the long tubular bones and is rare in other benign tumors or infectious lesions that involve the epiphysis.[2089] Based on data derived from bone scintigraphy and MR imaging, periostitis appears to represent a response to the inflammatory process that may accompany chondroblastomas.[2089]

In sites other than the tubular bones, the radiographic features of chondroblastomas are less specific, although a propensity to affect epiphyseal-equivalent areas, such as the posterior region of the calcaneus,[484] should be recognized (Figs. 83–102 and 83–103).

Other Imaging Techniques. Other imaging methods may be used to evaluate these tumors (Figs. 83–104 to 83–106). Scintigraphy reveals hypervascularity with avid accumulation of the bone-seeking radiopharmaceutical agent,[501] although an extended pattern of radionuclide uptake beyond the true limits of the lesion has been documented, especially in association with periosteal reaction.[495, 2089] Conventional tomography generally is not required; in some instances, areas of calcification and metaphyseal extension are well delineated with this technique. Similarly, CT rarely is necessary and is best reserved for aggressive or recurrent neoplasms; the observation of a fluid level within a chondroblastoma depicted by CT is of interest,[502] although this finding is not diagnostic, having been encountered with other tumors, including aneurysmal bone cysts, giant cell tumors, and even telangiectatic osteosarcomas. Angiograms may be entirely normal or reveal hypervascularity in the soft tissues and the absence of neoplastic vessels.[495]

MR imaging has been used to study chondroblastomas and other cartilaginous tumors.[2089, 2091, 2092] Chondroblastomas are of low signal intensity in T1-weighted spin echo MR images and of variable (and often low) signal intensity in T2-weighted spin echo MR images. The absence of high signal intensity in T2-weighted images in some chondroblastomas may relate to a prominent cellular stroma and

differs from the high signal intensity characteristic of foci of hyaline cartilage present in enchondromas, osteochondromas, and well-differentiated chondrosarcomas. Although this MR imaging feature in some chondroblastomas may have diagnostic significance, the signal intensity of clear cell chondrosarcomas (whose radiographic features simulate those of chondroblastomas) in T2-weighted spin echo MR images appears to be variable and, furthermore, the inflammatory response occurring about chondroblastomas is associated with high signal intensity in T2-weighted spin echo MR images.[2089, 2509]

Pathologic Abnormalities. On *macroscopic examination,* chondroblastomas are delineated sharply by the surrounding cancellous bone; blue-gray to gray-white in color with focal areas of gritty, yellow calcification or necrosis; soft, firm, rubbery or friable in consistency; and commonly lobular in configuration.[477, 478, 503–507] Cystic areas, many of which are hemorrhagic, may be present and, in 5 to 8 per cent of cases, the entire lesion is cystic, resembling a simple or aneurysmal bone cyst.[500, 508] Intra-articular extension of the tumor relates either to direct, transchondral invasion or to cortical perforation with ligamentous spread.[473, 477, 479, 509] Chondroblastomas also may involve the soft tissues, either as a result of iatrogenic implantation at the time of surgery or as a consequence of transcortical extension.[510] They vary in size from 1 to 19 cm, with most being between 3 and 5 cm. The larger tumors are found in the flat bones.

The *histomorphology* of chondroblastoma (Fig. 83–107) is characterized by broad areas of round, oval, or polyhedral chondroblasts that have well-defined cytoplasmic borders.[473, 477, 478, 503, 506] The cytoplasm is eosinophilic and may be quite dense. The nuclei are oval, round, or reniform, frequently are indented or cleaved, and contain one or two small nucleoli. Occasionally larger cells are found with more prominent and hyperchromatic nuclei. Significant nuclear atypia, however, is lacking. Mitotic figures usually are scarce but, in some cases, they may be quite numerous.[511] Multinucleated osteoclast-type giant cells are found dispersed among the chondroblasts or concentrated about areas of hemorrhage or necrosis.[509, 511] These giant cells are smaller and less numerous than those in giant cell tumors.[30] Hemorrhagic foci and cystic blood spaces, lined by chon-

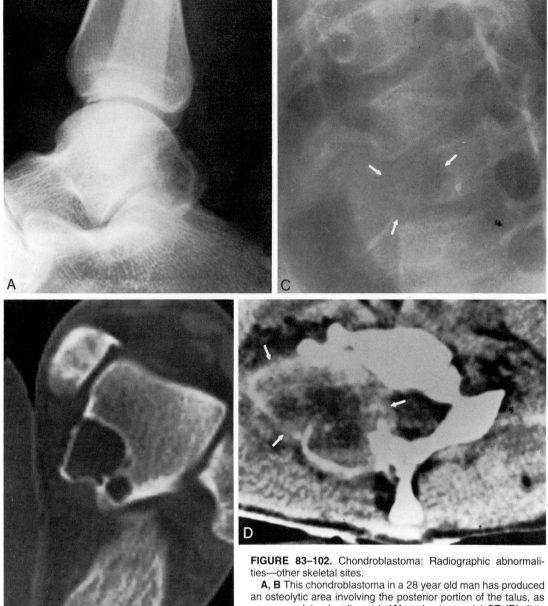

FIGURE 83–102. Chondroblastoma: Radiographic abnormalities—other skeletal sites.

A, B This chondroblastoma in a 28 year old man has produced an osteolytic area involving the posterior portion of the talus, as seen on a lateral radiograph **(A)** and a transaxial CT **(B).** It is well defined without calcification. (Courtesy of Regional Naval Medical Center, San Diego, California.)

C, D An oblique radiograph **(C)** and transaxial CT scan **(D)** in a 16 year old boy reveal a chondroblastoma involving the body and posterior osseous elements of a cervical vertebra (arrows). It is osteolytic and expansile. (Courtesy of T. Yochum, D.C., Denver, Colorado.)

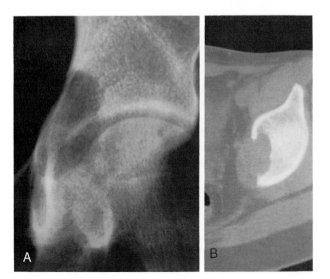

FIGURE 83–103. Chondroblastoma: Radiographic abnormalities—other skeletal sites. In an 18 year old man, routine radiography **(A)** and transaxial CT scan **(B)** reveal an osteolytic lesion in the acetabulum with a soft tissue mass.

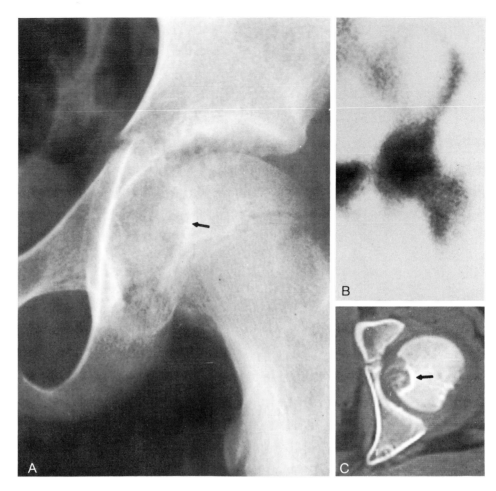

FIGURE 83–104. Chondroblastoma: Scintigraphic and CT abnormalities.

This 9 year old girl had hip pain of several weeks' duration. The radiograph **(A)** reveals a small osteolytic lesion in the medial aspect of the femoral head, possessing a sclerotic margin (arrow). Bone scintigraphy **(B)** shows an extended pattern of abnormal uptake of the radionuclide in the acetabulum and femoral head and neck. Transaxial CT **(C)** reveals the precise location of the tumor (arrow) and calcification within it.

(A–C, Courtesy of Regional Naval Medical Center, San Diego, California.)

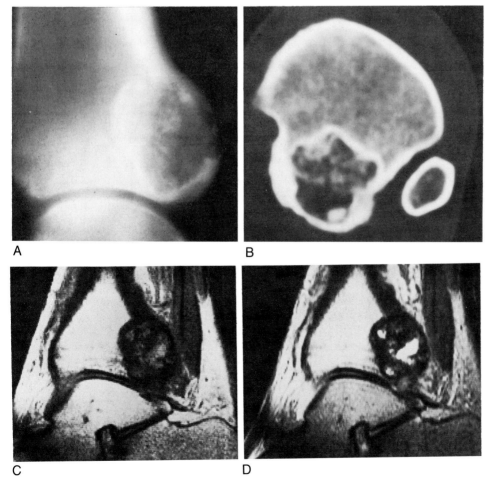

FIGURE 83–105. Chondroblastoma: CT and MR imaging abnormalities. This 16 year old boy developed progressive swelling in the posterior aspect of the ankle. A conventional tomogram **(A)** shows a lobulated, radiolucent lesion in the posterior aspect of the tibia, adjacent to the joint. It is slightly expansile, contains calcification, and possesses a sclerotic margin. A transaxial CT scan **(B)** defines the extent of the lesion, as well as its central calcifications and sclerotic margin. The lesion has low signal intensity in a T1-weighted sagittal MR image **(C)**, and it has some regions of higher signal intensity in a T2-weighted sagittal MR image **(D)**.

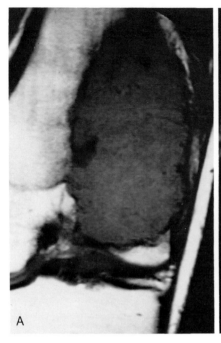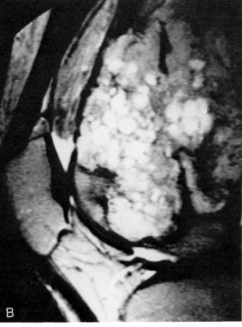

FIGURE 83–106. Chondroblastoma: MR imaging abnormalities. In a 16 year old boy with a 6 month history of knee pain, a coronal T1-weighted (TR/TE, 700/20) spin echo MR image **(A)** shows the lesion of the metaphyseal and epiphyseal portions of the femur. It is sharply defined and of low signal intensity. In a sagittal T2-weighted (TR/TE, 2000/80) spin echo MR image **(B),** the tumor is inhomogeneous in signal intensity. Rounded foci of high signal intensity are evident, however. A joint effusion is present.

droblasts and multinucleated giant cells that simulate those in an aneurysmal bone cyst, are reported in 15 to 25 per cent of chondroblastomas.[33] Such cases have been termed cystic chondroblastomas by some investigators.[478]

Lichtenstein[420] has emphasized the variability of the histologic pattern of chondroblastoma, a finding that he attributes to stages in the evolution of the lesion. The initially highly cellular tumor subsequently develops necrosis, resorption, reparative fibrosis, and chondroid and osseous metaplasia. Foci of cellular necrosis associated with dystrophic calcification frequently are identified. Deposition of calcium has a characteristic lacelike arrangement, creating, in two thirds of cases, a meshwork resembling chicken wire.[33] The necrotic foci resolve and are replaced by fibrous or chondroid areas in which spindle cells reside. Actual hyaline cartilage may form owing to maturation of the chondroid tissue. Focal areas of metaplastic bone may be so abundant that, when combined with the rich vascularity of chondroblastoma, they simulate the pattern of an osteoblastoma. According to some authors, chondroid differentiation or calcification must be present for chondroblastoma to be correctly diagnosed.[2457]

The close relationship of chondroblastoma with chondromyxoid fibroma is indicated by the occurrence in some chondroblastomas of areas indistinguishable from those of a chondromyxoid fibroma; furthermore, some chondromyxoid fibromas contain regions similar to those of a chondroblastoma such that, at times, the differential diagnosis between these two lesions on purely histologic grounds is difficult.

With *electron microscopy,* the tumor cells reveal prominent nuclear and cytoplasmic protrusions and invaginations and, along the inner nuclear membrane, a dense fibrous lamina.[421, 512–514] Similar features are also found in the cells of chondromyxoid fibromas, chondromas, and even chondrosarcomas.

Schajowicz and Gallardo,[478] on the basis of light microscopic, tissue culture, and histochemical studies, believed that chondroblastomas are reticulohistiocytic in nature. Al-

though other investigators have supported a histiocytic origin,[504] most believe that chondroblastomas are chondroid tumors that are derived from cartilage cell precursors that have varying degrees of differentiation.[421, 506, 512–514] Recent immunohistochemical studies have demonstrated the presence of S-100 protein, which also is found in normal human chondrocytes, and the lack of reactivity for histiocytic markers in the cells of chondroblastomas.[515–517] Rare cytokeratin positivity also has been reported in chondroblastomas.[2458, 2459]

Natural History. Although intraosseous recurrences of chondroblastoma have occurred following curettage of the neoplasm, the vast majority of these tumors behave in a benign fashion. Occasionally, however, chondroblastomas pursue a more aggressive course, with invasion of joint spaces, soft tissues, or adjacent bones[489, 518, 519, 1831, 1899] (Fig. 83–108). In fact, metastatic foci of chondroblastoma have been identified in the lungs of patients, usually subsequent to some form of surgical therapy for the primary bone tumor[520, 521, 2093] (Fig. 83–109). In these instances, removal of the pulmonary lesions has resulted in long-term survival, the histologic appearance of the metastatic foci has been identical to that of a conventional chondroblastoma, and some pulmonary metastases left in situ have failed to grow. These observations suggest that the tumoral behavior may not be truly malignant but, rather, the occurrence of pulmonary metastases may indicate that a benign osseous neoplasm has gained access to the vascular system owing to the surgical manipulation. The designation of benign or quasimalignant has been used to describe this simple transport system.[30] Rarely, even before operative intervention for a chondroblastoma, lesions appear in the lung and enlarge progressively, and skeletal foci of tumor develop.[522] These findings are consistent with the view that a variety of chondroblastoma exists that is capable of aggressive behavior in the form of either widespread invasion of soft tissue structures (including neurovascular bundles and lymphatic channels, with extension into adjacent bones) or distant metastases involving not only the lung but other organ

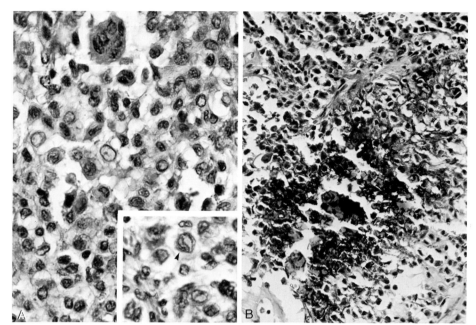

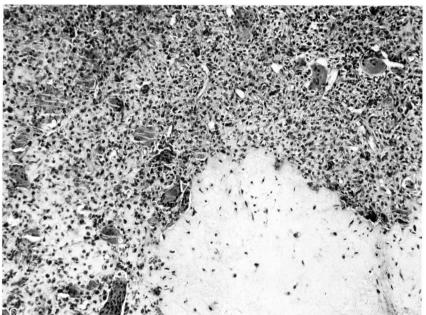

FIGURE 83–107. Chondroblastoma: Microscopic abnormalities.

A The cells of the neoplasm are oval or round. A multinucleated osteoclast-type giant cell is noted at the top of the photomicrograph. The inset at the bottom right reveals some nuclei that are folded or cleaved (arrowhead). (600×.)

B A focus of dystrophic calcification is shown. In one area, individual chondroblasts are surrounded by a thin rim of calcification. (300×.)

C Chondroblasts are intermixed with multinucleated giant cells. A large island of chondroid material is present at the lower right portion of the photomicrograph. (150×.)

systems as well.[522–524] Whether this variety of tumor should be regarded as a malignant chondroblastoma or a chondroblastoma-like chondrosarcoma[28] is not clear. What is certain, however, is that the occurrence of such aggressive behavior by a chondroblastoma is extremely rare and that no methods currently exist that allow an accurate prediction of which chondroblastomas will metastasize.[522]

Differential Diagnosis. The classic radiographic features of a chondroblastoma, which consist of a small radiolucent lesion, with or without calcification or periostitis, in an epiphysis or an apophysis of a tubular bone in the immature skeleton, are relatively specific, although other diagnostic considerations occasionally include infection and eosinophilic granuloma.[525] These last two disorders more frequently lead to metaphyseal or diaphyseal abnormalities, although epiphyseal or apophyseal localization is documented. The roentgenographic features of chondroblastoma generally are easily differentiated from those typical of a

giant cell tumor (epiphyseal lesion without calcification in the mature skeleton) and chondromyxoid fibroma (metaphyseal lesion with coarse trabecular pattern); however, in occasional cases, radiographic differentiation among these tumors as well as others, such as an enchondroma, osteoblastoma,[2094] and chondrosarcoma, may be difficult, and histologic verification of a specific diagnosis is required. Microscopically, although the cellular characteristics in certain chondroblastomas may resemble those of a giant cell tumor, chondroid tissue and hyaline cartilage are not found in the latter neoplasm. Similarly, the presence of such chondroid elements generally excludes the diagnosis of an osteoblastoma. A significant histologic problem in differential diagnosis arises owing to the recent descriptions of a specific type of chondrosarcoma, the clear cell chondrosarcoma, that may possess cartilaginous tissue and scattered, multinucleated giant cells similar to those in a chondroblastoma. Additional histologic characteristics of a clear cell

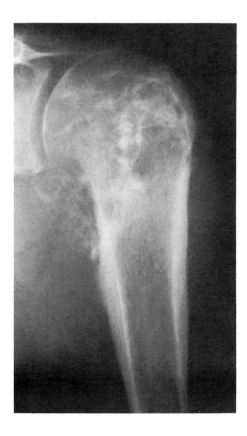

FIGURE 83–108. Chondroblastoma: Natural history—local recurrence and soft tissue extension. This recurrent chondroblastoma in the proximal portion of the humerus is associated with cortical violation and soft tissue extension. Mature periostitis also is seen. (Courtesy of A. D'Abreu, M.D., Porto Alegre, Brazil.)

chondrosarcoma generally allow its accurate identification (see later discussion).

Chondromyxoid Fibroma

The least common benign neoplasm of cartilage, chondromyxoid fibroma, was first identified as a distinctive lesion in 1948 by Jaffe and Lichtenstein,[526] having previously been considered a myxoma[527] or a myxomatous variant of giant cell tumor or mistaken for a malignant tumor, especially chondrosarcoma, chondromyxosarcoma, or myxosar-

coma.[528] Subsequently, a number of large series of chondromyxoid fibromas have been reported.[528–532, 2095, 2096]

Clinical Abnormalities. Although the reported ages of affected patients have varied considerably, this tumor is identified most typically in persons who are less than 30 years of age and is especially common in the second and third decades of life. The neoplasm may be slightly more frequent in men than in women. Slowly progressive pain, tenderness, swelling, and restriction of motion are observed, with a duration of symptoms usually varying from 1 week

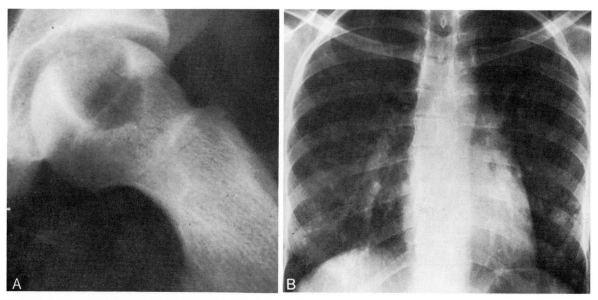

FIGURE 83–109. Chondroblastoma: Natural history—benign metastases.
  A The osteolytic lesion of the femoral head is well defined, with a sclerotic margin. Curettage documented that it was a chondroblastoma.
  B Four years later, multiple pulmonary nodules are evident.

or more to several years. A rapid onset of clinical abnormalities appears to be more characteristic of tumors developing in children.[533] Spontaneous fractures, which are infrequent, may be responsible for the patient's seeking medical attention.[529, 531] Rarely, the lesion is entirely asymptomatic.[530]

Skeletal Location. Chondromyxoid fibroma is observed most frequently in the long tubular bones, especially those in the lower extremity (70 per cent of cases). Involvement of the tibia or femur is evident in approximately 55 per cent of patients. Favored sites of tumor localization are the proximal end of the tibia, proximal and distal ends of the femur and fibula, and, less commonly, innominate bone and small bones of the foot (metatarsal bones, phalanges, calcaneus).[529, 534–536, 1832, 1900] The tumor is relatively rare in the spine, ribs, sternum, scapula, skull, carpal bones, mandible, and maxilla.[537–551, 2097–2100] Also rare is the occurrence of multicentric lesions.[552] In a tubular bone, a metaphyseal focus is favored, with extension into the adjacent epiphysis (in the presence of a closed physeal plate) or diaphysis.[528, 531] Primary localization in a diaphysis or an epiphysis is rare.[530, 532, 2095]

Although chondromyxoid fibromas and chondroblastomas share certain histologic features, their anatomic locations are somewhat different. Chondromyxoid fibroma is more frequent in the tibia than in the femur, whereas the reverse is true of chondroblastoma. Predilection for the tibial tuberosity has been observed in some cases of chondromyxoid fibroma.[2103, 2460] Furthermore, humeral involvement, which is relatively common in patients with chondroblastoma, is infrequent in cases of chondromyxoid fibroma. Most important, however, in the anatomic distinction be-

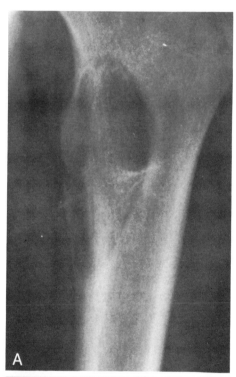

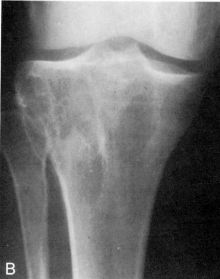

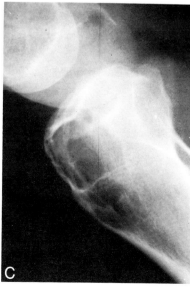

FIGURE 83–110. Chondromyxoid fibroma: Radiographic abnormalities—long tubular bones.

A Femur. An eccentric, osteolytic, slightly expansile lesion of the femoral metadiaphysis is evident. The expanded cortex is thinned and contains small perforations. Calcification and significant periostitis are absent.

B, C Tibia. An osteolytic, eccentric, slightly expansile lesion involves the anterior portion of the metaphysis and epiphysis of the bone and extends to the subchondral region. Slight trabeculation is evident. The lesion is well defined and contains no calcification. Periostitis is absent.

(**B, C,** Courtesy of O. J. Wollenman, M.D., Fort Worth, Texas.)

tween these two neoplasms is the epiphyseal localization that characterizes a chondroblastoma and the metaphyseal localization that typifies a chondromyxoid fibroma.

Radiographic Abnormalities. Although the roentgenographic findings usually are indicative of a benign tumor, they are variable, depending on the precise location of the neoplasm. When located in a long tubular bone, chondromyxoid fibromas generally are eccentrically situated, metaphyseal lesions that are radiolucent, of varying size (2 to 10 cm), and elongated in shape[2101–2104] (Fig. 83–110). Cortical expansion, exuberant endosteal sclerosis, and coarse trabeculation commonly are noted. Extensive periostitis and pathologic fractures are unusual, and calcification is rare.[530] Larger lesions may lead to complete penetration of the cortex; the resulting hemispherical osseous defect or ''bite,'' when unaccompanied by periostitis, is believed to be highly characteristic of a chondromyxoid fibroma.[531] It should be noted, however, that on the basis of the radiologic alterations, such lesions appear aggressive in behavior and may be diagnosed incorrectly as malignant tumors. Rarely, intracortical or periosteal chondromyxoid fibromas are encountered in the tubular bones, leading to exophytic growths, periosteal disruption, and a soft tissue mass.[553–555, 2096]

The possibility of a superimposed aneurysmal bone cyst should be considered in these instances.[554, 556]

In the flat and irregular bones, as well as the small bones of the hands and feet (Fig. 83–111), chondromyxoid fibromas lead to osteolysis, scalloped osseous erosions, bone expansion, and a coarse trabecular pattern. In some instances, they become massive, occupying much of the bone,[529] and their radiologic differentiation from a malignant neoplasm is difficult.

CT (Fig. 83–112) and MR imaging (Fig. 83–113) can be used to further define the extent of bone involvement.

Pathologic Abnormalities. The tumor usually is delineated sharply from the underlying bone and commonly has a scalloped or bosselated, sclerotic medullary border.[33, 34] Its orientation is parallel to the long axis of the tubular bone and, although classically it is eccentric in position, a chondromyxoid fibroma in the short tubular bones or fibula may be located centrally. Its surface is blue-gray to blue-white and resembles hyaline cartilage or fibrocartilage. Small cysts and mucoid areas may be evident. The consistency of the tumor may be firm, rubbery, or soft.

Chondromyxoid fibroma is characterized by several histologic patterns in which chondroid, myxomatous, and fi-

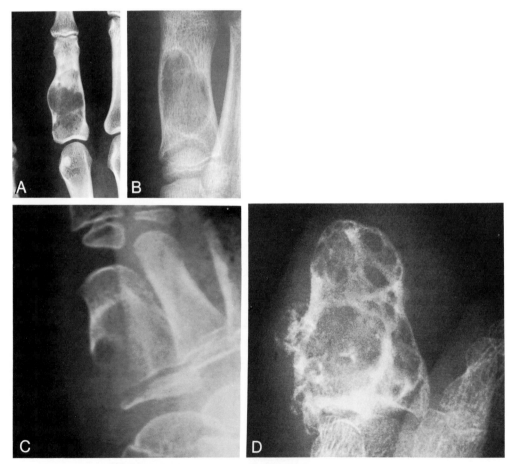

FIGURE 83–111. Chondromyxoid fibroma: Radiographic abnormalities—small bones of the hand and foot.

A Proximal phalanx of hand. The lesion is well defined, radiolucent, and slightly expansile and extends to the subchondral bone. It has a lobulated contour with endosteal erosion, and there is no calcification or periostitis.

B Metatarsal bone of foot. This well-marginated lesion involves the diaphysis and metaphysis of the bone. The inner portion of the cortex is eroded, and there is slight osseous expansion.

C Proximal phalanx of foot. A slightly more aggressive osteolytic lesion has led to cortical disruption. A sclerotic margin is apparent distally.

D Distal phalanx of foot. This aggressive lesion of the entire phalanx is characterized by thick trabeculation and calcification. Irregular calcific or ossific deposits are present in the soft tissues medially.

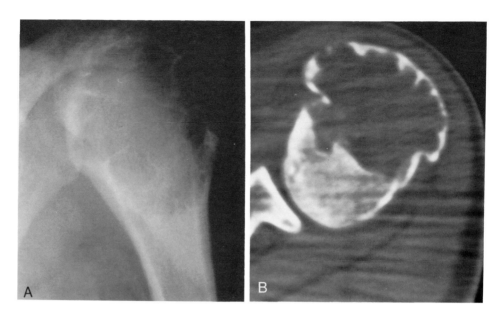

FIGURE 83–112. Chondromyxoid fibroma: CT abnormalities—long tubular bones.

A A routine radiograph in a 14 year old boy shows a trabeculated, osteolytic lesion involving the epiphysis and metaphysis of the proximal portion of the humerus.

B Transaxial CT reveals slight bone expansion and peripheral ridges of bone. There is no evidence of calcification. (Courtesy of T. Broderick, M.D., Orange, California.)

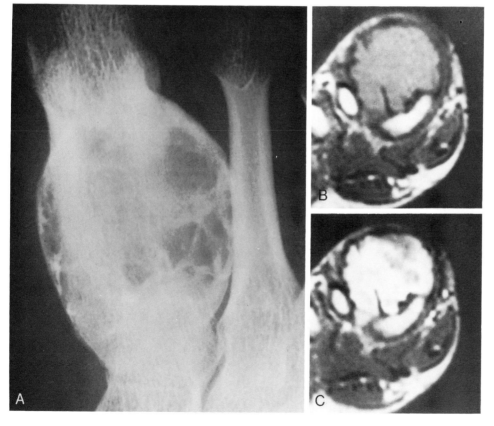

FIGURE 83–113. Chondromyxoid fibroma: MR imaging—small bones of the foot.

A An expansile, heavily trabeculated lesion of the first metatarsal bone is evident.

B, C Coronal T1-weighted (TR/TE, 650/20) spin echo MR images obtained before **(B)** and after **(C)** the intravenous injection of a gadolinium compound reveal the expansile tumor. It is of intermediate signal intensity in **B,** and there is diffuse enhancement of signal intensity in **C.** (Courtesy of H. S. Kang, M.D., Seoul, Korea.)

brous areas occur in varying proportions. Typically, the tumor is composed of well-defined or fused lobules in which reside round, oval, or stellate cells that have a dense, eosinophilic cytoplasm (Fig. 83–114A,B). In less mature neoplasms, the center of the lobules is composed predominantly of a loose myxoid stroma and stellate cells.[526, 532] With maturity, the stroma becomes more chondroid and the cells lie within lacunae. The lobules also may undergo progressive collagenization and form regions of fibrocartilage or actual fibrous nodules.[532] At the margin of the lobules, there is an increased concentration of cells that may be spindle-shaped and appear fibroblastic[532, 557] (Fig. 83–114C). The lobules are separated by thin, vascular, fibrous bands in which osteoid or bone may rarely be found. At the intersection of the individual lobules, the stroma may contain multinucleated osteoclast-like giant cells, hemosiderin pigment, and cartilage cells similar to those of a chondroblastoma.[30, 33, 34, 529] Areas consisting of dilated vascular sinusoidal spaces lined by multinucleated giant cells and tumor cells may be present, resembling the features of an aneurysmal bone cyst.[30] Some chondromyxoid fibromas contain foci of hyaline cartilage, similar to but less extensive than those found in an enchondroma. Focal calcification in chondromyxoid fibroma is not common, occurring in 5 to 27 per cent of cases. Mitotic figures are rare or nonexistent. In approximately one third of tumors, larger cells, some with two or three nuclei, are found; these nuclei, which may be irregular, hyperchromatic, and atypical in

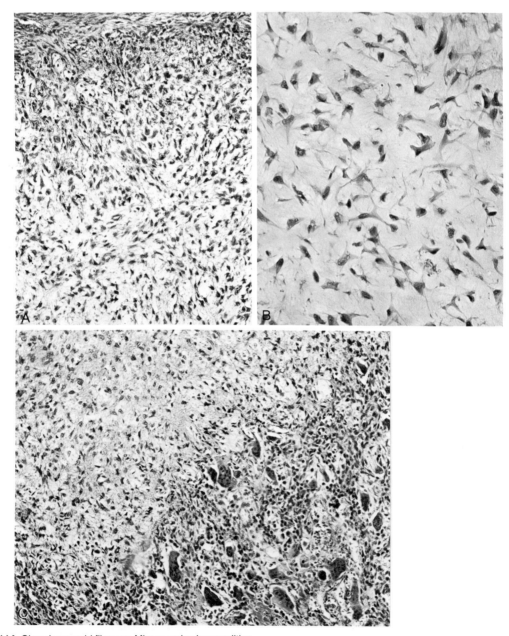

FIGURE 83–114. Chondromyxoid fibroma: Microscopic abnormalities.

  A A loose myxoid stroma is evident in which reside spindle and stellate tumor cells. The concentration of these cells increases from the center of the lobule (bottom) to its periphery (top). (150×.)

  B The stellate cells in a lobule of this neoplasm are shown at higher magnification. (300×.)

  C At the edge of a myxoid lobule of the tumor, the stroma contains multinucleated osteoclast-type giant cells and small cells with dense eosinophilic cytoplasm similar to those present in a chondroblastoma. (150×.)

appearance, are similar to those in the cells of a chondrosarcoma.

With electron microscopy, two cell types have been identified in chondromyxoid fibromas: fibroblast-like cells and cells with the fine structure of chondrocytes or chondroblasts.[421, 558, 559] Immunohistochemical studies have shown the presence of S-100 protein in the cells of chondromyxoid fibromas.[2461]

Natural History. Although there are reports that document the occurrence of locally aggressive behavior and tumor recurrence,[528, 530, 532, 533, 535, 560, 2105] the prevailing view is that chondromyxoid fibroma is a benign cartilaginous neoplasm and that its recurrence, which may take place in as many as 25 per cent of cases, relates to inadequate local excision.[561] Indeed, the recurrence of this tumor is most frequent when only curettage of the lesion is accomplished and is least frequent when wide local or block excision of the tumor is performed. Soft tissue involvement is rare and may indicate true tumor invasion or implantation of the neoplasm in the soft tissues at the time of surgery.[532, 561, 562, 2105] Those chondromyxoid fibromas that have been reported to produce metastases generally have been viewed as low grade chondrosarcomas that have been misinterpreted histologically as chondromyxoid fibromas.[530, 532] Rare documented cases of malignant transformation of this neoplasm do exist.[30]

Differential Diagnosis. The roentgenographic signs of chondromyxoid fibroma usually are those of a nonmalignant process, and accurate diagnosis depends on eliminating a variety of other benign lesions, including a simple or aneurysmal bone cyst, enchondroma, nonossifying fibroma, fibrous dysplasia, giant cell tumor, chondroblastoma, and osteoblastoma.[530] Accurate diagnosis of a chondromyxoid fibroma is least difficult when the osteolytic lesion is localized to the metaphyseal region of a tubular bone and reveals an eccentric position, endosteal sclerosis, and cortical expansion or violation with a bitelike configuration. The presence of radiographically detectable calcification within this tumor is rare, so that this finding should suggest alternative diagnoses, such as an enchondroma, chondroblastoma, or even fibrous dysplasia. The thick trabeculae that commonly are found in a chondromyxoid fibroma, which reflect the corrugation or grooving of adjacent bone by the lobulated periphery of the neoplasm, differ from the faint, thin trabeculae of a giant cell tumor or nonossifying fibroma. In nontubular bones, a precise radiographic diagnosis of a chondromyxoid fibroma is more difficult, as such lesions can be large and expansile. Alternative diagnoses in these cases include fibrous dysplasia and giant cell tumor as well as other lesions.

Considerable difficulty may be encountered in differentiating the pathologic features of a chondromyxoid fibroma from those of a chondrosarcoma. On macroscopic inspection, the former tumor appears more sharply demarcated than a chondrosarcoma, in which ill-defined, infiltrating neoplastic margins may be seen. Histologically, chondromyxoid fibroma lacks the cellular pleomorphism, necrosis, and mitotic activity that are evident in a typical chondrosarcoma. Furthermore, it is the variation in the histomorphologic pattern of chondromyxoid fibroma that distinguishes it from a chondrosarcoma, which possesses more homogeneous cartilaginous tissue. Histologic differentiation between a chondromyxoid fibroma and a chondroblastoma

also can be difficult, although chondroblastoma lacks the lobulated and peripheral condensation of cells found in chondromyxoid fibroma.

Osteochondroma

An osteochondroma can be considered a cartilage-covered osseous excrescence that arises from a surface of a bone. Osteochondromas may be solitary or multiple (hereditary multiple exostoses) or occur spontaneously or following accidental or iatrogenic injury or irradiation (see Chapter 73). Osteochondromas or osteochondroma-like lesions also may be encountered in certain other specific situations or locations (see later discussion).

Solitary Osteochondroma. The solitary osteochondroma, or osteocartilaginous exostosis, is a relatively frequent lesion. Its precise cause is not clear; some investigators consider the osteochondroma to be a true neoplasm and others believe it is a developmental physeal growth defect.[563] Osteochondromas develop in bones that form through the process of endochondral (enchondral) ossification and are intimately related to the physis.[2106] This anatomic localization has led to speculation that an osteochondroma arises from a portion of the physeal cartilage and that its subsequent growth, which occurs at approximately a 90 degree angle with respect to the axis of the physis, results from rotation of this portion of the physeal plate combined with the longitudinal endochondral growth of the parent bone.[563, 564] Alternatively, it has been suggested that osteochondromas arise from cartilaginous metaplasia within the periosteal membrane,[565] from defective modeling of the bone in which the absence of a periosteal ring about the physis allows the diaphyseal cartilage to expand in an abnormal direction,[566] from defective osseous remodeling and modified periosteal activity,[567] or from displacement of undifferentiated cells within the physeal growth plate to the surface of the bone.[568] Experimentally, it has been shown that osteochondromas can be produced by transplantation of fragments of the physeal plate,[569] supporting the concept that these lesions are derived in some manner from this plate, subsequently develop by endochondral ossification, and, with cessation of activity in the physis, stop growing.

Clinical Abnormalities. The majority of solitary osteochondromas are discovered in children and adolescents, with approximately 70 to 80 per cent of lesions occurring in patients who are younger than 20 years of age. A nontender, painless, slowly growing mass represents the most characteristic clinical manifestation. When large or at certain anatomic sites, osteochondromas may lead to additional and more significant symptoms and signs related to a fracture of the exostosis, irritation or damage of adjacent nerves or vessels, spinal cord compression, or even urinary tract obstruction (see later discussion).

Skeletal Location. Any bone that develops by endochondral ossification may be the site of an osteochondroma, although the long tubular bones (Fig. 83–115), especially the femur (30 per cent of cases), humerus (20 per cent of cases), and tibia (17 per cent of cases), are involved most frequently. Osteochondromas in certain long tubular bones, such as the radius and ulna, are distinctly unusual. The bones in the lower extremity are affected more frequently than those in the upper extremity, in a ratio of approximately 2 to 1. In the tubular bones, a metaphyseal localization is characteristic; osteochondromas are rare in the di-

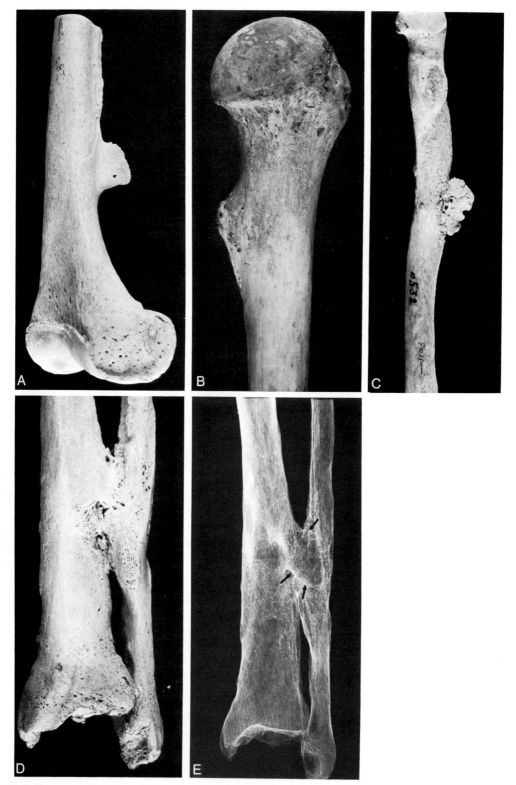

FIGURE 83–115. Solitary osteochondroma: Skeletal location—long tubular bones. Four examples are shown. In each case, note the osseous continuity between the osteochondroma and the parent bone. In **D** and **E,** note also the deformity of the fibula related to the tibial osteochondroma (arrows). **A,** Femur; **B,** humerus; **C,** radius; **D, E,** tibia.

aphysis, whereas those in the epiphysis, which also are rare, are considered to be indicative of a separate disorder, Trevor's disease or dysplasia epiphysealis hemimelica (see later discussion). Specific sites of predilection of osteochondromas are the distal metaphysis of the femur and proximal metaphyses of the humerus, tibia, and fibula. These regions correspond to areas of rapid bone growth.

The small bones of the hand and foot are involved in approximately 10 per cent of cases, and the innominate bone is involved in approximately 5 per cent of cases.[570, 571]

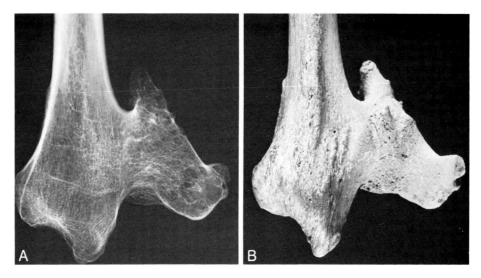

FIGURE 83–116. Solitary osteochondroma: Radiographic abnormalities—long tubular bones. The pedunculated osteochondroma arising from the distal metaphysis of the fibula contains spongiosa and cortex that are continuous with those of the parent bone. The metaphysis itself is slightly widened, a finding that is much more frequent and prominent in instances of multiple osteochondromas.

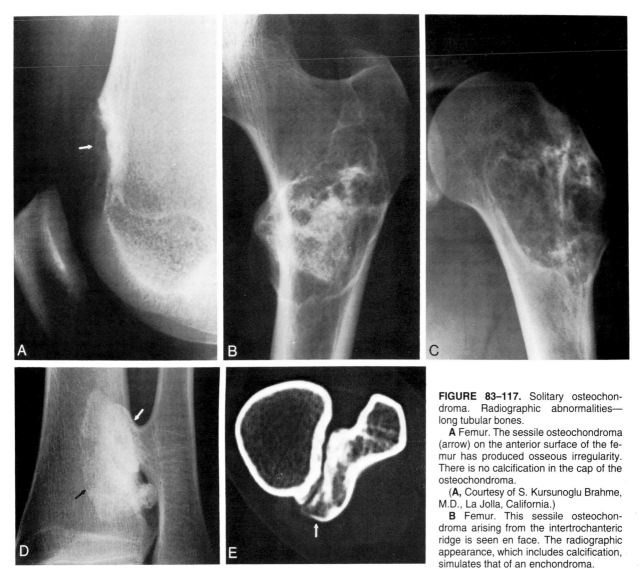

FIGURE 83–117. Solitary osteochondroma. Radiographic abnormalities—long tubular bones.

A Femur. The sessile osteochondroma (arrow) on the anterior surface of the femur has produced osseous irregularity. There is no calcification in the cap of the osteochondroma.

(**A,** Courtesy of S. Kursunoglu Brahme, M.D., La Jolla, California.)

B Femur. This sessile osteochondroma arising from the intertrochanteric ridge is seen en face. The radiographic appearance, which includes calcification, simulates that of an enchondroma.

C Humerus. Another sessile osteochondroma similar to that in **B** is shown.

(**C,** Courtesy of T. Broderick, M.D., Orange, California.)

D, E Fibula. Restricted motion in the ankle of this 61 year old man is related to a large pedunculated osteochondroma arising from the posteromedial surface of the fibula and wrapping itself about the tibia (arrows), as shown with routine radiography and transaxial CT. **E** is oriented to allow correlation with **D**.

Although the spine is affected infrequently (less than 2 per cent of cases), such involvement has received a great deal of attention owing to the possibility of compression of the spinal cord.[572–584, 1901, 2107–2110] Vertebral osteochondromas predominate in the posterior osseous elements, especially the spinous process, and the lumbar and cervical regions are involved most frequently. Osteochondromas of the cranial bones usually affect the base of the skull, particularly the sphenoid bone and parasellar region.[585–589] The gnathic bones, however, also may be involved.[2111] Scapular exostoses occur in approximately 4 per cent of cases and, especially when located on the anterior surface of the bone, can lead to malposition of the scapula or pain and audible snapping during movement.[590, 591] An osteochondroma arising from the scapula also may be misinterpreted as a pulmonary nodule during chest radiography. Clavicular osteochondromas are rare.[2112]

Radiographic Abnormalities. An osteocartilaginous exostosis is characterized radiographically by an osseous protuberance arising from the external surface of a long tubular bone and containing spongiosa and cortex that are continuous with those of the parent bone (Fig. 83–116). The outgrowths may be pedunculated (with a narrow stalk and bulbous tip) or sessile (with a broad, flat base) (Fig. 83–117). Commonly occurring in the metaphysis at osseous sites of tendinous or ligamentous attachment, osteochondromas grow according to the forces generated by these tendons and ligaments and, hence, typically point away from the nearby joint and toward the diaphysis. The metaphysis of the tubular bone may be widened, owing to failure of normal tubulation, although this finding is far more characteristic of multiple rather than solitary osteochondromas.

The tip of the osteochondroma is covered by a cap composed of hyaline cartilage. The degree of calcification within this cartilage is highly variable, although, owing to the occurrence of malignant transformation (see later discussion), this portion of the lesion must be evaluated carefully. If the cap is small and well defined, with regular, stippled calcification, the appearance is most compatible with a benign outgrowth; if it is large and poorly defined and contains irregular or incomplete calcification, malignant transformation should be given serious consideration. Between these two extremes exist radiographic patterns that are less diagnostic of a benign or malignant tumor, and the use of additional diagnostic methods may be required (see later discussion).

Osteochondromas arising in the innominate bone (Figs. 83–118 and 83–119A) frequently are large, leading to a soft tissue mass and displacement of adjacent structures, and the patterns of calcification are variable and commonly irregular. In this instance, differentiation of a benign osteochondroma from one that has undergone malignant transformation is extremely difficult. In the ribs (Fig. 83–119B), osteochondromas (as well as enchondromas) are particularly frequent at the costochondral junction owing to the presence in this area of normal cartilaginous tissue. Osteochondromas in the small tubular bones of the hand and foot lead to radiographic features that are similar to those evident in the long tubular bones. Those in the spine typically arise in the posterior osseous elements (Fig. 83–119C).

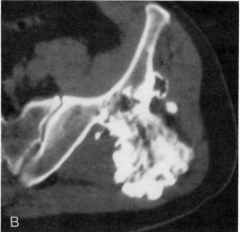

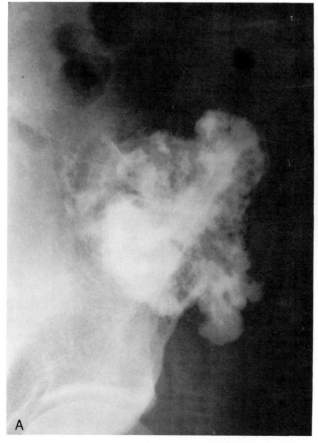

FIGURE 83–118. Solitary osteochondroma: Radiographic abnormalities—innominate bone. Routine radiography **(A)** and transaxial CT **(B)** show a large pedunculated osteochondroma arising from the posterior surface of the ilium. (Courtesy of R. Sweet, M.D., Pomona, California.)

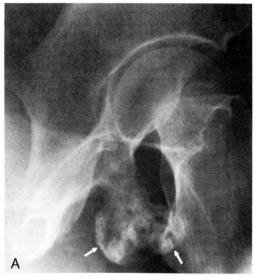

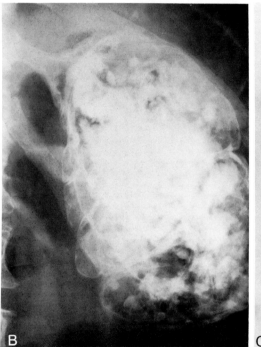

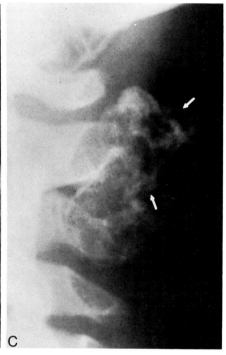

FIGURE 83–119. Solitary osteochondroma: Radiographic abnormalities—other osseous sites.

A Innominate bone. A pedunculated osteochondroma (arrows) arises from the pubic bone and contains a partially calcified cap.

B Ribs. A massive osteochondroma has led to gross deformity of a lower rib. Extensive calcification is apparent.

C Spine. This pedunculated osteochondroma (arrows) is arising from the spinous process of the third cervical vertebra. It extends upward, behind the spinous process of the axis.

Other Imaging Techniques. Conventional or computed tomography represents an additional imaging method that can be applied to the evaluation of osteochondromas, especially those that develop in regions of complex anatomy, such as the pelvis, shoulder, and spine[592, 593] (Fig. 83–120). It has been emphasized that CT (Fig. 83–121) has a role in differentiating between an osteochondroma and a peripheral chondrosarcoma by providing information regarding the relation of the lesion to the underlying bone, the type of lesional matrix, the pattern of mineralization within the outgrowth, and the thickness of the cartilaginous cap,[594] although such analysis is not without difficulty (see later discussion).[595] Scintigraphy with bone-seeking radiopharmaceutical agents also has been used for this differentiation (Fig. 83–121), but this method, too, is accompanied by diagnostic difficulty (see later discussion).[596, 597] Ultrasonography, too, may be applied to the analysis of the cartilaginous cap of an osteochondroma, although lesions that are

deeply situated and those oriented inwardly are not well evaluated with this method.[2113]

MR imaging represents an effective technique for further analysis of osteochondromas. The detection of continuity of the cortical and medullary bone in the outgrowth with that of the parent bone can be accomplished with MR imaging and is diagnostic of an osteochondroma (Fig. 83–122). Furthermore, the cartilaginous tissue in the cap of an osteochondroma is of high signal intensity in T2-weighted spin echo MR images and this tissue is covered with perichondrium that appears to be of low signal intensity in such images.[2114] These signal intensity characteristics allow precise identification and even measurement of the cap of an osteochondroma (Fig. 83–123). MR imaging, therefore, may supply information regarding the likelihood of malignant change and that may be useful in operative planning. The supplementary use of intravenous administration of gadolinium compounds as a means of differentiation of an

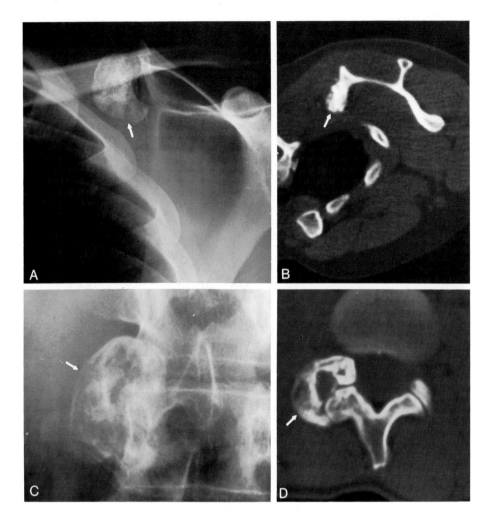

FIGURE 83–120. Solitary osteochondroma: CT abnormalities—regions of complex anatomy.

A, B Scapula. Although this osteochondroma is well seen (arrow) with routine radiography **(A)**, its attachment to the anterior surface of the medial portion of the scapula (arrow) is better shown with transaxial CT **(B)**, accomplished with the patient in the prone position.

C, D Lumbar spine. An expansile osseous outgrowth (arrow) is seen with conventional radiography **(C)**, but its attachment to the superior articular facet of the third lumbar vertebra (arrow) and its involvement of the inferior articular facet of the second lumbar vertebra are better shown with transaxial CT **(D)**.

(**C, D,** Courtesy of R. Kerr, M.D., Los Angeles, California.)

osteochondroma and a peripheral chondrosarcoma has been emphasized.[2115] The extent of enhancement of signal intensity following such administration in chondrosarcomas depends on their cellularity and extent of necrosis, but it may be profound. Even low grade chondrosarcomas may reveal enhancement of signal intensity in septae within the lesion. In cases of benign osteochondroma, such enhancement usually is limited to the fibrovascular tissue that covers the nonenhancing cartilage cap.[2115]

Pathologic Abnormalities. Osteochondromas vary considerably in size; the average size of those lesions arising in the long tubular bones is approximately 4 cm (in maximum dimension), whereas those occurring in the flat or irregular bones usually are larger and, in some instances, are greater than 40 cm in maximum dimension.[598, 599] The cortex and periosteum of the bone from which the osteochondroma arises are continuous with those of the lesion, and the external surface of the osteochondroma may be uniform and smooth or irregular and bosselated, creating a cauliflower-like appearance[600] (Fig. 83–124A).

When sectioned, the usual osteochondroma is found to contain a cartilaginous cap beneath which is cancellous bone that is in direct continuity with that of the parent bone (Fig. 83–124B,C). The chondral cap resembles normal cartilage, having a translucent gray to gray-white appearance, and it generally is only a few millimeters thick.[30, 33] The precise thickness of this cap correlates with the age of the patient.[180] In children and adolescents, in whom there is

active bone growth, the cap may be as thick as 3 cm; in adults, the cap may be entirely absent. This latter finding probably reflects progressive "wear and tear" following cessation of growth of the osteochondroma with a gradual loss of the cartilaginous cap owing to pressure and movement against adjacent structures. In adults, the occurrence of a cartilage cap that is thicker than 1 cm should raise the possibility of chondrosarcomatous transformation.[33, 34, 420, 595]

Examination of the cap of the osteochondroma shows that its histomorphology is similar to that of a physeal growth plate. During active growth, the cap is composed of hyaline cartilage (Fig. 83–125A), its chondrocytes arranged in clusters, with the cells in parallel rows that are perpendicular to the physeal cartilage. The peripheral chondrocytes usually have a single, small dark nucleus and rest in individual lacunae. In young patients, however, numerous binucleated chondrocytes may be found.[30, 33, 180] At its junction with the cancellous bone, the cartilage undergoes endochondral ossification with the formation of mature trabeculae (Fig. 83–125B); however, islands of nonossified or partially ossified cartilage may be found within the deeper, cancellous portion of the osteochondroma. If an osteochondroma is removed after general bone growth has ceased, the columnization of the chondrocytes is absent, and the interface between the cartilage and the cancellous bone appears quiescent, without any endochondral ossification.[28]

Natural History. Serial radiographic examinations provide information regarding the growth characteristics of an

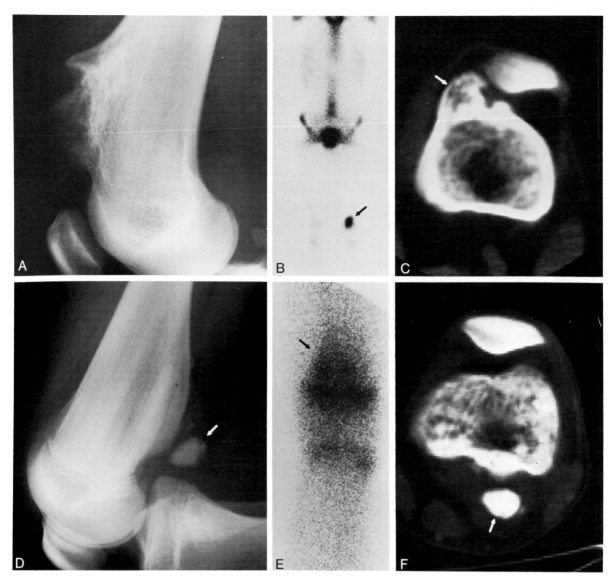

FIGURE 83–121. Solitary osteochondroma: CT and scintigraphic abnormalities.

A–C Femur. This 18 year old man developed an anterior mass above the knee over many years. It interfered with patellar movement. The conventional lateral radiograph **(A)** shows a sessile bone outgrowth with an irregular outline arising from the anterior surface of the distal portion of the femur. Bone scintigraphy **(B)** reveals intense accumulation of the radionuclide at the site of the lesion (arrow). Transaxial CT **(C)** reveals the osteochondroma (arrow), the absence of a prominent cartilage cap or soft tissue mass, and the presence of lateral displacement of the patella. Pathologic examination of the excised lesion documented a benign osteochondroma.

D–F Femur. This 17 year old boy had a mass behind the knee that he had noted for approximately 5 years. The lateral radiograph **(D)** reveals prominent thickening of the posterior femoral cortex and a large calcific focus (arrow). A frontal projection of the knee obtained during a bone scan **(E)** confirms increased uptake of the radionuclide at the site of the lesion (arrow). Transaxial CT **(F)** shows a thick femoral cortex and a calcified focus (arrow). There is no soft tissue mass. Although the possibility of a peripheral chondrosarcoma or parosteal osteosarcoma was considered unlikely, excisional biopsy was accomplished, documenting a benign osteochondroma.

FIGURE 83–122. Solitary osteochondroma: MR imaging abnormalities. A coronal T1-weighted (TR/TE, 600/15) spin echo MR image shows an osteochondroma (arrows) arising from the posterior surface of the tibia. Continuity of the cortical and medullary bone of the osteochondroma with that of the tibia is evident. (Courtesy of V. Chandani, M.D., Honolulu, Hawaii.)

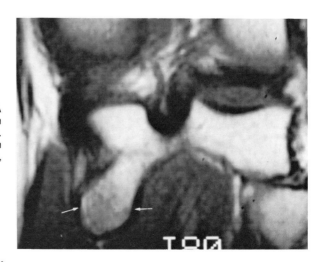

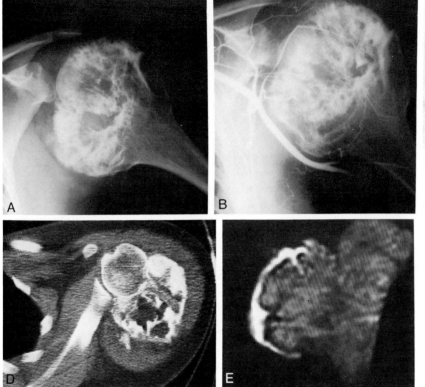

FIGURE 83–123. Solitary osteochondroma: CT, scintigraphic, angiographic, and MR imaging abnormalities. This 20 year old woman developed a mass in the shoulder. A previous biopsy had led to a histologic diagnosis of an enchondroma. As the mass persisted and was accompanied by increasing pain and decreasing range of motion of the shoulder, the patient was reevaluated. The conventional radiograph **(A)** shows a large, calcified lesion involving and extending from the proximal portion of the humerus. On an angiogram **(B),** displacement of vessels is apparent but there is no neovascularity. Intense uptake of the radionuclide at the site of the lesion is evident on a bone scan **(C).** Transaxial CT **(D)** confirms the extensive size of the calcified, posteriorly located lesion, which contains irregular radiolucent areas. A T2-weighted spin echo MR image **(E)** following surgical removal of the specimen reveals a relatively smooth and thin cartilaginous cap. The presence of a benign osteochondroma was confirmed histologically.

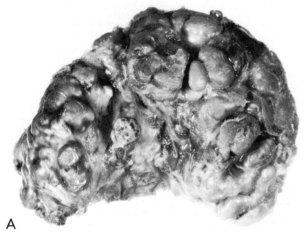

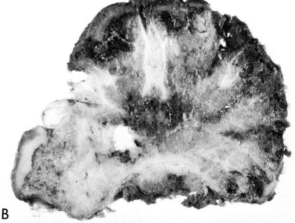

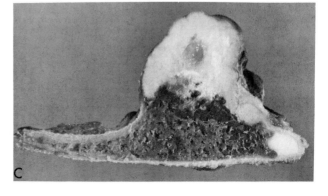

FIGURE 83–124. Solitary osteochondroma: Macroscopic abnormalities.

A The external surface of an osteochondroma may have a cauliflower-like appearance.

B A sagittal section of the osteochondroma in **A** shows that a portion of the lesion contains a cartilaginous cap, whereas elsewhere only irregular bone is present at its surface. White areas represent foci of calcified cartilage deep within the lesion.

C This sectioned osteochondroma of a rib possesses a well-formed cartilaginous cap. Note the continuity of cancellous and cortical bone of the rib and that of the osteochondroma.

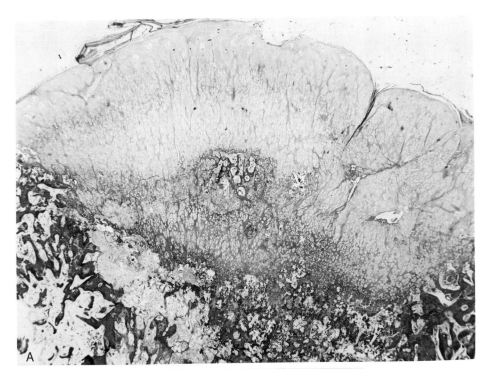

FIGURE 83–125. Solitary osteochondroma: Microscopic abnormalities.

A A low power photomicrograph of the periphery of an osteochondroma shows hyaline cartilage in the cap, overlying cancellous bone. (9.5×.)

B At higher power, note that the cartilage cap is covered by periosteum. The chondrocytes enlarge as they approach the zone of endochondral ossification (lower portion of the photomicrograph) with the formation of trabeculae. (150×.)

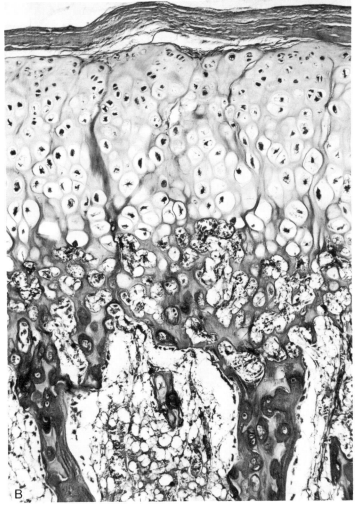

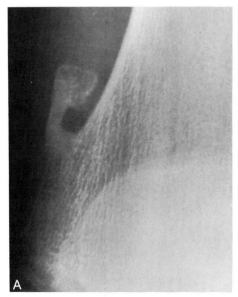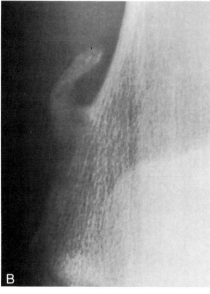

FIGURE 83–126. Solitary osteochondroma: Natural history—decrease in size. Radiographs obtained 1 year apart show an interval decrease in size of the tip of an osteochondroma and a change in its configuration. Such osteochondromas eventually may disappear. (Courtesy of J. Chalmers, M.D., Brownwood, Texas.)

osteochondroma. The lesions may continue to increase in size in the immature skeleton, although they may stop growing at any time, owing to the disappearance of the cartilage contained in the cap of the osteochondroma.[601] As such growth usually ceases at puberty with fusion of the adjacent growth plate, it has been emphasized repeatedly that osteochondromas that continue to enlarge after this time must be evaluated carefully for the possibility of malignant transformation. Alternatively, spontaneous resolution (Fig. 83–126) or even disappearance of an osteochondroma has been documented in children and adolescents, apparently related to the incorporation of the lesion into the enlarging metaphyseal bone or to active bone resorption.[602–605, 2116] Such regression of an osteochondroma also has occurred following its fracture.[602]

Complications. Potential complications of an osteochondroma (or multiple exostoses) include fracture, osseous deformity, vascular injury, neurologic compromise, bursa formation, malignant transformation, and miscellaneous complications.

Fracture. This complication is not frequent but also is not unexpected (Fig. 83–127). Those osteochondromas that are large or pedunculated are more likely to reveal fractures following an injury. There is no evidence to suggest a significant tendency for delayed union or nonunion of the

fracture despite its occasional occurrence.[2117] Of interest is the report of one patient in whom partial resolution of an osteochondroma followed its fracture.[602]

Osseous Deformity. In addition to failure of normal tubulation that may lead to a widened metaphysis, osseous deformity may occur as a complication of an osteochondroma in an adjacent bone. This finding is associated more frequently with large exostoses and those that arise in one of two anatomically intimate tubular bones. The typical situation in which this abnormality is encountered is a tibial osteochondroma that produces pressure deformity in the nearby fibula.[2118] As osteochondromas are metaphyseal lesions, such deformities may be accompanied by alterations in an adjacent articulation. Growth disturbances also may be identified (Fig. 83–128).

Vascular Injury. The ability of an osteochondroma to displace vessels, particularly those about the knee, is well recognized and relatively common; more severe vascular complications, including arterial or venous stenosis, vessel rupture, and pseudoaneurysms, are less frequent but again well documented.[606–618, 1902, 2119–2223] Such vascular injuries usually are seen in male patients and in late adolescence. The appearance of this complication near the end of normal skeletal growth may relate to the loss of a smooth, protective cartilaginous cap in the exostosis, which typically oc-

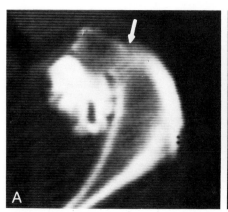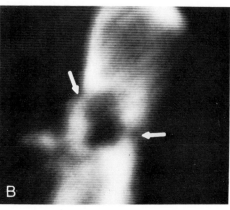

FIGURE 83–127. Solitary osteochondroma: Complications—fracture. This 44 year old man fell to the ground, striking his ilium. Two transaxial CT scans show a pedunculated osteochondroma arising from the inner surface of the ilium with a fracture at its base that extends through the parent bone (arrows).

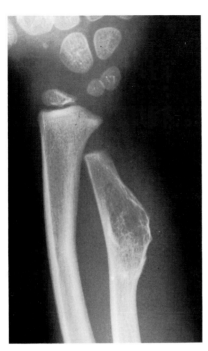

FIGURE 83–128. Solitary osteochondroma: Complications—osseous deformity. In a 4 year old boy, an osteochondroma in the distal portion of the ulna has led to shortening of the bone with deformity of the wrist.

curs at this time, and the contact of the artery with the irregular, bare osseous surface of the osteochondroma. Arterial pulsation or movements of the joint lead to repetitive trauma to the artery, producing abrasion and, eventually, laceration of the vascular wall. Pseudoaneurysm formation results. Almost all the pseudoaneurysms complicating osteochondromas have arisen in the proximal portion of the popliteal artery, although a similar complication has been noted in the posterior tibial artery associated with osteochondromas of the proximal end of the tibia[606, 615, 619] and in the brachial artery related to exostoses of the proximal portion of the humerus.[606, 620, 2122] Such pseudoaneurysms tend to occur in the popliteal region for two reasons: (1) the most common locations for osteochondromas are the lower metaphysis of the femur and the upper metaphysis of the tibia; and (2) the proximal end of the popliteal artery is fixed as it passes through an opening in the adductor magnus muscle, and the distal end of this artery is tethered by its divisions into the anterior and posterior tibial arteries. The lack of mobility of the proximal and distal portions of the popliteal artery causes it to be "bow-stringed" over the adjacent osteochondroma.

Clinical manifestations of these vascular complications are variable. A history of trauma, a soft tissue mass that may be pulsatile, and a change in the distal arterial pulses are helpful but inconstant findings. Rather, the clinical data may be misinterpreted as evidence of malignant transformation of an osteochondroma. Correct diagnosis relies on arteriography (see Chapter 14).

Neurologic Compromise. Although neurologic injury is a theoretical complication of any large osteochondroma (particularly one associated with hereditary multiple exostoses), it is that related to exostoses of the spine or, rarely, the head of a rib that has received the greatest attention.[578, 580, 583, 2107, 2109] Such a lesion may lead to compression of the

spinal cord or nerve roots or, in the case of lower spinal osteochondromas, the cauda equina. Myelography, CT scanning, and MR imaging represent the diagnostic methods of choice. Cranial and peroneal palsy also have been reported as complications of osteochondromas.[2124, 2125, 2462]

Bursa Formation. An additional complication of an osteochondroma is the formation of a bursal compartment surrounding the tip of the lesion.[621–624, 2126, 2127] This finding is particularly frequent when the osteochondroma is large and when it occurs at sites where friction exists with surrounding, unyielding structures such as the scapula and distal portion of the femur.[621, 2126, 2127, 2463] These bursae may become inflamed, painful, and distended with fluid, giving them a firm consistency, especially when they contain fibrin or chondral bodies.[622] When aspirated, the bursal fluid is found to be mucinous.

As the clinical manifestations associated with this complication may simulate those accompanying malignant transformation, accurate diagnosis assumes great importance. Routine radiography may reveal a soft tissue mass, new areas of calcification, and irregularities in the osteochondroma, findings again reminiscent of malignant transformation.[622] Although CT, MR imaging (Fig. 83–129), and angiography have been used as additional diagnostic methods, ultrasonography may be particularly helpful, documenting an anechoic cystic mass that may contain multiple intrabursal bodies.[622, 624] The latter reflect the presence of secondary synovial chondrometaplasia in the bursal lining with resultant osteocartilaginous nodules. These nodules may be malignant histologically in cases in which a bursal sac surrounds a chondrosarcoma arising in the osteochondroma.[623]

Malignant Transformation. Estimates of the risk of ma-

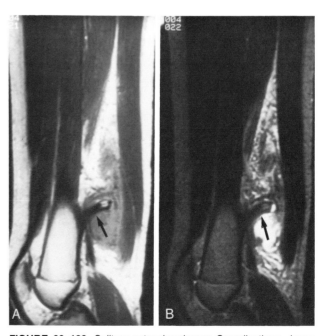

FIGURE 83–129. Solitary osteochondroma: Complications—bursa formation. Sagittal T1-weighted **(A)** and T2-weighted **(B)** spin echo MR images reveal an osteochondroma (arrows) surrounded by a soft tissue mass, which is of high signal intensity in **B.** Pathologic examination demonstrated an osteochondroma with a bursal sac that was thickened and showed chondroid metaplasia. (From Griffiths HJ, et al: Skel Radiol 20:513, 1991.)

lignant transformation of an osteochondroma vary from 1 to 25 per cent depending on whether the patient has a solitary exostosis or multiple osteocartilaginous exostoses.[30, 623] What is clear is that the likelihood of such transformation is greater in patients with multiple osteochondromas and that the resulting malignant tumor most commonly is a chondrosarcoma, although examples of malignant fibrous histiocytoma and osteosarcoma occurring in this setting are documented.[30, 625, 626, 2128, 2129] It appears likely that a more accurate estimate of the risk of malignant transformation of a solitary osteochondroma is about 1 per cent.[627]

Although there are clinical guidelines (such as pain, swelling, and a soft tissue mass) and routine radiologic findings (such as the growth of a previously stable osteochondroma, bone erosion, and irregular or scattered calcification) (Fig. 83–130) that aid in the identification of such malignant transformation, they are not entirely reliable.[628, 629] Scintigraphy accomplished with bone-seeking radionuclides represents an effective method for defining those osteochondromas that are active metabolically (Fig. 83–131) but does not allow differentiation of the endochondral ossification occurring in a benign osteochondroma and the hyperemia and osteoblastic reaction occurring in a peripheral chondrosarcoma.[596, 597] A normal bone scan, however, virtually excludes the diagnosis of malignant transformation of an exostosis. CT (Figs. 83–131 and 83–132) has met with variable success as a method allowing differentiation of a benign from a malignant osteochondroma.[594, 595] The reliability of this method to determine the thickness of the cartilage cap is inconsistent owing to similar attenuation values of cartilage and muscle, CT artifacts created by volume averaging, and the varying orientation of the image plane with respect to the osteochondroma.[595] MR imaging, as previously indicated, appears to be the method of choice in the assessment of the cartilage cap.[2114, 2115] There appears to be a significant degree of correlation between the thickness of the cartilage cap and the histologic composition of the osteochondroma. In general, peripheral chondrosarcomas possess a cartilage cap that is thicker than 1 cm and commonly greater than 2 cm, whereas in benign exostoses, the thickness is usually less than 1 cm.[420] Reported variations in the thicknesses of the cartilage cap in both the benign and the malignant lesions, however, have led to the belief that there are no criteria related to the size of the cap that consistently allow differentiation of a benign osteochondroma and a peripheral chondrosarcoma.[627] Ultimately, it is the microscopic finding of increased cellularity, associated with enlarged chondrocyte nuclei, binucleation, and occasional mitotic figures, that represents the strongest evidence of malignancy.

Miscellaneous Complications. Additional complications of solitary osteochondromas are rare. Reports of spontaneous hemarthrosis[2130] and necrosis of the osseous and marrow components of the lesion[2131] have appeared, however.

Differential Diagnosis. The radiographic features of a solitary osteochondroma usually are diagnostic. A sessile or pedunculated osseous excrescence arising from the metaphyseal region of a long tubular bone, directed away from the nearby joint, containing cortical and medullary bone that is continuous with that of the parent bone and variable amounts of calcification, is easily differentiated from other causes of osseous outgrowth, including an osteoma, osteophyte, and enthesophyte, and from heterotopic ossification

and a parosteal osteosarcoma. Osteochondromas or osteochondroma-like lesions are encountered occasionally in systemic disorders, such as pseudohypoparathyroidism, pseudopseudohypoparathyroidism, and myositis (fibrodysplasia) ossificans progressiva, and in various congenital diseases (see Chapter 88).

The major difficulty in differential diagnosis arises in distinguishing between a benign osteochondroma and a peripheral chondrosarcoma. This difficulty is accentuated in those instances in which a benign exostosis is unusually large or involves an atypical site, or in which a chondrosarcoma is small and produces minor radiographic alterations in the subjacent osteochondroma. The value of additional diagnostic methods in such cases has been emphasized in the previous section of this chapter, and the entire spectrum of peripheral chondrosarcoma will be addressed in a subsequent portion of this chapter.

Hereditary Multiple Exostoses. Hereditary multiple exostoses, an autosomal dominant disorder that also is discussed in Chapter 88, leads to clinical abnormalities in the first or second decade of life and characteristic radiographic alterations.[630, 631] Palpable osseous protuberances or masses, secondary deformities due to shortening and bowing of bones, and joint restriction are common. The masses relate to the osteochondromas, which typically are bilateral and symmetric in distribution, and which may number more than 100.[632] Typical sites of involvement are the distal and proximal portions of the femur, tibia, and fibula and the proximal portion of the humerus (Fig. 83–133). In fact, it is virtually impossible to establish the diagnosis of this disease if exostoses are not present in the bones about the knee. Slightly less common is localization to the distal regions of the radius and ulna. When compared with the distribution of solitary osteochondromas, there is a greater tendency for involvement of the scapula (Fig. 83–133), innominate bone (Figs. 83–134 and 83–135), and ribs in cases of multiple exostoses.[630, 633]

Highly characteristic of this disease is the occurrence of defects in normal modeling of bone and osseous deformities (Fig. 83–136). Of particular note is the presence of bilateral coxa valga and widening of the proximal femoral metaphysis[634, 635] (Fig. 83–135A), and of bilateral and progressive changes about the wrist, consisting of ulnar deviation, relative shortening of the ulna, bowing of either or both of the bones of the forearm, and shortening of the forearm[636, 2132, 2133] (Fig. 83–137). Clearly, an effective roentgenographic survey designed to delineate some of the more dramatic findings of hereditary multiple exostoses would include frontal radiographs of the knees (to demonstrate the osteochondromas), the pelvis (to define the metaphyseal changes in the femora), and the wrist (to document the presence of osseous deformities). A more complete radiographic survey would be required to serve as a baseline in view of the widespread nature of the osteochondromas as well as the modeling defects and deformities of bone, which include dislocations of the radial heads, obliquity of the distal tibial articular surface, and valgus alignment of the tibia.[631] This survey could be supplemented with bone scintigraphy as a method that would identify those lesions that are active metabolically.[637, 1833]

The complications associated with hereditary exostoses are identical in scope to but generally more frequent than the complications that accompany solitary osteochondro-

Text continued on page 3741

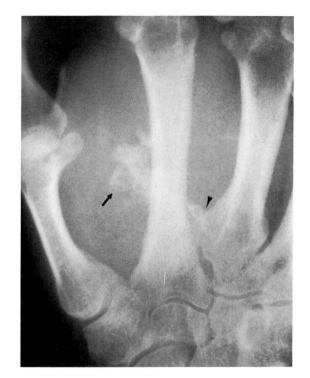

FIGURE 83–130. Solitary osteochondroma: Complications—malignant transformation. This chondrosarcoma (arrow) arose from a preexisting osteochondroma that originated from the base of the third metacarpal bone (arrowhead). A large soft tissue mass and irregular calcification are clues supporting the diagnosis of malignant transformation. More importantly, a significant interval change had occurred when comparison was made with earlier radiographs.

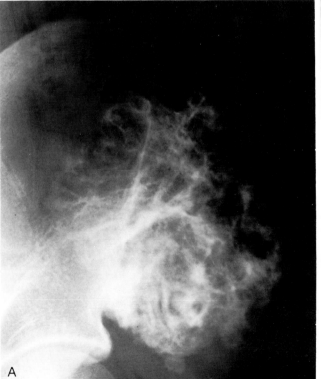

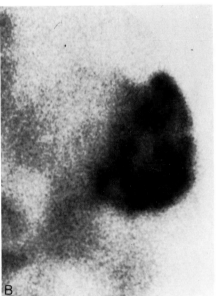

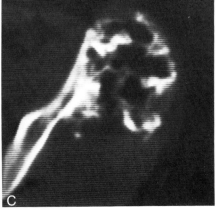

FIGURE 83–131. Solitary osteochondroma: Complications—malignant transformation.

    A The routine radiograph shows a large sessile outgrowth arising from the ilium in a 23 year old man.

    B A bone scan reveals nonuniform increased accumulation of the radionuclide in the lesion.

    C Transaxial CT shows that the posteriorly located lesion is irregular in outline and contains multiple regions of low attenuation. Biopsy confirmed the presence of a chondrosarcoma.

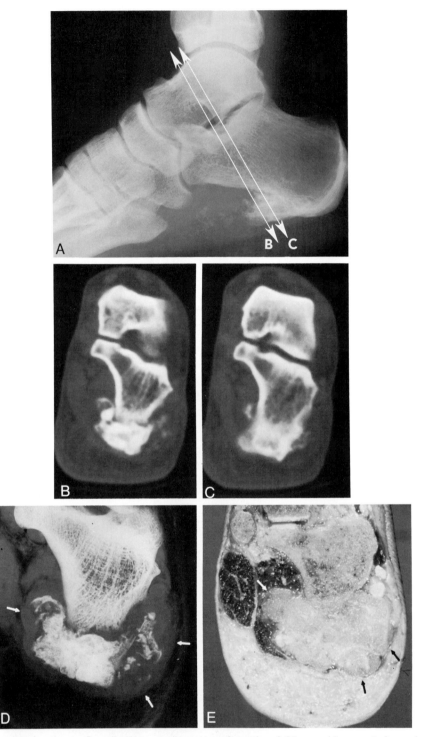

FIGURE 83–132. Solitary osteochondroma: Complications—malignant transformation. A 35 year old man noted an enlarging mass in his heel.

A A lateral radiograph shows an osseous outgrowth extending from the plantar aspect of the calcaneus. Distally, soft tissue prominence and calcification are evident.

B, C Two coronal CT scans at the approximate levels indicated in **A** reveal the extent of the lesion. More distally **(B),** an irregular pattern of calcification in a soft tissue component is evident. More proximally **(C),** the lesion is attached to the plantar surface of the calcaneus.

D, E A radiograph **(D)** and photograph **(E)** of a coronal section of the amputated specimen that corresponds to the plane in **B** reveal a large soft tissue component (arrows) that only is partially calcified. A low grade chondrosarcoma was the final histologic diagnosis.

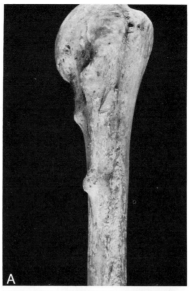

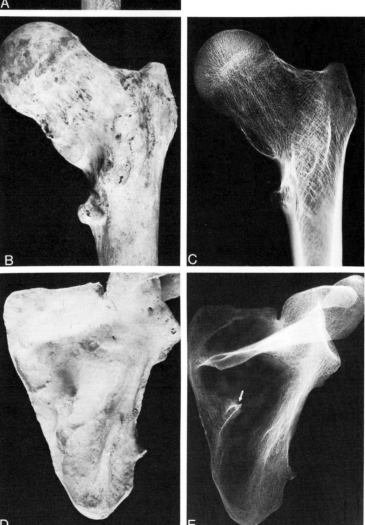

FIGURE 83–133. Hereditary multiple exostoses: Sites of involvement—tubular bones and scapula.

　A Humerus. Note multiple osteochondromas and metaphyseal widening.

　B, C Femur. In addition to the osteochondromas, widening of the femoral neck is a highly characteristic feature of this disease.

　D, E Scapula. Multiple osteochondromas are present. One (arrow) projects from the anterior margin of the bone and was better demonstrated on a lateral radiograph.

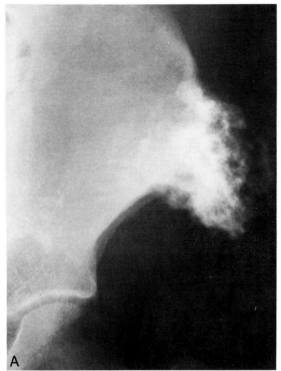

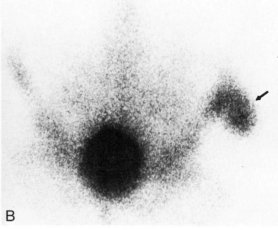

FIGURE 83–134. Hereditary multiple exostoses: Sites of involvement—innominate bone. An osteochondroma had previously been removed from the femur of this 28 year old woman. She noted an increasing mass above her hip.

A An irregular exostosis projects from the ilium.

B A bone scan reveals increased accumulation of the radionuclide (arrow). The lesion was excised, revealing a benign osteochondroma.

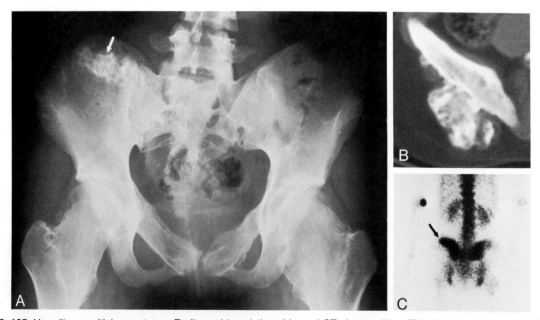

FIGURE 83–135. Hereditary multiple exostoses: Radiographic, scintigraphic, and CT abnormalities. This 19 year old woman had previously undergone resections of osteochondromas about the left and right knees and right shoulder. She noted pain and an enlarging mass in her low back.

A The radiograph reveals bilateral coxa valga deformity, widening of the femoral metaphyses, and multiple osteochondromas in the femora and innominate bones. Observe a large lesion (arrow) arising from the ilium.

B Transaxial CT documents the posterior location of the lesion and the absence of an adjacent soft tissue mass.

C A bone scan shows increased accumulation of the radionuclide at the site of the lesion (arrow). A benign osteochondroma was subsequently removed from the ilium.

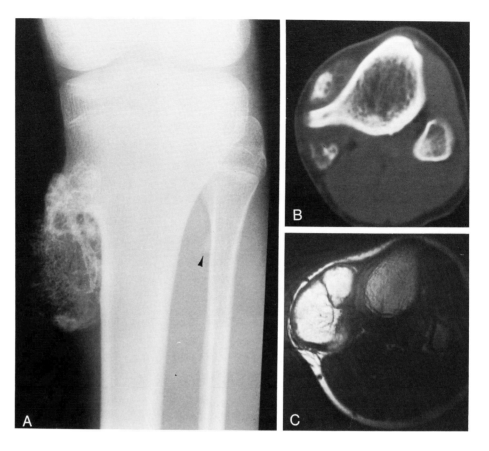

FIGURE 83–136. Hereditary multiple exostoses: Radiographic, CT, and MR imaging abnormalities. A 16 year old man developed a mass in the medial aspect of his lower leg.

A A radiograph shows widening of the tibial metaphysis, a small osteochondroma (arrowhead) in the fibula, and a large outgrowth arising from the proximal portion of the tibia.

B Transaxial CT reveals the tibial lesion and adjacent calcification.

C A transaxial T1-weighted (TR/TE, 500/32) spin echo MR image shows a bright signal in the bone outgrowth, perhaps representing marrow elements. A benign osteochondroma was documented following removal of the lesion.

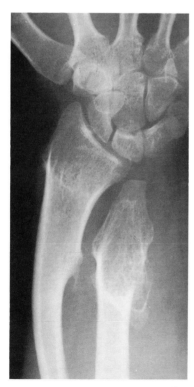

FIGURE 83–137. Hereditary multiple exostoses: Radiographic abnormalities. Wrist deformity is characterized by osteochondromas of the radius and ulna with shortening of the ulna, an angular articular surface of the radius, and bowing of the radius. There was shortening of multiple metacarpal bones. (Courtesy of T. Broderick, M.D., Orange, California.)

mas and include (in addition to the osseous deformity) fracture, vascular injury, neurologic compromise, bursa formation, and malignant transformation[638–641, 2134, 2135] (Figs. 83–138 and 83–139). The frequency of the last complication has been stated to be between 2 and 27 per cent, is probably about 5 per cent, and certainly is greater than the frequency of malignant transformation in solitary osteochondromas.[30, 642] The resulting chondrosarcomas are especially frequent in the femur, humerus, tibia, and innominate bone,[642, 643] and the diagnostic difficulties in such cases are identical to those encountered with malignant transformation of a solitary osteochondroma. Less commonly, osteosarcomas, dedifferentiated chondrosarcomas, malignant fibrous histiocytomas, or spindle cell sarcomas result from malignant transformation in patients with hereditary exostoses.

Dysplasia Epiphysealis Hemimelica (Trevor's Disease). Trevor's disease, which also is discussed in Chapter 84, was reported originally in 1926 by Mouchet and Belot[644] and subsequently in 1950 by Trevor.[645] Many additional accounts of this disease now exist.[646–651]

Dysplasia epiphysealis hemimelica usually becomes evident in children and young adults and is more common in men than in women in a ratio of approximately 3 to 1. Typical clinical manifestations include swelling and, less commonly, pain and deformity, which, with rare exceptions,[652] are localized to one side of the body. Lower extremity involvement is far more frequent than upper extremity involvement, although the latter is well documented.[653] The talus, distal portion of the femur, and distal and proximal regions of the tibia are principal sites

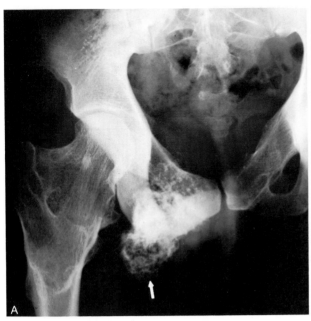

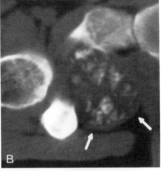

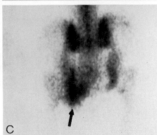

FIGURE 83–138. Hereditary multiple exostoses: Complications—malignant transformation.

A Observe multiple exostoses of the femur and innominate bones and widening of the femoral neck. A large and irregular lesion (arrow) is seen adjacent to the ischium.

B Transaxial CT documents the size of the lesion (arrows) and internal calcification.

C The bone scan shows increased scintigraphic activity at the site of the lesion (arrow). A chondrosarcoma was the final histologic diagnosis.

(Courtesy of T. Broderick, M.D., Orange, California.)

of abnormality[654–656, 2136, 2377, 2378]; less commonly or rarely, involvement of the proximal portion of the femur or humerus, patella, carpal bones, innominate bone, ulna, scapula, or other sites is evident.[657–662, 1834, 2379] Multiple bones (in a single extremity) are affected in 60 to 70 per cent of cases. This has led to the designations of a localized form (monostotic involvement), a classic form (more than one area of osseous involvement in a single extremity), and a generalized, or severe, form (involvement of an entire extremity).[658] In any form, as the name of the disease would imply, dysplasia epiphysealis hemimelica involves primarily one side of an epiphysis; the medial side is affected approximately twice as often as the lateral side. Examples of diffuse epiphyseal alterations, however, have been reported.[647, 649, 652]

The radiographic findings are characteristic. In an infant or young child, small, multifocal, irregular ossifications are seen adjacent to one side of an ossifying epiphysis (or carpal or tarsal bone) (Figs. 83–140 and 83–141). The adjacent metaphysis may be widened. Subsequently, the ossifications become confluent with the adjacent bone, eventually appearing as a lobulated osseous mass protruding from the epiphysis (or carpal or tarsal bone).[649] The final appearance resembles that of an osteochondroma with the affected area (or areas) remaining large and irregular. Arthrography and MR imaging have been used to further document the size and configuration of the exostosis,[1835, 2136] although these procedures are not required routinely. In severe cases,

muscle wasting, growth disturbance, and joint deformity are identified.[651, 663]

On macroscopic examination, the lesion either is found to be a pedunculated mass with a cartilaginous cap or is indistinguishable from the remainder of the epiphysis.[649] The histologic features of the lesion are identical to those of an osteochondroma, consisting of a base of normal bone and a cap of hyaline cartilage and exhibiting endochondral ossification. Of interest in this regard are reports of intracapsular chondromas and other benign cartilage tumors occurring in patients with a familial disorder resembling dysplasia epiphysealis hemimelica.[664]

Although the prognosis of this disease generally is regarded as good, with benefit derived from local excision of the lesion(s) or, rarely, arthrodesis,[651] persistent deformities and secondary osteoarthritis are evident in some cases. Malignant transformation of the osteochondroma is not encountered.

Other Osteochondromas or Osteochondroma-Like Lesions. A *subungual exostosis* is an uncommon, benign bone tumor arising in the distal phalanx of a digit, beneath or adjacent to the nailbed.[665] Almost invariably it is a solitary lesion, usually occurring in patients who are in the second or third decade of life and leading to clinical manifestations that include pain, swelling, and ulcerations of the nailbed or surrounding tissue with secondary infection.[666–669, 2137] The great toe is involved in 70 to 80 per cent of cases, followed in order of frequency by involvement of other

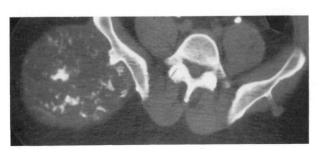

FIGURE 83–139. Hereditary multiple exostoses: Complications—malignant transformation. Transaxial CT in a 30 year old man with a buttock mass shows bilateral osteochondromas arising from the posterior surface of the ilii and a calcified mass on the right side, representing a chondrosarcoma. (Courtesy of R. Stiles, M.D., Atlanta, Georgia.)

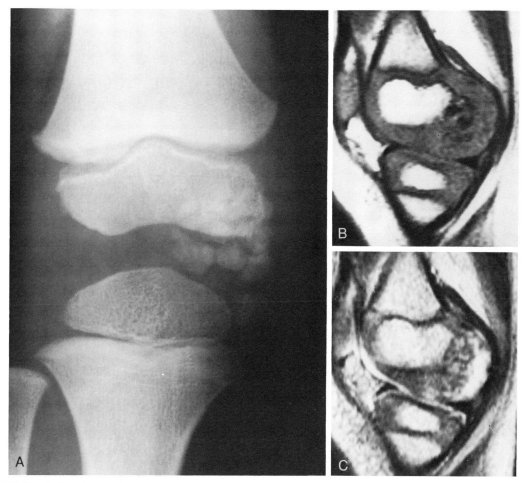

FIGURE 83–140. Dysplasia epiphysealis hemimelica (Trevor's disease): Radiographic abnormalities—long tubular bones.
A In a 3 year old boy, note the irregular ossifications about the medial aspect of the distal femoral and proximal tibial epiphyses.
B In a sagittal T1-weighted (TR/TE, 650/20) spin echo MR image, the cartilage in the medial aspect of the femoral epiphysis is enlarged posteriorly and contains foci of low signal intensity.
C In a sagittal T2-weighted (TR/TE, 2000/80) spin echo MR image, this cartilage now is of high signal intensity. (Courtesy of H. S. Kang, M.D., Seoul, Korea.)

toes and of fingers (usually the thumb or index finger).[665] Radiographically, the lesion is approximately 1 cm in diameter and projects from the dorsal or dorsomedial aspect of the distal portion of a terminal phalanx (Fig. 83–142). It is composed of mature bone with either a broad or narrow attachment to the phalanx.[1903] The terminal portion of the exostosis may be flat or cupped and smooth or irregular. Histologically, the lesion consists of a base of trabecular bone with a proliferating fibrocartilaginous cap, features that differ from those of a typical osteochondroma. In the cartilage cap, hypercellularity, frequent mitotic figures, and dark-staining nuclei may be apparent.[665] Although such histologic features may be misinterpreted as evidence of malignant potential, subungual exostoses are uniformly benign and local excision is the treatment of choice. Recurrences are common, however.

A *turret exostosis* is an infrequent osseous excrescence that typically arises on the dorsal surface of a proximal or middle phalanx in a finger.[670] Clinically, a history of trauma, perhaps a small puncture wound, is common, and the traumatic event is followed by pain and soft tissue swelling or a lump, which may be tender to palpation. The mass may grow for a period of months, become firm, and

lead to loss of flexion of a joint or joints distal to the exostosis (presumably related to limitation of excursion of the extensor tendon).[671] Radiographs reveal an initial soft tissue swelling and immature periostitis and a subsequent development of a broad-based bone protuberance on the dorsal surface of the affected phalanx. This osseous growth may be demarcated from the underlying bone by a faint radiolucent line. On the basis of the histologic findings, it is likely that a turret exostosis represents an ossifying, subperiosteal hematoma.

Additional osteochondroma-like lesions involving the small bones of the hands and feet include a reactive lesion of the great toe,[2138] florid reactive periostitis,[2139] and bizarre parosteal osteochondromatous proliferation.[2140–2143] A *reactive bone excrescence* commonly is seen in the medial portion of the base of the distal phalanx of the great toe (Fig. 83–143). It appears after closure of the adjacent physeal plate and rarely is symptomatic. The size of the excrescence is variable but it typically points distally. *Florid reactive periostitis* occurs in the small bones in the hands and feet, appearing as laminated or mature periosteal reaction, paraosseous calcification, and a normal cortical surface. A relationship to trauma is suggested but remains uncertain (see

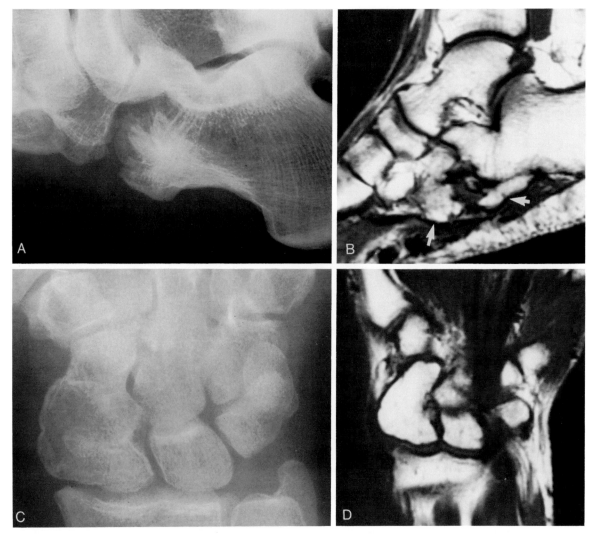

FIGURE 83–141. Dysplasia epiphysealis hemimelica (Trevor's disease): Radiographic abnormalities—small and irregular bones.

A, B In a 38 year old man, a lateral radiograph **(A)** shows irregular enlargement of the distal, plantar aspect of the calcaneus and the cuboid bone. In a sagittal T1-weighted (TR/TE, 500/18) spin echo MR image **(B),** the abnormal bone excrescences (arrows) containing marrow are evident. (Courtesy of S. K. Brahme, M.D., La Jolla, California.)

C, D In a 28 year old man, the routine radiograph **(C)** shows an enlarged and irregular scaphoid bone. The coronal T1-weighted (TR/TE, 550/20) spin echo MR image **(D)** reveals signal intensity in the enlarged scaphoid bone that is the same as normal marrow. (Courtesy of J. Blasinghame, M.D., La Jolla, California.)

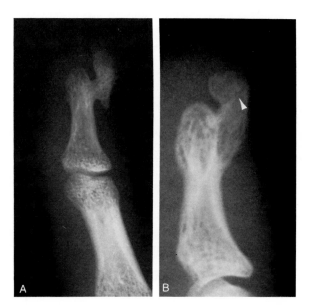

FIGURE 83–142. Subungual exostosis: Radiographic abnormalities. Two examples are shown. In **B,** a fracture line (arrowhead) extends through the distal portion of the lesion.

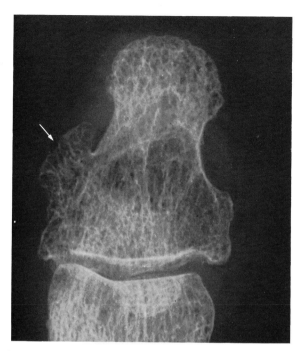

FIGURE 83–143. Reactive bone excrescence of the terminal phalanx of the great toe: Radiographic abnormalities. Note the broad excrescence (arrow) arising from the medial aspect of the terminal phalanx. The lesion points distally.

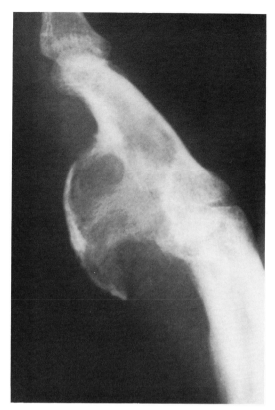

FIGURE 83–144. Bizarre parosteal osteochondromatous proliferation (Nora's lesion): Radiographic abnormalities. Note the irregular excrescence arising from the volar aspect of the middle phalanx of a finger. (Courtesy of A. Stauffer, M.D., Mission Viejo, California.)

Chapter 95). *Bizarre parosteal osteochondromatous proliferation,* or Nora's lesion, is observed most commonly in the bones in the hands and feet but also occurs in the long tubular bones and, rarely, the skull. A well-marginated mass of heterotopic ossification arises from the cortical surface of the affected bone (Fig. 83–144). There is no medullary continuity between the lesion and the adjacent bone. The sessile or pedunculated mass usually lies adjacent to the metaphyseal segment of the bone. The lesion, which appears in men and women of any age, is characterized histologically by a large amount of hypercellular cartilage showing maturation to trabecular bone, features that resemble those of a parosteal osteosarcoma.[2143] Although a history of trauma is evident in some affected patients, it is not constant and the cause of this lesion is not clear. A relationship between florid reactive periostitis and bizarre parosteal osteochondromatous proliferation is suggested[2144] but remains unproved.

A *supracondylar (supracondyloid) process of the humerus* represents an outgrowth of bone that occurs on the anteromedial surface of the distal portion of the humerus, approximately 5 to 7 cm above the medial epicondyle[672] (Fig. 83–145). It has been estimated that this process is present in less than 3 per cent of the general population and is more frequent in white than in black patients.[673, 674] It is believed to represent a phylogenetic vestige of the supracondyloid foramen found in reptiles and some mammals.[672] The supracondylar process is variable in size, and its apex may be roughened or irregular. The process may afford insertion to a persistent part of the coracobrachialis muscle as well as an anomalous origin of the pronator teres muscle.[672] A band of fibrous tissue, the ligament of Struthers, may join the tip of the supracondylar process and the medial epicondyle. The median nerve and brachial artery or

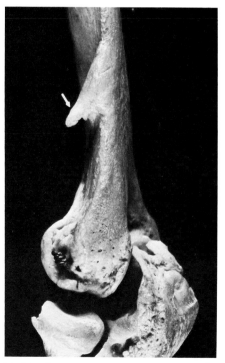

FIGURE 83–145. Supracondylar (supracondyloid) process of the humerus: Macroscopic abnormalities. Note the outgrowth (arrow) arising from the anterior surface of the humerus at a short distance from the elbow.

one of its branches usually pass from a medial to lateral direction through the arcade formed by the process and the fibrous band,[672] and this anatomic arrangement may explain the occurrence of neurologic compromise in patients with the anomaly.[675, 676] Although the ulnar nerve may be involved,[675] it is compression of the median nerve, owing to contraction of the pronator teres muscle, that is much more characteristic. Other causes of symptoms and signs in persons with this anomaly relate to compression of the brachial artery or one of its branches or a fracture of the process itself.

Bone outgrowths in the medial aspect of the proximal portion of the tibia sometimes are referred to as *pes anserinus spurs*.[2145] Their cause is not certain, although they may represent enthesophytes. They are identical in appearance to osteochondromas, but no cartilaginous cap is detected (Fig. 83–146).

Malignant Tumors

Chondrosarcoma

As was the case for osteosarcoma, the systems used to classify malignant cartilage tumors of the skeleton have undergone extensive modification in recent years. Such neoplasms may be categorized according to their precise location within the bone (central, peripheral, and juxtacortical chondrosarcomas), their occurrence as an initial (de novo) lesion (primary chondrosarcoma) or as a lesion superimposed on a preexistent process, such as an osteochondroma or enchondroma (secondary chondrosarcoma), their degree of cellular differentiation (low grade, medium grade, and high grade chondrosarcomas), the presence of unusual histologic characteristics (clear cell and mesenchymal chondrosarcomas), and the occurrence of changes in these histologic characteristics (dedifferentiated chondrosarcoma). In the following discussion, these malignant cartilage tumors are designated conventional chondrosarcomas (including central and peripheral types), juxtacortical (periosteal) chondrosarcomas, clear cell chondrosarcomas, mesenchymal chondrosarcomas, and dedifferentiated chondrosarcomas.

Conventional Chondrosarcoma. In this category can be considered those malignant tumors that arise within the medullary cavity either de novo or as a secondary complication of a preexisting enchondroma (central chondrosarcoma) and those that arise near the surface of the bone (peripheral chondrosarcoma). Peripheral chondrosarcomas sometimes are divided further into two groups: those developing from a preexisting osteochondroma (exostotic chondrosarcomas) and those originating from the periosteal membrane (juxtacortical or periosteal chondrosarcomas). The relative frequencies of central and peripheral chondrosarcomas are difficult to define as data contained in large series of patients with chondrosarcomas are conflicting.[677-683] At times, especially in well-advanced tumors in the flat bones, it may be impossible to determine if the chondrosarcoma developed in a central or a peripheral location.[684] Whether the separation of such tumors into these two categories (or three categories if juxtacortical chondrosarcoma is considered independently) has prognostic significance is not clear, although there is evidence indicating that the precise location of the chondrosarcoma within a particular bone is related to patient survival.[677]

Clinical Abnormalities. Conventional chondrosarcomas occur more frequently in men than in women in an approximate ratio of 3 to 2.[683, 685] Although the age range of affected patients is wide, varying from the first to ninth decades of life, the average age of persons with chondrosarcoma is approximately 40 to 45 years, and patients with this tumor generally are between the ages of 30 and 60 years. Those patients with peripheral chondrosarcomas tend to be slightly younger than those with central chondrosarcomas.[683] Chondrosarcomas are rare in children, but when

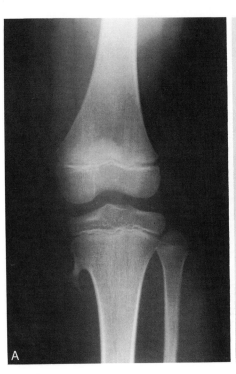
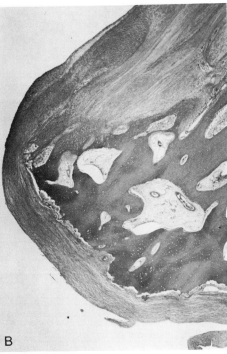

FIGURE 83–146. Pes anserinus spurs: Radiographic and pathologic abnormalities.

A In a 7 year old girl, note the osteochondroma-like lesion arising from the medial portion of the tibial metaphysis.

B A photomicrograph (hematoxylin and eosin, ×20) reveals that the lesion has no cartilaginous tissue on its surface. Rather, it is covered with a thin layer of periosteum. (From Ugai K, et al: Clin Orthop 231:130, 1988.)

the neoplasm is present in this age group, the clinical manifestations may be particularly rapid in onset,[686] a greater frequency of involvement of the facial bones may be evident,[2146] and a greater prevalence of mesenchymal chondrosarcomas may be noted.[2146]

Pain is the most characteristic presenting symptom of a chondrosarcoma. It may occur alone or, less frequently, in association with soft tissue prominence. A pathologic fracture is the initial manifestation in approximately 3 per cent of patients.[685] The average duration of the symptoms is 1 to 2 years. Physical findings include a tender soft tissue mass and increased warmth and erythema in the region of the tumor.

Skeletal Location. The long tubular bones are the sites of involvement in approximately 45 per cent of cases, with the femur being the most commonly affected bone (approximately 25 per cent of all cases).[30, 34, 139, 683, 687–689] The bones in the lower extremity are involved in approximately 35 per cent of chondrosarcomas, and those in the upper extremity are involved in 14 per cent of such neoplasms. Other common locations of these tumors are the innominate bone (25 per cent of cases) and the ribs (8 per cent of cases). Less frequent sites of involvement are the vertebrae (7 per cent), scapula (5 per cent), and sternum (2 per cent), and rarely affected sites include the skull, mandible, maxilla, fibula, radius, ulna, clavicle, patella, and small bones of the hand and foot.[2147–2151]

Most chondrosarcomas in the long tubular bones are located in the metaphysis, but, with closure of the physis, tumor extension into the epiphysis is encountered. Primary involvement of the diaphysis or epiphysis[2152, 2153] is infrequent. In the femur, tibia, humerus, and fibula, the proximal portion of the bone is affected more commonly than the distal portion. Chondrosarcomas are distinctly unusual in the distal region of the humerus.[678]

Excluding hematologic tumors, chondrosarcomas are the most frequent malignant neoplasm of the scapula, ribs, sternum, and small bones of the hand.[690–693] Chondrosarcomas in the ribs or sternum typically arise near the costochondral junction.[413, 694] Those arising in the hand predominate in the proximal phalanges and metacarpal bones, with rare localization to the distal phalanges or carpus.[695–704] Chondrosarcomas are relatively rare in the bones distal to the ankle, with the exception of the talus and calcaneus.[705–707] Maxillary involvement is slightly more frequent than mandibular involvement, and other sites of chondrosarcomas in the facial bones are the nasal turbinates, alae and septum, and paranasal sinuses.[708–719] Chondrosarcomas arising in the skull, especially in its base, are reported,[720, 721, 2148] although, in some cases, the tumors may have represented chondroid chordomas (see later discussion). Vertebral chondrosarcomas occur at every spinal level but are most common in the thoracic region. They have a propensity to involve the neural arches and spinous process.[722–725, 2149] Obviously, virtually any bone of the skeleton may be the site of a chondrosarcoma, and even the laryngeal cartilages may be the site of origin of this tumor.[726]

As histologically the differentiation between low grade, well-differentiated chondrosarcoma and benign enchondroma may be quite difficult, it is instructive to compare the anatomic distribution of these two neoplasms. In marked contrast to the common occurrence of enchondromas in the bones of the hands and feet, such localization is infrequent with chondrosarcomas. The innominate bone and femur are more characteristic sites of involvement of chondrosarcomas than of enchondromas, and chondrosarcomas are about twice as frequent in the long bones than are enchondromas.

Radiographic Abnormalities. The evaluation of malignant cartilaginous tumors of the skeleton using routine radiography (as well as other imaging techniques) is accomplished with two goals in mind: to allow precise diagnosis of chondrosarcoma; and to provide information regarding the aggressive or non-aggressive behavioral characteristics of the lesion. Both of these goals can be accomplished in many such tumors. The precise radiographic diagnosis of chondrosarcoma depends on a number of characteristic features, the most important of which is tumoral calcification. Other changes, including the patterns of bone destruction, cortical violation, and periostitis, are more variable. The importance of the second goal is underscored by the inexplicable and seemingly capricious manner in which chondrosarcomas behave.[727] The identification of roentgenographic alterations that imply tumor aggressiveness, therefore, has received a great deal of attention (see Chapter 82),[728] and, with regard to chondrosarcomas, such alterations relate to the pattern of calcification, the nature of the tumoral margin, and the size of the soft tissue mass. Although the application of other diagnostic methods, such as CT, MR imaging, and angiography, may further define these features (see later discussion), the importance of conventional radiography (and tomography) cannot be denied. It is well recognized that a relationship exists between the pattern and density of calcification in chondrosarcoma and the degree of malignancy.[727] Well-organized calcific rings within cartilage usually signify a low grade tumor.[729] High grade chondrosarcomas, which may contain a greater amount of myxoid material, frequently are associated with large areas of noncalcified tumor matrix.[730, 731] Furthermore, when calcification occurs within high grade chondrosarcomas, it typically is amorphous, punctate, scattered, or irregular.[727] With regard to the margins of the tumors, as would be expected, an ill-defined boundary with a long zone of transition between the abnormal and normal portions of the bone is indicative of an aggressive or high grade chondrosarcoma.[728] The size and nature of the soft tissue component of the tumor are less useful predictors of its malignant potential.[727] In all cases, close correlation of the radiographic and pathologic abnormalities, and cooperation among radiologist, pathologist, and orthopedic surgeon, ultimately are required to ensure appropriate diagnosis and management of bone tumors.[732]

The radiographic features of chondrosarcomas are influenced by the anatomic location of the tumor. In the following discussion, central and peripheral chondrosarcomas are considered independently. The description of a third type of tumor, the juxtacortical (periosteal) chondrosarcoma, whose very existence as a distinct entity is debated, is contained in a later segment of this chapter.

Central Chondrosarcoma. Central chondrosarcomas occur in both the tubular bones (particularly the femur and the humerus) and the flat and irregular bones (especially those in the pelvis). With involvement of the appendicular skeleton, radiographs typically reveal an elongated, slightly expansile, multilobulated osteolytic lesion accompanied by periosteal bone formation, cortical thickening, endosteal

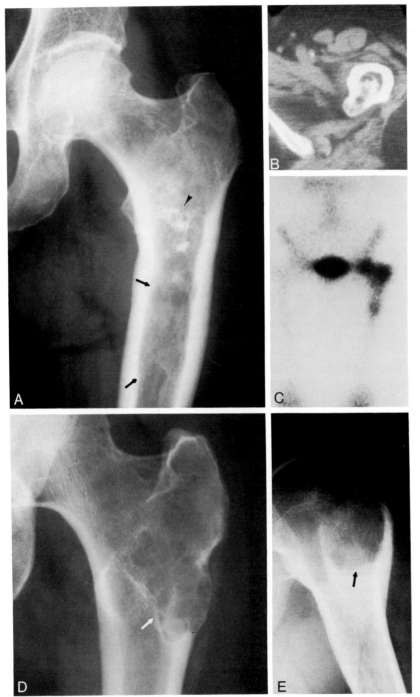

FIGURE 83–147. Conventional chondrosarcoma, central type: Radiographic abnormalities—long tubular bones.

A–C An 82 year old woman had pain in the left hip of several years' duration. The routine radiograph **(A)** reveals an elongated, central lesion of the diaphysis of the femur. Proximally it contains calcification (arrowhead), whereas distally osteolysis is evident without calcification (between arrows). Note endosteal erosion of the cortex. Incidental chondrocalcinosis in the hip also is evident. Transaxial CT **(B)** at the level of the lesser trochanter shows calcification in the medullary canal. A bone scan **(C)** reveals nonuniform increased uptake of the radionuclide in the proximal epiphysis, metaphysis, and diaphysis of the femur. A needle biopsy disclosed a well-differentiated chondrosarcoma. Prior to surgery, the patient fell, resulting in a pathologic fracture through the lesion. The tumor subsequently was resected completely.

D In a second patient, a radiograph reveals a lobulated, well-defined radiolucent lesion (arrow) in the proximal portion of the femoral diaphysis. No calcification is apparent. A low grade chondrosarcoma was documented following biopsy of the lesion.

E In a third patient, a low grade chondrosarcoma has produced an osteolytic lesion (arrow) in the proximal metaphysis of the humerus. Subsequent to curettage and bone grafting of this lesion, which was initially interpreted as a chondromyxoid fibroma, local recurrences of the tumor and regional lymph node metastasis occurred.

bone erosion, and scattered stippled or irregular calcification[733] (Figs. 83–147 to 83–149). Such calcification is evident in approximately 60 to 70 per cent of cases, although conventional tomography or CT scanning may be required for its detection.[734, 735] Infrequently, the tumors are extensively calcified. The pattern of bone destruction is variable, including geographic, motheaten, and permeative varieties. In some cases, obvious features of aggressive behavior, such as poorly defined osteolysis, cortical violation, and a soft tissue mass, are observed; however, more frequently, the radiographic abnormalities are those of a slowly evolving process, making the accurate diagnosis of a malignant tumor difficult.[734] In the flat and irregular bones (Figs. 83–150 to 83–152), chondrosarcomas reveal similar radiographic features, although soft tissue involvement may be more pronounced.

Peripheral Chondrosarcoma. Peripheral chondrosarcomas most commonly arise from a preexisting osteochondroma or, rarely, from the periosteal membrane in the form of a juxtacortical chondrosarcoma (see later discussion), and they may occur in flat, irregular, or tubular bones. The difficulty in distinguishing between a benign osteochondroma and one that has undergone malignant transformation already has been addressed. Such differentiation relies on the analysis of data derived from routine radiography, ultrasonography, scintigraphy, CT scanning, and MR imaging.[594–597, 2113–2115] Features suggestive of malignancy are a bulky cartilaginous cap, an irregular or indistinct surface to the calcified tissue beneath the cartilaginous cap, scattered calcifications in the cartilaginous part of the tumor, focal areas of radiolucency in the interior of the osteochondroma, a significant soft tissue mass, and destruction or pressure erosion of the adjacent bone[628] (Fig. 83–153). None of these imaging features is present uniformly, so that in an individual case, supplementation with histologic data is required; however, the presence of a soft tissue mass and, particularly, scattered and irregular calcification is a strong indicator of malignancy.[628] Furthermore, rapid growth of an osteochondroma, although not diagnostic of malignant transformation, is an ominous sign requiring surgical removal of the lesion.[629]

Other Imaging Techniques. Radionuclide scanning with bone-seeking radiopharmaceutical agents has been used in the evaluation of both central[734, 736] and peripheral[596, 597] chondrosarcomas. In the former situation, increased accumulation of the radionuclide at the site of tumor is uniformly present, and an extended pattern of scintigraphic activity beyond the true limits of the neoplasm is unusual. Therefore, it appears that this imaging method is reliable in identifying the boundaries of a central chondrosarcoma and sites of occult tumor spread.[736] In cases of peripheral chondrosarcoma, bone scanning allows documentation of those

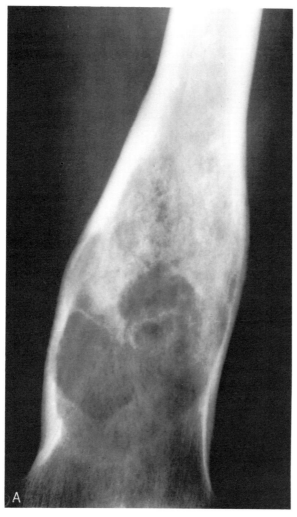

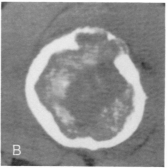

FIGURE 83–148. Conventional chondrosarcoma, central type: Radiographic abnormalities—long tubular bones. In a 37 year old man, routine radiography **(A)** shows an expansile lesion of the femoral diaphysis. The proximal portion of the lesion is calcified; the distal portion is not. Transaxial CT **(B)** reveals internal calcifications and cortical erosion.

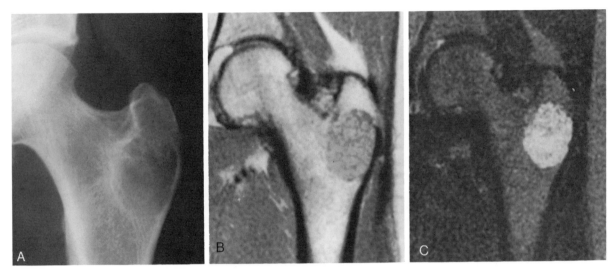

FIGURE 83–149. Conventional chondrosarcoma, central type: Radiographic abnormalities—long tubular bones. In a 38 year old woman, an osteolytic lesion in the greater trochanter of the femur reveals geographic bone destruction **(A)**. CT (not shown) confirmed that the lesion was calcified. Coronal proton density–weighted (TR/TE, 2500/20) **(B)** and T2-weighted (TR/TE, 2500/80) **(C)** spin echo MR images show the full extent of the tumor. It is inhomogeneous but mainly of high signal intensity in **C**.

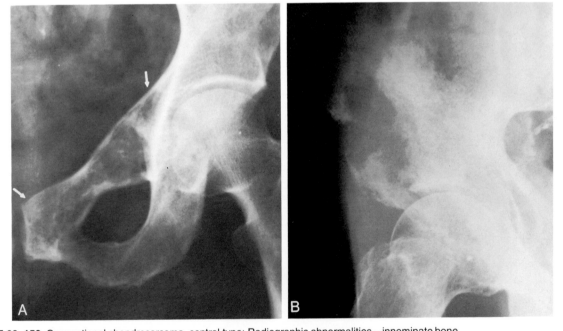

FIGURE 83–150. Conventional chondrosarcoma, central type: Radiographic abnormalities—innominate bone.
　A The elongated osteolytic lesion (between arrows) contains focal calcification. Note erosion of the cortex.
　B In a second case, a large, mixed osteolytic and osteosclerotic lesion in the ilium is associated with articular involvement and a pathologic fracture.

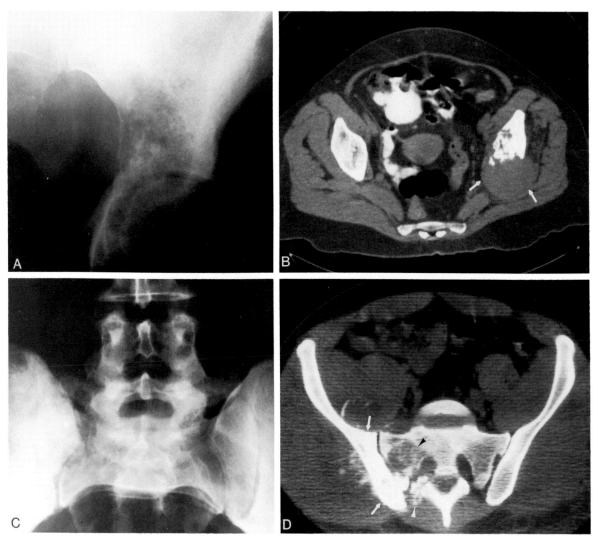

FIGURE 83–151. Conventional chondrosarcoma, central type: Radiographic abnormalities—innominate bone.

A, B In this 50 year old woman, the routine radiograph **(A)** shows an osteolytic lesion of the para-acetabular bone with a prominent soft tissue mass. Transaxial CT **(B)** documents the destruction of the acetabular roof, possible calcification, and a large soft tissue mass (arrows).

C, D In a 32 year old man with a 1 month history of low back pain and weakness in the right leg, a routine radiograph **(C)** reveals prominent osteosclerosis in the right ilium adjacent to the sacroiliac joint. Transaxial CT **(D)** confirms the iliac sclerosis (arrows) and, additionally, calcification or ossification in the soft tissues. Note also the involvement of the sacrum (arrowheads). Myelography (not shown) revealed an extradural defect at the lumbosacral level. During decompression laminectomy, it was observed that the tumor extended into the spinal canal.

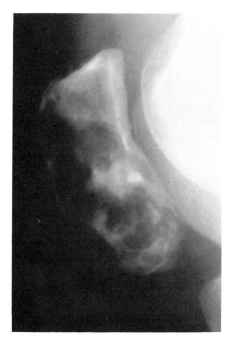

FIGURE 83–152. Conventional chondrosarcoma, central type: Radiographic abnormalities—patella. A low grade chondrosarcoma of the patella is associated with osteolysis, calcification, and a pathologic fracture.

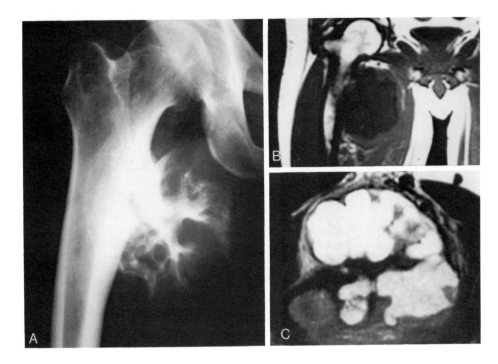

FIGURE 83–153. Conventional chondrosarcoma, peripheral type: Radiographic abnormalities—long tubular bones. In a 30 year old man with a firm, nontender mass in the medial aspect of the thigh, routine radiography **(A)** shows an irregular excrescence arising from the medial aspect of the femur. Its appearance is not that of a typical osteochondroma. The cortex of the subjacent femur is thickened. A coronal T1-weighted (TR/TE, 500/10) spin echo MR image **(B)** reveals a mass of low signal intensity. In a transaxial T2-weighted (TR/TE, 2000/80) spin echo MR image **(C),** a lobulated tumor of high signal intensity is evident. Vascular displacement and compression also are seen.

osteochondromas that are metabolically active but is unreliable in differentiating between those tumors that are benign and those that are malignant. Absence of uptake of the bone-seeking agent virtually eliminates the possibility of malignant transformation of an osteochondroma.[596]

CT scanning also has been used in the analysis of central[727, 734, 1836, 1837] and peripheral[594, 595, 628, 727] chondrosarcomas (Figs. 83–154 and 83–155). In either case, this method provides important information regarding the intraosseous and soft tissue extent of the neoplasm. It has been suggested that eccentric, lobular growth of a soft tissue mass generally indicates a low grade tumor and presumably relates to neoplastic extension along the path of least resistance; high grade chondrosarcomas more characteristically extend in all directions within the soft tissue and do not respect anatomic boundaries.[727] In peripheral chondrosarcomas, CT has been

used with varying degrees of success to define the thickness of the cartilage cap of the underlying osteochondroma.[594, 595]

MR imaging has been applied to the assessment of both central and peripheral chondrosarcomas[2115, 2154–2156] (Figs. 83–155 to 83–157). The technique is very useful in defining the full extent of the tumor in anatomically complex regions such as the spine and base of the skull. An inhomogeneous or homogeneous lesion of high signal intensity is typical in T2-weighted spin echo MR images. Enhancement of signal intensity in a focal or diffuse fashion within the tumor is evident following the intravenous administration of gadolinium compounds, and the extent of such enhancement may be greater in higher grade neoplasms. The diagnostic value of patterns of enhancement of signal intensity within the tumor following gadolinium administration is not agreed on, however.[2425, 2426] Although regions of tumor calcification may be seen with MR imaging, calcification is detected more easily with CT scanning.

Angiography represents one additional technique that may be applied to the assessment of chondrosarcomas. Reports have indicated some correlation between the angiographic abnormalities and the degree of malignancy,[737] although a more appropriate use of this method is to define preoperatively the extent of the tumor and its relationship to adjacent vasculature.[734, 738]

Pathologic Abnormalities. Chondrosarcomas tend to be relatively bulky tumors (Fig. 83–158A), most being over 4 cm in diameter with some as large as 25 or 35 cm and weighing many pounds.[627, 739–741] In one report, over 50 per cent of chondrosarcomas were larger than 10 cm.[685] The most extensive neoplasms occur in the flat and irregular bones, particularly the innominate bone, ribs, and scapula, where they may grow to a large size before producing symptoms. Even those chondrosarcomas in the more confined spaces of the hands or feet occasionally may be 10 cm or more in maximum dimension.[698, 704, 705] Central chondrosarcomas frequently erode the cortex and extend into the soft tissue, an important feature distinguishing them from enchondromas. Peripheral chondrosarcomas that arise from

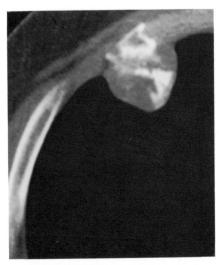

FIGURE 83–154. Conventional chondrosarcoma, peripheral type: CT abnormalities—rib. Transaxial CT reveals a calcified lesion arising from the anterior aspect of the rib.

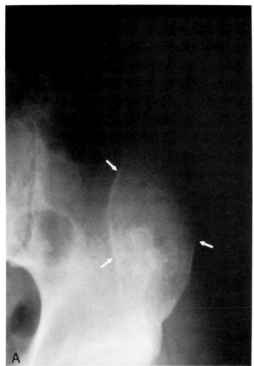

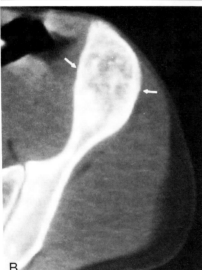

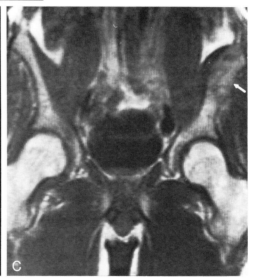

FIGURE 83–155. Conventional chondrosarcoma, central type: CT and MR imaging abnormalities—innominate bone. A 40 year old woman was involved in an automobile accident with an injury to the pelvis. During intravenous pyelography, a lesion of the ilium was identified.

A A radiograph reveals a large lesion of the ilium (arrows) with a hazy interior and calcification.

B Transaxial CT shows the calcification within the lesion and osseous expansion (arrows).

C A coronal T1-weighted (TR/TE, 550/30) spin echo MR image documents that the iliac lesion has decreased signal intensity (arrow). A biopsy and subsequent excision of the lesion confirmed a low grade chondrosarcoma.

malignant transformation of an osteochondroma are predominantly extraosseous, large, bosselated masses that appear relatively well delineated even though they have invaded the soft tissues. The cartilaginous caps of these tumors commonly are greater than 2 cm in thickness; such caps in a benign osteochondroma in an adult usually are less than 1 cm thick, whereas in children and adolescents, the thickness of the cartilaginous cap of a benign exostosis may be as great as 2.5 or 3 cm. The cartilage cap of a benign osteochondroma typically is uniform and smooth, and that of a peripheral chondrosarcoma may be irregular, rough, or granular.[627]

When sectioned, chondrosarcomas have a lobular bluegray to gray-white translucent appearance with a glistening surface typical of hyaline cartilage.[34, 681] Their consistency generally is firm, yet those regions unassociated with calcification can easily be cut with the blade of a scalpel. Soft

mucinous (Fig. 83–158B) or myxoid foci or cysts may be prominent in some chondrosarcomas[30, 34, 740]; in such cases, thick mucinous material may be discharged when the tumor is cut. The medullary limits of central chondrosarcomas are difficult to determine on macroscopic examination as the borders commonly are fuzzy and indistinct. This is in contrast to osteosarcoma, in which the gross extent of the tumor usually is clearly defined. In the better differentiated chondrosarcomas, flecks or spicules of yellow to yellow-white foci of calcification frequently are present (Fig. 83–158C).

Paradoxically, chondrosarcomas are among the easiest and the most difficult of primary bone tumors to diagnose correctly on the basis of histologic abnormalities. This paradox is explained by the ease with which high grade or poorly differentiated chondrosarcomas may be diagnosed but the great difficulty of distinguishing low grade, well-

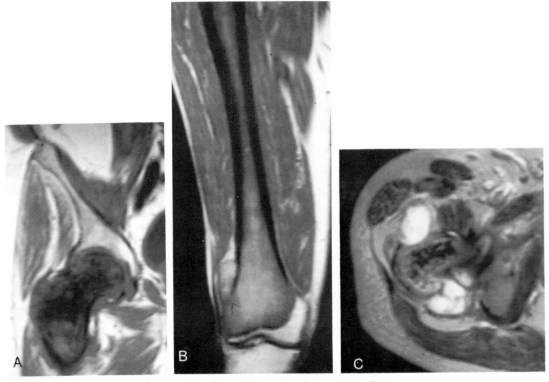

FIGURE 83–156. Conventional chondrosarcoma, central type: MR imaging abnormalities—femur.

A, B In a 71 year old man, coronal T1-weighted (TR/TE, 800/20) spin echo MR images show a tumor involving almost the entire femur. It is of low signal intensity and reveals extraosseous extension both superiorly and interiorly.

C A transaxial T2-weighted (TR/TE, 2000/70) spin echo MR image through the proximal portion of the femur reveals extraosseous extension of the tumor, which is of high signal intensity. (Courtesy of M. Mitchell, M.D., Halifax, Nova Scotia, Canada.)

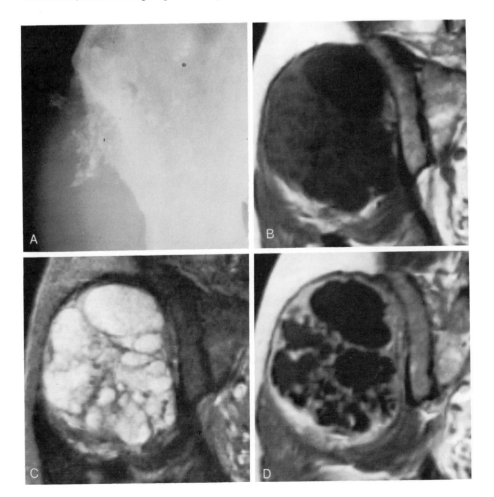

FIGURE 83–157. Conventional chondrosarcoma, peripheral type: MR imaging abnormalities—innominate bone.

A Routine radiography reveals a calcified lesion extending from the ilium.

B Note the large size of the tumor and its low signal intensity in a coronal T1-weighted (TR/TE, 700/15) spin echo MR image.

C In a coronal T2-weighted (TR/TE, 2500/90) spin echo MR image, the tumor is lobulated, is mainly of high signal intensity, and contains septations of low signal intensity.

D Following the intravenous administration of a gadolinium compound, a coronal T1-weighted (TR/TE, 700/15) spin echo MR image shows irregular enhancement of signal intensity in portions of the tumor.

(Courtesy of J. Kramer, M.D., Vienna, Austria.)

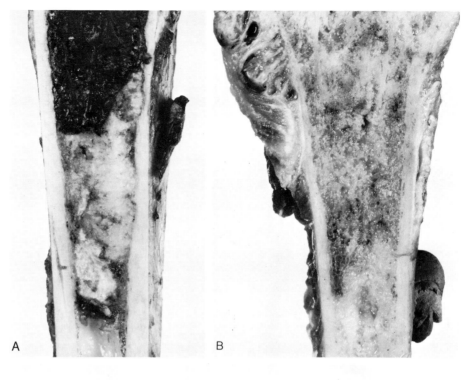

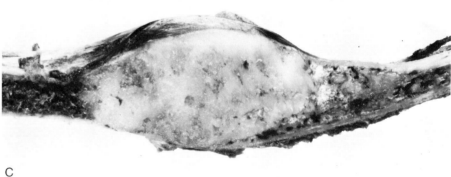

FIGURE 83–158. Conventional chondrosarcoma: Macroscopic abnormalities.

A A sagittal section of a large central chondrosarcoma of the tibia reveals calcification (white areas) and endosteal erosion of the cortex.

B A section of a central myxoid chondrosarcoma of the tibia shows indistinct tumor margins, a glistening surface with small cystic areas filled with mucinous material, and a prominent extraosseous neoplastic component (upper left portion of the photograph).

C A section of a central chondrosarcoma of a rib shows that the tumor has destroyed the cortices. Its surface is homogeneous with scattered foci of calcification (white areas).

differentiated chondrosarcomas and enchondromas. Various systems of grading the histologic features of these neoplasms have been proposed, on the basis of such characteristics as cellularity of the tumor, the apparent differentiation of the cells, and the degree of mitotic activity.[678, 679, 687, 742, 743] Chondrosarcomas usually are classified into four grades, I to IV, with the lower numbers indicating the better differentiated or less aggressive tumors; based on two large series of patients,[685, 687] most chondrosarcomas are classified as grade I or II. Non-numerical grading systems also exist in which the neoplasms are considered to be well, moderately, or poorly differentiated; in such a system the majority of chondrosarcomas would be considered to be in the first two categories.[689, 741]

In general, chondrosarcomas contain many round to oval cells with plump nuclei with a distinct chromatin pattern, numerous binucleated cells, and giant tumor cells with single or multiple large nuclei (Fig. 83–159A,B). The cells of higher grade tumors are more pleomorphic (Fig. 83–159B). Mitotic figures may be found, but even high grade chondrosarcomas may lack significant mitotic activity as, apparently, the tumor cells proliferate by amitotic division.[685, 704, 744] The usual criteria for the diagnosis of a chondrosar-

coma—namely, hypercellularity, plump tumor cells with enlarged nuclei, and frequent cells with double or triple nuclei—do not apply to those cartilaginous tumors in the bones of the hands and feet. Enchondromas in these sites, despite their benign character, may have the cellular features of a grade II chondrosarcoma.[678]

Chondrosarcomas usually are composed of lobules of cartilage; these lobules lack the peripheral encasement by woven or lamellar bone that is found in benign enchondromas (Fig. 83–159C). The lobules also are confluent, with no intervening marrow elements.[28, 688] In benign enchondromas, the lobules of hyaline-like cartilage are separated from the normal trabeculae by fibrous or fibrovascular connective tissue; in chondrosarcomas, however, the malignant cartilage invades the intertrabecular marrow space, and the advancing tumor entraps and surrounds the existing trabeculae.

Low grade, well-differentiated chondrosarcomas contain an abundance of hyaline-like cartilage, although some of these tumors have lobules with a myxoid or mucinous character similar to that found in the enchondromas in Ollier's disease and Maffucci's syndrome. Myxoid chondrosarcomas, however, are observed more frequently in the soft

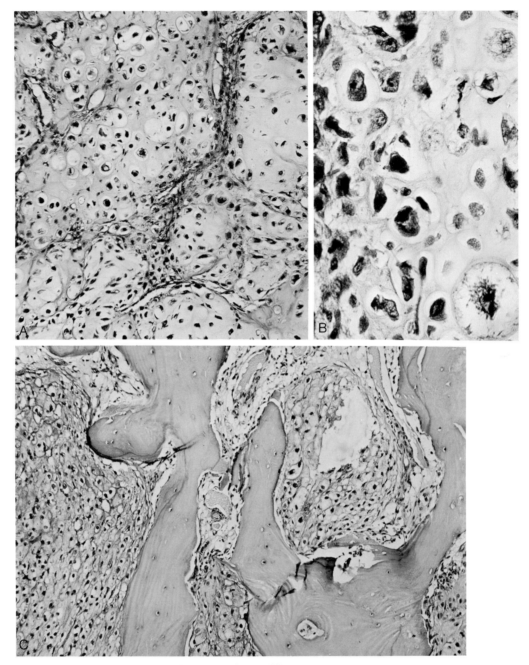

FIGURE 83–159. Conventional chondrosarcoma: Microscopic abnormalities.

A In a moderately differentiated chondrosarcoma, the tumor has a lobular configuration. There is marked variation in the size of the tumor cells, although many are large. (150×.)

B At higher magnification, enlarged cells are seen, with atypical nuclei that reside in lacunae. A large, bizarre tumor cell is seen in the lower portion of the photomicrograph. (600×.)

C The growth pattern of a chondrosarcoma is characterized by neoplastic invasion between preexisting trabeculae. (150×.)

tissues than in bone. Well-differentiated chondrosarcomas also possess areas of calcification and degeneration; such calcification is less frequent in the poorly differentiated neoplasms. In the areas not obscured by calcification, the occurrence of individual cell necrosis is an important clue to the diagnosis of a chondrosarcoma.[28]

The histologic differentiation between a chondrosarcoma that develops in an osteochondroma and a benign osteochondroma depends on the more haphazard arrangement of cells in the chondrosarcoma compared with the more structured columns of chondrocytes that are found in the simple osteochondroma.[627] Such secondary chondrosarcomas also

are more cellular than the usual osteochondroma in which the chondrocytes are widely separated from each other, are small with dotlike nuclei, and reside in individual lacunae.[627]

The cells of well-differentiated chondrosarcomas have electron microscopic features that are similar to those in the cells of a variety of benign lesions of cartilage and of nonneoplastic hyaline cartilage.[745–749]

Natural History. The natural history and ultimate prognosis of chondrosarcomas are extremely variable as such neoplasms, although often considered to be a fairly homogeneous group of tumors, are widely divergent both in their histologic and in their biochemical alterations.[689, 730] It is well recognized that chondrosarcomas have the potential to be locally infiltrative and, in some cases, to metastasize through the blood stream to distant organs,[750] especially the lungs but also the skeleton, liver, kidneys, heart, and other organs.[2427] The desirability of identifying clinical, imaging, histologic, and chemical markers that could gauge the behavioral characteristics of each individual tumor reliably is obvious. Locally aggressive manifestations of chondrosarcoma include focal or uniform intraosseous extension,[751] transarticular spread,[752] and soft tissue invasion. These manifestations as well as systemic metastasis increase in frequency with higher grades of neoplasms.[688] Tumor recurrence (Fig. 83–160) also is correlated with histologic grade and adequacy of treatment; although recurrent chondrosarcomas usually maintain the same degree of differentiation as that of the initial lesion, an increase in malignant potential is observed in approximately 10 per cent of such recurrences, accompanied by dedifferentiation of the tumor into a high grade spindle cell sarcoma (see later discussion). The reported overall rate of survival for a period of 10 years following treatment has varied from 30 to 70 per cent, with the risk of death being greatest for patients with spinal tumors and with high grade chondrosarcomas.[688]

Differential Diagnosis. The diagnosis of a chondrosarcoma based solely on the radiographic findings is not always possible. The presence in a tubular bone of an osteolytic lesion with a geographic or motheaten pattern of bone destruction, a lobulated contour, endosteal cortical erosion, periostitis, and calcification is indicative of a cartilaginous tumor and is most compatible with the diagnosis of a chondrosarcoma. The differentiation of a central chondrosarcoma and an enchondroma may be extremely difficult, although ill-defined osteolysis, a soft tissue mass, and the absence of calcification in a part of the lesion are roentgenographic findings more compatible with a chondrosarcoma. Similarly, the differentiation of a peripheral chondrosarcoma and a simple osteochondroma commonly is not possible on the basis of the conventional radiographic examination, requiring supplementation with other imaging techniques.

In the flat or irregular bones, a large osteolytic lesion with a soft tissue mass in an adult patient is compatible with a variety of lesions, including a chondrosarcoma, plasmacytoma, lymphoma, solitary skeletal focus of metastasis, and even an unusual infection, such as echinococcosis. More specific in such cases is the identification of calcification, although its differentiation from ossification, as might be seen in an osteosarcoma, may not be accomplished easily.

Considerable difficulty in accurate diagnosis of a chondrosarcoma may await the pathologist's analysis of the histologic findings. Much of the difficulty resides in the distinction of an enchondroma from a low grade chondrosarcoma, particularly when only a small sample of tissue is available. Patterns of tumor growth, rather than cytologic features, may aid in the accurate identification of chondrosarcomas by histologic means.[2464] Multinucleation and enlargement of cells, nuclear atypia, and prominent mitotic activity generally are signs of malignancy, but these microscopic abnormalities must be correlated with clinical and radiologic data. The histologic distinction between chondrosarcoma and chondromyxoid fibroma also may be difficult. In particular, the latter tumor may possess enlarged cells with irregular and atypical nuclei, a lobular configuration, and a myxoid matrix similar to the findings of a myxoid chondrosarcoma. Of diagnostic importance, the lobules of a chondromyxoid fibroma are not confluent and are separated by fibrous tissue septa with areas consisting of osteoclast- and chondroblast-type cells.

In chondrosarcomas, bone may develop within the cartilaginous lobules owing to the occurrence of endochondral ossification; therefore, the possibility of an osteosarcoma might be considered on initially reviewing the histologic material. Chondrosarcomas with such areas of ossification differ from chondroblastic osteosarcomas in the absence of direct production of osteoid by the malignant spindle cells and in the lack of tissue alkaline phosphatase activity.[688]

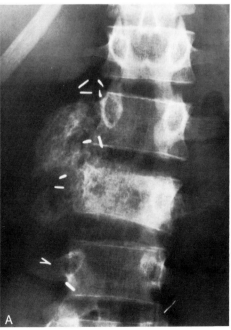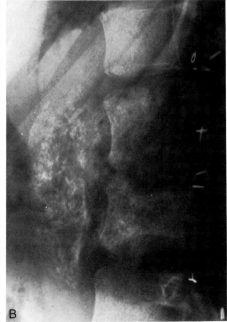

FIGURE 83–160. Conventional chondrosarcoma: Natural history—tumor recurrence. This 13 year old girl had had previous surgery to remove a chondrosarcoma originating in the lumbar spine. Frontal **(A)** and lateral **(B)** radiographs document tumor recurrence with both osseous and soft tissue involvement. Note prominent paravertebral calcification. (Courtesy of C. Resnik, M.D., Baltimore, Maryland.)

Juxtacortical (Periosteal) Chondrosarcoma. Although initial reports of malignant cartilaginous tumors of periosteal origin were provided by Lichtenstein[753] in 1955 and Jaffe[754] in 1958, it was the description of seven such neoplasms in 1977 by Schajowicz[755] that represented the first detailed account of this lesion, which is designated a juxtacortical (periosteal) chondrosarcoma. In almost all cases, the clinical and radiologic appearance of these tumors is similar to that of a periosteal osteosarcoma, leading many investigators to the conclusion that they are identical neo-

plasms. A long tubular bone, especially the femur, typically is affected, and the roentgenographic alterations include a small lesion on the osseous surface accompanied by spotty calcification, radiating bone spicules, and a typical Codman's triangle[221] (Fig. 83–161). Macroscopic examination confirms the tumor's origin in the external portion of the cortex. The lesion is covered by a thick fibrous layer that is a continuation of the periosteum.[347, 755, 756] The long axis of the tumor is parallel to the long axis of the bone. The length of the neoplasm varies from 3.5 cm to 20 cm and is gener-

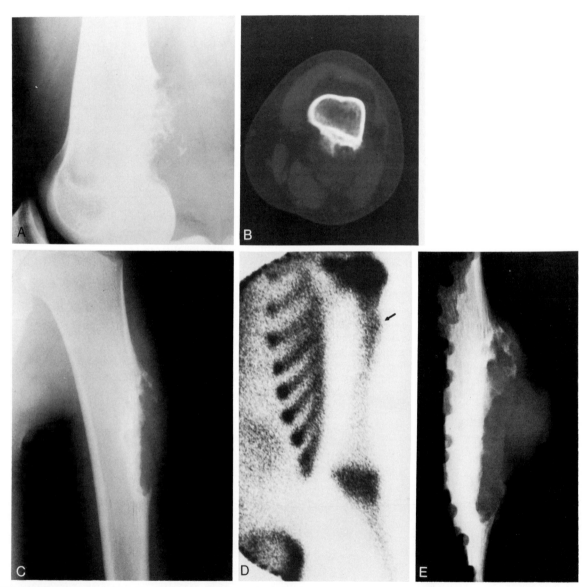

FIGURE 83–161. Juxtacortical (periosteal) chondrosarcoma: Radiographic, scintigraphic, and CT abnormalities.
   A, B A young adult woman developed pain and an enlarging mass posteriorly above the knee. A lateral radiograph **(A)** reveals calcification adjacent to the posterior surface of the distal metaphysis of the femur with cortical thickening and a Codman's triangle above. Transaxial CT **(B)** shows the lesion behind the femur containing calcification and a periosteal response. The tumor was removed and studied by several pathologists. The consensus was that it represented a juxtacortical (periosteal) chondrosarcoma, although both radiographically and histologically it resembled a periosteal osteosarcoma. (Courtesy of S. Kursunoglu Brahme, M.D., San Diego, California.)
   C–E This 10 year old girl had a 5 week history of an enlarging, painless, firm mass adjacent to the proximal portion of the humerus. On palpation, it measured 3 × 2 × 2 cm and was located beneath the osseous insertion of the deltoid muscle. The radiograph **(C)** shows an eccentric osteolytic lesion eroding the external surface of the cortex. The endosteal margin of the cortex is thickened and there is mature periosteal elevation at the superior and inferior margins of the tumor. A bone scan **(D)** shows a moderate increase in accumulation of the radionuclide at the site of the lesion (arrow). The radiographic diagnosis was a periosteal (juxtacortical) chondroma. This was confirmed following needle biopsy of the lesion. An en bloc excision supplied a specimen **(E)** whose external surface contained aggressive cartilaginous tissue with infiltration into the adjacent muscular stroma. After much deliberation by many pathologists, the consensus was that this lesion represented a grade II juxtacortical (periosteal) chondrosarcoma.

ally greater than 5 cm. The peripheral margin of a juxtacortical chondrosarcoma is soft and its central areas are firm or even hard. The subjacent cortex may be partially eroded but, characteristically, the medullary cavity is visibly free of tumor.[347, 755, 756]

It is the microscopic nature of this lesion that has promoted the debate between those investigators who consider it a malignant cartilage neoplasm and those who consider it an osteosarcoma. Undeniably, chondroblastic elements are the dominant abnormality, with tumor osteoid and bone being conspicuously absent[221]; however, the production of osteoid by a periosteal osteosarcoma may be very limited, and the ultimate classification of the neoplasm as a periosteal osteosarcoma or juxtacortical chondrosarcoma depends on the manner in which the cartilaginous and osseous tissue is interpreted. As in cases of periosteal osteosarcoma, the prognosis of juxtacortical chondrosarcoma is favorable despite its frequently ominous histologic characteristics.

Clear Cell Chondrosarcoma. In 1976, Unni and associates[757] described 16 patients with a low grade cartilaginous neoplasm that possessed a distinctive histologic appearance, terming it a clear cell chondrosarcoma on the basis of the configuration of its constituent tumor cells. Subsequent reports have further documented the clinical, radiographic, and histologic characteristics of this rare form of chondrosarcoma.[758–768, 2157–2160, 2465–2467]

Clinical Abnormalities. Clear cell chondrosarcoma occurs more frequently in men; it may be evident at any age but usually is seen in the third, fourth, or fifth decade of life. Symptoms are variable, of long duration, and include mild, localized pain and limited range of motion in the adjacent articulation. Pathologic fractures are not infrequent, occurring in approximately 25 per cent of cases, and may be the cause of the patient's seeking medical attention.

Skeletal Location. Clear cell chondrosarcomas predominate in the long tubular bones (approximately 85 per cent of cases), particularly the femur (approximately 55 per cent of cases) and the humerus (approximately 15 to 20 per cent of cases). The bones about the knee are involved in about 10 to 15 per cent of cases. Involvement of flat or irregular bones is unusual, in sharp contrast to the distribution of conventional chondrosarcomas. Rare sites of involvement include the vertebrae, ribs, scapula, skull, maxilla, pubic bone, and small bones of the hand and foot. In the tubular bones, epiphyseal localization is the rule, although, with larger lesions, tumor extension into the metaphysis is frequent; primary involvement of the metaphysis is unusual and that of the diaphysis is exceedingly rare.[765] This pattern of distribution is similar to that of a chondroblastoma and differs from that of a conventional chondrosarcoma, which more often is metaphyseal in origin.

It is the proximal end of the bone that is affected in approximately 90 per cent of cases; the most common site of involvement is the proximal portion of the femur, followed in order of decreasing frequency by the proximal portions of the humerus and the tibia. Multiple osseous sites of involvement are encountered infrequently and occur either simultaneously or metachronously[757]; therefore, these patterns of involvement may reflect the presence of either multifocal primary tumors or skeletal metastases.

Radiographic Abnormalities. Clear cell chondrosarcomas are predominantly osteolytic and slightly expansile.

The margin of the tumor may be either poorly defined or well defined, with a sclerotic border.[766] The reported frequency of calcification has varied (calcification probably occurs in about 35 per cent of cases), although, in some cases, such calcification is prominent. It has been suggested that the pattern of calcification, which has been described as soft and fluffy, resembles that of a chondroblastoma rather than a chondrosarcoma.[765] Endosteal erosion, cortical violation, pathologic fracture, and a soft tissue mass represent additional radiographic findings that are evident in some cases.

The radiographic features as well as the typical epiphyseal location in a tubular bone (Fig. 83–162) are identical to those of a chondroblastoma, and differentiation of these two neoplasms on the basis of roentgenographic abnormalities may be extremely difficult. The presence of metaphyseal involvement and the absence of periostitis are findings that favor the diagnosis of a clear cell chondrosarcoma.[766] The tumor is of low signal intensity in T1-weighted spin echo MR images (Fig. 83–163). High signal intensity in T2-weighted spin echo MR images may be more common in clear cell chondrosarcomas than in chondroblastomas.[2091]

Pathologic Abnormalities. Clear cell chondrosarcomas may be relatively small and confined to the epiphysis or large enough to replace the entire epiphysis and extend into the metaphysis. Macroscopically, these tumors do not have a typical cartilaginous appearance. Rather, they are soft, granular, white or red neoplasms that may reveal small or large cysts containing clear or hemorrhagic fluid.

Clear cell chondrosarcomas are histologically distinctive, with areas of closely compact cells arranged in sheets or separated into faint lobules by thin fibrovascular septa. The tumor cells have an abundant clear, glycogen-rich cytoplasm with distinct borders (Fig. 83–164A). Nuclei tend to be located centrally and hyperchromatic; they may be small or large, with little or no atypia. Mitotic figures are uncommon.

In some cases, the histologic features of clear cell chondrosarcoma resemble those of other neoplasms. In fact, regions of conventional chondrosarcoma are found in approximately 50 per cent of these tumors,[757, 758, 761, 765] although the occurrence of scattered, benign-appearing, multinucleated giant cells is a microscopic feature of clear cell chondrosarcoma that is virtually never found in a conventional chondrosarcoma. In clear cell chondrosarcomas, thin strands of calcium may be evident between the cartilage cells, creating a chicken-wire pattern, as is evident in chondroblastoma,[761] or the stromal cells of the neoplasm may produce seams of lacelike osteoid, as in an osteosarcoma[765] (Fig. 83–164B). Additional histologic abnormalities of these tumors may resemble those of an aneurysmal bone cyst or osteoblastoma.

Electron microscopy has shown that the tumor cells of this rare variety of chondrosarcoma have the fine structural features of either chondrocytes or chondroblasts.[758, 759, 762, 768, 1875]

Natural History. Clear cell chondrosarcomas are relatively slow growing, low grade malignant tumors with a much better prognosis than that of conventional chondrosarcomas. Local extension into the soft tissues and even the adjacent articulation[769] is encountered. Tumor recurrence (Fig. 83–165) is reported, particularly in those cases in which surgery was conservative, consisting of only curet-

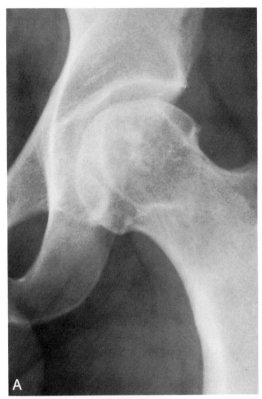
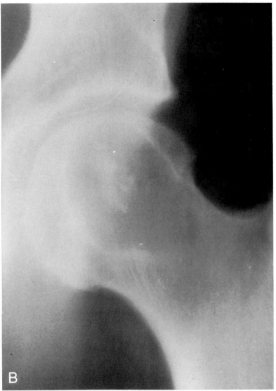

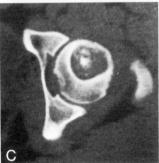

FIGURE 83–162. Clear cell chondrosarcoma: Radiographic and CT abnormalities. A 50 year old man developed progressive hip pain.

A, B A routine radiograph **(A)** and conventional tomogram **(B)** delineate a large, well-defined osteolytic lesion involving the femoral head and extending into the femoral neck. It contains central calcification and a peripheral sclerotic margin and has led to subtle collapse of the articular surface.

C A transaxial CT scan shows the calcified lesion in the femoral head. A bone scan (not shown) revealed increased accumulation of the radionuclide in the femoral head and neck. The tumor was resected, and a diagnosis of a clear cell chondrosarcoma was established.

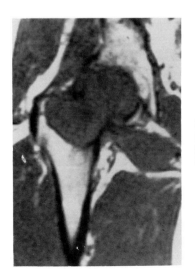

FIGURE 83–163. Clear cell chondrosarcoma: MR imaging abnormalities. A coronal T1-weighted (TR/TE, 400/20) spin echo MR image shows a tumor of low signal intensity occupying the proximal portion of the right femur with extension to the subchondral bone. (Courtesy of J. Gerharter, M.D., Denver, Colorado.)

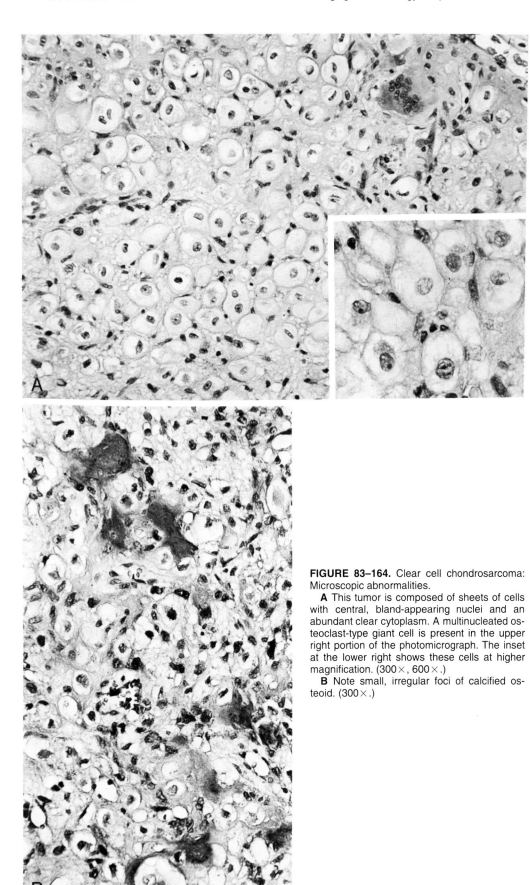

FIGURE 83–164. Clear cell chondrosarcoma: Microscopic abnormalities.

  A This tumor is composed of sheets of cells with central, bland-appearing nuclei and an abundant clear cytoplasm. A multinucleated osteoclast-type giant cell is present in the upper right portion of the photomicrograph. The inset at the lower right shows these cells at higher magnification. (300×, 600×.)

  B Note small, irregular foci of calcified osteoid. (300×.)

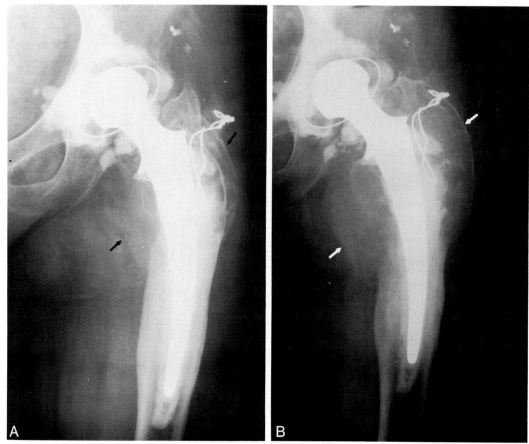

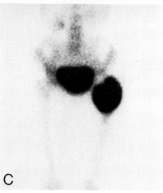

FIGURE 83–165. Clear cell chondrosarcoma: Natural history—tumor recurrence. A 61 year old woman requested evaluation of a painful total hip arthroplasty. Eleven years prior to this evaluation, she had developed a pathologic fracture of the left femoral neck, although the nature of the lesion producing the fracture was not known. This lesion recurred 1 year later, 10 years before her current evaluation, and a total hip arthroplasty had been performed. At the time of surgery, the diagnosis of an osteoblastoma was considered.

A, B Radiographs obtained 4 years before her current evaluation **(A)** and at the time of this evaluation **(B)** show an enlarging mass (arrows) with hazy radiodensity about the femoral component.

C A bone scan accomplished at the same time as the radiograph in **B** shows intense accumulation of the radionuclide in the proximal portion of the femur. Surgery confirmed the diagnosis of a clear cell chondrosarcoma, presumably a recurrence of the lesion that first appeared 11 years previously.

tage of the lesion.[757] Tumor resection appears to be curative. Disseminated metastases in the lungs, brain, and bones may be seen.[759, 766]

Differential Diagnosis. Bone lesions that radiographically may resemble clear cell chondrosarcoma are chondroblastoma, aneurysmal bone cyst, osteoblastoma, giant cell tumor, plasmacytoma, skeletal metastasis, and the brown tumor of hyperparathyroidism.[766] Furthermore, those clear cell chondrosarcomas that are large and aggressive produce roentgenographic features that are similar to those of a fibrosarcoma, malignant fibrous histiocytoma, or osteosarcoma.[765] Of all of these diagnostic considerations, it is the differentiation of clear cell chondrosarcoma and chondroblastoma that is most difficult; an older age of onset, the presence of metaphyseal involvement, and the absence of periostitis are more characteristic of the former tumor. Histopathologically, these two neoplasms are clearly distin-

guishable in the majority of cases. Chondroblastomas do not contain the tumor cells with clear cytoplasm, nor the areas of overt chondrosarcoma that are found in clear cell chondrosarcomas. Although malignant transformation of a chondroblastoma has been described (see previous discussion), the resulting tumor has histologic features that resemble those of a conventional chondrosarcoma rather than a clear cell chondrosarcoma. Clear cells may be evident in a site of bone metastasis from renal cell carcinoma, but additional histologic characteristics in these carcinomatous deposits and in clear cell chondrosarcoma allow their identification. Of importance, the presence of cartilaginous differentiation clearly excludes renal cell carcinoma as a diagnostic possibility.

Mesenchymal Chondrosarcoma. Although relatively rare, mesenchymal chondrosarcomas are particularly noteworthy in two respects: They represent one of the few primary malignant tumors of bone that not infrequently also arise in the soft tissues (30 to 75 per cent of cases)[30, 770–772, 1876]; and their histologic appearance is characteristic owing to an array of chondroid tissue in various stages of differentiation, intermixed with cellular areas of small, anaplastic, commonly spindly cells often in a perivascular arrangement.[773]

Clinical Abnormalities. Men and women are affected in approximately equal numbers; the age range of involved patients is great, although the majority are in the second, third, and fourth decades of life (average age of 25 years).[773–775] It should be noted, therefore, that patients with mesenchymal chondrosarcomas typically are younger than those with conventional chondrosarcomas and similar in age to those with conventional osteosarcomas. Pain, which is of several months to years in duration, swelling, a soft tissue mass, and stiffness are the most typical clinical manifestations. The size of the lesion on initial physical examination often is quite large.

Skeletal Location. The most frequent sites of involvement are the femur (15 per cent of skeletal cases), ribs (12 per cent), and spine (11 per cent), followed in order of decreasing frequency by the skull, maxilla, innominate bone, sacrum, humerus, tibia, mandible, calcaneus, and other bones.[773–785, 2161–2163, 2468–2470] Approximately 25 per cent of osseous tumors affect the lower extremity, 20 per cent originate in the craniofacial bones, and 10 per cent occur in the bones of the pelvis.[773] Mesenchymal chondrosarcomas can arise in any portion of a tubular bone, although a diaphyseal location has been emphasized in some reports.[770] Of interest are occasional descriptions of periosteal mesenchymal chondrosarcomas as well as multicentric bone involvement.[770, 776, 777, 785]

Radiographic Abnormalities. Osteolysis, a permeative pattern of bone destruction, an irregular outline, bone sclerosis, periostitis, and intralesional calcification are among the most characteristic of the varied roentgenographic features of this neoplasm[773] (Fig. 83–166). The pattern of calcification within the osseous or soft tissue component of the lesion usually is stippled, similar to that of a conventional chondrosarcoma (Fig. 83–167). In fact, all of the roentgenographic abnormalities resemble those of a typical chondrosarcoma; it is the relatively young age of the patient that may allow a more specific diagnosis of a mesenchymal chondrosarcoma. Certainly, the radiographic pattern of this neoplasm generally is that of a malignant process, with expansion of bone, cortical violation, irregular periosteal bone formation, and, possibly, soft tissue extension.

Pathologic Abnormalities. Mesenchymal chondrosarcomas are variable in size (2 to 18 cm in maximum dimension) with a lobulated or bosselated outline. Soft tissue components of the lesion may possess a fibrous pseudocapsule.[784]

Soft tissue and skeletal mesenchymal chondrosarcomas have an identical histomorphology.[770, 771, 776, 1876] An accurate microscopic diagnosis depends on the presence of two components: undifferentiated stromal cells and islands of cartilage. The former are small, with relatively little cytoplasm (Fig. 83–168A), and are arranged in sheets and clusters. Their nuclei are round to spindle-shaped and hyperchromatic. The cells are fairly uniform in size with no significant degree of pleomorphism and with a morphology simi-

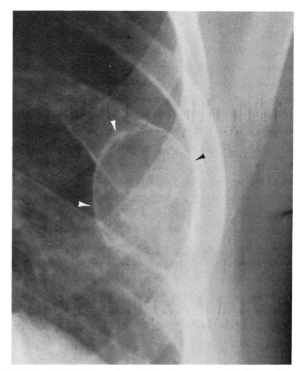

FIGURE 83–166. Mesenchymal chondrosarcoma: Radiographic abnormalities. An expansile, partially calcified lesion (arrowheads) of a rib is evident in this 65 year old man. Establishment of a precise radiographic diagnosis of mesenchymal chondrosarcoma would not be possible in this case as the features are compatible with a conventional chondrosarcoma. (Courtesy of J. Vilar, M.D., Valencia, Spain.)

lar to the cells of a Ewing's sarcoma. Some cells may contain cytoplasmic glycogen, but this is not abundant. Special stains show a meshwork of reticulin fibers about clusters of cells or about individual cells. Mitotic figures are variable in number. The tumors contain an extensive thin-walled vascular network intimately associated with undifferentiated small tumor cells (Fig. 83–168B); the resulting histologic pattern is strikingly similar to that found in hemangiopericytomas. Cartilaginous foci (Fig.

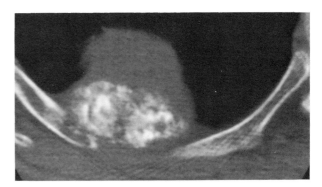

FIGURE 83–167. Mesenchymal chondrosarcoma: CT abnormalities. In a 51 year old woman with a 1 month history of right rib pain, transaxial CT shows a calcified tumor arising from the posterolateral aspect of the right eighth rib. A chest wall resection confirmed the presence of a mesenchymal chondrosarcoma.

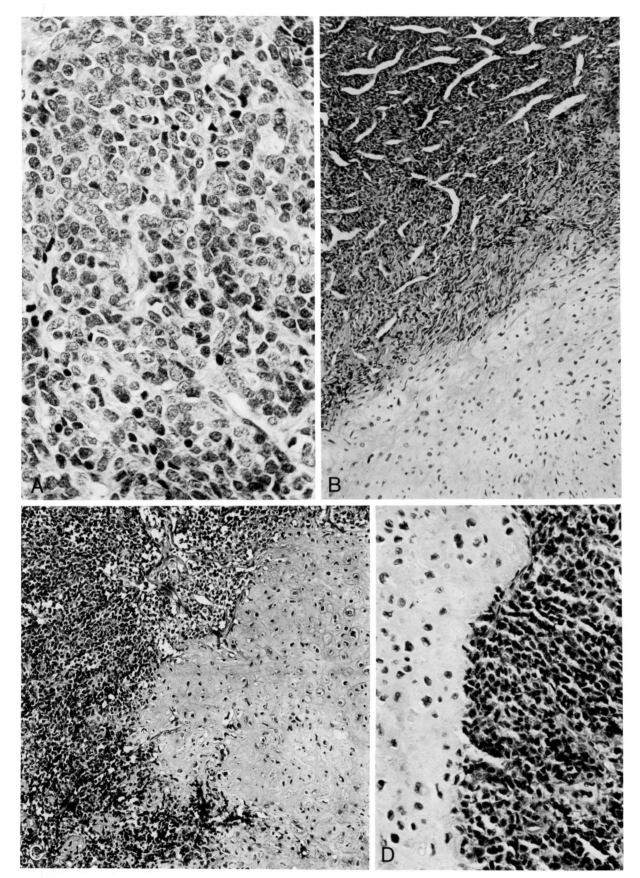

FIGURE 83–168. Mesenchymal chondrosarcoma: Microscopic abnormalities.

  A The undifferentiated tumor cells show little variation in size or shape, and their nuclear chromatin is diffuse and fine. Darker hyperchromatic nuclei probably reflect the presence of cellular degeneration. (600×.)

  B The vascular network consists of branching, thin-walled vessels creating an appearance similar to that of a hemangiopericytoma. A benign-appearing chondroid lobule is evident in the lower portion of the photomicrograph. (150×.)

  C The cells in this cartilage island lack significant atypia. The cartilage is well delineated from the stromal cells. (150×.)

  D Note the abrupt transition between the stromal cells and the adjacent cartilage, whose cells lack overt malignant features. (300×).

83–168C, D) in mesenchymal chondrosarcomas may be sparse or abundant and occur as well-marginated islands surrounded by the small stromal cells. The transition zone between the small cells and the islands of cartilage may be abrupt or gradual. Those cells within the cartilage islands lie in lacunae, are larger than the stromal cells, and appear to be chondroblasts or chondrocytes. They usually are bland in appearance, typically but not invariably lacking chondrosarcomatous features. Calcification frequently is found within the center of these cartilaginous islands, with many islands also showing endochondral ossification.[30]

Electron microscopy has shown that despite a hemangiopericytoma-like appearance by light microscopy, these tumors do not contain pericytes.[786–788] Rather, they are composed of primitive mesenchymal cells as well as those that show cartilaginous differentiation. The tumor stromal cells are considered to be precartilaginous mesenchymal cells. Immunohistochemically, the cells within the cartilage islands are reactive for S-100 protein, whereas the small stromal cells are nonreactive in this regard.

Natural History. Mesenchymal chondrosarcomas represent an aggressive variant of chondrosarcoma characterized by a poor prognosis. Local recurrences typify the clinical course, and these may precede the appearance of disseminated metastases, underscoring the significance of adequate local therapy.[773] The tendency of this tumor to metastasize to regional and distant lymph nodes and to other bones is quite uncharacteristic of ordinary chondrosarcoma.[773]

Differential Diagnosis. As the radiographic findings of mesenchymal chondrosarcoma are those of an aggressive tumor that contains calcification, it generally is not possible to differentiate this neoplasm from a conventional chondrosarcoma. The fact that mesenchymal chondrosarcomas are observed in relatively young patients assumes some diagnostic importance. Histologically, the differential diagnosis of such chondrosarcomas includes Ewing's sarcoma, hemangiopericytoma, small cell osteosarcoma, and dedifferentiated chondrosarcoma.

Dedifferentiated Chondrosarcoma. Chondrosarcoma with dedifferentiated foci represents a variant of conventional chondrosarcoma of bone in which a highly anaplastic sarcoma is associated with a borderline or low grade malignant cartilage tumor.[789] The term dedifferentiation is not ideally suited to describe this association, as differentiated malignant cells do not dedifferentiate; rather, the presence of primitive components is indicative of a lack of cellular differentiation. In any case, however, the importance of recognizing this dedifferentiated neoplasm relates to its frequency of occurrence (approximately 10 per cent of all chondrosarcomas), its locally aggressive behavior, and, ultimately, its poor prognosis.[1904] The phenomenon of dedifferentiation was initially described in detail in 1971 by Dahlin and Beabout[790]; additional accounts of this anaplastic change appeared subsequently and, currently, over 100 cases of dedifferentiated chondrosarcomas have been reported.[791–804, 1838, 2164–2168] Although the histologic features of the anaplastic zones have varied, the presence of a bimorphic pattern of low grade cartilage in direct association with a high grade sarcoma remains essential to the diagnosis.[801] Dedifferentiation may be identified in the initial biopsy sample or resected specimen (de novo pattern) or, less frequently, in recurrences of low grade chondrosarcomas

(interval pattern).[801] In all instances, the survival rate of affected persons is poor.[1838]

Clinical Abnormalities. Men and women in the fifth, sixth, and seventh decades of life generally are affected; the average age of these persons is approximately 60 years, and most are older than 50 years of age. Pain is the most frequent symptom, and its duration is variable but often protracted. Soft tissue swelling or a mass and pathologic fractures (10 to 40 per cent of cases) are additional, common clinical manifestations. In general, a preexisting cartilaginous tumor is not identified.[789]

Skeletal Location. Dedifferentiated chondrosarcomas reveal a similar distribution to that of conventional chondrosarcomas.[790] The femur, humerus, and innominate bone account for the majority of cases. In the long tubular bones, the proximal segments are far more frequently affected than the distal segments. The most characteristic sites of involvement are the proximal portion and diaphysis of the femur and the proximal portions of the humerus and tibia. The distal region of the humerus is selected infrequently.[794] Other uncommon sites of involvement include the scapula, vertebrae, and ribs.

Radiographic Abnormalities. These neoplasms frequently are accompanied by radiographic abnormalities that allow precise diagnosis.[1905] Typically, an osteolytic lesion with motheaten bone destruction is observed; the lesion is partially calcified, although, in one region, such calcification is sparse or entirely absent. These noncalcified areas commonly reveal the most aggressive bone destruction, with erosion and penetration of the cortex, soft tissue swelling, and, in some cases, a pathologic fracture. Periostitis is not prominent.

It should be emphasized that the accurate radiographic diagnosis of a dedifferentiated chondrosarcoma relies on the identification within the lesion of two characteristic patterns. The first is indicative of a low grade chondrosarcoma; the second is indicative of the dedifferentiated and more aggressive portion of the tumor. If these two patterns are evident, the radiographic diagnosis of a dedifferentiated chondrosarcoma generally is correct, although the second possibility of a sarcoma developing in an area of osteonecrosis also must be considered.

Pathologic Abnormalities. The gross morphology of dedifferentiated chondrosarcoma differs from that of a conventional chondrosarcoma. Although typical translucent gray to gray-white lobules of hyaline cartilage are present, they are found within the central portion of the tumor, whereas the peripheral areas are composed of nonspecific soft, fleshy, encapsulated, pink or white tumor tissue that is sharply delineated from the cartilage.[790, 794] At times, the majority of the tumor is composed of noncartilaginous tissue.

Histologically, dedifferentiated chondrosarcomas contain evidence of a low grade conventional chondrosarcoma and, in juxtaposition, an anaplastic sarcoma[780] (Fig. 83–169). The transition between these two tumoral components is usually, but not invariably, sharp. The specific characteristics of the primitive or anaplastic tissue may be indicative of a fibrosarcoma, osteosarcoma (fibroblastic or osteoblastic), malignant fibrous histiocytoma, angiosarcoma, rhabdomyosarcoma, or leiomyosarcoma in order of decreasing frequency.[1838]

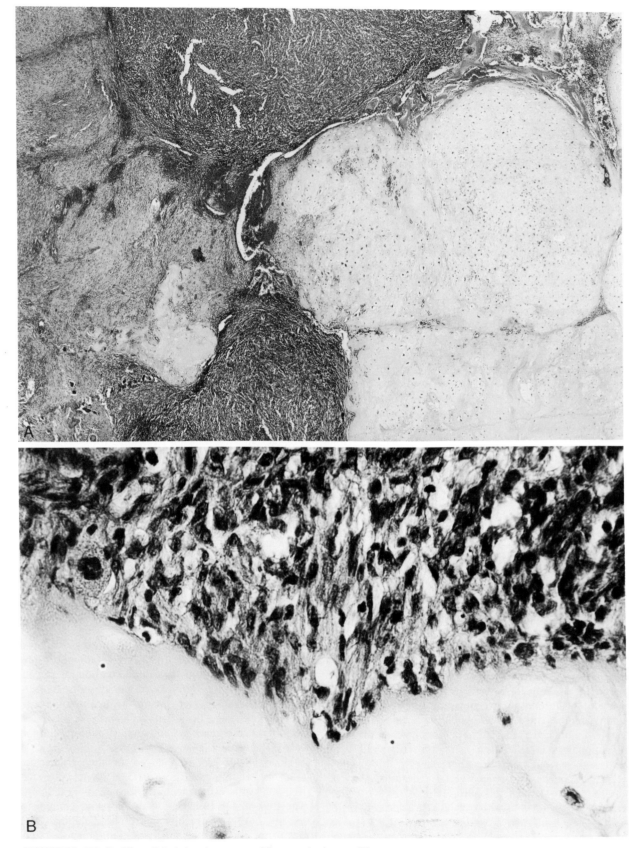

FIGURE 83–169. Dedifferentiated chondrosarcoma: Microscopic abnormalities.
  A Note that two types of tissue are present: a nodule of low grade chondrosarcoma and a highly anaplastic sarcoma. (31 ×.)
  B The interface between these two types of tissue is sharp. (600 ×.)

TUMORS ARISING FROM OR FORMING FIBROUS CONNECTIVE TISSUE

Benign Tumors

Nonossifying Fibroma

Nonossifying fibroma and the related fibrous cortical (fibrocortical) defect are common lesions composed histologically of whorled bundles of connective tissue cells. Precise definitions of these two conditions do not exist, and, in fact, in many reported investigations, the terms nonossifying fibroma and fibrous cortical defect are used interchangeably. It generally is agreed that the former designation is more appropriately applied to a larger and, perhaps, symptomatic lesion, whereas the latter designation is more suited for the description of a smaller, asymptomatic osseous abnormality. The issue of classification is further clouded owing to the existence of other terms, such as nonosteogenic fibroma, fibroxanthoma, and histiocytic fibroma, that have been used to describe such abnormalities, and to the erratic behavior of the fibrous cortical defect, which may either involute spontaneously and disappear completely or enlarge, assuming the characteristics of a nonossifying fibroma.

The origin and histogenesis of these lesions have been a source of great interest and speculation. In 1955, Caffey[805] provided a thorough account of fibrous defects in the cortical walls of growing tubular bones in which the issues of cause and pathogenesis were addressed. An unrecognized, local traumatic insult (or insults) to the periosteum, resulting in focal hemorrhage and edema, is consistent with both the natural history of fibrous cortical defects and their propensity to occur at osseous sites of muscular attachment, although such site selection is not uniformly apparent. Evidence for an inflammatory or neoplastic cause is less compelling, although proponents of either etiologic background can be found. Ultimately, it was Caffey's opinion that such lesions should be classified as variants of normal growth until a causal agent could be identified definitively.

The issue of histogenesis has led investigators to the electron microscope in an attempt to identify the earliest cellular aberrations that are responsible for a fibrous cortical defect or nonossifying fibroma.[806–810] The data provided by these investigations have been conflicting, supporting either a histiocytic, a fibroblastic, or a lipoblastic origin of the lesions. Such disagreement has resulted in further difficulty and conflict in tumor classification, with the segregation by some investigators of an additional variety of neoplasm, the benign fibrous histiocytoma (see later discussion). Others would consider a common origin for nonossifying fibromas and fibrous histiocytomas.[810]

Clinical Abnormalities. There is uniformity of opinion with regard to the clinical features of fibrous cortical defects and nonossifying fibromas. Small, cortical fibrous lesions in the tubular bones are encountered regularly during radiographic examination of healthy children. It has been estimated that one or more cortical defects are apparent in more than 50 per cent of boys and 20 per cent of girls who are older than 2 years of age.[805, 811] The reported frequency of fibrous cortical defects, however, is quite variable, with some investigators indicating their presence in only 2 per cent of persons under 20 years of age.[812] Generally, the lesions are silent clinically, being discovered on roentgenograms obtained for incidental reasons. Their rarity in children less than 2 years of age is consistent with the belief that muscle pull during weight-bearing and walking is important in their pathogenesis,[805] and their infrequency in adults supports the concept that most lesions heal by being replaced by normal bone,[813] although some become quite large and may lead to pathologic fracture (see later discussion). It is in these latter instances that symptoms and signs may appear, eventually necessitating surgical intervention.

Skeletal Location. Analysis of reported data related to the skeletal distribution of fibrous cortical defects and nonossifying fibromas is made more difficult because of the absence of uniformly accepted criteria that distinguish between the two lesions. In fact, many investigators have included both lesions together in their evaluations. It generally is believed that the anatomic locations of fibrous cortical defects are very similar or identical to those of nonossifying fibromas.[30, 33, 34, 139, 813–815] The smaller lesions (fibrous cortical defects), however, may occur at either a single site or in multiple locations in one or more bones, whereas the larger lesions (nonossifying fibromas) are far less commonly multifocal[33, 813, 816] and, when multiple, may or may not be accompanied by other clinical manifestations (see later discussion).[2169] Symmetry of involvement is characteristic of a bilateral distribution.[805]

The long tubular bones are affected predominantly (approximately 90 per cent of cases). The tibia (43 per cent) and the femur (38 per cent) are the most frequent sites of involvement; the fibula is involved in approximately 8 per cent of cases. Fibrous cortical defects and nonossifying fibromas in the bones of the upper extremity are uncommon (approximately 8 per cent of cases); in this situation, it is the humerus (5 per cent of cases) that is the most typical site of involvement, whereas radial or ulnar lesions are rare. Also rare is involvement of the ribs, innominate bone, clavicle, skull, mandible, scapula, and small bones of the hand and foot.[817–821, 1839]

In the tubular bones, fibrous cortical defects and nonossifying fibromas predominantly are metaphyseal lesions arising close to the physeal plate.[30, 805, 813, 815, 822–825] With continued growth of the parent bone, these lesions become situated at some distance from the physis and, if they do not involute, they may extend into the diaphysis. Epiphyseal localization or extension is distinctly unusual, except in cases of multifocal osseous involvement or, perhaps, of fibrous histiocytoma. In the femur, the vast majority (80 per cent) of lesions affect the distal metaphyseal region with the remainder distributed equally in the proximal and middle segments of the bone. In the tibia, the proximal and distal metaphyses are involved with similar frequency (45 per cent), with the remaining 10 per cent of tibial lesions located in the diaphysis. Other sites of predilection are the proximal segment of the fibula and the proximal and distal segments of the humerus. The bones about the knee account for about 55 per cent of all lesions. Fibrous cortical defects and nonossifying fibromas usually arise from the posterior wall of the tubular bone and affect the medial (rather than the lateral) osseous surface far more frequently.

Radiographic Abnormalities. Fibrous cortical defects and nonossifying fibromas are associated with characteristic radiographic abnormalities[805, 824, 826] (Fig. 83–170). The smaller lesions produce focal, superficial, shallow radiolucent areas in the cortex with normal or sclerotic adjacent bone and, in some instances, a blister-like peripheral osse-

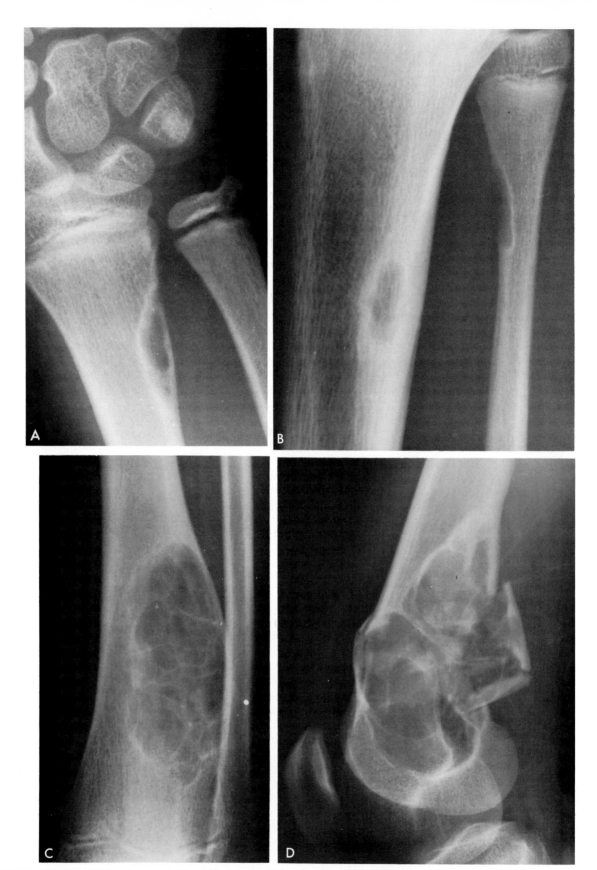

FIGURE 83–170. Nonossifying fibroma: Radiographic abnormalities—spectrum of changes.

   A This eccentric, radiolucent lesion in the radius possesses a sclerotic inner margin. It is located a short distance from the physis.

   B Nonossifying fibromas (or fibrous cortical defects) are identified in the proximal portions of the tibia and the fibula. Note their eccentric location and the geographic bone destruction. The nonossifying fibroma of the fibula is located a short distance from the neighboring growth plate.

   C A large, nonossifying fibroma of the distal portion of the tibia has produced deformity of the adjacent fibula. Note the eccentric location, geographic bone destruction, radiolucent lesion with lobulated trabeculation, internal sclerotic border, and cortical expansion. This lesion, too, is located a short distance from the neighboring physis.

   D This large nonossifying fibroma of the distal portion of the femur has led to a spontaneous fracture. Its upper border indicates its eccentric location.

3768

ous shell.[805] The lesions are circular or oval in shape, are well delineated, with smooth or lobulated edges, and are not accompanied by significant periostitis. Characteristically, they arise in the metaphysis at a short distance from the physis or, less commonly, adjacent to the physeal plate. With growth of the tubular bone, apparent shaftward migration of the lesion may be accompanied by segmental sclerosis within a portion of the osseous defect. Larger lesions are more elongated, with a multiloculated appearance; cortical thinning or slight expansion may be evident. These lesions as well as smaller ones in thinner tubular bones (such as the fibula) may assume a more central location, although careful analysis of radiographs obtained in multiple projections will generally confirm that the osseous defects have an eccentric origin.

These radiographic abnormalities are virtually diagnostic of a fibrous cortical defect or nonossifying fibroma, obviating the need for skeletal biopsy. Reports of scintigraphic features (Fig. 83–171), which include minimal to mild accumulation of bone-seeking radiopharmaceutical agents indicative of a benign process,[827] are of interest, but imaging methods other than conventional radiography generally are not required owing to the specificity of the roentgenographic abnormalities. An eccentric, well-defined, radiolucent lesion arising in the metaphysis of a tubular bone, at a short distance from the physis, in a child or adolescent almost is diagnostic of a fibrous cortical defect or nonossifying fibroma. Other tumors and tumor-like lesions generally can be excluded, including an osteoid osteoma (a smaller radiolucent area in the cortex with more extensive cortical thickening), bone abscess (a lesion in the medullary or cortical bone with a thicker rim of sclerosis), periosteal chondroma (an eccentrically placed lesion leading to erosion of the external surface of the cortex and, perhaps, possessing calcification), chondromyxoid fibroma (a larger,

trabeculated lesion abutting on the metaphysis that may extend into the epiphysis or diaphysis), avulsive cortical irregularity, or periosteal desmoid (a saucer-like radiolucent defect in the cortex with adjacent sclerosis and periostitis), desmoplastic fibroma (an aggressive osteolytic lesion with destruction of medullary bone, cortical erosion and expansion, and trabeculation), focal fibrocartilaginous dysplasia (a radiolucent defect found in the medial aspect of the proximal portion of the tibia in association with tibia vara), herniation pit (a radiolucent lesion found in the lateral aspect of the femoral neck that generally is stable but occasionally may enlarge gradually), and aneurysmal bone cyst (a more expansile osteolytic lesion). In other sites, such as the flat and irregular bones (Fig. 83–172), or when they are unusually large, nonossifying fibromas are more difficult to diagnose on the basis of the radiographic findings alone. In such cases, histologic analysis may be required.

The role of CT scanning (Figs. 83–172 and 83–173) and MR imaging (Figs. 83–174 and 83–175) in the assessment of fibrous cortical defects and nonossifying fibromas is limited. Delineation of the extent of the lesion in anatomically complex regions can be accomplished with these methods. With MR imaging, these fibrous processes show variability in signal intensity characteristics; although they typically are of low signal intensity in T1-weighted spin echo MR images, they may reveal low or high signal intensity in T2-weighted spin echo MR images.

Pathologic Abnormalities. Owing to the benign nature of fibrous cortical defects and nonossifying fibromas, few specimens have been made available for analysis of the macroscopic features of these lesions.[828] Fibrous cortical defects are small, varying in size from a few millimeters to several centimeters but rarely exceeding 3 cm.[829, 830] When sectioned, they are found to possess a scalloped border and usually are yellow with tan or brown foci. Nonossifying

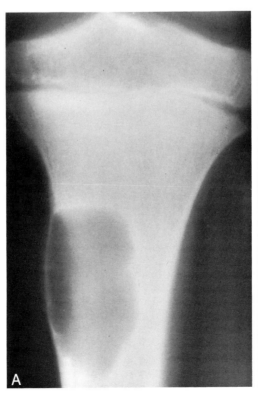
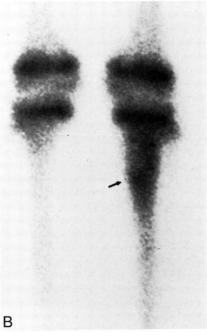

FIGURE 83–171. Nonossifying fibroma: Radiographic and scintigraphic abnormalities—long tubular bones. This lesion of the tibia was discovered as an incidental finding during the evaluation of an acute injury to the knee in a 10 year old boy.

A A conventional tomogram shows an eccentric, well-defined osteolytic lesion in the proximal portion of the tibia. It has a hazy interior and sclerotic margin; there is mild osseous expansion.

B A bone scan shows increased accumulation of the radionuclide at the site of the lesion (arrow). An extended pattern of radionuclide uptake is evident. These findings illustrate the difficulty in distinguishing between benign and malignant processes on the basis of the radionuclide study alone.

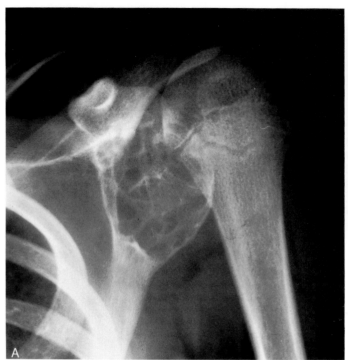

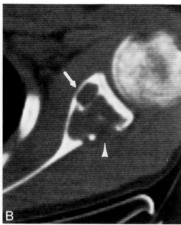

FIGURE 83–172. Nonossifying fibroma: Radiographic and CT abnormalities—flat bones. A 13 year old girl had a 10 month history of shoulder pain that began after exercise. A biopsy of the lesion had been accomplished prior to these imaging studies.

A A trabeculated, osteolytic lesion of the scapula is associated with osseous expansion. In addition to a nonossifying fibroma, an aneurysmal bone cyst and a chondroblastoma would represent diagnostic possibilities.

B Transaxial CT shows the precise location of the lesion with expansion of the anterior surface of the scapula (arrow). A defect in the posterior cortex of the bone (arrowhead) is indicative of the previous biopsy site. The histologic diagnosis was nonossifying fibroma.

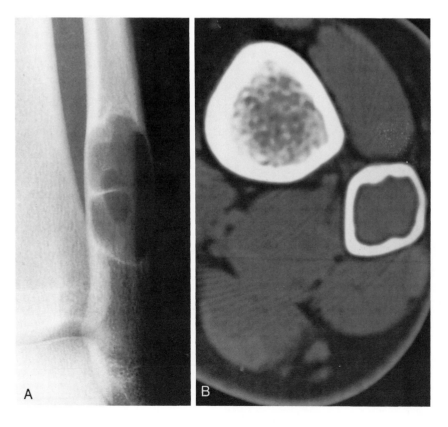

FIGURE 83–173. Nonossifying fibroma: CT abnormalities—long tubular bones. In a 14 year old girl, routine radiography **(A)** and transaxial CT **(B)** show a sharply defined lesion in the distal fibular metaphysis. Note its central location in **B,** with endosteal erosion. Eccentric lesions such as nonossifying fibroma may appear in a more central location in thin tubular bones such as the fibula. At surgery, the cortex about this nonossifying fibroma was markedly thinned.

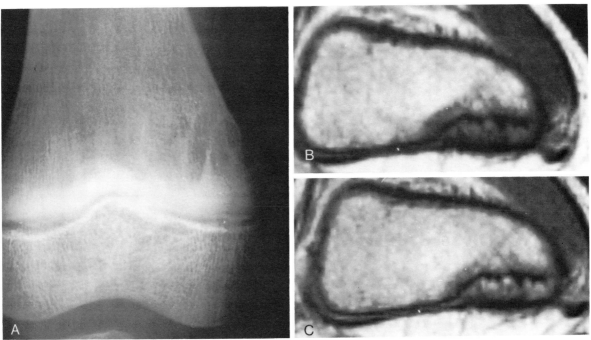

FIGURE 83–174. Nonossifying fibroma (fibrous cortical defect): MR imaging abnormalities—long tubular bones.
  A Routine radiography reveals a septated, radiolucent lesion in the femoral metaphysis.
  B, C Transaxial T1-weighted (TR/TE, 500/40) **(B)** and proton density–weighted (TR/TE, 1500/40) **(C)** spin echo MR images reveal an eccentric location of this lesion, which is of increased signal intensity in **C**. (Courtesy of M. Solomon, San Jose, California.)

FIGURE 83–175. Nonossifying fibroma (fibrous cortical defect): MR imaging abnormalities—long tubular bones.
  A Tibia. A coronal T1-weighted (TR/TE, 600/25) spin echo MR image in this 18 year old boy documents an elongated eccentric lesion (arrow) in the lateral aspect of the tibia. It is sharply defined and of low signal intensity. It remained of low signal intensity in T2-weighted spin echo MR images. (Courtesy of A. Peck, M.D., Portland, Oregon.)
  B, C Femur. Multiple eccentric lesions (arrows) in the distal femoral metaphysis are well delineated in transaxial T1-weighted (TR/TE, 400/20) **(B)** and T2-weighted (TR/TE, 2000/80) **(C)** spin echo MR images in this 14 year old boy. One of the lesions shows an increase in signal intensity in **C**. (Courtesy of P. VanderStoep, M.D., St. Cloud, Minnesota.)

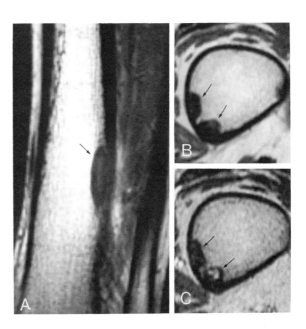

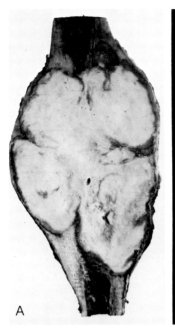
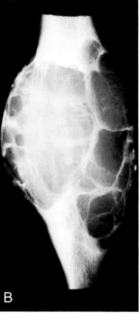

FIGURE 83–176. Nonossifying fibroma: Macroscopic abnormalities.

A A longitudinal section of a nonossifying fibroma in the fibula reveals that the well-marginated lesion involves the entire transverse diameter of the bone with expansion of the cortical surfaces. It still is covered by an intact periosteum. The tumor is solid, with a uniform cream-yellow color.

B A radiograph of the specimen in **A** shows the honeycomb appearance of the lesion that resulted from residual trabeculae.

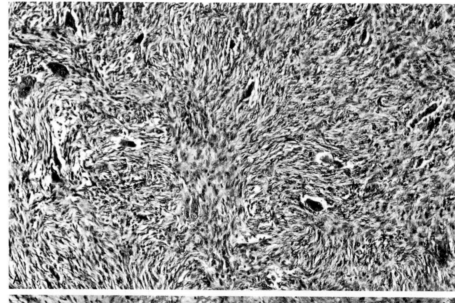

FIGURE 83–177. Nonossifying fibroma: Microscopic abnormalities.

A Note spindle-shaped fibroblasts arranged in a storiform pattern. Small, multinucleated osteoclast-type giant cells are distributed throughout the lesion (150 ×.)

B Clusters of bland-appearing foam cells are located between interlacing bands of fibroblasts. (150 ×.)

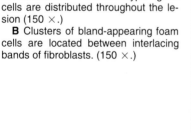

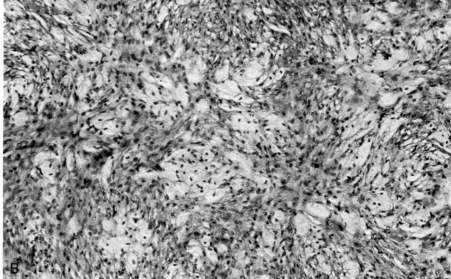

fibromas are larger lesions, usually between 3 and 9 cm in size. Even when larger than this, nonossifying fibromas generally do not extend completely across the diameter of the bone except in thin bones, such as the fibula, in which fusiform enlargement of the osseous contour may be seen (Fig. 83–176). Nonossifying fibromas are soft or rubbery and yellow with scattered tan or brown regions.

Both fibrous cortical defects and nonossifying fibromas have an identical histomorphology. They are composed of uniform, benign-appearing, spindle-shaped fibroblasts that are arranged in intersecting bands, creating a whorled or storiform pattern (Fig. 83–177A). Scattered within this fibrous stroma are multinucleated giant cells. Foam cells occur in 30 to 50 per cent of cases and are more common in older lesions (Fig. 83–177B). Cholesterol crystals and hemosiderin pigment also may be identified. Little or no mitotic activity is present. Occasionally foci of metaplastic bone or osteoid are evident, perhaps reflecting a reparative process following infraction.[30, 831] Stromal hemorrhage is frequent, and the occurrence of osteoclast giant cells about the hemorrhagic areas may simulate the appearance of a giant cell reparative granuloma.[832]

Natural History. It must be emphasized that fibrous cortical defects and nonossifying fibromas are to be considered benign processes. In many instances, an orderly sequence of evolution and involution occurs, although serial roentgenographic examinations are required for its documentation.[833, 2170] The initially small radiolucent lesions arising in the metaphysis may enlarge (Fig. 83–178), migrate shaftward, shrink, develop sclerotic borders (beginning in their diaphyseal aspect), and finally disappear, although this sequence is not uniform, nor is the duration of the natural life of these tumors constant.[805] The relative infrequency of fibrous cortical defects and nonossifying fibromas in the mature skeleton compared with those in the immature skeleton, however, supports their typically self-limited nature. Modifications in this behavior include a persistent potential to grow in a slow or rapid fashion[834] and disappearance with subsequent recurrence(s) of the lesion.[811] It generally is accepted that fibrous cortical defects and nonossifying fibromas do not appear for the first time in adults.[805] Furthermore, multiple, symmetric fibrous cortical defects in paired bones (e.g., femora) of a single person exhibit striking constancy in their rates of formation, regression, and recurrence when comparison is made between the two sides of the body, although those defects in one particular bone tend to behave independently with respect to those in a different bone.[805]

What is clear is that the lability of cortical defects and nonossifying fibromas and their tendencies to undergo sudden or gradual expansion, subdivision, multiplication, and recurrence may be misleading from the standpoint of prognosis.[805] Although reports exist of malignant transformation of a fibrous cortical defect or nonossifying fibroma,[835] they are subject to criticism. Similarly, although an association of these lesions with malignant neoplasms of bone has been

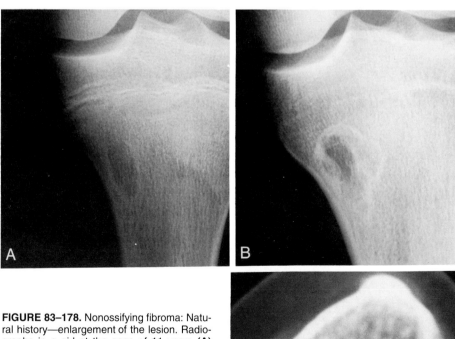

FIGURE 83–178. Nonossifying fibroma: Natural history—enlargement of the lesion. Radiographs in a girl at the ages of 11 years **(A)** and 14 years **(B)** reveal an enlarging nonossifying fibroma in the tibia. In both radiographs, the lesion reveals geographic bone destruction; in **B,** a thicker sclerotic margin is evident. A transaxial CT scan **(C)** obtained at the same time as **B** reveals the posteriorly located, multilocular lesion with a thick rim of bone sclerosis.

described,[836–839] this phenomenon probably occurs by chance alone. Ultimately, fibrous cortical defects and nonossifying fibromas should be regarded as benign conditions.

Complications. Although infrequent, several potential complications of fibrous cortical defects and nonossifying fibromas should be noted.

Pathologic Fracture. The occurrence of pathologic fractures through larger nonossifying fibromas is well documented.[824, 825, 840–842] This complication may be seen following minor trauma and is observed most frequently in the bones of the lower extremity (Fig. 83–179), especially the tibia but also the femur and the fibula; in the upper extremity, the humerus is affected most commonly. Such fractures generally heal in a normal fashion.[816] On the basis of an analysis of 23 patients with pathologic fractures through nonossifying fibromas, Arata and colleagues[843] concluded that those lesions in bones other than the fibula that were less than 33 mm long and occupied less than 50 per cent of the width of the bone were not likely to fracture, and that those lesions in the fibula that led to fracture might be smaller. Cortical defects rarely fracture.[1906, 1907]

Osteomalacia and Rickets. As indicated in Chapter 53, hypophosphatemic vitamin D–refractory rickets and osteomalacia have been associated with a variety of soft tissue and osseous neoplasms, both in children and in adults. Nonossifying fibroma represents one of the bone neoplasms that can lead to these conditions.[844, 845] In patients with oncogenic osteomalacia or rickets, hypophosphatemia is believed to be caused by a humoral substance elaborated by the tumor that decreases the threshold for renal reabsorption of phosphorus,[846] although the hypothetical substance has

yet to be characterized and its mode of action is a matter of speculation.[845] Of great importance, the findings of rickets or osteomalacia disappear following removal of the tumor.

Extraskeletal Anomalies (Jaffe-Campanacci Syndrome). In 1983, Campanacci and collaborators[847] described a syndrome consisting of multiple nonossifying fibromas (at least three) and extraskeletal congenital anomalies, including café-au-lait spots, mental retardation, hypogonadism or cryptorchidism, ocular abnormalities, and cardiovascular malformations. Some of these findings, such as café-au-lait spots, had previously been associated with multiple nonossifying fibromas by Jaffe,[754] leading to the designation of the Jaffe-Campanacci syndrome for this constellation of abnormalities.[832] Radiographically, large, osteolytic lesions are observed in the long tubular bones (Fig. 83–180); although these usually involve the metaphysis and diaphysis, as in ordinary nonossifying fibromas, epiphyseal localization also is encountered.[847] When widely disseminated with bilateral alterations, symmetry of involvement is the rule. In general, the natural history of the skeletal abnormalities is characterized by spontaneous resolution, although aggressive behavior of the lesions and pathologic fractures may be seen.[2171]

The precise relationship of this condition to neurofibromatosis is not clear.[1840, 2172, 2173] Although such a relationship has been suggested by some investigators,[847] others[832] indicate that no clinical or pathologic evidence of neurofibromas can be found in affected patients. The histopathology of the osseous lesions also is not clear. The observation that additional areas of osteolysis in these patients may occur in the bones of the jaw and that such lesions resemble giant

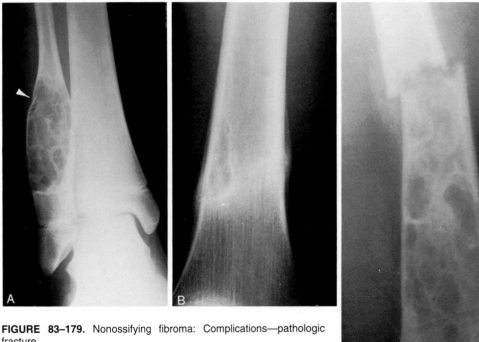

FIGURE 83–179. Nonossifying fibroma: Complications—pathologic fracture.

   A Fibula. A subtle depression of the cortical surface (arrowhead) is indicative of a fracture through this nonossifying fibroma.

   B Femur. A subacute fracture through a small nonossifying fibroma is associated with periostitis.

   C Femur. A subacute, transverse pathologic fracture has occurred at the superior margin of a large nonossifying fibroma. Periostitis is evident.

   (**B,** Courtesy of M. Dalinka, M.D., Philadelphia, Pennsylvania.)

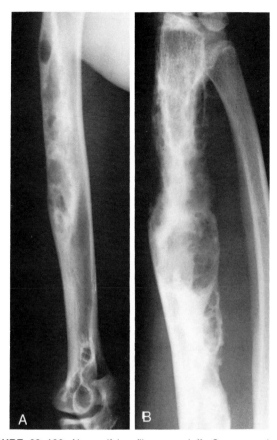

FIGURE 83–180. Nonossifying fibromas: Jaffe-Campanacci syndrome. Note eccentric radiolucent lesions of variable size involving the humerus **(A)** and ipsilateral radius **(B).** (Courtesy of P. Ellenbogen, M.D., Dallas, Texas.)

cell reparative granulomas suggests a relationship between these granulomas and nonossifying fibromas of bone.[832]

Multiple nonossifying fibromas may occur in the absence of café-au-lait spots and extraskeletal anomalies.[2174] The lesions may be large and distributed symmetrically. Such cases should be considered as distinct from the Jaffe-Campanacci syndrome.

Periosteal (Juxtacortical) Desmoid

As discussed in Chapter 90, a periosteal desmoid represents a tumor-like alteration of the periosteum characterized by fibroblastic proliferation analogous to that which occurs in a desmoplastic fibroma (see later discussion). It usually is apparent in patients between the ages of 15 and 20 years and may show a slight male predilection. Almost all cases are localized to the posteromedial cortex of the distal end of the femur, adjacent to the femoral condyle.[848–850] Most patients are asymptomatic, although mild pain occasionally is present.[2175] A history of local trauma is frequent. The radiographic characteristics (Fig. 83–181) of a periosteal desmoid include soft tissue swelling and a saucer-like defect of the cortex with adjacent sclerosis and periostitis. The periosteal response can be exuberant and irregular in outline, leading to an appearance which, for the radiologist unfamiliar with the lesion, might be mistaken for a malignant tumor (Fig. 83–181A).

The periosteal desmoid probably is not a neoplasm but a reaction to trauma occurring at the musculotendinous inser-

tion site of the adductor magnus muscle or, less commonly, of the medial head of the gastrocnemius muscle (Fig. 83–181B,C). MR imaging may be used to define the relationship of the osseous lesion and adjacent musculature (Fig. 83–181).

Desmoplastic Fibroma

This is a rare benign neoplasm of bone, originally described by Jaffe[754] in 1958, that is characterized by abundant collagen formation and the absence of both significant cellularity and pleomorphism.[33] The histologic characteristics of this lesion resemble those in soft tissue desmoids, central fibromas and nonodontogenic fibromas of the jaws, juvenile aponeurotic fibromas, and, in some cases, low grade fibrosarcomas.

Clinical Abnormalities. The clinical characteristics of these neoplasms have been defined in only a limited number of reports, most confined to descriptions of one or two patients.[851–874, 1841, 1842, 2176–2181, 2471] Desmoplastic fibromas are most common in the second and third decades of life, with approximately 75 per cent of tumors occurring in patients below the age of 30 years. Men and women are affected with equal frequency. Pain and swelling of weeks to months in duration are the major clinical manifestations, and patients may have a pathologic fracture as a presenting feature, a finding that is present in about 10 per cent of cases.

Skeletal Location. Desmoplastic fibromas most typically arise in the mandible,[1908] long tubular bones (femur, humerus, tibia, and radius), and innominate bone (ilium).[2510] Less frequent sites of involvement are the maxilla, scapula, vertebrae, ulna, fibula, clavicle, and ribs; the small bones of the hand and foot rarely are affected.[1842] In the tubular bones, a central location in the metaphysis is most characteristic, although a few examples of diaphyseal involvement are reported.[754, 856, 862, 872, 874] Epiphyseal extension of the neoplasm is unusual.[851, 855, 859, 874]

Radiographic Abnormalities. Desmoplastic fibromas are osteolytic lesions with a trabeculated, soap-bubble, or honeycomb pattern (Figs. 83–182 to 83–184). Endosteal erosion and limited periosteal bone formation may be accompanied by osseous expansion, with an appearance that may resemble that of nonossifying fibroma, chondromyxoid fibroma, giant cell tumor, aneurysmal bone cyst, or fibrous dysplasia. Although generally well-delineated, desmoplastic fibromas occasionally become large and possess a more aggressive appearance, with permeative bone destruction, irregular and coarse trabeculation, cortical erosion, soft tissue mass, and pathologic fracture. In these instances, the possibility of a malignant tumor (e.g., fibrosarcoma, skeletal metastasis from thyroid or renal carcinoma) may be considered on the basis of the radiographic alterations.

Pathologic Abnormalities. Macroscopically, the desmoplastic fibroma is variable in size, with some lesions measuring more than 10 cm in maximum dimension. It is white or gray in color (Fig. 83–185) and has a firm or rubbery consistency.[854, 856, 875] Although the tumor usually is solid and homogeneous, small cysts or slit-like spaces containing clear or yellow fluid are found occasionally.[180, 851, 854, 872] The lesion usually is separated easily from the bone. The cortex is thin, expanded, and, in some cases, completely eroded with tumor extension into the soft tissues.

Histologically, desmoplastic fibroma may be considered

Text continued on page 3780

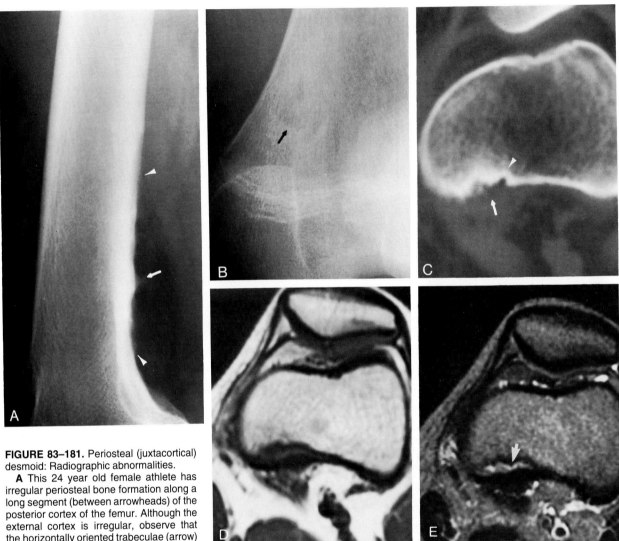

FIGURE 83–181. Periosteal (juxtacortical) desmoid: Radiographic abnormalities.

A This 24 year old female athlete has irregular periosteal bone formation along a long segment (between arrowheads) of the posterior cortex of the femur. Although the external cortex is irregular, observe that the horizontally oriented trabeculae (arrow) that extend from the surface of the bone are thick, supporting the role of chronic stress as a causative factor.

B, C Routine radiography **(B)** and transaxial CT **(C)** in an athletic patient reveal an area of cortical osteolysis (arrows) with endosteal bone formation (arrowhead). This lesion has occurred at the osseous site of attachment of the medial head of the gastrocnemius muscle, supporting a traumatic pathogenesis.

(**B, C,** Courtesy of T. Goergen, M.D., San Diego, California.)

D, E In a third patient whose routine radiographs revealed a lesion similar to that in **B**, a transaxial T1-weighted (TR/TE, 400/20) spin echo MR image **(D)** and a transaxial T2-weighted (TR/TE, 4500/90) fast spin echo MR image obtained with fat suppression **(E)** reveal cortical irregularity in the posteromedial portion of the femur and, in **E**, high signal intensity (arrow) at the base of the lesion.

(**D, E,** Courtesy of D. Witte, M.D., Memphis, Tennessee.)

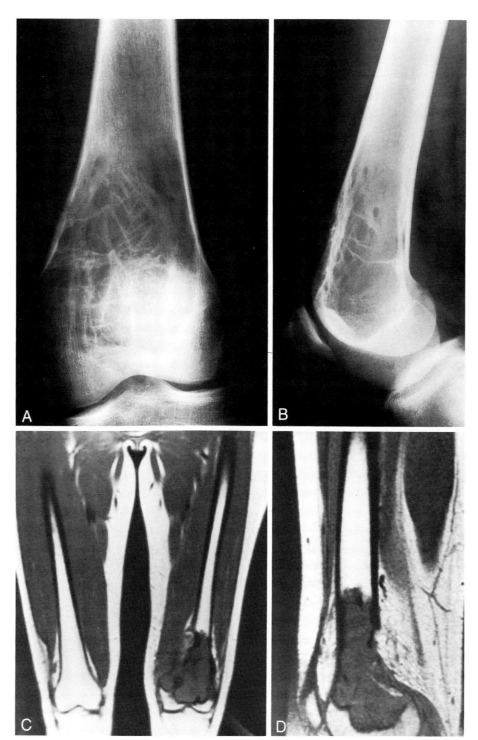

FIGURE 83–182. Desmoplastic fibroma: Radiographic abnormalities—long tubular bones.

A, B Anteroposterior **(A)** and lateral **(B)** radiographs of the femur in an 18 year old man reveal a large, trabeculated, osteolytic lesion in the metaphysis and diaphysis of the bone. The endosteal margin of the cortex is eroded and there is minimal periosteal response. The relatively central location of this lesion is more compatible with desmoplastic fibroma than with nonossifying fibroma or chondromyxoid fibroma.

C, D In a different patient, a 23 year old woman with a desmoplastic fibroma in almost an identical location, coronal **(C)** and sagittal **(D)** T1-weighted (TR/TE, 600/20) spin echo MR images show a large lesion with decreased signal intensity. The cortex is eroded. In T2-weighted spin echo MR images, which are not shown, an increase in signal intensity was observed.

(Courtesy of W. Peck, M.D., Orange, California.)

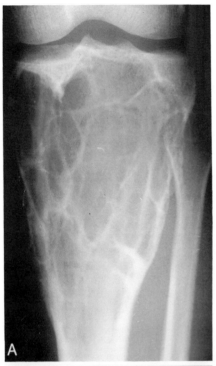

FIGURE 83–183. Desmoplastic fibroma: Radiographic abnormalities—long tubular bones.

A Tibia. This osteolytic lesion involving the metaphyseal and epiphyseal segments of the bone possesses coarse trabeculae. (Courtesy of B. Flanagan, M.D., Los Angeles, California.)

B, C Radius. In this child, the routine radiograph **(B)** demonstrates an eccentric metaphyseal and diaphyseal lesion with thick trabeculae. In a sagittal T2-weighted (TR/TE, 2000/70) spin echo MR image **(C),** inhomogeneous signal intensity, including linear regions of low signal intensity, is seen. Note the expansile nature of the tumor. **(B, C** Courtesy of G. Gundry, M.D., Minneapolis, Minnesota.)

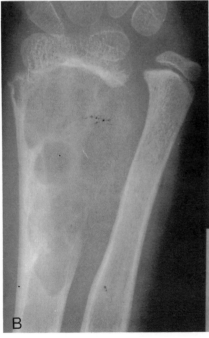

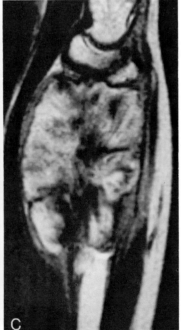

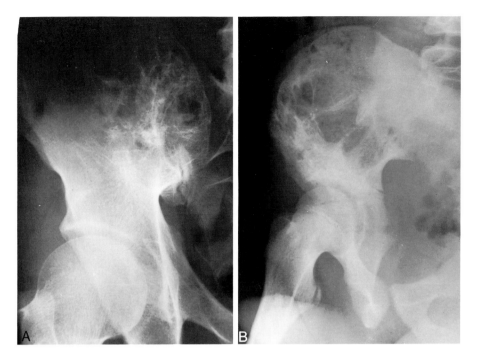

FIGURE 83–184. Desmoplastic fibroma: Radiographic abnormalities—flat bones. Two examples are shown of tumors in the ilium. Note the prominent trabeculation associated with the predominantly osteolytic lesions. (**A,** Courtesy of L. Yuan, M.D., St. Louis, Missouri; **B,** courtesy of W. Rosenau, M.D., San Francisco, California.)

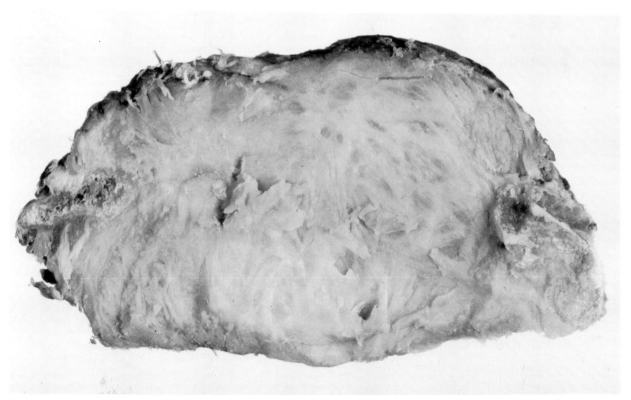

FIGURE 83–185. Desmoplastic fibroma: Macroscopic abnormalities. This mandibular lesion has been sectioned. Note its uniform surface and thick white bands of fibrous tissue that criss-cross the lesion. A portion of the destroyed mandible is present at the lower right area of the photograph.

to be the intraosseous counterpart of the soft tissue desmoid tumor. A typical lesion is composed of uniform, small, spindle-shaped fibroblasts that have oval or elongated nuclei.[754, 856, 857, 867] The cells lack any significant degree of hyperchromasia, pleomorphism, or atypia, and mitotic figures are either absent or extremely scarce.[180, 856, 867, 872] The cells are separated by an abundant, collagenized stroma in which dense collagen bands may be arranged in intersecting patterns (Fig. 83–186).

The degree of cellularity of desmoplastic fibromas is variable. In tumors in which hypercellularity is present, differentiation from a fibrosarcoma may be difficult.[34, 857] Fibrosarcoma typically is more cellular than desmoplastic fibroma, its component cells are larger, plumper, and hyperchromatic, and mitotic activity is more common. The fibroblasts of fibrosarcoma also may be arranged in a herringbone pattern, a feature not found in desmoplastic fibroma.[856] Similarly, with tumors in the mandible or maxilla, the distinction between odontogenic fibroma and desmoplastic fibroma may be extremely difficult.[876, 877] Desmoplastic fibroma rarely may arise in lesions of fibrous dysplasia.

Electron microscopy has revealed three principal cell types in desmoplastic fibromas: fibroblasts, myofibroblasts, and undifferentiated mesenchymal cells.[856, 869, 874, 875, 1842]

Natural History. Although tumor recurrence (with histologic features identical to those of the primary neoplasm) may be evident following conservative surgery,[875] wide resection of the lesion usually is curative.

Malignant Tumors

Fibrosarcoma

Fibrosarcoma, a rare malignant tumor of bone, is characterized histologically by poorly differentiated to well-differentiated fibrous tissue proliferation that is not associated with the production of cartilage, osteoid, or bone. Fibrosarcomas in bone can occur de novo or as a secondary phenomenon in areas of Paget's disease, osteonecrosis, or chronic osteomyelitis, following irradiation, or related to dedifferentiation of other neoplasms, especially chondrosarcoma.[30, 34, 878] An additional malignant tumor of bone, malignant fibrous histiocytoma (see later discussion), which contains both histiocytic and fibroblastic features, only recently has been differentiated from fibrosarcoma of bone, although it is certain that some of the previous descriptions of the latter tumor contained examples of malignant fibrous histiocytoma as well. Furthermore, the importance of distinguishing fibrosarcoma of bone from that of soft tissue relates, in part, to the poorer prognosis associated with the intraosseous neoplasm.[879]

Clinical Abnormalities. Fibrosarcomas of bone are observed in men and women with approximately equal frequency and are most common in the third, fourth, fifth, and sixth decades of life, although the age range of affected patients is wide, with documented examples of this tumor involving children[1843] as well as persons who are older than 80 years of age. Clinical manifestations include local pain, swelling, and limitation of motion, in order of decreasing frequency, which usually are of short duration (less than 6 months). Pathologic fractures are present at the time of the initial evaluation in approximately 33 per cent of patients.

Skeletal Location. The skeletal distribution of fibrosarcoma is similar to that of osteosarcoma and malignant fibrous histiocytoma.[30, 880, 881] The long tubular bones are involved in 70 per cent of cases; specific sites of involvement, in order of decreasing frequency, are the femur (40 per cent of cases), tibia (16 per cent), humerus (10 per cent), fibula (3 per cent), radius (1 per cent), and ulna (0.5 per cent).[30, 33, 34, 881–884] Those bones about the knee account for 33 to 80 per cent of fibrosarcomas.[880, 881, 885–887] The small bones of the hands and feet rarely are affected,[180, 888] and the osseous pelvis is involved in approximately 9 per cent of cases. The mandible (5 per cent of cases) and the maxilla (2 per cent of cases) are uncommon sites of fibrosarcomas,[889–893, 1877] and these tumors are rare in the skull in the absence of an underlying disorder such as Paget's disease or previous irradiation.[894, 895]

In the tubular bones, a metaphyseal or metadiaphyseal location is the preferred site.[884] Epiphyseal extension of a metaphyseal tumor is not infrequent.[881] Although fibrosarcomas are considered to arise as solitary tumors in the medullary bone, periosteal[896] and multifocal[897–899] lesions are described.

Radiographic Abnormalities. Fibrosarcomas are characterized radiographically by (1) osteolytic foci with a geographic, motheaten, or permeative pattern of bone destruction and, generally, a wide zone of transition between normal and abnormal bone, and (2) little osteosclerosis or periostitis[879] (Figs. 83–187 and 83–188). Indeed, the degree of bone destruction and the absence of significant osseous reaction can be striking. When present, periosteal bone formation is variable in appearance, revealing lamellar or spiculated patterns or a Codman's triangle.[900] Cortical destruction and soft tissue masses are seen. Visible tumor matrix is not evident, although dystrophic calcification and sequestered bone fragments may be encountered, perhaps related to pathologic fracture.

In the tubular bones, fibrosarcomas may be central or eccentric in position. It has been suggested that those tumors in the tubular bones that are eccentric in location, that exhibit a geographic pattern of bone destruction, and that involve only a portion of the cortex have a more favorable prognosis than those tumors that do not have these features.[900]

The radiographic abnormalities of fibrosarcomas of bone are not specific. Rather, they generally indicate an aggressive or malignant process. The absence of tumoral calcification or ossification in fibrosarcomas assumes diagnostic importance as such findings are evident in chondrosarcomas and conventional osteosarcomas. Malignant fibrous histiocytoma, telangiectatic osteosarcoma, lymphoma, plasma cell myeloma, desmoplastic fibroma, and skeletal metastasis remain reasonable differential diagnostic possibilities in many cases of fibrosarcoma, however. Although other imaging methods, such as scintigraphy, angiography, CT scanning, and MR imaging (Fig. 83–187), may provide information regarding the extent of the lesion or the presence of additional sites of involvement, they are unable to delineate features allowing specific diagnosis.

Pathologic Abnormalities. Fibrosarcomas are large (1.5 to 20 cm in size), destructive, and infiltrating tumors[180, 879, 885] (Fig. 83–189). Their macroscopic appearance depends on their size and histologic differentiation. Well-

Text continued on page 3785

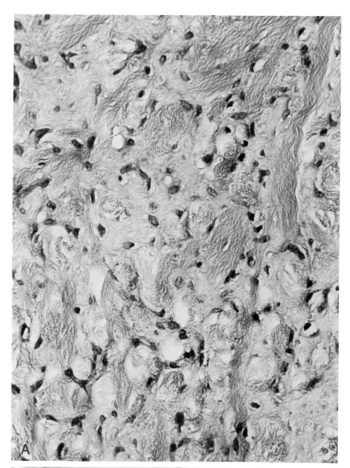

FIGURE 83–186. Desmoplastic fibroma: Microscopic abnormalities.

A Widely separated fibroblasts are present within an abundant fibrous stroma. Dense bands of collagen course through the lesion. (300×.)

B At higher magnification, note fibroblasts with bland, oval to spindle-shaped nuclei. Dense collagen bundles are present. (600×.)

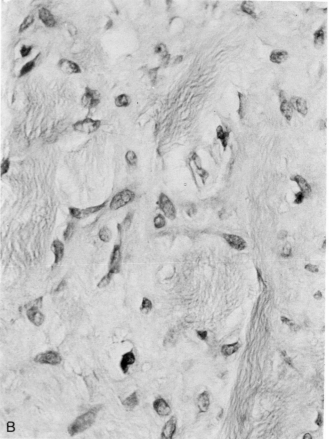

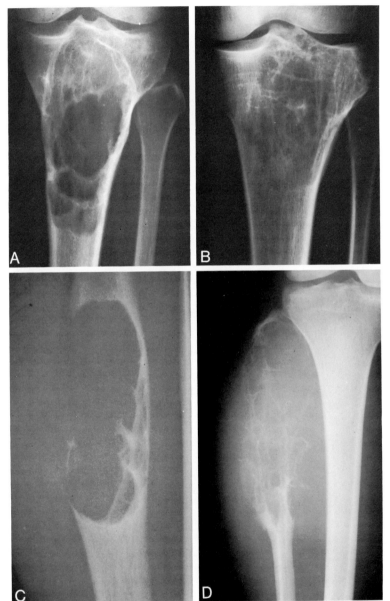

FIGURE 83–187. Fibrosarcoma: Radiographic abnormalities—long tubular bones.

A–C Tibia. Three examples are shown. The epiphyseal and metaphyseal segments **(A, B)** or the diaphyseal segment **(C)** is affected. The lesions are osteolytic and in these cases possess a pattern of geographic bone destruction. Note the relative absence of periostitis, particularly in **C.** Also in **C** observe a large tissue mass. (**A,** Courtesy of I. D. Wheeler, M.D., Flint, Michigan; **B,** courtesy of B. B. Harriman, M.D., Phoenixville, Pennsylvania.)

D Fibula. This lesion also is osteolytic, with a large soft tissue mass. A bizarre osseous response is apparent. (**D,** Courtesy of H. J. Linn, M.D., Royal Oak, Michigan.)

Illustration continued on opposite page

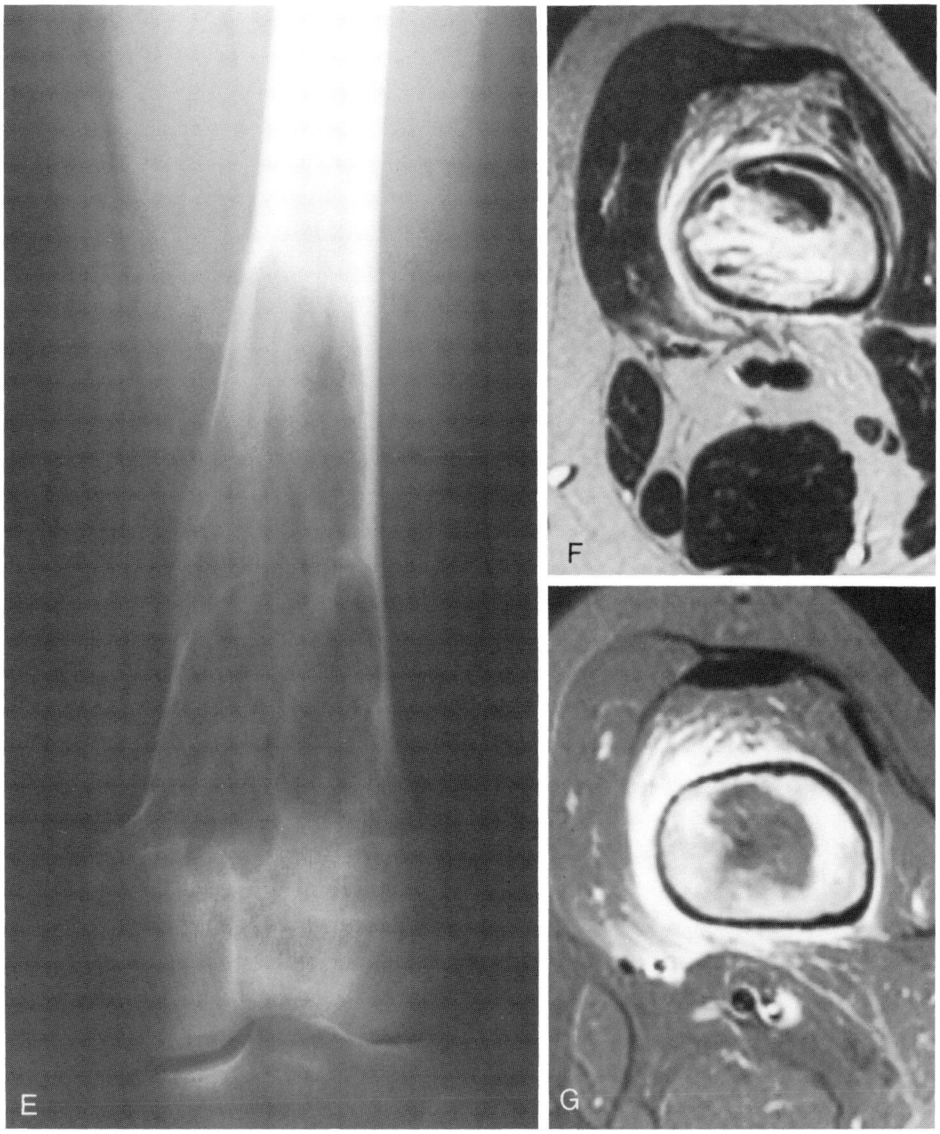

FIGURE 83–187 *Continued* **E–G**
Femur. In a 22 year old woman, the routine radiograph **(E)** shows a long osteolytic lesion of the metadiaphyseal portion of the femur. A transaxial T2-weighted (TR/TE, 2000/80) spin echo MR image **(F)** shows high signal intensity in the bone and surrounding soft tissue. The cortex is eroded. In a transaxial fat-suppressed T1-weighted (TR/TE, 583/12) spin echo MR image obtained after the intravenous injection of a gadolinium compound **(G)**, high signal intensity (representing enhancement) is evident in portions of the tumor. Similar high signal intensity is seen in the soft tissues, related to tumor, edema, or both.

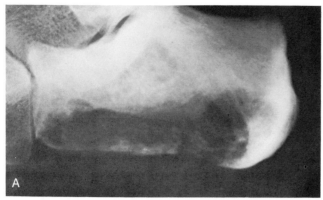

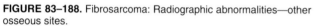

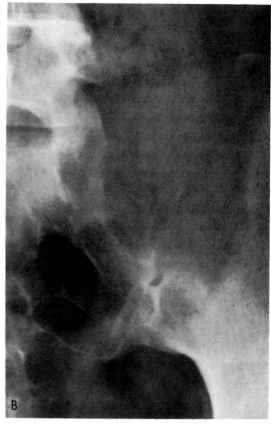

FIGURE 83–188. Fibrosarcoma: Radiographic abnormalities—other osseous sites.

A Calcaneus. A large osteolytic lesion involves the plantar aspect of the bone. Surrounding bone sclerosis is apparent. Periostitis is absent.

B Ilium and sacrum. An osteolytic lesion of both bones can be seen. No osseous reaction is identified.

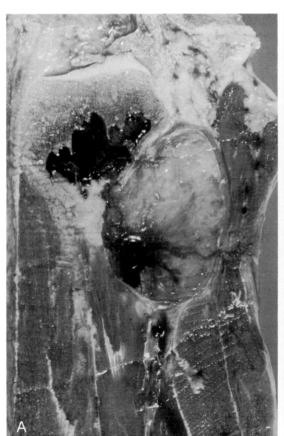

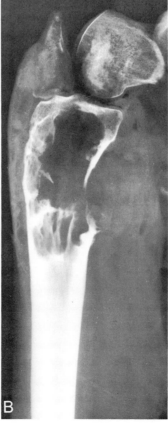

FIGURE 83–189. Fibrosarcoma: Macroscopic abnormalities. A photograph **(A)** and radiograph **(B)** of a section of the tibial tumor illustrated in Figure 83–187**A** reveal a large lesion that has extended through the posterior cortex. The adjacent soft tissue mass is homogeneous, with cystic, hemorrhagic degeneration. (Courtesy of I. D. Wheeler, M.D., Flint, Michigan.)

differentiated neoplasms produce more abundant collagen than do poorly differentiated tumors and are white or gray-white and firm, with a rubbery consistency. Poorly differentiated fibrosarcomas are softer, with a fleshy consistency and myxoid foci.[880, 881, 885, 896] Most fibrosarcomas are homogeneous, but very large tumors may have hemorrhagic and necrotic areas. They may appear pseudoencapsulated, facilitating their separation from the parent bone. Although electron microscopic studies may reveal occasional myofibroblasts, fibrosarcomas are a tumor of malignant fibroblasts. Histologically, fibrosarcomas may be categorized as well-differentiated, moderately differentiated, or poorly differentiated neoplasms[34, 180, 880, 883] or divided into four grades, I to IV, with the higher grades representing the less differentiated tumors.[884, 885, 888] Most of the criteria that are used for placement of the tumor in a specific category or grade are subjective and are based on an assessment of cellularity, mitotic activity, collagen production, nuclear morphology, and overall histologic pattern. As would be expected, however, patient survival rates are lower for the higher grade tumors. The majority of fibrosarcomas are either moderately or poorly differentiated.[28, 888]

Well-differentiated fibrosarcomas are composed of elongated and spindle-shaped tumor cells with small and uniform tapered nuclei (Fig. 83–190A,B). The cytoplasm usually is poorly defined, with indistinct borders. Intercellular collagen formation may be so abundant that the tumor may be interpreted as a desmoplastic fibroma.[881, 888] The tumor cells characteristically are arranged in intersecting fascicles, producing a herringbone pattern (Fig. 83–190C). Rarely, a storiform configuration, as in malignant fibrous histiocytoma, is evident.[28, 884, 888] In less well differentiated fibrosarcomas, there is increased cellularity, with the cells being more closely arranged, and a corresponding decrease in the amount of collagen. The nuclei are larger, ovoid or round, and more irregular. The chromatin is coarse, clumped, and more irregularly distributed. Nucleoli are more common and more prominent, and mitotic activity is increased. The herringbone pattern is less evident and may be absent. Necrosis and hemorrhage are more common in the poorly differentiated fibrosarcomas.

The histologic features of fibrosarcoma must be distinguished from those of nonossifying fibroma, fibrous dysplasia, desmoplastic fibroma, malignant fibrous histiocytoma, fibroblastic osteosarcoma, and metastatic spindle cell carcinoma.

Natural History. Osseous fibrosarcomas are aggressive tumors with a tendency for one or more recurrences. The rate of such recurrence as well as the likelihood of patient survival correlates with the histologic grade of the neoplasm. Fibrosarcomas of bone carry a poorer prognosis than those of soft tissue and are similar in behavior to malignant fibrous histiocytomas.[880, 883]

HISTIOCYTIC OR FIBROHISTIOCYTIC TUMORS

Benign Tumors

Fibrous Histiocytoma

Fibrous histiocytoma (fibroxanthoma) (Fig. 83–191) is a term that has been used to describe a benign tumor of bone that histologically is similar or identical to nonossifying

fibroma. Its existence as a separate lesion is not accepted uniformly. Those investigators who distinguish between fibrous histiocytoma and nonossifying fibroma emphasize their different clinical manifestations.[30, 33, 901–903, 1909, 2182–2184] Almost all of the reported fibrous histiocytomas have occurred in patients older than 20 years of age, and many are accompanied by pain, localize in the sacrum or ilium, and involve epiphyseal and diaphyseal segments of the tubular bones; nonossifying fibromas are virtually confined to patients younger than 20 years of age, are painless, and predominate in the metaphyseal regions of tubular bones.[904] Those investigators who consider fibrous histiocytoma and nonossifying fibroma to be identical tumors emphasize a histiocytic origin common to both lesions.[810]

Destouet and collaborators[902] provided a comprehensive literature review of previously described lesions that could be considered fibrous histiocytomas of bone. The designations applied to these lesions were variable and, in addition to fibrous histiocytoma and nonossifying fibroma, included xanthofibroma, fibroxanthoma, xanthoma, and xanthogranuloma.[817, 818, 820, 824, 905] Analysis of these cases as well as those that have appeared subsequently indicates that fibrous histiocytomas are most frequent in the innominate and long tubular bones, ribs, and clavicle, although other sites, such as the mandible, spine, and scapula, may be affected. Multifocal lesions occurring in association with a giant cell tumor have been observed in a single patient.[2185] The radiographic findings are variable and not diagnostic; osteolysis, trabeculation and bone sclerosis are seen, and the resulting radiographic pattern may resemble that in nonossifying fibroma, fibrous dysplasia, enchondroma, eosinophilic granuloma, osteoblastoma, and chondromyxoid fibroma.

The importance of defining the true nature of fibrous histiocytoma is underscored by occasional descriptions in which the lesion behaves in an aggressive fashion, with a potential for local spread and distant dissemination.[30]

Locally Aggressive Tumors

Giant Cell Tumor*

This relatively common and locally aggressive lesion is composed of connective tissue, stromal cells, and giant cells, which vary in amount and appearance. It is the giant cell itself from which the name of this lesion is derived, but such cells are not specific for a giant cell tumor, being observed in a large number of neoplastic and non-neoplastic skeletal disorders (Table 83–3). Initial descriptions of bone tumors placed great emphasis on giant cells, leading to the classification as a giant cell tumor of nearly every lesion that contained such cells. The result was the consolidation of a heterogeneous group of neoplasms with widely varying clinical, radiographic, and prognostic features.[906] In 1940, Jaffe and colleagues[907] began a systematic analysis of those lesions that contained giant cells and, by emphasizing additional histologic features, were able, during the next 10 years, to define the specific characteristics of a giant cell tumor and to separate this neoplasm from other giant cell–containing tumors and tumor-like lesions, such as nonossifying fibroma, aneurysmal bone cyst, and chondroblastoma.

---

*The placement of giant cell tumor in this portion of the chapter is done in an arbitrary fashion as the precise origin of this lesion is not clear.

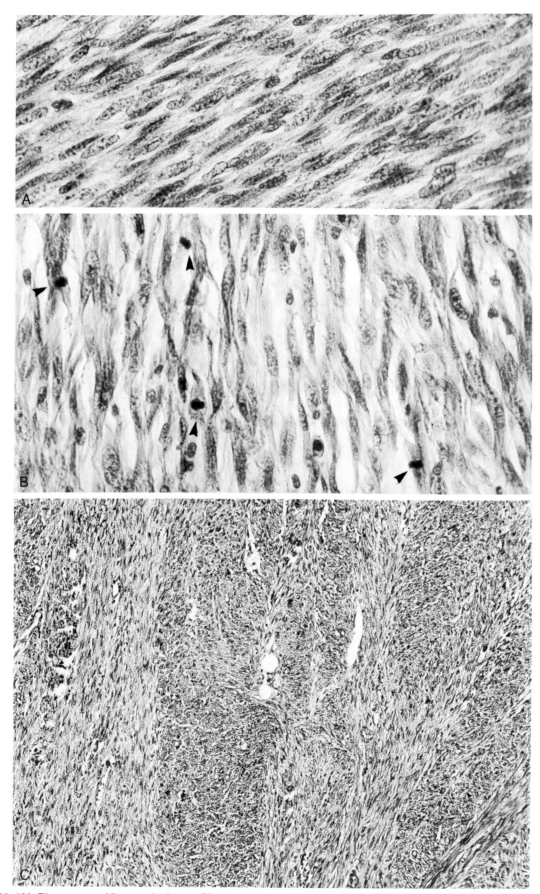

FIGURE 83–190. Fibrosarcoma: Microscopic abnormalities.

A Observe spindle-shaped fibroblasts with elongated nuclei and a fine chromatin pattern. The cytoplasmic borders are poorly defined. (600×.)

B Numerous mitotic figures are seen (arrowheads). This degree of mitotic activity combined with the cellularity and atypia of the nuclei helps distinguish a fibrosarcoma from a desmoplastic fibroma. (600×.)

C The herringbone pattern is shown, characterized by the presence of intersecting fascicles. (150×.)

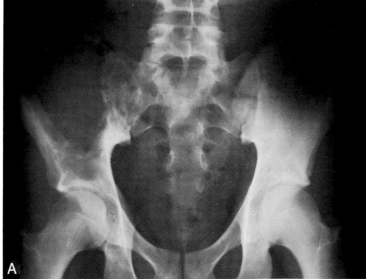

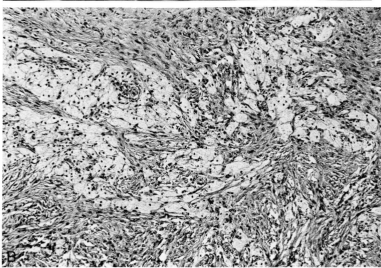

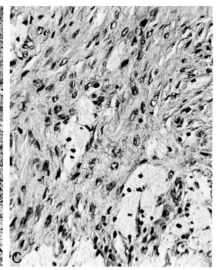

FIGURE 83–191. Fibrous histiocytoma: Radiographic and histologic abnormalities.
  A A large, osteolytic lesion of the ilium is associated with sclerosis in the inferior aspect of the bone adjacent to the sacroiliac joint. The radiographic findings are not specific. (Courtesy of H.F. Holman, M.D., Maryville, Illinois.)
  B, C Bland foam cells are scattered within a fibrous stroma. The lesion is histologically similar to a nonossifying fibroma. (150×, 350×.)

The description of osteoblastoma provided by Dahlin and Johnson[130] in 1954 represented another important step in the isolation and classification of various neoplasms that contain giant cells.

In most situations, the giant cell appears to be a multinucleated macrophage that works in conjunction with mononuclear macrophages and lymphocytes as an important part of the cell-mediated immune system to protect the host from invasive and potentially destructive antigens.[906] Giant cells are identified as a histologic component of the body's reaction to the stimulus provided by a foreign object, crystalline material (such as monosodium urate), infectious agents (such as mycobacteria and fungi), abnormal levels of hormones (such as the excess of parathyroid hormone that occurs in hyperparathyroidism), and neoplasms, of which giant cell tumor is but one. Attempts to identify specific staining techniques that would allow the pathologist to differentiate among these diverse stimuli generally have been unrewarding.[908]

Although there is general agreement that successful classification of those neoplasms containing giant cells depends on histologic evaluation of the stromal tissue rather than the giant cells themselves, the issue of whether such cells are true tumor cells or host-response macrophages is less clear. Data provided by investigations using tissue culture media and immunofluorescence generally support a non-neoplastic origin of the giant cells.[906] The specific stimulus that provokes the proliferation and accumulation of such cells in giant cell tumors also is not known, although the identification of paramyxovirus-like filamentous intranuclear inclusions in these tumors (in patients without Paget's disease of bone) is of interest.[909–911] Similar inclusions have been described in the osteoclasts in Paget's disease of bone and in the giant cells of the giant cell tumors that are associated with this disease (see Chapter 54). As, to date, no firm evidence exists to implicate paramyxoviruses in oncogenesis, the presence of these inclusions in giant cell tumors does not necessarily indicate a direct cause-and-effect relationship between them and the tumor but rather may indicate that giant cells are carriers of the virus-like particles.[911]

Clinical Abnormalities. Giant cell tumors usually are discovered in the third and fourth decades of life (60 to 70 per cent of all tumors), although they may appear in older patients and in younger patients who have not yet ceased growing.[912–921, 2186, 2187] The frequency of giant cell tumors is greater in women than in men.

TABLE 83–3. Differential Diagnosis of Giant Cell Lesions of Bone*

	Most Common Age Group	Location in Bone	Radiologic Appearance	Gross Features	Microscopic Features	
					Giant Cells	Stromal Cells
Giant cell tumor	Third and fourth decades	Epiphysis or metaphysis	Eccentric expanded radiolucent area	Fleshy soft tissue	Abundant number uniformly distributed	Plump and polyhedral cells with abundant cytoplasm
Nonossifying fibroma	First decade	Metaphysis	Eccentric oval defects	Fleshy soft tissue	Focal distribution, small with few nuclei	Slender and spindly cells with little cytoplasm; whorled pattern
Aneurysmal bone cyst	First and second decades	Vertebral column or metaphysis of long bone	Eccentric blow-out "soap bubble" appearance	Cavity filled with blood	Focal around vascular channels or hemorrhage	Large vascular channels; slender to plump cells with hemosiderin granules; metaplastic bone
Brown tumor of hyper-parathyroid-ism	Any age	Anywhere in bone	Subperiosteal, subchondral, and subligamentous resorption of bone	Fleshy tissue or cystic spaces	Focal around hemosiderin pigment or hemorrhage	Fibrous stroma with slender spindle cells
Simple bone cyst	First and second decades	Metaphysis	Trabeculations in radiolucent area	Cyst filled with clear fluid	Focal around cholesterol clefts	Cyst wall of fibrous tissue; metaplastic bone
Chondro-blastoma	Second decade	Epiphysis	Radiolucency with spotty opacities	Firm to fleshy tissue	Few and focal	Plump, and round or ovoid cells with pericellular calcifications
Fibrous dysplasia	First and second decades	Metaphysis	Ground-glass appearance	Firm and gritty	Few and focal	Woven bone and whorled fibrous tissue; no osteoblasts
Giant cell reparative granuloma	Second and third decades	Maxilla and mandible	Radiolucent focus	Soft fleshy tissue	Focal around hemosiderin pigment or hemorrhage	Slender or plump spindle cells
Ossifying fibroma	Second and third decades	Maxilla and mandible	Radiopaque	Firm and gritty	Few and focal	Lamellar bony trabeculae in fibrous tissue; osteoblastic rimming
Osteosarcoma	Second and third decades	Metaphysis	Radiolucent	Soft, firm, or hard	Focal distribution	Malignant cells with direct osteoid formation
Chondromyx-oid fibroma	Second and third decades	Metaphysis	Eccentric with expanded cortex	Soft to firm	Focal distribution	Chondroid, myxoid, and fibrous lobules
Osteoblastoma	Second and third decades	Vertebral column; diaphysis of long bone	Radiolucent or dense	Hemorrhagic, gritty	Focal distribution	Abundant osteoid trabeculae with osteoblasts

*Modified from Ghandur-Mnaymneh L, Mnaymneh WA: J Med Liban 25:91, 1972.

Pain is the most common symptom, followed in order of frequency by local swelling and limitation of motion in the adjacent articulation. The pain generally is of several months' duration, is not severe, and is aggravated by activity and relieved by bedrest. A pathologic fracture with an abrupt onset or aggravation of pain and swelling may be evident at the time of clinical presentation in approximately 10 per cent of patients. Neurologic symptoms may accompany spinal or sacral lesions.

Tenderness to palpation is a consistent physical finding. Muscle atrophy and a decreased range of joint motion also may be evident during the clinical examination.

Skeletal Location. Giant cell tumors predominate in the long tubular bones (75 to 90 per cent of all cases), especially the femur (approximately 30 per cent of cases), tibia (25 per cent of cases), radius (10 per cent of cases), and humerus (6 per cent of cases).[913, 915–919] The distal portions of the femur and radius and the proximal portion of the tibia are the most characteristic sites of involvement (approximately 50 per cent of cases). The bones about the knee are affected in 50 to 65 per cent of giant cell tumors. These neoplasms arise more commonly in the bones of the lower extremity than in those of the upper extremity, in a ratio of about 3 to 1.

The spine (7 per cent of cases) and innominate bone (4 per cent of cases), particularly the ilium, are involved occasionally.[2428] In the vertebral column, it is the sacrum that is the most typical site of localization; giant cell tumors arising at spinal levels above the sacrum are uncommon and involve, in order of decreasing frequency, the thoracic, cervical, and lumbar vertebrae.[922–928, 2188, 2189]

Giant cell tumors are relatively rare in the skull, although, when present, they most typically arise in the sphenoid and temporal bones.[929–931] As giant cell tumors more commonly occur in bones that develop by endochondral ossification, their relative absence in the cranial bones (which, in large part, are derived from intramembranous ossification) is not surprising.[930, 931] In the skull and the facial bones, giant cell tumors may be accompanied by

Paget's disease (see Chapter 54) and, furthermore, in these locations, the identification of a giant cell tumor is complicated by the occurrence of a similar lesion, the giant cell reparative granuloma (see later discussion).[932–939]

Approximately 5 per cent of giant cell tumors localize in the bones of the hands or, less commonly, the feet.[940–944, 1910, 2190, 2191, 2472] In the hand and wrist, metacarpal involvement predominates, followed closely by involvement of the phalanges (especially the proximal phalanx) and less closely by that of the carpal bones. In the foot, sites of involvement, in order of decreasing frequency, are the tarsal bones, metatarsal bones, and phalanges.

Rarely, giant cell tumors occur in other locations, includ-

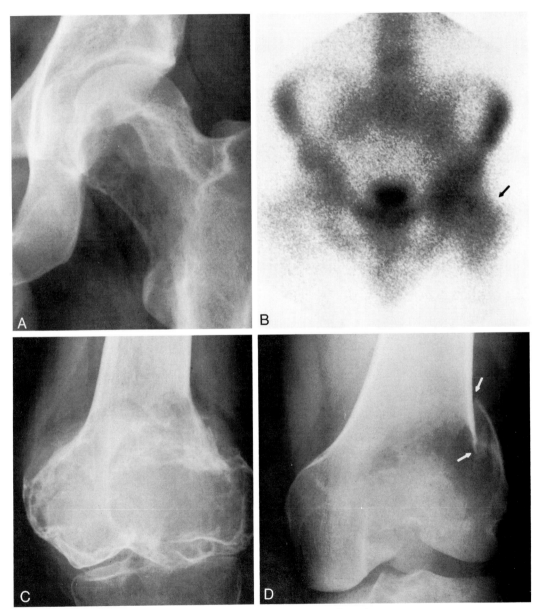

FIGURE 83–192. Giant cell tumor: Radiographic abnormalities—long tubular bones (femur).

A, B In a 29 year old man, the routine radiograph **(A)** reveals an eccentric, osteolytic lesion involving the metaphysis and epiphysis in the proximal portion of the femur. At this time, it does not extend to the subchondral bone. Bone scintigraphy **(B)** shows increased accumulation of the radionuclide at the site of the lesion (arrow).

C In a second patient, note a large, trabeculated, osteolytic lesion involving the metaphysis and epiphysis of the distal portion of the femur. It extends to the subchondral region. The bone is expanded, and there is collapse of the articular surface.

D Following a fall, this 29 year old man suffered a pathologic fracture (arrows) through an eccentric osteolytic lesion in the distal portion of the femur.

ing the ribs, scapula, patella, clavicle, ulna, ischium, and sternum.[945–947, 2192–2194]

In the *tubular bones,* giant cell tumors had long been considered an epiphyseal lesion, although, more recently, a metaphyseal origin has been emphasized.[1911] In either case, however, the presence of extensive epiphyseal involvement (as well as that of the metaphysis) at the time of initial evaluation is fundamental to correct identification of the tumor. As the vast majority of giant cell tumors occur in patients who are skeletally mature, with closed physeal plates, the combination of epiphyseal and metaphyseal components of the tumor does not firmly support the origin in one segment of the bone as opposed to the other. More helpful in the evaluation of tumor origin is the analysis of those relatively uncommon giant cell tumors that occur in the immature bones of the child or adolescent. In these instances, metaphyseal localization (with or without subsequent transphyseal spread) has been documented repeatedly,[948–951] with only rare descriptions of isolated epiphyseal involvement.[952, 953] Indeed, purely metaphyseal giant cell tumors occasionally have been encountered in skeletally mature patients.[30, 913, 915, 916, 919, 920] Very rarely, diaphyseal giant cell tumors are seen, usually in the femur or tibia.[954, 955, 2195, 2196]

Despite the controversy regarding the epiphyseal or metaphyseal origin of giant cell tumors, the importance of epiphyseal involvement with extension to subchondral bone in the accurate diagnosis of these tumors is undeniable. The localization of giant cell tumors in subchondral regions in flat or irregular bones, such as the sternum, clavicle, scapula, ribs, and innominate bone, also can provide a decisive diagnostic clue.

Multicentric giant cell tumors are well documented and are discussed in a later section of this chapter.

Radiographic Abnormalities. The radiographic appearance of a giant cell tumor is highly characteristic. In a long tubular bone (Figs. 83–192 to 83–196), an eccentric osteolytic lesion extending to the subchondral bone is seen, producing cortical thinning and expansion, and possessing a delicate trabecular pattern.[2197, 2198] The margins of the lesion may be well or poorly defined, although an extensive sclerotic rim and periostitis generally are not evident. Involvement of a portion of the metaphysis also is characteristic, and, as indicated previously, isolated metaphyseal lesions may be encountered in the child or adolescent. Similarly, extension of the tumor into the diaphysis commonly is evident. The aggressive nature of giant cell tumors is underscored not only by their potentially large intraosseous components but also by their violation of the cortical surface and spread into the adjacent soft tissues. It should be emphasized, however, that the radiographic characteristics generally are a poor guide to the histologic composition and clinical behavior of the lesion. Therefore, attempts to classify or grade the radiographic abnormalities[956] usually are not successful in defining the subsequent course of the tumor.

In the short tubular bones of the hands (Fig. 83–197) and feet, the radiographic features of giant cell tumors are similar to those in the long tubular bones. Epiphyseal involvement, subchondral extension, osteolysis, delicate trabeculae, and osseous expansion are among the characteristics of such neoplasms. Involvement of the head of a metacarpal bone or the base of the proximal phalanx in the hand should be emphasized. In the carpal and tarsal bones, poorly or well-defined osteolytic lesions of variable size are encountered.

There is less uniformity in the radiographic characteris-

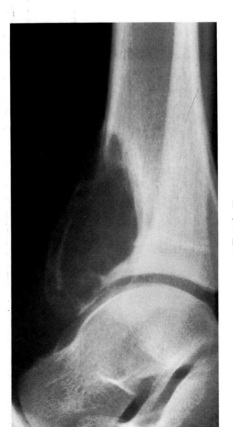

FIGURE 83–193. Giant cell tumor: Radiographic abnormalities—long tubular bones (tibia). A 16 year old girl had a 6 month history of ankle pain following a minor injury. The lateral radiograph shows an expansile, faintly trabeculated, eccentric osteolytic lesion in the distal portion of the tibia extending to subchondral bone and accompanied by minor periostitis. (Courtesy of R. Richley, M.D., San Diego, California.)

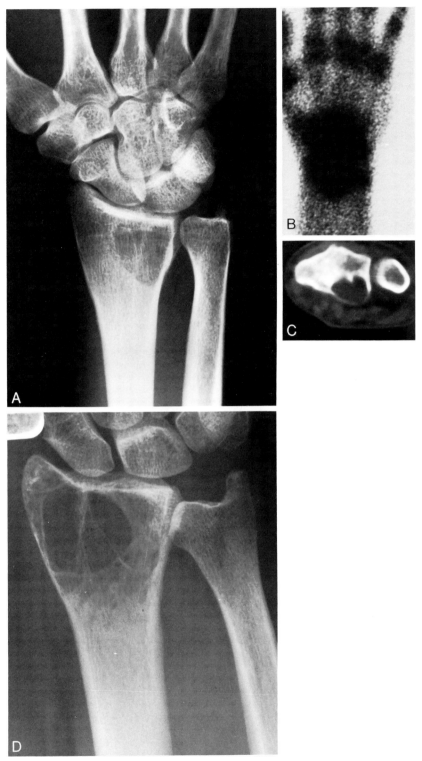

FIGURE 83–194. Giant cell tumor: Radiographic abnormalities—long tubular bones (radius).

   A–C A 22 year old man developed pain in the wrist following a fall. No mass could be palpated. The radiograph **(A)** shows an eccentric, osteolytic lesion involving the metaphysis and epiphysis of the distal portion of the radius and extending to subchondral bone. Its margins are well defined. A bone scan **(B)** shows intense uptake of the radionuclide in the wrist. A transaxial CT scan **(C)** demonstrates the volarly located osteolytic lesion that is expanding into the region of the pronator quadratus muscle. This giant cell tumor was treated with resection and insertion of a fibular graft.

   D In a 47 year old woman with a painful, tender, nonswollen wrist, a giant cell tumor in the distal portion of the radius reveals all the classic radiographic features: It is osteolytic, eccentric, trabeculated, and metaphyseal and epiphyseal in location with extension to subchondral bone.

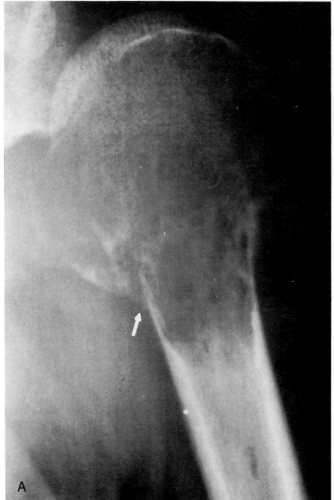

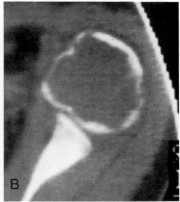

FIGURE 83–195. Giant cell tumor: Radiographic abnormalities—long tubular bones (humerus). This 22 year old woman came to medical attention following a fall with a pathologic fracture through a giant cell tumor of the proximal portion of the humerus. The radiograph **(A)** reveals a large, trabeculated, osteolytic lesion involving the greater tuberosity (seen en face owing to internal rotation of the humerus), lesser tuberosity, and metaphysis and epiphysis of the humerus. A pathologic fracture is identified (arrow). A transaxial CT scan **(B)** reveals osseous expansion with endosteal cortical erosion.

tics of giant cell tumors of flat and irregular bones (Fig. 83–198). Sternal[946] and sacral[957] lesions are osteolytic and, owing to a large size and a soft tissue component, may simulate the appearance of a malignant neoplasm. In the sacrum (and, occasionally, in other locations), transarticular extension of the tumor may be noted. In the innominate bone, an epiphyseal equivalent area, such as the bone adjacent to the sacroiliac or hip articulation, commonly is affected. In the spine (Fig. 83–198*B*), destruction of a vertebral body is more frequent than that of the posterior osseous elements (differing from the posterior involvement that characterizes an aneurysmal bone cyst or osteoblastoma), and the neoplasm may lead to vertebral collapse or extend into the intervertebral disc, adjacent vertebral body, spinal canal, or paraspinal soft tissues.[924, 958–960, 2188, 2189]

Other Imaging Techniques. Scintigraphy, with bone-seeking radiopharmaceutical agents, has been used to evaluate patients with giant cell tumors.[961, 962] Although intense accumulation of the radionuclide around the periphery of the neoplasm produces a characteristic doughnut configuration, an extended pattern of activity beyond the true limits of the tumor and the failure to define reliably the soft tissue extension of the process limit the usefulness of this technique.[1844] The uptake of ^{67}Ga-citrate by giant cell tumors occurs in an inconsistent manner.[962]

CT (with or without contrast enhancement) represents an imaging method that allows evaluation of the extraosseous

and, to a lesser degree, the intraosseous extent of the tumor and its relationship to major vessels and nerves[927, 961, 963, 964, 2199] (Figs. 83–199 and 83–200). The identification with CT (as well as with MR imaging) of a fluid level within a giant cell tumor (Figs. 83–201 and 83–202) is of interest,[965, 2200] although neither this finding nor other CT abnormalities allow a specific diagnosis of giant cell tumor to be made. Furthermore, CT alone may define inadequately the intra-articular spread of this neoplasm; evaluation of transchondral extension of a giant cell tumor is better accomplished with arthrography combined with conventional tomography, CT,[961, 963, 966] or MR imaging.

The role of angiography in patients with giant cell tumors includes the preoperative evaluation of tumor extent into the soft tissues and of regional vascular anatomy[961, 963, 967] and, perhaps, transcatheter arterial embolization using Gelfoam particles in instances of unresectable neoplasm.[968] Specific angiographic features, including the number and type of tumor vessels, do not correlate well with the degree of cellular differentiation evident on histologic analysis,[967] nor does angiography provide a specific diagnosis, although it may differentiate between a giant cell tumor and an aneurysmal bone cyst.[969] Furthermore, the presence of synovial hyperemia within a joint adjacent to a giant cell tumor may produce angiographic features that erroneously suggest extraosseous extension of the neoplasm.[970]

The primary role of MR imaging in cases of giant cell

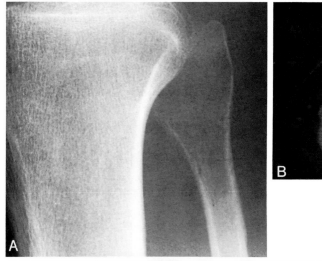

FIGURE 83–196. Giant cell tumor: Radiographic abnormalities—long tubular bones (fibula).

A, B A 25 year old woman had pain in the lateral aspect of the knee. A region of motheaten osteolysis in the metaphysis and epiphysis of the proximal portion of the fibula is evident on the radiograph **(A)**. A transaxial CT scan **(B)** reveals uniform expansion of the cortex of the involved fibula. A giant cell tumor was documented after biopsy and subsequent resection of the lesion.

C, D This 17 year old man had a 3 month history of leg pain. On physical examination, diffuse swelling was found over the lateral aspect of the knee and proximal portion of the fibula. A radiograph **(C)** shows an expansile, osteolytic lesion with a pathologic fracture (not well seen on this reproduction). CT (not shown) revealed no evidence of soft tissue extension. At surgery, a 5 × 4 × 4 cm cystic and hemorrhagic giant cell tumor was removed. A radiograph of the specimen **(D)** illustrates the classic features of a giant cell tumor.

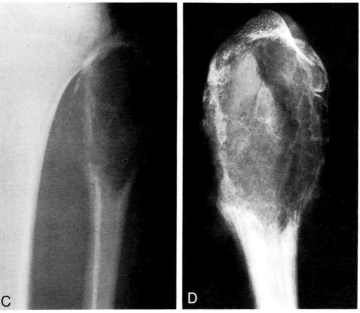

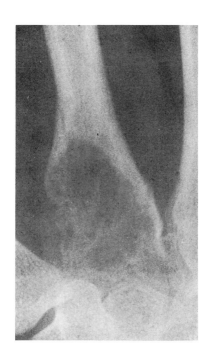

FIGURE 83–197. Giant cell tumor: Radiographic abnormalities—short tubular bones. In a 15 year old girl with pain and swelling in the hand, note the slightly expansile, trabeculated, osteolytic lesion of the second metacarpal bone that extends to its base.

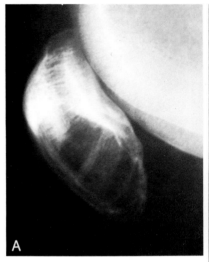
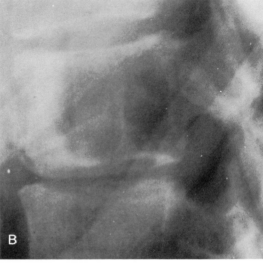

FIGURE 83–198. Giant cell tumor: Radiographic abnormalities—flat and irregular bones.

A Patella. A well-defined, trabeculated radiolucent lesion is seen.

B Spine. Osteolysis affects the posterior two thirds of a thoracic vertebral body. There is increased radiodensity in the anterior one third of the body.

(**A, B,** Courtesy of Regional Naval Medical Center, San Diego, California.)

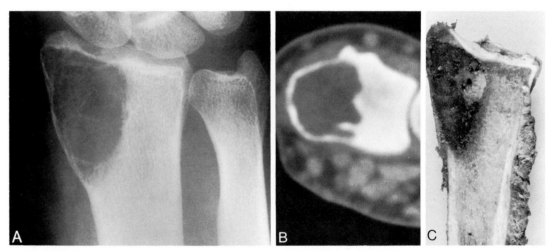

FIGURE 83–199. Giant cell tumor: CT abnormalities. This lesion in the radius was discovered as an incidental finding on a radiograph obtained in a 36 year old man who had injured his wrist.

A The routine radiograph demonstrates the classic features of a giant cell tumor, including subchondral extension, faint trabeculation, and mild osseous expansion.

B A transaxial CT scan shows that the lesion expands the bone, with marked thinning of the cortex.

C A coronal section of the radius demonstrates the giant cell tumor. Compare its location to that shown in **A**.

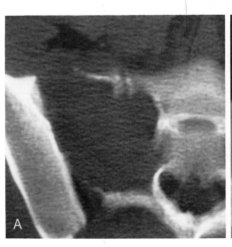
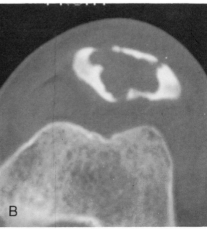

FIGURE 83–200. Giant cell tumor: CT abnormalities.

A Sacrum. Note the osteolytic lesion of the sacrum in this transaxial CT scan. The lesion extends to the region of the sacroiliac joint and into the anterior soft tissues. The neural foramen is destroyed. (Courtesy of K. Kortman, M.D., San Diego, California.)

B Patella. A transaxial CT scan shows an osteolytic lesion of the patella with a pathologic fracture. (Courtesy of G-S. Huang, M.D., Taipei, Taiwan.)

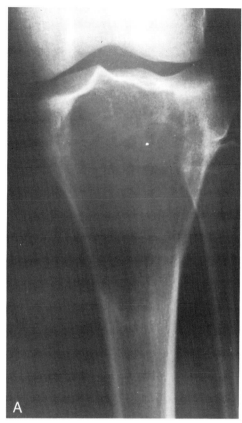

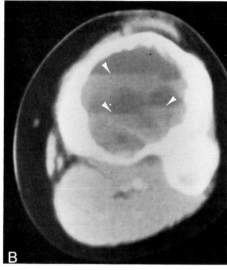

FIGURE 83–201. Giant cell tumor: CT abnormalities—fluid level. Routine radiography **(A)** in a 14 year old girl reveals a large osteolytic lesion of the tibia. A transaxial CT scan **(B)** through the lesion with the patient in a supine position shows multiple fluid levels (arrowheads). (Courtesy of P. Kaplan, M.D., Charlottesville, Virginia.)

tumor is to define the intraosseous, intra-articular, and soft tissue extent of the lesion[971, 2201] (Figs. 83–203 and 83–204). Typically the tumor is of low signal intensity in T1-weighted spin echo MR images and of high signal intensity in T2-weighted spin echo MR images, and it generally is well defined.[2202] Inhomogeneity of signal intensity and a poorly delineated tumor margin may be encountered, however.[2203] Such inhomogeneity may relate to the presence of necrotic and cystic regions within the tumor. Fluid-fluid levels are identified in MR images of some giant cell tumors,[2204] but the finding is much more characteristic of aneurysmal bone cysts.

Pathologic Abnormalities. Giant cell tumors are fairly large; their maximum dimension in a long tubular or flat bone may exceed 12 cm, and an entire small tubular bone in the hand or foot may be involved. In the tubular bones, the tumor is located eccentrically within the metaphysis and epiphysis and almost invariably extends to the articular cartilage[908, 920] (Fig. 83–205A). The cartilaginous tissue, however, rarely is perforated by the tumor. The cortical bone is thin and expanded, creating a bulge in the bony contour, but in the majority of cases the tumor still is contained by a thin layer of cortical or new bone and periosteum (Fig. 83–205B). The color of the neoplastic tissue is variable (gray, red, brown, yellow, or orange) and depends on the amount of hemorrhage or necrosis that has occurred.[920, 972] White, fibrotic areas may be present, especially in recurrent lesions or in those with previous fracture. These fibrotic foci may be in the form of either solid areas or bands that traverse the tumor and are firm owing to the presence of reactive osteoid or bone within them.[33, 34] The tumor itself commonly is soft, fleshy, and friable. Small or

large cystic areas filled with fresh or clotted blood or serosanguineous fluid are not uncommon, particularly in larger or recurrent tumors. In unusual circumstances, the joint space may contain tumor tissue, and the neoplasm may extend to adjacent bones.[33, 180] Cortical erosion with soft tissue extension is detected in 20 to 50 per cent of cases. Pathologic fracture, observed in 10 to 35 per cent of cases, may contribute to the soft tissue or articular[1911] tumor component.

Owing to the occurrence of osteoclast-type giant cells in a large number of tumors and tumor-like lesions, the microscopic appearance of a giant cell tumor may not, in itself, be diagnostic and must be correlated closely with clinical and radiographic data. Giant cell tumors typically contain an abundant number of homogeneously distributed giant cells (Fig. 83–206A) mixed with ovoid, round, and spindle-shaped stromal cells that have ill-defined cytoplasmic borders.[914, 920] The giant cells vary in size and are characterized by an abundant eosinophilic, granular cytoplasm containing centrally located nuclei that vary in number from dozens to 100 or more. These nuclei are regular in outline, may have a small nucleolus, and are similar in appearance to those in the adjacent stromal cells (Fig. 83–206B,C). Vacuolization of the giant cell cytoplasm may be present and, at times, quite prominent. Mitotic figures occasionally may be found in the stromal cells (Fig. 83–206B) but virtually never in the multinucleated giant cells. Vascular sinuses frequently are evident that may be either plugged or lined with the tumor cells; such vascular invasion has no prognostic significance.[973] Additional findings may include recent and old stromal hemorrhage with hemosiderin deposits in the cytoplasm of the stromal cells and nests of lipid-

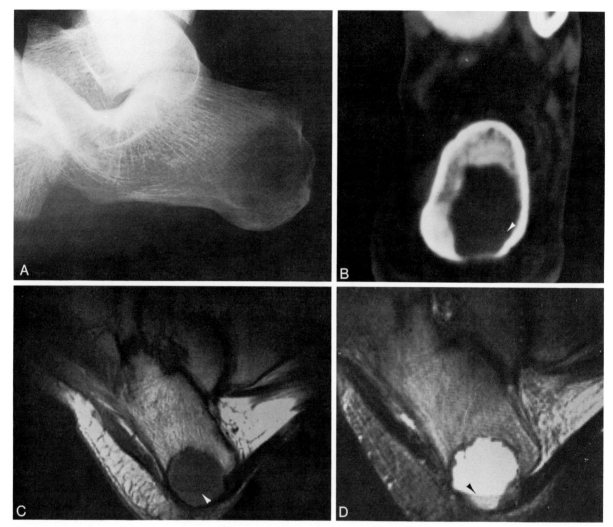

FIGURE 83–202. Giant cell tumor: CT and MR imaging abnormalities—fluid level. A 21 year old man reported 1 year of increasing pain in his heel.

A The lateral radiograph shows a well-defined osteolytic lesion of the posterior surface of the calcaneus.

B A direct coronal CT scan with the patient supine and the knees flexed reveals the extent of the lesion in the calcaneus and, although not well shown in this reproduction, a fluid level (arrowhead) within it.

C, D T1-weighted **(C)** and T2-weighted **(D)** sagittal spin echo MR images with the patient in a supine position and the knees flexed show that the tumor has low signal intensity in **C** and high signal intensity in **D**. A fluid level is evident (arrowheads). At surgery, this giant cell tumor contained serosanguineous fluid.

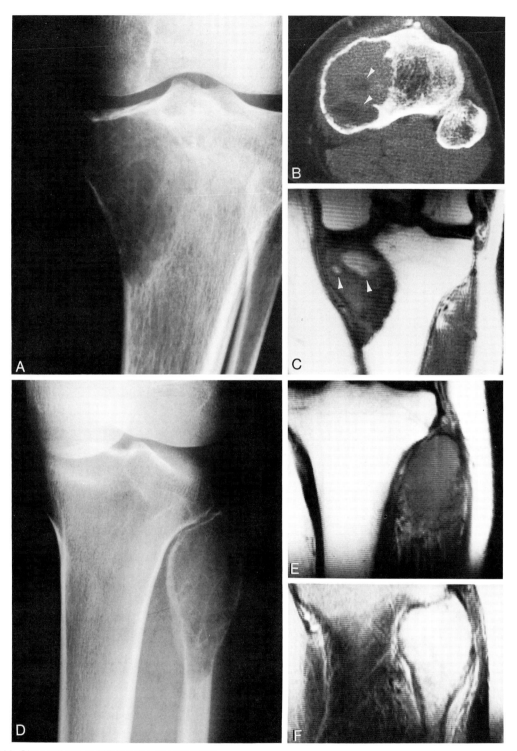

FIGURE 83–203. Giant cell tumor: MR imaging abnormalities.
   A–C Tibia. This 37 year old man had pain in his knee of several months' duration. The routine radiograph **(A)** shows an eccentric, slightly trabeculated osteolytic lesion in the proximal metaphysis and epiphysis of the tibia. Transaxial CT **(B)** demonstrates the lesion containing areas of low attenuation (arrowheads) and permeating the cortex. A coronal T1-weighted (TR/TE 500/32) spin echo MR image **(C)** reveals a lesion with low signal intensity containing regions of higher intensity (arrowheads). Histologic confirmation of a giant cell tumor with foci of hemorrhage was obtained.
   D–F Fibula. A 34 year old woman developed knee pain over a 6 month period. The routine radiograph **(D)** shows a classic giant cell tumor in the proximal portion of the fibula. A coronal T1-weighted (TR/TE, 500/32) spin echo MR image **(E)** indicates low signal intensity within the lesion. A coronal T2-weighted (TR/TE, 2000/60) spin echo MR image **(F)** shows increased signal intensity in the tumor. Presence of a giant cell tumor was confirmed following surgery.

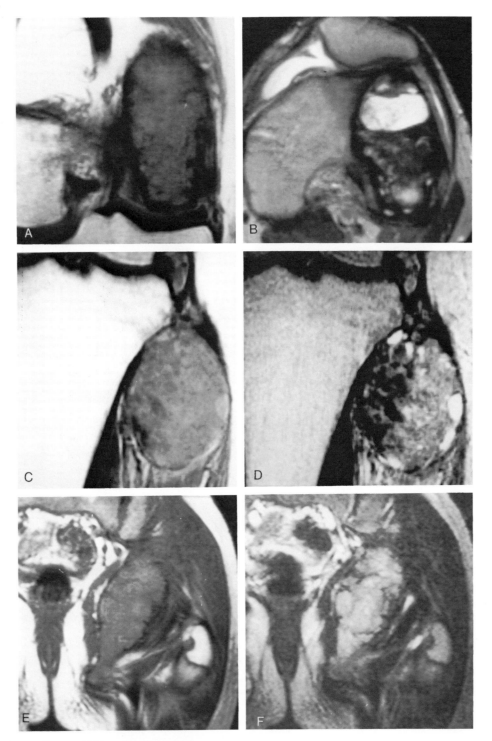

FIGURE 83–204. Giant cell tumor: MR imaging abnormalities.

A, B Femur. In a 26 year old man, a coronal T1-weighted (TR/TE, 775/20) spin echo MR image **(A)** reveals the tumor of low signal intensity involving the lateral femoral condyle. In a transaxial T2-weighted (TR/TE, 2000/70) spin echo MR image **(B)** the tumor is of inhomogeneous signal intensity; there is high signal intensity anteriorly and mainly low signal intensity posteriorly. A joint effusion is present. (Courtesy of M. Mitchell, M.D., Halifax, Nova Scotia, Canada.)

C, D Fibula. In a 27 year old woman, a coronal proton density–weighted (TR/TE, 2000/20) spin echo MR image **(C)** shows a tumor of inhomogeneous but mainly low signal intensity replacing and expanding the proximal portion of the fibula. With T2 weighting (TR/TE, 2000/80) in the coronal plane **(D)**, a tumor with inhomogeneous signal intensity is evident.

E, F Innominate bone. In a 14 year old child, a giant cell tumor occupies and expands the ilioischial bone column about the left hip. In a coronal T1-weighted (TR/TE, 533/26) spin echo MR image **(E)**, it is of low signal intensity; in a coronal T2-weighted (TR/TE, 2000/100) spin echo MR image **(F)**, the tumor is of intermediate to high signal intensity with septations of low signal intensity. A small hip effusion is present. (Courtesy of A. Motta, M.D., Cleveland, Ohio.)

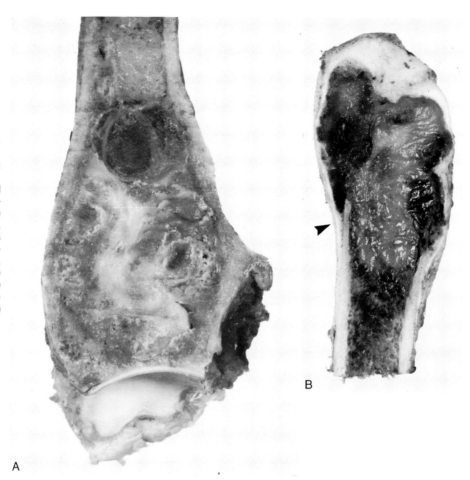

FIGURE 83–205. Giant cell tumor: Macroscopic abnormalities.

A This giant cell tumor in the distal portion of the tibia appears almost entirely solid, with a central fibrotic (white) zone. At the upper aspect of the lesion, a cystic area filled with clotted blood is present. The tumor extends to the subchondral bone and expands the cortex.

B This giant cell tumor extends to the distal portion of the ulna. Although the cortices have been perforated, an intact periosteal membrane (arrowhead) can be identified over the neoplasm.

A

B

laden, foamy macrophages.[974] Areas with features of an aneurysmal bone cyst are not uncommon, especially in larger tumors.

Bands of fibrous tissue or large collagenized foci are evident in most giant cell tumors. In these regions, spindle-shaped cells predominate and few, if any, giant cells are present. Osteoid foci also are evident in 20 to 50 per cent of cases, occurring about areas of hemorrhage, within the fibrous septa, or within the callus about a fracture.[975] Cartilage is not detected in giant cell tumors except as part of such callus.[180, 976] The presence of chondroid foci in a giant cell–containing tumor should suggest an alternative diagnosis, such as a chondroblastoma.

Histochemical, immunohistochemical, and electron microscopic studies have provided some information regarding the cellular characteristics and histogenesis of giant cell tumors, although debate on these issues continues.[906, 977–988, 2473–2475]

Natural History. Giant cell tumors should not be regarded as innocent lesions. Local extension, regional and systemic tumor implantation, and malignant transformation with widespread metastases are among the reported manifestations of these neoplasms that are indicative of their aggressive and unpredictable nature. The variations in the biologic behavior of giant cell tumors have led to considerable controversy regarding the manner in which they should be classified (benign, locally aggressive, or low grade malignant neoplasms); to an ongoing dispute regarding what should be considered appropriate therapy[1845]; and to repeated attempts to define histologic (and occasionally

radiologic) characteristics that could serve as reliable prognostic indicators.[2205] Initial interest in assigning a numerical grade to giant cell tumors based on the microscopic appearance of the stromal cells[33, 913, 920, 989] subsequently waned owing to the documentation of tumor recurrence and metastasis even in those neoplasms that were interpreted as histologically benign.[30, 33, 34, 908, 990] Although the histologic appearance of a giant cell tumor represents the most important indicator of its behavior, analysis of additional data provided by the clinical and radiographic examinations and the gross pathologic features of this neoplasm is essential for appropriate management of the patient.[1845, 1846]

The rate of *recurrence* of a giant cell tumor is quite high, with estimates generally in the range of 40 to 60 per cent.[221, 914, 921] The likelihood of such recurrence may be particularly great in those tumors that are located in the distal end of the femur and the proximal portion of the tibia.[914] Recurrent giant cell tumors generally are observed within the first 2 years following treatment of the neoplasm, although recurrences occasionally may be seen more than 5 years after such treatment.[991, 2206] The recurrent neoplasm usually occurs at the site of the primary giant cell tumor, with reportable exceptions in which a nearby bone is affected (e.g., carpal bone involvement following an initial tumor in the distal portion of the radius)[992] or more distal soft tissues are involved owing to tumor tissue emboli.[993]

The radiographic abnormalities associated with recurrent giant cell tumors are characteristic (Fig. 83–207). With regard to intraosseous recurrence, osteolysis adjacent to the

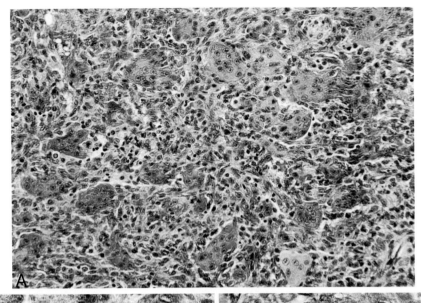

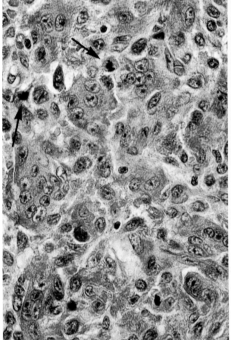

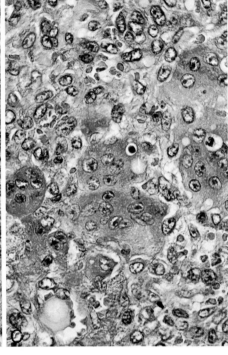

FIGURE 83–206. Giant cell tumor: Microscopic abnormalities.

A Note the even distribution of multinucleated giant cells whose nuclei contain small nucleoli. Among the giant cells are small stromal cells that are not well seen at this magnification. (300×.)

B, C Higher magnification reveals that the giant cells and intervening stromal cells have similar-appearing nuclei. Many of the stromal cells appear to fuse with the giant cells. A few mitotic figures in the stromal cells are seen in **B** (arrows). (600×.)

area of surgical resection or delayed resorption of a bone graft may be evident.[918, 994] Similar resorption may indicate physiologic reaction to or infection of the graft.[2207, 2476] At the time of surgery, local implantation of giant cell tumor in the adjacent soft tissues (or even in the soft tissues at the bone graft donor site if proper operative technique is not used[995]) can occur. In these instances, it is clear that the cells of the giant cell tumor can survive in the soft tissues and later lead to invasion of the adjacent bone. The soft tissue implants may remain radiographically invisible, although they also may appear as enlarging masses with peripheral ossification in the form of a radiodense thin shell or thick rind.[996, 2208, 2209]

Tumor implantation at distant sites, typically the lungs, in patients with benign giant cell tumors has been documented repeatedly.[997–1002, 1912, 2210–2214] This phenomenon,

which also is evident in cases of chondroblastoma (see previous discussion), relates to simple or passive vascular transport of neoplastic tissue from the primary musculoskeletal site to a remote location rather than true malignant metastasis. It typically occurs within 2 to 5 years following surgical manipulation of the primary neoplasm. Distant implantation of tumor appears to be more common in cases of giant cell tumor that involve the distal portion of the radius and that are associated with recurrent local disease.[2214] The pulmonary lesions are identical histologically to the primary giant cell tumor, appear to grow to a certain maximum size, and then ossify; they generally do not lead relentlessly to the demise of the patient,[997] although the behavior of the metastatic foci is somewhat unpredictable.[1000]

The frequency of *malignant giant cell tumor* (or malig-

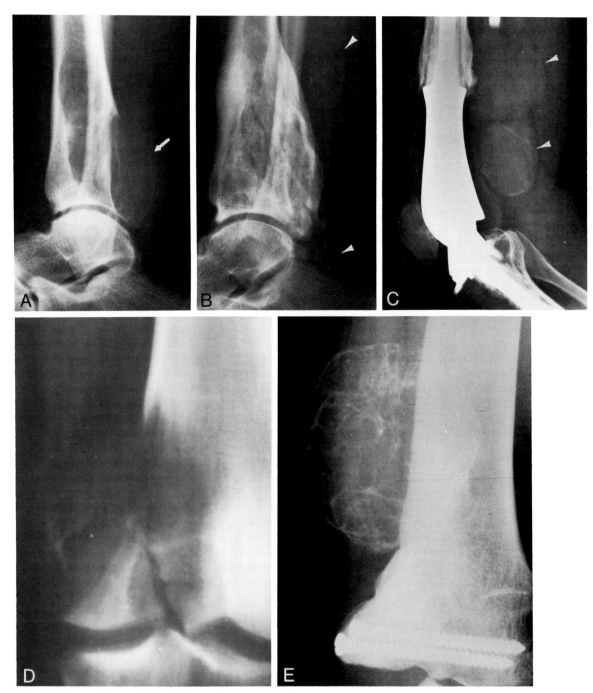

FIGURE 83–207. Giant cell tumor: Natural history—intraosseous and extraosseous recurrence.

A, B This 30 year old man developed a giant cell tumor of the distal portion of the tibia that was curetted with the insertion of a bone graft. Several years later **(A),** a recurrent intraosseous lesion is apparent, with bone destruction at the site of surgical resection (arrow). Four years after **A,** following further tumor resection and grafting **(B),** ossified nodules of giant cell tumor are apparent in the soft tissues (arrowheads). The soft tissue nodules contained ossified shells and subsequently were excised. Their histologic appearance was identical to that of the original osseous lesion, with the exception that osteoid and bone were present at the periphery of the soft tissue implants. (Courtesy of K. L. Cooper, M.D., Rochester, Minnesota.)

C This 36 year old man had a giant cell tumor of the distal portion of the femur that was treated by curettage and grafting. Five months later, further curettage was required, and the lesion was packed with methylmethacrylate. A pathologic fracture later developed, requiring resection of bone and a custom total knee arthroplasty. A soft tissue tumor deposit was found in one of the surgical scars at the time of the arthroplasty. Two years following this surgical procedure, as shown on the lateral radiograph, ossified soft tissue masses (arrowheads) were present. (From Cooper, K. L., et al.: Radiology *153:*597, 1984.)

D, E These radiographs were obtained 3 years apart. Initially **(D),** a giant cell tumor with a pathologic fracture of the distal portion of the femur is seen, and, subsequently **(E),** there is a large ossified soft tissue tumor recurrence. (Courtesy of J. Vilar, M.D., Valencia, Spain.)

nant transformation of a benign giant cell tumor) is difficult to ascertain because, in the past, many different types of bone sarcomas containing giant cells were diagnosed improperly as true giant cell tumors. Although some available data suggest that malignancy eventually occurs in as many as 30 per cent of all giant cell tumors, a more appropriate estimate appears to be 5 to 10 per cent.[30, 33, 914, 921] To be certain of the diagnosis of malignant giant cell tumor, the pathologist must be able to delineate (1) obviously sarcomatous stroma; and (2) zones of typical benign giant cell tumor in the neoplasm under appraisal or in tissue obtained earlier from the same neoplasm.[30] The vast majority (but not all[2215]) of malignant giant cell tumors develop following irradiation of the original giant cell tumor[1003] and reveal a histologic pattern consistent with fibrosarcoma, osteosarcoma, or, less commonly, malignant fibrous histiocytoma.[921, 1913] Such neoplasms are best considered radiation-induced sarcomas rather than malignant giant cell tumors.[33] It is because of this that the subject of malignant giant cell tumor is hotly debated.[28] Osteosarcomas with numerous osteoclast-type giant cells and malignant fibrous histiocytomas with malignant tumor giant cells probably account for most of the so-called primary malignant giant cell tumors. True primary malignant giant cell tumors apparently exist but are rare.[2477]

Multicentric Involvement. The presence of more than one primary giant cell tumor in the same patient (Fig. 83–208) is an unusual event that has been documented in only a limited number of publications.[915, 920, 921, 940, 1004–1011, 2478] The estimated frequency of this finding in cases of giant cell tumor is 0.5 to 5 per cent, but such estimates are difficult to analyze owing to the possibility that multifocal involvement in some cases may be a manifestation of metastasis rather than indicative of more than one independent tumor. The additional possibility of implantation of tissue from one giant cell tumor to a second contiguous osseous site also must be considered.[992, 1011] Furthermore, careful analysis of the patient is required to exclude the presence of hyperparathyroidism (with brown tumors) whenever the diagnosis of multiple giant cell tumors is being considered (Fig. 83–209).

Multicentric giant cell tumors may appear simultaneously or metachronously.[1914] In some instances, an interval of 10 years or more may elapse between the appearance of the first giant cell tumor and that of additional tumors; remarkable cases have been documented in which nine or more independent giant cell tumors have developed over the course of 15 years or more.[1007, 1009] Although the clinical, radiographic, and histologic features of each giant cell tumor in patients with multifocal involvement generally are similar to those of a typical giant cell tumor, certain modifications of these features may be encountered. First, the bones of the hand are affected more frequently in multicentric disease than in solitary giant cell tumors.[1010] Second, there is an increased propensity for metaphyseal involvement and for pathologic fracture in patients with multifocal lesions.[1007, 2478] Third, an abundance of spindle cells in the tumor may be encountered in persons with multiple giant cell tumors.[1010] Finally, the Goltz syndrome, consisting of focal dermal hypoplasia, ocular defects, and skeletal anomalies, has been associated with multifocal giant cell tumors,[1012] although it also has been observed in the presence of a solitary giant cell tumor.[1013]

Differential Diagnosis. Generally, the radiographic di-

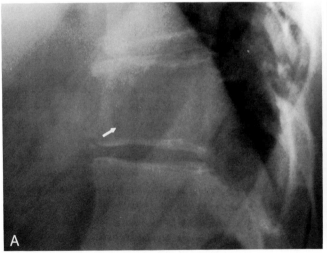
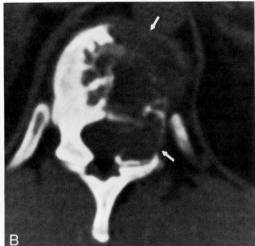
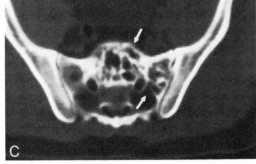

FIGURE 83–208. Giant cell tumor: Multicentric involvement. Two giant cell tumors developed in this 27 year old man. One is located in the spine, affecting a thoracic vertebra. The vertebral body and posterior osseous elements are involved (arrows), as shown with routine radiography **(A)** and transaxial CT **(B).** The second giant cell tumor is located in the sacrum (arrows), as shown with transaxial CT **(C).** Note the similarity in the CT abnormalities in **B** and **C.** (Courtesy of T. Broderick, M.D., Orange, California.)

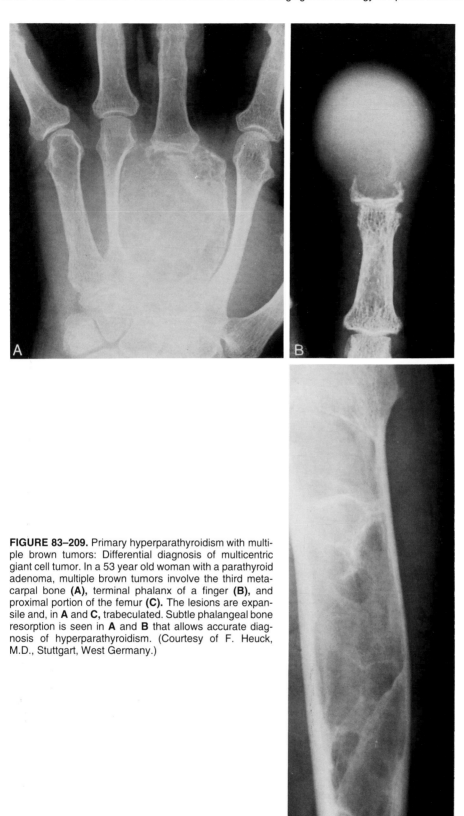

FIGURE 83–209. Primary hyperparathyroidism with multiple brown tumors: Differential diagnosis of multicentric giant cell tumor. In a 53 year old woman with a parathyroid adenoma, multiple brown tumors involve the third metacarpal bone **(A),** terminal phalanx of a finger **(B),** and proximal portion of the femur **(C).** The lesions are expansile and, in **A** and **C,** trabeculated. Subtle phalangeal bone resorption is seen in **A** and **B** that allows accurate diagnosis of hyperparathyroidism. (Courtesy of F. Heuck, M.D., Stuttgart, West Germany.)

agnosis of a giant cell tumor is straightforward, particularly when an eccentric, well or poorly defined osteolytic lesion containing faint or delicate trabeculation is discovered in the metaphysis or epiphysis of a long tubular bone and extends to the subchondral region. Although chondroblas-

toma, intraosseous ganglion, and a variety of cystic lesions can affect the epiphysis, clinical and radiologic characteristics usually allow the differentiation of a giant cell tumor from these other entities. Chondroblastoma typically occurs in the immature skeleton of a child or adolescent and may contain calcifications. An intraosseous ganglion is observed most frequently in the medial malleolus of the tibia, in the carpal bones, or in periarticular regions such as the hip (Fig. 83–210). It may be multilocular in appearance, with a sclerotic margin, and accompanied by a soft tissue ganglion. Although a variety of articular processes can lead to subchondral cysts, including rheumatoid arthritis, gout, calcium pyrophosphate dihydrate crystal deposition disease, hemophilia, and pigmented villonodular synovitis, such cysts commonly are multiple, communicate with the joint, and are associated with additional articular abnormalities. Further differential diagnostic considerations in patients with giant cell tumors include aneurysmal bone cyst, fibrous dysplasia (Fig. 83–211), eosinophilic granuloma, the brown tumor of hyperparathyroidism, and giant cell reparative granuloma. Most of these can be eliminated through close evaluation of the radiographs, although the last two deserve special emphasis. In any patient with multiple osseous lesions that have the characteristics of a giant cell tumor, the possibility of hyperparathyroidism must be considered, and careful clinical and chemical analysis is required. The problem of differentiating a giant cell tumor from a giant cell reparative granuloma can be considerable, especially when evaluating a bone lesion in the face or hand, and will be addressed independently later in this discussion of differential diagnosis.

Giant cell tumors with aggressive radiographic characteristics and those that occur in flat or irregular bones present unique diagnostic challenges. In the former situation, the exclusion of a malignant neoplasm, such as a fibrosarcoma,

malignant fibrous histiocytoma, chondrosarcoma, or osteosarcoma, may be accomplished when additional data derived from clinical and histologic evaluations are examined. In the innominate bone, giant cell tumors may possess radiographic abnormalities that are sufficient for accurate diagnosis, especially when a lesion extends to the subchondral bone about the hip or sacroiliac joint. In fact, sacral giant cell tumors may violate the articular space and involve a contiguous portion of the ilium. In the spine, the predilection for involvement of the vertebral body is a feature of giant cell tumors that differs from the localization in the posterior vertebral elements that characterizes an osteoblastoma or aneurysmal bone cyst.

Histologically, the accurate diagnosis of a giant cell tumor is made difficult in some cases owing to the large number of tumor and tumor-like processes that may contain osteoclast-type giant cells. Included among these are osteosarcoma, especially those that arise in patients with Paget's disease, in which the stromal cells show a greater degree of atypia and anaplasia than in giant cell tumors, and malignant osteoid or chondroid tissue may be identified. Other conditions include chondroblastoma (the cartilaginous or fibrocartilaginous tissue of this tumor is not found in a giant cell tumor), nonossifying fibroma and fibrous dysplasia (the whorled fibrous stroma of these lesions is not present in a giant cell tumor), osteoblastoma (this tumor is characterized by florid osteoid and bone production), aneurysmal bone cyst (the abundance and homogeneous distribution of giant cells that typify a giant cell tumor usually are not seen in an aneurysmal bone cyst, and the latter has a predominantly

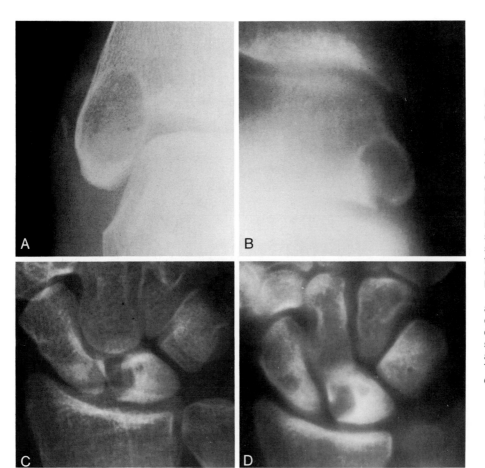

FIGURE 83–210. Intraosseous ganglion: Differential diagnosis of single or multicentric giant cell tumor.

A, B This 42 year old woman developed multiple tender nodules about the ankle. Aspiration of one of the nodules led to the recovery of cloudy, gelatinous material. Radiographs reveal well-defined osteolytic lesions, with sclerotic margins in the medial malleolus of the tibia **(A)** and in the talus **(B)**. Observe soft tissue swelling containing small osseous spicules in **A** and communication with the talocalcaneonavicular joint in **B**. (Courtesy of J. Scavulli, M.D., San Diego, California.)

C, D This 29 year old woman had a 6 month history of wrist pain. Several cystic lesions in the lunate, accompanied by bone sclerosis, are shown with routine radiography **(C)** and conventional tomography **(D)**. The large lunate lesion communicates with the radiocarpal articulation.

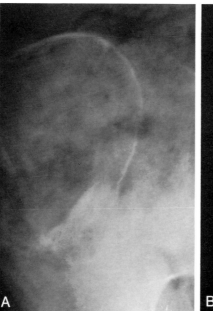 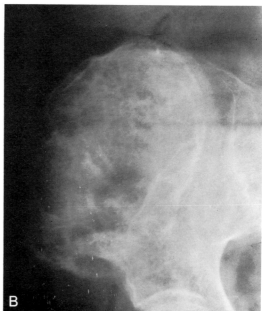

FIGURE 83–211. Fibrous dysplasia: Differential diagnosis of single or multicentric giant cell tumor. This 72 year old woman had had pain in her flank for approximately 1 or 2 years. She had received treatment during the previous 15 months for osteoporosis with fluoride and estrogen. A radiograph obtained prior to the initiation of treatment **(A)** shows an expansile, osteolytic lesion of the ilium. Two years later **(B),** after receiving estrogen, the lesion has increased dramatically in size. Also, at this time, the patient reported an enlarging abdominal mass. Surgery confirmed osseous fibrous dysplasia and benign fibromas in the ovaries. (Courtesy of P. Major, M.D., Winnipeg, Manitoba, Canada.)

fibrous spindle cell stroma), brown tumor of hyperparathyroidism (chemical analysis provides the most important clue to correct diagnosis in this lesion), and giant cell reparative granuloma (see following discussion).

The *giant cell reparative granuloma* is an uncommon bone lesion that has slightly different histologic characteristics and a more benign clinical course than a giant cell tumor. Its name was introduced in 1953 by Jaffe[1014] in a description of intraosseous lesions of the mandible and maxilla that contained prominent giant cells. It was Jaffe's belief that the lesions represented a response to intraosseous hemorrhage and were not true neoplasms. Subsequent reports of giant cell granulomas have indicated their proclivity to affect the facial bones and sinuses[1015–1020] and only a incidental relationship to trauma.[1015] The inconstant association of this lesion with injury has led to the elimination by some investigators of the word reparative from its name.[1021] There is uniform agreement, however, that the giant cell reparative granuloma is distinct from a true giant cell tumor and that it represents one of several giant cell–containing lesions of the face and sinuses, others being a true giant cell tumor, the brown tumor of hyperparathyroidism, aneurysmal bone cyst, fibrous dysplasia, and cherubism. Giant cell reparative granulomas represent less than 10 per cent of all benign tumors of the jaw and, in this location, demonstrate a female preponderance, a tendency to affect young patients, and a variety of clinical manifestations, including localized swelling, pain, headache, diplopia, and epistaxis[1022] that may be exacerbated during pregnancy.[1023] Radiographically, the giant cell reparative granuloma in the facial bones appears as a round or oval, radiolucent lesion that may be trabeculated and expansile and that may contain ossification.

Owing to the documented occurrence of giant cell reparative granulomas in most of the bones of the face and even the skull,[1024, 2216] it is not unexpected that these lesions also might affect the appendicular skeleton. Such involvement in the bones of the hands and feet was first described by Ackerman and Spjut[1025] in 1962. Subsequent reports con-

firmed that giant cell reparative granulomas could involve not only the bones of the hands and feet but also the carpal and tarsal bones.[1026–1031, 1847, 1878, 2217–2220] Rarely, long tubular bones may be involved.[2221] Such lesions also have been designated giant cell reactions,[1032, 1033, 1878, 1915] and some examples of the solid type of aneurysmal bone cyst (see later discussion) are considered to be giant cell reparative granulomas.

Giant cell reparative granulomas arising in the hands and feet occur more commonly in women than in men. The age range of affected patients is wide (6 to 53 years of age). A history of trauma is infrequent. Clinical manifestations include pain, discomfort, swelling, and tenderness, and the bone may feel enlarged when palpated. The phalanges of the hand are the most common site of involvement, followed in order of decreasing frequency by the metacarpal, metatarsal, carpal, and tarsal bones and the phalanges of the foot. Multifocal osseous involvement is encountered.[1027, 1030, 2219] Radiographically, the lesions are osteolytic, trabeculated, and slightly expansile and involve the metaphysis and diaphysis, although they may extend to the epiphysis and subchondral bone (Fig. 83–212). Cortical violation and periostitis are rare. Although giant cell reparative granulomas are not aggressive, recurrence of the lesion is seen if initial surgery is inadequate.[1847]

Accurate radiographic diagnosis in cases of giant cell reparative granuloma in the bones of the hands and feet is difficult, as similar radiographic features may occur in a variety of processes, including enchondroma, aneurysmal bone cyst, and true giant cell tumor. Giant cell reparative granulomas do not calcify (as opposed to enchondromas) and usually occur following closure of the physeal plate (which is not a typical characteristic of an aneurysmal bone cyst). Their differentiation, however, from giant cell tumors may be impossible solely on the basis of the radiographic features. Involvement of the distal phalanges in the hand is more frequent in cases of giant cell reparative granuloma than in cases of giant cell tumor.[1847] Histologically, giant cell reparative granulomas generally can be differentiated

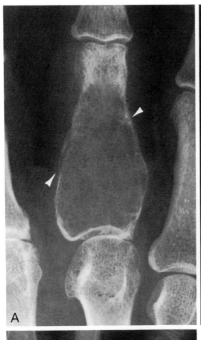

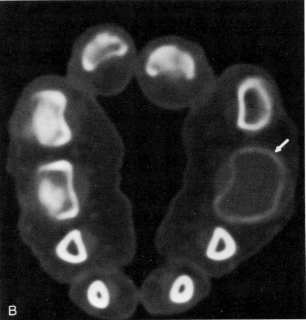

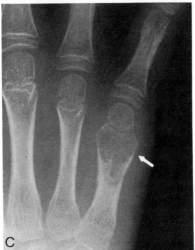

FIGURE 83–212. Giant cell reparative granuloma: Differential diagnosis of single or multicentric giant cell tumor.

A, B This 65 year old woman fell, hurting her hand. A radiograph (not shown) revealed a phalangeal lesion that was believed to be benign and to require only conservative management. One year later, a radiograph **(A)** shows an expansile, trabeculated lesion involving the proximal three quarters of the proximal phalanx of a finger. There appears to be a subtle pathologic fracture (arrowheads). The radiographic appearance is similar to that of a giant cell tumor. Transaxial CT **(B),** accomplished with the ulnar aspect of the hands in a dependent position, reveals the uniform expansion of the diametaphyseal portion of the phalanx (arrow). The cortex is thinned, but there is no soft tissue involvement. A biopsy revealed hemorrhagic fluid with pink and gray tissue, leading to an initial diagnosis of an aneurysmal bone cyst. Subsequently, curettage provided more ample tissue for analysis, resulting in a revised diagnosis of giant cell reparative granuloma.

C A 9 year old girl had a 4 month history of pain and swelling over her fifth metacarpal bone. The radiograph shows a slightly expansile, trabeculated lesion (arrow) affecting the diaphysis and metaphysis of the metacarpal bone. The epiphysis is uninvolved. CT (not shown) demonstrated that the lesion violated the cortex of the bone. Surgical excision led to a final diagnosis of a giant cell reparative granuloma.

from true giant cell tumors by their prominent fibroblastic stroma, granuloma-like arrangement around areas of stromal hemorrhage, smaller and more angulated giant cells and prominent osteoid; furthermore, giant cell reparative granulomas lack the diffuse sheets of giant cells and polygonal mononuclear cells that are seen in true giant cell tumors.[1027] Giant cell reparative granulomas are indistinguishable both radiographically and histologically from the brown tumors of hyperparathyroidism.

The precise cause and pathogenesis of this lesion are not known. Currently, giant cell reparative granulomas are considered a reactive process, perhaps in response to intraosseous hemorrhage.

Malignant Tumors

Malignant Fibrous Histiocytoma

In discussing malignant fibrous histiocytoma of bone, it is not the authors' intention to provide a comprehensive historical review of this rare tumor, as such is already available to the interested reader,[1034] nor can the controversy be resolved that even today surrounds its origin and classification. Certain aspects are clear, however: that the segregation of fibrous histiocytomas from the broad spectrum of histiocytic lesions evolved as a result of extensive investigation by Stout and many of his colleagues in the 1960s[1035–1038]; that malignant fibrous histiocytomas arise far more frequently in the soft tissues than in the bones; and that the diagnosis is established most firmly on the basis of conventional light microscopy, tissue culture, and ultrastructural studies. The occurrence of fibrous histiocytoma in bone was first emphasized by Feldman and Norman[1034] in 1972. In the ensuing 15 years, numerous additional accounts of this osseous neoplasm have appeared. Although it seems reasonable that considerable attention would be directed toward malignant fibrous histiocytomas of the soft tissue owing to their relative frequency and diverse locations in the human body, the high level of interest in malignant fibrous histiocytomas in bone is a bit surprising in view of the rarity of the tumor, and may indicate also that, in some instances, the diagnosis is incorrectly applied to other primary sarcomas of bone.[221] The concept of a histiocytic origin of a malignant (or benign) osseous (or soft tissue) neoplasm is based on the assumption that histiocytes may act as facultative fibroblasts[1038] or that primitive mesenchymal elements may give rise to both fibroblasts and histiocytes.[1039, 1040] Although it generally is held that histiocytes are derived from blood monocytes originating in the bone marrow[1041] some histochemical evidence exists that supports a close relationship between these cells and fibroblasts.[1042–1044] A recent study, however, has cast doubt on the histiocytic nature of this tumor.[1879]

Currently, certain histologic criteria that were applied originally to the diagnosis of fibrous histiocytoma of soft tissue[1035] are required for the identification of similar tumors arising in bone: bundles of fibrous and spindle-shaped fibroblast-like cells arranged in a storiform or cartwheel pattern and showing mitotic activity and nuclear atypism; round cells exhibiting features of histiocytes with ovoid, often indented or grooved nuclei and well-defined cytoplasmic borders; and typical and atypical multinucleated tumor giant cells of the osteoclastic type.[221]

Malignant fibrous histiocytoma of bone can occur de novo, in association with other osseous abnormalities, including bone infarction, intraosseous lipoma, and Paget's disease (see Chapters 54 and 80),[28, 1045] and after radiation therapy.[1880]

Clinical Abnormalities. Malignant fibrous histiocytoma of bone occurs in men more frequently than in women (in an approximate ratio of 3 to 2) and in patients of any age, although the majority of affected persons are in the fifth, sixth, and seventh decades of life.[1034, 1045–1050, 1848] Pain, tenderness, and an enlarging mass are the predominant symptoms and usually develop slowly over a period of months or even years. A more acute onset of these clinical manifestations may be indicative of a pathologic fracture (which may occur eventually in 30 to 50 per cent of patients). Discomfort and limitation of joint motion are associated with intra-articular extension of the neoplasm. A palpable and tender mass is the most common physical finding associated with malignant fibrous histiocytoma of bone.

Skeletal Location. The skeletal distribution of malignant fibrous histiocytomas is similar to that of osteosarcoma, with the ends of the long tubular bones chiefly affected (approximately 75 per cent of cases).[1046, 1051–1062] The bones in the lower extremity are involved more frequently than those in the upper extremity, in a ratio of approximately 6 to 1. The femur (approximately 45 per cent of cases), tibia (20 per cent), and humerus (9 per cent) are the most common sites of tumor localization. The innominate bone is affected in approximately 10 per cent of cases; other sites of involvement are the skull and facial bones (4 per cent), ribs (3 per cent), and, less frequently, fibula, spine, scapula, and clavicle.[1063–1072, 1881, 2222] Rarely affected are the patella[2223] and the bones of the hands and feet.

Within the long tubular bones, metaphyseal localization is the rule, with frequent extension of the tumor into the epiphysis or diaphysis, or both. The bones about the knee account for approximately 50 per cent of all tumors involving the tubular bones.

Subperiosteal[1051, 2224] and multifocal lesions in one or more bones[1059, 1069, 1073, 1074, 1916, 2225] are additional rare manifestations of malignant fibrous histiocytoma.

Radiographic Abnormalities. Osteolysis with a moth-eaten or permeative pattern of bone destruction, cortical erosion, limited periostitis, and a soft tissue mass represent the most characteristic radiographic abnormalities of a malignant fibrous histiocytoma (Fig. 83–213). The lesions are variable in size but may extend from the epiphysis to the diaphysis of a tubular bone, throughout the innominate bone, or between the body and posterior osseous elements of the vertebra. Osseous expansion is unusual but may be observed in the flat and irregular bones, such as the ribs, scapula, and sternum.[1050] Pathologic fractures are relatively frequent (Fig. 83–214).

It should be emphasized that these radiographic features indicate an aggressive skeletal process but are not specific in nature. In addition to malignant fibrous histiocytoma, osseous metastasis (especially from carcinoma of the lung or breast), plasmacytoma, lymphoma, osteolytic osteosarcoma, and fibrosarcoma are lesions that produce such abnormalities. In some instances, the age of the affected patient and additional clinical features will allow differentiation between a malignant fibrous histiocytoma and one (or more) of these other tumors; as an example, osteosarcoma usually is evident in younger persons and may be accompanied by an elevated serum level of alkaline phosphatase. Furthermore, the presence of a pathologic fracture and the absence of extensive periostitis are more compatible with a malignant fibrous histiocytoma than with an osteosarcoma. A most difficult diagnostic problem arises in attempting to differentiate between malignant fibrous histiocytoma and fibrosarcoma of bone. The similarities of the radiographic features of these two neoplasms have been emphasized repeatedly,[900] although it has been suggested that malignant fibrous histiocytomas are the more aggressive and rapidly growing of the two lesions.[1050]

Other Imaging Techniques. As in the case of most malignant neoplasms of bone, CT, MR imaging, and angiography[1075] can be used to assess the intraosseous or extraosseous extent of malignant fibrous histiocytomas. Of these methods, MR imaging probably is best at defining the size of the intraosseous tumoral component, whereas all three methods are beneficial to some degree in delineating soft tissue involvement and the relationship of the tumor to adjacent vessels or nerves. In no instance are the findings specific for malignant fibrous histiocytoma.

Pathologic Abnormalities. Macroscopically, malignant fibrous histiocytoma usually is located centrally within the bone, producing little or no osseous expansion.[1046] Cortical destruction with extension of the tumor into the soft tissue is found in 80 to 100 per cent of cases.[1045, 1055] The soft tissue component of the tumor may appear multinodular and pseudoencapsulated.[1050] The neoplasm generally is between 2 and 10 cm in size (some are larger than 20 cm)[1076] and varies in color and consistency depending on the relative proportions of fibroblastic and histiocytic cells that are present and their lipid content. It may be gray, brown, yellow, or orange and fleshy, soft, firm, or rubbery. Hemorrhagic zones are common (Fig. 83–215).

The histologic diagnosis of malignant fibrous histiocytoma frequently is one of exclusion, and it cannot be made with assurance when only a limited amount of biopsy tissue is available for analysis.[28] A spectrum of histomorphologic

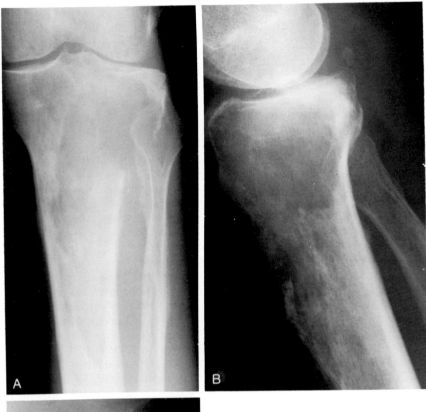

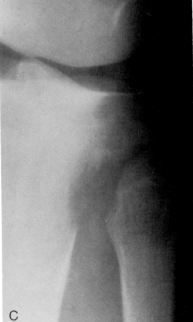

FIGURE 83–213. Malignant fibrous histiocytoma: Radiographic abnormalities—long tubular bones.

A, B Tibia. Frontal and lateral radiographs reveal motheaten bone destruction in the diaphysis, metaphysis, and epiphysis of the proximal portion of the tibia. The cortex is eroded, and a soft tissue mass and scalloped deformity of the adjacent fibula are seen. Limited periostitis is evident. (Courtesy of I. S. Tolod, M.D., Alton, Illinois.)

C Tibia. This eccentric, poorly defined osteolytic lesion involves the lateral aspect of the metaphyseal region of the tibia and is accompanied by subtle erosion of the fibula.

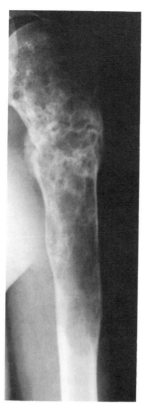

FIGURE 83–214. Malignant fibrous histiocytoma: Radiographic abnormalities—long tubular bones. An extensive osteolytic lesion of the proximal half of the humerus is seen. It is trabeculated and a pathologic fracture is seen proximally. An original biopsy was interpreted as evidence of fibrous dysplasia, but two years later, at the time of this radiograph, the diagnosis of malignant fibrous histiocytoma was documented histologically. (Courtesy of A. G. Bergman, M.D., Stanford, California.)

features, no one of which is specific or diagnostic, is evident. Although malignant fibrous histiocytomas do not have a uniform histologic pattern, they all share common light microscopic features marked by the presence, in varying amounts, of cells with fibroblastic or histiocytic characteristics, or both. The spindle-shaped fibroblasts that are evident in the fibrous regions of a malignant fibrous histiocytoma are not arranged in the classic herringbone pattern of a fibrosarcoma but, rather, the cells radiate outward in a spiral array from a central focus, producing the appearance of a nebula. In highly fibrous tumors, extensive fibrous foci create an overall mat-like or storiform appearance (Fig. 83–216A). Such storiform areas are found in about 80 per cent of the tumors, but in the more histiocytic-like varieties of malignant fibrous histiocytoma, such areas may be very scarce and may require an extensive search to be found. It should be noted, however, that the presence of the storiform pattern is not specific for malignant fibrous histiocytoma, as it also may be found in a variety of benign and malignant lesions, including osteosarcoma, leiomyosarcoma, neurosarcoma, nonossifying fibroma, and fibrous dysplasia. The fibroblast-like tumor cells also reveal a greater degree of nuclear atypism and irregularity than is seen in a conventional fibrosarcoma (Fig. 83–216B,C). Large pleomorphic multinucleated cells with abnormal mitotic figures usually are found scattered throughout these fibrous regions of malignant fibrous histiocytoma.

The histiocytic areas of malignant fibrous histiocytoma are more diverse histologically than the fibroblastic regions. In histiocytic areas, the cells may be small and oval, with grooved or reniform nuclei having clumped, irregularly distributed nuclear chromatin, prominent nucleoli, and little visible cytoplasm; they may resemble the cells of a histiocytic lymphoma.[1051, 1059, 1060] Other regions contain large, anaplastic-appearing mononuclear cells that have an abundant foamy or granular eosinophilic cytoplasm (Fig. 83–216D) frequently containing phagocytized debris or red blood cells. Cells with two or three nuclei with prominent, round eosinophilic nucleoli are present that may mimic Reed-Sternberg cells.[1059] In the more pleomorphic malignant fibrous histiocytomas, also designated fibroxanthosarcomas,[1077] there are numerous multinucleated bizarre giant cells with an abundant, dense, glassy, eosinophilic cytoplasm.

Additional histologic findings encountered in malignant fibrous histiocytomas include inflammatory cells (lymphocytes, plasma cells, eosinophils, polymorphonuclear leukocytes), foam cells, siderophages, and benign osteoclast-type giant cells. Thin bands of collagen that simulate osteoid may course between the tumor cells, making difficult the differentiation of a malignant fibrous histiocytoma and an osteosarcoma.[1051] Indeed, in decalcified sections it may be impossible to distinguish this collagen from true osteoid and, hence, to determine whether or not the tumor is an

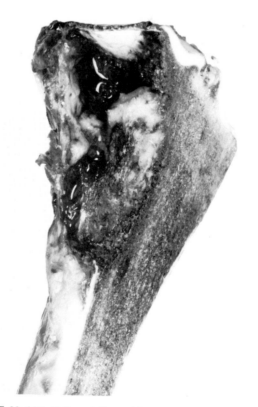

FIGURE 83–215. Malignant fibrous histiocytoma: Macroscopic abnormalities. A photograph of the lateral surface of the tibial lesion illustrated in Figure 83–213**C** reveals a partially cystic tumor that has extended to the articular cartilage. Hemorrhagic degeneration beneath the cartilaginous surface is evident. More solid neoplastic tissue also is apparent.

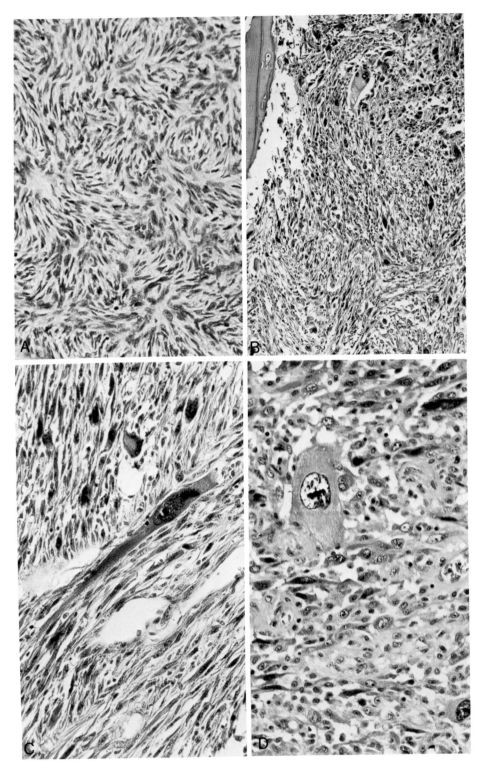

FIGURE 83–216. Malignant fibrous histiocytoma: Microscopic abnormalities.

A A highly fibrous type of tumor shows a mat-like or storiform arrangement of the spindle tumor cells. (300×.)

B Note bizarre giant tumor cells and spindle cells arranged in a whorled pattern. (150×.)

C In this fibroblastic region, the cells are spindle-shaped and vary greatly in size with malignant-appearing nuclei. This degree of nuclear pleomorphism is not found in a fibrosarcoma. (300×.)

D A predominantly histiocytic region contains round or oval tumor cells with more abundant granular cytoplasm. Large bizarre giant cells, as shown here, are quite common in the more pleomorphic (fibroxanthosarcomatous) malignant fibrous histiocytomas. (300×.)

osteosarcoma. In undecalcified material, the presence of calcification within these eosinophilic bands indicates that this is osteoid and that the tumor is in fact an osteosarcoma. Immunohistochemical stains for osteocalcin also may be helpful, being positive in osteosarcoma and negative in malignant fibrous histiocytoma.[2479]

The variability of the microscopic abnormalities of malignant fibrous histiocytomas has led to the subdivision of the soft tissue tumors into myxoid, inflammatory, angiomatoid, and pleomorphic varieties.[1078–1080] In most reports,

however, the osseous lesions are designated simply as malignant fibrous histiocytomas. Studies of these tumors using electron microscopy have allowed identification of three major types of cells: fibroblast-like cells, histiocyte-like cells, and primitive, undifferentiated mesenchymal cells.[1053, 1056, 1059, 1061, 1065, 1069, 1073, 1074, 1076, 1081] Myofibroblasts, foam cells, and multinucleated osteoclast-type giant cells also have been observed.

Natural History. The aggressive nature of malignant fibrous histiocytoma in bone is underscored by the frequency of local recurrence (as high as 80 per cent of tumors) and of metastasis to regional lymph nodes and distant sites (especially the lungs but also the liver, brain, heart, kidneys, intestines, and adrenal glands). Although the reported rate of 5 year survival in patients with this neoplasm has varied considerably (from zero to approximately 70 per cent),[28, 30, 180, 1045, 1046, 1049, 1052, 1061] the malignant nature of this tumor is not questioned, especially in older patients and in those with an underlying osseous abnormality (e.g., osteonecrosis).[1048]

TUMORS OF FATTY DIFFERENTIATION

Benign Tumors

Lipoma

Lipomas are among the most common of soft tissue lesions but among the more unusual of osseous lesions. As adipose tissue is present in abundance as a normal constit-

uent in the marrow cavity, the infrequency of lipomas of bone is surprising but may be explained, in part, by (1) the benign radiographic appearance of the lesions, which may lessen the need for surgical confirmation of the diagnosis; and (2) the classification of osseous lipomas as other processes, including ischemic necrosis, simple (unicameral) or aneurysmal bone cysts, or fibrous dysplasia on the basis of their radiographic or histologic characteristics, or both. When microscopic analysis reveals large collections of mature lipocytes, the diagnosis of a lipoma is most secure; when such analysis discloses myxomatous cells, cystic degeneration, or fat necrosis, alternative diagnoses may be offered by the pathologist. In fact, the true nature of the osseous lipoma is a subject of considerable controversy. It has been considered either a neoplasm or a degenerative phenomenon related to trauma, infection, or vascular compromise. Undeniable, however, are the unique radiographic abnormalities that accompany many of these lesions and that allow their precise identification.

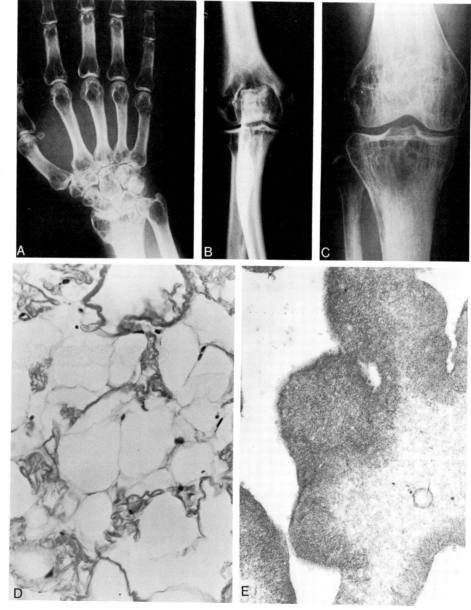

FIGURE 83–217. Membranous lipodystrophy. This rare hereditary disorder of adipose tissue affects principally the bones and central nervous system. Clinical manifestations related to pathologic fractures usually begin in the second or third decade of life; subsequently, progressive neuropsychiatric symptoms, dementia, and seizures may be evident, and the patients commonly die by the age of 50 years.

A–C The radiographic hallmark of this disease is symmetric, cystic lesions in the bones of the appendicular skeleton.

D Histologic evaluation of the bone reveals replacement of normal fat cells by numerous membranous structures with an eosinophilic, cystic appearance.

E Electron microscopy reveals a distinctive structure in the membranes. See Chapter 61 for a more detailed analysis of this disorder.

(Courtesy of I. Sugiura, M.D., Nagoya, Japan.)

Lipomas can be categorized according to their location in the bone as intraosseous, cortical, or parosteal lesions. Each of these will be considered in the following discussion. The reader should refer to Chapters 84 and 95 for information related to soft tissue lipomas and to Chapter 61 for an analysis of membranous lipodystrophy (Fig. 83–217).

Intraosseous Lipoma. Most of the descriptions of this rare lesion are based on observations in a single patient,[1082–1106, 1849, 1882, 2226–2228, 2237] although a few reports exist in which a series of affected patients have been evaluated.[30, 34, 1107–1111, 2229, 2236]

Clinical Abnormalities. Intraosseous lipomas are observed in men and women with about equal frequency and in patients of all ages (5 to 75 years of age), although most are identified in persons in the fourth, fifth, or sixth decade of life. These lesions may be entirely asymptomatic; however, approximately two thirds of patients with intraosseous lipomas have localized pain and variable amounts of soft tissue swelling. The pain may be short or long in duration, aching in character, constant or intermittent in nature, and possibly aggravated by activity.[1112] Tenderness to palpation and, rarely, manifestations related to compression of adjacent neurovascular structures are evident.

Skeletal Location. Intraosseous lipomas occur most commonly in the long tubular bones, especially the fibula (20 per cent of cases), femur (15 per cent), and tibia (13 per cent), and calcaneus (15 per cent). Other reported sites have included the ribs, skull, sacrum, ilium, ischium, coccyx, thoracolumbar spine, mandible, maxilla, and the bones in the hands and feet and about the shoulders and elbows. Involvement of the bones in the lower extremity is far more frequent than that in the upper extremity in a ratio of approximately 6 to 1. In the tubular bones, a metaphyseal localization is characteristic; diaphyseal involvement is unusual. Multifocal lesions are exceedingly rare,[1113] although patients are described in whom more than 10 bones have been affected (lipomatosis).[1114, 2230] Hyperlipoproteinemia may be an associated abnormality in such patients.[1113]

Radiographic Abnormalities. Intraosseous lipomas typically appear as osteolytic lesions that are surrounded by a thin, well-defined sclerotic border. Lobulation or internal osseous ridges frequently are present, and, in bones of small

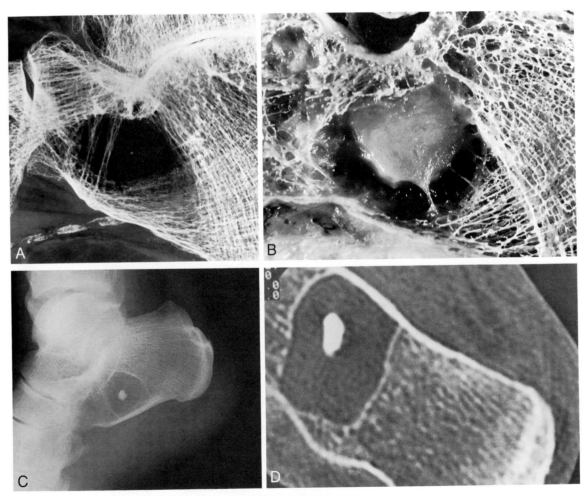

FIGURE 83–218. Intraosseous lipoma: Radiographic abnormalities—calcaneus.

A, B A radiograph **(A)** and photograph **(B)** of a sagittal section of the calcaneus show the classic location of an intraosseous lipoma. Note localization of the lesion in the triangular area between the major trabecular groups at the junction of the anterior and middle thirds of the bone. This location is identical to that in which simple cysts are found.

C, D A classic lipoma is shown with radiography **(C)** and transaxial CT **(D)**. The lesion is well defined, radiolucent, and surrounded by a thin sclerotic margin, and it contains a central radiodense focus. The documentation of fat in the lesion can be accomplished with measurements of attenuation derived from CT data.

(C, D, Courtesy of J. Castello, M.D., Madrid, Spain.)

caliber such as the fibula or the ribs, osseous expansion may be evident. Cortical destruction and periosteal reaction are notably absent. Rarely, an aggressive radiographic appearance is seen.[1086]

The aforementioned radiographic features are not entirely specific, but in two locations—the calcaneus and the proximal portion of the femur—the constellation of roentgenographic alterations is virtually diagnostic. In the calcaneus, intraosseous lipomas occur almost invariably in the triangular area between the major trabecular groups, in the same location as simple cysts (Fig. 83–218). An osteolytic area with sclerotic margins and, often, a central calcified or ossified nidus is evident. In the proximal portion of the femur (Fig. 83–219), an intraosseous lipoma is characterized by marked ossification involving a large portion of the lesional margin.[1100, 1110] In this site, lipomas most typically occur along the intertrochanteric line or in the femoral neck above the trochanters. Elsewhere, a sharply defined radiolucent lesion is typical (Fig. 83–220).

With regard to differential diagnosis, the radiographic

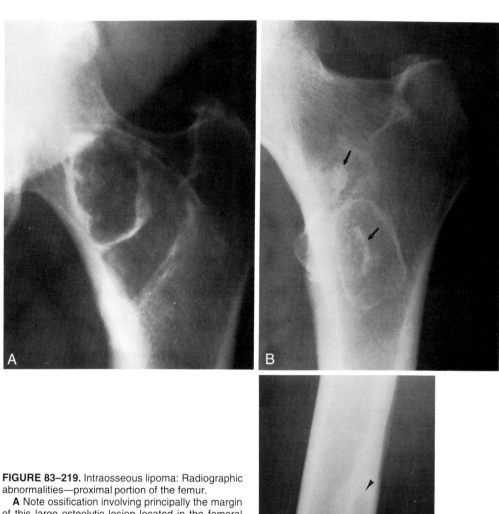

FIGURE 83–219. Intraosseous lipoma: Radiographic abnormalities—proximal portion of the femur.

A Note ossification involving principally the margin of this large osteolytic lesion located in the femoral neck above the intertrochanteric line.

B, C In a different patient, a radiograph of the proximal portion of the femur **(B)** reveals two lesions with features similar to those in **A.** A radiodense focus (arrows) is identified in the center of each of these lesions. CT (not shown) documented the fatty nature of these radiolucent foci. A lateral radiograph of the distal portion of the same femur **(C)** shows two intracortical radiolucent lesions (arrowheads), presumably representing additional lipomas.

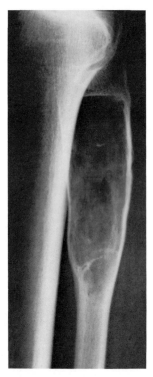

FIGURE 83–220. Intraosseous lipoma: Radiographic abnormalities—fibula. Note the slightly expansile, osteolytic lesion of the proximal portion of the fibula. (Courtesy of P. Sirotta, M.D., Seattle, Washington.)

features of an intraosseous lipoma in locations other than the calcaneus and proximal portion of the femur resemble those of other benign lesions. The major alternative diagnostic possibilities when considering intraosseous lipomas of the calcaneus are variations in the normal trabecular pattern (Fig. 83–221) and a simple bone cyst; in the proximal portion of the femur, intraosseous lipomas must be differentiated from fibrous dysplasia, a simple bone cyst, and, perhaps, a cementoma of bone. The last lesion, which may be related to a bone cyst, is considered later in this chapter.

Other Imaging Techniques. Although generally it is not necessary, CT is able to identify the fatty component of an intraosseous (or parosteal) lipoma definitively owing to the characteristic low attenuation value of such tissue[1109, 1111, 1849, 2238] (Figs. 83–222 and 83–223). It should be noted, however, that other lesions, such as those containing histiocytes laden with fat vacuoles or areas of fatty degeneration resulting from infarction, may yield comparably low CT values.[1111] Furthermore, the demonstration of a fluid level within a lesion on CT does not necessarily mean that it contains fat; fluid-fluid levels have been described in aneurysmal bone cysts, giant cell tumors, and chondroblastomas, and gas-fluid levels have been encountered in solitary bone cysts.

MR imaging represents an additional method that is capable of demonstrating fatty tissue exquisitely,[1917] although it has been applied principally to the evaluation of soft tissue lesions.[1115] The intrinsic relaxation parameters (T1, T2, and spin density) are the same for lipomas and normal fat owing to the presence in both cases of an identical type of cell. Therefore, benign lipomas and normal adipose tis-

sue yield signals of comparable intensity regardless of the echo and repetition times that are selected (Figs. 83–224 and 83–225). The differentiation between benign lipomas and old hematomas and between benign lipomas and liposarcomas in the soft tissues is possible with MR imaging, and this imaging method also is applied successfully to the evaluation of intraosseous lipomas.

Pathologic Abnormalities. Intraosseous lipomas vary in size (2 to 13 cm), with most measuring 5 to 6 cm in maximum dimension. They usually are pale or bright yellow and appear well demarcated, occasionally possessing a thin fibrous capsule.[1082, 1087, 1092, 1116] The lesions are divided into lobules of various sizes by delicate fibrous septa. Their cut surface is greasy and may reveal oily droplets.[1085, 1112] As with extraosseous lipomas, intraosseous lipomas are soft, but, unlike their extraosseous counterparts, they are somewhat gritty when sectioned owing to the presence of scattered small trabeculae within their substance. Central areas of the lesion may contain white calcified foci.

The basic histomorphology of an intraosseous lipoma is identical to that of an extraosseous lipoma.[1106] The tumor is composed of mature, adult fat cells separated into lobules by thin fibrovascular septa. In addition, intraosseous lipomas usually contain a few small, irregular, atrophic trabeculae. These trabeculae may appear either necrotic, as manifested by the lack of osteocytes in the bone lacunae, or normal (Fig. 83–226). In only a few reported cases have these trabeculae been absent or not mentioned.[1084, 1086, 1089, 1105, 1107] Occasionally, central areas of hyalinized fibrous tissue are found, as well as necrotic foci containing dystrophic calcification. These latter areas account for the sclerotic central regions that are noted on radiographs. Some reported cases of intraosseous lipoma have had increased vascularity and are best considered angiolipomas.[1093, 1101]

Histologically, it may not be possible to differentiate between a necrotic intraosseous lipoma and a bone infarct.

Intracortical Lipoma. The intracortical lipoma appears to represent the rarest of all osseous lipomas, with only one well-documented case being recorded.[1117] The patient, a 34 year old woman, developed a long, septate lesion in the posterolateral surface of the diaphysis of the femur, leading to cortical expansion (Fig. 83–227). A number of small spheroid and linear radiolucent areas were present within the lipoma.

Parosteal Lipoma. Although this rare lesion has been described on numerous occasions,[1086, 1111, 1118–1120, 2231–2233] it should be noted that a soft tissue lipoma that abuts on the bone cannot easily be distinguished from a lipoma that truly arises in the periosteal membrane and, indeed, parosteal and soft tissue lipomas may occur together.[2232] Parosteal lipomas show no specific age or sex predilection and generally are asymptomatic, although rarely they may lead to a soft tissue mass. Usually a long tubular bone is affected, most commonly the femur, humerus, or tibia. The diagnosis of this lesion can be suggested on the basis of the radiographic findings when a radiolucent mass (of fat density) is adherent to the external osseous surface in combination with cortical hyperostosis or periostitis (see Chapter 95). Such cortical changes, which may produce an osteochondroma-like configuration,[1118, 2232] are observed in approximately 10 per cent of cases. Additional radiographic abnormalities include bowing of the bone and cortical erosion. As with intraosseous lipoma, CT, and MR imaging (Fig. 83–228)

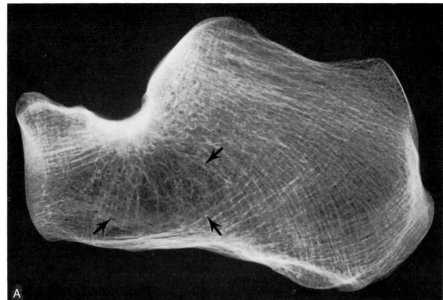

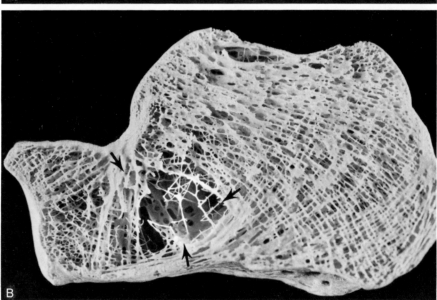

FIGURE 83–221. Normal calcaneal trabecular pattern: Differential diagnosis of intraosseous lipoma. A radiograph **(A)** and photograph **(B)** of a sagittal section of the calcaneus show the normal trabecular thinning (arrows) that may be encountered. The radiolucent area that is created by such thinning is usually less prominent and less well marginated than that related to an intraosseous lipoma or simple cyst.

can document the fatty tissue within the parosteal lesion.[1111, 2232, 2233, 2480, 2481] With MR imaging, foci of fibrous and cartilaginous tissue and muscle atrophy (related to nerve impingement) also may be evident.[2481]

Malignant Tumors

Liposarcoma

Liposarcoma rarely arises in bone. There only are a few reported descriptions of this occurrence, and the presence of osteosarcomatous foci in some of these reported examples probably would lead to their reclassification as osteosarcoma or malignant mesenchymoma on the basis of current diagnostic criteria.[1121–1124] An analysis of additional reported examples of intraosseous liposarcomas is made difficult owing to the unavailability of adequate histologic data[1125–1134]; the possibility of misdiagnosis becomes more likely in those instances in which a limited amount of biopsy tissue was available for microscopic evaluation,[1135, 1136]

as osteosarcoma and malignant fibrous histiocytoma may contain liposarcoma-like foci. In one report,[2235] histologic evidence of liposarcoma (or malignant fibrous histiocytoma) in association with benign intraosseous lipomas was found in four patients.

Liposarcomas of bone appear to be slightly more frequent in men than in women and may be seen in patients of all ages. They almost invariably occur in the long tubular bones, including the tibia, femur, and, less commonly, fibula, humerus, and ulna.[1137–1145, 2234, 2235] The diaphysis, metaphysis, or epiphysis may be affected, and large tumors may extend from one of these segments to an adjacent one. Very rarely, a nontubular bone is affected.[2381] Radiographically, a nonspecific, well-defined or poorly defined area of osteolysis is observed. Scalloped erosion of the external surface of the bone may accompany juxtacortical liposarcomas.[2234]

Macroscopically, intraosseous liposarcomas are soft, friable, lobulated, yellow tumors of variable size that may lead to thinning or erosion of the cortex, cortical violation,

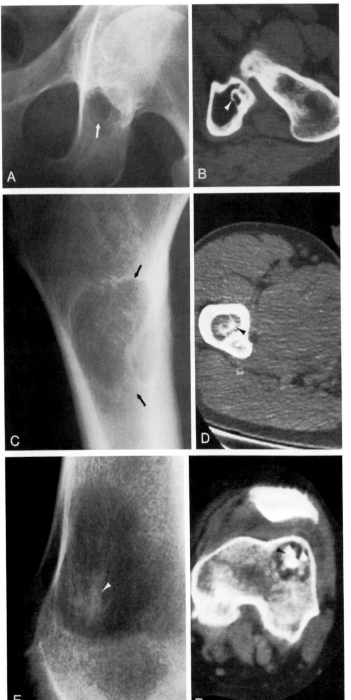

FIGURE 83–222. Intraosseous lipoma: CT abnormalities.

A, B Ischium. This radiolucent lesion (arrow) was discovered incidentally on a radiograph **(A).** With transaxial CT, its fatty nature and ossific component (arrowhead) are evident.

C, D Proximal portion of the femur. In a 36 year old man with several months of hip pain, a radiograph **(C)** reveals a well-defined lesion (arrows) of the metadiaphysis of the bone. Transaxial CT **(D)** shows its fatty nature and ossific component (arrowhead). Surgery confirmed the presence of a fatty lesion with trabecular necrosis.

E, F Distal portion of the femur. Knee pain in a 55 year old woman was accompanied by swelling, warmth, and redness. A radiograph **(E)** shows a large radiolucent lesion containing ossification (arrowhead). These features, including the ossification (arrowhead), are better seen with transaxial CT **(F).** A lipoma was documented after surgical removal of the lesion.

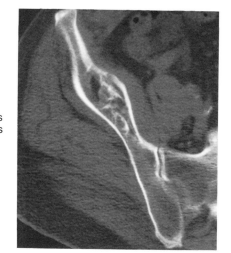

FIGURE 83–223. Intraosseous lipoma: CT abnormalities. In this case, transaxial CT reveals an ossified, slightly expansile radiolucent lesion of the ilium. Biopsy confirmed an intraosseous lipoma. (Courtesy of T. Broderick, M.D., Orange, California.)

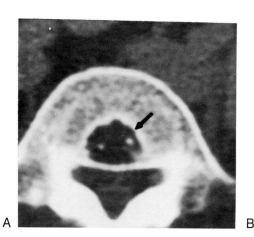

A

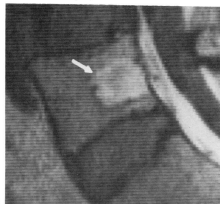

B

FIGURE 83–224. Intraosseous lipoma: MR imaging abnormalities. Transaxial CT **(A)** shows a radiolucent lesion (arrow) containing calcific foci. A sagittal T1-weighted (TR/TE, 200/20) spin echo MR image **(B)** confirms the fatty nature of the lesion (arrow).

FIGURE 83–225. Intraosseous lipoma: MR imaging abnormalities. In this sagittal T2-weighted (TR/TE, 2000/80) spin echo MR image, note the fatty nature of the partially ossified lesion of the calcaneus (arrow). (Courtesy of A. Newberg, M.D., Boston, Massachusetts.)

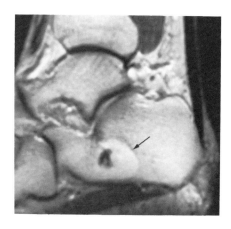

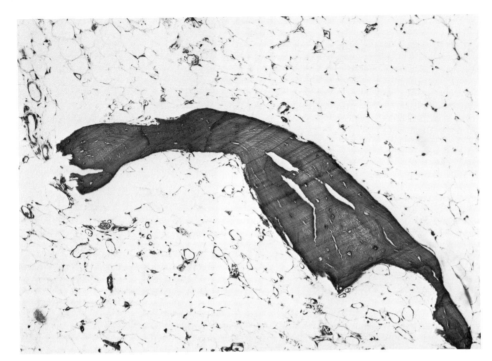

FIGURE 83–226. Intraosseous lipoma: Microscopic abnormalities. An isolated trabeculum of normal bone is surrounded by mature fat cells. (150×.)

FIGURE 83–227. Intracortical lipoma: Radiographic abnormalities. Note the area of localized cortical thickening containing serpentine-like radiolucent regions. (From Downey EF Jr, et al: Skel Radiol *10:*189, 1983.)

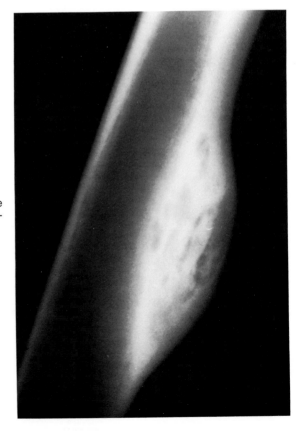

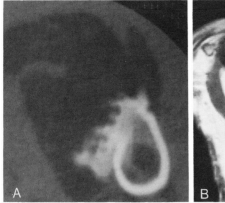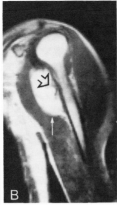

FIGURE 83–228. Parosteal lipoma: CT and MR imaging abnormalities. In a 32 year old man with a slowly enlarging mass in the shoulder, transaxial CT **(A)** confirms the fatty nature of the mass and subjacent hyperostosis and bone proliferation in the humerus. In a coronal T1-weighted (TR/TE, 500/16) spin echo MR image **(B),** the fatty composition of the mass (solid arrow) is confirmed. Irregular bone spicules (open arrow) of low signal intensity are evident. (Courtesy of M. Murphey, M.D., Washington, D.C.)

and soft tissue extension. Microscopically, the pleomorphic and myxoid varieties of liposarcoma have features in common with the pleomorphic and myxoid types of malignant fibrous histiocytoma.[1146] Pleomorphic (Fig. 83–229) or well-differentiated liposarcomas predominate. The former are characterized by irregular cells with abundant eosinophilic cytoplasm and bizarre anaplastic-appearing nuclei with prominent nucleoli. Many of the tumor cells are multinucleated, and numerous multivacuolated and univacuolated lipoblasts are present. Mitoses are frequent. In some regions, tumor cells may be spindle-shaped and arranged in a storiform pattern. The well-differentiated liposarcomas possess cells that resemble adult adipocytes, except for their irregular, hyperchromatic, atypical nuclei, or that contain large, centrally located nuclei surrounded by numerous cytoplasmic vacuoles. Electron microscopy of intraosseous liposarcomas indicates that these tumors have the same fine

structural cellular features that are found in soft tissue liposarcomas.[1142, 1143]

To establish a firm diagnosis of an intraosseous liposarcoma, two criteria must be met. The tumor must have the histologic features of liposarcoma, and a soft tissue origin or metastatic neoplasm must be excluded.[1140] Among the metastatic tumors, those arising from renal cell carcinoma most closely simulate liposarcoma.[1141]

TUMORS OF MUSCLE DIFFERENTIATION

Benign Tumors

Leiomyoma

This neoplasm of smooth muscle is well recognized in extraskeletal sites, such as the uterus, ovary, gastrointestinal tract, bladder, and lung. It also may occur in the superficial soft tissues of the extremity in close relationship to blood vessels or hair follicles, and, on rare occasions, a leiomyoma apparently can arise in the periosteal membrane[1147] or in bone.[2482]

Malignant Tumors

Leiomyosarcoma

Leiomyosarcoma is a malignant neoplasm of smooth muscle cells that occurs predominantly in the uterus and gastrointestinal tract. Such extraosseous tumors, especially those in the uterus, subsequently may metastasize to distant sites, including the lung, liver, kidney, brain, skin, and, less commonly, bone.[1148, 1149] Although the occurrence of skeletal metastasis as an initial manifestation of a leiomyosarcoma is rare, it is important to exclude such a possibility whenever leiomyosarcomatous tissue is discovered in bone.[1150]

Leiomyosarcomas originating in bone are exceedingly rare. The diagnosis is established by the exclusion of a primary malignant neoplasm in an extraosseous site; the presence within the bone of the bulk of the tumor; and the

FIGURE 83–229. Liposarcoma: Histologic abnormalities.

A In this pleomorphic tumor, lipoblasts with malignant nuclei and multivacuolated cytoplasm are seen. The cytoplasmic vacuoles indent and cause scalloping of the nuclei. (300×.)

B This pleomorphic tumor is characterized by the presence of bizarre giant cells that have abundant, glassy, eosinophilic cytoplasm. Such cells may also be found in malignant fibrous histiocytoma and osteosarcoma. Multivacuolated lipoblasts are seen in the lower left side of the photomicrograph. (350×.)

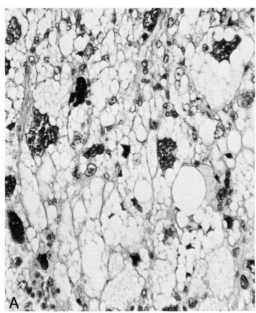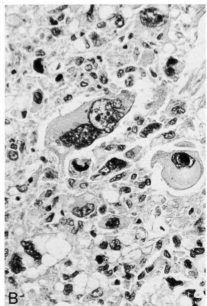

documentation of characteristic histopathologic features.[1151] In these instances, it generally is assumed that the leiomyosarcoma arose from preexisting smooth muscle cells. As bone is a tissue poor in smooth muscle, it is those cells in the media of the intraosseous blood vessels that are considered to be the point of neoplastic departure.[1151] Alternatively, a close relationship may exist between fibroblasts and smooth muscle cells such that an intermediate cellular form, the myofibroblast, may give rise to the leiomyosarcoma.[1151]

There are only a few documented cases of primary leiomyosarcoma of bone.[1151–1159, 1918, 2239, 2382, 2383] On the basis of these reports, it appears that primary leiomyosarcomas of bone occur in men and women with approximately equal frequency and at any age (although most commonly in elderly patients). Pain and swelling of months to years in duration are the most common manifestations. The lesions predominate in the tubular bones, especially the femur and the tibia, and involvement of the bones about the knee is particularly characteristic. Metaphyseal or, less commonly, epiphyseal or diaphyseal abnormalities typically consist of a poorly defined osteolytic lesion (Fig. 83–230A), with or without a soft tissue mass and, rarely, periostitis or intralesional calcification. A pathologic fracture and intra-articular extension are additional potential manifestations of this tumor.[1151] Less common sites of leiomyosarcoma include the gnathic bones, clavicle, acetabular region, ribs, and small bones of the hand and foot.

Macroscopically, intramedullary (Fig. 83–230B) and soft tissue extension of the tumor is seen. Its size is variable, with the greatest dimension of the neoplasm usually being between 3 and 12 cm. Microscopically, skeletal leiomyosarcoma consists of intersecting bundles of spindle-shaped cells that have elongated, blunt-ended, central nuclei residing within a scant fibrillar cytoplasm.[1157] This cytoplasm becomes intensely red with the use of trichrome stains. The cells vary in appearance within a single tumor, with some cells showing little or no nuclear atypia and others revealing highly pleomorphic, irregular, enlarged, and hyperchromatic nuclei (Fig. 83–231). Some tumor cells have prominent paranuclear vacuoles that are rich in glycogen. Multinucleated tumor cells with bizarre nuclei and prominent nucleoli are common. In some regions, the nuclei are round and plump, creating an epithelioid appearance. The stroma varies from areas in which little or no stroma is visible to broad hyalinized fibrous zones or edematous myxoid regions in which the cells are loosely arranged. Mitotic figures usually are easily found. Electron microscopy may reveal features suggestive of a smooth muscle origin.[1159]

The subsequent course of osseous leiomyosarcomas is variable; rapid local extension and widespread metastases

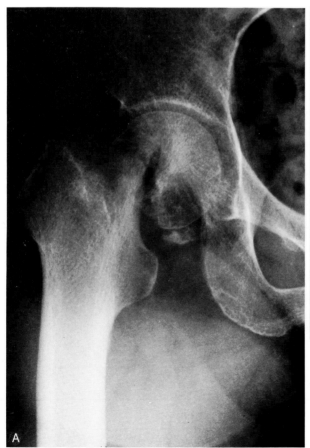

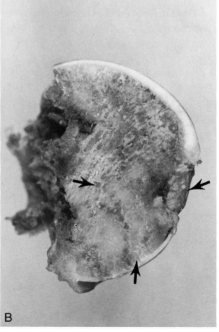

FIGURE 83–230. Leiomyosarcoma: Radiographic and macroscopic abnormalities. A 60 year old woman developed a mass in the right hip following a fall. Two months after the injury, a radiograph **(A)** shows an osteolytic lesion in the femoral neck and head with a pathologic fracture. A replacement of the femoral head was performed. The cut surface of the specimen **(B)** reveals tumor (arrows) extending to the subchondral bone and into the cartilage. Histologic evaluation confirmed the presence of a leiomyosarcoma apparently originating in bone. (From Kawai T, et al: Arch Pathol Lab Med 107:433, 1983. Copyright 1983 by the American Medical Association.)

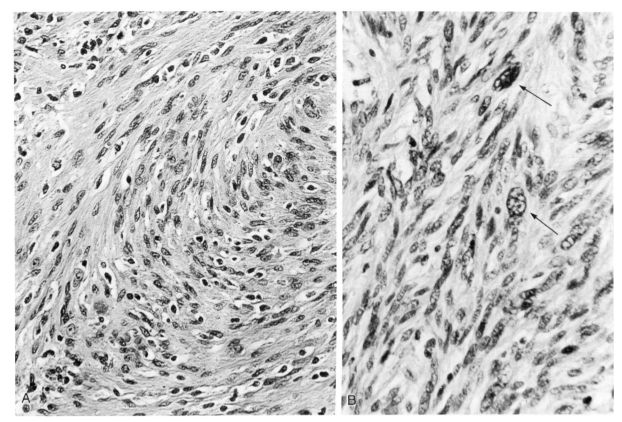

FIGURE 83–231. Leiomyosarcoma: Microscopic abnormalities.
A Spindle-shaped cells with bizarre nuclei are seen. (300×).
B At higher magnification, note the elongated nuclei. Two enlarged, atypical nuclei also are present (arrows). Similar nuclear atypia may be evident in benign smooth muscle cells. (600×.)

are evident in some cases, whereas in others, appropriate therapy has led to long-term patient survival.

Rhabdomyosarcoma

Although rhabdomyosarcoma is a common malignant tumor in children, arising principally in the soft tissues of the head and neck, the urogenital tract, and the retroperitoneum, its occurrence as a primary neoplasm of bone is exceedingly rare.[1160, 1850] Primary rhabdomyosarcoma of bone must be differentiated from an extraskeletal rhabdomyosarcoma that has metastasized to bone or one that originates in the periosseous soft tissue and secondarily invades bone.[1161, 1162] As striated muscle is not a normal constituent of bone, a primary intraosseous rhabdomyosarcoma must arise from other types of tissue, perhaps undifferentiated mesenchymal cells.[1163]

TUMORS OF VASCULAR DIFFERENTIATION

Benign Tumors

Hemangioma

Hemangiomas of bone are infrequent lesions composed of vascular channels that are cavernous, capillary, or venous in type.

Clinical Abnormalities. Osseous hemangiomas usually are identified in middle-aged patients, particularly those in the fourth and fifth decades of life. Women are affected about twice as frequently as men. Many such hemangiomas

are insignificant clinically, being discovered as incidental findings on radiographs obtained for unrelated reasons. Some, however, may be associated with soft tissue swelling or pain, particularly in the presence of a pathologic fracture. On rare occasions, vertebral hemangiomas may be accompanied by symptoms and signs of spinal cord compression owing to extension of the lesions into the epidural space, expansion of the involved vertebrae leading to narrowing of the spinal canal, epidural hemorrhage arising from the lesions, compression fractures of the involved vertebrae, or combinations of these causes.[1164–1166,1851] Asymptomatic hemangiomas of the vertebral column may become symptomatic during pregnancy owing to rapid expansion of the tumor or vertebral collapse.[2240, 2241] Single or multiple osseous hemangiomas (with or without soft tissue hemangiomas) also may lead to hemihypertrophy of an extremity.[1167]

Skeletal Location. Single lesions predominate, although examples of multiple primary hemangiomas of bone are recorded.[1167, 1168] The two most common sites of involvement are the vertebrae and the skull or facial bones. It has been estimated that hemangiomas can be found in approximately 10 per cent of spines that are examined carefully at the time of autopsy.[1169] In the spine, hemangiomas are most frequent in the thoracic segment and in the vertebral body, but cervical or lumbar regions may be affected, and hemangiomas may extend into or localize primarily in the posterior osseous elements of the vertebrae.[1170–1176] Most vertebral hemangiomas are small and asymptomatic. Although hemangiomas in the skull are less frequent than those in the

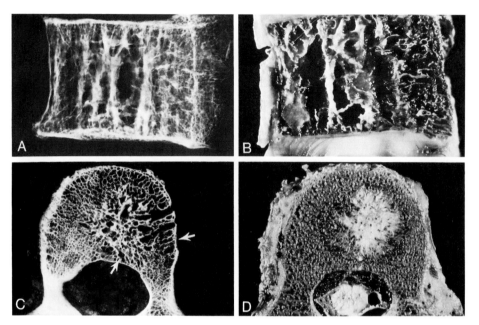

FIGURE 83–232. Hemangioma: Radiographic abnormalities—spine.

A, B A radiograph and photograph of a sagittal section of a thoracic vertebral body show a hemangioma. A corduroy appearance on the radiograph relates to thickening of some of the vertical trabeculae with dissolution of horizontal trabeculae. In this case, most of the vertebral body is affected.

C, D A radiograph and photograph of a transverse section of a vertebra show a hemangioma involving one portion of the vertebral body. Note the radiographic appearance that, in this plane, is characterized by focal cystic areas interspersed with regions of trabecular thickening (arrows). This appearance should be compared with that evident in the transaxial CT scans shown in Figure 83–233.

FIGURE 83–233. Hemangioma: Radiographic and CT abnormalities—spine.

A, B Cervical spine. In a 23 year old woman with neck pain, a radiograph **(A)** shows the characteristic coarse trabecular pattern of a hemangioma. Note that, in this case, the involved vertebral body is partially collapsed. Transaxial CT **(B)** shows the thick vertical trabeculae, appearing as radiodense foci, in the vertebral body. Surgery confirmed the presence of a hemangioma. (Courtesy of R. Linovitz, M.D., San Diego, California.)

C, D Lumbar spine. This elderly patient had hemangiomas in multiple vertebral bodies. A lateral radiograph **(C)** shows osteopenia of the fifth lumbar vertebral body (arrow) and pedicles. The transaxial CT scan **(D)** through this vertebra documents hemangiomatous involvement of the vertebral body and at least the left pedicle. (Courtesy of V. Vint, M.D., San Diego, California.)

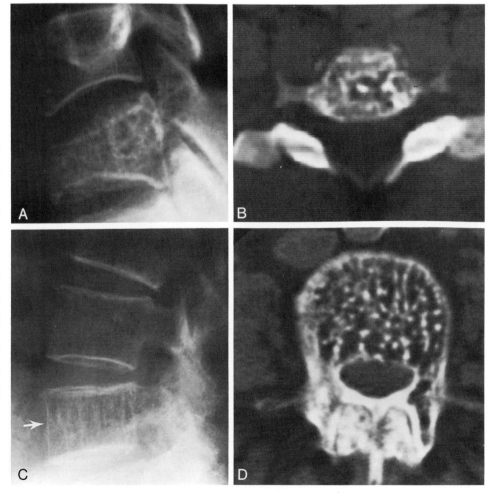

spine, they typically are more significant clinically.[30, 139, 1177] The frontal and parietal bones are affected most commonly.[1178–1182] In the facial bones, hemangiomas predominate in the mandible and, less commonly, the maxilla, although other sites may be affected.[1183–1198, 1852, 2242]

Hemangiomas in the long tubular bones are uncommon and usually are observed in the epiphyseal and metaphyseal regions, especially in the femur, tibia, and humerus.[33, 1199–1201, 2243] It is in such bones that intracortical and periosteal hemangiomas also are observed (see later discussion). Hemangiomas in the short tubular bones of the hands and feet also are uncommon.[1202, 2244] Rare sites of involvement are the patella, scapula, ribs, clavicle, sternum, and innominate, carpal, and tarsal bones.[1203–1205, 2245]

Radiographic Abnormalities. Hemangiomas in the spine produce diagnostic radiographic alterations (Figs. 83–232 to 83–234). A coarse, vertical trabecular pattern, the corduroy appearance, is identified in the vertebral body and may extend into the pedicles and laminae.[1919] The trabeculae are more prominent than those that accompany osteoporosis, and their vertical orientation differs from the subchondral, horizontally arranged trabecular condensation that

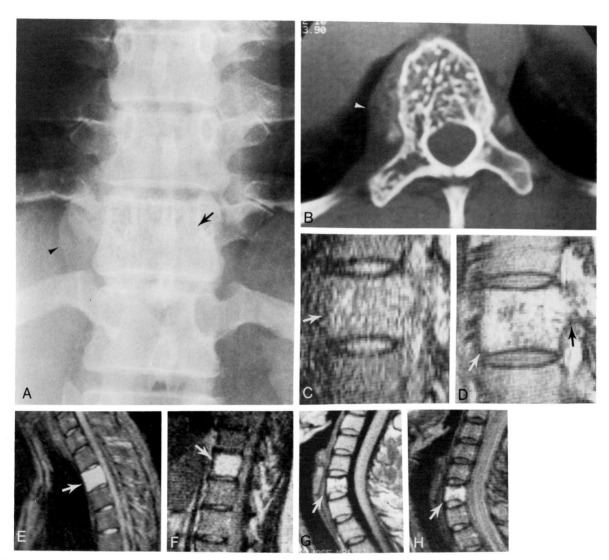

FIGURE 83–234. Hemangioma: Radiographic, CT, and MR imaging abnormalities—spine.

A–D A 37 year old woman developed back pain. A frontal radiograph **(A)** shows an osteopenic thoracic vertebral body (arrow) with accentuation of its vertical trabeculae. Note, in addition, the paraspinal mass (arrowhead) on the right side of the affected vertebral body. A bone scan (not shown) revealed increased uptake of the radionuclide at the site of the lesion. Transaxial CT **(B)** reveals the typical intraosseous findings of a hemangioma involving both the vertebral body and the posterior osseous elements on the right and a small paraspinal mass containing calcification or ossification (arrowhead). Sagittal spin echo MR images with T1 weighting **(C)** and T2 weighting **(D)** reveal increased signal intensity in the involved vertebral body and pedicle (arrows) that is more dramatic in **D**. Although the lesion was not biopsied, the findings are compatible with an intraosseous hemangioma associated with either tumor extension or hemorrhage in the soft tissues.

E, F Sagittal spin echo MR images with T2 weighting in two different hemangiomas of the thoracic vertebral bodies (arrows) show a bright signal at the site of the lesions.

(**E,** Courtesy of M. Modic, M.D., Cleveland, Ohio; **F,** courtesy of M. Solomon, M.D., San Jose, California.)

G, H T1- **(G)** and T2- **(H)** weighted sagittal spin echo MR images show a hemangioma (arrows) involving the sixth cervical vertebral body. The lesion has a bright signal on both imaging sequences.

(**G, H,** Courtesy of M. Solomon, M.D., San Jose, California.)

typifies Paget's disease (the picture-frame vertebral body) or renal osteodystrophy (the rugger-jersey vertebral body). It should be emphasized, however, that hemangiomas need not involve an entire vertebral body, but, rather, may lead to focal radiolucent areas with coarse trabeculae arranged in a honeycomb or cartwheel configuration, and that such lesions rarely may localize in a posterior osseous element of the vertebra without involvement of the vertebral body. Vertebral fracture is unusual (Fig. 83–235); however, extension of the lesion into the paraspinal soft tissues and spinal canal may be evident, resulting in radiographic abnormalities that simulate those of a malignant neoplasm (e.g., skeletal metastasis, lymphoma, plasmacytoma, and chordoma).[1919]

In extraspinal sites, the radiographic findings associated with hemangiomas are less characteristic, although a radiolucent, slightly expansile, and well-defined intraosseous lesion, possessing a radiating, lattice-like or weblike trabecular pattern, is highly suggestive of the diagnosis (Figs. 83–236 and 83–237). Cortical thinning and osseous expansion may be seen, but extensive periostitis or a soft tissue mass is rare. Rare also is the demonstration of osteosclerosis as a dominant radiologic abnormality.[1204] In all locations, it is the distinctive trabecular pattern of a hemangioma that represents the most helpful diagnostic clue. Although this finding is not uniformly present or entirely specific,[1206, 1207] its frequency and specificity should not be underestimated.

Intracortical[1176, 1208, 1209] and *periosteal*[1210–1213, 2243, 2246, 2247] hemangiomas, although rare, represent a definite diagnostic challenge. Both predominate in the diaphysis of a long tubular bone, especially the tibia or the fibula. Radiographically, intracortical hemangiomas are associated with a well-defined, osteolytic area with or without cortical thickening and periostitis, which is identical to the findings in an osteoid osteoma or, perhaps, cortical fibrous dysplasia, ossifying fibroma, or a Brodie's abscess. Similarly, a periosteal hemangioma leads to cortical thickening and periostitis in association with a cup-shaped or saucer-like depression in the outer surface of the cortex, resembling an osteoid osteoma, juxtacortical chondroma, parosteal lipoma,

neurofibroma, or a low grade malignant periosteal neoplasm.

Other Imaging Techniques. Bone scintigraphy may be used to evaluate skeletal hemangiomas, although the results are variable. Hemangiomas may be accompanied by no accumulation or moderate accumulation of the bone-seeking radionuclide, and a photopenic region at the site of tumor also may be evident.[2248] CT is most useful for assessment of hemangiomas in the spine, demonstrating the full extent of tumor. MR imaging typically reveals areas of high signal intensity in T1- and T2-weighted spin echo MR images, which have been related to accumulation of fat within the tumor[2249] (Figs. 83–238 and 83–239). Such signal intensity characteristics are not seen uniformly, however, and the soft tissue components of the tumor may reveal low signal intensity in the T1-weighted spin echo MR images.[2249] The presence of low signal intensity in T1-weighted spin echo MR images in the intraosseous component of a hemangioma also may be evident and has been associated with more aggressive tumor behavior.[2250] Enhancement of signal intensity following the intravenous administration of a gadolinium compound is typical of an hemangioma (Fig. 83–239).

Pathologic Abnormalities. In the skull, hemangiomas produce a hard excrescence on the surface of the bone.[1176, 1179] When sectioned, they appear as purple or red masses composed of a meshwork of small vascular spaces or cysts traversed by spicules of bone (Fig. 83–240). These osseous spicules may have no particular orientation, but frequently they are arranged perpendicular to the surface of the bone, accounting for a sunburst pattern that may be noted on the roentgenograms. In the long tubular bones, the cortex may be thinned or even bulged, but it still is covered by an intact periosteum. When sectioned, the hemangioma has a dark red or purple color, may appear spongelike, and may exude blood. In fact, during biopsy, hemangiomas may produce massive bleeding, leading to the patient's demise from exsanguination.[1183, 1184, 1189, 1190, 1214] In the vertebrae, most hemangiomas are 1 cm or less in maximum dimension (compared with those in the skull, which may vary from 1

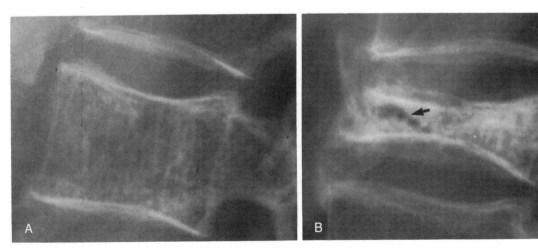

FIGURE 83–235. Hemangioma: Radiographic abnormalities—spine. Fracture with intraosseous gas formation. Two lateral radiographs of the spine reveal a hemangioma of a lumbar vertebra. In **A,** note the typical corduroy appearance with involvement also of the pedicles. Four months later **(B),** in films taken because of an increase in back pain that occurred without a history of spinal injury, the involved vertebral body has collapsed. Note loss of height of both the anterior and the middle bone columns. Note also a linear radiolucent collection (arrow) representing gas, within the involved vertebral body. This type of intraosseous gas, designated a vacuum vertebral body, rarely is associated with tumor.

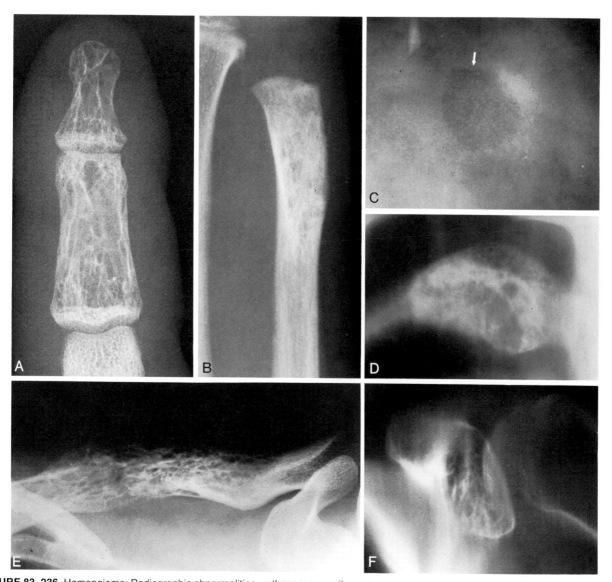

FIGURE 83–236. Hemangioma: Radiographic abnormalities—other osseous sites.

A Phalanges of the hand. Note osteopenia of the middle and distal phalanges of a finger with a weblike trabecular pattern. Hemangiomas in the adjacent soft tissues have led to swelling.

B Ulna. The trabecular pattern in the distal portion of the bone is prominent, and there is mild osseous expansion.

C Skull. Note a well-defined radiolucent area (arrow) containing trabeculation in the frontal bone.

D Rib. The posterior portion of this rib is expanded and contains a coarsely trabeculated lesion.

E Clavicle. An elongated lesion of the midportion of the clavicle is associated with osseous expansion and a lattice-like trabecular pattern.

F Scapula. On this frontal tomogram, note the radiolucent, trabeculated lesion of the glenoid area of the scapula.

(**E,** Courtesy of J. Knickerbocker, M.D., Vancouver, British Columbia, Canada.)

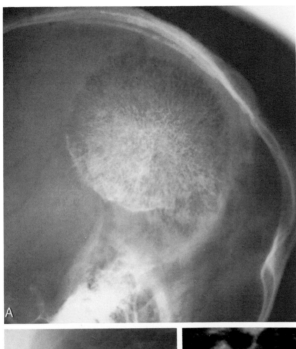

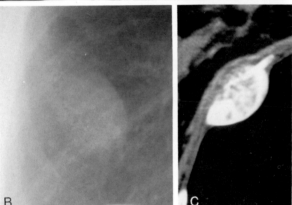

FIGURE 83–237. Hemangioma: Radiographic and CT abnormalities—other osseous sites.

A Skull. Note the large, sharply marginated lesion with a honeycomb or cartwheel configuration. (Courtesy of V. Wing, M.D., Pasadena, California.)

B, C Rib. A routine radiograph **(B)** shows a mass overlying the right lung. Transaxial CT **(C)** confirms osseous expansion of the fourth rib and prominent internal trabeculae.

FIGURE 83–238. Hemangioma: MR imaging abnormalities—tibia. A transaxial T2-weighted (TR/TE, 2000/90) spin echo MR image at the level of the proximal portion of the tibia shows a lesion with multiple channel-like regions of high signal intensity. The appearance is typical of a hemangioma. (Courtesy of M. Pathria, M.D., San Diego, California.)

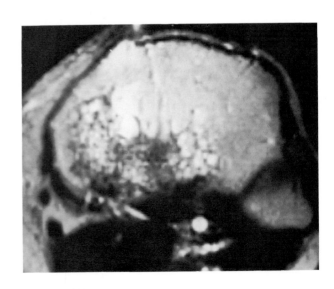

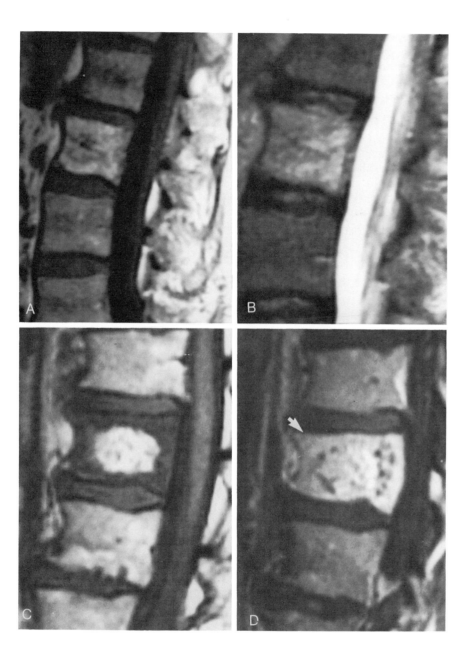

FIGURE 83–239. Hemangioma: MR imaging abnormalities—spine.

A, B A sagittal T1-weighted (TR/TE, 500/11) spin echo MR image **(A)** and a sagittal T2-weighted (TR/TE, 3800/144) fast spin echo MR image **(B)** reveal a hemangioma involving the second lumbar vertebral body, which reveals high signal intensity in both images. The lesion is more obvious in **B.**

C, D Sagittal T1-weighted (TR/TE, 500/20) spin echo MR images obtained before **(C)** and after **(D)** the intravenous injection of a gadolinium compound and, in **D,** in combination with chemical presaturation of fat (ChemSat) show a hemangioma in the first lumbar vertebral body in a second patient. This lesion (arrow) reveals enhancement of signal intensity in **D.**

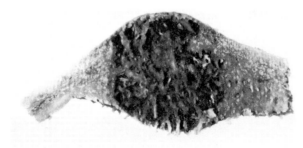

FIGURE 83–240. Hemangioma: Macroscopic abnormalities. A section of a hemangioma of the frontal bone reveals that the tumor has expanded the inner and outer tables of the skull and consists of vascular spaces through which pass wormlike spicules of bone.

to 7 cm in size). Hemangiomas as large as 14 cm occasionally are found in the ilium or ribs.[1200]

Hemangiomas of bone do not differ in their histomorphology from those in the skin or soft tissues. Cavernous and capillary hemangiomas are most frequent. The cavernous variety is composed of large, gaping, thin-walled vessels that are lined by flat endothelial cells and filled with fresh blood (Fig. 83–241A,B). Capillary hemangiomas are composed of similar but smaller vessels with narrow lumens (Fig. 83–241C). Mixed hemangiomas containing both cavernous and capillary vessels also may be encountered. Some hemangiomas contain vessels with thicker walls composed of smooth muscle, and these are termed venous hemangiomas.[33] In any situation, the vascular channels may either be directly juxtaposed to the trabeculae that course through the lesion or be separated from the bone by a band of fibrous connective tissue. The trabeculae usually are abundant and contain both osteoclasts and osteoblasts.[1179, 1200]

Cavernous hemangiomas are most common in the skull, whereas capillary hemangiomas are more frequent in the vertebrae. In general, however, the majority of osseous hemangiomas are cavernous in type.[180]

Natural History. Solitary or multiple hemangiomas represent benign lesions that may progress slowly in size. Clinical manifestations, when present, are related to the local effects of the hemangioma, such as osseous expansion, soft tissue extension, or hemorrhage. Malignant degeneration is not encountered.

Cystic Angiomatosis

This rare skeletal disorder, which also has been designated diffuse angiomatosis, hemangiomatosis, and heman-

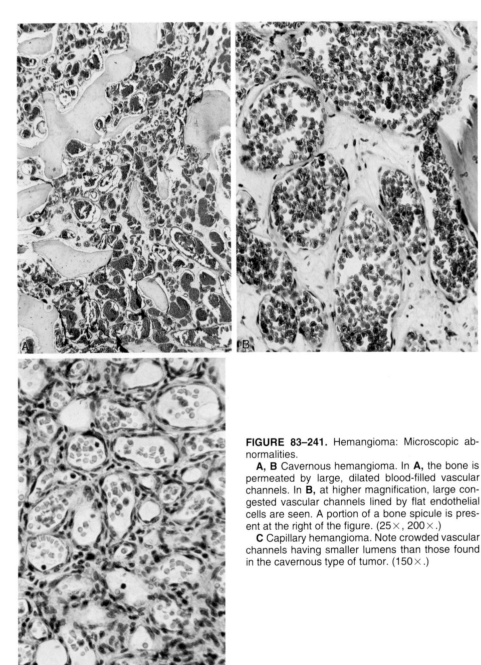

FIGURE 83–241. Hemangioma: Microscopic abnormalities.

A, B Cavernous hemangioma. In **A,** the bone is permeated by large, dilated blood-filled vascular channels. In **B,** at higher magnification, large congested vascular channels lined by flat endothelial cells are seen. A portion of a bone spicule is present at the right of the figure. (25×, 200×.)

C Capillary hemangioma. Note crowded vascular channels having smaller lumens than those found in the cavernous type of tumor. (150×.)

giolymphangiomatosis, is characterized by widespread cystic lesions of bone that frequently are combined with visceral involvement.[1215–1217] It is the latter involvement, which occurs in approximately 60 to 70 per cent of cases,[1218, 1219] that usually is responsible for the patient's symptoms and signs, although the skeletal lesions themselves can produce pain and swelling, especially if a pathologic fracture has developed or neighboring soft tissues are altered. This disease should be distinguished from massive osteolysis, or Gorham's disease, and from single or multiple (but otherwise typical) hemangiomas of bone. The lesions of cystic angiomatosis are differentiated from multiple primary hemangiomas of bone by the fact that the latter condition is associated with lesions that are localized to one or two bones, typically in an extremity, and that lack a cystic radiologic appearance. The precise relationship of cystic angiomatosis and lymphangiomatosis is not clear, as skeletal lesions resembling lymphangiomas are described in some patients with cystic angiomatosis.[2511]

Clinical Abnormalities. Patients usually are in the first, second, or third decade of life, although the disorder has been observed in persons of all ages. Men are affected about twice as often as women. A familial history of disease rarely is evident.[2251] The clinical manifestations and the course of the disease depend largely on the presence or absence of visceral involvement. In those patients in whom visceral lesions are not found, symptoms and signs may be entirely absent, or nonspecific low back pain and localized pain and swelling related to a pathologic fracture are observed. In these instances, the course of cystic angiomatosis is a relatively benign one that is not incompatible with a long life. In those persons with both visceral and osseous involvement, dramatic clinical abnormalities related to lesions in the soft tissues, spleen, liver, lungs, kidneys, thymus gland, peritoneal, pleural and pericardial membranes,

lymph nodes, larnyx, and other organs or tissues may be evident, and affected patients may die at an early age. Hemoptysis, dyspnea, cyanosis, ascites, anemia, congestive heart failure, splenomegaly, hepatomegaly, adenopathy, and soft tissue masses are among the reported clinical findings.[1216–1218, 1220–1228] The Rendu-Osler-Weber syndrome may be an associated abnormality.[1229, 1230]

Skeletal Location. The femur, ribs, vertebrae, skull, innominate bone, humerus, scapula, tibia, radius, fibula, and clavicle, in order of decreasing frequency, are involved most typically, although other osseous sites also may be affected.[1219, 1231, 2251, 2483] Involvement of the axial skeleton, therefore, is most characteristic, although even the small bones in the hands and feet rarely may be the sites of the angiomatous lesions.[1232, 2484] Such lesions may develop simultaneously or metachronously, sometimes over a period of many years.[1233–1235] Of interest, spontaneous regression of the angiomas in one site may occur while other lesions progress in size.[1217, 1222, 1223, 1236]

The lesions of cystic angiomatosis may be located anywhere within the bone. In the long bones, they occur in the epiphysis, metaphysis, or diaphysis in close proximity to the nutrient foramina. The lesions tend to involve the medullary portion of the bone and may be central or eccentrically placed, although occasionally lesions may be intracortical in location. They appear oval and are oriented in the long axis of the bone. In flat bones, such as a rib, the cortex may be quite thin, bulge in a fusiform fashion, and have a reddish color.

Radiographic Abnormalities. Well-defined, round or ovoid, osteolytic lesions of variable size usually are seen, surrounded by a rim of sclerotic bone[1237, 1238] (Figs. 83–242 and 83–243). Medullary involvement predominates, and cortical invasion, osseous expansion, and periostitis are unusual. In some instances, osteosclerotic lesions, simulating

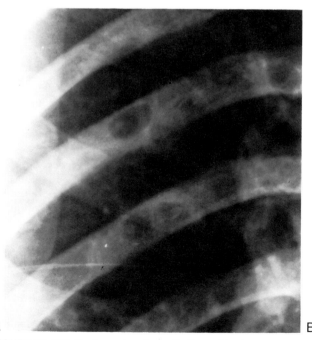 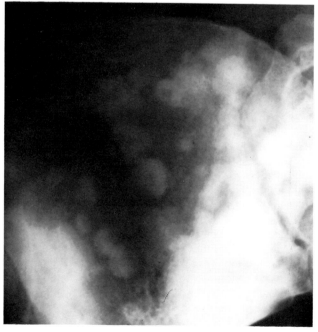

A   B

FIGURE 83–242. Cystic angiomatosis: Radiographic abnormalities. In this adult patient, note widespread skeletal lesions. Within the ribs **(A),** the lesions are well defined and osteolytic in nature, surrounded by a rim of sclerotic bone. In the pelvis **(B),** the circular lesions appear more radiodense but possess a central radiolucent zone.

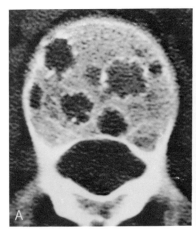 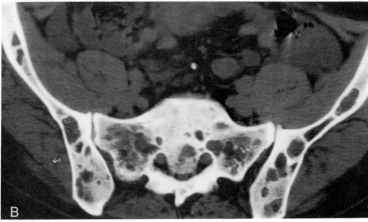

FIGURE 83–243. Cystic angiomatosis: CT abnormalities. Transaxial CT scans of a lumbar vertebra **(A)** and the pelvis **(B)** in an adult patient reveal multiple osteolytic lesions of variable size, each well circumscribed with a sclerotic margin. A symmetric distribution is apparent in **B**. (Courtesy of D. Levey, M.D., Corpus Christi, Texas.)

skeletal metastases from carcinoma of the prostate, are observed.[2512] Pathologic fractures also are encountered, especially in the presence of large areas of bone destruction.

The major differential diagnostic considerations include eosinophilic granuloma and other histiocytoses, hyperparathyroidism, fibrous dysplasia, lipomatosis, lymphangiomatosis, neurofibromatosis, skeletal metastasis, plasma cell myeloma, mastocytosis, sarcoidosis, and lymphoma. Of these, the first three deserve emphasis. Skeletal lesions in the histiocytoses generally are not accompanied by a peripheral sclerotic rim and usually are associated with periosteal reaction. Similarly, in hyperparathyroidism, a rim of bone sclerosis is unusual, and, furthermore, additional features such as subperiosteal resorption of bone commonly are noted. Polyostotic fibrous dysplasia can lead to skeletal abnormalities that closely resemble those of cystic angiomatosis.

Pathologic Abnormalities. When sectioned, the lesion may resemble a simple bone cyst, possessing a single, large cavity lined by a gray-yellow membrane.[1215, 1220] Alternatively, multiple communicating cysts of varying size are evident; these cysts may be empty or contain clear fluid or blood. They are separated by thickened trabeculae, producing a honeycomb appearance.

The lesions of cystic angiomatosis do not differ histologically from cavernous or capillary hemangiomas or even from lymphangiomas.[1221–1223, 1230] Most contain numerous, dilated, cavernous thin-walled vascular channels that are lined by flat endothelial cells. These channels fill the intertrabecular spaces and rest against the adjacent trabeculae. Some lesions reveal features of both capillary and cavernous hemangiomas.[1217] Blood or eosinophilic, proteinaceous fluid is evident within the cystic lesions. In the latter instance, the distinction between a hemangioma and a lymphangioma may be impossible. Patients with cystic angiomatosis have been described who have a lymphangioma at one site and typical hemangiomas in other areas. Owing to the contamination of the vascular spaces by blood during either the operative procedure or the histologic processing of fresh material, the channels of lymphangioma may become filled with blood and be indistinguishable from the vascular spaces of a hemangioma. Similarly, the blood contained within the vascular spaces of a cavernous heman-

gioma may empty during tissue processing, and the resultant empty channels mimic those of a lymphangioma. It has been found that, of all the bones that appear to be involved radiologically, it is the rib that provides the highest diagnostic yield in establishing a histologic diagnosis.

Lymphangioma and Lymphangiomatosis

Lymphangioma of bone can appear as one or more isolated lesions or in a more diffuse form as part of the spectrum of either cystic angiomatosis or massive osteolysis (Gorham's disease). It should be emphasized, however, that solitary lymphangiomas are extremely rare, only a few documented cases being known. Localized intraosseous lymphangiomas are most frequent in children or adolescents, although older patients also have been affected.[1239–1246] The most typical sites of involvement are the tibia, humerus, ilium, skull, mandible, vertebrae, and small bones in the hand. Clinical manifestations are variable in type and severity, although pain and swelling may be prominent, especially in the presence of a pathologic fracture, and neurologic findings may accompany spinal lesions. Radiographic abnormalities are not specific; an osteolytic lesion arising in the medullary portion of the bone is most characteristic. A multiloculated, septate, or bubble-like appearance is encountered, similar to that of a hemangioma.

Multiple intraosseous lymphangiomas can occur in several situations: involvement of two or more widely separated bones (Fig. 83–244A,B); involvement of two or more bones in one region of the body (e.g., shoulder girdle or spine) (Fig. 83–245); or diffuse involvement of many bones[1247–1267] (Fig. 83–244C). An analysis of cases in which multiple intraosseous lymphangiomas have been present indicates predilection for both the long tubular bones and the flat or irregular bones. The femur, ribs, humerus, tibia, skull, vertebrae, scapula, innominate bone, fibula, and clavicle, in order of decreasing frequency, are the favored sites of involvement. In patients with multifocal osseous alterations, many of whom are children, additional lymphangiomatous lesions may be evident in the soft tissues or viscera and may lead to a variety of findings, including chylothorax, chylopericardium, hepatosplenomegaly, lymphedema, and cystic hygromas. In these patients, the extraosseous manifestations can lead to considerable morbidity as

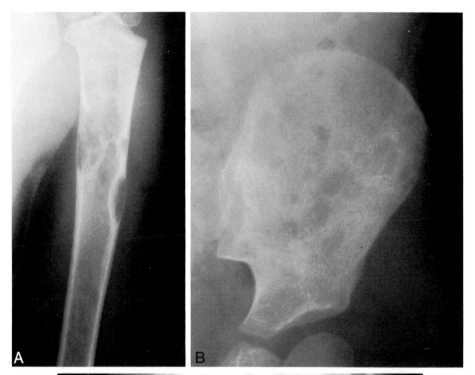

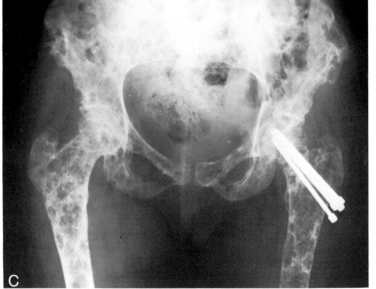

FIGURE 83–244. Lymphangioma and lymphangiomatosis: Radiographic abnormalities.

A, B This 3 year old boy had a neck mass, which on biopsy represented a cystic hygroma, and skeletal pain. Radiographs of the humerus **(A)** and ilium **(B)** show flame-shaped osteolytic lesions of variable size situated in both the medullary and cortical bone. Sclerotic margins are evident about some of the lesions.

C This adult had lesions scattered throughout the skeleton. A pathologic fracture of the left femoral neck, treated with multiple orthopedic lag screws, had occurred. The radiographic appearance, consisting of poorly defined osteolytic lesions, resembles that in plasma cell myeloma or skeletal metastases.

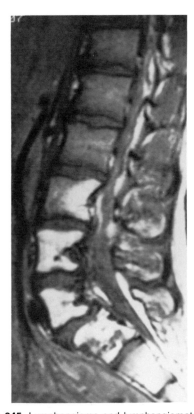

FIGURE 83–245. Lymphangioma and lymphangiomatosis: MR imaging abnormalities. In this 16 year old boy with a long history of documented lymphangiomatosis (or hemangiomatosis) of the lumbar spine, a sagittal T1-weighted (TR/TE, 617/20) spin echo MR image shows involvement of the third, fourth, and fifth lumbar vertebral bodies and sacrum, manifested as high signal intensity. Involvement of the epidural space was more apparent in other images. Enhancement of signal intensity in the involved regions was seen following the intravenous administration of a gadolinium compound (not shown). (Courtesy of R. Linovitz, M.D., San Diego, California.)

well as an early demise. The bone lesions again are primarily osteolytic and septate but may be associated with involvement of the adjacent soft tissues (which do not contain phleboliths) or a contiguous bone. A specific diagnosis can be provided by lymphangiography owing to the accumulation of the contrast material in the intraosseous lymphangiomas[1253, 1264, 1265, 1268] (Fig. 83–246). This finding suggests the possibility that lymphangiomas of bone are produced by insufficiency and agenesis of the valves within dysplastic, subcutaneous lymph vessels that lead to lymphatic backflow into bone.[1265] The slow, continuous progression of the osteolytic changes that is a characteristic but inconsistent feature of osseous lymphangiomas may relate to steadily increasing dilatation of the lymphatic cavities within the bone. Consistent with this hypothesis is the predominance of visible osteolysis in the second or third decade of life and the documentation of communication between the lymphatic channels in bone and those in lymphedematous soft tissues prior to the appearance of radiographically evident osseous lesions.[1269]

On macroscopic examination, skeletal lymphangiomas vary greatly in size and, occasionally, may involve an entire bone, such as the ilium. When sectioned, they are poorly defined and may ooze turbid, milky, or clear fluid.[1262, 1263] Unilocular or multilocular cystic spaces, separated by trabeculae, are evident. Microscopically, the features of a lym-

phangioma are similar to those of a cavernous hemangioma,[1244, 1247] consisting of widely patent, thin-walled vascular spaces that are lined by flat endothelial cells (Fig. 83–247). Typically, in a lymphangioma, these spaces are filled with eosinophilic, granular, proteinaceous fluid and do not contain red blood cells.[1241, 1244]

It should be noted that variations exist in the microscopic appearance of a lymphangioma so that its differentiation from a hemangioma may become extremely difficult or impossible. It is because of this that hemangioma, lymphangioma, cystic angiomatosis, hemangiomatosis (Fig. 83–248), and even massive osteolysis (Gorham's disease) (Fig. 83–249) are sometimes considered part of the spectrum of a single disease process despite attempts to sort out features that allow differentiation among these disorders.[1270] The interested reader should refer to Chapter 94 for a detailed description of massive osteolysis of Gorham.

Glomus Tumor

Although rare, the glomus tumor (angioglomoid tumor) has received considerable attention owing to its characteristic clinical manifestations and typical location in the tips of the fingers. The lesion arises from the neuromyoarterial glomus, which is located normally in some of the internal organs of the body, such as the stomach, and in the dermis and superficial subcutaneous tissues in the extremities, particularly the palmar and plantar areas and the fingertips in the region of the nailbed. The normal glomus, whose name is derived from the Latin word for ball or spherical mass, consists of a specialized vascular anastomotic complex sur-

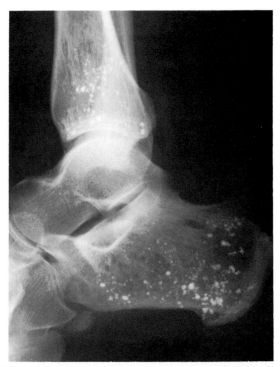

FIGURE 83–246. Lymphangioma and lymphangiomatosis: Radiographic abnormalities. A lateral radiograph of the ankle indicates the presence of lymphangiomas, especially in the distal portion of the tibia and calcaneus. They have produced small cystic lesions within the bone. The radiodense areas represent contrast material that had collected within the lymphangiomas during a previous lymphangiogram.

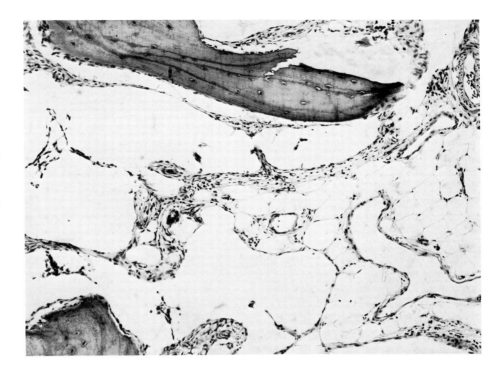

FIGURE 83–247. Lymphangioma and lymphangiomatosis: Microscopic abnormalities. Note widely dilated, empty vascular spaces between trabeculae. The spaces are lined by flat endothelial cells. (150×.)

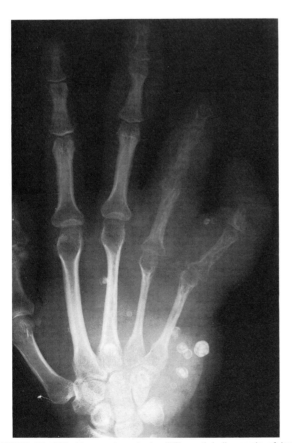

FIGURE 83–248. Hemangiomatosis: Differential diagnosis of lymphangiomatosis. In this patient, observe hemangiomatous involvement of both the bones and the soft tissues. The coarse trabecular pattern within the involved bones, particularly well shown in the phalanges of the fourth and fifth digits, and the calcifications (phleboliths) in the soft tissues allow a specific diagnosis of hemangiomatosis.

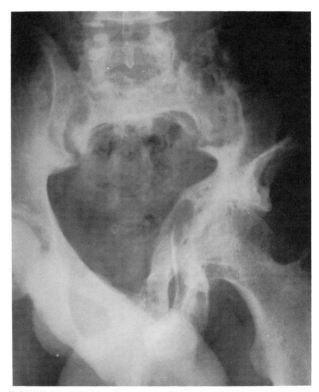

FIGURE 83–249. Massive osteolysis (Gorham's disease): Differential diagnosis of lymphangiomatosis. Note intraosseous lesions of the left innominate bone and left femur, which have led to considerable deformity, including acetabular protrusion. (Courtesy of M. Pathria, M.D., San Diego, California.)

rounded by nerve elements and functions as a regulator of body temperature.

Glomus tumors are far more common as extraosseous lesions than as intraosseous lesions. They may be encountered in such diverse locations as the stomach, mediastinum, penis, eyelid, nasal fossa, and even the synovial membrane.[1271, 1272] In the extremities, glomus tumors most frequently are evident in the region of the fingertips or nailbeds,[1273] with approximately 75 per cent of such lesions appearing in the upper extremities. Bone involvement usually is a secondary manifestation related to invasion of the bone by a soft tissue glomus tumor, with rare exceptions in which a true intraosseous lesion exists.

Clinical Abnormalities. Glomus tumors can be observed in patients of any age, although many persons are in the fourth or fifth decade of life. The tumors typically are small lesions in the soft tissues that are not palpable or visible on physical examination. Occasionally, a tiny pink or blue nodule may be observed beneath the nail. Characteristically, aching pain and exquisite point tenderness are present.[2485] Exposure to cold or minimal trauma may induce severe paroxysmal attacks of pain, a finding that is highly suggestive of a glomus tumor. This lesion is benign, and excision of the tumor is curative, although incomplete removal can result in local recurrence, frequently within a few months following surgery.

Skeletal Location. Secondary involvement of a bone adjacent to a soft tissue glomus tumor is observed in 15 to 65 per cent of cases, especially in the hand, although in other sites as well.[1273–1279] Primary intraosseous glomus tumors also are characteristically observed in the hand, particularly in a distal phalanx[2252] but rarely in a proximal or middle phalanx[1920] or a metacarpal bone, or even in a long tubular bone such as the femur, ulna, or fibula.[30, 33, 34, 1280–1284, 2253, 2486]

One instance of multiple glomus tumors has been described involving the bones of the hands and feet, but it is not clear whether the lesions arose primarily in the bone or in the soft tissues.[1285] This difficulty in identifying the precise site of origin of a glomus tumor is encountered in several of the reported cases of intraosseous lesions.[1276, 1286]

Reports describing glomus tumors in the pericoccygeal tissues associated with chronic coccygodynia[1275, 1287] have led to some controversy regarding the exact nature of the lesion. As the coccygeal body (glomus coccygeum) is situated in this region between the middle sacral vein and artery, it is possible that this normal tissue has previously been misinterpreted as a tumor.[1288, 2254]

Radiographic Abnormalities. Soft tissue glomus tumors produce shallow, well-marginated erosions in the subjacent bone, usually the dorsal, medial, or lateral surface in the tuft of a terminal phalanx. A sclerotic margin may be apparent about the erosion. In some instances, a partial shell of bone extends into the soft tissue, making difficult the distinction between a soft tissue and an intraosseous lesion. The latter appears as a well-defined, osteolytic region encased by cortical bone, again usually in a terminal phalanx. The resulting radiographic appearance resembles that of an inclusion cyst (Fig. 83–250A). Intraosseous glomus tumors in other phalanges or the metacarpal bones lead to roentgenographic alterations that are similar to those in an aneurysmal bone cyst or enchondroma (Figs. 83–250B and 83–251). The absence of calcification in an intraosseous glomus tumor assumes diagnostic importance, as calcific regions may be evident in an enchondroma. In all instances, the radiographic findings are those of a slowly growing, nonaggressive process, such that alternative diagnoses, including a metastatic focus arising from a bronchogenic carcinoma, rarely are appropriate. Additional diagnostic considerations regarding

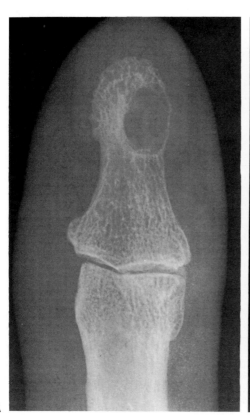

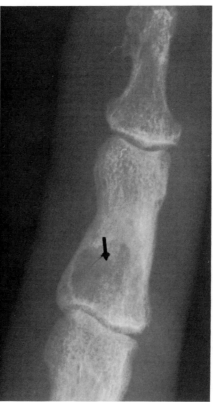

FIGURE 83–250. Glomus tumor: Radiographic abnormalities.

A Terminal phalanx. An eccentric, osteolytic lesion of the distal phalanx in a finger is characterized by geographic bone destruction. This is the typical appearance of a glomus tumor originating in or involving bone.

B Middle phalanx. This biopsy-proved glomus tumor (arrow) has a radiographic appearance identical to that of an enchondroma so that accurate diagnosis depends on analysis of clinical manifestations. The lesion is well defined and osteolytic. No calcification is apparent. This is an unusual appearance of a glomus tumor originating in bone.

A   B

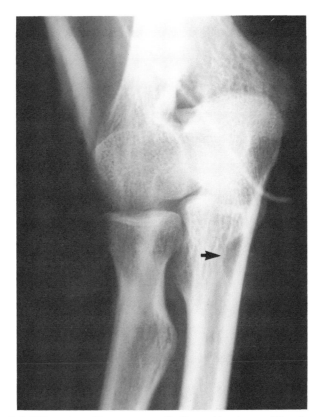

FIGURE 83–251. Glomus tumor: Radiographic abnormalities. In a 24 year old woman with a 2 year history of progressive elbow pain and an enlarging soft tissue mass, a small osteolytic lesion (arrow) is seen in the proximal portion of the ulna. At surgery, soft, friable hemorrhagic tissue was encountered lying within a cavity in the cortical surface of the ulna. A glomus tumor was confirmed histologically. (From Rozmaryn LM, et al: Clin Orthop 220:126, 1987.)

intraosseous glomus tumors of the hand are sarcoidosis, aneurysmal bone cyst, giant cell tumor, and tuberous sclerosis; these generally can be eliminated quite easily through the combination of the radiographic and clinical abnormalities.

Other Imaging Techniques. Ultrasonography, CT, and MR imaging represent additional imaging methods that can be used to detect glomus tumors.[2255, 2256, 2264] With ultrasonography, a hypoechoic mass is typical, although small, flattened subungual lesions may escape detection. MR imaging, during which the glomus tumor is of high signal intensity in T2-weighted spin echo images (Fig. 83–252), may be useful in the initial detection of the lesion and in the identification of tumor recurrence following surgery.

Pathologic Abnormalities. Extraosseous and intraosseous glomus tumors usually are only a few millimeters in maximum dimension.[1271, 1275, 1284, 1289] The cortex of the involved bone is extremely thin, and beneath it is located a red or violet, soft, friable lesion that may appear jellylike.[1280, 1281]

Glomus tumors usually are composed of various-sized vascular channels lined by flat or cuboidal endothelial cells that are cuffed by masses of polyhedral tumor (glomus) cells (Fig. 83–253). These cells are compact, have an epithelioid appearance, usually are round, and contain a finely granular eosinophilic cytoplasm with a central nucleus.[1271, 1281, 1290] Some of the cells are spindle-shaped and may show

morphologic characteristics that resemble those of smooth muscle cells.[1281]

The stroma varies from one that is loose, fibrillar, or hyalinized to one with a predominantly myxoid pattern, in which the vascular channels and their cuff of cells are widely separated from one another. In some cases, the tumor is composed predominantly of solid areas, where the glomus cells are diffusely distributed and tightly packed with a minimal amount of stroma.[1291] In glomus tumors of the soft tissue, a more vascular variant is found, termed a glomangioma.[1271]

Electron microscopic studies of both osseous and soft tissue glomus tumors have shown that the glomus cells have many of the features of smooth muscle cells, including the presence of myofilaments.[1291–1294] Nonmyelinated nerve fibers also may be evident.[1280]

Benign or Malignant Tumors

Hemangiopericytoma

The hemangiopericytoma is an uncommon tumor of pericytes with a propensity to involve soft tissues and to behave in an erratic or unpredictable fashion, leading to its designation as a benign or malignant neoplasm or one with behavioral characteristics intermediate between these two categories. Hemangiopericytomas arising in bone are rare, with only a limited number of documented examples having been reported.[1295–1308, 2487]

Clinical Abnormalities. Most affected patients are men or women who are middle-aged or elderly (in the fifth, sixth, or seventh decade of life), although adolescents and young adults may harbor this neoplasm. Nonspecific symptoms and signs are present, including local pain and swelling. Rarely, the findings of hypophosphatemic osteomalacia (oncogenic osteomalacia) are evident (see Chapter 53).

Skeletal Location. Involvement of the axial skeleton or proximal long bones is most characteristic; the humerus, the spine or sacrum, the femur, and the mandible are the bones affected most frequently. The long tubular bones are

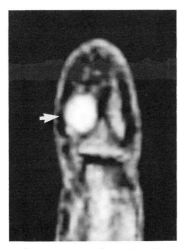

FIGURE 83–252. Glomus tumor: MR imaging abnormalities. In a 67 year old woman, a coronal multiplanar gradient recalled (MPGR) MR image (TR/TE, 500/15; flip angle, 30 degrees) shows a lesion (arrow) of high signal intensity applied to the radial aspect of the terminal phalanx of the fifth finger. (Courtesy of W. Glenn, M.D., Long Beach, California.)

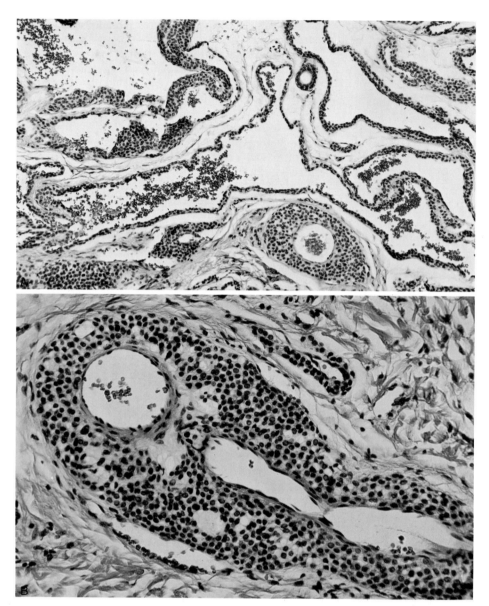

FIGURE 83–253. Glomus tumor: Microscopic abnormalities.

A Observe widely dilated vascular channels separated by a loose stroma. The vessels are lined by endothelial cells and encased by epithelioid-type tumor cells. (150×.)

B At higher magnification, note that the vascular channels are lined by flat endothelial cells and cuffed by bland epithelioid glomus cells. (300×.)

involved in approximately 40 per cent of cases, and the innominate bone is involved in approximately 10 per cent of cases. Within the tubular bones, a diaphyseal or metaphyseal location is the preferred site. Less frequently, the ribs, clavicle, sternum, scapula, skull, and small bones of the hand and foot are affected. As opposed to hemangioendothelioma (angiosarcoma) of bone, which may be multicentric, a solitary skeletal focus is typical of a hemangiopericytoma.

Radiographic Abnormalities. The nonspecific radiographic appearance of hemangiopericytoma of bone (Fig. 83–254) is characterized by osteolysis, delicate trabeculation with a honeycomb appearance, mild osseous expansion, and, in tumors of the sternum, spine, and calcaneus, significant bone sclerosis.[1304] Periostitis is exceedingly rare. More aggressive radiographic characteristics, including poor definition of the bone lesion, cortical violation, and a soft tissue mass, generally correlate with more sinister histologic features, and, in these cases, it may be difficult to determine if the tumor originates in bone or in soft tissues.

Pathologic Abnormalities. Variability in size, a solid or spongy texture, a granular or friable consistency, and a gray, white, or pink color are among the macroscopic features of osseous hemangiopericytoma.[1296, 1298, 1301, 1306, 1309] Large tumors may possess hyalinized, sclerotic foci.[1304]

The microscopic identification of hemangiopericytoma is difficult owing to the absence of distinctive cytologic features that are specific for pericytes and must rest on the overall architectural pattern of the lesion.[1300, 1302, 1304, 1308, 1310–1312] Hemangiopericytoma of bone or soft tissue is characterized by the presence of abundant, ramifying thin-walled blood vessels surrounded by closely packed, plump, round to spindle-shaped stromal cells that have relatively scant cytoplasm and indistinct cell borders (Fig. 83–255). Nuclei also are round, oval, or spindle-shaped and range from vesicular to hyperchromatic. The size and shape of the cells and their nuclei do not vary greatly within any single tumor. By electron microscopy these tumor cells have been shown to have the features of pericytes, cells that normally are found surrounding capillaries or postcapillary vessels.[1300, 1302, 1310–1312]

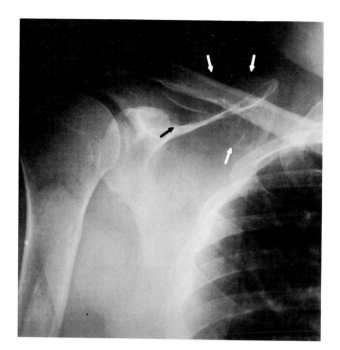

FIGURE 83–254. Hemangiopericytoma: Radiographic abnormalities. A nonspecific osteolytic lesion with a soft tissue mass (arrows) involves the superomedial aspect of the scapula. (Courtesy of J. D. Bauer, M.D., St. Louis, Missouri.)

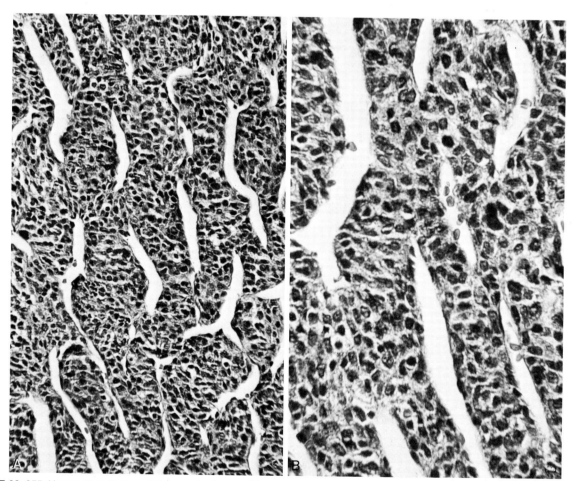

FIGURE 83–255. Hemangiopericytoma: Microscopic abnormalities.
   A Open vascular channels are surrounded by pericytes. Some of the channels branch at acute angles. (300×.)
   B At higher magnification, note that the pericytes contain round to oval nuclei, most of which are fairly uniform in size and shape. The cell borders are indistinct. (600×.)

The vascular channels are lined by flat, normal-appearing endothelial cells. The caliber of the vessels varies from large, widely dilated, cavernous spaces to narrow capillary slits. In highly cellular areas, the tumor stromal cells are so compact that they compress the channels to such a degree that these foci may appear to be composed only of compact cells without vessels. Reticulin stains, however, demonstrate the presence of the vascular channels clearly. Reticulin fibers surround and lie outside each vessel and enmesh each individual tumor cell. The endothelial cells lack such an investment, the reticulin network being external to them. In those regions in which the vascular channels are not obscured by tumor cells, the angles at which the vessels branch, combined with knob-like protrusions of the stromal cells against their walls, cause the vascular lumens to have a "staghorn" or "antler-like" appearance when the tissue sections are viewed under low power magnification. Despite these protrusions of tumor cells, a basement membrane actually separates the endothelial cells from the surrounding tumor cells.

The absolute diagnosis of an intraosseous hemangiopericytoma may rest with the identification of pericytes with electron microscopy, owing to the lack of specificity of the light microscopic studies and the existence of similar histologic alterations in a variety of other sarcomas, including mesenchymal chondrosarcoma, congenital fibrosarcoma, liposarcoma, synovial sarcoma, Ewing's sarcoma, and malignant fibrous histiocytoma.[1304, 1309, 1313]

Natural History. Controversy exists regarding the value of classifying or grading soft tissue hemangiopericytomas in terms of their malignant potential,[1304, 1309, 1314, 1315] although it has been suggested that such classification is more useful when considering hemangiopericytomas of bone.[1304] What is clear is that these osseous neoplasms, as well as their soft tissue counterparts, reveal a broad spectrum of behavioral features and that predicting the subsequent course of any single tumor on the basis of its radiographic or histologic characteristics, or both, may be possible but certainly is difficult. Radiographic abnormalities that include cortical violation or destruction and a soft tissue mass usually are indicative of a more aggressive hemangiopericytoma of bone. Histologic abnormalities that include a significant degree of cytologic atypia associated with marked cellularity, the presence of areas of necrosis and hemorrhage, and a mitotic rate of 4 mitoses or more per 10 high power fields generally are indicative of malignant potential.[1309] Unfortunately, there are no absolute criteria that uniformly distinguish between benign and malignant hemangiopericytomas, which accounts for the occurrence of metastases from lesions that were considered histologically benign.[1316] The designation of some hemangiopericytomas as intermediate in type (without definitive features of benignancy or malignancy) further underscores the difficulty that arises in assessing the aggressive potential of any individual neoplasm.[1304, 1316] Tumor recurrence or metastasis may develop years after initial therapy of hemangiopericytoma, indicating that long-term follow-up observations are required to test the accuracy of any proposed classification system. As a general rule, however, the presence of histologic alterations suggesting malignancy is more significant in predicting the final outcome of a hemangiopericytoma than is the absence of such alterations.

Malignant Tumors

Angiosarcoma (Hemangioendothelioma)

Hemangioendothelioma, a rare malignant tumor of bone, is composed of irregular anastomosing vascular channels lined by one or several layers of atypical endothelial cells.[33] It is the endothelial nature of the proliferating cell that distinguishes this lesion from a hemangiopericytoma, in which pericytes represent the cell of origin. Hemangioendotheliomas of bone also have been referred to as angiosarcomas (a designation that is used here) and hemangioendothelial sarcomas. Low grade or well-differentiated hemangioendotheliomas of bone sometimes are referred to as epithelioid hemangioendotheliomas or histiocytoid hemangiomas (see later discussion).

Clinical Abnormalities. Osseous angiosarcomas are more frequent in men than in women, in a ratio of approximately 2 to 1.[1317–1319] The lesions are observed in patients of all ages, although the majority of affected persons are in the third, fourth, or fifth decade of life. Those with multifocal disease usually are about 10 years younger than those possessing single lesions.[33] Local pain and, less commonly, swelling are the two most characteristic clinical findings and may be of weeks', months', or even years' duration. Cranial or spinal angiosarcomas are associated with severe headaches, back pain, or neurologic manifestations. Pathologic fractures, which are observed in approximately 10 per cent of patients, lead to more abrupt and prominent symptoms and signs. Less frequent or rare clinical abnormalities include constitutional symptoms, such as weight loss, weakness, anorexia, dyspnea, and malaise,[1320] microangiopathic hemolytic anemia, consumption coagulopathy, and high output cardiac failure owing to arteriovenous shunting of blood.[1321–1323]

Skeletal Location. Angiosarcomas predominate in the long tubular bones, especially those in the lower extremity.[28, 30, 34, 1324–1328] The long bones are affected in approximately 60 per cent of cases, with preferential involvement of the tibia (approximately 23 per cent of cases), femur (18 per cent), and humerus (13 per cent). A metaphyseal or diaphyseal location is typical, with rare instances of primary epiphyseal tumors.[1317, 1321] Of the flat bones, those in the pelvis (7 per cent of cases) and skull (4 per cent) are altered most commonly. The mandible is involved more frequently than the maxilla, although localization of an angiosarcoma in either of these two sites is unusual.[1329–1336] The ribs are affected in approximately 5 per cent of cases, and the vertebrae are involved in approximately 10 per cent of cases.[1337–1341] Rare sites of involvement are the scapula, clavicle, sternum, radius, patella, and the small bones of the hand and foot.[1342, 1343]

One of the characteristic features of angiosarcoma is synchronous or metachronous multicentric disease, a phenomenon that is observed in 20 to 50 per cent of cases. Multiple lesions may occur in a single bone, or one or more tumor foci may be apparent in multiple bones in a single extremity (especially the lower extremity) or throughout the skeleton. A regional pattern of involvement of a tubular bone of an extremity should be emphasized as one important diagnostic sign of this neoplasm, and modifications in this pattern include localization of the disease in several contiguous vertebral bodies, in all components of the innominate bone, or in the osseous structures about the shoulder or hip.

Angiosarcomas may develop in bones with preexisting abnormalities, such as chronic osteomyelitis, osteonecrosis, or other neoplasms, or at sites of metallic fixation devices.[1317, 1328, 1344]

Radiographic Abnormalities. The principal radiographic pattern is one of osteolysis that, uncommonly, is accompanied by osteosclerosis (Fig. 83–256A). Bone sclerosis alone is not evident. The lesions are variable in size, may localize in the cortex or the medullary bone, and possess either well-delineated or poorly defined margins. Cortical thinning and mild or moderate osseous expansion are additional radiographic features of angiosarcomas, and periostitis is infrequent. Extensive periosteal bone formation, cortical violation, and a soft tissue mass are indicative of more aggressive tumors.

Multifocal involvement is an important roentgenographic pattern of this neoplasm. It may be manifested as two or more osteolytic lesions involving a long segment of a single bone or osteolysis in contiguous bones (Fig. 83–256B,C). The radiographic demonstration of multiple neoplastic foci in the cortical bone or spongiosa, or both, leading to a bubble-like appearance and osseous expansion without periostitis in a tubular bone (or bones) of a lower extremity is highly characteristic, although other diagnostic considerations include skeletal metastasis, plasma cell myeloma, cystic angiomatosis, histiocytosis, Kaposi's sarcoma, bacillary angiomatosis, and fungal or tuberculous osteomyelitis. Bone scintigraphy also may be useful in confirming involvement of the bones of a single extremity in patients with angiosarcomas (Fig. 83–257). In the flat or irregular bones, a similar osteolytic pattern may be demonstrated

(Fig. 83–258). Angiosarcomas may lead to extensive destruction of several carpal or tarsal bones or, rarely, phalanges or metacarpal and metatarsal bones[1345, 1346] (Fig. 83–259). In the spine, osteolysis in contiguous vertebral bodies with narrowing of the intervening intervertebral disc(s) simulates the appearance of infection.[1337, 1339, 1340]

Pathologic Abnormalities. Macroscopically, angiosarcomas vary from 3 to 10 cm in maximum dimension and, when sectioned, are found either to be well circumscribed or to possess irregular and indistinct borders (Fig. 83–260). The tumor has a surface that usually appears bright red or purple, resembling currant jelly,[180] and a consistency that is soft or fleshy. The cortex may be partially or totally destroyed.

The two fundamental histologic criteria that are required for the diagnosis of an angiosarcoma were set forth in 1943 by Stout[1347]; these are (1) the formation of atypical endothelial cells in greater numbers than would be required to line vessels with a simple endothelial membrane; and (2) the formation of vascular tubes and channels that possess a delicate framework of reticulin fibers and commonly anastomose (Fig. 83–261). Subsequently, investigators have attempted to define histologic characteristics that were indicative of the malignant potential of angiosarcomas, using the designations of well-differentiated or poorly differentiated tumors or a grading system consisting of three numerical categories, I to III, with the last including the most aggressive neoplasms.[1317, 1319, 1326] These classification systems generally use the degree of vasoformative activity, atypia of the endothelial cells, and the frequency of mitotic activity as signs predictive of the tumor's malignant potential.

Very well differentiated angiosarcomas usually contain numerous blood vessels whose endothelial cells show only

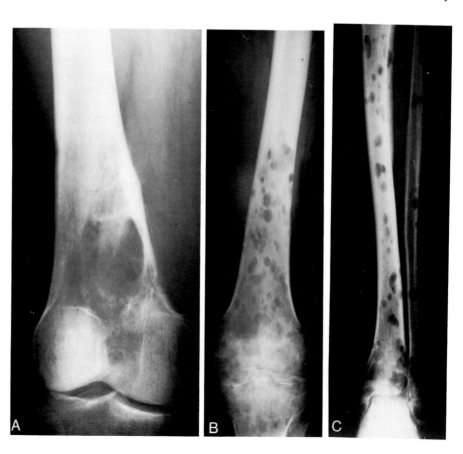

FIGURE 83–256. Angiosarcoma: Radiographic abnormalities—long tubular bones.

A Femur. A radiograph reveals a large osteolytic lesion involving the diaphysis and metaphysis in the distal portion of the femur. The bone is slightly expanded owing to the presence of periostitis, and there is an area of calcification or ossification at the upper margin of the lesion.

B, C Femur, tibia, and fibula. In a second patient, note multiple, well-defined, small osteolytic lesions scattered throughout the tibia, fibula, and femur. This type of regional distribution represents one of the characteristic patterns of angiosarcoma.

(**B, C,** Courtesy of H. J. Spjut, M.D., Houston, Texas.)

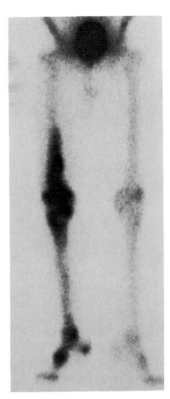

FIGURE 83–257. Angiosarcoma: Scintigraphic abnormalities—long tubular bones. Note abnormal accumulation of the bone-seeking radionuclide in the femur, tibia, and tarsal bones in the right leg. (Courtesy of A. Nemcek, M.D., Chicago, Illinois.)

minimal nuclear atypia, such that the lesions are difficult to distinguish from hemangiomas. In higher grade angiosarcomas, the endothelial cells are crowded together and are plump, are round or oval, and have an abundant eosinophilic granular cytoplasm, large vesicular nuclei, and prominent nucleoli.[33, 1317, 1318, 1325, 1348] These cells bulge into the lumina of the vascular channels, creating a hobnail pattern.[1297] Papillary tufts within the vascular channels may be seen, but, unlike extraosseous angiosarcomas, in which this feature is quite common, such tufts are found less frequently in skeletal angiosarcomas.

In more poorly differentiated tumors, spindle-shaped cells that clearly are pleomorphic may be evident. In some instances, the tumor cells grow as solid sheets and assume an epithelial appearance, resembling hepatocytes.[1317–1319, 1325] Such solid areas possess little or no visible vasoformative activity and may be interpreted as evidence of metastatic disease, especially that arising from a carcinoma of the kidney or thyroid gland, synovial sarcoma, or adamantinoma.[1349, 1350] The vascular channels may be reduced to slitlike spaces or be so compressed by the spindle cells that an erroneous diagnosis of fibrosarcoma is suggested. Areas of necrosis and chronic inflammatory reaction with nodules of lymphocytes are additional, inconsistent histologic features of aggressive angiosarcomas.

Angiosarcomas have been studied using immunohistochemical methods[1351–1354] as well as electron microscopy.[1354, 1355] Immunohistochemical methods have demonstrated two endothelial cell markers, factor VIII–related antigen and *Ulex europaeus* I lectin, in the tumor cells of angiosarcoma. Stains for the Ulex lectin marker apparently are more sensitive but less specific. Guarda and associates,[1351] using stains for factor VIII antigen in 28 angiosarcomas, found positive results in 23 of the cases. The five tumors that were negative were predominantly solid, whereas among the positive cases the areas that stained most strongly were those with the greatest vasoformative activity. In a series of 27 angiosarcomas reported by Ordóñez and Batsakis,[1353] all were positive for Ulex lectin whereas only 20 of the 27 cases stained for factor VIII–related antigen. Electron microscopic studies of angiosarcomas have demonstrated Weibel-Palade bodies, morphologic markers for endothelial cells, in some angiosarcomas, as well as fine, 5 to 10 nm cytoplasmic filaments, located about the nucleus in dense irregular bundles.

Epithelioid Variant of Hemangioendothelioma (Hemangioma). The accurate diagnosis of hemangioendothelioma has been complicated somewhat by the recent introduction of data that support the concept of an additional neoplasm, a *histiocytoid hemangioma,* or epithelioid hemangioendothelioma (hemangioma), that is characterized by an apparently histologically distinct population of endothelial cells.[1356] An analysis of reported cases of histiocytoid hemangioma[1356–1360, 2257–2263] indicates the following features: typical occurrence in adult men and women; involvement of the tubular or flat and irregular bones, including the vertebrae, sacrum, and clavicle; rare multicentric disease; associated skin lesions (angiolymphoid hyperplasia with eosinophilia); radiographically evident poorly marginated and occasionally expansile regions; soft tissue involvement in some cases; and, histologically, the presence of proliferation of histiocytic-like or epithelial-like cells that, on electron microscopy, possess characteristics of endothelial cells; the presence of stromal inflammatory cells; and the absence of anastomosing blood channels (Fig. 83–262). It has been further suggested that some of the previously described low grade or well-differentiated angiosarcomas of bone that were associated with a more favorable prognosis represented, in reality, histiocytoid hemangiomas.[1356, 2263] Histiocytoid hemangiomas of bone, indeed, appear to be benign, although tumor recurrence after surgery may be encountered.

Natural History. The ultimate prognosis in patients with angiosarcoma of bone depends largely on the histologic grade of the tumor. Well-differentiated or low grade neoplasms are associated with a more favorable prognosis; patients do well following surgical excision of such lesions. On the opposite end of the spectrum, high grade angiosarcomas of bone must be treated early and aggressively, although the prognosis for long-term survival in these cases remains grave. Although it has been observed that patients with multifocal lesions have a better prognosis than those with unifocal disease,[33, 1325] this is not a constant finding.[1319]

TUMORS OF NEURAL DIFFERENTIATION

Primary osseous tumors of neurogenic origin are rare. Unfortunately, as with their soft tissue counterparts, problems arise owing to inconsistencies in the terminology used to describe these neoplasms. The designation of schwannoma has been applied by some investigators to both of the major benign neural tumors, neurilemoma and neurofibroma, whereas others use schwannoma as a synonym for

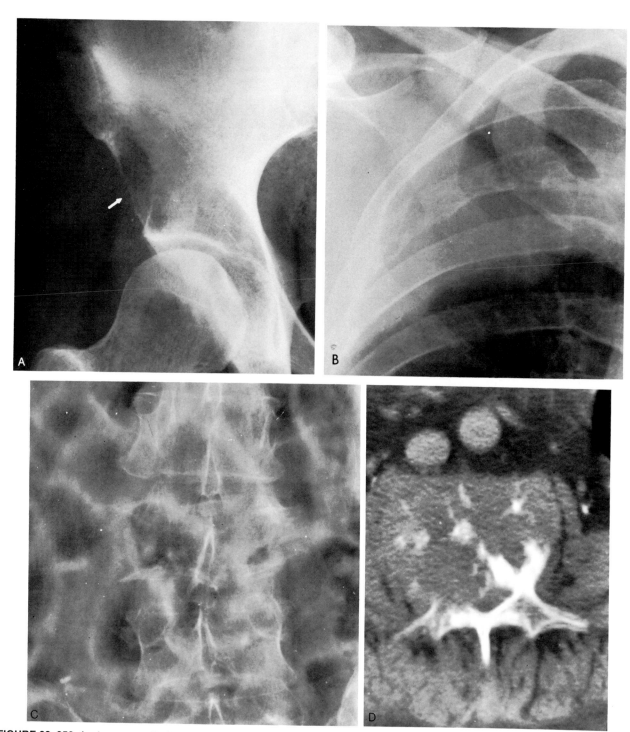

FIGURE 83–258. Angiosarcoma: Radiographic abnormalities—flat and irregular bones.

A Ilium. A nonspecific motheaten, osteolytic lesion is present in the ilium above the acetabulum (arrow).

B Ribs. An ill-defined lesion of the posterior aspect of the fourth rib is associated with a coarsened trabecular pattern and a large soft tissue mass. The osseous changes are consistent with a vascular lesion. The extent of the soft tissue involvement would suggest an aggressive process.

C, D Spine. In a 43 year old man with low back pain, a frontal radiograph of the lumbar spine **(C)** shows osteolysis of the third lumbar vertebral body and right pedicle. The adjacent intervertebral disc spaces are preserved. Transaxial CT **(D)** reveals complete dissolution of the vertebral body and right pedicle with involvement of a portion of the adjacent lamina and transverse process.

(C, D, Courtesy of R. Kerr, M.D., Los Angeles, California.)

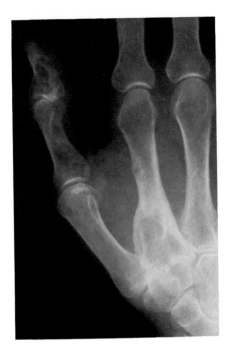

FIGURE 83–259. Angiosarcoma: Radiographic abnormalities—small bones of the hand. Note osteolytic lesions in the terminal phalanx of the thumb and the base of the second metacarpal bone. (Courtesy of M. Mitchell, M.D., Halifax, Nova Scotia, Canada.)

neurilemoma alone. Certainly, the two lesions have many features in common, and both are believed to originate from the Schwann cell and, perhaps, the perineural fibroblast. Nonetheless, neurofibromas and neurilemomas have histologic characteristics that are easily distinguished from one another and should be regarded as distinct entities.

The malignant counterpart of these lesions has been designated a neurogenic sarcoma or malignant schwannoma. In this case, disagreement exists regarding the precise origin of the neoplasm. Although many investigators consider this lesion to be of Schwann cell origin, some maintain that the tumor is not truly related to nerve tissue but arises from fibrous elements (fibrosarcoma) or fascial and other tissue adjacent to the nerve.

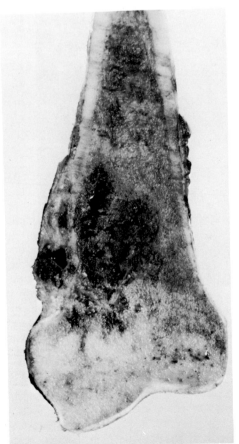

FIGURE 83–260. Angiosarcoma: Macroscopic abnormalities. This granular-appearing, hemorrhagic tumor in the metaphysis and epiphysis of the distal portion of the femur has indistinct margins and extends through the cortex.

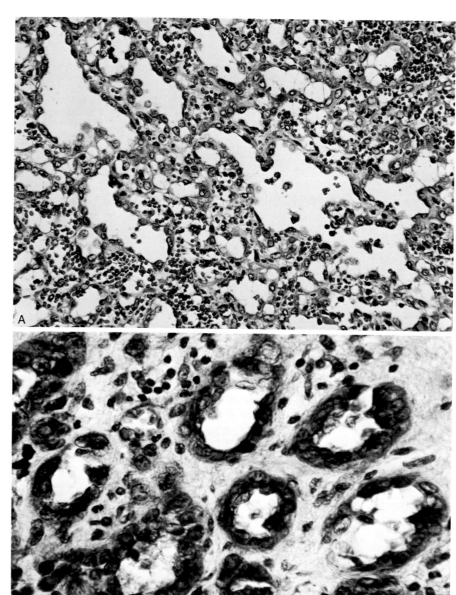

FIGURE 83–261. Angiosarcoma: Microscopic abnormalities.

A A well-differentiated angiosarcoma of bone shows intercommunicating vascular channels lined by mildly atypical, plump, endothelial cells that protrude into the lumina. (300×.)

B In a moderately differentiated angiosarcoma, the lining endothelial cells are more numerous and are crowded together. Their nuclei are plump, irregular, and hyperchromatic. (600×.)

Benign Tumors

Solitary Neurofibroma

Although multiple neurogenic tumors are well recognized as part of neurofibromatosis (see Chapter 92), solitary neurofibromas are uncommon. These lesions generally occur in persons between the ages of 25 and 45 years, originating from the cranial, peripheral, and sympathetic nerves. Neurofibromas arising from peripheral nerves and appearing in the soft tissues are discussed in Chapter 95. When occurring adjacent to a bone, these tumors as well as those arising in the periosteum or at the outer portion of the osseous neurovascular foramina may lead to eccentric bone erosion. True intraosseous neurofibromas are indeed rare. Clinical manifestations usually are mild owing to the slow growth of the neoplasms and include local pain, swelling, and tenderness. In certain locations, such as the sacrum, more prominent symptoms and signs, including both local and radiating pain, may be evident.

The mandible is the bone that is affected most typically, being involved in approximately two thirds of cases; other sites of involvement, in order of decreasing frequency, include the maxilla, vertebral column (especially the sacrum), tibia, fibula, and humerus.[1361–1369] It is the posterior portion of the mandible in which neurofibromas generally appear. Central or eccentric osteolytic lesions are encountered, which may result in cortical destruction and periosteal reaction. When the tumors are large and accompanied by a soft tissue mass, it may be difficult to determine whether they arose in bone, on the surface of the bone, or in the soft tissues. Intraosseous neurofibromas can be associated with neurofibromatosis[1362, 1365] as well as with congenital bowing of a tubular bone (see Chapter 90).[1370]

Macroscopically, osseous neurofibromas vary in size (generally being between 2.5 and 10 cm in maximum dimension), are soft and nonencapsulated, and have a gray, white, or brown surface. Histologically, these tumors of bone are similar to those of soft tissues (Fig. 83–263), being

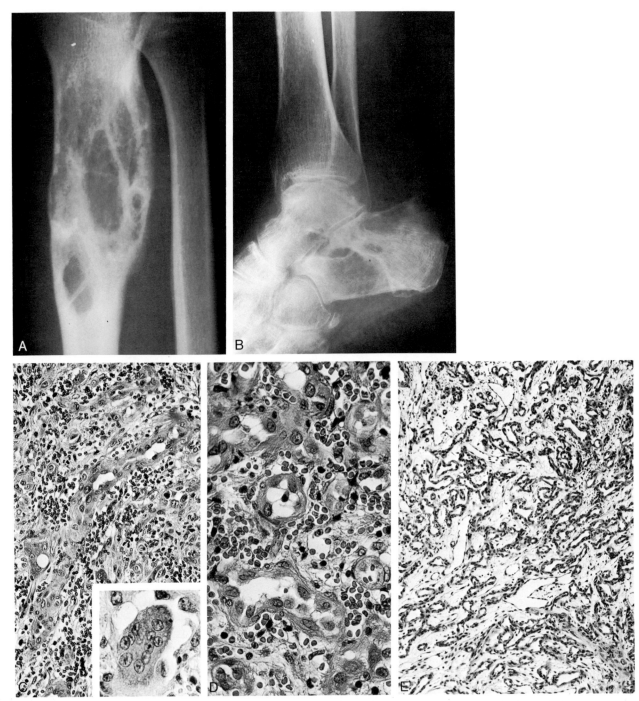

FIGURE 83–262. Histiocytoid hemangioma (epithelioid hemangioendothelioma): Radiographic and microscopic abnormalities.

A, B In these two examples, note the presence of poorly defined, slightly expansile osteolytic lesions in the distal portion of the radius **(A)** and the calcaneus **(B)**.

C This histiocytoid hemangioma shows strands of cells with granular eosinophilic cytoplasm. The cells of these strands or cores contain cytoplasmic vacuoles, the fusion of which leads to the formation of lumina of blood vessels. The stroma contains extravasated red blood cells. In the inset at the bottom right, note a multinucleated histiocytic cell with peripheral vacuolization of its cytoplasm. The vacuoles have partially fused, leading to the formation of a vascular lumen. (300×, 600×.)

D With regard to the developing vessels in a histiocytoid hemangioma, the lining cells have abundant cytoplasm and the bland nuclei protrude into the lumina of the vessels. Scattered chronic inflammatory cells are present in the stroma. (600×.)

E Florid proliferation of blood vessels lined by histiocytoid endothelial cells is seen. Unlike angiosarcoma, these vessels do not form interconnecting channels. (150×.)

Illustration continued on opposite page

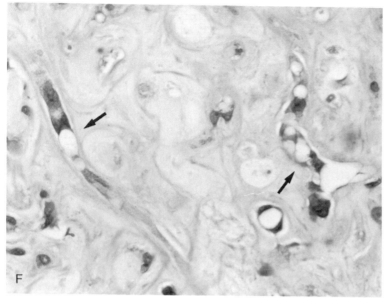

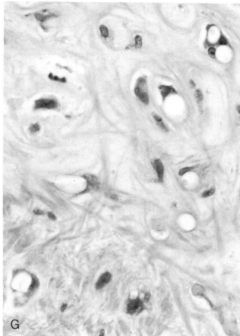

FIGURE 83–262 *Continued* **F** View of epithelioid hemangioendothelioma shows fibrochondroid type matrix with dispersed cells. Two foci of primitive blood vessel formation are present (arrows). The cells show cytoplasmic vacuoles.

G Cells of epithelioid hemangioendothelioma within a fibrochondroid matrix. Cells show blister-type cytoplasmic vacuolization.

FIGURE 83–263. Solitary neurofibroma: Microscopic abnormalities. Note the haphazard arrangement of collagen bundles separated by a loose stroma in which Schwann cells proliferate. The two insets at the bottom right show the occasional atypical nuclei that may be found in neurofibromas. Such cells, in themselves, are not indicative of malignancy. (150×, 600×.)

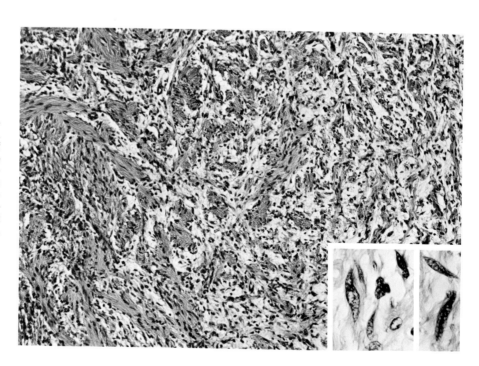

composed of spindle-shaped or stellate cells that have elongated, wavy, or twisted nuclei. Diffusely distributed collagen bundles or fibers are evident, and the stroma is edematous and widely separates the individual tumor cells. This stroma stains strongly for mucopolysaccharide. Occasionally a neurofibroma contains cells with pleomorphic nuclei, but such cells presumably are related to degenerative changes and, in the absence of considerable mitotic activity, are not indicative of malignancy.

Neurilemoma

Neurilemomas, which arise from a nerve sheath, rarely originate in bone. Men and women of all ages are affected, although most are in the second, third, fourth, or fifth decade of life.[1361, 1371] Clinical manifestations include pain, swelling, and, less frequently, impairment of sensory and motor function. Rarely, the presenting symptoms and signs relate to a pathologic fracture.

The most frequent sites of involvement are the mandible, sacrum, maxilla, femur, and humerus, in order of descending frequency, although virtually any bone may be affected.[1371–1396, 2265–2267] It is of interest that the mandible and sacrum represent bones that normally contain lengthy nerve segments, perhaps explaining the predilection of neurilemomas (and neurofibromas) to affect these sites. Mandibular tumors predominate in the posterior portion of the bone[1362]; lesions in the long tubular bones are evident in the diaphysis or metaphysis, or both, with rare exceptions involving the epiphysis.

The radiographic characteristics of neurilemomas are not specific. Three modes of presentation are encountered: central involvement characterized as a cystic osteolytic focus with a sclerotic margin; localization to the nutrient canal with production of a dumbbell lesion; and periosteal involvement leading to cortical erosion or excavation.[1390]

On macroscopic inspection, neurilemomas are variable in size (less than 1 cm to more than 10 cm in maximum dimension), are soft or rubbery, and are well delineated and encapsulated. Their surface is variegated and may be pink, gray, yellow, or brown. Larger tumors may contain cystic regions filled with mucoid material or hemorrhagic fluid.

Classically, neurilemomas are composed of compact cellular areas in combination with loosely arranged hypocellular regions, the former being termed Antoni A areas and the latter Antoni B areas. This biphasic pattern, so common in soft tissue neurilemomas, may not be so clearly present in intraosseous neurilemomas.[1373] In the Antoni A areas (Fig. 83–264A), bipolar spindle cells are aligned in either interweaving fascicles or palisading patterns (Fig. 83–264B). The spindle cells also may be grouped in organoid structures termed Verocay bodies.[1373] In Antoni B areas (Fig. 83–264A), tumor cells are separated by a watery type of matrix that, unlike the matrix of neurofibroma, stains weakly or not at all for acid mucopolysaccharide. Neurilemomas are vascular lesions; the stroma may contain areas of fresh or old hemorrhage with hemosiderin pigment, macrophages, and lymphocytes.[1361] Neurites are not found in a neurilemoma, and malignant degeneration of an intraosseous lesion is not reported.[1373] Some neurilemomas may contain cells with large, irregular, hyperchromatic and bizarre nuclei. Such cells occasionally have led to a misdiagnosis of neurosarcoma. These tumors have been termed "ancient neurilemomas" and the atypical cells are a manifestation of degeneration.

Electron microscopy confirms the Schwann cell nature of this tumor.[1373, 1387, 1393, 1394]

Malignant Tumors

Neurogenic Sarcoma (Malignant Schwannoma)

Neurogenic sarcomas (malignant peripheral nerve sheath tumors) are unusual lesions that have a variable histologic appearance, perhaps related to the versatility of Schwann cells, which, through metaplasia, can produce cartilage, bone, fat, and muscle.[420] The malignant schwannoma of bone usually appears in a patient in the third, fourth, or fifth decade of life as an ill-defined osteolytic process with soft tissue extension.[1397] It may be seen in patients with generalized neurofibromatosis.

TUMORS OF NOTOCHORD ORIGIN

Locally Aggressive or Malignant Tumors

Chordoma

Chordoma is a rare lesion of notochord origin characterized by a lobular arrangement and composed of highly vacuolated (physaliferous) cells and mucoid intercellular material.[33] It is a locally aggressive tumor that grows slowly, invades surrounding soft tissue structures, and metastasizes infrequently. Diagnosis often is delayed, such that the lesions commonly are large when first discovered and amenable only to palliative treatment.

It is the origin of the neoplasm in vestigial remnants of the embryonic notochord that governs its characteristic localization to the vertebral column. During its early development, the cephalad portion of the notochord pursues a convoluted course, giving rise to dendritic tracts that penetrate the anlagen of the cranial bones and ramify beneath the nasopharyngeal mucosa, extending into the parapharyngeal space and regions of the paranasal sinuses.[1398–1401] By the fifth week of embryonic development, the notochord becomes encased in the anlagen of the bones of the skull (as well as those of the vertebral column) and gradually disappears.[1401–1403] Microscopic vestiges of the notochord are found in 0.5 to 2 per cent of cadavers at the time of autopsy, however[1402–1404]; such vestiges most frequently are apparent in the midline in the region of the spheno-occipital synchondrosis, where they have been termed ecchondrosis or ecchordosis physaliphora spheno-occipitalis.[1405, 1406] They also have been found in the maxilla and mandible,[1399] the sacral and coccygeal region,[1407] and the thoracolumbar vertebrae.[1408] Observations in fetuses have confirmed the presence of ectopic vestiges of notochord, most commonly located in the spheno-occipital and sacrococcygeal areas.[1398] These data regarding the distribution of notochord rests derived from investigations in the fetus and the adult are compatible with the well-documented preference for chordomas to involve the spheno-occipital and sacrococcygeal regions and, less typically, other spinal regions and with the concept that chordomas arise specifically from such vestigial tissue.

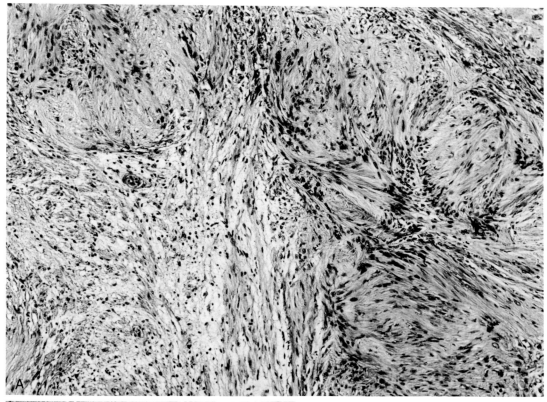

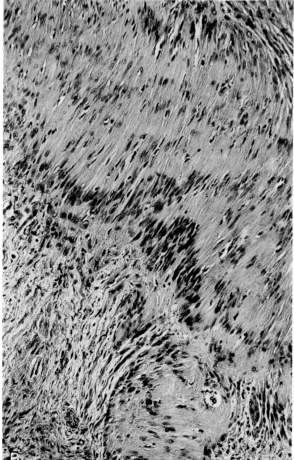

FIGURE 83–264. Neurilemoma: Microscopic abnormalities.

A Antoni A areas are well shown at the top and right of this photomicrograph. They are composed of elongated spindle-shaped Schwann cells. To the center and left of this photomicrograph, observe an area of loosely arranged cells with a watery type of matrix. Such degenerative foci are termed Antoni B regions. (150×.)

B Note nuclear palisading created by the parallel arrangement of the Schwann cell nuclei. (150×.)

Clinical Abnormalities. Chordomas can become evident in men and women of all ages, including elderly persons as well as neonates,[1409, 2268] although most patients are in the fourth, fifth, sixth, or seventh decade of life. Chordomas occurring in children, which are rare, appear to be more aggressive than those in adults, with rapid tumor growth and a propensity to metastasize. Sacrococcygeal lesions arise in men more commonly than in women, in a ratio of approximately 2 to 1, and have their greatest frequency in persons between the ages of 40 and 70 years; spheno-occipital chordomas have an equal sex distribution and generally occur in persons between the ages of 30 and 60 years.[1410]

Clinical manifestations relate to the precise location of the chordoma, although they initially may be mild and nonspecific, leading to considerable delay in the patient's seeking medical attention. Chordomas arising in the *sacrococcygeal region* produce gradually progressive perineal pain and numbness. Additional manifestations depend on the pressure exerted by the tumor on surrounding structures, including the rectum (constipation and bleeding), the bladder (frequency and urgency of urination, incontinence), and the emerging nerve roots (paresthesias and anesthesia).[1410] Physical findings include the presence of a firm and fixed presacral tumor mass on rectal examination, diminished perianal sensation, and cutaneous and rectal ulceration.[30, 1399, 1411]

Spheno-occipital chordomas lead to an increase in intracranial pressure and encroachment on adjacent structures and are manifested as headaches, blurred vision, diplopia, weakness, memory loss, and emotional instability.[1410] Dysfunction of the pituitary gland may be accompanied by amenorrhea, sterility, loss of libido, and visual disturbances. Additional abnormalities result from involvement of the cranial nerves and obstruction of the nasal passages.[1411–1413]

Vertebral chordomas involve the adjacent spinal cord and nerve roots progressively, resulting in pain, numbness, motor weakness, and, eventually, paralysis.[1414, 1415]

Skeletal Location. Favored locations of chordomas are the sacrococcygeal region (50 to 60 per cent of cases), spheno-occipital region (25 to 40 per cent), and remaining portions of the vertebral column (15 to 20 per cent)[1416–1425, 1853, 2269]; of the vertebrae above the sacrum, those in the cervical region (particularly the second cervical vertebra) are affected most commonly, followed in order of frequency by the lumbar and thoracic vertebrae.[1418, 1424–1427, 2270–2272] In some reported series, however, the lumbar spine has been involved most commonly.[2271] In children and young adults, spheno-occipital chordomas are more frequent than sacrococcygeal and vertebral chordomas.[1428]

Although cranial chordomas predominate in the spheno-occipital region, especially in the clivus,[1429, 1430] these lesions rarely may occur in the nasopharynx, maxilla, or paranasal sinuses.[1430–1434] Sacrococcygeal tumors develop as retrorectal masses that frequently extend into the buttocks[1410]; chordomas are the most common aggressive retrorectal neoplasm, accounting for as many as 38 per cent of such tumors.[1435] Spinal chordomas generally arise in the vertebral body, although they may extend into (or, rarely, arise in) the posterior osseous elements of the vertebra. Very rarely, chordomas develop in the epidural space.[2273] Chordomas may lead to large posterior mediastinal masses that are not contiguous with lesions in the bone.[1436, 1437]

Additional infrequent or rare manifestations of chordoma

are multicentric involvement (e.g., both the sacrum and the base of the skull),[1438] multifocal deposits in the spinal cord,[1439] nodules of tumor in subcutaneous tissue and muscles[1440] (such nodules actually may represent hamartomatous lesions of fibroblastic derivation), and involvement of other bones, such as the scapula.[1409] The last-mentioned occurrence probably represents a chordoid chondrosarcoma rather than a true chordoma.

Radiographic and Other Imaging Abnormalities. Osteolysis with or without calcification, cortical violation, and a soft tissue mass are the predominant radiographic findings, although additional abnormalities may be observed, depending on the specific location of the chordoma.

Sacrococcygeal Tumors. The fundamental radiographic features of these chordomas are irregular destruction of bone, osseous expansion, and an anterior soft tissue mass. Calcification (50 to 70 per cent of cases) and osteosclerosis are additional abnormalities (Fig. 83–265A) that are prominent in some cases.[1421, 1441] It has been emphasized repeatedly that although these tumors may be large, their detection with routine radiography is made difficult owing to obscuration of bone by overlying soft tissue and gaseous shadows. Conventional tomography may clarify the osseous abnormalities[1441]; however, other methods, including CT[1441–1444, 1853, 1921] and MR imaging[1444, 1445] appear to be more useful (Fig. 83–266). CT may define the extent of the tumor, particularly its soft tissue component, and detect calcification in as many as 90 per cent of cases.[1443] Such calcification is amorphous and predominates in the periphery of the tumor. MR imaging appears to be at least equal to and probably better than CT in delineating the osseous and soft tissue components of chordomas, especially in instances of recurrent tumor. Excellent contrast between the neoplasm and the surrounding soft tissue is provided by T2-weighted spin echo images; the relative brightness of the chordoma on these images results from its markedly prolonged T2 values, a property that this tumor shares with the nucleus pulposus of the intervertebral disc.[1444] Myelography, scintigraphy, and angiography represent additional techniques that can be applied to the evaluation of sacrococcygeal chordomas.[1441] Photon-deficient (or ''cold'') lesions have been reported to be typical of the scintigraphic findings of sacrococcygeal chordomas.[2274]

With regard to the differential diagnosis of the radiographic features, an expansile lesion of the sacrum may also indicate a giant cell tumor, plasmacytoma, chondrosarcoma, neurogenic tumors, meningocele, or skeletal metastasis (Fig. 83–267).

Spheno-occipital Tumors. Destruction of the clivus and sella turcica, osseous expansion, a soft tissue mass, and extension of tumor to the petrous and sphenoid bones as well as the nasopharynx may be evident.[1421, 1429] Reticular, nodular, or scattered calcifications within the lesion are detected in 20 to 70 per cent of cases.[1446] Of interest in this regard is the identification of a specific variety of chordoma, the *chondroid chordoma,* that exhibits cartilaginous features, represents approximately one third of all chordomas in this region, and is accompanied by a better prognosis (see later discussion).[1416]

Conventional and computed tomography,[1443] angiography,[1421, 1429] and MR imaging[1447, 2275–2277] are additional methods that allow further evaluation of spheno-occipital chordomas. With regard to MR imaging, spheno-occipital

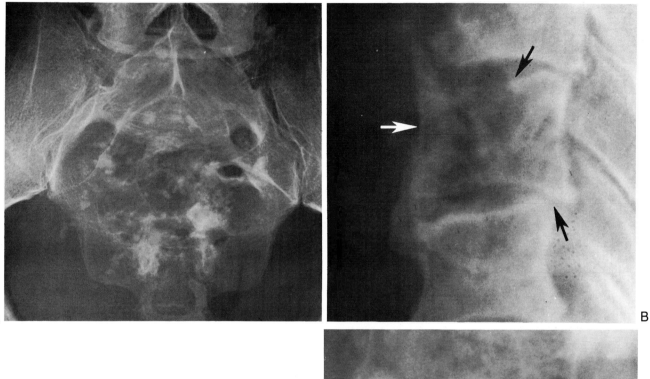

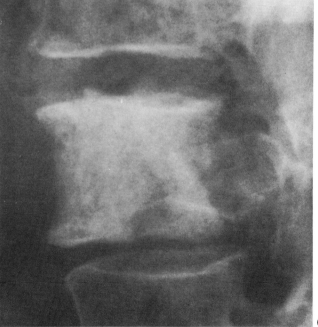

FIGURE 83–265. Chordoma: Radiographic abnormalities.

A Sacrococcygeal tumor. Within the sacrum, this large chordoma had led to osteolysis with prominent calcification.

B Vertebral tumor. This chordoma of a cervical vertebral body is associated with osteolysis (arrows). The adjacent intervertebral discs appear slightly narrowed.

C Vertebral tumor. Osteosclerosis is the predominant abnormality in this chordoma of a vertebral body. Note erosion of the posterior aspect of the vertebral body and narrowing of the intervertebral disc above the involved vertebra.

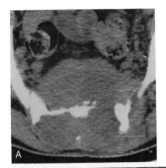

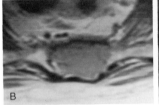
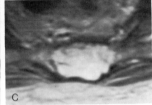

FIGURE 83–266. Chordoma: CT and MR imaging abnormalities.

A Sacrococcygeal tumor. Transaxial CT scan shows a large tumor that has destroyed the sacrum and led to a prominent soft tissue mass.

B, C Sacrococcygeal tumor. In a different patient, transaxial proton density–weighted (TR/TE, 2500/20) **(B)** and T2-weighted (TR/TE, 2500/70) **(C)** spin echo MR images show an intraosseous lesion of low to intermediate signal intensity in **B** and high signal intensity in **C**.

(Courtesy of K. Kortman, M.D., San Diego, California.)

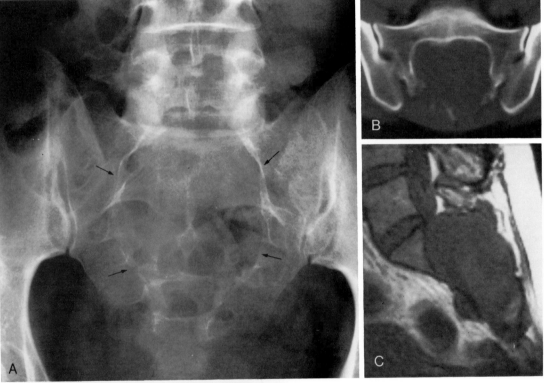

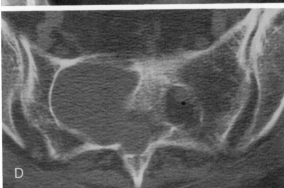

FIGURE 83–267. Chordoma: Differential diagnosis.

A–C Ependymoma. In a 28 year old woman with low back pain of several years' duration and a normal neurologic examination, routine radiography **(A)** reveals an osteolytic lesion (arrows) in the sacrum. Transaxial CT scan **(B)** confirms its central location and posterior extension. A sagittal T1-weighted (TR/TE, 300/50) spin echo MR image **(C)** shows its large size, posterior extension, and low signal intensity. The tumor was of high signal intensity in T2-weighted spin echo MR images (not shown). Histologic analysis confirmed a myxopapillary ependymoma that did not communicate with the dural sac.

D Meningocele. Transaxial CT scan shows a right-sided sacral lesion that has led to distortion of the neural foramen. It is sharply delineated with a sclerotic margin. (Courtesy of P. Kindynis, M.D., Geneva, Switzerland.)

chordomas typically reveal low to intermediate signal intensity in T1-weighted spin echo MR images and lobulated regions of high signal intensity with septations of low signal intensity in T2-weighted spin echo MR images. Disagreement exists regarding the ability to differentiate typical chordomas and chondroid chordomas on the basis of the MR imaging findings.[2275, 2276] MR imaging appears to be superior to CT in demonstrating the relationship of the tumor to the cavernous internal carotid artery and the vertebral and basilar arteries; CT appears to be superior in defining the presence and extent of tumoral calcification.[2276] Intravenous administration of gadolinium-based contrast agents can be used as a supplementary MR imaging technique (Fig. 83–268).

The differential diagnosis of these tumors includes craniopharyngioma, meningioma, osteochondroma, chondrosarcoma, pituitary neoplasms, aneurysm, optic glioma, nasopharyngeal carcinoma, and metastasis.[1421]

Vertebral Tumors. Initially, destruction of the vertebral body is unaccompanied by loss of height of the adjacent intervertebral disc[1426] (Fig. 83–265B). Subsequently, osteosclerosis and soft tissue abnormalities may become prominent (Fig. 83–265C) and contiguous vertebral bodies may be affected, with involvement of the intervertebral discs.[1418, 1420, 1448, 1449] Cervical lesions appear most likely to involve contiguous vertebrae.[2270] Calcification in an anterior soft tissue mass occurs in approximately 30 per cent of cases. Vertebral collapse, radiodense vertebral bodies (ivory vertebrae), and enlarged neural foramina are additional manifestations of this lesion.[1450, 1451, 2271, 2272] Intraspinal extension is readily apparent during myelography. Angiography, CT,

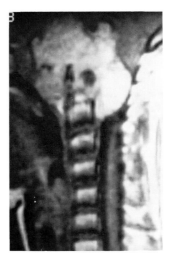

FIGURE 83–268. Chordoma: MR imaging abnormalities. In a 12 year old child, a sagittal T1-weighted (TR/TE, 600/20) spin echo MR image obtained after the intravenous injection of a gadolinium compound shows a large lesion in the base of the skull with inferior extension into the upper cervical vertebrae and spinal canal. The tumor is of high signal intensity, representing enhancement related to the injected contrast agent. It is lobulated, and there appear to be septations of low signal intensity. (Courtesy of S. K. Brahme, M.D., La Jolla, California.)

and MR imaging (Fig. 83–269) also can be used to evaluate spinal chordomas.[1427, 1452] The last two methods are particularly helpful in defining the anterior or lateral extent of the soft tissue mass, the degree of bone destruction, and, with regard to CT, the presence of calcification. MR imaging

FIGURE 83–269. Chordoma: Radiographic and MR imaging abnormalities. This 46 year old man complained of low back pain of 3 weeks' duration. The pain began as he attempted to lift a heavy object, became more intense, and radiated to the left foot.

A Routine radiograph shows subtle regions of osteolysis (arrows) involving the first and second lumbar vertebral bodies.

B, C Sagittal T1-weighted (TR/TE, 600/18) **(B)** and T2-weighted (TR/TE, 3000/80) **(C)** spin echo MR images show the tumorous involvement (arrows) of these two vertebral bodies. The lesions are of low signal intensity in **B** and high signal intensity in **C**. Extension of the tumor in front of the second lumbar vertebral body is seen. Discal involvement at the L1-L2 spinal level is not well shown in these images.

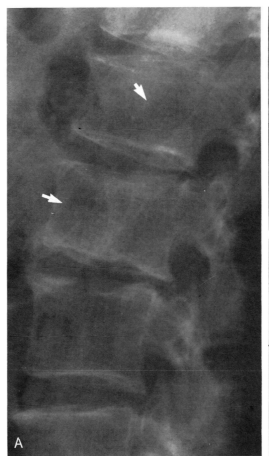

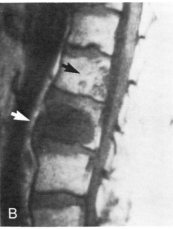

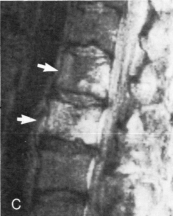

combined with intravenous administration of a gadolinium compound is useful in the assessment of epidural extension of the tumor.[2270]

Spinal chordomas produce radiographic findings that also are evident in skeletal metastasis, plasma cell myeloma, lymphoma, chondrosarcoma, giant cell tumor, and infection.

Pathologic Abnormalities. The size of chordomas is extremely variable. Those of the sacrococcygeal region may be enormous, measuring more than 30 cm in maximum dimension and weighing as much as 80 pounds.[28, 1399] The typical size of chordomas in this region is 5 to 20 cm. Spheno-occipital chordomas may be as small as 2 or 3 mm or large enough to fill the entire middle cranial fossa.[1410, 1423] Vertebral chordomas are small or moderate in size.

The macroscopic features of chordomas include a lobulated configuration, a variable texture depending upon the relative proportions of chondroid and mucinous material that are present, a gelatinous consistency, and a gray or blue color.[1410, 1423, 1424, 1453] Focal areas of hemorrhage and cyst formation may be evident. Soft tissue components of the neoplasm (Fig. 83–270) generally are well-defined, possessing a pseudocapsule.

The most prominent histologic feature of a chordoma is its abundant production of intracellular and extracellular mucin.[1423, 1426, 1454] Most chordomas have a distinct lobular pattern, at least focally, that is produced by crisscrossing fibrous tissue septa.[34] These lobules consist of either solid masses of tumor cells or pools of mucin in which reside fragments of the neoplasm and individual tumor cells (Fig. 83–271A,B). The latter are stellate, polygonal, or spindle-shaped and have abundant, eosinophilic, vacuolated cytoplasm.[1416, 1423] Many of the cells have an epithelioid appearance, resembling the cells in adenocarcinoma. Their nuclei are plump and oval, with a diffuse chromatin pattern, and they may contain a small nucleolus (Fig. 83–271B). Binucleated and a few multinucleated tumor cells occasionally are seen, and in some chordomas, hyperchromatic and pleomorphic cells also are found.

As intracellular mucin accumulates, the cytoplasmic vacuoles become larger and more numerous, displacing the nucleus peripherally, and creating a signet-ring appearance.[1416, 1419] Larger cells with central nuclei and an abundant vacuolated and reticulated cytoplasm, termed physaliferous cells, characteristically are found in chordomas (Fig. 83–271C,D), although they rarely represent the dominant

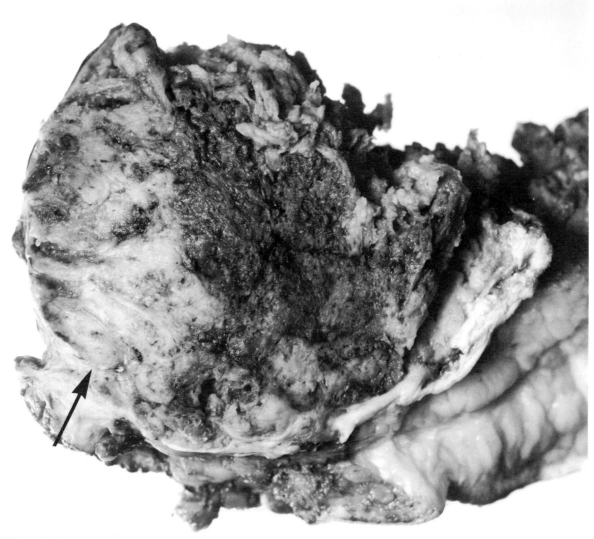

FIGURE 83–270. Chordoma: Macroscopic abnormalities. In this sacrococcygeal chordoma, soft tissue extension is apparent. The tumor is well delineated and divided into lobules by connective tissue septa (arrow). Much of this neoplasm has undergone hemorrhagic degeneration.

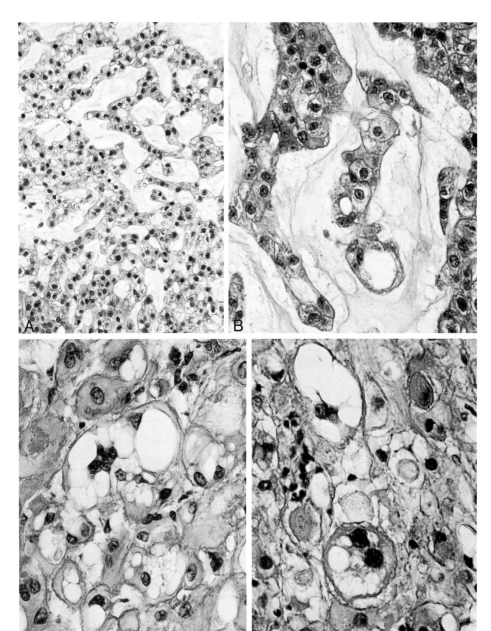

FIGURE 83–271. Chordoma: Microscopic abnormalities.

A Branching strands of chordoma epithelial cells reside in a pool of mucin. The nuclei are small, dark, and uniform. (300×.)

B At higher magnification, the cells have well-defined borders and their nuclei are located centrally, some having a small nucleolus. The cytoplasm is abundant, with a foamy appearance. The stringy material is mucin. (600×.)

C, D Central multivacuolated physaliferous cavities are seen. The cells in **C** resemble multivacuolated lipoblasts with scalloping of the nuclei by the cytoplasmic vacuoles. Other nonvacuolated tumor cells show cytoplasm with well-defined borders. (600×, 600×.)

cellular pattern. Syncytial cords of smaller cells lying within the pools of mucin are equally characteristic of this tumor. The tumor cells stain positively not only for mucin but also for cytoplasmic glycogen.[1410, 1423, 1426] In most chordomas, mitotic activity is either absent or scarce. Chordomas in children, however, may be pleomorphic, with large sarcomatoid foci.

Electron microscopic studies have shown that the cells of chordomas resemble those of the developing notochord.[1455, 1456] They consist of undifferentiated stellate cells, physaliferous cells, and cells with morphologic features intermediate between these two types.[1455] It has been suggested that it is the stellate cells that proliferate, not the physaliferous cells.[1453] The vacuoles consist of either dilated endoplasmic reticulum or invaginations or herniations into the cytoplasm of the extracellular interstitial material.[1459–1461] Immunohistochemical methods have shown cytokeratin and S-100 protein in the chordoma cells.[1883] The interested reader should refer to additional sources.[2488–2491]

Natural History. The prognosis of a chordoma is variable, depending on the location of the neoplasm and its extent at the time it is first discovered. Unfortunately, many chordomas are massive when evaluated initially and, owing to their locally aggressive behavior, have infiltrated adjacent structures. In these instances, palliative surgery is the only option. Masses of tumor are, by necessity, left behind, eventually leading to recurrence of the clinical abnormalities.[1410] In primary or recurrent tumors or in those that have been irradiated, large areas of sarcomatous-appearing cells may develop similar to those of malignant fibrous histiocytoma, fibrosarcoma, chondrosarcoma, or osteosarcoma.[1462–1464, 1884, 2278, 2279] Tumors with these cellular components have been referred to as dedifferentiated chordomas or those with a malignant spindle cell component.[2429]

Hematogenous metastases (to such sites as the lungs, liver, skeleton, skin, subcutaneous tissue, muscle, peritoneum, heart, pleura, spleen, adrenal glands, kidneys, urinary bladder, and pancreas)[1854] eventually may be evident in 10 to 40 per cent of chordomas.[30, 1426, 2280] This phenomenon is far more frequent in cases of chordoma of the sacrococcygeal region or spine than of the base of the skull. Significant in this regard is the frequent occurrence of a specific type of chordoma, the chondroid chordoma, in the spheno-occipital region. This tumor, which has been reported to be less aggressive than the conventional chordoma, deserves special emphasis (see following discussion).

Chondroid Chordoma

In 1973, Heffelfinger and collaborators[1416] emphasized that some chordomas arising in the base of the skull possessed a chondroid component that could even be the dominant histologic characteristic. These investigators suggested that such neoplasms should be classified as a distinct variant of conventional chordomas, owing to their indolent course and relatively good prognosis. It has been suggested further that the existence of tumor with cartilaginous and chordoid features is consistent with the known embryology of the notochord, in which certain stages of development are characterized by an intimate relationship of cartilaginous and notochordal tissue.[1465] Chondroid chordomas rarely are evident in other sites, such as the sacrococcygeal region,[1416, 1464] but their predominance in the spheno-occipital area is undeniable. In fact, it is estimated that approximately 33 per cent of chordomas in the base of the skull are chondroid in type.[1425, 1428] Although, in the past, some investigators have grouped together chondromas and chordomas that occur in the clival region owing to their clinical, radiologic, and pathologic similarities,[1413] it seems more appropriate to differentiate chondroid chordomas from chondromas (as well as chondrosarcomas) because such chordomas are associated with distinctive behavioral characteristics, revealing a proclivity to invade bone and entwine themselves around vital structures.[1466]

Chondroid chordomas are slightly more frequent in women than in men and usually are observed in patients below the age of 40 years. Radiographic and gross morphologic features are similar to those of typical chordomas, although calcification is particularly prominent. Histologically, the cartilaginous foci in chondroid chordomas may resemble those of a chondroma or a low grade chondrosarcoma.[1416] Reticulin stains have been emphasized as a technique that allows differentiation of chondroid chordomas (or other chordomas) and chondrosarcomas, owing to the positive nature of the staining response in chondrosarcoma and the absence of this response in chordoma,[1467] but the results of this technique are inconsistent.[1425, 1431] Additional methods, including immunohistochemical, electron microscopic, and enzymatic analyses, appear more promising in the differentiation of these two neoplasms.[1468–1471, 2281]

TUMORS OF HEMATOPOIETIC ORIGIN

Malignant Tumors

Non-Hodgkin's Lymphomas, Hodgkin's Disease, Leukemias

The skeletal manifestations of these tumors are discussed in Chapter 62.

PLASMA CELL DYSCRASIAS

Locally Aggressive or Malignant Tumors

Plasmacytoma, Multiple Myeloma

These and other plasma cell dyscrasias are discussed in Chapter 60.

TUMORS AND TUMOR-LIKE LESIONS OF MISCELLANEOUS OR UNKNOWN ORIGIN

Benign Tumors

Simple (Solitary or Unicameral) Bone Cyst

The simple bone cyst is a common lesion of unknown cause and pathogenesis. Early suggestions that this cystic lesion represented a true neoplasm[1472] or occurred secondary to osteomyelitis[1473] have not stood the test of time. It was the belief of Jaffe and Lichtenstein,[1474] as proposed in 1942, that simple bone cysts were dysplastic lesions related to a disturbance in endochondral bone formation resulting from trauma. This hypothesis, too, is no longer favored. In 1960 and 1970, Cohen[1475, 1476] demonstrated that the chemical constituents of the fluid in these cysts were similar to those of serum and, furthermore, that stasis of contrast material was apparent following its direct injection into the cystic lesions. These observations were used to support the concept that venous obstruction within bone was a primary factor in the development of simple bone cysts. More recent evidence has supported the importance of venous obstruction and of the blocking of drainage of interstitial fluid in a rapidly growing and remodeling area of cancellous bone in the pathogenesis of such cysts,[1477–1479] and, indeed, this hypothesis has been used as a guide to the formulation of appropriate treatment strategies in dealing with these lesions.[1480] Still, the precise pathogenesis of the simple bone cyst has yet to be firmly established.

Clinical Abnormalities. That simple bone cysts are predominantly a lesion of the young is not debated. Most of these cysts are discovered in the first and second decades of life and affect boys with greater frequency than girls (ratio of 2 to 1). In those patients below the age of 20 years, cysts generally are observed in the tubular bones, particularly the proximal ends of the humerus (mean age at presentation, 8 years; age range, 1 to 25 years) and the femur (mean age at presentation, 20 years; age range, 3 to 54 years).[1479] After the age of 20 years, cysts reveal predilection for the innominate bone and the calcaneus.[1481] In any site, simple bone cysts rarely are symptomatic unless a pathologic fracture has occurred.[1482] Such fractures usually result from minor trauma and are minimally displaced; local growth retardation may be a significant sequela of this complication.[1477, 1483]

Skeletal Location. The simple bone cyst is observed most frequently in a long tubular bone (approximately 90 to 95 per cent of cases).[1484–1489] The humerus (56 per cent of cases), the femur (27 per cent), and the tibia (6 per cent) are involved most commonly, and lesions in the fibula (2 per cent), radius (1 per cent), and ulna (0.5 per cent) are infrequent.[1490] With the exception of the calcaneus,[2282, 2283] which is affected in approximately 3 per cent of cases, simple bone cysts are rare in the small bones of the hand and foot.[2284, 2285] In the osseous pelvis, it is the ilium (2 per cent) that usually is involved. Rare sites of localization are the ischium, sacrum, pubic bone, ribs, patella, scapula, clavicle, and spine.[1491–1494, 1922, 2286–2290] As indicated previously, simple bone cysts discovered in adult patients, when compared with those in young patients, more commonly are localized in the flat or irregular bones or the bones in the hand or foot.[1481] Rarely, more than one simple bone cyst is evident in a single patient[1481, 1485, 2284, 2291, 2292] (see Fig. 83–276).

With regard to the long tubular bones, a metaphyseal location is the preferred site. Approximately 85 per cent of humeral cysts and 83 per cent of femoral cysts are located in the region of the proximal metaphysis. Diaphyseal involvement occurs in 4 to 12 per cent of lesions in the tubular bones. Epiphyseal localization or extension is exceedingly rare; simple bone cysts involving the epiphysis typically are observed in young adults and in the proximal portion of the femur or, less commonly, the humerus.[1495–1497, 1855] Simple bone cysts located in the metaphysis adjacent to the growth plate have been considered active because of their capacity for growth, whereas those that have "migrated" away from the plate have been considered latent.[1498–1500] This division of simple bone cysts into active and latent forms based on location in the bone is not entirely accurate; examples of active cysts in the diaphysis are recorded.[1481] Such activity appears to correlate better with the age of the patient; the recurrence rate of these lesions is much greater in patients below the age of 10 years.[1481, 1486, 1498]

Radiographic Abnormalities. Although small radiodense lesions occasionally have been documented as an early finding of a simple bone cyst,[1501, 1502] a centrally located radiolucent lesion with cortical thinning and mild osseous expansion should be regarded as the radiographic hallmark of this lesion. Some cysts may possess a multilocular appearance. A thin, sclerotic margin is a frequent finding, producing a classic pattern of geographic bone destruction with a short zone of transition from abnormal to normal bone. In a long tubular bone, additional radiographic features include a lesion mainly confined to the metaphysis, juxtaposed to the physis, and an elongated shape with the longitudinal axis of the lesion parallel to that of the parent bone (Fig. 83–272). On the basis of these roentgenographic findings, the accurate diagnosis of a simple bone cyst in a long tubular bone is not difficult, particularly when it is the proximal portion of the humerus or the femur in a child or adolescent that is affected. In some cases, other diagnoses, such as an aneurysmal bone cyst, enchondroma, and fibrous dysplasia, must be considered.

A pathologic fracture through a simple bone cyst is a common associated abnormality (see later discussion) and should not lead to the choice of one of these alternative diagnoses. Furthermore, such a fracture may be accompanied by a vertical fragment within the cyst that migrates to a dependent portion of the lesion owing to its fluid content. This finding (Fig. 83–273), which has been designated the fallen fragment sign,[1503, 1856, 2293] virtually ensures the accurate analysis of the roentgenograms. It usually is evident in

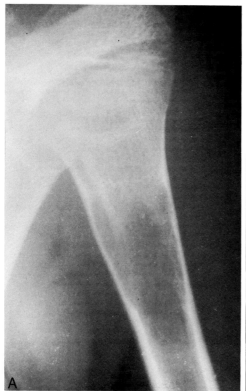
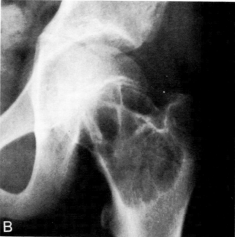
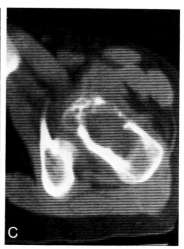

FIGURE 83–272. Simple (solitary or unicameral) bone cyst: Radiographic abnormalities—long tubular bones.

A Humerus. A relatively well defined, central osteolytic lesion in the proximal metaphysis of the humerus in this 8 year old boy is virtually diagnostic of simple bone cyst. Note the elongated shape of the lesion and endosteal bone erosion.

B, C Femur. In an 11 year old girl with the spontaneous onset of hip pain and a normal physical examination, a radiograph **(B)** shows a well-marginated, osteolytic metaphyseal lesion juxtaposed to the physis. Transaxial CT **(C)** documents the extent of the cyst, which had an attenuation value of 30 Hounsfield units. A percutaneous biopsy of the lesion led to the recovery of dark amber fluid. The histologic diagnosis was a simple bone cyst.

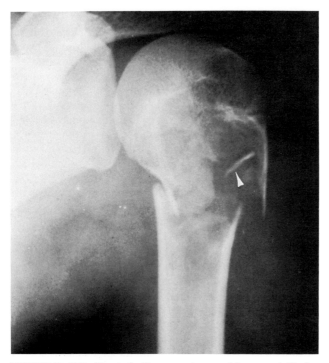

FIGURE 83–273. Simple (solitary or unicameral) bone cyst: Radiographic abnormalities—long tubular bones. A transverse pathologic fracture through a cystic lesion of the humerus is evident. Note the piece of cortex (arrowhead) that lies within the lesion. (Courtesy of D. Pate, D.C., San Diego, California.)

cases of fractured cysts that occur in children and in tubular bones. Of interest is the further documentation of the principle that a heavier object is able to move freely in a lighter environment that is provided by a description of a tumbling bullet within a posttraumatic bone cyst.[1504]

Simple cysts that involve the diaphysis or epiphysis of a long tubular bone also can be diagnosed on the basis of the radiographic abnormalities. In some instances, diaphyseal lesions are large, multiloculated, and slightly expansile (Fig. 83–274), resembling the appearance of fibrous dysplasia, chondromyxoid fibroma, desmoplastic fibroma, and eosinophilic granuloma. Features of a simple bone cyst, including a central location, an elongated shape, and prominent radiolucency, usually allow its differentiation from these other processes. With epiphyseal involvement or extension, the cyst may produce radiographic abnormalities simulating those of chondromyxoid fibroma or chondroblastoma, or, owing to considerable deformity of the articular surface,[1495] the cyst may resemble ischemic necrosis of bone.

Simple cysts in sites other than the long tubular bones may present a greater diagnostic challenge, although those in the calcaneus possess characteristic abnormalities.[1505, 1506] In this site, the cyst is a well-defined and radiolucent lesion, almost invariably occurring in the base of the calcaneal neck just inferior to the anterior portion of the posterior facet (Fig. 83–275). Its anterior margin usually is straight and vertical, whereas the posterior border of the lesion typically is curvilinear, paralleling the trabeculae in the posterior portion of the calcaneus.[1505] Infrequent osseous expansion, intraosseous extension (Fig. 83–276), absent periostitis, and a lateral location on tangential radiographic projections represent additional features of this lesion. Frac-

ture of a simple cyst in the calcaneus is rare.[1857] The major differential diagnostic considerations are a lipoma (see previous discussion) and thinning of trabeculae that normally occurs in this portion of the calcaneus.

Simple cysts of the talus may lead to prominent radiolucent regions that involve large portions of the superior surface of the bone and extend to the subchondral area adjacent to the tibiotalar articulation.[1507, 1508] They may resemble ischemic necrosis of bone or chondroblastomas. Simple bone cysts of the short tubular bones in the hands and feet resemble those of the long tubular bones (Fig. 83–276).

Simple cysts of the ilium also may be large. Radiographically, they are well defined and radiolucent, and they possess commonly a sclerotic margin (Fig. 83–277). Osseous expansion may be evident, although this finding is better documented using CT.[1509] Fibrous dysplasia is the primary differential diagnostic consideration. Simple bone cysts in the spine may localize in the vertebral body[1510, 2290] or posterior osseous elements.[1491] Although generally well marginated and radiolucent, these lesions are difficult to diagnose accurately solely on the basis of the radiographic abnormalities.

Other Imaging Techniques. As routine radiography allows accurate diagnosis of the vast majority of simple bone cysts, other imaging methods rarely are required. CT can be used to evaluate the extent of lesions in anatomically complex areas such as the spine or osseous pelvis[1509] (Fig. 83–278). Of interest, CT analysis of simple bone cysts and

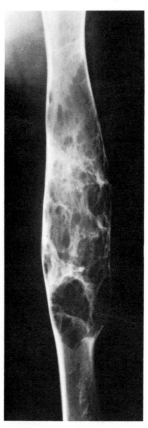

FIGURE 83–274. Multilocular bone cyst: Radiographic abnormalities—long tubular bones. Observe this multiloculated, expansile, osteolytic lesion in the diaphysis of the humerus. (Courtesy of A. D'Abreu, M.D., Porto Alegre, Brazil.)

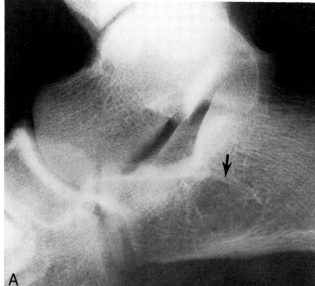

FIGURE 83–275. Simple (solitary or unicameral) bone cyst: Radiographic and CT abnormalities—calcaneus.

A Note the typical appearance and location of this simple bone cyst (arrow).

B, C Coronal **(B)** and transverse **(C)** CT displays show the well-defined border of this lesion (arrows).

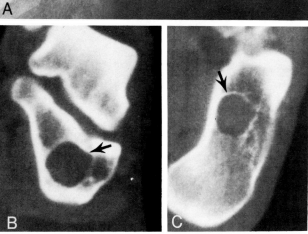

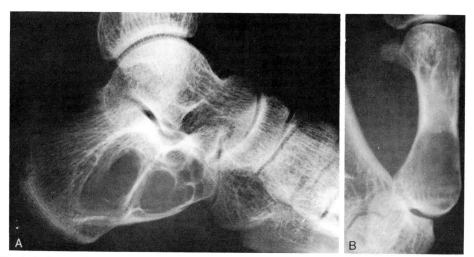

FIGURE 83–276. Simple (unicameral) bone cysts: Radiographic abnormalities—multiple lesions and involvement of the small bones of the hands and feet. This 22 year old Japanese man developed cystic lesions of multiple bones, including those of the hands and feet. Biopsy confirmed the presence of simple bone cysts.

A A lateral radiograph shows a large cyst involving more than 50 per cent of the calcaneus. It is sharply defined and multiloculated.

B The simple bone cyst in the first metacarpal bone also is sharply defined.

(From Chigira M, et al: Arch Orthop Trauma Surg *106*:390, 1987.)

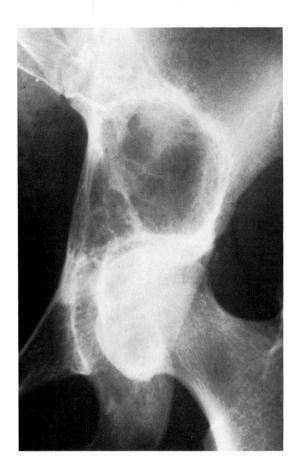

FIGURE 83–277. Simple (solitary or unicameral) bone cyst: Radiographic abnormalities—ilium. A large, osteolytic lesion of the ilium, possessing a sclerotic margin, in a 21 year old woman proved to be a simple bone cyst.

FIGURE 83–278. Simple (solitary or unicameral) bone cyst: CT abnormalities.

A, B During an intravenous pyelogram in a 25 year old man, this iliac lesion was discovered. Radiography **(A)** documents its large size, well-defined margins, and osteolytic nature. Transaxial CT **(B)** reveals the lesion (arrow), which had an attenuation value of 20 Hounsfield units. There is no soft tissue mass. A bone scan (not shown) was normal. The lesion was not biopsied, although its features are consistent with the diagnosis of a simple bone cyst.

C, D In a 15 year old boy, the routine radiograph **(C)** shows an osteolytic lesion (arrows) in the ilium. A transaxial CT scan **(D)** reveals its eccentric location and an ossified shell (arrow), findings typical of a simple bone cyst at this site.

(**C, D,** Courtesy of J. Healy, M.D., San Diego, California.)

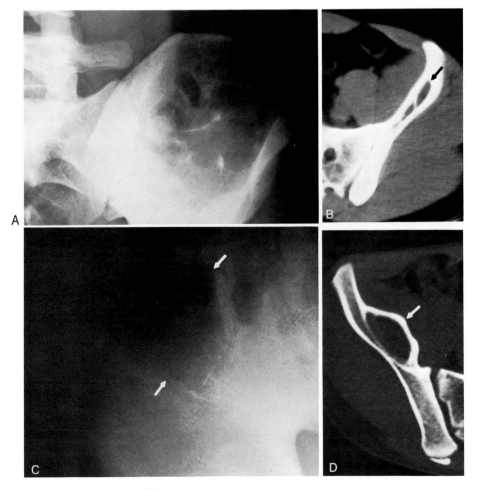

other cystic lesions of bone occasionally has demonstrated intralesional gas (pneumatocyst),[1511] gas-fluid levels,[1512] or fluid-fluid levels.[2294] MR imaging can confirm the fluid content of a simple bone cyst, documenting that the lesion has prolonged T1 and T2 relaxation times[1513, 1858] (Fig. 83–279). Although the MR imaging characteristics of a simple bone cyst usually differ from those of an aneurysmal bone cyst[1858] fluid-fluid levels may be detected in either lesion[2294] (Fig. 83–280). Enhancement of signal intensity in the peripheral portion of the cyst or within internal septations is evident following the intravenous injection of gadolinium-based contrast agents (Fig. 83–281).

Pathologic Abnormalities. On macroscopic examination, the affected bone has an expanded cortex, resembling an eggshell, that is covered by an intact periosteum. The cyst usually contains fluid that is clear, yellow, orange, red, or brown, depending upon whether a previous fracture with hemorrhage has occurred. Cases are encountered, however, in which no fluid is present, the cyst apparently being filled only with gas.[1514] A membrane generally lines the cystic cavity. This membrane may be barely visible to the naked eye, or it may be as thick as 1 cm,[28] particularly when a fracture has led to reparative callus or reactive fibrosis.[1479] The membrane is gray or brown, the latter indicating the deposition of hemosiderin pigment.[180] The membrane may bleed when touched by the surgeon. The endosteal bone not infrequently shows incomplete grooves or ridges. Fibrous septa may form following a fracture and traverse the cavity, creating a multilocular appearance.[1515] Solid cysts are reported in older patients.[1516]

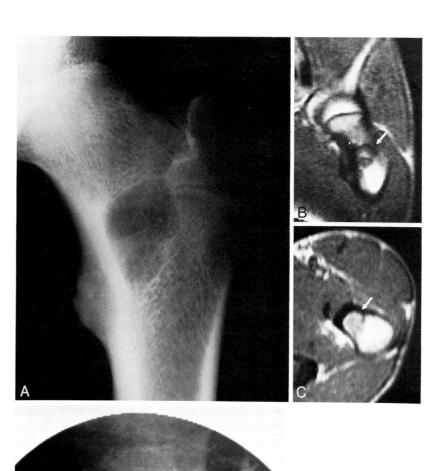

FIGURE 83–279. Simple (solitary or unicameral) bone cyst: MR imaging abnormalities. In a 16 year old man this lesion of the proximal portion of the femur was discovered as an incidental radiographic finding. The routine radiograph **(A)** reveals the characteristic features of a simple bone cyst. Coronal **(B)** and transaxial **(C)** T1-weighted spin echo MR images reveal decreased signal intensity (arrows) at the site of the lesion. Percutaneous aspiration of the lesion led to the recovery of clear, yellow fluid. A corticosteroid preparation and radiopaque contrast material were then injected, documenting the cystic nature of the abnormality **(D)**. An opacified vein is also evident.

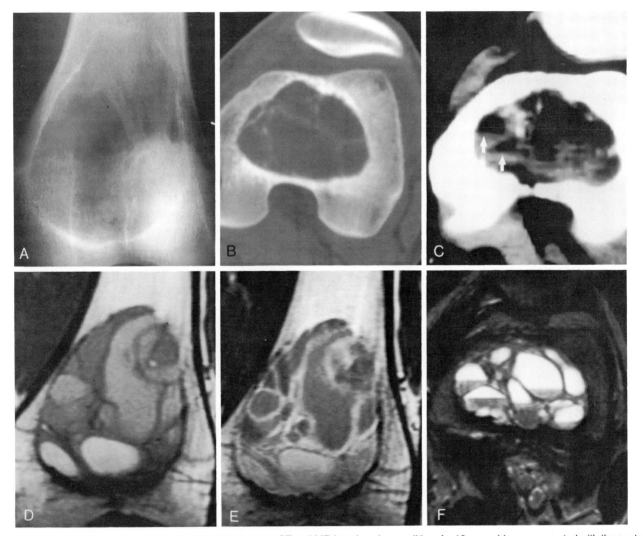

FIGURE 83–280. Simple (solitary or unicameral) bone cysts: CT and MR imaging abnormalities. An 18 year old man presented with the acute onset of pain and swelling in the knee. There was no history of injury.

    A Routine radiograph shows a large osteolytic lesion of the distal femoral metaphysis with extension into the epiphysis. A fine sclerotic border is evident.

    B Transaxial CT image, filmed with bone windowing, shows the full extent of the lesion and internal septations.

    C Transaxial CT scan, filmed with soft tissue windowing, reveals fluid levels (arrows) in the lesion.

    D Coronal T1-weighted (TR/TE, 810/15) spin echo MR image demonstrates multiple lobules of varying signal intensity.

    E After the intravenous injection of a gadolinium compound, a coronal T1-weighted (TR/TE, 810/15) spin echo MR image reveals enhancement of signal intensity in the thin septations separating the lobules.

    F Transaxial T2-weighted (TR/TE, 2200/90) spin echo MR image shows multiple fluid levels. At surgery, a gray, soft friable mass containing multiple cystic spaces was found. A histologic diagnosis of unicameral bone cyst was made.

    (From Burr VA, et al: J Comput Assist Tomogr *17*:134, 1993.)

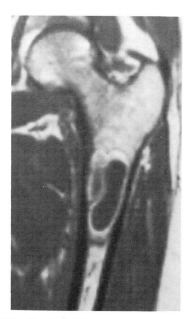

FIGURE 83–281. Simple (solitary or unicameral) bone cysts: MR imaging abnormalities. A coronal T1-weighted (TR/TE, 500/15) spin echo MR image obtained after the intravenous injection of a gadolinium compound shows enhancement of signal intensity in the peripheral portion of this simple bone cyst of the femur. (Courtesy of J. Kramer, M.D., Vienna, Austria.)

Microscopically, the wall of the cyst is thin, consisting of well-vascularized new bone produced by the overlying periosteum and of a loose network of trabeculae separated by dilated vascular channels.[180, 1517] The membrane lining the cyst contains a fibrous stroma in which are located spicules of metaplastic bone or osteoid, multinucleated giant cells, hemosiderin pigment, and chronic inflammatory cells (Fig. 83–282). Some cysts also contain incomplete fibrous septa that are lined by fibroblasts and giant cells, creating an appearance that may be indistinguishable from an aneurysmal bone cyst.[1518]

Natural History. The natural history of simple bone cysts

is not entirely clear. Although, as stated earlier, those that are located in the metaphysis in contact with the physis have been considered to be active, with a propensity for growth, and those that have "migrated" into the diaphysis have been designated inactive, these concepts, while emphasizing the potential for simple bone cysts to increase in size, are not without exception (Fig. 83–283). As indicated previously, aggressive growth potential and a higher frequency of recurrence following treatment appear to be characteristic of lesions that are discovered in children or adolescents; these features are less dependent on the precise anatomic location of the bone cyst within the bone. Although bone cysts rarely may undergo spontaneous regression,[1481, 1482, 1485, 1517] even after fracture,[1519] the usual approach to the management of simple bone cysts has been based not on the principle of "wait and watch" but rather on one of surgical intervention, particularly curettage and packing or, recently, intramedullary nailing or more radical surgery.[1479, 1486, 1498, 2295] Hence, the fact that simple bone cysts are relatively frequent in children and adolescents and infrequent in adults may be the result of aggressive treatment of these lesions, not of a tendency for them to regress spontaneously. Depending on the type of surgical procedure that is employed, as many as 40 per cent of simple bone cysts may recur.

An alternative method of treatment that has been advocated in recent years is the injection of steroid preparations (methylprednisolone acetate) directly into the simple cyst,[1488, 1489, 1515, 1520–1522, 2292, 2296, 2297] a technique that also has been employed successfully for the treatment of eosinophilic granulomas of bone. This injection method has been reported to be effective in 70 to 95 per cent of cases of simple bone cysts, although recurrences of the lesion are evident in 10 to 20 per cent of cases and additional steroid injections are required in some patients. The precise mechanism by which the steroid preparations induce healing of the simple bone cyst is not clear, although a reparative response to the minor injury of the injection process may be a factor. Indeed, simple drilling of the bone may be accompanied by similar healing.[1885] Healing of the lesion

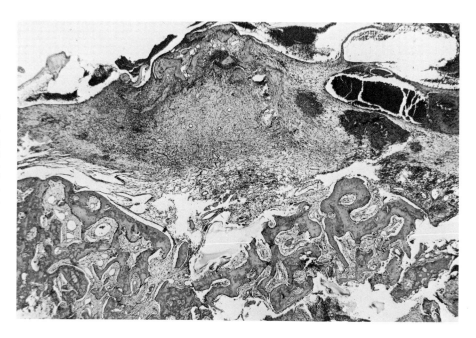

FIGURE 83–282. Simple (solitary or unicameral) bone cyst: Microscopic abnormalities. The lining of the cyst rests on the bone of the neocortex (which is located at the bottom of the photomicrograph) and is composed of vascular fibrous tissue. A few fragments of metaplastic bone may be seen at the superior aspect of the membrane. (25×.)

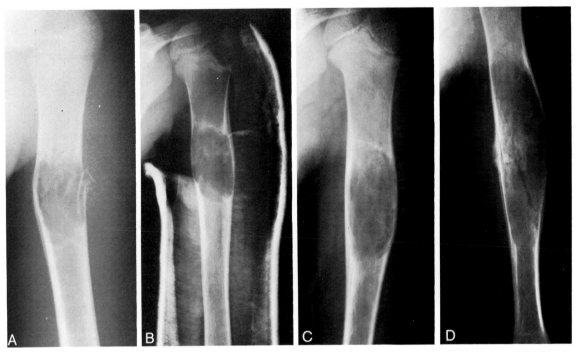

FIGURE 83–283. Simple (solitary or unicameral) bone cyst: Natural history—enlargement of the lesion. This 8 year old girl had an acute fracture through a simple bone cyst in the humerus **(A)**. The lesion was aspirated with the recovery of clear, straw-colored fluid; it then was injected with methylprednisolone acetate, and the arm was placed in a cast. One month after **A**, the pathologic fracture has healed **(B)**. One year after **B**, the lesion is somewhat larger **(C)**. It was reinjected with methylprednisolone acetate. Eighteen months after **C** (31 months after **A**), the lesion has grown dramatically and contains a second pathologic fracture **(D)**.

following the injection of steroids into a simple bone cyst also has been related to the antiprostaglandin activity of the hydrocortisone[2296] or a direct effect on the cellular component of the cyst.[2297] Radiographic signs of a favorable response include reduced size of the cystic cavity, increased radiodensity within the cyst, cortical thickening, and osseous remodeling.[1522] The instillation of radiopaque contrast material at the time of injection of the methylprednisolone has been used by some investigators as a means of identifying those cysts that are more likely to heal following the procedure.[1515] The presence of an increased number of septa within the lesion, as demonstrated by the contrast agent, usually is associated with an increased risk of recurrence, presumably related to the inability to obtain a uniform distribution of the corticosteroid preparation. Other factors indicative of a poor response to this procedure are large lesions and those with radiographically evident septations.

Complications. Several potential complications of simple bone cysts deserve emphasis.

Fracture. Although the frequency of this complication in patients with simple bone cysts is difficult to define owing to the probability that many cysts that do not fracture are never discovered, there is no question that fracture represents a significant sequela of simple bone cysts and one that generally results in the patient's seeking medical attention (Fig. 83–284). In some instances, however, incomplete infractions of bone about the cyst occur that are characterized by minor clinical and radiologic manifestations.[1477] Complete fractures are readily apparent on the radiographs and may be accompanied by the fallen fragment sign (see previous discussion). Osseous displacement at the fracture site is infrequent and of minor degree, and complete healing is expected following appropriate conservative management.

Subsequent complications include refracture, articular or osseous deformity, and growth disturbance.[1483, 1523]

Cementoma. Acellular, amorphous, granular fibrin-like material that is surrounded by osteoblasts has been identified histologically in approximately 10 to 15 per cent of simple bone cysts.[28, 30, 34, 1485, 1516, 1524–1528] The material may undergo calcification and ossification, producing a substance that by ordinary light microscopy resembles odontogenic cementum. In some instances, the term cementoma or cementifying fibroma has been been applied to lesions containing this material.[2298] This material apparently is a unique feature of simple bone cysts.

The precise relationship of simple cysts and cementomas (or cementifying fibromas) of bone is not entirely clear, although evidence currently indicates that they probably are related entities. The frequency of cementum-like material in proved simple bone cysts (Fig. 83–285), especially in those that are observed in older patients,[1516] and electron microscopic findings that document differences between this material and true cementum[1525] are consistent with the view that cementomas of bone are not a distinct lesion but rather a form of simple bone cyst in which a peculiar, poorly cellular type of osseous tissue, mimicking cementum, is produced.

Cementum-like bone production is most frequent in those simple bone cysts that develop in the proximal portion of the femur. Such lesions appear as radiolucent areas containing variable amounts of calcification or ossification. These radiographic findings are reminiscent of those of fibrous dysplasia and ossifying lipoma.

Malignant Transformation. There are rare reports of malignant tumors occurring in simple bone cysts. These neoplasms have included chondrosarcoma, liposarcoma, osteo-

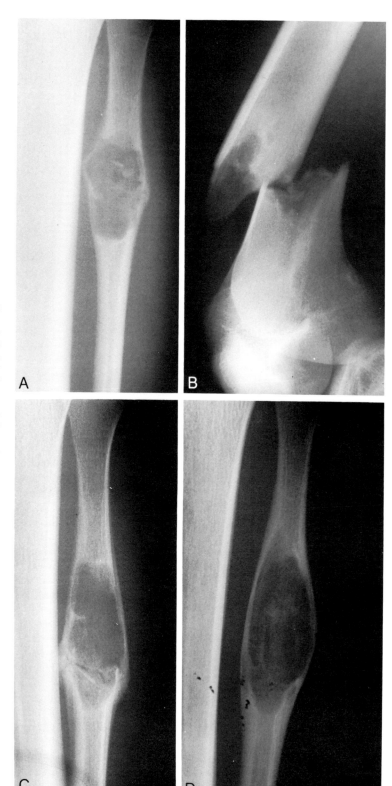

FIGURE 83–284. Simple (solitary or unicameral) bone cyst: Complications—pathologic fracture.

A This 11 year old girl had progressive pain in the lower leg 3 weeks after an injury. Focal tenderness was evident on physical examination. A radiograph shows a subacute fracture through an osteolytic lesion in the diaphysis of the fibula. The lesion was biopsied, and the final histologic diagnosis was a simple bone cyst with hemorrhage because of a recent fracture.

B In a 16 year old boy, a displaced pathologic fracture through a simple bone cyst in the diaphysis of the femur is evident.

C, D In a third patient, radiographs obtained 4 months apart show, initially, a subacute fracture involving a simple bone cyst in the fibula **(C)** and, subsequently, growth of the lesion and complete healing of the fracture **(D).**

(C, D, Courtesy of V. Vint, M.D., San Diego, California.)

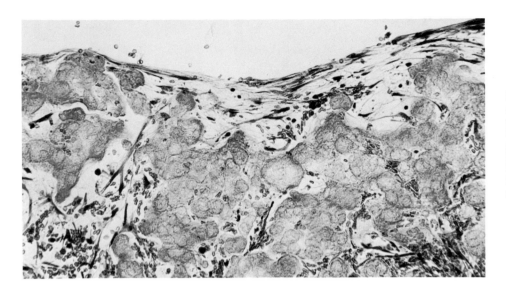

FIGURE 83–285. Simple (solitary or unicameral) bone cyst: Complications—production of cementum-like material. Amorphous, acellular granular material, which resembles cementum, is evident in the lining of a simple bone cyst. Osteoblasts about this material are not evident. (300×.)

sarcoma, fibrosarcoma, and Ewing's sarcoma.[30, 1477, 1529–1531] In some instances, irradiation had been employed in the treatment of the cyst, suggesting that the malignancy was a complication not of the cyst itself but of the therapeutic method. If a true association exists between simple bone cysts and malignancy, it must be exceedingly rare.

Epidermoid Cyst

Epidermoid cysts of bone are uncommon. Although their pathogenesis is debated, a history of blunt or penetrating trauma is evident in most affected patients, suggesting that such an injury may lead to intraosseous implantation of ectodermal tissue and the subsequent development of an epidermoid cyst. This concept is consistent with the typical localization of the lesion to superficially situated bones. Men are affected more frequently than women, and patients are usually in the second, third, or fourth decade of life. Clinical manifestations may include pain and swelling.

Intraosseous epidermoid cysts arise almost exclusively in the skull and phalanges of the hand, with the former being the most common site of involvement.[1532–1549] In the hands, the terminal phalanx is involved in almost all cases; in those instances in which an epidermoid cyst develops in a more proximal phalanx, preexisting trauma or surgery generally has occurred, leading to amputation of the digit with the subsequent localization of the cyst in the stump of the injured or resected bone.[1535, 1540, 1541] In the hands, the left side and the middle finger represent preferred sites of involvement; multiple lesions developing metachronously have been described.[1538–1540] Involvement of the phalanges in the foot is encountered occasionally.[1538, 1541, 1544] Rare sites of epidermoid cysts are the metacarpal bones, tibia, ulna, femur, sacrum, and sternum.[28, 1550–1552, 2299, 2492] Any bone of the skull can be affected, with the frontal and parietal bones representing the most typical locations. In the temporal bone, it may be difficult to differentiate between true epidermoid cysts and cysts that develop secondary to infections of the middle ear.[30, 1538] Epidermoid cysts also are observed in the mandible and maxilla.[1553] Furthermore, in any site, it may be difficult to distinguish between a primary intraosseous epidermoid cyst and one that arises adjacent to the bone, with subsequent osseous erosion and invasion.

The radiographic findings are highly characteristic. In the terminal phalanges of the fingers or toes, a well-defined, osteolytic lesion possessing a sclerotic margin is observed (Fig. 83–286). Soft tissue swelling also can be evident. The findings are not unlike those of an enchondroma, although the latter tumor rarely localizes in the terminal phalanx. One other differential diagnostic consideration is a glomus tumor. In the skull, a well-marginated radiolucent lesion is seen. The characteristically sharp edge of an epidermoid cyst differs from the pattern of poorly defined osteolysis that accompanies skeletal infection or metastasis. Furthermore, the lack of a beveled lesional margin, as may be apparent in eosinophilic granuloma, is a radiographic finding that aids in the identification of an epidermoid cyst. CT or MR imaging rarely is required.[1545] Epidermoid cysts in the long tubular bones produce less diagnostic radiographic features.

With regard to gross morphology, those cysts arising in the terminal phalanx rarely exceed 2 cm in maximum dimension and lead to mild expansion of bone and cortical thinning; a microfracture may be present but adjacent periosteal reaction is unusual. In the skull, epidermoid cysts may be limited to the diploic area or extend through one or both tables, with possible involvement of the dura.[1538] They usually are 1 to 5 cm in maximum dimension. In either area, the interior of the bone is filled with soft, white, cheesy, keratinous debris.[1533, 1536, 1537] A tough connective tissue membrane, 1 to 5 mm in thickness, forms the wall of the cyst and can be peeled easily from the adjacent bone.

Microscopically, sections of the cyst wall reveal stratified squamous epithelium, usually only a few cells thick, supported by a dense fibrous tissue stroma; a hyperkeratotic and parakeratotic layer is found that blends with the debris in the center of the cyst (Fig. 83–287A). The squamous epithelium may show pseudoepitheliomatous proliferation to such a degree that the lesion is mistaken for an epidermoid carcinoma.[1537–1539] The contents of the cyst may rupture into the connective tissue stroma and elicit an intense inflammatory and foreign body reaction to the liberated keratin (Fig. 83–287B). Cholesterol granulomas also may be present within this zone of reaction. Resulting accumulation of giant cells at first may suggest the diagnosis of a giant cell tumor or a giant cell reparative granuloma.

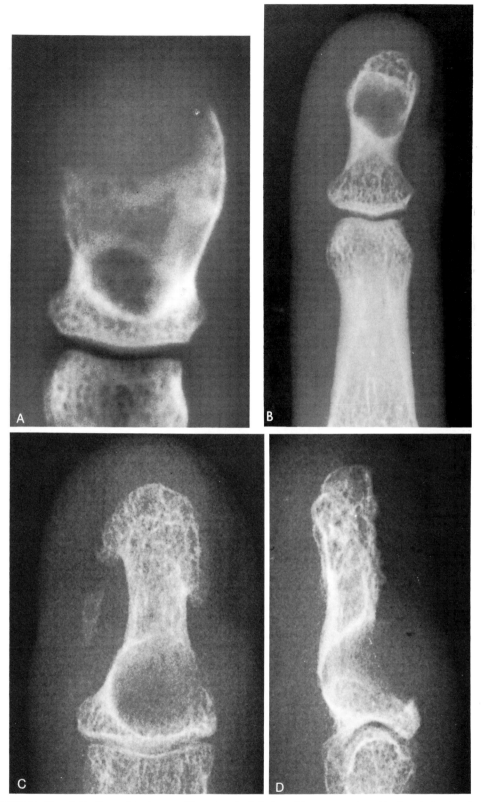

FIGURE 83–286. Epidermoid cyst: Radiographic abnormalities—terminal phalanx. Three examples of lesions in the hand are shown. In **A,** a large, well-defined osteolytic lesion possesses a sclerotic margin. The distal cortex is incomplete. In **B,** a smaller lesion has a sclerotic rim. In **C** and **D,** frontal and lateral radiographs reveal an epidermoid cyst involving the base of a terminal phalanx. Note again the sclerotic margin and the interruption of the cortex dorsally.

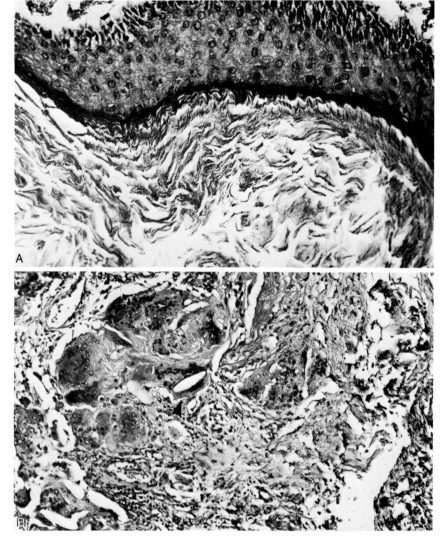

FIGURE 83–287. Epidermoid cyst: Microscopic abnormalities.

A The stratified squamous epithelium of the cyst is several cells thick with a granular layer at its surface. Exfoliated anucleated squames fill the cavity of the cyst. (300×.)

B A marked foreign body reaction has been caused by rupture of an epidermoid cyst into the surrounding soft tissues. Multinucleated giant cells have engulfed keratin debris. The arrowhead shows a space in the cytoplasm of one of these cells where a squame had been present. There is associated chronic inflammation. (150×.)

Aneurysmal Bone Cyst

An aneurysmal bone cyst is an expansile lesion containing thin-walled, blood-filled cystic cavities. It generally is regarded as non-neoplastic in nature, resembling in some of its radiographic or histologic features such reactive processes as giant cell reparative granuloma and hyperparathyroidism.[1554] Trauma appears to be important in the pathogenesis of some aneurysmal bone cysts, with well-documented examples of this lesion developing subsequent to acute fracture or other injuries.[1555–1557, 2300, 2302] This has led to speculation that local alterations of hemodynamics related to venous obstruction or arteriovenous fistulae that occur following an injury are important in the pathogenesis of an aneurysmal bone cyst, a concept that is supported by angiographic data.[1555] It also is well documented that lesions resembling aneurysmal bone cysts accompany a variety of benign processes of the skeleton, including chondroblastoma, chondromyxoid fibroma, nonossifying fibroma, osteoblastoma, giant cell tumor, giant cell reparative granuloma, fibrous histiocytoma, brown tumor, solitary cyst, and fibrous dysplasia, and, less frequently, some malignant tumors, such as osteosarcoma, chondrosarcoma, fibrosarcoma, malignant fibrous histiocytoma, and hemangioendothelioma.[1554, 1558–1564, 2301, 2493] The coexistence of aneurysmal bone cyst and a companion lesion again is consistent with the concept that a precursor tumor or event (e.g., trauma) leads to local hemodynamic changes, providing the ideal environment for the superimposition of a secondary aneurysmal bone cyst.[1565–1568] It also is possible that alterations in osseous hemodynamics resulting from the companion process give rise to rapid enlargement of an already existing aneurysmal bone cyst.[1559]

Whether one adheres to the belief that aneurysmal bone cysts commonly occur as a secondary event in association with another osseous abnormality or, alternatively, to the belief that such cysts are coexistent lesions whose behavior as an "innocent bystander" is significantly modified by the adjacent process, the association of aneurysmal bone cysts and other lesions is undeniable. This phenomenon assumes significance in clinical, radiologic, and pathologic analyses: Rapidly developing clinical manifestations in a patient with a known primary disorder such as fibrous dysplasia or chondroblastoma need not indicate malignant transformation of the lesion but, rather, are consistent with the development or enlargement of an aneurysmal bone cyst; the radiographic characteristics of the combination process (consisting of an aneurysmal bone cyst and another disorder) may be dominated by those of the coexisting lesion rather than the aneurysmal bone cyst; and histologic documentation of features of an aneurysmal bone cyst alone does not exclude the possibility of an associated malignancy.[1563] It should be emphasized, however, that most aneurysmal bone cysts are found without histologic evidence of any underlying lesion.

Clinical Abnormalities. Aneurysmal bone cysts usually are observed in the first, second, or third decade of life. Approximately 80 per cent of affected patients are less than 20 years of age.[1554, 1563, 1569–1572, 1859, 1860, 2303, 2304] Such lesions have been identified in children as young as 3 years of age as well as in persons as old as 70 years. There appears to be a slight female predominance in patients with aneurysmal bone cysts. Local findings including pain and swelling of weeks to years in duration are dominant. Other clinical manifestations depend on the specific site of involvement; aneurysmal bone cysts in the spine may be accompanied by neurologic abnormalities, those in the skull may be associated with moderate or severe headaches, lesions in the flat or irregular bones may lead to prominent, enlarging masses, and aneurysmal bone cysts in the tubular bones and the spine may result in pathologic fracture with acute, severe pain and tenderness. Additional symptoms and signs include an increase in local skin temperature and restriction of movement in an adjacent articulation.

Skeletal Location. Although virtually any bone of the skeleton may be affected, aneurysmal bone cysts are most frequent in the long tubular bones and spine, which, together, account for approximately 60 to 70 per cent of cases.[1554, 1566, 1573–1578] Specific sites of involvement include, in order of decreasing frequency, the tibia (approximately 15 per cent of cases), vertebrae (14 per cent), femur (13 per cent), humerus (9 per cent), innominate bone (9 per cent), fibula (7 per cent), ulna (4 per cent), clavicle (3 per cent), radius (3 per cent), ribs (3 per cent), scapula (2 per cent), skull (2 per cent), and mandible and maxilla (2 per cent); the small bones in the feet and, less frequently, the hands are affected in approximately 10 to 14 per cent of cases.[34, 1554, 1576, 1577, 1579–1590, 2305–2307] Rare sites of involvement include the sacrum and acetabular region.

Within the long tubular bones, aneurysmal bone cysts are seen almost exclusively in a metaphysis; there is an approximately equal distribution of aneurysmal bone cysts in the proximal and distal metaphyses of the tibia as well as of the femur, the fibula, and the humerus. Isolated or predominant involvement of the diaphysis occurs in about 8 per cent of cases. Epiphyseal extension of a metaphyseal aneurysmal bone cyst is uncommon and usually (but not invariably) is apparent following closure of the growth plate.[1574, 1576–1578, 1591, 2303] In such cases, the possibility of an associated lesion, such as a chondroblastoma, should be considered.[1576] Rarely, aneurysmal bone cysts arise within the cortex of a tubular bone.[2494]

In the spine, involvement of the thoracic, lumbar, cervical or sacral level, in order of decreasing frequency, is seen.[1584] Vertebral aneurysmal bone cysts generally arise in the posterior osseous elements, including the neural arches, laminae, and transverse and spinous processes; the vertebral bodies are affected less frequently, and rarely does this occur in isolation without posterior osseous abnormalities.[1566, 1574, 1575, 1584, 1592–1596] Involvement of both the vertebral body and posterior osseous elements was observed in 90 per cent of spinal aneurysmal bone cysts in one study.[2303] Aneurysmal bone cysts may extend from one vertebra to

another, to an adjacent rib, or to paraspinal soft tissues, simulating the appearance of infection or a malignant tumor.

Radiographic Abnormalities. Although osteolysis and osseous expansion are the dominant radiographic abnormalities of aneurysmal bone cysts (Fig. 83–288), it is instructive to consider these lesions in categories based on the site of involvement.

Tubular Bones. An eccentric, osteolytic, occasionally trabeculated process centered in a metaphysis of a long tubular bone represents the classic appearance of an aneurysmal bone cyst (Fig. 83–289). The inner margin of the lesion usually is well defined, with or without a rim of bone sclerosis, and the cortical surface of the affected bone is expanded or ballooned. The loss of cortical definition and the apparent extension of the lesion into the adjacent soft tissue are alarming features that simulate the appearance of a malignant tumor. More correctly, these abnormalities should be considered indications of an aggressive and rapidly expansile intraosseous process that are not diagnostic of malignancy. Lifting of the periosteum accompanies the osseous extension of an aneurysmal bone cyst; eventually, it is the stimulation of the periosteal membrane with resultant bone formation that provides the radiographic clues that are necessary for accurate interpretation. Horizontally oriented trabeculae extending into the soft tissue component of the lesion from the parent bone and a partial or complete osseous shell at the margin of this component are features that are fundamental for precise analysis of the radiographs.[2308] It must be emphasized, however, that until these alterations appear and become prominent, additional diagnostic considerations that include a variety of sarcomas and, particularly, telangiectatic osteosarcoma[326] are reasonable.

Although a more central location of an aneurysmal bone cyst leading to symmetric expansion of the entire metaphysis occasionally is evident in a long tubular bone[1569] (Fig. 83–290), this pattern is more frequent in short tubular bones in the hands and feet.[1563, 1570, 1597–1599] In this location, a long segment of a metatarsal or metacarpal bone or a phalanx may be affected; cortical thinning or violation, osseous expansion, trabeculation or septation, periosteal reaction, pathologic fracture, and epiphyseal extension are all recognized features of aneurysmal bone cysts in these sites[1561, 1563, 1591] (Figs. 83–291 and 83–292). The radiographic features may resemble those of a giant cell tumor (which more characteristically involves the epiphysis), enchondroma (which is less expansile and contains calcification), giant cell reparative granuloma, brown tumor of hyperparathyroidism, osteoblastoma and, rarely, infection.

Spine. The typical spinal lesion is osteolytic and expansile and involves either the posterior osseous elements (Fig. 83–293A) or both the posterior elements and the vertebral body (Fig. 83–293B,C). When an aneurysmal bone cyst is confined to the spinous or transverse process in a child or adolescent, an accurate diagnosis generally is possible on the basis of the radiographic alterations, although osteoblastoma and even hemangioma represent reasonable alternative choices. In a pedicle or lamina, osseous expansion may be less dramatic, and accurate radiologic analysis becomes more difficult. It is in the vertebral body, however, where the radiographic findings of an aneurysmal bone cyst are least specific. Involvement of adjacent vertebral bodies owing to violation of the intervening intervertebral disc, ver-

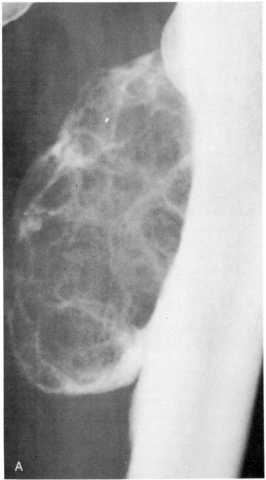

FIGURE 83–288. Aneurysmal bone cyst: Radiographic abnormalities—spectrum of disease.

A Femur. An eccentric, heavily trabeculated lesion arises from the surface of the bone.

B Humerus. Observe the expansile, osteolytic lesion of the proximal metaphysis and diaphysis of the humerus in a child. It is trabeculated and enclosed by a shell of bone.

C Metacarpal bone. This aggressive lesion is associated with osteolysis and a soft tissue mass. A calcific shell (arrowheads) surrounds the mass, and faint horizontal trabeculae (open arrow) are evident. These features suggest the diagnosis of an aneurysmal bone cyst.

(**C,** Courtesy of Regional Naval Medical Center, San Diego, California.)

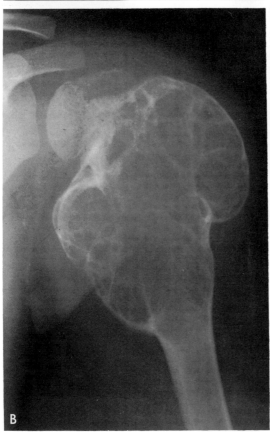

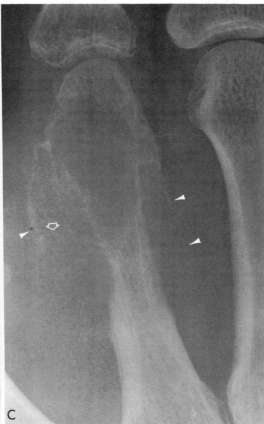

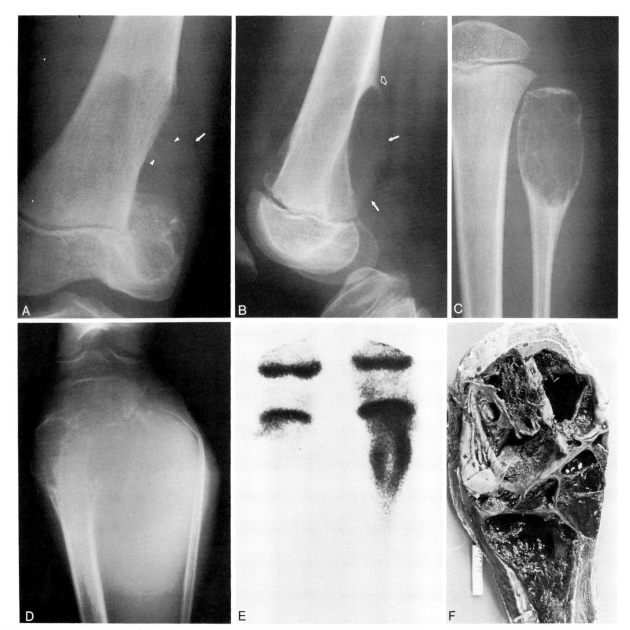

FIGURE 83–289. Aneurysmal bone cyst: Radiographic abnormalities—long tubular bones.

A, B In this 11 year old boy with progressive knee pain, anteroposterior **(A)** and lateral **(B)** radiographs show an aggressive, eccentric osteolytic lesion. Observe a soft tissue mass (solid arrows), a Codman's triangle (open arrow), and faint trabeculae extending from the bone into the soft tissue mass (arrowheads). Although these features suggest the diagnosis of an aneurysmal bone cyst, a malignant tumor cannot be entirely excluded.

C In a young child, a centrally located aneurysmal bone cyst of the proximal metaphysis of the fibula is osteolytic, expansile, and trabeculated, and it is accompanied by periostitis and a ossific shell.

(C, Courtesy of W. Ewing, M.D., Pueblo, Colorado.)

D–F This 16 year old boy had a rapidly enlarging mass in his leg. The frontal radiograph **(D)** shows an extraordinary soft tissue mass associated with an osteolytic process in the proximal metaphysis of the tibia and deformity and displacement of the fibula. The bone scan **(E)** reveals an inhomogeneous increase in uptake of the radionuclide at the site of the lesion. At surgery, a blood-filled cystic lesion was identified and removed **(F).** An aneurysmal bone cyst was the final histologic diagnosis.

(D–F, Courtesy of D. Fraser, M.D., Halifax, Nova Scotia, Canada.)

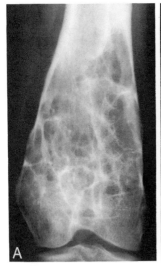
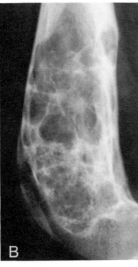

FIGURE 83–290. Aneurysmal bone cyst: Radiographic abnormalities—long tubular bones. Frontal **(A)** and lateral **(B)** radiographs show a more central lesion of the femur that is heavily trabeculated and slightly expansile.

FIGURE 83–291. Aneurysmal bone cyst: Radiographic abnormalities—short tubular bones.

A Metacarpal bone. This central aneurysmal bone cyst is metaphyseal in location, osteolytic, and expansile. There is transphyseal extension of the process to involve a small segment of the epiphysis. The differential diagnosis would include an osteoblastoma and giant cell reparative granuloma, in addition to an aneurysmal bone cyst.

B Middle phalanx. An expansile, trabeculated lesion involves the entire phalanx.

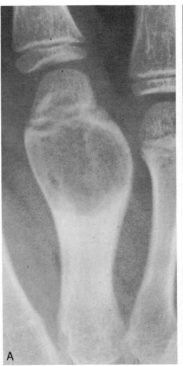
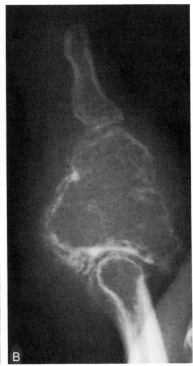

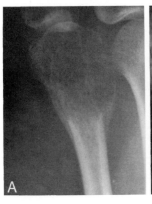
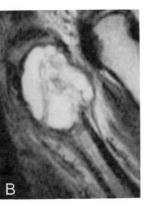

FIGURE 83–292. Aneurysmal bone cyst: Radiographic abnormalities—short tubular bones. A routine radiograph **(A)** of the hand in a 24 year old man reveals an osteolytic lesion involving the metaphyseal and epiphyseal segments of the second metacarpal bone, with osseous expansion, trabeculation, periosteal reaction, and extension to subchondral bone. A coronal T2-weighted (TR/TE, 2000/70) spin echo MR image **(B)** shows an expansile lesion of high signal intensity with internal septations of low signal intensity. (Courtesy of M. Zlatkin, M.D., Hollywood, Florida.)

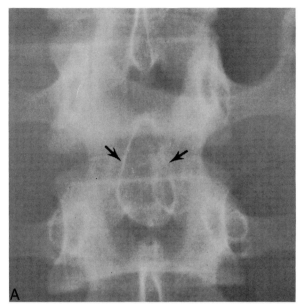

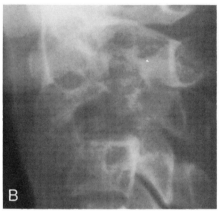
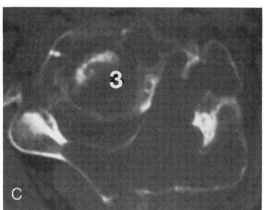

FIGURE 83–293. Aneurysmal bone cyst: Radiographic abnormalities—spine.

A Uniform enlargement of the spinous process of a lumbar vertebra is seen (arrows). (Courtesy of D. Pate, D.C., San Diego, California.)

B, C In this child, routine radiography **(B)** shows an expansile, osteolytic lesion of the body and posterior elements of the third cervical vertebra. Transaxial CT **(C)** confirms the extent of involvement and the expansile nature of the lesion. (Courtesy of L. Pinckney, M.D., San Diego, California.)

tebral collapse, or extension into the spinal canal, ribs, and paraspinal soft tissues, or all of these, are findings of this lesion that resemble those of many others, including eosinophilic granuloma, malignant tumors, and infection.[1584]

Other Sites. In the innominate bone (Fig. 83–294A,B), osteolysis and bone expansion are present. Although a sclerotic margin about the lesion may indicate the nonmalignant nature of the process, soft tissue extension with displacement of viscera, such as the bladder, in some aneurysmal bone cysts makes difficult their differentiation from a sarcoma.[1569] Similar difficulties are encountered during the interpretation of radiographs in patients with aneurysmal bone cysts of the ribs (owing to the potential for extraosseous extension with the development of an extrapleural mass)[1600] (Fig. 83–295), scapula (where soft tissue extension and even calcification may be observed)[1601] (Fig. 83–294C,D), and sternum (in which malignant neoplasms are more frequent than benign tumors).[1586] In other locations, such as the patella,[1602] and in the tarsal and carpal regions,[1603] aneurysmal bone cysts may lead to osteolysis of an entire bone. Lesions of the skull typically reveal osseous expansion with involvement of the inner and outer tables and intracranial extension,[1604–1606] and those of the mandible or maxilla appear as multilocular, expansile osteolytic lesions predominating in the region of the molar teeth.[1607, 1608]

Other Imaging Techniques. It is not entirely unexpected

that, owing to the presence of nonspecific radiographic findings in some aneurysmal bone cysts and to the possibility that such findings may simulate those of malignancy, interest has developed in evaluating these lesions using other imaging techniques. In general, however, these supplementary methods are more useful in defining the intraosseous and extraosseous extent of the process than in providing clues to a specific diagnosis.

Angiography represents one of these techniques. Aneurysmal bone cysts usually are described as hypovascular lesions with localized regions of hypervascularity.[1609, 1610] These features may have diagnostic importance in differentiating aneurysmal bone cysts from more aggressive lesions, such as osteosarcoma and giant cell tumor, in which abundant tumor vessels are more characteristic. Furthermore, it has been suggested that the hypervascular regions provide information regarding the prognosis of an aneurysmal bone cyst, as their number and size are correlated positively with the likelihood of lesional recurrence.[1610]

Scintigraphy has only a limited role in the evaluation of aneurysmal bone cysts. The predominant pattern noted on the bone scan is accumulation of the radiopharmaceutical agent at the periphery of the lesion with little activity in its center,[1611, 1612] a finding that is evident in approximately 65 per cent of cases.[1611] This scintigraphic pattern lacks specificity, being evident not only in cystic lesions of bone but

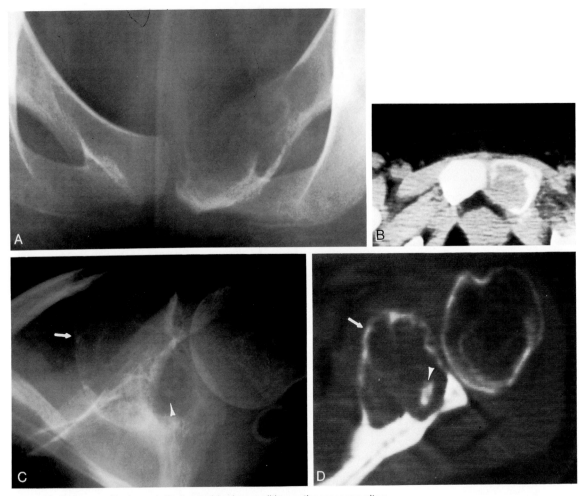

FIGURE 83–294. Aneurysmal bone cyst: Radiographic abnormalities—other osseous sites.

A, B Pubic bone. An expansile, osteolytic lesion is evident on routine radiography **(A)** and transaxial CT **(B).** There is no soft tissue mass.

C, D Scapula. As shown with conventional radiography **(C)** and transaxial CT **(D),** this aneurysmal bone cyst is markedly expansile (arrows) and appears to contain calcification (arrowheads). In such cases, the possibility of a coexistent lesion, such as a chondroblastoma, must be considered.

(**C, D,** Courtesy of T. Broderick, M.D., Orange, California.)

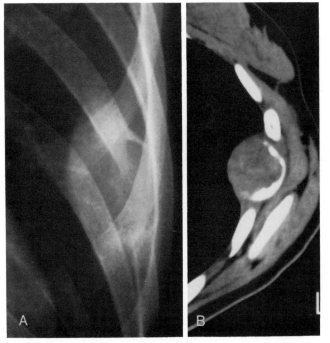

FIGURE 83–295. Aneurysmal bone cyst: Radiographic abnormalities—ribs. In this 28 year old woman with a painful, enlarging mass of 5 months' duration, routine radiography **(A)** shows an expansile lesion with a soft tissue component arising from a rib. Transaxial CT scan **(B)** better localizes the lesion and clearly indicates an intraosseous origin.

also in giant cell tumors and chondrosarcomas. Furthermore, there is no apparent correlation between the intensity and pattern of radionuclide uptake and the size of the lesions, the type and amount of fluid contained within the cysts, or the degree and distribution of osteoblastic activity, new bone formation, or any other identifiable histologic abnormality.[1611]

CT is most useful in delineating the size and location of the intraosseous and extraosseous components of an aneurysmal bone cyst, especially in anatomically complex areas, such as the spine (where CT may be combined with myelography) and osseous pelvis, and in the skull.[1604] In these and other locations, the CT abnormalities usually provide little diagnostic information, although the detection of fluid levels with CT (as well as with MR imaging) in some aneurysmal bone cysts is of interest[1614, 1615] (Fig. 83–296). This finding, which is independent of the type of fluid present in the aneurysmal bone cyst (bloody, serosanguineous, or serous), is evident only when the patient has been held motionless for a period of time (approximately 10 min), allowing the fluid to settle, and when imaging is accomplished in a plane perpendicular to the fluid level. Such fluid levels also are apparent in other osseous lesions, including giant cell tumor, simple bone cyst, and chondro-

blastoma, but the finding is most suggestive of the diagnosis of an aneurysmal bone cyst.

MR imaging also has been applied to the evaluation of aneurysmal bone cysts.[1616–1618, 2309–2313] This method is valuable in defining the full extent of the lesion, especially in anatomically complex areas such as the spine (Fig. 83–297). An expansile and lobulated or septated lesion is typical. The internal septations create cystic cavities whose walls contain diverticulum-like projections.[1618] A thin, well-defined rim of low signal intensity about an aneurysmal bone cyst is common.[2311] The signal intensity characteristics within this rim are variable (Fig. 83–298). Although high signal intensity commonly is evident in portions of an aneurysmal bone cyst in T2-weighted spin echo MR images, it is not present uniformly.[2309] Inhomogeneity of signal intensity is encountered, and individual lobules of the lesion may reveal markedly different signal intensity characteristics.[2311] In general, however, the signal intensity of an aneurysmal bone cyst increases with increasing T2 weighting.[2311] Fluid levels also may be identified[1617, 2309, 2311] (Fig. 83–299). Although such levels are not diagnostic of an aneurysmal bone cyst (occurring also in giant cell tumors, simple bone systs, chondroblastomas, and telangiectatic osteosarcomas), they are most compatible with the diagnosis of aneurysmal

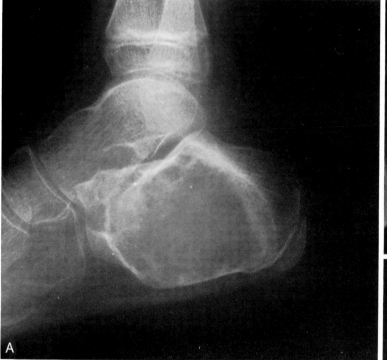

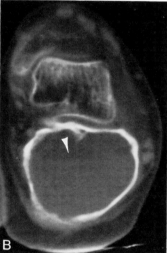

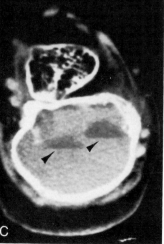

FIGURE 83–296. Aneurysmal bone cyst: CT abnormalities—fluid levels. The initial radiograph **(A)** in this 11 year old boy shows an expansile, trabeculated lesion of the calcaneus. Direct coronal CT scans obtained with the patient supine and the knees flexed using bone **(B)** and soft tissue **(C)** window settings reveal the expansile lesion with fluid levels (arrowheads). The histologic diagnosis was an aneurysmal bone cyst. (Courtesy of T. Broderick, M.D., Orange, California.)

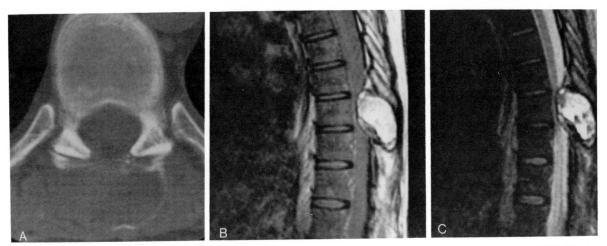

FIGURE 83–297. Aneurysmal bone cyst: CT and MR imaging abnormalities—spine. In a 52 year old man, transaxial CT **(A)** shows an expansile lesion of the spinous process of the ninth thoracic vertebra. A calcified or ossified shell is evident about a portion of this lesion. Sagittal proton density–weighted (TR/TE, 2000/30) **(B)** and T2-weighted (TR/TE, 2000/90) **(C)** spin echo MR images show the lesion, which is inhomogeneous but mainly of high signal intensity. Fluid levels are present in **A** and **C**.

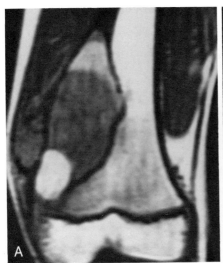
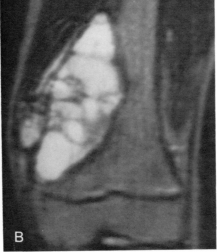

FIGURE 83–298. Aneurysmal bone cyst: MR imaging abnormalities—long tubular bones. This expansile lesion in the distal portion of the femur is well evaluated with coronal T1-weighted (TR/TE, 600/25) **(A)** and T2-weighted (TR/TE, 2500/70) **(B)** spin echo MR images. In **A,** the lesion reveals inhomogeneous signal intensity; the uppermost portion is of intermediate to high signal intensity, the middle portion is of low signal intensity, and the lowest portion is of high signal intensity. A rim of low signal intensity about the lesion is evident. In **B,** the full extent of the lesion and internal septation are more evident. High signal intensity regions are separated by linear and branching areas of low signal intensity. (Courtesy of A. Newberg, M.D., Boston, Massachusetts, and M. Dalinka, M.D., Philadelphia, Pennsylvania.)

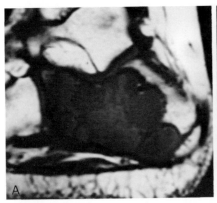
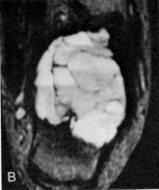
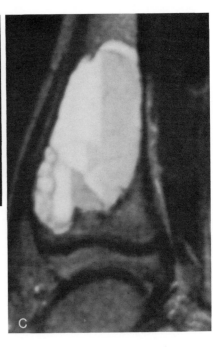

FIGURE 83–299. Aneurysmal bone cyst: MR imaging abnormalities—fluid levels.

   A, B In the evaluation of an aneurysmal bone cyst in the calcaneus, a sagittal T1-weighted (TR/TE, 700/11) spin echo MR image **(A)** and a transverse T2-weighted (TR/TE, 2000/80) spin echo MR image **(B)** reveal involvement of a large portion of the bone. Note multiple fluid levels in **B.**

   C In a second patient, a sagittal T2-weighted (TR/TE, 2000/90) spin echo MR image shows an aneurysmal bone cyst in the distal tibial metaphysis with multiple fluid levels.

bone cyst. Fluid levels in aneurysmal bone cysts (and, less commonly, in other lesions) may be solitary or multiple.

Pathologic Abnormalities. On external examination, an aneurysmal bone cyst creates an oval bulge in the contour of the metaphysis with its major dimension in the long axis of the tubular bone.[1566] The lesion is covered by an intact, thin periosteum beneath which may be a thin layer of new bone.[1565, 1619] Aneurysmal bone cysts vary considerably in size.[1563, 1620] Although generally they are less than 10 cm in maximum dimension,[1576, 1577] some cysts, especially those in the ilium, scapula, or skull, measure 30 cm or more.[1581]

When a typical aneurysmal bone cyst is sectioned, blood exudes slowly from its surface. The lesion may contain a single large cystic cavity with a few fragments of friable red tissue on its wall or, more commonly, a meshwork of multiple cysts varying in maximum dimension from a few millimeters to several centimeters[1621] (Fig. 83–300). The walls of these cysts are formed by thin fibrous septa between which is located solid, soft, friable or granular, gray, white, or brown tissue. The resulting appearance is that of a blood-filled sponge.[1621] Although the solid component of an aneurysmal bone cyst usually constitutes no more than half of its bulk, an entire lesion occasionally may consist of solid tissue without visible cysts. These latter lesions have been designated the solid variant of aneurysmal bone cysts (see later discussion).[1622]

Microscopically, the cavernous blood-filled cysts (Fig. 83–301) that characterize the gross morphology of an aneurysmal bone cyst do not represent true vascular channels but, rather, are lined by fibroblasts and multinucleated osteoclast-type giant cells. They lack both an endothelial lining and the elastic tissue or smooth muscle that is found in the walls of normal blood vessels. Fibrous septa appear as incomplete strands that have a sinusoidal shape and contain

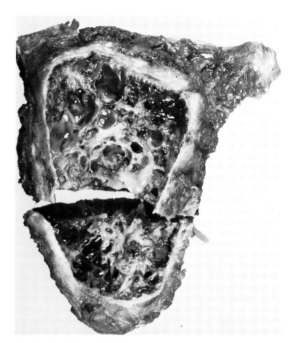

FIGURE 83–300. Aneurysmal bone cyst: Macroscopic abnormalities. A section of an aneurysmal bone cyst in the scapula shows that the well-marginated lesion involves a major portion of the bone. It is composed of a sponge-like array of variably sized cysts, many filled with blood.

trabeculae of osteoid and woven or lamellar bone, multinucleated giant cells, histiocytes, and hemosiderin deposits.[1623] The cysts may be filled with fresh blood or appear empty owing to draining during histologic processing. Fibrin clots rarely are found.[1577]

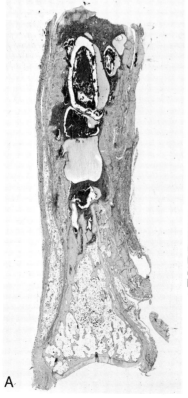

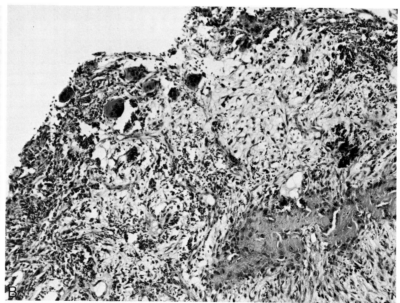

FIGURE 83–301. Aneurysmal bone cyst: Microscopic abnormalities.
  A A portion of the metaphysis of a phalanx has been replaced by cystic, hemorrhagic blood spaces. (3×.)
  B The fibrous wall of an aneurysmal bone cyst contains a strand of metaplastic new bone. Multinucleated giant cells and fibroblasts line the cyst, which lacks endothelial cells. Extravasated blood is present diffusely in the stroma. (150×.)
  (Courtesy of B. Cruickshank, M.D., Toronto, Ontario, Canada.)

The solid portions of the lesion are composed predominantly of fibrous tissue that frequently contains numerous multinucleated giant cells, mimicking the appearance of a giant cell tumor. These giant cells are concentrated about areas of stromal hemorrhage similar to foci that are found in a giant cell reparative granuloma.[1621] Metaplastic bone may be abundant, forming a meshwork of interconnecting trabeculae.[1624] Mitotic figures in the stromal fibroblasts vary from few to as many as 20 to 25 per 50 high power fields.[1577]

Electron microscopic studies of aneurysmal bone cysts confirm that they lack endothelial cells or basement membranes. Cells with the structural features of fibroblasts, myofibroblasts, osteoblasts, histiocytes, and multinucleated giant cells are found.[1625, 1626]

With regard to accurate histologic analysis, difficulty arises owing to the known association of aneurysmal bone cysts with other osseous lesions. Furthermore, even in primary aneurysmal bone cysts, three conditions, solitary bone cyst, giant cell tumor and, most importantly, telangiectatic osteosarcoma, pose significant diagnostic challenges to the pathologist.

Natural History. Although aneurysmal bone cyst is a non-neoplastic condition with no propensity to metastasize, its potential for rapid growth, considerable destruction of bone, and extension into adjacent soft tissue[1627] generally has led to aggressive therapy, despite the existence of reports that have documented spontaneous regression or regression following simple biopsy of the lesion[1628, 2313] (Fig. 83–302). Such regression appears to be a rare phenomenon, perhaps related to thrombosis and fibrosis of the aneurysmal bone cyst; a similar sequence of events following transcatheter embolization techniques may have therapeutic significance.[1629, 2314, 2315] A more conventional therapeutic approach has consisted of either surgery or radiotherapy,[1568, 1630, 1631] although the choice of the latter

technique for the treatment of a benign condition has been considered by some investigators to be an unreasonable alternative owing to its carcinogenic potential.[1554, 1628] One or more recurrences of an aneurysmal bone cyst occur in approximately 10 to 20 per cent of patients,[2495] particularly when the location of the lesion is such that its complete surgical removal is difficult. Although malignant change occasionally is attributed to aneurysmal bone cysts, such lesions may represent telangiectatic osteosarcomas rather than true aneurysmal bone cysts.

Additional Types of Lesions. A *solid variant* of aneurysmal bone cyst has been identified.[1622, 1632, 2303, 2316] This lesion sometimes is referred to as extragnathic giant cell reparative granuloma. As with typical aneurysmal bone cysts, boys and girls in the first or second decade of life usually are affected (although young and middle-aged adults also may be affected). However, there appears to be a preference for axial involvement (e.g., spine and innominate bone) by solid aneurysmal bone cysts compared with the distribution of the classic type of lesion. The long tubular bones, especially the femur, also may be involved.[2316] Radiographically, the solid variant of aneurysmal bone cyst is characterized by a spectrum of abnormalities consisting of, at one end, lesions that are indistinguishable from a classic aneurysmal bone cyst (Figs. 83–303 and 83–304) and, at the other end, lesions, especially in the axial skeleton, that are highly aggressive, with motheaten bone destruction, cortical violation, and soft tissue extension.[1632] Conventional or computed tomography may reveal a rim of bone at the periphery of the process, usually allowing its differentiation from a malignant tumor. Histologically, florid fibroblastic or fibrohistiocytic proliferation, osteoblastic differentiation with osteoid production, areas rich in osteoclast-type giant cells, and occasional foci of calcified fibromyxoid tissue with a chondroid appearance are seen.[1622] The typical aneurysmal sinusoids of conventional aneurysmal bone cysts

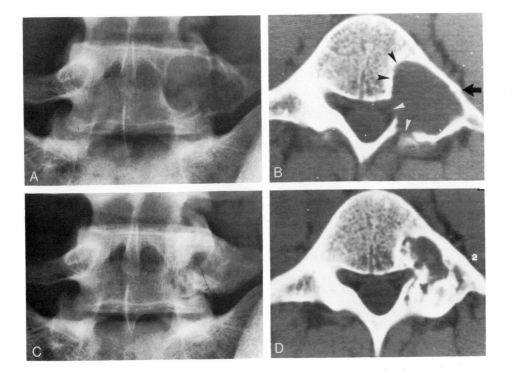

FIGURE 83–302. Aneurysmal bone cyst: Spontaneous regression of lesion. An 18 year old man had a 2 week history of low back pain. An initial radiograph **(A)** and transaxial CT scan **(B)** show an expansile lesion of the transverse process of the fifth lumbar vertebra. In **B**, note the sharply marginated lesion (black arrowheads) and defects in the anterior (arrow) and posterior (white arrowheads) aspects of the lesion. Similar radiographic **(C)** and CT **(D)** images seen 22 months later show partial reossification of the lesion. (From Malghem J, et al: J Bone Joint Surg [Br] 71:645, 1989.)

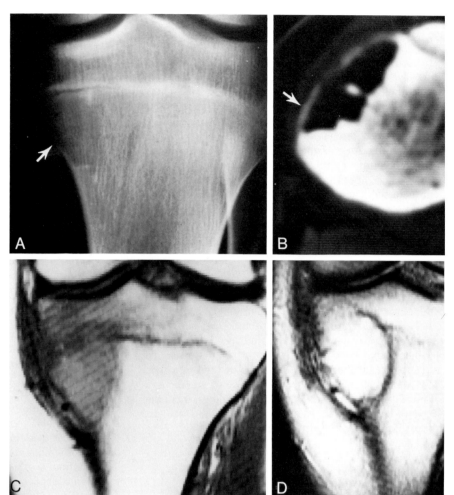

FIGURE 83–303. Aneurysmal bone cyst: Solid variant. This 12 year old girl had pain and a soft tissue mass below the knee, of several weeks' duration.

A A conventional tomogram defines a small, eccentric lesion in the proximal metaphysis of the tibia (arrow).

B Transaxial CT shows that the lesion contains a rim of increased attenuation (arrow) and an internal ossific focus. A biopsy provided tissue that was interpreted as a solid variant of an aneurysmal bone cyst.

C, D Three months later, coronal T1-weighted (TR/TE, 500/32) **(C)** and T2-weighted (TR/TE, 2000/60) **(D)** spin echo MR images reveal that the lesion, which has low signal intensity in **C** and high signal intensity in **D,** is somewhat larger and involves the epiphysis.

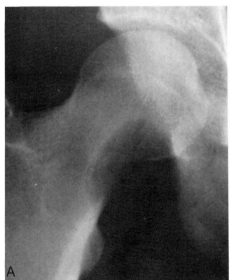

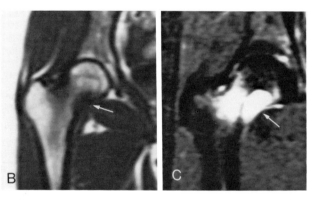

FIGURE 83–304. Aneurysmal bone cyst: Solid variant. This 13 year old girl developed hip pain.

A A routine radiograph shows an eccentric, well-marginated lesion in the medial portion of the femoral neck.

B In a coronal T1-weighted (TR/TE, 400/20) spin echo MR image, the lesion (arrow) is of low signal intensity.

C The coronal short tau inversion recovery (STIR) MR image (TR/TE, 2000/40; inversion time, 150 msec) reveals the lesion in the medial portion of the femoral neck, which is of high signal intensity (arrow). The high signal intensity within the remainder of the femoral neck is indicative of the overestimation of the extent of the lesion that may be seen with STIR imaging. (Courtesy of C. Gundry, M.D., Minneapolis, Minnesota.)

may or may not be present. Intralesional excision (curettage) or marginal resection of the lesion generally is curative.

Aneurysmal bone cysts associated with other skeletal lesions have been designated secondary aneurysmal bone cysts, although, as indicated previously, this designation may not be ideal or even accurate. The associated osseous lesions have included chondroblastoma (Fig. 83–305), chondromyxoid fibroma, fibrous dysplasia, giant cell tumor (Fig. 83–306), osteoblastoma, simple bone cyst, hemangioma, brown tumor of hyperparathyroidism, telangiectatic osteosarcoma, fibrosarcoma, malignant fibrous histiocytoma, hemangioendothelioma, giant cell reparative granuloma, and nonossifying fibroma.[1554, 1558, 1563, 1574, 1576, 1577, 1590, 2301, 2317–2319] It is difficult to define precisely the relative frequency of primary aneurysmal bone cysts and those associated with another lesion; estimates of the incidence of a precursor lesion in cases of aneurysmal bone cyst have varied from less than 1 per cent[1567, 1574, 1577] to greater than 30 per cent,[1576, 2301] or even as high as 80 per cent.[1590] Much of this variation relates to the amount of material that is examined histologically and the strictness of the criteria used to designate the microscopic findings as those of a true aneurysmal bone cyst.[28] It should be noted that the radiographic characteristics of the associated lesion, particularly when malignant, may obscure those of the aneurysmal bone cyst.[1563] Similarly, the clinical findings, including the age of onset, are related more closely to the associated lesion rather than to the aneurysmal bone cyst.[2301]

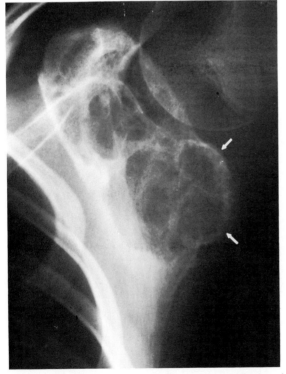

FIGURE 83–305. Aneurysmal bone cyst associated with other skeletal lesions: Chondroblastoma. A documented chondroblastoma of the scapula in a 28 year old patient was removed but subsequently recurred and the tumor enlarged rapidly. The radiograph reveals that the lower portion of the lesion is expansile and trabeculated (arrows). Presence of an aneurysmal bone cyst was documented histologically. (Courtesy of J. Smith, M.D., New York, New York.)

Intraosseous Ganglion Cyst

Intraosseous ganglion cysts appear to represent frequent lesions of uncertain pathogenesis that predominate in the subchondral regions of tubular bones, in the acetabulum, and in the carpal bones, especially the lunate. Their true prevalence, however, is difficult to define owing to inconsistencies in terminology and, in many instances, to the absence of histologic verification of the diagnosis. Most investigators regard the intraosseous ganglion cyst as an entity that can be separated from posttraumatic and degenerative cysts of bone (see Chapter 39). The precise pathogenesis of an intraosseous ganglion cyst is not clear, however. Although the lesion appears to arise de novo within bone, intraosseous ganglion cysts, cutaneous myxoid cysts, and soft tissue ganglion cysts are identical histologically. Furthermore, the simultaneous occurrence of intraosseous and periosseous ganglion cysts is well recognized, leading to an alternative theory that intraosseous ganglion cysts relate to the extension of an adjacent soft tissue ganglion into bone. Continuity between the soft tissue and osseous lesions is consistent with gradual erosion of the bone surface as a cause of an intraosseous ganglion cyst. Intraosseous ganglia and soft tissue ganglia may occur independently, however (see Chapter 95), clouding the issue of the pathogenesis of the intraosseous lesion. Indeed, the pathogenesis of the more common soft tissue ganglion cyst is not agreed upon, with existing theories being well summarized by Feldman and Johnston.[2384] These theories include their development from outpouching of the synovium of a joint capsule or tendon sheath or from synovial remnants that are derived from developing periarticular tissues; from connective tissue degeneration with subsequent liquefaction; or from metaplasia or proliferation of connective tissue.

Intraosseous ganglion cysts occur in persons of all ages, although most are discovered in adults between the ages of 20 and 60 years.[2385] A slight male predominance has been cited in many reports of these lesions.[2386, 2387] Intraosseous ganglia often are clinically silent; however, chronic pain, which sometimes increases with physical activity, may be evident.[2384, 2385] Those lesions associated with soft tissue ganglion cysts may be accompanied by swelling or a mass. Although solitary lesions predominate, multiple and bilateral intraosseous ganglion cysts are encountered.[2384, 2385, 2388] A subchondral lesion in a long tubular bone (e.g., tibia, femur, radius, and ulna) is most characteristic. Common sites of involvement are the femoral head, distal portions of the radius and ulna, distal portion of the femur, proximal aspect of the tibia, and medial malleolus.[2384, 2385, 2389–2391] Any long tubular bone may be affected, however, including the phalanges and metacarpal and metatarsal bones.[2392, 2393] The acetabulum is a frequent site of involvement,[2385, 2394, 2395] with the glenoid region of the scapula being affected less commonly.[2396, 2397] Carpal involvement is more characteristic than tarsal involvement; of the carpal bones, the lunate and scaphoid bones are involved most commonly, although intraosseous ganglion cysts may occur in any of the carpus.[2398–2401]

Radiographically, intraosseous ganglia are osteolytic lesions of variable size, which are well demarcated and sharply circumscribed (Figs. 83–307 and 83–308). They may be solitary or multiple and, when multiple, may be localized to a single bone or adjacent bones. A sclerotic

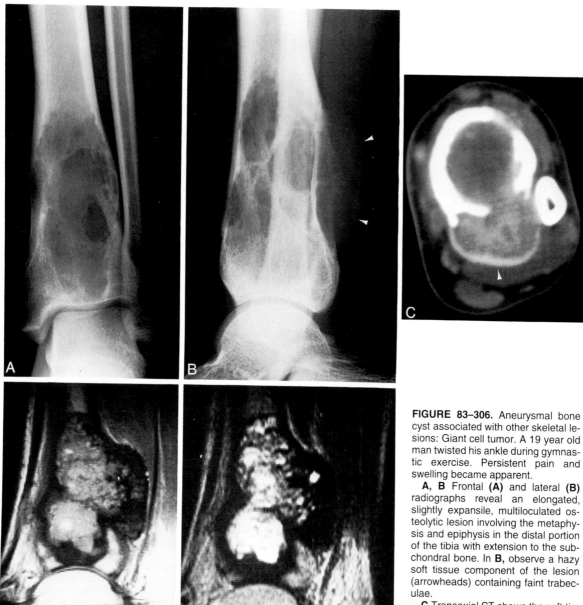

FIGURE 83–306. Aneurysmal bone cyst associated with other skeletal lesions: Giant cell tumor. A 19 year old man twisted his ankle during gymnastic exercise. Persistent pain and swelling became apparent.

A, B Frontal **(A)** and lateral **(B)** radiographs reveal an elongated, slightly expansile, multiloculated osteolytic lesion involving the metaphysis and epiphysis in the distal portion of the tibia with extension to the subchondral bone. In **B,** observe a hazy soft tissue component of the lesion (arrowheads) containing faint trabeculae.

C Transaxial CT shows the soft tissue component with a rim of increased attenuation (arrowhead).

D A sagittal T1-weighted (TR/TE, 500/30) spin echo MR image shows the full extent of the lesion. Although it is predominantly of low signal intensity, this lesion reveals small cystic regions of higher signal intensity.

E A sagittal T2-weighted (TR/TE, 2000/120) spin echo MR image reveals cystic regions with increased signal intensity within the lesion. At surgery, a cystic lesion containing considerable hemorrhage and little tissue was found. The initial histologic diagnosis was an aneurysmal bone cyst. Subsequently, additional evidence of a giant cell tumor was found.

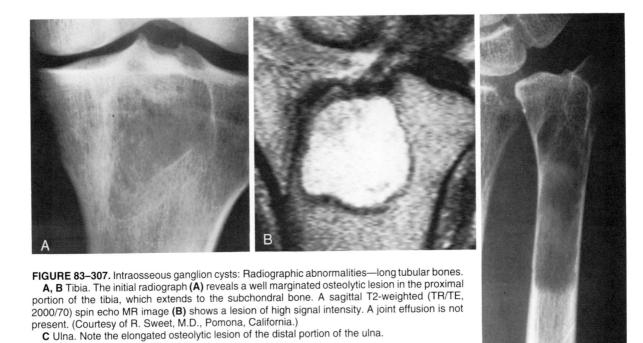

FIGURE 83–307. Intraosseous ganglion cysts: Radiographic abnormalities—long tubular bones.
   A, B Tibia. The initial radiograph **(A)** reveals a well marginated osteolytic lesion in the proximal portion of the tibia, which extends to the subchondral bone. A sagittal T2-weighted (TR/TE, 2000/70) spin echo MR image **(B)** shows a lesion of high signal intensity. A joint effusion is not present. (Courtesy of R. Sweet, M.D., Pomona, California.)
   C Ulna. Note the elongated osteolytic lesion of the distal portion of the ulna.

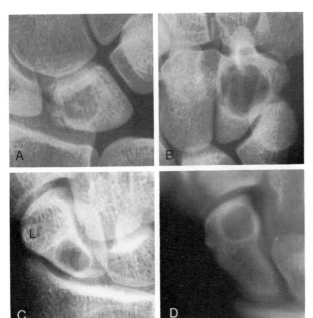

FIGURE 83–308. Intraosseous ganglion cysts: Radiographic abnormalities—carpal bones.
   A Lunate bone. A focal radiolucent region affects the radial aspect of the lunate bone.
   B Hamate bone. A similar lesion of the hamate bone is evident.
   C Scaphoid bone. Note this well-marginated osteolytic lesion in the ulnar aspect of the scaphoid bone. (Courtesy of R. Kerr, M.D., Los Angeles, California.)
   D Scaphoid bone. This ganglion cyst involves the distal portion of the bone.

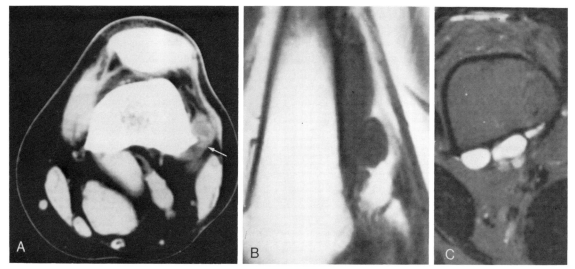

FIGURE 83–309. Subperiosteal ganglion cysts: CT and MR imaging abnormalities.
   A Femur. Transaxial CT scan shows a lesion adjacent to the lateral aspect of the femur (arrow). The lesion reveals low attenuation centrally with a rim of higher attenuation. The subjacent portion of the bone shows proliferation.
   B, C Femur. A sagittal T1-weighted (TR/TE, 600/20) spin echo MR image **(B)** reveals a lobulated lesion of low signal intensity applied to the posterior margin of the femur. In a transaxial T2-weighted (TR/TE, 2500/90) spin echo MR image **(C)**, the lesion is of high signal intensity. (Courtesy of T. Pope, M.D., Winston-Salem, North Carolina.)

margin about the lesion often is evident. Pathologic fractures and soft tissue masses (representing ganglion cysts) are additional findings. In a long tubular bone, an intraosseous ganglion generally is eccentric in location, often extending to the subchondral bone plate. Although the bone plate may appear intact, tomographic techniques not uncommonly reveal that it is violated. Larger lesions may extend into the metaphysis, leading to mild expansion of bone. Isolated involvement of the metaphyseal or diaphyseal portion of the bone is uncommon but is encountered (see later discussion). Acetabular lesions may affect the weight-bearing or non–weight-bearing portion of the bone. They rarely are accompanied by additional lesions in the femoral head. Intraosseous ganglion cysts of the lunate bone often abut the scapholunate interosseous space. In any para-articular location, gas may be evident in the intraosseous (as well as the soft tissue) ganglion cyst (see later discussion).

Subperiosteal ganglion cysts are observed in the long tubular bones.[2402–2406, 2408] The tibia, femur, and radius are involved most commonly. Diaphyseal or metaphyseal localization is typical. A soft tissue mass, cortical erosion, and thick bone spicules extending outwardly from the cortex are typical radiographic findings (Fig. 83–309). Intracortical ganglion cysts are very rare.[2407]

Bone scintigraphy, CT, and MR imaging may be used in the assessment of intraosseous ganglion cysts.[2409–2411] The radionuclide examination shows increased accumulation of the bone-seeking agent. With MR imaging, a lesion of low signal intensity in T1-weighted spin echo MR images and high signal intensity in T2-weighted spin echo MR images is evident (Fig. 83–310).

Pathologically, intraosseous ganglia most often are located at the end of the bone, with normal-appearing adjacent articular cartilage. The ganglion cyst may communicate with the joint. The cyst is smooth and round or oval, and it may reveal a bluish color.[2384] The cyst typically contains thick, gelatinous material, differing from the

clearer, less viscid synovial fluid or from the serous or serosanguineous contents of a simple or aneurysmal bone cyst.[2384] Multiple small or large cavities that communicate or are separated by connective tissue septa are evident. Histologically, the structure of the intraosseous ganglion cyst is identical to that of soft tissue ganglia. Surrounding the major cyst is a connective tissue membrane formed by parallel fascicles of collagen fibers with relatively few fibroblasts; these cells cover the inner surface of the cavity in a discontinuous fashion and often are flattened, acquiring an appearance similar to that of synovium.[2385] A continuous synovial layer is not present, however. Numerous foci of myxoid transformation of the connective tissue, with stellate cells separated by abundant mucoid ground substance, are apparent.[2385] These foci appear to represent newly formed cystic lesions. The cancellous bone that surrounds the cyst contains regions of osteoclastic resorption, as well as areas of new bone formation, accounting for a rim of bone sclerosis.[2385]

Curetage or excision of the bone lesion (with excision of any accompanying soft tissue lesion) usually is curative, although recurrent lesions develop in some cases.

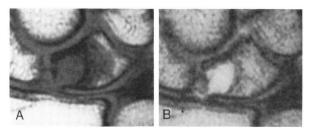

FIGURE 83–310. Intraosseous ganglion cysts: MR imaging abnormalities—lunate. Coronal T1-weighted (TR/TE, 600/20) **(A)** and T2-weighted (TR/TE, 2000/80) **(B)** spin echo MR images reveal a well-marginated lesion involving the radial aspect of the lunate bone. The lesion is of low signal intensity in **A** and of high signal intensity in **B**. Surrounding edema of the bone marrow is evident.

The differential diagnosis of intraosseous ganglion cysts includes a variety of lesions, such as giant cell tumor and chondroblastoma, that lead to epiphyseal and subchondral radiolucent foci. The sclerotic margin about the ganglion cyst and the absence of calcification generally allow its differentiation from these tumors. Intraosseous ganglion cysts, however, share many radiographic features with the subchondral cysts of osteoarthritis (see Chapter 39). The relatively normal appearance of the adjacent articulation in cases of intraosseous ganglia is not a finding of osteoarthritis. Subchondral radiolucent lesions containing gas, designated intraosseous pneumatocysts, are encountered in the ilium, sacrum, vertebral body and, rarely, other sites.[2412, 2413] The relationship of these lesions, which are described in Chapters 39 and 40, to intraosseous ganglion cysts is not clear. Indeed, such ganglion cysts, as well as those occurring in the soft tissues, also may contain gas, which is identified more easily in CT scans than in routine radiographs. The gas that collects in ganglion cysts, as well as in intraosseous pneumatocysts, is believed to have originated from the adjacent joint space, extending through cartilage fissures into the bone lesions and through channels into the soft tissue ganglion cysts (see Chapter 95).

Locally Aggressive or Malignant Tumors

Adamantinoma (Angioblastoma)

Adamantinoma, an extremely rare, locally aggressive or malignant lesion, is composed of rows of epithelium-like cells in a dense fibrous stroma.[1633] The initial classic description of this tumor was provided in 1913 by Fischer,[1634] who used the term primary adamantinoma of the tibia because of its similarity to the more common adamantinoma of the bones of the jaw. Subsequently, the tumor of the mandible and maxilla was redesignated an ameloblastoma (see later discussion); although there is little evidence to suggest that a close relationship exists between adamantinoma of the appendicular skeleton and ameloblastoma of the jaw, even today the two occasionally are classified as one lesion.[1635]

The pathogenesis of adamantinoma is controversial. Proposed concepts of this pathogenesis have been well summarized by Moon and Mori.[1635] The initial belief was that adamantinoma originated in fetal rest cells[1634] or represented a basal cell carcinoma of traumatic origin.[1636] In 1957, Changus and collaborators[1637] suggested a mesodermal origin of the tumor, emphasizing that the angioblast or primitive vascular cell was its primary component. The application of ultrastructural techniques to the evaluation of adamantinoma was initiated by Albores Saavedra and coworkers[1638] in 1968, who believed that the tumor was epithelial in nature. Further investigations using electron microscopy have been reported during the last 20 or 25 years and, in general, have confirmed an epithelial origin, with rare exceptions in which an angioblastic neoplasm was favored.[1639–1643] Immunohistochemical analysis has provided additional evidence that adamantinomas represent epithelial tumors.[1641, 1644, 1645]

A discussion of the origin of adamantinoma would not be complete without reference to the relationship of this neoplasm to other lesions. In some instances, adamantinoma contains Ewing's sarcoma–like tumor cells,[1646, 1647]

and in other adamantinomas, peripheral zones are composed of tissue resembling that of fibrous dysplasia or ossifying fibroma.[1648–1650] This latter phenomenon may explain the reported association of adamantinoma and fibrous dysplasia.[1651] It also has led to the suggestion that the cells of origin in an adamantinoma are able to undergo both epithelial and mesenchymal differentiation with the latter reflected in the fibrous dysplasia–like regions.[1649]

In 1989, Schajowicz and Santini-Araujo[2320] emphasized the difficulty in differentiating adamantinoma and fibrous dysplasia in a description of three cases of intracortical adamantinoma of the tibia, two of which occurred in children less than 10 years of age. In each of the three patients, radiographic features were characteristic of intracortical fibrous dysplasia, and in two of three, histologic findings initially suggested the diagnosis of osteofibrous dysplasia (ossifying fibroma). These authors suggested that adamantinoma of the tibia in children less than 10 years of age is not as rare as has been reported in the literature. Furthermore, they believed that some cases of osteofibrous dysplasia with aggressive behavior (e.g., tumor recurrence following excision) in children that had been described in the literature were, in reality, examples of adamantinoma of the tibia. In the same year, Czerniak and coworkers[2321] used immunohistochemical assays in 7 of 25 cases of adamantinoma in long tubular bones. A new type of adamantinoma, differentiated adamantinoma, that could be distinguished from classic adamantinoma, was identified. Differentiated adamantinoma predominated in the first two decades of life, revealed an intracortical location, and exhibited an osteofibrous dysplasia-like histologic pattern. The authors postulated that the predominance of this histologic pattern was the result of a secondary reparative process that led to the elimination of recognizable tumor cells. Further, they postulated that osteofibrous dysplasia of long bones, in some cases, represented the evolution of an underlying adamantinoma. In 1992, Ishida and associates[2322] reported the results of a clinicopathologic and immunohistochemical study of 12 cases of osteofibrous dysplasia, two cases of differentiated adamantinoma, and five cases of adamantinoma of long bones. The authors concluded that these three lesions shared the same histogenic origin and that classic adamantinoma was a more progressive form of differentiated adamantinoma, as evidenced by tumor invasiveness, metastatic potential, and absence of spontaneous regression. Furthermore, these authors indicated that Ewing's-like adamantinoma was a distinct variant of classic adamantinoma, with different histogenic, radiologic, histologic, and histochemical features.

Clinical Abnormalities. Adamantinomas are slightly more common in men than in women (in a ratio of approximately 5 to 4). Although the age range of patients with this lesion is variable, most are in the second, third, fourth, or fifth decade of life. Females with this tumor are between 11 and 30 years of age, and males are between 30 and 50 years of age.[1635] Rare examples of adamantinoma in young children[1652] and elderly patients[1653] have been documented. A history of trauma is frequent, and many affected persons describe local swelling with or without pain as the major clinical finding. Not infrequently, this finding is present for a period of years before the patient seeks medical attention.

Skeletal Location. It is the striking predilection for the long tubular bones (97 per cent of cases) and, specifically,

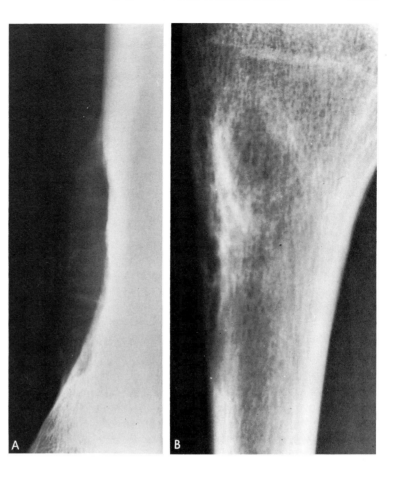

FIGURE 83–311. Adamantinoma (angioblastoma): Radiographic abnormalities.

A In this 35 year old man with an enlarging mass in the medial aspect of his lower leg, a radiograph shows an expansile lesion arising from the distal tibial surface. The external portion of the cortex is eroded and trabeculae extend into the soft tissue component of the lesion. Minimal periostitis is seen.

B In a different patient, an eccentric, predominantly osteolytic lesion involves the proximal metaphysis of the tibia. Bone sclerosis also is apparent, and periostitis is absent.

(**B,** Courtesy of R. Freiberger, M.D., New York, New York.)

the tibia (80 to 85 per cent of cases) that represents the most characteristic feature of this tumor. Other bones that are involved, in order of decreasing frequency, include the humerus (6 per cent), ulna (4 per cent), femur (3 per cent), fibula (3 per cent), and radius (1 per cent), with rare localization to the innominate bone, ribs, spine, and small bones of the hand and foot.[1654–1674, 2323, 2325] Multifocal lesions may rarely develop in a single bone[1662] or in two or more bones (e.g., tibia and fibula; tibia and femur; pubis and ischium; humerus, ribs, and spine).[34, 420, 1635, 1641, 1648, 1669, 1672, 2324] Multiple osseous sites of adamantinoma may represent synchronously or metachronously developing primary tumors or metastases.

Within a long tubular bone, diaphyseal localization predominates, although metaphyseal extension of lesions within the diaphysis or isolated involvement of a metaphysis is encountered occasionally.[33, 180] Epiphyseal abnormalities are uncommon.[1645, 1661] Additional unusual or rare manifestations of adamantinoma include involvement of an entire bone,[1648, 1654] transarticular extension (e.g., tibia to femur across the knee),[1657] and soft tissue, periosteal, or juxtacortical localization.[420, 1675, 1676, 2326, 2327]

Radiographic Abnormalities. In the tibia, adamantinoma usually is localized in the middle third of the bone and appears as a central or eccentric, multilocular, slightly expansile, sharply or poorly delineated osteolytic lesion (Fig. 83–311). Reactive bone sclerosis and small satellite radiolucent foci in direct continuity with the major lesion may be identified. In fact, lesions in the adjacent fibula may be seen[2324] (Fig. 83–312). Periostitis usually is not apparent in the absence of a pathologic fracture. Occasionally, cortical

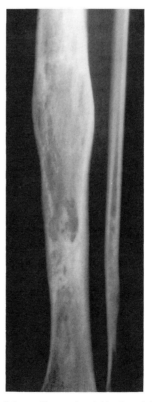

FIGURE 83–312. Adamantinoma (angioblastoma): Radiographic abnormalities. In this case, lesions accompanied by both bone sclerosis and lysis are observed in the tibia and fibula. (Courtesy of R. Kerr, M.D., Los Angeles, California.)

destruction, exuberant periostitis, and a soft tissue mass are noted. Although adamantinomas are rare tumors, an accurate radiographic diagnosis is possible when a typical tibial lesion is encountered. Fibrous dysplasia, nonossifying or ossifying fibroma, aneurysmal or simple bone cyst, chondromyxoid fibroma, chondrosarcoma, hemangioendothelioma, and eosinophilic granuloma are reasonable alternative diagnoses in some cases.

The radiographic features of adamantinomas that are located in other tubular bones generally are similar to those of lesions in the tibia. Unusual abnormalities, including cortical violation with a large soft tissue component, extensive bone sclerosis, and marked osseous expansion, are possible.

Radiographically, the differentiation of adamantinoma, fibrous dysplasia, and osteofibrous dysplasia may be very difficult.[2328] In one study of 46 patients with fibrous dysplasia and 22 patients with adamantinoma in the tibia, the most important findings suggesting a diagnosis of fibrous dysplasia were found to be, in order of decreasing importance, a young age, the presence of a ground-glass appearance with or without additional opacifications, the absence of multilayered periosteal reaction and motheaten bone destruction, and the presence of anterior bowing of the tibia.[2329] The presence of infantile or congenital pseudarthrosis of the tibia, although an infrequent finding of fibrous dysplasia, allows the exclusion of the diagnosis of adamantinoma.[2329] Except for this finding, however, no clinical or radiologic features exist that allow separation of cases of adamantinoma and those of fibrous dysplasia. Similarly, the features of adamantinoma and osteofibrous dysplasia of the tibia generally are indistinguishable and, as indicated earlier, some reported cases of osteofibrous dysplasia, in actuality, may have represented differentiated (or juvenile) adamantinoma.

Although CT and MR imaging (Fig. 83–313) have been used to study the lesions of adamantinoma,[2330, 2331] the findings are not specific. The tumor usually displays low signal intensity in T1-weighted spin echo MR images and high signal intensity in T2-weighted spin echo MR images.

Pathologic Abnormalities. Macroscopically, the lesions are between 3 and 15 cm in maximum dimension and may be located in the medullary or cortical bone. They usually are confined by the periosteal membrane. Single or multiple discrete foci of tumor are evident and, in some instances, the entire bone is involved. When sectioned, a pale gray or white neoplasm containing cystic areas with watery, yellow, or hemorrhagic fluid is observed. Additional characteristics of this lesion include a firm and rubbery or soft and fleshy consistency, a lobulated contour, and, when palpated, a gritty texture related to the presence of bone spicules.

The microscopic pattern generally is one in which epithelial-like cells assuming a variety of forms reside within a fibrous stroma.[1677–1679] Four basic forms are found in varying combinations: basaloid, squamous, spindle, and tubular. The basaloid pattern consists of nests of cells that resemble those of a basal cell carcinoma[1672]; the squamous pattern (Fig. 83–314*A,B*) is characterized by collections of squamous cells that may contain keratohyalin granules and intercellular bridges[1649, 1677]; the spindle pattern consists of islands or whorled areas of small spindle-shaped cells without evidence of peripheral palisading[33]; and the tubular pattern (Fig. 83–314*C,D*) is characterized by cuboidal or flat

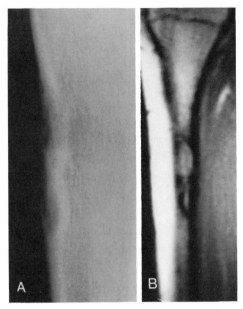

FIGURE 83–313. Adamantinoma (angioblastoma): MR imaging abnormalities.

A A frontal radiograph shows cortical lesions involving the metadiaphyseal portion of the tibia.

B A sagittal T1-weighted (TR/TE, 256/11) spin echo MR image shows that the lesion is of intermediate signal intensity. It was of high signal intensity in T2-weighted spin echo images (not shown).

cells that are aligned along tubular channels that, occasionally, are filled with erythrocytes, simulating the appearance of a true vessel.[33] The fibrous stroma commonly consists of benign-appearing fibroblasts that are arranged in a cartwheel or storiform pattern similar to that found in fibrous histiocytoma, ossifying fibroma, or fibrous dysplasia. These storiform areas, which frequently are found at the periphery of the tumor, may contain metaplastic bone or osteoid and mimic fibrous dysplasia or ossifying fibroma.

Natural History. Adamantinomas are a locally aggressive tumor with the potential to metastasize.[2332, 2333] Although the growth of the initial tumor may be slow, this feature should not lead to a cavalier approach regarding the need for appropriate treatment.[1635] Recurrence of tumor is frequent following inadequate therapy, and the behavior of the recurrent neoplasm resembles more and more that of a sarcoma. Although 10 year patient survival rate has been estimated to be as high as 65 per cent,[1680] a figure of less than 10 per cent appears more accurate.[1635] Despite the potential of some of these neoplasms to metastasize, even years after initial therapy,[1861] it remains difficult to identify clinical, radiographic, or histologic characteristics that can predict reliably the ultimate behavior of any individual tumor. It should be noted, however, that some investigators believe that the Ewing's sarcoma–like variant of conventional adamantinoma, characterized by the presence of small dark cells containing cytoplasmic glycogen, is accompanied by more aggressive behavior and a poorer prognosis.[1647]

Malignant Tumors

Ewing's Sarcoma

This relatively common malignant tumor derives its name from Ewing who, in 1921, provided the first compre-

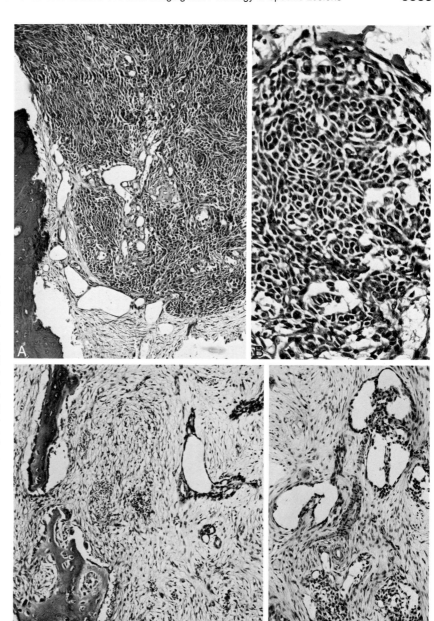

FIGURE 83–314. Adamantinoma (angioblastoma): Microscopic abnormalities.

A, B Squamous pattern. In **A,** a large, well-circumscribed nest of epithelial cells is evident within the bone. In **B,** at higher magnification, the cells are loosely joined with small microcystic areas, creating a reticulated appearance. (150×, 300×.)

C, D Tubular pattern. In **C,** several blood vessel–like channels, lined by flat epithelial cells, are present. The spindle cell stroma is loosely arranged in a whorled pattern. Newly formed irregularly shaped trabeculae lined by osteoblasts are associated with the epithelial cells. The stroma and bone simulate an ossifying fibroma. In **D,** some solid nests of epithelial cells are seen, as are foci where the tumor has formed vessel-like channels. (150×, 150×.)

hensive description of the neoplasm, designating it a diffuse endothelioma of bone (and, later, an endothelial myeloma), and distinguishing it from osteosarcoma.[1681] In 1939, Parker and Jackson[1682] further evaluated this neoplasm and segregated it from reticulum cell sarcoma. Although many subsequent reports of Ewing's sarcoma verified its prominent position among the malignant neoplasms of bone, its histogenesis has remained unresolved despite the numerous histochemical, immunohistochemical, and ultrastructural studies published in recent years.[221] Proposed origins of Ewing's sarcoma have included mesenchymal cells of the bone marrow,[1683] immature reticulum cells,[1684] vascular[1685] or myelogenic[1686] elements,[33] or undifferentiated mesenchymal cells of the bone marrow,[1687–1689] with some data de-

rived from electron microscopy and immunofluorescence analysis being interpreted as supportive of an endothelial origin.[1690] Recent immunohistochemical and cytogenic studies have provided results that suggest a neuroectodermal origin of the tumor.[2496, 2497] There is no disagreement, however, that considerable difficulty in differential diagnosis results in distinguishing histologically between Ewing's sarcoma and other malignant small round cell tumors involving bone, including lymphomas and neuroblastoma (Table 83–4). Indeed, in some of the early reports, tumors were encountered that had the histologic features of Ewing's sarcoma but, at autopsy, were found to represent other neoplasms, especially neuroblastoma. Careful analysis of chemical, radiographic, light and electron microscopic, and

TABLE 83–4. Differential Diagnosis of Some Small Cell Tumors of Bone in Children*

Ewing's Sarcoma	Non-Hodgkin's Lymphoma
Most common in second decade (but frequently occurs below 10 years of age)	No age or race predilection in children
Rare in blacks	Long bones most common (femur and tibia)
Pain is most common presenting symptom	Diffuse metaphyseal lesion, usually mixed osteolytic and osteosclerotic areas
Flat bones (ribs, scapula, pelvis) are common sites	Lymphadenopathy and splenomegaly may be present
Femur is most common site	Early diffuse bone marrow involvement in children
Metadiaphyseal lesion in long bones	Reticulum fibers demonstrable with special stain
Diffuse osteolytic lesion	Cell nuclei somewhat larger and rounder than in Ewing's sarcoma
Large soft tissue mass	Negative PAS reaction for glycogen
Positive PAS reaction for glycogen	
Negative reaction to reticulin stain	

Metastatic Neuroblastoma	Embryonal Rhabdomyosarcoma
Usually in children less than 5 years of age	Lesions of the trunk and extremity may frequently involve bone
Long bones frequently are symmetrically involved	Usually presents with soft tissue swelling rather than pain as the predominant symptom
Lytic lesions may be very extensive with a paucity of soft tissue mass	The soft tissue mass usually invades bone secondarily
Bone marrow aspiration may show cells in rosettes	Systemic symptoms are rare
Presence of primary tumor; abnormal intravenous pyelogram or paraspinal mass	Lesions in the head and neck area are usually primary, not metastatic
Urine may be positive for vanillylmandelic acid or catecholamine metabolites	Cells have a predominance of pink cytoplasm, and may exhibit striations on higher magnification

*Modified from Rosen G: Pediatr Clin North Am 23:183, 1976.

histochemical abnormalities has confirmed important differences between Ewing's sarcoma and neuroblastoma,[1693–1695] and postmortem examinations have further underscored the validity of Ewing's sarcoma as a distinct neoplasm.[1696–1698] The recent description of a primary neuroectodermal tumor of bone that shares clinical, radiologic, and histologic features with Ewing's sarcoma[1699] (see later discussion), however, emphasizes again the close relationship that exists between Ewing's sarcoma and neuroblastoma and suggests that Ewing's sarcoma actually may be neuroectodermal in nature.[1862]

Clinical Abnormalities. Ewing's sarcoma usually is identified in patients in the first, second, or third decade of life; approximately 90 per cent of persons with this neoplasm are between the ages of 5 and 30 years at the time of clinical presentation,[1700] and the highest frequency of this sarcoma occurs in patients between the ages of 10 and 15 years.[1701] Instances of Ewing's sarcoma in infancy and early childhood[2334] as well as in middle-aged and elderly patients are encountered but are rare. There is a slight male predilection (approximately 60 per cent are men) and an overwhelming predominance of white patients (95 per cent). The rarity of Ewing's sarcoma in blacks deserves emphasis (1 or 2 per cent of patients). Localized pain and swelling may be combined with fever, weight loss, anemia, and leukocytosis, simulating the clinical findings of an infection. Other manifestations depend on the specific site of involvement; as examples, neurologic symptoms and signs or headaches accompany a spinal or cranial lesion, a limp or other abnormality of gait may indicate a tumor in the long or short tubular bones of the leg or foot, paresthesias and dental abnormality may indicate a Ewing's sarcoma in the mandible and maxilla, and pleuritic manifestations are

compatible with the diagnosis of involvement of the ribs. Ewing's sarcoma occurring in the end of a tubular bone may lead to articular complaints similar to those of septic arthritis,[1702, 2335] and Ewing's sarcoma arising in the ilium or sacrum may produce clinical findings that simulate those of sacroiliitis.[2336, 2337]

Skeletal Location. Although Ewing's sarcoma may develop in virtually any bone in the human body, it affects principally the lower segment of the skeleton, with the sacrum, innominate bone, and bones in the lower extremity accounting for approximately two thirds of all cases.[1701, 1703–1705, 2430] The most frequent sites of involvement are the femur (approximately 22 per cent of cases), ilium (12 per cent), tibia (11 per cent), humerus (10 per cent), fibula (9 per cent), and ribs (8 per cent); Ewing's sarcoma is relatively uncommon in the vertebrae above the sacrum (6 per cent), scapula (5 per cent), bones of the forearm (3 per cent) and hand and foot (3 per cent), mandible and maxilla (2 per cent), and clavicle (2 per cent), and it is rare in the skull (1 per cent), facial bones (0.5 per cent), and sternum (0.2 per cent).[1706–1737]

It has classically been taught that in the long tubular bones, Ewing's sarcoma is diaphyseal in location.[1705, 1738] More often, however, it is metadiaphyseal or, less commonly, metaphyseal rather than purely diaphyseal.[1739, 1740] Estimates of the frequency of isolated involvement of the diaphysis in cases of Ewing's sarcoma in the tubular bones have included 20 and 35 per cent.[1706, 1741] Although epiphyseal extension of Ewing's sarcoma may be observed in as many as 10 per cent of such cases,[1738] isolated involvement of the epiphysis is rare.[1742] Localization in the proximal segment of a tubular bone is more frequent than that in the distal segment, in a ratio of approximately 5 to 3.

Involvement of the bones in the feet is much more common than that of the bones in the hands, in a ratio of approximately 4 to 1. Although tarsal, metatarsal, metacarpal, and phalangeal abnormalities may be seen,[2338-2344] the authors are not aware of any cases of Ewing's sarcoma localized to a carpal bone.

In the vertebral column, sacral involvement dominates, followed in order of decreasing frequency by the lumbar, thoracic, cervical, and coccygeal regions. The vertebral body is affected primarily, although the neoplasm not infrequently extends from this region to the posterior osseous elements of the vertebra.[1707, 1863] It should be noted that despite the relatively infrequent localization to the spine of primary Ewing's sarcoma, this site (as well as the skull) commonly is altered in instances of metastases derived from this sarcoma.[180, 1743]

With regard to the thoracic cage, Ewing's sarcoma predominates in the ribs with less common or rare involvement of the scapula, clavicle, and sternum.[1742, 1744, 1745, 2334, 2345, 2346] With regard to the bones of the jaw, mandibular lesions are more frequent than those of the maxilla, in a ratio of approximately 3 to 1.[1708, 1712, 1864, 2347-2349]

It should also be noted that rare descriptions of Ewing's sarcoma in the soft tissues rather than in the bones exist, although the accuracy in interpretation of the precise site of origin in some of these reports is subject to question (see later discussion). Periosteal localization of the tumor also is rare.[2498]

Radiographic Abnormalities. The fundamental radiographic findings in Ewing's sarcoma reflect the aggressive nature of this lesion and include osteolysis, cortical erosion or violation, periostitis, and a soft tissue mass. The bone destruction generally is permeative or motheaten in appearance; the periosteal response often is exuberant and may consist of multiple layers of new bone (the laminated, onion-skin, or onion-peel pattern) or horizontally oriented thin osseous strands extending at right angles to the parent bone (the hair-on-end pattern). Although classically Ewing's sarcoma is a medullary lesion, changes in the cortex of the bone may be dominant, including longitudinal cortical striations, or tunneling, and external cortical saucerization.[2350]

Reinus and collaborators[1741] divided the radiographic features of Ewing's sarcoma as studied in 373 patients into three categories based on frequency. Common manifestations included poorly marginated bone destruction (96 per cent), frequently classified as permeative in type (76 per cent), soft tissue involvement (80 per cent), laminated periostitis (57 per cent), and osteosclerosis (40 per cent). The last finding apparently resulted from reactive bone formation and osteoid deposition on foci of necrotic bone, perhaps related to the tumor's outgrowing its blood supply.[1746] Uncommon manifestations included spiculated (hair-on-end or sunburst) periostitis (28 per cent), thickening (21 per cent) or violation (19 per cent) of the cortex, pure osteolysis (19 per cent), pathologic fracture (15 per cent), osseous expansion (13 per cent), and cystic abnormality (12 per cent). Rare manifestations included soft tissue calcification (9 per cent), cortical saucerization (6 per cent), and a honeycomb (6 per cent) or well-marginated (4 per cent) appearance. Of interest, three of the patients had entirely normal findings on routine radiographs, and, in at least one of these, an intraosseous (rather than an extraosseous) neoplasm was documented.

Tubular Bones. A poorly defined, osteolytic, metadiaphyseal lesion in a long tubular bone accompanied by cortical erosion, periostitis, and a soft tissue mass is the classic description[1723] (Fig. 83–315). Bone sclerosis in some cases resembles that seen in an osteosarcoma.[1746] Similar abnormalities are observed in Ewing's sarcoma in the metacarpal and metatarsal bones and in the phalanges (Fig. 83–316). It has been suggested that an aggressive radiographic pattern is more frequent in these peripheral locations than in more typical sites of involvement and that, with the exception of bone sclerosis, osseous reaction (in the form of cortical thickening or periostitis, or both) in the bones of the hands and feet is rare.[1714] Conversely, osteolysis alone, pathologic fracture, osseous expansion, and cystic change (with a honeycomb appearance) are more frequent in those Ewing's sarcomas that develop in the hands and feet.[1714, 1715, 1724] The major differential diagnostic considerations are osteosarcoma, lymphoma, and infection.

Vertebral Column. A Ewing's sarcoma in a vertebral body leads to bone destruction, which may be followed by fracture and collapse (vertebra plana) (Fig. 83–317). Less frequently, osteosclerosis of a vertebral body or even a pedicle or other posterior osseous element is observed.[1707, 1747, 1748] Extension of the process into the paraspinal[1713] and intraspinal[1707, 1748] tissues is well described. Additional patterns of vertebral involvement include extension to an adjacent vertebral body with loss of height of the intervening intervertebral disc and spread to the pedicles, laminae, and transverse and spinous processes.[1707] In the sacrum, osteolysis, cortical destruction, and a soft tissue mass are encountered. The differential diagnosis of a Ewing's sarcoma in the vertebral column includes pyogenic or tuberculous osteomyelitis, lymphoma, leukemia, histiocytoses, and metastatic disease.

Innominate Bone. Although the radiographic abnormalities accompanying Ewing's sarcoma in any of the bones constituting the innominate bone is similar to that occurring in other involved skeletal sites, a large soft tissue mass containing calcification may be evident (Fig. 83–318). When combined with significant alterations in the bone itself, the resulting radiographic appearance easily is misinterpreted as evidence of an osteosarcoma or chondrosarcoma.

Other Sites. In the ribs (Fig. 83–319A–C), Ewing's sarcomas produce lesions that are either predominantly osteolytic or osteosclerotic or reveal both osteolysis and osteosclerosis. The direction of tumor growth tends to be intrathoracic, resulting in an adjacent extrapleural mass and, usually, a relatively insignificant soft tissue component in the chest wall itself.[1749] The large size of the extrapleural mass in comparison to the subtle rib destruction can be striking.[1750]

In the mandible or maxilla, permeative bone destruction, periosteal reaction, and an extraosseous soft tissue component are most typical.[1708] Similar alterations occur in other osseous sites (Fig. 83–319D).

Other Imaging Techniques. As in most aggressive osseous neoplasms, scintigraphy using a bone-seeking radiopharmaceutical agent generally shows increased uptake of the radionuclide in foci of Ewing's sarcoma (Figs. 83–319 and 83–320), with reportable exceptions in which a photon deficient region (''cold'' lesion) is evident.[1751] Gallium scanning represents an additional radionuclide technique

Text continued on page 3893

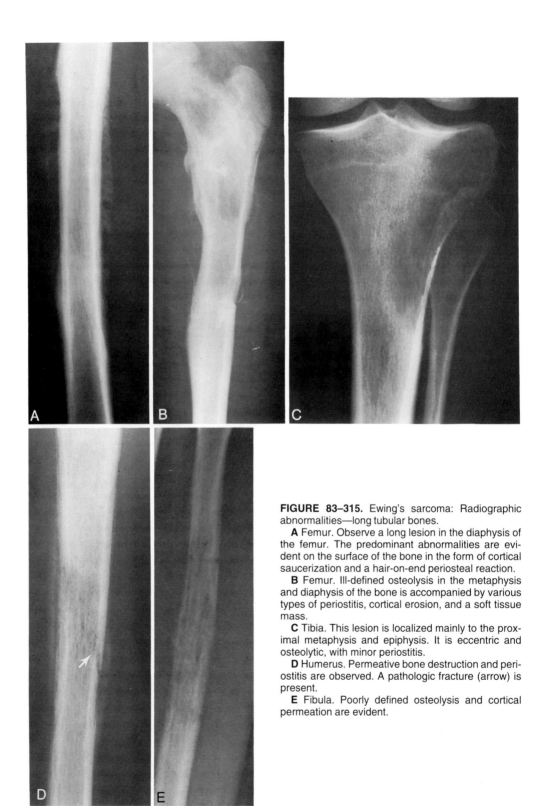

FIGURE 83–315. Ewing's sarcoma: Radiographic abnormalities—long tubular bones.

A Femur. Observe a long lesion in the diaphysis of the femur. The predominant abnormalities are evident on the surface of the bone in the form of cortical saucerization and a hair-on-end periosteal reaction.

B Femur. Ill-defined osteolysis in the metaphysis and diaphysis of the bone is accompanied by various types of periostitis, cortical erosion, and a soft tissue mass.

C Tibia. This lesion is localized mainly to the proximal metaphysis and epiphysis. It is eccentric and osteolytic, with minor periostitis.

D Humerus. Permeative bone destruction and periostitis are observed. A pathologic fracture (arrow) is present.

E Fibula. Poorly defined osteolysis and cortical permeation are evident.

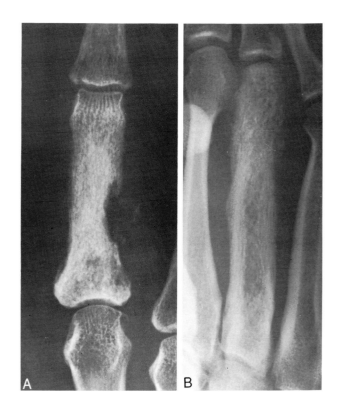

FIGURE 83–316. Ewing's sarcoma: Radiographic abnormalities—short tubular bones of the hands and feet.

A Proximal phalanx of hand. Observe considerable osteosclerosis, cortical permeation, and minor periostitis. The large cortical defect and soft tissue radiodense shadows relate to a previous biopsy. (Courtesy of J. Rausch, M.D., Fort Wayne, Indiana.)

B Metatarsal bone. The distal two thirds of the bone is affected. Osteosclerosis, ill-defined osteolysis, and cortical permeation are evident.

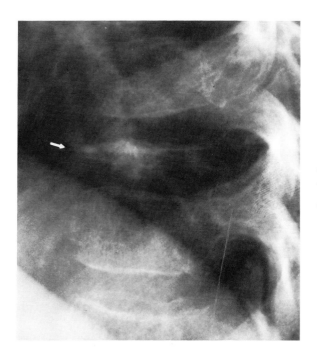

FIGURE 83–317. Ewing's sarcoma: Radiographic abnormalities—vertebral column. Note the complete collapse of a thoracic vertebral body (arrow). Although this abnormality occurred as a result of skeletal metastasis from Ewing's sarcoma, a similar change is observed with primary Ewing's sarcomas.

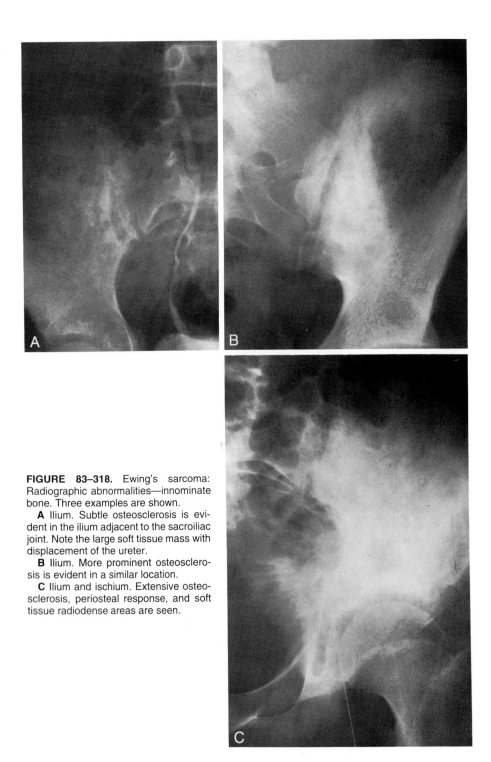

FIGURE 83–318. Ewing's sarcoma: Radiographic abnormalities—innominate bone. Three examples are shown.

A Ilium. Subtle osteosclerosis is evident in the ilium adjacent to the sacroiliac joint. Note the large soft tissue mass with displacement of the ureter.

B Ilium. More prominent osteosclerosis is evident in a similar location.

C Ilium and ischium. Extensive osteosclerosis, periosteal response, and soft tissue radiodense areas are seen.

FIGURE 83–319. Ewing's sarcoma: Radiographic abnormalities—other osseous sites.

A–C Ribs. This 28 year old man had a 3 year history of an enlarging mass in the right side of the chest. A radiograph **(A)** shows the mass as well as osteolysis involving the anterior portion of the right third rib. Transaxial CT **(B)** reveals the extensive destruction of the rib and an anterior (arrowhead) and, to a lesser extent, posterior soft tissue mass. A bone scan **(C)** shows a region of increased radionuclide uptake (arrowhead) with central photopenia in the right third rib. Histologic analysis confirmed the diagnosis of Ewing's sarcoma.

D Clavicle. In a 3 year old child, a long area of permeative osteolysis in the distal portion of the clavicle is evident.

(D, Courtesy of T. Broderick, M.D., Orange, California.)

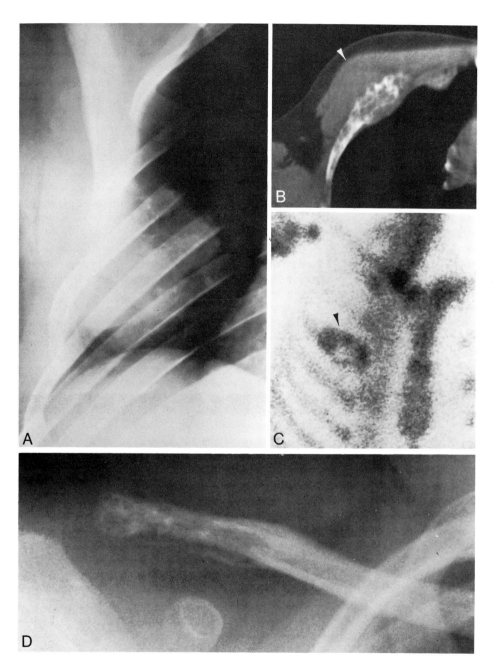

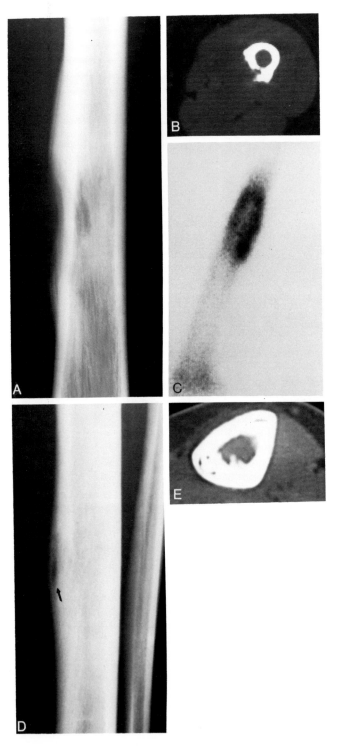

FIGURE 83–320. Ewing's sarcoma: Scintigraphic and CT abnormalities.

A–C This 20 year old woman complained of increasing pain in the thigh. A radiograph **(A)** shows saucerization of the cortex in the diaphysis of the femur, associated with laminated periostitis. Transaxial CT **(B)** demonstrates the cortical erosion and saucerization. A soft tissue mass was more evident on other CT scans. Bone scintigraphy **(C)** shows increased accumulation of the radionuclide in the femur at the site of the lesion. A Ewing's sarcoma was confirmed after biopsy and histologic evaluation.

D, E This 23 year old woman had mild pain over the tibia of approximately 3 months' duration. Five years previously, she had lacerated the skin over this region. On physical examination, local soft tissue tenderness and thickening were apparent. The radiograph **(D)** shows an elongated radiolucent area within the cortex (arrow) and poorly defined osteolysis. Transaxial CT **(E)** reveals the cortical radiolucent area as well as increased attenuation in the bone marrow. Although the preoperative diagnosis was osteomyelitis, biopsy disclosed a Ewing's sarcoma.

that allows the identification of this neoplasm as an area of increased scintigraphic activity and that can be used to monitor the tumor's response to therapy.[2351]

CT (Figs. 83–320 and 83–321) is best used to define the extraosseous extent of a Ewing's sarcoma, especially in the skull, spine, ribs, and pelvis.[1752–1754, 1865] This technique also is helpful in the delineation of the precise portals to be used during radiation therapy and in the evaluation of the tumor's response to irradiation or chemotherapy.

MR imaging provides information similar to that obtainable with CT.[2352] This technique allows assessment of the extent of intraosseous and soft tissue involvement, revealing a process that is of low signal intensity in T1-weighted spin echo MR images and high signal intensity in T2-weighted spin echo MR images (Figs. 83–322 and 83–323). With standard MR imaging or that combined with intravenous administration of a gadolinium compound, differentiation of tumor and surrounding edema may be difficult.

Available data regarding the role of MR imaging in the evaluation of the response of Ewing's sarcoma to chemotherapy are not uniform. Lemmi and coworkers[2353] indicated that an increase in signal intensity of the bone marrow in T2-weighted images reflected a favorable response to chemotherapy and that changes in signal intensity in the adjacent soft tissue were not useful prognostically. Holscher and associates,[2354] in an evaluation of patients with Ewing's sarcoma or osteosarcoma who had undergone chemotherapy, found that a decrease in tumor volume and a decrease in signal intensity of the soft tissue component in T2-weighted spin echo MR images were indicative of a favorable response. MacVicar and coworkers,[2355] in a study of patients with Ewing's sarcoma who had undergone chemotherapy, indicated that areas of high signal intensity in T2-weighted spin echo MR images could represent tumor necrosis, cystic hemorrhagic areas, and fibroblastic repair tissue, but that such a pattern also was consistent with the presence of active tumor. Fletcher and coworkers,[2356] in an analysis of the chemotherapeutic response of Ewing's and other sarcomas, used dynamic MR imaging following the

intravenous administration of a gadolinium compound. The rate of gadolinium accumulation (and, hence, increased signal intensity) in the area of the treated lesion was reduced in tumors that responded to chemotherapy when compared with those that did not respond. These authors concluded that such dynamic MR imaging allowed more accurate analysis of tumor response than standard T2-weighted spin echo MR images or static gadolinium-enhanced T1-weighted spin echo MR images.

Pathologic Abnormalities. Ewing's sarcomas are relatively large at the time of initial clinical evaluation, frequently measuring between 5 and 10 cm in maximum dimension[1755, 1756] (Fig. 83–324). When intact tumors are examined pathologically, they frequently are found to be more extensive than expected owing to radiographic underestimation of their size.[1757] An associated extraosseous neoplastic component is present in 80 to 100 per cent of cases[1758] and commonly is larger than the intraosseous component of the tumor. Pathologic fractures are evident in 2 to 15 per cent of cases.[1714, 1721, 1741] When sectioned, Ewing's sarcomas typically are soft, friable, and pink or gray with hemorrhagic and necrotic foci. A semiliquid consistency is common.[1757–1759]

Ewing's sarcoma is composed essentially of small, round, undifferentiated tumor cells (Fig. 83–325A,B). These cells have little visible cytoplasm, and their borders are indistinct; nuclei are round with stippled chromatin and one or two small nucleoli.[1759, 1760] The cells generally are uniform in appearance, with little variation in either size or shape.[1761] Scattered among these principal tumor cells are smaller cells with folded or wrinkled nuclei that have a condensed, pyknotic-appearing chromatin pattern; these dark cells are thought to represent degenerated principal cells.[1761]

The tumor cells usually are crowded together in sheets or segregated in lobules by fine fibrovascular septa.[1687] A "filigree" pattern has been described in which these cells are arranged in bicellular strands separated by a filmy fibrovascular stroma.[1701] Special stains indicate the absence of

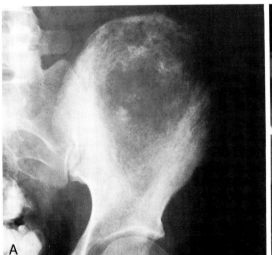
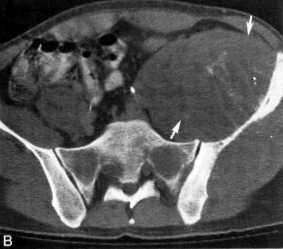

FIGURE 83–321. Ewing's sarcoma: CT abnormalities. A 30 year old man developed pain and tenderness in the low back and hip. A radiograph **(A)** shows a mixed osteolytic and osteosclerotic lesion involving the entire ilium. Although a soft tissue mass is observed extending into the pelvis, it is better seen (arrows) with transaxial CT **(B).** Note the periosteal response and ossification in the intrapelvic soft tissue mass.

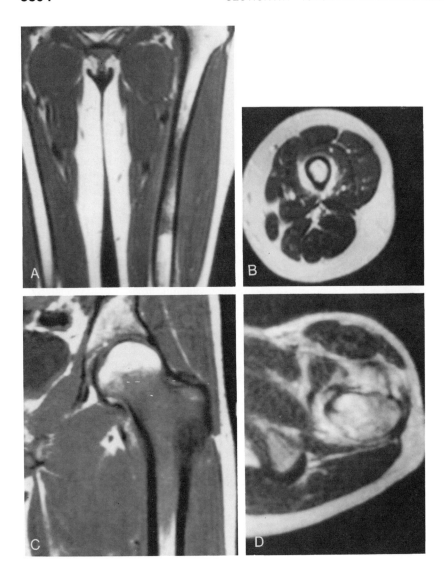

FIGURE 83–322. Ewing's sarcoma: MR imaging abnormalities—long tubular bones.

A, B In a 20 year old woman, the tumor in the diaphysis of the femur is of low signal intensity in a coronal T1-weighted (TR/TE, 600/20) spin echo MR image **(A)**. Metastatic foci (skip metastases) involving the proximal portion of the bone were better seen in other T1-weighted spin echo MR images. A transaxial T2-weighted (TR/TE, 2200/80) spin echo MR image **(B)** shows the tumor within the femoral diaphysis as a region of high signal intensity. Note the high signal intensity also in the periosseous tissue, indicative of tumor extension, edema, or both processes. (Courtesy of B. Martin, M.D., Paris, France.)

C, D In an 18 year old man, a Ewing's sarcoma in the proximal portion of the femur appears as an intraosseous region of low signal intensity in a coronal T1-weighted (TR/TE, 750/20) spin echo MR image **(C)**. Soft tissue abnormalities are not well demonstrated in this image however. Both the intraosseous and extraosseous components of the tumor are evident in a transaxial T2-weighted (TR/TE, 2100/70) spin echo MR image **(D)** although, with regard to the extraosseous abnormalities, differentiation of tumor and edema is difficult. (Courtesy of M. Mitchell, M.D., Halifax, Nova Scotia, Canada.)

reticulin fibers within the tumor except for those in the reticulin sheath around blood vessels and in the fibrovascular septa. Mitotic activity varies greatly, although most Ewing's sarcomas do not contain numerous mitotic figures.

Although Ewing's sarcomas usually are vascular, with frequent hemorrhagic areas, extensive necrosis is common. The necrotic tumor cells typically lose their nuclei but retain their cytoplasm, creating a ghost-cell appearance[1701] (Fig. 83–325C). Rosette or rosette-like foci (Fig. 83–325D), similar to those of neuroblastoma,[1762] may be found in a minority of Ewing's tumors, but the presence of these structures are an indication of neural differentiation and such tumors currently would be considered neuroectodermal tumors.

The diagnostic value of detecting glycogen granules in the cytoplasm of the tumor cells in Ewing's sarcoma was first emphasized by Schajowicz[1763] in 1959. By light microscopy, PAS positivity for glycogen is found in 70 to 100 per cent of cases. It should be noted, however, that glycogen granules may not be distributed uniformly in a Ewing's sarcoma, being more abundant in those cells that are closest to blood vessels.[1764] Furthermore, material to be examined must be fixed correctly, preferably in alcohol.[221] Glycogen granules are absent in malignant lymphoma and, with rare exceptions,[221, 1765, 1766] in metastatic neuroblastoma. The

presence of glycogen, however, occurs in other small cell tumors including neuroectodermal tumors.

Numerous cytogenic and immunohistochemical studies of Ewing's sarcomas have been undertaken in recent years to define more precisely features that allow separation of these tumors from neuroectodermal tumors. A discussion of the results of such studies is beyond the scope of this chapter.

Natural History. Ewing's sarcoma is regarded as a highly aggressive tumor with the propensity to invade local tissues and disseminate throughout the body.[1767] It has been estimated that between 15 and 30 per cent of patients with Ewing's sarcoma have metastatic disease. The use of both radiation therapy and chemotherapy, sometimes in combination with surgery, in recent years has had a dramatic favorable impact on the prognosis of patients with this type of cancer. The major objective of radiation or surgical therapy regarding the primary tumor is optimal local control.[1700] With regard to radiographic findings of Ewing's sarcoma that may be predictive of a favorable response to therapy, small size, involvement of sites other than the innominate bone, femur, or humerus, and a honeycombed appearance were emphasized in one report.[2357] Tumor recurrences at or near the site of origin are frequent, however, with estimates ranging from 12 to 25 per cent.

FIGURE 83–323. Ewing's sarcoma: MR imaging abnormalities—innominate bone.

A, B During the investigation of hip pain in a 14 year old boy, a transaxial T1-weighted (TR/TE, 417/12) spin echo MR image **(A)** was obtained that reveals a large tumor arising from the iliopubic bone column and extending medially, displacing the bladder. It is of low signal intensity. In a coronal short tau inversion recovery (STIR) MR image (TR/TE, 2900/27; inversion time, 160 msec) **(B),** the tumor is inhomogeneous in appearance but mainly of high signal intensity. Note its extension into the pelvis and thigh. A hip effusion is evident.

C, D In a 12 year old boy with hip pain, coronal proton density–weighted (TR/TE, 2000/30) **(C)** and T2-weighted (TR/TE, 2000/90) **(D)** spin echo MR images document a massive tumor arising from the ischium and extending medially and interiorly. The lesion is of intermediate signal intensity in **C** and high signal intensity in **D.** Irregular enhancement of signal intensity was apparent in MR images obtained after the intravenous administration of a gadolinium compound (not shown).

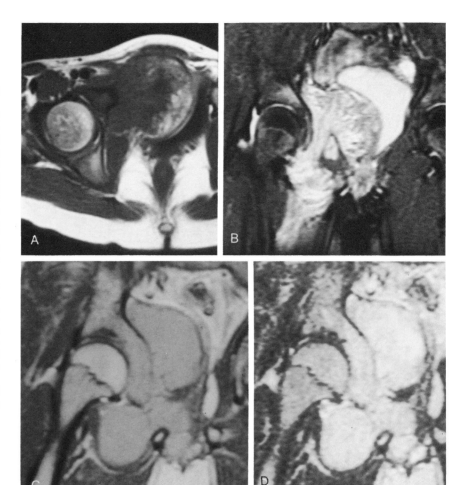

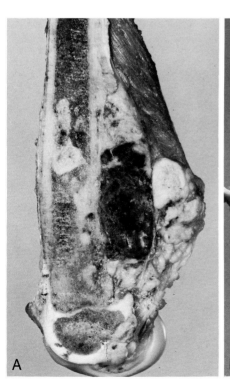
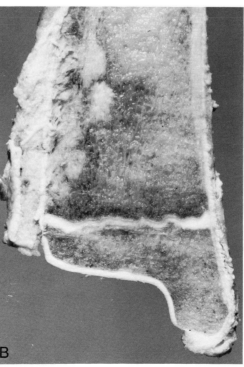

FIGURE 83–324. Ewing's sarcoma: Macroscopic abnormalities.

A This tumor in the distal portion of the femur has extended through the cortex and has formed a large, partially hemorrhagic mass beneath the periosteum. Nodular collections of tumor are present in the adjacent skeletal muscle.

B Note the poorly defined tumor (white) in the distal portion of the tibia. It, too, has extended through the cortex and infiltrated the periosteum.

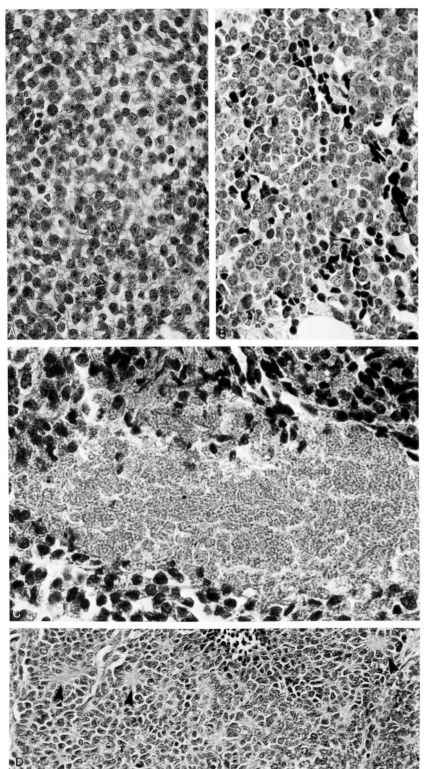

FIGURE 83–325. Ewing's sarcoma: Microscopic abnormalities.

A The cells are small and round, and their nuclei have fine nuclear chromatin and occasionally a micronucleolus. In this focus, the cells have more distinct cytoplasmic borders than is usually seen, and the cytoplasm appears pale owing to its glycogen content. The cells are fairly uniform in their overall appearance. (600×.)

B The borders of the principal tumor cells are indistinct, and there is little or no cytoplasm. In addition to these cells, smaller, "dark" degenerate cells are intermixed. (600×.)

C In this necrotic focus, a few ghost cells can be recognized. (600×.)

D Rosette formation (arrowheads) is evident. The centers of the rosettes contain material indistinguishable from the neurofibrillary material that is found in a neuroblastoma. It would not be possible to distinguish between these two tumors based on this photomicrograph alone.(600×.)

Routine radiography can be used to evaluate patients who have received treatment for a Ewing's sarcoma. Radiographic changes suggesting healing occur within a period of months, and include maturation of the periosteal response, reconstitution of the cortex, and increasing bone sclerosis (Fig. 83–326); those suggesting recurrent or persistent disease also occur within months and include failure of the predicted healing pattern to develop or progression of the initial neoplastic changes.[1768]

The lungs and bones[1866, 2358] are common locations for metastases, requiring careful examination for effective surveillance of tumor progression.[1767] Imaging techniques that have been used for this purpose are bone and gallium scintigraphy, chest radiography, conventional and computed tomography, and MR imaging (see previous discussion). The late development (measured in years) of a secondary neoplastic tumor, such as osteosarcoma, in the field of irradiation is well documented. Disorganized osteoblastic changes superimposed on areas of osseous healing are indicative of the radiation-induced osteosarcoma.[1768]

Additional Types of Lesion. A *large cell (atypical) type* of Ewing's sarcoma has been described, representing approximately 6 to 13 per cent of all such sarcomas.[28, 1769] In addition to being of greater size, the tumor cells in this type of Ewing's sarcoma are more polymorphic, with conspicuous nucleoli and less diffuse nuclear chromatin. The large cell sarcoma usually is observed in patients in the first or second decade of life and is more common in males than in

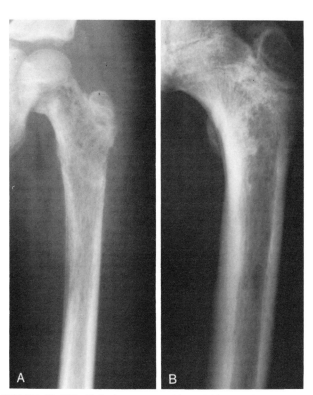

FIGURE 83–326. Ewing's sarcoma: Natural history—favorable response of tumor following radiation therapy.
A An initial radiograph shows the classic features of a Ewing's sarcoma in the diaphysis of the femur. These include permeative bone destruction, cortical erosion, and periostitis.
B The tumor was irradiated, and 6 years later, a routine radiograph shows reconstitution of the cortex and medullary bone sclerosis. (Courtesy of R. Stiles, M.D., Atlanta, Georgia.)

females. Localization in a tubular bone is most frequent (Fig. 83–327), and a permeative pattern of osteolysis is the dominant radiographic abnormality.[1769] Some examples of this tumor appear to represent neuroectodermal tumors.

A soft tissue neoplasm resembling Ewing's sarcoma *(extraskeletal Ewing's sarcoma)* also has been described.[1770–1777, 2359] Both men and women are affected, and the age of involved patients has varied from approximately 1 year to 60 or 65 years. Common sites of involvement are the thigh, paravertebral region, pelvis, and lower extremity (Figs. 83–328 and 83–329). Although a soft tissue mass represents the hallmark of the lesion, osseous changes including bone sclerosis and periosteal reaction may be evident. Owing to these changes in the bone, it is not always clear in an individual case whether the tumor originated in an extraosseous, periosteal,[1923] or intraosseous site (Fig. 83–330). Although the cytologic, histochemical (i.e., abundant cytoplasmic glycogen), and ultrastructural features of this neoplasm are similar to those of Ewing's sarcoma, it is the belief of some investigators[221] that until the histogenesis of this soft tissue tumor is clarified, it should not be termed a Ewing's sarcoma. Indeed, many of these extraskeletal tumors have been shown by immunohistochemistry or electron microscopy to represent soft tissue peripheral neuroectodermal tumors.

Neuroectodermal tumors initially were described by Askin and coworkers[2414] in 1979 as neoplasms of neuroectodermal origin that arose from the thoracopulmonary soft tissues in children and adolescents. Subsequent descriptions of this tumor (i.e., Askin tumor) documented its occurrence in the retroperitoneum and the soft tissues of the pelvis and extremities,[2415–2420] although a variety of terms (e.g., peripheral neuroblastoma, malignant neuroepithelioma, peripheral neuroepithelioma, and malignant peripheral neuroectodermal tumor) were used to describe it. In most reports, the identification of an intraosseous component of the lesion was believed to result from local invasion of the soft tissue neoplasm or from skeletal metastasis related to a distant neuroblastoma.

Primary (primitive) neuroectodermal tumors (PNET) of bone were described initially by Jaffe and collaborators[1699] in 1984. In their report, four patients between the ages of 3 and 12 years developed bone tumors that, in two cases, were unassociated with a soft tissue component. Although the neoplasms resembled Ewing's sarcoma on histologic analysis, their cells contained neuron-specific enolase and only a sparse amount of glycogen. Furthermore, when grown in tissue culture, each tumor was shown to produce neurite processes, a feature not seen in Ewing's sarcoma. The similarities between PNET and Ewing's sarcoma are great, however, and evidence exists that neuroectodermal-associated antigens may be found on Ewing's sarcoma cell lines.[2421] In experimental situations, neuronal expressions may be induced from the cells of a Ewing's sarcoma.[2422] Indeed, Ewing's sarcoma may constitute a more undifferentiated form of PNET of bone.[2422, 2423]

Analysis of available data indicate that PNET of bone affects mainly children, adolescents, and young adults. A male predominance appears likely. Common clinical manifestations include pain, a palpable mass, and in some cases fever. A relentless downhill course characterized by local recurrences of tumor following surgical excision, distant

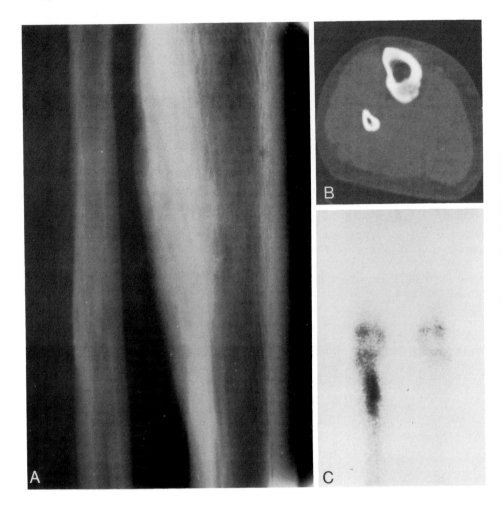

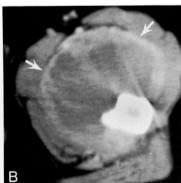

FIGURE 83–327. Ewing's sarcoma: Large cell (atypical) type. A 15 year old girl had calf pain of 8 months' duration. Physical examination revealed tenderness to palpation of the calf. A radiograph **(A)** shows cortical thickening and irregularity in the posterior surface of the diaphysis of the tibia. Transaxial CT **(B)** documents thickening of the cortex, radiolucent cortical regions, and increased attenuation in the marrow cavity. On the bone scan **(C)**, note increased accumulation of the radionuclide in the tibia. Biopsy confirmed the presence of a large cell type of Ewing's sarcoma.

FIGURE 83–328. Ewing's sarcoma: Extraskeletal soft tissue origin. This 20 year old woman developed an enlarging mass in the thigh. An oblique radiograph **(A)** shows the mass (arrows) containing ill-defined radiolucent areas. The femur appears normal. Transaxial CT **(B)** following the introduction of intravenous contrast material reveals enhancement of the margin of the soft tissue tumor (arrows). At surgery, the bone was found to be uninvolved. Microscopic and ultrastructural analysis documented the presence of an extraskeletal Ewing's sarcoma. (Courtesy of T. Broderick, M.D., Orange, California.)

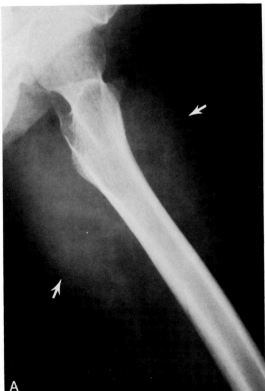

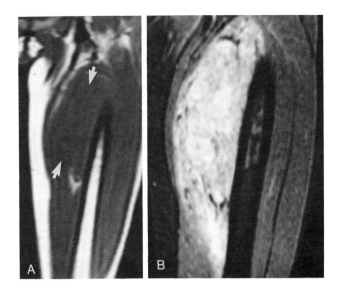

FIGURE 83–329. Ewing's sarcoma: Extraskeletal soft tissue origin. A prominent soft tissue mass developed gradually in the medial portion of the thigh in a 20 year old woman.

A A coronal T1-weighted (TR/TE, 600/16) spin echo MR image shows the mass (arrows) of low signal intensity.

B In a coronal short tau inversion recovery (STIR) MR image (TR/TE, 2000/20; inversion time, 150 msec), the tumor is of in-homogeneous but mainly high signal intensity. The femur appears to be uninvolved.

(Courtesy of M. Schweitzer, M.D., Philadelphia, Pennsylvania.)

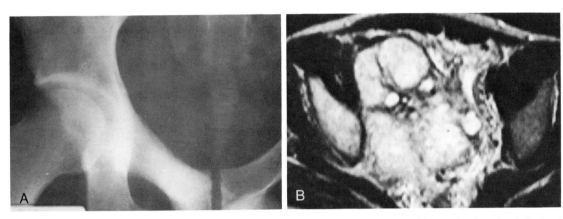

FIGURE 83–330. Ewing's sarcoma: Extraskeletal soft tissue versus skeletal origin. This 22 year old man developed pain in the right thigh, buttock, groin, and knee that progressed over an 18 month period. On physical examination, the mass was palpated easily.

A The routine radiograph shows bone sclerosis involving the right pubic bone and acetabular region.

B A transaxial T2-weighted (TR/TE, 2000/120) spin echo MR image shows the tumor of high signal intensity both in the soft tissues of the pelvis and in the acetabulum. Although the surgeon interpreted the operative findings as indicative of a soft tissue origin of the tumor, the precise site of origin in this case is not clear.

FIGURE 83–331. Primitive neuroectodermal tumor (PNET) of bone: Radiographic abnormalities—long tubular bones.

A A routine radiograph shows osteolytic lesions in the distal metaphysis and diaphysis of the tibia, associated with cortical erosion and soft tissue calcifications.

B In a sagittal T1-weighted (TR/TE, 400/20) spin echo MR image, the extent of the soft tissue involvement is more apparent. The intraosseous and extraosseous portions of the tumor are of low signal intensity.

(From Rousselin B, et al: Skel Radiol *18:*115, 1989.)

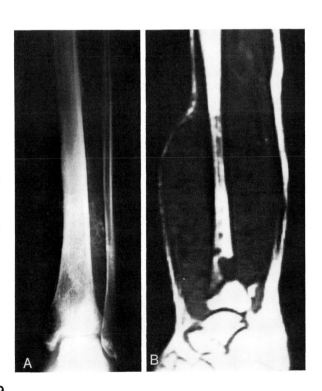

metastases (especially in the lungs and bones), and death is typical.

The most complete radiologic assessment of these tumors is provided in a report by Rousselin and associates.[2422] Involvement of the long tubular bones (40 per cent of cases), innominate bones and sacrum (30 per cent of cases), and ribs (20 per cent of cases) is most frequent. Involvement of the lower extremity is more common than that of the upper extremity, although scapular involvement occurs in about 5 per cent of cases. The imaging features resemble those of Ewing's sarcoma,[2424] with permeative bone destruction, periostitis, a soft tissue mass, and pathologic fracture encountered regularly (Figs. 83–331 to 83–333). When compared with Ewing's sarcoma, PNET of bone may reveal more frequent epiphyseal involvement and pathologic fractures and more frequent metastases.[2422, 2499–2505]

Neuroectodermal tumors may have a light microscopic morphology that is indistinguishable from Ewing's sarcoma with principal and dark cells, and cells with uniform, round to oval nuclei with powdery diffuse nuclear chromatin, indistinct cell borders, and cytoplasmic glygogen.[2502, 2503] However, most examples of neuroectodermal tumor contain cells with more atypical nuclei that are larger, with irregular contours and indentations, have a coarser and more irregularly distributed chromatin, and have nucleoli that may be prominent (Fig. 83–333E). The cells are compact and frequently divided into nests, lobules, or cords by fibrovascular septa. Some of the cases described as large cell or atypical variants of Ewing's sarcoma would currently be considered as examples of neuroectodermal tumor. Another characteristic histologic feature of neuroectodermal tumor is the occurrence of true rosettes and pseudorosettes (Fig. 83–333F–H). Although such rosette structures were described in Ewing's sarcoma and also occur in neuroblastomas, their presence would, under the correct clinical situation, indicate that the bone tumor is not a Ewing's tumor. Current opinion is that these rosettes are an indication of neural differentiation, which should not occur in classic Ewing's sarcoma because the latter is considered a primitive, undifferentiated tumor.

Electron microscopy of neuroectodermal tumors shows morphologic features of neural differentiation, including dendritic cell processes, abundant cytoplasmic organelles, intermediate filaments, microtubule formation, and neurosecretory granules. Immunohistochemical studies show reactivity of the tumor cells for a variety of neural markers.[2503–2505] However, because of the variable specificities of some of these markers, the exact immunohistochemical criteria required for the diagnosis of a neuroectodermal tumor still are unresolved. Some would require the presence of at least two different neural markers in the tumor in order for it to be designated as neuroectodermal in origin. The recently introduced antibody HBA-71 is reactive, as it is in Ewing's sarcoma, in over 90 per cent of neuroectodermal tumors, and this positivity helps to distinguish these two tumors from other small cell tumors, such as neuroblastoma, which are nonreactive with this antibody. Other antibodies common to Ewing's sarcoma and neuroectodermal tumor,[2506] as well as one that may distinguish between these two tumors,[2507] have been reported. Cytogenetic studies show that both Ewing's sarcoma and neuroectodermal tumor share a common chromosomal translocation.

Because Ewing's sarcoma and neuroectodermal tumor may, as indicated, share common light microscopic features, the diagnosis of neuroectodermal tumor of bone often depends on immunohistochemical or electron microscopic studies. This distinction is of clinical importance, as the prognosis of neuroectodermal tumor is poorer than that of Ewing's sarcoma.

TUMORS OF DENTAL ORIGIN AND RELATED LESIONS

The accurate analysis of tumors and tumor-like lesions in the mandible or maxilla presents a unique challenge. These bones may be affected by many of the neoplastic and neoplastic-like disorders that have been described throughout this chapter. Furthermore, the mandible and maxilla and the adjacent soft tissues are the specific locations for a diverse group of odontogenic and nonodontogenic tumors and cysts that have been described eloquently and in great detail in a number of textbooks of oral pathology.[1778–1782] Diagnostic difficulty in such cases relates not only to the seemingly overwhelming variety of processes but also to disagreement in their classification and to problems in obtaining adequate images of these bones. Routine radiography, panoramic techniques,[1783] conventional and computed tomography, and MR imaging are among the methods that have been advocated for delineating mandibular and maxillary lesions.

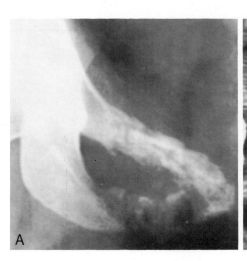
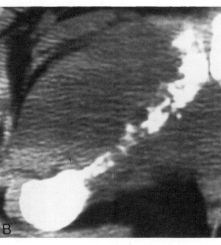

FIGURE 83–332. Primitive neuroectodermal tumor (PNET) of bone: Radiographic abnormalities—innominate bone.

A Note the osteolytic lesion of the pubic bone with pathologic fractures and a soft tissue mass.

B These features are better seen with transaxial CT.

(From Rousselin B, et al: Skel Radiol *18:*115, 1989.)

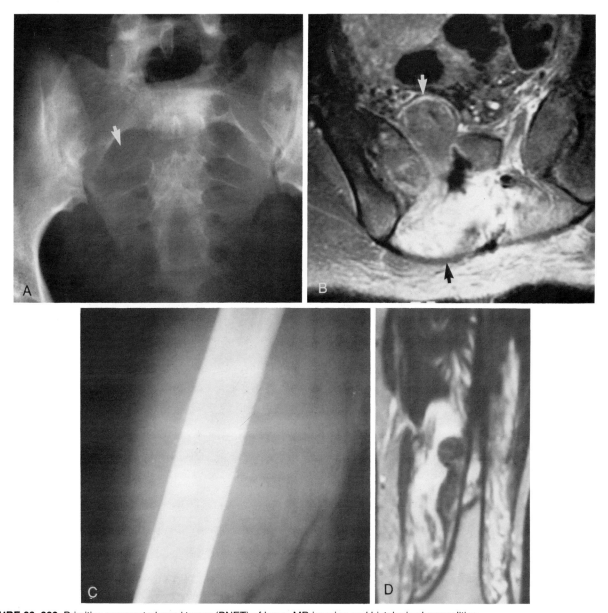

FIGURE 83–333. Primitive neuroectodermal tumor (PNET) of bone: MR imaging and histologic abnormalities.

A, B Sacrum. An initial radiograph **(A)** in a 17 year old girl shows subtle destruction (arrow) in the right side of the sacrum. A transaxial T1-weighted (TR/TE, 600/20) spin echo MR image **(B)** obtained with chemical presaturation of fat (ChemSat) after the intravenous injection of a gadolinium compound shows the extent of the tumor (arrows), which is of inhomogeneous signal intensity. When compared with its appearance prior to administration of a contrast agent, the tumor revealed definite enhancement of signal intensity.

C, D Femur. In a 20 year old man, a lateral radiograph **(C)** of the femur shows a large soft tissue mass extending both anteriorly and posteriorly, with minimal bone involvement. A coronal T2-weighted (TR/TE, 2550/90) spin echo MR image **(D)** reveals inhomogeneous but mainly high signal intensity in both the soft tissues and the bone. **(C, D** Courtesy of J. Kramer, M.D., Vienna, Austria.)

Illustration continued on following page

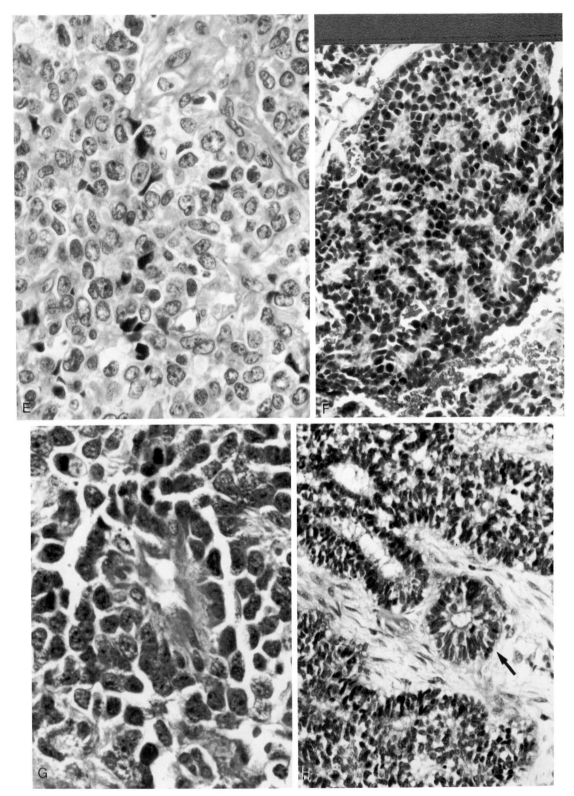

FIGURE 83–333 *Continued* **E** Cells in neuroectodermal tumor show nuclear variability in size and shape. Some nuclei have prominent nucleoli and nuclear grooves or indentations.

F Another example of neuroectodermal tumor with a field composed of several Homer-Wright pseudorosettes.

G View of pseudorosette shows circle of small, undifferentiated appearing cells with a central core of interdigitating fibrillary cytoplasmic projections.

H Neuroectodermal tumor with "true" rosettes (Flexner-Wintersteiner type) having a central lumen about which are cytoplasmic projections from the surrounding tumor cells (arrow).

It is beyond the scope of this chapter to describe in detail the many tumors and tumor-like lesions that affect these bones and adjacent soft tissues, and the interested reader should refer to other sources for such information. Rather, a few points of differential diagnosis are outlined and one tumor, the ameloblastoma, is emphasized owing to its relative frequency and characteristic radiographic abnormalities.

The roentgenographic approach to lesions of the jawbones generally is based on the precise location or radiographic characteristics of the process, or both. The diagnostic value provided by the location of the lesions is best exemplified by considering those that develop in intimate association with a tooth. Periapical processes (originating close to the apex or root of a tooth) include acute or chronic infections such as caries, abscesses, or granulomas; apical or radicular cysts (radiolucent lesions surrounded by a sclerotic margin); and condensing osteitis or sclerosing osteomyelitis (a small region of osteolysis and a wider zone of osteosclerosis). Pericoronal processes (arising about the crown of an erupting or unerupted tooth) (Fig. 83–334) are best represented by the dentigerous cyst (follicular or eruption cyst) that originates in the reduced enamel epithelium

about the crown of an unerupted or impacted tooth, often a third molar or cuspid.[1783] It produces a well-defined radiolucent area distributed symmetrically or asymmetrically about the crown and may become quite prominent and even expansile. Less common examples of pericoronal processes[1783] include ameloblastic fibromas, ameloblastic fibro-odontomas (Fig. 83–334A), calcifying epithelial odontogenic tumors (Pindborg tumor),[1784] adenomatoid odontogenic tumor (adenoameloblastoma), and keratinizing and calcifying odontogenic cysts[1785, 1786] (Fig. 83–334B).

The second diagnostic approach, based on the principal radiographic appearance of the process, has been well summarized by Eversole and Rovin.[1787] Lesions that contain predominantly radiolucent areas, those that contain predominantly radiopacified areas, and those that have both types of regions can be identified. A number of specific cystic lesions produce single or multiple radiolucent areas with relatively distinct borders. Among these are the Stafne developmental cyst (a stable, well-defined, round or elliptical cavity occurring in the angle of the mandible that may contain salivary gland tissue)[1788, 1789] (Fig. 83–335A), the primordial cyst (a round or oval, well-marginated lesion that arises from cystic degeneration of a developing tooth,

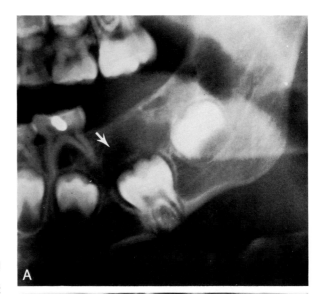

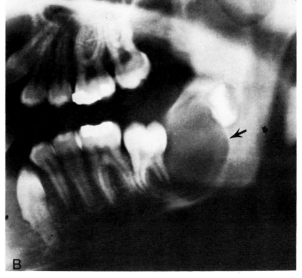

FIGURE 83–334. Gnathic tumors and tumor-like lesions: Pericoronal processes—mandible.

A Ameloblastic fibro-odontoma. Note a large pericoronal radiolucent area (arrow) about an unerupted tooth.

B Calcifying odontogenic cyst (Gorlin's cyst). A large, well-defined radiolucent lesion is observed (arrow).

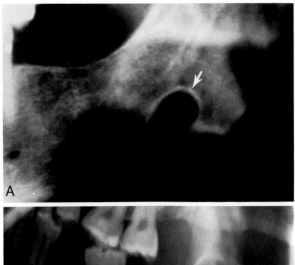

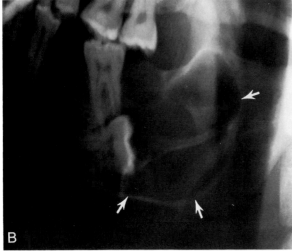

FIGURE 83–335. Gnathic tumors and tumor-like lesions: Single or multiple radiolucent areas—mandible.

A Stafne developmental cyst. A well-marginated lesion (arrow) is located in the posterior portion of the mandible.

B Odontogenic keratocyst. A large lesion (arrows) arises adjacent to an impacted molar tooth.

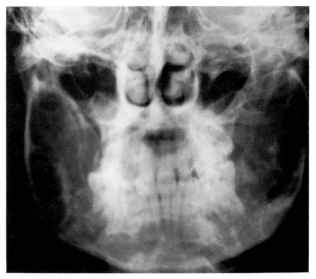

FIGURE 83–336. Gnathic tumors and tumor-like lesions: Single or multiple radiolucent areas—mandible. Cherubism. Note bilateral, symmetric expansile lesions of the mandible. (Courtesy of M. Pathria, M.D., San Diego, California.)

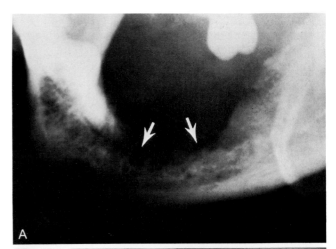

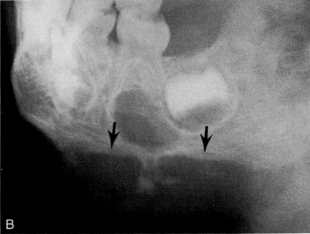

FIGURE 83–337. Gnathic tumors and tumor-like lesions: Ill-defined radiolucent areas—mandible.

A Squamous cell carcinoma. Poorly defined osteolysis (arrows) relates to invasion from a neighboring squamous cell carcinoma.

B Juvenile fibromatosis. Note erosion of the inferior surface of the mandible (arrows).

(Courtesy of D. J. Sartoris, M.D., San Diego, California.)

especially in the region of the third molar of the mandible and at sites of supernumerary teeth),[1783] the incisive canal cyst or median anterior maxillary cyst (a heart-shaped radiolucent lesion located between the roots of the central incisors of the maxilla),[1783] the median mandibular cyst (a well-defined cystic lesion located between the central incisors of the mandible),[1790, 1791] and the globulomaxillary cyst (a lesion that arises between the roots of the maxillary lateral incisors and cuspids).

Multilocular cystic areas may be related to osteomyelitis, fibrous dysplasia, traumatic cysts, odontogenic keratocyst (Fig. 83–335B) or nonkeratocyst, ameloblastoma (see later discussion), aneurysmal bone cyst, hemangioma, cherubism (familial fibrous dysplasia transmitted as an autosomal dominant trait that becomes manifest in childhood as bilateral osseous expansion and usually stabilizes in adolescence)[1792, 1793, 1867] (Fig. 83–336), giant cell reparative granuloma, and additional lesions described previously in this chapter.

Ill-defined regions of osteolysis in the mandible or maxilla may indicate osteomyelitis, skeletal metastasis (relatively rare in the jawbones), histiocytosis, plasma cell myeloma, radiation necrosis, lymphoma, leukemia, adjacent squamous cell carcinoma (Fig. 83–337A), fibromatosis (Fig. 83–337B), and primary bone sarcomas.[1794]

Periapical lesions that are opacified include focal condensing osteitis, hypercementosis (related to excessive deposition of cementum on the roots of the teeth, occurring on an idiopathic basis or in association with Paget's disease or Gardner's syndrome), benign cementoblastoma or true cementoma (of variable size, although sometimes large, occurring in adolescents and young adults, and leading to either a mixed radiolucent and radiodense focus or a purely opacified area)[1795] (Fig. 83–338A), and cemento-ossifying fibroma (arising in young adults, slowly progressing, and

involving the mandible in the area of the molar teeth)[1783] (Fig. 83–338B).

Multiple discrete or diffuse radiopaque regions may relate to sclerosing osteomyelitis, osteomas (with or without Gardner's syndrome), osteosarcoma, Paget's disease, fibrous dysplasia (Fig. 83–339), skeletal metastases, primary bone sarcomas (e.g., osteosarcoma, chondrosarcoma), and congenital disorders (e.g., osteopetrosis, van Buchem's disease, craniometaphyseal dysplasias). Trabecular abnormalities may accompany hemangiomas (Fig. 83–340A) and odontogenic myxomas (Fig. 83–340B,C).

The odontomas, which consist of several different types, usually are encountered in young patients. Although this lesion is partly radiolucent, central opaque regions may be identified owing to the capability of the tumor cells to elaborate dental tissues, including dentin, pulp, and cementum.[1783] The radiographic appearance is variable; initially, the lesion may be entirely osteolytic, but subsequently it becomes partially opacified (target lesion consisting of a central radiodense area and a radiolucent halo) or completely opacified (Fig. 83–341).

Locally Aggressive or Malignant Tumors

Ameloblastoma

An ameloblastoma is an invasive tumor of unknown origin that affects the mandible (in the region of the molar teeth and ramus or, less commonly, the symphysis) and, far less frequently, the maxilla (in the area of the maxillary sinus).[1796] Most patients with this tumor are adults, and many are in the fourth and fifth decades of life; however, children are affected not infrequently. The lesion is seen with approximately equal frequency in men and women. Clinical findings include a gradually enlarging mass with or without pain. Early diagnosis is important as invasion of surrounding structures, distant metastasis, and progressive facial deformity may occur. If left untreated, the tumor may become massive.[1797, 1868, 2360]

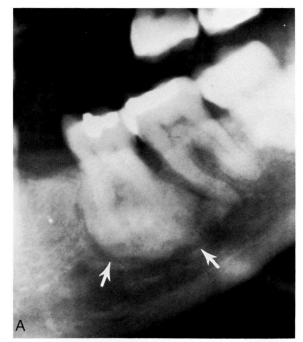

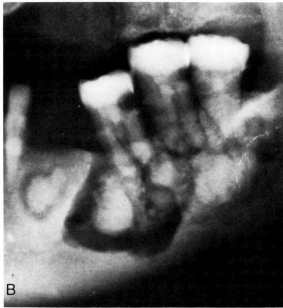

FIGURE 83–338. Gnathic tumors and tumor-like lesions: Single or multiple radiodense areas—mandible.

A Benign cementoblastoma. Observe a well-defined region of increased density (arrows) fused to the apex of a vital first molar tooth. There is a thin radiolucent band about the lesion.

B Cemento-ossifying fibroma. This bizarre lesion is associated with multiple radiodense foci in the region of the molar teeth.

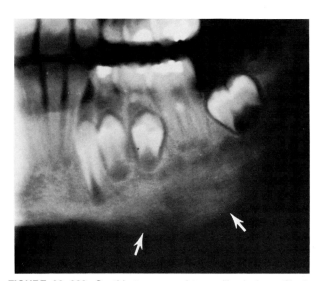

FIGURE 83–339. Gnathic tumors and tumor-like lesions: Single, multiple, or diffuse radiodense areas—fibrous dysplasia (mandible). A hazy, radiodense, expansile lesion (arrows) represents fibrous dysplasia.

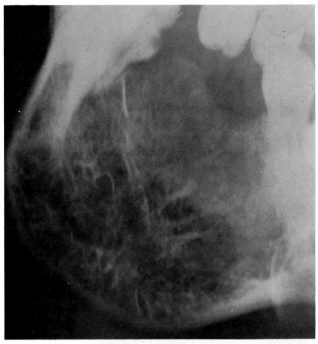

FIGURE 83–340. Gnathic tumors and tumor-like lesions: Trabeculated areas—mandible.

A Hemangioma. A large, expansile lesion contains a radiating trabecular pattern.

B, C Odontogenic myxoma. A similar radiographic pattern **(B)** to that in **A** is seen. A sagittal T2-weighted spin echo MR image **(C)** shows increased signal intensity within the lesion.

A

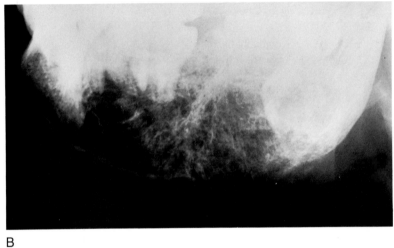

B

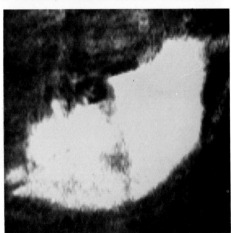

C

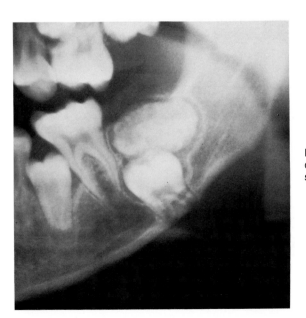

FIGURE 83–341. Gnathic tumors and tumor-like lesions: Odontoma—mandible. A radiodense lesion arises adjacent to an unerupted molar tooth. It is surrounded by a radiolucent band.

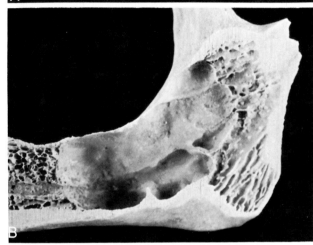

FIGURE 83–342. Ameloblastoma: Radiographic abnormalities. A radiograph **(A)** and photograph **(B)** of a sagittal section of the mandible show a multilocular, slightly expansile, cystic lesion in the angle of the bone.

A radiolucent, unilocular or multilocular cystic lesion with cortical expansion (Fig. 83–342) is typical.[1798, 1799] The margin of the lesion may be scalloped, and resorption of the root or roots of neighboring teeth may be identified. Recurrent lesions may appear even more aggressive, with

perforation of the cortical plate. CT may allow more precise delineation of the full extent of the primary or recurrent tumor[1800] (Fig. 83–343). MR imaging may reveal a multilocular or unilocular lesion with a mixed pattern of solid and cystic components.[2361] Although low signal intensity in

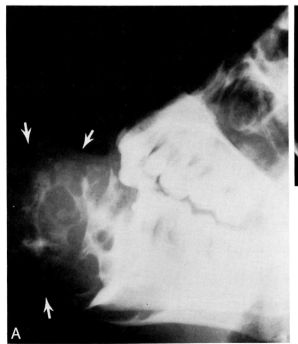

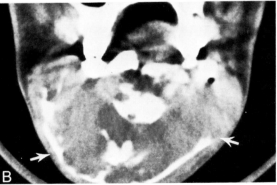

FIGURE 83–343. Ameloblastoma: Radiographic and CT abnormalities. This 28 year old man had a 2 year history of painless swelling of the anterior portion of the mandible. He sought cosmetic relief. Routine radiography **(A)** and a coronal CT scan **(B)** show a large, very expansile, trabeculated lesion (arrows). Biopsy and subsequent resection of the tumor confirmed the presence of an ameloblastoma.

T1-weighted spin echo MR images and high signal intensity in T2-weighted spin echo MR images are typical features of the cystic areas, high signal intensity in T1-weighted images also is encountered. Following the intravenous administration of a gadolinium compound, enhancement of signal intensity in the solid portions of the tumor, including papillary projections, walls, and septa, is seen.[2361]

There are five major histologic types of ameloblastoma: follicular, plexiform, basal cell, acanthomatous, and granular cell[1783]; the follicular type usually is reported to be the most common,[1799] the plexiform type occurs more frequently in the maxilla,[1783] and the granular cell type represents the lesion that is most capable of metastasizing.[1801] There generally is little correlation between the radiographic and the histologic appearance of the lesion; however, it has been suggested that follicular ameloblastomas are multilocular, and plexiform ameloblastomas are unilocular.[1869]

The source of the cells within this tumor is unknown; they may originate from the epithelial lining of an odontogenic cyst, the dental lamina or enamel, the stratified squamous epithelium of the oral cavity, or the dental epithelial remnants.[1802, 1803]

SUMMARY

Many tumors and tumor-like lesions may involve bone. Accurate diagnosis of these lesions requires close cooperation among the orthopedic surgeon, radiologist, and pathologist. The patient's age and the site of skeletal localization are fundamental to the proper interpretation of the abnormalities as detected with routine radiography and specialized imaging techniques. In many instances, however, a single diagnosis cannot be offered on the basis of such abnormalities, and careful histologic analysis is required.

References

1. Steel HH: Calcified islands in medullary bone. J Bone Joint Surg [Am] 32:405, 1950.
2. Kim SK, Barry WF Jr: Bone island. AJR 92:1301, 1964.
3. Onitsuka H: Roentgenologic aspects of bone islands. Radiology 123:607, 1977.
4. Ackerman W, Schwarz GS: Non-neoplastic sclerosis in vertebral bodies. Cancer 11:703, 1958.
5. Broderick TW, Resnick D, Goergen TG, et al: Enostosis of the spine. Spine 3:167, 1978.
6. Smith J: Giant bone islands. Radiology 107:35, 1973.
7. Ngan H: Growing bone islands. Clin Radiol 23:199, 1972.
8. Blank N, Lieber A: The significance of growing bone islands. Radiology 85:508, 1965.
9. Resnick D, Nemcek AA Jr, Haghighi P: Spinal enostoses (bone islands). Radiology 147:373, 1983.
10. Lagier R, Nussle D: Anatomy and radiology of a bone island. ROFO 128:261, 1978.
11. Lagier R, Mbakop A, Bigler A: Osteopoikilosis: A radiological and pathological study. Skel Radiol 11:161, 1984.
12. Jaffe HL: Osteoid osteoma, a benign osteoblastic tumor composed of osteoid and atypical bone. Arch Surg 31:709, 1935.
13. Schajowicz F, Lemos C: Osteoid osteoma and osteoblastoma: Closely related entities of osteoblastic derivation. Acta Orthop Scand 41:272, 1970.
14. Orlowski JP, Mercer RD: Osteoid osteoma in children and young adults. Pediatrics 59:526, 1977.
15. Habermann ET, Stern RE: Osteoid-osteoma of the tibia in an eight-month-old boy. A case report. J Bone Joint Surg [Am] 56:633, 1974.
16. Cohen MD, Harrington TM, Ginsbury WW: Osteoid osteoma: 95 cases and a review of the literature. Semin Arthritis Rheum 12:265, 1983.
17. Wiss DA, Reid BS: Painless osteoid osteoma of the fingers. Report of three cases. J Hand Surg 8:914, 1983.
18. Golding JSR: The natural history of osteoid osteoma with a report of twenty cases. J Bone Joint Surg [Br] 36:218, 1954.
19. Sherman MS, McFarland G: Mechanism of pain in osteoid osteoma. South Med J 58:163, 1965.
20. Schulman L, Dorfman HD: Nerve fibers in osteoid osteoma. J Bone Joint Surg [Am] 52:1351, 1970.
21. Esquerdo J, Fernandez CF, Gomar F: Pain in osteoid osteoma: Histological facts. Acta Orthop Scand 47:520, 1976.
22. Halperin N, Gadoth N, Reif R, et al: Osteoid osteoma of the proximal femur simulating spinal root compression. Clin Orthop 162:191, 1982.
23. Jaffe HL: Osteoid-osteoma of bone. Radiology 45:319, 1945.
24. Jaffe HL: Osteoid-osteoma. Proc R Soc Med 46:1007, 1953.
25. Byers PD: Solitary benign osteoblastic lesions of bone. Osteoid osteoma and benign osteoblastoma. Cancer 22:43, 1968.
26. Dias L, Forst HM: Osteoid osteoma—osteoblastoma. Cancer 33:1075, 1974.
27. Swee RG, McLeod RA, Beabout JW: Osteoid osteoma. Detection, diagnosis, and localization. Radiology 130:117, 1979.
28. Mirra JM: Bone tumors. Diagnosis and treatment. Philadelphia, JB Lippincott Co, 1980.
29. Jackson RP, Reckling FW, Mantz FA: Osteoid osteoma and osteoblastoma. Similar histologic lesions with different natural histories. Clin Orthop 128:303, 1977.
30. Dahlin DC: Bone Tumors. General Aspects and Data on 6,221 Cases. 3rd Ed. Springfield, Ill, Charles C Thomas, 1978.
31. Sherman MS: Osteoid osteoma associated with changes in adjacent joint. Report of two cases. J Bone Joint Surg 29:483, 1947.
32. Freiberger RH, Loitman BS, Helpern M, et al: Osteoid osteoma: A report on 80 cases. AJR 82:194, 1959.
33. Huvos AG: Bone Tumors. Diagnosis, Treatment and Prognosis. Philadelphia, WB Saunders Co, 1979.
34. Schajowicz F: Tumors and Tumorlike Lesions of Bones and Joints. New York, Springer-Verlag, 1981.
35. Maclellan DI, Wilson FC: Osteoid osteoma of the spine. A review of the literature and report of six new cases. J Bone Joint Surg [Am] 49:111, 1967.
36. Paus BC, Kim TK: Osteoid osteoma of the spine. Acta Orthop Scand 33:24, 1963.
37. Keim HA, Reina EG: Osteoid-osteoma as a cause of scoliosis. J Bone Joint Surg [Am] 57:159, 1975.
38. Heiman ML, Cooley CJ, Bradford DS: Osteoid osteoma of a vertebral body. Report of a case with extension across the intervertebral disk. Clin Orthop 118:159, 1976.
39. Fielding JW, Keim HA, Hawkins RJ, et al: Osteoid osteoma of the cervical spine. Clin Orthop 128:163, 1977.
40. Francis WR Jr, Einhorn T, Fielding JW: Osteoid osteoma of the thoracic spine: Report of a case. Clin Orthop 149:175, 1980.
41. Janin Y, Epstein JA, Carras R, et al: Osteoid osteomas and osteoblastomas of the spine. Neurosurgery 8:31, 1981.
42. Zwimpfer TJ, Tucker WS, Faulkner JF: Osteoid osteoma of the cervical spine: Case reports and literature review. Can J Surg 25:637, 1982.
43. Kirwan EO, Hutton PAN, Pozo JL, et al: Osteoid osteoma and benign osteoblastoma of the spine. J Bone Joint Surg [Br] 66:21, 1984.
44. Carroll RE: Osteoid osteoma in the hand. J Bone Joint Surg [Am] 35:888, 1953.
45. Giannikas A, Papachristou G, Tiniakos G, et al: Osteoid osteoma of the terminal phalanges. Hand 9:295, 1977.
46. Ghiam GF, Bora FW Jr: Osteoid osteoma of the carpal bones. J Hand Surg 3:280, 1978.
47. Shereff MJ, Cullivan WT, Johnson KA: Osteoid-osteoma of the foot. J Bone Joint Surg [Am] 65:638, 1983.
48. Levy Y, Rosenheck S, Torok G, et al: Osteoid osteoma of the distal phalanx of the thumb. Acta Orthop Scand 50:667, 1979.
49. Herndon JH, Eaton RG, Littler JW: Carpal-tunnel syndrome. An unusual presentation of osteoid-osteoma of the capitate. J Bone Joint Surg [Am] 56:1715, 1974.
50. Riester J, Mosher JF: Osteoid osteoma of the capitate: A case report. J Hand Surg [Am] 9:278, 1984.
51. Szabo RM, Smith B: Possible congenital osteoid-osteoma of a phalanx. A case report. J Bone Joint Surg [Am] 67:815, 1985.
52. Lamb DW, Del Castillo F: Phalangeal osteoid osteoma in the hand. Hand 13:291, 1981.
53. Hundley JD: Osteoid osteoma of the trapezium. Clin Orthop 116:170, 1976.
54. Rosenfeld K, Bora FW, Lane JM: Osteoid osteoma of the hamate. A case report and review of the literature. J Bone Joint Surg [Am] 55:1085, 1973.
55. Bordelon RL, Cracco A, Book MK: Osteoid-osteoma producing premature fusion of the epiphysis of the distal phalanx of the big toe. A case report. J Bone Joint Surg [Am] 57:120, 1975.
56. Jensen EG: Osteoid osteoma of the capitate bone. Hand 11:102, 1979.
57. Prabhakar B, Reddy R, Dayananda B, et al: Osteoid osteoma of the skull. J Bone Joint Surg [Br] 54:146, 1972.
58. Daly JG: Osteoid osteoma of the skull. Br J Radiol 46:392, 1973.
59. Munk J, Peyser E, Gellei B: Osteoid osteoma of the frontal bone. Br J Radiol 33:328, 1960.
60. Foss EL, Dockerty MB, Good CA: Osteoid osteoma of the mandible. Cancer 8:592, 1955.
61. Klein MJ, Lusskin R, Becker MH, et al: Osteoid osteoma of the clavicle. Clin Orthop 143:162, 1979.
62. Gamba JL, McCollum DE, Martinez S: Osteoid osteoma of the clavicle: A case report and review of the literature. Rev Interam Radiol 8:65, 1983.

63. Kehl DK, Alonso JE, Lovell WW: Scoliosis secondary to an osteoid-osteoma of the rib. A case report. J Bone Joint Surg [Am] 65:701, 1983.
64. McGuire MH, Mankin HJ: Osteoid osteoma: An unusual presentation as a rib lesion. A case report. Orthopedics 7:305, 1984.
65. Worland RL, Dick HM: Osteoid-osteoma of the radius. Report of a case. Clin Orthop 106:189, 1975.
66. Greenspan A, Elguezabel A, Bryk D: Multifocal osteoid osteoma. A case report and review of the literature. AJR 121:103, 1974.
67. Glynn JJ, Lichtenstein L: Osteoid-osteoma with multicentric nidus. A report of two cases. J Bone Joint Surg [Am] 55:855, 1973.
68. Alcalay M, Clarac JP, Bontoux D: Double osteoid-osteoma in adjacent carpal bones. A case report. J Bone Joint Surg [Am] 64:799, 1982.
69. O'Dell CW Jr, Resnick D, Niwayama G, et al: Osteoid osteomas arising in adjacent bones: Report of a case. J Can Assoc Radiol 27:298, 1976.
70. Apple DF, Loughlin EC Jr: Osteoid osteoma of the ankle in an athlete. Am J Sports Med 9:254, 1981.
71. Beerman PJ, Crowe JE, Summer TE, et al: Case report 164. Skel Radiol 7:71, 1981.
72. Seitz WH Jr, Dick HM: Intraepiphyseal osteoid osteoma of the distal femur in an 8-year-old girl. J Pediatr Orthop 3:505, 1983.
73. Giustra PE, Freiberger RH: Severe growth disturbance with osteoid osteoma. A report of two cases involving the femoral neck. Radiology 96:285, 1970.
74. Norman A, Dorfman HD: Osteoid-osteoma inducing pronounced overgrowth and deformity of bone. Clin Orthop 110:233, 1975.
75. Kattapuram SV, Kushner DC, Phillips WC, et al: Osteoid osteoma: An unusual cause of articular pain. Radiology 147:383, 1983.
76. Corbett JM, Wilde AH, McCormack LJ, et al: Intra-articular osteoid osteoma. A diagnostic problem. Clin Orthop 98:225, 1974.
77. Cronemeyer RL, Kirchmer NA, DeSmet AA, et al: Intra-articular osteoid-osteoma of the humerus simulating synovitis of the elbow. A case report. J Bone Joint Surg [Am] 63:1172, 1981.
78. Snarr JW, Abell MR, Martel W: Lymphofollicular synovitis with osteoid osteoma. Radiology 106:557, 1973.
79. Séruzier E, Simonin JL, Ducastelle C, et al: Ostéome Ostéoïde avec synovite. A propos de deux observations. Rev Rhum Mal Osteoartic 43:521, 1976.
80. Bussiere JL, Sauvezie B, Lopitaux R, et al: Ostéome ostéoïde avec synovite d'allure rhumatöide. Rev Rhum Mal Osteoartic 43:651, 1976.
81. Norman A, Abdelwahab IF, Buyon K, et al: Osteoid osteoma of the hip simulating an early onset of osteoarthritis. Radiology 158:417, 1986.
82. Goldberg VM, Jacobs B: Osteoid osteoma of the hip in children. Clin Orthop 106:41, 1975.
83. Clark CR, Ozonoff MB, Drennan JC: Case report 157. Skel Radiol 6:286, 1981.
84. Caldicott WJH: Diagnosis of spinal osteoid osteoma. Radiology 92:1192, 1969.
85. Mehta MH: Pain provoked scoliosis. Observations on the evolution of the deformity. Clin Orthop 135:58, 1978.
86. Mehta MH, Murray RO: Scoliosis provoked by painful vertebral lesions. Skel Radiol 1:223, 1977.
87. Ransford AO, Pozo JL, Hutton PAN, et al: The behavior pattern of the scoliosis associated with osteoid osteoma or osteoblastoma of the spine. J Bone Joint Surg [Br] 66:16, 1984.
88. McConnell JR, Daneman A: Fatty replacement of muscles adjacent to spinal osteoid osteoma. J Comput Assist Tomogr 8:147, 1984.
89. Gamba JL, Martinez S, Apple J, et al: Computed tomography of axial skeletal osteoid osteomas. AJR 142:769, 1984.
90. Nelson OA, Greer RB III: Localization of osteoid-osteoma of the spine using computerized tomography. A case report. J Bone Joint Surg [Am] 65:263, 1983.
91. Blery M, LeRoux B: Ostéome ostéoïde vertébral. A propos de six cas. Ann Radiol 21:59, 1978.
92. Lundeen MA, Herring JA: Osteoid-osteoma of the spine: Sclerosis in two levels. J Bone Joint Surg [Am] 62:476, 1980.
93. Fehring TK, Green NE: Negative radionuclide scan in osteoid osteoma. A case report. Clin Orthop 185:245, 1984.
94. Smith FW, Gilday DL: Scintigraphic appearances of osteoid osteoma. Radiology 137:191, 1980.
95. Lisbona R, Rosenthall L: Role of radionuclide imaging in osteoid osteoma. AJR 132:77, 1979.
96. Gore DR, Mueller HA: Osteoid-osteoma of the spine with localization aided by 99mTc-polyphosphate bone scan. Case report. Clin Orthop 113:132, 1975.
97. Winter PF, Johnson PM, Hilal SK, et al: Scintigraphic detection of osteoid osteoma. Radiology 122:177, 1977.
98. Helms CA, Hattner RS, Vogler JB III: Osteoid osteoma: Radionuclide diagnosis. Radiology 151:779, 1984.
99. Israeli A, Zwas ST, Horoszowski H, et al: Use of radionuclide method in preoperative and intraoperative diagnosis of osteoid osteoma of the spine. Case report. Clin Orthop 175:194, 1983.
100. Rinsky LA, Goris M, Bleck EE, et al: Intraoperative skeletal scintigraphy for localization of osteoid-osteoma in the spine. Case report. J Bone Joint Surg [Am] 62:143, 1980.
101. Simons GW, Sty J: Intraoperative bone imaging in the treatment of osteoid osteoma of the femoral neck. J Pediatr Orthop 3:399, 1983.
102. Sty J, Simons G: Intraoperative 99m-technetium bone imaging in treatment of benign osteoblastic tumors. Clin Orthop 165:223, 1982.

103. Ghelman B, Thompson FM, Arnold WD: Intraoperative radioactive localization of osteoid osteoma. J Bone Joint Surg [Am] 63:826, 1981.
104. Ghelman B, Vigorita VJ: Postoperative radionuclide evaluation of osteoid osteomas. Radiology 146:509, 1983.
105. O'Brien TM, Murray TE, Malone LA, et al: Osteoid osteoma: Excision with scintimetric guidance. Radiology 153:543, 1984.
106. Papanicolaou N: Osteoid osteoma: Operative confirmation of complete removal by bone scintigraphy. Radiology 154:821, 1985.
107. Omojola MF, Cockshott WP, Beatty EG: Osteoid osteoma: An evaluation of diagnostic modalities. Clin Radiol 32:199, 1981.
108. Gamba JL, Apple JS, Martinez S: Current concepts in the radiographic evaluation of osteoid osteoma. Rev Interam Radiol 8:53, 1983.
109. Howie JL: CT of osteoid osteoma of the femoral neck: The value of oblique reformatting. J Can Assoc Radiol 36:254, 1985.
110. Kumar SJ, Harcke HT, MacEwan GD, et al: Osteoid osteoma of the proximal femur: New techniques in diagnosis and treatment. J Pediatr Orthop 4:669, 1984.
111. Herrlin K, Ekelund L, Lovdahl R, et al: Computed tomography in suspected osteoid osteoma of tubular bones. Skel Radiol 9:92, 1982.
112. Lechner G, Riedl P, Knahr K, et al: Das angiographische Bild des Osteoid-Osteoms. ROFO 122:323, 1975.
113. Lechner G, Knahr K, Riedl P: Das osteoid-osteom. ROFO 128:511, 1978.
114. O'Hara JP III, Tegtmeyer C, Sweet DE, et al: Angiography in the diagnosis of osteoid-osteoma of the hand. J Bone Joint Surg [Am] 57:163, 1975.
115. Lateur L, Baert AL: Localization and diagnosis of osteoid osteoma of the carpal area by angiography. Skel Radiol 2:75, 1977.
116. Tanaka C, Fujiwara Y, Yamamuro T, et al: Intraperiosteal osteoid osteoma. A case report. Clin Orthop 175:190, 1983.
117. Ponseti I, Barta CK: Osteoid osteoma. J Bone Joint Surg 29:767, 1947.
118. Sherman MS: Osteoid osteoma. Review of the literature and report of thirty cases. J Bone Joint Surg 29:918, 1947.
119. Pritchard JE, McKay JW: Osteoid osteoma. Can Med Assoc J 58:567, 1948.
120. Jaffe HL, Lichtenstein L: Osteoid-osteoma: Further experience with this benign tumor of bone. J Bone Joint Surg 22:645, 1940.
121. Steiner GC: Ultrastructure of osteoid osteoma. Hum Pathol 7:309, 1976.
122. Broderick T, Resnick D, Usselman J: Case report 123. Skel Radiol 5:193, 1980.
123. Norman A: Persistence or recurrence of pain: A sign of surgical failure in osteoid-osteoma. Clin Orthop 130:263, 1978.
124. Morrison GM, Hawes LE, Sacco JJ: Incomplete removal of osteoid-osteoma. Am J Surg 80:476, 1950.
125. Worland RL, Ryder CT, Johnston AD: Recurrent osteoid-osteoma. Report of a case. J Bone Joint Surg [Am] 57:277, 1975.
126. Sim FH, Dahlin DC, Beabout JW: Osteoid-osteoma: Diagnostic problems. J Bone Joint Surg [Am] 57:154, 1975.
127. Saville PD: A medical option for the treatment of osteoid osteoma. Arthritis Rheum 23:1409, 1980.
128. Vickers SW, Pugh DC, Ivins JC: Osteoid osteoma: A 15 year follow-up of an untreated patient. J Bone Joint Surg [Am] 41:357, 1959.
129. Moberg E: The natural course of osteoid osteoma. J Bone Joint Surg [Am] 33:166, 1951.
130. Dahlin DC, Johnson EW Jr: Giant osteoid osteoma. J Bone Joint Surg [Am] 36:559, 1954.
131. Golding JSR, Sissons HA: Osteogenic fibroma of bone. Report of 2 cases. J Bone Joint Surg [Br] 36:428, 1954.
132. Kirkpatrick HJR, Murray RC: Osteogenic fibroma of bone: Report of a case. J Bone Joint Surg [Br] 37:606, 1955.
133. Jaffe HL: Benign osteoblastoma. Bull Hosp J Dis 17:141, 1956.
134. Lichtenstein L: Benign osteoblastoma: Category of osteoid- and bone-forming tumors other than classical osteoid osteoma, which may be mistaken for giant-cell tumor or osteogenic sarcoma. Cancer 9:1044, 1956.
135. McLeod RA, Dahlin DC, Beabout JW: The spectrum of osteoblastoma. AJR 126:321, 1976.
136. Tonai M, Campbell CJ, Ahn GH, et al: Osteoblastoma: Classification and report of 16 patients. Clin Orthop 167:222, 1982.
137. Marsh BW, Bonfiglio M, Brady LP, et al: Benign osteoblastoma: Range of manifestations. J Bone Joint Surg [Am] 57:1, 1975.
138. Dorfman HD, Weiss SW: Borderline osteoblastic tumors: Problems in the differential diagnosis of aggressive osteoblastoma and low-grade osteosarcoma. Semin Diagn Pathol 1:215, 1984.
139. The Netherlands Committee on Bone Tumours: Radiological Atlas of Bone Tumors. Vols I and II. The Hague, Mouton and Co, 1966, 1973.
140. Giannestras NJ, Diamond JR: Benign osteoblastoma of the talus. A review of the literature and report of a case. J Bone Joint Surg [Am] 40:469, 1958.
141. Schein AJ: Osteoblastoma of the scapula. A case report. J Bone Joint Surg [Am] 41:359, 1959.
142. Rosensweig J, Pintar K, Mikail M, et al: Benign osteoblastoma (giant osteoid osteoma): Report of an unusual rib tumour and review of the literature. Can Med Assoc J 89:1189, 1963.
143. Yllanes H, Compere EL: Benign osteoblastoma. A rare tumor involving the humerus of a 5-year-old boy. Clin Orthop 42:147, 1965.
144. Kent JN, Castro HF, Girotti WR: Benign osteoblastoma of the maxilla. Case report and review of the literature. Oral Surg 27:209, 1969.
145. Tulloh HP, Harry D: Osteoblastoma in a rib in childhood. Clin Radiol 20:337, 1969.

146. DiGiglia JW, Bradford JK, Leonard GL, et al: Benign osteoblastoma of the rib: Report of a case. South Med J 64:624, 1971.

147. Brady CL, Browne RM: Benign osteoblastoma of the mandible. Cancer 30:329, 1972.

148. Fu YS, Perzin KH: Non-epithelial tumors of the nasal cavity, paranasal sinuses, and nasopharynx: A clinicopathologic study. II. Osseous and fibro-osseous lesions, including osteoma, fibrous dysplasia, ossifying fibroma, osteoblastoma, giant cell tumor, and osteosarcoma. Cancer 33:1289, 1974.

149. Greenspan A, Elquezabal A, Bryk D: Benign osteoblastoma of a rib. J Can Assoc Radiol 26:208, 1975.

150. Freedman SR: Benign osteoblastoma of the ethmoid bone. Report of a case. Am J Clin Pathol 63:391, 1975.

151. Farman AG, Nortje CJ, Grotepass F: Periosteal benign osteoblastoma of the mandible. Report of a case and review of the literature pertaining to benign osteoblastic neoplasms of the jaw. Br J Oral Surg 14:12, 1976.

152. Khermosh O, Schujman E: Benign osteoblastoma of the calcaneus. Clin Orthop 127:197, 1977.

153. Greer RO Jr, Berman DN: Osteoblastoma of the jaws: Current concepts and differential diagnosis. J Oral Surg 36:304, 1978.

154. Chatterji P, Purohit GN, Bikaner INR: Benign osteoblastoma of the maxilla (periosteal). J Laryngol Otol 92:337, 1978.

155. Black JA, Levick RK, Sharrard WJW: Osteoid osteoma and benign osteoblastoma in childhood. Arch Dis Child 54:459, 1979.

156. Tom LWC, Lowry LD, Quinn-Bogard A: Benign osteoblastoma of the maxillary sinus. Otolaryngol Head Neck Surg 88:397, 1980.

157. Potter C, Conner GH, Sharkey FE: Benign osteoblastoma of the temporal bone. Am J Otol 4:318, 1983.

158. Fabris D, Trainiti G, DiComun M, et al: Scoliosis due to rib osteoblastoma: Report of two cases. J Pediatr Orthop 3:370, 1983.

159. Denis F, Armstrong GWD: Scoliogenic osteoblastoma of the posterior end of the rib. A case report. Spine 9:74, 1984.

160. Adler CP: Case report 255. Osteoblastoma of the lesser trochanter of the left femur. Skel Radiol 11:65, 1984.

161. Clutter DJ, Leopold DA, Gould LV: Benign osteoblastoma. Report of a case and review of the literature. Arch Otolaryngol 110:334, 1984.

162. Goldman RL: The periosteal counterpart of benign osteoblastoma. Am J Clin Pathol 56:73, 1971.

163. Lichtenstein L, Sawyer WF: Benign osteoblastoma: Further observations and report of twenty additional cases. J Bone Joint Surg [Am] 46:755, 1964.

164. Davis NA, Dooley BJ, Bardsley A: Benign osteoblastoma. Aust NZ J Surg 46:37, 1976.

165. Dias LDS, Frost HM: Osteoblastoma of the spine. A review and report of eight new cases. Clin Orthop 91:141, 1973.

166. Griffin JB: Benign osteoblastoma of the thoracic spine. Case report with fifteen-year follow-up. J Bone Joint Surg [Am] 60:833, 1978.

167. Akbarnia BA, Rooholamini SA: Scoliosis caused by benign osteoblastoma of the thoracic or lumbar spine. J Bone Joint Surg [Am] 63:1146, 1981.

168. Lindholm TS, Snellman O, Osterman K: Scoliosis caused by benign osteoblastoma of the lumbar spine. A report of three patients. Spine 2:276, 1977.

169. von Ronnen JR: Case report 4. Skel Radiol 1:61, 1976.

170. Gelberman RH, Olson CO: Benign osteoblastoma of the atlas. A case report. J Bone Joint Surg [Am] 56:808, 1974.

171. Williams RN, Boop WC Jr: Benign osteoblastoma of the skull. Case report. J Neurosurg 41:769, 1974.

172. Doron Y, Gruszkiewicz J, Gelli B, et al: Benign osteoblastoma of vertebral column and skull. Surg Neurol 7:86, 1977.

173. von Ronnen JR: Case report 2. Skel Radiol 1:57, 1976.

174. Berciano J, Perez-Lopez JL, Fernandez F, et al: Voluminous benign osteoblastoma of the skull. Surg Neurol 20:383, 1983.

175. Gutjahr P, Meyer WW, Spranger J: Case report 28. Skel Radiol 1:253, 1977.

176. Tehranzadeh J, Jenkins JJ III, Horton JA: Case report 249. Skel Radiol 10:276, 1983.

177. Smith RA, Hansen LS, Resnick D, et al: Comparison of the osteoblastoma in gnathic and extragnathic sites. Oral Surg 54:285, 1982.

178. Remagen W, Prein J: Benign osteoblastoma. Oral Surg 39:279, 1975.

179. Marcove RC, Alpert M: A pathologic study of benign osteoblastoma. Clin Orthop 30:175, 1963.

180. Spjut HJ, Dorfman HD, Fechner RE, et al: Tumors of Bone and Cartilage. Atlas of Tumor Pathology. Second Series, Fascicle 5. Washington, DC, Armed Forces Institute of Pathology, 1971.

181. Mirra JM, Kendrick RA, Kendrick RE: Pseudomalignant osteoblastoma versus arrested osteoblastoma. A case report. Cancer 37:2005, 1976.

182. Merryweather R, Middlemiss JH, Sanerkin NG: Malignant transformation of osteoblastoma. J Bone Joint Surg [Br] 62:381, 1980.

183. Dorfman HD: Malignant Transformation of Benign Bone Lesions. Proceedings of the 7th National Cancer Conference. Philadelphia, JB Lippincott Co, 1973, p 901.

184. Mayer L: Malignant degeneration of so-called benign osteoblastoma. Bull Hosp Joint Dis 28:4, 1967.

185. Dalinka MK, Chunn SP: Osteoblastoma—benign or malignant precursor? Report of a case. J Can Assoc Radiol 23:214, 1972.

186. Seki T, Fukuda H, Ishii Y, et al: Malignant transformation of benign osteoblastoma. A case report. J Bone Joint Surg [Am] 57:424, 1975.

187. Jackson JR, Bell MEA: Spurious ''benign osteoblastoma.'' A case report. J Bone Joint Surg [Am] 59:397, 1977.

188. Jackson RP: Recurrent osteoblastoma. A review. Clin Orthop 131:229, 1978.

189. Steiner GC: Ultrastructure of osteoblastoma. Cancer 39:2127, 1977.

190. Gertzbein SD, Cruickshank B, Hoffman H, et al: Recurrent benign osteoblastoma of the second thoracic vertebra. A case report. J Bone Joint Surg [Br] 55:841, 1973.

191. Eisenbrey AB, Huber PJ, Rachmaninoff N: Benign osteoblastoma of the spine with multiple recurrences. J Neurol 31:468, 1969.

192. Marsh HO, Choi C: Primary osteogenic sarcoma of the cervical spine originally mistaken for benign osteoblastoma. J Bone Joint Surg [Am] 52:1467, 1970.

193. Kenan S, Floman Y, Robin GC, et al: Aggressive osteoblastoma. A case report and review of the literature. Clin Orthop 195:294, 1985.

194. Schajowicz F, Lemos C: Malignant osteoblastoma. J Bone Joint Surg [Br] 58:202, 1976.

195. Schajowicz F: Current trends in the diagnosis and treatment of malignant bone tumors. Clin Orthop 180:220, 1983.

196. Bertoni F, Unni KK, McLeod RA, et al: Osteosarcoma resembling osteoblastoma. Cancer 55:416, 1985.

197. Revell PA, Scholtz CL: Aggressive osteoblastoma. J Pathol 127:195, 1979.

198. Roessner A, Metze K, Heymer B: Aggressive osteoblastoma. Pathol Res Pract 179:433, 1985.

199. Waldron CA: Fibro-osseous lesions of the jaws. J Oral Maxillofac Surg 43:249, 1985.

200. Eversole LR, Sabes WR, Rovin S: Fibrous dysplasia: A nosologic problem in the diagnosis of fibro-osseous lesions of the jaws. J Oral Pathol 1:189, 1972.

201. Eversole LR, Leider AS, Nelson K: Ossifying fibroma: A clinicopathologic study of sixty-four cases. Oral Surg 60:505, 1985.

202. Budal J: The surgical removal of large osteofibromas. Oral Surg 30:303, 1970.

203. Damjanov I, Maenza RM, Snyder GG III, et al: Juvenile ossifying fibroma: an ultrastructural study. Cancer 42:2668, 1978.

204. Walter JM, Terry BC, Small EW, et al: Aggressive ossifying fibroma of the maxilla: Review of the literature and report of a case. J Oral Surg 37:276, 1979.

205. Kempson RL: Ossifying fibroma of the long bones. A light and electron microscopic study. Arch Pathol 82:218, 1966.

206. Campanacci M: Osteofibrous dysplasia of long bones. A new clinical entity. Ital J Orthop Traumatol 2:221, 1976.

207. Goergen TG, Dickman PS, Resnick D, et al: Long bone ossifying fibromas. Cancer 39:2067, 1977.

208. Markel SF: Ossifying fibroma of long bone. Its distinction from fibrous dysplasia and its association with adamantinoma of long bone. Am J Clin Pathol 69:91, 1978.

209. Capusten BM, Rochon L, Rosman MA, et al: Osteofibrous dysplasia. J Can Assoc Radiol 31:50, 1980.

210. Campanacci M, Laus M: Osteofibrous dysplasia of the tibia and fibula. J Bone Joint Surg [Am] 63:367, 1981.

211. Klein M, Becker MH, Genieser NB, et al: Case report 161. Skel Radiol 6:307, 1981.

212. Schoenecker PL, Swanson K, Sheridan JJ: Ossifying fibroma of the tibia. Report of a new case and review of the literature. J Bone Joint Surg [Am] 63:483, 1981.

213. Batory I: Beitrag zur Klinik, Pathologie und Therapie des ossifizierenden Fibroms in langen Röhrenknochen. Z Orthop 119:475, 1981.

214. Elliot AJ: Ossifying fibroma of the peripheral skeleton. Case of a rare bone tumor in an 18-year-old girl is reported. RI Med J 65:151, 1982.

215. Campbell CJ, Hawk T: A variant of fibrous dysplasia (osteofibrous dysplasia). J Bone Joint Surg [Am] 64:231, 1982.

216. Nakashima Y, Yamamuro T, Fujiwara Y, et al: Osteofibrous dysplasia (ossifying fibroma of long bones). A study of 12 cases. Cancer 52:909, 1983.

217. Alguacil-Garcia A, Alonso A, Pettigrew NM: Osteofibrous dysplasia (ossifying fibroma) of the tibia and fibula and adamantinoma. A case report. Am J Clin Pathol 82:470, 1984.

218. Labrune M, Guinard J, Rengeval JP, et al: L'ostéofibrodysplasie des os longs à évolution régressive. A propos de 3 observations. Arch Franç Pediatr 36:134, 1979.

219. Sanerkin NG: Definition of osteosarcoma, chondrosarcoma, and fibrosarcoma of bone. Cancer 46:178, 1980.

220. Schajowicz F, Cabrini RL: Histochemical studies of bone in normal and pathologic conditions with special reference to alkaline phosphatase, glycogen, and mucopolysaccharides. J Bone Joint Surg [Br] 36:474, 1954.

221. Schajowicz F: Current trends in the diagnosis and treatment of malignant bone tumors. Clin Orthop 180:220, 1983.

222. Prior ES, Wilbur JR, Dmochowski L: Immunofluorescence tests on sera of patients with osteogenic sarcoma. J Natl Cancer Inst 46:1299, 1971.

223. Eilber FR, Morton DL: Sarcoma-specific antigens: Detection by complement fixation with serum from sarcoma patients. J Natl Cancer Inst 44:651, 1970.

224. Farrands PA, Perkins A, Sully L, et al: Localization of human osteosarcoma by antitumour monoclonal antibody. J Bone Joint Surg [Br] 65:638, 1983.

225. Ohno T, Abe M, Tateishi A, et al: Osteogenic sarcoma. A study of one hundred and thirty cases. J Bone Joint Surg [Am] 57:397, 1975.

226. Wu KK, Guise ER, Frost HM, et al: Osteogenic sarcoma. Report of one hundred and fifty-seven cases. Henry Ford Hosp Med J 24:213, 1976.

227. Enneking WF, Springfield DS: Osteosarcoma. Orthop Clin North Am 8:785, 1977.

228. Levy ML, Jaffe N: Osteosarcoma in early childhood. Pediatrics 70:302, 1982.

229. Siegel GP, Dahlin DC, Sim FH: Osteoblastic osteogenic sarcoma in a 35-month-old girl: Report of a case. Am J Pathol 63:886, 1975.

230. de Santos LA, Rosengren JE, Wooten WB, et al: Osteogenic sarcoma after the age of 50: A radiographic evaluation. AJR *131:*481, 1978.
231. Miller CW, McLaughlin RE: Osteosarcoma in siblings. Report of two cases. J Bone Joint Surg [Am] *59:*261, 1977.
232. Swaney JJ: Familial osteogenic sarcoma. Clin Orthop *97:*64, 1973.
233. Dahlin DC, Coventry MB: Osteogenic sarcoma. A study of six hundred cases. J Bone Joint Surg [Am] *49:*101, 1967.
234. Campanacci M, Cervellati G: Osteosarcoma. A review of 345 cases. Ital J Orthop Traumatol *1:*5, 1975.
235. Dahlin DC, Unni KK: Osteosarcoma of bone and its important recognizable varieties. Am J Surg Pathol *1:*61, 1977.
236. Uribe-Botero G, Russell WO, Sutow WW, et al: Primary osteosarcoma of bone. A clinicopathologic investigation of 243 cases, with necropsy study in 54. Am J Clin Pathol *67:*427, 1977.
237. Cohen P: Osteosarcoma of the long bones. Clinical observations and experiences in the Netherlands. Eur J Cancer *14:*995, 1978.
238. Patel DV, Hammer RA, Levin B, et al: Primary osteogenic sarcoma of the spine. Skel Radiol *12:*276, 1984.
239. Barwick KW, Huvos AG, Smith J: Primary osteogenic sarcoma of the vertebral column. A clinicopathologic correlation of ten patients. Cancer *46:*595, 1980.
240. Huvos AG, Sundaresan N, Bretsky SS, et al: Osteogenic sarcoma of the skull. A clinicopathologic study of 19 patients. Cancer *56:*1214, 1985.
241. Benson JE, Goske M, Brodkey JS, et al: Primary osteogenic sarcoma of the calvaria. Am J Neuroradiol *5:*810, 1984.
242. Goodman MA, McMaster JH: Primary osteosarcoma of the skull. Clin Orthop *120:*110, 1976.
243. Nora FE, Unni KK, Pritchard DJ, et al: Osteosarcoma of extragnathic craniofacial bones. Mayo Clin Proc *58:*268, 1983.
244. Wang YC, Shih CJ, Leu FJ, et al: Primary osteogenic sarcoma of the skull: Case report. Neurosurgery *9:*307, 1981.
245. Fleegler EJ, Marks KE, Sebek BA, et al: Osteosarcoma of the hand. Hand *12:*316, 1980.
246. Sneppen O, Dissing I, Schiodt T: Osteosarcoma of the metatarsal bones. Review of the literature and report of a case. Acta Orthop Scand *49:*220, 1978.
247. Amini M, Colacecchi C: An unusual case of primary osteosarcoma of the talus. Clin Orthop *150:*217, 1980.
248. Carroll RE: Osteogenic sarcoma in the hand. J Bone Joint Surg [Am] *39:*325, 1957.
249. Drompp BW: Bilateral osteosarcoma in the phalanges of the hand. A solitary case report. J Bone Joint Surg [Am] *43:*199, 1961.
250. Ellman H, Gold RH, Mirra JM: Roentgenographically ''benign'' but rapidly lethal diaphyseal osteosarcoma. A case report. J Bone Joint Surg [Am] *56:*1267, 1974.
251. Gold RH, Ellman H, Mirra JM: Case report 23. Skel Radiol *1:*235, 1977.
252. Kozlowski K: Osteosarcoma with unusual clinical and/or radiographic appearances. Pediatr Radiol *9:*167, 1980.
253. Haworth JM, McCall IW, Park WM, et al: Sclerotic medullary spread in diaphyseal osteosarcoma. Skel Radiol *4:*212, 1979.
254. Haworth JM, Watt I, Park WM, et al: Diaphyseal osteosarcoma. Br J Radiol *54:*932, 1981.
255. Simon MA, Bos GD: Epiphyseal extension of medullary osteosarcoma in skeletally immature individuals. J Bone Joint Surg [Am] *62:*195, 1980.
256. Unni KK: Case report 214. Skel Radiol *9:*129, 1982.
257. Mink JH, Gold RH, Mirra JM, et al: Case report 65. Skel Radiol *3:*69, 1978.
258. de Santos LA, Edeiken BS: Subtle early osteosarcoma. Skel Radiol *13:*44, 1985.
259. de Santos LA, Edeiken B: Purely lytic osteosarcoma. Skel Radiol *9:*1, 1982.
260. Azouz EM, Esseltine DW, Chevalier L, et al: Radiologic evaluation of osteosarcoma. J Can Assoc Radiol *33:*167, 1982.
261. Fauré C, Boccon-Gibod L, Bercovy M: Case report 257. Skel Radiol *11:*73, 1984.
262. Chew FS, Hudson TM: Radionuclide bone scanning of osteosarcoma: Falsely extended uptake patterns. AJR *139:*49, 1982.
263. Kirks DR, McCook TA, Merten DF, et al: The value of radionuclide bone imaging in selected patients with osteogenic sarcoma metastatic to lung. Pediatr Radiol *9:*139, 1980.
264. Goldstein H, McNeil BJ, Zufall E, et al: Changing indication for bone scintigraphy in patients with osteosarcoma. Radiology *135:*177, 1980.
265. McNeil BJ, Hanley J: Analysis of serial radionuclide bone images in osteosarcoma and breast carcinoma. Radiology *135:*171, 1980.
266. Sandler MS, Heyman S, Watts H: Localization of ^{99m}TC methylene diphosphonate within synovial fluid in osteosarcoma. AJR *143:*349, 1984.
267. Yaghmai I: Angiographic features of osteosarcoma. AJR *129:*1073, 1977.
268. Rittenberg GM, Schabel SI, Vujic I, et al: The vascular ''sunburst'' appearance of osteosarcoma: A new angiographic finding. Skel Radiol *2:*243, 1978.
269. Coffre C, Vanel D, Contesso G, et al: Problems and pitfalls in the use of computed tomography for the local evaluation of long bone osteosarcoma: Report on 30 cases. Skel Radiol *4:*137, 1979.
270. Hudson TM, Schiebler M, Springfield DS, et al: Radiologic imaging of osteosarcoma: Role in planning surgical treatment. Skel Radiol *10:*137, 1983.
271. Destouet JM, Gilula LA, Murphy WA: Computed tomography of long-bone osteosarcoma. Radiology *131:*439, 1979.
272. de Santos LA, Bernardino ME, Murray JA: Computed tomography in the

273. Shirkhoda A, Jaffe N, Wallace S, et al: Computed tomography of osteosarcoma after intraarterial chemotherapy. AJR *144:*95, 1985.
274. Dahlin DC: Pathology of osteosarcoma. Clin Orthop *111:*23, 1975.
275. Enneking WF, Kagan A II: Transepiphyseal extension of osteosarcoma: Incidence, mechanism, and implications. Cancer *41:*1526, 1978.
276. Ghandur-Mnaymneh L, Mnaymneh WA, Puls S: The incidence and mechanism of transphyseal spread of osteosarcoma of long bones. Clin Orthop *177:*210, 1983.
277. Larsson SE, Lorentzon R, Wedren H, et al: Osteosarcoma. A multifactorial clinical and histopathological study with special regard to therapy and survival. Acta Orthop Scand *49:*571, 1978.
278. Upshaw JE, McDonald JR, Ghormley RK: Extension of primary neoplasms of bone to bone marrow. Surg Gynecol Obstet *89:*704, 1949.
279. Lewis RJ, Lotz MJ: Medullary extension of osteosarcoma. Implications for rational therapy. Cancer *33:*371, 1974.
280. Enneking WF, Kagan A: ''Skip'' metastases in osteosarcoma. Cancer *36:*2192, 1975.
281. Malawer MM, Dunham WK: Skip metastases in osteosarcoma: Recent experience. J Surg Oncol *22:*236, 1983.
282. Huvos AG, Butler A, Bretsky SS: Osteogenic sarcoma associated with Paget's disease of bone. A clinicopathologic study of 65 patients. Cancer *52:*1489, 1983.
283. Huvos AG, Woodard HQ, Cahan WG, et al: Postradiation osteogenic sarcoma of bone and soft tissues. A clinicopathologic study of 66 patients. Cancer *55:*1244, 1985.
284. Troup JB, Dahlin DC, Coventry MB: The significance of giant cells in osteogenic sarcoma: Do they indicate a relationship between osteogenic sarcoma and giant cell tumor of bone? Mayo Clin Proc *35:*179, 1960.
285. Meister P, Konrad E, Lob G, et al: Osteosarcoma: Histological evaluation and grading. Arch Orthop Trauma Surg *94:*91, 1979.
286. Paschall HA, Paschall MM: Electron microscopic observations of 20 human osteosarcomas. Clin Orthop *111:*42, 1975.
287. Williams AH, Schwinn CP, Parker JW: The ultrastructure of osteosarcoma. A review of twenty cases. Cancer *37:*1293, 1976.
288. Ferguson RJ, Yunis EJ: The ultrastructure of human osteosarcoma. A study of nine cases. Clin Orthop *131:*234, 1978.
289. Katenkamp D, Stiller D, Waldmann G: Ultrastructural cytology of human osteosarcoma cells. Virchows Arch (Pathol Anat) *381:*49, 1978.
290. Reddick RL, Michelitch HJ, Levin AM, et al: Osteogenic sarcoma. A study of the ultrastructure. Cancer *45:*64, 1980.
291. Grundmann E, Roessner A, Immenkamp M: Tumor cell types in osteosarcoma as revealed by electron microscopy. Implications for histogenesis and subclassification. Virchows Arch (Cell Pathol) *36:*257, 1981.
292. Garbe LR, Monges GM, Pellegrin EM, et al: Ultrastructural study of osteosarcomas. Hum Pathol *12:*891, 1981.
293. Aho AJ, Aho HJ: Ultrastructure of human osteosarcoma. Malignant transformation of a multipotential connective tissue cell. Pathol Res Pract *174:*53, 1982.
294. Aparisi T, Stark A, Ericsson JLE: Human osteogenic sarcoma. Study of the ultrastructure, with special notes on the localization of alkaline and acid phosphatase. Int Orthop (SICOT) *6:*171, 1982.
295. Stark A, Aparisi T: Human osteogenic sarcoma: Fine structure of the osteoblastic type. Ultrastruct Pathol *4:*311, 1983.
296. Marquart KH: Intranuclear vermicellar bodies in human osteosarcoma and ossifying fibroma cells. J Cancer Res Clin Oncol *106:*74, 1983.
297. Stark A, Aparisi T, Ericsson JL: Human osteogenic sarcoma: Fine structure of the chondroblastic type. Ultrastruct Pathol *6:*51, 1984.
298. Chuang VP, Benjamin R, Jaffe N, et al: Radiographic and angiographic changes in osteosarcoma after intraarterial chemotherapy. AJR *139:*1065, 1982.
299. Smith J, Heelan RT, Huvos AG, et al: Radiographic changes in primary osteogenic sarcoma following intensive chemotherapy. Radiological-pathological correlation in 63 patients. Radiology *143:*355, 1982.
300. Mail JT, Cohen MD, Mirkin LD, et al: Response of osteosarcoma to preoperative intravenous high-dose methotrexate chemotherapy: CT evaluation. AJR *144:*89, 1985.
301. Pho RWH, Lim SML, Satku K: Late metastases from osteogenic sarcoma. A case report. J Bone Joint Surg [Am] *67:*147, 1985.
302. Campanacci M, Laus M: Local recurrence after amputation for osteosarcoma. J Bone Joint Surg [Br] *62:*201, 1980.
303. Tobias JD, Pratt CB, Parham DM, et al: The significance of calcified regional lymph nodes at the time of diagnosis of osteosarcoma. Orthopedics *8:*49, 1985.
304. Madsen EH: Lymph node metastases from osteoblastic osteogenic sarcoma visible on plain films. Skel Radiol *4:*216, 1979.
305. Forsted DH, Dalinka MK, Kaplan F, et al: Case report 48. Skel Radiol *2:*179, 1978.
306. Miki T, Yamamuro T, Kotoura Y, et al: Osteosarcoma with multiple intramuscular metastases. A case report. Acta Orthop Scand *56:*92, 1985.
307. Goldstein C, Ambos MA, Bosniak MA: Multiple ossified metastases to the kidney from osteogenic sarcoma. AJR *128:*148, 1977.
308. Kragh LV, Dahlin DC, Erich JB: Osteogenic sarcoma of the jaws and facial bones. Am J Surg *96:*496, 1958.
309. Hofmann WB: Osteogenic sarcoma of the mandible. Arch Otolaryngol *84:*439, 1966.

310. Garrington GE, Scofield HH, Cornyn J, et al: Osteosarcoma of the jaws. Analysis of 56 cases. Cancer 20:377, 1967.

311. Roca AN, Smith JL Jr, Jing BS: Osteosarcoma and parosteal osteogenic sarcoma of the maxilla and mandible: Study of 20 cases. Am J Clin Pathol 54:625, 1970.

312. Caron AS, Hajdu SI, Strong EW: Osteogenic sarcoma of the facial and cranial bones. A review of forty-three cases. Am J Surg 122:719, 1971.

313. Curtis ML, Elmore JS, Sotereanos GC: Osteosarcoma of the jaws: Report of case and review of the literature. J Oral Surg 32:135, 1974.

314. Windle-Taylor PC: Osteosarcoma of the upper jaw. J Maxillofac Surg 5:62, 1977.

315. Li Volsi VA: Osteogenic sarcoma of the maxilla. Arch Otolaryngol 103:485, 1977.

316. Russ JE, Jesse RH: Management of osteosarcoma of the maxilla and mandible. Am J Surg 140:572, 1980.

317. Clark JL, Unni KK, Dahlin DC, et al: Osteosarcoma of the jaw. Cancer 51:2311, 1983.

318. Vener J, Rice DH, Newman AN: Osteosarcoma and chondrosarcoma of the head and neck. Laryngoscope 94:240, 1984.

319. Nora FE, Unni KK, Pritchard DH, et al: Osteosarcoma of extragnathic cranio-facial bones. Mayo Clin Proc 58:268, 1983.

320. Matsuno T, Unni KK, McLeod RA, et al: Telangiectatic osteogenic sarcoma. Cancer 38:2538, 1976.

321. Campanacci M, Pizzoferrato A: Osteosarcoma emorragico. Chir Organi Mov 60:409, 1971.

322. Ruiter DJ, Cornelisse CJ, van Rijssel ThG, et al: Aneurysmal bone cyst and telangiectatic osteosarcoma. A histopathological and morphometric study. Virchows Arch (Pathol Anat) 373:311, 1977.

323. Larsson SE, Lorentzon R, Boquist L: Telangiectatic osteosarcoma. Acta Orthop Scand 49:589, 1978.

324. Roessner A, Hobik HP, Immenkamp M, et al: Ultrastructure of telangiectatic osteosarcoma. J Cancer Res Clin Oncol 95:197, 1979.

325. Adler CP: Case report 111. Skel Radiol 5:56, 1980.

326. Kaufman RA, Towbin RB: Telangiectatic osteosarcoma simulating the appearance of an aneurysmal bone cyst. Pediatr Radiol 11:102, 1981.

327. Huvos AG, Rosen G, Bretsky SS, et al: Telangiectatic osteogenic sarcoma: A clinicopathologic study of 124 patients. Cancer 49:1679, 1982.

328. Farr GH, Huvos AG, Marcove RC, et al: Telangiectatic osteogenic sarcoma. A review of twenty-eight cases. Cancer 34:1150, 1974.

329. Heaston DK, Gelman MI: Case report 41. Skel Radiol 2:117, 1977.

330. Sim FH, Unni KK, Beabout JW, et al: Osteosarcoma with small cells simulating Ewing's tumor. J Bone Joint Surg [Am] 61:207, 1979.

331. Martin SE, Dwyer A, Kissane JM, et al: Small-cell osteosarcoma. Cancer 50:990, 1982.

332. Roessner A, Immenkamp M, Hiddemann W, et al: Case report 331. Skel Radiol 14:216, 1985.

333. Unni KK, Dahlin DC, McLeod RA, et al: Intraosseous well-differentiated osteosarcoma. Cancer 40:1337, 1977.

334. Campanacci M, Bertoni F, Capanna R, et al: Central osteosarcoma of low grade malignancy. Ital J Orthop Traumatol 7:71, 1981.

335. Lodwick GS: Case report 169. Skel Radiol 7:139, 1981.

336. Xipell JM, Rush J: Case report 340. Skel Radiol 14:312, 1985.

337. Unni KK: Case report 136. Skel Radiol 6:65, 1981.

338. Jaffe HL: Intraosseous osteogenic sarcoma. Bull Hosp J Dis 21:189, 1960.

339. Kyriakos M: Intracortical osteosarcoma. Cancer 46:2525, 1980.

340. Picci P, Gherlinzoni F, Guerra A: Intracortical osteosarcoma: Rare entity or early manifestation of classical osteosarcoma? Skel Radiol 9:255, 1983.

341. Vigorita VJ, Jones JK, Ghelman B, et al: Intracortical osteosarcoma. Am J Surg Pathol 8:65, 1984.

342. Wold LE, Unni KK, Beabout JW, et al: High-grade surface osteosarcoma. Am J Surg Pathol 8:181, 1984.

343. Sonneland PRL, Unni KK: Case report 258. Skel Radiol 11:77, 1984.

344. Unni KK, Dahlin DC, Beabout JW: Periosteal osteogenic sarcoma. Cancer 37:2476, 1976.

345. Lawson JP, Barwick KW: Case report 162. Skel Radiol 7:63, 1981.

346. Sundaram M, Burdge RW, Martin SA, et al: Case report 142. Skel Radiol 6:131, 1981.

347. Bertoni F, Boriani S, Laus M, et al: Periosteal chondrosarcoma and periosteal osteosarcoma. Two distinct entities. J Bone Joint Surg [Br] 64:370, 1982.

348. Martinez-Tello FJ, Navas-Palacios JJ: The ultrastructure of conventional, parosteal, and periosteal osteosarcoma. Cancer 50:949, 1982.

349. Zarbo RJ, Regezi JA, Baker SR: Periosteal osteogenic sarcoma of the mandible. Oral Surg 57:643, 1984.

350. Levine E, de Smet AA, Huntrakoon M: Juxtacortical osteosarcoma: A radiologic and histologic spectrum. Skel Radiol 14:38, 1985.

351. Hall RB, Robinson LH, Malawar MM, et al: Periosteal osteosarcoma. Cancer 55:165, 1985.

352. de Santos LA, Murray JA, Finklestein JB, et al: The radiographic spectrum of periosteal osteosarcoma. Radiology 127:123, 1978.

353. Dahlin DC: Case report 27. Skel Radiol 1:249, 1977.

354. Smith J, Ahuja SC, Huvos AG, et al: Parosteal (juxtacortical) osteogenic sarcoma. A roentgenological study of 30 patients. J Can Assoc Radiol 29:167, 1978.

355. Farr GZH, Huvos AG: Juxtacortical osteogenic sarcoma. An analysis of fourteen cases. J Bone Joint Surg [Am] 54:1205, 1972.

356. Luck JV Jr, Luck JV, Schwinn CP: Parosteal osteosarcoma: A treatment-oriented study. Clin Orthop 153:92, 1980.

357. Campanacci M, Picci P, Gherlinzoni F, et al: Parosteal osteosarcoma. J Bone Joint Surg [Br] 66:313, 1984.

358. Lorentzon R, Larsson SE, Boquist L: Parosteal (juxtacortical) osteosarcoma. A clinical and histopathological study of 11 cases and a review of the literature. J Bone Joint Surg [Br] 62:86, 1980.

359. Unni KK, Dahlin DC, Beabout JW, et al: Parosteal osteogenic sarcoma. Cancer 37:2466, 1976.

360. Edeiken J, Farrell C, Ackerman LV, et al: Parosteal sarcoma. AJR J 111:579, 1971.

361. Solomon MP, Biernacki J, Slippen M, et al: Parosteal osteogenic sarcoma of the mandible. Existence masked by diffuse periodontal inflammation. Arch Otolaryngol 101:754, 1975.

362. Newland JR, Ayala AG: Parosteal osteosarcoma of the maxilla. Oral Surg 43:727, 1977.

363. Banerjee SC: Juxtacortical osteosarcoma of mandible: Review of literature and report of case. J Oral Surg 39:535, 1981.

364. Green PWB, Ilardi CF, Bitter JJ, et al: Case report 260. Skel Radiol 11:141, 1984.

365. Farmlet E, Fishman EK: Case report 300. Skel Radiol 13:89, 1985.

366. van der Heul RO, Von Ronnen JR: Juxtacortical osteosarcoma. Diagnosis, differential diagnosis, treatment, and an analysis of eighty cases. J Bone Joint Surg [Am] 49:415, 1967.

367. Dwinnell LA, Dahlin DC, Ghormley RK: Parosteal (juxtacortical) osteogenic sarcoma. J Bone Joint Surg [Am] 36:732, 1954.

368. Scaglietti O, Calandriello B: Ossifying parosteal sarcoma. J Bone Joint Surg [Am] 44:635, 1962.

369. Ahuja SC, Villacin AB, Smith J, et al: Juxtacortical (parosteal) osteogenic sarcoma. Histologic grading and prognosis. J Bone Joint Surg [Am] 59:632, 1977.

370. Hudson TM, Springfield DS, Benjamin M, et al: Computed tomography of parosteal osteosarcoma. AJR 144:961, 1985.

371. Orcutt J, Ragsdale BD, Curtis DJ, et al: Misleading CT in parosteal osteosarcoma. AJR 136:1233, 1981.

372. Kricun ME, Stead J: Case report 289. Skel Radiol 12:227, 1984.

373. Bertoni F, Present D, Hudson T, et al: The meaning of radiolucencies in parosteal osteosarcoma. J Bone Joint Surg [Am] 67:901, 1985.

374. Copeland MM, Geschickter CF: The treatment of parosteal osteosarcoma of bone. Surg Gynecol Obstet 108:537, 1959.

375. Geschickter CF, Copeland MM: Parosteal osteosarcoma of bone: A new entity. Ann Surg 133:790, 1951.

376. Dunham WK, Wilborn WH, Zarzour RJ: A large parosteal osteosarcoma with transformation to high-grade osteosarcoma. A case report. Cancer 44:1495, 1979.

377. Wold LE, Unni KK, Beabout JW, et al: Dedifferentiated parosteal osteosarcoma. J Bone Joint Surg [Am] 66:53, 1984.

378. Vuletin JC: Myofibroblasts in parosteal osteogenic sarcoma. Arch Pathol Lab Med 101:272, 1977.

379. Reddick RL, Popovsky MA, Fantone JC, et al: Parosteal osteogenic sarcoma. Ultrastructural observations in three cases. Hum Pathol 11:373, 1980.

380. Thayer C, Rogers LF: Unicentric osteosarcoma of bone with subsequent skeletal metastases. Skel Radiol 4:148, 1979.

381. Mahoney DH, Shepherd DA, DePuey EG, et al: Childhood multifocal osteosarcoma: Diagnosis by 99m-technetium bone scan. A case report. Med Pediatr Oncol 6:347, 1979.

382. Parham DM, Pratt CB, Parvey LS, et al: Childhood multifocal osteosarcoma. Clinicopathologic and radiologic correlates. Cancer 55:2653, 1985.

383. Amstutz HC: Multiple osteogenic sarcomata: Metastatic or multicentric? Report of two cases and review of the literature. Cancer 24:923, 1969.

384. Lowbeer L: Multifocal osteosarcomatosis: A rare entity. Bull Pathol 9:52, 1968.

385. Mahoney JP, Spanier SS, Morris JL: Multifocal osteosarcoma. A case report with review of the literature. Cancer 44:1897, 1979.

386. Reider-Grosswasser I, Grunebaum M: Metaphyseal multifocal osteosarcoma. Br J Radiol 51:671, 1978.

387. Gherlinzoni F, Antoci B, Canale V: Case report 250. Skel Radiol 10:281, 1983.

388. Fitzgerald RH, Dahlin DC, Sim FH: Multiple metachronous osteogenic sarcoma. Report of twelve cases with two long-term survivors. J Bone Joint Surg [Am] 55:595, 1973.

389. Simodynes EE, Jardon OM, Connolly JF: Multiple metachronous osteosarcoma with eleven-year survival. J Bone Joint Surg [Am] 63:317, 1981.

390. Jaffe HL, Lichtenstein L: Solitary benign enchondroma of bone. Arch Surg 46:480, 1943.

391. Takigawa K: Chondroma of the bones of the hand. A review of 110 cases. J Bone Joint Surg [Am] 53:1591, 1971.

392. McFarland GB, Morden ML: Benign cartilaginous lesions. Orthop Clin North Am 8:737, 1977.

393. Adler CP: Differential diagnosis of cartilage tumors. Pathol Res Pract 166:45, 1979.

394. Shellito JG, Dockerty MB: Cartilaginous tumors of the hand. Surg Gynecol Obstet 86:465, 1948.

395. Boriani S, Laus M: Chondromas and chondromatosis (a study of 265 cases, 200 with long term follow-up). Ital J Orthop Traumatol 4:353, 1978.

396. Adler CP, Klumper A, Wenz W: Enchondrome aus radiogischer und pathologisch-anatomischer Sicht. Radiologe 19:341, 1979.
397. Noble J, Lamb DW: Enchondromata of the hand bones. Ann Chir 28:855, 1974.
398. Jewusiak EM, Spence KF, Sell KW: Solitary benign enchondroma of the long bones of the hand. Results of curettage and packing with freeze-dried cancellous-bone allograft. J Bone Joint Surg [Am] 53:1587, 1971.
399. Takigawa K: Carpal chondroma. Report of a case. J Bone Joint Surg [Am] 53:1601, 1971.
400. Noble J, Lamb DW: Enchondromata of bones of the hand. A review of 40 cases. Hand 6:275, 1974.
401. Stephenson WH: Enchondroma of patella. Br J Radiol 26:156, 1953.
402. Kragh LV, Dahlin DC, Erich JB: Cartilaginous tumors of the jaws and facial regions. Am J Surg 99:852, 1960.
403. Lammot TR III: Enchondroma of the patella. A case report. J Bone Joint Surg [Am] 50:1230, 1968.
404. Falconer MA, Bailey IC, Duchen LW: Surgical treatment of chordoma and chondroma of the skull base. J Neurosurg 29:261, 1968.
405. Katz S: Sternal chondroma. Dis Chest 55:166, 1969.
406. Minagi H, Newton TH: Cartilaginous tumors of the base of skull. AJR 105:308, 1969.
407. Faccini JM, William JL: Nasal chondroma. J Laryngol Otol 87:811, 1973.
408. Tomich CE, Hutton CE: Chondroma of the anterior nasal spine. J Oral Surg 34:911, 1976.
409. Bernard TN, Haddad RJ Jr: Enchondroma of the proximal clavicle. An unusual cause of pathologic fracture-dislocation of the sternoclavicular joint. Clin Orthop 167:239, 1982.
410. Sarwar M, Swischuk LE, Schechter MM: Intracranial chondromas. AJR 127:973, 1976.
411. Schacter IB, Wortzman G, Noyek AM: The clinical and radiological diagnosis of cartilaginous tumors of the base of the skull. Can J Otolaryngol 4:364, 1975.
412. Minagi H, Newton TH: Cartilaginous tumors of the base of the skull. AJR 105:308, 1969.
413. Marcove RC, Huvos AG: Cartilaginous tumors of the ribs. Cancer 27:794, 1971.
414. Sabanathan S, Salama FD: Cartilaginous tumours of rib. J R Coll Surg Edinb 29:363, 1984.
415. Tomita K, Nomura S, Nanri Y: Thoracic cord compression from chondroma of rib. A case report. Spine 9:535, 1984.
416. Keating RB, Wright PW, Staple TW: Enchondroma protuberans of the rib. Skel Radiol 13:55, 1985.
417. Pandey S: Giant chondroma arising from the ribs. A report of four cases. J Bone Joint Surg [Br] 57:519, 1975.
418. Caballes RL: Enchondroma protuberans masquerading as osteochondroma. Hum Pathol 13:734, 1982.
419. Schiller AL: Diagnosis of borderline cartilage lesions of bone. Semin Diagn Pathol 2:42, 1985.
420. Lichtenstein L: Bone Tumors. 5th Ed. St Louis, CV Mosby Co, 1977.
421. Steiner GC: Ultrastructure of benign cartilaginous tumors of intraosseous origin. Hum Pathol 10:71, 1979.
422. Wu KK, Frost HM, Guise EE: A chondrosarcoma of the hand arising from an asymptomatic benign solitary enchondroma of 40 years duration. J Hand Surg 8:317, 1983.
423. Sanerkin NG: Fibrosarcomata and malignant fibrous histiocytomata arising in relation to enchondromata. J Bone Joint Surg [Br] 61:366, 1979.
424. Rockwell MA, Enneking WF: Osteosarcoma developing in a solitary enchondroma of the tibia. J Bone Joint Surg [Am] 53:341, 1971.
425. Bonfiglio M, Platz CE: Case report 141. Skel Radiol 6:127, 1981.
426. Ollier M: De la dyschondroplasie. Bull Soc Chir Lyon 3:22, 1899–1900.
427. Shapiro F: Ollier's disease. An assessment of angular deformity, shortening, and pathological fracture in twenty-one patients. J Bone Joint Surg [Am] 64:95, 1982.
428. Mosher JF: Multiple enchondromatosis of the hand. A case report. J Bone Joint Surg [Am] 58:717, 1976.
429. Manizer F, Minagi H, Steinbach HL: The variable manifestations of multiple enchondromatosis. Radiology 99:377, 1971.
430. Fairbank HAT: Dyschondroplasia. Synonyms—Ollier's disease, multiple enchondromatosis. J Bone Joint Surg [Br] 30:689, 1948.
431. Goodman SB, Bell RS, Fornasier VL, et al: Ollier's disease with multiple sarcomatous transformations. Hum Pathol 15:91, 1984.
432. Braddock GTF, Hadlow VD: Osteosarcoma in enchondromatosis (Ollier's disease). J Bone Joint Surg [Br] 48:145, 1966.
433. Spranger J, Kemperdieck H, Bakowski H, et al: Two peculiar types of enchondromatosis. Pediatr Radiol 7:215, 1978.
434. Bender BL, Yunis E: Fibrocartilaginous lesions of bone and hemangiomas and lipomas of soft tissue resembling Maffucci's syndrome. A case report. J Bone Joint Surg [Am] 61:1104, 1979.
435. Kaibara N, Mitsuyasu M, Katsuki I, et al: Generalized enchondromatosis with unusual complications of soft tissue calcifications and hemangiomas. Follow-up for over a twelve-year period. Skel Radiol 8:43, 1982.
436. Schorr S, Legum C, Ochshorn M: Spondyloenchondrodysplasia. Enchondromatosis with severe platyspondyly in two brothers. Radiology 118:133, 1976.
437. Bassett GS, Cowell HR: Metachondromatosis. Report of four cases. J Bone Joint Surg [Am] 67:811, 1985.
438. Beals RK: Metachondromatosis. Clin Orthop 169:167, 1982.
439. Wickenhauser J, Raff M, Canigiani G, et al: Seltene Entwicklungsstorungen des mittleren Keimblattes an der Extremitaten. ROFO 118:52, 1973.
440. Maffucci A: Di un caso di enchondroma ed angioma multiplo. Mov Med Chir Nap 3:399, 565, 1881.
441. Sun TC, Swee RG, Shives TC, et al: Chondrosarcoma in Maffucci's syndrome. J Bone Joint Surg [Am] 67:1214, 1985.
442. Lewis RJ, Ketcham AS: Maffucci's syndrome: Functional and neoplastic significance. Case report and review of the literature. J Bone Joint Surg [Am] 55:1465, 1973.
443. Cook PL, Evans PG: Chondrosarcoma of the skull in Maffucci's syndrome. Br J Radiol 50:833, 1977.
444. Banna M, Parwani GS: Multiple sarcomas in Maffucci's syndrome. Br J Radiol 42:304, 1969.
445. Chen VT: Maffucci's syndrome. Hand 10:292, 1978.
446. Anderson IF: Maffucci's syndrome. South Afr Med J 39:1066, 1965.
447. Loewinger RJ, Lichtenstein JR, Dodson WE, et al: Maffucci's syndrome: A mesenchymal dysplasia and multiple tumour syndrome. Br J Dermatol 96:317, 1977.
448. Kuzma JF, King JM: Dyschondroplasia with hemangiomatosis (Maffucci's syndrome) and teratoid tumor of the ovary. Arch Pathol 46:74, 1948.
449. Lichtenstein L, Hall JE: Periosteal chondroma: A distinctive benign cartilage tumor. J Bone Joint Surg [Am] 34:691, 1952.
450. Boriani S, Bacchini P, Bertoni F, Campanacci M: Periosteal chondroma. A review of twenty cases. J Bone Joint Surg [Am] 65:205, 1983.
451. Nojima T, Unni KK, McLeod RA, et al: Periosteal chondroma and periosteal chondrosarcoma. Am J Surg Pathol 9:666, 1985.
452. Fornasier VL, McGonigal D: Periosteal chondroma. Clin Orthop 124:233, 1977.
453. Rockwell MA, Saiter ET, Enneking WF: Periosteal chondroma. J Bone Joint Surg [Am] 54:102, 1972.
454. de Santos LA, Spjut HJ: Periosteal chondroma: A radiographic spectrum. Skel Radiol 6:15, 1981.
455. Bauer TW, Dorfman HD, Latham JT Jr: Periosteal chondroma. A clinico-pathologic study of 23 cases. Am J Surg Pathol 6:631, 1982.
456. Jaffe HL: Juxtacortical chondroma. Bull Hosp Joint Dis 17:20, 1956.
457. Marmor L: Periosteal chondroma (juxtacortical chondroma). Clin Orthop 37:150, 1964.
458. Grayson A, Bain M: Juxtacortical chondroma of the hyoid bone. Report of a case. Arch Otolaryngol 86:679, 1967.
459. Calderone A, Naimark A, Schiller AL: Case report 196. Skel Radiol 8:160, 1982.
460. Kirchner SG, Pavlov H, Heller RM, et al: Periosteal chondromas of the anterior tibial tubercle: two cases. AJR 131:1088, 1978.
461. Wheelhouse WW, Griffin PP: Periosteal chondroma. South Med J 75:1003, 1982.
462. Cooke GM, Pearce JG: Periosteal chondroma. Report of two cases with atypical radiologic features. J Can Assoc Radiol 27:301, 1976.
463. Pazzaglia UE, Ceciliani L: Periosteal chondroma of the humerus leading to shortening. A case report. J Bone Joint Surg [Br] 67:290, 1985.
464. Merlino AF, Nixon JE: Periosteal chondroma. Report of an atypical case and review of the literature. Am J Surg 107:773, 1964.
465. Cary GR: Juxtacortical chondroma. A case report. J Bone Joint Surg [Am] 47:1405, 1965.
466. Feinberg SB, Wilber MC: Periosteal chondroma. A report of two cases. Radiology 66:383, 1956.
467. Dahlin DC, Salvador AH: Cartilaginous tumors of the soft tissues of the hands and feet. Mayo Clin Proc 49:721, 1974.
468. Chung EB, Enzinger FM: Chondroma of soft parts. Cancer 41:1414, 1978.
469. Zlatkin MB, Lander PH, Begin LR, et al: Soft-tissue chondromas. AJR 144:1263, 1985.
470. Ewing J: Neoplastic Diseases. A Treatise on Tumors. 3rd Ed. Philadelphia, WB Saunders Co, 1928.
471. Kolodny A: Bone sarcoma; the primary malignant tumor of the bone and giant cell tumor. Surg Gynecol Obstet 44(Suppl 1):1, 1927.
472. Codman EA: Epiphyseal chondromatous giant cell tumors of the upper end of the humerus. Surg Gynecol Obstet 52:543, 1931.
473. Jaffe HL, Lichtenstein L: Benign chondroblastoma of bone. A reinterpretation of the so-called calcifying or chondromatous giant cell tumor. Am J Pathol 18:969, 1942.
474. Kingsley TC, Markel SF: Extraskeletal chondroblastoma: A report of the first recorded case. Cancer 27:203, 1971.
475. Abdul FW, Ayala Ag, Spjut HJ: Case report 321. Skel Radiol 14:73, 1985.
476. McBryde A Jr, Goldner JL: Chondroblastoma of bone. Ann Surg 36:94, 1970.
477. Dahlin DC, Ivins JC: Benign chondroblastoma. A study of 125 cases. Cancer 30:401, 1972.
478. Schajowicz F, Gallardo H: Epiphyseal chondroblastoma of bone. A clinicopathological study of sixty-nine cases. J Bone Joint Surg [Br] 52:205, 1970.
479. Springfield DS, Capanna R, Gherlinzoni F, et al: Chondroblastoma. A review of seventy cases. J Bone Joint Surg [Am] 67:748, 1985.
480. Aprin H: Benign chondroblastoma. Orthopedics 4:1134, 1981.
481. Aronsohn RS, Hart WR, Martel W: Metaphyseal chondroblastoma of bone. AJR 127:686, 1976.
482. Fechner RE, Wilde HD: Chondroblastoma in the metaphysis of the femoral neck. A case report and review of the literature. J Bone Joint Surg [Am] 56:413, 1974.
483. Hatcher CH, Campbell JC: Benign chondroblastoma of bone. Its histologic

variations and a report of late sarcoma in the site of one. Bull Hosp Joint Dis 12:411, 1951.

484. Kricun ME, Kricun R, Haskin ME: Chondroblastoma of the calcaneus: Radiographic features with emphasis on location. AJR 128:613, 1977.

485. Neviaser RJ, Wilson JN: Benign chondroblastoma in the finger. J Bone Joint Surg [Am] 54:389, 1972.

486. Moore TM, Roe JB, Harvey JP: Chondroblastoma of the talus. A case report. J Bone Joint Surg [Am] 59:830, 1977.

487. Assor D: Chondroblastoma of the rib. J Bone Joint Surg [Am] 55:208, 1973.

488. Harner SG, Cody DTR, Dahlin DC: Benign chondroblastoma of the temporal bone. Otolaryngol Head Neck Surg 87:229, 1979.

489. Hull MT, Gonzalez-Crussi F, DeRosa GP, et al: Aggressive chondroblastoma. Report of a case with multiple bone and soft tissue involvement. Clin Orthop 126:261, 1977.

490. Feely M, Keohane C: Chondroblastoma of the skull. J Neurol Neurosurg Psychiatry 47:1348, 1984.

491. Buraczewski J, Lysakowska J, Rudowski W: Chondroblastoma (Codman's tumour) of the thoracic spine. J Bone Joint Surg [Br] 39:705, 1957.

492. Wellmann KF: Chondroblastoma of the scapula. A case report with ultrastructural observations. Cancer 24:408, 1969.

493. Remagen W, Schafer R, Roggatz J: Chondroblastoma of the patella. Arch Orthop Trauma Surg 96:157, 1980.

494. Roberts PF, Taylor JG: Multifocal benign chondroblastomas: Report of a case. Hum Pathol 11:296, 1980.

495. Hudson TM, Hawkins IF: Radiological evaluation of chondroblastoma. Radiology 139:1, 1981.

496. Nolan DJ, Middlemiss H: Chondroblastoma of bone. Clin Radiol 26:343, 1975.

497. McLeod RA, Beabout JW: The roentgenographic features of chondroblastoma. AJR 118:464, 1973.

498. Bloem JL, Mulder JD: Chondroblastoma: A clinical and radiological study of 104 cases. Skel Radiol 14:1, 1985.

499. Gravanis MB, Giansanti JS: Benign chondroblastoma. Report of four cases with a discussion of the presence of ossification. Am J Clin Pathol 55:624, 1971.

500. Alexander C: Case report 5. Skel Radiol 1:63, 1976.

501. Humphrey A, Gilday DL, Brown RG: Bone scintigraphy in chondroblastoma. Radiology 137:497, 1980.

502. Kahmann R, Gold RH, Eckardt JJ, Mirra JM: Case report 337. Skel Radiol 14:301, 1985.

503. Huvos AG, Marcove RC: Chondroblastoma of bone. A critical review. Clin Orthop 95:300, 1973.

504. Higaki S, Takeyama S, Tateishi A, et al: Clinicopathological study of twenty-two cases of benign chondroblastoma. Nippon Seikeigeka Gakkai Zasshi 55:647, 1981.

505. Kunkel MG, Dahlin DC, Young HH: Benign chondroblastoma. J Bone Joint Surg [Am] 38:817, 1956.

506. Huvos AG, Marcove RC, Erlandson RA, et al: Chondroblastoma of bone. A clinicopathologic and electron microscopic study. Cancer 29:760, 1972.

507. Valls J, Ottolenghi CE, Schajowicz F: Epiphyseal chondroblastoma of bone. J Bone Joint Surg [Am] 33:997, 1951.

508. Campanacci M, Giunti A, Martucci E, et al: Epiphyseal chondroblastoma (a study of 39 cases). Ital J Orthop Traumatol 3:67, 1977.

509. Sundaram TKS: Benign chondroblastoma. J Bone Joint Surg [Br] 48:92, 1966.

510. Coleman SS: Benign chondroblastoma with recurrent soft-tissue and intra-articular lesions. Report of a case. J Bone Joint Surg [Am] 48:1554, 1966.

511. Lichtenstein L, Bernstein D: Unusual benign and malignant chondroid tumors of bone. A survey of some mesenchymal cartilage tumors and malignant chondroblastic tumors, including a few multicentric ones, as well as many atypical benign chondroblastomas and chondromyxoid fibromas. Cancer 12:1142, 1959.

512. Welsh RA, Meyer AT: A histogenetic study of chondroblastoma. Cancer 17:578, 1964.

513. Levine GD, Bensch KG: Chondroblastoma—the nature of the basic cell. A study by means of histochemistry, tissue culture, electron microscopy, and autoradiography. Cancer 29:1546, 1972.

514. Povysil C, Matejovsky A: Ultrastructure of benign chondroblastoma. Pathol Res Pract 166:80, 1979.

515. Cocchia D, Lauriola L, Stolfi VM, et al: S-100 antigen labels neoplastic cells in liposarcoma and cartilaginous tumours. Virchows Arch (Pathol Anat) 402:139, 1983.

516. Nakamura Y, Becker LE, Marks A: S-100 protein in tumors of cartilage and bone. An immunohistochemical study. Cancer 52:1820, 1983.

517. Monda L, Wicks MR: S-100 protein immunostaining in the differential diagnosis of chondroblastoma. Hum Pathol 16:287, 1985.

518. McLaughlin RE, Sweet DE, Webster T, et al: Chondroblastoma of the pelvis suggestive of malignancy. Report of an unusual case treated by wide pelvic excision. J Bone Joint Surg [Am] 57:549, 1975.

519. Mirra JM, Ulich TR, Eckardt JJ, et al: ''Aggressive'' chondroblastoma. Light and ultramicroscopic findings after en bloc resection. Clin Orthop 178:276, 1983.

520. Green P, Whittaker RP: Benign chondroblastoma. Case report with pulmonary metastases. J Bone Joint Surg [Am] 57:416, 1975.

521. Riddell RJ, Louis CJ, Bromberger NA: Pulmonary metastases from chondroblastoma of the tibia. Report of a case. J Bone Joint Surg [Br] 55:848, 1973.

522. Kyriakos M, Land VJ, Penning L, et al: Metastatic chondroblastoma. Report

of a fatal case with a review of the literature on atypical, aggressive, and malignant chondroblastoma. Cancer 55:1770, 1985.

523. Reyes CV, Kathuria S: Recurrent and aggressive chondroblastoma of the pelvis with late malignant neoplastic changes. Am J Surg Pathol 3:449, 1979.

524. Kahn LB, Wood FM, Ackerman LV: Malignant chondroblastoma. Report of two cases and review of the literature. Arch Pathol 88:371, 1969.

525. Leeson MC, Smith A, Carter JR, et al: Eosinophilic granuloma of bone in the growing epiphysis. J Pediatr Orthop 5:147, 1985.

526. Jaffe HL, Lichtenstein L: Chondromyxoid fibroma of bone: A distinctive benign tumor likely to be mistaken especially for chondrosarcoma. Arch Pathol 45:541, 1948.

527. Bloodgood JC: Bone tumors: Myxoma. Ann Surg 80:817, 1924.

528. Schajowicz F, Gallardo H: Chondromyxoid fibroma (fibromyxoid chondroma) of bone. A clinico-pathological study of thirty-two cases. J Bone Joint Surg [Br] 53:198, 1971.

529. Gherlinzoni F, Rock M, Picci P: Chondromyxoid fibroma. The experience at the Instituto Ortopedico Rizzoli. J Bone Joint Surg [Am] 65:198, 1983.

530. Feldman F, Hecht HL, Johnston AD: Chondromyxoid fibroma of bone. Radiology 94:249, 1970.

531. Beggs IG, Stoker DJ: Chondromyxoid fibroma of bone. Clin Radiol 33:671, 1982.

532. Rahimi A, Beabout JW, Ivins JC, et al: Chondromyxoid fibroma: A clinico-pathologic study of 76 cases. Cancer 30:726, 1972.

533. Scaglietti O, Stringa G: Myxoma of bone in childhood. J Bone Joint Surg [Am] 43:67, 1961.

534. Kreicbergs A, Lonnquist PA, Willems J: Chondromyxoid fibroma. A review of the literature and a report on our own experience. Acta Pathol Microbiol Immunol Scand (A) 93:189, 1985.

535. Dahlin DC: Chondromyxoid fibroma of bone, with emphasis on its morphological relationship to benign chondroblastoma. Cancer 9:195, 1956.

536. Norman A, Steiner GC: Case report 66. Skel Radiol 3:115, 1978.

537. Lawson JP, Barwick KW: Case report 209. Skel Radiol 9:53, 1982.

538. Nunez C, Bennett T, Bohlman HH: Chondromyxoid fibroma of the thoracic spine. Case report and review of the literature. Spine 7:436, 1982.

539. Standefer M, Hardy RW Jr, Marks K, et al: Chondromyxoid fibroma of the cervical spine—a case report with a review of the literature and a description of an operative approach to the lower anterior cervical spine. Neurosurgery 11:288, 1982.

540. Zeman SC, Hurley EJ: Chondromyxoid fibroma of the rib initially seen as a pulmonary lesion. JAMA 242:2588, 1979.

541. Ramani PS: Chondromyxoid fibroma: A rare cause of spinal cord compression. Case report. J Neurosurg 40:107, 1974.

542. Mayer BS: Chondromyxoid fibroma of lumbar spine. J Can Assoc Radiol 29:271, 1978.

543. Klein GM: Chondromyxoid fibroma: An unusual location. Clin Orthop 164:249, 1982.

544. Miyamoto E, Kuriyama T, Iwamoto M, et al: Cranial chondromyxoid fibroma. Case report. J Neurosurg 55:1001, 1981.

545. Teitelbaum SL, Bessone L: Resection of a large chondromyxoid fibroma of the sternum. Report of the first case and review of the literature. J Thorac Cardiovasc Surg 57:333, 1969.

546. Merli GA, Angiari P, Botticelli A, et al: Chondromyxoid fibroma with spinal cord compression. Surg Neurol 10:123, 1978.

547. Thompson SH, Weathers DR, Vatral JJ: Chondromyxoid fibroma of the jaws. Head Neck Surg 4:330, 1982.

548. Shulman L, Bale P, de Silva M: Sacral chondromyxoid fibroma. Pediatr Radiol 15:138, 1985.

549. Prichard RW, Stoy RP, Barwick JTF: Chondromyxoid fibroma of the scapula. Report of a case. J Bone Joint Surg [Am] 46:1759, 1964.

550. Kearney V: Chondromyxoid fibroma of the mandible. Br J Oral Surg 21:304, 1983.

551. Blair WF, Robinson RA, Buckwalter JA: Chondromyxoid fibroma in carpal bone. Clin Orthop 188:199, 1984.

552. Munzenberg KJ, Cremer H: Mutlizentrisches Chondromyxoidfibrom des Knochens mit extraskeletaler Beteiligung. Z Orthop 115:355, 1977.

553. Andrew T, Kenwright J, Woods C: Periosteal chondromyxoid fibroma of the tibia. A case report. Acta Orthop Scand 53:467, 1982.

554. Bialik V, Kedar A, Ben-Arie Y, et al: Case report 315. Skel Radiol 13:323, 1985.

555. Chacha PB, Tan KK: Periosteal myxoma of the femur. J Bone Joint Surg [Am] 54:1091, 1972.

556. Adler CP: Case report 338. Skel Radiol 14:305, 1985.

557. Ralph LL: Chondromyxoid fibroma of bone. J Bone Joint Surg [Br] 44:7, 1962.

558. Montaguti A, Esposito C, Segato P, et al: Chondromyxoid fibroma of the iliac bone: A case report with ultrastructural observations. Tumori 70:89, 1984.

559. Tornberg DN, Rice RW, Johnston AD: The ultrastructure of chondromyxoid fibroma. Its biologic and diagnostic implications. Clin Orthop 95:295, 1973.

560. Norman A, Steiner GC: Case report 38. Skel Radiol 2:105, 1977.

561. Kyriakos M: Soft tissue implantation of chondromyxoid fibroma. Am J Surg Pathol 3:363, 1979.

562. Mikilowski P, Ostberg G: Recurrent chondromyxoid fibroma. Acta Orthop Scand 42:385, 1971.

563. Milgran JW: The origins of osteochondromas and enchondromas. A histopathologic study. Clin Orthop 174:264, 1983.

564. Hume JB: The causation of multiple exostoses. Br J Surg 17:236, 1929.

565. Muller E: Uber hereditäre multiple cartilaginare Exostosen und Echondrosen. Beitr Pathol Anat Allg Pathol 57:232, 1913–1914.

566. Keith A: Studies on the anatomical changes which accompany certain growth disorders of the human body. I. The nature of the structural alterations in the disorder known as multiple exostoses. J Anat 54:101, 1920.

567. Jaffe HL: Hereditary multiple exostosis. Arch Pathol 36:335, 1943.

568. Langenskiold A: Normal and pathologic bone growth in the light of the development of cartilaginous foci in chondrodysplasia. Acta Chir Scand 95:367, 1947.

569. D'Ambrosia R, Ferguson AB Jr: The formation of osteochondroma by epiphyseal cartilage transplantation. Clin Orthop 61:103, 1968.

570. Heiple KG: Carpal osteochondroma. J Bone Joint Surg [Am] 43:861, 1961.

571. Ghormley RK, Meyerding HW: Osteochondromata of the pelvic bones. J Bone Joint Surg 28:40, 1946.

572. Gokay H, Bucy PC: Osteochondroma of the lumbar spine. Report of a case. J Neurosurg 12:72, 1955.

573. Bell MS: Benign cartilaginous tumours of the spine. A report of one case together with a review of the literature. Br J Surg 58:707, 1971.

574. Fielding JW, Ratzan S: Osteochondroma of the cervical spine. J Bone Joint Surg [Am] 55:640, 1973.

575. Twersky J, Kassner EG, Tenner MS, et al: Vertebral and costal osteochondromas causing spinal cord compression. AJR 124:124, 1975.

576. Inglis AE, Rubin RM, Lewis RJ, et al: Osteochondroma of the cervical spine. Case report. Clin Orthop 126:127, 1977.

577. Wu KK, Guise ER: Osteochondroma of the atlas: A case report. Clin Orthop 136:160, 1978.

578. Julien J, Riemens V, Vital C, et al: Cervical cord compression by solitary osteochondroma of the atlas. J Neurol Neurosurg Psychiatry 41:479, 1978.

579. MacGee EE: Osteochondroma of the cervical spine: A cause of transient quadriplegia. Neurosurgery 4:259, 1979.

580. Palmer FJ, Blum PW: Osteochondroma with spinal cord compression. Report of three cases. J Neurosurg 52:842, 1980.

581. Novick GS, Pavlov H, Bullough PG: Osteochondroma of the cervical spine: Report of two cases in preadolescent males. Skel Radiol 8:13, 1982.

582. Karian JM, DeFilipp G, Buchheit WA, et al: Vertebral osteochondroma causing spinal cord compression. Case report. Neurosurgery 14:483, 1984.

583. Linkowski GD, Tsai FY, Recher L, et al: Solitary osteochondroma with spinal cord compression. Surg Neurol 23:388, 1985.

584. Esposito PW, Crawford AH, Vogler C: Solitary osteochondroma occurring on the transverse process of the lumbar spine. A case report. Spine 10:398, 1985.

585. List CF: Osteochondromas arising from the base of the skull. Surg Gynecol Obstet 76:480, 1943.

586. King LS, Butcher J: Osteochondroma of the base of the skull. Arch Pathol 37:282, 1944.

587. Gabrielsen TO, Kingman AF Jr: Osteocartilaginous tumors of the base of the skull. Report of a unique case and review of the literature. AJR 91:1016, 1964.

588. Bakdash H, Alksne JF, Rand RW: Osteochondroma of the base of the skull causing an isolated oculomotor nerve paralysis. Case report emphasizing microsurgical techniques. J Neurosurg 31:230, 1969.

589. Fon G, Sage MR: Osteochondroma of the clivus. Australas Radiol 23:46, 1979.

590. Cooley LH, Torg JS: "Pseudowinging" of the scapula secondary to subscapular osteochondroma. Clin Orthop 162:119, 1982.

591. Parsons TA: The snapping scapula and subscapular exostoses. J Bone Joint Surg [Br] 55:345, 1973.

592. Trotter D, Zindrick M, Ibrahim K: An unusual presentation of an osteochondroma. Report of a case. J Bone Joint Surg [Am] 66:299, 1984.

593. Lanzieri CF, Solodnik P, Sacher M, et al: Computed tomography of solitary spinal osteochondromas. J Comput Assist Tomogr 9:1042, 1985.

594. Kenney PJ, Gilula LA, Murphy WA: The use of computed tomography to distinguish osteochondroma and chondrosarcoma. Radiology 139:129, 1981.

595. Hudson TM, Springfield DS, Spanier SS, et al: Benign exostoses and exostotic chondrosarcoma: Evaluation of cartilage thickness by CT. Radiology 152:595, 1984.

596. Lange RH, Lange TA, Rao BK: Correlative radiographic, scintigraphic, and histological evaluation of exostoses. J Bone Joint Surg [Am] 66:1454, 1984.

597. Hudson TM, Chew FS, Manaster BJ: Scintigraphy of benign exostoses and exostotic chondrosarcoma. AJR 140:581, 1983.

598. Hopkins SM, Freitas EL: Bilateral osteochondroma of the ribs in an infant: An unusual case of cyanosis. J Thorac Cardiovasc Surg 49:247, 1965.

599. Chrisman OD, Goldenberg RR: Untreated solitary osteochondroma. Report of two cases. J Bone Joint Surg [Am] 50:508, 1968.

600. Meyerding HW: Exostosis. Radiology 8:282, 1927.

601. Harsha WN: The natural history of osteocartilaginous exostoses (osteochondroma). Am Surg 20:65, 1954.

602. Copeland RL, Meehan PL, Morrissy RT: Spontaneous regression of osteochondromas. Two case reports. J Bone Joint Surg [Am] 67:971, 1985.

603. Merle P, Rougier JL, Duclos AM, et al: Exostose évanescente. Un cas. J Radiol 61:291, 1980.

604. Callan JE, Wood VE: Spontaneous resolution of an osteochondroma. J Bone Joint Surg [Am] 57:723, 1975.

605. Paling MR: The "disappearing" osteochondroma. Skel Radiol 10:40, 1983.

606. Vallance R, Hamblen DL, Kelly IG: Vascular complications of osteochondroma. Clin Radiol 36:639, 1985.

607. Greenway G, Resnick D, Bookstein JJ: Popliteal pseudoaneurysm as a com-

plication of an adjacent osteochondroma: Angiographic diagnosis. AJR 132:294, 1979.

608. Manner R, Makinen E: Angiographic findings in a false popliteal aneurysm due to osteochondroma of the femur. Pediatr Radiol 3:244, 1975.

609. Solhaugh JH, Olerud SE: Pseudoaneurysm of the femoral artery caused by osteochondroma of the femur. J Bone Joint Surg [Am] 57:867, 1975.

610. Cassie GF, Dawson AS, Sheville E: False aneurysm of femoral artery from cancellous exostosis of the femur. J Bone Joint Surg [Br] 57:379, 1975.

611. Hovelius L: Aneurysm of popliteal artery caused by cartilaginous exostosis. Acta Orthop Scand 46:836, 1975.

612. Schoene HR, Berthelsen S, Ahn C: Aneurysm of femoral artery secondary to osteochondroma. J Bone Joint Surg [Am] 55:847, 1973.

613. Hershey SL, Landsen FT: Osteochondromas as a cause of false popliteal aneurysms. J Bone Joint Surg [Am] 54:1765, 1972.

614. Kover JH, Schwalbe N, Levowitz BS: Popliteal aneurysm due to osteochondroma in athletic injury. NY State J Med 70:3001, 1970.

615. Chalstrey LJ: Aneurysm of the posterior tibial artery due to a tibial osteochondroma. Br J Surg 57:151, 1970.

616. Ferriter P, Hirschy J, Kesseler H, et al: Popliteal pseudoaneurysm. A case report. J Bone Joint Surg [Am] 65:695, 1983.

617. Ennker J, Freyschmidt J, Reilmann H, et al: False aneurysm of the femoral artery due to an osteochondroma. Arch Orthop Trauma Surg 102:206, 1984.

618. Han SK, Henein MHG, Novin N, et al: An unusual arterial complication seen with a solitary osteochondroma. Am J Surg 43:471, 1977.

619. Lemaire R, Beaujean M: Popliteal aneurysm complicating an osteogenic exostosis of the tibia. Acta Orthop Belg 41:625, 1975.

620. Cachera JP, Letournel E, Kieffer E: A case of arterial aneurysm complicating an osteogenic exostosis of the upper extremity or the humerus. J Chir (Paris) 99:39, 1970.

621. Borges AM, Huvos AG, Smith J: Bursa formation and synovial chondrometaplasia associated with osteochondromas. Am J Clin Pathol 75:648, 1981.

622. El-Khoury GY, Bassett GS: Symptomatic bursa formation with osteochondromas. AJR 133:895, 1979.

623. Josefczyk MA, Smith J, Huvos AG, et al: Bursa formation in secondary chondrosarcoma with intrabursal chondrosarcomatosis. Am J Surg Pathol 9:309, 1985.

624. Voegeli E, Laissue J, Kaiser A, et al: Case report 143. Skel Radiol 6:134, 1981.

625. Anderson RL Jr, Popowitz L, Li JKH: An unusual sarcoma arising in a solitary osteochondroma. J Bone Joint Surg [Am] 51:1199, 1969.

626. Schweitzer G, Pirie D: Osteosarcoma arising in a solitary osteochondroma. S Afr Med J 45:810, 1971.

627. Garrison RC, Unni KK, McLeod RA, et al: Chondrosarcoma arising in osteochondroma. Cancer 49:1890, 1982.

628. Norman A, Sissons HA: Radiographic hallmarks of peripheral chondrosarcoma. Radiology 151:589, 1984.

629. Stoker DJ, Pringle J: Case report 168. Skel Radiol 7:135, 1981.

630. Solomon L: Hereditary multiple exostosis. J Bone Joint Surg [Br] 45:292, 1963.

631. Shapiro F, Simon S, Glimcher MJ: Hereditary multiple exostoses. Anthropometric, roentgenographic, and clinical aspects. J Bone Joint Surg [Am] 61:815, 1979.

632. Ehrenfried A: Hereditary deforming chondrodysplasia—multiple cartilaginous exostoses. A review of the American literature and report of twelve cases. JAMA 68:502, 1917.

633. Stark JD, Adler NN, Robinson WH: Hereditary multiple exostoses. Radiology 59:212, 1952.

634. Weiner DS, Hoyt WA Jr: The development of the upper end of the femur in multiple hereditary exostosis. Clin Orthop 137:187, 1978.

635. Gierse H: Das gemeinsame Auftreten von Coxa valga und multiplen kartilagrnairen Exostosen. Z Orthop 124:4, 1983.

636. Fogel GR, McElfresh EC, Peterson HA, et al: Management of deformities of the forearm in multiple hereditary osteochondromas. J Bone Joint Surg [Am] 66:670, 1984.

637. Epstein DA, Levin EJ: Bone scintigraphy in hereditary multiple exostoses. AJR 130:331, 1978.

638. Roman G: Hereditary multiple exostoses. A rare cause of spinal cord compression. Spine 3:230, 1978.

639. Signargout J, Guégan Y, Le Marec B, et al: Les paraplégies de la maladie des exostoses multiples. A propos de deux observations. J Radiol Electrol 54:403, 1973.

640. Vinstein AL, Franken EA Jr: Hereditary multiple exostoses. Report of a case with spinal cord compression. AJR 112:405, 1971.

641. Becker MH, Epstein F: Case report 77. Skel Radiol 3:197, 1978.

642. Solomon L: Chondrosarcoma in hereditary multiple exostosis. S Afr Med J 48:671, 1974.

643. El-Khoury GAY, Bonfiglio M: Case report 60. Skel Radiol 3:49, 1978.

644. Mouchet A, Belot J: La tarsomegalie. J Radiol Electrol 10:289, 1926.

645. Trevor D: Tarso-epiphyseal aclasis. Congenital error of epiphyseal development. J Bone Joint Surg [Br] 32:204, 1950.

646. Keats T: Dysplasia epiphysealis hemimelica. Radiology 68:558, 1957.

647. Fairbank TJ: Dysplasia epiphysealis hemimelica (tarso-epiphyseal aclasis). J Bone Joint Surg [Br] 38:237, 1956.

648. Fasting OJ, Bjerkreim I: Dysplasia epiphysealis hemimelica. Acta Orthop Scand 47:217, 1976.

649. Kettelkamp DB, Campbell CJ, Bonfiglio M: Dysplasia epiphysealis hemime-

lica. A report of fifteen cases and a review of the literature. J Bone Joint Surg [Am] 48:746, 1966.

650. Barta O, Schanzl A, Szepesi J: Dysplasia epiphysealis hemimelica. Acta Orthop Scand 44:702, 1973.

651. Connor JM, Horan FT, Beighton P: Dysplasia epiphysealis hemimelica. A clinical and genetic study. J Bone Joint Surg [Br] 65:350, 1983.

652. Wiedermann HR, Mann M, Kreudenstein PS: Dysplasia epiphysealis hemimelica—Trevor disease. Severe manifestations in a child. Eur J Pediatr 136:311, 1981.

653. Azous EM, Slomic AM, Archambault H: Upper extremity involvement in Trevor disease. J Can Assoc Radiol 35:209, 1984.

654. Oates E, Cutler JB, Miyamoto EK, et al: Case report 305. Skel Radiol 13:174, 1985.

655. Fisher MR, Hernandez RJ, Poznanski AK, et al: Case report 262. Skel Radiol 11:147, 1984.

656. Wolfgang GL, Heath RD: Dysplasia epiphysealis hemimelica. A case report. Clin Orthop 116:32, 1976.

657. Bigliani LU, Neer CS II, Parisien M, et al: Dysplasia epiphysealis hemimelica of the scapula. A case report. J Bone Joint Surg [Am] 62:292, 1980.

658. Azouz EM, Slomic AM, Marton D, et al: The variable manifestations of dysplasia epiphysealis hemimelica. Pediatr Radiol 15:44, 1985.

659. Enriquez J, Quiles M, Torres C: A unique case of dysplasia epiphysealis hemimelica of the patella. Clin Orthop 160:168, 1981.

660. Buckwalter JA, El-Khoury GY, Flatt AE: Dysplasia epiphysealis hemimelica of the ulna. Clin Orthop 135:36, 1978.

661. Lamesch AJ: Dysplasia epiphysealis hemimelica of the carpal bones. J Bone Joint Surg [Am] 65:398, 1983.

662. Stockley I, Smith TWD: Dysplasia epiphysealis hemimelica. An unusual case of macrodactyly of the thumb. J Hand Surg [Br] 10:249, 1985.

663. Carlson DH, Wilkinson RH: Variability of unilateral epiphyseal dysplasia (dysplasia epiphysealis hemimelica). Radiology 133:369, 1979.

664. Hensinger RN, Cowell HR, Ramsey PL, et al: Familial dysplasia epiphysealis hemimelica, associated with chondromas and osteochondromas. J Bone Joint Surg [Am] 56:1513, 1974.

665. Landon GC, Johnson KA, Dahlin DC: Subungual exostoses. J Bone Joint Surg [Am] 61:256, 1979.

666. Brenner MA, Montgomery RM, Kalish SR: Subungual exostosis. Cutis 25:518, 1980.

667. Kurtz AD: Subungual exostoses. Surg Gynecol Obstet 43:488, 1926.

668. Cohen HJ, Frank SB, Minkin W, et al: Subungual exostoses. Arch Dermatol 107:431, 1973.

669. Bennett RG, Gammer S: Painful callus of the thumb due to phalangeal exostosis. Arch Dermatol 108:826, 1973.

670. Wissinger HA, McClain EJ, Boyes JH: Turret exostosis. J Bone Joint Surg [Am] 48:105, 1966.

671. Lee BS, Kaplan R: Turret exostosis of the phalanges. Clin Orthop 100:186, 1974.

672. Engber WD, McBeath AA, Cowle AE: The supracondylar process. Clin Orthop 104:228, 1974.

673. Parkinson C: The supracondyloid process. Radiology 62:556, 1954.

674. Terry RJ: On the racial distribution of the supracondyloid variation. Am J Phys Anthropol 14:459, 1930.

675. Thomsen PB: Processus supracondyloidea humeri with concomitant compression of the median nerve and the ulnar nerve. Acta Orthop Scand 48:391, 1977.

676. Delahaye RP, Metges PJ, Lomazzi R, et al: Apophyse susepitrochléene. J Radiol Electrol 57:341, 1976.

677. Campanacci M, Guernelli N, Leonessa C, et al: Chondrosarcoma: A study of 133 cases, 80 with long term follow-up. Ital J Orthop Traumatol 1:387, 1975.

678. O'Neal LW, Ackerman LV: Chondrosarcoma of bone. Cancer 5:551, 1952.

679. Lindbom Å, Söderberg G, Spjut HJ: Primary chondrosarcoma of bone. Acta Radiol 55:81, 1961.

680. Henderson ED, Dahlin DC: Chondrosarcoma of bone—a study of two hundred and eighty-eight cases. J Bone Joint Surg [Am] 45:1450, 1963.

681. Goldenberg RR: Chondrosarcoma. Bull Hosp Joint Dis 25:30, 1964.

682. Salib PI: Chondrosarcoma. A study of the cases at the Massachusetts General Hospital in twenty-seven years (1937–1963). Am J Orthop 9:240, 1967.

683. Gitelis S, Bertoni F, Picci P, et al: Chondrosarcoma of bone. The experience at the Istituto Ortopedico Rizzoli. J Bone Joint Surg [Am] 63:1248, 1981.

684. Marcove RC, Miké V, Hutter RVP, et al: Chondrosarcoma of the pelvis and upper end of the femur. An analysis of factors influencing survival time in one hundred and thirteen cases. J Bone Joint Surg [Am] 54:561, 1972.

685. Pritchard DJ, Lunke RJ, Taylor WF, et al: Chondrosarcoma: A clinicopathologic and statistical analysis. Cancer 45:149, 1980.

686. Aprin H, Riseborough EJ, Hall JE: Chondrosarcoma in children and adolescents. Clin Orthop 166:226, 1982.

687. Evans HL, Ayala AG, Romsdahl MM: Prognostic factors in chondrosarcoma of bone. A clinicopathologic analysis with emphasis on histologic grading. Cancer 40:818, 1977.

688. Sanerkin NG, Gallagher P: A review of the behaviour of chondrosarcoma of bone. J Bone Joint Surg [Br] 61:395, 1979.

689. Mankin HJ, Cantley KP, Lippiello L, et al: The biology of human chondrosarcoma. I. Description of the cases, grading, and biochemical analyses. J Bone Joint Surg [Am] 62:160, 1980.

690. Pascuzzi CA, Dahlin DC, Clagett OT: Primary tumors of the ribs and sternum. Surg Gynecol Obstet 104:390, 1957.

691. Smith J, McLachlan DL, Huvos AG, et al: Primary tumors of the clavicle and scapula. AJR 124:113, 1975.

692. Palmieri TJ: Chondrosarcoma of the hand. J Hand Surg [Am] 9:332, 1984.

693. Sabanathan S, Salama FD: Cartilaginous tumours of rib. J R Coll Surg Edinb 29:363, 1984.

694. O'Neal LW, Ackerman LV: Cartilaginous tumors of ribs and sternum. J Thorac Surg 21:71, 1951.

695. Gottschalk RG, Smith RT: Chondrosarcoma of the hand. Report of a case with radioactive sulphur studies and review of literature. J Bone Joint Surg [Am] 45:141, 1963.

696. Miki T, Yamamuro T, Oka M, et al: Chondrosarcoma developed in the distal phalangeal bone of the third toe. A case report. Clin Orthop 136:241, 1978.

697. Lansche WE, Spjut HJ: Chondrosarcoma of the small bones of the hand. J Bone Joint Surg [Am] 40:1139, 1958.

698. Dahlin DC, Salvador AH: Chondrosarcomas of bones of the hands and feet—a study of 30 cases. Cancer 34:755, 1974.

699. Patel MR, Pearlman HS, Engler J, et al: Chondrosarcoma of the proximal phalanx of the finger. Review of the literature and report of a case. J Bone Joint Surg [Am] 59:401, 1977.

700. Habal MB, Snyder HH Jr, Murray JE: Chondrosarcoma of the hand. Am J Surg 125:775, 1973.

701. Granberry WM, Bryan W: Chondrosarcoma of the trapezium: A case report. J Hand Surg 3:277, 1978.

702. Scott WW Jr, Fishman EK, Lubbe WJ: Case report 259. Skel Radiol 11:137, 1984.

703. Trias A, Basora J, Sanchez G, et al: Chondrosarcoma of the hand. Clin Orthop 134:297, 1978.

704. Roberts PH, Price CHG: Chondrosarcoma of the bones of the hand. J Bone Joint Surg [Br] 59:213, 1977.

705. Pachter MR, Alpert M: Chondrosarcoma of the foot skeleton. J Bone Joint Surg [Am] 46:601, 1964.

706. DeBenedetti MJ, Waugh TR, Evanski PM, et al: Chondrosarcoma of the talus. A case report. Clin Orthop 136:234, 1978.

707. Wiss DA: Chondrosarcoma of the first metatarsal. J Surg Oncol 23:110, 1983.

708. Batsakis JG, Dito WR: Chondrosarcoma of the maxilla. Arch Otolaryngol 75:55, 1962.

709. Arlen M, Tollefsen HR, Huvos AG, et al: Chondrosarcoma of the head and neck. Am J Surg 120:456, 1970.

710. Curphey JE: Chondrosarcoma of the maxilla: Report of case. J Oral Surg 29:285, 1971.

711. Lanier VC Jr, Rosenfeld L, Wilkinson HA: Chondrosarcoma of the mandible. South Med J 64:711, 1971.

712. Paddison GM, Hanks GE: Chondrosarcoma of the maxilla. Report of a case responding to supervoltage irradiation and review of the literature. Cancer 28:616, 1971.

713. Sato K, Nukaga H, Horikoshi T: Chondrosarcoma of the jaws and facial skeleton: A review of the Japanese literature. J Oral Surg 35:892, 1977.

714. Martis C: Chondrosarcoma of the mandible: Report of case. J Oral Surg 36:227, 1978.

715. Berktold R, Krespi YP, Bytell DE, et al: Chondrosarcoma of the maxilla. Otolaryngol Head Neck Surg 92:484, 1984.

716. Gallagher TM, Strome M: Chondrosarcomas of the facial region. Laryngoscope 82:978, 1972.

717. McCoy JM, McConnel FMS: Chondrosarcoma of the nasal septum. Arch Otolaryngol 107:125, 1981.

718. Bailey CM: Chondrosarcoma of the nasal septum. J Laryngol Otol 96:459, 1982.

719. Nishizawa S, Fukaya T, Inouye K: Chondrosarcoma of the nasal septum: A report of an uncommon lesion. Laryngoscope 94:550, 1984.

720. Grossman RI, Davis KR: Cranial computed tomographic appearance of chondrosarcoma of the base of the skull. Radiology 141:403, 1981.

721. Bahr AL, Gayler BW: Cranial chondrosarcomas. Report of four cases and review of the literature. Radiology 124:151, 1977.

722. Blaylock RL, Kempe LG: Chondrosarcoma of the cervical spine. Case report. J Neurosurg 44:500, 1976.

723. Smith FW, Nandi SC, Mills K: Spinal chondrosarcoma demonstrated by Tc-99m-MDP bone scan. Clin Nucl Med 7:111, 1982.

724. Hermann G, Sacher M, Lanzieri CF, et al: Chondrosarcoma of the spine: an unusual radiographic presentation. Skel Radiol 14:178, 1985.

725. Camins MB, Duncan AW, Smith J, et al: Chondrosarcoma of the spine. Spine 3:202, 1978.

726. Anderson DE, Davidson JK: Case report 117. Skel Radiol 5:129, 1980.

727. Rosenthal DI, Schiller AL, Mankin HJ: Chondrosarcoma: Correlation of radiological and histological grade. Radiology 150:21, 1984.

728. Lodwick GS, Wilson AJ, Farrell C, et al: Determining growth rates of focal lesions of bone from radiographs. Radiology 134:577, 1980.

729. Lodwick GS: The radiologist's role in the management of chondrosarcoma. Radiology 150:275, 1984.

730. Mankin HJ, Cantley KP, Schiller AL, et al: The biology of human chondrosarcoma. II. Variation in chemical composition among types and subtypes of benign and malignant cartilage tumors. J Bone Joint Surg [Am] 62:176, 1980.

731. Sweet DE, Madewell JE, Ragsdale BD: Radiologic and pathologic analysis of solitary bone lesions. Part III: Matrix patterns. Radiol Clin North Am 19:785, 1981.

732. Freiberger R: Thoughts on the diagnosis of bone tumors. Radiology 150:276, 1984.

733. Reiter FB, Ackerman LV, Staple TW: Central chondrosarcoma of the appendicular skeleton. Radiology 105:525, 1972.

734. Hudson TM, Manaster BJ, Springfield DS, et al: Radiology of medullary chondrosarcoma: Preoperative treatment planning. Skel Radiol 10:69, 1983.

735. Middlemiss JH: Cartilage tumors. Br J Radiol 37:277, 1964.

736. Hudson TM, Chew FS, Manaster BJ: Radionuclide bone scanning of medullary chondrosarcoma. AJR 139:1071, 1982.

737. Yaghmai I: Angiographic features of chondromas and chondrosarcomas. Skel Radiol 3:91, 1978.

738. Menanteau BP, Dilenge D: Considerations semilogiques sur l'aspect angiographique des chondrosarcomes. J Can Assoc Radiol 28:193, 1977.

739. Barnes R, Catto M: Chondrosarcoma of bone. J Bone Joint Surg [Br] 48:729, 1966.

740. Phelan JT, Cabrera A: Chondrosarcoma of bone. Surg Gynecol Obstet 119:42, 1964.

741. Kaufman JH, Douglass HO Jr, Blake W, et al: The importance of initial presentation and treatment upon the survival of patients with chondrosarcoma. Surg Gynecol Obstet 145:357, 1977.

742. Dahlin DC, Henderson ED: Chondrosarcoma, a surgical and pathological problem. Review of 212 cases. J Bone Joint Surg [Am] 38:1025, 1956.

743. Kreicbergs A, Slezak E, Söderberg G: The prognostic significance of different histomorphologic features in chondrosarcoma. Virchows Arch (Pathol Anat) 390:1, 1981.

744. Lichtenstein L, Jaffe HL: Chondrosarcoma of bone. Am J Pathol 19:553, 1943.

745. Erlandson RA, Huvos AG: Chondrosarcoma: A light and electron microscopic study. Cancer 34:1642, 1974.

746. Schajowicz F, Cabrini RL, Simes RJ, et al: Ultrastructure of chondrosarcoma. Clin Orthop 100:378, 1974.

747. Aparisi T, Arborgh B, Ericsson JLE, et al: Contribution to the knowledge of the fine structure of chondrosarcoma of bone. With a note on the localization of alkaline phosphatase and ATPase. Acta Pathol Microbiol Immunol Scand (A) 86:157, 1978.

748. Ghadially FN, Lalonde JMA, Yong NK: Amianthoid fibres in a chondrosarcoma. J Pathol 130:147, 1980.

749. Martinez-Tello FJ, Navas-Palacios JJ: Ultrastructural study of conventional chondrosarcomas and mycoid- and mesenchymal-chondrosarcomas. Virchows Arch (Pathol Anat) 396:197, 1982.

750. Meachim G: Histological grading of chondrosarcomata. J Bone Joint Surg [Br] 61:393, 1979.

751. Pope TL Jr, McLaughlin R, Wanebo HJ, et al: Case report 281. Skel Radiol 12:134, 1984.

752. Pinstein ML, Sebes JI, Scott RL: Transarticular extension of chondrosarcoma. AJR 142:779, 1984.

753. Lichtenstein L: Tumors of periosteal origin. Cancer 8:1060, 1955.

754. Jaffe HL: Tumors and Tumorous Conditions of the Bones and Joints. Philadelphia, Lea & Febiger, 1958.

755. Schajowicz F: Juxtacortical chondrosarcoma. J Bone Joint Surg [Br] 59:473, 1977.

756. Wu KK, Kelly AP: Periosteal (juxtacortical) chondrosarcoma: Report of a case occurring in the hand. J Hand Surg 2:314, 1977.

757. Unni KK, Dahlin DC, Beabout JW, et al: Chondrosarcoma: Clear-cell variant. J Bone Joint Surg [Am] 58:676, 1976.

758. Volpe R, Mazabraud A, Thiery JP: Clear cell chondrosarcoma. Report of a new case and review of the literature. Pathologica 75:775, 1983.

759. Le Charpentier Y, Forest M, Postel M, et al: Clear-cell chondrosarcoma. A report of five cases including ultrastructural study. Cancer 44:622, 1979.

760. Slootweg PJ: Clear-cell chondrosarcoma of the maxilla. Oral Surg 50:233, 1980.

761. Campanacci M, Bertoni F, Laus M: Clear cell chondrosarcoma. Ital J Orthop Traumatol 6:365, 1980.

762. Faraggiana T, Sender B, Glicksman P: Light- and electron-microscopic study of clear cell chondrosarcoma. Am J Clin Pathol 75:117, 1981.

763. Salzer-Kuntschik M: Clear-cell chondrosarcoma. J Cancer Res Clin Oncol 101:171, 1981.

764. Faraggiana T, Sender B, Glicksman P: Light- and electron-microscopic study of clear cell chondrosarcoma. Am J Clin Pathol 75:117, 1981.

765. Bjornsson J, Unni KK, Dahlin DC, et al: Clear cell chondrosarcoma of bone. Observations in 47 cases. Am J Surg Pathol 8:223, 1984.

766. Kumar R, David R, Cierney G: Clear cell chondrosarcoma. Radiology 154:45, 1985.

767. Dahlin DC: Case report 54. Skel Radiol 2:247, 1978.

768. Angervall L, Kindblom LG: Clear-cell chondrosarcoma. A light and electron microscopic and histochemical study of two cases. Virchows Arch (Pathol Anat) 389:27, 1980.

769. Duparc J, Badelon O, Bocquet L, et al: Un cas inhabituel de chondrosarcome à cellules claires avec des localisations tumorales intra-synoviales. Rev Chir Orthop 71:127, 1985.

770. Salvador AH, Beabout JW, Dahlin DC: Mesenchymal chondrosarcoma—observations on 30 new cases. Cancer 28:605, 1971.

771. Guccion JG, Font FL, Enzinger FM, et al: Extraskeletal mesenchymal chondrosarcoma. Arch Pathol 95:336, 1973.

772. Tonai M, Hizawa K: Extraskeletal mesenchymal chondrosarcoma: A case report of extraskeletal case with review of the literature. Tokushima J Exp Med 25:193, 1978.

773. Huvos AG, Rosen G, Dabska M, et al: Mesenchymal chondrosarcoma. A clinicopathologic analysis of 35 patients with emphasis on treatment. Cancer 51:1230, 1983.

774. Harwood AR, Krajbich JI, Fornasier VL: Mesenchymal chondrosarcoma: A report of 17 cases. Clin Orthop 158:144, 1981.

775. Pepe AJ, Kuhlmann RF, Miller DB: Mesenchymal chondrosarcoma. A case report. J Bone Joint Surg [Am] 59:256, 1977.

776. Bertoni F, Picci P, Bacchini P, et al: Mesenchymal chondrosarcoma of bone and soft tissues. Cancer 52:533, 1983.

777. Steiner GC, Mirra JM, Bullough PG: Mesenchymal chondrosarcoma. A study of the ultrastructure. Cancer 32:926, 1973.

778. Mazabraud A: Le chondrosarcome mesenchymateux. Rev Chir Orthop 60:197, 1974.

779. Pittman MR, Keller EE: Mesenchymal chondrosarcoma. Report of case. J Oral Surg 32:443, 1974.

780. Mikata A, Iri H, Inuyama Y: Mesenchymal chondrosarcoma—a case report with an ultrastructural study and review of Japanese literatures. Acta Pathol Jpn 27:93, 1977.

781. Bloch DM, Bragoli AJ, Collins DN, et al: Mesenchymal chondrosarcomas of the head and neck. J Laryngol Otol 93:405, 1979.

782. Caravolas JJ, Pierce JM, Andrews JE, et al: Mesenchymal chondrosarcoma of the mandible. Oral Surg 52:478, 1981.

783. Christensen RE Jr: Mesenchymal chondrosarcoma of the jaws. Oral Surg 54:197, 1982.

784. Dabska M, Huvos AG: Mesenchymal chondrosarcoma in the young. A clinicopathologic study of 19 patients with explanation of histogenesis. Virchows Arch (Pathol Anat) 399:89, 1983.

785. Dahlin DC, Henderson ED: Mesenchymal chondrosarcoma. Further observations on a new entity. Cancer 15:410, 1962.

786. Fu YS, Kay S: A comparative ultrastructural study of mesenchymal chondrosarcoma and myxoid chondrosarcoma. Cancer 33:1531, 1974.

787. Scheithauer BW, Rubinstein LJ: Meningeal mesenchymal chondrosarcoma. Report of 8 cases with review of the literature. Cancer 42:2744, 1978.

788. Rollo JL, Green WR, Kahn LB: Primary meningeal mesenchymal chondrosarcoma. Arch Pathol Lab Med 103:239, 1979.

789. McCarthy EF, Dorfman HD: Chondrosarcoma of bone with dedifferentiation: A study of eighteen cases. Hum Pathol 13:36, 1982.

790. Dahlin DC, Beabout JW: Dedifferentiation of low grade chondrosarcomas. Cancer 28:461, 1971.

791. Mirra JM, Marcove RC: Fibrosarcomatous dedifferentiation of primary and secondary chondrosarcoma. Review of five cases. J Bone Joint Surg [Am] 56:285, 1974.

792. Kahn LB: Chondrosarcoma with dedifferentiated foci. A comparative and ultrastructural study. Cancer 37:1365, 1976.

793. McFarland GB, McKinley LM, Reed RJ: Dedifferentiation of low grade chondrosarcomas. Clin Orthop 122:157, 1977.

794. Campanacci M, Bertoni F, Capanna R: Dedifferentiated chondrosarcomas. Ital J Orthop Traumatol 5:331, 1979.

795. Jaworski RC: Gibson M: Test and teach. Number forty-three. Part 1. Pathology 15:364, 504, 1983.

796. Bertoni F, Present D, Picci P, et al: Case report 301. Skel Radiol 13:228, 1985.

797. Astorino RN, Tesluk H: Dedifferentiated chondrosarcoma with rhabdomyosarcomatous component. Hum Pathol 16:318, 1985.

798. Rywlin AM: Chondrosarcoma of bone with "dedifferentiation." Letter to the editor. Hum Pathol 13:963, 1982.

799. Robb JA: Chondrosarcoma of the bone with "dedifferentiation." Letter to the editor. Hum Pathol 13:964, 1982.

800. Jaworski RC: Dedifferentiated chondrosarcoma. An ultrastructural study. Cancer 53:2674, 1984.

801. Frassica FJ, Unni KK, Sim FH: Case report 347. Skel Radiol 15:77, 1986.

802. Dahlin DC: Case report 71. Skel Radiol 3:133, 1978.

803. Hertz I, Hermann G, Shafir M, et al: Case report 239. Skel Radiol 10:126, 1983.

804. Sissons HA: Case report 83. Skel Radiol 3:257, 1979.

805. Caffey J: On fibrous defects in cortical walls of growing tubular bones: Their radiologic appearance, structure, prevalence, natural course, and diagnostic significance. Adv Pediatr 7:13, 1955.

806. Ide F, Kusuhara S, Onuma H, et al: Xanthic variant of non-ossifying fibroma (so-called xanthofibroma) of the mandible. An ultrastructural study. Acta Pathol Jpn 32:135, 1982.

807. Bosch AL, Olaya AP, Fernandez AL: Non-ossifying fibroma of bone. A histochemical and ultrastructural characterization. Virchows Arch (Pathol Anat) 362:13, 1974.

808. Steiner GC: Fibrous cortical defect and nonossifying fibroma of bone. A study of the vetrastructure. Arch Pathol 97:205, 1974.

809. Lazarus SS, Trombetta LD: Non-ossifying fibroma or benign lipoblastoma of bone—an electron-microscopic and histochemical study. Histopathology 6:793, 1982.

810. Herrera GA, Reimann BEF, Scully TJ, et al: Nonossifying fibroma. Electron microscopic examination of two cases supporting a histiocytic rather than a fibroblastic origin. Clin Orthop 167:269, 1982.

811. Sontag LW, Pyle SI: The appearance and nature of cyst-like areas in the distal femoral metaphysis of children. AJR 46:185, 1941.

812. Freyschmidt J, Saure D, Dammenhain S: Der fibrose metaphysare Defekt (fibroser Kurtikalisdefekt, nicht ossifizierendes Knochenfibrom). ROFO 134:169, 1981.

813. Hatcher CH: The pathogenesis of localized fibrous lesions in the metaphysis of long bones. Ann Surg 122:1016, 1945.

814. Compere CL, Coleman SS: Nonosteogenic fibroma of bone. Surg Gynecol Obstet 105:588, 1957.

815. Laus M, Vicenzi G: Histiocytic fibroma of bone (a study of 170 cases). Ital J Orthop Traumatol 5:343, 1979.

816. Cunningham JB, Ackerman LV: Metaphyseal fibrous defects. J Bone Joint Surg [Am] 38:797, 1956.

817. Palmieri AJ, Kovarik JL: Nonosteogenic fibroma of the rib. Am Surg 28:794, 1962.

818. Rudy HN, Scheingold SS: Solitary xanthogranuloma of the mandible. Report of a case. Oral Surg 18:262, 1964.

819. Elzay RP, Mills S, Kay S: Fibrous defect (nonossifying fibroma) of the mandible. Oral Surg 58:402, 1984.

820. Magliato HJ, Nastasi A: Non-osteogenic fibroma occurring in the ilium. J Bone Joint Surg [Am] 49:384, 1967.

821. Gardiner GA: Clavicular nonosteogenic fibroma. An old tumor in a new location. Am J Dis Child 127:734, 1974.

822. Maudsley RH, Stansfeld AG: Non-osteogenic fibroma of bone (fibrous metaphyseal defect). J Bone Joint Surg [Br] 38:714, 1956.

823. Jaffe HL, Lichtenstein L: Non-osteogenic fibroma of bone. Am J Pathol 18:205, 1942.

824. Purcell WM, Mulcahy F: Non-osteogenic fibroma of bone. Clin Radiol 11:51, 1960.

825. Campbell CJ, Harkess J: Fibrous metaphyseal defect of bone. Surg Gynecol Obstet 104:329, 1957.

826. Allman RA: RPC of the month from the AFIP. Radiology 93:167, 1969.

827. Brenner RJ, Hattner RS, Lilien DL: Scintigraphic features of nonosteogenic fibroma. Radiology 131:727, 1979.

828. Mubarak S, Saltzstein SL, Daniel DM: Non-ossifying fibroma. Report of an intact lesion. Am J Clin Pathol 61:697, 1974.

829. Selby S: Metaphyseal cortical defects in the tubular bones of growing children. J Bone Joint Surg [Am] 43:395, 1961.

830. Phelan JT: Fibrous cortical defect and nonosseous fibroma of bone. Surg Gynecol Obstet 119:807, 1964.

831. Morton KS: Bone production in non-osteogenic fibroma. J Bone Joint Surg [Br] 46:233, 1964.

832. Mirra JM, Gold RH, Rand F: Disseminated nonossifying fibromas in association with café-au-lait spots (Jaffe-Campanacci syndrome). Clin Orthop 168:192, 1982.

833. Ponseti IV, Friedman B: Evolution of metaphyseal fibrous defects. J Bone Joint Surg [Am] 31:582, 1949.

834. Young JWR, Levine AM, Dorfman HD: Case report 293. Skel Radiol 12:294, 1984.

835. Bhagwandeen SB: Malignant transformation of a non-osteogenic fibroma of bone. J Pathol Bacteriol 92:562, 1966.

836. Katz JF, Marek FM: Case of coexistent benign and malignant bone tumors. J Mt Sinai Hosp 17:187, 1950.

837. Koppers B, Rakow D, Schmid L: Monostotische kombination eines osteogenen sarkoms mit einem nicht-ossifizierenden knochenfibrom. Roentgenblaetter 30:261, 1977.

838. Kyriakos M, Murphy WA: Concurrence of metaphyseal fibrous defect and osteosarcoma. Skel Radiol 6:179, 1981.

839. Hastrup J, Jensen TS: Osteogenic sarcoma arising in a non-osteogenic fibroma of bone. Acta Pathol Microbiol Scand 63:493, 1965.

840. Devlin JA, Bowman HE, Mitchell CL: Non-osteogenic fibroma of bone. A review of the literature with the addition of six cases. J Bone Joint Surg [Am] 37:472, 1955.

841. Drennan DB, Maylahn DJ, Fahey JJ: Fracture through large nonossifying fibromas. Clin Orthop 103:82, 1974.

842. Peterson HA, Fitzgerald EM: Fractures through nonossifying fibromata in children. Minn Med 63:139, 1980.

843. Arata MA, Peterson HA, Dahlin DC: Pathological fractures through nonossifying fibromas. Review of the Mayo Clinic experience. J Bone Joint Surg [Am] 63:980, 1981.

844. Asnes RS, Berdon WE, Bassett CA: Hypophosphatemic rickets in an adolescent cured by excision of a nonossifying fibroma. Clin Pediatr 20:646, 1981.

845. Leehey DJ, Ing TS, Daugirdas JT: Fanconi syndrome associated with a nonossifying fibroma of bone. Am J Med 78:708, 1985.

846. Salassa RM, Jowsey J, Arnaud CD: Hypophosphatemic osteomalacia associated with "nonendocrine" tumors. N Engl J Med 283:65, 1970.

847. Campanacci M, Laus M, Boriani S: Multiple non-ossifying fibromata with extraskeletal anomalies: A new syndrome? J Bone Joint Surg [Br] 65:627, 1983.

848. Barnes GR Jr, Gwinn JL: Distal irregularities of the femur simulating malignancy. AJR 122:180, 1974.

849. Brower AC, Culver JE Jr, Keats TE: Histological nature of the cortical irregularity of the medial posterior distal femoral metaphysis in children. Radiology 99:389, 1971.

850. Resnick D, Greenway G: Distal femoral cortical defects, irregularities, and excavations. A critical review of the literature with the addition of histologic and paleopathologic data. Radiology 143:345, 1982.

851. Whitesides TE Jr, Ackerman LV: Desmoplastic fibroma. A report of three cases. J Bone Joint Surg [Am] 42:1143, 1960.

852. Dahlin DC, Hoover NW: Desmoplastic fibroma of bone. Report of two cases. JAMA 188:685, 1964.

853. Cohen P, Goldenberg RR: Desmoplastic fibroma of bone. Report of two cases. J Bone Joint Surg [Am] 47:1620, 1965.

854. Rabhan WN, Rosai J: Desmoplastic fibroma. Report of ten cases and review of the literature. J Bone Joint Surg [Am] 50:487, 1968.

855. Nilsonne U, Göthlin G: Desmoplastic fibroma of bone. Acta Orthop Scand 40:205, 1969.

856. Bertoni F, Calderoni P, Bacchini P, et al: Desmoplastic fibroma of bone. A report of six cases. J Bone Joint Surg [Br] 66:265, 1984.

857. Gebhardt MC, Campbell CJ, Schiller AL, et al: Desmoplastic fibroma of bone. A report of eight cases and review of the literature. J Bone Joint Surg [Am] 67:732, 1985.

858. Scheer GE, Kuhlman RE: Vertebral involvement by desmoplastic fibroma. Report of a case. JAMA 185:669, 1963.

859. Godinho FS, Chiconelli JR, Lemos C: Desmoplastic fibroma of bone. Report of a case. J Bone Joint Surg [Br] 49:560, 1967.

860. Hardy R, Lehrer H: Desmoplastic fibroma vs desmoid tumor of bone. Two cases illustrating a problem in differential diagnosis and classification. Radiology 88:899, 1967.

861. Hinds EC, Kent JN, Fechner RE: Desmoplastic fibroma of the mandible: Report of case. J Oral Surg 27:271, 1969.

862. Scudese VA: Desmoplastic fibroma of the radius. Report of a case with segmental resection. Clin Orthop 79:141, 1971.

863. Triantafyllou NM, Triantafyllou DN, Antonados DN: Desmoid tumors of the bone. Int Surg 57:793, 1972.

864. Cunningham CD, Enriquez P, Smith RO, et al: Desmoplastic fibroma of the mandible. A case report. Ann Otol Rhinol Laryngol 84:125, 1975.

865. Nussbaum GB, Terz JJ, Joy ED Jr: Desmoplastic fibroma of the mandible in a 3-year-old child. J Oral Surg 34:1117, 1976.

866. Freedman PD, Cardo VA, Kerpel SM, et al: Desmoplastic fibroma (fibromatosis) of the jawbones. Report of a case and review of the literature. Oral Surg 46:386, 1978.

867. Taguchi N, Kaneda T: Desmoplastic fibroma of the mandible: Report of case. J Oral Surg 38:441, 1980.

868. Green TL, Gaffney E: Desmoplastic fibroma of the mandible. J Oral Med 36:47, 1981.

869. Thirupathi RG, Vuletin JC, Wadwa R, et al: Desmoplastic fibroma of the ulna. A case report. Clin Orthop 179:231, 1983.

870. Graudal N: Desmoplastic fibroma of bone. Case report and literature review. Acta Orthop Scand 55:215, 1984.

871. Eisen MZ, Butler HE: Desmoplastic fibroma of the maxilla: Report of case. J Am Dent Assoc 108:608, 1984.

872. Lichtman EA, Klein MJ: Case report 302. Skel Radiol 13:160, 1985.

873. Beskin JL, Haddad RJ Jr: Desmoplastic fibroma of the first metatarsal area. A case report. Clin Orthop 195:299, 1985.

874. Lagacé R, Bouchard HL, Delage C, et al: Desmoplastic fibroma of bone. An ultrastructural study. Am J Surg Pathol 3:423, 1979.

875. Sugiura I: Desmoplastic fibroma. Case report and review of the literature. J Bone Joint Surg [Am] 58:126, 1976.

876. Martis C, Karakasis D: Central fibroma of the mandible: Report of case. J Oral Surg 30:758, 1972.

877. Slootweg PJ, Müller H: Central fibroma of the jaw, odontogenic or desmoplastic. A report of five cases with reference to differential diagnosis. Oral Surg 56:61, 1983.

878. Wilner D: Radiology of Bone Tumors and Allied Disorders. Philadelphia, WB Saunders Co, 1982.

879. Larsson SE, Lorentzon R, Boquist L: Fibrosarcoma of bone. A demographic, clinical and histopathological study of all cases recorded in the Swedish cancer registry from 1958 to 1968. J Bone Joint Surg [Br] 58:412, 1976.

880. Pritchard DJ, Sim FH, Ivins JC, et al: Fibrosarcoma of bone and soft tissues of the trunk and extremities. Orthop Clin North Am 8:869, 1977.

881. Bertoni F, Capanna R, Calderoni P, et al: Primary central (medullary) fibrosarcoma of bone. Semin Diagn Pathol 1:185, 1984.

882. Eyre-Brook AL, Price CHG: Fibrosarcoma of Bone. Review of fifty consecutive cases from the Bristol bone tumour registry. J Bone Joint Surg [Br] 51:20, 1969.

883. Jeffree GM, Price CHG: Metastatic spread of fibrosarcoma of bone. A report on forty-nine cases, and a comparison with osteosarcoma. J Bone Joint Surg [Br] 58:418, 1976.

884. Taconis WK, Van Rijssel TG: Fibrosarcoma of long bones. A study of the significance of areas of malignant fibrous histiocytoma. J Bone Joint Surg [Br] 67:111, 1985.

885. McLeod JJ, Dahlin DC, Ivins JC: Fibrosarcoma of bone. Am J Surg 94:431, 1957.

886. Gilmer WS Jr, MacEwen GD: Central (medullary) fibrosarcoma of bone. J Bone Joint Surg [Am] 40:121, 1958.

887. Cunningham MP, Arlen M: Medullary fibrosarcoma of bone. Cancer 21:31, 1968.

888. Dahlin DC, Ivins JC: Fibrosarcoma of bone. A study of 114 cases. Cancer 23:35, 1969.

889. Hoggins GS, Brady CL: Fibrosarcoma of maxilla. Report of a case. Oral Surg 15:34, 1962.

890. Van Blarcom CW, Masson JK, Dahlin DC: Fibrosarcoma of the mandible. A clinicopathologic study. Oral Surg 32:428, 1971.

891. MacFarlane WI: Fibrosarcoma of the mandible with pulmonary metastases: A case report. Br J Oral Surg 10:168, 1972.

892. Richardson JF, Fine MA, Goldman HM: Fibrosarcoma of the mandible. A clinicopathologic controversy: Report of case. J Oral Surg 30:664, 1972.

893. Slootweg PJ, Müller H: Fibrosarcoma of the jaws. A study of 7 cases. J Maxillofac Surg 12:157, 1984.
894. Mansfield JB: Primary fibrosarcoma of the skull. Case report. J Neurosurg 47:785, 1977.
895. Arita N, Ushio Y, Hayakawa T, et al: Primary fibrosarcoma of the skull. Surg Neurol 14:381, 1980.
896. Huvos AG, Higinbotham NL: Primary fibrosarcoma of bone. A clinicopathologic study of 130 patients. Cancer 35:837, 1975.
897. Steiner PH: Multiple diffuse fibrosarcoma of bone. Am J Pathol 20:877, 1944.
898. Nielsen AR, Poulsen H: Multiple diffuse fibrosarcomata of the bones. Acta Pathol Microbiol Scand 55:265, 1962.
899. Hernandez FJ, Fernandez BB: Multiple diffuse fibrosarcoma of bone. Cancer 37:939, 1976.
900. Taconis WK, Mulder JD: Fibrosarcoma and malignant fibrous histiocytoma of long bones: Radiographic features and grading. Skel Radiol 11:237, 1984.
901. Bertoni F, Capanna R, Calderoni P, et al: Case report 223. Skel Radiol 9:225, 1983.
902. Destouet JM, Kyriakos M, Gilula LA: Fibrous histiocytoma (fibroxanthoma) of a cervical vertebra. A report with a review of the literature. Skel Radiol 5:241, 1980.
903. Roessner A, Immenkamp M, Wiedner A, et al: Benign fibrous histiocytoma of bone. Light- and electron-microscopic observations. J Cancer Res Clin Oncol 101:191, 1981.
904. Clark TD, Stelling CB, Fechner RE: Case report 328. Skel Radiol 14:149, 1985.
905. Ruffoni R: Solitary bone xanthoma. Panminerva Med 3:416, 1981.
906. Johnston J: Giant cell tumor of bone. The role of the giant cell in orthopedic pathology. Orthop Clin North Am 8:751, 1977.
907. Jaffe HL, Lichtenstein L, Portis RB, Giant cell tumor of bone. Its pathologic appearance, grading, supposed variants and treatment. Arch Pathol 30:993, 1940.
908. Schajowicz F: Giant-cell tumors of bone (osteoclastoma). J Bone Joint Surg [Am] 43:1, 1961.
909. Schajowicz F, Ubios AM, Araujo ES, et al: Virus-like intranuclear inclusions in giant cell tumor of bone. Clin Orthop 201:247, 1985.
910. Welsh RA, Meyer AT: Nuclear fragmentations and associated fibrils in giant cell tumor of bone. Lab Invest 22:63, 1970.
911. Fornasier VL, Flores L, Hastings D, et al: Virus-like filamentous intranuclear inclusions in a giant-cell tumor, not associated with Paget's disease of bone. A case report. J Bone Joint Surg [Am] 67:333, 1985.
912. McGrath PJ: Giant-cell tumor of bone. An analysis of fifty-two cases. J Bone Joint Surg [Br] 54:216, 1972.
913. Goldenberg RR, Campbell CJ, Bonfiglio M: Giant-cell tumor of bone. An analysis of two hundred and eighteen cases. J Bone Joint Surg [Am] 52:619, 1970.
914. Larsson SE, Lorentzon R, Boquist L: Giant-cell tumor of bone. A demographic, clinical, and histopathological study of all cases recorded in the Swedish Cancer Registry for the years 1958 through 1968. J Bone Joint Surg [Am] 57:167, 1975.
915. Dahlin DC, Cupps RE, Johnson EW Jr: Giant-cell tumor: A study of 195 cases. Cancer 25:1061, 1970.
916. McGrath PJ: Giant-cell tumour of bone. An analysis of fifty-two cases. J Bone Joint Surg [Br] 54:216, 1972.
917. Campanacci M, Giunti A, Olmi R: Giant-cell tumours of bone. A study of 209 cases with long-term follow-up in 130. Ital J Orthop Traumatol 1:249, 1975.
918. McInerney DP, Middlemiss JH: Giant-cell tumour of bone. Skel Radiol 2:195, 1978.
919. Sung HW, Kuo DP, Shu WP, et al: Giant-cell tumor of bone: Analysis of two hundred and eight cases in Chinese patients. J Bone Joint Surg [Am] 64:755, 1982.
920. Jaffe HL: Giant-cell tumour (osteoclastoma) of bone: Its pathologic delimitation and the inherent clinical implications. Ann R Coll Surg Engl 13:343, 1953.
921. Dahlin DC: Giant cell tumor of bone: Highlights of 407 cases. AJR 144:955, 1985.
922. Hutter RVP, Worcester JN Jr, Francis KC, et al: Benign and malignant giant cell tumors of bone. A clinicopathological analysis of the natural history of the disease. Cancer 15:653, 1962.
923. Cohen DM, Dahlin DC, MacCarty CS: Vertebral giant-cell tumor and variants. Cancer 17:461, 1964.
924. Dahlin DC: Giant-cell tumor of vertebrae above the sacrum. A review of 31 cases. Cancer 39:1350, 1977.
925. Di Lorenzo N, Spallone A, Nolletti A, et al: Giant cell tumors of the spine: A clinical study of six cases, with emphasis on the radiological features, treatment, and follow-up. Neurosurgery 6:29, 1980.
926. Larsson SE, Lorentzon R, Boquist L: Giant-cell tumors of the spine and sacrum causing neurological symptoms. Clin Orthop 111:201, 1975.
927. Savini R, Gherlinzoni F, Morandi M, et al: Surgical treatment of giant-cell tumor of the spine. The experience at the Istituto Ortopedico Rizzoli. J Bone Joint Surg [Am] 65:1283, 1983.
928. Shirakuni T, Tamaki N, Matsumoto S, et al: Giant cell tumor in cervical spine. Surg Neurol 23:148, 1985.
929. Johnston AD: Giant cell lesions of bone. Prog Surg Pathol 4:217, 1982.
930. Wolfe JT III, Schiethauer BW, Dahlin DC: Giant-cell tumor of the sphenoid bone. Review of 10 cases. J Neurosurg 59:322, 1983.
931. Motomochi M, Handa Y, Makita Y, et al: Giant cell tumor of the skull. Surg Neurol 23:25, 1985.
932. Smith GA, Ward PH: Giant-cell lesions of the facial skeleton. Arch Otolaryngol 104:186, 1978.
933. Brooke RI: Giant cell tumor in patients with Paget's disease. Oral Surg 30:230, 1970.
934. Jacobs TP, Michelsen J, Polay JS, et al: Giant cell tumor in Paget's disease of bone. Familial and geographic clustering. Cancer 44:742, 1979.
935. Upchurch KS, Simon LS, Schiller AL, et al: Giant cell reparative granuloma of Paget's disease of bone: A unique entity. Ann Intern Med 98:35, 1983.
936. Schajowicz F, Slullitel I: Giant-cell tumor associated with Paget's disease of bone. A case report. J Bone Joint Surg [Am] 48:1340, 1966.
937. Nusbacher N, Sclafani SJ, Birla SR: Case report 155. Skel Radiol 6:233, 1981.
938. Mirra JM, Gold RH: Case report 186. Skel Radiol 8:67, 1982.
939. Hutter RVP, Foot FW Jr, Frazell EL, et al: Giant cell tumors complicating Paget's disease of bone. Cancer 16:1044, 1963.
940. Averill RM, Smith RJ, Campbell CJ: Giant-cell tumors of the bones of the hand. J Hand Surg 5:39, 1980.
941. Henard DC: Giant cell tumor of the thumb metacarpal in an elderly patient: A case report. J Hand Surg [Am] 9:343, 1984.
942. Wold LE, Swee RG: Giant cell tumor of the small bones of the hands and feet. Semin Diagn Pathol 1:173, 1984.
943. Mechlin MB, Kricun ME, Stead J, et al: Giant cell tumor of tarsal bones. Report of three cases and review of the literature. Skel Radiol 11:266, 1984.
944. McGeoch CM, Varian JPW: Osteoclastoma of the first metacarpal. J Hand Surg [Br] 10:129, 1985.
945. Kelikian H, Clayton I: Giant-cell tumor of the patella. J Bone Joint Surg [Am] 39:414, 1957.
946. Sundaram M, Martin SA, Johnson FE, et al: Case report 198. Skel Radiol 8:225, 1982.
947. Tuli SM, Gupta IM, Kumar S: Giant-cell tumor of the scapula treated by total scapulectomy. A case report. J Bone Joint Surg [Am] 56:836, 1974.
948. Bogumill GP, Schultz MA, Johnson LC: Giant-cell tumor—a metaphyseal lesion. J Bone Joint Surg [Am] 54:1558, 1972.
949. Peison B, Feigenbaum J: Metaphyseal giant-cell tumor in a girl of 14. Radiology 118:145, 1976.
950. Picci P, Manfrini M, Zucchi V, et al: Giant-cell tumor of bone in skeletally immature patients. J Bone Joint Surg [Am] 65:486, 1983.
951. Rietveld LAC, Mulder JD, de la Riviere GB, et al: Giant cell tumor: Metaphyseal or epiphyseal origin. Diagn Imaging 50:289, 1981.
952. Kaufman RA, Wakely PE, Greenfield DJ: Case report 224. Skel Radiol 9:218, 1983.
953. Jacobs P: The diagnosis of osteoclastoma (giant-cell tumour): A radiological and pathological correlation. Br J Radiol 45:121, 1972.
954. Wilkerson JA, Cracchiolo A III: Giant-cell tumor of the tibial diaphysis. J Bone Joint Surg [Am] 51:1205, 1969.
955. Ogihara Y, Tsuruta T: A case of giant-cell tumour of femoral shaft origin. Australas Radiol 26:79, 1982.
956. Erens AC: Giant cell tumour of bone. Radiological characteristics. Radiol Clin Biol 42:385, 1973.
957. Smith J, Wixon D, Watson RC: Giant-cell tumor of the sacrum. Clinical and radiologic features in 13 patients. J Can Assoc Radiol 30:34, 1979.
958. Schwimer SR, Bassett LW, Mancuso AA, et al: Giant cell tumor of the cervicothoracic spine. AJR 136:63, 1981.
959. Heuck F: Case report 43. Skel Radiol 2:121, 1977.
960. Mirra JM, Rand F, Rand R, et al: Giant-cell tumor of the second cervical vertebra treated by cryosurgery and irradiation. Clin Orthop 154:228, 1981.
961. Hudson TM, Schiebler M, Springfield DS, et al: Radiology of giant cell tumors of bone: Computed tomography, arthro-tomography, and scintigraphy. Skel Radiol 11:85, 1984.
962. Levine E, De Smet AA, Neff JR, et al: Scintigraphic evaluation of giant cell tumor of bone. AJR 143:343, 1984.
963. Levine E, De Smet AA, Neff JR: Role of radiologic imaging in management planning of giant cell tumor of bone. Skel Radiol 12:79, 1984.
964. de Santos LA, Murray JA: Evaluation of giant cell tumor by computerized tomography. Skel Radiol 2:205, 1978.
965. Resnik CS, Steffe JW, Wang SE: Case report 353. Skel Radiol 15:175, 1986.
966. De Smet AA, Levine E, Neff JR: Tumor involvement of peripheral joints other than the knee: Arthrographic evaluation. Radiology 156:597, 1985.
967. Prando A, de Santos LA, Wallace S, et al: Angiography in giant-cell bone tumors. Radiology 130:323, 1979.
968. Chuang VP, Soo CS, Wallace S, et al: Arterial occlusion: Management of giant cell tumor and aneurysmal bone cyst. AJR 136:1127, 1981.
969. Gunterberg B, Kindblom LG, Laurin S: Giant-cell tumor of bone and aneurysmal bone cyst. A correlated histologic and angiographic study. Skel Radiol 2:65, 1977.
970. de Santos LA, Prando A: Synovial hyperemia in giant cell tumor of bone: Angiographic pitfall. AJR 133:281, 1979.
971. Brady TJ, Gebhardt MC, Pykett IL, et al: NMR imaging of forearms in healthy volunteers and patients with giant-cell tumor of bone. Radiology 144:549, 1982.
972. Stewart MJ, Richardson TR: Giant-cell tumor of bone. J Bone Joint Surg [Am] 34:372, 1952.

973. Sladden RA: Intravascular osteoclasts. J Bone Joint Surg [Br] 39:346, 1957.

974. Williams RR, Dahlin DC, Ghormley RK: Giant-cell tumor of bone. Cancer 7:764, 1954.

975. Marcove RC, Weis LD, Vaghaiwalla MR, et al: Cryosurgery in the treatment of giant cell tumors of bone. A report of 52 consecutive cases. Cancer 41:957, 1978.

976. Murphy WR, Ackerman LV: Benign and malignant giant-cell tumors of bone. A clinical-pathological evaluation of thirty-one cases. Cancer 9:317, 1956.

977. Troup JB, Dahlin DC, Coventry MB: The significance of giant cells in osteogenic sarcoma: Do they indicate a relationship between osteogenic sarcoma and giant cell tumor of bone? Proc Staff Meet Mayo Clin 35:179, 1960.

978. Aparisi T, Arborgh B, Ericsson JLE: Giant cell tumor of bone. Fine structural localization of acid phosphatase. Virchows Arch (Pathol Anat) 376:299, 1977.

979. Aparisi T, Arborgh B, Ericsson JLE: Giant cell tumor of bone. Fine structural localization of alkaline phosphatase. Virchows Arch (Pathol Anat) 378:287, 1978.

980. McCarthy EF, Serrano JA, Wasserkrug HL, et al: The ultrastructural localization of secretory acid phosphatase in giant cell tumor of bone. Clin Orthop 141:295, 1979.

981. Yoshida H, Akeho M, Yumoto T: Giant cell tumor of bone. Enzyme histochemical, biochemical and tissue culture studies. Virchows Arch (Pathol Anat) 395:319, 1982.

982. Burmester GR, Winchester RJ, Dimitriu-Bona A, et al: Delineation of four cell types comprising the giant cell tumor of bone. Expression of Ia and monocyte-macrophage lineage antigens. J Clin Invest 71:1633, 1983.

983. Roessner A, Bassewitz DB, Schlake W, et al: Biologic characterization of human bone tumors. III. Giant cell tumor of bone. A combined electron microscopical, histochemical, and autoradiographical study. Pathol Res Pract 178:431, 1984.

984. Hanaoka H, Friedman B, Mack RP: Ultrastructure and histogenesis of giant-cell tumor of bone. Cancer 25:1408, 1970.

985. Steiner GC, Ghosh L, Dorfman HD: Ultrastructure of giant cell tumors of bone. Hum Pathol 3:569, 1972.

986. Boquist L, Larsson SE, Lorentzon R: Genuine giant-cell tumour of bone; a combined cytological, histopathological and ultrastructural study. Pathol Eur 11:117, 1976.

987. Aparisi T, Arborgh B, Ericsson JLE: Giant cell tumor of bone. Detailed fine structural analysis of different cell components. Virchows Arch (Pathol Anat) 376:273, 1977.

988. Aparisi T, Arborgh B, Ericsson JLE: Giant cell tumor of bone. Variations in patterns of appearance of different cell types. Virchows Arch (Pathol Anat) 381:159, 1979.

989. Mnaymneh WA, Dudley HR, Mnaymneh LG: Giant-cell tumor of bone. An analysis and follow-up study of the forty-one cases observed at the Massachusetts General Hospital between 1925 and 1961. J Bone Joint Surg [Am] 46:63, 1964.

990. Johnson EW Jr, Dahlin DC: Treatment of giant-cell tumor of bone. J Bone Joint Surg [Am] 41:895, 1959.

991. Laurin S, Ekelund L, Persson B: Late recurrence of giant-cell tumor of bone: Pharmacoangiographic evaluation. Skel Radiol 5:227, 1980.

992. Osterman AL, Dalinka MK, Thompson JJ: Case report 210. Skel Radiol 9:56, 1982.

993. Joly MA, Vazquez JJ, Martinez A, et al: Blood-borne spread of a benign giant cell tumor from the radius to the soft tissue of the hand. Cancer 54:2564, 1984.

994. Harris WR, Lehmann ECH: Recurrent giant-cell tumour after en block excision of the distal radius and fibular autograft replacement. J Bone Joint Surg [Br] 65:618, 1983.

995. Joynt GHC, Ortved WE: The accidental operative transplantation of benign giant cell tumor. Ann Surg 127:1232, 1948.

996. Cooper KL, Beabout JW, Dahlin DC: Giant cell tumor: Ossification in soft-tissue implants. Radiology 153:597, 1984.

997. Mirra JM, Ulich T, Magidson J, et al: A case of probable benign pulmonary ''metastases'' or implants arising from a giant cell tumor of bone. Clin Orthop 162:245, 1982.

998. Bertoni F, Present D, Enneking WF: Giant-cell tumor of bone with pulmonary metastases. J Bone Joint Surg [Am] 67:890, 1985.

999. Vanel D, Contesso G, Rebibo G, et al: Benign giant-cell tumours of bone with pulmonary metastases and favourable prognosis. Report on two cases and review of the literature. Skel Radiol 10:221, 1983.

1000. Rock MG, Pritchard DJ, Unni KK: Metastases from histologically benign giant-cell tumor of bone. J Bone Joint Surg [Am] 66:269, 1984.

1001. Caballes RL: The mechanism of metastasis in the so-called ''benign giant cell tumor of bone.'' Hum Pathol 12:762, 1981.

1002. Hall FM, Frank HA, Cohen RB, et al: Ossified pulmonary metastases from giant cell tumor of bone. AJR 127:1046, 1976.

1003. Nascimento AG, Huvos AG, Marcove RC: Primary malignant giant cell tumor of bone. A study of eight cases and review of the literature. Cancer 44:1393, 1979.

1004. Tornberg DN, Dick HM, Johnston AD: Multicentric giant-cell tumors in the long bones. A case report. J Bone Joint Surg [Am] 57:420, 1975.

1005. Sybrandy S, De La Fuente AA: Multiple giant-cell tumor of bone. Report of a case. J Bone Joint Surg [Br] 55:350, 1973.

1006. Kaufman SM, Isaac PC: Multiple giant cell tumors. South Med J 70:105, 1977.

1007. Sim FH, Dahlin DC, Beabout JW: Multicentric giant-cell tumor of bone. J Bone Joint Surg [Am] 59:1052, 1977.

1008. Feldman F: Case report 115. Skel Radiol 5:119, 1980.

1009. Singson R, Feldman F: Case report 229. Skel Radiol 9:276, 1981.

1010. Peimer CA, Schiller AL, Mankin HJ, et al: Multicentric giant-cell tumor of bone. J Bone Joint Surg [Am] 62:652, 1980.

1011. Deburge A, de Grandmaison P: Tumeur à cellules géantes bifocale. Un cas. Rev Chir Orthop 66:323, 1980.

1012. Selzer G, David R, Revach M, et al: Goltz syndrome with multiple giant-cell tumor-like lesions in bones. A case report. Ann Intern Med 80:714, 1974.

1013. Joannides T, Pringle JAS, Shaw DG, et al: Giant cell tumour of bone in focal dermal hypoplasia. Br J Radiol 56:684, 1983.

1014. Jaffe HL: Giant-cell reparative granuloma, traumatic bone cyst, and fibrous (fibro-osseous) dysplasia of the jawbones. Oral Surg 6:159, 1953.

1015. Waldron CA, Shafer WG: The central giant cell reparative granuloma of the jaws. Am J Clin Pathol 15:437, 1966.

1016. Shklar G, Meyer I: Giant-cell tumors of the mandible and maxilla. Oral Surg 14:809, 1961.

1017. Austin LT Jr, Dahlin DC, Royer RQ: Giant-cell reparative granuloma and related conditions affecting the jawbones. Oral Surg 12:1285, 1959.

1018. Schlorf RA, Koop SH: Maxillary giant cell reparative granuloma. Laryngoscope 87:10, 1977.

1019. Som PM, Lawson W, Cohen BA: Giant-cell lesions of the facial bones. Radiology 147:129, 1983.

1020. Rhea JT, Weber AL: Giant-cell granuloma of the sinuses. Radiology 147:135, 1983.

1021. Brooke RI: Giant-cell tumor in patients with Paget's disease. Oral Surg 30:230, 1970.

1022. Rogers LF, Mikhael M, Christ M, et al: Case report 276. Skel Radiol 12:48, 1984.

1023. Littler BO: Central giant-cell granuloma of the jaw—a hormonal influence. Br J Oral Surg 17:43, 1979.

1024. Hirschl S, Katz A: Giant cell reparative granuloma outside the jaw bone. Diagnostic criteria and review of the literature with the first case described in the temporal bone. Hum Pathol 5:171, 1974.

1025. Ackerman LV, Spjut HJ: Giant cell reaction. In Tumors of Bone and Cartilage. Washington DC, Armed Forces Institute of Pathology, 1962, pp 282, 345.

1026. Lorenzo JC, Dorfman HD: Giant-cell reparative granuloma of short tubular bones of the hands and feet. Am J Surg Pathol 4:551, 1980.

1027. Glass TA, Mills SE, Fechner RE, et al: Giant-cell reparative granuloma of the hands and feet. Radiology 149:65, 1983.

1028. Bertheussen KJ, Holck S, Schiodt T: Giant cell lesion of bone of the hand with particular emphasis on giant cell reparative granuloma. J Hand Surg 8:46, 1983.

1029. Strasberg Z, Kirkpatrick D, Tuttle RJ: Case report 86. Skel Radiol 4:47, 1979.

1030. Caskey PM, Wolf MD, Fechner RE: Multicentric giant cell reparative granuloma of the small bones of the hand. A case report and review of the literature. Clin Orthop 193:199, 1985.

1031. Lingg G, Roessner A, Fiedler V, et al: Das reparative Riesenzellgranulom der Extremitaten. ROFO 142:185, 1985.

1032. Jernstrom P, Stark HH: Giant cell reaction of a metacarpal. Am J Clin Pathol 55:77, 1971.

1033. D'Alonzo RT, Pitcock JA, Milford LW: Giant-cell reaction. Report of two cases. J Bone Joint Surg [Am] 45:1267, 1972.

1034. Feldman F, Norman D: Intra- and extraosseous malignant histiocytoma (malignant fibrous xanthoma). Radiology 104:497, 1972.

1035. Stout AP, Lattes R: Tumors of soft tissues. Atlas of Tumor Pathology, Fascicle 1, Second Series. Washington DC, Armed Forces Institute of Pathology, 1967, p 38.

1036. O'Brien JE, Stout AP: Malignant fibrous xanthomas. Cancer 17:1445, 1964.

1037. Kauffman SL, Stout AP: Histiocytic tumors (fibrous xanthoma and histiocytoma) in children. Cancer 14:469, 1961.

1038. Ozzello L, Stout AP, Murray MR: Cultural characteristics of malignant histiocytomas and fibrous xanthomas. Cancer 16:331, 1963.

1039. Seiss SW, Enzinger FM: Malignant fibrous histiocytoma: An analysis of 200 cases. Cancer 41:2250, 1978.

1040. Fu YS, Gabbiani G, Kaye GI, et al: Malignant soft tissue tumors of probable histiocytic origin (MFH): General considerations and electron microscopic and tissue culture studies. Cancer 35:176, 1975.

1041. Van Furth R: Origin and kinetics of monocytes and macrophages. Semin Hematol 17:125, 1970.

1042. Golde DW, Hocking WG, Quan SG, et al: Origin of human bone marrow fibroblasts. Br J Haematol 44:183, 1980.

1043. Groopman JE, Golde DW: The histiocytic disorders: A pathophysiologic analysis. Ann Intern Med 94:95, 1981.

1044. Kosima M: Tumor growth of the reticuloendothelial system. Acta Pathol Jpn 263:273, 1976.

1045. Spanier SS: Malignant fibrous histiocytoma of bone. Orthop Clin North Am 8:947, 1977.

1046. Capanna R, Bertoni F, Bacchini P, et al: Malignant fibrous histiocytoma of bone. The experience at the Rizzoli Institute: Report of 90 cases. Cancer 54:177, 1984.

1047. Ros PR, Viamonte M Jr, Rywlin AM: Malignant fibrous histiocytoma: Mesenchymal tumor of ubiquitous origin. AJR 142:753, 1984.

1048. Huvos AG, Heilweil M, Bretsky SS: The pathology of malignant fibrous histiocytoma of bone. A study of 130 patients. Am J Surg Pathol 9:853, 1985.

1049. Yuen WWH, Saw D: Malignant fibrous histiocytoma of bone. J Bone Joint Surg [Am] 67:482, 1985.
1050. Feldman F, Lattes R: Primary malignant fibrous histiocytoma (fibrous xanthoma) of bone. Skel Radiol 1:145, 1977.
1051. Dahlin DC, Unni KK, Matsuno T: Malignant (fibrous) histiocytoma of bone—fact or fancy? Cancer 39:1508, 1977.
1052. Spanier SS, Eneking WF, Enriquez P: Primary malignant fibrous histiocytoma of bone. Cancer 36:2084, 1975.
1053. Nakashima Y, Morshita S, Kotoura Y, et al: Malignant fibrous histiocytoma of bone. A review of 13 cases and an ultrastructural study. Cancer 55:2804, 1985.
1054. Newland RC, Harrison MA, Wright RG: Fibroxanthosarcoma of bone. Pathology 7:203, 1975.
1055. Huvos AG: Primary malignant fibrous histiocytoma of bone. Clinicopathologic study of 18 patients. NY State J Med 76:552, 1976.
1056. Inada O, Yumoto T, Furuse K, et al: Ultrastructural features of malignant fibrous histiocytoma of bone. Acta Pathol Jpn 26:491, 1976.
1057. Kahn LB, Webber B, Mills E, et al: Malignant fibrous histiocytoma (malignant fibrous xanthoma: xanthosarcoma) of bone. Cancer 42:640, 1978.
1058. Takechi H, Taguchi K: Malignant fibrous histiocytoma with skeletal involvement. Acta Med Okayama 32:343, 1978.
1059. McCarthy EF, Matsuno T, Dorfman HD: Malignant fibrous histiocytoma of bone: A study of 35 cases. Hum Pathol 10:57, 1979.
1060. Martinez-Tello FJ, Navas-Palacios JJ, Calvo-Asensio M, et al: Malignant fibrous histiocytoma of bone. A clinicopathological and electronmicroscopical study. Pathol Res Pract 173:141, 1981.
1061. Ghandur-Mnaymneh L, Zych G, et al: Primary malignant fibrous histiocytoma of bone: Report of six cases with ultrastructural study and analysis of the literature. Cancer 49:698, 1982.
1062. Kristensen IB, Jensen OM: Malignant fibrous histiocytoma of bone. A clinicopathologic study of 9 cases. Acta Pathol Microbiol Scand (A) 92:205, 1984.
1063. Barney PL: Atypical fibrous histiocytoma (fibroxanthoma) of the temporal bone. Trans Am Acad Ophthalmol Otolaryngol 76:1392, 1972.
1064. Yumoto T, Mori Y, Inada O, et al: Malignant fibrous histioctyoma of bone. Acta Pathol Jpn 26:295, 1976.
1065. Johnson WW, Coburn TP, Pratt CB, et al: Ultrastructure of malignant histiocytoma arising in the acromion. Hum Pathol 9:199, 1978.
1066. Nunnery EW, Kahn LB, Guilford WB: Locally aggressive fibrous histiocytoma of bone. S Afr Med J 55:763, 1978.
1067. Dunham WK, Wilborn WH: Malignant fibrous histiocytoma of bone. Report of two cases and review of the literature. J Bone Joint Surg [Am] 61:939, 1979.
1068. Chitale VS, Sundaresan N, Helson L, et al: Malignant fibrous histiocytoma of the temporal bone with intracranial extension. Acta Neurochir 59:239, 1981.
1069. Katenkamp D, Stiller D: Malignant fibrous histiocytoma of bone. Light microscopic and electron microscopic examination of four cases. Virchows Arch (Pathol Anat) 391:323, 1981.
1070. Kessler HP, Callihan MD: Case for diagnosis. Milit Med 146:193, 1981.
1071. Shuman LS, Chuang VP, Wallace S, et al: Intraarterial chemotherapy of malignant fibrous histiocytoma of the pelvis. Radiology 142:343, 1982.
1072. Blitzer A, Lawson W, Zak FG, et al: Clinical-pathological determinants in prognosis of fibrous histiocytomas of head and neck. Laryngoscope 91:1, 1981.
1073. Chen KTK: Multiple fibroxanthosarcoma of bone. Cancer 42:770, 1978.
1074. Shapiro F: Malignant fibrous histiocytoma of bone: An ultrastructural study. Ultrastruct Pathol 2:33, 1981.
1075. Hudson TM, Hawkins IF, Spanier SS, et al: Angiography of malignant fibrous histiocytoma of bone. Radiology 131:9, 1979.
1076. Saito R, Caines MJ: Atypical fibrous histiocytoma of the humerus. A light and electron microscopic study. Am J Clin Pathol 68:409, 1977.
1077. Kempson RL, Kyriakos M: Fibroxanthosarcoma of the soft tissues. A type of malignant fibrous histiocytoma. Cancer 29:961, 1972.
1078. Kyriakos M, Kempson RL: Inflammatory fibrous histiocytoma. An aggressive and lethal lesion. Cancer 37:1584, 1976.
1079. Enzinger FM: Angiomatoid malignant fibrous histiocytoma. A distinct fibrohistiocytic tumor of children and young adults simulating a vascular neoplasm. Cancer 44:2147, 1979.
1080. Poon MC, Durant JR, Norgard MJ, et al: Inflammatory fibrous histiocytoma: An important variant of malignant fibrous histiocytoma highly responsive to chemotherapy. Ann Intern Med 97:858, 1982.
1081. Taxy JB, Battifora H: Malignant fibrous histiocytoma. An electron microscopic study. Cancer 40:254, 1977.
1082. Hart JAL: Intraosseous lipoma. J Bone Joint Surg [Br] 55:624, 1973.
1083. Leeson MC, Kay D, Smith BS: Intraosseous lipoma. Clin Orthop 181:186, 1983.
1084. Oringer MJ: Lipoma of the mandible. Oral Surg 1:1134, 1948.
1085. Dickson AB, Ayres WW, Mason MW, et al: Lipoma of bone of intra-osseous origin. J Bone Joint Surg [Am] 33:257, 1951.
1086. Caruolo JE, Dahlin DC: Lipoma involving bone and simulating malignant bone tumor: Report of case. Mayo Clin Proc 28:361, 1953.
1087. Cowdell RH: Intra-osseous lipoma of rib. Br J Surg 41:664, 1954.
1088. Child PL: Lipoma of the os calcis. Report of a case. Am J Clin Pathol 25:1050, 1955.
1089. Newman CW: Fibrolipoma of the mandible: Report of case. J Oral Surg 15:251, 1957.

1090. Skinner GB, Fraser RG: Medullary lipoma of bone. J Can Assoc Radiol 8:19, 1957.
1091. Smith WE, Fienberg R: Intraosseous lipoma of bone. Cancer 10:1151, 1957.
1092. Mueller MC, Robbins JL: Intramedullary lipoma of bone. Report of a case. J Bone Joint Surg [Am] 42:517, 1960.
1093. Johnson EC: Intraosseous lipoma: Report of case. J Oral Surg 27:868, 1969.
1094. Zorn DT, Cordray DR, Randels PH: Intraosseous lipoma of bone involving the sacrum. J Bone Joint Surg [Am] 53:1201, 1971.
1095. Appenzeller J, Weitzner S: Intraosseous lipoma of os calcis. Case report and review of literature of intraosseous lipoma of extremities. Clin Orthop 101:171, 1974.
1096. Hanelin LG, Sclamberg EL, Bardsley JL: Intraosseous lipoma of the coccyx. Report of a case. Radiology 114:343, 1975.
1097. Specchiulli F, Florio U, Mori F: Intraosseous lipoma. Ital J Orthop Traumatol 2:290, 1976.
1098. Poussa M, Holmström T: Intraosseous lipoma of the calcaneus. Acta Orthop Scand 47:570, 1976.
1099. Small ML, Green WR, Johnson LC: Lipoma of the frontal bone. Arch Ophthalmol 97:129, 1979.
1100. DeLee JC: Intra-osseous lipoma of the proximal part of the femur. J Bone Joint Surg [Am] 61:601, 1979.
1101. Lewis DM, Brannon RB, Isaksson B, et al: Intraosseous angiolipoma of the mandible. Oral Surg 50:156, 1980.
1102. Lagier R: Case report 128. Skel Radiol 5:267, 1980.
1103. Matsubayashi T, Makajima M, Tsukada M: Case report 118. Skel Radiol 5:131, 1980.
1104. Mohan V, Gupta SK, Cherian J, et al: Intra-osseous lipoma of the calcaneum. J Postgrad Med 27:127, 1981.
1105. Miller WB, Ausich JE, McDaniel RK, et al: Mandibular intraosseous lipoma. J Oral Maxillofac Surg 40:594, 1982.
1106. Goldman AB, Marcove RC, Huvos AG, et al: Case report 280. Skel Radiol 12:209, 1984.
1107. Gunterberg B, Kindblom LG: Intraosseous lipoma. A report of two cases. Acta Orthop Scand 49:95, 1978.
1108. Döhler R, Harms D: Intraossäre Lipome. Z Orthop 119:138, 1981.
1109. Ketyer S, Brownstein S, Cholankeril J: CT diagnosis of intraosseous lipoma of the calcaneus. J Comput Assist Tomgr 7:546, 1983.
1110. Milgram JW: Intraosseous lipomas with reactive ossification in the proximal femur. Skel Radiol 7:1, 1981.
1111. Ramos A, Castello J, Sartoris DJ, et al: Osseous lipoma: CT appearance. Radiology 157:615, 1985.
1112. Lauf E, Mullen BR, Ragsdale BD, et al: Intraosseous lipoma of distal fibula. Biomechanical considerations for successful treatment. J Am Podiatry Assoc 74:434, 1984.
1113. Freiberg RA, Air GW, Glueck CJ, et al: Multiple intraosseous lipomas with type IV hyperlipoproteinemia. J Bone Joint Surg [Am] 56:1729, 1974.
1114. Döhler R, Poser HL, Harms D, et al: Systemic lipomatosis of bone. A case report. J Bone Joint Surg [Br] 64:84, 1982.
1115. Dooms GC, Hricak H, Sollitto RA, et al: Lipomatous tumors and tumors with fatty component: MR imaging potential and comparison of MR and CT results. Radiology 157:479, 1985.
1116. Moorefield WG Jr, Urbaniak JR, Gonzalvo AAA: Intramedullary lipoma of the distal femur. South Med J 69:1210, 1976.
1117. Downey EE Jr, Brower AC, Holt RB: Case report 243. Skel Radiol 10:189, 1983.
1118. Fleming RJ, Alpert M, Garcia A: Parosteal lipoma. AJR 87:1075, 1962.
1119. Demos TC, Bruno E, Armin A, et al: Parosteal lipoma with enlarging osteochondroma. AJR 143:365, 1984.
1120. Steiner M, Gould AR, Rasmussen J, et al: Parosteal lipoma of the mandible. Oral Surg 52:51, 1981.
1121. Ross CF, Hadfield G: Primary osteo-liposarcoma of bone (malignant mesenchymoma). Report of a case. J Bone Joint Surg [Br] 50:639, 1968.
1122. Bertoni F, Laus M: Primary malignant mesenchymoma of bone (case report). Ital J Orthop Traumatol 4:105, 1978.
1123. Cremer H, Koischwitz D, Tismer R: Primary osteoliposarcoma of bone. J Cancer Res Clin Oncol 101:203, 1981.
1124. Downey EF Jr, Worsham GF, Brower AC: Liposarcoma of bone with osteosarcomatous foci: Case report and review of the literature. Skel Radiol 8:47, 1982.
1125. Stewart FW: Primary liposarcoma of bone. Am J Pathol 7:87, 1931.
1126. Barnard L: Primary liposarcoma of bone. Arch Surg 29:560, 1934.
1127. Rehbock DJ, Hauser H: Liposarcoma of bone. Report of two cases and review of literature. Am J Cancer 27:37, 1936.
1128. Duffy J, Stewart FW: Primary liposarcoma of bone. Report of a case. Am J Pathol 14:621, 1938.
1129. Williford HB, Fatherree TJ: Primary liposarcoma of bone. Report of a case. Naval Med Bull 46:1750, 1946.
1130. Agerholm-Christensen AJ: Liposarcoma humeri—behandlet med excision og acrylprothese. Ugeskr Laeger 114:1768, 1952.
1131. Dawson EK: Liposarcoma of bone. J Pathol Bacteriol 70:513, 1955.
1132. Cohen C: Primary liposarcoma of bone. The angiographic findings and doubts as to its intramedullary origin. Br J Radiol 31:442, 1958.
1133. Coste F, Lapresle J, Basset F: Un case de liposarcome. Presse Med 67:834, 1959.
1134. Retz LD: Primary liposarcoma of bone. Report of a case and review of the literature. J Bone Joint Surg [Am] 43:123, 1961.

1135. Agarwal PN, Mishra SD, Pratap VK: Primary liposarcoma of the mastoid. J Laryngol Otol 89:1079, 1975.

1136. Srivastava KP, Chandra H, Sharma RD, et al: Primary liposarcoma of the skull. Int Surg 61:234, 1976.

1137. Mastragostino S: Tumori lipoblastici primitivi dello scheletro. Chir Organi Mov 44:18, 1957.

1138. Catto M, Stevens J: Liposarcoma of bone. J Pathol Bacteriol 86:248, 1963.

1139. Goldman RL: Primary liposarcoma of bone. Report of a case. Am J Clin Pathol 42:503, 1964.

1140. Schwartz A, Shuster M, Becker SM: Liposarcoma of bone. Report of a case and review of the literature. J Bone Joint Surg [Am] 52:171, 1970.

1141. Larsson SE, Lorentzon R, Boquist L: Primary liposarcoma of bone. Acta Orthop Scand 46:869, 1975.

1142. Schneider HM, Wunderlich T, Puls P: The primary liposarcoma of the bone. Arch Orthop Trauma Surg 96:235, 1980.

1143. Pardo-Mindan FJ, Ayala H, Joly M, et al: Primary liposarcoma of bone: Light and electron microscopic study. Cancer 48:274, 1981.

1144. Addison AK, Payne SR: Primary liposarcoma of bone. Case report. J Bone Joint Surg [Am] 64:301, 1982.

1145. Torok G, Meller Y, Maor E: Primary liposarcoma of bone. Case report and review of the literature. Bull Hosp Joint Dis Orthop Inst 43:28, 1983.

1146. Enzinger FM: Case 5. Liposarcoma vs. malignant fibrous histiocytoma. In Management of Primary Bone and Soft Tissue Tumors. Chicago, Year Book Medical Publishers, 1977, p 453.

1147. Taxy JB, Conklin J, Mann JJ, et al: Case report 147. Skel Radiol 6:153, 1981.

1148. Boutselis JG, Ullery JC: Sarcoma of the uterus. Obstet Gynecol 20:23, 1962.

1149. Spiro RH, Koss LG: Myosarcoma of the uterus: A clinicopathological study. Cancer 18:571, 1965.

1150. Fornasier VL, Paley D: Leiomyosarcoma in bone: Primary or secondary? A case report and review of the literature. Skel Radiol 10:147, 1983.

1151. von Hochstetter AR, Eberle H, Ruttner JR: Primary leiomyosarcoma of extragnathic bones. Case report and review of literature. Cancer 53:2194, 1984.

1152. Evans DMD, Sanerkin NG: Primary leiomyosarcoma of bone. J Pathol Bacteriol 90:348, 1965.

1153. Overgaard J, Frederiksen P, Helmig O, et al: Primary leiomyosarcoma of bone. Cancer 39:1664, 1977.

1154. Meister P, Konrad E, Gokel JM, et al: Case report 59. Skel Radiol 2:265, 1978.

1155. Sanerkin NG: Primary leiomyosarcoma of the bone and its comparison with fibrosarcoma: A cytological, histological and ultrastructural study. Cancer 44:1375, 1979.

1156. Shamsuddin AK, Reyes F, Harvey JW, et al: Primary leiomyosarcoma of bone. Hum Pathol 1(Suppl):581, 1980.

1157. Angervall L, Berlin O, Kindblom LG, et al: Primary leiomyosarcoma of bone. A study of five cases. Cancer 46:1270, 1980.

1158. Wang T, Erlandson RA, Marcove RC, et al: Primary leiomyosarcoma of bone. Arch Pathol Lab Med 104:100, 1980.

1159. Kawai T, Suzuki M, Mukai M, et al: Primary leiomyosarcoma of bone. An immunohistochemical and ultrastructural study. Arch Pathol Lab Med 107:433, 1983.

1160. Pasquel PM, Levet SN, De Leon B: Primary rhabdomyosarcoma of bone. A case report. J Bone Joint Surg [Am] 58:1176, 1976.

1161. Calinog TA, Cushing W, Merkow LP, et al: Rhabdomyosarcoma of the sternum. The surgical management and the availability of techniques of sternal reconstruction. J Thorac Cardiovasc Surg 61:811, 1971.

1162. El-Gothamy B, Fujita S, Hayden RC Jr: Rhabdomyosarcoma—a temporal bone report. Arch Otolaryngol 98:106, 1973.

1163. Min KW, Gyorkey F, Halpert B: Primary rhabdomyosarcoma of the cerebrum. Cancer 35:1405, 1975.

1164. Graham JJ, Yang WC: Vertebral hemangioma with compression fracture and paraperis treated with preoperative embolization and vertebral resection. Spine 9:97, 1984.

1165. Zito G, Kadis GN: Multiple vertebral hemangiomas resembling metastases with spinal cord compression. Arch Neurol 37:247, 1980.

1166. Krieger AJ: Hemangioma of fifth cervical vertebra with intermittent spinal cord dysfunction. South Med J 70:1008, 1977.

1167. Cohen J, Cashman WF: Hemihypertrophy of lower extremity associated with multifocal intraosseous hemangioma. Clin Orthop 109:155, 1975.

1168. Karlin CA, Brower AC: Multiple primary hemangiomas of bone. AJR 129:162, 1977.

1169. Schmorl G, Junghanns H: The Human Spine in Health and Disease. Translated by EF Besemann. New York, Grune & Stratton, 1971, p 325.

1170. Ghormley RK, Adson AW: Hemangioma of vertebrae. J Bone Joint Surg 23:887, 1941.

1171. McAllister VL, Kendall BE, Bull JWD: Symptomatic vertebral haemangiomas. Brain 98:71, 1975.

1172. Bergstrand A, Höök O, Lidvall H: Vertebral haemangiomas compressing the spinal cord. Acta Neurol Scand 39:59, 1963.

1173. Nelson DA: Spinal cord compression due to vertebral angiomas during pregnancy. Arch Neurol 11:408, 1964.

1174. Greenspan A, Klein MJ, Bennett AJ, et al: Case report 242. Skel Radiol 10:183, 1983.

1175. Sherman RS, Wilner D: The roentgen diagnosis of hemangioma of bone. AJR 86:1146, 1961.

1176. Dorfman HD, Steiner GC, Jaffe HL: Vascular tumors of bone. Hum Pathol 2:349, 1971.

1177. Thomas A: Vascular tumors of bone. A pathological and clinical study of twenty-seven cases. Surg Gynecol Obstet 74:777, 1942.

1178. Rowbotham GF: Haemangiomata arising in the bones of the skull. Br J Surg 30:1, 1942.

1179. Wyke BD: Primary hemangioma of the skull: A rare cranial tumor. Review of the literature and report of a case, with special reference to the roentgenographic appearances. AJR 61:302, 1949.

1180. Holmes EM, Sweet WH, Kelemen G: Hemangiomas of the frontal bone. Report of three cases. Ann Otol Rhinol 61:45, 1952.

1181. Sargent EN, Reilly EB, Posnikoff J: Primary hemangioma of the skull. Case report of an unusual tumor. AJR 95:874, 1965.

1182. Overend TD: Haemangioma of the occipital bone. Br J Radiol 6:626, 1933.

1183. Smith HW: Hemangioma of the jaws. Arch Otolaryngol 70:579, 1959.

1184. Lund BA, Dahlin DC: Hemangiomas of the mandible and maxilla. J Oral Surg Anesth 22:234, 1964.

1185. James JN: Cavernous haemangioma of the mandible. Proc R Soc Med 57:797, 1964.

1186. Davies D: Cavernous hemangioma of the mandible. Plast Reconstr Surg 33:457, 1964.

1187. Walker EA, McHenry LC: Primary hemangioma of the zygoma. Arch Otolaryngol 81:199, 1965.

1188. Siegelman SS, Frankel TN, Lewin ML: Hemangioma of the nasal bone. Report of a case. Arch Otolaryngol 88:269, 1968.

1189. Baum SM, Pochaczevsky R, Sussman R, et al: Central hemangioma of the maxilla. J Oral Surg 30:885, 1972.

1190. Macansh JD, Owen MD: Central cavernous hemangioma of the mandible: Report of cases. J Oral Surg 30:293, 1972.

1191. Gamez-Araujo JJ, Toth BB, Luna MA: Central hemangioma of the mandible and maxilla: review of a vascular lesion. Oral Surg 37:230, 1974.

1192. Bridger MWM: Haemangioma of the nasal bones. J Laryngol Otol 90:191, 1976.

1193. Azaz B, Lustmann J: Central hemangioma of the maxilla. Int J Oral Surg 5:240, 1976.

1194. Zizmor J, Robbett WF, Spiro RH, et al: Tawfik B: Hemangioma of the nasal bones: Radiographic appearance. Ann Otol 87:360, 1978.

1195. Schvarcz LW: Giant cavernous haemangioma of the nasal bones. Br J Plast Surg 32:315, 1979.

1196. Marshak G: Hemangioma of the zygomatic bone. Arch Otolaryngol 106:581, 1980.

1197. Sadowsky D, Rosenberg RD, Kaufman J, et al: Central hemangioma of the mandible. Literature review, case report, and discussion. Oral Surg 52:471, 1981.

1198. Stassi J, Rao VM, Lowry L: Hemangioma of bone arising in the maxilla. Skel Radiol 12:187, 1984.

1199. Wold LE, Swee RG, Sim FH: Vascular lesions of bone. Pathol Annu (Part 2) 20:101, 1985.

1200. Bucy PC, Capp CS: Primary hemangioma of bone with special reference to roentgenologic diagnosis. AJR 23:1, 1930.

1201. Geschickter CF, Maseritz IH: Primary hemangioma involving bones of the extremities. J Bone Joint Surg 20:888, 1938.

1202. Martin LFW, Rafferty E: Hemangioma of a metacarpal: A case report. J Can Assoc Radiol 33:50, 1982.

1203. Bansal VP, Singh R, Grewal DS: Haemangioma of the patella. A report of two cases. J Bone Joint Surg [Br] 56:139, 1974.

1204. Feldman F: Case report 104. Skel Radiol 4:245, 1979.

1205. Ekerot L, Jonsson K, Eiken O, et al: Hemangioma of the lunate (Klippel-Trénaunay syndrome). Case report. Scand J Plast Reconstr Surg 15:153, 1981.

1206. Subbarao K: Case report 228. Skel Radiol 9:273, 1983.

1207. Stevens J, Love S, Davis C, et al: Capillary hemangioblastoma of bone resembling a vertebral haemangioma. Br J Radiol 56:571, 1983.

1208. Willinsky RA, Rubenstein JD, Cruickshank B: Case report 216. Skel Radiol 9:137, 1982.

1209. Schajowicz F, Rebecchini AC, Bosch-Mayol G: Intracortical haemangioma simulating osteoid osteoma. J Bone Joint Surg [Br] 61:94, 1979.

1210. Loxley SS, Thiemeyer JS Jr, Ellsasser JC: Periosteal hemangioma. A report of two cases. Clin Orthop 85:151, 1972.

1211. Sugiura I: Tibial periosteal hemangioma. Clin Orthop 106:242, 1975.

1212. Pena JM, Calone JA, Ortega F, et al: Case report 324. Skel Radiol 14:133, 1985.

1213. Hall FM, Goldberg RP, Kasdon EJ, et al: Case report 131. Skel Radiol 5:275, 1980.

1214. Suss RA, Kumar AJ, Dorfman HD, et al: Capillary hemangioma of the sphenoid bone. Skel Radiol 11:102, 1984.

1215. Jacobs JE, Kimmelstiel P: Cystic angiomatosis of the skeletal system. J Bone Joint Surg [Am] 35:409, 1953.

1216. Seckler SG, Rubin H, Rabinowitz JG: Systemic cystic angiomatosis. Am J Med 37:976, 1964.

1217. Boyle WJ: Cystic angiomatosis of bone. A report of three cases and review of the literature. J Bone Joint Surg [Br] 54:626, 1972.

1218. Gutierrez RM, Spjut HJ: Skeletal angiomatosis. Report of three cases and review of the literature. Clin Orthop 85:82, 1972.

1219. Graham DY, Gonzales J, Kothari SM: Diffuse skeletal angiomatosis. Skel Radiol 2:131, 1979.

1220. Ritchie G, Zeier FG: Hemangiomatosis of the skeleton and the spleen. J Bone Joint Surg [Am] 38:115, 1956.

1221. Koblenzer PJ, Bukowski MJ: Angiomatosis (hamartomatous hem-lymphangiomatosis). Report of a case with diffuse involvement. Pediatrics 28:65, 1961.
1222. Lidholm SO, Lindbom Å, Spjut HJ: Multiple capillary hemangiomas of the bones of the foot. Acta Pathol Microbiol Scand 51:9, 1961.
1223. Spjut HJ, Lindbom Å: Skeletal angiomatosis. Report of two cases. Acta Pathol Microbiol Scand 55:49, 1962.
1224. Moseley JE, Starobin SG: Cystic angiomatosis of bone: Manifestation of a hamartomatous disease entity. AJR 91:1114, 1964.
1225. Waldron RL II, Zeller JA: Diffuse skeletal hemangiomatosis with visceral involvement. J Can Assoc Radiol 20:119, 1969.
1226. Dadash-Zadeh M, Czapek EE, Schwartz AD: Skeletal and splenic hemangiomatosis with consumption coagulopathy: Response to splenectomy. Pediatrics 57:803, 1976.
1227. Schajowicz F, Aiello CL, Francone MV, et al: Cystic angiomatosis (hamartous haemolymphangiomatosis) of bone. A clinicopathological study of three cases. J Bone Joint Surg [Br] 60:100, 1978.
1228. Moore WH, Dhekne RD: Radiotracer imaging in a case of diffuse skeletal hemangiomatosis. Clin Nucl Med 6:405, 1981.
1229. Czerniak P, Schorr S: Hereditary hemorrhagic telangiectasis with involvement of bone. AJR 74:299, 1955.
1230. Mirra JM, Arnold WD: Skeletal hemangiomatosis in association with hereditary hemorrhagic telangiectasia. A case report. J Bone Joint Surg [Am] 55:850, 1973.
1231. Wallis LA, Asch T, Maisel BW: Diffuse skeletal hemangiomatosis. Report of two cases and review of literature. Am J Med 37:545, 1964.
1232. Tuñon JB, Gonzalez FP: Angiomatosis of the metacarpal skeleton. Hand 9:88, 1977.
1233. Parsons LG, Ebbs JH: Generalized angiomatosis presenting the clinical characteristics of storage reticulosis with some observations of the reticuloendothelioses. Arch Dis Child 15:129, 1940.
1234. Ackerman AJ, Hart MS: Multiple primary hemangioma of the bones of the extremity. AJR 48:47, 1942.
1235. Neidhart JA, Roach RW: Successful treatment of skeletal hemangioma and Kasabach-Merritt syndrome with aminocaproic acid. Is fibrinolysis "defensive?" Am J Med 73:434, 1982.
1236. Pierson JW, Farber G, Howard JE: Multiple hemangiomas of bone, probably congenital. JAMA 116:2145, 1941.
1237. Brower AC, Culver JE Jr, Keats TE: Diffuse cystic angiomatosis of bone. Report of two cases. AJR 118:456, 1973.
1238. Zenny JC, Leclere J, Boccon-Gibod L, et al: L'angiomatose kystique diffuse des os ou ectasies capillaires intra-osseuses. J Radiol 62:43, 1981.
1239. Shopfner CE, Allen RP: Lymphangioma of bone. Radiology 76:449, 1961.
1240. Bickel WH, Broders AC: Primary lymphangioma of the ilium. J Bone Joint Surg 29:517, 1947.
1241. Falkmer S, Tilling G: Primary lymphangioma of bone. Acta Orthop Scand 26:99, 1956.
1242. Kooperman M, Antoine JE: Primary lymphangioma of the calvarium. AJR 121:118, 1974.
1243. Bullough PG, Goodfellow JW: Solitary lymphangioma of bone. A case report. J Bone Joint Surg [Am] 58:418, 1976.
1244. Ellis GL, Brannon RB: Intraosseous lymphangiomas of the mandible. Skel Radiol 5:253, 1980.
1245. Jumbelic M, Feuerstein IM, Dorfman HD: Solitary intraosseous lymphangioma. A case report. J Bone Joint Surg [Am] 66:1479, 1984.
1246. Rosenquist CJ, Wolfe DC: Lymphangioma of bone. J Bone Joint Surg [Am] 50:158, 1968.
1247. Cohen J, Craig JM: Multiple lymphangiectases of bone. J Bone Joint Surg [Am] 37:585, 1955.
1248. Tucker SM: Bilateral chylothorax with multiple osteolytic lesions? Generalized abnormality of lymphatic system. Proc R Soc Med 60:17, 1967.
1249. Najman E, Facečić-Sabadi V, Temmer B: Lymphangioma in the inguinal region with cystic lymphangiomatosis of bone. J Pediatr 71:561, 1967.
1250. Goldstein MR, Benchimol A, Cornell W, et al: Chylopericardium with multiple lymphangioma of bone. N Engl J Med 280:1034, 1969.
1251. Steiner GM, Farman J, Lawson JP: Lymphangiomatosis of bone. Radiology 93:1093, 1969.
1252. Morphis LG, Arcinue EL, Krause JR: Generalized lymphangioma in infancy with chylothorax. Pediatrics 46:566, 1970.
1253. Winterberger AR: Radiographic diagnosis of lymphangiomatosis of bone. Radiology 102:321, 1972.
1254. Reilly BJ, Davidson JW, Bain H: Lymphangiectasis of the skeleton. A case report. Radiology 103:385, 1972.
1255. Asch MJ, Cohen AH, Moore TC: Hepatic and splenic lymphangiomatosis with skeletal involvement: Report of a case and review of the literature. Surgery 76:334, 1974.
1256. Chu JY, Graviss ER, Danis RK, et al: Lymphangiography and bone scan in the study of lymphangiomatosis. Pediatr Radiol 6:46, 1977.
1257. Bell KA, Simon BK: Chylothorax and lymphangiomas of bone: Unusual manifestations of lymphatic disease. South Med J 71:459, 1978.
1258. Siegel MJ, McAlister WH, Askin FN: Lymphangiomas in children: Report of 121 cases. J Can Assoc Radiol 30:99, 1979.
1259. Ducharme JC, Bélanger R, Simard P, et al: Chylothorax, chylopericardium with multiple lymphangioma of bone. J Pediatr Surg 17:365, 1982.
1260. Watts MA, Gibbons JA, Aaron BL: Mediastinal and osseous lymphangiomatosis: Case report and review. Ann Thorac Surg 34:324, 1982.

1261. Tsyb AF, Mukhamedzhanov IK, Guseva LI: Lymphangiomatosis of bone and soft tissue (results of lymphangiographic examinations). Lymphology 16:181, 1983.
1262. Harris R, Prandoni AG: Generalized primary lymphangiomas of bone: Report of case associated with congenital lymphedema of forearm. Ann Intern Med 33:1302, 1950.
1263. Hayes JT, Brody GL: Cystic lymphangiectasis of bone. A case report. J Bone Joint Surg [Am] 43:107, 1961.
1264. Nixon GW: Lymphangiomatosis of bone demonstrated by lymphangiography. AJR 110:582, 1970.
1265. Hafner E, Fuchs WA, Kuffer F: Lymphangiography in lymphangiomatosis of bone. Lymphology 5:129, 1972.
1266. Rogers HM, Chou SN: Lymphangioma of the craniocervical junction. Case report. J Neurosurg 38:510, 1973.
1267. Oppermann HC, Greinacher I, Ball F, et al: Die Knochenlymphangiomatose im Kindesalter. ROFO 131:60, 1979.
1268. Wenz W, Reichelt A, Rau WS, et al: Lymphographischer Nachweis eines Wirbellymphangioms. Radiologe 24:381, 1984.
1269. Abe R: Lymphatico-osseous communication and primary lymphedema. Radiology 129:375, 1978.
1270. Edwards WH Jr, Thompson RC Jr, Varsa EW: Lymphangiomatosis and massive osteolysis of the cervical spine. A case report and review of the literature. Clin Orthop 177:222, 1983.
1271. Shugart RR, Soule EH, Johnson EW: Glomus tumor. Surg Gynecol Obstet 117:334, 1963.
1272. Apfelberg DB, Teasley JL: Unusual locations and manifestations of glomus tumors (glomangiomas). Am J Surg 116:62, 1968.
1273. Riveros M, Pack GT: The glomus tumor. Report of twenty cases. Ann Surg 133:394, 1951.
1274. Carroll RE, Berman AT: Glomus tumors of the hand. J Bone Joint Surg [Am] 54:691, 1972.
1275. Ho KL, Pak MSY: Glomus tumor of the coccygeal region. Case report. J Bone Joint Surg [Am] 62:141, 1980.
1276. Mackenzie DH: Intraosseous glomus tumours. Report of two cases. J Bone Joint Surg [Br] 44:648, 1962.
1277. Harris WR: Erosion of bone produced by glomus tumour. Can Med Assoc J 70:684, 1954.
1278. Camirand P, Giroux JM: Subungual glomus tumor. Radiological manifestations. Arch Dermatol 102:677, 1970.
1279. Mathis WH Jr, Schulz MD: Roentgen diagnosis of glomus tumors. Radiology 51:71, 1948.
1280. Sugiura I: Intra-osseous glomus tumour. A case report. J Bone Joint Surg [Br] 58:245, 1976.
1281. Lattes R, Bull DC: A case of glomus tumor with primary involvement of bone. Ann Surg 127:187, 1948.
1282. Lehman W, Kraissl C: Glomus tumor within bone. Surgery 25:118, 1949.
1283. Chan CW: Intraosseous glomus tumor—case report. J Hand Surg 6:368, 1981.
1284. Serra JM, Muirragui A, Tadjalli H: Glomus tumor of the metacarpophalangeal joint: A case report. J Hand Surg [Am] 10:142, 1985.
1285. Bergstrand H: Multiple glomic tumors. Am J Cancer 29:470, 1937.
1286. Siegel MW: Intraosseous glomus tumor. A case report. Am J Orthop 9:68, 1967.
1287. Pambakian H, Smith MA: Glomus tumours of the coccygeal body associated with coccydynia. A preliminary report. J Bone Joint Surg [Br] 63:424, 1981.
1288. Bell RS, Goodman SB, Fornasier VL: Coccygeal glomus tumors: A case of mistaken identity. J Bone Joint Surg [Am] 64:595, 1982.
1289. Horton C, Maguire C, Georgiade N, et al: Glomus tumors. An analysis of twenty-five cases. Arch Surg 71:712, 1955.
1290. Blanchard AJ: The pathology of glomus tumors. Can Med Assoc J 44:357, 1941.
1291. Tsuneyoshi M, Enjoji M: Glomus tumor. A clinicopathologic and electron microscopic study. Cancer 50:1601, 1982.
1292. Venkatachalam MA, Greally JG: Fine structure of glomus tumor: Similarity of glomus cells to smooth muscle. Cancer 23:1176, 1969.
1293. Toker C: Glomangioma. An ultrastructural study. Cancer 23:487, 1969.
1294. Harris M: Ultrastructure of a glomus tumor. J Clin Pathol 24:520, 1971.
1295. Stout AP, Murray MR: Hemangiopericytoma. A vascular tumor featuring Zimmermann's pericytes. Ann Surg 116:26, 1942.
1296. Marcial-Rojas RA: Primary hemangiopericytoma of bone. Review of the literature and report of the first case with metastases. Cancer 13:308, 1960.
1297. Unni KK, Ivins JC, Beabout JW, et al: Hemangioma, hemangiopericytoma, and hemangioendothelioma (angiosarcoma) of bone. Cancer 27:1403, 1971.
1298. Dunlop J: Primary haemangiopericytoma of bone. Report of two cases. J Bone Joint Surg [Br] 55:854, 1973.
1299. Sciortino R: Contributo casistico allo studio dell'emangiopericitoma dell'osso. Chir Organi Mov 65:335, 1979.
1300. Stern MB, Grode ML, Goodman MD: Hemangiopericytoma of the cervical spine: Report of an unusual case. Clin Orthop 151:201, 1980.
1301. Vang PS, Falk E: Haemangiopericytoma of bone. Review of the literature and report of a case. Acta Orthop Scand 51:903, 1980.
1302. Nunnery EW, Kahn LB, Reddick RL, et al: Hemangiopericytoma: A light microscopic and ultrastructural study. Cancer 47:906, 1981.
1303. Giunti A, Calderoni P, Martucci E: Haemangiopericytoma of bone. Ital J Orthop Traumatol 8:345, 1982.
1304. Wold LE, Unni KK, Cooper KL, et al: Hemangiopericytoma of bone. Am J Surg Pathol 6:53, 1982.

1305. Bohndorf K, Vogel P: Radiologisches Bild eines Hämangiopericytoms an der Schädelbasis. Radiologe 22:405, 1982.

1306. Genet PE, Bernstein ML, Alpert B, et al: Vascular lesion of the mandible. J Oral Maxillofac Surg 42:537, 1984.

1307. Vathana P: Primary hemangiopericytoma of bone in the hand: A case report. J Hand Surg [Am] 9:761, 1984.

1308. Kahn LB, Nunnery EW, Lipper S, et al: Case report 144. Primary hemangiopericytoma of the right radius. Skel Radiol 6:139, 1981.

1309. Enzinger FM, Smith BH: Hemangiopericytoma. An analysis of 106 cases. Hum Pathol 7:61, 1976.

1310. Battifora H: Hemangiopericytoma: Ultrastructural study of five cases. Cancer 31:1418, 1973.

1311. Murad TM, von Haam E, Murthy MSN: Ultrastructure of a hemangiopericytoma and a glomus tumor. Cancer 22:1239, 1968.

1312. Waldo ED, Vuletin JC, Kaye GI: The ultrastructure of vascular tumors: Additional observations and a review of the literature. Pathol Annu 12:279, 1977.

1313. Tsuneyoshi M, Daimaru Y, Enjoji M: Malignant hemangiopericytoma and other sarcomas with hemangiopericytoma-like pattern. Pathol Res Pract 178:446, 1984.

1314. McMaster MJ, Soule EH, Ivins JC: Hemangiopericytoma. A clinicopathologic study and long-term followup of 60 patients. Cancer 36:2232, 1975.

1315. Backwinkel KD, Diddamis JA: Hemangiopericytoma. Report of a case and comprehensive review of the literature. Cancer 25:896, 1970.

1316. Angervall L, Kindblom LG, Nielsen JM, et al: Hemangiopericytoma. A clinicopathologic, angiographic and microangiographic study. Cancer 42:2412, 1978.

1317. Campanacci M, Boriani S, Giunti A: Hemangioendothelioma of bone: A study of 29 cases. Cancer 46:804, 1980.

1318. Volpe R, Mazabraud A: Hemangioendothelioma (angiosarcoma) of bone: A distinct pathologic entity with an unpredictable course? Cancer 49:727, 1982.

1319. Wold LE, Unni KK, Beabout JW, et al: Hemangioendothelial sarcoma of bone. Am J Surg Pathol 6:59, 1982.

1320. Wu KK, Guise ER: Malignant hemangioendothelioma of bone: A clinical analysis of 11 cases treated at Henry Ford Hospital. Orthopedics 4:58, 1981.

1321. Srinivasan CK, Patel MR, Pearlman HS, et al: Malignant hemangioendothelioma of bone. Review of the literature and report of two cases. J Bone Joint Surg [Am] 60:696, 1978.

1322. Benisch BM, Alpert LT: Malignant hemangioendothelioma and consumption coagulopathy. N Engl J Med 258:804, 1971.

1323. Price AC, Coran AG, Mattern AL, et al: Hemangioendothelioma of the pelvis. A cause of cardiac failure in the newborn. N Engl J Med 286:647, 1972.

1324. Bundens WD, Brighton CT: Malignant hemangioendothelioma of bone. Report of two cases and review of the literature. J Bone Joint Surg [Am] 47:762, 1965.

1325. Otis J, Hutter RVP, Foote RW Jr, et al: Hemangioendothelioma of bone. Surg Gynecol Obstet 127:295, 1968.

1326. Garcia-Moral CA: Malignant hemangioendothelioma of bone. Review of world literature and report of two cases. Clin Orthop 82:70, 1972.

1327. Schoepf R, Zaunbauer W, Schmid U, et al: Case report 283. Skel Radiol 12:142, 1984.

1328. Larsson SE, Lorentzon R, Boquist L: Malignant hemangioendothelioma of bone. J Bone Joint Surg [Am] 57:84, 1975.

1329. Toto PD, Lavieri J: Primary hemangiosarcoma of the jaw. Oral Surg 12:1459, 1959.

1330. Gandhi RK, Kinare SG, Parulkar GB, et al: Hemangiosarcoma (malignant hemangioendothelioma) of the mandible in a child. Oral Surg 22:359, 1966.

1331. Mladick RA, Georgiade NG, Williams TG, et al: Angiosarcoma of the mandible. Case report. Plast Reconstr Surg 43:92, 1969.

1332. Singh J, Sidhu BS, Kanta S: Hemangioendothelioma of the mandible: Report of case. J Oral Surg 35:673, 1977.

1333. Zachariades N, Papadakou A, Koundouris J, et al: Primary hemangioendotheliosarcoma of the mandible: Review of the literature and report of case. J Oral Surgery 38:288, 1980.

1334. McClatchey KD, Batsakis JG, Rice DH, et al: Angiosarcoma of the maxillary sinus: Report of a case. J Oral Surg 34:1019, 1976.

1335. Bankaci M, Myers EN, Barnes L, et al: Angiosarcoma of the maxillary sinus: Literature review and case report. Head Neck Surg 1:274, 1979.

1336. Sharma BG, Nawalkha PL: Angiosarcoma of the maxillary antrum: Report of a case with brief review of literature. J Laryngol Otol 93:181, 1979.

1337. Sweterlitsch PR, Torg JS, Watts H: Malignant hemangioendothelioma of the cervical spine. A case report. J Bone Joint Surg [Am] 52:805, 1970.

1338. Stjernvall L: Vertebral angiosarcoma. A case report. Acta Orthop Scand 41:165, 1970.

1339. Glenn JN, Reckling FW, Mantz FA: Malignant hemangioendothelioma in a lumbar vertebra. A rare tumor in an unusual location. J Bone Joint Surg [Am] 56:1279, 1974.

1340. Dalinka MK, Brennan RE, Patchefsky AS: Case report 3. Skel Radiol 1:59, 1976.

1341. Konrad EA, Meister P: Multifokales Angiosarkom der Wirbelsäule und des Sternums mit viszeralen Metastasen. Arch Orthop Trauma Surg 93:249, 1979.

1342. Pollak A: Angiosarcoma of the sternum. Am J Surg 77:522, 1949.

1343. Finsterbush A, Husseini N, Rousso M: Multifocal hemangioendothelioma of bones in the hand—a case report. J Hand Surg 6:353, 1981.

1344. Dube VE, Fisher DE: Hemangioendothelioma of the leg following metallic fixation of the tibia. Cancer 30:1260, 1972.

1345. Ekerot L, Eiken O, Jonsson K, et al: Malignant hemangioendothelioma of metacarpal bones. Case report. Scand J Plast Reconstr Surg 15:73, 1981.

1346. Bohn LE, Dehner LP, Walker HC Jr: Case report 204. Skel Radiol 8:303, 1982.

1347. Stout AP: Hemangio-endothelioma: A tumor of blood vessels featuring vascular endothelial cells. Ann Surg 118:445, 1943.

1348. Hartmann WH, Stewart FW: Hemangioendothelioma of bone. Unusual tumor characterized by indolent course. Cancer 15:846, 1962.

1349. Beabout JW: Case report 11. Skel Radiol 1:121, 1976.

1350. Rosai J, Sumner HW, Kostianovsky M, et al: Angiosarcoma of the skin. A clinicopathologic and fine structural study. Hum Pathol 7:83, 1976.

1351. Guarda LA, Ordóñez NG, Smith JL, et al: Immunoperoxidase localization of factor VIII in angiosarcomas. Arch Pathol Lab Med 106:515, 1982.

1352. Miettinen M, Holthofer H, Veli-Pekka L, et al: Ulex europaeus I lectin as a marker for tumors derived from endothelial cells. Am J Clin Pathol 79:32, 1983.

1353. Ordóñez NG, Batsakis JG: Comparison of Ulex europaeus I lectin and factor VIII-related antigen in vascular lesions. Arch Pathol Lab Med 108:129, 1984.

1354. Capo V, Ozzello L, Fenoglio CM, et al: Angiosarcomas arising in edematous extremities: Immunostaining for factor VIII-related antigen and ultrastructural features. Hum Pathol 16:144, 1985.

1355. Carstens PHB: The Weibel-Palade body in the diagnosis of endothelial tumors. Ultrastruct Pathol 2:315, 1981.

1356. Rosai J, Gold J, Landy R: The histiocytoid hemangiomas. A unifying concept embracing several previously described entities of skin, soft tissue, large vessels, bone, and heart. Hum Pathol 10:707, 1979.

1357. Fornasier VL, Finkelstein S, Gardiner GW, et al: Angiolymphoid hyperplasia with eosinophilia: A bone lesion pathologically resembling Kimura's disease of skin. A report of two cases. Clin Orthop 166:243, 1982.

1358. Cone RO, Hudkins P, Nguyen V, et al: Histiocytoid hemangioma of bone: A benign lesion which may mimic angiosarcoma. Report of a case and review of the literature. Skel Radiol 10:165, 1983.

1359. Ose D, Vollmer R, Shelburne J, et al: Histiocytoid hemangioma of the skin and scapula. A case report with electron microscopy and immunohistochemistry. Cancer 51:1656, 1983.

1360. Viñuela A, Fernandez-Rojo F, Gonzales-Nuñez A: Hemangioendothelioma of bone. A case report with massive tissular necrosis. Pathol Res Pract 178:297, 1984.

1361. Gordon EJ: Solitary intraosseous neurilemmoma of the tibia. Review of intraosseous neurilemmoma and neurofibroma. Clin Orthop 117:271, 1976.

1362. Ellis GL, Abrams AM, Melrose RJ: Intraosseous benign neural sheath neoplasms of the jaws. Report of seven new cases and review of the literature. Oral Pathol 44:731, 1977.

1363. Friedman MM: Neurofibromatosis of bone. AJR 51:623, 1944.

1364. Pescott GH, White RE: Solitary, central neurofibroma of the mandible: Report of case and review of the literature. J Oral Surg 28:305, 1970.

1365. Lorson EL, DeLong PE, Osbon DB, et al: Neurofibromatosis with central neurofibroma of the mandible: Review of the literature and report of case. J Oral Surg 35:733, 1977.

1366. Larsson Å, Praetorius F, Hjörting-Hansen E: Intraosseous neurofibroma of the jaws. Int J Oral Surg 7:494, 1978.

1367. Gnepp DR, Keyes GG: Central neurofibromas of the mandible: Report of two cases. J Oral Surg 39:125, 1981.

1368. Brady GL, Schaffner DL, Joy ED Jr, et al: Solitary neurofibroma of the maxilla. J Oral Maxillofac Surg 40:43, 1982.

1369. Gross P, Bailey FR, Jacox HW: Primary intramedullary neurofibroma of the humerus. Arch Pathol 28:716, 1939.

1370. Baldwin DM, Weiner DS: Congenital bowing and intraosseous neurofibroma of the ulna. A case report. J Bone Joint Surg [Am] 56:803, 1974.

1371. Wirth WA, Bray CB: Intra-osseous neurilemmoma. Case report and review of thirty-one cases from the literature. J Bone Joint Surg [Am] 59:252, 1977.

1372. DeSanto DA, Burgess E: Primary and secondary neurilemmoma of bone. Surg Gynecol Obstet 71:454, 1940.

1373. DeLaMonte SM, Dorfman HD, Chandra R, et al: Intraosseous schwannoma: Histologic features, ultrastructure, and review of the literature. Hum Pathol 15:551, 1984.

1374. Conley AH, Miller DS: Neurilemmoma of bone. A case report. J Bone Joint Surg 24:684, 1942.

1375. Jones HM: Neurilemmoma of bone. Br J Surg 41:63, 1953.

1376. Hart MS, Basom WC: Neurilemoma involving bone. J Bone Joint Surg [Am] 40:465, 1958.

1377. Samter TG, Vellios F, Shafer WG: Neurilemmoma of bone. Report of 3 cases with a review of the literature. Radiology 75:215, 1960.

1378. Seth HN, Rao BDP, Kathpalia PML: Neurilemmoma of bone. Report of a case. J Bone Joint Surg [Br] 45:382, 1963.

1379. Morton KS, Vassar PS: Neurilemmoma in bone. Report of a case. Can J Surg 7:187, 1964.

1380. Cucolo GF, Pearlman HS, Ramachandran VS: Neurilemmoma of os calcis. NY State J Med 64:3015, 1964.

1381. Friedman M: Intraosseous schwannoma. Report of a case. Oral Surg 18:90, 1964.

1382. Dickson JH, Waltz TA, Fechner RE: Intraosseous neurilemoma of the third lumbar vertebra. J Bone Joint Surg 53:349, 1971.

1383. Jacobs RL, Fox TA: Neurilemoma of bone. A case report with a review of the literature. Clin Orthop 87:248, 1971.

1384. Shimura K, Allen EC, Kinoshita Y, et al: Central neurilemoma of the mandible: Report of case and review of the literature. J Oral Surg 31:363, 1973.

1385. Agha FP, Lilienfeld RM: Roentgen features of osseous neurilemmoma. Diagn Radiol 102:325, 1972.

1386. Lewis HH, Kobrin HI: Neurilemoma of the first metacarpal. A case report. Clin Orthop 82:67, 1972.

1387. Sugimura M, Shirasuna K, Yoshimura Y, et al: A case of neurilemmoma in the mandible. Int J Oral Surg 3:194, 1974.

1388. Polkey CE: Intraosseous neurilemmoma of the cervical spine causing paraparesis and treated by resection and grafting. J Neurol Neurosurg Psychiatry 38:776, 1975.

1389. Dalinka MK, Cannino C, Patchefsky AS, et al: Case report 12. Skel Radiol 1:123, 1976.

1390. Morrison MJ, Ivins JC: Case report 47. Skel Radiol 2:177, 1978.

1391. Ord RA, Rennie JS: Central neurilemmoma of the maxilla. Report of a case and review of the literature. Int J Oral Surg 10:137, 1981.

1392. Schofield IDF, Gardner DG: Central neurilemmoma of the mandible. Can Dent Assoc J 3:175, 1981.

1393. Rengachary SS, O'Boynick P, Batnitzky S, et al: Giant intrasacral schwannoma: Case report. Neurosurgery 9:573, 1981.

1394. Satterfield SD, Elzay RP, Mercuri L: Mandibular central schwannoma: Report of case. J Oral Surg 39:776, 1981.

1395. Fawcett KJ, Dahlin DC: Neurilemmoma of bone. Am J Clin Pathol 47:759, 1967.

1396. Hibri NS, El-Khoury GY: Case report 113. Skel Radiol 5:112, 1980.

1397. Peers JH: Primary intramedullary neurogenic sarcoma of the ulna. Am J Pathol 10:811, 1934.

1398. Horwitz T: Chordal ectopia and its possible relation to chordoma. Arch Pathol 31:354, 1941.

1399. Utne JR, Pugh DG: The roentgenologic aspects of chordoma. AJR 74:593, 1955.

1400. Wright D: Nasopharyngeal and cervical chordoma—some aspects of their development and treatment. J Laryngol Otol 81:1337, 1967.

1401. Shugar JMA, Som PM, Krespi YP, et al: Primary chordoma of the maxillary sinus. Laryngoscope 90:1825, 1980.

1402. Mills RP: Chordomas of the skull base. J R Soc Med 77:10, 1984.

1403. Berryhill BH, Armstrong BW: Extracranial presentation of craniocervical chordoma. Laryngoscope 94:1063, 1984.

1404. Windeyer BW: Chordoma. Proc R Soc Med 52:1088, 1959.

1405. Luschka H: Die Altersveraenderungen der Zwischenwirbelknorpel. Virchows Arch (Pathol Anat) 9:311, 1856.

1406. Steward M, Burrow F: Ecchordosis physaliphora spheno-occipitalis. J Neurol Psychopathol 4:218, 1923.

1407. Congdon C: Benign and malignant chordomas. A clinico-anatomical study of twenty-two cases. Am J Pathol 28:793, 1952.

1408. Ulich TR, Mirra JM: Ecchordosis physaliphora vertebralis. Clin Orthop 163:282, 1982.

1409. Higinbotham NL, Phillips RF, Farr HW, et al: Chordoma. Thirty-five year study at Memorial Hospital. Cancer 20:1841, 1967.

1410. Mindell ER: Chordoma. J Bone Joint Surg [Am] 63:501, 1981.

1411. Mabrey RE: Chordoma: A study of 150 cases. Am J Cancer 25:501, 1935.

1412. Adson AW, Kernohan JW, Woltman HW: Cranial and cervical chordomas. A clinical and histologic study. Arch Neurol Psychiatry 33:247, 1935.

1413. Falconer MA, Bailey IC, Duchen LW: Surgical treatment of chordoma and chondroma of the skull base. J Neurosurg 29:261, 1968.

1414. Kamrin RP, Potanos JN, Pool JL: An evaluation of the diagnosis and treatment of chordoma. J Neurol Neurosurg Psychiatry 27:157, 1964.

1415. Dahlin DC, MacCarty CS: Chordoma. A study of fifty-nine cases. Cancer 5:1170, 1952.

1416. Heffelfinger MJ, Dahlin DC, MacCarty CS, et al: Chordomas and cartilaginous tumors at the skull base. Cancer 32:410, 1973.

1417. Krayenbühl H, Yasargil MG: Cranial chordomas. Prog Neurol Surg 6:380, 1975.

1418. Stoker DJ, Pringle J: Case report 205. Skel Radiol 8:306, 1982.

1419. Volpe R, Mazabraud A: A clinicopathologic review of 25 cases of chordoma (a pleomorphic and metastasizing neoplasm). Am J Surg Pathol 7:161, 1983.

1420. Davidson JK, Mucci B: Case report 322. Skel Radiol 14:76, 1985.

1421. Firooznia H, Pinto RS, Lin JP, et al: Chordoma: Radiologic evaluation of 20 cases. AJR 127:797, 1976.

1422. Paavolainen P, Teppo L: Chordoma in Finland. Acta Orthop Scand 47:46, 1976.

1423. Eriksson B, Gunterberg B, Kindblom LG: Chordoma. A clinicopathologic prognostic study of a Swedish national series. Acta Orthop Scand 52:49, 1981.

1424. Chetiyawardana AD: Chordoma: Results of treatment. Clin Radiol 35:159, 1984.

1425. Rich TA, Schiller A, Suit HD, et al: Clinical and pathological review of 48 cases of chordoma. Cancer 56:182, 1985.

1426. Sundaresan N, Galicich JH, Chu FCH, et al: Spinal chordomas. J Neurosurg 50:312, 1979.

1427. Meyer JE, Lepke RA, Lindfors KK, et al: Chordomas: Their CT appearance in the cervical thoracic and lumbar spine. Radiology 153:693, 1984.

1428. Wold LE, Laws ER Jr: Cranial chordomas in children and young adults. J Neurosurg 59:1043, 1983.

1429. Schechter MM, Liebeskin AL, Azar-Kia B: Intracranial chordomas. Neuroradiology 8:67, 1974.

1430. Eisemann ML: Sphenooccipital chordoma presenting as a nasopharyngeal mass. A case report. Ann Otol 89:271, 1980.

1431. Batsakis JG, Kittleson AC: Chordomas. Otorhinolaryngologic presentation and diagnosis. Arch Otolaryngol 78:168, 1963.

1432. Berdal P, Myhre E: Cranial chordomas involving the paranasal sinuses. J Laryngol Otol 78:906, 1964.

1433. Richter HJ Jr, Batsakis JG, Boles R: Chordomas: Nasopharyngeal presentation and atypical long survival. Ann Otol 84:327, 1975.

1434. Campbell WM, McDonald TJ, Unni KK, et al: Nasal and paranasal presentations of chordomas. Laryngoscope 90:612, 1980.

1435. Cody HS III, Marcove RC, Quan SH: Malignant retrorectal tumors: 28 years' experience at Memorial Sloan-Kettering Cancer Center. Dis Colon Rectum 24:501, 1981.

1436. Levowitz BS, Khan MY, Rand E, et al: Thoracic vertebral chordoma presenting as a posterior mediastinal tumor. Ann Thorac Surg 2:75, 1966.

1437. Stratt B, Steiner RM: The radiologic findings in posterior mediastinal chordoma. Skel Radiol 5:171, 1980.

1438. Anderson WB, Meyers HI: Multicentric chordoma. Report of a case. Cancer 21:126, 1968.

1439. Marigil MA, Pardo-Mindan FJ, Joly M: Diagnosis of chordoma by cytologic examination of cerebrospinal fluid. Am J Clin Pathol 80:402, 1983.

1440. Tang TT, Dunn DK, Hodach AE, et al: Subcutaneous and skeletal chordomoid nodules in an infant. Am J Dermatopathol 3:303, 1981.

1441. Hudson TM, Galceran M: Radiology of sacrococcygeal chordoma. Difficulties in detecting soft tissue extension. Clin Orthop 175:237, 1983.

1442. Hertzanu Y, Glass RBJ, Mendelsohn DB: Sacrococcygeal chordoma in young adults. Clin Radiol 34:327, 1983.

1443. Krol G, Sundaresan N, Deck M: Computed tomography of axial chordomas. J Comput Assist Tomogr 7:286, 1983.

1444. Rosenthal DI, Scott JA, Mankin HJ, et al: Sacrococcygeal chordoma: Magnetic resonance imaging and computed tomography. AJR 145:143, 1985.

1445. Pettersson H, Hudson T, Hamlin D, et al: Magnetic resonance imaging of sacrococcygeal tumors. Acta Radiol Diagn 26:161, 1985.

1446. Lindgren E, DiChiro G: Suprasellar tumours with calcification. Acta Radiol 36:173, 1951.

1447. Mapstone TB, Kaufman B, Ratcheson RA: Intradural chordoma without bone involvement: Nuclear magnetic resonance (NMR) appearance. Case report. J Neurosurg 59:535, 1983.

1448. Murali R, Rovit RL, Benjamin MV: Chordoma of the cervical spine. Neurosurgery 9:253, 1981.

1449. Heaston DK, Gelman MI: Case report 74. Skel Radiol 3:186, 1978.

1450. Hagenlocher HU, Ciba K: Radiologische Aspekte des zervikalen Chordoms. ROFO 125:228, 1976.

1451. Wang AM, Joachim CL, Shillito J Jr, et al: Cervical chordoma presenting with intervertebral foramen enlargement mimicking neurofibroma: CT findings. J Comput Assist Tomogr 8:529, 1984.

1452. Pinto RS, Lin JP, Firooznia H, et al: The osseous and angiographic features of vertebral chordomas. Neuroradiology 9:231, 1975.

1453. Cummings BJ, Esses S, Harwood AR: The treatment of chordomas. Cancer Treat Rev 9:299, 1982.

1454. Birrell JHW: Chordomata. A review of nineteen cases of chordomata including five vertebral cases. Aust NZ J Surg 22:258, 1953.

1455. Spjut HJ, Luse SA: Chordoma: An electron microscopic study. Cancer 17:643, 1964.

1456. Murad TM, Murthy MSN: Ultrastructure of a chordoma. Cancer 25:1204, 1970.

1457. Mikuz G, Mydla F, Gütter W: Chordoma: Ultrastructural, biochemical and cytophotometric findings. Beitr Pathol 161:150, 1977.

1458. Pardo-Mindan FJ, Guillen FJ, Villas C, et al: A comparative ultrastructural study of chondrosarcoma, chordoid sarcoma, and chordoma. Cancer 47:2611, 1981.

1459. Fu YS, Pritchett PS, Young HF: Tissue culture study of a sacrococcygeal chordoma with further ultrastructural study. Acta Neuropathol (Berl) 32:225, 1975.

1460. Peña CE, Horvat BL, Fisher ER: The ultrastructure of chordoma. Am J Clin Pathol 53:544, 1970.

1461. Kay S, Schatzki PF: Ultrastructural observations of a chordoma arising in the clivus. Hum Pathol 3:403, 1972.

1462. Fox JE, Batsakis JG, Owano LR: Unusual manifestations of chordoma. A report of two cases. J Bone Joint Surg [Am] 50:1618, 1968.

1463. Knechtges TC: Sacrococcygeal chordoma with sarcomatous features (spindle cell metaplasia). Am J Clin Pathol 53:612, 1970.

1464. Kaiser TE, Pritchard DJ, Unni KK: Clinicopathologic study of sacrococcygeal chordoma. Cancer 53:2574, 1984.

1465. Cappell DF: Chordoma of the vertebral column with three new cases. J Pathol 31:797, 1928.

1466. Clark WC, Robertson JH, Lara R: Chondroid chordoma. Case report. J Neurosurg 57:842, 1982.

1467. Crawford T: The staining reactions of chordoma. J Clin Pathol 11:110, 1958.

1468. Bottles K, Beckstead JH: Enzyme histochemical characterization of chordomas. Am J Surg Pathol 8:443, 1984.

1469. Miettinen M, Lehto VP, Dahl D, et al: Differential diagnosis of chordoma, chondroid, and ependymal tumors as aided by anti-intermediate filament antibodies. Am J Pathol 112:160, 1983.

1470. Salisbury JR, Isaacson PG: Demonstration of cytokeratins and an epithelial membrane antigen in chordomas and human fetal notochord. Am J Surg Pathol *9:*791, 1985.

1471. Nakamura Y, Becker LE, Marks A: S100 protein in human chordoma and human and rabbit notochord. Arch Pathol Lab Med *107:*118, 1983.

1472. Monckeberg G: Ueber Cystenbildung bei Ostitis fibrosa. Verh Dtsch Pathol Geb *7:*232, 1904.

1473. Phemister DB, Gordon JE: The etiology of solitary bone cyst. JAMA *87:*1429, 1926.

1474. Jaffe HL, Lichtenstein L: Solitary unicameral bone cyst: With emphasis on the roentgen picture, the pathologic appearance and the pathogenesis. Arch Surg *44:*1004, 1942.

1475. Cohen J: Simple bone cysts. Studies of cyst fluid in six cases with a theory of pathogenesis. J Bone Joint Surg [Am] *42:*609, 1960.

1476. Cohen J: Etiology of simple bone cyst. J Bone Joint Surg [Am] *52:*1493, 1970.

1477. Cohen J: Unicameral bone cysts. A current synthesis of reported cases. Orthop Clin North Am *8:*715, 1977.

1478. Guyton AC, Taylor AE, Brace RA: A synthesis of interstitial fluid regulation and lymph formation. Fed Proc *35:*1881, 1976.

1479. Neer CS, Francis KC, Johnston AD, et al: Current concepts on the treatment of solitary unicameral bone cyst. Clin Orthop *97:*40, 1973.

1480. Chigira M, Maehara S, Arita S, et al: The aetiology and treatment of simple bone cysts. J Bone Joint Surg [Br] *65:*633, 1983.

1481. Norman A, Schiffman M: Simple bone cysts: Factors of age dependency. Radiology *124:*779, 1977.

1482. Garceau GJ, Gregory CF: Solitary unicameral bone cyst. J Bone Joint Surg [Am] *36:*267, 1954.

1483. Moed BR, LaMont RL: Unicameral bone cyst complicated by growth retardation. Report of three cases. J Bone Joint Surg [Am] *64:*1379, 1982.

1484. Neer CS II, Francis KC, Marcove RC, et al: Treatment of unicameral bone cyst. A follow-up study of one hundred seventy-five cases. J Bone Joint Surg [Am] *48:*731, 1966.

1485. Boseker EH, Bickel WH, Dahlin DC: A clinicopathologic study of simple unicameral bone cysts. Surg Gynecol Obstet *127:*550, 1968.

1486. Spence KF Jr, Bright RW, Fitzgerald SP, et al: Solitary unicameral bone cyst: Treatment with freeze-dried crushed cortical-bone allograft. A review of one hundred and forty-four cases. J Bone Joint Surg [Am] *58:*636, 1976.

1487. McKay DW, Nason SS: Treatment of unicameral bone cysts by subtotal resection without grafts. J Bone Joint Surg [Am] *59:*515, 1977.

1488. Capanna R, Dal Monte A, Gitelis S, et al: The natural history of unicameral bone cyst after steroid injection. Clin Orthop *166:*204, 1982.

1489. Scaglietti O, Marchetti PG, Bartolozzi P: Final results obtained in the treatment of bone cysts with methylprednisolone acetate (depo-medrol) and a discussion of results achieved in other bone lesions. Clin Orthop *165:*33, 1982.

1490. Porat S, Lowe J, Rousso M: Solitary bone cyst in the infant radius. A case report. Clin Orthop *135:*132, 1978.

1491. Wu KK, Guise ER: Unicameral bone cyst of the spine. A case report. J Bone Joint Surg [Am] *63:*324, 1981.

1492. Shulman HS, Wilson SR, Harvie JN, et al: Unicameral bone cyst in a rib of a child. AJR *128:*1058, 1977.

1493. Watanabe R: Solitary bone cyst of the rib. Arch Jpn Chir *46:*68, 1977.

1494. Wientroub SH, Salama R, Baratz M, et al: Unicameral bone cyst of the patella. Clin Orthop *140:*159, 1979.

1495. Cztirom AA, Pritzker KPH: Simple bone cyst causing collapse of the articular surface of the femoral head and incongruity of the hip joint. A case report. J Bone Joint Surg [Am] *62:*842, 1980.

1496. Nelson JP, Foster RJ: Solitary bone cyst with epiphyseal involvement. A case report. Clin Orthop *118:*147, 1976.

1497. Malawer MM, Markle B: Unicameral bone cyst with epiphyseal involvement: Clinicoanatomic analysis. J Pediatr Orthop *2:*71, 1982.

1498. Fahey JJ, O'Brien ET: Subtotal resection and grafting in selected cases of solitary unicameral bone cyst. J Bone Joint Surg [Am] *55:*59, 1973.

1499. Lodwick GS: Juvenile unicameral bone cyst. A roentgen reappraisal. AJR *80:*495, 1958.

1500. Hagberg S, Mansfeld L: The solitary bone cyst. A follow-up study of 24 cases. Acta Chir Scand *133:*25, 1967.

1501. Broder HM: Possible precursor of unicameral bone cysts. J Bone Joint Surg [Am] *50:*503, 1968.

1502. Weisel A, Hecht HL: Development of a unicameral bone cyst. Case report. J Bone Joint Surg [Am] *62:*664, 1980.

1503. Reynolds J: The "fallen fragment sign" in the diagnosis of unicameral bone cysts. Radiology *92:*949, 1969.

1504. Taxin RN, Feldman F: The tumbling bullet sign in a post-traumatic bone cyst. AJR *123:*140, 1975.

1505. Smith RW, Smith CF: Solitary unicameral bone cyst of the calcaneus. A review of twenty cases. J Bone Joint Surg [Am] *56:*49, 1974.

1506. Van Linthoudt D, Lagier R: Calcaneal cysts. A radiological and anatomico-pathological study. Acta Orthop Scand *49:*310, 1978.

1507. Ogden JA, Griswold DM: Solitary cyst of the talus. A case report. J Bone Joint Surg [Am] *54:*1309, 1972.

1508. Paaby H: Solitary cysts of the talus. Report of two operated cases. Acta Orthop Scand *44:*560, 1973.

1509. Blumberg ML: CT of iliac unicameral bone cysts. AJR *136:*1231, 1981.

1510. Dawson EG, Mirra JM, Yuhl ET, et al: Solitary bone cyst of the cervical spine. Clin Orthop *119:*141, 1976.

1511. Ramirez H Jr, Blatt ES, Cable HF, et al: Intraosseous pneumatocysts of the ilium. Findings on radiographs and CT scans. Radiology *150:*503, 1984.

1512. Hahn PF, Rosenthal DI, Ehrlich MG: Case report 286. Skel Radiol *12:*214, 1984.

1513. Lemmens JAM, Huynen CHJN, van Horn JR, et al: MR imaging of a cystic lesion of the bone. A case report. ROFO *143:*362, 1985.

1514. Johnson LC: The anatomy of bone cyst. J Bone Joint Surg [Am] *40:*1440, 1958.

1515. Capanna R, Albisinni U, Caroli GC, et al: Contrast examination as a prognostic factor in the treatment of solitary bone cyst by cortisone injection. Skel Radiol *12:*97, 1984.

1516. Adler CP: Tumour-like lesions in the femur with cementum-like material. Does a "cementoma" of long bone exist? Skel Radiol *14:*26, 1985.

1517. Graham JJ: Solitary unicameral bone cyst. A follow-up study of thirty-one cases with proven pathological diagnoses. Bull Hosp Joint Dis *13:*106, 1952.

1518. Sanerkin NG: Old fibrin coagula and their ossification in simple bone cysts. J Bone Joint Surg [Br] *61:*194, 1979.

1519. Robins PR, Peterson HA: Management of pathologic fractures through unicameral bone cysts. JAMA *222:*80, 1972.

1520. Robbins H: The treatment of unicameral or solitary bone cysts by the injection of corticosteroids. Bull Hosp Joint Dis *42:*1, 1982.

1521. Campos OP: Treatment of bone cysts by intracavitary injection of methylprednisolone acetate. A message to orthopedic surgeons. Clin Orthop *165:*43, 1982.

1522. Fernbach SK, Blumenthal DH, Poznanski AK, et al: Radiographic changes in unicameral bone cysts following direct injection of steroids: A report on 14 cases. Radiology *140:*689, 1981.

1523. Khermosh O, Weissman SL: Coxa vara, avascular necrosis and osteochondritis dissecans complicating solitary bone cysts of the proximal femur. Clin Orthop *126:*143, 1977.

1524. Friedman NB, Goldman RL: Cementoma of long bones. An extra-gnathic odontogenic tumor. Clin Orthop *67:*243, 1969.

1525. Mirra JM, Bernard GW, Bullough PG, et al: Cementum-like bone production in solitary bone cysts (so-called "cementoma" of long bones). Report of three cases. Electron microscopic observations supporting a synovial origin to the simple bone cyst. Clin Orthop *135:*295, 1978.

1526. Stelling CB, Martin W, Fechner RE, et al: Case report 150. Skel Radiol *6:*213, 1981.

1527. Kolar JJ, Horn V, Zidkova H, et al: Cementifying fibroma (so-called "cementoma") of tibia. Br J Radiol *54:*989, 1981.

1528. Horn V, Bozdech Z, Macek M, et al: Cementoma-like tumours of bone. Arch Orthop Trauma Surg *100:*267, 1982.

1529. Grabias S, Mankin HJ: Chondrosarcoma arising in histologically proved unicameral bone cyst. A case report. J Bone Joint Surg [Am] *56:*1501, 1974.

1530. Johnson LC, Vetter H, Putschar WGJ: Sarcomas arising in bone cysts. Virchows Arch (Pathol Anat) *335:*428, 1962.

1531. Steinberg GG: Ewing's sarcoma arising in a unicameral bone cyst. J Pediatr Orthop *5:*97, 1985.

1532. Rand CW, Reeves DL: Dermoid and epidermoid tumors (cholesteatomas) of the central nervous system. Report of twenty-three cases. Arch Surg *46:*350, 1943.

1533. Carroll RE: Epidermoid (epithelial) cyst of the hand skeleton. Am J Surg *85:*327, 1953.

1534. Haig PV: Primary epidermoids of the skull including a case with malignant change. AJR *76:*1076, 1956.

1535. Fisher ER, Gruhn J, Skerrett P: Epidermal cyst in bone. Cancer *11:*643, 1958.

1536. Skandalakis JE, Godwin JT, Mabon RF: Epidermoid cyst of the skull. Report of four cases and review of the literature. Surgery *43:*990, 1958.

1537. Sieracki JC, Kelly AP: Traumatic epidermoid cysts involving digital bones. Epidermoid cysts of the distal phalanx. Arch Surg *78:*597, 1959.

1538. Roth SI: Squamous cysts involving the skull and distal phalanges. J Bone Joint Surg [Am] *46:*1442, 1964.

1539. Byers P, Mantle J, Salm R: Epidermal cysts of phalanges. J Bone Joint Surg [Br] *48:*577, 1966.

1540. Lerner MR, Southwick WO: Keratin cysts in phalangeal bones. Report of an unusual case. J Bone Joint Surg [Am] *50:*365, 1968.

1541. Schwajowicz F, Aiello CL, Slullitel I: Cystic and pseudocystic lesions of the terminal phalanx with special reference to epidermoid cysts. Clin Orthop *68:*84, 1970.

1542. Svenes KJ, Halleraker B: Epidermal bone cyst of the finger. A case report. Acta Orthop Scand *48:*29, 1977.

1543. Rengachary S, Kishore PRS, Watanabe I: Intradiploic epidermoid cyst of the occipital bone with torcular obstruction. J Neurosurg *48:*475, 1978.

1544. Hoessly M, Lagier R: Anatomico-radiological study of intraosseous epidermoid cysts. ROFO *137:*48, 1982.

1545. Garcia J, Lagier R, Hoessly M: Case report. Computed tomography-pathology correlation in skull epidermoid cyst. J Comput Assist Tomogr *6:*818, 1982.

1546. Abedi E, Frable MA: Epidermoid cyst of the frontal bone masquerading as frontal sinusitis. Laryngoscope *94:*545, 1984.

1547. Constans JP, Meder JF, De Divitiis E, et al: Giant intradiploic epidermoid cysts of the skull. Report of two cases. J Neurosurg *62:*445, 1985.

1548. Roquiz PM, Susann PW: Painful mass of the phalanx following trauma. Milit Med *150:*144, 1985.

1549. Trias A, Beauregard G: Epidermoid cyst of bone. Can J Surg *17:*1, 1974.

1550. Exner G, Hort W, Böger A: Epidermoidzyste der tibia. Z Orthop *116:*362, 1978.

1551. Maritz NGJ, De Bruin B: Epidermal cysts of the femur. A case report. S Afr Med J *58:*779, 1980.

1552. Mollan RAB, Wray AR, Hayes D: Traumatic epidermoid cyst of the ulna. Report of a case. J Bone Joint Surg [Br] *64:*456, 1982.

1553. Pons J, Gaume B, Lombard JP, et al: Les Kystes epidermoides de la mandibule. Six observations. Rev Stomat (Paris) *70:*374, 1969.

1554. Dahlin DC, McLeod RA: Aneurysmal bone cyst and other nonneoplastic conditions. Skel Radiol *8:*243, 1982.

1555. Ginsburg LD: Congenital aneurysmal bone cyst. Case report with comments on the role of trauma in the pathogenesis. Radiology *110:*175, 1974.

1556. Dabezies EJ, D'Ambrosia RD, Chuinard RG, et al: J Bone Joint Surg [Am] *64:*617, 1982.

1557. Kushner DC, Vance Z, Kirkpatrick JA Jr: Case report 103. Skel Radiol *4:*240, 1979.

1558. Levy WM, Miller AS, Bonakdarpour A, et al: Aneurysmal bone cyst secondary to other osseous lesions. Report of 57 cases. Am J Clin Pathol *63:*1, 1975.

1559. Diercks RL, Sauter AJM, Mallens WMC: Aneurysmal bone cyst in association with fibrous dysplasia. A case report. J Bone Joint Surg [Br] *68:*144, 1986.

1560. Buraczewski J, Dabska M: Pathogenesis of aneurysmal bone cyst: Relationship between aneurysmal bone cyst and fibrous dysplasia of bone. Cancer *28:*597, 1971.

1561. Clough JR, Price CHG: Aneurysmal bone cysts: Review of 12 cases. J Bone Joint Surg [Br] *50:*116, 1968.

1562. Oliver LP: Aneurysmal bone cyst: Report of a case. Oral Surg *35:*67, 1973.

1563. Bonakdarpour A, Levy WM, Aegerter E: Primary and secondary aneurysmal bone cyst: A radiological study of 75 cases. Radiology *126:*75, 1978.

1564. El Deeb M, Sedano HO, Waite DE: Aneurysmal bone cyst of the jaws: Report of a case associated with fibrous dysplasia and review of the literature. Int J Oral Surg *9:*301, 1980.

1565. Jaffe HL: Aneurysmal bone cyst. Bull Hosp Joint Dis *11:*3, 1950.

1566. Donaldson WF Jr: Aneurysmal bone cyst. J Bone Joint Surg [Am] *44:*25, 1962.

1567. Lichtenstein L: Aneurysmal bone cyst: Further observations. Cancer *6:*1228, 1953.

1568. Clough JR, Price CHG: Aneurysmal bone cyst: Pathogenesis and long term results of treatment. Clin Orthop *97:*52, 1973.

1569. Carlson DH, Wilkinson RH, Bhakkaviziam A: Aneurysmal bone cysts in children. AJR *116:*644, 1972.

1570. Slowick FA Jr, Campbell CJ, Kettelkamp DB: Aneurysmal bone cyst. An analysis of thirteen cases. J Bone Joint Surg [Am] *50:*1142, 1968.

1571. Koskinen EVS, Visuri TI, Holmstrom T, et al: Aneurysmal bone cyst. Evaluation of resection and of curettage in 20 cases. Clin Orthop *118:*136, 1976.

1572. Kozlowski K, Middleton RWD: Aneurysmal bone cysts—review of 10 cases. Aust Radiol *24:*170, 1980.

1573. Lichtenstein L: Aneurysmal bone cyst. Observations on fifty cases. J Bone Joint Surg [Am] *39:*873, 1957.

1574. Tillman BP, Dahlin DC, Lipscomb PR, et al: Aneurysmal bone cyst: An analysis of ninety-five cases. Mayo Clin Proc *43:*478, 1968.

1575. Dabska M, Buraczewski J: Aneurysmal bone cyst. Pathology, clinical course and radiologic appearances. Cancer *23:*371, 1969.

1576. Biesecker JL, Marcove RC, Huvos AG, et al: Aneurysmal bone cysts. A clinicopathological study of 66 cases. Cancer *26:*615, 1970.

1577. Ruiter DJ, van Rijssel ThG, van der Velde EA: Aneurysmal bone cysts. A clinicopathological study of 105 cases. Cancer *9:*2231, 1977.

1578. Capanna R, Springfield DS, Biagini R, et al: Juxtaepiphyseal aneurysmal bone cyst. Skel Radiol *13:*21, 1985.

1579. Sherman RS, Soong KY: Aneurysmal bone cyst: Its roentgen diagnosis. Radiology *68:*54, 1957.

1580. Bhaskar SN, Bernier JL, Godby F: Aneurysmal bone cyst and other giant cell lesions of the jaws: Report of 104 cases. J Oral Surg *17:*30, 1959.

1581. Odeku EL, Mainwaring AR: Unusual aneurysmal bone cyst. A case report. J Neurosurg *22:*172, 1965.

1582. Srivastava KK, Ahuja SC, Hochhar VL: Aneurysmal bone cyst of the patella. Aust NZ J Surg *43:*52, 1973.

1583. Hurvitz JS, Harrison MR, Weitzman JJ: Aneurysmal bone cyst mimicking Ewing's sarcoma of the rib. J Pediatr Surg *12:*1067, 1977.

1584. Hay MC, Paterson D, Taylor TKF: Aneurysmal bone cysts of the spine. J Bone Joint Surg [Br] *60:*406, 1978.

1585. Ishinada Y, Yabe H, Ogoshi E, et al: Aneurysmal bone cyst of the sternum. Ann Thorac Surg *27:*254, 1979.

1586. Klein GM, Spector HL, Nernoff J III: Case report 203. Skel Radiol *8:*299, 1982.

1587. DeLuccia VC, Reyes EC: Aneurysmal cyst of the rib. NY State J Med *82:*1077, 1982.

1588. Hertzanu Y, Mendelsohn DB, Gottschalf F: Aneurysmal bone cyst of the calcaneus. Radiology *151:*51, 1984.

1589. Gingell JC, Levy BA, Beckerman T, et al: Aneurysmal bone cyst. J Oral Maxillofac Surg *42:*527, 1984.

1590. Struthers PJ, Shear M: Aneurysmal bone cyst of the jaws (II). Pathogenesis. Int J Oral Surg *13:*92, 1984.

1591. Dryer R, Stelling CB, Fechner RE: Epiphyseal extension of an aneurysmal bone cyst. AJR *137:*172, 1981.

1592. Beeler JW, Helman CH, Campbell JA: Aneurysmal bone cysts of spine. JAMA *163:*914, 1957.

1593. Capanna R, Albisinni U, Picci P, et al: Aneurysmal bone cyst of the spine. J Bone Joint Surg [Am] *67:*527, 1985.

1594. Schaffer L, Kranzler LI, Siqueira EB: Aneurysmal bone cyst of the spine. A case report. Spine *10:*390, 1985.

1595. Faure C, Boccon-Gibod L, Herve J, et al: Case report 154. Skel Radiol *6:*229, 1981.

1596. Shacked I, Tadmor R, Wolpin G, et al: Aneurysmal bone cyst of a vertebral body with acute paraplegia. Paraplegia *19:*294, 1981.

1597. El-Khoury GY, Seaman RW: Case report 125. Skel Radiol *5:*201, 1980.

1598. Chalmers J: Aneurysmal bone cysts of the phalanges. A report of three cases. Hand *13:*296, 1981.

1599. Erseven A, Garti A, Weigl K: Aneurysmal bone cyst of the first metatarsal bone mimicking malignant tumor. Clin Orthop *181:*171, 1983.

1600. Robinson AE, Thomas RL, Monson DM: Aneurysmal bone cyst of the rib. A report of two unusual cases. AJR *100:*526, 1967.

1601. Gold RH, Mirra JM: Case report 234. Skel Radiol *10:*57, 1983.

1602. Faris WF, Rubin BD, Fielding JW: Aneurysmal bone cyst of the patella. A case report. J Bone Joint Surg [Am] *60:*711, 1978.

1603. Soreff J: Aneurysmal bone cyst of the talus. Acta Orthop Scand *47:*358, 1976.

1604. Luccarelli G, Fornari M, Savoiardo M: Angiography and computerized tomography in the diagnosis of aneurysmal bone cyst of the skull. Case report. J Neurosurg *53:*113, 1980.

1605. Bilge T, Coban O, Ozden B, et al: Aneurysmal bone cysts of the occipital bone. Surg Neurol *20:*227, 1983.

1606. Cacdac MA, Malis LI, Anderson PJ: Aneurysmal parietal bone cyst. Case report. J Neurosurg *37:*237, 1972.

1607. Struthers PJ, Shear M: Aneurysmal bone cyst of the jaws (I). Clinicopathological features. Int J Oral Surg *13:*85, 1984.

1608. Oliver LP: Aneurysmal bone cyst. Report of a case. Oral Surg *35:*67, 1973.

1609. Lindbom A, Soderberg G, Spjut HJ, Sunnquist O: Angiography of aneurysmal bone cyst. Acta Radiol Diagn *55:*12, 1961.

1610. de Santos L, Murray JA: The value of arteriography in the management of aneurysmal bone cyst. Skel Radiol *2:*137, 1978.

1611. Hudson TM: Scintigraphy of aneurysmal bone cysts. Am J Roentgenol *142:*761, 1984.

1612. Makhija MC: Bone scanning in aneurysmal bone cyst. Clin Nucl Med *6:*500, 1981.

1613. Haney P, Gellad F, Swartz J: Aneurysmal bone cyst of the spine: Computed tomographic appearance. J Comput Tomogr *7:*319, 1983.

1614. Hudson TM: Fluid levels in aneurysmal bone cysts: A CT feature. Am J Roentgenol *141:*1001, 1984.

1615. Hertzanu Y, Mendelsohn DB, Gottschalk F: Aneurysmal bone cyst of the calcaneus. Radiology *151:*51, 1984.

1616. Zimmer WD, Berquist TH, Sim FH, et al: Magnetic resonance imaging of aneurysmal bone cyst. Mayo Clin Proc *59:*633, 1984.

1617. Hudson TM, Hamlin DJ, Fitzsimmons JR: Magnetic resonance imaging of fluid levels in an aneurysmal bone cyst and in anticoagulated human blood. Skel Radiol *13:*267, 1985.

1618. Beltran J, Simon DC, Levy M, et al: Aneurysmal bone cysts: MR imaging at 1.5T. Radiology *158:*689, 1986.

1619. Lichtenstein L: Aneurysmal bone cyst. A pathological entity commonly mistaken for giant-cell tumor and occasionally for hemangioma and osteogenic sarcoma. Cancer *3:*279, 1950.

1620. Hadders HN, Oterdoom HJ: The identification of aneurysmal bone cyst with haemangioma of the skeleton. J Pathol Bacteriol *71:*193, 1956.

1621. Reed RJ, Rothenberg M: Lesions of bone that may be confused with aneurysmal bone cyst. Clin Orthop Rel Res *35:*150, 1964.

1622. Sanerkin NG, Mott MG, Roylance J: An unusual intraosseous lesion with fibroblastic, osteoclastic, osteoblastic, aneurysmal and fibromyxoid elements. "Solid" variant of aneurysmal bone cyst. Cancer *51:*2278, 1983.

1623. Besse BE Jr, Dahlin DC, Bruwer A, Svien HJ, Ghormley RK: Aneurysmal bone cyst. Proc Staff Meet Mayo Clin *28:*249, 1953.

1624. Thompson PC: Subperiosteal giant-cell tumor. Ossifying subperiosteal hematoma-aneurysmal bone cyst. J Bone Joint Surg [Am] *36:*281, 1954.

1625. Steiner GC, Kantor EB: Ultrastructure of aneurysmal bone cyst. Cancer *40:*2967, 1977.

1626. Aho HJ, Aho AJ, Einola S: Aneurysmal bone cyst, a study of ultrastructure and malignant transformation. Virchows Arch (Pathol Anat) *395:*169, 1982.

1627. Kaernbach A, Strecker EP, Schafer JH: Aggressive aneurysmale Knochencyste der Wirbelsaule im Kindesalter. Radiologe *18:*279, 1978.

1628. McQueen MM, Chalmers J, Smith GD: Spontaneous healing of aneurysmal bone cysts. A report of two cases. J Bone Joint Surg [Br] *67:*310, 1985.

1629. Murphy WA, Strecker WB, Schoenecker PL: Transcatheter embolisation therapy of an ischial aneurysmal bone cyst. J Bone Joint Surg [Br] *64:*166, 1982.

1630. Nobler MP, Higinbotham NL, Phillips RF: The cure of aneurysmal bone cyst. Irradiation superior to surgery in an analysis of 33 cases. Radiology *90:*1185, 1968.

1631. Marks RD Jr, Scruggs HJ, Wallace KM, et al: Megavoltage therapy in patients with aneurysmal bone cysts. Radiology *118:*421, 1976.

1632. Buirsky G, Watt I: The radiological features of "solid" aneurysmal bone cysts. Br J Radiol *57:*1057, 1984.

1633. Huvos AG, Marcove RC: Adamantinoma of long bones. A clinicopathological study of fourteen cases with vascular origin suggested. J Bone Joint Surg [Am] *57:*148, 1975.

1634. Fischer B: Uber ein primäres Adamantinom der Tibia. Z Pathol *12:*422, 1913.
1635. Moon NF, Mori H: Adamantinoma of the appendicular skeleton—updated. Clin Orthop *204:*215, 1986.
1636. Ryrie BJ: Adamantinoma of the tibia: Aetiology and pathogenesis. Br Med J *2:*1000, 1932.
1637. Changus GW, Speed JS, Stewart FW: Malignant angioblastoma of bone. Cancer *10:*540, 1957.
1638. Albores Saavedra J, Diaz Gutierrez D, Altamirano Dimas M: Adamantinoma de la tibia. Observaciones ultraestructurales. Rev Med Hosp Gen *31:*241, 1968.
1639. Yoneyama T, Winter WG, Milsow L: Tibial adamantinoma: Its histogenesis from ultrastructural studies. Cancer *40:*1138, 1977.
1640. Llombart-Bosch A, Ortuño-Pacheco G: Ultrastructural findings supporting the angioblastic nature of the so-called adamantinoma of the tibia. Histopathology *2:*189, 1978.
1641. Mori H, Yamamoto S, Hiramatsu K, et al: Adamantinoma of the tibia. Ultrastructural and immunohistochemic study with reference to histogenesis. Clin Orthop *190:*299, 1984.
1642. Eisenstein W, Pitcock JA: Adamantinoma of the tibia. An eccrine carcinoma. Arch Pathol Lab Med *108:*246, 1984.
1643. Pověyšil C, Matějovský Z: Ultrastructure of adamantinoma of long bones. Virchows Arch (Pathol Anat) *393:*233, 1981.
1644. Rosai J, Pinkus GS: Immunohistochemical demonstration of epithelial differentiation in adamantinoma of the tibia. Am J Surg Pathol *6:*427, 1982.
1645. Perez-Atayde AR, Kozakewich HPW, Vawter GF: Adamantinoma of the tibia. An ultrastructural immunohistologic study. Cancer *55:*1015, 1985.
1646. Meister P, Konrad E, Hübner G: Malignant tumor of humerus with features of "adamantinoma" and Ewing's sarcoma. Pathol Res Pract *166:*112, 1979.
1647. Lipper S, Kahn LB: Case report 235. Skel Radiol *10:*61, 1983.
1648. Unni KK, Dahlin DC, Beabout JW, et al: Adamantinomas of long bones. Cancer *34:*1796, 1974.
1649. Weiss SW, Dorfman HD: Adamantinoma of long bone. An analysis of nine new cases with emphasis on metastasizing lesions and fibrous dysplasia-like changes. Hum Pathol *8:*141, 1977.
1650. Konrad EA, Meister P, Stotz S: "Adamantinom" der Tibia und reaktive Knochenveränderungen. Arch Orthop Trauma Surg *92:*297, 1978.
1651. Cohen DM, Dahlin DC, Pugh DG: Fibrous dysplasia associated with adamantinoma of the long bones. Cancer *15:*515, 1962.
1652. Sadykhov AG, Brodskiĭ SR, Badoeva FI: Adamantinoma dlinnykh trubchatykh kosteĭ. Vestn Khir *117:*138, 1976.
1653. Hicks JD: Synovial sarcoma of the tibia. J Pathol Bacteriol *67:*151, 1954.
1654. Anderson CE, Saunders JBD: Primary adamantinoma of the ulna. Surg Gynecol Obstet *75:*351, 1942.
1655. Bell AL: A case of adamantinoma of the femur. Br J Surg *30:*81, 1942–1943.
1656. Halpert B, Dohn HP: Adamantinoma in the tibia. Arch Pathol *43:*313, 1947.
1657. Mangalik VS, Mehrotra RML: Adamantinoma of the tibia. Report of a case. Br J Surg *39:*429, 1951–1952.
1658. Diepeveen WP, Hjort GH, Pock-Steen OC: Adamantinoma of the capitate bone. Acta Radiol *53:*377, 1960.
1659. Rosen RS, Schwinn CP: Adamantinoma of limb bone. Malignant angioblastoma. AJR *97:*727, 1966.
1660. Besemann EF, Perez MA: Malignant angioblastoma, so-called adamantinoma, involving the humerus. A case report. AJR *100:*538, 1967.
1661. Rosai J: Adamantinoma of the tibia. Electron microscopic evidence of its epithelial origin. Am J Clin Pathol *51:*786, 1969.
1662. Bullough PG, Goldberg VM: Multicentric origin of adamantinoma of the tibia. A case report. Rev Hosp Spec Surg *1:*71, 1971.
1663. Shah IC, Castro EB, Miller TR, et al: Malignant angioblastoma (so-called adamantinoma) of humerus. Int Surg *57:*753, 1972.
1664. Zand A, Chambers GH, Street DM: So-called "adamantinoma of long bone." Clin Orthop *86:*178, 1972.
1665. Braidwood AS, McDougall A: Adamantinoma of the tibia. Report of two cases. J Bone Joint Surg [Br] *56:*735, 1974.
1666. Thurner VJ, Marcacci M: A so-called adamantinoma of the right femur. Zentralbl Allg Pathol *120:*398, 1976.
1667. Lasda NA, Hughes EC: Adamantinoma of the ischium. Case report. J Bone Joint Surg [Am] *61:*599, 1979.
1668. Hierton T, Kolstad K, Lindgren A, et al: Adamantinoma tibiae. Acta Orthop Scand *50:*97, 1979.
1669. Schneider H, Enderle A: Zur Differentialdiagnose eines metastasierenden Adamantinoms der Tibia und Fibula. Arch Orthop Trauma Surg *94:*143, 1979.
1670. Dameron TB Jr: Adamantinoma of the appendicular skeleton. Johns Hopkins Med J *145:*107, 1979.
1671. Johansen S, Wennberg E: Adamantinoma tibiae. A report of a new case. Acta Orthop Scand *51:*971, 1980.
1672. Campanacci M, Giunti A, Bertoni F, et al: Adamantinoma of the long bones. The experience at the Istituto Ortopedico Rizzoli. Am J Surg Pathol *5:*533, 1981.
1673. Knapp RH, Wick MR, Scheithauer BW, et al: Adamantinoma of bone. An electron microscopic and immunohistochemical study. Virchows Arch (Pathol Anat) *398:*75, 1982.
1674. Pieterse AS, Smith PS, McClure J: Adamantinoma of long bones: Clinical, pathological and ultrastructural features. J Clin Pathol *35:*780, 1982.
1675. Bambirra EA, Margarida A, Nogueira MF, et al: Adamantinoma of the soft tissue of the leg. Arch Pathol Lab Med *107:*500, 1983.
1676. Mills SE, Rosai J: Adamantinoma of the pretibial soft tissue. Clinicopathologic features, differential diagnosis, and possible relationship to intraosseous disease. Am J Clin Pathol *83:*108, 1985.
1677. Baker PL, Dockerty MB, Coventry MB: Adamantinoma (so-called) of the long bones. Review of the literature and a report of three new cases. J Bone Joint Surg [Am] *36:*704, 1954.
1678. Baker AH, Hawksley LM: A case of primary adamantinoma of the tibia. Br J Surg *18:*415, 1930.
1679. Donner R, Dikland R: Adamantinoma of the rib. A long-standing case with unusual histological features. J Bone Joint Surg [Br] *48:*138, 1966.
1680. Mandard JC, Le Gal Y, Fievez M: "L'adamantinome" des os longs. Ann Anat Pathol *16:*483, 1971.
1681. Ewing J: Diffuse endothelioma of bone. Proc NY Pathol Soc *21:*17, 1921.
1682. Parker F Jr, Jackson H Jr: Primary reticulum cell sarcoma of bone. Surg Gynecol Obstet *68:*45, 1939.
1683. Llombart-Bosch A, Blache R, Peydro-Olaya A: Ultrastructural study of 28 cases of Ewing's sarcoma: Typical and atypical forms. Cancer *41:*1362, 1978.
1684. Friedman B, Gold H: Ultrastructure of Ewing's sarcoma of bone. Cancer *22:*307, 1968.
1685. Povysil C, Matejovsky Z: Ultrastructure of Ewing's tumour. Virchows Arch (Pathol Anat) *374:*303, 1977.
1686. Kadin ME, Bensch KG: On the origin of Ewing's tumor. Cancer *27:*257, 1971.
1687. Navas-Palacios JJ, Aparicio-Duque R, Valdés MD: On the histogenesis of Ewing's sarcoma. An ultrastructural, immunohistochemical, and cytochemical study. Cancer *53:*1882, 1984.
1688. Dickman PS, Liotta LA, Triche TJ: Ewing's sarcoma. Characterization in established cultures and evidence of its histogenesis. Lab Invest *47:*375, 1982.
1689. Miettinen M, Lehto VP, Virtanen I: Histogenesis of Ewing's sarcoma. An evaluation of intermediate filaments and endothelial cell markers. Virchows Arch (Cell Pathol) *41:*277, 1982.
1690. Roessner A, Voss B, Rauterberg J, et al: Biologic characterization of human bone tumors. I. Ewing's sarcoma. A comparative electron and immunofluorescence microscopic study. J Cancer Res Clin Oncol *104:*161, 1982.
1691. Colville HC, Willis RA: Neuroblastoma metastases in bones, with a criticism of Ewing's endothelioma. Am J Pathol *9:*421, 1933.
1692. Willis RA: Metastatic neuroblastoma in bone presenting the Ewing syndrome, with a discussion of "Ewing's sarcoma." Am J Pathol *16:*317, 1940.
1693. Ynuis EJ, Agostini RM Jr, Walpusk JA, et al: Glycogen in neuroblastomas. A light- and electron-microscopic study of 40 cases. Am J Surg Pathol *3:*313, 1979.
1694. Triche TJ: Round cell tumors in childhood: The application of newer techniques to the differential diagnosis in perspectives. *In* HS Rosenberg, J Bernstein (eds): Pediatric Pathology. Vol 7, New York, Masson 1982, p 270.
1695. Horn RC Jr, Koop CE, Kiesewetter WB: Neuroblastoma in childhood. Clinicopathologic study of forty-four cases. Lab Invest *5:*106, 1956.
1696. Lumb G, Mackenzie DH: Round-cell tumours of bone. Br J Surg *43:*380, 1955–1956.
1697. Marsden HB, Steward JK: Ewing's tumours and neuroblastomas. J Clin Pathol *17:*411, 1964.
1698. Telles NC, Rabson AS, Pomeroy TC: Ewing's sarcoma: An autopsy study. Cancer *41:*2321, 1978.
1699. Jaffe R, Santamaria M, Yunis EJ, et al: The neuroectodermal tumor of bone. Am J Surg Pathol *8:*885, 1984.
1700. Neff JR: Nonmetastatic Ewing's sarcoma of bone: The role of surgical therapy. Clin Orthop *204:*111, 1986.
1701. Kissane JM, Askin FB, Foulkes M, et al: Ewing's sarcoma of bone: Clinicopathologic aspects of 303 cases from the intergroup Ewing's sarcoma study. Hum Pathol *14:*773, 1983.
1702. McGirr EE, Edmonds JP: Ewing's sarcoma presenting as monoarthritis. J Rheumatol *11:*534, 1984.
1703. Wang CC, Schulz MD: Ewing's sarcoma. A study of fifty cases treated at the Massachusetts General Hospital, 1930–1952 inclusive. N Engl J Med *248:*571, 1953.
1704. Falk S, Alpert M: The clinical and roentgen aspects of Ewing's sarcoma. Am J Med Sci *250:*492, 1965.
1705. Campanacci M, Bacci G, Boriani S, et al: Ewing's sarcoma (a review of 195 cases). Ital J Orthop Traumatol *5:*293, 1979.
1706. Vohra VG: Roentgen manifestations in Ewing's sarcoma. A study of 156 cases. Cancer *20:*727, 1967.
1707. Whitehouse GH, Griffiths GJ: Roentgenologic aspects of spinal involvement by primary and metastatic Ewing's tumor. J Can Assoc Radiol *27:*290, 1976.
1708. de Santos LA, Jing BS: Radiographic findings of Ewing's sarcoma of the jaws. Br J Radiol *51:*682, 1978.
1709. Pilepich MV, Vietti TJ, Nesbit ME, et al: Ewing's sarcoma of the vertebral column. Int J Radiat Oncol Biol Phys *7:*27, 1981.
1710. Russin LA, Robinson MJ, Engle HA, et al: Ewing's sarcoma of the lumbar spine: A case report of long-term survival. Clin Orthop *164:*126, 1982.
1711. Mansfield JB: Primary Ewing's sarcoma of the skull. Surg Neurol *18:*286, 1982.
1712. Arafat A, Ellis GL, Adrian JC: Ewing's sarcoma of the jaws. Oral Surg *55:*589, 1983.
1713. Weinstein JB, Siegel MJ, Griffith RC: Spinal Ewing sarcoma: Misleading appearances. Skel Radiol *11:*262, 1984.
1714. Reinus WR, Gilula LA, Shirley SK, et al: Radiographic appearance of Ewing sarcoma of the hands and feet: Report from the Intergroup Ewing Sarcoma Study. AJR *144:*331, 1985.

1715. Shirley SK, Askin FB, Gilula LA, et al: Ewing's sarcoma in bones of the hands and feet: A clinicopathologic study and review of the literature. J Clin Oncol 3:686, 1985.

1716. Baird RJ, Krause VW: Ewing's tumor: A review of 33 cases. Can J Surg 6:136, 1963.

1717. Boyer CW Jr, Brickner TJ, Perry RH: Ewing's sarcoma. Case against surgery. Cancer 20:1602, 1967.

1718. Potdar GG: Ewing's tumor. Clin Radiol 22:528, 1971.

1719. Larsson SE, Boquist L, Bergdahl L: Ewing's sarcoma. A consecutive series of 64 cases diagnosed in Sweden 1958–1967. Clin Orthop 95:263, 1973.

1720. Macintosh DJ, Price CHG, Jeffree GM: Ewing's tumour. A study of behaviour and treatment in forty-seven cases. J Bone Joint Surg [Br] 57:331, 1975.

1721. Gasparini M, Barni S, Lattuada A, et al: Ten years experience with Ewing's sarcoma. Tumori 63:77, 1977.

1722. Chan RC, Sutow WW, Lindberg RD, et al: Management and results of localized Ewing's sarcoma. Cancer 43:1001, 1979.

1723. Lavallee G, Lemarbre L, Bouchard R, et al: Ewing's sarcoma in adults. J Can Assoc Radiol 30:223, 1979.

1724. Dick HM, Francis KC, Johnston AD: Ewing's sarcoma of the hand. J Bone Joint Surg [Am] 53:345, 1971.

1725. Dunn EJ, Yuska KH, Judge DM, et al: Ewing's sarcoma of the great toe. A case report. Clin Orthop 116:203, 1976.

1726. Dryer RF, Buckwalter JA, Flatt AE, et al: Ewing's sarcoma of the hand. J Hand Surg 4:372, 1979.

1727. Wientroub S, Michels H, Baratz M, et al: Ewing's tumor of the cuboid bone simulating avascular necrosis. Report of a case. J Bone Joint Surg [Am] 61:951, 1979.

1728. Chen KTK, McGann PD, Flam MS: Ewing's sarcoma of the phalangeal bone. J Surg Oncol 22:92, 1983.

1729. Kedar A, Bialik V, Fishman J: Ewing sarcoma of the hand: Literature review and a case report of nonsurgical management. J Surg Oncol 25:25, 1984.

1730. Fitzer PM, Steffey WR: Brain and bone scans in primary Ewing's sarcoma of the petrous bone. Case report. J Neurosurg 44:608, 1976.

1731. Roca AN, Smith JL, MacComb WS, et al: Ewing's sarcoma of the maxilla and mandible. Study of six cases. Oral Surg 25:194, 1968.

1732. Hunsuck EE: Ewing's sarcoma of the maxilla. Report of a case. Oral Surg 25:923, 1968.

1733. Brownson RJ, Cook RP: Ewing's sarcoma of the maxilla. Ann Otol Rhinol Laryngol 78:1299, 1969.

1734. Potdar GG: Ewing's tumors of the jaws. Oral Surg 29:505, 1970.

1735. Dehner LP: Tumors of the mandible and maxilla in children. II. A study of 14 primary and secondary malignant tumors. Cancer 32:112, 1973.

1736. Borghelli RF, Barros RE, Zampieri J: Ewing sarcoma of the mandible: Report of case. J Oral Surg 36:473, 1978.

1737. Ferlito A: Primary Ewing's sarcoma of the maxilla: A clinicopathological study of four cases. J Laryngol Otol 92:1007, 1978.

1738. Sherman RS, Soong KY: Ewing's sarcoma: Its roentgen classification and diagnosis. Radiology 66:529, 1956.

1739. Dahlin DC, Coventry MB, Scanlon PW: Ewing's sarcoma. A critical analysis of 165 cases. J Bone Joint Surg [Am] 43:185, 1961.

1740. Bhansali SK, Desai PB: Ewing's sarcoma. Observations of 107 cases. J Bone Joint Surg [Am] 45:541, 1963.

1741. Reinus WR, Gilula LA, the IESS Committee: Radiology of Ewing's sarcoma: Intergroup Ewing's Sarcoma Study (IESS). RadioGraphics 4:929, 1984.

1742. Schifter S, Vendelbo L, Jensen OM: Ewing's tumor following bilateral retinoblastoma. A case report. Cancer 57:1746, 1983.

1743. Pritchard DJ, Dahlin DC, Dauphine RT, et al: Ewing's sarcoma. A clinicopathological and statistical analysis of patients surviving five years or longer. J Bone Joint Surg [Am] 57:10, 1975.

1744. Ochsner A Jr, Lucas GL, McFarland GB Jr: Tumors of the thoracic skeleton. Review of 134 cases. J Thorac Cardiovasc Surg 52:311, 1966.

1745. Kedar A, Ghoorah J, Thomas PRM, et al: Primary Ewing's sarcoma of the sternum: A case report. Med Pediatr Oncol 7:163, 1979.

1746. Shirley SK, Gilula LA, Siegal GP, et al: Roentgenographic-pathologic correlation of diffuse sclerosis in Ewing sarcoma of bone. Skel Radiol 12:69, 1984.

1747. Vacher H, Vacher-Lavenu MC, Sauvegrain J: Etude anatomo-radioclinique des sarcomes d'Ewing du rachis lombaire. J Radiol 62:425, 1981.

1748. Wooten WB, Sumner TE, Crowe JE, et al: Case report 64. Skel Radiol 3:65, 1978.

1749. Levine E, Levine C: Ewing tumor of rib: Radiologic findings and computed tomography contribution. Skel Radiol 9:227, 1983.

1750. Staalman CR: Ewing's sarcoma in rib. J Belge Radiol 65:329, 1982.

1751. Bushnell D, Shirazi P, Khedkar N, et al: Ewing's sarcoma seen as a "cold" lesion on bone scans. Clin Nucl Med 8:173, 1983.

1752. Ginaldi S, de Santos LA: Computed tomography in the evaluation of small round cell tumors of bone. Radiology 134:441, 1980.

1753. Vanel D, Contesso G, Couanet D, et al: Computed tomography in the evaluation of 41 cases of Ewing's sarcoma. Skel Radiol 9:8, 1982.

1754. Turoff NB, Becker M, Lewis M: Ewing's sarcoma: Unusual presentation delineated by computerized tomography. Report of a case. J Bone Joint Surg [Am] 60:1109, 1978.

1755. Thomas PRM, Foulkes MA, Gilula LA, et al: Primary Ewing's sarcoma of the ribs. A report from the Intergroup Ewing's Sarcoma Study. Cancer 51:1021, 1983.

1756. Mendenhall CM, Marcus RB Jr, Enneking WF, et al: The prognostic significance of soft tissue extension of Ewing's sarcoma. Cancer 51:913, 1983.

1757. Phelan JT, Cabrera A: Ewing's sarcoma. Surg Gynecol Obstet 118:795, 1964.

1758. Stout AP: A discussion of the pathology and histogenesis of Ewing's tumor of bone marrow. AJR 50:334, 1943.

1759. McCormack LJ, Dockerty MB, Ghormley RK: Ewing's sarcoma. Cancer 5:85, 1952.

1760. Llombart-Bosch A, Blache R, Peydro-Olaya A: Round-cell sarcomas of bone and their differential diagnosis (with particular emphasis on Ewing's sarcoma and reticulosarcoma). A study of 233 tumors with optical and electron microscopic techniques. Pathol Annu 17 (Part 2):113, 1982.

1761. Llombart-Bosch A, Peydro-Olaya A: Scanning and transmission electron microscopy of Ewing's sarcoma of bone (typical and atypical variants). An analysis of nine cases. Virchows Arch (Pathol Anat) 398:329, 1983.

1762. Lichtenstein L, Jaffe HL: Ewing's sarcoma of bone. Am J Pathol 23:43, 1947.

1763. Schajowicz F: Ewing's sarcoma and reticulum-cell sarcoma of bone with special reference to the histochemical demonstration of glycogen as an aid to differential diagnosis. J Bone Joint Surg [Am] 41:349, 1959.

1764. Pomeroy TC, Johnson RE: Combined modality therapy of Ewing's sarcoma. Cancer 35:36, 1975.

1765. Triche TJ, Ross WE: Glycogen-containing neuroblastoma with clinical and histopathologic features of Ewing's sarcoma. Cancer 41:1425, 1978.

1766. Ushigome S, Takakuwa T, Takagi M, et al: Case report 263. Skel Radiol 11:151, 1984.

1767. Dwyer AJ, Glaubiger DL, Ecker JG, et al: The radiographic follow-up of patients with Ewing's sarcoma: A demonstration of a general method. Radiology 145:327, 1982.

1768. Taber DS, Libshitz HI, Cohen MA: Treated Ewing sarcoma: Radiographic appearance in response, recurrence, and new primaries. AJR 140:753, 1983.

1769. Nascimento AG, Unni KK, Pritchard DJ, et al: A clinicopathologic study of 20 cases of large-cell (atypical) Ewing's sarcoma of bone. Am J Surg Pathol 4:29, 1980.

1770. Angervall L, Enzinger FM: Extraskeletal neoplasm resembling Ewing's sarcoma. Cancer 36:240, 1975.

1771. Wigger HJ, Salazar GH, Blanc WA: Extraskeletal Ewing sarcoma. An ultrastructural study. Arch Pathol Lab Med 101:446, 1977.

1772. Soule EH, Newton W Jr, Moon TE, et al: Extraskeletal Ewing's sarcoma. A preliminary review of 26 cases encountered in the Intergroup Rhabdomyosarcoma study. Cancer 42:259, 1978.

1773. Meister P, Gokel JM: Extraskeletal Ewing's sarcoma. Virchows Arch (Pathol Anat) 378:173, 1978.

1774. Mahoney JP, Alexander RW: Ewing's sarcoma. A light- and electron-microscopic study of 21 cases. Am J Surg Pathol 2:283, 1978.

1775. Gillespie JJ, Roth LM, Wills ER, et al: Extraskeletal Ewing's sarcoma. Histologic and ultrastructural observations in three cases. Am J Surg Pathol 3:99, 1979.

1776. Rose JS, Hermann G, Mendelson DC, et al: Extraskeletal Ewing sarcoma with computed tomography correlation. Skel Radiol 9:234, 1983.

1777. Bignold LP: So-called "extraskeletal" Ewing's sarcoma. Am J Clin Pathol 73:142, 1980.

1778. Bernier J: The Management of Oral Disease. 2nd Ed. St Louis, CV Mosby Co, 1959.

1779. Shafer WG, Hine MK, Levy BM et al: Textbook of Oral Pathology. 4th Ed. Philadelphia, WB Saunders Co, 1983.

1780. Gorlin RJ, Goldman HM: Thomas' Oral Pathology. 6th ed. St Louis, CV Mosby Co, 1970.

1781. Tiecke RW: Oral Pathology. New York, McGraw-Hill, 1965.

1782. Pindborg JJ: Pathology of the Dental Hard Tissue. Philadelphia, WB Saunders Co, 1970.

1783. Langland OE, Langlais RP, Morris CR: Principles and Practice of Panoramic Radiology, Including Intraoral Radiographic Interpretation. Philadelphia, WB Saunders Co, 1982.

1784. Krolls SO, Allman RM: Calcifying epithelial odontogenic tumor of the mandible (Pindborg tumor). Radiology 105:439, 1972.

1785. Sauk JJ Jr: Calcifying and keratinizing odontogenic cyst. J Oral Surg 30:893, 1972.

1786. Schwimmer AM, Barr CE, Grauer SJ: Keratinizing and calcifying odontogenic cyst of the mandible: Literature review and a case report. Mt Sinai J Med 50:501, 1983.

1787. Eversole LR, Rovin S: Differential radiographic diagnosis of lesions of the jawbones. Radiology 105:277, 1972.

1788. Stafne EC: Bone cavities situated near the angle of the mandible. J Am Dent Assoc 29:1969, 1942.

1789. Adra NA, Barakat N, Melhem RE: Salivary gland inclusions in the mandible: Stafne's idiopathic bone cavity. AJR 134:1082, 1980.

1790. White DK, Lucas RM, Miller AS: Median mandibular cyst: Review of the literature and report of two cases. J Oral Surg 33:372, 1975.

1791. Tenca JI, Giunta JL, Norris LH: The median mandibular cyst and its endodontic significance. Oral Surg 60:316, 1985.

1792. Cornelius EA, McClendon JL: Cherubism—hereditary fibrous dysplasia of the jaws. Roentgenographic features. AJR 106:136, 1969.

1793. Lawrence D'A, Nogrady MB, Cloutier AM: Cherubism. A case report. AJR 108:468, 1970.

1794. Baker CG, Tishler JM: "Malignant disease in the jaws." J Can Assoc Radiol 28:129, 1977.

1795. Lyons AJ, Babajews AV: Gigantiform cementoma—an unusual incidental finding. Br J Radiol 59:277, 1986.

1796. Sehdev MK, Huvos AG, Strong EW, et al: Ameloblastoma of maxilla and mandible. Cancer 33:324, 1974.
1797. Rambo VB, Davies NE: Giant ameloblastomas. JAMA 238:418, 1977.
1798. McIvor J: The radiological features of ameloblastoma. Clin Radiol 25:237, 1974.
1799. Sirichitra V, Dhiravarangkura P: Intrabony ameloblastoma of the jaws. An analysis of 147 Thai patients. Int J Oral Surg 13:187, 1984.
1800. Hertzanu Y, Mendelsohn DB, Cohen M: Computed tomography of mandibular ameloblastoma. J Comput Assist Tomogr 8:220, 1984.
1801. Takahashi K, Kitajima T, Lee M, et al: Granular cell ameloblastoma of the mandible with metastasis to the third thoracic vertebra. A case report. Clin Orthop 197:171, 1985.
1802. Hinds EC, Pleasants JE, Snyder PL: Management of ameloblastoma. Oral Surg 7:1169, 1954.
1803. Gorlin RJ, Chaudhry AP, Pindborg JJ: Odontogenic tumors. Cancer 14:73, 1961.
1804. Senac MO Jr, Isaacs H, Gwinn JL: Primary lesions of bone in the 1st decade of life: Retrospective survey of biopsy results. Radiology 160:491, 1986.
1805. Malghem J, Maldague B: L'ostéome ostéoide indolore (ou primitivement indolore). Ann Radiol 28:475, 1985.
1806. Healey JH, Ghelman B: Osteoid osteoma and osteoblastoma. Current concepts and recent advances. Clin Orthop 204:76, 1986.
1807. Iceton J, Rang M: An osteoid osteoma in an open distal femoral epiphysis. A case report. Clin Orthop 206:162, 1986.
1808. Fassier F, Duhaime M, Marton D, et al: Un cas d'ostéome ostéoide de l'epiphysis de la tête fémorale chez un enfant de 9 ans. Rev Chir Orthop 72:215, 1986.
1809. Nuñez-Samper M, Fashho SN, Muñoz JL, et al: Osteoid osteoma of the hamate bone. Case report and review of the literature. Clin Orthop 207:146, 1986.
1810. Brabants K, Geens S, van Damme B: Subperiosteal juxta-articular osteoid osteoma. J Bone Joint Surg [Br] 68:320, 1986.
1811. Lynch MC, Dorgan JC: Osteoid osteoma of a rib as a cause of scoliosis. A case report. Spine 11:480, 1986.
1812. Pettine KA, Klassen RA: Osteoid-osteoma and osteoblastoma of the spine. J Bone Joint Surg [Am] 68:354, 1986.
1813. Ayala AG, Murray JA, Erling MA, et al: Osteoid-osteoma: Intraoperative tetracycline-fluorescence demonstration of the nidus. J Bone Joint Surg [Am] 68:747, 1986.
1814. Mahboubi S: CT appearance of nidus in osteoid osteoma versus sequestration in osteomyelitis. J Comput Assist Tomogr 10:457, 1986.
1815. Pitman MI, Norman A: Value of CT scanning in differential pain diagnosis in runners. Am J Sports Med 14:324, 1986.
1816. Weatherley CR, Jaffray D, O'Brien JP: Radical excision of an osteoblastoma of the cervical spine. A combined anterior and posterior approach. J Bone Joint Surg [Br] 68:325, 1986.
1817. Abdelwahab IF, Frankel VH, Klein MJ: Case report 351. Skel Radiol 15:164, 1986.
1818. Mitchell ML, Ackerman LV: Metastatic and pseudomalignant osteoblastoma: A report of two unusual cases. Skel Radiol 15:213, 1986.
1819. Huvos AG: Osteogenic sarcoma of bones and soft tissues in older patients. A clinicopathologic analysis of 117 patients older than 60 years. Cancer 57:1442, 1986.
1820. Shives TC, Dahlin DC, Sim FH, et al: Osteosarcoma of the spine. J Bone Joint Surg [Am] 68:660, 1986.
1821. Huvos AG, Sundaresan N, Bretsky SS, et al: Osteogenic sarcoma of the skull. A clinicopathologic study of 19 patients. Cancer 56:1214, 1985.
1822. Lane JM, Hurson B, Boland PJ, et al: Osteogenic sarcoma. Clin Orthop 204:93, 1986.
1823. Mazabraud A, Perdereau B, Gongora R, et al: Classification of osteosarcoma by 85-Sr scintimetry. Acta Orthop Scand 57:74, 1986.
1824. Zimmer WD, Berquist TH, McLeod RA, et al: Magnetic resonance imaging of osteosarcomas. Comparison with computed tomography. Clin Orthop 208:289, 1986.
1825. Kumpan W, Lechner G, Wittich GR, et al: The angiographic response to osteosarcoma following pre-operative chemotherapy. Skel Radiol 15:96, 1986.
1826. Bathurst N, Sanerkin N, Watt I: Osteoclast-rich osteosarcoma. Br J Radiol 59:667, 1986.
1827. Sundaram M, Herbold DR, McGuire MH: Case report 370. Skel Radiol 15:338, 1986.
1828. Remagen W, Nidecker A, Dolane B: Case report 368. Skel Radiol 15:330, 1986.
1829. Smith GD, Chalmers J, McQueen MM: Osteosarcoma arising in relation to an enchondroma. A report of three cases. J Bone Joint Surg [Br] 68:315, 1986.
1830. Blauth W, Sönnichsen S: Enchondromatosen der Hand. Z Orthop 124:165, 1986.
1831. Ohno T, Kadoya H, Park P, et al: Case report 382. Skel Radiol 15:478, 1986.
1832. Anderson WJ, Bowers WH: Chondromyxoid fibroma of the proximal phalanx. A tumor that may be confused with chondrosarcoma. J Hand Surg [Br] 11:144, 1986.
1833. Bouvier JF, Chassard JL, Brunat-Mentigny M, et al: Radionuclide bone imaging in diaphyseal aclasis with malignant change. Cancer 57:2280, 1986.
1834. Sherlock DA, Benson MKD: Dysplasia epiphysialis hemimelica of the hip. A case report. Acta Orthop Scand 57:173, 1986.
1835. Ho AMW, Blane CE, Kling TF Jr: The role of arthrography in the management of dysplasia epiphysealis hemimelica. Skel Radiol 15:224, 1986.

1836. Healey JH, Lane JM: Chondrosarcoma. Clin Orthop 204:119, 1986.
1837. Buirski G, Ratliff AHC, Watt I: Cartilage-cell-containing tumours of the pelvis: A radiological review of 40 patients. Br J Radiol 59:197, 1986.
1838. Johnson S, Tetu B, Ayala AG, et al: Chondrosarcoma with additional mesenchymal component (dedifferentiated chondrosarcoma). I. A clinicopathologic study of 26 cases. Cancer 58:278, 1986.
1839. Remagan W, Nidecker A, Prein J: Case report 359. Skel Radiol 15:251, 1986.
1840. Fauré C, Laurent JM, Schmit P, et al: Multiple and large non-ossifying fibromas in children with neurofibromatosis. Ann Radiol 29:369, 1986.
1841. Richter R, Mohr W, Richter Th, et al: Desmoplastiches fibrom. ROFO 144:236, 1986.
1842. Hadjipavlou A, Lander PH, Begin LR, et al: Desmoplastic fibroma of a metatarsal. Case report. J Bone Joint Surg [Am] 68:459, 1986.
1843. Lysko JE, Guilford WB, Siegal GP: Case report 362. Skel Radiol 15:268, 1986.
1844. Van Nostrand D, Madewell JE, McNeish LM, et al: Radionuclide bone scanning in giant cell tumor. J Nucl Med 27:329, 1986.
1845. Eckardt JJ, Grogan TJ: Giant cell tumor of bone. Clin Orthop 204:45, 1986.
1846. Present D, Bertoni F, Hudson T, et al: The correlation between the radiologic staging studies and histopathologic findings in aggressive stage 3 giant cell tumor of bone. Cancer 57:237, 1986.
1847. Picci P, Baldini N, Boriani S, et al: Giant cell reparative granuloma and other giant cell lesions of the bones of the hands and feet. Skel Radiol 15:415, 1986.
1848. Boland PJ, Huvos AG: Malignant fibrous histiocytoma of bone. Clin Orthop 204:130, 1986.
1849. Crone-Münzebrock W, Rehder U: Computertomographische Diagnose eines Knochenlipoms. ROFO 144:363, 1986.
1850. Hsueh S, Hsih S-N, Kuo T: Primary rhabdomyosarcoma of long bone. A case report. Orthopedics 9:705, 1986.
1851. Baker ND, Greenspan A, Neuwirth M: Symptomatic vertebral hemangiomas: A report of four cases. Skel Radiol 15:458, 1986.
1852. Pope TL Jr, Fechner RE, Keats TE: Case report 367. Skel Radiol 15:327, 1986.
1853. Sundaresan N: Chordomas. Clin Orthop 204:135, 1986.
1854. Abdelwahab IF, O'Leary PF, Steiner GC, et al: Case report 357. Skel Radiol 15:242, 1986.
1855. Capanna R, Van Horn J, Ruggieri P, et al: Epiphyseal involvement in unicameral bone cysts. Skel Radiol 15:428, 1986.
1856. McGlynn FJ, Mickelson MR, El-Khoury GY: The fallen fragment sign in unicameral bone cyst. Clin Orthop 156:157, 1981.
1857. Grumbine NA, Clark GD: Unicameral bone cyst in the calcaneus with pathologic fracture. A literature review and case report. J Am Podiatr Med Assoc 76:96, 1986.
1858. Lemmens JAM, van Horn JR, Ruijs JHJ: Case study. 1.5 tesla MR imaging of juvenile bone cysts. Medicamundi 30:93, 1985.
1859. Morton KS: Aneurysmal bone cyst: A review of 26 cases. Can J Surg 29:110, 1986.
1860. Campanacci M, Capanna R, Picci P: Unicameral and aneurysmal bone cysts. Clin Orthop 204:25, 1986.
1861. Cohn BT, Brahms MA, Froimson AI: Metastasis of adamantinoma sixteen years after knee disarticulation. Report of a case. J Bone Joint Surg [Am] 68:772, 1986.
1862. Yunis EJ: Ewing's sarcoma and related small round cell neoplasms in children. Am J Surg Pathol 10(Suppl 1):54, 1986.
1863. Kornberg M: Primary Ewing's sarcoma of the spine. A review and case report. Spine 11:54, 1986.
1864. Bacchini P, Marchetti C, Mancini L, et al: Ewing's sarcoma of the mandible and maxilla. Oral Surg 61:278, 1986.
1865. Bassoulet J, Labrune P, Delmer A, et al: Tumeurs d'Ewing à localisation costale place de la scanographie. Sem Hôp Paris 62:2183, 1986.
1866. Coombs RJ, Zeiss J, McCann K, et al: Case report 360. Skel Radiol 15:254, 1986.
1867. Ramon Y, Engelberg IS: An unusually extensive case of cherubism. J Oral Maxillofac Surg 44:325, 1986.
1868. Pramulio THS, Said HM, Kozlowski K: Huge ameloblastoma of the jaw. (Report of three cases.) Australas Radiol 29:308, 1985.
1869. Ueno S, Nakamura S, Mushimoto K, et al: A clinicopathologic study of ameloblastoma. J Oral Maxillofac Surg 44:361, 1986.
1870. Beyer WF, Kühn H: Can an osteoblastoma become malignant? Virchows Arch (A) 408:297, 1985.
1871. Rosen G, Huvos AG, Marcove R, et al: Telangiectatic osteogenic sarcoma. Improved survival with combination chemotherapy. Clin Orthop 207:164, 1986.
1872. Mirra JM, Gold R, Downs J, et al: A new histologic approach to the differentiation of enchondroma and chondrosarcoma of the bones. A clinicopathologic analysis of 51 cases. Clin Orthop 201:214, 1985.
1873. Sotelo-Avila C, Sundaram M, Kyeiakos M, et al: Case report 373. Skel Radiol 15:387, 1986.
1874. Kahmann R, Gold RH, Eckardt JJ, et al: Case report 337. Skel Radiol 14:301, 1985.
1875. Ohno T, Park P, Oquro K, et al: Ultrastructural study of a clear cell chondrosarcoma. Ultrastruct Pathol 10:321, 1986.
1876. Nakashima Y, Unni KK, Shives TC, et al: Mesenchymal chondrosarcoma of bone and soft tissue. A review of 111 cases. Cancer 57:2444, 1986.

1877. Taconis WK, van Rijssel ThG: Fibrosarcoma of the jaws. Skel Radiol *15:*10, 1986.

1878. Wold LE, Dobyns JH, Swee RG, et al: Giant cell reaction (giant cell reparative granuloma) of the small bones of the hands and feet. Am J Surg Pathol *10:*491, 1986.

1879. Wood GS, Beckstead JH, Turner RR, et al: Malignant fibrous histiocytoma tumor cells resemble fibroblasts. Am J Surg Pathol *10:*323, 1986.

1880. Huvos AG, Woodard HQ, Heilweil M: Postradiation malignant fibrous histiocytoma of bone. A clinicopathologic study of 20 patients. Am J Surg Pathol *10:*9, 1986.

1881. Abdul-Karim FW, Ayala AG, Chawla SP, et al: Malignant fibrous histiocytoma of jaws. A clinicopathologic study of 11 cases. Cancer *56:*1590, 1985.

1882. Hall FM, Cohen RB, Grumbach K: Case report 377. Skel Radiol *15:*401, 1986.

1883. Abenoza P, Sibley RK: Chordoma: an immunohistologic study. Hum Pathol *17:*744, 1986.

1884. Belza MG, Urich H: Chordoma and malignant fibrous histiocytoma. Evidence for transformation. Cancer *58:*1082, 1986.

1885. Chigira M, Shimizu T, Arita S, et al: Radiological evidence of healing of a simple bone cyst after hole drilling. Arch Orthop Trauma Surg *105:*150, 1986.

1886. Mullin DM, Rodan BA, Bean WJ, et al: Osteoid osteoma in unusual locations: Detection and diagnosis. South Med J *79:*1299, 1986.

1887. Kind M, Diard F, Germaneau J, et al: Ostéome ostéoïde du col du fémur avec synovite simulant une monoarthrite chronique de hanche. Arch Fr Pediatr *43:*417, 1986.

1888. Jones DA: Osteoid osteoma of the atlas. J Bone Joint Surg [Br] *69:*149, 1987.

1889. Szypryt EP, Hardy JG, Colton CL: An improved technique of intraoperative bone scanning. J Bone Joint Surg [Br] *68:*643, 1986.

1890. Lander PH, Azouz M, Marton D: Subperiosteal osteoid osteoma of the talus. Clin Radiol *37:*491, 1986.

1891. Byrd T, Gleis GE, Johnson JR: Primary osteogenic sarcoma of the clavicle. A case report. Orthopedics *9:*1717, 1986.

1892. Schreiman J S, Crass JR, Wick MR, et al: Osteosarcoma: Role of CT in limb-sparing treatment. Radiology *161:*485, 1986.

1893. Sundaram M, McGuire MH, Herbold DR: Magnetic resonance imaging of osteosarcoma. Skel Radiol *16:*23, 1987.

1894. Boyko OB, Cory DA, Cohen MD, et al: MR imaging of osteogenic and Ewing's sarcoma. AJR *148:*317, 1987.

1895. Lindqvist C, Teppo L, Sane J, et al: Osteosarcoma of the mandible: Analysis of nine cases. J Oral Maxillofac Surg *44:*759, 1986.

1896. Lindell MM Jr, Shirkhoda A, Raymond AK, et al: Parosteal osteosarcoma: Radiologic-pathologic correlation with emphasis on CT. AJR *148:*323, 1987.

1897. Picci P, Campanacci M, Bacci G, et al: Medullary involvement in parosteal osteosarcoma. A case report. J Bone Joint Surg [Am] *69:*131, 1987.

1898. Mitchell ML, Ackerman LV: Case report 405. Skel Radiol *16:*61, 1987.

1899. Akai M, Tateishi A, Machinami R, et al: Chondroblastoma of the sacrum. A case report. Acta Orthop Scand *57:*378, 1986.

1900. Van Horn JR, Lemmens JAM: Chondromyxoid fibroma of the foot. A report of a missed diagnosis. Acta Orthop Scand *57:*375, 1986.

1901. Malat J, Virapongse C, Levine A: Solitary osteochondroma of the spine. Spine *11:*625, 1986.

1902. Kraus RA, Macke JC, Crawford AH, et al: Popliteal vein compression by a fibular osteochondroma. A case report. Pediatr Radiol *6:*173, 1986.

1903. Muse G, Rayan G: Subungual exostosis. Orthopedics *9:*997, 1986.

1904. Frassica FJ, Unni KK, Beabout JW, et al: Dedifferentiated chondrosarcoma. A report of the clinicopathological features and treatment of seventy-eight cases. J Bone Joint Surg [Am] *68:*1197, 1986.

1905. de Lange EE, Pope TL Jr, Fechner RE: Dedifferentiated chondrosarcoma: Radiographic features. Radiology *160:*489, 1986.

1906. Hoeffel JC, Voinchet A, Brasse F, et al: Fracture parcellaire sur lacunes fibreuses fémorales inférieures. A propos d'une observation. Clin Pediatr *27:*108, 1986.

1907. Kumar R, Swischuk LE, Madewell JE: Benign cortical defect: Site for an avulsion fracture. Skel Radiol *15:*553, 1986.

1908. Schultz E, Hermann G, Irwin GAL, et al: Case report 380. Skel Radiol *15:*560, 1986.

1909. Bertoni F, Calderoni P, Bacchini P, et al: Benign fibrous histiocytoma of bone. J Bone Joint Surg [Am] *68:*1225, 1986.

1910. Louis DS, Hankin FM, Braunstein EM: Giant cell tumors of the triquetrum. J Hand Surg [Br] *11:*279, 1986.

1911. Campanacci M, Baldini N, Boriani S, et al: Giant-cell tumor of bone. J Bone Joint Surg [Am] *69:*106, 1987.

1912. Present DA, Bertoni F, Springfield D, et al: Giant cell tumor of bone with pulmonary and lymph node metastases. A case report. Clin Orthop *209:*286, 1986.

1913. Rock MG, Sim FH, Unni KK, et al: Secondary malignant giant-cell tumor of bone. Clinicopathological assessment of nineteen patients. J Bone Joint Surg [Am] *68:*1073, 1986.

1914. Wu KK, Ross PM, Mitchell DC, et al: Evolution of a case of multicentric giant cell tumor over a 23-year period. Clin Orthop *213:*279, 1986.

1915. Capozzi JD, Green S, Levy RN, et al: Giant cell reaction of small bones. Clin Orthop *214:*181, 1987.

1916. Castillo M, Tehranzadeh J, Becerra J, et al: Case report 408. Skel Radiol *16:*74, 1987.

1917. Hajek PC, Baker LL, Goobar JRE, et al: Focal fat deposition in axial bone marrow: MR characteristics. Radiology *162:*245, 1987.

1918. Hilpert PL, Radecki PD, Edmonds P, et al: Case report 392. Skel Radiol *15:*570, 1986.

1919. Laredo J-D, Reizine D, Bard M, et al: Vertebral hemangiomas: Radiologic evaluation. Radiology *161:*183, 1986.

1920. Bjorkengren AG, Resnick D, Haghighi P, et al: Intraosseous glomus tumor: Report of a case and review of the literature. AJR *147:*739, 1986.

1921. Smith J, Ludwig RL, Marcove RC: Sacrococcygeal chordoma. A clinicoradiological study of 60 patients. Skel Radiol *16:*37, 1986.

1922. Brodsky AE, Khalil M, vanDeventer L: Unicameral bone cyst of a lumbar vertebra. A case report. J Bone Joint Surg [Am] *68:*1283, 1986.

1923. Bator SM, Bauer TW, Marks KE, et al: Periosteal Ewing's sarcoma. Cancer *58:*1781, 1986.

1924. Morton KS, McGraw RW: Osteoid-osteoma. Report of a case in a sixty-seven-year-old man. J Bone Joint Surg [Am] *69:*449, 1987.

1925. Hasegawa T, Hirose T, Sakamoto R, et al: Mechanism of pain in osteoid osteomas: an immunohistochemical study. Histopathol *22:*487, 1993.

1926. Klein MH, Shankman S: Osteoid osteoma: radiologic and pathologic correlation. Skel Radiol *21:*23, 1992.

1927. Kransdorf MJ, Stull MA, Gilkey FW, et al: Osteoid osteoma. RadioGraphics *11:*671, 1991.

1928. Khurana JS, Mayo-Smith W, Kattapuram SV: Subtalar arthralgia caused by juxtaarticular osteoid osteoma. Clin Orthop *252:*205, 1990.

1929. Capanna R, Ayala A, Bertoni F, et al: Sacral osteoid osteoma and osteoblastoma: a report of 13 cases. Arch Orthop Trauma Surg *105:*205, 1986.

1930. Bettelli G, Capanna R, van Horn JR, et al: Osteoid osteoma and osteoblastoma of the pelvis. Clin Orthop *247:*261, 1989.

1931. Gille P, Gross Ph, Brax P, et al: Osteoid osteoma of the acetabulum: Two cases. J Pediatr Orthop *10:*416, 1990.

1932. Mosheiff R, Liebergall M, Ziv I, et al: Osteoid osteoma of the scapula. A case report and review of the literature. Clin Orthop *262:*129, 1991.

1933. Nelson MC, Brower AC, Ragsdale BD: Case report 448. Skel Radiol *16:*601, 1987.

1934. Mehdian H, Summers B, Eisenstein S: Painful scoliosis secondary to an osteoid osteoma of the rib. Clin Orthop *230:*273, 1988.

1935. de la Roque Ph M, Chabannier MH, Laffitte A, et al: Ostéome ostéoïde costal. A propos d'un cas. Revue de la littérature. Rev Rhum *58:*43, 1991.

1936. Fromm B, Martini A, Schmidt E: Osteoid osteoma of the radial styloid mimicking stenosing tenosynovitis. J Hand Surg [Br] *17:*236, 1992.

1937. Shaw JA: Osteoid osteoma of the lunate. J Hand Surg [Am] *12:*128, 1987.

1938. Ambrosia JM, Wold LE, Amadio PC: Osteoid osteoma of the hand and wrist. J Hand Surg [Am] *12:*794, 1987.

1939. Kozlowski K, Azouz EM, Campbell J, et al: Primary bone tumours of the hand. Pediatr Radiol *18:*140, 1988.

1940. Muren C, Höglund M, Engkvist O, et al: Osteoid osteomas of the hand. Report of three cases and review of the literature. Acta Radiologica *32:*62, 1991.

1941. Savornin C, Valenti Ph, Daunois O, et al: L'ostéome ostéoïde du semi-lunaire. A propos d'un cas. Intérêt de la tomodensitométrie. Ann Radiol *34:*210, 1991.

1942. van Horn JR, Karthaus RP: Epiphyseal osteoid osteoma. Two case reports. Acta Orthop Scand *60:*625, 1989.

1943. Brody JM, Brower AC, Shannon FB: An unusual epiphyseal osteoid osteoma. AJR *158:*609, 1992.

1944. Kruger GD, Rock MG: Osteoid osteoma of the distal femoral epiphysis. A case report. Clin Orthop *222:*203, 1987.

1945. Destian S, Hernanz-Schulman M, Raskin K, et al: Case report 468. Skel Radiol *17:*141, 1988.

1946. Chen SC, Caplan H: An unusual site of osteoid osteoma in the proximal phalanx of a finger. J Hand Surg [Br] *14:*341, 1989.

1947. Meng Q, Watt I: Phalangeal osteoid osteoma. Br J Radiol *62:*321, 1989.

1948. Marck KW, Dhar BK, Spauwen PHM: A cryptic cause of monarthritis in the hand: the juxta-articular osteoid osteoma. J Hand Surg [Br] *13:*221, 1988.

1949. Bowen CVA, Dzus AK, Hardy DA: Osteoid osteomata of the distal phalanx. J Hand Surg [Br] *12:*387, 1987.

1950. McCarten GM, Dixon PL, Marshall DR: Osteoid osteoma of the distal phalanx: A case report. J Hand Surg [Br] *12:*391, 1987.

1951. Schlesinger AE, Hernandez RJ: Intracapsular osteoid osteoma of the proximal femur: Findings on plain film and CT. AJR *154:*1241, 1990.

1952. Moser RP Jr, Kransdorf MJ, Brower AC, et al: Osteoid osteoma of the elbow. A review of six cases. Skel Radiol *19:*181, 1990.

1953. Lafforgue P, Senbel E, Boucraut J, et al: Elbow synovitis related to an intra-articular osteoid osteoma of the humerus, with immunologic and histochemical data. J Rheumatol *19:*633, 1992.

1954. Cassar-Pullicino VN, McCall IW, Wan S: Intra-articular osteoid osteoma. Clin Radiol *45:*153, 1992.

1955. Chouc PY, Germain D, Grimaldi F, et al: Arthrites satellites d'ostéomes ostéoïdes. Intérêts diagnostique et physiopathogénique. Sem Hôp Paris *67:*329, 1991.

1956. Bauer TW, Zehr RJ, Belhobek GH, et al: Juxta-articular osteoid osteoma. Am J Surg Path *15:*381, 1991.

1957. Carpentier E, Saragaglia D, Farizon F, et al: L'apophyse épineuse lombaire. Localisation exceptionnelle de l'ostéome ostéoide. Rev Rhum *55:*1001, 1988.

1958. Keret D, Harcke HT, MacEwen GD, et al: Multiple osteoid osteomas of the fifth lumbar vertebra. A case report. Clin Orthop *248:*163, 1989.

1959. Larsen LJ, Mall JC, Ichtertz DF: Metachronous osteoid-osteomas. J Bone Joint Surg [Am] *73:*612, 1991.

1960. Helms CA: Osteoid osteoma. The double density sign. Clin Orthop *222:*167, 1987.

1961. Kumar R, Swischuk LE, Schreiber MH: Role of indium-111 chloride imaging in osteoid osteoma. Clin Nucl Med *11:*721, 1986.

1962. Todd BD, Godfrey LW, Bodley RN: Intraoperative radioactive localization of an osteoid osteoma: a useful variation in technique. Br J Radiol *62:*187, 1989.

1963. Steinberg GG, Coumas JM, Breen T: Preoperative localization of osteoid osteoma: A new technique that uses CT. AJR *155:*883, 1990.

1964. Glass RBJ, Poznanski AK, Fisher MR, et al: MR imaging of osteoid osteoma. J Comput Assist Tomogr *10:*1065, 1986.

1965. Bulas RV, Hayes CW, Conway WF, et al: Case report 738. Skel Radiol *21:*326, 1992.

1966. Thompson GH, Wong KM, Konsens RM, et al: Magnetic resonance imaging of an osteoid osteoma of the proximal femur: A potentially confusing appearance. J Pediatr Orthop *10:*800, 1990.

1967. Assoun J, de Haldat F, Richardi G, et al: Magnetic resonance imaging in osteoid osteoma. Rev Rhum [Engl Ed] *60:*29, 1993.

1968. Biebuyck J-C, Katz LD, McCauley T: Soft tissue edema in osteoid osteoma. Skel Radiol *22:*37, 1993.

1969. Woods ER, Martel W, Mandell SH, et al: Reactive soft-tissue mass associated with osteoid osteoma: Correlation of MR imaging features with pathologic findings. Radiology *186:*221, 1993.

1970. Goldman AB, Schneider R, Pavlov H: Osteoid osteomas of the femoral neck: Report of four cases evaluated with isotopic bone scanning, CT, and MR imaging. Radiology *186:*227, 1993.

1971. Lee DH, Malawer MM: Staging and treatment of primary and persistent (recurrent) osteoid osteoma. Evaluation of intraoperative nuclear scanning, tetracycline fluorescence, and tomography. Clin Orthop *281:*229, 1992.

1972. Ziegler DN, Scheid DK: A method for location of an osteoid-osteoma of the femur at operation. A case report. J Bone Joint Surg [Am] *74:*1549, 1992.

1973. Graham HK, Laverick MD, Cosgrove AP, et al: Minimally invasive surgery for osteoid osteoma of the proximal femur. J Bone Joint Surg [Br] *75:*115, 1993.

1974. Kohler R, Mazoyer JF, Besse JL, et al: The treatment of osteoid osteoma by percutaneous drill resection under CT scanning control. A study of five cases. Fr J Orthop Surg *4:*251, 1990.

1975. Mazoyer JF, Kohler R, Bossard D: Osteoid osteoma: CT-guided percutaneous treatment. Radiology *181:*269, 1991.

1976. Assoun J, Railhac J-J, Bonnevialle P, et al: Osteoid osteoma: Percutaneous resection with CT guidance. Radiology *188:*541, 1993.

1977. Rosenthal DI, Alexander A, Rosenberg AE, et al: Ablation of osteoid osteomas with a percutaneously placed electrode: A new procedure. Radiology *183:*29, 1992.

1978. Kneisl JS, Simon MA: Medical management compared with operative treatment for osteoid-osteoma. J Bone Joint Surg [Am] *74:*179, 1992.

1979. Regan MW, Galey JP, Oakeshott RD: Recurrent osteoid osteoma. Case report with a ten-year asymptomatic interval. Clin Orthop *253:*221, 1990.

1980. Bettelli G, Tigani D, Picci P: Recurring osteoblastoma initially presenting as a typical osteoid osteoma. Report of two cases. Skel Radiol *20:*1, 1991.

1981. Apergis E, Tsamouri M, Theodoratos G, et al: Osteoblastoma of the hamate bone: A case report. J Hand Surg [Am] *18:*137, 1993.

1982. Lin E, Oliver S, Lieberman Y, et al: Osteoblastoma of the sternum. Arch Orthop Trauma Surg *106:*132, 1987.

1983. Albinana J, Grueso FSP, Barea FL, et al: Rib osteoblastoma: A clinical manifestation. Spine *13:*212, 1988.

1984. De Coster E, van Tiggelen R, Shahabpour M, et al: Osteoblastoma of the patella. Case report and review of the literature. Clin Orthop *243:*216, 1989.

1985. Kroon HM, Schurmans J: Osteoblastoma: Clinical and radiologic findings in 98 new cases. Radiology *175:*783, 1990.

1986. Boriani S, Capanna R, Donati D, et al: Osteoblastoma of the spine. Clin Orthop *278:*37, 1992.

1987. Myles ST, MacRae ME: Benign osteoblastoma of the spine in childhood. J Neurosurg *68:*884, 1988.

1988. Ellis BI, Shier CK, Gaba AR, et al: Case report 538. Skel Radiol *18:*228, 1989.

1989. Weinberg S, Katsikeris N, Pharoah M: Osteoblastoma of the mandibular condyle: Review of the literature and report of a case. J Oral Maxillofac Surg *45:*350, 1987.

1990. Gentry JF, Schechter JJ, Mirra JM: Case report 574. Skel Radiol *18:*551, 1989.

1991. Paige ML, Michael AS, Brodin A: Case report 647. Skel Radiol *20:*54, 1991.

1992. Bertoni F, Unni KK, Lucas DR, et al: Osteoblastoma with cartilaginous matrix. An unusual morphologic presentation in 18 cases. Am J Surg Pathol *17:*69, 1993.

1993. Bisset GS, Kaufman RA, Towbin R, et al: Case report 452. Skel Radiol *16:*666, 1987.

1994. Morton KS, Quenville NF, Beauchamp CP: Aggressive osteoblastoma. A case previously reported as a recurrent osteoid osteoma. J Bone Joint Surg [Br] *71:*428, 1989.

1995. Crim JR, Mirra JM, Eckardt JJ, et al: Widespread inflammatory response to osteoblastoma: The flare phenomenon. Radiology *177:*835, 1990.

1996. O'Connell JX, Rosenthal DI, Mankin HJ, et al: A unique multifocal osteoblastoma-like tumor of the bones of a single lower extremity. Report of a case. J Bone Joint Surg [Am] *75:*597, 1993.

1997. Wang J-W, Shih C-H, Chen W-J: Osteofibrous dysplasia (ossifying fibroma of long bones). A report of four cases and review of the literature. Clin Orthop *278:*235, 1992.

1998. Anderson MJ, Townsend DR, Johnston JO, et al: Osteofibrous dysplasia in the newborn. Report of a case. J Bone Joint Surg [Am] *75:*265, 1993.

1999. Abdelwahab IF, Hermann G, Zawin J, et al: Case report 543. Skel Radiol *18:*249, 1989.

2000. Castellote A, Garcia-Peña P, Lucaya J, et al: Osteofibrous dysplasia. A report of two cases. Skel Radiol *17:*483, 1988.

2001. Smith NM, Byard RW, Foster B, et al: Congenital ossifying fibroma (osteofibrous dysplasia) of the tibia—a case report. Pediatr Radiol *21:*449, 1991.

2002. Kumar R, David R, Madewell JE, et al: Radiographic spectrum of osteogenic sarcoma. AJR *148:*767, 1987.

2003. Fahey M, Spanier SS, Vander Griend RA: Osteosarcoma of the pelvis. A clinical and histopathological study of twenty-five patients. J Bone Joint Surg [Am] *74:*321, 1992.

2004. Miller TT, Abdelwahab IF, Hermann G, et al: Case report 735. Skel Radiol *21:*277, 1992.

2005. Greenspan A, Unni KK, Mann J: Case report 804. Skel Radiol *22:*469, 1993.

2006. Kim H, Park C, Lee YB, et al: Case report 643. Skel Radiol *19:*609, 1990.

2007. Mirra JM, Kameda N, Rosen G, et al: Primary osteosarcoma of toe phalanx: First documented case. Review of osteosarcoma of short tubular bones. Am J Surg Pathol *12:*300, 1988.

2008. Moss CS, Williams C, Ellis BI, et al: Case report 523. Skel Radiol *18:*70, 1989.

2009. López-Barea F, Contreras F, Sanchez-Herrera S: Case report 540. Skel Radiol *18:*237, 1989.

2010. Okada K, Wold LE, Beabout JW, et al: Osteosarcoma of the hand. A clinicopathologic study of 12 cases. Cancer *72:*719, 1993.

2011. Tsuneyoshi M, Dorfman HD: Epiphyseal osteosarcoma: Distinguishing features from clear cell chondrosarcoma, chondroblastoma, and epiphyseal enchondroma. Hum Pathol *18:*644, 1987.

2012. Paltiel HJ, Wilkinson RH, Kozakewich HPW: Case report 507. Skel Radiol *17:*527, 1988.

2013. Knop J, Delling G, Heise U, et al: Scintigraphic evaluation of tumor regression during preoperative chemotherapy of osteosarcoma. Correlation of ^{99m}Tc-methylene diphosphonate parametric imaging with surgical histopathology. Skel Radiol *19:*165, 1990.

2014. Menendez LR, Fideler BM, Mirra J: Thallium-201 scanning for the evaluation of osteosarcoma and soft-tissue sarcoma. A study of the evaluation and predictability of the histological response to chemotherapy. J Bone Joint Surg [Am] *75:*526, 1993.

2015. Carrasco CH, Charnsangavej C, Raymond AK, et al: Osteosarcoma: Angiographic assessment of response to preoperative chemotherapy. Radiology *170:*839, 1989.

2016. Hermann G, Leviton M, Mendelson D, et al: Osteosarcoma: Relation between extent of marrow infiltration on CT and frequency of lung metastases. AJR *149:*1203, 1987.

2017. de Baere T, Vanel D, Shapeero LG, et al: Osteosarcoma after chemotherapy: Evaluation with contrast material-enhanced subtraction MR imaging. Radiology *185:*587, 1992.

2018. Bonnerot V, Charpentier A, Frouin F, et al: Factor analysis of dynamic magnetic resonance imaging in predicting the response of osteosarcoma to chemotherapy. Invest Radiol *27:*847, 1992.

2019. Holscher HC, Bloem JL, Vanel D, et al: Osteosarcoma: Chemotherapy-induced changes at MR imaging. Radiology *182:*839, 1992.

2020. O'Flanagan SJ, Stack JP, McGee HMJ, et al: Imaging of intramedullary tumour spread in osteosarcoma. A comparison of techniques. J Bone Joint Surg [Br] *73:*998, 1991.

2021. Fletcher BD: Response of osteosarcoma and Ewing sarcoma to chemotherapy: Imaging evaluation. AJR *157:*825, 1991.

2022. Seeger LL, Widoff BE, Bassett LW, et al: Preoperative evaluation of osteosarcoma: Value of gadopentetate dimeglumine-enhanced MR imaging. AJR *157:*347, 1991.

2023. Erlemann R, Sciuk J, Bosse A, et al: Response of osteosarcoma and Ewing sarcoma to preoperative chemotherapy: Assessment with dynamic and static MR imaging and skeletal scintigraphy. Radiology *175:*791, 1990.

2024. Pan G, Raymond AK, Carrasco CH, et al: Osteosarcoma: MR imaging after preoperative chemotherapy. Radiology *174:*517, 1990.

2025. Redmond OM, Stack JP, Dervan PA, et al: Osteosarcoma: Use of MR imaging and MR spectroscopy in clinical decision making. Radiology *172:*811, 1989.

2026. Shramek JK, Kassner EG, White SS: MR appearance of osteogenic sarcoma of the calvaria. AJR *158:*661, 1992.

2027. Gillespy T III, Manfrini M, Ruggieri P, et al: Staging of intraosseous extent of osteosarcoma: Correlation of preoperative CT and MR imaging with pathologic macroslides. Radiology *167:*765, 1988.

2028. Seeger LL, Eckardt JJ, Bassett LW: Cross-sectional imaging in the evaluation of osteogenic sarcoma: MRI and CT. Semin Roentgenol *24:*174, 1989.

2029. Ballance WA Jr, Mendelsohn G, Carter JR, et al: Osteogenic sarcoma. Malignant fibrous histiocytoma subtype. Cancer *62:*763, 1988.

2030. Schajowicz F, de Próspero JD, Cosentino E: Case report 641. Skel Radiol *19:*603, 1990.

2031. Povysil O, Matejovsky Z, Zidkova H: Osteosarcoma with a clear-cell component. Virch Arch Pathol Anat Histopathol *412:*273, 1988.

2032. English R, Dicks-Mireaux C, Malone M, et al: Osteosarcoma—presumed lymph node metastases in two cases. Skel Radiol *18:*289, 1989.

2033. Vanel D, Lacombe M-J, Couanet D, et al: Musculoskeletal tumors: follow-up with MR imaging after treatment with surgery and radiation therapy. Radiology *164:*243, 1987.

2034. Hanna SL, Fletcher BD, Fairclough DL, et al: Use of dynamic Gd-DTPA enhanced MRI in musculoskeletal malignancies. Magn Res Imaging 8(Suppl):9, 1990.

2035. Lee Y-Y, Van Tassel P, Nauert C, et al: Craniofacial osteosarcomas: Plain film, CT, and MR findings in 46 cases. AJR 150:1397, 1988.

2036. Vanel D, Tcheng S, Contesso G, et al: The radiological appearances of telangiectatic osteosarcoma. A study of 14 cases. Skeletal Radiol 16:196, 1987.

2037. Chan CW, Kung TM, Lily MA: Telangiectatic osteosarcoma of the mandible. Cancer 58:2110, 1986.

2038. Edeiken J, Raymond AK, Ayala AG, et al: Small-cell osteosarcoma. Skel Radiol 16:621, 1987.

2039. Ayala AG, Ro JY, Raymond AK, et al: Small cell osteosarcoma. A clinico-pathologic study of 27 cases. Cancer 64:2162, 1989.

2040. Kyriakos M, Gilula LA, Becich MJ, et al: Intracortical small cell osteosarcoma. Clin Orthop 279:269, 1992.

2041. Sanjay B, Raj GA, Vishwakama G: A small-cell osteosarcoma with multiple skeletal metastasis. Arch Orthop Trauma Surg 107:58, 1988.

2042. Ellis JH, Siegel CL, Martel W, et al: Radiologic features of well-differentiated osteosarcoma. AJR 151:739, 1988.

2043. Bertoni F, Bacchini P, Fabbri N, et al: Osteosarcoma. Low-grade intraosseous-type osteosarcoma, histologically resembling parosteal osteosarcoma, fibrous dysplasia, and desmoplastic fibroma. Cancer 71:338, 1993.

2044. Iemoto Y, Ushigome S, Fukunaga M, et al: Case report 679. Skel Radiol 20:379, 1991.

2045. Anderson RB, McAlister JA Jr, Wrenn RN: Case report 585. Skel Radiol 18:627, 1989.

2046. López-Barea F, Rodriguez-Peralto JL, González-López J, et al: Intracortical osteosarcoma. A case report. Clin Orthop 268:218, 1991.

2047. Mirra JM, Dodd L, Johnston W, et al: Case report 700. Skel Radiol 20:613, 1991.

2048. Sim FH, Kurt A-M, McLeod RA, et al: Case report 628. Skel Radiol 19:457, 1990.

2049. Kenan S, Abdelwahab IF, Klein MJ, et al: Lesions of juxtacortical origin (surface lesions of bone). Skel Radiol 22:337, 1993.

2050. Raymond AK: Surface osteosarcoma. Clin Orthop 270:140, 1991.

2051. Schajowicz F, McGuire MH, Araujo ES, et al: Osteosarcomas arising on the surfaces of long bones. J Bone Joint Surg [Am] 70:555, 1988.

2052. Hermann G, Abdelwahab IF, Kenan S, et al: Case report 795. Skel Radiol 22:383, 1993.

2053. Ritts GD, Pritchard DJ, Unni KK, et al: Periosteal osteosarcoma. Clin Orthop 219:299, 1987.

2054. Oda Y, Hashimoto H, Tsuneyoshi M, et al: Case report 793. Skel Radiol 22:375, 1993.

2055. Xipell JM, McConchie I, Wallis PL: Case report 447. Skel Radiol 16:597, 1987.

2056. Marks MP, Marks SC, Segall HD, et al: Case report 420. Skel Radiol 16:246, 1987.

2057. Iemoto Y, Ushigome S, Ikegami M, et al: Case report 648. Skel Radiol 20:59, 1991.

2058. Kumar R, Moser RP Jr, Madewell JE, et al: Parosteal osteogenic sarcoma arising in the cranial bones: Clinical and radiologic features in eight patients. AJR 155:113, 1990.

2059. Hermann G, Abdelwahab IF, Klein MJ, et al: Case report 711. Skel Radiol 21:69, 1992.

2060. Müller-Miny H, Erlemann R, Wuisman P, et al: Röntgenmorphologie des parossalen Osteosarkoms (POS). ROFO 155:165, 1991.

2061. Sauer DD, Chase DR: Case report 461. Skel Radiol 17:72, 1988.

2062. Kavanagh TG, Cannon SR, Pringle J, et al: Parosteal osteosarcoma. Treatment by wide resection and prosthetic replacement. J Bone Joint Surg [Br] 72:959, 1990.

2063. Ritschl P, Wurnig C, Lechner G, et al: Parosteal osteosarcoma. 2-23-year follow-up of 33 patients. Acta Orthop Scand 62:195, 1991.

2064. Benedikt RA, Kransdorf MJ, Jelinek JS, et al: Case report 722. Skel Radiol 21:187, 1992.

2065. Olson PN, Prewitt L, Griffiths HJ, et al: Case report 703. Skel Radiol 20:624, 1991.

2066. Hopper KD, Haseman DB, Moser RP Jr, et al: Case report 634. Skel Radiol 19:535, 1990.

2067. Hopper KD, Moser RP Jr, Haseman DB, et al: Osteosarcomatosis. Radiology 175:233, 1990.

2068. McCarthy EF, Tolo VT, Dorfman HD: Case report 446. Skel Radiol 16:592, 1987.

2069. Sim FH, DeVries EMG, Miser JS, et al: Case report 760. Skel Radiol 21:543, 1992.

2070. Bonnevialle P, Mansat M, Durroux R, et al: Les chondromes de la main. Étude d'un série de trente-cinq cas. Ann Chir Main 7:32, 1988.

2071. Masada K, Fujiwara K, Yoshikawa H, et al: Chondroma of the scaphoid. J Bone Joint Surg [Br] 71:705, 1989.

2072. Crim JR, Mirra JM: Enchondroma protuberans. Report of a case and its distinction from chondrosarcoma and osteochondroma adjacent to an enchondroma. Skel Radiol 19:431, 1990.

2073. Resnik CS, Levine AM, Aisner SC, et al: Case report 522. Skel Radiol 18:66, 1989.

2074. Lewis MM, Kenan S, Yabut SM, et al: Periosteal chondroma. A report of ten cases and review of the literature. Clin Orthop 256:185, 1990.

2075. Rubenstein DJ, Harkavy L, Glantz L: Case report 518. Skel Radiol 18:47, 1989.

2076. Mora R, Guerreschi F, Fedeli A, et al: Two cases of periosteal chondroma. Acta Orthop Scand 59:723, 1988.

2077. Greenspan A, Unni KK, Matthews J II: Periosteal chondroma masquerading as osteochondroma. J Canad Assoc Radiol 44:205, 1993.

2078. Abdelwahab IF, Hermann G, Lewis MM, et al: Case report 588. Skel Radiol 19:59, 1990.

2079. Dwaik M, Devlin PB: Case report: Metadiaphyseal chondroblastoma. Clin Radiol 45:131, 1992.

2080. Ochsner PE, von Hochstetter AR, Hilfiker B: Chondroblastoma of the talus: Natural development over 9.5 years. Case report. Arch Orthop Trauma Surg 107:122, 1988.

2081. Abdelwahab IF, Hermann G, Klein MJ, et al: Case report 696. Skel Radiol 20:547, 1991.

2082. Matsuno T, Hasegawa I, Masuda T: Chondroblastoma arising in the triradiate cartilage. Report of two cases with review of the literature. Skel Radiol 16:216, 1987.

2083. Mayo-Smith W, Rosenberg AE, Khurana JS, et al: Chondroblastoma of the rib. A case report and review of the literature. Clin Orthop 251:230, 1990.

2084. Sundaram M, McGuire MH, Naunheim K, et al: Case report 467. Skel Radiol 17:136, 1988.

2085. Martinez-Madrigal F, Vanel D, Luboinski B, et al: Case report 670. Skel Radiol 20:299, 1991.

2086. Howe JW, Baumgard S, Yochum TR, et al: Case report 449. Skel Radiol 17:52, 1988.

2087. Hoeffel JC, Brasse F, Schmitt M, et al: About one case of vertebral chondroblastoma. Pediatr Radiol 17:392, 1987.

2088. Moser RP Jr, Brockmole DM, Vinh TN, et al: Chondroblastoma of the patella. Skel Radiol 17:413, 1988.

2089. Brower AC, Moser RP, Kransdorf MJ: The frequency and diagnostic significance of periostitis in chondroblastoma. AJR 154:309, 1990.

2090. Pignatti G, Nigrisoli M: Case report 537. Skel Radiol 18:225, 1989.

2091. Fobben ES, Dalinka MK, Schiebler ML, et al: The magnetic resonance imaging appearance at 1.5 Tesla of cartilaginous tumors involving the epiphysis. Skel Radiol 16:647, 1987.

2092. Cohen EK, Kressel HY, Frank TS, et al: Hyaline cartilage-origin bone and soft-tissue neoplasms: MR appearance and histologic correlation. Radiology 167:477, 1988.

2093. van Horn JR, Vincent JG, Wiersma-van Tilburg AM, et al: Late pulmonary metastases from chondroblastoma of the distal femur. A case report. Acta Orthop Scand 61:466, 1990.

2094. Raymond AK, Raymond PG, Edeiken J: Case report 531. Skel Radiol 18:143, 1989.

2095. Zillmer DA, Dorfman HD: Chondromyxoid fibroma of bone: Thirty-six cases with clinicopathologic correlation. Hum Pathol 20:952, 1989.

2096. Wilson AJ, Kyriakos M, Ackerman LV: Chondromyxoid fibroma: Radiographic appearance in 38 cases and in a review of the literature. Radiology 179:513, 1991.

2097. Tang J, Gold RH, Mirra JM: Case report 454. Skel Radiol 16:675, 1987.

2098. Mitchell M, Sartoris DJ, Resnick D: Case report 713. Skel Radiol 21:252, 1992.

2099. Tsuchiya H, Tomita K, Tsuchida T, et al: Case report 741. Skel Radiol 21:339, 1992.

2100. Frank E, Deruaz J-P, de Tribolet N: Chondromyxoid fibroma of the petrous-sphenoid junction. Surg Neurol 27:182, 1987.

2101. Adams MJ, Spencer GM, Totterman S, et al: Quiz: Case report 776. Skel Radiol 22:358, 1993.

2102. Davey HA, Cremin BJ, Smith CS: Case report 625. Skel Radiol 19:395, 1990.

2103. Schajowicz F: Chondromyxoid fibroma: Report of three cases with predominant cortical involvement. Radiology 164:783, 1987.

2104. Müller-Miny H, Erlemann R, Roessner A, et al: Röntgenmorphologie des Chondromyxoid fibroms. ROFO 150:390, 1989.

2105. Troncoso A, Ro JY, Edeiken J, et al: Case report 798. Skel Radiol 22:445, 1993.

2106. Burgess RC: Physeal osteochondroma of a phalanx. South Med J 83:1087, 1990.

2107. Tajima K, Nishida J, Yamazaki K, et al: Case report 545. Skel Radiol 18:306, 1989.

2108. Kozlowski K, Scougall J, Stevens M: Solitary osteochondroma of the spine. Report of two unusual cases in children. ROFO 146:462, 1987.

2109. Marchand EP, Villemure J-G, Rubin J, et al: Solitary osteochondroma of the thoracic spine presenting as spinal cord compression. A case report. Spine 11:1033, 1986.

2110. Fanney D, Tehranzadeh J, Quencer RM, et al: Case report 415. Skel Radiol 16:170, 1987.

2111. Loftus MJ, Bennett JA, Fantasia JE: Osteochondroma of the mandibular condyles. Oral Surg Med Path 61:221, 1986.

2112. Alman BA, Goldberg MJ: Solitary osteochondroma of the clavicle. J Pediatr Orthop 11:181, 1991.

2113. Malghem J, Vande Berg B, Noël H, et al: Benign osteochondromas and exostotic chondrosarcomas: evaluation of cartilage cap thickness by ultrasound. Skel Radiol 21:33, 1992.

2114. Lee JK, Yao L, Wirth CR: MR imaging of solitary osteochondromas: Report of eight cases. AJR 149:557, 1987.

2115. Geirnaerdt MJA, Bloem JL, Eulderink F, et al: Cartilaginous tumors: Correlation of gadolinium-enhanced MR imaging and histopathologic findings. Radiology 186:813, 1993.

2116. Montgomery DM, LaMont RL: Resolving solitary osteochondromas. A report of two cases and literature review. Orthopedics 12:861, 1989.

2117. Davids JR, Glancy GL, Eilert RE: Fracture through the stalk of pedunculated osteochondromas. A report of three cases. Clin Orthop 271:258, 1991.

2118. Danielsson LG, El-Haddad I, Quadros O: Distal tibial osteochondroma deforming the fibula. Acta Orthop Scand 61:469, 1990.

2119. Harrington I, Campbell V, Valazques R, et al: Pseudoaneurysm of the popliteal artery as a complication of an osteochondroma. A review of the literature and a case report. Clin Orthop 270:283, 1991.

2120. Lizama VA, Zerbini MA, Gagliardi RA, et al: Popliteal vein thrombosis and popliteal artery pseudoaneurysm complicating osteochondroma of the femur. AJR 148:783, 1987.

2121. Marcove RC, Lindeque BG, Silane MF: Pseudoaneurysm of the popliteal artery with an unusual arteriographic presentation. A case report. Clin Orthop 234:142, 1988.

2122. Nevelsteen A, Pype P, Broos P, et al: Brachial artery rupture due to an exostosis: Brief report. J Bone Joint Surg [Br] 70:672, 1988.

2123. Matthews MG: Unilateral oedema of the lower limb caused by an osteochondroma. J Bone Joint Surg [Br] 69:339, 1987.

2124. Slavotinek JP, Brophy BP, Sage MR: Bony exostosis of the atlas with resultant cranial nerve palsy. Neuroradiol 33:453, 1991.

2125. Watson LW, Torch MA: Peroneal nerve palsy secondary to compression from an osteochondroma. Orthopedics 16:707, 1993.

2126. Shogry MEC, Armstrong P: Case report 630. Skel Radiol 19:465, 1990.

2127. Griffiths HJ, Thompson RC Jr, Galloway HR, et al: Bursitis in association with solitary osteochondromas presenting as mass lesions. Skel Radiol 20:513, 1991.

2128. van Lerberghe E, van Damme B, van Holsbeeck M, et al: Case report 626. Skel Radiol 19:594, 1990.

2129. Nojima T, Yamashiro K, Fujita M, et al: A case of osteosarcoma arising in a solitary osteochondroma. Acta Orthop Scand 62:290, 1991.

2130. Hanrahan PS, Edelman J, Brash S: Spontaneous hemarthrosis associated with an exostosis of the talus. J Rheumatol 14:171, 1987.

2131. Unger EC, Gilula LA, Kyriakos M: Case report 430. Skel Radiol 16:416, 1987.

2132. Bock GW, Reed MH: Forearm deformities in multiple cartilaginous exostoses. Skel Radiol 20:483, 1991.

2133. Burgess RC, Cates H: Deformities of the forearm in patients who have multiple cartilaginous exostosis. J Bone Joint Surg [Am] 75:13, 1993.

2134. Shapiro SA, Javid T, Putty T: Osteochondroma with cervical cord compression in hereditary multiple exostoses. Spine 15:600, 1990.

2135. Matsuno T, Ichioka Y, Yagi T, et al: Spindle-cell sarcoma in patients who have osteochondromatosis. A report of two cases. J Bone Joint Surg [Am] 70:137, 1988.

2136. Keret D, Spatz DK, Caro PA, et al: Dysplasia epiphysealis hemimelica: Diagnosis and treatment. J Pediatr Orthop 12:365, 1992.

2137. Miller-Breslow A, Dorfman HD: Dupuytren's (subungual) exostosis. Am J Surg Pathol 12:368, 1988.

2138. Lee M, Hodler J, Haghighi P, et al: Bone excrescence at the medial base of the distal phalanx of the first toe: normal variant, reactive change, or neoplasia. Skel Radiol 21:161, 1992.

2139. Spjut HJ, Dorfman HD: Florid reactive periostitis of the tubular bones of the hands and feet. A benign lesion which may simulate osteosarcoma. Am J Surg Pathol 5:423, 1981.

2140. Nora FE, Dahlin DC, Beabout JW: Bizarre parosteal osteochondromatous proliferations of the hands and feet. Am J Surg Pathol 7:245, 1983.

2141. de Lange EE, Pope TL Jr, Fechner RE, et al: Case report 428. Skel Radiol 16:481, 1987.

2142. Davies CWT: Bizarre parosteal osteochondromatous proliferation in the hand. A case report. J Bone Joint Surg [Am] 67:648, 1985.

2143. Meneses MF, Unni KK, Swee RG: Bizarre parosteal osteochondromatous proliferation of bone (Nora's lesion). Am J Surg Pathol 17:691, 1993.

2144. Yuen M, Friedman L, Orr W, et al: Proliferative periosteal processes of phalanges: a unitary hypothesis. Skel Radiol 21:301, 1992.

2145. Ugai K, Sato S, Matsumoto K, et al: A clinicopathologic study of bony spurs on the pes anserinus. Clin Orthop 231:130, 1988.

2146. Huvos AG, Marcove RC: Chondrosarcoma in the young. A clinicopathologic analysis of 79 patients younger than 21 years of age. Am J Surg Pathol 11:930, 1987.

2147. Schneider HJ, Weinstein AS: Case report 470. Skel Radiol 17:148, 1988.

2148. Boorstein JM, Spizarny DL: Case report 476. Skel Radiol 17:208, 1988.

2149. Shives TC, McLeod RA, Unni KK, et al: Chondrosarcoma of the spine. J Bone Joint Surg [Am] 71:1158, 1989.

2150. Sivridis E, Verettas D: Chondrosarcoma in the distal phalanx of the ring finger. A case report. Acta Orthop Scand 61:183, 1990.

2151. Nelson DL, Abdul-Karim FW, Carter JR, et al: Chondrosarcoma of small bones of the hand arising from enchondroma. J Hand Surg [Am] 15:655, 1990.

2152. Young CL, Sim FH, Unni KK, et al: Case report 559. Skel Radiol 18:403, 1989.

2153. Greenfield GB, Cardenas C, Dawson PJ, et al: Case report 650. Skel Radiol 20:67, 1991.

2154. Varma DGK, Ayala AG, Carrasco CH, et al: Chondrosarcoma: MR imaging with pathologic correlation. RadioGraphics 12:687, 1992.

2155. Meyers SP, Hirsch WL Jr, Curtin HD, et al: Chondrosarcomas of the skull base: MR imaging features. Radiology 184:103, 1992.

2156. Oot RF, Melville GE, New PFJ, et al: The role of MR and CT in evaluating clival chordomas and chondrosarcomas. AJNR 9:715, 1988.

2157. Present DA, Bonar SFM, Greenspan A, et al: Clear-cell chondrosarcoma. An unusual case complicated by a microinfiltrative pattern of bone marrow involvement and postsurgical myositis ossificans. Clin Orthop 237:164, 1988.

2158. Weiss A-PC, Dorfman HD: Clear-cell chondrosarcoma: A report of ten cases and review of the literature. Skel Radiol 1:123, 1984.

2159. Present D, Bacchini P, Pignatti G, et al: Clear cell chondrosarcoma of bone. A report of 8 cases. Skel Radiol 20:187, 1991.

2160. Bagley L, Kneeland JB, Dalinka MK, et al: Unusual behavior of clear cell chondrosarcoma. Skel Radiol 22:279, 1993.

2161. Mainwaring BL, Khoury MB, Khodadoust K: Case report 484. Skel Radiol 17:295, 1988.

2162. Bertoni F, Bacchini P, Picci P, et al: Case report 517. Skel Radiol 18:221, 1989.

2163. Nguyen BD, Daffner RH, Dash N, et al: Case report 790. Skel Radiol 22:362, 1993.

2164. Lee JK, Yao L, Phelps CT: Case report 459. Skel Radiol 17:60, 1988.

2165. Munk PL, Connell DG, Quenville NF: Dedifferentiated chondrosarcoma of bone with leiomyosarcomatous mesenchymal component: A case report. J Can Assoc Radiol 39:218, 1988.

2166. Daly PJ, Sim FH, Wold LE: Dedifferentiated chondrosarcoma of bone. Orthopedics 12:763, 1989.

2167. Capanna R, Bertoni F, Bettelli G, et al: Dedifferentiated chondrosarcoma. J Bone Joint Surg [Am] 70:60, 1988.

2168. Sissons HA, Matlen JA, Lewis MM: Dedifferentiated chondrosarcoma. Report of an unusual case. J Bone Joint Surg [Am] 73:294, 1991.

2169. Moser RP Jr, Sweet DE, Haseman DB, et al: Multiple skeletal fibroxanthomas: radiologic-pathologic correlation of 72 cases. Skel Radiol 16:353, 1987.

2170. Ritschl P, Karnel F, Hajek P: Fibrous metaphyseal defects—determination of their origin and natural history using a radiomorphological study. Skel Radiol 17:8, 1988.

2171. Blau RA, Zwick DL, Westphal RA: Multiple non-ossifying fibromas. A case report. J Bone Joint Surg [Am] 70:299, 1988.

2172. Gross ML, Soberman N, Dorfman HD, et al: Case report 556. Skel Radiol 18:389, 1989.

2173. Erlemann R, Fischedick A-R, Edel G, et al: Neurofibromatose und multiple nicht-ossifizierende knochenfibrome. ROFO 147:20, 1987.

2174. Kozlowski K, Harrington C, Lees R: Multiple, symmetrical non-ossifying fibromata without extraskeletal anomalies: report of two related cases. Pediatr Radiol 23:311, 1993.

2175. Hoeffel JC, Voinchet A, Ligier JN: Avulsion fracture on benign cortical defect of the distal femur. ROFO 149:336, 1988.

2176. Fuji T, Hamada H, Masuda T, et al: Desmoplastic fibroma of the axis. A case report. Clin Orthop 234:16, 1988.

2177. Greenspan A, Unni KK: Case report 787. Skel Radiol 22:296, 1993.

2178. Young JWR, Aisner SC, Levine AM, et al: Computed tomography of desmoid tumors of bone: desmoplastic fibroma. Skel Radiol 17:333, 1988.

2179. Hufnagel TJ, Artiles C, Piepmeier J, et al: Desmoplastic fibroma of parietal bone simulating eosinophilic granuloma. Case report. J Neurosurg 67:449, 1987.

2180. Bridge JA, Rosenthal H, Sanger WG, et al: Desmoplastic fibroma arising in fibrous dysplasia. Chromosomal analysis and review of the literature. Clin Orthop 247:272, 1989.

2181. Kumar R, Madewell JE, Lindell MM, et al: Fibrous lesions of bones. RadioGraphics 10:237, 1990.

2182. Matsuno T: Benign fibrous histiocytoma involving the ends of long bones. Skel Radiol 19:561, 1990.

2183. Hermann G, Steiner GC, Sherry HH: Case report 465. Skel Radiol 17:195, 1988.

2184. Campanacci M, Baldini N, Boriani S, et al: Giant-cell tumor of bone. J Bone Joint Surg [Am] 69:106, 1987.

2185. Wuisman P, Roessner A, Härle A, et al: Case report 503. Skel Radiol 17:592, 1989.

2186. Schütte HE, Taconis WK: Giant cell tumor in children and adolescents. Skel Radiol 22:173, 1993.

2187. Kransdorf MJ, Sweet DE, Buetow PC, et al: Giant cell tumor in skeletally immature patients. Radiology 184:233, 1992.

2188. Biagini R, De Cristofaro R, Ruggieri P, et al: Giant-cell tumor of the spine. A case report. J Bone Joint Surg [Am] 72:1102, 1990.

2189. Sanjay BKS, Sim FH, Unni KK, et al: Giant-cell tumours of the spine. J Bone Joint Surg [Br] 75:148, 1993.

2190. McDonald DJ, Schajowicz F: Giant cell tumor of the capitate. A case report. Clin Orthop 279:264, 1992.

2191. Gould ES, Cooper JM, Potter HG, et al: Case report 740. Skel Radiol 21:335, 1992.

2192. Hanna RM, Kyriakos M, Quinn SF: Case report 757. Skel Radiol 21:482, 1992.

2193. Aoki J, Moser RP Jr, Vinh TN: Giant cell tumor of the scapula. A review of 13 cases. Skel Radiol 18:427, 1989.

2194. Beg MH, Ansari MM, Uddin R, et al: A case of giant-cell tumor of the clavicle. Acta Orthop Scand 60:122, 1989.

2195. Visscher DW, Alexander RW, Dempsey TR: Case report 472. Skel Radiol 17:285, 1988.

2196. Fain JS, Unni KK, Beabout JW, et al: Nonepiphyseal giant cell tumor of the long bones. Clinical, radiologic, and pathologic study. Cancer 71:3514, 1993.

2197. Moser RP Jr, Kransdorf MJ, Gilkey FW, et al: Giant cell tumor of the upper extremity. RadioGraphics 10:83, 1990.

2198. Manaster BJ, Doyle AJ: Giant cell tumors of bone. Radiol Clin North Am 31:299, 1993.

2199. Bidwell JK, Young JWR, Khalluff E: Giant cell tumor of the spine: Computed tomography appearance and review of the literature. CT 11:307, 1987.

2200. Kaplan PA, Murphey M, Greenway G, et al: Fluid-fluid levels in giant cell tumors of bone: Report of two cases. CT 11:151, 1987.

2201. Herman SD, Mesgarzadeh M, Bonakdarpour A, et al: The role of magnetic resonance imaging in giant cell tumor of bone. Skel Radiol 16:635, 1987.

2202. Tehranzadeh J, Murphy BJ, Mnaymneh W: Giant cell tumor of the proximal tibia: MR and CT appearance. J Comput Assist Tomogr 13:282, 1989.

2203. Yao L, Mirra JM, Seeger LL, et al: Case report 715. Skel Radiol 21:124, 1992.

2204. Buetow PC, Newman S, Kransdorf MJ: Giant-cell tumor of the tibia in a child presenting as an expansile metaphyseal lesion with fluid-fluid levels on MR. Magn Res Imag 8:341, 1990.

2205. Komiya S, Inoue A, Nakashima M, et al: Prognostic factors in giant cell tumor of bone. A modified histological grading system useful as a guide to prognosis. Arch Orthop Trauma Surg 105:67, 1986.

2206. Gitelis S, Wang J-W, Quast M, et al: Recurrence of a giant-cell tumor with malignant transformation to a fibrosarcoma twenty-five years after primary treatment. A case report. J Bone Joint Surg [Am] 71:757, 1989.

2207. Kattapuram SV, Phillips WC, Mankin HJ: Giant cell tumor of bone: Radiographic changes following local excision and allograft replacement. Radiology 161:493, 1986.

2208. Ehara S, Nishida J, Abe M, et al: Ossified soft tissue recurrence of giant cell tumor of bone. Clin Imag 16:168, 1992.

2209. Hefti FL, Gächter A, Remagen W, et al: Recurrent giant-cell tumor with metaplasia and malignant change, not associated with radiotherapy. A case report. J Bone Joint Surg [Am] 74:930, 1992.

2210. Bertoni F, Present D, Sudanese A, et al: Giant-cell tumor of bone with pulmonary metastases. Six case reports and a review of the literature. Clin Orthop 237:275, 1988.

2211. Scott SM, Pritchard DJ, Unni KK, et al: "Benign" metastasizing giant cell tumor: Evaluation of nuclear DNA patterns by flow cytometry. J Orthop Res 7:463, 1989.

2212. Maloney WJ, Vaughan LM, Jones HH, et al: Benign metastasizing giant-cell tumor of bone. Report of three cases and review of the literature. Clin Orthop 243:208, 1989.

2213. Wray CC, MacDonald AW, Richardson RA: Benign giant cell tumour with metastasis to bone and lung. One case studied over 20 years. J Bone Joint Surg [Br] 72:486, 1990.

2214. Tubbs WS, Brown LR, Beabout JW, et al: Benign giant-cell tumor of bone with pulmonary metastases: Clinical findings and radiologic appearance of metastasis in 13 cases. AJR 158:331, 1992.

2215. Meis JM, Dorfman HD, Nathanson SD, et al: Primary malignant giant cell tumor of bone: "Dedifferentiated" giant cell tumor. Modern Pathol 2:541, 1989.

2216. Tesluk H, Senders CW, Dublin AB: Case report 562. Skel Radiol 18:599, 1989.

2217. Dahlin DC: Giant-cell-bearing lesions of bone of the hands. Hand Clin 3:291, 1987.

2218. Wenner SM, Johnson K: Giant cell reparative granuloma of the hand. J Hand Surg [Am] 12:1097, 1987.

2219. Robinson D, Hendel D, Halperin N, et al: Multicentric giant-cell reparative granuloma. A case in the foot. Acta Orthop Scand 60:232, 1989.

2220. Ratner V, Dorfman HD: Giant-cell reparative granuloma of the hand and foot bones. Clin Orthop 260:251, 1990.

2221. Hermann G, Abdelwahab IF, Klein MJ, et al: Case report 603. Skel Radiol 19:367, 1990.

2222. Akai M, Ohno T, Sugano I, et al: Case report 601. Skel Radiol 19:154, 1990.

2223. López-Barea F, Rodríguez-Peralto JL, Burgos-Lizalde E, et al: Case report 639. Skel Radiol 20:125, 1991.

2224. Kemp HBS, Byers PD: Case report 444. Skel Radiol 16:584, 1987.

2225. Finci R, Günhan O, Ucmakli E, et al: Multiple and familial malignant fibrous histiocytoma of bone. A report of two cases. J Bone Joint Surg [Am] 72:295, 1990.

2226. Ehara S, Kattapuram SV, Rosenberg AE: Case report 619. Skel Radiol 19:375, 1990.

2227. Gero MJ, Kahn LB: Case report 498. Skel Radiol 17:443, 1988.

2228. Latham PD, Athanasou NA: Intraosseous lipoma within the femoral head. A case report. Clin Orthop 265:228, 1991.

2229. Milgram JW: Intraosseous lipomas: Radiologic and pathologic manifestations. Radiology 167:155, 1988.

2230. Szendroi M, Karlinger K, Gonda A: Intraosseous lipomatosis. A case report. J Bone Joint Surg [Br] 73:109, 1991.

2231. Jones JG, Habermann ET, Dorfman HD: Case report 553. Skel Radiol 18:537, 1989.

2232. Goldman AB, DiCarlo EF, Marcove RC: Case report 774. Skel Radiol 22:138, 1993.

2233. Kawashima A, Magid D, Fishman EK, et al: Parosteal ossifying lipoma: CT and MR findings. J Comput Assist Tomogr 17:147, 1993.

2234. Kenan S, Klein M, Lewis MM: Juxtacortical liposarcoma. A case report and review of the literature. Clin Orthop 243:225, 1989.

2235. Milgram JW: Malignant transformation in bone lipomas. Skel Radiol 19:347, 1990.

2236. Milgram JW: Intraosseous lipomas. A clinicopathologic study of 66 cases. Clin Orthop 231:277, 1988.

2237. Buckley SL, Burkus JK: Intraosseous lipoma of the ilium. A case report. Clin Orthop 228:297, 1988.

2238. Reig-Boix V, Guinot-Tormo J, Risent-Martinez F, et al: Computed tomography of intraosseous lipoma of os calcis. Clin Orthop 221:286, 1987.

2239. Berlin O, Angervall L, Kindblom L-G, et al: Primary leiomyosarcoma of bone. A clinical, radiographic, pathologic-anatomic, and prognostic study of 16 cases. Skel Radiol 16:364, 1987.

2240. Liu C-L, Yang D-J: Paraplegia due to vertebral hemangioma during pregnancy. A case report. Spine 13:107, 1988.

2241. Tekkök IH, Acikgöz B, Saglam S, et al: Vertebral hemangioma symptomatic during pregnancy—report of a case and review of the literature. Neurosurg 32:302, 1993.

2242. Bunel K, Sindet-Pedersen S: Central hemangioma of the mandible. Oral Surg Med Pathol 75:565, 1993.

2243. Kenan S, Abdelwahab IF, Klein MJ, et al: Hemangiomas of the long tubular bone. Clin Orthop 280:256, 1992.

2244. Thomas AMC, Mulligan PJ, Jones EL: Benign haemangioma of bone in a middle phalanx. J Hand Surg [Br] 15:484, 1990.

2245. Boker SM, Cullen GM, Swank M, et al: Case report 593. Skel Radiol 19:77, 1990.

2246. Yao L, Lee JK: Case report 494. Skel Radiol 17:378, 1988.

2247. Kenan S, Bonar S, Jones C, et al: Subperiosteal hemangioma. A case report and review of the literature. Clin Orthop 232:279, 1988.

2248. Makhija M, Bofill ER: Hemangioma, a rare cause of photopenic lesion on skeletal imaging. Clin Nucl Med 13:661, 1988.

2249. Ross JS, Masaryk TJ, Modic MT, et al: Vertebral hemangiomas: MR imaging. Radiology 165:165, 1987.

2250. Laredo J-D, Assouline E, Gelbert F, et al: Vertebral hemangiomas: Fat content as a sign of aggressiveness. Radiology 177:467, 1990.

2251. Reid AB, Reid IL, Johnson G, et al: Familial diffuse cystic angiomatosis of bone. Clin Orthop 238:211, 1989.

2252. Simmons TJ, Bassler TJ, Schwinn CP, et al: Case report 749. Skel Radiol 21:407, 1992.

2253. Rozmaryn LM, Sadler AH, Dorfman HD: Intraosseous glomus tumor in the ulna. A case report. Clin Orthop 220:126, 1987.

2254. Albrecht S, Zbieranowski I: Incidental glomus coccygeum. When a normal structure looks like a tumor. Am J Surg Pathol 14:922, 1990.

2255. Fornage BD: Glomus tumors in the fingers: Diagnosis with US. Radiology 167:183, 1988.

2256. Kneeland JB, Middleton WD, Matloub HS, et al: High resolution MR imaging of glomus tumor. J Comput Assist Tomogr 11:351, 1987.

2257. Carmody E, Loftus B, Corrigan J, et al: Case report 759. Skel Radiol 21:538, 1992.

2258. Abrahams TA, Bula W, Jones M: Epithelioid hemangioendothelioma of bone. A report of two cases and review of the literature. Skel Radiol 21:509, 1992.

2259. Tsuneyoshi M, Dorfman HD, Bauer TW: Epithelioid hemangioendothelioma of bone. A clinicopathologic, ultrastructural, and immunohistochemical study. Am J Surg Pathol 10:754, 1986.

2260. Martinez-Tello FJ, Marcos-Robles J, Blanco-Lorenzo F: Case report 520. Skel Radiol 18:55, 1989.

2261. Jaffe JW, Mesgarzadeh M, Bonakdarpour A, et al: Case report 519. Skel Radiol 18:50, 1989.

2262. De Smet AA, Inscore D, Neff JR: Case report 521. Skel Radiol 18:60, 1989.

2263. O'Connell JX, Kattapuram SV, Mankin HJ, et al: Epithelioid hemangioma of bone. A tumor often mistaken for low-grade angiosarcoma or malignant hemangioendothelioma. Am J Surg Pathol 17:610, 1993.

2264. Hou S-M, Shih T T-F, Lin M-C: Magnetic resonance imaging of an obscure glomus tumour in the fingertip. J Hand Surg [Br] 18:482, 1993.

2265. Marzola C, Borguetti MJ, Consolaro A: Neurilemmoma of the mandible. J Oral Maxillofac Surg 46:330, 1988.

2266. Abdelwahab IF, Hermann G, Stollman A, et al: Case report 564. Skel Radiol 18:466, 1989.

2267. Sanado L, Ruiz JL, Laidler L, et al: Femoral intraosseous neurilemoma. Arch Orthop Trauma Surg 110:212, 1991.

2268. Kaneko Y, Sato Y, Iwaki T, et al: Chordoma in early childhood: A clinicopathological study. Neurosurg 29:442, 1991.

2269. Smith J, Reuter V, Demas B: Case report 576. Skel Radiol 18:561, 1989.

2270. Le Pointe HD, Brugieres P, Chevalier X, et al: Imagerie des chordomes du rachis mobile. J Neuroradiol 18:267, 1991.

2271. de Bruine FT, Kroon HM: Spinal chordoma: Radiologic features in 14 cases. AJR 150:861, 1988.

2272. Roddie M, Adam A, Lambert H, et al: Case report 516. Skel Radiol 17:611, 1989.

2273. Yuh WTC, Lozano RL, Flickinger FW, et al: Lumbar epidural chordoma: MR findings. J Comput Assist Tomogr 13:508, 1989.

2274. Suga K, Tanaka N, Nakanishi T, et al: Bone and gallium scintigraphy in sacral chordoma. Report of four cases. Clin Nucl Med 17:206, 1992.

2275. Sze G, Uichanco LS III, Brant-Zawadski MN, et al: Chordomas: MR imaging. Radiology 166:187, 1988.

2276. Oot RF, Melville GE, New PFJ, et al: The role of MR and CT in evaluating clival chordomas and chondrosarcomas. AJR 151:567, 1988.

2277. Chaljub G, Van Fleet R, Guinto FC Jr, et al: MR imaging of clival and paraclival lesions. AJR 159:1069, 1992.

2278. Miettiner M, Karaharju E, Jarvinen H: Chordoma with a massive spindle-cell sarcomatous transformation. A light- and electron-microscopic and immuno-histological study. Am J Surg Pathol 11:563, 1987.

2279. Meis JM, Raymond AK, Evans HL, et al: "Dedifferentiated" chordoma. A clinicopathologic and immunohistochemical study of three cases. Am J Surg Pathol 11:516, 1987.

2280. Resnik CS, Young JWR, Levine AM, et al: Case report 544. Skel Radiol 18:303, 1989.

2281. Wojno KJ, Hruban RH, Garin-Chesa P, et al: Chondroid chordomas and low-grade chondrosarcomas of the craniospinal axis. An immunohistochemical analysis of 17 cases. Am J Surg Pathol 16:1144, 1992.

2282. Abdelwahab IF, Lewis MM, Klein MJ, et al: Case report 515. Skel Radiol 17:607, 1989.

2283. Södergard J, Karaharju EO: Calcaneal cysts: diagnosis and treatment. Fr J Orthop Surg 4:424, 1990.

2284. Jasan J, House JH, Brand JC: Bilateral unicameral bone cysts in the hamate bones. J Hand Surg [Am] 15:888, 1990.

2285. Gordon SL, Denton JR, McCann PD, et al: Unicameral bone cyst of the talus. Clin Orthop 215:201, 1987.

2286. Ruggieri P, Biagini R, Picci P: Case report 437. Skel Radiol 16:493, 1987.

2287. Abdelwahab IF, Hermann G, Lewis MM, et al: Case report 534. Skel Radiol 18:157, 1989.

2288. Abdelwahab IF, Hermann G, Norton KI, et al: Simple bone cysts of the pelvis in adolescents. A report of four cases. J Bone Joint Surg [Am] 73:1090, 1991.

2289. Ehara S, Rosenberg AE, El-Khoury GY: Sacral cysts with exophytic compo-nents. A report of two cases. Skel Radiol 19:117, 1990.

2290. Matsumoto K, Fujii S, Mochizuki T, et al: Solitary bone cyst of a lumbar vertebra. A case report and review of literature. Spine 15:605, 1990.

2291. Chigira M, Takehi Y, Nagase M, et al: A case of multiple simple bone cysts with special reference to their etiology and treatment. Arch Orthop Trauma Surg 106:390, 1987.

2292. Keret D, Kumar SJ: Unicameral bone cysts in the humerus and femur in the same child. J Pediatr Orthop 7:712, 1987.

2293. Struhl S, Edelson C, Pritzker H, et al: Solitary (unicameral) bone cyst. The fallen fragment sign revisited. Skel Radiol 18:261, 1989.

2294. Burr BA, Resnick D, Syklawer R, et al: Fluid-fluid levels in a unicameral bone cyst: CT and MR findings. J Comput Assist Tomogr 17:134, 1993.

2295. Santori F, Ghera S, Castelli V: Treatment of solitary bone cysts with intramed-ullary nailing. Orthopedics 11:873, 1988.

2296. Shindell R, Connolly JF, Lippiello L: Prostaglandin levels in a unicameral bone cyst treated by corticosteroid injection. J Pediatr Orthop 7:210, 1987.

2297. Yu C, D'Astous J, Finnegan M: Simple bone cysts. The effects of methylpred-nisolone on synovial cells in culture. Clin Orthop 262:34, 1991.

2298. Black DL, De Smet AA, Neff JR, et al: Case report 695. Skel Radiol 20:543, 1991.

2299. Oda Y, Hashimoto H, Tsuneyoshi M, et al: Case report 742. Skel Radiol 21:343, 1992.

2300. Dagher AP, Magid D, Johnson CA, et al: Aneurysmal bone cyst developing after anterior cruciate ligament tear and repair. AJR 158:1289, 1992.

2301. Martinez V, Sissons HA: Aneurysmal bone cyst. A review of 123 cases including primary lesions and those secondary to other bone pathology. Can-cer 61:2291, 1988.

2302. Ratcliffe PJ, Grimer RJ: Aneurysmal bone cyst arising after tibial fracture. A case report. J Bone Joint Surg [Am] 75:1225, 1993.

2303. De Dios AMV, Bond JR, Shives TC, et al: Aneurysmal bone cyst. A clinico-pathologic study of 238 cases. Cancer 69:2921, 1992.

2304. Arlet V, Rigault P, Padovani JP, et al: Aneurysmal bone cysts in children. A study of 28 cases. Fr J Orthop Surg 3:240, 1987.

2305. Mortensen NHM, Kuur E: Aneurysmal bone cyst of the proximal phalanx. J Hand Surg [Br] 15:482, 1990.

2306. Kashuk KB, Hanft JR, Schabler JA, et al: Aneurysmal bone cyst of the cuboid. J Am Podiatr Med Assoc 80:588, 1990.

2307. Frassica FJ, Amadio PC, Wold LE, et al: Aneurysmal bone cyst: Clinicopatho-logic features and treatment of ten cases involving the hand. J Hand Surg [Am] 13:676, 1988.

2308. Burnstein MI, De Smet AA, Hafez GR, et al: Case report 611. Skel Radiol 19:294, 1990.

2309. Sigmund G, Vinée Ph, Dosch JC, et al: MRT der aneurysmalen knochenzyste. ROFO 155:289, 1991.

2310. Caro PA, Mandell GA, Stanton RP: Aneurysmal bone cyst of the spine in children. MRI imaging at 0.5 tesla. Pediatr Radiol 21:114, 1991.

2311. Munk PL, Helms CA, Holt RG, et al: MR imaging of aneurysmal bone cysts. AJR 153:99, 1989.

2312. Daffner RH, Linetsky L, Zabkar JH: Case report 433. Skel Radiol 16:428, 1987.

2313. Malghem J, Maldague B, Esselinckx W, et al: Spontaneous healing of aneu-rysmal bone cysts. A report of three cases. J Bone Joint Surg [Br] 71:645, 1989.

2314. Cory DA, Fritsch SA, Cohen MD, et al: Aneurysmal bone cysts: Imaging findings and embolotherapy. AJR 153:369, 1989.

2315. DeRosa GP, Graziano GP, Scott J: Arterial embolization of aneurysmal bone cyst of the lumbar spine. A report of two cases. J Bone Joint Surg [Am] 72:777, 1990.

2316. Bertoni F, Bacchini P, Capanna R, et al: Solid variant of aneurysmal bone cyst. Cancer 71:729, 1993.

2317. Abdelwahab IF, Hermann G, Klein MJ, et al: Case report 635. Skel Radiol 19:539, 1990.

2318. Crim JR, Gold RH, Mirra JM, et al: Case report 748. Skel Radiol 21:403, 1992.

2319. Vade A, Wilbur A, Pudlowski R, et al: Case report 566. Skel Radiol 18:475, 1989.

2320. Schajowicz F, Santini-Araujo E: Adamantinoma of the tibia masked by fibrous dysplasia. Report of three cases. Clin Orthop 238:294, 1989.

2321. Czerniak B, Rojas-Corona RR, Dorfman HD: Morphologic diversity of long bone adamantinoma. The concept of differentiated (regressing) adamantinoma and its relationship to osteofibrous dysplasia. Cancer 64:2319, 1989.

2322. Ishida T, Iijima T, Kikuchi F, et al: A clinicopathological and immunohisto-chemical study of osteofibrous dysplasia, differentiated adamantinoma, and adamantinoma of long bones. Skel Radiol 21:493, 1992.

2323. Keeney GL, Unni KK, Beabout JW, et al: Adamantinoma of long bones. A clinicopathologic study of 85 cases. Cancer 64:730, 1989.

2324. Letourneau JG, Day DL, Crass JR, et al: Adamantinoma involving the distal tibia and fibula. AJR 148:1049, 1987.

2325. Nerubay J, Chechick A, Horoszowski H, et al: Adamantinoma of the spine. A case report. J Bone Joint Surg [Am] 70:467, 1988.

2326. Bertoni F, Zucchi V, Mapelli S, et al: Case report 506. Skel Radiol 17:522, 1988.

2327. Ishida T, Kikuchi F, Oka T, et al: Case report 727. Skel Radiol 21:205, 1992.

2328. Adler C-P: Case report 587. Skel Radiol 19:55, 1990.

2329. Bloem JL, van der Heul RO, Schuttevaer HM, et al: Fibrous dysplasia vs. adamantinoma of the tibia: Differentiation based on discriminant analysis of clinical and plain film findings. AJR 156:1017, 1991.

2330. Young JWR, Aisner SC, Resnik CS, et al: Case report 660. Skel Radiol 20:152, 1991.

2331. Tehranzadeh J, Fanney D, Ghandur-Mnaymneh L, et al: Case report 517. Skel Radiol 17:614, 1989.

2332. Clarke RP, Leonard JR, von Kuster L, et al: Adamantinoma of the humerus with early metastases and death. A case report with autopsy findings. Ortho-pedics 12:1121, 1989.

2333. Gebhardt MC, Lord FC, Rosenberg AE, et al: The treatment of adamantinoma of the tibia by wide resection and allograft bone transplantation. J Bone Joint Surg [Am] 69:1177, 1987.

2334. Maygarden SJ, Askin FB, Siegal GP, et al: Ewing sarcoma of bone in infants and toddlers. Cancer 71:2109, 1993.

2335. Halla JT, Hirsch V: Monoarthritis as the presenting manifestation of localized Ewing's sarcoma in an older patient. J Rheumatol 14:628, 1987.

2336. Pouchot J, Barge J, Marchand A, et al: Ewing's sarcoma of the ilium mimick-ing an infectious sacroiliitis. J Rheumatol 19:1318, 1992.

2337. Adelman HM, Wallach PM, Flannery MT: Ewing's sarcoma of the ilium presenting as unilateral sacroiliitis. J Rheumatol 18:1109, 1991.

2338. Strege DW, Hanel DP, Vogler C, et al: Ewing sarcoma in a phalanx of an infant's finger. A case report. J Bone Joint Surg [Am] 71:1262, 1989.

2339. Lacey SH, Danish EH, Thompson GH, et al: Ewing sarcoma of the proximal phalanx of a finger. A case report. J Bone Joint Surg [Am] 69:931, 1987.

2340. Leeson MC, Smith MJ: Ewing's sarcoma of the foot. Foot Ankle 10:147, 1989.

2341. Goodwin MI: A case of metatarsal Ewing's sarcoma. Acta Orthop Scand 61:187, 1990.

2342. Escobedo EM, Bjorkengren AG, Moore SG: Ewing's sarcoma of the hand. AJR 159:101, 1992.

2343. Hoeffel JC: Ewing's sarcoma of the hand. AJR 160:1362, 1993.

2344. Coombs RJ, Zeiss J, Paley KJ, et al: Case report 802. Skel Radiol 22:460, 1993.

2345. Kozlowski K, Campbell J, Morris L, et al: Primary rib tumours in children. (Report of 27 cases with short literature review). Australas Radiol 33:210, 1989.

2346. Moser RP Jr, Davis MJ, Gilkey FW, et al: Primary Ewing sarcoma of rib. RadioGraphics 10:899, 1990.

2347. Wood RE, Nortje CJ, Hesseling P, et al: Ewing's tumor of the jaw. Oral Surg Med Pathol 69:120, 1990.

2348. Narasimhan A, Sundaram M, Chandy SM, et al: Case report 786. Skel Radiol 22:293, 1993.

2349. Siegal GP, Oliver WR, Reinus WR, et al: Primary Ewing's sarcoma involving the bones of the head and neck. Cancer 60:2829, 1987.

2350. Kolár J, Zidkova H, Matějovský Zd, et al: Periosteal Ewing's sarcoma. ROFO 150:179, 1989.

2351. Estes DN, Magill HL, Thompson EI, et al: Primary Ewing sarcoma: Follow-up with Ga-67 scintigraphy. Radiology 177:449, 1990.

2352. Frouge C, Vanel D, Coffre C, et al: The role of magnetic resonance imaging in the evaluation of Ewing sarcoma. A report of 27 cases. Skel Radiol 17:387, 1988.

2353. Lemmi MA, Fletcher BD, Marina NM, et al: Use of MR imaging to assess results of chemotherapy for Ewing sarcoma. AJR 155:343, 1990.

2354. Holscher HC, Bloem JL, Nooy MA, et al: The value of MR imaging in monitoring the effect of chemotherapy on bone sarcomas. AJR 154:763, 1990.

2355. MacVicar AD, Olliff JFC, Pringle J, et al: Ewing sarcoma: MR imaging of chemotherapy-induced changes with histologic correlation. Radiology 184:859, 1992.

2356. Fletcher BD, Hanna SL, Fairclough DL, et al: Pediatric musculoskeletal tumors: Use of dynamic, contrast-enhanced MR imaging to monitor response to chemotherapy. Radiology 184:243, 1992.

2357. Reinus WR, Gehan EA, Gilula LA, et al: Plain radiographic predictors of survival in treated Ewing's sarcoma. Skel Radiol 21:287, 1992.

2358. Plowman PN: Bone metastases from Ewing's sarcoma radiologically recapitulate the features of a primary Ewing's tumour. Clin Radiol 40:498, 1989.

2359. Rud NP, Reiman HM, Pritchard DJ, et al: Extraosseous Ewing's sarcoma. A study of 42 cases. Cancer 64:1548, 1989.

2360. Pérez JS, Arias JLR, Rivera EA: Ameloblastoma gigante. Rev Mex Radiol 43:26, 1989.

2361. Minami M, Kaneda T, Yamamoto H, et al: Ameloblastoma in the maxillomandibular region: MR imaging. Radiology 184:389, 1992.

2362. Pravda J, Dorfman HD: Radiologic manifestations of Ollier's disease. Einstein Quart J Biol Med 7:80, 1989.

2363. Bessler W, Grauer W, Allemann J: Case report 726. Skel Radiol 21:201, 1992.

2364. Liu J, Hudkins PG, Swee RG, et al: Bone sarcomas associated with Ollier's disease. Cancer 59:1376, 1987.

2365. Nakajima H, Ushigome S, Fukuda J: Case report 482. Skel Radiol 17:289, 1988.

2366. Bendel CJA, Gelmers HJ: Multiple enchondromatosis (Ollier's disease) complicated by malignant astrocytoma. Europ J Radiol 12:135, 1991.

2367. Asivatham R, Rooney RJ, Watts HG: Ollier's disease with secondary chondrosarcoma associated with ovarian tumor. A case report. Internat Orthop (SICOT) 15:393, 1991.

2368. LeGall C, Bouvier R, Chappuis J, et al: Maladie d'Ollier et tumeur de la granulosa ovarienne de type juvénile. Arch Fr Pediatr 48:115, 1991.

2369. Robinson D, Tieder M, Copeliovitch L, et al: Spondyloenchondrodysplasia. A rare cause of short-trunk syndrome. Acta Orthop Scand 62:375, 1991.

2370. Paterson DC, Morris LL, Binns GF, et al: Generalized enchondromatosis. A case report. J Bone Joint Surg [Am] 71:133, 1989.

2371. Azouz EM: Case report 418. Skel Radiol 16:236, 1987.

2372. Lerman-Sagie T, Grunebaum M, Mimouni M: Case report 416. Skel Radiol 16:175, 1987.

2373. Ben-Itzhak I, Denolf FA, Versfeld GA, et al: The Maffucci syndrome. J Pediatr Orthop 8:345, 1988.

2374. Howie FMC, Davidson JK: Case report 492. Skel Radiol 17:368, 1988.

2375. Harris WR: Chondrosarcoma complicating total hip arthroplasty in Maffucci's syndrome. Clin Orthop 260:212, 1990.

2376. Lawson JP, Scott G: Case report 602. Skel Radiol 19:158, 1990.

2377. Weltevrede HJ, Jansen BRH: Dysplasia epiphysealis hemimelica—three different types in the ankle joint. Arch Orthop Trauma Surg 107:89, 1988.

2378. Graves SC, Kuester DJ, Richardson EG: Dysplasia epiphysealis hemimelica (Trevor disease) presenting as peroneal spastic flatfoot deformity: A case report. Foot Ankle 12:55, 1991.

2379. Mendez AA, Keret D, MacEwen GD: Isolated dysplasia epiphysealis hemimelica of the hip joint. J Bone Joint Surg [Am] 70:921, 1988.

2380. Tourniaire J, Bossard D, Gleize B, et al: Case report 801. Skel Radiol 22:457, 1993.

2381. Kenan S, Lewis MM, Abdelwahab IF, et al: Case report 652. Skel Radiol 20:73, 1991.

2382. Young CL, Wold LE, McLeod RA, et al: Primary leiomyosarcoma of bone. Orthopedics 11:615, 1988.

2383. Abdelwahab IF, Hermann G, Kenan S, et al: Case report 794. Skel Radiol 22:379, 1993.

2384. Feldman F, Johnston A: Intraosseous ganglion. AJR 118: 328, 1973.

2385. Schajowicz F, Sainz MC, Slullitel JA: Juxta-articular bone cysts (intra-osseous ganglia). A clinicopathological study of eighty-eight cases. J Bone Joint Surg [Br] 61:107, 1979.

2386. Hicks JD: Synovial cysts in bone. Aust N Z J Surg 26:138, 1956.

2387. Woods CG: Subchondral bone cysts. J Bone Joint Surg [Br] 43:758, 1961.

2388. Crabbe WA: Intra-osseous ganglia of bone. Brit J Surg 53:15, 1966.

2389. Richter R, Richter Th, Heine M: Das intraossäre Ganglion des Tibiakopfes. Akt Rheumatol 13:140, 1988.

2390. Yaghmai I, Foster WC: Case report 404. Skel Radiol 16:153, 1987.

2391. Kambolis C, Bullough PG, Jaffe HL: Ganglionic cystic defects of bone. J Bone Joint Surg [Am] 55:496, 1973.

2392. Kenan S, Graham S, Lewis M, et al: Intraosseous ganglion in the first metacarpal bone. J Hand Surg [Am] 12:471, 1987.

2393. Posner MA, Green SM: Intraosseous ganglion of a phalanx. J Hand Surg [Am] 9:280, 1984.

2394. Stark DD, Genant HK, Spring DB: Primary cystic arthrosis of the hip. Skel Radiol 11:124, 1984.

2395. Oliete S, Castaño-Llaneza JC, Asensio MC, et al: Ganglion intraóseo de preferente localización supraacetubular. Radiologia 23:221, 1981.

2396. Graf L, Freyschmidt J: Die subchondrale Synovialzyste (intraossäres Ganglion). ROFO 148:398, 1988.

2397. Freundlich BD, Pascal PE: Juxta-articular bone cyst of the glenoid. Case report. Clin Orthop 188:196, 1984.

2398. Eiken O, Jonsson K: Carpal bone cysts. A clinical and radiographic study. Scand J Reconstr Surg 14:285, 1980.

2399. Iwahara T, Hirayama T, Takemitu Y: Intraosseous ganglion of the lunate. J Hand Surg [Br] 15:297, 1983.

2400. Helal B, Vernon-Roberts B: Intraosseous ganglion of the pisiform bone. J Hand Surg [Br] 8:150, 1976.

2401. Jonsson K, Eiken O: Development of carpal bone cysts as revealed by radiography. Acta Radiol Diagn 24:231, 1983.

2402. McCarthy EF, Matz S, Steiner GC, et al: Periosteal ganglion: A cause of cortical bone erosion. Skel Radiol 10:243, 1983.

2403. Grange WJ: Subperiosteal ganglion. A case report. J Bone Joint Surg [Br] 60:124, 1978.

2404. Kenan S, Mobley K, Steiner GC: Periosteal ganglion. Case report and review of the literature. Bull Hosp J Dis 47:46, 1987.

2405. Barry M, Heyse-Moore GH: Acute hemorrhage into a subperiosteal ganglion. J Bone Joint Surg [Br] 72:519, 1990.

2406. Kolář J, Zídková H, Matějovský 2d: Periosteal ganglion. ROFO 144:234, 1986.

2407. Menendez LR, Chandler DR, Moore TM, et al: Diaphyseal intraosseous ganglion. Clin Orthop 227:310, 1988.

2408. Heyse-Moore GH, Grange WJ: Case report 82. Skel Radiol 3:255, 1979.

2409. Makhija MC, Lopano AJ: Intraosseous ganglion. Bone imaging with Tc-99m MDP. Clin Nucl Med 8:54, 1983.

2410. Yamato M, Saotome K, Tamai K, et al: Case report 783. Skel Radiol 22:227, 1993.

2411. Dungan DH, Seeger LL, Mirra JM: Case report 555. Skel Radiol 18:385, 1989.

2412. Ramirez H Jr, Blatt ES, Cable HF, et al: Intraosseous pneumatocysts of the ilium. Findings on radiographs and CT scans. Radiology 150:503, 1984.

2413. Weinberg S, Schneider H: Case report 211. Skel Radiol 9:61, 1982.

2414. Askin FB, Rosai J, Sibley PK, et al: Malignant small cell tumor of the thoracopulmonary region in childhood: a distinctive clinicopathological entity of uncertain histogenesis. Cancer 43:2438, 1979.

2415. Fink IJ, Kurtz TW, Casenave L, et al: Malignant thoracopulmonary small cell (Askin) tumor. AJR 145:517, 1985.

2416. Hashimoto M, Enjoji M, Nakajima T, et al: Malignant neuroepithelioma (peripheral neuroblastoma). A clinicopathological study of 15 cases. Am J Surg Pathol 7:309, 1983.

2417. Jurgens H, Bier V, Harms D, et al: Malignant peripheral neuroectodermal tumors. A retrospective analysis of 42 patients. Cancer 61:349, 1988.

2418. Enjoji M, Hashimoto H: Diagnosis of soft tissue sarcomas. Pathol Res Pract 178:215, 1984.

2419. Voss BC, Pyscher TJ, Humphrey GB: Peripheral neuroepithelioma in childhood. Cancer 54:3059, 1984.

2420. Miser JS, Kinsella TJ, Triche M, et al: Treatment of peripheral neuroepithelioma in children and young adults. J Clin Oncol 5:1752, 1987.

2421. Lipinski M, Braham K, Philip I, et al: Neuroectoderm associated antigens on Ewing's sarcoma cell lines. Cancer Res 47:183, 1987.

2422. Rousselin B, Vanel D, Terrier-Lacombe MJ, et al: Clinical and radiologic analysis of 13 cases of primary neuroectodermal tumors of bone. Skel Radiol 18:115, 1989.

2423. Llombart-Bosch A, Lacombe MJ, Peydro-Olaya A, et al: Malignant peripheral neuroectodermal tumors of bone other than Askin's neoplasm: an analysis of 14 cases with immunohistochemical and electron microscopic support. Virchows Arch 412:421, 1982.

2424. Moran RE, Govoni AF, Brandwein M: A 21-year-old man with a 2 year history of low back pain. Clin Imag 14:341, 1990.

2425. Crim JR, Seeger LL: Diagnosis of low-grade chondrosarcoma. Radiology 189:503, 1993.

2426. Geirnaerdt MJA, Bloem JL, Eulderink F, et al: Reply. Radiology 189:504, 1993.

2427. Disler DG, Rosenberg AE, Springfield D, et al: Extensive skeletal metastases from chondrosarcoma without pulmonary involvement. Skel Radiol 22:595, 1993.

2428. Sanjay BKS, Frassica FJ, Frassica DA, et al: Treatment of giant-cell tumor of the pelvis. J Bone Joint Surg [Am] 75:1466, 1993.

2429. Fleming GF, Heimann PS, Stephens JK, et al: Dedifferentiated chordoma. Response to aggressive chemotherapy in two cases. Cancer 72:714, 1993.

2430. Frassica FJ, Frassica DA, Pritchard DJ, et al: Ewing sarcoma of the pelvis. Clinicopathological features and treatment. J Bone Joint Surg [Am] 75:1457, 1993.

2431. Hasegawa T, Hirose T, Sakamoto R, et al: Mechanism of pain in osteoid osteomas: an immunohistochemical study. Histopathology 22:487, 1993.

2432. Bergeron P, Beauregard CG, Gagnon S, et al: Case report 831. Skeletal Radiol 23:161, 1994.

2433. Malghem J, Vande Berg B, Clapuyt P, et al: Osteoid osteomas of the femoral neck: Evaluation with US. Radiology 190:905, 1994.

2434. Greenspan A: Benign bone-forming lesions: osteoma, osteoid osteoma, and osteoblastoma. Skeletal Radiol 22:485, 1993.

2435. Assoun J, Richardi G, Railhac J-J, et al: Osteoid osteoma: MR imaging versus CT. Radiology 191:217, 1994.

2436. Stroz PM, Rubenstein J, Gershater R, et al: Case report 838. Skeletal Radiol 23:241, 1994.

2437. Azouz EM: Bone marrow edema in osteoid osteoma. Skeletal Radiol 23:53, 1994.

2438. Leone CR Jr, Lawton AW, Leone RT: Benign osteoblastoma of the orbit. Ophthalmology 95:1154, 1988.

2439. Lowder CY, Berlin AJ, Cox WA, et al: Benign osteoblastoma of the orbit. Ophthalmology 93:1351, 1986.

2440. Bertoni F, Unni KK, Lucas DR, et al: Osteoblastoma with cartilaginous matrix. An unusual morphologic presentation in 18 cases. Am J Surg Pathol *17*:69, 1993.

2441. Loizaga JM, Calvo M, Barea FL, et al: Osteoblastoma and osteoid osteoma. Clinical and morphological features of 162 cases. Pathol Res Pract *189*:33, 1993.

2442. Miyayama H, Sakamoto K, Ide M, et al: Aggressive osteoblastoma of the calcaneus. Cancer *71*:346, 1993.

2443. Sweet DE, Vinh TN, Devaney K: Cortical osteofibrous dysplasia of long bones and its relationship to adamantinoma. A clinicopathologic study of 30 cases. Am J Surg Pathol *16*:282, 1992.

2444. Holscher HC, van der Woude H-J, Hermans J, et al: Magnetic resonance relaxation times of normal tissue in the course of chemotherapy: a study in patients with bone sarcoma. Skeletal Radiol *23*:181, 1994.

2445. Bjornsson J, Inwards CY, Wold LE, et al: Prognostic significance of spontaneous tumour necrosis in osteosarcoma. Virchows Arch *423*:195, 1993.

2446. Raymond AK, Chawla SP, Carrasco CH, et al: Osteosarcoma chemotherapy effect: A prognostic factor. Semin Diagn Pathol *4*:212, 1987.

2447. Benedict WF, Xu H-J, Takahashi R: Role of the retinoblastoma gene in the initiation and progression of human cancer. J Clin Invest *85*:988, 1990.

2448. Tokito T, Ushijima M, Hara N, et al: Case report 812. Skeletal Radiol *22*:549, 1993.

2449. Kurt AM, Unni KK, McLeod RA, et al: Low-grade intraosseous osteosarcoma. Cancer *65*:1418, 1990.

2450. Kenan S, Abdelwahab IF, Klein MJ, et al: Case report 835. Skeletal Radiol *23*:229, 1994.

2451. Okada K, Frassica FJ, Sim FH, et al: Parosteal osteosarcoma. A clinicopathological study. J Bone Joint Surg [Am] *76*:366, 1994.

2452. Hinton CE, Turnbull AE, O'Donnell HDT, et al: Parosteal osteosarcoma of the skull. Histopathology *14*:322, 1989.

2453. Van Der Walt JD, Ryan JF: Parosteal osteosarcoma of the hand. Histopathology *16*:75, 1990.

2454. Ippolito V, Mirra JM, Fedenko A, et al: Case report 827. Skeletal Radiol *23*:143, 1994.

2455. Morard M, de Tribolet N, Janzer RC: Chondromas of the spine: Report of two cases and review of the literature. Br J Neurosurg *7*:551, 1993.

2456. Bertoni F, Unni KK, Beabout JW, et al: Chondroblastoma of the skull and facial bones. Am J Clin Pathol *88*:1, 1987.

2457. Kurt AM, Unni KK, Sim FH, et al: Chondroblastoma of bone. Hum Pathol *20*:965, 1989.

2458. Brecher ME, Simon MA: Chondroblastoma: An immunohistochemical study. Hum Pathol *19*:1043, 1988.

2459. Semmelink HJF, Pruszczynski M, Tilburg AW-V, et al: Cytokeratin expression in chondroblastomas. Histopathology *16*:257, 1990.

2460. Kenan S, Abdelwahab IF, Klein MJ, et al: Case report 837. Skeletal Radiol *23*:237, 1994.

2461. Bleiweiss IJ, Klein MJ: Chondromyxoid fibroma: Report of six cases with immunohistochemical studies. Mod Pathol *3*:664, 1990.

2462. Gallagher-Oxner K, Bagley L, Dalinka MK, et al: Case report 822. Skeletal Radiol *23*:71, 1994.

2463. Schofield TD, Pitcher JD, Youngberg R: Synovial chondromatosis simulating neoplastic degeneration of osteochondroma: Findings on MRI and CT. Skeletal Radiol *23*:99, 1994.

2464. Mirra JM, Gold R, Downs J, et al: A new histologic approach to the differentiation of enchondroma and chondrosarcoma of the bones. A clinicopathologic analysis of 51 cases. Clin Orthop *201*:214, 1985.

2465. Ding J, Hashimoto H, Tsuneyoshi M, et al: Clear cell chondrosarcoma: A case report with topographic analysis. Acta Pathol Jpn *39*:533, 1989.

2466. Lian-tang W, Tze-chun L: Clear cell chondrosarcoma of bone. A report of three cases with immunohistochemical and affinity histochemical observations. Pathol Res Pract *189*:411, 1993.

2467. Ohno T, Park P, Oguro K, et al: Ultrastructural study of a clear cell chondrosarcoma. Ultrastruct Pathol *10*:321, 1986.

2468. Bagchi M, Husain N, Goel MM, et al: Extraskeletal mesenchymal chondrosarcoma of the orbit. Cancer *72*:2224, 1993.

2469. Chetty R: Extraskeletal mesenchymal chondrosarcoma of the mediastinum. Histopathology *17*:261, 1990.

2470. Salmo NAM, Shukur ST, Abulkhail A: Mesenchymal chondrosarcoma of the maxilla: Report of a case. J Oral Maxillofac Surg *46*:887, 1988.

2471. Inwards CY, Unni KK, Beabout JW, et al: Desmoplastic fibroma of bone. Cancer *68*:1978, 1991.

2472. Aaron AD, Kenan S, Klein MJ, et al: Case report 810. Skeletal Radiol *22*:543, 1993.

2473. Doussis IA, Puddle B, Athanasou NA: Immunophenotype of multinucleated and mononuclear cells in giant cell lesions of bone and soft tissue. J Clin Pathol *45*:398, 1992.

2474. Goldring SR, Roelke MS, Petrison KK, et al: Human giant cell tumors of bone. Identification and characterization of cell types. J Clin Invest *79*:483, 1987.

2475. Mii Y, Miyauchi Y, Morishita T, et al: Osteoclast origin of giant cells in giant cell tumors of bone: Ultrastructural and cytochemical study of six cases. Ultrastruct Pathol *15*:623, 1991.

2476. Mund DF, Yao L, Fu Y-S, et al: Case report 826. Skeletal Radiol *23*:139, 1994.

2477. Meis JM, Dorfman HD, Nathanson SD, et al: Primary malignant giant cell tumor of bone: "Dedifferentiated" giant cell tumor. Mod Pathol *2*:541, 1989.

2478. Hindman BW, Seeger LL, Stanley P, et al: Multicentric giant cell tumor: Report of five new cases. Skeletal Radiol *23*:187, 1994.

2479. Ushigome S, Shimoda T, Fukunaga M, et al: Immunocytochemical aspects of the differential diagnosis of osteosarcoma and malignant fibrous histiocytoma. Surg Pathol *1*:347, 1988.

2480. Rodriguez-Peralto J, Lopez-Barea F, Gonzalez-Lopez J, et al: Case report 821. Skeletal Radiol *23*:67, 1994.

2481. Murphey MD, Johnson DL, Bhatia PS, et al: Parosteal lipoma: MR imaging characteristics. AJR *162*:105, 1994.

2482. MacLeod SPR, Mitchell DA, Miller ID: Intraosseous leiomyoma of the mandible: Report of a case. Br J Oral Maxillofac Surg *31*:187, 1993.

2483. Morshed A, Mohit P: Cystic angiomatosis of the skull presenting with extradural pneumocephalus. J Neurosurg *72*:968, 1990.

2484. Toxey J, Achong DM: Skeletal angiomatosis limited to the hand: Radiographic and scintigraphic correlation. J Nucl Med *32*:1912, 1991.

2485. Murphy RX Jr, Rachman RA: Extradigital glomus tumor as a cause of knee pain. Plast Reconstr Surg *92*:1371, 1993.

2486. Sunderraj S, Al-Khalifa AA, Pal AK, et al: Primary intra-osseous glomus tumor. Histopathology *14*:532, 1988.

2487. Tang JSH, Gold RH, Mirra JM, et al: Hemangiopericytoma of bone. Cancer *62*:848, 1988.

2488. Coindre J-M, Rivel J, Trojani M, et al: Immunohistological study in chordomas. J Pathol *150*:61, 1986.

2489. Karabela-Bouropoulou V, Kontogeorgos G, Papamichales G, et al: S-100 protein and neutron specific enolase (NSE) expression by chordomas in relation to the composition of their stromal mucosubstances. Pathol Res Pract *183*:256, 1988.

2490. Meis JM, Giraldo AA: Chordoma. An immunohistochemical study of 20 cases. Arch Pathol Lab Med *112*:553, 1988.

2491. Mitchell A, Scheithauer BW, Unni KK, et al: Chordoma and chondroid neoplasms of the spheno-occiput. An immunohistochemical study of 41 cases with prognostic and nosologic implications. Cancer *72*:2943, 1993.

2492. Adachi H, Yoshida H, Yumoto T, et al: Intraosseous epidermal cyst of the sacrum. A case report. Acta Pathol Jpn *38*:1561, 1988.

2493. Wojno KJ, McCarthy EF: Fibro-osseous lesions of the face and skull with aneurysmal bone cyst formation. Skeletal Radiol *23*:15, 1994.

2494. Okada K, Masuda H, Shozawa T, et al: A small aneurysmal bone cyst restructed to the cortical bone of the femur resembling so-called subperiosteal giant cell tumor or subperiosteal osteoclasia. Acta Pathol Jpn *39*:539, 1989.

2495. Scully SP, Temple HT, O'Keefe RJ, et al: Case report 830. Skeletal Radiol *23*:157, 1994.

2496. Cavazzana AO, Magnani JL, Ross RA, et al: Ewing's sarcoma is an undifferentiated neuroectodermal tumor. Adv Neuroblastoma Res *2*:487, 1988.

2497. Cavazzano AO, Miser JS, Jefferson T, et al: Experimental evidence for a neural origin of Ewing's sarcoma of bone. Am J Pathol *127*:507, 1987.

2498. Kenan S, Abdelwahab IF, Klein MJ, et al: Case report 819. Skeletal Radiol *23*:59, 1994.

2499. Mitchell CS, Wood BP, Shimada H: Neonatal disseminated primitive neuroectodermal tumor. AJR *162*:1160, 1994.

2500. Hoffer FA, Gianturco LE, Fletcher JA, et al: Percutaneous biopsy of peripheral primitive neuroectodermal tumors and Ewing's sarcomas for cytogenetic analysis. AJR *162*:1141, 1994.

2501. Llombart-Bosch A, Lacombe MJ, Contesso G, et al: Small round blue cell sarcoma of bone mimicking atypical Ewing's sarcoma with neuroectodermal features. An analysis of five cases with immunohistochemical and electron microscopic support. Cancer *60*:1570, 1987.

2502. Schmidt D, Herrmann C, Jürgens H, et al: Malignant peripheral neuroectodermal tumor and its necessary distinction from Ewing's sarcoma. Cancer *68*:2251, 1991.

2503. Shishikura A, Ushigome S, Shimoda T: Primitive neuroectodermal tumors of bone and soft tissue: Histological subclassification and clinicopathologic correlations. Acta Pathol Jpn *43*:176, 1993.

2504. Tsuneyoshi M, Yokoyama R, Hashimoto H, et al: Comparative study of neuroectodermal tumor and Ewing's sarcoma of the bone. Histopathologic, immunohistochemical, and ultrastructural features. Acta Pathol Jpn *39*:573, 1989.

2505. Ushigome S, Shimoda T, Nikaido T, et al: Primitive neuroectodermal tumors of bone and soft tissue. With reference to histologic differentiation in primary or metastatic foci. Acta Pathol Jpn *42*:483, 1992.

2506. Kahn HJ, Thorner PS: Monoclonal antibody MB2: A potential marker for Ewing's sarcoma and primitive neuroectodermal tumor. Pediatr Pathol *9*:153, 1989.

2507. Hara S, Ishii E, Tanaka S, et al: A monoclonal antibody specifically reactive with Ewing's sarcoma. Br J Cancer *60*:875, 1989.

2508. Kroon HM, Bloem JL, Holscher HC, et al: MR imaging of edema accompanying benign and malignant bone tumors. Skeletal Radiol *23*:261, 1994.

2509. Weatherall PT, Maale GE, Mendelsohn DB, et al: Chondroblastoma: Classic and confusing appearance at MR imaging. Radiology *190*:467, 1994.

2510. Taconis WK, Schütte HE, van der Heul RO: Desmoplastic fibroma of bone: A report of 18 cases. Skeletal Radiol *23*:283, 1994.

2511. Devaney K, Vinh TN, Sweet DE: Skeletal-extraskeletal angiomatosis. J Bone Joint Surg [Am] *76*:878, 1994.

2512. Ishida T, Dorfman HD, Steiner GC, et al: Cystic angiomatosis of bone with sclerotic changes mimicking osteoblastic metastasis. Skeletal Radiol *23*:247, 1994.

84

Tumors and Tumor-Like Lesions in or about Joints*

John E. Madewell, M.D., and Donald E. Sweet, M.D.

Numerous tumors and tumor-like lesions of the soft tissues with a variety of clinical and radiographic patterns have been described.[1–15, 658] They range from the common (lipoma and liposarcoma) to the rare (glomus tumor) and are summarized in a publication in which the extensive experience of the Armed Forces Institute of Pathology is detailed.[610] A number of these lesions are of interest because of their dominant clinical features, such as the production of pain (glomus tumors, leiomyomas, and multiple, painful lipomatosis). The soft tissue tumors may be benign or malignant and may vary greatly in size, especially the fatty tumors. Each lesion usually has a characteristic clinical, pathologic, and radiographic pattern. In this chapter those soft tissue tumors and tumor-like lesions that are manifested as masses in or about the joint are discussed. Their routine radiographic features are emphasized. A more complete discussion of the CT scanning and MR imaging abnormalities of these lesions is contained in Chapter 95 and elsewhere in this book.

DIAGNOSTIC TECHNIQUES

Soft tissue tumors and tumor-like lesions usually first appear as a soft tissue mass or swelling. A variety of im-

---

*The opinions or assertions contained herein are the private views of the authors and are not to be construed as official or as reflecting the views of the United States Departments of the Army, Air Force, Navy, or Defense.

aging techniques are useful in evaluation of the mass.[16-19] All techniques assist in determination of the anatomic extent and effect on structures adjacent to the lesion. Such findings, which are predicted accurately by radiographic techniques, are extremely helpful in planning management, which usually is surgical.[20-28, 659, 660] A definite diagnosis using radiographic features alone usually is not possible. Specific radiographic findings, however, such as phleboliths, fat, and cartilage mineralization, are very important clues to the lesion's identity.

Plain Film Radiography

The plain film radiographs, when obtained with technical excellence and special attention to soft tissue detail, are most helpful in showing soft tissue masses and their effect on bone.[19, 29-31] Overpenetrated views may be helpful in demonstrating less obvious abnormalities of the adjacent bone. Conventional tomography also is of assistance by delineating soft tissue abnormalities adjacent to complex bony structures (pelvis and shoulder), and it augments but does not replace the plain film examination.[19, 32] The plain film is still superior to other techniques in predicting the presence and nature of bone involvement.[32] When bone is involved by a slow-growing soft tissue mass, local pressure by the mass results in a scalloped appearance with a well-defined sclerotic margin. This is seen most frequently in benign processes. Irregular cortical destruction usually is associated with fast-growing and frequently malignant lesions. Obliteration or displacement, or both, of the normal fascial planes due to soft tissue infiltration is common in both benign and malignant tumors. Occasionally the interface may be lobulated and smooth, suggesting an encapsulated tumor. This usually is pseudoencapsulation, because most of the lesions will invade locally. Thus, the margin about soft tissue tumors, either benign or malignant, can be deceptive, and inaccurate information may be disseminated if the presence of a smooth margin always is equated with benign, noninfiltrating tumors. In the evaluation of patients with soft tissue masses, an integration of radiographic procedures plus clinical correlation is necessary for adequate diagnosis and management.

Xeroradiography and Arthrography

Xeroradiography and arthrography may characterize the soft tissue mass by the process of edge enhancement. Xeroradiographs demonstrate fine structures adjacent to the soft tissue lesion, especially fascial planes and musculotendinous structures.[33, 34, 611-613] This definition enables the xeroradiogram to show soft tissue displacement by the tumor. It still is questionable, however, whether the information is greater than that obtained with conventional radiography under optimal techniques.[19] Arthrography also is a useful radiographic technique for demonstrating synovial lesions and secondary involvement of the synovium by adjacent soft tissue or bony tumors (see Chapter 13).

Radionuclide Scanning

Radionuclide scanning with phosphate agents may demonstrate uptake in soft tissue tumors. Results are inconsistent, however, and if isotopic uptake occurs, the margins and local extent of the lesion are poorly defined.[32, 35-43, 614, 615] The involvement of contiguous bone about the tumor may be detected by radionuclide techniques, and the resulting information can be crucial in determining the resectability of the neoplasm.[616] Scanning also is helpful in demonstrating additional skeletal or soft tissue lesions that may not be detected on conventional radiographs.[32] Such findings are significant for patient management, because they may alter the therapeutic procedure.

Sonography

Sonography provides an accurate method of determining the size of soft tissue masses and distinguishes fluid collections from more solid masses in the extremities.[32, 617] It is less reliable when the mass occurs in a complex location, such as the pelvis, or is located deep in the soft tissue adjacent to bone. With the sonographic image, the precise anatomic relationships and tumor margins have less detail than with other techniques, such as angiography or CT scanning. Ultrasonography can be very useful in following the size of a soft tissue mass on serial studies or the response of the mass to treatment by nonsurgical means, such as chemotherapy or radiation therapy.[32]

Angiography

Angiography is most helpful in evaluating soft tissue masses, especially those in the peripheral portions of the extremities, where fatty tissue is sparse.[19, 22, 32, 44-56] It provides information about the anatomic extent of the tumor, its effect on adjacent structures, the vascular anatomy, and the venous drainage. These features influence the choice of operative procedure and thus conventional angiography and even digital subtraction angiography are valuable adjuncts in patient management.[22, 618] Malignant soft tissue tumors frequently are heterogeneous, with areas appearing histologically benign, hemorrhagic, and necrotic. If these sites are biopsied, confusing and erroneous data may be obtained. These sites tend to be less vascular on angiography, whereas the most malignant sites tend to have the greatest vascularity.[51, 55, 432] Thus, angiography can be helpful in localizing an area within the soft tissue tumor that will be likely to yield the most accurate biopsy data. Unsuspected satellite tumors may be uncovered by this method.[53] Although certain angiographic patterns are suggestive of specific histologic diagnoses (hemangiomas), an absolute pathologic diagnosis cannot be made. It also is difficult to differentiate benign from malignant soft tissue tumors definitely.[19, 22, 56] Thus, biopsy and histologic confirmation of the suspected diagnosis remain essential.

Computed Tomography

CT scanning has proved to be extremely helpful in planning the management of soft tissue tumors.[32, 37-67, 619-624, 661-665] CT is most useful in defining the extent of the soft tissue mass and its relationship to adjacent structures, even in complex bony areas like the pelvis. Occasionally it may help establish a diagnosis, especially with regard to fatty tumors. Contrast enhancement is of value in determining the vascularity of the soft tissue mass.

In the surgical management of soft tissue tumors of an extremity, several factors are important and influence the choice of operative procedure and its results. These factors include histologic diagnosis, determination of anatomic extent of the tumor, and prevention of tumor spread during the operative procedure.[22] Data pertaining to the last two factors are best obtained through use of the multiple diagnostic imaging systems outlined previously. The integration of these procedures will be of great importance in future soft tissue tumor studies.[18]

It is important to understand that even though all of these techniques assist in obtaining significant morphologic information about the soft tissue mass, the preoperative diagnosis remains speculative and, almost invariably, a biopsy is required to establish a histologic diagnosis.

Magnetic Resonance Imaging

The role of MR imaging in the evaluation of soft tissue tumors (and other processes) is discussed in Chapters 10, 70, and 95. MR imaging usually is the imaging method of choice for soft tissue tumors because of their intrinsic contrast differences as displayed in T1-weighted and T2-weighted spin echo images.[666–675] MR imaging does not allow visualization of calcification and ossification as well as plain films and CT. As with other imaging techniques, MR imaging is most useful in defining the extent of soft

tissue involvement, the relationship of the tumor to the adjacent bone and, in some cases, the specific histologic nature of the neoplasm.[654–657] Contrast enhanced MR imaging provides the ability to distinguish cystic and necrotic areas from cellular regions and evaluate the lesion's vascularity.[676–679] However these features are not specific for benign or malignant soft tissue tumors. Thus, biopsy remains the definitive diagnostic procedure.

BENIGN SOFT TISSUE TUMORS

Lipomatous Tumors

Lipomas. Lipomas arise from fatty tissue and are among the most common and widely distributed soft tissue tumors of mesenchymal origin.[14, 68–70] They usually are solitary but occasionally cases of multiple lipomas have been encountered. Lipomas may occur in any soft tissue that contains fat, such as subcutaneous fat,[70] muscle,[71, 72] nerves,[73, 74] or synovium,[75] or adjacent to bone in the periosteum.[76–79] Lipomas located deep within the limb grow within muscles (intramuscular type) or between muscles (intermuscular type).[71] Lipomas most commonly occur in the extremities of women as a movable, soft, compressible, asymptomatic, slow-growing, subcutaneous soft tissue mass[1] (Fig. 84–1). They are infrequent in the hands or feet[80–82] and if present are rarely identified prior to surgery.[83] Lipomas are uncom-

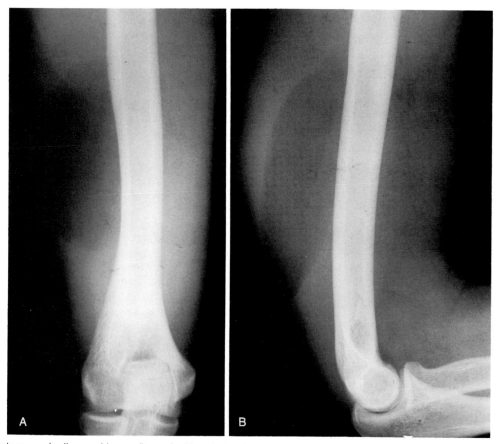

FIGURE 84–1. Intermuscular lipoma. Lipoma (in arm) with typical radiographic appearance and changing shape. This patient had a palpable soft tissue mass.
A Anteroposterior radiograph shows a sharply circumscribed, homogeneous, radiolucent fatty mass.
B On the lateral radiograph the shape of the lipoma changes with muscular contraction.
(Armed Forces Institute of Pathology Neg. Nos. 72-6580-1,2.)

mon in children[14, 81] and rarely are congenital or familial.[84, 85]

Rarely, lipomas may be painful (lipoma dolorosa).[86] This type usually is associated with multiple nonsymmetric lipomatosis, in which one tumor after another becomes symptomatic. Lipomas occurring in dependent areas tend to become large and pedunculated.[87] Lipomas occasionally may be associated with nerve paralysis,[76, 88] macrodactyly,[89, 90] osseous deformity,[625] and carpal tunnel syndrome.[91] Deep lipomas in the extremities, which occur commonly in the shoulder or thigh, are recognized less readily by clinical examination[71] (Fig. 84–2). These tumors usually change shape with muscular contraction and rarely cause dysfunction of the involved muscle.[71] If they develop in a closed fascial space, however, a firm mass may be palpable even when the muscle is relaxed. This contrasts with the typical pliable consistency of most lipomas.

Lipomas represent a local collection of adipose tissue, and some appear related to disturbances in fat metabolism.[14] The adipose tissue in lipomas is similar histologically and chemically to normal fat, but it is not available for normal metabolism, as evidenced by the fact that it maintains its size or amount during starvation.[1, 92] Grossly, intermuscular and subcutaneous lipomas usually are well-defined masses with smooth rounded or lobular surfaces, which may grow to considerable size[71, 87, 93, 94] (Fig. 84–3). In contrast, grossly, intramuscular lipomas are poorly defined lesions with extensive infiltration both locally and into adjacent muscles[71] (Fig. 84–4). Huge lipomas, which may weigh more than the patient, seldom occur in the extremities. The lipoma is arranged in lobules with many fibrous septa and is surrounded by a delicate capsule. The latter, which is the boundary between the lipoma and surrounding tissue, may be indistinct and difficult to identify in surgery, especially when it is located within normal adipose tissue.

Microscopically, lipomas consist of aggregates of mature fat cells with trabeculated fibrous septa. They occasionally may contain bone (ossifying lipoma),[95–98] cartilage,[99] or bone marrow (myelolipoma).[100] An admixture of other mesenchymal structures can occur, such as embryonic fat, blood vessels, and fibrous tissue. Whether they are deep or subcutaneous, lipomas rarely undergo malignant change.[14, 101–103]

An interesting form of lipoma is the spindle cell lipoma.[104] In contrast to most lipomas, it occurs chiefly in men over the age of 45 years. The spindle cell lipoma has a predilection for the shoulder and posterior aspect of the neck, although it occasionally is seen in the extremities. This tumor usually first appears in the dermis or subcutaneous tissue as a slow-growing, well-circumscribed, painless mass. Histologically, it contains an intricate mixture of lipocytes with uniform spindle cells and a matrix of mucinous material traversed by birefringent collagen fibers.[104] This pattern easily can be mistaken for a liposarcoma. The spindle cell lipomas have a uniformly favorable clinical course, however.

The lipomas, either subcutaneous or deep, are of special radiographic interest because of their fat density. When these fatty tumors are surrounded by tissues of water density, as in deep locations, the radiograph shows a pathognomonic homogeneous radiolucent mass with sharp margins (Fig. 84–1). Lipomas in the usual subcutaneous location showing characteristic clinical findings are not a diagnostic problem and may not need to be studied radio-

graphically. The radiograph can easily confirm the fatty nature of the mass, however. The deep lipomas of the intermuscular or intramuscular type are not identified as readily by clinical examination but are diagnosed easily radiologically.[16, 71] They are more radiolucent than the surrounding tissue and have two patterns. The intermuscular lipoma is a well-circumscribed, homogeneous, radiolucent mass with only occasional focal irregularity of the margin[71, 105] (Fig. 84–3). Intramuscular lipomas frequently have an inhomogeneous radiolucent appearance because they may contain streaks of muscle bundles of higher density that traverse the mass (Fig. 84–4). Because the lipomas, either in the subcutaneous or in the deeper soft tissue, are soft, muscular contraction or local compression may change the lipoma's shape and be documented on soft tissue radiographs (Fig. 84–1).

The homogeneous radiolucency of lipomas may be disturbed by metaplastic bone or cartilage formation.[96–99] The mineralized matrix can appear plaquelike or as a homogeneous dense area. The latter is seen in the ossifying lipoma and is due to extensive bone formation. The demonstration of bone and cartilage within the lipoma is not an indication of malignancy[97]; however, bone and cartilage probably are more frequent in liposarcomas.[16]

The nonhomogeneous fatty tumor, whether resulting from collagen or muscle of water density or from calcified cartilage or bone, always presents a bothersome pattern on radiography. An identical inhomogeneous pattern frequently is seen in liposarcomas and, therefore, when it is encountered, histologic confirmation of the nature of the mass is essential. Arteriograms of the lipoma, whether superficial or deep in location, reveal displacement of normal vessels and absent neovascularity, early venous filling, or hypervascularity.[71, 106] Lipomas usually appear on CT scans as homogeneous, sharply marginated, low-density masses with attenuation numbers usually in the range of −50 to −60 Hounsfield units (Fig. 84–2). Occasionally the fibrous capsule separating the fatty mass from the adjacent soft tissue may be seen with CT scanning. These lesions are not enhanced on postcontrast CT scans.[61] MR imaging represents an additional technique that allows accurate diagnosis of a lipoma owing to its unique signal intensity characteristics.[626, 691–693]

Synovial lipomas are rare and occur almost exclusively in the knee joint, producing nonspecific symptoms.[75, 107, 108] They are solitary round to oval masses of mature fat located intra-articularly, with a covering synovium. The gross specimen reveals the fatty nature of the mass, and osseous metaplasia can be encountered.[75] On plain films, synovial lipomas appear as a swelling about the knee, and fat may be seen. Arthrography demonstrates a smooth, lobular synovial mass. CT or MR imaging confirms the fatty nature of the tumor. This lesion is different from the more common lipoma arborescens, which also is monoarticular and is found most commonly in the knee[109] (Fig. 84–5). Lipoma arborescens is characterized by numerous swollen synovial villous projections of fatty tissue. It may begin de novo but frequently is associated with degenerative joint disease, chronic rheumatoid arthritis, or posttraumatic conditions.[75, 109, 112] The plain film radiograph shows soft tissue swelling that may or may not be radiolucent, and the lesion may be seen only on arthrography as multiple, sharply marginated filling defects.[110]

Text continued on page 3947

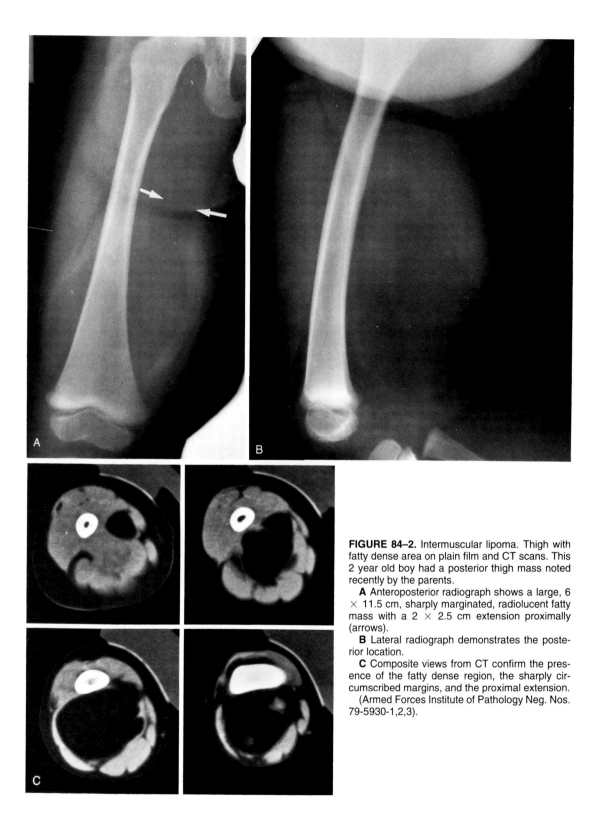

FIGURE 84–2. Intermuscular lipoma. Thigh with fatty dense area on plain film and CT scans. This 2 year old boy had a posterior thigh mass noted recently by the parents.

A Anteroposterior radiograph shows a large, 6 × 11.5 cm, sharply marginated, radiolucent fatty mass with a 2 × 2.5 cm extension proximally (arrows).

B Lateral radiograph demonstrates the posterior location.

C Composite views from CT confirm the presence of the fatty dense region, the sharply circumscribed margins, and the proximal extension.

(Armed Forces Institute of Pathology Neg. Nos. 79-5930-1,2,3).

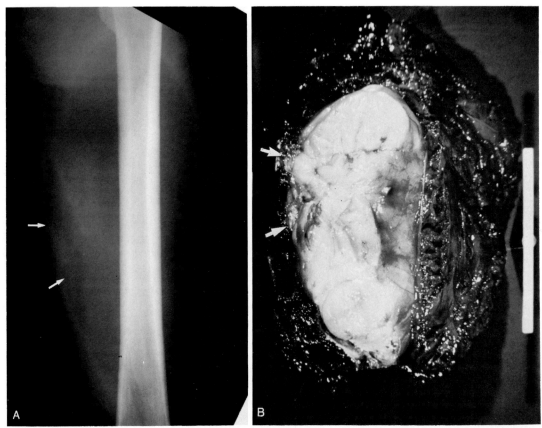

FIGURE 84–3. Intermuscular lipoma. Thigh with focal poorly defined margin. This 38 year old man had progressive swelling of the thigh of 15 months' duration.

A Oblique radiograph shows a fatty mass that is sharply circumscribed except for a poorly defined medial border (arrows). Note the area of water density adjacent to the poorly defined margin.

B Gross specimen confirms these findings, with focal infiltration into adjacent muscle (arrows). The well-defined margin and pseudocapsule also are appreciated about most of the lesion.

(Armed Forces Institute of Pathology Neg. Nos. 74-5340-2, 74-5656-1.)

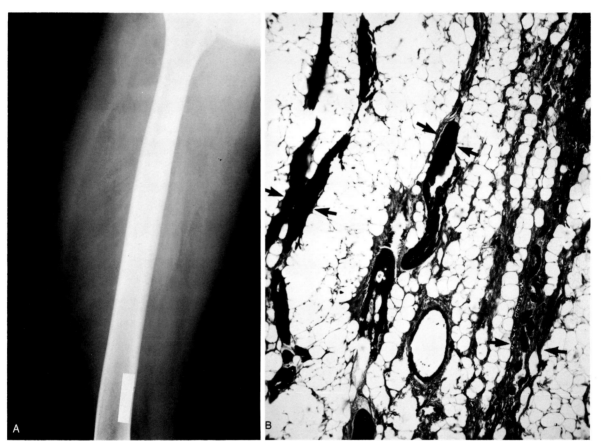

FIGURE 84–4. Intramuscular lipoma. Thigh with nonhomogeneous radiolucent mass. This 37 year old woman had a painless mass in the thigh.

A Oblique radiograph demonstrates a well-circumscribed, nonhomogeneous fatty mass with oblique streaks of water density.

B Photomicrograph (63×) reveals the fatty tumor to have infiltrated and entrapped muscle bundles (arrows). This pattern is reflected in the radiograph by the water-dense streaks.

(Armed Forces Institute of Pathology Neg. Nos. 69-5538, 79-16648.)

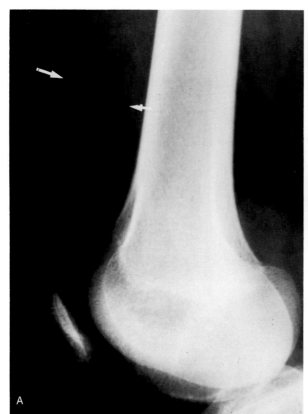

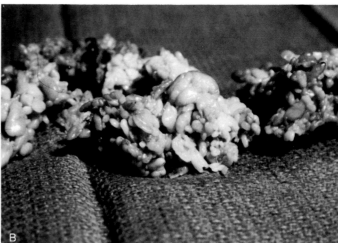

FIGURE 84–5. Lipomatosis of synovium (lipoma arborescens). This 18 year old man had right knee pain and effusion. There was no evidence of rheumatoid arthritis, osteoarthritis, or trauma.

A Lateral radiograph shows a fatty, radiolucent suprapatellar swelling (arrows).

B Gross specimen demonstrates prominent villous projections of variable size.

C Low power photomicrograph (3×) reveals fatty infiltration throughout the synovium and adjacent capsule.

D High power photomicrograph (15×) confirms the fatty engorgement of villi.

(Armed Forces Institute of Pathology Neg. Nos. 79-2792-5, 80-231, 80-225, 80-226.)

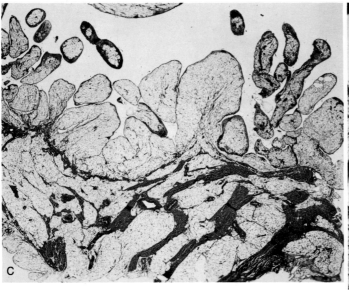

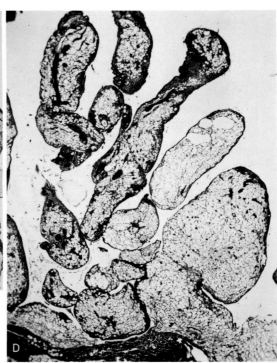

Lipomas originating in the periosteum also are rare (Fig. 84–6). They appear as large soft tissue masses and occasionally are accompanied by nerve paralysis.[76, 78, 88, 113] The plain film radiograph has a characteristic appearance, with a deep, radiolucent soft tissue mass adjacent to bone, which frequently is associated with cortical hyperostosis.[113] Calcifications may be present as broad spicules extending out into the fatty mass or as patchy homogeneous bony dense areas with a trabecular appearance. The dense shadows are due to osteoid formation with mineralization.

Angiolipomas. The angiolipomas are rare benign fatty tumors with a distinct cellular composition.[114–120] They are composed of mature lipocytes with many areas of angiomatous elements interposed within normal tissue. Most commonly the lesions are found in young adults. Firmness is more apparent in these lesions than in the ordinary lipoma. The tumors have been divided into noninfiltrating and infiltrating types.[118] The noninfiltrating type is more common and usually is located in subcutaneous tissue. These tumors appear as firm, painful, and sometimes multiple masses in the upper extremity. A thin capsule frequently is found. Enucleation of the mass is appropriate, and recurrence is rare. The infiltrating type of angiolipoma usually is found within the deep soft tissue and is less common than the noninfiltrating type. These tumors are poorly defined masses with infiltration of adjacent structures. Although the lesions are benign histologically, local invasion and recurrence are a problem,[116, 118] and wide excision usually is necessary.

Radiographically, the angiolipoma, especially the infiltrating type, appears as a soft tissue mass with an inhomogeneous appearance owing to intermixed tissues of water and fatty density, and it has poorly defined margins. Ossification[61] and phleboliths have been noted. Unlike typical lipomas, angiolipomas have coarse, irregular hypervascularity, show mottled staining during the capillary phase of arteriography, and lack precapillary arteriovenous shunts.[121] Although they are benign, angiolipomas may be misdiagnosed as malignant on arteriography. CT scanning demonstrates a poorly defined, heterogeneous mass with elements of both fat and water density and infiltration of the mass into adjacent tissue.[61] Contrast-enhanced studies may confirm the hypervascularity of the mass.

Hibernomas. Hibernomas are an interesting variant of benign lipoma (Fig. 84–7). They are thought to be a manifestation of a vestigial fat storage organ analogous to the dorsal fat pad of hibernating animals.[122–126, 680] They usually present in the 30 to 50 year age group as a firm, movable, asymptomatic mass that occurs more frequently in women. Occasionally, the prominent vascularity of the tumor will

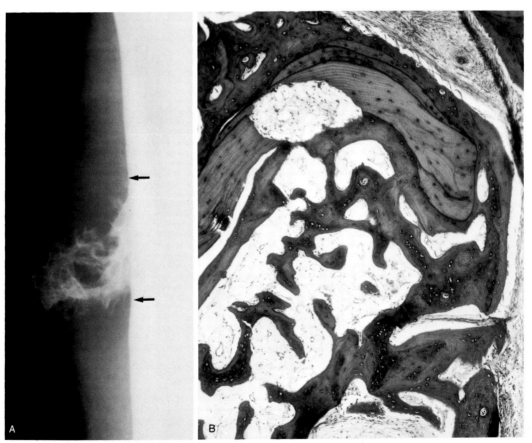

FIGURE 84–6. Lipoma of the periosteum of the femur. This 51 year old man had symptoms of local pressure due to a thigh mass since childhood.

A Anteroposterior coned radiograph of the proximal thigh shows a 9 × 4 cm, sharply marginated, radiolucent fatty mass with a central area of structured density. This dense area has both cortical margins and trabeculae, representing mature bone formation. Note its origin from the bony surface and secondary cortical scalloping (arrows).

B Photomicrograph (15×) is characterized by a centrally located trabecula of mature lamellar bone encased by successive layers of less mature bone. Note the focus of active bone resorption within the mature trabecula.

(Armed Forces Institute of Pathology Neg. Nos. 68-7665, 80-219.)

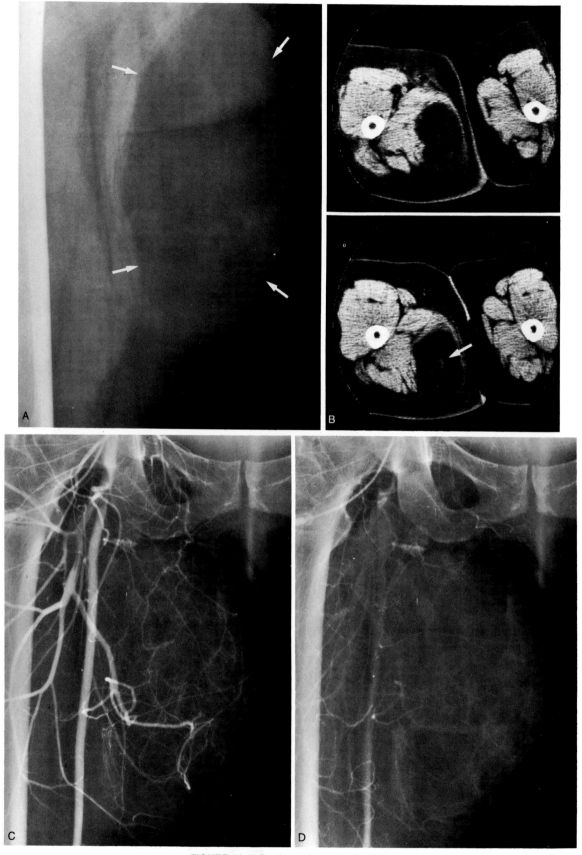

FIGURE 84–7 *See legend on opposite page*

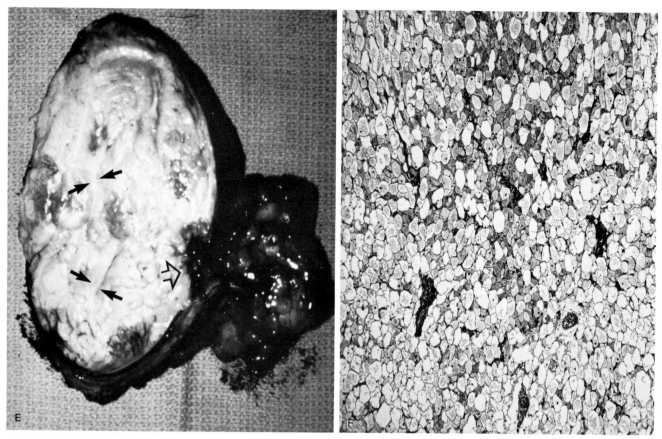

FIGURE 84–7. Hibernoma of the thigh. This 30 year old woman had recent dull, aching pain in a thigh mass that had been present for several years.

A Anteroposterior radiograph shows a poorly defined, nonhomogeneous mass of less than water density (arrows) in the medial thigh.

B Composite CT scans demonstrate a low attenuation coefficient (fatty) mass with well-delineated but not sharply circumscribed margins. The nonhomogeneous dense area is characterized by water-dense streaks throughout the lesion (arrow).

C A hypervascular lesion with neovascularity is noted on the arteriogram (arterial phase).

D Arteriogram (late arterial phase) reveals a nonhomogeneous parenchymal blush within the mass.

E The fatty nature of the lesion is confirmed on the gross specimen. Note the well-delineated margin and streaks (arrows) of fibrovascular tissue seen on the radiographic studies. An old biopsy site also is seen (open arrow).

F Photomicrograph (63×) shows the typical large, polyhedral cells with vacuolated, coarsely granular cytoplasm.

(Armed Forces Institute of Pathology Neg. Nos. 79-2565-1,2,3,4; 79-14847-2; 80-230.)

be detected in the overlying skin as an area of warmth compared with the adjacent normal skin.[127] Hibernomas grow slowly, but rapid enlargement can occur.[128] Microscopically, they are composed of large, polyhedral cells with vacuolated, coarsely granular cytoplasm and central nuclei. On plain films, the hibernoma resembles an inhomogeneous lipoma. On angiography, however, the hibernoma is seen to be very vascular, with irregular vessels, an intense homogeneous vascular blush during the capillary phase,[71, 127] and early venous filling. With these findings the hibernoma may be misdiagnosed as malignant preoperatively. CT also demonstrates the inhomogeneity and fairly well defined margins of the lesion. Malignant degeneration has not been described in this entity.

Lipomatosis

Multiple lipomas (lipomatosis) usually are distributed randomly throughout the soft tissue. Rarely, however, they are deposited symmetrically and in this case are referred to as multiple symmetric lipomatosis.[14, 129] Affected patients have a striking, bizarre appearance, with masses resembling overdeveloped and unusually located muscles.[14, 627] Lipomas also may be multiple and nonsymmetric in distribution, and these are called nonsymmetric lipomatosis. Some patients may have lipoma dolorosa, characterized by pain that develops in one lipoma after another.[14] The cause of this pain is unknown.

Diffuse Lipomatosis. Diffuse lipomatosis is a disorder of fat tissue in which part or all of a limb may be infiltrated extensively by adipose tissue.[130–132] This fatty infiltration may extend into subcutaneous tissue, muscle, fascia, or even bone.[133] Diffuse lipomatosis is found most frequently in children and rarely occurs in adults. It is considered a congenital disorder and frequently is manifested clinically with overgrowth of the soft tissues and bone of the affected limb[89, 90, 130, 132, 134–143, 628] (Fig. 84–8). The overgrowth is referred to as macrodystrophia lipomatosa. It is progressive and involves all mesenchymal elements, with a disproportionate increase in fibroadipose tissue. Macrodystrophia lipomatosa usually is found at birth, and growth is variable. Cessation of growth occurs at puberty. Usually one or more adjacent digits are involved in the affected extremity.

Radiographically, diffuse lipomatosis is neither circum-

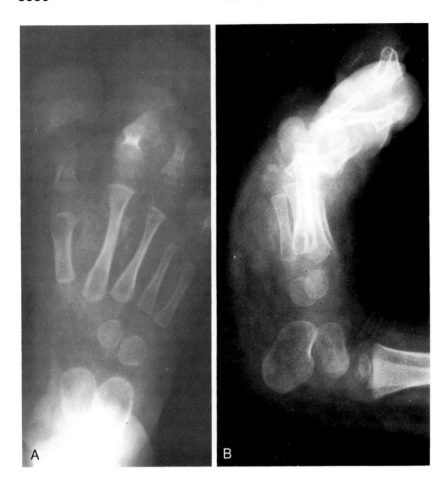

FIGURE 84–8. Diffuse lipomatosis in foot with macrodystrophia lipomatosa. Eleven month old girl with deformity of the right foot since birth.
A Anteroposterior radiograph shows a disproportionately enlarged foot consisting of both soft tissue and bony overgrowth.
B Lateral radiograph (oriented to facilitate comparison with **A**) more clearly demonstrates the nonhomogeneous consistency (fatty and water density) of the soft tissue.
(Armed Forces Institute of Pathology Neg. Nos. 73-3477-1,2.)

scribed nor homogeneous. Diffuse swelling of the soft tissue and overgrowth of the bone with severe deformity are frequent. Mottled lucent areas usually are apparent in the soft tissue. An unusual form of diffuse lipomatosis may affect the leg after poliomyelitis,[133] with diffuse infiltration of fat into subcutaneous tissue, muscle, fascia, and bone, and associated enlargement of the osseous elements.

Lipoblastomatosis. Lipoblastomatosis is a rare type of embryonal fatty tumor.[84, 144–148] These tumors are limited predominantly to the pediatric age group, especially during the first year of life, and are rare in adults.[14, 145] In most instances the tumor is located superficially in the extremities[144] and appears as a soft tissue swelling (Fig. 84–9). It may be confused with liposarcoma on histologic examination, but liposarcoma is extremely rare in children. These lesions may appear as circumscribed or diffuse swellings. Recurrence and continued growth of the tumor after surgery are a particular problem, especially in the diffuse form of the tumor.

Vascular Tumors

The cause and classification of vascular lesions are complicated problems, and agreement on them is not universal.[14, 18, 149–159] The most common vascular tumor is the hemangioma, which occurs in all tissues but is especially common in the skin, where it usually is seen at birth or within the first several years of life.[14] The majority of these cutaneous hemangiomas are asymptomatic and regress spontaneously before the seventh year of life. These lesions

infrequently are studied radiographically because of their obvious clinical manifestations. The less common, deeper soft tissue hemangiomas, however, can be recognized and studied easily radiographically.

Hemangiomas. The majority of deeper soft tissue hemangiomas are asymptomatic and usually remain so until late childhood or early adult life. Less commonly, they may appear prior to the age of 30 years with nonspecific symptoms, such as a mass, pain, or swelling, perhaps requiring cosmetic correction.[149, 155] On rare occasions, in the female adult, they will become clinically apparent during pregnancy.[154] The lesions frequently are associated with overlying skin abnormalities, such as reddish-blue discoloration, enlarged veins, or even cutaneous hemangiomas.[156, 160] The mass may vary its size spontaneously, independently of position. Occasionally enlargement with a color change will occur in the dependent position, and rarely pulsations and bruits may be found.[161] The deeper soft tissue hemangiomas may involve any soft tissue, such as muscle, tendon, connective tissue, fatty tissue, synovium, or bone, and involvement of a combination of these sites is not uncommon[162–176] (Fig. 84–10). Hemangiomas are relatively common in skeletal muscle, with the highest prevalence in young women, particularly in the third decade of life[149, 154, 155, 177–180] (Fig. 84–11). A predilection for the limbs, especially distal to the elbows and knees, is noted.[149, 155] These lesions usually are cured by local excision; however, recurrence can take place.[181]

Hemangiomas are associated with a variety of clinical problems, such as consumption coagulopathy, cardiac decompensation, gangrene, discrepancies in extremity growth, osteomalacia, varicose veins, massive osteolysis, Maffucci's syndrome, and Klippel-Trenaunay-Weber syndrome. In 1940, Kasabach and Merritt described a syndrome bearing their names, marked by the association of capillary hemangiomas with extensive purpura.[182] This syndrome usually affects infants up to 1 year of age. It is characterized by an asymptomatic hemangioma, commonly located in the extremities, which suddenly increases in size and is accompanied by a generalized bleeding tendency, usually manifested by bruising, petechiae, and purpura. Thrombocytopenia and hypofibrinogenemia are noted.[183] The vascular lesion may be either a cavernous or a capillary hemangioma or even a hemangioendothelioma.[183–191] The clinical and laboratory findings result from trapping of platelets and deposition of fibrin clot in the vascular spaces of the tumor, which provoke intravascular hemolysis and red cell fragmentation.[192–195] Massive precapillary arteriovenous shunting of blood may result in cardiac decompensation[153, 196, 197] as well as cyanosis and, on rare occasions, even gangrene of the soft tissue distal to the lesion.[153] Growth discrepancies associated with vascular lesions are not uncommon, frequently reflected by overgrowth and, less commonly, atrophy or shortening of the involved extremity.[153, 197–199] This feature may be seen as a part of the Klippel-Trenaunay-Weber syndrome (varicose veins, soft tissue and bony hypertrophy, and cutaneous hemangiomas).[200] On physical examination, these extremities typically are found to be warm, with dilated superficial veins and cutaneous hemangiomas. The bony hypertrophy is manifested clinically by discrepancy in leg length.[197, 201, 202] Other bony changes can be noted with hemangiomas, such as osteomalacia,[203–207] massive osteolysis,[208, 209] and Maffucci's syndrome.[210]

The hemangioma manifested as a soft tissue mass may be characterized as a poorly circumscribed, localized or diffuse swelling on gross inspection. These tumors vary in size from less than 4 cm to over 20 cm, but most are less than 9 cm in diameter.[149] Hemangiomas may recur locally but do not metastasize.

Hemangiomas are benign lesions classically divided into capillary and cavernous types,[14] depending on their composition. Capillary hemangiomas are composed of capillaries with a sparse fibrous stroma and that are arranged haphazardly, whereas cavernous hemangiomas are composed of large, dilated, blood-filled spaces lined by flat endothelium. In fact, a large number of hemangiomas exhibit a continuous spectrum ranging from pure capillary hemangiomas through mixed cavernous and capillary types to the pure cavernous type of hemangioma.[149]

Hemangioendotheliomas are rare tumors that occur most frequently in infants and young children but may present in the adult.[1, 14] A thick endothelial layer is found within the capillaries. This layer is formed by proliferation of endothelial cells, which assume a rounded to cuboidal shape instead of the typical flattened shape. This results in a relatively solid mass of large cells about narrow blood channels, which needs to be distinguished from a malignant tumor.

Radiographically, hemangiomas appear as a nonhomo-

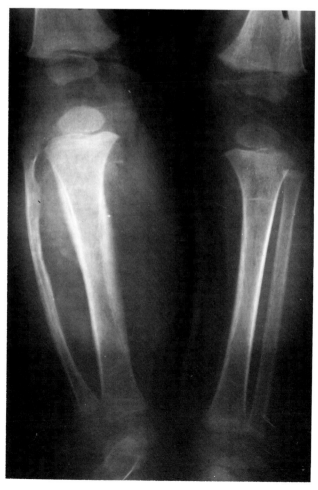

FIGURE 84–9. Lipoblastomatosis of the right calf. This 9 month old boy had an increasing right calf size. Anteroposterior radiograph shows large, poorly defined, nonhomogeneous mass with deformity, erosion, and periosteal new bone formation in the adjacent tibia and fibula. (Armed Forces Institute of Pathology Neg. No. 76-11506-2.)

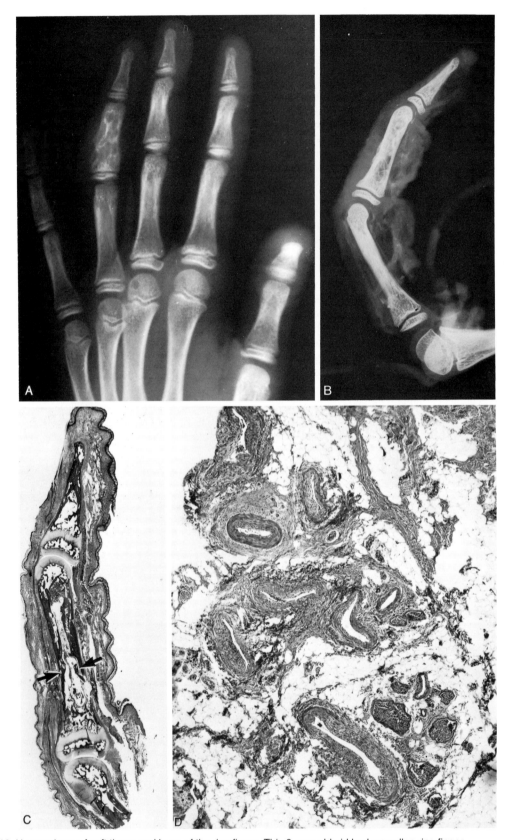

FIGURE 84–10. Hemangioma of soft tissue and bone of the ring finger. This 8 year old girl had a swollen ring finger.

  A Oblique radiograph shows multiple, sharply circumscribed lytic lesions involving the middle phalanx, with sclerotic margins and extension into the adjacent soft tissue.

  B Specimen radiograph confirms the presence of intraosseous lysis.

  C Macrophotomicrograph (1.5×) shows the intraosseous hemangioma (arrows). Note the areas of cortical thickening (distally) and thinning (proximally).

  D Photomicrograph (25×) demonstrates a cluster of thickened vessels of varying sizes in the adjacent soft tissue.

  (Armed Forces Institute of Pathology Neg. Nos. 78-6162-1, 78-6162-2, 80-221, 80-220.)

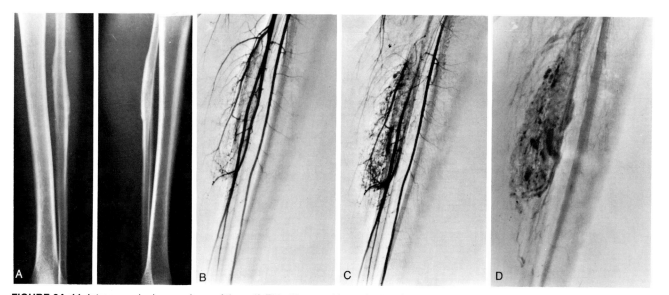

FIGURE 84–11. Intramuscular hemangioma of the calf. This 19 year old man had calf pain on ambulation.
A Composite anteroposterior and lateral radiographs show cortical hyperostosis of the fibula.
B Arteriogram (arterial phase) shows vessel displacement with hypervascularity.
C Arteriogram (late arterial phase) demonstrates tumor blush and involvement of adjacent fibular cortex.
D Arteriogram (venous phase) reveals arteriovenous shunting and puddling of contrast material in small venous channels.
(Armed Forces Institute of Pathology Neg. Nos. 79-1343-1,2,3,4.)

geneous mass of water density or a swelling that may be localized or diffuse. Single or multiple focal discrete nodules may be seen. These usually vary in size and are due to focal proliferation of hemangiomatous tissue. The margin typically is poorly defined, especially in the diffuse type, but occasionally a sharp interface between the tumor and adjacent soft tissue is seen. Tortuous channels of water density representing the arterial supply and venous drainage of the tumor occasionally may be demonstrated radiographically within the adjacent subcutaneous fat. Calcification within the hemangioma is common and may be of three types. The nonspecific type is either amorphous or, at times, curvilinear. The second type, which is more specific and is the most frequent (49 per cent) type of calcification, is the phlebolith[161, 211–213] (Fig. 84–12). Phleboliths are rounded calcific masses frequently demonstrating a laminated structure. Occasionally, metaplastic ossification may be found in hemangiomas, and this is the third type of calcification.[155, 629] Adjacent smooth bone erosions can occur, especially with the deep hemangiomas. This may be due to the localized pressure effect of the adjacent consolidated mass or the hypertrophied vessels of the soft tissue, periosteum, cortex, or marrow cavity (Fig. 84–10).[630] Overgrowth of the bone and soft tissue of the extremity is seen with hemangiomas, especially if they are diffuse or extensive. In patients so affected, bone scans usually show increased activity in the growth plates on the involved side.[197] Rarely, periosteal new bone, cortical hyperostosis, or regional osteoporosis may be found.

Arteriography in vascular tumors is extremely helpful in patient management by defining the lesion's extent, degree of vascularity, and vascular supply.[22, 153, 156, 214–217] It also helps in differentiating among the several types of vascular masses: hemangiomas, arteriovenous malformations, and venous malformations.[156] These types have been referred to under the broad descriptive term "angiodysplasia."[153, 218]

Regardless of the terms applied, arteriography is a helpful tool in the evaluation of vascular tumors.

Hemangiomas are hypervascular, usually with fine-caliber vessels, and reveal homogeneous contrast opacification or staining (Fig. 84–11). These features also are seen with MR imaging.[681–683] Occasionally coarse, irregular vessels are seen on angiograms, and the vascular pattern may be indistinguishable from that of malignant soft tissue tumors.[156] Large hemangiomas may be painful, and partial embolization has been successful in controlling pain in unresectable lesions.[219]

Arteriovenous malformations are composed of large tortuous and coarse arterial and venous vessels and thick-walled capillaries. Arteriographically, large vessels with densely opacified vascular spaces and early filling of draining veins are seen[153, 156, 631] (Fig. 84–13). The vessels of the arteriovenous malformations also are seen in MR images.[684] These vessels may be arranged regularly and parallel to each other along the fiber bundle axis of an involved muscle. This striation suggests benignancy, because malignant tumors rarely leave muscle bundles intact.[151]

Venous malformations consist of large dilated venous spaces, which have very slow blood flow within the enlarged vascular spaces, and the feeding vessels may be thrombosed. These two features may explain why venous malformations are seen uncommonly on arteriography. Venography, including direct injection, may be necessary to demonstrate the lesion and determine its extent.[153] These vascular deformities commonly are associated with lymphatic abnormalities, which may be related to secondary hypertrophy or which may be part of the original vessel anomaly or neoplasm.[220] Thus, lymphangiography may be helpful and frequently demonstrates hypoplasia or aplasia of lymph vessels, vesicles, lymph fistulae, and cysts. These findings usually are seen when the venous elements are dominant and in conjunction with the Klippel-Trenaunay-

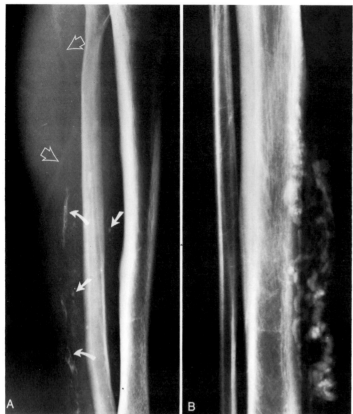

FIGURE 84–12. Intramuscular hemangioma of the calf with phleboliths. This 25 year old man had recurrent swelling and calf pain.

A Lateral radiograph shows two patterns of calcification: small circular dense lesions (straight arrows) and linear dense areas with a central lucent core (curved arrows). Both are due to dystrophic calcification **(D)** of organized thrombi (phlebolith). The channels of water density (open arrows) result from dilated subcutaneous veins. Note the smooth pressure erosion of the tibia posteriorly.

B Arteriogram (late arterial phase) demonstrates arteriovenous shunting into tortuous dilated venous channels, which are patent and do not contain phleboliths. Their close proximity to bone occasionally may cause pressure erosion **(A)**.

C Specimen radiograph confirms the phleboliths as small calcifications—one lamellated and two with central lucent cores.

D Photomicrograph displays large dilated venous channels with thrombi in different stages of organization. The largest thrombus is attached in part to the vessel wall. Spotty dystrophic calcification (straight arrows) is present in the old organized portion of the thrombus. Note the propagating clot (curved arrow) emanating from a more recently organized portion of the thrombus. The eventual dystrophic calcification within the propagating thrombus produces the linear density pattern **(A)**.

(Armed Forces Institute of Pathology Neg. Nos. 75-2058-3, 75-2058-2, 75-2059, 79-16646.)

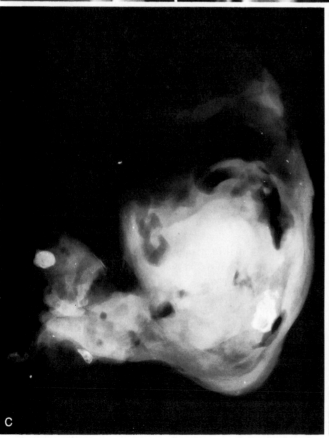

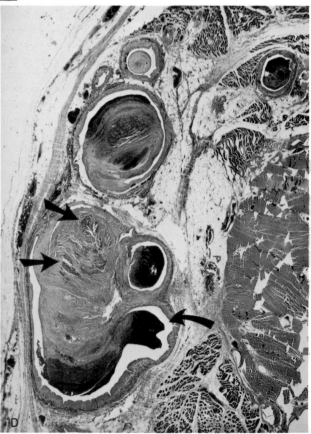

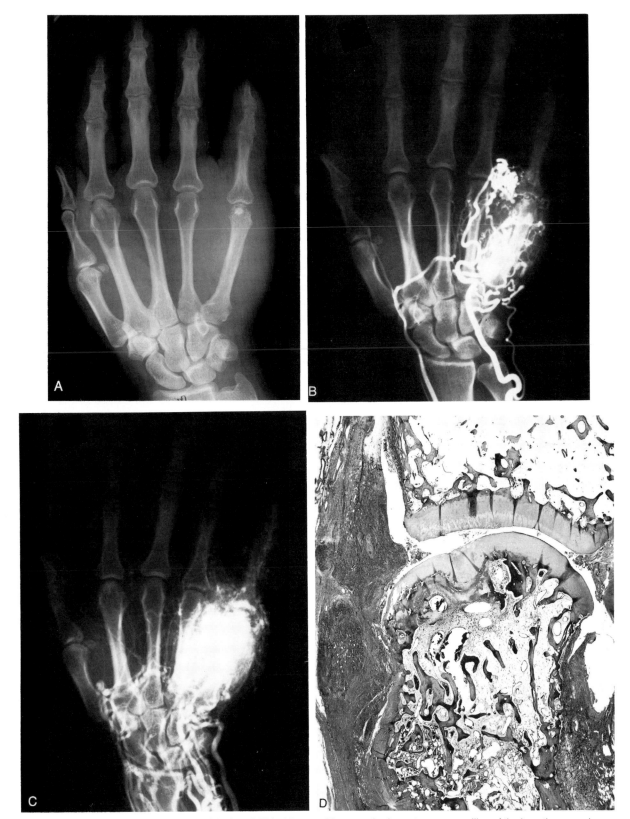

FIGURE 84–13. Arteriovenous malformation of the hand. This 36 year old woman had spontaneous swelling of the hypothenar eminence and little finger.

   A Frontal film shows diffuse soft tissue swelling about the fifth metacarpal bone and phalanges in association with erosions and osteoporosis of the underlying bone.

   B Arteriogram (arterial phase) demonstrates an enlarged ulnar artery and mass of tortuous vessels predominantly about the fifth metacarpal bone.

   C Arteriogram (late arterial phase) reveals an intense blush, with arteriovenous shunting. Note the extensive hypervascularity extending beyond the blush into adjacent soft tissue and to the tip of the little finger.

   D Photomicrograph (7×) of the metacarpophalangeal joint shows densely packed small vessels with extensive involvement of the periarticular soft tissue and synovium. These findings are responsible for the intense arteriographic blush and cortical erosions. The dilated intraosseous vascular channels account for the localized areas of trabecular loss.

   (Armed Forces Institute of Pathology Neg. Nos. 78-8767-3, 78-8767-2, 78-8767-7, 80-227.)

Weber syndrome. Hyperplastic lymph pathways on lymphangiography typically are seen in the arteriovenous shunts and malformations.

CT scanning, especially with contrast enhancement, augments the arteriographic findings by displaying tumor extent and relationship to adjacent structures as well as prominent areas of vascularity. It also shows the infiltrative margins of the tumor. Sometimes contrast enhanced CT scanning of hemangiomas may show no recognizable change when compared with nonenhanced studies.[66]

Synovial Hemangiomas. Hemangiomas of the synovium are uncommon tumors, occurring most frequently in the knee. They invariably are unilateral (Fig. 84–14) and rarely are found in other joints or in synovial tendon sheaths.[202, 221–223] Synovial hemangiomas usually occur in adolescent girls or young women and frequently are symptomatic, with pain, swelling, and decreased range of motion. They commonly are associated with adjacent cutaneous and deeper soft tissue hemangiomas.[224]

Pathologically, two morphologic patterns are seen. One is the localized, pedunculated synovial mass, which may cause mechanical problems with locking of the joint[225] and which is excised easily. The other pattern is diffuse, with intermittent pain, hemarthrosis, and occasionally increase in limb length. These lesions are difficult to excise, may recur, and also may be associated with visceral and cutaneous vascular lesions. The synovial proliferation accompanying the diffuse synovial hemangioma can be quite similar to that seen in hemophilia.[202, 226]

The plain film radiographs usually show soft tissue swelling or a mass about the involved joint,[222, 227–229] occasionally with phleboliths[227–229] (Fig. 84–14). Advanced maturity of the epiphysis, discrepancy in limb length, periosteal new bone, and articular destruction may be seen[229] (see Chapter 63). Arthrography usually shows the intra-articular mass as multiple filling defects with a villous configuration. The lesions are hypervascular on arteriography, with a fine vascular pattern and staining.[230] Thermography also may help in assessing the hemangioma's extrasynovial extent when it is unsuspected clinically.[231]

Hemangiopericytomas. Hemangiopericytomas are vascular tumors of the soft tissue that are believed to originate from the pericytes of Zimmerman, which surround the capillary wall[14, 232–237] (Fig. 84–15). These tumors most frequently appear in adults and are located in the deep soft tissue of the thigh.[237–241] A slowly growing, painless mass (with a median size of 6.5 cm) is the most frequent clinical symptom. Because of the tumor's striking hypervascularity, its surgical removal frequently is complicated by hemorrhage. The majority of hemangiopericytomas act in a benign fashion, although occasionally malignant lesions have been encountered. Grossly, the hemangiopericytoma is a well-circumscribed mass with a frequent covering of large plexiform vessels about its periphery. Microscopically, rounded or elongated cells proliferate just outside of the capillary reticular sheath. This relation is best seen on silver reticulin stain.

The plain film radiograph is nonspecific, revealing a focal homogeneous soft tissue mass with a variable margin. The tumors occasionally may demonstrate calcification and bone erosion. Arteriography demonstrates an extremely hypervascular tumor with lobular growth, tumor vessels, and striking heterogeneous blush[242–248, 632] (Fig. 84–15). Occa-

sionally, the tumor can function as an arteriovenous shunt.[249]

A closer look at the pattern of hypervascularity demonstrates that the main arteries, early in the arterial phase, are displaced by the tumor. Later, the feeding arteries spread around the tumor before entering it. Occasionally, the vessels will coalesce into a vascular pedicle and enter the outer margin of the mass, whereupon the vessels branch and encircle the tumor. This peripheral distribution of arteries correlates well with the gross findings of a plexiform meshwork of vessels covering the tumor.[238] This angiographic pattern is highly suggestive of hemangiopericytoma.[248]

Lymphangiomas. Lymphangiomas are rare tumors composed of multiple lymph-filled vessels and cystic spaces, with occasional foci of lymphoid tissue.[250–252] They usually occur in the skin and subcutaneous tissue and frequently are noted at birth or by 1 year of age. Local invasion into adjacent tissues is common, and recurrence rate is high after local excision. Wide excision is recommended, leaving a margin of normal tissue.[250] The lesions are poorly defined, with infiltrative margins, and only rarely are localized. Inspection of the gross tissue shows a diffuse, spongy, compressible mass. Microscopically, there is proliferation of lymph vessels with dilated lymph channels, which may form cysts.[14] The plain film radiograph is nonspecific but may demonstrate a diffuse, poorly defined, poorly marginated mass.

Cartilage Tumors

Chondromas may occur as cartilage proliferations of the soft tissue, usually composed of well-differentiated hyaline cartilage and frequently demonstrating endochondral bone formation. They most commonly arise from synovium of joints and occasionally from a tendon sheath or bursa. In these sites they are referred to as (idiopathic) synovial (osteo)chondromatosis.[8, 253–262] Less commonly, benign cartilage proliferations (chondromas) of other soft parts are encountered. The exact origin of these latter tumors is unknown, but they commonly are attached to a tendon and also could represent a tenosynovial process.[263–266]

Synovial (Osteo)Chondromatosis. Idiopathic synovial chondromatosis represents cartilage formation by the synovial membrane.[8, 258] The cause is unknown, but it most likely represents a metaplasia or neoplasia.[254, 267] This disorder almost invariably is a monoarticular disease with a chronic progressive course.[258] Rarely, spontaneous regression has been reported.[253, 268, 269] The most commonly affected joints are the knee, hip, and elbow.[259] The disorder is twice as common in men as in women and usually is found in the third to fifth decades of life.[267] Clinically, patients show a several-year history of joint pain with limitation of motion.[259] Joint effusion is rare but when present may be bloody. Intra-articular loose body formation is common and may lead to mechanical destruction of the articular cartilage, with resultant osteoarthritis.[254, 267, 295–297] Joint instability also can occur and be responsible for pain.[294] Focal recurrence after surgery is not uncommon and usually necessitates many surgical procedures. Synovial chondromatosis rarely may become malignant.[260, 267, 297–302, 587]

The synovium in idiopathic synovial chondromatosis is hyperplastic, with foci of cartilage metaplasia. Grossly, the synovium has many villous or nodular projections. These

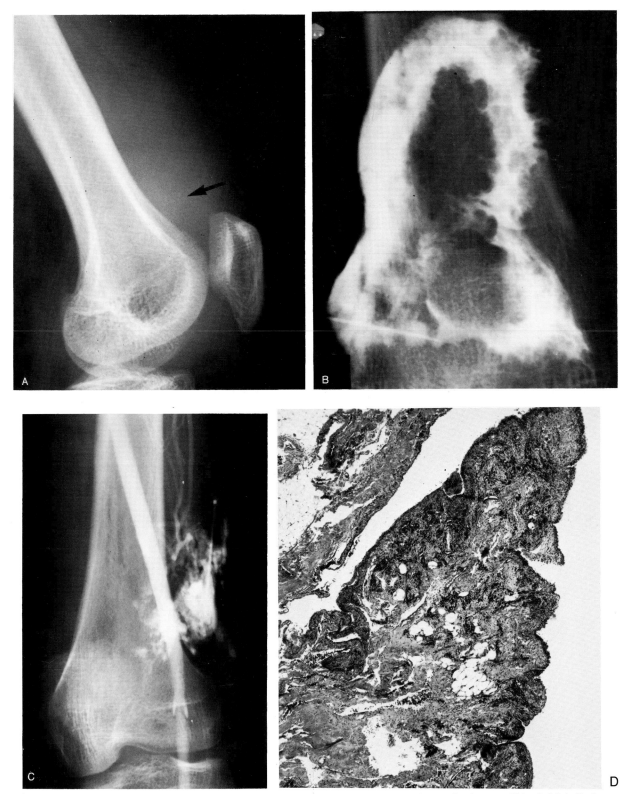

FIGURE 84–14. Hemangioma of the synovium of the knee. This 18 year old man had a painful, swollen knee and bloody joint effusion.

A Lateral radiograph shows soft tissue swelling about the knee, especially in the suprapatellar space. Note the faint, small calcification (phlebolith) (arrow).

B The arthrogram demonstrates a villonodular pattern.

C Direct injection of contrast medium into the mass indicates a hypervascular lesion and venous shunting.

D Photomicrograph (40×) of the synovium shows a villus with proliferation of the synovial membrane, increased vascularity, and extensive hemosiderin deposition.

(Armed Forces Institute of Pathology Neg. Nos. 77-4645-7, 77-4645-6, 77-4645-2, 80-223, 80-222.)

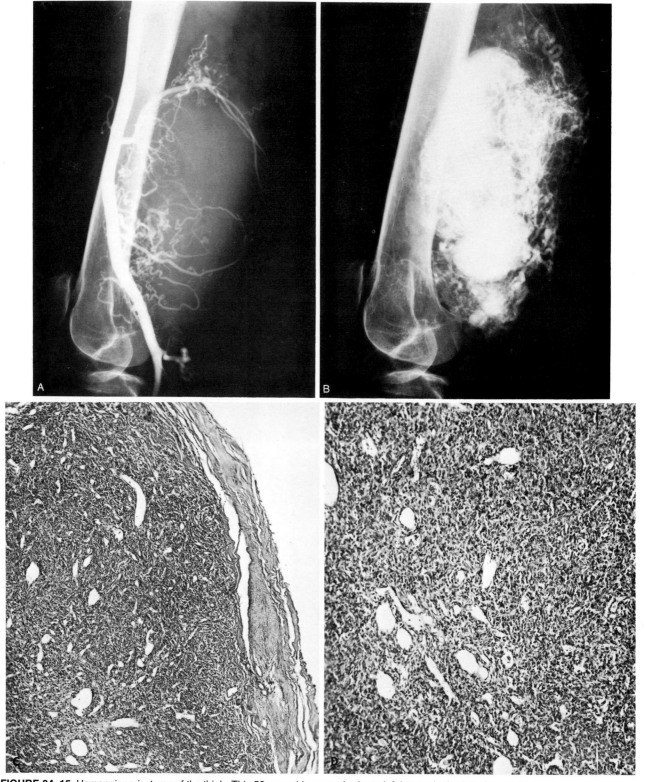

FIGURE 84–15. Hemangiopericytoma of the thigh. This 58 year old woman had a painful mass in the leg of 1 year's duration.

A Arteriogram (arterial phase) shows a large hypervascular mass displacing the femoropopliteal artery anteriorly. The vascularity is concentrated around the periphery in a plexiform arrangement.

B Arteriogram (late arterial phase) demonstrates a dense heterogeneous blush, neovascularity, and a lobular configuration, which also was seen in the gross specimen.

C Photomicrograph (low power view) reveals cellular proliferation about vascular spaces of varying sizes.

D Photomicrograph (63×) shows an intricate network of small, thin-walled branching vascular channels separated by rounded and sometimes elongated cells.

(Armed Forces Institute of Pathology Neg. Nos. 69-11422-1,2; 71-2102-1; 80-232.)

cartilage nodules usually have an upper limit of 2 to 3 cm in size. Rarely, a large dominant nodule will be found.[303] As these cartilage nodules continue to grow, they may project into the joint space by means of a delicate pedicle. Endochondral bone formation within these cartilage nodules occurs frequently and requires an intact blood supply through the pedicle. With slight trauma, the pedicle breaks and the nodule becomes a loose body.[259, 297] The loose bodies are white to gray in color and oval to round or faceted in shape.[304–306] Although the body is free within the joint space with its vascular supply disrupted, the cartilage component may increase in size by continuous cartilage proliferation on the surface, which is nourished by synovial fluid. The loose body may become reattached to the thickened synovium.[259] With reestablishment of a vascular supply at this new site, the nodule again may grow and form bone or be resorbed. The cartilage nodules may extend through the joint capsule and continue to proliferate within the adjacent soft tissue.[267, 298] Microscopically, numerous circumscribed nodules of cartilage may be myxoid in type but more commonly are composed of hyaline cartilage. Mineralization of chondroid matrix is common and bone, when present, frequently develops fatty marrow. Considerable cellular proliferation with atypical nuclei is common in the subcapsular cartilage areas, and although this often is misinterpreted as a sign of aggressiveness, this pattern still is compatible with a benign process.[267, 307–309]

Radiographically, synovial chondromatosis commonly demonstrates multiple juxta-articular radiodense shadows (Fig. 84–16). They range in size from a few millimeters to several centimeters and show varying degrees of mineralization (chondrification or ossification) within each lesion.[275, 296, 310–316] The typical pattern of mineralization ranges from small specks of calcification to large calcified bodies with peripheral linear dense areas and radiolucent centers. Bony trabeculation can be seen in the mature osteoid areas of the nodules. Some nodules may be of water density and seen only as soft tissue masses in or about the joint. The nodules may cause erosions of the adjacent bone and widening of the joint space (Fig. 84–17). Noncalcified lesions are best seen on arthrography as they displace the contrast medium and produce multiple filling defects (Fig. 84–18). CT alone or in combination with arthrography is useful in documenting the intra-articular location of the nodules, bone erosion, and capsular constriction or adhesive capsulitis.[633, 634] In the late stages, many loose bodies will be found, and secondary osteoarthritis is common. The joint space at this time will be narrow, with eburnation and osteophyte formation consistent with secondary osteoarthritis.

Soft Tissue Chondromas. Chondromas of the soft parts are less common than idiopathic synovial chondromatosis.[263–266, 317, 318, 635] They occur more frequently in men and are seen predominantly in the third and fourth decades of life. The tumors are slow-growing masses that are lobular and well demarcated and almost invariably occur in the extremities, especially in the hands and feet.[263] These masses shell out easily at surgery, which thus attests to their having circumscribed margins. They are rubbery to firm in consistency and rarely exceed 2 cm in size. Microscopically, they are composed of adult type hyaline cartilage with some areas of ossification and calcification. They may have spindle-shaped nuclei that vary in size and shape, as

well as mitotic figures. This pattern may be confused with chondrosarcoma if the pathologist is not aware of the range of histologic findings in this lesion.[263]

Radiographs show a nonspecific soft tissue mass, often with coarse specks of calcification. Occasionally, a lacy or trabecular pattern, which corresponds to areas of ossification, will be demonstrated. The mass also can cause extrinsic pressure erosion of the adjacent bone, with scalloping and a sclerotic margin.

Fibrous Tumors

Fibrous tumors of soft tissue represent a numerous and heterogeneous group of lesions, which have been supplied with a variety of terms and classifications.[14, 319–325] Benign forms of fibrous proliferative ''tumors'' are encountered with some frequency in the deeper soft and subcutaneous tissues. They have been termed ''fibromatosis'' to distinguish them from persistent hyperplasia or reparative scar tissue. Such hyperplasia or scar tissue usually is self-limiting. Two principal groups of fibromatosis are recognized.[322, 323] In one group the disorder occurs as a congenital lesion or is diagnosed during childhood. From this group, some lesions can be differentiated by anatomic location and microscopic appearance into specific diagnoses, such as juvenile aponeurotic fibroma, infantile dermal fibromatosis, aggressive infantile fibromatosis, and congenital generalized fibromatosis.[320, 323] These lesions are discussed in more detail because of their frequency of presentation in the extremities. The other group of lesions may occur at any time during life but usually are found in the adult. In this group of cellular fibroblastic lesions, it is difficult to separate specific diagnostic types and, in some cases, to differentiate them on a morphologic basis from adult fibrosarcoma.

Juvenile Aponeurotic Fibromas. Juvenile aponeurotic fibroma is a specialized form of fibromatosis that occurs in children or adolescents, with a male predominance.[14, 326–336] It usually arises in the aponeurotic tissue of the hands and feet, especially in the palms and soles,[326, 329] and is manifested as a painless, poorly circumscribed soft tissue mass, which frequently is firm and fixed. The tumor grows slowly with infiltration and tends to calcify.[636] The mass usually is less than 4 cm in diameter, and local recurrence is common as a result of its infiltrative nature.[326, 331]

Infantile Dermal Fibromatosis. Infantile dermal fibromatosis is a benign fibrous proliferative lesion that involves the extensor surfaces of fingers and toes almost exclusively.[321, 337–343] It appears within the first 2 years of life and frequently is discovered at birth. Boys are affected predominantly. Classically, several digits are involved by multiple nodules, which are well circumscribed and firmly attached to skin. If they are large enough, they also may attach to the adjacent fascia or periosteum. Clinically, there may be a reddish appearance to the nodules. Grossly, they are whitish and usually less than 1 cm in diameter. The histologic appearance typically is of uniformly arranged interlacing bundles of fibroblasts, compressed by abundant birefringent collagen with incorporated adnexal structures.[321] Recurrence is frequent after surgery.

Radiologically, multiple soft tissue masses or swellings are noted on the extensor surface of the digits. The fingers may be deformed with flexion contractures, and rarely bone erosions are found.[344]

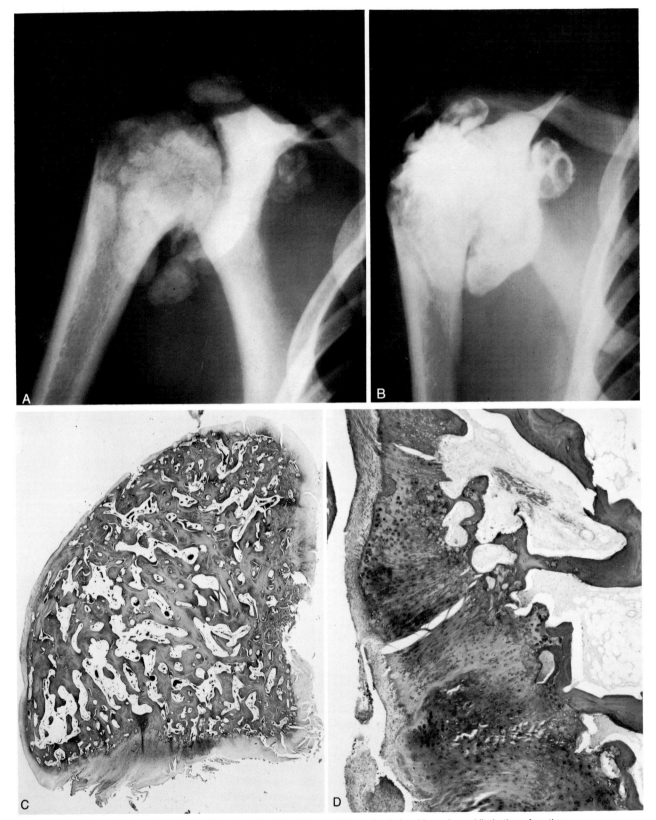

FIGURE 84–16. Synovial chondromatosis of the shoulder. This 20 year old man had shoulder pain and limitation of motion.

A Frontal radiograph shows multiple calcific nodules distributed throughout the joint. These nodules have smooth margins with a nonhomogeneous trabeculated pattern. Note the extensive secondary osteoarthritis with joint space narrowing, eburnation, and osteophytes.

B Arthrography reveals a multinodular pattern, confirming the intra-articular location of the nodules.

C Macroslide of an intra-articular nodule shows a coarse trabecular pattern encased by a predominantly smooth fibrocartilaginous capsule.

D Photomicrograph (43×) of the capsule documents its cartilaginous nature. Areas of hyaline cartilage with endochondral bone formation and fibrocartilage are noted.

(Armed Forces Institute of Pathology Neg. Nos. 76-268-2,5; 79-16663; 80-224.)

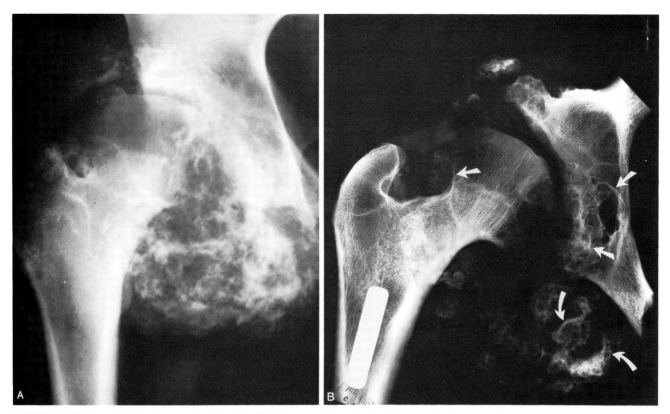

FIGURE 84–17. Synovial chondromatosis of the hip. This 29 year old man had a slow-growing hip mass of 15 years' duration.

A Anteroposterior radiograph shows a large joint mass with stipples, rings, and arcs of calcification. The femoral head is displaced laterally and osteoarthritic changes are present. Bony erosions also are noted.

B Specimen radiograph demonstrates bony erosions (arrows) and bone formation (curved arrows) within the mass.

Illustration continued on following page

Aggressive Infantile Fibromatosis. Aggressive infantile fibromatosis appears as painless soft tissue swellings or masses in the extremities, usually during the first 2 years of life (Fig. 84–19). They are slightly more prominent in boys. The tumor rarely metastasizes[321, 345]; however, these tumors are locally aggressive, infiltrating into muscles, vessels, nerves, fasciae, tendons, and subcutaneous fat. Microscopically, the level of mitotic activity varies greatly among the interlacing bundles of fusiform and spindle-shaped cells and reticulin and collagen fibers. The histologic features make differentiation from fibrosarcoma difficult.[321] The lesions tend to recur after surgery. The radiographs demonstrate a soft tissue mass or swelling with an occasional bone deformity and scalloped defect.

Infantile Myofibromatosis. Infantile myofibromatosis (originally termed congenital generalized fibromatosis) is a disseminated disease that develops in utero and usually is fatal shortly after birth, if the infant is not stillborn.[321, 346–356, 610, 641] It consists of multiple nodular lesions of fibroblastic proliferation in superficial soft tissue, muscle, viscera, and bone. It has been reported in a solitary form.[350–352] Familial occurrences have been noted.[14, 357] The nodules are subcutaneous, firm, unencapsulated, and yellowish to white when removed from the body. Microscopically, there are curving fascicles of comparatively large elongated fibroblasts with a somewhat immature appearance.[321] The radiograph shows soft tissue swelling or masses and frequently multiple lytic lesions in bone.[358–360] Another form with no visceral involvement is now known (congenital multiple fibromatosis); it has a much better prognosis.[354–356] Regres-

sion with resolution of the lytic bone lesions in this type can occur[354, 356] (see Chapter 95).

Other Benign Soft Tissue Tumors

Although many additional soft tissue tumors exist (see Chapter 95), a few deserve special emphasis.

Ganglion Cysts. Ganglion cysts are cystic masses, usually attached to tendon sheaths of the hands and feet.[14] Occasionally they may be found within tendons, muscles, subcutaneous tissue at the fingertips, and semilunar cartilages. These lesions are characterized by unilocular or multilocular cystic spaces with a myxoid matrix. The lesions rarely communicate with the synovium of a tendon sheath or a joint in the unoperated patient, and they are not lined by synovium. Radiographically, they appear as soft tissue masses, and if large enough, the fluid-filled space may be demonstrated by sonography, CT scanning, or MR imaging (see Chapter 95). Angiography shows the mass to be avascular.[51]

Myxomas. Myxomas are soft, gelatinous growths; most frequently they are encountered in the heart, but not uncommonly they occur in subcutaneous soft tissues or within muscular structures.[14, 361–364] They usually are painless masses, appearing in the 50 to 60 year old age range. These lesions are uncommon in young adults and rare in children. The mass is poorly defined and unencapsulated, and it infiltrates adjacent structures, for which reason it may be difficult to eradicate. Microscopically, there is a fairly uniform consistency of poorly vascular, richly mucoid tumor, containing scattered stellate cells and minimal fibrosis. In con-

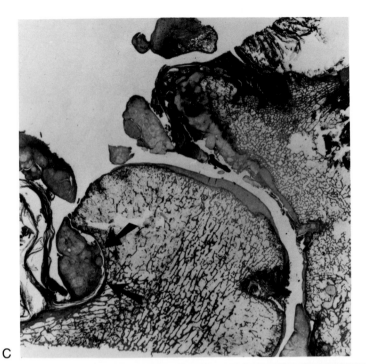

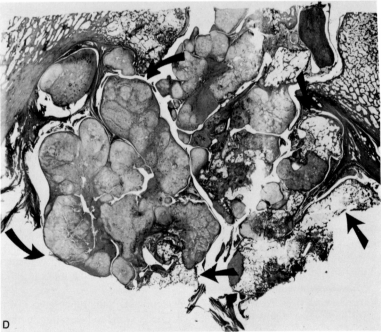

FIGURE 84–17. *Continued*

   C Macroslide of the upper femur and acetabulum shows evidence of joint remodeling
and cartilage nodules in the adjacent soft tissue, one of which is causing a smooth bony
erosion (arrows).

   D Macroslide of the lower femur and inferior
portion of the mass reveals the characteristic
multilobular pattern of cartilage proliferation
with (straight arrows) and without (curved arrows) bone formation.

   (Armed Forces Institute of Pathology Neg.
Nos. 74-12924-2,1; 76-5768-1; 76-5769.)

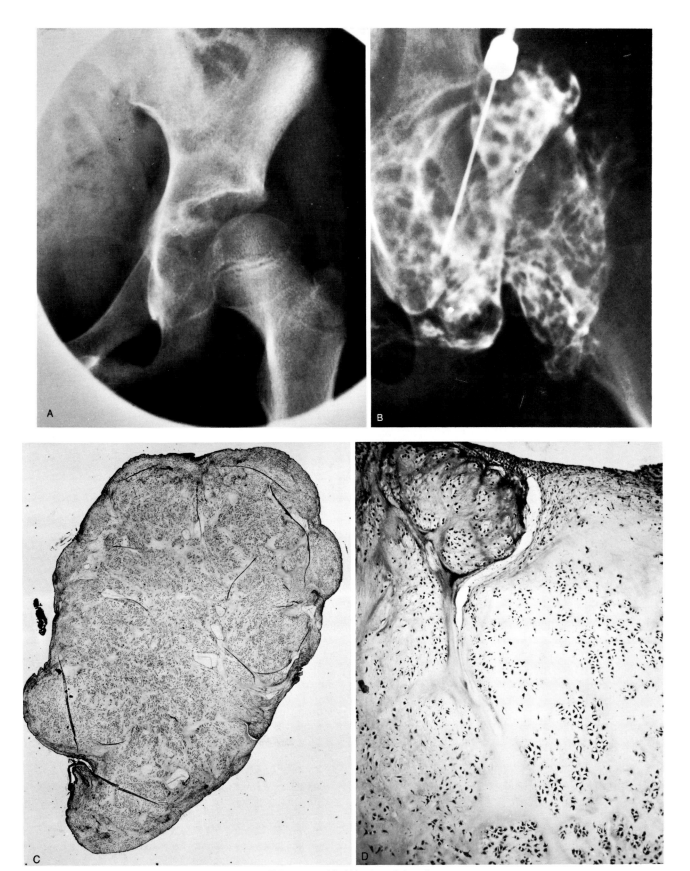

FIGURE 84–18. Synovial chondromatosis of the hip. This 7 year old girl had a painless limp.

  A Anteroposterior radiograph of the hip shows a widened joint space with lateral displacement of the femoral head. There is no evidence of soft tissue calcification.

  B Arthrogram demonstrates multiple noncalcified nodules filling the joint.

  C Photomicrograph (7×) of a single nodule shows the lobulated appearance of proliferating cartilage.

  D Photomicrograph (63×) of the nodule's surface reveals the increased cellularity and variability of the cartilage.

  (Armed Forces Institute of Pathology Neg. Nos. 79-2001-1,2; 80-229; 80-228.)

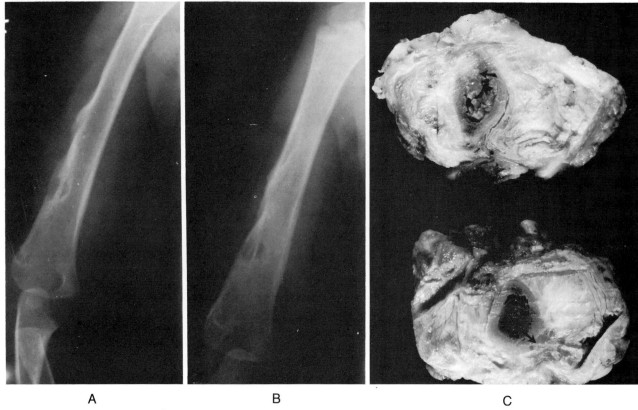

| A | B | C |

FIGURE 84–19. Aggressive infantile fibromatosis of the upper arm. This 5 month old female infant had a rapidly growing mass attached to the periosteum.
A, B Anteroposterior and oblique radiographs show bony erosions with areas of cortical hyperostosis.
C Gross specimen demonstrates the large soft tissue mass and its extension into bone (arrows).
(Armed Forces Institute of Pathology Neg. Nos. 67-6597-1, 67-6444.)

trast to ganglia, myxomas rarely are cystic. The radiograph usually demonstrates a nonspecific, poorly defined soft tissue mass. With CT, myxomas appear as well-demarcated and homogeneous masses with attenuation coefficients in the range of 10 to 60 Hounsfield units.[637]

Leiomyomas. Leiomyomas are uncommon outside of the uterus and gastrointestinal tract but may be found in the skin and subcutaneous soft tissue.[14, 365–367] One type, the vascular leiomyoma, arises from small blood vessels of smooth muscle. These tumors may be solitary or multiple and usually are seen in the skin or deep soft tissues. The superficial lesions may cause paroxysmal pain. Because of the tumor's prominent vascularity, radiographic techniques, such as arteriography or contrast-enhanced CT scanning or MR imaging, may demonstrate the lesion.

Other Tumors. Other lesions occurring in soft tissue include histiocytoma,[368] xanthomatosis,[369, 370] rhabdomyoma,[371–373] and myoblastoma.[14, 371] These lesions have no specific radiographic findings (see Chapter 95).

MALIGNANT SOFT TISSUE TUMORS

Malignant Fibrous Histiocytomas

Malignant fibrous histiocytoma is the most common soft tissue sarcoma occurring in late adult life (50 to 70 years of age).[14, 368, 452–455, 610, 638, 639] It is rare in children or in patients under 20 years of age. Its histogenesis remains controversial, but the tumor generally is regarded as arising from primitive mesenchymal cells that demonstrate partial

histiocytic (phagocytosis) and fibroblastic (collagen production) differentiation. Many histologic appearances are found, necessitating the separation of the neoplasm into five subtypes: (1) storiform-pleomorphic (most common), (2) myxoid, (3) giant cell, (4) inflammatory, and (5) angiomatoid. The lesion predominates in white men and is most frequent in the deep soft tissue of the extremities (especially in the legs) and retroperitoneum. Notable exceptions to this preferred site occur in the inflammatory type of tumor, which is seen most commonly in the retroperitoneum, and in the angiomatoid type of tumor, which most frequently arises in the extremities in the superficial tissues, including the subcutis and hypodermis. Another distinguishing feature of the angiomatoid malignant fibrous histiocytoma is its occurrence in patients less than 20 years old.

Clinically, a patient with a malignant fibrous histiocytoma in the extremity typically comes to medical attention with a painless mass of several months' duration. Retroperitoneal malignant fibrous histiocytomas are associated with constitutional symptoms, such as malaise, weight loss, and anorexia, and, occasionally, a palpable mass. An unusual symptom complex including fever and leukocytosis with neutrophilia or eosinophilia can be seen, especially in the inflammatory type of tumor. After removal of the neoplasm, these symptoms usually disappear.

Grossly, the mass is multinodular, circumscribed, and about 5 to 10 cm in diameter. It frequently spreads between muscles and along fascial planes with local extension, which probably explains its high recurrence rate. Focal hemorrhage and necrosis are common within the primary tumor; in some instances, these latter findings produce a fluctuant, clinically palpable mass, which, when removed, has a dominant cystic appearance with hemorrhage. Metastases are frequent, usually involving the lungs, lymph nodes, liver, and bones. The primary tumor usually will be obvious when metastatic disease is noted. This finding is helpful diagnostically when the pathologist is evaluating an isolated spindle cell neoplasm in the lung or lymph node.

Radiologic evaluation shows a well-defined, homogeneous soft tissue mass that may calcify[640] and, rarely, erode bone. CT scanning demonstrates a mass with some areas that reveal enhancement (vascularly intact tumor) and others that are nonenhancing, corresponding to sites of necrosis with cystic and hemorrhagic spaces. The malignant fibrous histiocytoma usually is hypervascular during angiography.[452] MR imaging findings are not specific.[694]

Liposarcomas

Liposarcoma is a common soft tissue malignancy.[1, 14, 374–387] It is seen most frequently in adults (fifth decade) but may occur at any age.[642] Young children have a more favorable prognosis.[377, 388] The tumors usually are located in the fat-containing or deep soft tissues of the buttock, thigh, lower leg, and retroperitoneum, and there is a slight male predominance.[1, 14] Clinically these lesions are either poorly defined or well-circumscribed swellings or masses. Recurrence after surgery is common. Although the duration of symptoms may be long, thus suggesting origin from an antecedent benign lesion as a possibility, it generally is agreed that liposarcomas arise de novo rather than from benign lipomas.[1, 14] The usual treatment is surgery, but local recurrence is common. The most common sites for metastasis are the lungs, pleurae, and liver.[14]

Liposarcomas often are large, bulky tumors. They not infrequently appear grossly as a circumscribed or encapsulated lesion, but usually they infiltrate into adjacent soft tissue[14, 92] (Fig. 84–20). Several different histologic types occur. The most common type found in the extremities, especially the thigh and popliteal area, is the well-differentiated myxoid form of liposarcoma.[1, 376–378, 388]

Radiographically, the liposarcoma usually presents as a nonhomogeneous, poorly defined mass that may calcify.[19, 61] The mass may be well circumscribed, however, with obvious fatty content on plain films. The latter finding is seen most frequently in the well-differentiated liposarcoma[61, 389] (Fig. 84–21). CT scanning may demonstrate the fatty character as a nonhomogeneous, fat-containing mass, with structures of water density and with poor margins[620] (Fig. 84–22). The portions of water density usually will show enhancement on CT scans after intravenous injection of contrast medium; these regions correspond to the hypervascular areas. Liposarcomas may contain little or no fat in MR images.[668] When fat is present it usually is irregular, with thick septa, solid components, and masses that are mostly isointense to muscle in T1-weighted and hyperintense to muscle in T2-weighted spin echo MR images.[668, 685, 686, 691] Occasionally, nonlipogenic tumors may infiltrate normal fat tissue, trapping the fat and producing a mottled appearance. This pattern can be confused with liposarcoma; however, it usually does not have the bulky fatty component seen in well-differentiated liposarcoma.

Synovial Sarcomas

Synovial sarcoma is an uncommon malignant tumor, which is located most frequently in the soft tissue of the extremities[390–399] (Fig. 84–23). The lower extremities are affected more commonly than the upper extremities, with the knee, ankle, and foot involved most frequently. The neoplasms generally arise adjacent to a joint, bursa, or tendon sheath. Fewer than 10 per cent are located primarily within the joint cavity, however.[377] Occasionally the synovial membrane is involved by direct extension. Synovial sarcomas occur at all ages but are most frequent in the young adult and rare in infants.[14, 400, 401, 643]

Clinically, patients have a painful swelling or mass. Rarely, cutaneous pain will be present without a palpable tumor mass.[402, 403] The tumor usually grows slowly, with the duration of symptoms from onset to death varying from 5 months to 16 years.[14, 404, 405] Metastasis, when present, usually occurs to the lungs. Local recurrence after surgery is common and is associated with a poor prognosis.[1]

The tumors are grossly solid, with sharply circumscribed margins, appearing encapsulated. Adjacent soft tissue structures usually are displaced, and local extension occurs. Microscopically, the tumors usually have a biphasic histologic appearance.[14, 406–408] One phase demonstrates slightly enlarged polygonal cells and occasional cylindrical cells growing in cords arranged around clefts or slits, resulting in an adenomatous or pseudoglandular appearance. The other phase shows spindle-shaped cells (fibrous-appearing) filling in the areas between the slits.[14] Occasionally, one cell type will predominate, giving the tumor a monophasic appearance. These histologic patterns have been subclassified into (1) pseudoglandular, (2) fibrosarcoma, and (3) endothelioid types. The first two patterns may have a more favorable prognosis.[377]

Radiographically, a soft tissue mass possessing a variable peripheral margin, ranging from smooth to indistinct, usually is present.[409, 410, 644–646] Spotty calcification is common, occurring in about one third of lesions.[390, 411] The tumor also can cause adjacent osteoporosis or bone destruction. In slow-growing lesions, bone destruction appears as an extrinsic pressure erosion (Fig. 84–23). If the bone has been invaded, however, an aggressive pattern of irregular destruction is seen. Arteriography in synovial sarcoma usually demonstrates a hypervascular lesion with neovascularity and nonhomogeneous staining. Occasionally the lesion is hypovascular. CT scanning shows a soft tissue mass, which may infiltrate adjacent structures. Because of its extensive vascular supply, the synovial sarcoma enhances after injection of contrast medium. With MR imaging, a mass of low signal intensity in T1-weighted spin echo MR images and of high signal intensity in T2-weighted spin echo images is typical. Fluid levels may be observed.

Rhabdomyosarcomas

Rhabdomyosarcoma is a common malignant soft tissue tumor of muscle origin, which has an exceedingly poor prognosis.[412–422] Two distinct groups exist, one found in children and the other in adults. In children, the mass frequently is found in the head and neck or genitourinary tract. Tumors in adult patients most commonly occur in the deep

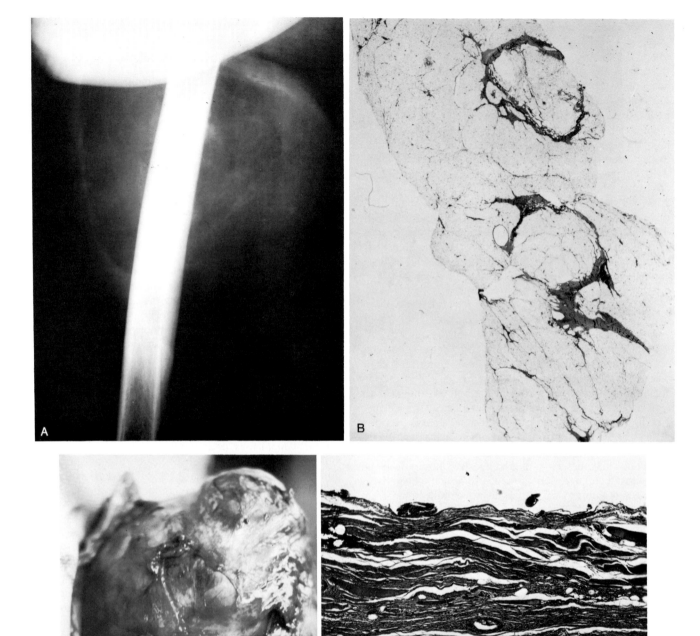

FIGURE 84–20. Liposarcoma of the thigh, well-differentiated type. This 44 year old woman had a progressively enlarging thigh mass of 2 years' duration.

   A Oblique radiograph shows a large, sharply circumscribed, nonhomogeneous fatty mass with a linear component of water density.

   B Photomicrograph (low power view) confirms the fatty nature and fibrous septa of the tumor. The latter cause the nonhomogeneous radiographic feature.

   C Gross specimen demonstrates the sharp, well-delineated peripheral margin.

   D Photomicrograph (high power view) reveals a fibrous pseudocapsule about the periphery of the tumor.

(Armed Forces Institute of Pathology Neg. Nos. 73-11119-1, 76-5775-1, 73-11241-1, 76-5785-1.)

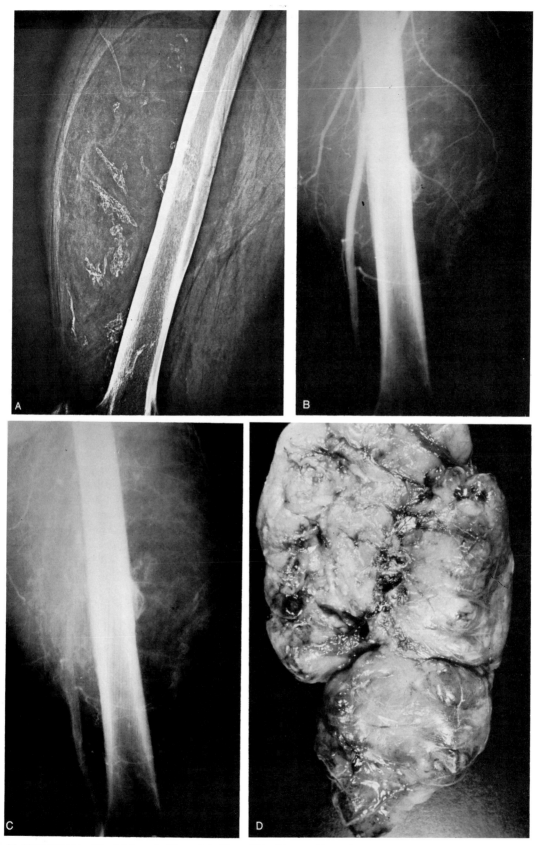

FIGURE 84–21. Liposarcoma of the thigh, well-differentiated type. This 45 year old man had a rapidly growing soft tissue mass in the thigh.

A Lateral xeroradiograph shows the sharply circumscribed, fatty mass with multiple calcifications. Some dense areas have a trabecular pattern and represent ossification.

B Arteriogram (arterial phase) demonstrates a relatively hypervascular lesion with vessel displacement and neovascularity.

C Arteriogram (late arterial phase) reveals a nonhomogeneous blush.

D Gross specimen demonstrates the well-delineated tumor margin.

(Armed Forces Institute of Pathology Neg. Nos. 77-7859-4,2,3; 77-7820.)

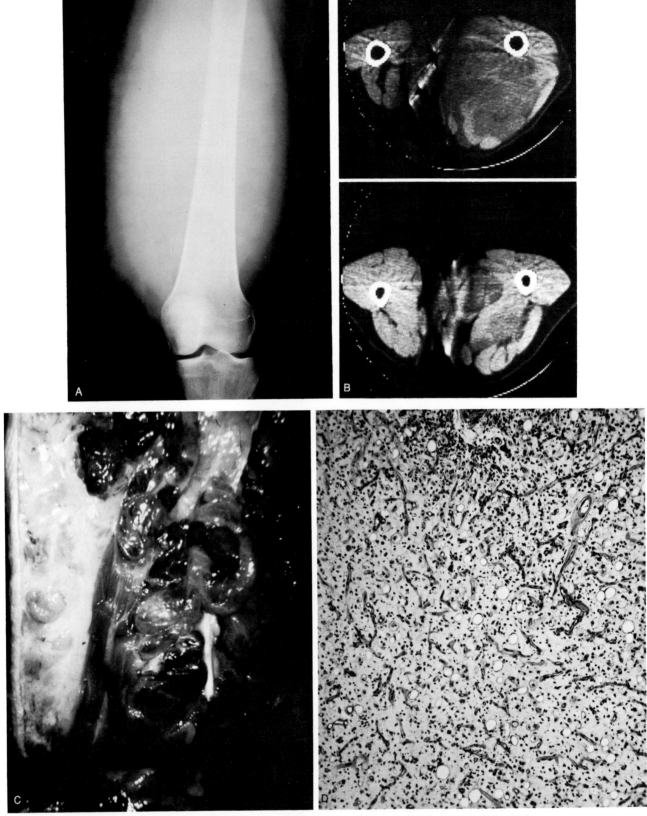

FIGURE 84–22. Liposarcoma of the thigh, myxoid type. This 30 year old woman had a large, hard mass in the thigh.

  A Anteroposterior radiograph shows a large mass of water density with a poorly defined margin medially.

  B A nonhomogeneous, low attenuation coefficient mass is noted on CT. This finding suggests a fatty component not appreciated on plain film **(A)**. The margin is irregular, with infiltration into adjacent soft tissue.

  C Gross specimen confirms the fatty nature and infiltrative features of the tumor.

  D Photomicrograph (63×) demonstrates delicate vascular channels, loose myxoid stroma, and lipoblasts.

  (Armed Forces Institute of Pathology Neg. Nos. 77-9059-4,7; 77-7931-5; 79-16670.)

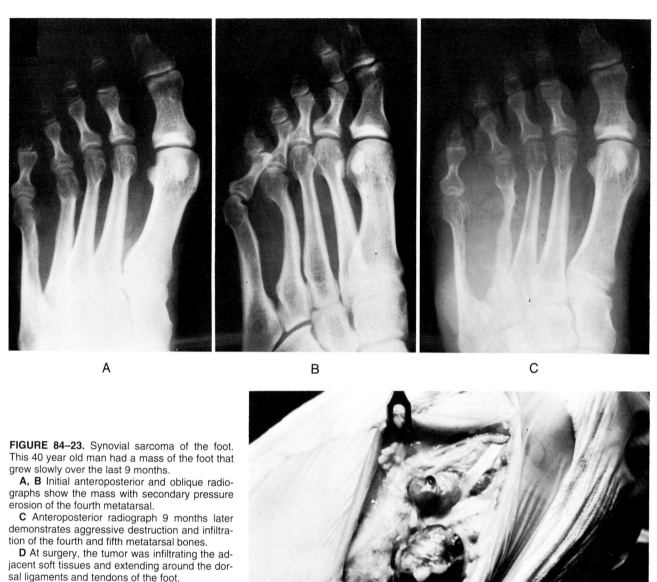

A   B   C

D

FIGURE 84–23. Synovial sarcoma of the foot. This 40 year old man had a mass of the foot that grew slowly over the last 9 months.

A, B Initial anteroposterior and oblique radiographs show the mass with secondary pressure erosion of the fourth metatarsal.

C Anteroposterior radiograph 9 months later demonstrates aggressive destruction and infiltration of the fourth and fifth metatarsal bones.

D At surgery, the tumor was infiltrating the adjacent soft tissues and extending around the dorsal ligaments and tendons of the foot.

(Armed Forces Institute of Pathology Neg. Nos. 74-19670-1,2; 74-12420-3,6.)

soft tissues of the extremities. Grossly, the lesions have a soft consistency. Infiltration of local tissues is common and probably is responsible for the frequent recurrence after initial surgery. Distant spread to the lungs and occasionally lymph nodes also is common. Three histologic types occur: embryonic, alveolar, and pleomorphic. The embryonic type is the most common type and typically occurs in children. This histologic pattern is uncommon in the extremities. The alveolar type tends to affect older children and young adults and frequently is found in the extremities. The pleomorphic type is the least common and predominates in the skeletal muscles of adults. Radiographically, these tumors appear as poorly defined soft tissue masses. They tend to involve adjacent bone by local extension, resulting in either destruction or saucerization, or, occasionally, sclerosis of the cortex. Calcification within the tumor also may occur and is more common than is generally appreciated.[16, 417] The rhabdomyosarcoma usually is hypervascular on arteriography.

Fibrosarcomas

Fibrosarcoma appears as a swelling or mass among the fibrous supportive structures of muscles, tendons, ligaments, and fasciae.[423–427] The tumor is most frequent in the external soft tissues of the extremities, such as the thighs,[428] and occasionally develops in cicatrices after trauma or irradiation.[14] Fibrosarcoma is found in both adults and children and has a male predominance. It is less often fatal when present in children.[429, 430] The tumor infiltrates the adjacent soft tissue, and therefore recurrence after surgery is frequent.

Grossly, fibrosarcomas are firm, with poorly defined margins, and vary widely in size. The histologic distinction between fibromatosis and well-differentiated fibrosarcoma can be difficult.[14] In the latter tumor, fewer fibers are present; disproportionate cell size and mitoses are found without difficulty.

The fibrosarcoma appears as a nonspecific soft tissue mass on the plain film radiograph. Infiltration into adjacent bone with destruction and calcification, although not common, can be seen. Arteriography demonstrates hypervascularity with neovascularity. The angioarchitecture usually is uneven owing to the heterogeneous arrangement of the fibrosarcoma.[428] The more vascular tumors generally reflect a higher grade sarcoma and a poorer prognosis.[428, 431, 432]

The fibrosarcomas in infants are unique and differ from the fibrosarcomas of adults.[429, 430, 433–437, 647, 648] They usually occur within the first 2 years of life, frequently at birth, and have a better prognosis (Fig. 84–24). These tumors are more common in boys and chiefly affect the distal areas of the lower and upper extremities. Like the adult type, they are poorly marginated and infiltrate adjacent tissues. After treatment, which usually is wide local excision or amputation, late recurrence and metastatic disease can occur. Thus, long-term follow-up is necessary. Radiographically, a soft tissue mass is seen, and frequently severe deformity and marked erosions of adjacent bone are noted (Fig. 84–24).

Other Malignant Soft Tissue Tumors

Other malignant soft tissue tumors may be considered in the differential diagnosis of soft tissue masses in and about the joint; among these are malignant schwannoma,[1] leiomyosarcoma,[1, 438–441, 649, 650] extraskeletal osteosarcoma,[14, 442–444] extraskeletal chondrosarcoma,[14, 443–451] mesenchymoma,[1, 14] and epithelioid sarcoma[1] (see Chapter 95).

The malignant schwannoma and leiomyosarcoma are found uncommonly in the extremities, with the exception of malignant schwannoma associated with neurofibromatosis.[1] Extraskeletal osteosarcoma and extraskeletal chondrosarcoma occur in the deeper soft tissues of the extremities. Mineralized osteoid with a homogeneous pattern may be seen in the former, and a stippled calcification pattern, suggesting chondroid matrix, may be seen in the latter. The mesenchymoma and epithelioid sarcoma also will be found in the extremities. These lesions are associated with no specific radiographic findings, however.

SOFT TISSUE TUMOR–LIKE LESIONS

Myositis Ossificans

Localized myositis ossificans is a tumor-like heterotopic formation of bone and cartilage in soft tissue, usually muscles, but also tendons, ligaments, fasciae, aponeuroses, and joint capsules.[1, 14, 456–467] Patients of any age or either sex may be affected. They usually develop a mass after trauma, although ossification also is encountered with some frequency, especially about the knee, thigh, and hip, in paraplegic patients.[1, 462] The mass may be doughy, painful, and warm during its early development. With time, the lesion shrinks to a firm and definable mass attached to the adjacent soft tissues or bone.[1, 459] Growth of the mass occurs during this active proliferative phase and is self-limited.[14] Although lesions usually are small, occasionally they may be quite large—up to 10 cm in diameter.[14] The proliferating tissue, including osteoid, interdigitates with the muscle bundles. During this active phase, the florid osteoblastic repair tissue may be mistaken for an osteosarcoma on biopsy.[14, 456, 468] Rarely an osteosarcoma may arise from this otherwise

benign process.[469, 470] Eventually, the lesion develops into a mass of mature bone with a cortical shell surrounding central cancellous, less mature tissue.[471]

Serial radiographs are required to appreciate a dynamic changing pattern[49, 468, 472–475] (Fig. 84–25). Initially, a nonspecific, poorly defined soft tissue mass without calcification is seen. As cell proliferation and maturation occur, the peripheral zone produces osteoid, which in turn will mineralize. This change appears from 4 to 6 weeks after injury and results in a well-developed ossified shell surrounding a central radiolucent, usually cystic area (Fig. 84–26) from 8 to 10 weeks post injury. Sonography data are similar to those obtained with plain film radiography.[472] Myositis ossificans, if associated with a deep injury, may involve the periosteum and attach to bone with superficial erosion or thickening of the cortex (Fig. 84–26). If adjacent bones are closely apposed, myositis ossificans in the intervening soft tissue may produce bony struts with synostosis. Joint ligaments and capsules also may be involved, producing external ankylosis. Arteriographic findings in myositis ossificans vary during the different phases of the disease.[474] In the acute phase, the lesion is hypervascular with fine vessels and staining on late films. In the healing phase, the lesion usually is avascular. MR imaging findings similarly are variable, depending on the stage of the process (see Chapter 95).

Villonodular Synovitis

Villonodular synovitis is a proliferative disorder of the synovium, which frequently is localized or nodular.[476–498] The mass is thought to arise in the synovial lining of joints, tendon sheaths, fascial planes, or ligamentous tissue. It usually involves young adults and is slightly more common in men. The lesions appear as nonpainful soft tissue masses, frequently located in the digits of the hands and feet (Fig. 84–27). Other joints, especially the knees,[586] and tendon sheaths can be involved. A monoarticular distribution is the rule, but rare polyarticular involvement occurs. The cause is unknown[499–502]; some investigators consider it an inflammatory response,[503] whereas others consider it a neoplasm.[14]

Grossly, localized villonodular synovitis is a firm, nodular mass, with a gray or yellowish appearance. Microscopically, considerable variability is seen in the histologic pattern. Low power views reflect an accentuated villous and nodular morphologic appearance. Higher magnification reveals extensive cellular (stromal cell) proliferation in association with fibroblastic tissue, multinucleated giant cells, xanthoma cells, lymphocytes, and variable amounts of hemosiderin deposition. The varying histologic features have resulted in a number of synonyms, such as giant cell tumor, fibroma, fibroxanthoma, or xanthoma of the tendon sheath.

The localized nodular lesion described previously probably should be differentiated from a more diffuse pigmented villonodular synovitis.[504, 505] The latter is less common and usually involves the larger joints, especially the knee. Grossly, the specimen is brown, owing to extensive hemosiderin deposition. It often is associated with hemorrhagic effusions and is thought by some observers to represent a vascular anomaly,[505] distinguishing it from villonodular synovitis, which may be either a reactive or a true neoplastic process. Such differentiation between villonodular syno-

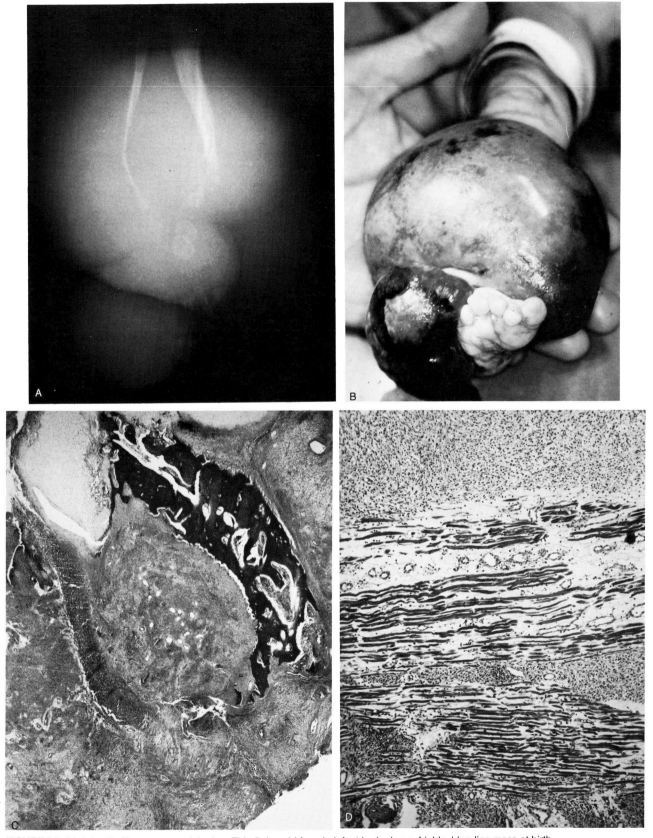

FIGURE 84–24. Infantile fibrosarcoma of the leg. This 3 day old female infant had a large, friable, bleeding mass at birth.
A Conventional tomography of the leg shows a large water-density mass with displacement, deformity, and erosion of the tibia and fibula.
B The mass with its bleeding surface is seen on the clinical photograph.
C Photomicrograph (15×) demonstrates the tumor infiltrating bone, as seen in the radiograph **(A)**.
D Photomicrograph (63×) taken from the soft tissue component of the mass shows tumor infiltrating muscle.
(Armed Forces Institute of Pathology Neg. Nos. 77-477-9, 77-432-2, 79-16668, 79-16665.)

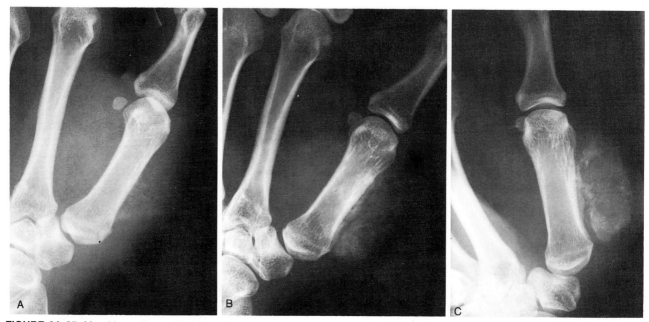

FIGURE 84–25. Myositis ossificans (florid reactive periostitis) of the hand with serial radiographic changes. This 24 year old woman had swelling adjacent to the first metacarpal bone of 2 months' duration. The evolving radiographic characteristics of this lesion are consistent with myositis ossificans or florid reactive periostitis (see Chapter 95).
  A Initial film shows soft tissue swelling with poorly defined calcification.
  B Follow-up film 3 weeks later demonstrates an organized calcification pattern. The lesion has a peripheral shell of increased density with a less dense center. Also noted is periosteal reaction and attachment of the process to the adjacent bone.
  C The attachment and peripheral shell of bone are best seen on this oblique radiograph.
  (Armed Forces Institute of Pathology Neg. Nos. 73-3602-2,5,1.)

vitis and pigmented villonodular synovitis is not always possible on histologic grounds.[504] Thus, some authorities use the term pigmented villonodular synovitis to encompass all of these various synovial processes[506] (see Chapter 95).

On radiographs, localized villonodular synovitis appears as a soft tissue mass, frequently associated with bony erosions[507–514] (Fig. 84–27). These erosions have well-defined sclerotic margins and are a sign not of malignancy but of direct extension and pressure effect.[515] Diffuse intra-articular pigmented villonodular synovitis produces a joint effusion. Usually, the joint space is normal in width and osteoporosis is absent or mild. Bony erosions can occur in juxta-articular locations and are variable in size. Such osseous defects are more frequent in "tight" joints, such as the hip, the elbow, and the wrist. Calcification is not typical, although cartilaginous and osseous metaplasia of the synovial lining has been encountered on rare occasions. If hemosiderin deposition is extensive, it can be demonstrable on CT scans as increased attenuation values.[516] MR imaging also will demonstrate the joint effusion, bone erosions, and hemosiderin-laden tissue[687–690] (see Chapter 95). Arteriography usually shows a hypervascular lesion. In the late stages, or if fibrosis dominates, however, the lesion may appear avascular. Arthrography likewise will show the lesion and its extent as a localized nodule or a diffuse villonodular mass.[517–520]

The differential diagnosis of the radiographic features of localized nodular synovitis includes other soft tissue tumors and tumor-like lesions. Diffuse pigmented villonodular synovitis must be differentiated from idiopathic synovial osteochondromatosis (in which calcification and ossification may appear), infection (in which osteoporosis, joint space loss, and poorly defined bony erosions may be seen), and other articular disorders.

Idiopathic Tumoral Calcinosis

Idiopathic tumoral calcinosis is a rare condition, consisting of calcium salt deposition in extracapsular soft tissues about joints[521–527] (Fig. 84–28). The masses are painless and occur most frequently in children and adolescents. An increased prevalence in blacks and a familial tendency are recognized.[529] These lesions are found most commonly about the shoulders, hips, and elbows. They are considered idiopathic, but metabolic defects, collagen vascular disorders, and trauma have been suggested in their pathogenesis.[528] Because the masses are extracapsular, there is little limitation of motion at the joint unless the tumors are exceedingly large. The cutaneous surface over the masses occasionally breaks down, and a draining sinus with chalky material will be found. This draining sinus may become infected secondarily if it is not treated adequately. The deposits tend to grow and recur after incomplete excision. Rarely, the serum alkaline phosphatase and phosphate levels will be elevated.[530–532]

At surgery, the masses are found to be encapsulated, multilocular spaces with dense, fibrous walls. The spaces are filled with very viscous semifluid calcium salts and white particles. Microscopically, these cysts are lined by giant cells with adjacent lymphocytic infiltration.[10, 533–535]

These masses of tumoral calcinosis usually appear extremely dense, homogeneous, and loculated on the radiographs[536–541] (Fig. 84–28). Initially, however, only faint calcification may be seen within the multiloculated lesions,

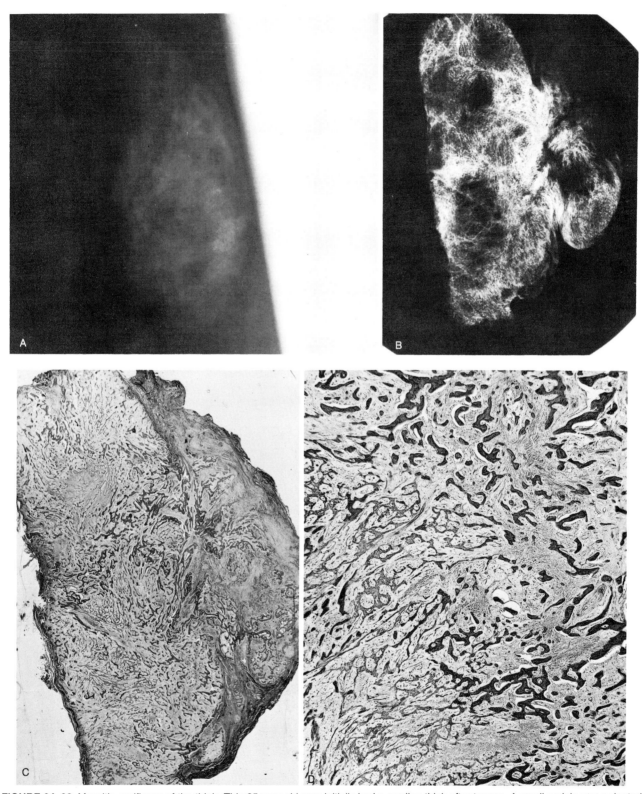

FIGURE 84–26. Myositis ossificans of the thigh. This 25 year old man initially had a swollen thigh after trauma. A small nodule was palpated several months later.
   A Anteroposterior radiograph taken several months after the injury shows an oval calcified soft tissue mass with a peripheral shell.
   B The peripheral shell, bony trabecular pattern, and less dense (lucent) areas are noted on the specimen radiograph.
   C Macroslide shows an admixture of fibrous tissue and varying degrees of maturing bone trabeculae surrounded by a bony shell.
   D Photomicrograph (11×) more clearly demonstrates varying degrees of bone maturation.
   (Armed Forces Institute of Pathology Neg. Nos. 74-8835-1,3; 75-3853; 75-3852.)

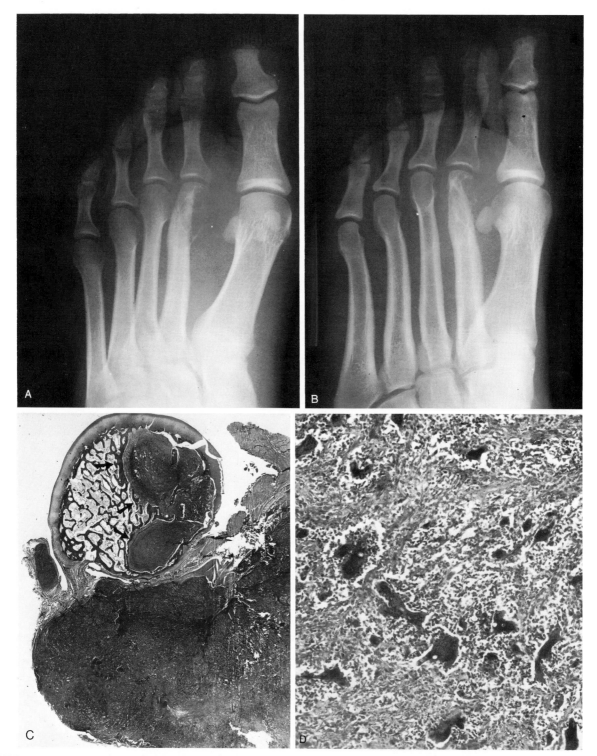

FIGURE 84–27. Villonodular synovitis of the foot. This 17 year old man had a mass on the plantar aspect of the foot.

A Anteroposterior radiograph shows a soft tissue mass widening the space between the first and second metatarsal bones and bone erosions.

B Oblique radiograph reveals multiple, well-circumscribed bone erosions with sclerotic margins involving the second metatarsal head.

C Macroscopic coronal cut through the distal second metatarsal head demonstrates the large plantar mass with erosion into bone. Note the sclerotic bony margins (arrows) about the intraosseous extension.

D Photomicrograph (63×) documents the proliferative stromal cells, giant cells, and fibrous components that characterize this lesion.

(Armed Forces Institute of Pathology Neg. Nos. 66-2598-1,2; 71-3116-1; 71-3118.)

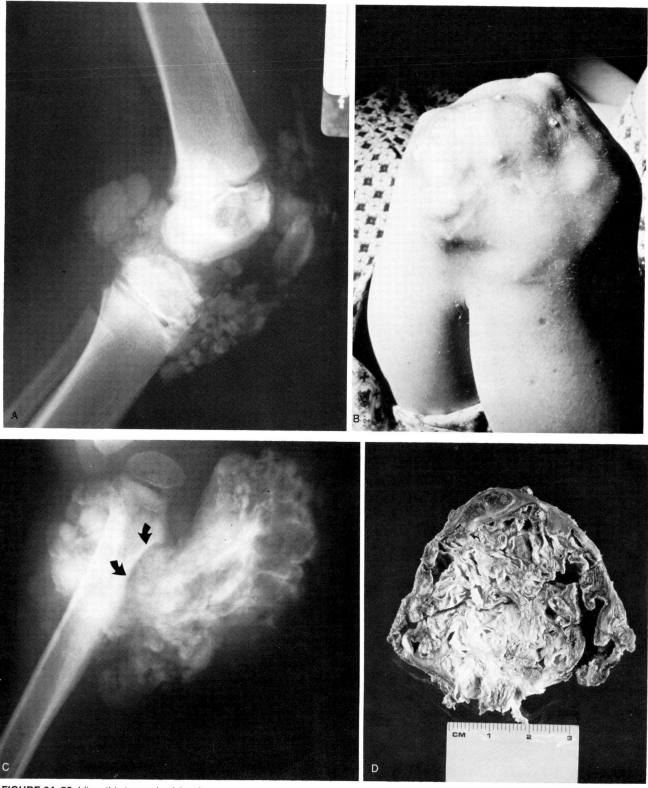

FIGURE 84–28. Idiopathic tumoral calcinosis.
   A, B Knee. This 7 year old boy had a swollen knee of 2 years' duration. There was no evidence of pain, trauma, or infection. **A,** Lateral radiograph shows homogeneous calcific dense nodules about the knee joint. **B,** The clinical photograph demonstrates the knee in a flexed position, indicating little limitation of motion. Note the nodular surface of the skin, with areas of draining sinus tracts, old cutaneous scars, and pointing of a few nodules. These represent cutaneous complications from the subcutaneous nodules.
   C, D Shoulder. This patient is a 2 year old child with a shoulder mass of 6 months' duration. **C,** Axillary radiograph demonstrates a nonhomogeneous, dense, multilocular-appearing mass about the shoulder with humeral erosions (arrows). **D,** Gross specimen confirms the multilocular configuration, fibrous septa, and grumous material within these locules.
   (Armed Forces Institute of Pathology Neg. Nos. 74-8966-2, 74-11906-1, 78-1059-2, 77-8127-2.)

with radiolucent septa of water density separating the lobules of calcification. The peripheral margin is smooth and bosselated. Fluid calcium layers on an upright film or CT scan may be seen rarely.[542, 543] Adjacent bone erosion from pressure by the mass occurs but is rare.

Aneurysms

Popliteal artery aneurysm is the most common aneurysm found in the extremities.[544–547] Patients usually first come to medical attention in the fifth or sixth decade of life with pain and claudication; however, ischemia and swelling in the lower leg and neurologic symptoms resulting from pressure on the sciatic nerve also can be noted. Rarely a patient is asymptomatic. The aneurysm usually is palpated on physical examination. It commonly is associated with additional aneurysms, especially of the contralateral popliteal artery or of the abdominal aorta. Complications usually are arterial in origin, such as thrombosis, rupture of the aneurysm, or embolic occlusion of the artery distal to the aneurysm.

Radiographically, the aneurysm appears as a pulsatile soft tissue mass in the popliteal space. Curvilinear calcification may be noted in the aneurysm wall. The aneurysm also may erode adjacent bone, causing scalloping of the cortex. Arteriography is extremely helpful in evaluating the arterial and venous vascular beds and in demonstrating the vascular origin of the soft tissue mass. Occasionally partial occlusion by venous thrombosis of the popliteal vein may be demonstrated. Sonography, Doppler studies, radionuclide venography, MR imaging, and CT scanning also may establish the diagnosis (see Chapters 70 and 95).

Granulomatous Synovitis

Advanced granulomatous synovitis, especially tuberculous synovitis, which results from chronic infection, produces such a proliferative granulomatous pannus that it may cause a soft tissue mass in or about the joint (Fig. 84–29). The process is insidious and progressive, with ultimate destruction of the joint. The organisms usually reach the joint by hematogenous spread but occasionally extend directly from an adjacent bony or bursal focus. The primary site usually is the lung. The chest radiograph frequently fails to show extensive disease, however.[548, 549]

The patients have a painful, swollen, tender, doughy joint and occasionally a draining sinus tract. This clinical setting easily can be misinterpreted as evidence of a tumor, because these patients usually do not have toxic symptoms. Granulomatous synovitis is a monoarticular disease most commonly involving the hip, knee, elbow, or ankle.

The gross appearance may resemble an infiltrating tumor, with a mass that involves a joint and extends into the adjacent soft tissue, causing extensive tissue destruction and fibrotic reaction. Microscopic evaluation, however, will document the granulomatous nature of the process and therefore characterize the lesion correctly.

The radiographic findings depend on the stage of development.[550–554] Early disease is manifested as nonspecific soft tissue swelling. Arteriography at this time may show a hypervascular inflammatory synovitis (Fig. 84–29). With progression, however, the findings become more specific, with a soft tissue mass, juxta-articular osteoporosis, and

marginal bony erosions in the non–weight-bearing surfaces. Eventually, the articular cartilage and subarticular bone plate will be destroyed. With repair, the extensive soft tissue, articular, and bone destruction may heal, with subsequent soft tissue calcification and bony ankylosis.

Synovial Cysts

A variety of cystic lesions may be found about a joint, especially the knee, including a synovial cyst, a distended bursa (with or without communication with the adjacent articulation), and a meniscal cyst (see Chapters 70 and 95). The term ''synovial cyst'' describes a continuation or herniation of the synovial membrane through the joint capsule. The common popliteal cyst is most identifiable, owing to its location in the posterior aspect of the knee. It results from a communication of the joint with the gastrocnemio-semimembranosus bursa.[588–591] Similar lesions at other locations (shoulder, elbow, hip, hand, foot, and ankle) can be seen but are less frequent.[592, 593] Synovial cysts commonly contain fluid and often are associated with traumatic, degenerative, or inflammatory processes in the joint.[594–596] Rheumatoid arthritis is the most recognized cause of large synovial cysts.

Synovial cysts are of clinical significance because they may appear as a periarticular mass, cause pain or limitation of joint mobility, or compress adjacent neurovascular structures; they also may rupture acutely or dissect or become infected secondarily.[597–600]

Grossly, synovial cysts can be unilocular or multilocular. The wall of the cyst is composed of predominantly acellular dense fibrous tissue. Rarely, dystrophic calcification within the fibrous wall may be demonstrated.[601] If the cysts are not infected or traumatized severely, they are lined with flat or cuboidal cells. With regard to imaging techniques, the identification of the fluid-filled cystic mass can be accomplished with arthrography (particularly if the cyst communicates with the nearby joint), sonography, MR imaging, and CT scanning.[602–608] Occasionally synovial cysts may produce smooth erosions and sclerosis in the adjacent bone.[609]

Small cysts about the knee may be associated with meniscal tears. These are referred to as meniscal cysts, and typically they involve the lateral aspect of the joint (see Chapters 13 and 70).

BONE TUMORS

Benign Bone Tumors

Bone tumors may involve the adjacent soft tissue and should be a consideration in the differential diagnosis of soft tissue tumors in and about the joint. Usually obvious bony change on the radiograph will indicate the origin of the lesion. These bony changes may be seen in both benign and malignant bone tumors. Benign bone tumors involving soft tissue usually arise from the bone surface and include osteochondroma, periosteal (juxtacortical) chondroma, articular chondroma (Trevor's disease), and osteoid osteoma. Occasionally benign intraosseous lesions such as giant cell tumor (Fig. 84–30) and chondroblastoma will extend beyond the confines of the bony cortex into the adjacent soft tissue. Postoperative recurrences of benign bone tumors frequently will involve the soft tissue and are seen most commonly with giant cell tumors.

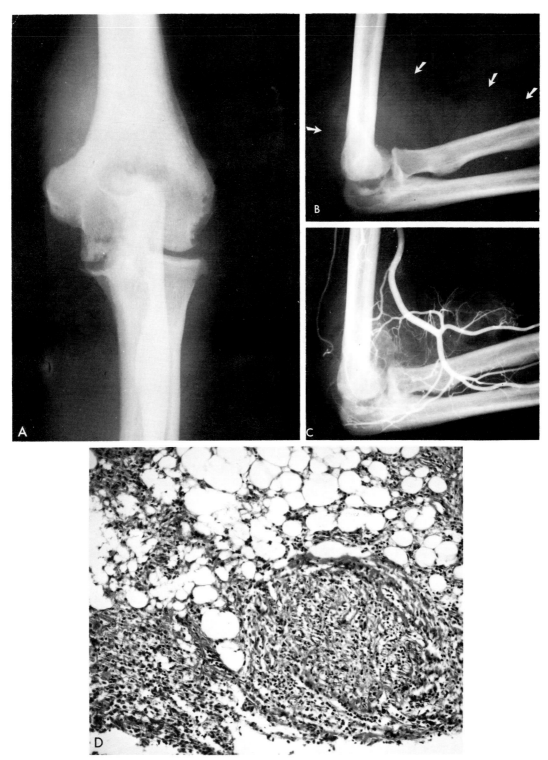

FIGURE 84–29. Tuberculous synovitis of the elbow. This 61 year old man had pain and a doughy mass about the elbow of 6 months' duration.
A Anteroposterior radiograph shows para-articular bony erosions with relative sparing of the joint space.
B Lateral radiograph demonstrates a large mass (arrows) and bony erosions.
C The mass is hypervascular, with neovascularity and vessel displacement demonstrated on arteriography.
D Photomicrograph (157×) confirms the presence of a granulomatous synovitis.
(Armed Forces Institute of Pathology Neg. Nos. 73-7980-3,4,2; 80-233.)

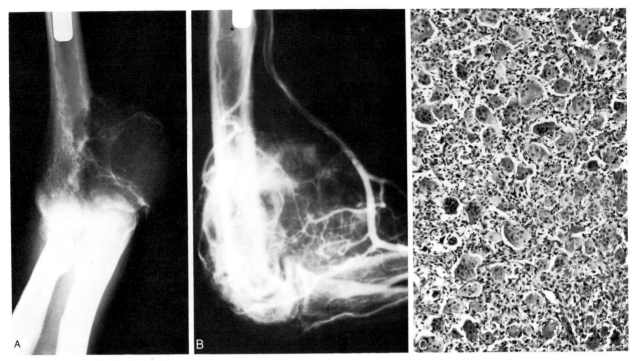

FIGURE 84–30. Giant cell tumor of the humerus. This 37 year old man had pain and swelling in the elbow of 5 years' duration. The mass had increased in size during the last year, with limitation of motion.
  A Anteroposterior radiograph shows an expansile "bubbly" lytic lesion with bony septa and extension to the subarticular bony plate.
  B Arteriogram (arterial phase) demonstrates a hypervascular mass with neovascularity, blushing, and vessel displacement.
  C Photomicrograph (100×) demonstrates the typical pattern of this tumor.
  (Armed Forces Institute of Pathology Neg. Nos. 73-7980-1,2,3; 79-16651.)

Benign cartilage tumors of bone arising as proliferative lesions from the bony cortex, periosteum, or articular cartilage are labeled osteochondroma, periosteal chondroma, and articular chondroma (Trevor's disease), respectively.

Osteochondromas. Osteochondromas consist of hyperplastic displaced or aberrant growth plate cartilage and are characterized by a cartilage cap, perichondrium, and bony stalk. The lesions may be solitary or multiple and usually are located in the metaphyseal end of the long bone. The patients usually are asymptomatic, unless the adjacent soft tissue structures are disturbed or traumatized. The lesions are found most commonly about the knee and usually point away from the joint. Pain and rapid growth suggest malignancy, especially after the third decade of life. These symptoms also may be associated with symptomatic bursitis[555, 556] or pseudoaneurysm, especially of the popliteal artery, however.[557, 558] Grossly, osteochondromas can be of two types, sessile or pedunculated. The cortex and spongiosa of the lesion are derived from the growing cartilage cap and are in direct continuity with the parent bone. The cartilage cap may be considerably thickened or may demonstrate endochondral bone formation with mineralization. The radiograph usually shows a bony projection from the normal bone with a varying-sized cartilage cap (Fig. 84–31). The latter may have areas of stippled calcification.

Periosteal (Juxtacortical) Chondromas. Periosteal chondromas result from the growth of displaced or metaplastic cartilage within the periosteum.[559–566] They are found most frequently about the hand and foot, ankle, and proximal portions of the humerus, tibia, and femur and usually are discovered in the third to fifth decades of life. Pathologically, these lesions are located on the cortical surface of bone and are covered by a fibrous capsule (perichondrium). Microscopically, myxoid degeneration, pleomorphism, and double nuclei are found and underscore the importance of the pathologist's being aware of the presence of the tumor, as it frequently resembles more ominous cartilaginous neoplasms.

Radiographs show a soft tissue mass, with scalloping of the adjacent bony cortex. The intact cortical margin is sclerotic and separates the lesion from the adjacent marrow cavity. A small periosteal buttress on either side of the lesion is frequent. Stippled calcification within the mass also is common.

Articular Chondromas. Articular chondromas, often referred to as dysplasia epiphysealis hemimelica or Trevor's disease[567–572, 651] (see Chapter 88), also represent a form of cartilage proliferation. The lesion is an osteocartilaginous growth involving single or multiple epiphyses on one side of the body. It is more frequent in boys and usually is discovered during the first decade of life. Deformity, limitation of motion, and joint pain are common symptoms. The lesions usually occur on the talus and distal femoral or distal tibial epiphysis. Severe deformity and even joint fusion may occur postoperatively.[568] The condition may be hereditary and associated with chondromas elsewhere in the skeleton.[570] Grossly, the focal overgrowth or pedunculated mass of hyaline cartilage involving the epiphysis results in a misshapen articular surface. Microscopically, the findings are identical to those of other osteocartilaginous masses. Radiographically, a lobular mass is observed arising from the epiphysis, usually with calcification[652, 653] (Fig. 84–32). Initially mineralized portions of the lesion may be separated from the underlying bone by nonmineralized cartilage. As

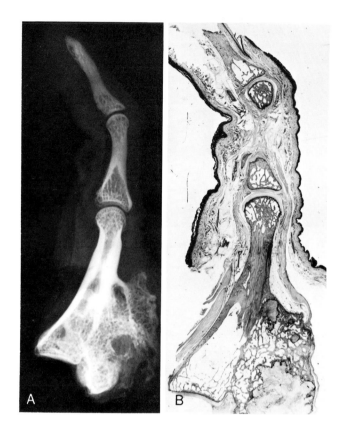

FIGURE 84–31. Osteochondroma of the proximal phalanx. A mass of long duration on the finger had shown recent growth.

A Lateral specimen radiograph shows a bony growth with an irregular surface and lucent areas. Note the trabecular pattern of the lesion and its continuity with the adjacent normal marrow space of the involved phalanx.

B Macroslide demonstrates an exophytic growth consisting of a bony stalk (trabecular pattern) and foci of cartilage of varying sizes (lucent areas).

(Armed Forces Institute of Pathology Neg. Nos. 59-6685, 72-3066.)

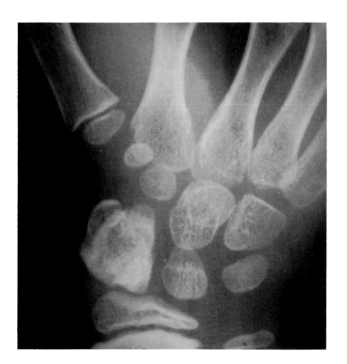

FIGURE 84–32. Trevor's disease. Note the asymmetric enlargement of the scaphoid. Histologically, the findings were virtually identical to those of an osteochondroma. More frequently, the bones about the knee or ankle are affected. (Courtesy of R. Freiberger, M.D., New York, New York.)

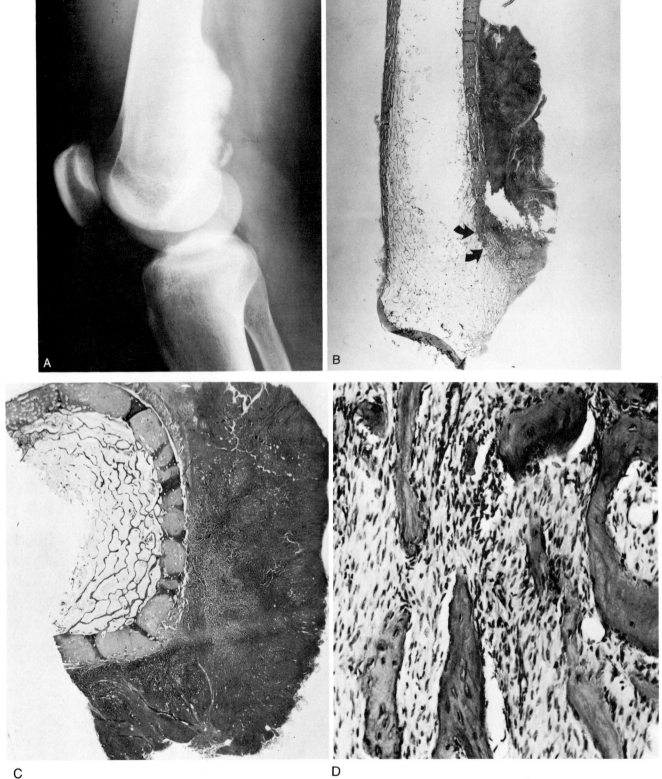

FIGURE 84–33. Parosteal osteosarcoma of the femur. This 24 year old man had pain and tenderness on the posterior aspect of the knee of 1 year's duration.

A Lateral radiograph shows a dense homogeneous mass with an irregular margin arising from the posterior surface of the distal aspect of the femur.

B Sagittal cut macroslide corresponding to the radiograph in **A** demonstrates a tumor mass arising from the posterior femoral cortical surface with minimal growth (arrows) into the bone distally. This location is typical of parosteal osteosarcomas.

C A cross-sectional macroslide confirms the bone nature of the lesion, which accounts for the homogeneous dense area on the radiograph.

D Photomicrograph (165×) reveals irregular and slightly atypical bone trabeculae separated by an excessively cellular spindle cell pattern. This also is typical of parosteal osteosarcomas.

(Armed Forces Institute of Pathology Neg. Nos. 52-7554, 72-4251, 72-4253, 72-4254.)

the lesion matures, the calcification becomes confluent with the adjacent epiphyseal bone, as is seen in osteochondromas. The ossification centers may appear prematurely in affected bones.

Osteoid Osteomas. Osteoid osteoma is a common benign bone lesion of unknown cause that usually arises in the midshaft of long bones and has as its presenting symptom intermittent local pain, particularly at night.[573–580] It may produce joint swelling if it involves a segment of bone confined by a joint capsule. Under this circumstance, the lesion will appear as a monoarticular arthritis with an inflammatory synovitis and loss of range of motion. It is more frequent in men, usually occurring during the second or third decade of life. Pathologically, osteoid osteoma is characterized by a central nidus of atypical-appearing osteoid and adjacent sclerotic bone formation.

On radiographs, extra-articular cortical lesions evoke a significant degree of reactive sclerosis, although intra-articular osteoid osteomas may appear as very subtle lucent areas with little or no adjacent sclerosis. The joint is swollen, and periarticular osteoporosis is common if symptoms have been present for some time. The nidus may be difficult to see on plain films but is readily apparent on bone scan as a photodense area[581–583] or on the arteriogram as a small hypervascular focus.[584, 585] CT scanning and MR imaging also allow accurate diagnosis (see Chapter 83).

Malignant Bone Tumors

Malignant bone tumors frequently extend into the adjacent soft tissue. This extension commonly is seen with primary skeletal malignancies, such as osteosarcoma, chondrosarcoma, and Ewing's tumor, and it reflects the aggressive growth characteristics. The extraosseous extension can be evaluated by plain films, arteriography, CT scanning, and MR imaging and easily is differentiated from primary soft tissue lesions. Parosteal sarcoma, a malignant tumor developing from the periosteum, may be confused with soft tissue tumor, however. Typically it is a slow-growing, low-grade malignancy; however, rapid aggressive growth with early death can occur. These lesions have few symptoms and usually appear as gradually enlarging masses. They most commonly involve the posterior aspect of the distal end of the femur. Grossly, these tumors are attached to cortical bone and grow into the adjacent soft tissue. Most parosteal sarcomas demonstrate some degree of osseous, cartilaginous, or collagenous matrix production. This provides the basis for labeling them parosteal osteosarcoma, parosteal chondrosarcoma, or parosteal fibrosarcoma. The matrix patterns may appear very mature in some areas and frankly malignant in others.

Radiographically, parosteal osteosarcoma is the most common tumor and usually shows a dense, homogeneous calcific mass on the cortical surface of the distal end of the femur (Fig. 84–33). Calcification extends into the adjacent soft tissue, with an irregular margin. The tumor occasionally may grow into the adjacent medullary space.

SUMMARY

A discussion of tumors and tumor-like lesions that appear about joints emphasizes the diverse nature of the processes that can lead to periarticular masses. In most cases, careful evaluation of the clinical history and routine radiographs provides a single, most likely diagnosis, although at times additional techniques, such as scintigraphy, sonography, arteriography, CT scanning, and MR imaging, must be used. These lesions also are considered in Chapters 13, 70, and 95.

References

1. Aegerter E, Kirkpatrick JA Jr: Orthopedic Diseases: Physiology, Pathology, Radiology. 4th Ed. Philadelphia, WB Saunders Co, 1975, p. 721.
2. Brindley HH: Malignant tumors of the soft tissues of the extremity. South Med J 56:868, 1963.
3. Collins DH: The Pathology of Articular and Spinal Diseases. Baltimore, Williams & Wilkins Co, 1950.
4. Enzinger FM, Lattes R, Torloni H: Histological Typing of Soft Tissue Tumors. International Classification of Tumors, No. 3. Geneva, World Health Organization, 1969.
5. Gerner RE, Moore GE, Pickren JW: Soft tissue sarcomas. Ann Surg 181:803, 1975.
6. Hare HF, Cerny MD Jr: Soft tissue sarcoma. A review of 200 cases. Cancer 16:1332, 1963.
7. Horn RC Jr: Sarcomas of soft tissues. JAMA 183:511, 1963.
8. Jaffe HL: Tumors and Tumorous Conditions of the Bones and Joints. Philadelphia, Lea & Febiger, 1958, p 502.
9. Pack GT, Anglem TJ: Tumors of the soft somatic tissues in infancy and childhood. J Pediatr 15:372, 1939.
10. Spjut HJ, Dorfman HD, Fechner RE, et al: Tumors of Bone and Cartilage. Atlas of Tumor Pathology. Second Series, Fascicle 5. Washington, DC, Armed Forces Institute of Pathology, 1971, p 391.
11. Suit HD, Russell WO, Martin RG: Sarcoma of soft tissue—clinical and histopathologic parameters and response to treatment. Cancer 35:1478, 1975.
12. Stout AP: Pathology and classification of tumors of the soft tissues. AJR 66:903, 1951.
13. Stout AP: Sarcomas of the soft parts. J Mo Med Assoc 44:329, 1947.
14. Stout AP, Lattes R: Tumors of the Soft Tissues. Atlas of Tumor Pathology. Second Series, Fascicle 1. Washington DC, Armed Forces Institute of Pathology, 1967, p 11.
15. Thompson DE, Frost HM, Hendrick JW, et al: Soft tissue sarcomas involving the extremities and limb girdles: A review. South Med J 64:33, 1971.
16. Cavanagh RC: Tumors of the soft tissues of the extremities. Semin Roentgenol 8:73, 1973.
17. Forrester DM, Becker TS: The radiology of bone and soft tissue sarcomas. Orthop Clin North Am 8:973, 1977.
18. Levine E, Lee KR, Neff JR, et al: Comparison of computed tomography and other imaging modalities in the evaluation of musculoskeletal tumors. Radiology 131:431, 1979.
19. Martel W, Abell MR: Radiologic evaluation of soft tissue tumors. Cancer 32:352, 1973.
20. Das Gupta TK, Ghosh BC: Principles of diagnosis and management of soft tissue sarcomas. Surg Annu 7:115, 1975.
21. Fortner JG, Kim DK, Shiu MH: Limb-preserving vascular surgery for malignant tumors of the lower extremity. Arch Surg 112:391, 1977.
22. Hudson TM, Hass G, Enneking WF, et al: Angiography in the management of musculoskeletal tumors. Surg Gynecol Obstet 141:11, 1975.
23. Krementz ET, Shaver, JO: Behavior and treatment of soft tissue sarcomas. Ann Surg 157:770, 1963.
24. Morton DL, Eilber FR, Townsend CM Jr, et al: Limb salvage from a multidisciplinary treatment approach for skeletal and soft tissue sarcomas of the extremity. Ann Surg 184:268, 1976.
25. Rosenberg JC: The value of arteriography in the treatment of soft tissue tumors of the extremities. J Int Coll Surg 41:405, 1964.
26. Shiu MH, Castro ER, Hajdu SI, et al: Surgical treatment of 297 soft tissue sarcomas of the lower extremity. Ann Surg 182:597, 1975.
27. Simon MA, Enneking WF: The management of soft tissue sarcomas of the extremities. J Bone Joint Surg [Am] 58:317, 1976.
28. Suit HD, Russell WO, Martin RG: Management of patients with sarcomas of soft tissue in an extremity. Cancer 31:1247, 1973.
29. Frantzell A: Soft tissue radiography. Acta Radiol Suppl 85:1, 1951.
30. Melson GL, Staple TW, Evens RG: Soft tissue radiographic technique. Semin Roentgenol 8:19, 1973.
31. Pirkey EL, Hurt J: Roentgen evaluation of the soft tissues in orthopedics. AJR 82:271, 1959.
32. Levine E, Lee KR, Neff JR, et al: Comparison of computed tomography and other imaging modalities in the evaluation of musculoskeletal tumors. Radiology 131:431, 1979.
33. Nessi R: La xeroradiografia nello studio delle parti molli. Radiol Med (Torino) 63:1083, 1977.
34. Wolfe JN: Xeroradiography of the bones, joints, and soft tissues. Radiology 93:583, 1969.
35. Blatt CJ, Hayt DB, Desai M, et al: Soft tissue sarcomas imaged with technetium-99m pyrophosphate. NY State J Med 77:2118, 1977.

36. Chaudhuri JK, Chaudhuri TK, Go RT, et al: Uptake of ^{87}Sr by liver metastasis from carcinoma of colon. J Nucl Med 14:293, 1973.

37. Matsui K, Yamada H, Chiba K, et al: Visualization of soft tissue malignancies by using ^{99m}Tc polyphosphate, pyrophosphate and diphosphonate (^{99m}TcP). J Nucl Med 14:632, 1973.

38. Nolan NG: Intense uptake of ^{99m}Tc-diphosphonate by an extra-osseous neurofibroma. J Nucl Med 15:1207, 1974.

39. Papavasiliou C, Kostamis P, Angelakis P, et al: Localization of ^{87m}Sr in extra-osseous tumors. J Nucl Med 12:265, 1971.

40. Rosenthall L, Hawkins D: Radionuclide joint imaging in the diagnosis of synovial disease. Semin Arthritis Rheum 7:49, 1977.

41. Samuels LD: Detection and localization of extraskeletal malignant neoplasms of children with strontium-87m. AJR 115:777, 1972.

42. Telfer N: Nuclear medicine in the management of musculoskeletal tumors. Orthop Clin North Am 8:1011, 1977.

43. Wenzel WW, Heasty RG: Uptake of ^{99m}Tc-stannous polyphosphate in an area of cerebral infarction. J Nucl Med 15:207, 1974.

44. Cockshott WP, Evans KT: The place of soft tissue arteriography. Br J Radiol 37:367, 1964.

45. Finck EJ, Moore TM: Angiography for mass lesions of bone, joint, and soft tissue. Orthop Clin North Am 8:999, 1977.

46. Gronner AT: Muscle necrosis simulating a malignant tumor angiographically. Case report. Radiology 103:309, 1972.

47. Hawkins IF Jr, Hudson T: Priscoline in bone and soft-tissue angiography. Radiology 110:541, 1974.

48. Herzberg DL, Schreiber MH: Angiography in mass lesions of the extremities. AJR 111:541, 1971.

49. Hutcheson J, Klatte EC, Kremp R: The angiographic appearance of myositis ossificans circumscripta. A case report. Radiology 102:57, 1972.

50. Lagergren C, Lindbom A: Angiography of peripheral tumors. Radiology 79:371, 1962.

51. Levin DC, Watson RC, Baltaxe HA: Arteriography in the diagnosis and management of acquired peripheral soft-tissue masses. Radiology 104:53, 1972.

52. Margulis AR, Murphy TO: Arteriography in neoplasms of extremities. AJR 80:330, 1958.

53. Stanley P, Miller JA: Angiography of extremity masses in children. AJR 130:1119, 1978.

54. Steckel RJ: Usefulness of extremity arteriography in special situations. Radiology 86:293, 1966.

55. Templeton AW, Stevens E, Jansen C: Arteriographic evaluation of soft tissue masses. South Med J 59:1255, 1966.

56. Viamonte M Jr, Roen S, Le Page J: Nonspecificity of abnormal vascularity in the angiographic diagnosis of malignant neoplasms. Radiology 106:59, 1973.

57. Berger PE, Kuhn JP: Computed tomography of tumors of the musculoskeletal system in children. Radiology 127:171, 1978.

58. deSantos LA, Goldstein HM, Murray JA, et al: Computed tomography in the evaluation of musculoskeletal neoplasms. Radiology 128:89, 1978.

59. Heelan RT, Watson RC, Smith J: Computed tomography of lower extremity tumors. AJR 132:933, 1979.

60. Hermann G, Rose JS: Computed tomography in bone and soft tissue pathology of the extremities. J Comput Assist Tomogr 3:58, 1979.

61. Hunter JC, Johnston WH, Genant HK: Computed tomography evaluation of fatty tumors of the somatic soft tissues: Clinical utility and radiologic-pathologic correlation. Skel Radiol 4:79, 1979.

62. Levinsohn EM, Bryan PJ: Computed tomography in unilateral extremity swelling of unusual cause. J Comput Assist Tomogr 3:67, 1979.

63. Levitt RG, Sagel SS, Stanley RJ, et al: Computed tomography of the pelvis. Semin Roentgenol 13:193, 1978.

64. McLeod RA, Gisvold JJ, Stephens DH, et al: Computed tomography of soft tissues and breast. Semin Roentgenol 13:267, 1978.

65. Schumacher IM, Genant HK, Korobkin M, et al: Computed tomography: Its use in space-occupying lesions of the musculoskeletal system. J Bone Joint Surg [Am] 60:600, 1978.

66. Wilson JS, Korobkin M, Genant HK, et al: Computed tomography of musculoskeletal disorders. AJR 131:55, 1978.

67. Weinberger G, Levinsohn EM: Computed tomography in evaluation of sarcomatous tumors of the thigh. AJR 130:115, 1978.

68. Regan JM, Bickel WH, Broders AC: Infiltrating benign lipomas of the extremities. West J Surg Obstet Gynecol 54:87, 1946.

69. Geschickter CF: Lipoid tumors. Am J Cancer 27:617, 1934.

70. Robbins SL, Cotran RS: Pathologic Basis of Disease. 2nd Ed. Philadelphia, WB Saunders Co, 1979.

71. Kindblom LG, Angervall L, Stener B, et al: Intermuscular and intramuscular lipomas and hibernomas, a clinical, roentgenologic, histologic, and prognostic study of 46 cases. Cancer 33:754, 1974.

72. Dempster WH: Intermuscular lipomata. Br J Radiol 25:553, 1952.

73. Rowland SA: Case report: Ten year follow-up of lipofibroma of the median nerve in the palm. J Hand Surg 2:316, 1977.

74. Terzis JK, Daniel RK, Williams HB, et al: Benign fatty tumors of the peripheral nerves. Ann Plast Surg 1:193, 1978.

75. Pudlowski RM, Gilula LA, Kyriakos M: Intra-articular lipoma with osseous metaplasia: Radiographic pathologic correlation. AJR 132:471, 1979.

76. Berry JB, Moiel RH: Parosteal lipoma producing paralysis of the deep radial nerve. South Med J 66:1298, 1973.

77. Kenin A, Levine J, Spinner M: Parosteal lipoma, a report of two cases with associated bone changes. J Bone Joint Surg [Am] 41:1122, 1959.

78. Khan AA: Parosteal lipoma. J Indian Med Assoc 63:285, 1974.

79. Rosen H: Parosteal lipoma. Bull Hosp Joint Dis 20:96, 1959.

80. Booher RJ: Lipoblastic tumors of the hands and feet. Review of the literature and report of thirty-three cases. J Bone Joint Surg [Am] 47:727, 1965.

81. Kalisman M, Beck AR: Lipoma of the thumb in a child. Ann Plast Surg 2:165, 1979.

82. Leffert RD: Lipomas of the upper extremity. J Bone Joint Surg [Am] 54:1262, 1972.

83. Straus FH: Deep lipomas of the hand. Ann Surg 94:269, 1931.

84. Kauffman SL, Stout AP: Lipoblastic tumors of children. Cancer 12:912, 1959.

85. Elsahy NI, Lorimer A: Congenital fibrolipomata in both heels. Case report. Plast Reconstr Surg 59:434, 1977.

86. Wohl MG, Pastor N: Adiposis dolorosa (Dercum's disease); treatment of asthenic phase with prostigmine and aminoacetic acid. JAMA 110:1261, 1938.

87. Bellemore C: Massive pedunculated lipoma. Aust NZ J Surg 32:83, 1962.

88. Wu KT, Jordan FR, Eckert C: Lipoma, a cause of paralysis of deep radial (posterior interosseous) nerve: Report of a case and review of the literature. Surgery 75:790, 1974.

89. Goldman AB, Kaye JJ: Macrodystrophia lipomatosa: Radiographic diagnosis. AJR 128:101, 1977.

90. Yaghmai I, McKowne F, Alizadeh A: Macrodactylia fibrolipomatosis. South Med J 69:1565, 1976.

91. Engeron O, Stallings JO: An unusual cause of carpal tunnel syndrome. J Iowa Med Soc 65:25, 1975.

92. Wells HG: Adipose tissue, a neglected subject. JAMA 114:2177, 1940.

93. Bartis JR: Massive lipoma of the foot—a case report. J Am Podiatry Assoc 64:874, 1974.

94. Delamater J: Mammoth tumor. Cleveland Med Gaz 1:31, 1859.

95. Louis DS, Dick HM: Ossifying lipofibroma of the median nerve. J Bone Joint Surg [Am] 55:1082, 1973.

96. Murphy NB: Ossifying lipoma. Br J Radiol 47:97, 1974.

97. Plaut GS, Salm R, Trascott DE: Three cases of ossifying lipoma. J Pathol Bacteriol 78:292, 1959.

98. Robson PN: A large calcified lipoma of the thigh. Report of a case. J Bone Joint Surg [Br] 32:384, 1950.

99. McAndrews PG, Greenspan JS: Lipoma of the lip with cartilage formation. Br Dent J 140:239, 1976.

100. Dodge OG, Evans DM: Haemopoiesis in a presacral fatty tumour (myelolipoma). J Pathol Bacteriol 72:313, 1956.

101. Sampson CC, Saunders EH, Green WE, et al: Liposarcoma developing in a lipoma. Arch Pathol 69:506, 1960.

102. Sternberg SS: Liposarcoma arising within a subcutaneous lipoma. Cancer 5:975, 1952.

103. Wright CJE: Liposarcoma arising in a simple lipoma. J Pathol Bacteriol 60:483, 1948.

104. Enzinger FM, Harvey DA: Spindle cell lipoma. Cancer 36:1852, 1975.

105. Greenberg SD, Isensee C, Gonzalez-Angulo A, et al: Infiltrating lipomas of the thigh. Am J Clin Pathol 39:66, 1963.

106. Schobinger RA, Ruzicka FF Jr: Vascular Roentgenology. New York, Macmillan Co, 1964.

107. Jaffe H: Tumors and Tumorous Conditions of the Bones and Joints. Philadelphia, Lea & Febiger, 1974, p 574.

108. Smillie IS: Diseases of the Knee Joint. Edinburgh, Churchill Livingstone, 1974.

109. Arzimanoglu A: Bilateral arborescent lipoma of the knee—a case report. J Bone Joint Surg [Am] 39:976, 1957.

110. Burgan DW: Lipoma arborescens of the knee: Another cause of filling defects on knee arthrogram. Radiology 101:583, 1971.

111. Weitzman G: Lipoma arborescens of the knee. Report of a case. J Bone Joint Surg [Am] 47:1030, 1965.

112. Weston WJ: The intra-synovial fatty masses in chronic rheumatoid arthritis. Br J Radiol 46:213, 1973.

113. Jacobs P: Parosteal lipoma with hyperostosis. Clin Radiol 23:196, 1972.

114. Bradley RL, Klein MM: Angiolipoma. Am J Surg 108:887, 1964.

115. Dionne GP, Seemayer TA: Infiltrating lipomas and angiolipomas revisited. Cancer 33:732, 1974.

116. Gonzalez-Crussi F, Enneking WF, Arean VM: Infiltrating angiolipoma. J Bone Joint Surg [Am] 48:1111, 1966.

117. Howard WR, Helwig EB: Angiolipoma. Arch Dermatol 82:924, 1960.

118. Lin JJ, Lin F: Two entities in angiolipoma. A study of 459 cases of lipoma with review of literature on infiltrating angiolipoma. Cancer 34:720, 1974.

119. Räsänen O, Nohteri H, Dammert K: Angiolipoma and lipoma. Acta Chir Scand 133:461, 1967.

120. Stimpson N: Infiltrating angiolipomata of skeletal muscle. Br J Surg 58:464, 1971.

121. Finberg HJ, Levin DC: Angiolipoma: A rare benign soft tissue tumor with a malignant arteriographic appearance. AJR 128:697, 1977.

122. Angervall L, Björntorp P, Stener B: The lipid composition of hibernoma as

compared with that of lipoma and of mouse brown fat. Cancer Res 25:405, 1965.

123. Brines OA, Johnson MH: Hibernoma, a special fatty tumor: Report of a case. Am J Pathol 25:467, 1949.
124. Fentiman IS, Davies EE, Ramsay GS: Hibernoma of the thigh. Clin Oncol 1:71, 1975.
125. Hull D, Segall MM: Distinction of brown from white adipose tissue. Nature 212:469, 1966.
126. Rasmussen AT: The so-called hibernating gland. J Morphol 38:147, 1923.
127. McLane RC, Meyer LC: Axillary hibernoma: Review of the literature with report of a case examined angiographically. Radiology 127:673, 1978.
128. Lawson W, Biller HF: Cervical hibernoma. Laryngoscope 86:1258, 1976.
129. Kodish ME: Alsever RN, Block MB: Benign symmetric lipomatosis: Functional sympathetic denervation of adipose tissue and possible hypertrophy of brown fat. Metabolism 23:937, 1974.
130. Lewis D, Geschickter CF: Diffuse lipoma of the right upper extremity. Prolan A and B yielded by bio-assay of fat. Ann Surg 102:154, 1935.
131. Lippitt DA, Johnston JR: Diffuse lipomatosis of lower extremities. Report of a case. Bull Ayer Clin Lab Penn Hosp 4:55, 1954.
132. Oosthuizen SF, Barnetson J: Two cases of lipomatosis involving bone. Br J Radiol 20:426, 1947.
133. Kindblom L-G, Möller-Nielsen J: Diffuse lipomatosis in the leg after poliomyelitis. Acta Pathol Microbiol Scand (A) 83:339, 1975.
134. Barsky AJ: Macrodactyly. J Bone Joint Surg [Am] 49:1255, 1967.
135. Ben-Bassat M, Kaplan I, Laron Z, et al: Congenital macrodactyly: A case report with a three-year follow-up. J Bone Joint Surg [Br] 48:359, 1966.
136. Inglis K: Local gigantism (a manifestation of neurofibromatosis): Its relation to general gigantism and to acromegaly illustrating the influence of intrinsic factors in disease when development of the body is abnormal. Am J Pathol 26:1059, 1950.
137. Minkowitz S, Minkowitz F: A morphological study of macrodactylism: A case report. J Pathol 90:323, 1965.
138. Moore BH: Macrodactyly and associated peripheral nerve changes. J Bone Joint Surg 24:617, 1942.
139. Moore BH: Peripheral-nerve changes, associated with congenital deformities. J Bone Joint Surg 26:282, 1944.
140. Ranawat CS, Arora MM, Singh RG: Macrodystrophia lipomatosa with carpal-tunnel syndrome. A case report. J Bone Joint Surg [Am] 50:1242, 1968.
141. Thorne FL, Posch JL, Miladick RA: Megalodactyly. Plast Reconstr Surg 41:232, 1968.
142. Tuli SM, Khanna NN, Sinha GP: Congenital macrodactyly. Br J Plast Surg 22:237, 1969.
143. Adair FE, Pack GT, Farrior JH: Lipomas. Am J Cancer 16:1104, 1932.
144. Chung EB, Enzinger FM: Benign lipoblastomatosis. An analysis of 35 cases. Cancer 32:482, 1973.
145. Gibbs MK, Soule EH, Hayles AB, et al: Lipoblastomatosis: A tumor of children. Pediatrics 60:235, 1977.
146. Langloh JT, Reing CM, Chun BK, et al: Lipoblastomatosis: A case report. J Bone Joint Surg [Am] 60:130, 1978.
147. Paarlberg D, Linscheid RL, Soule EH: Lipomas of the hand: Including a case of lipoblastomatosis in a child. Mayo Clin Proc 47:121, 1972.
148. Vellios F, Baez J, Schumacker HB: Lipoblastomatosis: A tumor of fetal fat different from hibernoma. Am J Pathol 34:1149, 1958.
149. Allen PW, Enzinger FM: Hemangioma of skeletal muscle, an analysis of 89 cases. Cancer 29:8, 1972.
150. Andervont HB, Grady HG, Edwards JE: Induction of hepatic lesions, hepatomas, pulmonary tumors and hemangio-endotheliomas in mice with O-aminoazotoluene. J Natl Cancer Inst 3:131, 1942.
151. Angervall L, Nielsen JM, Stener B, et al: Concomitant arteriovenous vascular malformation in skeletal muscle: A clinical angiographic and histologic study. Cancer 44:232, 1979.
152. Ben-Menachem Y, Epstein MJ: Post-traumatic capillary hemangioma of the hand. A case report. J Bone Joint Surg [Am] 56:1741, 1974.
153. Bliznak J, Staple TW: Radiology of angiodysplasias of the limb. Radiology 110:35, 1974.
154. Goidanich IF, Campanacci M: Vascular hamartomata and infantile angioectatic osteohyperplasia of the extremities. J Bone Joint Surg [Am] 44:815, 1962.
155. Heitzman ER, Jones JB: Roentgen characteristics of cavernous hemangioma of striated muscle. Radiology 74:420, 1960.
156. Levin DC, Gordon DH, McSweeney J: Arteriography of peripheral hemangiomas. Radiology 121:625, 1976.
157. Thomas ML, Andress MR: Angiography in venous dysplasias of the limbs. AJR 113:722, 1971.
158. Malan E, Puglionisi A: Congenital angiodysplasias of the extremities. Note 2. Arterial, arterial and venous, and haemolymphatic dysplasias. J Cardiovasc Surg 6:255, 1975.
159. Malan E, Puglionisi A: Congenital angiodysplasias of the extremities. Note 1. Generalities and classification; venous dysplasias. J Cardiovasc Surg 5:87, 1964.
160. Fergusson ILC: Haemangiomata of skeletal muscle. Br J Surg 59:634, 1972.
161. Fulton MN, Sosman MC: Venous angiomas of skeletal muscle; report of 4 cases. JAMA 119:319, 1942.

162. Bendeck TE, Lichtenberg F: Cavernous hemangioma of striated muscle. Review of the literature and report of 2 cases. Ann Surg 146:1011, 1957.
163. Borden JI, Shea TP: Cavernous hemangioma of the foot. A case report and review. J Am Podiatry Assoc 66:484, 1976.
164. Brodsky AE: Synovial hemangioma of the knee joint. Bull Hosp Joint Dis 17:58, 1956.
165. Cobey MC: Hemangioma of joints. Arch Surg 46:465, 1943.
166. Harkins HN: Hemangioma of tendon or tendon sheath. Report of a case with a study of twenty-four cases from the literature. Arch Surg 34:12, 1937.
167. Jacobs, JE, Lee FW: Hemangioma of the knee joint. J Bone Joint Surg [Am] 31:831, 1949.
168. Karlholm S, Stjernswärd J: Hemangioma of the knee joint. Acta Orthop Scand 33:306, 1963.
169. Perras P, Boulianne P: Multiple congenital hemangiomatosis. J Can Assoc Radiol 24:231, 1973.
170. Politz MJ: Hemangioma of the digits. Two cases. J Am Podiatry Assoc 66:515, 1976.
171. Sugiura I: Tibial periosteal hemangioma. Clin Orthop 106:242, 1975.
172. Sutherland AD: Equinus deformity due to haemangioma of calf muscle. J Bone Joint Surg [Br] 57:104, 1975.
173. Stevens J, Katz PL, Archer FL, et al: Synovial hemangioma of the knee. Arthritis Rheum 12:647, 1969.
174. Szilagyi DE, Smith RF, Elliott JP, et al: Congenital arteriovenous anomalies of the limbs. Arch Surg 111:423, 1976.
175. Weaver JB: Hemangiomata of the lower extremities. With special reference to those of the knee-joint capsule and the phenomenon of spontaneous obliteration. J Bone Joint Surg 20:731, 1938.
176. Wind ES, Pillari G: Deep soft tissue hemangioma of infancy: Kasabach-Merritt syndrome. NY State J Med 79:373, 1979.
177. Jenkins HP, Delaney PA: Benign angiomatous tumors of skeletal muscles. Surg Gynecol Obstet 55:464, 1932.
178. Jones KG: Cavernous hemangioma of striated muscle—a review of the literature and a report of four cases. J Bone Joint Surg [Am] 35:717, 1953.
179. Scott JES: Hemangiomata in skeletal muscle. Br J Surg 44:496, 1957.
180. Shallow TA, Eger SA, Wagner FB Jr: Primary hemangiomatous tumors of skeletal muscle. Ann Surg 119:700, 1944.
181. Oldmixon WJ: Hemangioma. Case for diagnosis. Milit Med 142:434, 1977.
182. Kasabach HH, Merritt KK: Capillary hemangioma with extensive purpura. Report of a case. Am J Dis Child 59:1063, 1940.
183. Sutherland DA, Clark H: Hemangioma associated with thrombocytopenia. Report of a case and review of the literature. Am J Med 33:150, 1962.
184. Carnelli U, Bellini F, Ferrari M, et al: Giant hemangioma with consumption coagulopathy: Sustained response to heparin and radiotherapy. J Pediatr 91:504, 1977.
185. Dadash-Zadeh M, Czapek EE, Schwartz AD: Skeletal and splenic hemangiomatosis with consumption coagulopathy: Response to splenectomy. Pediatrics 57:803, 1976.
186. Evan J, Batchelor ADR, Stark G, et al: Haemangioma with coagulopathy: Sustained response to prednisone. Arch Dis Child 50:809, 1975.
187. Hagerman LJ, Czapek EE, Donnellan WL, et al: Giant hemangioma with consumption coagulopathy. J Pediatr 87:766, 1975.
188. Inceman S, Tangün Y: Chronic defibrination syndrome due to a giant hemangioma associated with microangiopathic hemolytic anemia. Am J Med 46:997, 1969.
189. Lee JH Jr, Kirk RF: Pregnancy associated with giant hemangiomata, thrombocytopenia, and fibrinogenopenia (Kasabach-Merritt syndrome). Report of a case. Obstet Gynecol 29:24, 1967.
190. Rodriguez-Erdmann F, Button L, Murray JE, et al: Kasabach-Merritt syndrome: Coagulo-analytical observations. Am J Med Sci 261:9, 1971.
191. Thompson LR, Umlauf HJ Jr: Hemangioma associated with thrombocytopenia: Report of two cases and review of the literature with emphasis on methods of therapy. Milit Med 129:652, 1964.
192. Blix S, Aas K: Giant hemangioma, thrombocytopenia, fibrinogenopenia, and fibrinolytic activity. Acta Med Scand 169:63, 1961.
193. Hillman RS, Phillips LL: Clotting—fibrinolysis in a cavernous hemangioma. Am J Dis Child 113:649, 1967.
194. Lozman J, Holmblad J: Cavernous hemangiomas associated with scoliosis and a localized consumption coagulopathy. A case report. J Bone Joint Surg [Am] 58:1021, 1976.
195. Propp RP, Scharfman WB: Hemangioma-thrombocytopenia syndrome associated with microangiopathic hemolytic anemia. Blood 28:623, 1966.
196. Keller L, Bluhm JF III: Diffuse neonatal hemangiomatosis. A case with heart failure and thrombocytopenia. Cutis 23:295, 1979.
197. Letts RM: Orthopaedic treatment of hemangiomatous hypertrophy of the lower extremity. J Bone Joint Surg [Am] 59:777, 1977.
198. Cohen J, Cashman WF: Hemihypertrophy of lower extremity associated with multifocal intraosseous hemangioma. Clin Orthop 109:155, 1975.
199. Milikow E, Asch T: Hemangiomatosis, localized growth disturbance and intravascular coagulation disorder presenting with an unusual arthritis resembling hemophilia. Radiology 97:387, 1970.
200. Klippel M, Trenaunay P: Du naevus variqueux ostéo-hypertrophique. Arch Gen Med 185:641, 1900.

201. Lindenauer SM: The Klippel-Trenaunay syndrome: Varicosity, hypertrophy and hemangioma with no arteriovenous fistula. Ann Surg *162*:303, 1965.

202. Resnick D, Oliphant M: Hemophilia-like arthropathy of the knee associated with cutaneous and synovial hemangiomas. Report of 3 cases and review of the literature. Radiology *114*:323, 1975.

203. Evans DJ, Azzopardi JG: Distinctive tumours of bone and soft tissue causing acquired vitamin D resistant osteomalacia. Lancet *1*:353, 1972.

204. Linovitz RJ, Resnick D, Keissling P, et al: Tumor-induced osteomalacia and rickets: A surgically curable syndrome, a report of two cases. J Bone Joint Surg [Am] *58*:419, 1976.

205. Renton P, Shaw DG: Hypophosphatemic osteomalacia secondary to vascular tumors of bone and soft tissue. Skel Radiol *1*:21, 1976.

206. Salassa RM, Jowsey J, Arnaud CD: Hypophosphatemic osteomalacia associated with ''nonendocrine tumors.'' N Engl J Med *283*:65, 1970.

207. Turner ML, Dalinka MK: Osteomalacia: Uncommon causes. AJR *133*:539, 1979.

208. Gorham LW, Stout AP: Hemangiomatosis and its relation to massive osteolysis. Trans Assoc Am Phys *67*:302, 1954.

209. Yamamoto K, Ueki J: Proceedings: Massive osteolysis with periosteal hemangiomatosis, report of a case. Calcif Tissue Res *15*:160, 1974.

210. Lewis RJ, Ketcham AS: Maffucci's syndrome: Functional and neoplastic significance. Case report and review of the literature. J Bone Joint Surg [Am] *55*:1456, 1973.

211. Schwartz A, Salz N: Cavernous hemangioma associated with phleboliths in the masseter muscle. Acta Radiol *43*:233, 1955.

212. Shallow TA, Eger SA, Wagner FB Jr: Primary hemangiomatous tumours of skeletal muscle. Ann Surg *119*:700, 1944.

213. Teller WH, Soliscohen T, Levine S: Cavernous hemangioma of the leg. Radiology *22*:369, 1934.

214. McNeill TW, Chan GE, Capek V, et al: The value of angiography in the surgical management of deep hemangiomas. Clin Orthop *101*:176, 1974.

215. Bartley O, Wickbom I: Angiography in soft tissue hemangiomas. Acta Radiol *51*:81, 1959.

216. Olcott C IV, Newton TH, Stoney RJ, et al: Intra-arterial embolization in the management of arteriovenous malformations. Surgery *79*:3, 1976.

217. Piyachon C: Radiology of peripheral arteriovenous malformations. Australas Radiol *21*:246, 1977.

218. Thomas ML, Andress MR: Angiography in venous dysplasias of the limbs. AJR *113*:722, 1971.

219. Mitty HA, Kleiger B: Partial embolization of large peripheral hemangioma for pain control. Radiology *127*:671, 1978.

220. Kinmonth JB, Young AE, Edwards JM, et al: Mixed vascular deformities of the lower limbs, with particular reference to lymphography and surgical treatment. Br J Surg *63*:899, 1976.

221. Larsen IJ, Landry RM: Hemangioma of the synovial membrane. J Bone Joint Surg [Am] *51*:1210, 1969.

222. Lewis RC Jr, Coventry MB, Sowle EH: Hemangioma of the synovial membrane. J Bone Joint Surg [Am] *41*:264, 1959.

223. Waddell GF: A haemangioma involving tendons. J Bone Joint Surg [Am] *49*:138, 1967.

224. Moon NF: Synovial hemangioma of the knee joint. A review of previously reported cases and inclusion of two new cases. Clin Orthop *90*:183, 1973.

225. Bennett GE, Cobey MC: Hemangioma of joints. Report of five cases. Arch Surg *38*:487, 1939.

226. Wynne-Roberts C, Anderson C: Synovial haemangioma of the knee: Light and electron microscopic findings. J Pathol *123*:247, 1977.

227. DePalma AF, Mauler GG: Hemangioma of synovial membrane. Clin Orthop *32*:93, 1964.

228. Forrest J, Staple TW: Synovial hemangioma of the knee. Demonstration by arthrography and arteriography. AJR *112*:512, 1971.

229. Halborg A, Hansen H, Sneppen HO: Haemangioma of the knee joint. Acta Orthop Scand *39*:209, 1968.

230. Mahadevan H, Ozonoff MB, Joki P: Arteriographic findings in synovial hemangioma of the knee. Radiology *106*:627, 1973.

231. McInerney D, Park WM: Thermographic assessment of synovial hemangioma. Clin Radiol *25*:469, 1978.

232. Kauffman SL, Stout AP: Hemangiopericytoma in children. Cancer *13*:695, 1960.

233. McCormack LJ, Gallivan WF: Hemangiopericytoma. Cancer *7*:595, 1954.

234. McMaster MJ, Soule EH, Ivins JC: Hemangiopericytoma. A clinico-pathologic study and long term follow-up of 60 patients. Cancer *36*:2232, 1975.

235. Stout AP: Hemangiopericytoma. A study of twenty-five new cases. Cancer *2*:1027, 1949.

236. Stout AP: Tumors featuring pericytes; glomus tumor and hemangiopericytoma. Lab Invest *5*:217, 1956.

237. Stout AP, Murray MR: Hemangiopericytoma. A vascular tumor featuring Zimmermann's pericytes. Ann Surg *116*:26, 1942.

238. Enzinger FM, Smith BH: Hemangiopericytoma. An analysis of 106 cases. Hum Pathol *7*:61, 1976.

239. Kennedy JC, Fisher JH: Haemangiopericytoma: its orthopaedic manifestations. J Bone Joint Surg [Br] *42*:80, 1960.

240. Reynolds FC, Lansche WE: Hemangiopericytoma of the lower extremity, a case report. J Bone Joint Surg [Am] *40*:921, 1958.

241. Daeke DA, Lindorfer DB: Malignant retroperitoneal hemangiopericytoma with associated hypoglycemia. Treatment via radiotherapy. Wis Med J *73*:S92, 1974.

242. Angervall L, Kindblom LG, Nielsen JM, et al: Hemangiopericytoma: A clinicopathologic, angiographic and microangiographic study. Cancer *42*:2412, 1978.

243. Ayella RJ: Hemangiopericytoma: A case report with arteriographic findings. Radiology *97*:611, 1970.

244. Gerstmann KE, Nimberg GA: Hemangiopericytoma with angiographic studies. A case report. Clin Orthop *68*:108, 1970.

245. Hoeffel IL, Chardot C, Parache R, et al: Radiologic patterns of hemangiopericytoma of the leg. Am J Surg *123*:591, 1972.

246. Joffe N: Haemangiopericytoma: Angiographic findings. Br J Radiol *33*:614, 1960.

247. Mujahed Z, Vasilas, A, Evans JA: Hemangiopericytoma; report of four cases with a review of the literature. AJR *82*:658, 1959.

248. Yaghmai I: Angiographic manifestations of soft-tissue and osseous hemangiopericytomas. Radiology *126*:653, 1978.

249. Gensler S, Caplan LH, Laufman H: Giant benign hemangiopericytoma functioning as an arteriovenous shunt. JAMA *198*:85, 1966.

250. Harkins GA, Sabiston DC Jr: Lymphangioma in infancy and childhood. Surgery *47*:811, 1960.

251. Hill JT, Briggs JD: Lymphangioma. West J Surg Obstet Gynecol *69*:78, 1961.

252. Nix JT: Lymphangioma. Essential data in forty-two cases from Charity Hospital of Louisiana at New Orleans. Am J Surg *20*:556, 1954.

253. Freund E: Chondromatosis of the joints. Arch Surg *34*:670, 1937.

254. Jeffreys TE: Synovial chondromatosis. J Bone Joint Surg [Br] *49*:530, 1967.

255. Lichtenstein L, Goldman RL: Cartilage tumors in soft tissue, particularly in the hand and foot. Cancer *17*:1203, 1964.

256. Mallory TB: A group of metaplastic and neoplastic bone- and cartilage-containing tumors of soft parts. Am J Pathol *9*:765, 1933.

257. Murphy AF, Wilson JN: Tenosynovial osteochondroma in the hand. J Bone Joint Surg [Am] *40*:1236, 1958.

258. Murphy FP, Dahlin DC, Sullivan CR: Articular synovial chondromatosis. J Bone Joint Surg [Am] *44*:77, 1962.

259. Mussey RD Jr, Henderson MS: Osteochondromatosis. J Bone Joint Surg [Am] *31*:619, 1949.

260. Nixon JE, Frank GR, Chambers G: Synovial osteochondromatosis with report of four cases, one showing malignant change. US Armed Forces Med J *11*:1434, 1960.

261. Symeonides P: Bursal chondromatosis. J Bone Joint Surg [Br] *48*:371, 1966.

262. Wilmoth CL: Osteochondromatosis. J Bone Joint Surg *23*:367, 1941.

263. Chung EB, Enzinger FM: Chondroma of soft parts. Cancer *41*:1414, 1978.

264. Dellon AL, Weiss SW, Mitch WE: Bilateral extraosseous chondromas of the hand in a patient with chronic renal failure. J Hand Surg *3*:139, 1978.

265. Sim FH, Dahlin DC, Ivins JC: Extra-articular synovial chondromatosis. J Bone Joint Surg [Am] *59*:492, 1977.

266. Wells TJ, Hooker SP, Roche WC: Osteochondroma cutis: Report of a case. J Oral Surg *35*:144, 1977.

267. Spjut HJ, Dorfman HD, Fechner RE, et al: Tumors of Bone and Cartilage. *In* Atlas of Tumor Pathology. Second Series, Fascicle 5. Washington DC, Armed Forces Institute of Pathology, 1971, p 391.

268. Someren A, Merrirt WH: Tenosynovial chondroma of the hand: A case report with a brief review of the literature. Hum Pathol *9*:476, 1978.

269. Swan EF, Owens WF Jr: Synovial chondrometaplasia, a case report with spontaneous regression and a review of the literature. South Med J *65*:1496, 1972.

270. Akhtar M, Mahajan S, Kott E: Synovial chondromatosis of the temporomandibular joint. Report of a case. J Bone Joint Surg [Am] *59*:266, 1977.

271. Bloom R, Pattinson JN: Osteochondromatosis of hip joint. J Bone Joint Surg [Br] *33*:80, 1954.

272. Brahms MA, Fumich RM: Chondroma within the flexor hallucis longus tendon sheath. A case report and literature review. Am J Sports Med *6*:143, 1978.

273. Christensen JH, Poulsen JO: Synovial chondromatosis. Acta Orthop Scand *46*:919, 1975.

274. Constant E, Harebottle NH, Davis DG: Synovial chondromatosis of the hand. Case report. Plast Reconstr Surg *54*:353, 1974.

275. Giustra PE, Furman RS, Roberts L, et al: Synovial chondromatosis involving the elbow. AJR *127*:347, 1976.

276. Ishizuki M, Isobe Y, Arai T, et al: Osteochondromatosis of the finger joints. Hand *9*:198, 1977.

277. Kettlekamp DB, Dolan J: Synovial chondromatosis of an interphalangeal joint of a finger. Report of a case. J Bone Joint Surg [Am] *48*:329, 1966.

278. Lewis MM, Marshall JL, Mirra JM: Synovial chondromatosis of the thumb. A case report and review of the literature. J Bone Joint Surg [Am] *56*:180, 1974.

279. Lynn MD, Lee J: Periarticular tenosynovial chondrometaplasia. Report of a case at the wrist. J Bone Joint Surg [Am] *54*:650, 1972.

280. Lyritis G: Synovial chondromatosis of the inferior radial ulnar joint. Acta Orthop Scand *47*:373, 1976.

281. McBryde AM Jr: Benign (intracapsular) tumors of the hip. *In* JP Ahstrom Jr (Ed): Current Practice in Orthopaedic Surgery, Vol 7. St Louis, CV Mosby Co, 1977, p 154.

282. Miller AS, Harwick RD, Daley DJ: Temporomandibular joint synovial chondromatosis: Report of a case. J Oral Surg *36*:467, 1978.

283. Mishra KP: Synovial chondromatosis of shoulder joint. A case report and review of literature. East Afr Med J 55:130, 1978.

284. Moazzez K: Osteochondromatosis of the hip joint. Report of a case. Acta Med Iran 18:35, 1975.

285. Mosher JF, Kettelkamp DB, Campbell CJ: Intracapsular or para-articular chondroma. A report of three cases. J Bone Joint Surg [Am] 48:1561, 1966.

286. Paul RG, Leach RE: Synovial chondromatosis of the shoulder. Clin Orthop 68:130, 1970.

287. Ronald JB, Keller EE, Weiland LH: Synovial chondromatosis of the temporomandibular joint. J Oral Surg 36:13, 1978.

288. Rosen PS, Pritzker KPH, Greenbaum J, et al: Synovial chondromatosis affecting the temporomandibular joint. Case report and literature review. Arthritis Rheum 20:736, 1977.

289. Szepesi J: Synovial chondromatosis of the metacarpophalangeal joint. Acta Orthop Scand 46:926, 1975.

290. Thomas S.: Synovial chondromatosis of the hip: Case with long-term follow up. SD J Med 30:7, 1977.

291. Tormes FR, Hardin NJ, Pledger SR: Synovial chondromatosis of the shoulder: Case report. Milit Med 143:872, 1978.

292. Trias A, Quintana O: Synovial chondrometaplasia: Review of world literature and a study of 18 Canadian cases. Can J Surg 19:151, 1976.

293. Varma BP, Ramakrishna YJ: Synovial chondromatosis of the shoulder. Aust NZ J Surg 46:44, 1976.

294. Weiss C, Averbuch PF, Steiner GC, et al: Synovial chondromatosis and instability of the proximal tibiofibular joint. Clin Orthop 108:187, 1975.

295. Collins DH: The Pathology of Articular and Spinal Diseases. Baltimore, Williams & Wilkins Co, 1950.

296. Jacob RA, Campbell WP, Niemann KMW: Synovial chondrometaplasia. A case report. Clin Orthop 109:152, 1975.

297. Jones HT: Loose body formation in synovial osteochondromatosis with specific reference to the etiology and pathology. J Bone Joint Surg 6:407, 1924.

298. Dunn AW, Whisler JH: Synovial chondromatosis of the knee with associated extracapsular chondromas. J Bone Joint Surg [Am] 55:1747, 1973.

299. Goldman RL, Lichtenstein L: Synovial chondrosarcoma. Cancer 17:1233, 1964.

300. King JW, Spjut HJ, Fechner RE, et al: Synovial chondrosarcoma of the knee joint. J Bone Joint Surg [Am] 49:1389, 1967.

301. Milgram JW, Addison RG: Synovial osteochondromatosis of the knee. Chondromatosis recurrence with possible chondrosarcomatous degeneration. J Bone Joint Surg [Am] 58:264, 1976.

302. Mullins F, Berard CW, Eisenberg SH: Chondrosarcoma following synovial chondromatosis. A case study. Cancer 18:1180, 1965.

303. Sarmiento A, Elkins RW: Giant intra-articular osteochondroma of the knee, a case report. J Bone Joint Surg [Am] 57:560, 1975.

304. Fisher AGT: A study of loose bodies composed of cartilage or of cartilage and bone occurring in joints. With special reference to their pathology and etiology. Br J Surg 8:493, 1921.

305. Halstead AE: Floating bodies in joints. Ann Surg 22:327, 1895.

306. Milgram JW: The classification of loose bodies in human joints. Clin Orthop 124:282, 1977.

307. Holm CL: Primary synovial chondromatosis of the ankle. A case report. J Bone Joint Surg [Am] 58:878, 1976.

308. Milgram JW: Synovial osteochondromatosis. A histopathological study of thirty cases. J Bone Joint Surg [Am] 59:792, 1977.

309. Strong ML Jr: Chondromas of the tendon sheath of the hand. Report of a case and review of the literature. J Bone Joint Surg [Am] 57:1164, 1975.

310. Crittenden JJ, Jones DM, Santarelli AG: Knee arthrogram in synovial chondromatosis. Radiology 94:133, 1970.

311. Goldberg RP, Genant HK: Calcified bodies in popliteal cysts: A characteristic radiographic appearance. AJR 131:857, 1978.

312. Henderson MS, Jones HT: Loose bodies in joints and bursae due to synovial osteochondromatosis. J Bone Joint Surg 5:400, 1923.

313. Leydig SM, Odell RT: Synovial osteochondromatosis. Surg Gynecol Obstet 89:457, 1949.

314. Noyek AM, Holgate RC, Fireman SM, et al: The radiologic findings in synovial chondromatosis (chondrometaplasia) of the temporomandibular joint. J Otolaryngol 6:45, 1977.

315. Prager RJ, Mall JC: Arthrographic diagnosis of synovial chondromatosis. AJR 127:344, 1976.

316. Zimmerman C, Sayegh V: Roentgen manifestations of synovial osteochondromatosis. AJR 83:680, 1960.

317. Dahlin DC, Salvador AH: Cartilaginous tumor of the soft tissues of the hands and feet. Mayo Clin Proc 49:721, 1974.

318. Shellito JG, Dockerty MB: Cartilaginous tumors of the hand. Surg Gynecol Obstet 86:465, 1948.

319. Allen PW: The fibromatoses: A clinicopathologic classification based on 140 cases. Am J Surg Pathol 1:255, 1977.

320. Dehner LP, Askin FB: Tumors of fibrous tissue origin in childhood. A clinicopathologic study of cutaneous and soft tissue neoplasms in 66 children. Cancer 38:888, 1976.

321. Enzinger FM: Fibrous tumors of infancy. In Tumors of Bone and Soft Tissue. 8th Annual Clinical Conference on Cancer, MD Anderson Hospital and Tumor Institute, 1963. Chicago, Year Book Medical Publishers, 1965, p 375.

322. MacKenzie DH: The fibromatoses—a clinicopathological concept. Br Med J 4:277, 1972.

323. MacKenzie DH: The Differential Diagnosis of Fibroblastic Disorders. Oxford, Blackwell Scientific Publications, 1970.

324. Stout AP: Juvenile fibromatoses. Cancer 7:953, 1954.

325. Stout AP: Fibrous tumors of the soft tissues. Minn Med 43:455, 1960.

326. Allen PW, Enzinger FM: Juvenile aponeurotic fibroma. Cancer 26:857, 1970.

327. Booher RJ, McPeak CJ: Juvenile aponeurotic fibromas. Surgery 46:924, 1959.

328. Goldman RL: The cartilage analogue of fibromatosis (aponeurotic fibroma). Further observations based on 7 new cases. Cancer 26:1325, 1970.

329. Keasbey LE: Juvenile aponeurotic fibroma (calcifying fibroma): A distinctive tumor arising in the palms and soles of young children. Cancer 6:338, 1953.

330. Keasbey LE, Fanselau HA: The aponeurotic fibroma. Clin Orthop 19:115, 1961.

331. Keller RB, Beaz-Giangreco A: Juvenile aponeurotic fibroma. Report of 3 cases and review of the literature. Clin Orthop 106:198, 1975.

332. Lichtenstein L, Goldman RL: The cartilage analogue of fibromatosis. A reinterpretation of the condition called ''juvenile aponeurotic fibroma.'' Cancer 17:810, 1964.

333. Rios-Dalenz JL, Kim JS, McDowell FW: The so-called ''juvenile aponeurotic fibroma.'' Am J Clin Pathol 44:632, 1965.

334. Zeide MS, Wiesel S, Terry RL: Juvenile aponeurotic fibroma, case report. Plast Reconstr Surg 61:922, 1978.

335. Arlen M, Koven L, Frieder M: Juvenile fascial fibromatosis of the forearm with osseous involvement. J Bone Joint Surg [Am] 51:591, 1969.

336. Karasick D, O'Hara AE: Juvenile aponeurotic fibroma. A review and report of a case with osseous involvement. Radiology 123:725, 1977.

337. Shapiro L: Infantile digital fibromatosis and aponeurotic fibroma. Case reports of two rare pseudosarcomas and review of the literature. Arch Dermatol 99:37, 1969.

338. Allen PW: Recurring digital fibrous tumours of childhood. Pathology 4:215, 1972.

339. Beckett JH, Jacobs AH: Recurring digital fibrous tumors of childhood: A review. Pediatrics 59:401, 1977.

340. Grunnet N, Genner J, Morgensen B, et al: Recurring digital fibrous tumor of childhood, case report and survey. Acta Pathol Microbiol Scand (A) 81:167, 1973.

341. Iwasaki H, Tsuneyoshi M, Enjoji M: Infantile digital fibromatosis histopathological and electron microscopic study with a review of the literature. Acta Pathol Jpn 24:717, 1974.

342. O'Gorman DJ, Fairburn EA: Infantile digital fibromatosis. Proc R Soc Med 67:880, 1974.

343. Reye RDK: Recurring digital fibrous tumors of childhood. Arch Pathol 80:228, 1965.

344. Bloem JJ, Vuzevski VD, Huffstadt AJC: Recurring digital fibroma of infancy. J Bone Joint Surg [Br] 56:746, 1974.

345. Siegal A: Aggressive fibromatosis (infantile fibrosarcoma). Difficulty of diagnostic and prognostic evaluation. Clin Pediatr 17:517, 1978.

346. Antine BE, Brown FM, Arisco MJ: Fibroma of the cornea. Report of a case associated with congenital generalized fibromatosis. Arch Ophthalmol 91:278, 1974.

347. Beatty EC Jr: Congenital generalized fibromatosis in infancy. Am J Dis Child 103:620, 1962.

348. Elliott DE: Congenital generalized fibromatosis. Birth Defects 11:355, 1975.

349. Familusi JB, Nottidge VA, Antia AN, et al: Congenital generalized fibromatosis. An African case with gingival hypertrophy and other unusual features. Am J Dis Child 130:1215, 1976.

350. Kindblom LG, Termen G, Säve-Söderbergh J, et al: Congenital solitary fibromatosis of soft tissues, a variant of congenital generalized fibromatosis. Two case reports. Acta Pathol Microbiol Scand (A) 85:640, 1977.

351. Kindblom LG, Angervall L: Congenital solitary fibromatosis of the skeleton. Case report of a variant of congenital generalized fibromatosis. Cancer 41:636, 1978.

352. Plaschkes J: Congenital fibromatosis: Localized and generalized forms. J Pediatr Surg 9:95, 1974.

353. Shnitka TK, Asp DM, Horner RH: Congenital generalized fibromatosis. Cancer 11:627, 1958.

354. Baer JW, Radkowski MA: Congenital multiple fibromatosis. A case report with review of the world literature. AJR 118:200, 1973.

355. Schaffzin EA, Chung SMK, Kaye R: Congenital generalized fibromatosis with complete spontaneous regression. A case report. J Bone Joint Surg [Am] 54:657, 1972.

356. Teng P, Warden MJ, Cohn WL: Congenital generalized fibromatosis (renal and skeletal) with complete spontaneous regression. J Pediatr 62:748, 1963.

357. Barlett RC, Otis RD, Laakso AO: Multiple congenital neoplasms of soft tissues. Report of 4 cases in one family. Cancer 14:913, 1961.

358. Condon VR, Allen RP: Congenital generalized fibromatosis. Case report with roentgen manifestations. Radiology 76:444, 1961.

359. Morettin LB, Mueller E, Schreiber M: Generalized hamartomatosis (congenital generalized fibromatosis). AJR 114:722, 1972.

360. Schlangen JT: Congenital generalized fibromatosis: A case report with roentgen manifestations of the skeleton. Radiol Clin North Am 45:18, 1976.

361. Dutz W, Stout AP: The myxoma in childhood. Cancer *14*:629, 1961.

362. Enzinger FM: Intramuscular myxoma. A review and follow-up study of 34 cases. Am J Clin Pathol *43*:104, 1965.

363. Stout AP: Myxoma; the tumor of primitive mesenchyme. Ann Surg *127*:706, 1948.

364. Sponsel KH, McDonald JR, Ghormley RK: Myxoma and myxosarcoma of the soft tissues of the extremities. J Bone Joint Surg [Am] *34*:820, 1952.

365. Fisher WC, Helwig EB: Leiomyomas of the skin. Arch Dermatol *88*:510, 1963.

366. Goodman AH, Briggs RC: Deep leiomyoma of an extremity. J Bone Joint Surg [Am] *47*:529, 1965.

367. Stout AP: Solitary cutaneous and subcutaneous leiomyoma. Am J Cancer *29*:435, 1937.

368. Kauffman SL, Stout AP: Histiocytic tumors (fibrous xanthoma and histiocytoma) in children. Cancer *14*:469, 1961.

369. Bloom D, Kaufman SR, Stevens RA: Hereditary xanthomatosis. Familial incidence of xanthoma tuberosum associated with hypercholesteremia and cardiovascular involvement, with report of several cases of sudden death. Arch Dermatol *45*:1, 1942.

370. Montgomery H: Cutaneous xanthomatosis. Ann Intern Med *13*:671, 1939.

371. Cappell DF, Montgomery GL: On rhabdomyoma and myoblastoma. J Pathol Bacteriol *44*:517, 1937.

372. Goldman RL: Multicentric benign rhabdomyoma of skeletal muscle. Cancer *16*:1609, 1963.

373. Parsons HG, Puro HE: Rhabdomyoma of skeletal muscle; report of a case. Am J Surg *89*:1187, 1955.

374. Ackerman LV, Wheeler P: Liposarcoma. South Med J *35*:156, 1942.

375. Adair, FE, Pack GT, Farrior JH: Lipomas. Am J Cancer *16*:1104, 1932.

376. Enterline HT, Culberson JD, Rochlin DB, et al: Liposarcoma: a clinical and pathological study of 53 cases. Cancer *13*:932, 1960.

377. Enzinger FM: Recent trends in soft tissue pathology. *In* Tumors of Bone and Soft Tissue. 8th Annual Clinical Conference on Cancer, MD Anderson Hospital and Tumor Institute, Houston, Texas, 1963. Chicago, Year Book Medical Publishers, 1965, p 315.

378. Holtz F: Liposarcomas. Cancer *11*:1103, 1958.

379. Hutton I: Liposarcoma of the thigh: Management. Proc R Soc Med *67*:655, 1974.

380. Kelly PC, Shramowiat M: Liposarcoma of the foot: A case report. J Foot Surg *17*:27, 1978.

381. Pack GT, Pierson JC: Liposarcoma: A study of 105 cases. Surgery *36*:687, 1954.

382. Phelan JT, Perez-Mesa C: Liposarcoma of the superficial soft tissues. Surg Gynecol Obstet *115*:609, 1962.

383. Quinonez GE: Liposarcoma of the lower extremity. A review of 30 cases from Ohio State University Hospitals from 1955 to 1970. Ohio State Med J *68*:942, 1972.

384. Reszel PA, Soule EH, Coventry MB: Liposarcoma of the extremities and limb girdles. A study of two hundred twenty-two cases. J Bone Joint Surg [Am] *48*:229, 1966.

385. Sawhney KK, McDonald JM, Jaffe HW: Liposarcoma of the hand. Am Surg *41*:117, 1975.

386. Shiu MA, Chu F, Castro EB, et al: Results of surgical and radiation therapy in the treatment of liposarcoma arising in an extremity. AJR *123*:577, 1975.

387. Stout AP: Liposarcoma—the malignant tumor of lipoblasts. Ann Surg *119*:86, 1944.

388. Enzinger FM, Winslow DJ: Liposarcoma. A study of 103 cases. Virchows Arch (Pathol Anat) *335*:367, 1962.

389. Kindblom LG, Angervall L, Svendsen P: Liposarcoma: A clinicopathologic, radiographic and prognostic study. Acta Pathol Microbiol Scand (A) Suppl *253*:1, 1975.

390. Cadman NL, Soule EH, Kelly PJ: Synovial sarcoma. An analysis of 134 tumors. Cancer *18*:613, 1965.

391. Cade S: Synovial sarcoma. J R Coll Surg Edinb *8*:1, 1962.

392. Galinski AW, Vlahos M: Malignant synovioma of the foot: A case report. J Am Podiatry Assoc *65*:175, 1975.

393. Gerner RE, Moore GE: Synovial sarcoma. Ann Surg *181*:22, 1975.

394. Haagensen CD, Stout AP: Synovial sarcoma. Ann Surg *120*:826, 1944.

395. Jaworek TA: Synovial sarcoma, a case report of foot involvement. J Am Podiatry Assoc *66*:544, 1976.

396. Madewell BR, Pool R: Neoplasms of joints and related structures. Vet Clin North Am *8*:511, 1978.

397. Murray JA: Synovial sarcoma. Orthop Clin North Am *8*:963, 1977.

398. Raina V: Synovial sarcoma. An analysis of 31 cases in 26 years. Indian J Cancer *15*:10, 1978.

399. Thunold J, Bang G: Synovial sarcoma: A case report. Acta Orthop Scand *47*:231, 1976.

400. Crocker DW, Stout AP: Synovial sarcoma in children. Cancer *12*:1123, 1959.

401. Lee SM, Hajdu SI, Exelby PR: Synovial sarcoma in children. Surg Gynecol Obstet *138*:701, 1974.

402. Ichinose H, Derbes VJ, Hoerner H: Cutaneous pain without tumor. A manifestation of occult synovioma. Cutis *21*:74, 1978.

403. Ichinose H, Hoerner H, Derbes VJ: Minute synovial sarcoma in the occult nonpalpable phase. A case report. J Bone Joint Surg [Am] *60*:836, 1978.

404. Cameron HU, Kostuik JP: A long-term follow-up of synovial sarcoma. J Bone Joint Surg [Br] *56*:613, 1974.

405. Sutro CJ: Synovial sarcoma of the soft parts in the 1st toe: Recurrence after a 35 year interval. Bull Hosp Joint Dis *37*:105, 1976.

406. Dische FE, Darby AJ, Howard ER: Malignant synovioma: Electron microscopical findings in 3 patients and review of the literature. J Pathol *124*:149, 1978.

407. Fernandez BB, Hernandez FJ: Poorly differentiated synovial sarcoma. A light and electron microscopic study. Arch Pathol Lab Med *100*:221, 1976.

408. Mackenzie DH: Monophasic synovial sarcoma—a histological entity? Histopathology *1*:151, 1977.

409. deSantos LA, Lindell MM Jr, Goldman AM, et al, Calcification within metastatic pulmonary nodules from synovial sarcoma. Orthopedics *1*:141, 1978.

410. Hale DE: Synovioma with special reference to the clinical and roentgenologic aspects. AJR *65*:769, 1951.

411. Lewis RW: Roentgen recognition of synovioma. AJR *44*:170, 1940.

412. Albores-Saavedra J, Martin RG, Smith JL Jr: Rhabdomyosarcoma: A study of 35 cases. Ann Surg *157*:186, 1963.

413. Enterline HT, Horn RC Jr: Alveolar rhabdomyosarcoma. A distinctive tumor type. Am J Clin Pathol *29*:356, 1958.

414. Enzinger FM, Shiraki M: Alveolar rhabdomyosarcoma. An analysis of 110 cases. Cancer *24*:18, 1969.

415. Horn RC Jr, Patton RB: Rhabdomyosarcoma. Clin Orthop *19*:99, 1961.

416. Horn RC Jr, Enterline HT: Rhabdomyosarcoma: A clinicopathological study and classification of 39 cases. Cancer *11*:181, 1958.

417. Linscheid RL, Soule EH, Henderson ED: Pleomorphic rhabdomyosarcomata of the extremities and limb girdles. J Bone Joint Surg [Am] *47*:715, 1965.

418. Moore O, Grossi C: Embryonal rhabdomyosarcoma of the head and neck. Cancer *12*:69, 1959.

419. Pack GT, Eberhart WF: Rhabdomyosarcoma of skeletal muscle: Report of 100 cases. Surgery *32*:1023, 1952.

420. Pinkel D, Pickren J: Rhabdomyosarcoma in children. JAMA *175*:293, 1961.

421. Stobbe GD, Dargeon HW: Embryonal rhabdomyosarcoma of head and neck in children and adolescents. Cancer *3*:826, 1950.

422. Stout AP: Rhabdomyosarcoma of skeletal muscles. Ann Surg *123*:447, 1946.

423. MacKenzie DH: Fibroma—a dangerous diagnosis. A review of 205 cases of fibrosarcoma of soft tissues. Br J Surg *51*:607, 1964.

424. Pritchard DJ, Soule EH, Taylor WF, et al: Fibrosarcoma—a clinicopathologic and statistical study of 199 tumors of the soft tissue of the extremities and trunk. Cancer *33*:888, 1974.

425. Pritchard DJ, Sim FH, Ivins JC, et al: Fibrosarcoma of bone and soft tissues of the trunk and extremities. Orthop Clin North Am *8*:869, 1977.

426. Stout AP: Fibrosarcoma. The malignant tumor of fibroblasts. Cancer *1*:30, 1948.

427. van der Werf-Messing B, van Unnik JAM: Fibrosarcoma of the soft tissues. A clinicopathologic study. Cancer *18*:1113, 1965.

428. Yaghmai I: Angiographic features of fibromas and fibrosarcomas. Radiology *124*:57, 1977.

429. Chung EB, Enzinger FM: Infantile fibrosarcoma. Cancer *38*:729, 1976.

430. Soule EH, Pritchard DJ: Fibrosarcoma in infants and children. A review of 110 cases. Cancer *40*:1711, 1977.

431. Kindblom LG, Merck, C, Svendsen P: Myxofibrosarcoma: A pathologicoanatomical, microangiographic and angiographic correlative study of 8 cases. Br J Radiol *50*:876, 1977.

432. Lagergren C, Lindblom A, Söderberg G: Vascularization of fibromatous and fibrosarcomatous tumors: Histopathologic, microangiographic and angiographic studies. Acta Radiol *53*:1, 1960.

433. Balsaver AM, Butler JJ, Martin RG: Congenital fibrosarcoma. Cancer *20*:1607, 1967.

434. Exelby PR, Knapper WH, Huvos AG, et al: Soft tissue fibrosarcoma in children. J Pediatr Surg *8*:415, 1973.

435. Horne CHW, Slavin G, McDonald AM: Late recurrence of juvenile fibrosarcoma. Br J Surg *55*:102, 1968.

436. Schvarcz LW: Congenital dermatofibrosarcoma protuberans of the hand. Hand *9*:182, 1977.

437. Stout AP: Fibrosarcoma in infants and children. Cancer *15*:1028, 1962.

438. Haug WA, Losli EJ: Primary leiomyosarcoma within the femoral vein. Report of a case and review of the literature. Cancer *7*:159, 1954.

439. Phelan JT, Sherer W, Mesa P: Malignant smooth-muscle tumors (leiomyosarcomas) of soft tissue origin. N Engl J Med *266*:1027, 1962.

440. Rising JA, Booth E: Primary leiomyosarcoma of the skin with lymphatic spread. Report of a case. Arch Pathol *81*:94, 1966.

441. Stout AP, Hill WT: Leiomyosarcoma of the superficial soft tissues. Cancer *11*:844, 1958.

442. Fine G, Stout AP: Osteogenic sarcoma of the extraskeletal soft tissues. Cancer *9*:1027, 1956.

443. Kauffman SL, Stout AP: Extraskeletal osteogenic sarcomas and chondrosarcomas in children. Cancer *16*:432, 1963.

444. Salm R: A case of primary osteogenic sarcoma of extraskeletal soft tissues. Br J Cancer *13*:614, 1959.

445. Enzinger FM, Shiraki M: Extraskeletal myxoid chondrosarcoma. An analysis of 34 cases. Hum Pathol *3*:421, 1972.

446. Lewis MM, Marcove RC, Bullough PG: Chondrosarcoma of the foot. A case report and review of the literature. Cancer 36:586, 1975.

447. Marcove RC: Chondrosarcoma: Diagnosis and treatment. Orthop Clin North Am 8:811, 1977.

448. Moore JP, Shannon E: Extraskeletal chondrosarcomas. Tex Med 70:65, 1974.

449. Ream JR, Corson JM, Holdsworth DE, et al: Chondrosarcoma of the extraskeletal soft tissue of the finger. Clin Orthop 97:148, 1973.

450. Smith MT, Farinacci CJ, Carpenter HA, et al: Extraskeletal myxoid chondrosarcoma. A clinicopathological study. Cancer 37:821, 1976.

451. Stout AP, Verner EW: Chondrosarcoma of the extraskeletal soft tissues. Cancer 6:581, 1953.

452. Feldman F, Norman D: Intra- and extraosseous malignant histiocytoma (malignant fibrous xanthoma). Radiology 104:497, 1972.

453. O'Brien JE, Stout AP: Malignant fibrous xanthomas. Cancer 17:1445, 1964.

454. Soule EH, Enriquez P: Atypical fibrous histiocytoma, malignant fibrous histiocytoma, malignant fibrous histiocytoma, and epithelioid sarcoma. A comparative study of 65 tumors. Cancer 30:128, 1972.

455. Weiss SW, Enzinger FM: Myxoid variant of malignant fibrous histiocytoma. Cancer 39:1672, 1977.

456. Ackerman LV: Extra-osseous localized non-neoplastic bone and cartilage formation (so-called myositis ossificans). Clinical and pathological confusion with malignant neoplasms. J Bone Joint Surg [Am] 40:279, 1958.

457. Angervall L, Stener B, Stener I, et al: Pseudomalignant osseous tumor of soft tissue. A clinical, radiological and pathological study of 5 cases. J Bone Joint Surg [Br] 51:654, 1969.

458. Chung BS: Drug-induced myositis ossificans circumscripta. JAMA 226:469, 1973.

459. Geschickter CF, Maseritz IH: Myositis ossificans. J Bone Joint Surg 20:661, 1938.

460. Gilmer WS Jr, Anderson LD: Reactions of soft somatic tissue which may progress to bone formation: Circumscribed (traumatic) myositis ossificans. South Med J 52:1432, 1959.

461. Gunn DR, Young WB: Myositis ossificans as a complication of tetanus. J Bone Joint Surg [Br] 41:535, 1959.

462. Heilbrun N, Kuhn WG Jr: Erosive bone lesions and soft-tissue ossifications associated with spinal cord injuries (paraplegia). Radiology 48:579, 1947.

463. Hughston JC, Whatley GS, Stone MM: Myositis ossificans traumatica (myoosteosis). South Med J 55:1167, 1962.

464. Jeffreys TE, Stiles PJ: Pseudomalignant osseous tumor of soft tissue. J Bone Joint Surg [Br] 48:488, 1966.

465. Kern WH: Proliferative myositis: A pseudosarcomatous reaction to injury. A report of 7 cases. Arch Pathol 69:209, 1960.

466. Lewis D. Myositis ossificans. JAMA 80:1281, 1923.

467. Skajaa T: Myositis ossificans. Acta Chir Scand 116:68, 1958.

468. Goldman AB: Myositis ossificans circumscripta: A benign lesion with malignant differential diagnosis. AJR 126:32, 1976.

469. Pack GT, Braund RR: The development of sarcoma in myositis ossificans. Report of three cases. JAMA 119:776, 1942.

470. Shanoff LB, Spira M, Hardy SB: Myositis ossificans: Evolution to osteogenic sarcoma. Report of a histologically verified case. Am J Surg 113:537, 1967.

471. Johnson LC: Histogenesis of myositis ossificans (Abstr). Am J Pathol 24:681, 1948.

472. Kramer FL, Kurtz AB, Rubin C, et al: Ultrasound appearance of myositis ossificans. Skel Radiol 4:19, 1979.

473. Norman A, Dorfman HD: Juxtacortical circumscribed myositis ossificans: Evolution and radiographic features. Radiology 96:301, 1970.

474. Yaghmai I: Myositis ossificans: Diagnostic value of arteriography. AJR 128:811, 1977.

475. Tibone J, Sakimura I, Nickel VL, et al: Heterotopic ossification around the hip in spinal cord-injured patients: A long-term follow-up study. J Bone Joint Surg [Am] 60:769, 1978.

476. Alguacil-Garcia A, Unni KK, Goellner JR: Giant cell tumor of tendon sheath and pigmented villonodular synovitis: An ultrastructural study. Am J Clin Pathol 69:6, 1978.

477. Barnard JD: Pigmented villonodular synovitis in the temporomandibular joint. A case report. Br J Oral Surg 13:183, 1975.

478. Carstens HB: Giant cell tumors of tendon sheath. An electron microscopical study of 11 cases. Arch Pathol Lab Med 102:99, 1978.

479. Chung SMK, Janes JM: Diffuse pigmented villonodular synovitis of the hip joint. Review of the literature and report of four cases. J Bone Joint Surg [Am] 47:293, 1965.

480. Byers PD, Cotton RE, Deacon OW, et al: The diagnosis and treatment of pigmented villonodular synovitis. J Bone Joint Surg [Am] 50:290, 1968.

481. Decker JP, Owen BJ: An invasive giant cell tumor of tendon sheath in the foot. Bull Ayer Clin Lab Penn Hosp 4:43, 1954.

482. Eisenstein R: Giant-cell tumor of tendon sheath: Its histogenesis as studied in the electron microscope. J Bone Joint Surg [Am] 50:476, 1968.

483. Eisenberg RL, Hedgcock MW: Bilateral pigmented villonodular synovitis of the hip. Br J Radiol 51:916, 1978.

484. Fletcher AG Jr, Horn RC Jr: Giant cell tumors of tendon sheath origin. A consideration of bone involvement and report of two cases with extensive bone destruction. Ann Surg 133:374, 1951.

485. Granowitz SP, Mankin HJ: Localized pigmented villonodular synovitis of the knee. Report of 5 cases. J Bone Joint Surg [Am] 49:122, 1967.

486. Granowitz SP, D'Antonio J, Mankin HL: The pathogenesis and longterm end results of pigmented villonodular synovitis. Clin Orthop 114:335, 1976.

487. Jones FE, Soule EH, Coventry MB: Fibrous xanthoma of synovium (giant-cell tumor of tendon sheath, pigmented nodular synovitis). A study of 118 cases. J Bone Joint Surg [Am] 51:76, 1969.

488. Kindblom LG, Gunterberg B: Pigmented villonodular synovitis involving bone. J Bone Joint Surg [Am] 60:830, 1978.

489. Kleinstiver BJ, Rodriguez HA: Nodular fasciitis: Study of 45 cases and review of literature. J Bone Joint Surg [Am] 50:1204, 1968.

490. Leszczynski J, Huckell JR, Percy JS, et al: Pigmented villonodular synovitis in multiple joints. Occurrence in a child with cavernous haemangioma of lip and pulmonary stenosis. Ann Rheum Dis 34:269, 1975.

491. Levine HA, Enrile F: Giant-cell tumor of patellar tendon coincident with Paget's disease. J Bone Joint Surg [Am] 53:335, 1971.

492. Lichtenstein L: Tumors of synovial joints, bursae and tendon sheaths. Cancer 8:816, 1955.

493. Schajowicz F, Blumenfeld I: Pigmented villonodular synovitis of the wrist with penetration into bone. J Bone Joint Surg [Am] 50:312, 1968.

494. Shafer SJ, Larmon WA: Pigmented villonodular synovitis. A report of seven cases. Surg Gynecol Obstet 92:574, 1951.

495. Sherry JB, Anderson W: The natural history of pigmented villonodular synovitis of tendon sheaths. J Bone Joint Surg [Am] 37:1005, 1955.

496. Torisu T, Iwabuchi R, Kamo Y: Pigmented villonodular synovitis of the elbow with bony erosion. Clin Orthop 94:275, 1973.

497. Woods C Jr, Alade CO, Anderson V, et al: Pigmented villonodular synovitis of the knee presenting as a loose body. A case report. Clin Orthop 129:230, 1977.

498. Yanklowitz BA: Giant cell tumor of tendon sheath: A literature review and case report. J Am Podiatry Assoc 68:706, 1978.

499. Hoaglund FT: Experimental hemarthrosis. The response of canine knees to injections of autologous blood. J Bone Joint Surg [Am] 49:285, 1967.

500. McCollum DE, Musser AW, Rhangos WC: Experimental villonodular synovitis. South Med J 59:966, 1966.

501. Roy S, Ghadially FN: Synovial membrane in experimentally-produced chronic haemarthrosis. Ann Rheum Dis 28:402, 1969.

502. Young JM, Hudacek AG: Experimental production of pigmented villonodular synovitis in dogs. Am J Pathol 30:799, 1954.

503. Jaffe HL, Lichtenstein L, Sutro CJ: Pigmented villonodular synovitis, bursitis and tenosynovitis. Arch Pathol 31:731, 1941.

504. Cavanagh RC, Schwamm HA: Localized nodular synovitis. RPC of the month from the AFIP. Radiology 100:409, 1971.

505. Johnson LC: Personal communication.

506. Byers PD, Cotton RE, Deacon OW, et al: The diagnosis and treatment of pigmented villonodular synovitis. J Bone Joint Surg [Br] 50:290, 1968.

507. Breimer CW, Freiberger RH: Bone lesions associated with villonodular synovitis. AJR 79:618, 1958.

508. Crosby EB, Inglis A, Bullough PG: Multiple joint involvement with pigmented villonodular synovitis. Radiology 122:671, 1977.

509. Gehweiler JA, Wilson JW: Diffuse biarticular pigmented villonodular synovitis. Radiology 93:845, 1969.

510. Greenfield MM, Wallace KM: Pigmented villonodular synovitis. Radiology 54:350, 1950.

511. Jergesen HE, Mankin HJ, Schiller AL: Diffuse pigmented villonodular synovitis of the knee mimicking primary bone neoplasms. J Bone Joint Surg [Am] 60:825, 1978.

512. Lewis RW: Roentgen diagnosis of pigmented villonodular synovitis and synovial sarcoma of the knee joint: Preliminary report. Radiology 49:26, 1947.

513. McMaster PE: Pigmented villonodular synovitis with invasion of bone. Report of six cases. J Bone Joint Surg [Am] 42:1170, 1960.

514. Smith JH, Pugh DG: Roentgenographic aspects of articular pigmented villonodular synovitis. AJR 87:1146, 1962.

515. Scott PM: Bone lesions in pigmented villonodular synovitis. J Bone Joint Surg [Br] 50:306, 1968.

516. Rosenthal DI, Aronow S, Murray WT: Iron content of pigmented villonodular synovitis detected by computed tomography. Radiology 133:409, 1979.

517. Goergen IG, Resnick D, Niwayama G: Localized nodular synovitis of the knee. A report of two cases with abnormal arthrograms. AJR 126:647, 1976.

518. Halpern A, Donovan TL, Horowitz B, et al: Arthrographic demonstration of pigmented villonodular synovitis of the knee. Clin Orthop 132:193, 1978.

519. Rein BI, Bilodeau LP, Johanson P: Arthrography and arteriography in pigmented villonodular synovitis of the knee. AJR 92:1322, 1964.

520. Wolfe RD, Giuliano VJ: Double-contrast arthrography in the diagnosis of pigmented villonodular synovitis of the knee. AJR 110:793, 1970.

521. Chater EH: Tumoral calcinosis. Br Med J 1:644, 1969.

522. Cooke RA: Tumoral calcinosis. Br Med J 4:174, 1969.

523. Inclan A, Leon P, Gomez Camejo M: Tumoral calcinosis. JAMA 121:490, 1943.

524. Maathuis JB, Koten JW: Kikuyu-bursa and tumoral calcinosis. Trop Geogr Med 21:389, 1969.

525. McClatchie S, Bremmer AD: Tumoral calcinosis—an unrecognized disease. Br Med J 1:153, 1969.

526. Najjar SS, Farah FS, Kurban AK, et al: Tumoral calcinosis and pseudoxanthoma elasticum. J Pediatr 72:243, 1968.

527. Slavin G, Klenerman L, Darby A, et al: Tumoral calcinosis in England. Br Med J 1:147, 1973.

528. Harkess JW, Peters HJ: Tumoral calcinosis. A report of six cases. J Bone Joint Surg [Am] 49:721, 1967.

529. Agnew CH: Tumoral calcinosis. A radiologic teaching method. J Kans Med Soc 62:100, 1961.

530. Albright F, Reifenstein EC Jr.: Parathyroid Glands and Metabolic Bone Disease. Baltimore, Williams & Wilkins Co, 1948.

531. Baldursson H, Evans EB, Dodge WF, et al: Tumoral calcinosis with hyperphosphatemia. A report of a family with incidence in four siblings. J Bone Joint Surg [Am] 51:913, 1969.

532. Poppel MH, Zeitel BE: Roentgen manifestations of milk drinker's syndrome. Radiology 67:195, 1956.

533. Hacihanefioğlu U: Tumoral calcinosis: A clinical and pathologic study of eleven unreported cases in Turkey. J Bone Joint Surg [Am] 60:1131, 1978.

534. Lafferty FW, Reynolds ES, Pearson OH: Tumoral calcinosis. A metabolic disease of obscure etiology. Am J Med 38:105, 1965.

535. Reed RJ, Hunt RW: Granulomatous (tumoral) calcinosis. Clin Orthop 43:233, 1965.

536. Barton DL, Reeves RJ: Tumoral calcinosis. Report of three cases and review of the literature. AJR 86:351, 1961.

537. Palmer PES: Tumoural calcinosis. Br J Radiol 39:518, 1966.

538. Riemenschneider PA, Ecker A: Sciatica caused by tumoral calcinosis. J Neurosurg 9:304, 1952.

539. Smit GG, Schmaman A: Tumoral calcinosis. J Bone Joint Surg [Br] 49:698, 1967.

540. Thomson JG: Calcifying collagenolysis (tumoural calcinosis). Br J Radiol 39:526, 1966.

541. Yaghmai I, Mirbod P: Tumoral calcinosis. AJR 111:573, 1971.

542. Hug I, Guncaga J: Tumoral calcinosis with sedimentation sign. Br J Radiol 47:734, 1974.

543. Kolawole TM, Bohrer SP: Tumoral calcinosis with ''fluid levels'' in the tumoral masses. AJR 120:461, 1974.

544. Bouhoutsos J, Martin P: Popliteal aneurysm: A review of 116 cases. Br J Surg 61:469, 1974.

545. Gifford RW Jr, Hines EA Jr, Janes JM: An analysis and follow-up study of one hundred popliteal aneurysms. Surgery 33:284, 1953.

546. Giustra PE, Root JA, Mason SE, et al: Popliteal vein thrombosis secondary to popliteal artery aneurysm. AJR 130:25, 1978.

547. Hardy JD, Tompkins WC Jr, Hatten LE, et al: Aneurysms of the popliteal artery. Surg Gynecol Obstet 140:401, 1975.

548. Hunt DD: Problems in diagnosing osteoarticular tuberculosis. JAMA 190:95, 1964.

549. Marwah V: Changing pattern of osteoarticular tuberculosis. J Indian Med Assoc 38:18, 1962.

550. Dickson FD: Differential diagnosis of tuberculous arthritis. JAMA 107:531, 1936.

551. Dickson FD: Differential diagnosis of tuberculous arthritis. J Lab Clin Med 22:35, 1936.

552. Houkom SS: Tuberculosis of the ankle joint; an end result of 25 cases. Surg Gynecol Obstet 76:438, 1943.

553. Phemister DB: Changes in the articular surfaces in tuberculosis and pyogenic infections of joints. AJR 12:1, 1924.

554. Phemister DB, Hatcher CH: Correlation of pathological and roentgenological findings in diagnosis of tuberculous arthritis. AJR 29:736, 1933.

555. El-Khoury GY, Bassett GS: Symptomatic bursa formation with osteochondromas. AJR 133:895, 1979.

556. Smithuis T: Exostosis bursata. Report of a case. J Bone Joint Surg [Br] 46:544, 1964.

557. Gomez-Reino JJ, Radin A, Gorevic PD: Pseudoaneurysm of the popliteal artery as a complication of an osteochondroma. Skel Radiol 4:26, 1979.

558. Greenway G, Resnick D, Bookstein JJ: Popliteal pseudoaneurysm as a complication of an adjacent osteochondroma: Angiographic diagnosis. AJR 132:294, 1979.

559. Cary GR: Juxtacortical chondroma, a case report. J Bone Joint Surg [Am] 47:1405, 1965.

560. Cooke GM, Pearce JG: Periosteal chondroma. Report of two cases with atypical radiologic features. J Can Assoc Radiol 27:301, 1976.

561. Fornasier VL, McGonigal D: Periosteal chondroma. Clin Orthop 124:233, 1977.

562. Jaffe HL: Juxtacortical chondroma. Bull Hosp Joint Dis 17:20, 1956.

563. Kirchner SG, Pavlov H, Heller RM, et al: Periosteal chondromas of the anterior tibial tubercle: Two cases. AJR 131:1088, 1978.

564. Lichtenstein L, Hall JE: Periosteal chondroma; a distinctive benign cartilage tumor. J Bone Joint Surg [Am] 34:691, 1952.

565. Nosanchuk JS, Kaufer H: Recurrent periosteal chondroma. Report of two cases and a review of the literature. J Bone Joint Surg [Am] 51:375, 1969.

566. Rockwell MA, Saiter ET, Enneking WF: Periosteal chondroma. J Bone Joint Surg [Am] 54:102, 1972.

567. Buckwalter JA, El-Khoury GY, Flatt AE: Dysplasia epiphysealis hemimelica of the ulna. Clin Orthop 135:36, 1978.

568. Carlson DH, Wilkinson RH: Variability of unilateral epiphyseal dysplasia (dysplasia epiphysealis hemimelica). Radiology 133:368, 1979.

569. Fairbank TJ: Dysplasia epiphysealis hemimelica (tarso-epiphyseal aclasis). J Bone Joint Surg [Br] 38:237, 1956.

570. Hensinger RN, Cowell HR, Ramsey PL, et al: Familial dysplasia epiphysealis hemimelica, associated with chondromas and osteochondromas. Report of a kindred with variable presentations. J Bone Joint Surg [Am] 56:1513, 1974.

571. Kettelkamp DB, Campbell CJ, Bonfiglio M: Dysplasia epiphysealis hemimelica. Report of fifteen cases and a review of the literature. J Bone Joint Surg [Am] 48:746, 1966.

572. Trevor D: Tarso-epiphyseal aclasis: A congenital error in epiphyseal development. J Bone Joint Surg [Br] 32:204, 1950.

573. Freiberger RH, Loitman BS, Helpern M, et al: Osteoid osteoma, a report of 80 cases. AJR 82:194, 1959.

574. Giustra PE, Freiberger RH: Severe growth disturbance with osteoid osteoma; a report of 2 cases involving the femoral neck. Radiology 96:285, 1970.

575. Johnson GF: Osteoid osteoma of the femoral neck. AJR 74:65, 1955.

576. Lawrie TR, Aterman K, Sinclair AM: Painless osteoid osteoma; a report of 2 cases. J Bone Joint Surg [Br] 52:1357, 1970.

577. Marcove RC, Freiberger RH: Osteoid osteoma of the elbow. A diagnostic problem: Report of 4 cases. J Bone Joint Surg [Am] 48:1185, 1966.

578. Sherman MS: Osteoid osteoma associated with changes in an adjacent joint. Report of two cases. J Bone Joint Surg 29:483, 1947.

579. Snarr JW, Abell MR, Martel W: Lymphofollicular synovitis with osteoid osteoma. Radiology 106:557, 1973.

580. Spence AJ, Lloyd-Roberts GC: Regional osteoporosis in osteoid osteoma. J Bone Joint Surg [Br] 43:501, 1961.

581. Lisbona R, Rosenthall L: Role of radionuclide imaging in osteoid osteoma. AJR 132:77, 1979.

582. Mitnick JS, Genieser NB: Osteoid osteoma of the hip; unusual isotopic appearance. AJR 133:322, 1979.

583. Winter PF, Johnson PM, Hilal SK, et al: Scintigraphic detection of osteoid osteoma. Radiology 122:177, 1978.

584. Lateur L, Baert AL: Localization and diagnosis of osteoid osteoma of the carpal area by angiography. Skel Radiol 2:75, 1977.

585. O'Hara JP III, Tegtmeyer C, Sweet DE, et al: Angiography in the diagnosis of osteoid-osteoma of the hand. J Bone Joint Surg [Am] 57:163, 1975.

586. Lowenstein MB, Smith JRV, Cole S: Infrapatellar pigmented villonodular synovitis: Arthrographic detection. AJR 135:279, 1980.

587. Kaiser TE, Ivins JC, Unni KK: Malignant transformation of extraarticular synovial chondromatosis: Report of a case. Skel Radiol 5:223, 1980.

588. Burleson RJ, Bickel WH, Dahlin DC: Popliteal cyst. A clinicopathological survey. J Bone Joint Surg [Am] 38:1265, 1956.

589. Fedullo LM, Bonakdarpour A, Moyer RA, et al: Giant synovial cysts. Skel Radiol 12:90, 1984.

590. Guerra J Jr, Newell JD, Resnick D, et al: Gastrocnemiosemimembranosus bursal region of the knee. AJR 136:593, 1981.

591. Sartoris DJ, Danzig L, Gilula L, et al: Synovial cysts of the hip joint and iliopsoas bursitis: A spectrum of imaging abnormalities. Skel Radiol 14:85, 1985.

592. Goode JD: Synovial rupture of the elbow joint. Ann Rheum Dis 27:604, 1968.

593. Halpern AA: Massive synovial cyst of the shoulder causing vascular compromise. Clin Orthop 143:151, 1979.

594. Bacon PA, Gerber NJ: Popliteal cysts and synovial rupture in osteoarthrosis. Rheumatol Rehabil 13:98, 1974.

595. Bowerman JW, Muhletaler C: Arthrography of rheumatoid synovial cysts of the knee and wrist. J Can Assoc Radiol 24:24, 1973.

596. Harvey JP, Corcos J: Large cysts in lower leg originating in the knee occurring in patients with rheumatoid arthritis. Arthritis Rheum 3:218, 1960.

597. Burt TB, MacCarter DK, Gelman MI, et al: Clinical manifestations of synovial cysts. West J Med 133:99, 1980.

598. Dixon AS, Grant C: Acute synovial rupture in rheumatoid arthritis. Clinical and experimental observations. Lancet 1:742, 1964.

599. Eyanson S, MacFarlane JD, Brandt KD: Popliteal cyst mimicking thrombophlebitis as the first indication of rheumatoid arthritis. Clin Orthop 144:215, 1979.

600. Kilcoyne RF, Imray TJ, Stewart ET: Ruptured Baker's cyst simulating acute thrombophlebitis. JAMA 240:1517, 1978.

601. Kattapuram SV: Case Report 181: Calcified popliteal cyst (Baker's cyst). Skel Radiol 7:279, 1982.

602. Carpenter JR, Hattery RR, Hunder GG, et al: Ultrasound evaluation of the popliteal space—comparison with arthrography and physical examination. Mayo Clin Proc 51:498, 1976.

603. Cooper RA: Computerized tomography (body scan) of Baker's cyst. J Rheumatol 5:184, 1978.

604. Gerber NJ, Dixon ASJ: Synovial cysts and juxta-articular bone cysts (geodes). Semin Arthritis Rheum 3:323, 1974.

605. Goldberg RP, Genant HK: Calcified bodies in popliteal cysts: A characteristic radiographic appearance. AJR 131:857, 1978.

606. Hermann G, Yeh H, Lehr-Janus C, et al: Diagnosis of popliteal cyst: Double contrast arthrography and sonography. AJR 137:369, 1981.

607. Lee KR, Tines MD, Price HI, et al: The computed tomographic findings of popliteal cysts. Skel Radiol 10:26, 1983.

608. Wolf RD, Colloff B: Popliteal cysts. An arthrographic study and review of the literature. J Bone Joint Surg [Am] 54:1057, 1972.
609. Rosenthal DI, Schwartz AN, Schiller AL: Case report 179: Subperiosteal synovial cyst of knee. Skel Radiol 7:142, 1981.
610. Enzinger FM, Weiss SW: Soft Tissue Tumors. 2nd Ed. St Louis, CV Mosby Company, 1988.
611. Nessi R, Coopmans de Yoldi G: Soft tissue xeroradiography. Radiol Clin (Basel) 47:157, 1978.
612. Nessi R, Gattoni F, Mazzoni R, et al: Lipoblastic tumours of somatic soft tissues: A xerographic evaluation of 67 cases. Skel Radiol 5:137, 1980.
613. Otto R, Pouliadis GP, Kumpe DA: The evaluation of pathologic alterations of juxtaosseous soft tissue by xeroradiography. Radiology 120:297, 1976.
614. Chew FS, Hudson TM: Radionuclide imaging of lipoma and liposarcoma. Radiology 136:741, 1980.
615. Johnson RJ, Garvie N: Case report 121: Synovioma (synovial sarcoma) of left knee. Skel Radiol 5:185, 1980.
616. Enneking WF, Chew FS, Springfield DS, et al: The role of radionuclide bonescan in determining the resectability of soft-tissue sarcomas. J Bone Joint Surg [Am] 63:249, 1981.
617. Braunstein EM, Silver TM, Martel W, et al: Ultrasonographic diagnosis of extremity masses. Skel Radiol 6:157, 1981.
618. Paushter DM, Borkowski GP, Buonocore E, et al: Digital subtraction angiography for preoperative evaluation of extremity tumors. AJR 141:129, 1983.
619. Bernardino ME, Jing B, Thomas JL, et al: The extremity soft-tissue lesion: A comparative study of ultrasound, computed tomography, and xeroradiography. Radiology 139:53, 1981.
620. Egund N, Ekelund L, Sako M, et al: CT of soft-tissue tumors. AJR 137:725, 1981.
621. Ekelund L, Herrlin K, Rydholm A: Comparison of computed tomography and angiography in the evaluation of soft tissue tumors of the extremities. Acta Radiol [Diagn] (Stockh) 23:15, 1982.
622. Golding SJ, Husband JE: The role of computed tomography in the management of soft tissue sarcomas. Br J Radiol 55:740, 1982.
623. Rosenthal DL: Computed tomography in bone and soft tissue neoplasm: application and pathologic correlation. CRC Crit Rev Diagn Imaging 18:243, 1982.
624. Weeks RG, McLeod RA, Reiman HM, et al: CT of soft-tissue neoplasms. AJR 144:355, 1985.
625. Sauer JM, Ozonoff MB: Congenital bone anomalies associated with lipomas. Skel Radiol 13:276, 1985.
626. Dooms GC, Hricak H, Sollitto RA, et al: Lipomatous tumors and tumors with fatty component: MR imaging potential and comparison of MR and CT results. Radiology 157:479, 1985.
627. Enzi G, Biondetti PB, Fiore D, et al: Computed tomography of deep fat masses in multiple symmetrical lipomatosis. Radiology 144:121, 1982.
628. Lachman RS, Finklestein J, Mehringer CM, et al: Congenital aggressive lipomatosis. Skel Radiol 9:248, 1983.
629. Engelstad BL, Gilula LA, Kyriakos M: Ossified skeletal muscle hemangioma: Radiologic and pathologic features. Skel Radiol 5:35, 1980.
630. Subbarao K: Case report 228, congenital venous dysplasia of the index finger involving soft tissue and bone. Skel Radiol 9:273, 1983.
631. Gilliland JD, Solonick DM, Whigham CJ, et al: Case report 327: Arteriovenous malformation eroding the right femoral neck. Skel Radiol 14:145, 1985.
632. McGahan JP, Hansen SK, Palmer PES: Case report 163: Hemangiopericytoma of the soft tissue in the area of the left scapula. Skel Radiol 7:66, 1981.
633. Ginaldi S: Computed tomography feature of synovial osteochondromatosis. Skel Radiol 5:219, 1980.
634. Lequesne M, Becker J, Bard M, et al: Capsular constriction of the hip: Arthrographic and clinical considerations. Skel Radiol 6:1, 1981.
635. Zlatkin MB, Lander PH, Begin LR, et al: Soft-tissue chondromas. AJR 144:1263, 1985.
636. Pringle J, Stoker DJ: Case report 110: Juvenile aponeurotic fibroma. Skel Radiol 5:53, 1980.
637. Ekelund L, Herrlin K, Rydholm A: Computed tomography of intramuscular myxoma. Skel Radiol 9:14, 1982.
638. Weiss SW, Enzinger FM: Malignant fibrous histiocytoma: An analysis of 200 cases. Cancer 41:2250, 1978.
639. Fischer HJ, Lois JF, Gomes AS, et al: Radiology and pathology of malignant fibrous histiocytomas of the soft tissues: A report of ten cases. Skel Radiol 13:202, 1985.
640. Dorfman HD, Bhagauan BS: Malignant fibrous histiocytoma of soft tissue with metaplastic bone and cartilage formation: A new radiologic sign. Skel Radiol 8:145, 1982.
641. Brill PW, Yandow DR, Langer LO, et al: Congenital generalized fibromatosis. Pediatr Radiol 12:269, 1982.
642. Shmookler BM, Enzinger FM: Liposarcoma occurring in children. Cancer 52:567, 1983.
643. Israels SJ, Chan HSL, Daneman A, et al: Synovial sarcoma in childhood. AJR 142:803, 1984.
644. Craig RM, Pugh DG, Soule EH: Roentgenologic manifestations of synovial sarcoma. Radiology 65:837, 1955.
645. Horowitz AL, Resnick D, Watson RC: The roentgen features of synovial sarcoma. Clin Radiol 24:481, 1973.
646. Sherman RS, Chu FCH: A roentgenographic study of synovioma. AJR 67:80, 1952.
647. Dahlin DC: Case report 189: Infantile fibrosarcoma (congenital fibrosarcoma-like fibromatosis). Skel Radiol 8:77, 1982.
648. Fauré C, Gruner M, Baccon-Gibod L: Case report 149: Infantile congenital fibrosarcoma of humerus. Skel Radiol 6:208, 1981.
649. Park JJ, Park HC, Chai SH: Leiomyosarcomas of the extremities: Angiography as a diagnostic aid. J Surg Oncol 10:407, 1978.
650. Ekelund L, Rydholm A: The value of angiography in soft tissue leiomyosarcomas of the extremities. Skel Radiol 9:201, 1983.
651. Connor JM, Horan FT, Beighton P: Dysplasia epiphysealis hemimelica. A clinical and genetic study. J Bone Joint Surg [Br] 65:350, 1983.
652. Goldstein WB: Dysplasia epiphysealis hemimelica with confirmation by knee arthrography. Br J Radiol 46:470, 1973.
653. Oates E, Cutler JB, Miyamoto EK, et al: Case report 305: Dysplasia epiphysealis hemimelica (Trevor disease) of left ankle with an associated osteochondral (post-traumatic) fracture fragment, probably arising from talus. Skel Radiol 13:174, 1985.
654. Sartoris DJ, Haghighi P, Resnick D: Painful swelling of the toe in a young boy. Invest Radiol 22:170, 1987.
655. Sundaram M, McGuire MH, Herbold DR, et al: High signal intensity soft tissue masses on T1 weighted pulsing sequences. Skel Radiol 16:30, 1987.
656. Beltran J, Simon DC, Katz W, et al: Increased MR signal intensity in skeletal muscle adjacent to malignant tumors: Pathologic correlation and clinical relevance. Radiology 162:251, 1987.
657. Steinbach L, Hellman D, Petri M, et al: Magnetic resonance imaging: a review of rheumatologic applications. Semin Arthritis Rheum 16:79, 1986.
658. Enzinger FM, Weiss SW: Soft Tissue Tumors. 2nd Ed. St. Louis, CV Mosby, 1988, p 43.
659. Bland KI, McCoyd M, Kinard RE, et al: Application of magnetic resonance imaging and computerized tomography as an adjunct to the surgical management of soft tissue sarcomas. Ann Surg 205:473, 1987.
660. Chang AE, Matory YL, Dwyer AJ, et al: Magnetic resonance imaging versus computed tomography in the evaluation of soft tissue tumors of the extremities. Ann Surg 205:340, 1987.
661. Demas BE, Heelan RT, Lane J, et al: Soft-tissue sarcomas of the extremities: Comparison of MR and CT in determining the extent of disease. AJR 150:615, 1988.
662. Petasnick JP, Turner DA, Charters JR, et al: Soft-tissue masses of the locomotor system: Comparison of MR imaging and CT. Radiology 160:125, 1986.
663. Weekes RG, Berquist TH, McLeod RA, et al: Magnetic resonance imaging of soft-tissue tumors: Comparison with computed tomography. Magn Reson Imaging 3:345, 1985.
664. Aisen AM, Martel W, Braunstein EM, et al: MRI and CT evaluation of primary bone and soft tissue tumors. AJR 146:749, 1986.
665. Tehranzadeh J, Mnaymneh W, Ghavam C, et al: Comparison of CT and MR imaging in musculoskeletal neoplasms. J Comput Assist Tomogr 13:466, 1989.
666. Berquist TH, Ehman RL, King BF, et al: Value of MR imaging in differentiating benign from malignant soft tissue masses: Study of 95 lesions. AJR 155:1251, 1990.
667. Kransdorf MJ, Jelinek JS, Moser RP, et al: Soft tissue masses: Diagnosis using MR imaging. AJR 153:541, 1989.
668. Sundaram M, McGuire MH, Herbold DR: Magnetic resonance imaging of soft tissue masses: An evaluation of fifty-three histologically proven tumors. Magn Reson Imaging 6:237, 1988.
669. Hudson TM, Hamlin DJ, Enneking WF, et al: Magnetic resonance imaging of bone and soft tissue tumors: Early experience in 31 patients compared to computed tomography. Skel Radiol 13:134, 1985.
670. Kilcoyne RF, Richardson ML, Porter BA, et al: Magnetic resonance imaging of soft tissue masses. Clin Orthop 228:13, 1988.
671. Richardson ML, Kilcoyne RF, Gillespy T, et al: Magnetic resonance imaging of musculoskeletal neoplasms. Radiol Clin North Am 24:259, 1986.
672. Potty WG, Murphy WA, Lee JKT: Soft-tissue tumors: MR imaging. Radiology 160:135, 1986.
673. Sundaram M, McGuire MH, Herbold DR, et al: High signal intensity soft tissue masses on T1-weighted pulsing sequences. Skel Radiol 16:30, 1987.
674. Sundaram M, McLeod RA: MR imaging of tumor and tumorlike lesions of bone and soft tissue. AJR 155:817, 1990.
675. Sundaram M, McGuire MH, Schajowicz F: Soft-tissue masses: Histologic basis for decreased signal (short T2) on T2-weighted MR images. AJR 148:1247, 1987.
676. Erlemann R, Reiser MF, Peters PE, et al: Musculoskeletal neoplasms: Static and dynamic Gd-DTPA-enhanced MR imaging. Radiology 171:767, 1989.
677. Erlemann R, Vassallo P, Bongartz G, et al: Musculoskeletal neoplasms: Fast low-angle shot imaging with and without Gd-DTPA. Radiology 176:489, 1990.
678. Petersson H, Eliasson J, Egund N, et al: Gadolinium-DTPA enhancement of soft tissue tumors in magnetic resonance imaging—preliminary clinical experience in five patients. Skel Radiol 17:319, 1988.
679. Beltran J, Chandnani V, McGhee RA, et al: Gadopentetate dimeglumine-enhanced MR imaging of the musculoskeletal system. AJR 156:457, 1991.
680. Nigrisoli M, Ruggieri P, Pecci P, et al: Hibernoma. Skel Radiol 17:435, 1988.

681. Buetow PC, Kransdorf MJ, Moser RP, et al: Radiologic appearance of intra-muscular hermangioma with emphasis on MR imaging. AJR *154*:563, 1990.

682. Cohen EK, Kressel HY, Perosio T, et al: MR imaging of soft-tissue hemangiomas: Correlation with pathologic findings. AJR *150*:1079, 1988.

683. Kaplan PA, Williams SM: Mucocutaneous and peripheral soft-tissue hemangiomas: MR imaging. Radiology *163*:163, 1987.

684. Cohen JM, Weinreb JC, Redman HC: Arteriovenous malformations of the extremities: MR imaging. Radiology *158*:475, 1986.

685. London J, Kim EE, Wallace S, et al: MR imaging of liposarcomas: Correlation of MR features and histology. J Comput Assist Tomogr *13*:832, 1989.

686. Sundaram M, Baron G, Merenda G, et al: Myxoid liposarcoma: Magnetic resonance imaging appearances with clinical and histologic correlation. Skel Radiol *19*:359, 1990.

687. Jelinek JS, Kransdorf MJ, Utz RT, et al: Imaging of pigmented villonodular synovitis with emphasis on MR imaging. AJR *152*:337, 1989.

688. Kottal RA, Vogler JB, Matamoros A, et al: Pigmented villonodular synovitis: A report of MR imaging in two cases. Radiology *163*:551, 1987.

689. Mandelbaum BR, Grant TT, Hartzman S, et al: The use of MRI to assist in diagnosis of pigmented villonodular synovitis of the knee joint. Clin Orthop *231*:135, 1988.

690. Spritzer CE, Dalinka MK, Kressel HY: Magnetic resonance imaging of pigmented villonodular synovitis: A report of two cases. Skel Radiol *16*:316, 1987.

691. Dooms GC, Hricak H, Sollitto RA, et al: Lipomatous tumors and tumors with fatty component: Comparison of MRI and CT results. Radiology *157*:479, 1985.

692. Bush CH, Spanier SS, Gillespy T: Imaging of atypical lipomas of the extremities: Report of three cases. Skel Radiol *17*:472, 1988.

693. Murphy WD, Hurst GC, Duerk JL, et al: Atypical appearance of lipomatous tumors on MR images: High signal intensity with fat-suppression STIR sequences. J Magn Reson Imaging. *1*:477, 1991.

694. Panicek DM, Casper ES, Brennan MF, et al: Hemorrhage simulating tumor growth in malignant fibrous histiocytoma at MR imaging. Radiology *181*:398, 1992.

85

Skeletal Metastases

Donald Resnick, M.D., and Gen Niwayama, M.D.

Metastasis is defined as "the transfer of disease from one organ or part to another not directly connected with it," a process that "may be due either to the transfer of pathogenetic microorganisms ... or to the transfer of cells, as in malignant tumors."[1] Metastatic spread of infectious diseases to the skeleton (or nearby soft tissues) is discussed in Chapters 64, 65, and 66. Any malignant neoplasm possesses the capacity to metastasize to the musculoskeletal system although some do so more frequently than others. Furthermore, nonmalignant tumors occasionally can metastasize if, through the erosion of the wall of a blood vessel, neoplastic cells enter the vascular system.

The subject of skeletal metastasis is complex. Entire books[2, 342] or large portions thereof[3] are devoted to it. In this chapter, an overview of the problem is presented. Emphasis is given to the pathogenesis of metastasis to the skeleton and adjacent soft tissues, radiographic-pathologic correlation of the resulting lesions, common and uncommon patterns of bone destruction, articular involvement in and complications of the metastatic process, and the use of other imaging methods in the evaluation of patients with suspected or proven metastatic foci in the musculoskeletal system.

GENERAL MECHANISMS OF METASTASIS

The basic mechanisms of metastasis have been well summarized by Gullino and Liotta,[4] Springfield,[5] and Grundmann.[6] Tumors are composed of a variety of neoplastic cells, each type possessing its own behavioral characteristics. Some of these cells are more capable of metastases than others, so that the cellular constituency of a metastatic site generally is not identical to that of the primary tumor.[5] Cells within the tumor are continually separating from the primary lesion and gain access to the circulation,[4] but few are capable of establishing a metastatic focus. It has been estimated that fewer than 0.1 per cent of all tumor cells that reach the vascular system survive the transportation process to a distant location.[7] As indicated by Springfield,[5] the successful metastatic spread of a tumor requires the completion of a series of events; neoplastic cells must separate from the primary tumor, gain access to an efferent lymphatic channel or blood capillary, survive the transport, attach to the endothelium of a distant capillary bed, exit the vessel, and develop a supporting blood supply of their own at the new site. That an ample blood supply to a distant site alone is not sufficient in promoting successful metastasis and that local factors at the distant target area are important in this process are exemplified by the situation in skeletal muscle, a tissue rich in vascularity yet one in which metastatic foci are relatively rare (see later discussion).

Of the potential pathways available for the dissemination of tumor, vascular channels are more important than lymphatic channels; extension of neoplastic cells through lymph vessels to regional lymph nodes generally is followed by entrance into the vascular system. Invasion of vessels is characteristic of aggressive neoplasms but is not a feature confined to malignant tumors. Venous invasion is more common than arterial invasion as the arterial wall exhibits striking immunity to tumor penetration in the absence of associated infection.[8] As summarized by Galasko,[8] tumor emboli that are liberated into the systemic venous circulation or main lymphatic trunks will be trapped in the lungs; those liberated within the portal venous system in the liver and those liberated from the lungs into the pulmonary veins will be trapped in the peripheral organs to which they are carried by the systemic arterial circulation. Three possible exceptions to these general rules of vascular dissemination are recognized[8]: paradoxic embolization, in which tumor emboli bypass the pulmonary circulation (as in the situation of a patent foramen ovale); retrograde venous embolization, in which the occlusion of a vein is followed by the development of collateral channels in which the direction of blood flow is reversed; and transpulmonary passage of malignant cells.

GENERAL MECHANISMS OF SKELETAL METASTASIS

The skeleton is one of the most frequent sites of tumor metastasis and, as in other locations, successful metastatic implantation requires both the transport of viable tumor cells to the bone and the interaction of these cells with the osseous tissue.

Routes Allowing Spread of Tumor to Bone

Several distinct routes allow tumors to metastasize to bone: direct extension or invasion from adjacent tissues; lymphatic spread; hematogenous dissemination; and intraspinal spread.

Direct Extension. Malignant neoplasms located in the soft tissues adjacent to a bone subsequently may penetrate that bone by direct extension. In some instances, such as the situation in which a squamous cell carcinoma of the skin involves an underlying bone, a carcinoma at the apex of the lung (Pancoast tumor) invades the ribs or cervical vertebrae (Fig. 85–1A), a tumor of the nasopharynx leads to destruction in the base of the skull, a carcinoma of the bladder or the rectum involves the bones of the pelvis (Fig. 85–1B,C), or a pancreatic carcinoma extends directly into the lower thoracic and lumbar vertebrae,[9] the mode of skeletal involvement does not precisely fit the definition of metastasis in that the intraosseous tumor is in direct continuity with the site of primary involvement. In other instances, contiguous spread of tumor into bone originates from a site that itself is distant from the primary tumor. Examples of this situation include carcinomas of the lung that extend into the mediastinum with subsequent involvement of the spine (Fig. 85–2), or a soft tissue metastatic deposit resulting from hematogenous or lymphatic dissemination that subsequently invades the adjacent osseous tissue.

In all of these situations, the final step leading to "metastatic" disease of the skeleton is the invasion of bone from a tumorous site adjacent to it. The resulting abnormalities, whether they be depicted on routine radiographs or by more sophisticated diagnostic techniques such as CT scanning or MR imaging, typically consist of a soft tissue mass (of variable size) and osseous destruction (of variable degree). This combination of findings also is observed in infectious lesions of the skeleton and primary malignant tumors of the skeleton or soft tissues; a large soft tissue mass is an infrequent manifestation of skeletal metastasis arising from hematogenous dissemination of tumor (see later discussion). Accurate interpretation of the imaging abnormalities requires, initially, a decision regarding the soft tissue or osseous origin of the process. Are the findings more compatible with a soft tissue process involving bone or an osseous process extending into the soft tissues? Determining whether the epicenter of the lesion lies in the soft tissues or bone aids in this decision. Furthermore, osseous invasion arising from a malignant tumor (or infection) lying outside the bone is accompanied by a sequence of steps commencing with invasion and stimulation of the periosteal membrane, followed by violation of the external surface of the cortex, penetration of the entire cortex, and extension into the medullary cavity. Conversely, an intraosseous tumor (or infection) first affects the inner portion of the cortex, then the periosteum and finally the soft tissues.

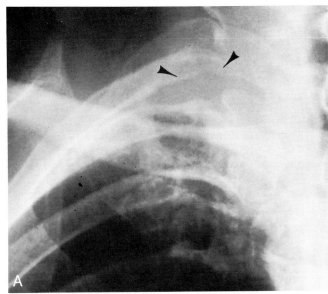

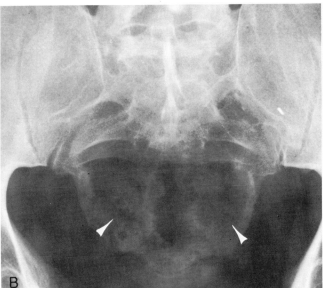

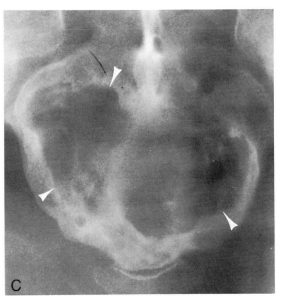

FIGURE 85–1. Routes of tumor spread to bone: Direct extension.

A Pancoast tumor. A carcinoma in the apex of the lung has led to destruction of the posterior portion of the second rib (arrowheads).

B, C Carcinoma of the rectum. Observe destruction of the sacrum (arrowheads) due to direct extension of the tumor. The abnormalities are difficult to detect on the routine radiograph **(B)** but are well shown on the conventional tomogram **(C).**

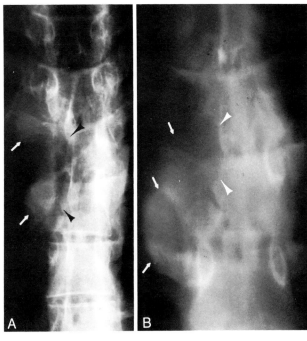

FIGURE 85–2. Routes of tumor spread to bone: Lymphatic spread with direct extension. A carcinoma of the lung has spread to paravertebral lymph nodes (arrows) with subsequent extension into several thoracic vertebrae (arrowheads). Note the pediculate destruction.

Although unusual examples are encountered, the typical imaging abnormalities associated with skeletal metastasis arising from a contiguous soft tissue neoplasm include the following: a soft tissue mass (unusual in cases of hematogenous extension of tumor to bone) with a well-defined, smooth or lobulated contour (unusual in cases of infection, in which an ill-defined border and obscuration of tissue planes are more characteristic); irregular erosion of the cortex (uncommon in benign processes of the soft tissues, in which pressure erosion leads to well-defined osseous scalloping); irregular or ''fluffy'' periosteal reaction (an inconstant feature influenced by the location of the skeletal process); and geographic, motheaten or permeative bone destruction (when the neoplastic process reaches the medullary canal).

Lymphatic Spread. Although the lymphatic system is relatively unimportant in the transportation of tumor cells to distant bones, metastatic deposits in regional draining lymph nodes secondarily can involve the adjacent osseous structures. In addition to the situation noted previously, in which mediastinal nodal involvement by malignant neoplasms in the lung is accompanied by spinal extension of tumor (Fig. 85–2), an important example of this phenomenon is the occurrence of vertebral destruction in cases of pelvic carcinomas arising in such sites as the prostate, bladder, cervix, and uterus.[10] A predilection for the lumbar spine and the absence of pulmonary metastasis in some of these cases are findings supporting the role of local spread of tumor via lymphatic or venous channels to paravertebral plexuses with subsequent spread to the vertebrae. Imaging studies demonstrate characteristic abnormalities, including a paravertebral soft tissue mass and scalloped erosions of one or more vertebral bodies.[11] Predominant involvement of the left side of the lumbar spine[12] is consistent with the fact that the lymph nodes on this side are closer to the spine than those on the right side, where the inferior vena cava and the aorta may be interposed.[13] Although these findings are suggestive of tumorous involvement of paravertebral lymph nodes, they are not specific for skeletal metastasis accompanying malignant tumors of the pelvis; similar abnormalities are observed in some patients with lymphomas and plasma cell myeloma. Furthermore, infectious lesions of the spine are accompanied by vertebral destruction and soft tissue masses; loss of height of intervertebral discs is more characteristic of infection than tumor.

Hematogenous Dissemination. The blood stream is the major pathway allowing dissemination of malignant neoplasms to the skeleton. Two potential vascular routes exist, the arterial system and the venous system, particularly the vertebral plexus of veins described by Batson in 1940.[14] Although the importance of the latter system in the spread of malignant tumors (as well as infections) has been emphasized repeatedly,[15–17] the relative roles of the arterial and venous routes in this dissemination are difficult to define. The predilection for metastases to affect the axial skeleton, especially the spine, and the presence of vertebral metastasis in the absence of pulmonary (or other organ) involvement are findings that support the significance of Batson's vertebral plexus in tumor spread, but other factors could contribute to these observations (see previous and later discussions). Certainly, additional vascular channels also allow dissemination of tumors, including the pulmonary veins, which permit transport of cancer cells from a malignancy in the lung to the systemic arterial circulation, and the portal venous system, which allows tumor cells to reach or even bypass the lung. As indicated previously, direct arterial invasion is unusual in the absence of infection.

The paravertebral plexus of veins consists of an intercommunicating system of thin-walled vessels with a low intraluminal pressure and, frequently, without valves; they lie outside the thoracoabdominal cavity and, unlike the veins therein, are not subject to the direct pressure of the thoracoabdominal muscular press.[8] These veins have extensive communications with veins in the spinal canal (Fig. 85–3) as well as those in the caval, portal, azygos, intercostal, pulmonary, and renal systems. The resulting venous pool, which also communicates with the veins of the breast, head, and neck, and major venae vasorum of the extremities, represents a large vascular reservoir in which the direction of blood flow is variable, influenced by shifts of pressures in any of its constituent vessels during such routine and daily activities as coughing, sneezing, straining, or physical exertion. It was Batson's belief that owing to the extensive communications of this venous system and to the variability of the direction of its blood flow, tumors arising in many sites, such as the pelvic organs, breast, and lung, release cells that could be deposited anywhere along the course of the vessels, including the skeleton, even in the absence of liver or lung involvement (Fig. 85–4). Thus, tumor cells from a carcinoma of the prostate, which under normal circumstances would be expected to enter the prostatic plexus and inferior vena cava, might pass into the vertebral venous plexus owing to increased intra-abdominal pressure; and those from a breast or thyroid carcinoma might enter the system via the intercostal and cervical veins.[8]

Experimental, clinical, radiologic, and pathologic data support a fundamental role of Batson's venous plexus in tumor dissemination[10, 17–19] although results have not been entirely uniform.[20] Not debated, however, is the importance of various components of the blood stream in providing the necessary channels that result in a high frequency of abnormal cells reaching the skeleton in malignant tumors of varying histologic composition and site of origin. Local factors subsequently govern the success of skeletal implantation of the neoplasm.

Intraspinal Spread. The cerebrospinal fluid represents an additional pathway for tumor dissemination, allowing secondary deposits in the spinal canal to develop in patients with intracranial neoplasms.[21–24] Subarachnoid seeding is related to several specific mechanisms, including fragmentation of a tumor bathed with cerebrospinal fluid,[25] ependymal breaching by the primary intracranial tumor or fissuring secondary to hydrocephalus,[22, 26] or shedding of portions of the tumor at the time of craniotomy.[22, 24, 27, 28] Children and adults are affected, and the types of tumors leading to subarachnoid spread (in children) are, in order of decreasing frequency, medulloblastoma, ependymoma, pineal neoplasms, astrocytoma, lymphoma, choroid plexus papilloma, and retinoblastoma.[24] Clinical manifestations of the spinal cord metastases may be minor, overshadowed by findings related to the primary neoplasm, and routine spinal radiographs generally are unremarkable, although osteoblastic lesions of the vertebrae (as well as the pelvis and elsewhere), occasionally are seen. Accurate diagnosis requires the use of other methods, especially myelography, CT, and

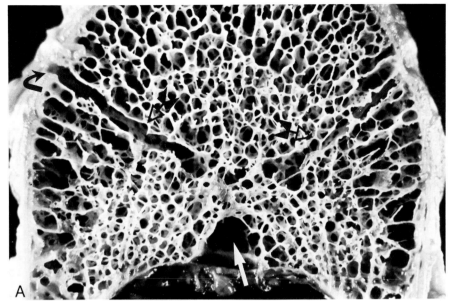

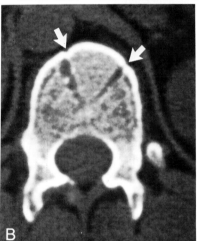

FIGURE 85–3. Routes of tumor spread to bone: Normal basivertebral veins.

A A photograph of a transverse section of the vertebral body illustrates the Y-shaped configuration of the major basivertebral venous channels, with a flared posterior channel (straight arrow) forming the base and more anterior channels (open arrows) composing the limbs. The well-defined osseous walls of the channels and the anterolateral cortical fenestration (curved arrow) are well demonstrated.

B On a transaxial CT image of a thoracic vertebra, observe a V-shaped configuration of the anterior venous channels with cortical fenestrations (arrows).

(From Sartoris DJ, et al: Radiology *155*:745, 1985.)

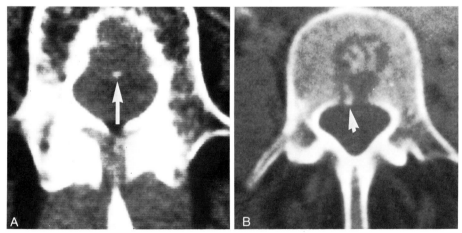

FIGURE 85–4. Routes of tumor spread to bone: Hematogenous dissemination via basivertebral veins.

A Renal cell carcinoma. A transaxial CT scan at the level of the third lumbar vertebra reveals involvement of the posterior portion of the vertebral body by the metastatic lesion. Observe tumor extension into the spinal canal with a small remnant of the posterior vertebral margin (arrow).

B Malignant melanoma. In a similar scan of the third lumbar vertebra, a metastatic focus of the tumor is present in the vertebral body. Its large size, poorly defined irregular margins, bone sequestration, and posterior extension (arrow) are apparent.

(From Sartoris DJ, et al: Radiology *155*:745, 1985.)

MR imaging (see later discussion).[24, 29, 343, 344] Nodularity and irregularity of the thecal sac, thickening of the nerve roots, obliteration of root sleeves, and narrowing of the subarachnoid space are among the reported myelographic alterations.[24] Predominant involvement of the lumbosacral region may reflect the effect of gravity.

It should be emphasized that dissemination of intracranial tumors by the cerebrospinal fluid represents only one of a number of mechanisms by which metastatic foci involve the spinal cord. Arterial or venous tumor emboli and direct extension of tumor from adjacent structures are additional pathways of spread,[30, 343, 344] accounting for the occurrence of spinal cord and leptomeningeal metastases from non-neurogenic tumors such as carcinoma of the lung (see later discussion).

Osseous Response to Metastatic Tumor

The response of bone to secondary deposits of tumor has been well described by Galasko,[31–33, 335] and others.[34, 345, 468] Various experimental animal models have been analyzed in an attempt to define cellular characteristics of the osseous response to malignant tumors; hematogenous metastasis in humans generally begins in the medullary cavity and secondarily involves the cortex, so that experimental studies usually have employed the intramedullary injection of tumor cell suspensions.[31] The osseous abnormalities in such studies, which appear to be duplicated in cases of human skeletal metastasis, can be classified broadly into two types: bone resorption and bone formation.

Bone Resorption. There is no single unifying mechanism that accounts for the increased bone resorption occurring in patients with malignant disease.[34] Humoral factors appear to be important, although the precise nature of these and their individual contribution to the osseous changes are not clear. The role of osteoclasts,[35] tumor cells,[35] and tumor cell extracts[36] in this process has experimental support, but additional factors, including resorption induced by monocytes[37] or macrophages,[38] may be important. A more generalized distribution of bone resorption as well as hypercalcemia has been observed in patients with tumors in whom skeletal metastasis is absent, suggesting that immobilization[39] or other humoral factors, such as parathyroid hormone, prostaglandins, or tumor-derived substances, are contributing to bone loss[40–43, 316, 317, 346, 347] (see later discussion).

Osteoclast-mediated osteolysis is suggested as an early and quantitatively important mechanism of bone loss accompanying skeletal metastasis.[32] A similar pattern of osteolysis is observed in patients with hematologic malignancies, including plasma cell myeloma and lymphoma, in which leukocytes produce an osteoclast activating factor.[44–46] In carcinomas, the humoral substance promoting local bone loss may be a prostaglandin, an osteoclast activating factor, alpha transforming growth factors, a parathyroid hormone-like substance, a tumor necrosis factor, or other as yet unidentified agents.[31, 42, 345, 347] In the late stage of bone destruction related to skeletal metastasis, osteoclastic activity decreases, and histologic inspection reveals an intimate association of residual spicules of bone and clusters of malignant cells.[32] A plausible explanation for this finding is that the malignant cells themselves are attracted to the osseous surface by chemotactic factors released by the bone[34] and that, once there, they secrete lytic enzymes responsible for the continued destruction of the bone.[32, 323]

Bone Formation. Two main mechanisms account for new bone formation associated with skeletal metastasis: stromal bone formation and reactive bone formation.[31–33] Experimentally, the earlier and quantitatively less important mechanism is the stromal variety, in which intramembranous ossification proceeds in areas of fibrous stroma within the tumor. In humans, stromal new bone formation occurs only in those skeletal metastases that are associated with the development of fibrous stroma, particularly those arising from carcinoma of the prostate; highly cellular tumors possess little or no stroma and are not accompanied by this type of bone formation.[32]

Reactive new bone occurs as a response to bone destruction and is similar to the callus that develops in fracture healing.[32] Immature woven bone is deposited initially, which is converted subsequently to more stable lamellar bone.[31] This process is seen to variable extent in virtually all malignant neoplasms, but it may be a minor or insignificant feature in highly anaplastic, rapidly growing tumors, in plasma cell myeloma, lymphomas, or leukemias, and in the late stages of the lesions when sheets of malignant cells surround the few remaining spicules of bone.[32]

The histologic components of the cancellous bone in many cases of skeletal metastasis reflect the ongoing processes of bone resorption and bone formation; these include increases in blood vessels and other stromal tissues and in both osteoblasts and osteoclasts, whose activities are unbalanced. The microscopic appearance has been termed carcinomatous osteodysplasia,[47] and it may resemble findings evident in primary and secondary hyperparathyroidism or myelofibrosis. The precise features of carcinomatous osteodysplasia are influenced by the type of tumor, the stage of the disease, and the effects of any therapeutic regimens.

GENERAL CLINICAL MANIFESTATIONS

Although the clinical findings accompanying skeletal metastasis are influenced by the age of the patient, the type of tumor, and the site or sites of bone involvement, certain general characteristics deserve emphasis. Bone pain is a common, although not invariable,[348] abnormality that can relate to cellular events, such as the release of prostaglandins,[48] or to elevation of medullary pressure, stretching of the periosteal membrane, the occurrence of a pathologic fracture, or compression and entrapment of adjacent neurologic structures. Thus, pain may be localized to the site of skeletal involvement or referred to a distant site, particularly when the lesion involves the spine.[349] Bone tenderness, a soft tissue mass, and deformity are additional possible manifestations.

Laboratory parameters of skeletal metastasis include elevation of the serum level of calcium, which, although not constant, is a well-recognized complication of tumors. As described previously, the hypercalcemia has a complex pathogenesis, is dependent on such factors as the degree of immobilization or bone resorption and destruction, and may relate to the secretion of a humoral substance, such as parathyroid hormone, prostaglandins, or osteolytic sterols by the tumor itself (see later discussion). Elevation of the serum level of alkaline phosphatase in patients with skeletal metastasis reflects the magnitude of osteoblastic activity in the absence of liver disease.[49] Such elevation is less constant in patients with purely osteolytic lesions and may appear only after widespread osseous involvement with pathologic fractures has occurred. An increase in hydroxyproline excretion in the urine and a myelophthisic anemia are additional laboratory abnormalities that may be evident. Measurement of serum acid phosphatase (and other enzymes) is useful in the evaluation of patients with prostatic carcinoma.

FREQUENCY AND DISTRIBUTION OF SKELETAL METASTASIS

Although it is well recognized that metastasis to the skeleton represents the most common type of malignant bone tumor, the determination of accurate statistics regarding the frequency of skeletal metastasis is extremely difficult. Such statistics are influenced dramatically by the choice of technique used to detect sites of bone involvement. The estimated frequency of skeletal metastasis determined on the basis of radiographic examination is obviously low owing to the relatively insensitive nature of this diagnostic technique (Fig. 85–5). Scintigraphy using bone-seeking radiopharmaceutical agents is a more sensitive method of analysis, although it, too, is beset with problems, including the known occurrence of falsely negative examinations in some types of malignant tumors, especially those that are extremely aggressive in their behavior, and in some persons, particularly those who are markedly debilitated; additionally, falsely positive examinations also occur related to the nonspecific nature of the radionuclide study, in which bone lesions other than metastases are detected in patients with malignant tumors. MR imaging also represents a sensitive diagnostic method, but a survey of the entire skeleton using this technique is impractical. Pathologic inspection at the time of autopsy potentially is an accurate method of detecting osseous metastasis, but severe

limitations of this technique are encountered owing to certain legal constraints that prevent analysis of all portions of the skeleton and to the meticulous and time-consuming process that is required if all sites of bone metastasis are to be discovered. Despite these limitations, adequate sampling of the skeleton, particularly the spine, pelvic bones, ribs, and sternum, accomplished during the postmortem examination represents the best method for detecting metastatic foci, although it is employed rarely; more typically, a cursory examination of the external surfaces of the bones and of sections of one or two vertebral bodies is performed.

Previous reports that relied on imaging or pathologic data,[50–57] although they varied considerably in individual statistics, generally confirmed the following observations:

1. The skeleton is a common site of metastasis in many types of primary malignant tumor.

2. In accordance with the relative frequency of various types of primary malignant tumors, carcinomas of the breast, prostate, and lung, in decreasing order, are the common sources of skeletal metastases in a general population; carcinomas of the prostate, lung, and bladder, in similar order, are the typical sources of such metastases in a male population; and carcinomas of the breast and uterus are common causes of skeletal metastases in a female population.

3. Based on an equal number of various types of primary malignant tumors, carcinomas of the prostate, breast, kidney, lung, and thyroid gland, in order of decreasing frequency, metastasize to the skeleton.

4. The vast majority of metastatic lesions in the skeleton are encountered in middle-aged and elderly patients.

5. Typical causes of skeletal metastasis in children are neuroblastoma, Ewing's sarcoma, osteosarcoma, and malignant tumors of soft tissues.

6. In adults carcinoma of the prostate, breast, kidney, and lung account for more than 75 per cent of cases of

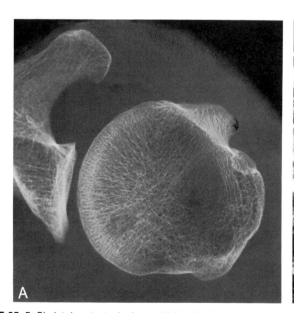
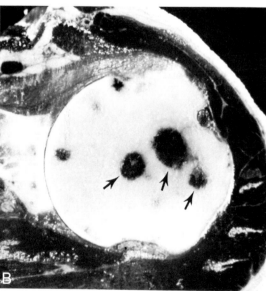

FIGURE 85–5. Skeletal metastasis: Insensitivity of radiographic examination—malignant melanoma. A radiograph **(A)** and photograph **(B)** of a transverse section of the shoulder dramatically illustrate the insensitivity of routine radiography in the detection of skeletal metastasis. Although this is a high quality radiograph of a thin cadaveric section, the multiple metastatic foci in the humeral head that are obvious in the specimen photograph (arrows) almost are invisible in the radiograph.

skeletal metastasis, carcinoma of the prostate is responsible for approximately 60 per cent of cases of such metastasis in men, and carcinoma of the breast accounts for approximately 70 per cent of cases of skeletal metastasis in women.[3]

Although the distribution of skeletal metastases is influenced by the specific type of primary malignant tumor, predominant involvement of the axial skeleton, a region rich in red marrow, is well known. Factors favoring the development of metastatic foci in sites of red marrow may include a large capillary network, a sluggish blood flow, and the suitability of this tissue for the growth of tumor emboli.[8] The vertebral column (thoracolumbar spine and sacrum), the bones of the pelvis, the ribs, the sternum, the femoral and humeral shafts, and the skull, in decreasing order, are the usual locations for skeletal metastasis. Spine involvement in the metastatic process should be emphasized,[336] with the frequency of metastasis being greatest in the lumbar region followed by the thoracic and cervical segments. Several explanations exist for the reported frequency of spinal metastasis: Batson's venous plexus provides direct communication between this area and numerous other locations in the body; a large amount of bone mass is found in the spine; and the spine is most accessible to inspection at the time of routine autopsy.[8] Metastatic foci are more common in the vertebral bodies than in the posterior osseous elements, although pediculate destruction is more frequent in cases of skeletal metastasis than in those of plasma cell myeloma.

Infrequent sites of skeletal metastasis are the mandible (a site more typically involved in plasma cell myeloma), the patella,[350, 351] and the bones of the extremities that are distal to the elbow and knee (Figs. 85–6 and 85–7). With regard to the distal portions of the extremities, potential explanations for the low frequency of skeletal metastasis are an afferent blood supply that virtually is limited to the arterial route and the relative absence of red marrow, a suitable ''soil'' in which metastatic tumors can grow.[3] In reported instances in which metastatic lesions have been encountered in the peripheral skeleton,[58–81, 324, 325, 352–355] bronchogenic carcinoma is the leading cause, perhaps related to the shedding of tumor cells into the pulmonary veins, from where they can reach the arterial side of the circulation. Such metastases usually, although not invariably, are accompanied by widespread skeletal lesions and are associated with heat, pain, and soft tissue swelling, simulating the findings of osteomyelitis or arthritis. The terminal phalanges and the metacarpal bones are most commonly affected in the hand,[74, 76] the scaphoid and lunate are the usual sites of involvement in the wrist,[74] and tarsal involvement, especially of the calcaneus, predominates in the foot.[69] In cases of skeletal metastasis in the foot, carcinomas of the colon and kidney as well as the lung are most frequent.[69, 353] The occurrence of skeletal metastasis in the foot originating from subdiaphragmatic neoplasms, such as gastrointestinal, renal, and uterine malignant tumors, may relate to retrograde spread of tumor emboli from the vertebral venous plexus down incompetent leg veins.[352]

In unusual circumstances, metastasis develops at an osseous site that already is altered by disease (osteomyelitis and Paget's disease) (Fig. 85–8A) or surgical manipulation

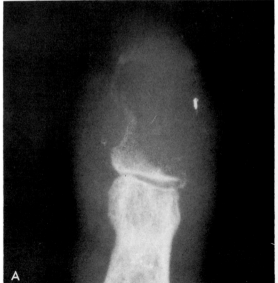
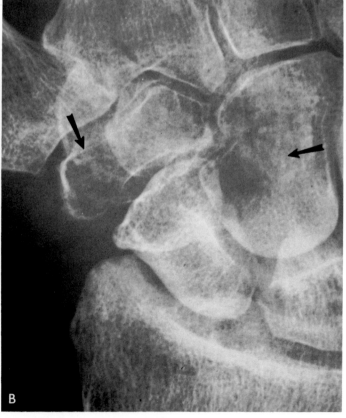

FIGURE 85–6. Skeletal metastasis: Hand and wrist.

A Bronchogenic carcinoma. Extensive lysis of the terminal phalanx of the finger is associated with considerable soft tissue swelling. The articular space appears uninvolved.

B Bronchogenic carcinoma. Note the lytic lesions of the capitate and trapezium (arrows), which are poorly defined and unassociated with sclerosis. The preservation of the joint spaces favors a diagnosis of tumor rather than pyogenic infection.

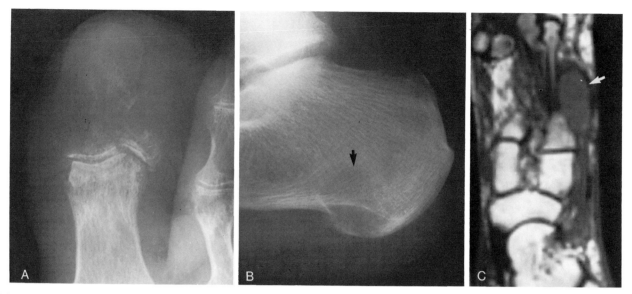

FIGURE 85–7. Skeletal metastasis: Foot.

　A Bronchogenic carcinoma. Complete destruction of the terminal phalanx of the great toe and soft tissue swelling are evident. A pathologic fracture is present.

　B Pharyngeal carcinoma. Note the osteolytic lesion (arrow) of the calcaneus.

　C Renal cell carcinoma. Metatarsal (arrow) and soft tissue involvement are apparent on this transverse T1-weighted (TR/TE, 600/15) spin echo MR image. (**C,** Courtesy of J. Kramer, M.D., Vienna, Austria.)

(metallic implants) (Fig. 85–8B,C).[356] The cause for this is not clear, although changes in local blood flow or tissue resistance may promote tumor growth.

RADIOGRAPHIC-PATHOLOGIC CORRELATION

The radiographic characteristics of skeletal metastases are highly variable and influenced by a number of factors, including the nature of the primary tumor, the age of the patient, the location of the metastatic lesion or lesions, and the timing of the roentgenographic examination. The relative insensitivity of this diagnostic technique compared with others such as scintigraphy and MR imaging accounts for the absence of radiologic findings in many cases in which metastatic foci exist in the skeleton. In certain locations, such as the spine, a great amount of bone destruction is required before lesions are detected by routine radiography.[82, 357, 358] This diagnostic problem is accentuated if metastatic foci are confined to the medullary space, in which relatively few trabeculae are found; destruction of the cortex is more readily apparent owing to the presence of larger amounts of bone that is compact in nature. Although the cancellous bone in the medullary canal generally is the initial site of hematogenously derived skeletal metastases, endosteal erosion of the cortex or, more rarely, small intracortical lesions (sometimes situated about nutrient vessels) may represent the first radiographic sign of the disease.[359, 360] Furthermore, the external cortical surface commonly is the initial site of osseous involvement in cases of skeletal metastasis arising from direct extension of an adjacent tumorous deposit.

Number of Lesions

Multiplicity is the general rule regarding sites of skeletal metastasis; however, solitary lesions certainly are encoun-

tered, especially in patients with carcinoma of the kidney or thyroid. Furthermore, in some instances, only one metastatic lesion is detected on routine radiographs at a time when scintigraphy or MR imaging indicates the presence of many such lesions. In cases of an apparently solitary focus of bone involvement, the radiographic differentiation of an osseous metastasis from a primary bone tumor can be difficult. When multiple lesions are detected on the roentgenograms, they commonly are of variable size as opposed to the uniformity of size that frequently is apparent in plasma cell myeloma.

Patterns of Bone Response

The radiographic appearance of skeletal metastases can be broadly classified as purely osteolytic (Fig. 85–9A,B), purely osteosclerotic (Fig. 85–9C,D), and mixed osteolytic-osteosclerotic, although histologically, a combination of both bone resorption and bone formation is present in the vast majority of lesions. Purely osteolytic lesions typically arise from carcinoma of the thyroid, kidney, adrenal gland, uterus, and gastrointestinal tract, as well as from Wilms' tumor, Ewing's tumor, pheochromocytoma, melanoma, hepatoma, squamous cell carcinoma of the skin, and certain tumors of the head, neck, and vascular and soft tissues; mixed osteolytic-osteosclerotic lesions generally occur in carcinomas of the lung, breast, and cervix, and in ovarian and testicular tumors; purely osteosclerotic lesions are encountered in carcinoma of the prostate, and, less constantly, in bronchial carcinoid tumor, bladder carcinoma involving the prostate, carcinomas of the nasopharynx and stomach, medulloblastoma, and neuroblastoma (Table 85–1). None of these patterns is without exception; for example, pancreatic carcinoma can lead to sclerotic changes in the thoracolumbar spine, colonic carcinoma and ovarian and testicular tumors can be purely osteosclerotic, and prostatic carcinoma in older persons and in the cervical spine can be

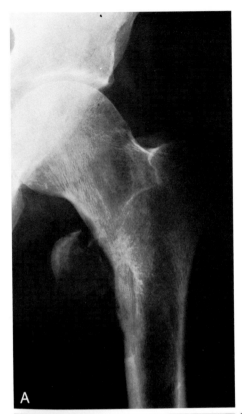

FIGURE 85–8. Skeletal metastasis: Involvement of previously abnormal sites.

A Paget's disease. An adenocarcinoma has metastasized to the region of the lesser trochanter, leading to its avulsion and dissolution. Observe the coarsened trabecular pattern in the femoral head and neck, consistent with Paget's disease. (Courtesy of J. Slivka, M.D., San Diego, California.)

B, C A metastatic lesion is responsible for the osteolysis in the medullary canal and cortex of the proximal portion of the femur (arrows) as well as the increased accumulation of the bone-seeking radiopharmaceutical agent (arrowhead) in a patient who has had previous surgery for a subcapital fracture. (Courtesy of J. A. Amberg, M.D., San Diego, California.)

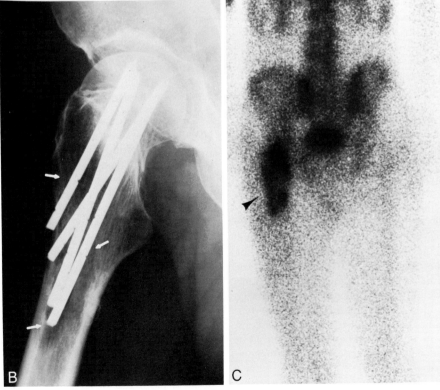

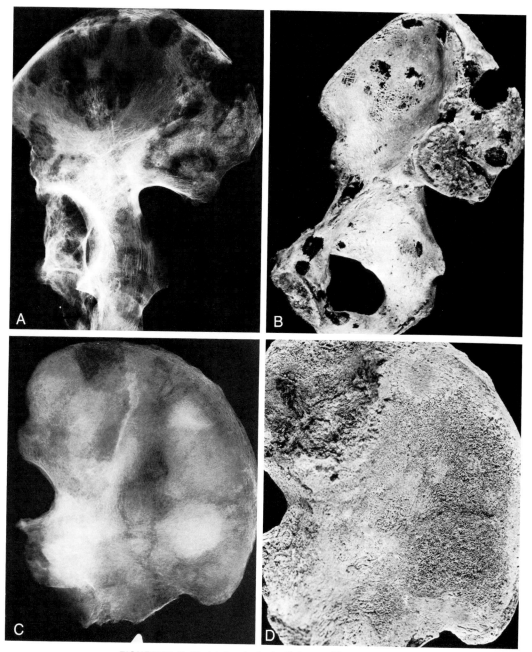

FIGURE 85–9. Skeletal metastasis: Patterns of bone response.
A, B Purely osteolytic.
C, D Purely osteosclerotic.

TABLE 85–1. Sites of Skeletal Metastases*

Primary Focus	Type of Skeletal Lesion	Relative Frequency (Percentage) of Skeletal Lesion		
		X-ray	Bone Scan	Autopsy
Common Primary Cancer				
Breast	Lytic; also mixed; frequently blastic	30 to 50	52 to 67	57 to 73
Lung	Lytic; also mixed; occasionally blastic	14 to 25	54 to 64	19 to 32
Kidney	Invariably lytic	20 to 32	33 to 60	23 to 45
Thyroid	Invariably lytic	8	43	19 to 50
Prostate	Usually blastic; occasionally lytic	33 to 35	62 to 92	57 to 84
Head and Neck				
Upper respiratory & digestive tract				
Nasal fossa and nasopharynx	Lytic; occasionally blastic	4		
Oral cavity and oropharynx	Lytic	14 to 21		
Endolarynx and hypopharynx	Lytic	1 to 2		
Maxillary sinuses	Lytic	12		
Salivary glands	Lytic	5		28
Other carcinomas of neck				
Parathyroid	Lytic	<1		
Central nervous system				
Brain tumors	Lytic; infrequently blastic	<1		
Paragangliomas	Lytic	<1		
Chordoma	Lytic	15		
Neuroblastoma	Lytic or mixed; occasionally blastic	35 to 75		
Chest				
Pleura and pericardium				
Mesothelioma	Lytic	<1		
Mediastinum				
Thymoma	Lytic; frequently blastic	<1		
Teratoma, etc.	Lytic	<1		
Gastrointestinal Tract			41	
Esophagus	Lytic or mixed	3 to 5		1 to 2
Stomach	Lytic or mixed; occasionally blastic	0 to 2.6		2 to 17.5
Colon	Lytic or mixed; infrequently blastic	0.5 to 1	57	9 to 11
Rectum	Lytic or mixed; infrequently blastic	6 to 10	61	
Pancreas	Lytic or mixed; occasionally blastic	1.3 to 3.5		
Liver	Lytic or mixed	<1		
Gall bladder and bile ducts	Lytic or mixed	<1		
Genitourinary Tract			37	
Urinary bladder	Lytic; infrequently blastic	5 to 11	43	13 to 26
Adrenal	Lytic			44
Reproductive System			29	
Uterine cervix	Lytic or mixed; occasionally blastic	3 to 4	56	8 to 15
Uterine corpus	Lytic	6		22
Ovary	Lytic; rarely blastic	2 to 7		6
Testis	Lytic; occasionally blastic	6	8	10 to 20
Skin				
Squamous and basal cell carcinoma	Lytic	<1		
Malignant melanoma	Lytic	2 to 7	57	44 to 57

TABLE 85–1. Sites of Skeletal Metastases* *Continued*

Primary Focus	Type of Skeletal Lesion	Relative Frequency (Percentage) of Skeletal Lesion		
		X-ray	Bone Scan	Autopsy
Primary Bone Tumors				
Osteosarcoma	Lytic or mixed; frequently blastic	4 to 14		
Chondrosarcoma	Lytic or mixed; occasionally blastic	2 to 18		
Fibrosarcoma	Lytic	2 to 23		
Malignant fibrous histiocytoma	Lytic	17		
Hemangioendothelial sarcoma	Lytic (frequently multifocal)	1 to 2		
Ewing's sarcoma	Lytic (permeative)	40 to 50		
Histiocytic lymphoma	Lytic (permeative)	49		
Primary Soft Tissue Tumors				
Fibrous histiocytoma, angiosarcoma, rhabdomyosarcoma, etc.	Lytic or mixed	10 or less	56	
Carcinoid Tumors				
Bronchial and abdominal carcinoids (other than appendix)	Blastic; frequently mixed, occasionally lytic	1 or less		

*From Wilner D: Radiology of Bone Tumors and Allied Disorders. Philadelphia, WB Saunders Co, 1982, p 3646.

predominantly osteolytic. Although the skeleton in any one patient generally responds in a single manner to metastatic foci, accounting for uniformity in the radiographic appearance of the lesions, this too is not constant. Thus, a purely osteosclerotic or mixed osteolytic-osteosclerotic lesion in one skeletal site may be accompanied by a purely osteolytic lesion in a different location; in such cases, the possibility of more than one type of malignant tumor always should, however, be considered.

Osteolytic lesions (Fig. 85–10) may be well circumscribed (geographic bone destruction) or poorly defined (motheaten or permeative bone destruction). These patterns reflect varying degrees of aggressiveness of the metastatic deposits; well-defined osteolytic foci with a short zone of transition from normal to abnormal bone generally are less aggressive than those that are poorly marginated, with a long zone of transition. A metastatic lesion may change its behavior during the course of the disease, influenced by local or systemic factors, including the type of therapeutic regimen (see later discussion).

Osteosclerotic lesions (Fig. 85–11) have been further classified as nodular deposits (rounded, discrete, fairly well circumscribed areas of uniform radiodensity, varying in size up to several centimeters); mottled deposits (irregular zones of bone sclerosis that are interspersed between areas of essentially normal appearing bone); and diffuse deposits (larger zones of increased radiodensity).[3]

Periosteal Reaction

As a general rule, periosteal new bone is either absent or of limited extent in metastatic lesions, a characteristic that differs from the extensive degree of periostitis that commonly accompanies primary malignant tumors of the skeleton. In unusual circumstances, exuberant periosteal reaction leading to bone spiculation and a sunburst appearance

is evident in cases of skeletal metastasis, especially those arising from prostatic carcinoma (Fig. 85–12*A,B*), gastrointestinal malignancies, retinoblastoma (Fig. 85–12*C*), and neuroblastoma (Fig. 85–12*D*).[83–86, 361, 362] Such periostitis typically is seen with involvement of long tubular bones, more commonly in the lower extremity, and with osteoblastic lesions. The resulting radiographic abnormalities are similar to those evident in osteosarcoma, Ewing's sarcoma, and certain anemias.

Bone Expansion

Either osteolytic or osteosclerotic metastatic lesions occasionally can lead to bone expansion. Carcinomas of the kidney[3, 87, 88] or thyroid[3] and hepatomas[89, 326] are among the primary malignant tumors that result in expansile, osteolytic skeletal foci. In some of these lesions, such as those arising from renal carcinoma, a distinctive septate appearance accompanies the osseous expansion (Fig. 85–13).

Large, expansile osteoblastic lesions are evident in some patients with metastatic prostatic carcinoma[90–93] (Fig. 85–14). On radiographic examination, such lesions may resemble Paget's disease or, when solitary, osteosarcoma. The abnormal accumulation of bone-seeking radiopharmaceutical agents confirms the expansile nature of the metastasis, although the scintigraphic appearance must be differentiated from the "blooming" phenomenon that produces a halo of increased activity about some lesions that are associated with intense uptake of the radiotracer.[92]

Soft Tissue Mass

As a general rule, prominent soft tissue masses are observed infrequently in association with skeletal metastasis, and the detection of such a mass favors the diagnosis of a primary malignant lesion of bone rather than a secondary

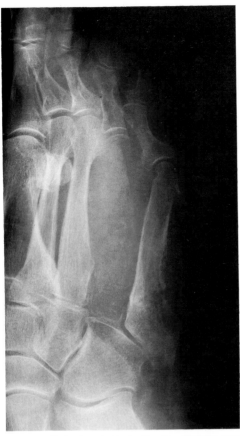

FIGURE 85–10. Skeletal metastasis: Purely osteolytic pattern. The entire fourth metatarsal bone reveals lytic destruction, and a similar lesion is present at the base of the fifth metatarsal bone. A poorly differentiated adenocarcinoma of unknown origin was responsible for the defects.

deposit. Exceptions to this rule are encountered in certain locations and with certain types of neoplasms. In the ribs, extrapleural extension of metastatic lesions leads to soft tissue masses of variable size, usually in association with obvious adjacent osseous abnormality. This combination of findings resembles that seen in plasma cell myeloma, although, in the latter disease, the degree of soft tissue abnormality sometimes is far greater than that in the bone. Carcinoma of the colon may metastasize to the bones of the pelvis, producing soft tissue masses that occasionally contain calcification.[94] Furthermore, metastasis to skeletal muscle, although rare, may lead to one or more painful soft tissue masses (see later discussion).[363, 364]

Soft Tissue Ossification

Ossification in sites of soft tissue metastases occurring with or without adjacent bone involvement has been identified, particularly with carcinoma of the colon,[95] gastric carcinoma,[96, 97] other gastrointestinal malignancies, transitional cell carcinoma of the bladder,[98, 99] carcinoma of the breast,[100] and bronchogenic carcinoma.[101] Osseous metaplasia also is identified in the primary tumor itself as well as in metastatic foci in many regions of the body, including the lymph nodes and lungs. The cause for such ossification is not entirely clear and probably varies according to the specific histologic composition of the malignant neoplasm.

Chalmers and collaborators[102] have indicated three conditions that are necessary for the induction of heterotopic bone formation: An osteogenic precursor cell must be present; an inducing agent also must be present; and a suitable environment must be established. The stromal elements of the tumor[103] or the tumor cells themselves,[95] alone or in combination, may represent the site of origin of the osseous metaplasia; the extraskeletal bone-inducing capability of transitional cell epithelium has been established in experimental situations.[98, 104, 105] Certain tissues, such as muscle and fascia, enhance osteogenesis, whereas others, such as the spleen and kidney, inhibit it.[96] Of interest in this regard are reports of extensive bone formation in muscles in association with metastatic deposits, especially from carcinoma of the stomach[96, 97] (Fig. 85–15).

The accurate radiographic diagnosis of ossifying metastases may be difficult. Such ossification in the soft tissues adjacent to an area of bone destruction simulates the appearance of an osteosarcoma of osseous origin, whereas isolated soft tissue ossific collections in metastases resemble findings in post-traumatic heterotopic ossification, pseudomalignant osseous tumor of soft tissue, an osteosarcoma of soft tissue origin, and ossification following burns and neurologic injuries.

Pathologic Fracture

Metastatic lesions in the skeleton lead to osseous weakening and, frequently, to pathologic fracture (Fig. 85–16). Metastases arising from breast carcinomas appear to be the leading cause of such fractures.[347] This complication is well recognized in the spine, where compression or collapse of a tumor-containing vertebral body is seen. Pathologic fractures accompanying metastases in tubular bones are evident most commonly in the proximal portion of the femur,[106] although other portions of this bone and other bones are involved as well.[107, 108, 369] Fractures occur more commonly

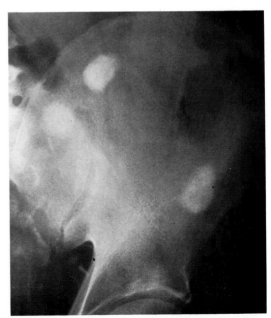

FIGURE 85–11. Skeletal metastasis: Purely osteosclerotic pattern. Carcinoma of the prostate resulted in multiple well-defined radiodense lesions of the ilium.

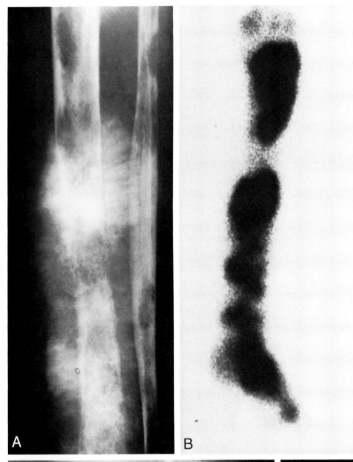

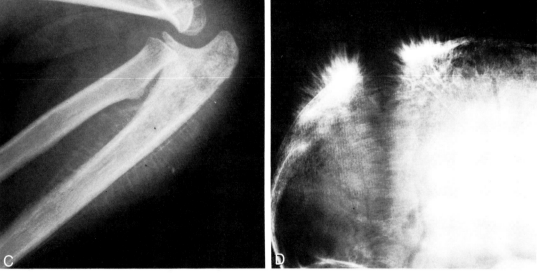

FIGURE 85–12. Skeletal metastasis: Periosteal reaction.

A, B Carcinoma of the prostate. An extremely unusual pattern of exuberant periostitis of the tibia, associated with a dramatic increase in the accumulation of a bone-seeking radionuclide in a 76 year old man, is shown. Osteolytic lesions are seen in the tibia and fibula. (Courtesy of A. Brower, M.D., Norfolk, Virginia.)

C Retinoblastoma. In a 3 year old girl, observe a sunburst periosteal reaction in the proximal portion of the ulna, accompanied by permeative bone destruction.

D Neuroblastoma. Findings include sutural widening and a sunburst pattern of periosteal bone formation. (Courtesy of T. Yochum, D.C., Denver, Colorado.)

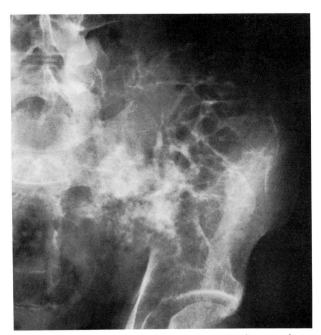

FIGURE 85–13. Skeletal metastasis: Bone expansion—carcinoma of the kidney. A large expansile, predominantly osteolytic lesion arises in the ilium. Note the septate appearance.

with lesions in the lower extremity than in the upper extremity. It is apparent that the likelihood of pathologic fracture in a tubular bone becomes more pronounced with increasing degrees of cortical destruction, and it is this likelihood, when combined with information regarding the site of osseous involvement, the type of tumor, and the patient's ultimate prognosis, that guides the orthopedic surgeon in the decision to use prophylactic internal fixation of the bone.[107, 109–111, 365–367] It is suggested that increasing pain and destruction of at least one half of the cortex are indications for such surgery[111] as the majority of pathologic fractures in long tubular bones occur when more than 50 per cent of the cortical surface has been destroyed.[112, 368] Unfortunately, estimates of cortical bone involvement generally are made on the basis of analysis of routine radiographs[113] and, in most instances, neglect the depth of the cortical erosion. CT represents a method that is more suitably applied to such analyses[327] (Fig. 85–17).

Although the potential for healing of pathologic fractures in patients with skeletal metastasis depends on many factors, including the age of the patient, the type of tumor, the site of the fracture, and the specific therapeutic techniques that are employed, estimates generally indicate solid bone union in less than 35 per cent of these fractures.[108, 114, 115] More favorable results are encountered in patients whose life expectancy is longer than 6 months and in those with prostatic or breast carcinoma; the short survival time of persons with bronchogenic carcinoma accounts for the reported low rate of healing of pathologic fractures related to skeletal metastasis of this tumor.[108, 116] Internal fixation usually improves the rate of fracture healing[108]; a total radio-

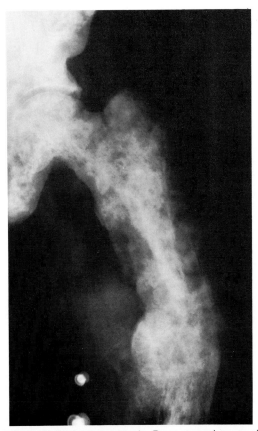

FIGURE 85–14. Skeletal metastasis: Bone expansion—carcinoma of the prostate. Exuberant new and abnormal bone cloaks the original femoral diaphysis in this patient with widespread osseous metastases. A previous pathologic fracture of the femoral shaft is apparent. The radiographic findings resemble those of Paget's disease.

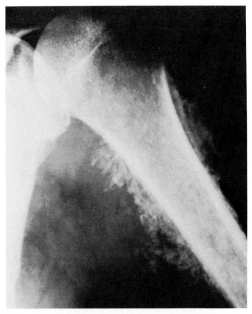

FIGURE 85–15. Skeletal metastasis: Soft tissue (muscle) ossification—carcinoma of the stomach. In this 54 year old man with progressive shoulder pain, soft tissue masses developed at several sites. A radiograph of the shoulder reveals heterotopic bone formation in the soft tissues adjacent to the humerus. A biopsy of the lesion in the left shoulder documented metastatic signet-ring adenocarcinoma. At autopsy, a primary gastric carcinoma was identified. Ossifying metastases were present in the muscles.

(Courtesy of L. Cooperstein, M.D., D. Obley, M.D., and L. H. Rosenbaum, M.D., Pittsburgh, Pennsylvania.)

FIGURE 85–16. Skeletal metastasis: Pathologic fracture.

A, B Carcinoma of the prostate. In this 82 year old man, a spontaneous fracture developed in the subcapital region of the femur (arrows). A transaxial CT image reveals increased radiodensity in the femoral neck (arrowhead) at the fracture site. At the time of internal fixation, tumor was found in this region.

C Carcinoma of the lung. In a 63 year old woman with carcinoma of the lung, a spontaneous fracture of the femoral neck occurred through an osteolytic lesion (arrows). At the time of internal fixation of the fracture, metastatic tumor was discovered.

D Carcinoma of the lung. An oblique fracture has occurred through a "motheaten" region of bone destruction in the diaphysis of the humerus.

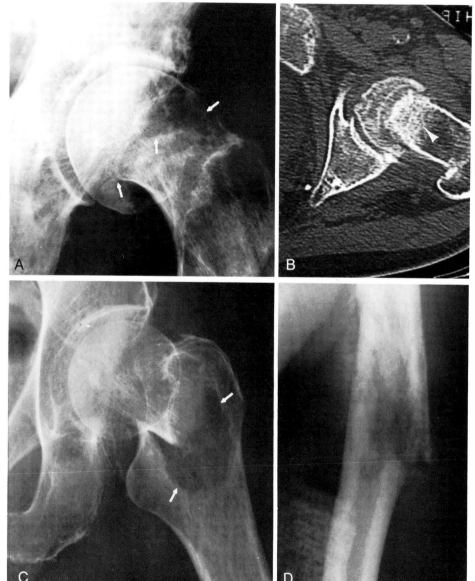

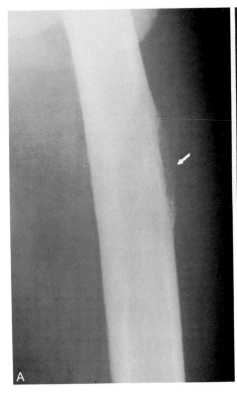

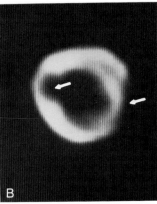

FIGURE 85–17. Skeletal metastasis: Amount of cortical destruction depicted with CT. A 51 year old man with carcinoma of the prostate developed leg pain.

A A radiograph of the femur shows an osteolytic lesion in the diaphysis with cortical involvement (arrow).

B A transaxial CT scan of this lesion better delineates the extent of cortical involvement (arrows).

therapy dose equal to or less than 3000 cGy (rad) does not inhibit callus formation[108] (although larger radiation doses may retard fracture repair)[117]; and polymethylmethacrylate, which commonly is used as an adjunct to therapy, does not interfere with osseous healing.[116]

SPECIFIC SITES OF OSSEOUS INVOLVEMENT

Skull

Single or multiple osteolytic lesions of variable size are evident. They typically possess ill-defined or irregular edges, without sclerotic margins, and involve the inner table, the outer table, or the diploic portion of the cranium alone or in combination. Perforation of the external surface of the bone may be associated with a soft tissue mass that requires tangential radiographic projections for detection. Rarely, a radiodense focus, the button sequestrum, exists in the center of the lesion[118] (Fig. 85–18), although this finding is more typical of eosinophilic granuloma and is observed also in radiation necrosis, tuberculosis and other infections, fibrous dysplasia, multiple myeloma, Paget's disease, and dermoid and epidermoid tumors.[118–122]

Other conditions that enter into the differential diagnosis of a solitary osteolytic metastatic lesion of the skull include an epidermoid or dermoid tumor (which appears as a small, well-defined, round or oval radiolucent diploic focus with a sclerotic margin),[123] hemangioma (which possesses a spiculated or reticular pattern), eosinophilic granuloma (which is an oval or lobulated lesion of the diploic portion of the cranium with differential involvement of the inner and outer tables that produces a beveled margin), fibrous dysplasia (which commonly has a ground-glass or sclerotic appearance, affecting the outer table to a greater degree than the

inner table), the doughnut lesion (of unknown cause, which produces one or more radiolucent areas, each surrounded by a sclerotic margin of variable thickness)[124–126] (Fig. 85–19), various infections, lymphomas, and sarcoidosis. Additional disorders that produce multiple osteolytic areas in the skull are multiple myeloma (in which uniformity of size and mandibular involvement are more characteristic), hy-

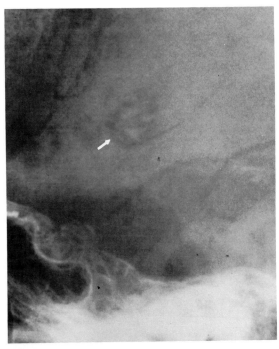

FIGURE 85–18. Skeletal metastasis: Skull—Button sequestrum. A metastasis from carcinoma of the breast has led to an osteolytic lesion (arrow) containing several small osseous spicules.

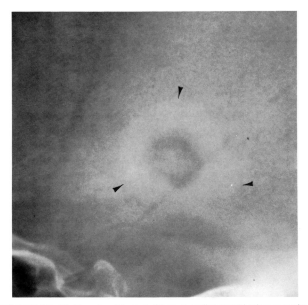

FIGURE 85–19. Doughnut lesion: Skull. A radiolucent lesion containing bone is surrounded by a rim of bone sclerosis (arrowheads). The radiologic findings are distinctive.

perparathyroidism (which produces the "salt and pepper" appearance), histiocytosis, radiation necrosis, prominent venous lakes,[127] and arachnoid granulations.[128]

Osteosclerotic metastatic lesions of the skull usually arise from carcinoma of the prostate. Any portion of the cranium may be affected, including the base.[129] Osteosclerosis of the base of the skull also is a well-recognized manifestation of nasopharyngeal carcinoma,[130, 131] and may become accentuated following radiotherapy of this tumor.[132] Additional causes of basal osteosclerosis include meningioma,[133] other tumors,[134] fibrous dysplasia,[135] and adjacent inflammatory processes; other disorders leading to multifocal or diffuse cranial osteosclerosis include Paget's disease, fibrous dysplasia, sarcoidosis, osteomas, syphilis, and a variety of congenital diseases.

Spine

The spine represents the most frequent site of skeletal metastasis. Involvement of the thoracic and lumbar levels predominates, although the sacrum often is affected. The cervical vertebrae are involved less typically.[136] Metastases more commonly occur in the vertebral bodies than in the posterior osseous elements. Of the malignant tumors that secondarily involve the spine, carcinomas of the lung, breast, and prostate (as well as lymphomas and plasma cell myeloma) are encountered most often.

Clinical manifestations associated with spinal metastasis are highly variable. In some instances, extensive tumorous deposits produce no symptoms, being discovered on routine radiographs or those obtained in patients with positive bone scans. When present, such manifestations commonly relate to an enlarging mass, fracture, vertebral instability, or compression of the spinal cord.[137] The last-mentioned finding has been observed in 5 to 10 per cent of persons with systemic cancer[138, 347] and is caused by extradural or, more rarely, intradural lesions, vertebral collapse with resulting spinal angulation, and pathologic fracture-dislocation.[137, 139]

Pain, muscle weakness, loss of sensation, and bowel and bladder dysfunction are among the clinical abnormalities that become apparent.

The radiographic findings of spinal involvement in cases of metastatic disease also are variable, although some characteristic patterns emerge.

Destruction and Collapse of Vertebral Body. Osteolysis of a vertebral body is difficult to detect with routine radiography until a large portion of the bone is destroyed.[357, 358, 370] An associated soft tissue or intraspinal mass is better delineated with myelography, CT, and MR imaging (Fig. 85–20); this finding is evident not only in metastatic disease but also in infectious diseases. Preservation of discal height is remarkable in many cases of skeletal metastasis, serving as a useful diagnostic aid in differentiating tumor from infection, although exceptions to this rule are encountered (see discussion later in this chapter).

Collapse of a vertebral body (or vertebral bodies) is an abnormality that occurs in skeletal metastasis, may be its presenting manifestation, and is evident in various other disorders as well, particularly osteoporosis, osteomalacia, and plasma cell myeloma.[57] Carcinomas of the breast, lung, and prostate, in order of decreasing frequency, represent the common causes of such collapse.[140] The level of spinal involvement varies somewhat according to the type of primary tumor (the second lumbar vertebral body most frequently is collapsed in breast carcinoma and the twelfth thoracic vertebral body most typically is collapsed in lung carcinoma),[57] and more than one vertebral body may collapse simultaneously or sequentially. Although some general radiographic rules exist that may permit differentiation of vertebral collapse related to tumor from that resulting from non-neoplastic disease,[328] such differentiation frequently is difficult; furthermore, it is reported that approximately one third of patients with malignancy and vertebral collapse have a nontumorous cause of the collapse.[140] Findings suggesting that a collapsed vertebral body has resulted from metastatic disease (or other malignant tumors) include involvement of the upper thoracic spine (a level of collapse infrequently observed in osteoporosis or osteomalacia); the presence of a soft tissue mass or pediculate destruction; and angular or irregular deformity of the vertebral endplates. Complicating the interpretation of the radiologic findings are the facts that the integrity of the adjacent intervertebral disc and the position of the vertebral body in the spinal column may influence the pattern of vertebral collapse and that cartilaginous (Schmorl's) nodes may produce focal and, sometimes, irregular regions of vertebral depression. Although uniform involvement of many vertebral bodies, leading to "fish" vertebrae, is typical of osteomalcia and nonuniform involvement of many vertebral bodies, again leading to "fish" vertebrae, is characteristic of osteoporosis, these conditions may coexist with metastatic disease in elderly persons. As there frequently is no specific routine radiographic pattern indicating tumorous vertebral collapse, CT and MR imaging have been used as additional diagnostic methods (see later discussion). A biopsy, however, ultimately is required for accurate diagnosis in many patients. Such biopsy generally is not necessary if skeletal alterations at additional sites are diagnostic of metastatic disease or if associated vertebral abnormalities permit a specific alternative diagnosis (such as an intraosseous vacuum phenome-

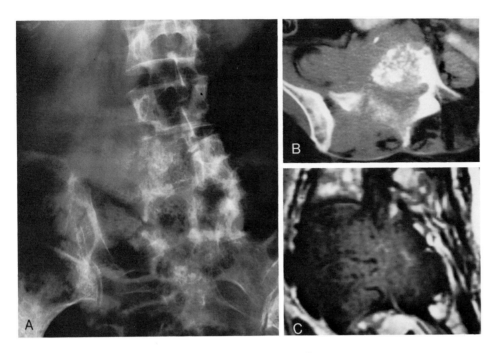

FIGURE 85–20. Skeletal metastasis: Spine—destruction of the vertebral body. Carcinoma of the cervix. In this 65 year old woman with a history of cervical carcinoma treated with irradiation five years previously, low back pain developed.

A Routine radiography reveals destruction of the fourth and fifth lumbar vertebrae and a right-sided soft tissue mass. Bone sclerosis also is evident.

B A transaxial CT scan at the level of L4 shows destruction of the vertebral body and posterior osseous elements with a large mass extending anteriorly, laterally, and posteriorly, as well as into the spinal canal.

C A sagittal T1-weighted (TR/TE, 400/10) spin echo MR image shows the full extent of bone and soft tissue involvement.

(Courtesy of G. Greenway, M.D., Dallas, Texas.)

non that is most compatible with ischemic necrosis of the vertebral body).

Sclerosis of Vertebral Body. The detection of inhomogeneous or homogeneous sclerotic areas in one or more vertebral bodies in an elderly man is most compatible with a diagnosis of metastatic disease arising from carcinoma of the prostate, although other metastatic tumors as well as lymphomas and, rarely, chordoma or plasma cell myeloma must be considered. Additional causes of vertebral osteosclerosis include chronic osteomyelitis (in which the intervertebral disc generally is affected), mastocytosis, tuberous sclerosis, myelofibrosis, Paget's disease, discogenic abnormalities, renal osteodystrophy, compression fractures (especially when associated with corticosteroid therapy), primary bone sarcomas (such as osteosarcoma and Ewing's sarcoma), enostosis, sarcoidosis, and a variety of congenital disorders. An entirely radiodense vertebral body (the ivory vertebral body) also is observed in cases of skeletal metastasis (Fig. 85–21), particularly carcinoma of the prostate, generally at more than a single level. An ivory vertebral body is a recognized manifestation of additional disorders, including lymphomas and, rarely, chordoma, plasmacytoma, and Paget's disease. It should be differentiated from the corduroy vertebral body (characterized by accentuated vertical striations) of a hemangioma (Fig. 85–22A), the rugger-jersey vertebral body (characterized by radiodense stripes at the top and the bottom of the vertebral body) of renal osteodystrophy (Fig. 85–22B), the picture-frame vertebral body (associated with condensation of bone along the margins of the vertebral body) of Paget's disease (Fig. 85–22C), and the sandwich vertebral body (accompanied by an extreme and uniform increase in radiodensity in the superior and inferior margins of the vertebral body) of osteopetrosis (Fig. 85–22D).

Pedicle Involvement. Destruction of one or both pedicles of a vertebra represents a well-known roentgenographic finding of skeletal metastasis (Fig. 85–23) that rarely is evident in plasma cell myeloma. It is best observed in the anteroposterior radiograph as an absence of one or both "eyes" of the vertebral body. Osteosclerosis of a pedicle is apparent in some patients with skeletal metastasis and is a reported (albeit rare) manifestation of Paget's disease.[371] It is simulated by pediculate hypertrophy that accompanies contralateral spondylolysis or congenital hypoplasia of the neural arch.

The diagnostic importance of pediculate destruction as a sign of skeletal metastasis has led to a misconception that pediculate localization is more frequent than that in the vertebral body in cases of metastatic disease. Such is not the case. Indeed, studies using CT[372] or MR imaging[373] clearly have shown that involvement of the pedicle usually occurs as a result of further extension of a tumorous deposit within the posterior portion of the vertebral body.

Pelvis

The bones of the pelvis frequently are involved in skeletal metastasis. Typical routes of tumor spread to this region are hematogenous dissemination and direct extension from the primary neoplastic site or from tumorous lymph nodes. Osteolytic (Fig. 85–24A), osteosclerotic (Fig. 85–24B), or mixed osteolytic-osteosclerotic lesions are seen. Diffuse osteosclerotic metastases, especially from carcinoma of the prostate, should be differentiated from other disorders leading to sclerosis in the pelvic bones (and spine), such as Paget's disease (Fig. 85–25A), sickle cell anemia, lymphomas, myelofibrosis, mastocytosis, tuberous sclerosis, fluorosis (Fig. 85–25B,C), and a number of congenital diseases.

Long Tubular Bones

Of the long tubular bones, it is the femur and the humerus that are involved most commonly in cases of skeletal metastasis. Metaphyseal localization predominates, al-

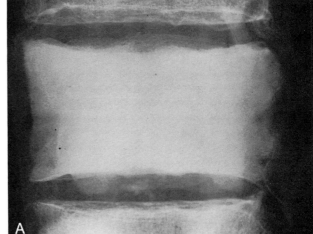

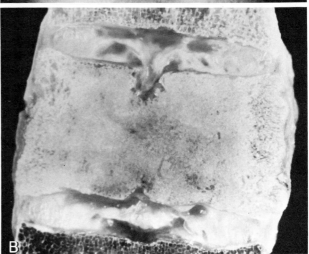

FIGURE 85–21. Skeletal metastasis: Spine—the ivory vertebral body. Carcinoma of the prostate.
A Observe the uniformly increased radiodensity of the entire vertebral body in this radiograph of a spinal specimen.
B Tumorous involvement of the vertebral body is evident. Cartilaginous (Schmorl's) nodes are apparent in both the top and the bottom of the vertebral body.

though diaphyseal (Fig. 85–26) or epiphyseal lesions are not infrequent. Preferential involvement of the metaphysis in the immature skeleton is consistent with the arterial vascular anatomy that promotes lodgment of tumor cells (or microorganisms) in this region.[141] Spongy bone in the medullary cavity typically is affected first with secondary involvement of the cortex in instances of hematogenous spread of tumor, although, as indicated previously, cortical destruction is more readily apparent on the roentgenograms. Unusual but characteristic osseous patterns of destruction that are observed with metastatic involvement of the long tubular bones include small cortical radiolucent foci near the entrance of the nutrient arteries and eccentrically located, scalloped erosions of the external surface of the cortex (cookie-bite sign) (Fig. 85–27), particularly in (but not limited to) cases of bronchogenic carcinoma (see later discussion).[142, 359, 360] As discussed previously, pathologic fractures are not infrequent, especially in the femur, and relate to the extent of cortical destruction.[374] The pathologic nature of such fractures is readily apparent when an adjacent osteolytic or, more rarely, osteosclerotic lesion is seen; fractures at certain sites, such as isolated avulsion of the lesser trochanter,[143, 375] or transversely oriented fracture lines suggest a pathologic fracture even in the absence of an obvious lesion.

A solitary metastatic focus in a long tubular bone (Fig. 85–26) may possess radiologic characteristics that simulate those of a primary locally aggressive or malignant osseous tumor, including giant cell tumor, fibrosarcoma, malignant fibrous histiocytoma, plasmacytoma, osteosarcoma, or chondrosarcoma.[3] The absence of both extensive periostitis and a prominent soft tissue mass in most metastatic lesions is helpful diagnostically.

Short Tubular and Irregular Bones

As indicated earlier in this chapter, metastatic lesions in the bones of the hands, wrists, and feet are infrequent, yet, they have received a great deal of attention.[58–81, 325, 352–355, 376] Bronchogenic, renal, and colonic carcinomas are the leading causes of such metastases (Fig. 85–28). Resulting multiple osteolytic lesions must be differentiated from those accompanying other disorders, including sarcoidosis, enchondromatosis, hemangiomatosis, lipomatosis, tuberous sclerosis, and multiple myeloma, as well as leukemias and lymphomas, infectious diseases, and fat necrosis; the differential diagnosis of a solitary metastatic focus in the peripheral portion of the skeleton includes a great number of possibilities, among which are primary bone neoplasms.

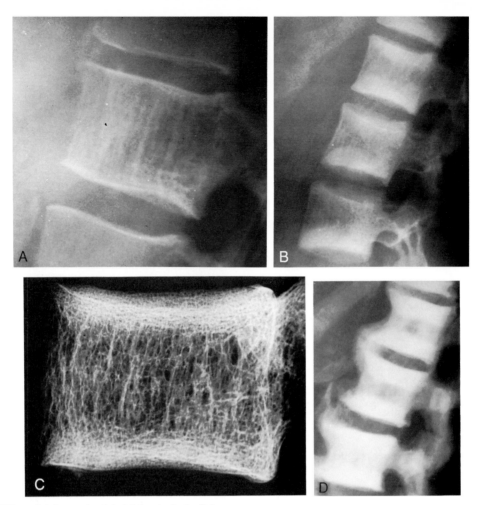

FIGURE 85–22. Differential diagnosis of skeletal metastasis: Spine.

A Hemangioma. The corduroy vertebral body is characterized by a spongy appearance and an accentuation of the vertical trabeculae.

B Renal osteodystrophy. The rugger-jersey appearance is accompanied by condensation of bone in the form of stripes at the top and bottom of each vertebral body.

C Paget's disease. A picture-frame appearance is characterized by trabecular thickening at the margins of the vertebral body.

D Osteopetrosis. Note the typical sandwich appearance of the vertebral bodies. (**D,** Courtesy of R. Dussault, M.D., Charlottesville, Virginia.)

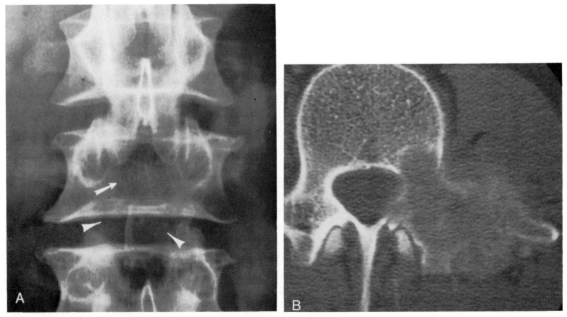

FIGURE 85–23. Skeletal metastasis: Spine—pedicle, transverse process, and lamina involvement.

A In this patient, osseous destruction (arrowheads) of a portion of the pedicles, the entire lamina, the inferior articulating processes, and the spinous process is seen. The appearance is that of an empty vertebral body (arrow).

B In a different patient, prostatic metastasis has led to destruction of the pedicle, lamina, transverse process, and posterior portion of the vertebral body. Pathologic fractures are present. (**B,** Courtesy of P. Kindynis, M.D., Geneva, Switzerland.)

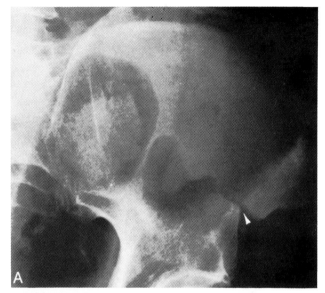

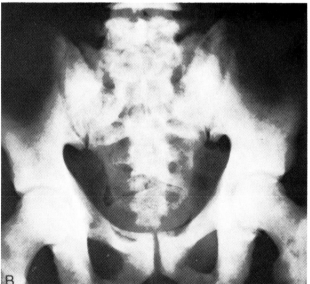

FIGURE 85–24. Skeletal metastasis: Pelvic bones.

  A An osteolytic lesion of the ilium is associated with a pathologic fracture (arrowhead).

  B Osteosclerotic foci throughout the bones of the pelvis (as well as the spine and proximal portion of the femora) are related to metastases from carcinoma of the prostate.

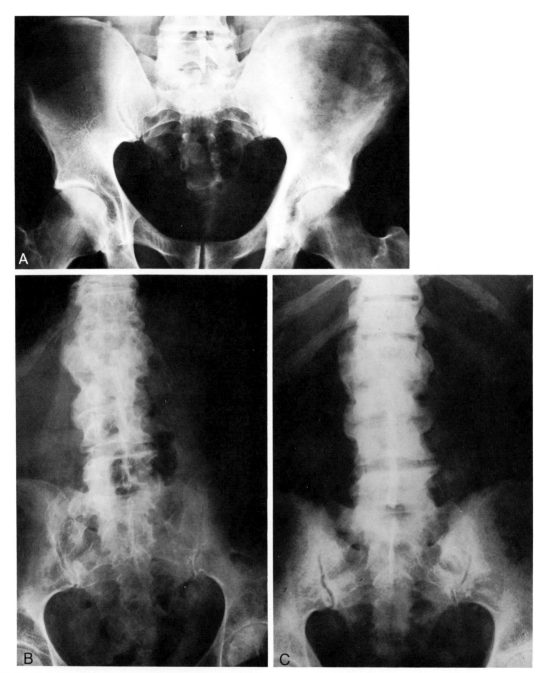

FIGURE 85–25. Differential diagnosis of skeletal metastasis: Pelvic bones.

A Paget's disease. The ilium and ischium on the left side are enlarged and radiodense. Although the findings simulate osteoblastic metastases, the unilateral nature of the diffuse process is much more characteristic of Paget's disease.

B, C Iatrogenic fluorosis. Radiographs obtained 4 years apart in this woman reveal the skeletal effects of fluoride treatment for osteoporosis. In the earlier film, taken at age 75 years **(B)**, osteopenia and vertebral collapse are identified. Subsequently at 79 years of age **(C)**, widespread osteosclerosis in the spine and pelvic bones is related to fluorosis.

(B, C, Courtesy of P. Berman, M.D., Ogdensburg, New York.)

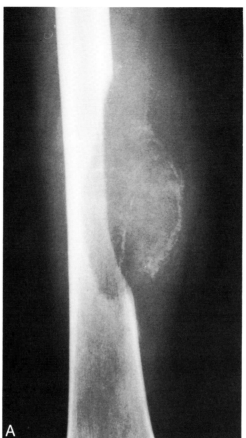 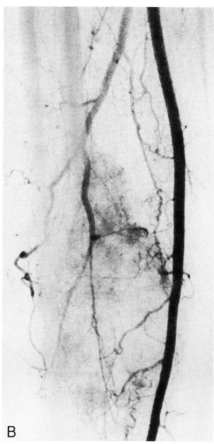

FIGURE 85–26. Skeletal metastasis: Long tubular bones. A 67 year old man developed pain in the upper portion of the leg over a 6 month period. On physical examination, a 7 cm mass was palpable.

A The radiograph shows an osteolytic lesion arising in the diaphysis of the femur with extensive cortical disruption. Ossification or calcification is present in the adjacent soft tissue mass. The findings resemble those of a primary malignant tumor of bone.

B The angiogram reveals tumor hypervascularity. A chest x-ray showed a nodule in the lung periphery. A bone biopsy documented poorly differentiated adenocarcinoma. The lung lesion was not biopsied.

(Courtesy of G. Greenway, M.D., Dallas, Texas.)

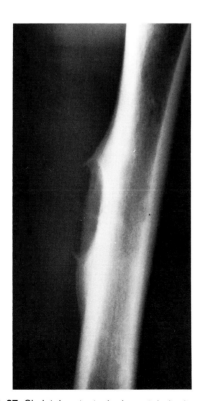

FIGURE 85–27. Skeletal metastasis: Long tubular bones—Cookie-bite sign in bronchogenic carcinoma. A well-circumscribed erosion of the external surface of the diaphysis of the femur is associated with periosteal reaction. (Courtesy of W. Murphy, M.D., St. Louis, Missouri.)

Sternum and Sacrum

These two bones are relatively common sites of metastasis. In both locations, routine radiographs often are suboptimal owing to overlying osseous and soft tissue structures, so that special techniques including oblique projections, conventional or computed tomography, or MR imaging are required (Fig. 85–29). Although primary tumors of the sternum are uncommon, most are malignant so that the differential diagnosis of an aggressive lesion in this bone encompasses, primarily, lymphomas, chondrosarcoma, and plasma cell myeloma in addition to skeletal metastasis.[144] Similarly, in the sacrum, such a lesion may indicate a chondrosarcoma, other sarcomas, plasmacytoma, chordoma, and giant cell tumor, as well as metastatic disease.

Chest Wall

Two principal mechanisms account for metastasis to the chest wall: hematogenous dissemination and direct extension of tumor. Hematogenously derived rib metastases most typically produce osteolytic or osteosclerotic lesions without an accompanying soft tissue mass, although the latter finding occasionally is evident, simulating the appearance of plasma cell myeloma. Pathologic fractures commonly are seen with such rib lesions. With regard to contiguous spread of tumor, invasion of the chest wall occurs in approximately 10 per cent of patients with adjacent pulmonary malignancies.[145, 146] A soft tissue mass in these patients relates to the tumor itself or to pleural thickening; the mass

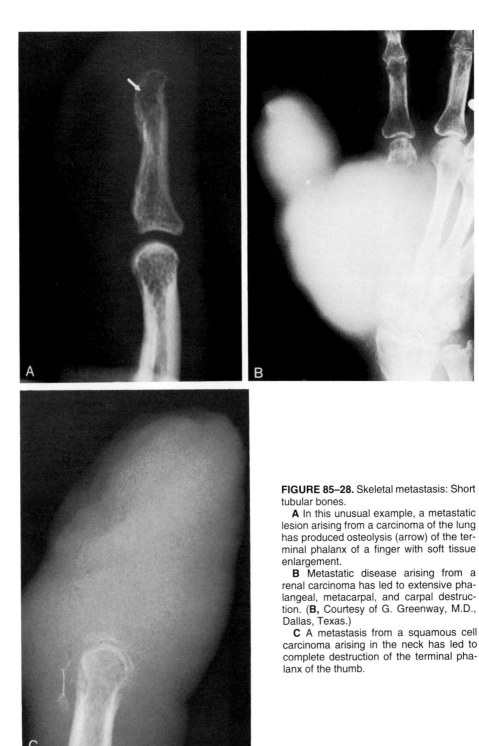

FIGURE 85–28. Skeletal metastasis: Short tubular bones.

A In this unusual example, a metastatic lesion arising from a carcinoma of the lung has produced osteolysis (arrow) of the terminal phalanx of a finger with soft tissue enlargement.

B Metastatic disease arising from a renal carcinoma has led to extensive phalangeal, metacarpal, and carpal destruction. (**B,** Courtesy of G. Greenway, M.D., Dallas, Texas.)

C A metastasis from a squamous cell carcinoma arising in the neck has led to complete destruction of the terminal phalanx of the thumb.

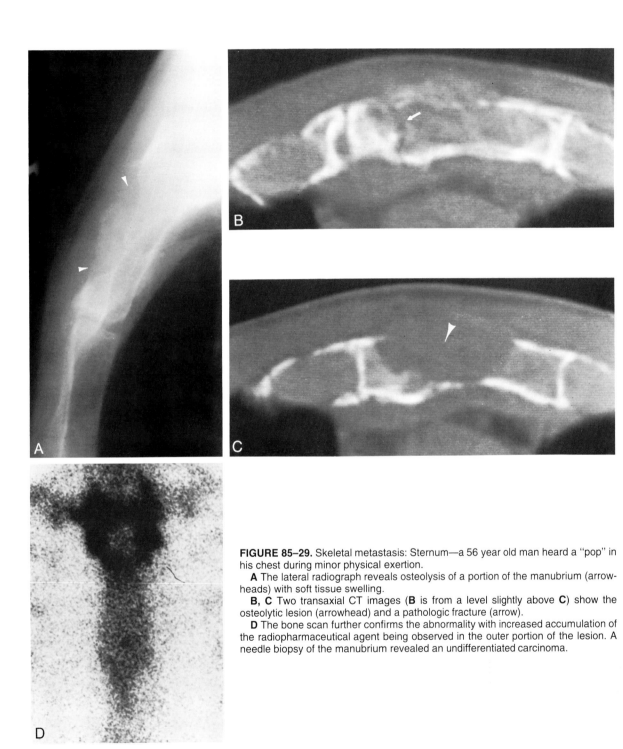

FIGURE 85–29. Skeletal metastasis: Sternum—a 56 year old man heard a "pop" in his chest during minor physical exertion.

A The lateral radiograph reveals osteolysis of a portion of the manubrium (arrowheads) with soft tissue swelling.

B, C Two transaxial CT images (**B** is from a level slightly above **C**) show the osteolytic lesion (arrowhead) and a pathologic fracture (arrow).

D The bone scan further confirms the abnormality with increased accumulation of the radiopharmaceutical agent being observed in the outer portion of the lesion. A needle biopsy of the manubrium revealed an undifferentiated carcinoma.

may be large or small and, in the latter case, its identification commonly requires routine radiography supplemented with fluoroscopy, conventional or computed tomography, or MR imaging.[147]

SPECIFIC TYPES OF TUMOR

It is beyond the scope of the current chapter to consider in great detail the many patterns of skeletal involvement associated with each of the neoplasms that may metastasize to bone; the interested reader should consult other sources that contain this information, including Wilner's textbook.[3] What follows is a brief summary of the major and distinctive osseous manifestations of metastasis found in some of the more important malignant tumors.

Carcinoma of the Breast

A common cause of hematogenous skeletal metastasis, this tumor usually produces osteolytic or mixed osteolytic-osteosclerotic lesions or, rarely, osteoblastic lesions, predominating in the axial skeleton and ribs. Pathologic fractures are frequent, particularly involving the femur, vertebrae, and ribs, and such fractures involving the odontoid process of the axis have been emphasized.[148] Metastatic breast carcinoma may remain confined to the skeleton without involvement of other organ systems for prolonged periods.[377, 378] Other types of breast tumors, including cystosarcoma phylloides,[149] also may metastasize to the skeleton.

Carcinoma of the Lung

Carcinoma of the lung, a common tumor, involves the skeleton owing to lymphatic spread to regional lymph nodes (mediastinal) with direct extension into bone, lymphatic spread through the diaphragm to regional lymph nodes (para-aortic) with direct osseous extension, and invasion of the pulmonary veins with dissemination via the arterial circulation (Figs. 85–30 and 85–31). Four major cell types of lung cancer are encountered: squamous cell (epidermoid) carcinoma, anaplastic large cell carcinoma, small cell (oat cell) carcinoma, and adenocarcinoma. Of these, small cell carcinoma is the most aggressive, followed

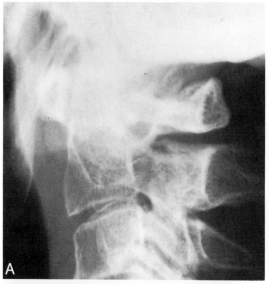

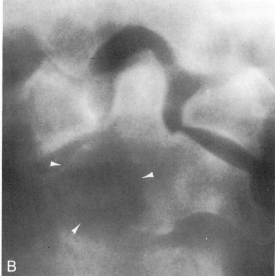

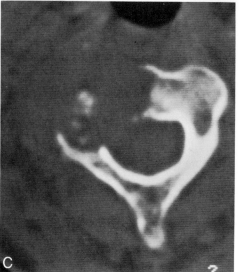

FIGURE 85–30. Skeletal metastasis: Carcinoma of the lung—involvement of the cervical spine.

A With the exception of soft tissue swelling, the lateral radiograph almost is normal, although there is increased radiolucency of the vertebral body and pediculate region of the axis.

B A frontal tomogram shows a large osteolytic lesion (arrowheads) in the body of the axis with extension to the region of the right lateral atlantoaxial joint.

C A transaxial CT scan at the level of the body of the axis reveals the degree of bone destruction and a soft tissue mass.

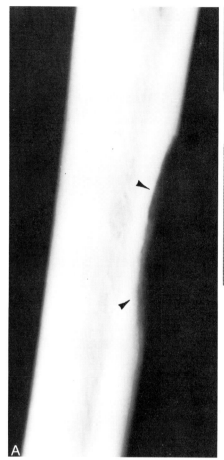
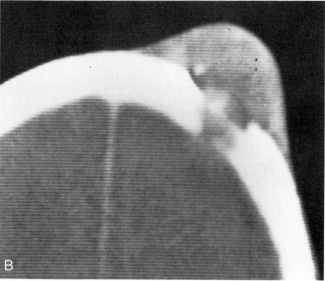

FIGURE 85–31. Skeletal metastasis: Carcinoma of the lung—Cookie-bite sign. Two examples of eccentric cortical metastatic lesions are shown. In **A,** a scalloped erosion (arrowheads) of the diaphysis of the femur is seen; in **B,** a soft tissue mass is accompanied by erosion of the outer table and diploic region and, to a lesser extent, the inner table of the skull. (**A,** From Deutsch A, Resnick D: Radiology *137*:49, 1980.)

by large cell carcinoma and adenocarcinoma, with squamous cell carcinoma being the least virulent.[3] In squamous cell and anaplastic large cell carcinomas, osteolytic or mixed osteolytic-osteosclerotic lesions predominate; in small cell carcinoma and adenocarcinoma, osteoblastic lesions may be visible.[150] The latter finding is apparent in fewer than 15 per cent of patients.[3]

Characteristic patterns of skeletal involvement include rib erosion related to a peripheral tumor of the lung, destruction of vertebrae in association with tumor-containing mediastinal lymph nodes, destruction of ribs and cervical vertebrae in response to a Pancoast tumor, eccentric cookie-bite excavation of the external surface of the cortex,[142, 150, 359, 360] and a soft tissue mass, containing bone, adjacent to the cortical surface,[151] typically in a femur, and rarely multifocal in a symmetric distribution.[152]

Carcinoid of the Bronchus (and Other Carcinoids)

Extra-appendiceal carcinoid tumors (argentaffinomas) commonly are malignant and have an ability to metastasize. Skeletal metastasis is relatively infrequent, arises from hematogenous dissemination, and, when present, is most likely to occur with tumors in the lung, stomach, pancreas, descending colon, and rectum, and with those that are large and locally invasive; the typical osseous sites of involvement, in order of decreasing frequency, are the vertebrae, pelvic bones, ribs, and femora.[3] Osteosclerotic lesions pre-

dominate.[153–157, 380] The osteoblastic response may be intense and, in some instances, leads to bone spiculation simulating that of an osteosarcoma.[157] Osseous expansion and periostitis are encountered in the spine, ribs, and tubular bones.[379]

Carcinoma of the Prostate

Carcinoma of the prostate is a common cause of osseous metastasis; potential routes allowing spread to the skeleton include Batson's venous plexus and extension from tumorous nodes in the pelvic and para-aortic regions. Osteoblastic metastases are characteristic, although not invariable, and predominate in the axial skeleton (Fig. 85–32). Recognized radiographic patterns of skeletal involvement are single or multiple, focal or diffuse areas of bone sclerosis; one or more ivory vertebral bodies; spinal lesions with narrowing of the intervening intervertebral disc space (see later discussion); and bone expansion (Fig. 85–33) simulating the appearance of Paget's disease.[90–92, 381]

Carcinoma of the Kidney

Renal cell carcinoma spreads principally in three ways: by direct extension, by involvement of lymphatic channels that ultimately drain into the paraaortic, hilar, paratracheal, and mediastinal regions, and by invasion of the renal veins with subsequent extension to the inferior vena cava, right atrium, and pulmonary vessels.[3] Metastasis to the skeleton is common and, infrequently, this occurs in the absence of

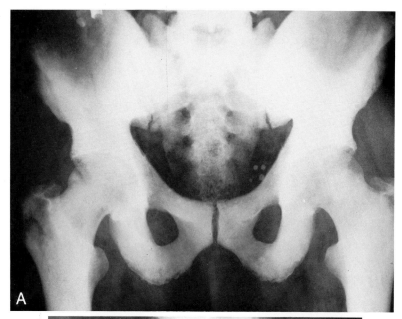

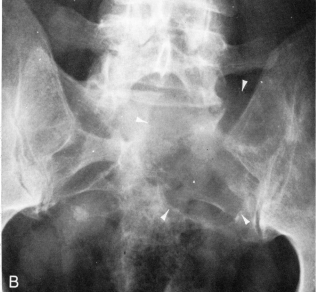

FIGURE 85–32. Skeletal metastasis: Carcinoma of the prostate.

A Osteoblastic type. The entire bony pelvis, proximal portion of the femora, and lower lumbar spine are involved. One osteolytic lesion is observed in the greater trochanter on the right side.

B Osteolytic type. A large lesion of the sacrum (arrowheads) might be missed if comparison with the opposite side were not accomplished.

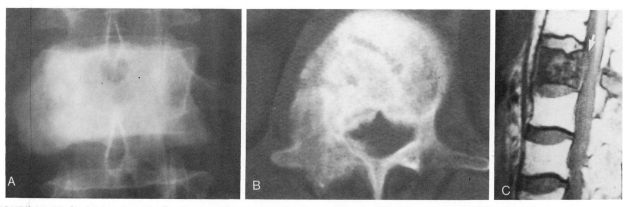

FIGURE 85–33. Skeletal metastasis: Carcinoma of the prostate. Routine radiogaphy **(A)** and transaxial CT **(B)** show an expansile osteoblastic lesion involving the vertebral body and posterior osseous elements. A sagittal T1-weighted (TR/TE, 800/25) spin echo MR image **(C)** reveals predominantly low signal intensity in the vertebral body and posterior extension of tumor (arrow) into the subarachnoid space. Small metastatic foci were evident elsewhere in the spine.

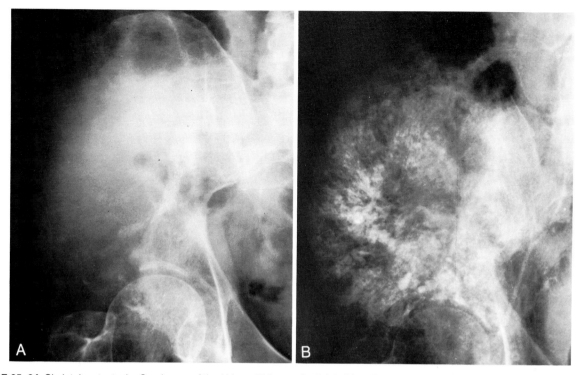

FIGURE 85–34. Skeletal metastasis: Carcinoma of the kidney. This man had right hip pain and a soft tissue mass.
A The initial radiograph reveals an expansile, osteolytic lesion of the right ilium extending to the subchondral acetabular bone.
B Angiography documents its vascular nature. Biopsy of the bone lesion documented the presence of renal carcinoma metastatic to the skeleton.

metastases in other organ systems.[158] Typical sites of involvement are the thoracolumbar spine, bones of the pelvis, ribs, and femora. Solitary osseous lesions are relatively frequent, and such lesions may occur in the pelvis, spine, and long tubular bones, especially the femora and humeri.[3, 158] Symptoms and signs related to skeletal metastasis may represent the initial clinical features of an occult renal cell carcinoma.[159] Conversely, bone lesions may occur years after the discovery or treatment of a carcinoma of the kidney.[160] Following nephrectomy, serial radiographs have revealed regression of the skeletal lesions.[87]

Osteolysis is the predominant radiographic finding (Fig. 85–34). Solitary or multiple, small or large areas of bone destruction are seen, and, in some cases, massive and expansile lesions are identified. Septation, a soft tissue mass, and a pathologic fracture are additional roentgenographic features of these metastases. Angiography reveals the hypervascular nature of the osseous lesions.[88] Very rarely, an osteosclerotic response in association with skeletal metastasis from renal cell carcinoma is evident.[161]

Wilms' Tumor

Skeletal metastasis in Wilms' tumor has been regarded as uncommon, with a reported frequency of less than 5 per cent in most series. The histologic features of the metastatic foci have been described as atypical of Wilms' tumor by some investigators, who believe that the term ''bone-metastasizing renal tumor of childhood'' is more accurate.[162] Those neoplasms with a polygonal or clear cell pattern more typically disseminate to bone, leading to their separation in some reports from nephroblastomas and rhabdomyo-

sarcomas[162]; in others, these tumors are all considered together as variants of Wilms' tumor.[163]

Bone metastases usually are osteolytic and have a widespread distribution in both the axial and the appendicular skeleton (Fig. 85–35). A honeycomb pattern of destruction sometimes is seen, and a button sequestrum, similar to that of an eosinophilic granuloma, has been identified in a lesion of the skull.[164] Osteosclerotic alterations rarely have been evident.[165]

Carcinoma of the Thyroid

Hematogenous dissemination of thyroid carcinoma to the skeleton results in solitary or multiple osteolytic lesions predominating in the axial skeleton (Fig. 85–36). An expansile nature, small calcific collections, a pathologic fracture, and a tendency to extend across articulations are features of thyroid metastases that have been emphasized previously.[3] Osteoblastic foci are exceedingly rare.[318]

Medullary carcinoma of the thyroid accounts for less than 10 per cent of malignancies of the thyroid gland, is a component of the multiple endocrine neoplasia (type II) syndrome, and is associated with the consistent production of a hormonal marker (thyrocalcitonin) and with calcification of both the primary tumor and the metastatic foci.[166] Although osseous metastases are infrequent, they are variable in appearance and may be entirely osteosclerotic.[167]

Carcinoma of the Bladder

Osseous lesions in carcinoma of the bladder arise either from direct extension from the primary neoplasm and tu-

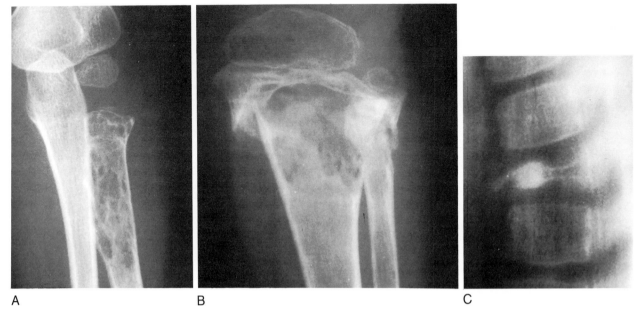

A   B   C

FIGURE 85–35. Skeletal metastasis: Wilms' tumor.

A, B In this 4 year old girl, osteolytic lesions are observed in the radius, tibia, and fibula. In the last two sites, pathologic fractures are evident. In the radius, a honeycomb pattern is apparent. The spine also was affected.

C In a different 4 year old girl with back pain and quadriplegia, a collapsed thoracic vertebral body, similar to that occurring in eosinophilic granuloma, containing a sclerotic focus is apparent. Biopsy of the bone lesion as well as a left renal neoplasm documented the presence of Wilms' tumor.

(**C,** Courtesy of A. D'Abreu, M.D., Porto Alegre, Brazil.)

morous lymph nodes (Fig. 85–37A,B) or from hematogenous dissemination (Fig. 85–37C). They are relatively infrequent and typically affect the thoracolumbar spine and bones of the pelvis, with less common involvement of other skeletal sites.[168–170] The frequency of bone metastases increases with the depth of invasion of the bladder wall and the degree of cellular dedifferentiation.[171] Osteolytic changes are characteristic, and heterotopic ossification in the adjacent soft tissues occasionally is observed.[96, 97] Osteosclerotic lesions may indicate prostatic invasion.[168, 172]

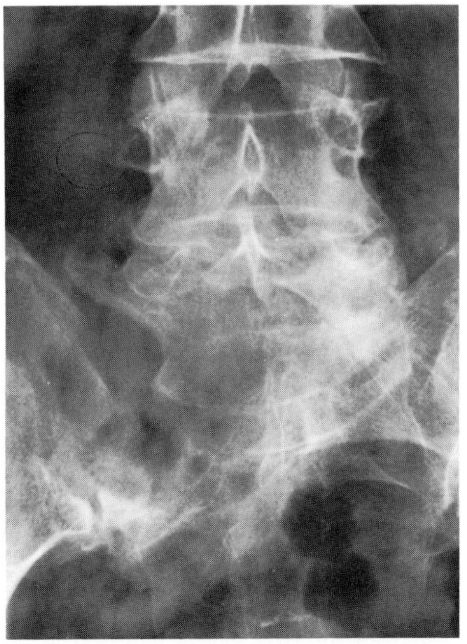

Malignant Melanoma

Skeletal metastasis from melanoma, arising as a result of hematogenous dissemination, is uncommon but not rare.[173] Osteolytic lesions, with or without adjacent soft tissue masses, are observed, principally in the spine, ribs, and bones of the pelvis,[382] although virtually any skeletal location may be involved (Figs. 85–38 and 85–39).[383] Fracture and collapse of one or more affected vertebral bodies are frequent. Unusual features of skeletal involvement by this tumor include expansile lesions similar to those arising from carcinoma of the thyroid and kidney,[3, 174] sclerosis about the lesional margins,[175] joint effusions in association with subchondral foci,[175] and paravertebral masses containing calcification.[176]

Carcinoma of the Uterine Cervix and Corpus

Carcinoma of the uterine cervix may extend to regional lymph nodes and from there to paravertebral and mediastinal lymph nodes; it also may disseminate via the portal and caval venous systems. Osseous involvement results from direct extension into the bones of the pelvis; from tumorous lymph nodes that erode the vertebrae (especially in the lumbar spine) and pelvic bones; or from venous and arterial tumor emboli to any portion of the skeleton[3] (Fig. 85–40). The thoracolumbar region of the vertebral column and the pelvic bones are the most frequent sites of metastasis. Characteristics of such metastases include erosion of the pubic bone, ilium, and sacrum with a contiguous soft tissue mass[177, 178] and unilateral destruction of vertebral bod-

FIGURE 85–36. Skeletal metastasis: Carcinoma of the thyroid.
In a 71 year old woman, a purely osteolytic lesion involves the right side of the sacrum. Compare with the normal left side.

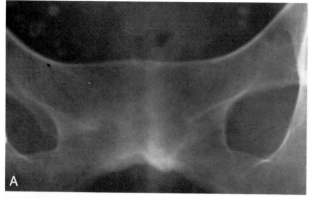
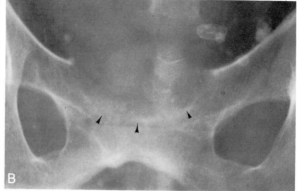
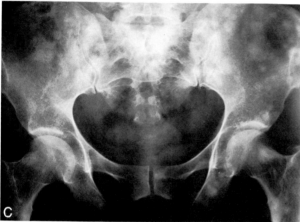

FIGURE 85–37. Skeletal metastasis: Carcinoma of the bladder.

A, B Direct extension. This 81 year old man had undergone multiple transurethral resections for carcinoma of the bladder. In **A**, observe osteitis pubis, which has resulted in complete bone ankylosis of the symphysis pubis. Five years later **(B)**, at the age of 86 years, direct invasion of the bone (arrowheads) by the tumor is evident. A soft tissue mass is seen.

C Hematogenous dissemination. In this patient, widespread focal osteosclerotic metastases have resulted from carcinoma of the bladder.

ies.[10–12] Purely osteolytic lesions are more typical than either mixed osteolytic-osteosclerotic or purely osteosclerotic foci whether they are located in the axial or the appendicular skeleton.

Adenocarcinoma of the uterine corpus rarely metastasizes to bone, and the sites of involvement generally are confined to the axial skeleton with reportable exceptions.[179] Hematogenous dissemination of the tumor to bone, rather than lymphatic spread, is the rule.[3] Again, osteolysis is typical.

Tumors of the Gastrointestinal System

Metastatic lesions arising from *carcinoma of the esophagus* are rare and of the osteolytic type.[3] A similar pattern of bone destruction is evident in cases of *gastric carcinoma,* although diffuse osseous sclerosis may be an initial feature of this tumor[180] (Fig. 85–41). Skeletal metastases from *carcinoma of the colon or rectum* generally are osteolytic or mixed osteolytic-osteosclerotic[181]; adjacent soft tissue masses containing calcification occasionally are evident.[94, 384]

Pancreatic carcinoma involves the skeleton as a result of posterior extension of the primary tumor into the lower thoracic and upper lumbar vertebral bodies or through hematogenous dissemination to the spine, pelvis, and ribs.[3] Although osteolytic lesions predominate,[319] sclerotic changes at the thoracolumbar junction (Fig. 85–42) and elsewhere are encountered.[182]

Hepatocellular carcinoma is a rare malignant tumor that may metastasize to the skeleton.[320] Clinical manifestations

related to such osseous metastases may be the initial findings of the disease.[89, 183] Osteolysis is the major radiographic characteristic, and large, expansile, and hypervascular lesions are seen. Pathologic fractures and soft tissue masses may be evident.[326, 385]

The *Zollinger-Ellison syndrome* consists of gastric hypersecretion, intractable peptic ulceration, and gastrin-secreting islet cell tumors of the pancreas.[184] Approximately 60 per cent of these tumors are malignant, and osteoblastic metastases have been reported in one patient.[184]

Nasopharyngeal Carcinoma

As indicated earlier in this chapter, carcinomas arising in the nasopharynx may extend directly into the base of the skull, leading to osteolytic destruction or, more rarely, osteosclerosis.[130–132] Distant skeletal metastases also are evident in some cases.[185]

Intracranial Tumors

Osseous metastasis is a known manifestation of several different types of brain tumors. The typical pathway of spread in such neoplasms is along the leptomeninges and, occasionally, via the cerebrospinal fluid into the spinal canal (see previous discussion).[21–24] In some instances, ventricular shunts provide a pathway for extraneural dissemination of tumor, and in other circumstances, generally but not invariably following a craniotomy, dural disruption allows more widespread intravascular and perineural lymphatic dissemination.

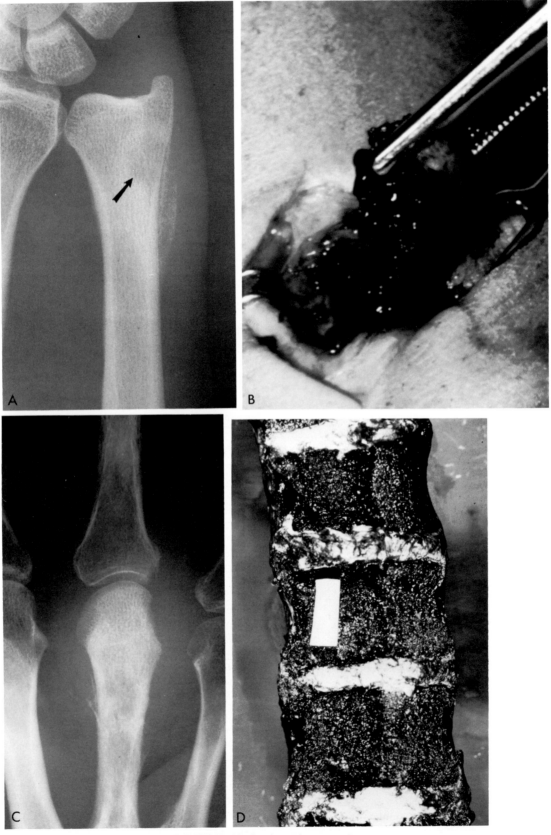

FIGURE 85–38. *See legend on opposite page*

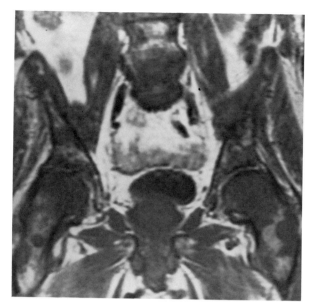

FIGURE 85–39. Skeletal metastasis: Malignant melanoma. In a 67 year old man with known melanoma and low back pain, routine radiographs of the lumbosacral spine (not shown) were normal. A coronal T1-weighted (TR/TE, 600/20) spin-echo MR image reveals metastatic lesions of low signal intensity in the lower spine, pelvic bones, and proximal femora.

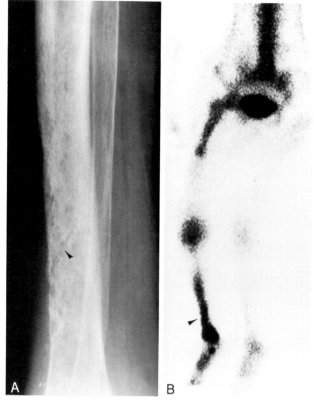

FIGURE 85–40. Skeletal metastasis: Carcinoma of the uterine cervix. An 89 year old woman developed right leg pain which progressed over a 1 year period. Three years previously, a diagnosis of stage 2 squamous cell carcinoma of the cervix and nodular lymphocytic lymphoma had been established. She had undergone irradiation to the pelvis.

A A roentgenogram shows permeative bone destruction in the lower one half of the tibia with a pathologic fracture (arrowhead). Minimal periostitis is evident. The radiologic findings are consistent with lymphoma.

B A bone scan reveals increased accumulation of the radionuclide in the distal half of the right tibia (arrowhead), in the region of a right hip arthroplasty, and in the proximal portion of the right tibia at the site of a previous tibial plateau fracture. A biopsy of the tibial lesion documented metastasis from carcinoma of the cervix.

(Courtesy of G. Greenway, M.D., Dallas, Texas.)

Medulloblastomas appear to represent the intracranial tumor that is most likely to spread outside the central nervous system, and systemic metastases from this tumor are more frequent in children and adolescents than in adults. Skeletal involvement is characterized by osteosclerotic, osteolytic, or mixed osteolytic-osteosclerotic lesions.[26, 27, 29, 186–193, 386–389] The vertebrae, pelvis, femora, and ribs are the typical sites of involvement (Fig. 85–43A,B), although more widespread involvement may be apparent (Fig. 85–43C). Myelography, CT, and MR imaging allow identification of neoplastic seeding of the spinal cord.[337]

Other intracranial neoplasms, including astrocytomas,[194] glioblastoma multiforme,[3] pinealoblastoma,[390] and meningiomas,[195, 196, 391] less commonly metastasize to the skeleton. With regard to meningiomas (Fig. 85–44), invasion of the dural sinuses may predispose to extracranial metastases, and bone involvement is associated with osteolysis, osseous expansion, and a soft tissue mass, especially in the axial skeleton.[195]

Neuroblastoma

Neuroblastoma, which represents a common malignant tumor in the young child, may arise from the medulla of the adrenal gland or anywhere in the sympathetic nervous system (see Chapter 58).[321] Characteristics of skeletal metastasis include symmetric involvement, osteolysis with permeative bone destruction (Fig. 85–45), sutural widening, and collapse of vertebral bodies with adjacent soft tissue masses.[392] Spinal cord compression is frequent.[197, 393] In rare circumstances, multifocal neuroblastomas relate not to metastasis but to multiple primary tumors, a phenomenom that may occur in families.[198]

FIGURE 85–38. Skeletal metastasis: Malignant melanoma. This 23 year old man had pain and swelling over the distal ulna. His pertinent history included the removal of a skin "cyst" several years previously.

A On initial evaluation, a motheaten or permeative destructive lesion with lysis and sclerosis of the distal ulna (arrow) is found to be associated with adjacent periosteal proliferation and soft tissue swelling. At this time, no other osseous lesions were identified, and a preoperative diagnosis of a primary malignant tumor, probably Ewing's sarcoma, was made.

B An operative photograph delineates a lesion of the distal ulna containing melanin (held by upper clamp), which on histologic evaluation was diagnosed as a malignant melanoma, presumably originating from the cutaneous lesion that previously had been removed. Within months, the patient developed widespread skeletal metastasis.

C A subsequent skeletal survey outlined a destructive mixed lytic-sclerotic lesion of the metacarpal and proximal phalanx of the third finger, with periostitis and soft tissue swelling, as well as additional osseous metastases.

D At the time of autopsy, diffuse involvement with melanotic lesions is evident on this photograph of a coronal section of the spine. Pigmentation extends into several of the intervertebral discs.

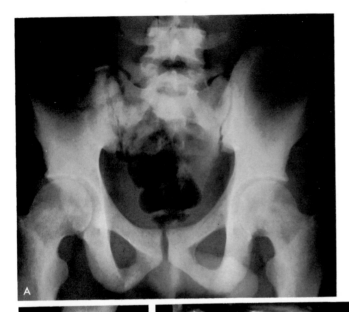

FIGURE 85–41. Skeletal metastasis: Carcinoma of the stomach. This 36 year old man with gastric carcinoma developed widespread osteoblastic skeletal lesions, predominating in the axial skeleton. The radiograph of the pelvis **(A)** demonstrates a uniform increase in radiodensity of all the bones. A radiograph **(B)** and photograph **(C)** of a sagittal section of the spine indicate the extent of osteoblastic metastasis. A photomicrograph **(D, 90×)** shows that the marrow spaces of a vertebral body are replaced by metastatic adenocarcinoma.

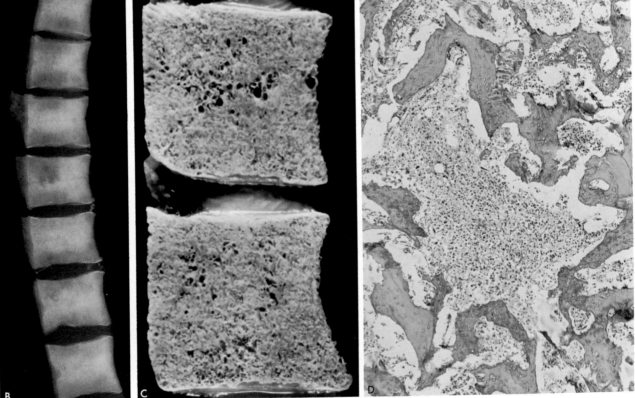

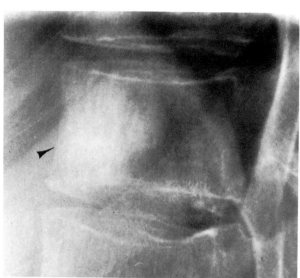

FIGURE 85–42. Skeletal metastasis: Carcinoma of the pancreas. A sclerotic region (arrowhead) in the anterior aspect of the vertebral body at the thoracolumbar junction is a recognized manifestation of extension from carcinoma of the pancreas. In this case, the twelfth thoracic vertebral body is affected in a 66 year old man.

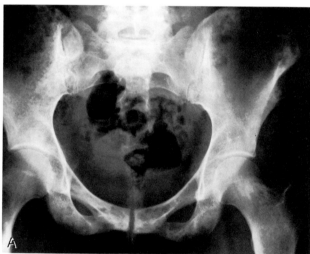

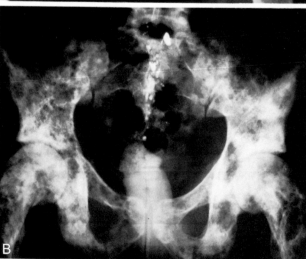

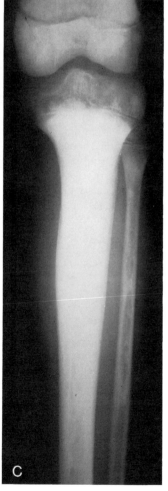

FIGURE 85–43. Skeletal metastasis: Medulloblastoma.

A This radiograph of the pelvis was obtained in a 23 year old woman 2 years following a craniotomy with excision of a medulloblastoma. Patchy osteosclerosis is evident in the left iliac crest, right acetabulum, symphyseal regions, ischial tuberosities, and left femoral neck.

B Following the removal of a medulloblastoma in a 20 year old man, extensive osteoblastic metastases developed in the spine and, as shown here, throughout the pelvic bones and proximal portions of the femora.

C In a 12 year old boy who had undergone excision of a medulloblastoma, widespread osteoblastic skeletal metastases developed, shown here in the tubular bones of the lower extremity.

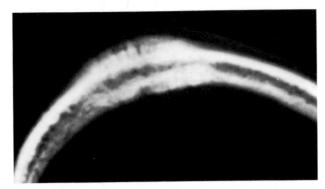

FIGURE 85–44. Skeletal metastasis: Parasagittal meningioma. In a 37 year old man who developed progressive headaches and a lump on his head over a 9 month period, a CT scan reveals expansion of the outer table of the skull, radiating osseous spicules, narrowing of the diploic portion, and osteosclerosis of the inner table. Other scans showed a parasagittal mass that was involving the superior sagittal sinus, being supplied by the middle meningeal artery.

Until recently, it has been maintained that osseous involvement with classic neuroblastoma always is a manifestation of metastatic disease from a visceral primary tumor.[394] It now is recognized that a neoplasm, primary primative neuroectodermal tumor, that strongly resembles neuroblastoma on histologic analysis may originate in the skeleton[395] (see Chapter 83). It also may metastasize to the skeleton (Fig. 85–46).

Retinoblastoma

Retinoblastoma arises from cells of the granular layer of the retina and represents a common primary tumor of childhood. The occurrence of this neoplasm in multiple family members occasionally is recognized, and bilateral and sometimes simultaneous involvement of both eyes is evident in approximately 30 per cent of cases.[3] Typical clinical manifestations are strabismus, persistent tearing, and visual disturbances with slowly developing blindness. Patterns of tumor spread include direct extension beyond the orbit with destruction of the facial bones and sinuses, subdural and subarachnoid invasion with extension to the spinal canal, and hematogenous dissemination throughout the body with

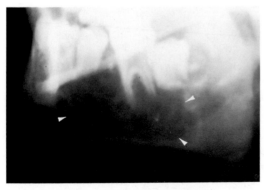

FIGURE 85–45. Skeletal metastasis: Neuroblastoma. Observe the osteolytic lesion (arrowheads) of the mandible in this 9 year old girl. Several teeth are partially destroyed and appear to be floating. The findings are similar to those of the histiocytoses.

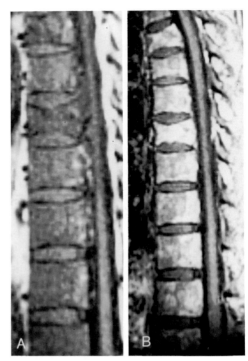

FIGURE 85–46. Skeletal metastasis: Primitive neuroectodermal tumor (PNET). In this 57 year old man, an initial sagittal T1-weighted (TR/TE, 500/12) spin echo MR image **(A)** reveals diffuse metastatic foci in the spine manifested as multiple collapsed vertebral bodies and signal intensity in the bone marrow that is lower than normal. Following intravenous administration of gadolinium, a sagittal T1-weighted (TR/TE, 800/12) spin echo MR image **(B)** shows enhancing spinal metastatic lesions.

involvement of the skeleton.[199–201] Osteolysis with a permeative pattern of bone destruction and periostitis are seen at one or more sites, commonly in a symmetric distribution. These radiographic features resemble those of neuroblastoma and medulloblastoma. Of interest in this regard, histologic similarities occur among these three tumors,[201] and, in both neuroblastoma and retinoblastoma, elevated urinary excretion of vanillylmandelic acid and homovanillic acid[202] as well as punctate calcification of the primary tumor[201] is observed. Furthermore, in neuroblastoma and retinoblastoma, spontaneous tumor regression or maturation, infiltration of the bone marrow, and dissemination to the meninges, liver, and lymph nodes are evident.[201]

Patients with retinoblastoma may subsequently develop secondary neoplasms. Radiation-induced sarcomas are reported in 1.5 per cent of cases[3] and lead to osseous destruction in the facial bones and a soft tissue mass. Familial cases of bilateral retinoblastomas have been associated with secondary malignant tumors, particularly osteosarcoma and, less frequently, fibrosarcoma, angiosarcoma, Ewing's sarcoma, rhabdomyosarcoma, Wilms' tumor and other neoplasms.[3, 396] The bones of the skull (Fig. 85–47) or the appendicular skeleton typically are affected.

Embryonal Rhabdomyosarcoma

Although rare, this neoplasm represents the most frequent soft tissue sarcoma of childhood. It may arise from

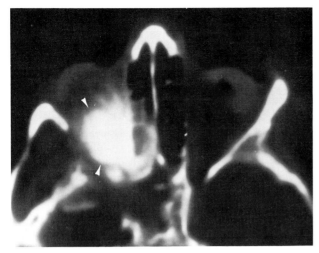

FIGURE 85–47. Bilateral retinoblastomas with secondary neoplasia. This 6 year old child had undergone treatment for bilateral retinoblastomas, including enucleation and radiation therapy. An osteosarcoma (arrowheads) subsequently developed. (Courtesy of T. Broderick, M.D., Orange, California.)

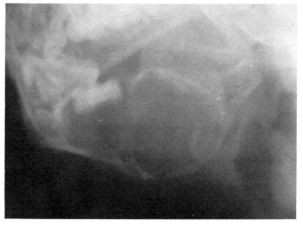

FIGURE 85–48. Skeletal metastasis: Embryonal rhabdomyosarcoma. Note extensive destruction of the mandible with "floating" teeth in a 2 year old child. (Courtesy of T. Broderick, M.D., Orange, California.)

striated muscle at many different sites, including the head and neck (35 to 50 per cent of cases), pelvis, thoracic and abdominal walls, and extremities.[3] The tumor is extremely malignant, with a tendency for local invasion, recurrence, and widespread dissemination to the lungs, liver, lymph nodes, and skeleton. Osseous involvement, which rarely may be the presenting manifestation of the disease,[469] may relate to direct extension from an adjacent soft tissue tumorous deposit or hematogenous spread, especially in the pelvis, spine, ribs, skull, and tubular bones.[3] Multiple lesions are common, and symmetric changes sometimes are encountered. Osteolysis with motheaten or permeative bone destruction predominates (Fig. 85–48).

Other Tumors

Virtually any malignant tumor may lead to metastasis with potential involvement of the musculoskeletal system. Primary bone tumors, such as osteosarcoma, chondrosarcoma, fibrosarcoma, chordoma, Ewing's sarcoma, and lymphomas, can spread from the initial osseous site to one or more distant locations in the skeleton (see Chapter 83). Malignant soft tissue tumors can lead to similar dissemination.[338] Infrequent or rare causes of skeletal metastasis include malignant mesothelioma, carcinomas of the oral cavity (Fig. 85–49A), salivary glands, urachus, larynx, trachea, oropharynx, and biliary system, ovarian and testicular tumors, squamous cell and basal cell carcinomas of the skin, tumors of the sweat glands, cardiac myxomas, leiomyosarcomas of the uterus and gastrointestinal tract, thymoma,

FIGURE 85–49. Skeletal metastasis: Other malignant tumors.

A Carcinoma of the tonsil. An osteolytic lesion of the proximal portion of the humerus is associated with a pathologic fracture (arrowhead).

B Chemodectoma. Note an osteoblastic lesion (arrowheads), which has replaced the body of the axis. The tip of the odontoid process still is visible.

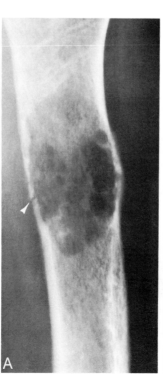

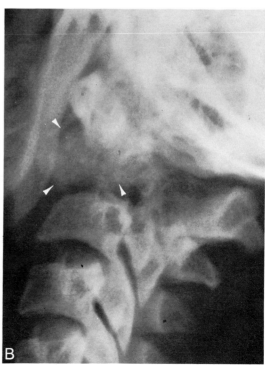

chemodectoma (Fig. 85–49*B*) and paraganglioma, and pheochromocytoma.[203–209, 339, 397–408, 464]

ARTICULAR INVOLVEMENT

The previous chapter has detailed the many neoplastic and pseudoneoplastic processes that can affect articular and periarticular tissue. Included in these processes are skeletal metastases. The manner in which metastatic lesions affect synovial and cartilaginous joints is further delineated in the following pages. A certain degree of overlap of material contained in these two chapters is provided for emphasis.

Synovial Joints

Skeletal Metastasis to Periarticular Bone. Metastases to periarticular foci about synovial joints are not infrequent. Such deposits typically are encountered in the hip,[210] the shoulder,[211] and the knee[212]; at these sites and others, tumors can lead to symptoms and signs simulating arthritis.[213–215, 409] The clinical manifestations may be derived from osseous foci that have not altered in any fashion the adjacent articulation, from foci that have led to disruption and collapse of the nearby articular surface, or from foci that have produced a non-neoplastic reaction within the neighboring articulation. (A fourth possibility, that of neoplastic involvement of the joint itself, is discussed later in this chapter.)

Roentgenograms reveal a lytic or sclerotic epiphyseal focus that may extend down to the subchondral bone (Figs. 85–50 to 85–52). Its appearance may be reminiscent of that of a subchondral "cyst," which may be observed in a variety of articular processes such as rheumatoid arthritis, osteoarthritis, pigmented villonodular synovitis, and gout, a primary bone tumor such as a giant cell tumor or chondroblastoma, plasma cell myeloma, or an intraosseous gan-

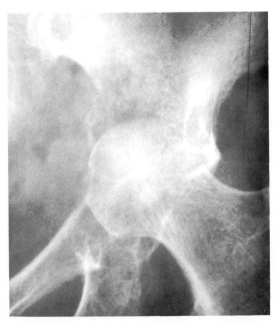

FIGURE 85–50. Skeletal metastasis to periarticular bone: Hip. This 65 year old woman developed a destructive lesion of the left hemipelvis, which was due to metastasis (or direct invasion) from a clear cell carcinoma of the uterus. The loss of acetabular support has allowed inward protrusion of the femoral head. (Courtesy of R. Taketa, M.D., Long Beach, California.)

glion. At times, weakening of bone beneath the cartilage, especially in a weight-bearing articulation, will promote osseous collapse and fragmentation identical to the findings in osteonecrosis or neuropathic osteoarthropathy. Accurate clinical and radiographic diagnosis frequently depends on the presence of a known primary tumor and the detection of additional sites of skeletal metastasis. Biopsy of the skeletal lesion may be required.

Inflammation of synovial tissue in proximity to metastatic tumor is unusual.[212, 409, 411] This finding should be differentiated from neoplastic involvement of the synovium and from synovial reaction in hypertrophic osteoarthropathy, although the histologic appearance of the synovial membrane in the latter condition may be identical to that associated with a neighboring skeletal metastatic site[216] (Fig. 85–53). A similar synovial reaction can be encountered in conjunction with neighboring benign tumors, such as osteoid osteoma, and malignant tumors, such as leukemia and lymphosarcoma.[217] On histologic examination, hypervascularity and cellular infiltration with lymphocytes and plasma cells are seen.[212] The synovial reaction may be related to tumor release of substances containing enzymatic or antigenic properties, a mechanism that also may be responsible for a rheumatoid arthritis-like carcinomatous polyarthritis that can be associated with a distant neoplastic focus (see discussion later in this chapter).[218]

Skeletal Metastasis to Periarticular Bone with Intraarticular Extension. A metastatic focus in subchondral bone may extend into the nearby articulation.[210, 219–227, 410, 412] Although this may occur at various locations, it appears to be especially frequent about the knee. In this site, patellar, femoral, or tibial lesions can disrupt the subchondral bone plate, leading to neoplastic involvement of the synovial membrane. On radiographs, the osteolytic or osteosclerotic process at any site commonly is combined with a joint effusion or mass. Arthrography may provide more direct visualization of the intra-articular extension of the tumor with nodular irregularities of the contrast-coated synovial membrane.[220] Cytologic study of the synovial fluid may detect cancer cells,[219, 224, 227–229] and the presence of intraarticular tumor is firmly established on histologic examination of the synovial membrane.[223, 225, 226]

Metastasis to Synovial Membrane. Hematogenous spread of tumor to the synovial membrane with or without adjacent osseous involvement occasionally is encountered.[210, 230] In these instances, monoarthritis may be unaccompanied by any osseous disruption, the radiographs revealing a joint effusion or mass. Analysis of synovial fluid may show malignant cells, and tissue examination confirms the presence of metastatic synovial deposits[231–233] (Fig. 85–54). A similar pattern of synovial extension has been observed in patients with leukemia.[234] Of tumors metastasizing to the synovium, those of the breast and lung do so most frequently. In most instances the existence of a malignancy is known at the time of synovial metastasis, although the subsequent joint manifestations may be misinterpreted as those of rheumatoid arthritis, gout, or infection.

Cartilaginous Joints

Osseous metastasis can occur in and around cartilaginous joints. Although this may be observed in relationship to the

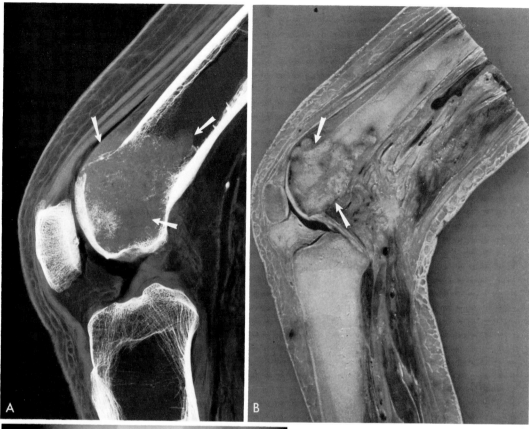

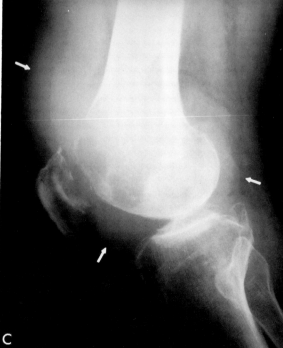

FIGURE 85–51. Skeletal metastasis to periarticular bone: Knee.

A, B An unexpected finding in this cadaver donated to an anatomy laboratory was an adenocarcinoma of the colon metastatic to the femur. A radiograph and photograph of a sagittal section of the femur, patella, and tibia indicate the extent of the lesion (arrows). It violates the anterior femoral cortex but does not extend distally into the joint. (Courtesy of M. Pitt, M.D., Birmingham, Alabama.)

C In another patient, a large osteolytic lesion of the distal femur is associated with a large joint effusion or mass (arrows). Biopsy indicated anaplastic carcinoma involving bone extending into the articular cavity with hemarthrosis. (Courtesy of V. Vint, M.D., La Jolla, California.)

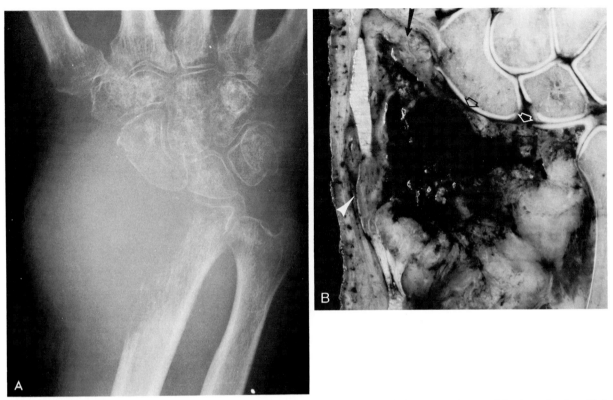

FIGURE 85–52. Skeletal metastasis to periarticular bone: Wrist. This 63 year old man with known carcinoma of the lung developed left arm and wrist pain and swelling. Because of the debilitating nature of the pain, the forearm was resected following radiation therapy.

A An initial radiograph reveals the extent of the radial lesion. It has produced permeative bone destruction and extends into the soft tissues, with considerable mass effect. Patchy osteoporosis of the carpus is identified.

B A photograph of the sectioned specimen demonstrates the extent of the radial tumor. Note that it has expanded the distal radius (solid arrow), destroyed a portion of the articular cartilage of the radius (open arrows), and enveloped surrounding tendons (arrowhead). The carpus is free of tumor.

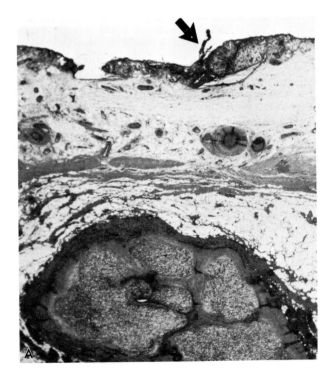

FIGURE 85–53. Synovial reaction to malignant tumors. Chondrosarcoma. A 70 year old man had a disarticulation for a chondrosarcoma of the inferior right femoral metaphysis. The subsynovial tissue is invaded by neoplasm, and the synovial lining is edematous with cellular hyperplasia and superficial fibrin deposits (arrow). (From Lagier R: J Rheumatol 4:65, 1977.)

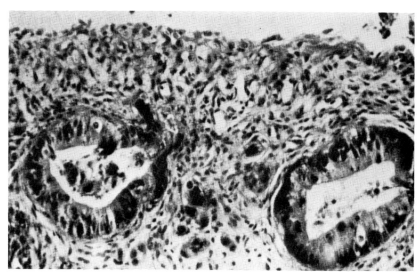

FIGURE 85–54. Synovial metastasis. This 62 year old man with adenocarcinoma of the sigmoid colon developed pain and swelling of the knee. Although radiographs were negative, synovial aspiration revealed malignant cells, and biopsy showed malignant invasion of the synovium with cells arranged in glandular formation (150×). (From Goldenberg DL, et al: Arthritis Rheum *18*:107, 1975.)

symphysis pubis or manubriosternal joint (Fig. 85–55), it is detected most commonly at the discovertebral junction. Metastatic deposits in the spine are very frequent; Fornasier and Horne[57] noted pathologic evidence of skeletal metastasis in the vertebral bodies of the thoracolumbar spine in 140 of 374 cases (38 per cent) of malignant neoplasm. The frequency of radiographically evident vertebral metastasis is lower, as it repeatedly has been emphasized that at least 30 to 50 per cent of bone loss in the vertebral bodies may

be required before an abnormality becomes detectable on the roentgenogram.

A basic radiographic and pathologic concept with regard to vertebral metastasis is that the intervertebral disc is relatively resistant to the spread of tumor; the presence of vertebral destruction in the absence of significant disc alteration is a reliable indication of tumor, whereas the presence of vertebral destruction and loss of intervertebral disc space suggests infection. This concept is extremely useful but not

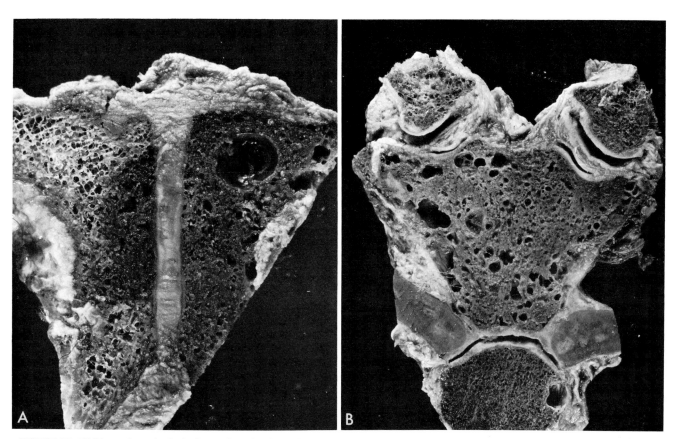

FIGURE 85–55. Tumor in periarticular bone: Symphysis pubis and manubriosternal joint. Observe the focal areas of bony destruction about the symphysis pubis and proximal portion of the sternum on these coronal sections. This appearance can occur with skeletal metastasis as well as with plasma cell myeloma and other neoplasms.

without exception. In unusual circumstances, tumor indeed may produce abnormality of an intervertebral disc. Discal destruction has been noted in association with plasma cell myeloma, chordoma,[235] and vertebral metastases[236, 237] (Fig. 85–56).

In a radiographic and pathologic study of the vertebral column in 25 cadavers with prostatic carcinoma and spinal metastases, Resnick and Niwayama[238] noted abnormalities of the intervertebral discs in six instances. The discal changes could be classified into three types: intervertebral disc degeneration (intervertebral [osteo]chondrosis); cartilaginous (Schmorl's) node formation; and discal invasion by tumor.

Intervertebral Disc Degeneration (Intervertebral [Osteo]Chondrosis). Intervertebral chondrosis and (osteo)chondrosis are terms applied to the various stages of disc degeneration that are frequent in older persons (see Chapter 40). Disc degeneration involves predominantly the nucleus pulposus and relates to physiologic or pathologic dehydration and desiccation of the nucleus, with progressive cleft formation, discal flattening, and necrosis. Concomitant vertebral changes consist of bone eburnation or sclerosis (Fig. 85–57).

The presence of intervertebral (osteo)chondrosis adjacent to sites of vertebral body metastasis may represent the coincidental occurrence of two not infrequent conditions. In some instances, however, the location and prominence of disc degeneration at only one level in the spine—adjacent to a vertebral body containing metastatic deposits—are noteworthy. Furthermore, as proper nutrition of the intervertebral disc depends, at least in part, on diffusion of fluid from the marrow space of the vertebral body through the endplates into the disc, it would appear that tumor within the vertebral body might interfere with proper disc nutrition and lead to its early degeneration. Intervertebral osteochondrosis should be particularly prominent when metastatic deposits within the vertebral body are intimate with the subchondral bone plate. The term secondary intervertebral (osteo)chondrosis is more appropriate in these patients to distinguish this type of discal abnormality from that of primary intervertebral (osteo)chondrosis, a process occurring as a result of gradual aging. The term secondary intervertebral (osteo)chondrosis already has been used to describe abnormality of disc tissue that may accompany primary changes outside the disc, such as instability of vertebral arches and alterations in spinal curvature.[239]

Cartilaginous (Schmorl's) Node Formation. Cartilaginous (Schmorl's) nodes represent protrusions of disc material into the adjacent vertebral body, which occur when defects exist in the cartilaginous endplate. Any disorder that weakens the osseous architecture of the vertebral body may lead to disruption of the cartilaginous endplate and cartilaginous node formation; this disruption may be accentuated by obvious or occult trauma. Tumor metastasis to the vertebral body can lead to cartilaginous node formation (Fig. 85–58). In these instances, defects within the vertebrae contain a combination of tumor and disc material. If extensive, discal displacement can produce radiographically and pathologically evident disc space loss. It has been suggested that such discal protrusion may predispose the adjacent disc to secondary intervertebral osteochondrosis,[239, 240] which could lead to further disc space loss.

Discal Invasion by Tumor. Neoplasm can locate within the intervertebral disc by (1) tumor implantation related to direct hematogenous spread within the intervertebral disc and (2) invasion of the intervertebral disc from a contiguous source of tumor within the vertebral body.[431, 432] Extensive involvement of the intervertebral disc by tumor may be observed; however, there rarely is evidence of discal metastatic foci without contiguous neoplasm in the vertebral body. Instances of bony metastasis adjacent to the subchondral bone plate with little or no alteration of the bony or cartilaginous endplate are identified. Additionally, examples can be noted of disruption of the bone plate (and, less frequently, the cartilaginous endplate) by tumor and discal extension of tumor through normal gaps where marrow is continuous with cartilage (Fig. 85–59). Although in almost all instances neoplastic involvement of the intervertebral discs appears to result from tumor invasion from the adjacent vertebral body, isolated tumor localization at the peripheral portion of a discovertebral junction can be identified on rare occasions. It also should be noted that the phenomenon of neoplastic invasion of a fibrocartilaginous disc from an adjacent osseous focus is not confined to the discovertebral junction. Similar findings are encountered at the symphysis pubis and manubriosternal joint.

The foregoing observations indicate that mechanisms for alteration of the intervertebral disc in association with vertebral metastasis include (1) intervertebral disc degeneration (intervertebral [osteo]chondrosis); (2) cartilaginous (Schmorl's) node formation; and (3) discal invasion by tumor. Intervertebral (osteo)chondrosis may occur as an incidental finding, unrelated to the presence of bony metastasis in a neighboring vertebral body. Adjacent vertebral metastatic foci apparently may interfere with proper diffusion of nutrients from the vertebral body to the intervertebral disc, however, and thus produce extensive disc degeneration. Cartilaginous node formation associated with vertebral metastasis is not unexpected. These discal protrusions relate to weakening of osseous structure and are more prevalent with increased destruction of the vertebral body. Discal invasion by tumor is not common, a fact that may relate to avascularity of the intervertebral disc and perhaps some additional inherent quality of cartilage that inhibits tumor growth.[241] When present within the intervertebral disc, tumor usually is associated with spread from a contiguous source within the vertebra rather than hematogenous spread directly to the intervertebral disc. Once neoplastic tissue reaches the intervertebral disc, the advancing tumor may use existing tears for further dissemination.

Although abnormalities of the intervertebral disc usually are related to metastases arising from carcinoma of the prostate,[238] similar abnormalities may be associated with vertebral metastasis of tumors derived from other primary sites. As hematogenous spread of metastasis from pelvic organs such as the prostate may relate to the peculiar anatomy of the venous plexus of the vertebral column,[14–16, 18] however, the frequency and distribution of vertebral metastasis may depend on whether the primary tumor is located within either a pelvic organ, such as the prostate, or a nonpelvic site. It has been suggested by Batson[14–16] and others[18] that tumors in nonpelvic organs, such as the breast, also may metastasize to the skeleton via connections with vertebral veins. In addition, the spread of tumor from adjacent soft tissues into the vertebral bodies and intervertebral

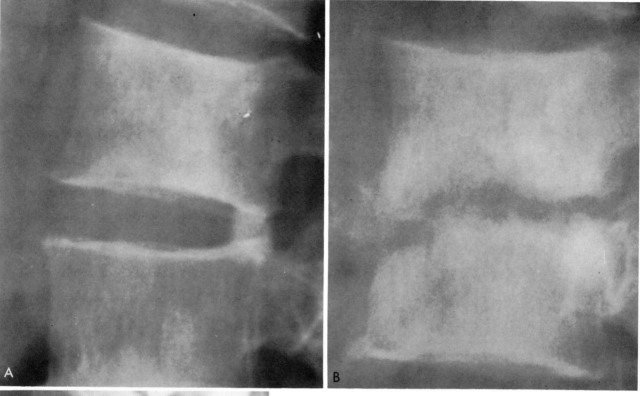

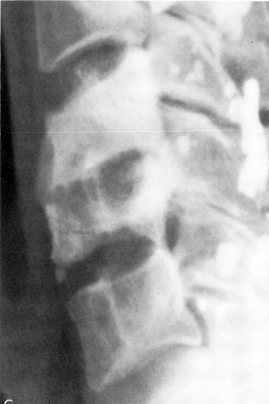

FIGURE 85–56. Abnormalities of the intervertebral discs in patients with skeletal metastasis.

A, B This 58 year old man had prostatic carcinoma and metastatic disease in two adjacent vertebral bodies. On the initial radiograph **(A),** sclerotic lesions are apparent within the vertebral bodies, and the intervertebral disc spaces appear normal. On a radiograph obtained 3 months later **(B),** the bony outlines are extremely irregular and the disc space is narrowed. Biopsies on numerous occasions, as well as subsequent postmortem examination, failed to document the presence of infection.

C In another patient with carcinoma of the prostate and metastatic disease in the cervical spine, sclerotic lesions of two adjacent vertebral bodies are recognized. Both demonstrate partial collapse. The intervertebral disc space appears narrowed and focally obliterated. A myelogram had been obtained previously. (From Resnick D, Niwayama G: Invest Radiol *13:*182, 1978.)

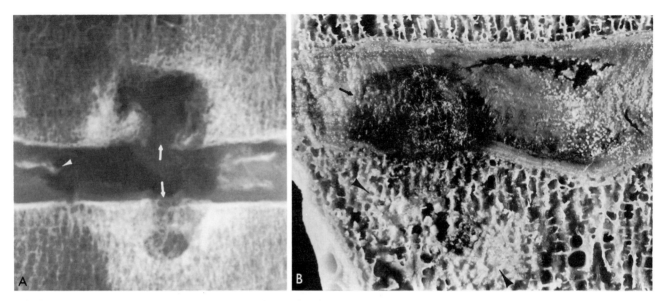

FIGURE 85–57. Vertebral metastasis with intervertebral osteochondrosis.

   A Intervertebral disc degeneration (intervertebral osteochondrosis) is evident in a cadaver with metastatic prostatic carcinoma and sclerotic lesions of two adjacent vertebral bodies. Findings include vacuum phenomena and disc calcification (arrowhead), disc space loss, and cartilaginous (Schmorl's) nodes (arrows). These nodes are surrounded by a thin margin of sclerosis, which merges with sclerotic metastatic foci.

   B In another cadaver, note the sclerotic metastatic deposits (arrowheads). These extend to the subchondral bone. Discoloration and degeneration of the intervertebral disc (arrow) can be seen, presumably related to discal necrosis. No evidence of neoplasm within the disc is seen.

   (From Resnick D, Niwayama G: Invest Radiol *13:*182, 1978.)

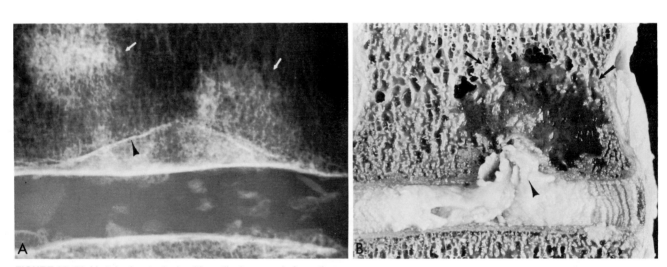

FIGURE 85–58. Vertebral metastasis with cartilaginous node formation.

   A Magnification radiograph outlines a cartilaginous node (arrowhead) producing a contour defect along the inferior surface of the vertebral body. Note the adjacent metastatic lesions (arrows).

   B In an additional cadaver, metastasis has produced considerable destruction of a large segment of the vertebral body (arrows). Note the displacement of intervertebral disc material into the osseous defect (arrowhead).

   (From Resnick D, Niwayama G: Invest Radiol *13:*182, 1978.)

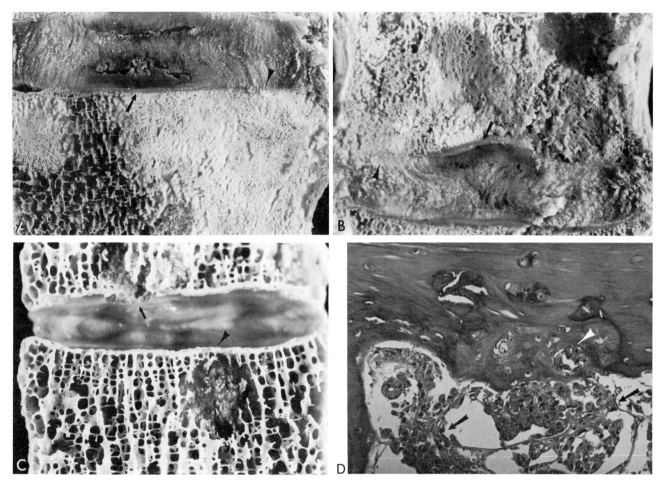

FIGURE 85–59. Vertebral metastasis with discal invasion by tumor.

   A Sclerotic metastatic foci are apparent. Observe that these lesions extend to the cartilaginous endplate. This latter structure appears intact in most areas (arrow). At the peripheral portion of the vertebral body, tumor has obscured the interface between intervertebral disc and bony plate (arrowhead).

   B In another cadaver, widespread metastatic lesions can be seen. Portions of the cartilaginous endplate appear intact (arrow), whereas the bone plate at the margins of the vertebra is destroyed (arrowhead).

   C Metastatic lesions in two adjacent vertebral bodies are associated with varying changes in the subchondral bone plate. In some locations, the plate appears intact (arrowhead); elsewhere, it is disrupted (arrow).

   D On a photomicrograph (140×), observe tumor infiltration into the junctional area between the intervertebral disc and the subchondral bone of the vertebral body. Tumor cells are readily identifiable within the bone (arrows) and extend into the cartilage (arrowhead).

   (**A–D,** From Resnick D, Niwayama G: Invest Radiol *13*:182, 1978.)

discs is well known. Metastasis in paravertebral lymph nodes or meninges and primary neoplasms of retroperitoneal tissues may advance into the vertebral structures.

Differential Diagnosis

The abnormalities occurring at synovial and cartilaginous articulations in patients with skeletal metastasis must be differentiated from additional joint manifestations that are associated indirectly with neoplastic disease.[242]

Secondary Hypertrophic Osteoarthropathy. Periosteal proliferation is associated with many neoplastic (and nonneoplastic) processes, principally those of the lungs and pleurae (see Chapter 93).[242] The findings commonly are bilateral and symmetric, affecting predominantly the tibiae, fibulae, radii, ulnae, metacarpals, metatarsals, phalanges, femora, and humeri (Fig. 85–60). Articular abnormalities can simulate those of rheumatoid arthritis, with clinically detectable morning stiffness, pain, warmth, and swelling, and radiographically evident soft tissue swelling, joint effusion, and osteoporosis. A nonspecific synovitis that does not require the presence of tumor within or around the involved joints may be evident.

Secondary Gout. Secondary hyperuricemia and gout may be encountered in patients with disseminated carcinoma and sarcoma (see Chapter 43). In these cases, radiographic abnormalities may be mild or absent, although occasionally asymmetric soft tissue swelling and eccentric erosion become apparent.

Carcinomatous Polyarthritis. A polyarthritis resembling rheumatoid arthritis can be an initial manifestation of malignancy.[218, 244–247] Articular findings may precede the oc-

currence of malignant neoplasm by a period of months to years. Differentiation from true rheumatoid arthritis may be accomplished on the basis of some unusual features: the sudden onset of symptoms and signs, asymmetric joint involvement, systemic manifestations such as fever and mental confusion, poor response to salicylates, and the absence of serum rheumatoid factor and rheumatoid nodules. Biopsy reveals a nonspecific synovitis. Rarely, a seropositive (rheumatoid factor) arthritis may accompany neoplastic disease.[246]

The cause and pathogenesis of the process and its relationship to rheumatoid arthritis and tumor are not clear. Adjacent neoplastic osseous foci are not required for the appearance of the polyarticular synovitis, suggesting that a generalized systemic aberration, rather than a local effect, is important. Surgical removal of the tumor may result in complete clinical remission, and regression of nodules and serum rheumatoid factor in those cases in which they are present.[248] Changes in cellular immunity and circulating immune complexes have been reported in some cases of malignancy,[244, 250] perhaps indicating a clue to the pathogenesis of carcinomatous polyarthritis,[218, 251] although these results are not uniform.[252, 253] The roentgenographic findings, which may consist of soft tissue swelling and osteoporosis, are not related to hypertrophic osteoarthropathy, gout, or joint and bone metastasis.

Pyogenic Arthritis. Pyogenic arthritis, due to intestinal flora, has been reported as a complication of advanced neoplastic disease.[254] In fact, the presence of bacteremia due to *Streptococcus bovis* or other enteric organisms causing endocarditis[255] or arthritis[256] may be the first sign of an occult colonic neoplasm. In this situation, neoplastic mu-

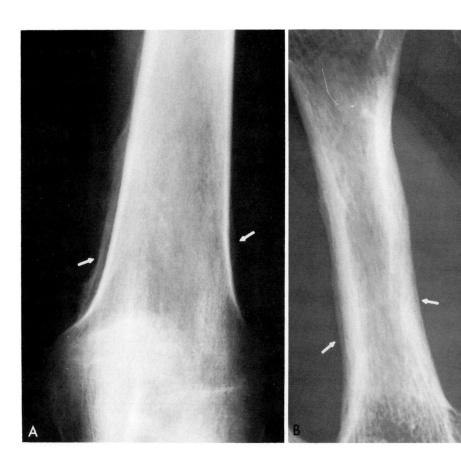

FIGURE 85–60. Secondary hypertrophic osteoarthropathy: Bronchogenic carcinoma.

A In the femur, solid periosteal bone formation is evident in the diaphyseal and metaphyseal segments (arrows).

B A magnification radiograph of an affected metacarpal bone indicates new bone formation in the diaphysis and metaphysis (arrows).

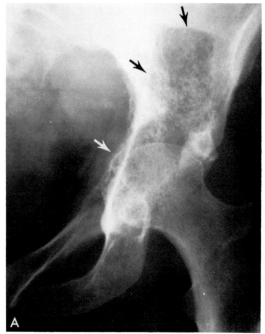

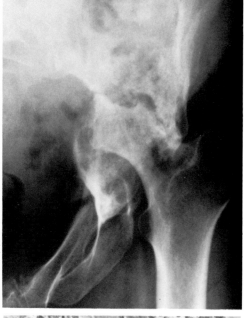

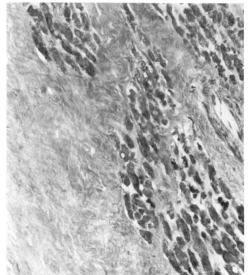

FIGURE 85–61. Irradiation effect. This 46 year old woman was admitted to the hospital for investigation of left flank and left hip pain. A pelvic mass was discovered encasing the distal left ureter, producing obstructive uropathy. A lytic bone lesion was also discovered in the left acetabulum at that time. Biopsy of the pelvic mass revealed a squamous cell carcinoma of undetermined origin, most probably from the cervix. Chemotherapy and radiotherapy were administered. The calculated total dose to the ilium was 6500 cGy (rad).

A A radiograph obtained prior to the radiation therapy indicates neoplastic infiltration of the periacetabular region (arrows) with intrapelvic protrusion of the femoral head.

B Two years following radiotherapy, considerable destruction of the acetabulum and femoral head with acetabular protrusion is consistent with irradiation effect. The presence of neoplasm is not required to produce this radiographic picture.

C A biopsy of the area indicates radiation fibrosis. Muscle bundles are surrounded by dense collagen fibers. A vessel at the right reveals intimal sclerosis (trichrome stain, 160×).

cosal ulceration may provide the portal of entry for the organisms.

Irradiation. Irradiation of sites of skeletal metastasis can lead to local osseous complications, including osteoporosis, osteonecrosis, and radiation-induced sarcoma (see Chapter 73). Knowledge of these complications is important so that the appearance of bony destruction following such treatment is not misinterpreted as evidence of progressive metastasis. This especially is pertinent in neoplasms about the pelvis; acetabular fracture, fragmentation, and protrusion can represent an osseous response to irradiation (Figs. 85–61 and 85–62).

Other Manifestations. Additional rheumatic disorders, such as Sjögren's syndrome, systemic lupus erythematosus, and dermatomyositis, may represent an initial manifestation of malignant disease.[257–259] Amyloidosis also may be associated with neoplasm, as can a Jaccoud-type arthropathy[413]

and the reflex sympathetic dystrophy syndrome.[247] Polymyalgia rheumatica rarely has been described in patients with underlying malignancies. Additionally, relapsing polychondritis and fat necrosis can be manifestations of neoplasms, the latter in association with pancreatic carcinoma. The occurrence of heterotopic ossification in the soft tissues, "malignant myositis ossificans," in relationship to metastases from certain tumors, such as gastric carcinoma, has been discussed previously.

MUSCLE INVOLVEMENT

Although direct extension of malignant tumors of bone to adjacent skeletal muscle commonly is encountered, especially in the chest wall and paravertebral locations, hematogenous metastatic foci in the skeletal muscle in either appendicular or axial sites are reported to be rare. As skel-

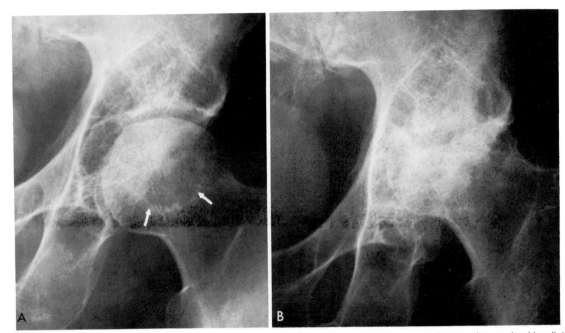

FIGURE 85–62. Irradiation effect. This 57 year old man with metastatic disease to the ilium from an unknown site received irradiation to the left hemipelvis.
  A Approximately 1½ years following irradiation, osteonecrosis of the femoral head (arrows) and local osteoporosis are evident.
  B Eighteen months after the radiograph in **A,** the collapse of the femoral head has progressed.

etal muscle represents tissue that is rich in vasculature, factors other than blood supply must be important in explaining the rarity of metastatic tumors in skeletal muscle. Such factors may include enzyme inhibitors, the acidic environment, or muscle contractions that may dislodge tumor cells.[414, 415] Furthermore, although skeletal muscle has an extensive vascular supply, the flow is extremely variable, increasing during physical exercise, and is under the influence of beta-adrenergic receptors.[364]

Primary tumors leading to skeletal muscle metastasis arise most frequently in the lung, colon, and pancreas,[364, 416] although other malignant tumors, including those in the breast[416] and kidney,[417] as well as many additional sites, and leukemia and lymphoma can lead to such metastasis.[418, 419] Although other foci of metastasis usually are apparent, skeletal muscle involvement may be the initial manifestation of a distant tumor.[363, 364, 416] Pain, tenderness, and a nodular mass may be evident; however, such involvement can remain asymptomatic. Indeed, at autopsy, metastatic foci in skeletal muscle may be apparent only microscopically. In

one autopsy study, 16 per cent of patients with a known carcinoma had histologically detectable metastases in skeletal muscle.[420]

Routine radiography generally does not contribute to the diagnosis of such metastasis. CT, ultrasonography, and MR imaging represent more effective diagnostic tools (Figs. 85–63 and 85–64).[363, 364] Bone scintigraphy also may be used.[416] Although abnormalities may be detected in any muscle, those of the pelvis, particularly the psoas muscle, are affected most commonly,[363] and multiple sites may be involved simultaneously.

RADIOGRAPHIC MONITORING OF TUMOR RESPONSE TO TREATMENT

The routine radiographic appearance of skeletal metastases encountered during the course of tumor therapy depends on a number of factors, including the effectiveness of the therapeutic regimen, the type of neoplasm, and the pattern of osseous abnormality that was present prior to the

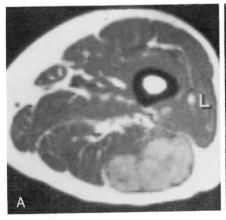
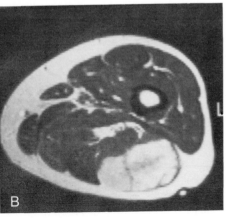

FIGURE 85–63. Muscle metastasis: Renal cell carcinoma. Transverse T1-weighted (TR/TE, 500/15) **(A)** and T2-weighted (TR/TE, 2000/60) **(B)** spin echo MR images reveal a metastatic focus infiltrating the biceps femoris muscle. The signal intensity of the tumor is slightly higher than muscle in **A** and increases in **B.** (Courtesy of J. Robbins, M.D., San Diego, California.)

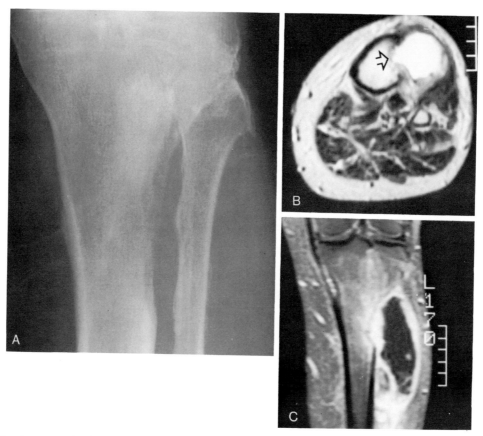

FIGURE 85–64. Muscle metastasis: Carcinoma of the prostate.

A A routine radiograph reveals irregular destruction of the proximal tibia with an adjacent, poorly seen soft tissue mass.

B A transaxial fast spin echo MR image (TR/TE, 3600/102) reveals the mass, of high signal intensity, occupying the tibialis anterior and extensor hallucis longus muscles and invading the tibia (arrow).

C A coronal T1-weighted (TR/TE, 500/12) spin echo MR image, obtained with fat suppression (ChemSat) after the intravenous administration of a gadolinium compound, shows enhancement of the periphery of the necrotic tumor, tibial invasion, and adjacent bone marrow edema.

initiation of the treatment program. When combined with the results of clinical, biochemical, and other imaging examinations, this appearance provides useful information that aids in the care of the cancer patient.[329]

As indicated in a number of reports,[260–263] the initial manifestation of a healing response of a purely osteolytic lesion to chemotherapy or radiation therapy is the development of a faint sclerotic rim in its periphery. Continued healing is manifested as progressive bone sclerosis proceeding from the outside of the lesion toward its center, the conversion of the osteolytic focus to one that is uniformly or predominantly osteosclerotic, and the eventual shrinkage and disappearance of the osteosclerotic area.[260] In some instances, a successful response to therapy is manifested as sclerotic zones in regions of the bones that initially were radiographically normal, apparently owing to the presence of prexisting osteolytic destruction that was not detected on the roentgenograms. Furthermore, in some instances, healing of an osteolytic lesion is accompanied by progressive ossification at its periphery, leading to a well-defined and sometimes expanded appearance (Fig. 85–65). Signs of disease progression are an increase in the size of the osteolytic area, the development of new zones of osteolysis, or progressive osteolytic destruction in an osseous lesion that was responding to the therapy in a normal fashion.[261]

With regard to a mixed osteolytic-osteosclerotic lesion, a successful response to chemotherapy or radiation therapy is its gradual conversion to a uniformly sclerotic area. Subsequent stages of the healing process are identical to those of purely osteolytic lesions. Radiographic signs of tumor progression include increasing osteolysis in sclerotic portions of the lesion and an increase in the overall size of the metastatic focus; the appearance of new mixed osteolytic-osteosclerotic lesions in the follow-up period is not prognostically helpful as this finding can indicate either tumor progression (with the development of additional skeletal metastases) or tumor response to therapy (with the identification of a sclerotic zone about a previously undetected lesion).[261]

It is the response to therapy of a purely osteosclerotic lesion that is most complex and difficult to analyze. In general, a decrease in size or complete disappearance of an osteoblastic focus is a favorable prognostic sign (Fig. 85–66), whereas increasing size of the osteosclerotic lesion and the development of osseous destruction within an osteosclerotic area are signs of tumor progression.[260, 261, 330] The differentiation between osteolytic conversion of an osteosclerotic area (a sign of tumor progression) and fading of an osteosclerotic lesion (a sign of tumor response) is difficult.[264, 265] Furthermore, although an increase in the

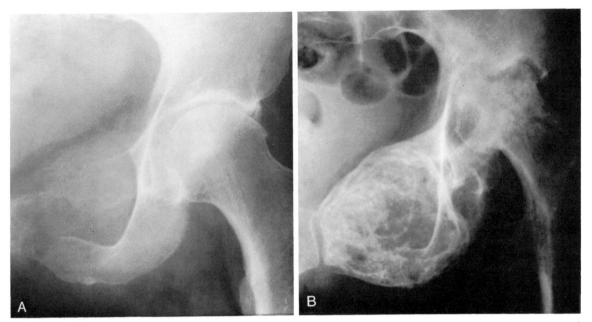

FIGURE 85–65. Osteolytic metastasis: Healing with irradiation effect. This 55 year old woman received radiation therapy for an endometrial carcinoma.

A Prior to therapy, osteolytic destruction of the pubic rami and a soft tissue mass are apparent. Minor changes of osteoarthritis are present in the left hip.

B Thirty months after completion of therapy, mature ossification is indicative of lesional healing. Note the irradiation effects about the left hip.

(Courtesy of H. Kroon, M.D., Leiden, The Netherlands.)

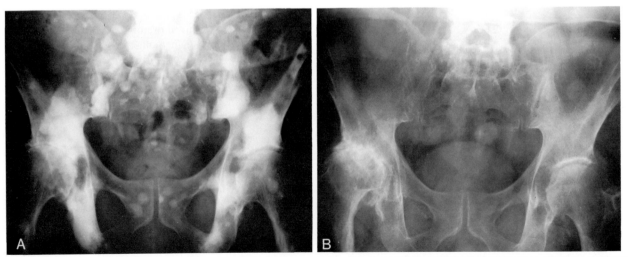

FIGURE 85–66. Osteosclerotic metastasis: Healing with chemotherapy. In this 67 year old patient with metastatic disease related to carcinoma of the prostate, an initial radiograph **(A)** obtained prior to chemotherapy and orchiectomy shows osteoblastic metastases. Thirty-two months after chemotherapy and orchiectomy **(B)**, dramatic improvement is apparent. Note the progression of osteoarthritis in the right hip.

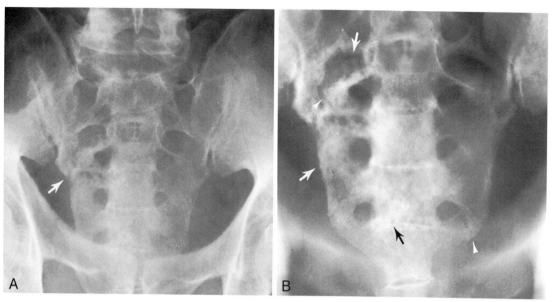

FIGURE 85–67. Irradiation effect. This 62 year old man underwent radiation therapy for an adenocarcinoma of the colon. Subsequent changes in the sacrum are consistent with irradiation effect.
  A Observe osteosclerosis involving the right side of the sacrum (arrow).
  B Six months later, more extensive osteosclerosis (arrows) and insufficiency fractures (arrowheads) are apparent. Changes such as these are difficult to distinguish from skeletal metastases.

number of osteoblastic foci usually indicates progression of the disease,[264] it also may signal a healing response of a preexisting lesion that initially was not identified on the roentgenograms. In fact, an osteoblastic reaction as part of a successful response to therapy can lead to a dramatic increase in both the size and the number of radiographically detectable tumor foci, findings that easily are misinterpreted as evidence of disease progression.[266] In some tumors, such as carcinoma of the prostate, osteosclerotic zones remain unchanged rather than decreasing in size during tumor remission.[266] Correlation of the radiographic changes with clinical and laboratory data as well as varying scintigraphic patterns (see later discussion) may allow more accurate interpretation of the patient's true status, although these results, too, are not analyzed without difficulty.[262]

Radiation therapy used in conjunction with skeletal metastasis, in itself, is associated with a number of osseous alterations that are discussed in Chapter 73. Such changes, which include osteopenia, coarsening of the trabecular pattern, insufficiency fractures, ischemic necrosis of bone, and secondary neoplasia, further complicate the accurate radiographic appraisal of the metastatic process (Fig. 85–67).

OTHER DIAGNOSTIC TECHNIQUES

It is beyond the scope of this chapter to consider in great detail the role of each of the diagnostic techniques used in the evaluation of skeletal metastasis; some of this information is available in other portions of this textbook (see Chapters 8, 10, 12, 15, and 16) and additional sources.[2, 3] An overview of the imaging approach to the detection of skeletal metastases and to the analysis of their response to therapy, as well as certain limitations of the diagnostic techniques, is provided here.

Conventional Radiographic Survey

The "metastatic bone survey" had long been a standard part of the radiographic protocols employed by most x-ray departments and still is in widespread use today, although the indications for this examination and the manner in which it is obtained have undergone modifications in recent years. This survey originally was designed to detect, with a limited number of radiologic projections, the majority of metastatic foci in the skeleton. Owing to the propensity of such lesions to be located in the axial skeleton, the typical survey consisted of films of the spine, skull, pelvis, thorax, and proximal tubular bones (femora and humeri). In certain situations, this imaging strategy still is required and can be fulfilled with the following series of roentgenograms: anteroposterior projection of the pelvis; anteroposterior and lateral projections of the thoracic spine and the lumbar spine; a lateral projection of the cervical spine; a lateral projection of the skull; an anteroposterior projection of the thorax; and an anteroposterior (and sometimes lateral) projection of each femur and humerus. Although the indications for this radiographic survey as an initial part of the patient's assessment vary from one institution to another, and its benefit relative to those of scintigraphy and MR imaging is a subject on which there is no uniform agreement (with opinions ranging from the extremes of using it as a standard method to its complete replacement by one or both of these other methods),[267] there exists a general consensus that, when used, the radiographic survey examination should be performed in conjunction with bone scintigraphy and that the latter examination is more appropriately obtained first so that its results can serve as a guide to the specific roentgenographic projections that are obtained subsequently. In certain tumors, such as carcinomas of the prostate, lung, and breast and lymphomas, scintigraphy

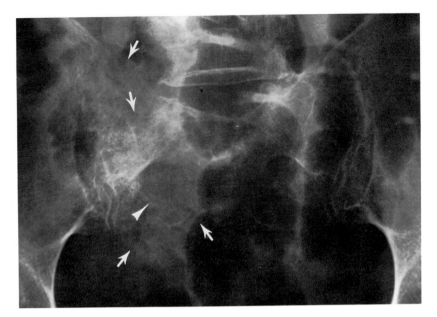

FIGURE 85–68. Skeletal metastasis: Conventional radiographic survey—problem area. Large lesions of the sacrum (arrows) easily are obscured by overlying structures. Distortion of the pelvic sacral foramina (arrowhead) is an important radiographic sign. Compare to the opposite (normal) side.

using bone-seeking radiopharmaceutical agents is a consistently sensitive means of detecting osseous sites of involvement; radiographic surveys of bones in these cases can be reasonably confined to areas of scintigraphic abnormality or, perhaps, to the pelvis when the bone scan is normal, in recognition of potential obscuration of a lesion in this region due to radionuclide activity in the bladder.[53] In other tumors in which results of bone scans are less uniform, a standard skeletal survey supplemented with radiographs of scintigraphically abnormal areas is useful. The insensitivity of the roentgenograms in the early detection of osseous destruction cannot be denied, and careful and thorough analysis of the radiographs is fundamental to the recognition of those lesions that are detectable. Although diagnostic difficulties can be encountered during the interpretation of radiographs of any skeletal site, typical problem areas include the following: lesions of the pelvic bones and sacrum that are partially obscured by adjacent soft tissues[322] (Fig. 85–68); regions of rib destruction that are poorly visualized owing to technical inadequacies or overlying osseous and soft tissue shadows; sternal lesions that are barely seen because of the difficulty of visualizing this bone adequately on the standard survey radiograph; the differentiation of a vertebral body that is collapsed because of metastatic disease from one whose deformity is related to osteoporosis or trauma; and erosion of the endosteal margin of the cortex as a response to a tumor in the medullary canal of a tubular bone that is misinterpreted as normal cortical scalloping.

The use of MR imaging as a substitute for survey radiographs also could be considered (see later discussion). The value of MR imaging, however, lies not in its application to the analysis of the entire skeleton but rather in its sensitivity and specificity when applied to a portion of the skeleton.[424] In this regard, it is far more practical to study selected skeletal regions such as the spine or pelvis using MR imaging when results of routine radiographic or scintigraphic analysis are not clear. In general, MR imaging has equal or greater sensitivity to the detection of osseous metastases than bone scintigraphy and has greater specificity.

Owing to the fact that radiographic manifestations of progression or healing of sites of skeletal metastasis are fairly constant from one region of the body to another, an abbreviated or shortened version of the survey examination may suffice when monitoring the tumor's response to therapy.[421] In patients having widespread skeletal involvement, radiographs of the pelvis, the spine, or both regions, may provide all necessary information and can be used effectively as a substitute for the more technically difficult, time-consuming and expensive "metastatic bone survey."

Scintigraphy

The sensitivity of the bone scan in detecting skeletal metastases (as well as other osseous lesions) can be attributed to its dependence on changes in regional blood flow and bone turnover that, even when of minor degree, ensure the delivery of an abnormal amount of the radiotracer to and its incorporation into sites of abnormality. Within minutes following the intravenous injection of a bolus of the bone-seeking radioisotope, the tracer diffuses through capillary pores at the edge of the tumor; subsequently, the radiopharmaceutical agent is selectively concentrated in the reactive new bone that accompanies the neoplasm.[268] These immediate and later scintigraphic patterns can be detected when three-phase bone scanning is employed,[269] a technique that has been used more extensively for infectious lesions of the skeleton; interpretation of the delayed static images is the general standard in the analysis of metastatic disease. On such images, the classic (although not invariable) finding of skeletal metastasis is a focus (or foci) of increased accumulation of the radionuclide ("hot" spot) (Fig. 85–69). Modifications in the abnormalities of a positive bone scan include an area of diminished uptake of the radiotracer ("cold" spot)—a phenomenon related primarily to the absence of blood perfusion to a localized region of bone (which is present in many different disease processes, including infection, ischemic necrosis, and radiation changes),[270–272] as well as to complete destruction of bone[273]; and an increased accumulation of the radiophar-

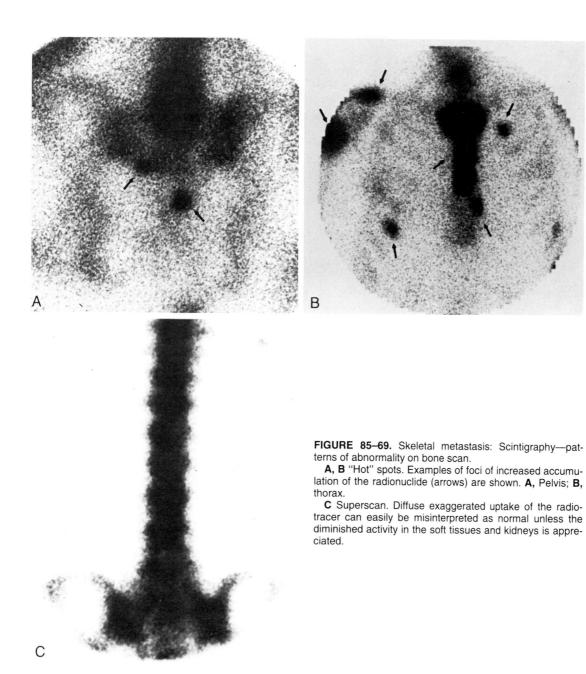

FIGURE 85–69. Skeletal metastasis: Scintigraphy—patterns of abnormality on bone scan.

A, B "Hot" spots. Examples of foci of increased accumulation of the radionuclide (arrows) are shown. **A,** Pelvis; **B,** thorax.

C Superscan. Diffuse exaggerated uptake of the radiotracer can easily be misinterpreted as normal unless the diminished activity in the soft tissues and kidneys is appreciated.

maceutical agent diffusely throughout the skeleton ("super-scan") (Fig. 85–69)—a phenomenon most frequent in cases of carcinoma of the prostate, in which the scintigraphic pattern easily is misinterpreted as normal unless the absence of renal uptake, the presence of diminished activity in the bones of the appendicular skeleton, and a high ratio of bone to soft tissue activity are recognized.[274–276, 331] A modification of the "superscan" pattern in which only the skull shows no evidence of increased radionuclide uptake, designated the "headless" bone scan, also suggests the diagnosis of skeletal metastasis derived from prostate carcinoma.[423]

Falsely negative bone scans are encountered, especially in certain situations. Any neoplasm that is unaccompanied by ongoing new bone formation may lead to a "cold" region on the bone scan (if there is a great deal of bone destruction) or to an apparently normal examination; this situation is encountered most commonly in plasma cell myeloma, leukemia, and highly aggressive anaplastic carcinomas. Furthermore, a poor host response in debilitated persons or in those who have undergone radiation therapy also accounts for falsely negative results in cases of skeletal metastasis.

Falsely positive bone scans reflect the nonspecific nature of the scintigraphic examination; a great number of skeletal disorders lead to an increase in accumulation of the radiotracer, mandating close radiographic-scintigraphic correlation. In those patients with a primary malignant tumor in whom a positive bone scan is combined with a negative radiographic examination, a diagnostic dilemma arises in which the cause of the scintigraphic abnormality must be ascertained by other means.[277, 340] Indirect signs of skeletal metastases in these persons are provided by clinical and laboratory manifestations that may include local pain and tenderness and changes in serum chemistry values; more direct evidence can be obtained with MR imaging and bone biopsy techniques (see later discussion).

The limitations in the specificity of the bone scan must be recognized by all physicians who would interpret its results. A reliance on the radionuclide study itself, in the belief that a particular scintigraphic pattern is diagnostic of skeletal metastasis and does not require radiographic correlation, will result in errors in diagnosis in many patients. The presence of multiple and widespread focal areas of increased accumulation of the radionuclide on the bone scan in a patient with a known primary malignant tumor is a pattern most suggestive of metastases, but it is one that occasionally is simulated by other conditions. The identification of a superscan in a patient with prostatic carcinoma is not entirely pathognomonic for skeletal metatastases, as a similar pattern may accompany hyperparathyroidism, osteomalacia, mastocytosis, and myelofibrosis.[276, 278–280] The accumulation of a bone-seeking radionuclide in the ribs of a patient with carcinoma of the breast immediately suggests skeletal metastasis, although increased radioisotopic uptake may be observed as a normal finding[332] or following a mastectomy in the ribs on the same side as the surgery.[281] Furthermore, nonpathologic rib fractures are frequent and may produce scintigraphic findings resembling those of metastatic disease; although criteria have been proposed to differentiate such fractures from foci of metastasis on the basis of the radionuclide study (a focal as opposed to a

linear pattern of activity, the involvement of two or more ribs in the same location, and a decrease in activity on serial examinations each suggest fracture),[282] correlative radiographs are required. As a general rule, solitary lesions of the ribs detected scintigraphically in patients with known primary malignant tumors most frequently are benign in causation and do not represent sites of skeletal metastases.[422] Indeed, even two areas of increased radionuclide uptake in the ribs or, for that matter, any skeletal site with the exception of the sternum, commonly denotes a non-malignant process in patients with cancer[425]; however, most sternal lesions are metastases in such patients,[426, 427] particularly those with carcinoma of the breast.

The sequential evaluation of patients with skeletal metastasis who are receiving chemotherapy or radiation therapy has been accomplished with bone scintigraphy, although, as in the case of conventional radiography, difficulties in interpretation of the results arise.[261, 262, 283–289] The beliefs that decreasing accumulation of a bone-seeking radionuclide implies tumor healing and that increasing accumulation of this radiotracer suggests tumor progression are both inaccurate. The degree of accumulation of the radiopharmaceutical agent is related to the amount of active bone reaction or deposition that is occurring at any given moment. Aggressive behavior of a metastatic focus in the skeleton is accompanied by increasing bone destruction, which may be associated with little or no bone formation; the radionuclide manifestation of such tumor progression is a decrease in activity of the lesion on the bone scan. As an extreme example of this paradox between tumor behavior and scintigraphic abnormality, a rapidly enlarging osteolytic lesion that completely destroys the adjacent osseous tissue and, with it, the ability to produce new bone is manifested on serial bone scans as a conversion of a "hot" lesion to one that may be entirely "cold." Conversely, an increase in the amount of accumulation of the bone-seeking radionuclide in a lesion, particularly during the early stages of therapy, may indicate tumor healing due to the presence of the "flare" phenomenon. Although infrequent, this phenomenon has been observed in 10 to 15 per cent of patients undergoing treatment for carcinoma of the breast[289, 290] and in 6 to 23 per cent of those receiving therapy for prostatic carcinoma.[285, 291] It relates either to an increase in regional blood flow or to an accentuation of bone turnover, or both, at the site of metastasis. Fortunately, the more typical healing response of such metastases as observed on serial bone scans is a decrease in radionuclide accumulation, a finding that is extremely useful in the evaluation of patients with carcinoma of the prostate in whom an increase in radiodensity about an osseous lesion or lesions on radiographs is easily misinterpreted as evidence of tumor progression.[283] It has been suggested that the discovery of new lesions on serial bone scintigraphy is a more reliable sign of tumor progression than is an increase in radionuclide uptake at the site of old lesions,[286] although this rule, too, is not without exception. A "flare" response may result in the appearance of apparently new foci of skeletal metastasis during the first months of therapy when, in fact, what has occurred is an osteoblastic reaction at involved sites not detected on the initial scans.[287]

Although quantitative analysis of serial bone scans may increase the accuracy of interpretation,[262, 284, 288] the results of the examinations should always be correlated with clinical and laboratory parameters as well as with changing radiographic patterns of disease.

Computed Tomography

In a summary of the role of CT in the evaluation of patients with suspected or proved skeletal metastases, several aspects deserve emphasis. This technique may be used to further delineate the nature of a scintigraphically positive osseous region in such patients (Fig. 85–70), especially if radiographs fail to document the existence of a metastatic focus.[430] In persons with known cancer, 50 per cent or fewer solitary lesions on bone scan relate to skeletal metastasis[277, 292]; however, following radiography, further analysis of these lesions is best accomplished with CT,

especially if a bone biopsy is being considered.[293, 294] Information provided by CT in these circumstances may alter the presumed diagnosis of metastatic disease and influence the decision regarding the need for bone biopsy. Furthermore, CT monitoring of the biopsy procedure itself can be employed.

In the spine, CT appears to be more sensitive than conventional radiography in the detection of metastatic lesions,[295, 296, 428] and it also may be more specific, documenting findings characteristic of malignant neoplasm, including pediculate destruction, multiple osteolytic foci in the vertebral body, and paravertebral masses with adjacent bone erosion,[293] or, alternately, abnormalities indicative of a nonneoplastic process.

In the tubular bones of the appendicular skeleton, CT allows detection of subtle changes in the attenuation co-

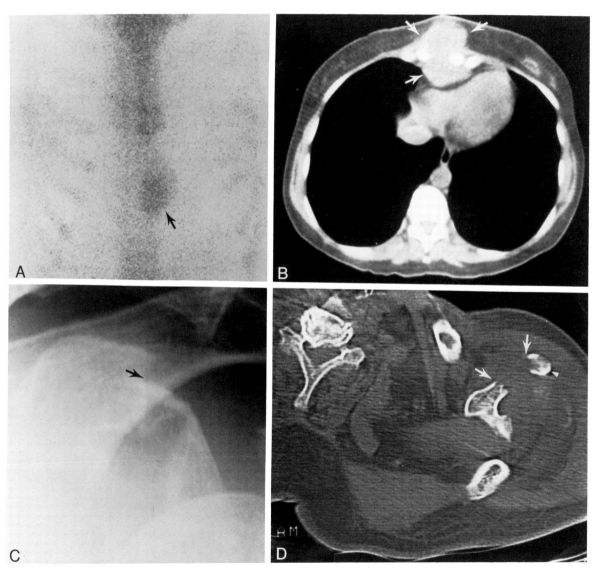

FIGURE 85–70. Skeletal metastasis: CT.

 A, B In a woman with carcinoma of the breast, abnormal accumulation (arrow) of a bone-seeking radionuclide **(A)** confirmed a subxiphoid lesion (which was not detected on conventional radiographs). A transaxial CT scan **(B)** in this area better delineates the lesion and the accompanying soft tissue mass (arrows).

 C, D A metastatic lesion in the scapula, arising from carcinoma of the lung, is poorly seen with conventional radiography **(C)**, although the tip of the coracoid process is amputated (arrow). The bone scan was abnormal, and a transaxial CT image **(D)** reveals a large osteolytic lesion of the coracoid process (arrows) leading to isolation of its tip (arrowhead).

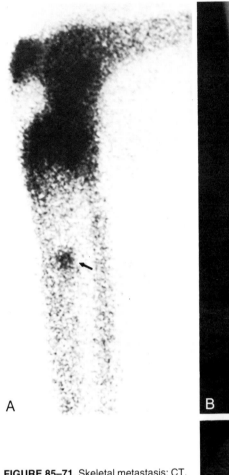

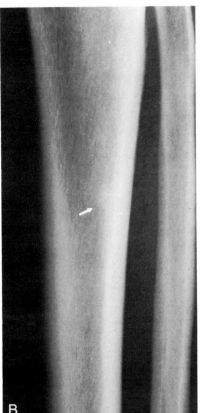

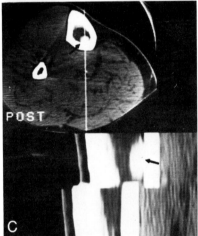

FIGURE 85–71. Skeletal metastasis: CT. As part of the evaluation of carcinoma of the prostate, a bone scan was obtained.

A An area of increased accumulation of the radionuclide in the tibia (arrow) is seen on this lateral image.

B A corresponding radiograph shows an osteosclerotic lesion in the tibia (arrow).

C A transaxial CT scan (above) with sagittal reformation of the image (below) documents the presence of a metastatic lesion (arrows).

efficient of the marrow that may indicate tumor infiltration[297, 298] (a finding also evident in infection) or, more specifically, tumorous marrow deposits not apparent on conventional radiographs (Fig. 85–71). Certain limitations in the interpretation of the attenuation values of the medullary cavity should be recognized: symmetric positioning of the limbs in the gantry of the CT scanner is required if comparison of values for the two sides is attempted; and incidental bone irregularities and ridges arising from the endosteal margin of the cortex can simulate metastatic processes. It has been suggested that a difference in CT numbers of greater than 20 Hounsfield units derived from the medullary canals of the paired bones is abnormal,[298] although the finding is not specific for metastasis. Furthermore, following radiation therapy or chemotherapy, tumor necrosis

may lead to a similar increase in marrow attenuation values.[297] This increase may not be apparent, however, until months after the radiotherapy has been completed. Indeed, some data do support the value of quantitative CT as a method for assessing the response of osteolytic metastatic lesions of the spine to radiotherapy; an initial decrease in bone density following such therapy may represent a favorable therapeutic sign.[429]

CT represents an excellent means of defining the extent of any metastatic lesion, especially those located at sites, such as the vertebral column and pelvis, that are difficult to evaluate with conventional imaging techniques. Paravertebral and intraspinal extension, transarticular spread, and soft tissue involvement with violation of neurovascular structures are examples of information that can be derived from the CT display. In certain locations, such as the bones of the thorax, the results of CT in cases of tumor metastasis or extension are less dramatic.[299]

Magnetic Resonance Imaging

Metastases, in common with lymphoma, leukemia, primary bone tumors and a variety of non-neoplastic conditions, lead to infiltration or replacement of normal marrow. It is this change in marrow constituency that is fundamental to the sensitivity of MR imaging in the detection of sites of skeletal metastasis. Identification of such sites using this technique requires the observer to recognize normal age-related marrow changes, particularly in regions such as the spine and pelvis[433, 434] that commonly are involved in the metastatic process. As discussed in detail elsewhere in this book, these changes relate to a predictable and orderly pattern of conversion of red to yellow marrow that occurs during growth and development.[435] Marrow conversion usually is complete with the establishment of an adult pattern by the time a person is 25 years of age. At this time, red marrow is concentrated predominantly in the axial skeleton (skull, vertebrae, ribs, sternum, and pelvis) and to a lesser degree in the proximal portions of the appendicular skeleton (proximal femora and humeri).[435] Although normal variations in the distribution of the two types of marrow are encountered and minor changes and fluctuations in this distribution take place throughout life and as a response to bodily demands, MR imaging can be employed effectively in the detection of disease processes, including metastasis, that modify marrow composition.

MR imaging has been used most extensively in the evaluation of metastasis in the vertebral column, for which it competes favorably with other techniques such as CT[300] and myelography.[436] Its advantages include superior demonstration of paravertebral tumor extension, identification of additional sites of osseous metastasis, and visualization of areas of spinal cord compression occurring between regions of myelographic blocks.[436, 437, 439] Furthermore, when compared with myelography, even when myelography is combined with CT, MR imaging has proven more sensitive, particularly with regard to the detection of extradural masses that do not lead to cord compression.[438, 440] Compar-

ison studies with bone scintigraphy have indicated superior sensitivity of MR imaging in cases of focal[424] or diffuse[441] spinal metastasis. MR imaging can provide further diagnostic information regarding spinal (or extraspinal) sites that are scintigraphically positive[442] as well as those that are normal on bone scans[443]; however, as a screening test for evaluating the entire skeleton, bone scintigraphy is more useful.[424]

The specific abnormalities seen on MR imaging related to spinal (and extraspinal) metastatic foci are dependent, foremost, upon the particular imaging parameters employed. Most investigations of spinal metastases have used standard spin echo sequences, relying predominantly on sagittal and transaxial MR images. On T1-weighted images, intravertebral lesions are of low signal intensity (Fig. 85–72), and these images are useful in demonstrating spinal cord compressions.[436] The signal characteristics of intravertebral lesions are more variable on T2-weighted spin echo MR images, although an increase in signal intensity is most characteristic. In some reports, the T2-weighted images have been judged superior to the T1-weighted images in showing extension of the tumor into the subarachnoid space in the absence of cord compression.[436] The appearance of spinal metastases on gradient echo sequences is influenced by the specific choice of imaging parameters (repetition time, echo time, flip angle); on those sequences emphasizing proton density or T2* weighting, high signal intensity of metastatic foci may be observed,[441] although gradient echo sequences are not optimal for demonstrating abnormalities of the bone marrow (Fig. 85–73).

It is important to recognize some diagnostic difficulties that may arise when standard spin echo sequences are employed to assess metastatic foci within the vertebral bodies. In adult patients, normal bone marrow in the spine contains significant fat. Therefore, tumorous foci with their high water content generally are conspicuous on the T1-weighted images; on T2-weighted images as well as on proton density images, however, this conspicuity may not be as apparent and, in some instances, the metastatic lesions become isointense with the bone marrow. In elderly patients whose marrow may appear heterogeneous in composition and in patients with chronic anemia in whom increased iron storage in the marrow results in decreased

FIGURE 85–72. Skeletal metastasis: MR imaging. Standard spin echo technique. Sagittal T1-weighted (TR/TE, 600/20) **(A)** and T2-weighted (TR/TE, 2000/80) **(B)** images reveal tumorous replacement of the fifth lumbar vertebral body (arrows) related to metastasis from an adenocarcinoma of the breast. A prominent epidural mass also is evident (arrowheads).

(Courtesy of M. Solomon, M.D., San Jose, California.)

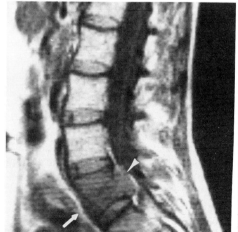

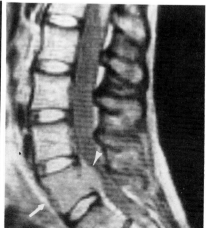

A

B

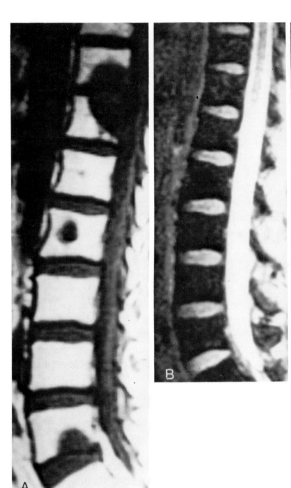
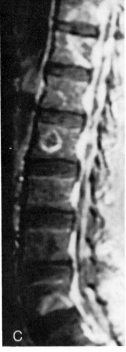

FIGURE 85–73. Skeletal metastasis: MR imaging. Insensitivity of gradient echo technique. This 47 year old woman with carcinoma of the breast developed osteosclerotic spinal metastases.

A On a sagittal T1-weighted (TR/TE, 416/11) spin echo MR image, the metastatic lesions are prominent and of low signal intensity.

B A sagittal multiplanar gradient recalled (MPGR) MR image (TR/TE, 400/15; flip angle: 15 degrees) fails to reveal the lesions.

C A sagittal T1-weighted (TR/TE, 650/11) spin echo MR image obtained with fat suppression (ChemSat) after the intravenous injection of a gadolinium compound shows enhancement of signal intensity at the periphery of the lesions.

marrow signal intensity on all spin echo sequences, variations in lesion conspicuity will be evident.[440] Furthermore, the richly hematopoietic bone marrow of the child's spine reveals low signal intensity on the T1-weighted images; metastatic foci may be difficult to detect when such images are used alone. This is particularly true in instances of diffuse spinal (and extraspinal) metastases in which homogeneous low signal intensity of the tumorous bone marrow on the T1-weighted images may simulate that of normal hematopoietic marrow. With T2-weighting, however, hyperintensity of the abnormal marrow becomes evident, a finding designated the flip-flop sign,[444] allowing accurate diagnosis (Fig. 85–74).

There has been considerable interest in the use of intravenous gadolinium administration to assess vertebral metastasis with or without extension into the epidural space.[445, 446] In general, the pattern and extent of tumor enhancement after such administration are variable; some metastatic lesions enhance markedly, others slightly, and still others not at all (Fig. 85–75).[440] Furthermore, enhancement may be homogeneous, initially peripheral with subsequent central spread, or random. In patients with multiple lesions, the pattern of enhancement may vary from one lesion to another.[440] Diagnostic difficulty may arise when T1-weighted gadolinium-enhanced MR images are used alone; metastatic lesions in the vertebral bone marrow may enhance so that their signal intensity may be similar to or identical with that of the marrow itself, decreasing significantly their conspicuity (Fig. 85–76). Because of this possibility, it is important to obtain precontrast spin echo MR images.[445] Short tau inversion recovery (STIR) sequences also can be used as an adjunct to the unenhanced and gadolinium-enhanced spin echo MR images.[446, 471]

The value of gadolinium-enhanced MR imaging may be increased with the supplementary use of fat-suppression techniques (Fig. 85–76). Fat suppression, when used alone without the intravenous administration of gadolinium, actually may lead to decreased lesion conspicuity on T1-weighted spin echo MR images. The signal intensity derived from the fat in the marrow of the vertebral body is depressed and, in some instances, will be identical to the low signal intensity of the lesion itself. When fat suppression is combined with gadolinium administration, however, the accentuated signal intensity in the metastatic focus is made more obvious owing to the suppression of signal intensity in the surrounding marrow.[440, 472] Fat suppression technique can be used effectively without gadolinium administration in some cases of skeletal metastasis when the method is combined with T2-weighted, rather than T1-weighted, images.[471]

Owing to the inadequacies of routine radiography, and even scintigraphy, in allowing differentiation between nontumorous and tumorous compression fractures of vertebral bodies, the role of MR imaging in this differentiation has

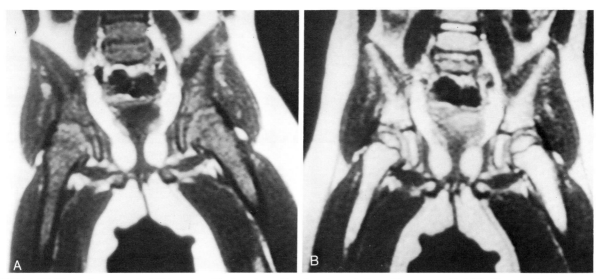

FIGURE 85–74. Skeletal metastasis: MR imaging. Flip-flop sign with spin echo technique. Three year old child with neuroblastoma.

A On this coronal T1-weighted (TR/TE, 500/30) spin echo MR image, diffusely hypointense marrow is seen in the innominate bones and femora. Routine radiographs (not shown) were normal.

B On the T2-weighted (TR/TE, 2000/60) spin echo MR image, hyperintensity of the marrow in these sites is evident.

(From C Ruzal-Shapiro, et al: Radiology *181*:587, 1991.)

been studied.[447, 448] Routine spin echo sequences generally allow discrimination between compression fractures related to skeletal metastasis (or other tumors) and those that are chronic in nature and are related to benign causes such as osteoporosis. Difficulty arises, however, in differentiating with MR imaging between tumorous fractures and those that are benign but more acute. The typical appearance of

chronic nontumorous or benign fractures of the vertebral body on spin echo sequences relates to the presence of signal intensity of the marrow in the affected vertebral body identical to that of the normal vertebrae (Fig. 85–77A,B).[447] Pathologic vertebral fractures caused by metastasis (and other tumors) reveal low signal intensity on T1-weighted images and high signal intensity on T2-weighted images (Fig. 85–77C,D), and similar but less pronounced changes in signal intensity accompany acute (less that 30 days old) benign compression fractures (Fig. 85–77E,F).[447] Chemical shift and STIR sequences can serve as effective supplementary techniques in these situations, as can intravenous gadolinium administration (Fig. 85–78).

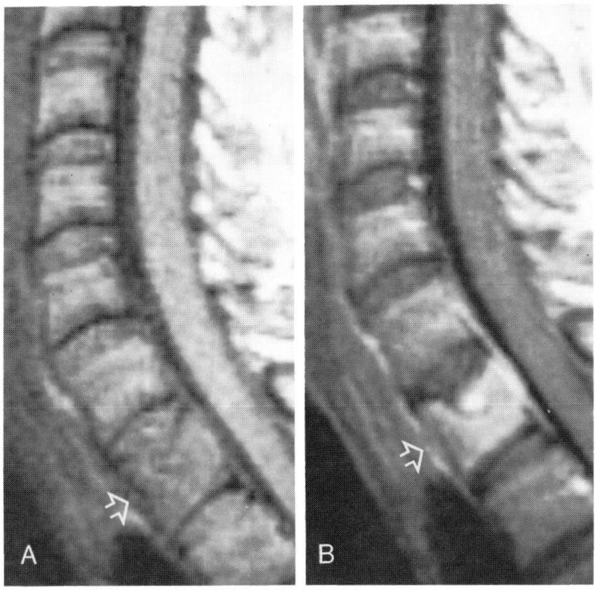

Although the great majority of metastases involving the spinal canal affect the epidural space and usually relate to bone involvement, intradural-extramedullary and intramedullary sites of metastasis also may be encountered. The MR imaging findings in both of these rarer sites have been well summarized by Kamholtz and Sze.[440] With regard to intra-dural-extramedullary metastases, subarachnoid spread of systemic cancer generally occurs late in the course of the disease. Usually such metastasis originates from tumors of the central nervous system, such as medulloblastomas, glioblastomas, ependymomas, and pinealomas (see previous discussion), although extracranial neoplasms, including carcinomas of the lung and breast, melanomas, lymphomas, and leukemias, also can spread into the subarachnoid space.[440] Focal nodular masses or diffuse involvement (i.e., leptomeningeal carcinomatosis) may be evident. Clinical findings may include headache, change of mental status, low back and leg pain, cranial and spinal nerve deficits, and gait disturbances.[344] Lumbar puncture and cytologic evaluation of the cerebrospinal fluid usually are diagnostic. Myelography with or without CT reveals intra-arachnoid nodular filling defects, longitudinal striations, prominent and crowded nerve roots of the cauda equina, and scalloping of the subarachnoid space.[344] Standard MR imaging has been reported to give inconsistent diagnostic results in this clini-

FIGURE 85–75. Skeletal metastasis: MR imaging. Gadolinium enhancement. A 37 year old man with renal cell carcinoma.

A In this unenhanced sagittal T1-weighted (TR/TE, 600/20) spin echo MR image, a metastatic lesion in the first thoracic vertebral body (arrow) appears as a region of low signal intensity, although the finding is subtle.

B Following the intravenous administration of a gadolinium compound, an identical MR image (TR/TE, 600/20) shows increased signal intensity in the involved vertebral body (arrow), increasing its conspicuity.

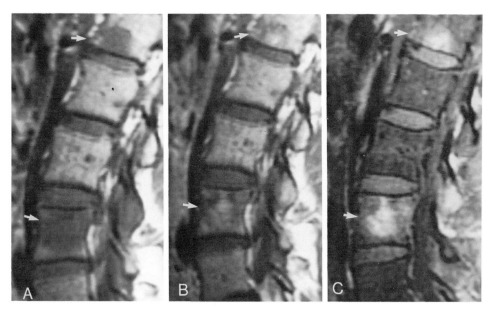

FIGURE 85–76. Skeletal metastasis: MR imaging. Gadolinium enhancement with and without fat suppression. A 31 year old woman with carcinoma of the lung.
A This unenhanced sagittal T1-weighted (TR/TE, 600/20) spin echo MR image shows several metastatic lesions (arrows) in the thoracolumbar spine, each revealing low signal intensity.
B Following the intravenous administration of a gadolinium compound, an identical MR image (TR/TE, 600/20) reveals less obvious metastatic lesions (arrows). Enhancement of signal intensity in the sites of metastasis has made it more difficult to distinguish them from the uninvolved bone marrow.
C With the combination of gadolinium enhancement and fat suppression (ChemSat), the metastatic foci (arrows) are readily apparent as regions of high signal intensity on this T1-weighted spin echo MR image (TR/TE, 600/20).

cal setting owing to poor contrast between the tumor and surrounding cerebrospinal fluid, the absence of surrounding edema, and technical difficulties related, in part, to the presence of pulsations of the cerebrospinal fluid that lead to motion artifact.[344, 440, 449] The supplementary use of gadolinium, delivered intravenously, can provide important diagnostic information (Figs. 85–79 and 85–80).[440, 450–452] T1-weighted MR images obtained after gadolinium administration show tumor enhancement, and the tumor, with its high signal intensity, becomes conspicuous owing to the low signal intensity of the cerebrospinal fluid. Nodular or diffuse tumor infiltration can be diagnosed in this fashion. In some reports, differences in enhancement patterns have been noted with regard to dural and leptomeningeal metastasis (Fig. 85–81).[453, 454]

Intramedullary metastases, although rare, may arise from malignant tumors of the central nervous system or from systemic cancers, particularly carcinomas of the lung (i.e., small cell carcinomas) and breast but also melanomas, lymphomas, leukemias, and carcinomas of the colon, rectum, and head and neck.[343] With regard to systemic tumors, intramedullary metastasis occurs most commonly in the thoracic cord, followed in frequency by the cervical cord,[455] although multiple segments of the cord may be affected simultaneously.[343] Pathologic findings include an enlarged and firm spinal cord with microscopic evidence of tumor infiltration, infarction, and necrosis.[455] Associated leptomeningeal and intradural involvement may be found.[343]

The mechanism of spread of tumor to the spinal cord varies according to whether the tumor originates in the central nervous system or outside it. Central nervous system tumors commonly spread into the cerebrospinal fluid path-

ways, and resulting leptomeningeal involvememt may lead to direct invasion of the spinal cord, with multiple dorsal nodular implants of varying size on the spinal cord and nerve roots and thickened leptomeninges. Non-neurogenic tumors are believed to reach the spinal cord through hematogenous arterial dissemination of tumor emboli or, less often, through dissemination of tumor via the vertebral venous plexus or direct extension from the nerve roots and cerebrospinal fluid.[343] Single tumors causing fusiform expansion of the cord are the typical manifestation of metastatic foci of such non-neurogenic neoplasms.

Clinical manifestations associated with metastasis to the spinal cord are variable, although they typically are of short duration and include pain, weakness, sensory loss, and bladder and bowel dysfunction.[343] Myelography may reveal intramedullary mass lesions with or without obstruction to the flow of contrast material or more subtle lobular excrescences protruding eccentrically from the widened spinal cord.[343] CT may show increased attenuation values in affected regions of the spinal cord, findings that may be more apparent when intravenous contrast-enhanced techniques are employed. MR imaging allows evaluation of the entire cord, and with routine methods, the tumor appears hypointense on T1-weighted images and hyperintense on T2-weighted images.[440] As edema of the spinal cord is an associated finding, unenhanced MR scans may not allow clear separation of tumor and edema. After the intravenous administration of gadolinium, however, MR imaging shows enhancing tumor nodules, often much smaller than the area of cord enlargement, that can be distinguished from surrounding edema.[440, 456] Although tumor enhancement generally is adequate on MR images obtained immediately

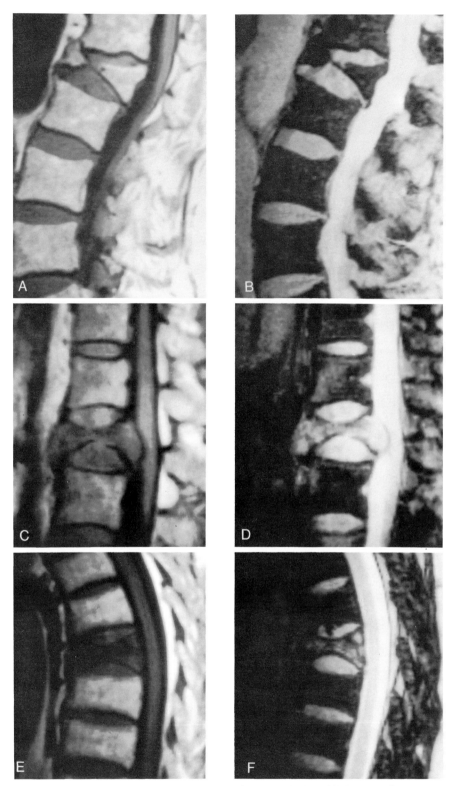

FIGURE 85–77. Nontumorous versus tumorous compression fractures of vertebral bodies: MR imaging. Spin echo and multiplanar gradient recalled (MPGR) techniques.

A, B Chronic nontumorous compression fracture. Sagittal T1-weighted (TR/TE, 800/20) **(A)** and MPGR (TR/TE, 400/15; flip angle, 15 degrees) **(B)** MR images. The signal intensity in the marrow of the collapsed vertebral body is identical to that in the uninvolved vertebral bodies.

C, D Tumorous compression fracture (carcinoma of the breast). Identical T1-weighted **(C)** and MPGR **(D)** MR images. Note the abnormally low signal intensity in the involved vertebral body in **C** and the abnormally high signal intensity in this vertebral body in **D**. Compression of the spinal cord is evident.

E, F Acute nontumorous compression fracture. Identical T1-weighted **(E)** and MPGR **(F)** MR images. Low signal intensity in the collapsed vertebral body in **E** and high signal intensity in this vertebral body in **F** are evident.

(Courtesy of L. L. Baker, M.D., La Jolla, California.)

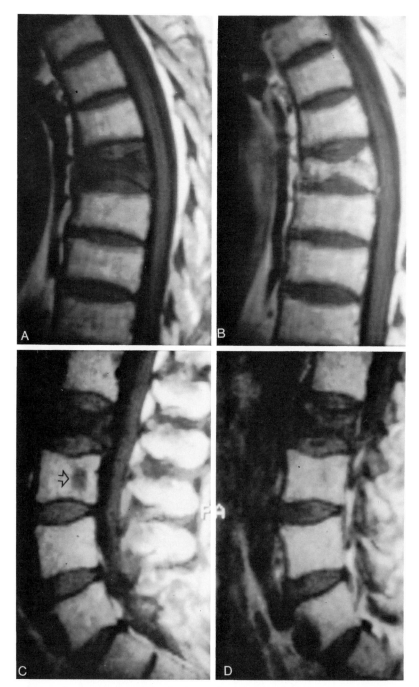

FIGURE 85–78. Nontumorous versus tumorous compression fractures of vertebral bodies: MR imaging. Spin echo technique with and without gadolinium enhancement.

A, B Acute nontumorous compression fracture. Sagittal T1-weighted (TR/TE, 800/20) spin echo MR images before **(A)** and after **(B)** intravenous administration of a gadolinium compound. Note diffuse enhancement of signal intensity in the collapsed vertebral body in **B.**

C, D Tumorous compression fracture (carcinoma of the breast). Identical nonenhanced **(C)** and enhanced **(D)** T1-weighted (TR/TE, 800/20) spin echo MR images to those in **A** and **B.** In **C,** observe low signal intensity in the collapsed vertebral body and in another metastatic lesion (arrow). In **D,** slight enhancement of signal intensity in the collapsed vertebral body has occurred. Owing to enhancement of signal intensity, the other metastatic lesion is less conspicuous.

(Courtesy of L. L. Baker, M.D., La Jolla, California.)

after gadolinium injection, tumors with extensive necrosis may demonstrate marked delayed enhancement.[457]

Although less attention has been given to the MR findings in cases of extraspinal metastatic disease, the general imaging concepts remain the same (Fig. 85–82). The need for gadolinium-enhanced and fat-suppressed techniques is influenced by the signal intensity characteristics of the marrow in the specific skeletal site being evaluated. Fat suppression, when combined with intravenous administration of gadolinium, is more advantageous when portions of the skeleton, such as the appendicular regions, that contain abundant fatty marrow are being assessed. In the proximal

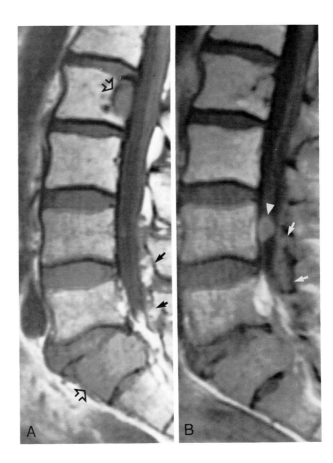

FIGURE 85–79. Intradural and extradural metastasis: MR imaging. Spin echo technique with and without gadolinium enhancement. This 56 year old man had renal cell carcinoma with known pelvic bone metastasis.

A A sagittal T1-weighted (TR/TE, 567/19) spin echo MR image demonstrates bone metastasis (open arrows) in the lumbosacral spine. Mottling of the fat posterior to the thecal sac at the L4 and L5 levels (closed arrows) is indicative of epidural metastasis. Anterior bulging of the L5-S1 intervertebral disc is evident.

B Following the intravenous administration of a gadolinium compound, a T1-weighted (TR/TE, 567/19) spin echo MR image shows an enhancing intradural metastasis (arrowhead) that was not well seen in **A.** Also note enhancement of the posterior epidural metastases (closed arrows) and the metastatic lesions in the vertebral body, which now are more difficult to see.

(Reproduced with permission from Lowe GM, Ramsey RG: MRI of spinal meningeal carcinomatosis. MRI Decisions 6:24–33, 1992. © 1992, Physicians World Communications Group. All rights reserved.)

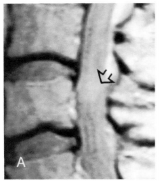
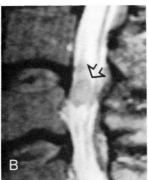
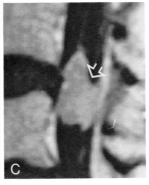

FIGURE 85–80. Intradural metastasis: MR imaging. Spin echo MR imaging technique with and without gadolimium enhancement. In this patient with metastatic bronchogenic carcinoma, proton density (TR/TE, 2500/21) **(A),** T2-weighted (TR/TE, 2500/105) **(B),** and gadolinium-enhanced T1-weighted (TR/TE, 500/15) **(C)** spin echo images show the site of lumbar metastasis (arrows), which is most obvious in **C.**

(Courtesy of R. Taketa, M.D., Long Beach, California.)

FIGURE 85–81. Intradural metastasis: MR imaging. Spin echo MR imaging technique with and without gadolinium enhancement. In this 72 year old woman with metastatic breast carcinoma, precontrast **(A)** and postcontrast **(B)** sagittal T1-weighted (TR/TE, 400/20) spin echo MR images are shown. The linear streak of enhancement along the dorsal surface of the spinal cord (arrows) in **B** represents the site of pial metastasis.

(From Lim V, et al: AJNR 11:975, 1990. © by American Society of Neuroradiology.)

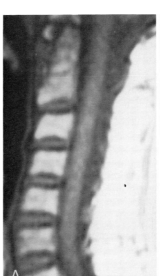
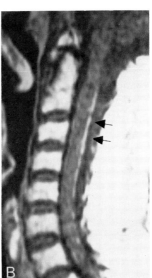

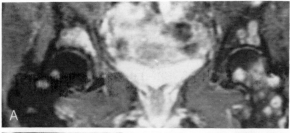

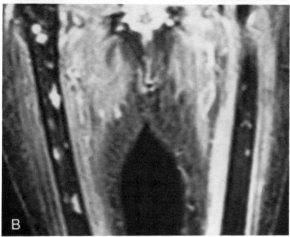

FIGURE 85–82. Skeletal metastasis: MR imaging. Extraspinal sites. Short tau inversion recovery (STIR) technique.

A Carcinoma of the breast. Lesions of high signal intensity are observed in the acetabuli and femora in this STIR image (TR/TE, 1500/40; inversion time, 150 msec).

B Carcinoma of the breast. Similar lesions of the femora are evident on this STIR image (TR/TE, 2000/25; inversion time, 160 msec).

portions of the femora and humeri and in the innominate bones considerable hematopoietic marrow may be present, even in adults; the use of gadolinium enhancement alone (without fat suppression) may be sufficient for diagnosis of metastatic lesions at these skeletal sites.

It should be emphasized that many of the MR imaging abnormalities associated with skeletal metastasis lack specificity, being simulated by findings seen in cases of primary tumors and infections of bone. Cortical violation and a soft tissue mass, when detected with MR imaging, usually are indicative of an aggressive bone tumor such as skeletal metastasis or primary malignant neoplasms, although infections and certain nonmalignant tumors or tumorlike lesions, including osteoid osteoma, chondroblastoma, and eosinophilic granuloma, may reveal similar features on MR imaging. Even acute nonpathologic fractures may cause diagnostic difficulty, particularly when MR imaging alone is employed as a diagnostic technique. Furthermore, CT competes favorably and even may be superior as an imaging method that provides information regarding cortical violation, calcific or ossific deposits, and pathologic fracture. Difficulties in accurate diagnosis of skeletal metastases using MR imaging may result from normal variations in the signal intensity of bone marrow,[433, 434, 458] sites of hyperplasia of hematopoietic bone marrow,[435, 459, 460] sites of reconversion of yellow to red marrow occurring as a response to an increased demand for hematopoiesis,[435] bone marrow edema resulting from trauma, stress, the reflex sympathetic dystrophy syndrome, or unknown cause, and bone marrow

ischemia. The differentiation of such metastasis and insufficiency fractures of the pelvis, proximal portions of the femur, or other locations with MR imaging can be particularly difficult (see Chapters 25, 51, and 67).

With regard to the differentiation of skeletal metastasis and sites of normal hematopoietic marrow, careful attention to the pattern of signal intensity in and about focal lesions may prove diagnostic.[473] On T1-weighted spin echo MR images, one or more areas of high signal intensity (equivalent to that of fat) within a lesion of low signal intensity, a pattern designated the bull's-eye sign, may be a specific indicator of hematopoietic marrow. Conversely, the presence of a halo sign, defined as a rim of high signal intensity about the lesion on T2-weighted spin echo images, appears to be a reliable indicator of skeletal metastasis, particularly when multiple such lesions are present in a patient with a known malignant tumor.[473]

Following radiation therapy, MR imaging may allow differentiation of osseous changes related to the treatment itself from those associated with tumor recurrence; in the former situation, areas of increased signal intensity during certain imaging strategies are consistent with either an absolute or a relative increase in fatty tissue (Fig. 85–83), whereas in the latter situation, a low signal intensity is more characteristic.[301, 333, 334] Some diagnostic pitfalls may be encountered, however (see Chapter 83).[465] In particular, the MR imaging features of the bone marrow after irradiation are time-dependent, with findings indicative of edema or hemorrhage appearing in the acute or subacute phase and of fatty replacement occurring in the chronic phase.[474]

Biopsy Techniques

Although biopsy methods are discussed in greater detail in Chapter 16, a few comments regarding skeletal biopsy procedures in patients with osseous metastases are appropriate here. These procedures may provide a rapid and accurate diagnosis in some persons with solitary or multiple aggressive bone lesions in whom skeletal metastasis is suspected.[463] It has been suggested that 3 to 30 per cent of all metastatic carcinomas have an unknown primary site, and osseous metastases occur in as many as 20 per cent of these cases.[302, 461] Whereas skeletal metastases of known origin commonly are found to originate in the breast, prostate, or lung, those of unknown origin may indicate an occult tumor of the lung, pancreas, liver, colon, or kidney.[302, 303, 462] Skeletal metastases from occult carcinomas have been reported to occur more often in men, with a high incidence of spinal lesions, cord compression, and pathologic fractures.[461] In some instances, pathologic characterization of the type of tumor (e.g., adenocarcinoma) does not identify the specific site of the primary tumor.[470] In these cases, an extensive workup may be required for complete diagnosis, although, in the view of some investigators, such diagnostic accuracy may not improve the length or the quality of the patient's life.[304, 462] As certain disseminated neoplasms are better controlled than others, the tissue removed during bone biopsy should be used as a guide for determining the need for further diagnostic studies; if the histologic diagnosis is one of adenocarcinoma (Fig. 85–84) or undifferentiated carcinoma, no additional diagnostic tests are required owing to the unlikelihood of identifying the site of the primary tumor and the expected short survival time of the patient.[302] The

FIGURE 85–83. Skeletal metastasis and irradiation effect: MR imaging.

A This 17 year old girl had received radiation therapy for lymphoma when she was a child. The sagittal T1-weighted (TR/TE, 500/12) spin echo MR image shows irradiation effect in the second through fifth lumbar vertebral bodies and sacrum with fat infiltration and decreased anteroposterior size of the vertebral bodies.

B A 40 year old man underwent surgery for the partial removal of a grade II astrocytoma involving the spinal cord at the level of the conus medullaris. He then received 5000 cGy (rad) of radiation treatment to the lower thoracic spinal cord over a 5 week period. Progressive weakness and numbness of the right leg developed subsequently. A sagittal T1-weighted (TR/TE, 530/30) spin echo MR image shows increased signal intensity of the tenth, eleventh, and twelfth thoracic vertebral bodies and a portion of the first lumbar vertebral body (between arrowheads) consistent with irradiation effect. No recurrent tumor is evident.

(**B**, From Ramsey RG, Zacharias CE: AJR *144*:1131, 1985. Copyright 1985, American Roentgen Ray Society.)

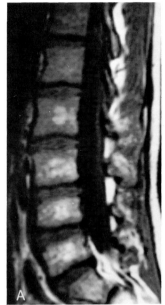
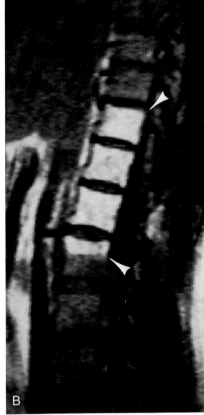

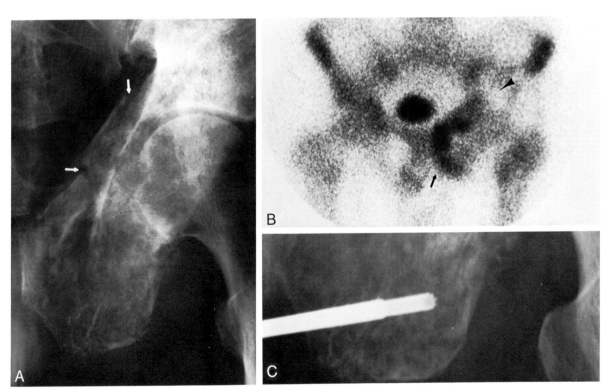

FIGURE 85–84. Skeletal metastasis: Biopsy techniques. This 55 year old alcoholic man had left hip pain.

A A radiograph demonstrates an expansile, mixed osteolytic-osteosclerotic lesion of the symphysis pubis, pubic rami, and ischium with pathologic fractures (arrows).

B A bone scan shows increased accumulation of the radionuclide in portions of the tumor (arrow) and decreased accumulation elsewhere (arrowhead).

C A Craig needle biopsy of the lesion documented adenocarcinoma. Although a probable origin of the primary tumor was the liver, no further workup was accomplished.

recovery of tissue interpreted as clear-cell carcinoma requires evaluation of the thyroid and kidney, whereas that diagnosed as squamous cell carcinoma should direct attention to the upper respiratory tract and lungs.[302] As intramedullary nailing represents an effective means of fixation for impending or documented pathologic fractures of the shafts of the long tubular bones, tissue biopsy can be combined with the surgical procedure.[305]

In the patient with a known primary tumor, single or multiple skeletal lesions discovered by conventional radiography, scintigraphy, CT, or MR imaging, or any combination of these, can be further evaluated with a bone biopsy, especially if the imaging features of the lesion(s) are not characteristic of metastasis. In this situation, the identification of a non-neoplastic cause for the osseous alterations may influence the subsequent treatment plan dramatically.

METABOLIC CONSEQUENCES OF SKELETAL METASTASIS

Hypercalcemia

Hypercalcemia is a well-recognized manifestation of cancer, occurring in as many as 10 to 20 per cent of patients. Although generally associated with detectable osseous metastasis, hypercalcemia can appear in patients with malignant tumors in whom metastatic involvement of the skeleton is absent,[306] a situation that has been termed pseudo-hyperparathyroidism. A decrease in the serum levels of calcium has been observed during successful treatment of the tumors, suggesting that the neoplasms themselves were involved in the synthesis and secretion of a humoral substance capable of producing hypercalcemia.[307] The nature of this substance is not clear; among the proposed humoral agents are parathyroid hormone, prostaglandin E_2, vitamin D metabolites, an osteolytic sterol unrelated to vitamin D, an osteoclast activating factor, transforming growth factors, and a parathyrotropic factor.[306, 307, 467] Surgical and autopsy examination of the parathyroid glands in some patients with hypercalcemia has revealed hyperplasia,[308] although the precise relationship of this change to the functional state of the parathyroid glands is not clear.[307] Morphologic alterations in the bones of such patients include osteoclastic resorption and fibroblastic proliferation in the marrow similar or identical to findings in hyperparathyroidism, but laboratory values suggest that a state of suppressed secretion of the parathyroid gland exists and that the humoral factor responsible for the hypercalcemia of malignancy resides elsewhere than in the parathyroid glands or the malignant tumor itself.[307]

Hypocalcemia

Hypocalcemia also is a well-recognized manifestation in cancer patients, occurring in as many as 16 per cent of persons who have osteoblastic metastases. In some cases, the laboratory aberration relates to uremia or hypoalbuminemia; in others, the cause is not clear, and associated abnormalities exist, including hypoparathyroidism, secondary hyperparathyroidism, defects in vitamin D metabolism, hypomagnesemia, and renal refractoriness to parathyroid hormone.[309] An unidentified humoral substance capable of stimulating osteoblasts has been proposed as a possible cause of the hypocalcemia,[309] although its exact nature and site of elaboration are not known.

Oncogenic Osteomalacia

In addition to hypocalcemia, hypophosphatemia and elevated serum levels of alkaline phosphatase are identified in some patients with extensive osteoblastic metastasis, particularly those arising from carcinoma of the prostate.[310, 311] The diagnosis of osteomalacia has been substantiated in these persons on the basis of histologic findings[312, 313] as well as depressed serum levels of 1,25-hydroxyvitamin D and normalization of clinical and laboratory abnormalities following administration of vitamin D derivatives.[314, 341] Oncogenic osteomalacia leads to generalized weakness and painful muscles and bones, clinical manifestations that easily are attributed to the metastases themselves. It is associated more typically with a number of primary bone and soft tissue neoplasms, including vascular (sclerosing hemangioma, hemangiopericytoma, cavernous hemangioma) and mesenchymal tumors as well as giant cell reparative granuloma, giant cell tumor, fibrous dysplasia, nonossifying fibroma, and osteoblastoma, in which case removal of the neoplasm is followed by rapid and dramatic reversal of the clinical and biochemical abnormalities.[315] Although variable in their histologic features, most of the reported tumors have contained giant cells and extreme vascularity.[466, 467] Either or both of these components may be important in the cause and pathogenesis of the osteomalacia, perhaps by elaborating a substance that gains quick access to the general circulation and depletes the body's phosphate concentrations.

SUMMARY

Metastatic disease of the skeleton can arise from direct extension, lymphatic or hematogenous dissemination, or intraspinal spread of tumor. The osseous response to the neoplasm consists of bone resorption or bone formation, or both. Such metastases predominate in the bones of the axial skeleton, although atypical patterns of distribution are encountered.

In synovial joints, neoplastic deposits in periarticular bone can lead to collapse and fragmentation with or without intra-articular extension of a tumor. Hematogenous seeding to the synovial membrane also can occur. In cartilaginous joints (discovertebral junction), intervertebral disc space narrowing can indicate adjacent vertebral metastatic lesions that are interfering with proper cartilage nutrition or that are associated with cartilaginous node formation or discal invasion by tumor. Additional ''articular'' syndromes include secondary hypertrophic osteoarthropathy, carcinomatous polyarthritis, pyogenic arthritis, irradiation effect, and associated rheumatic disorders.

A variety of diagnostic techniques, including scintigraphy, computed tomography, and magnetic resonance imaging, can be used in addition to routine radiography in the initial detection and subsequent monitoring of the metastatic foci.

References

1. Dorland's Illustrated Medical Dictionary. 25th Ed. Philadelphia, WB Saunders Co, 1974, p 945.
2. Weiss L, Gilbert HA: Bone Metastasis. Boston, GK Hall, 1981.
3. Wilner D: Radiology of Bone Tumors and Allied Disorders. Philadelphia, WB Saunders Co, 1982, p 3641.
4. Gullino PM, Liotta LA: Cell shedding by tumors. In L Weiss, HA Gilbert (Eds): Bone Metastasis. Boston, GK Hall, 1981, p 11.
5. Springfield DS: Mechanisms of metastasis. Clin Orthop 169:15, 1982.
6. Grundmann E: Rules in metastatic tumor spread. In Tumor Progression and Markers. Proceedings of the Sixth Meeting of the European Association for Cancer Research, Budapest, October 12–15, 1981. Amsterdam, Kugler Publications, 1982, p 71.
7. Fidler IJ: Tumor heterogeneity and the biology of cancer invasion and metastasis. Cancer Res 38:2651, 1978.
8. Galasko CSB: The anatomy and pathways of skeletal metasasis. In L Weiss, HA Gilbert (Eds): Bone Metastasis. Boston, GK Hall, 1981, p. 49.
9. Borak J: Roentgen examination of pancreatic tumors. Radiology 41:170, 1943.
10. Drury RAB, Palmer PH, Highman WJ: Carcinomatous metastasis to the vertebral bodies. J Clin Pathol 17:448, 1964.
11. Norgaard F: Bone destruction in carcinoma of the uterine cervix, by direct propagation or by lymphogenic or hematogenic metastasis. Acta Radiol 21:221, 1940.
12. Rubin P, Prabhasawat D: Characteristic bone lesions in post-irradiated carcinoma of the cervix. Radiology 76:703, 1961.
13. Fisher MS: Lumbar spine metastasis in cervical carcinoma: A characteristic pattern. Radiology 134:631, 1980.
14. Batson OV: The function of the vertebral veins and their role in the spread of metastases. Ann Surg 112:138, 1940.
15. Batson OV: The role of the vertebral veins in metastatic processes. Ann Intern Med 16:38, 1942.
16. Batson OV: The vertebral vein system. AJR 78:198, 1957.
17. Vider M, Maruyama Y, Narvaez R: Significance of the vertebral venous (Batson's) plexus in metastatic spread in colorectal carcinoma. Cancer 40:67, 1977.
18. Coman DR, De Long RP: The role of the vertebral venous system in the metastasis of cancer to the spinal column. Cancer 4:610, 1951.
19. Burns FJ, Plaff J: Vascular invasion in carcinoma of the colon and rectum. Am J Surg 92:704, 1956.
20. Willis RA: The Spread of Tumors in the Human Body. 3rd Ed. London, Butterworths, 1973.
21. Bryan P: CSF seeding of intra-cranial tumours: A study of 96 cases. Clin Radiol 25:355, 1974.
22. Cairns H, Russell DS: Intracranial and spinal metastasis in gliomas of the brain. Brain 54:377, 1931.
23. Svien JH, Gates EM, Kernohan JW: Spinal subarachnoid implantation associated with ependymoma. Arch Neurol Psychiatry 62:847, 1949.
24. Stanley P, Senac MO Jr, Segali HD: Intraspinal seeding from intracranial tumors in children. AJR 144:157, 1985.
25. Svien HJ, Mabon RF, Kernohan JW, et al: Ependymoma of the brain: Pathological aspects. Neurology 3:1, 1953.
26. Strang RR: Intraspinal metastases from medulloblastomas of the posterior fossa. Med J Aust 2:507, 1962.
27. Ingrahan FD, Bailey OT, Baker WF: Medulloblastoma cerebelli. N Engl J Med 238:171, 1948.
28. Tarlov IM, Davidoff LM: Subarachnoid and ventricular implants in ependymal and other gliomas. J Neuropathol Exp Neurol 5:213, 1946.
29. Dorwart RH, Wara WM, Norman D, et al: Complete myelographic evaluation of spinal metastases from medulloblastoma. Radiology 139:403, 1981.
30. Costigan DA, Winkelman MD: Intramedullary spinal cord metastasis. A clinicopathological study of 13 cases. J Neurosurg 62:227, 1985.
31. Galasko CSB: Bone metastases studied in experimental animals. Clin Orthop 155:269, 1981.
32. Galasko CSB: Mechanisms of lytic and blastic metastatic disease of bone. Clin Orthop 169:20, 1982.
33. Galasko CSB: The development of skeletal metastases. In L Weiss, HA Gilbert (Eds): Bone Metastasis. Boston, GK Hall, 1981, p 83.
34. Mundy GR, Spiro TP: The mechanisms of bone metastasis and bone destruction by tumor cells. In L Weiss, HA Gilbert (Eds): Bone Metastasis. Boston, GK Hall, 1981, p 64.
35. Galasko CSB: Mechanisms of bone destruction in the development of skeletal metastases. Nature 263:507, 1976.
36. Eilon G, Mundy GR: Direct resorption of bone by human breast cancer cells in vitro. Nature 276:726, 1978.
37. Mundy GR, Altman AJ, Gondek MD, et al: Direct resorption of bone by human monocytes. Science 196:1109, 1977.
38. Minkin C, Posek R, Newbrey J: Mononuclear phagocytes and bone resorption: Identification and preliminary characterization of a bone-derived macrophage chemotactic factor. Metab Bone Dis Rel Res 2:363, 1981.
39. Jaworski ZFG, Liskova-Kiar M, Uhtoff HK: Effect of long-term immobilization on the pattern of bone loss in older dogs. J Bone Joint Surg [Br] 62:104, 1978.
40. Stewart AF, Horst R, Deftos LJ, et al: Biochemical evaluation of patient with cancer-associated hypercalcemia. Evidence for humoral and non-humoral groups. N Engl J Med 303:1377, 1980.
41. Kukreja SC, Shemerdiak WP, Lad TE, et al: Elevated nephrogenous cyclic AMP with normal serum parathyroid hormone levels in patients with lung cancer. J Clin Endocrinol Metab 51:167, 1980.
42. Minkin C, Fredericks RS, Pokress S, et al: Bone resorption and humoral hypercalcemia of malignancy: Stimulation of bone resorption in vitro by tumor extracts is inhibited by prostaglandin synthesis inhibitors. J Clin Endocrinol Metab 53:941, 1981.
43. McDonnell GD, Dunstan CR, Evans RA, et al: Quantitative bone histology in the hypercalcemia of malignant disease. J Clin Endocrinol Metab 55:1066, 1982.
44. Mundy GR, Raisz LG, Cooper RA, et al: Evidence for the secretion of an osteoclast activating factor in myeloma. N Engl J Med 291:1041, 1974.
45. Mundy GR, Raisz LG: Big and little forms of osteoclast activating factor. J Clin Invest 60:122, 1977.
46. Horton JE, Raisz LG, Simmons HA, et al: Bone resorbing activity in supernatant fluid from cultured human peripheral blood leukocytes. Science 177:793, 1972.
47. Burkhardt R, Frisch B, Schlag R, et al: Carcinomatous osteodysplasia. Skel Radiol 8:169, 1982.
48. Collier HO, Schneider C: Nociceptive response to prostaglandins and analgesic actions of aspirin and morphine. Nature 236:141, 1972.
49. Taylor SJ, Haskell CM: The clinical and laboratory consequences of metastatic cancer in bone. In L Weiss, HA Gilbert (Eds): Bone Metastasis. Boston, GK Hall, 1981, p 114.
50. Abrams HL, Spiro R, Goldstein N: Metastases in carcinoma. Analysis of 1000 autopsied cases. Cancer 3:74, 1950.
51. Abrams HL: Skeletal metastases in carcinoma. Radiology 55:534, 1950.
52. Galasko CSB: The value of scintigraphy in malignant disease. Cancer Treat Rev 2:225, 1975.
53. Mall JC, Bekerman C, Hoffer PB, et al: A unified approach to the detection of skeletal metastases. Radiology 118:323, 1976.
54. Tofe AJ, Francis MD, Harvey WJ: Correlation of neoplasms with incidence and localization of skeletal metastases: An analysis of 1,355 diphosphonate bone scans. J Nucl Med 16:987, 1976.
55. Willis RA: A review of 500 consecutive cancer autopsies. Med J Aust 2:258, 1941.
56. Young JM, Funk FJ: Incidence of tumor metastasis to the lumbar spine, a comparative study of roentgenographic changes and gross lesions. J Bone Joint Surg [Am] 35:55, 1953.
57. Fornasier VL, Horne JG: Metastases to the vertebral column. Cancer 36:590, 1975.
58. Fragiadakis EG, Panayotopoulos G: Metastatic carcinoma of the hand. Hand 4:268, 1972.
59. Kerin R: Metastatic tumors of the hand. J Bone Joint Surg [Am] 40:263, 1958.
60. Bryan RS, Soule EH, Dobyns JH, et al: Metastatic lesions in the hand and forearm. Clin Orthop 101:167, 1974.
61. Mulvey RB: Peripheral bone metastasis. AJR 91:155, 1964.
62. Copeland MM: Bone metastases—a study of 334 cases. Radiology 16:198, 1931.
63. Fort WA: Cancer metastatic to bone. Radiology 24:96, 1935.
64. Gall RJ, Sim FH, Pritchard DJ: Metastatic tumors to the bones of the foot. Cancer 37:1492, 1976.
65. Barnett LS, Morris JM: Metastases of renal-cell carcinoma simutaneously to a finger and a toe. A case report. J Bone Joint Surg [Am] 51:773, 1969.
66. Bouvier M, Lejeune E, Robillard J, et al: Les metastases osseuses distales. Rev Lyon Med 19:811, 1970.
67. Uriburu IJF, Morchio FJ, Marin JC: Metastases of carcinoma of the larynx and thyroid gland to the phalanges of the hand. Report of two cases. J Bone Joint Surg [Am] 58:134, 1976.
68. Wu KK, Winkelman NZ, Guise ER: Metastatic bronchogenic carcinoma to the finger simulating acute osteomyelitis. Orthopedics 3:25, 1980.
69. Zindrick MR, Young MP, Daley RJ, et al: Metastatic tumors of the foot. Case report and literature review. Clin Orthop 170:219, 1982.
70. Bonvoisin B, Joasson JM, Bouvier M, et al: Metastase osseuse distale d'aspect inhabituel. Lyon Med 245:251, 1981.
71. Bouvier M, Lejeune E, Bonvoisin B, et al: Les metastases osseuses distales de membre superieur. Ann Radiol 25:359, 1982.
72. Cary PC, Helms CA, Genant HK: Metastatic disease to the carpus. Br J Radiol 54:992, 1981.
73. Khokhar N, Lee JD: Phalangeal metastasis: First clinical sign of bronchogenic carcinoma. South Med J 76:927, 1983.
74. Kerin R: Metastatic tumors of the hand. A review of the literature. J Bone Joint Surg [Am] 65:1331, 1983.
75. Rose BA, Wood FM: Metastatic bronchogenic carcinoma masquerading as a felon. J Hand Surg 8:325, 1983.
76. Chung TS: Metastatic malignancy to the bones of the hand. J Surg Oncol 24:99, 1983.
77. Ioia JV, Sumner JM, Gallagher T: Presentation of malignancy by metastasis to the carpal navicular bone. Clin Orthop 188:230, 1984.
78. Gottlieb PD, Parikh SJ, Singh JK: Case report 295. Skel Radiol 13:154, 1985.
79. Ghandur-Mnaymneh L, Mnaymneh W: Solitary bony metastasis to the foot with long survival following amputation. Clin Orthop 166:117, 1982.
80. Pirschel J, Metzger HOFJ, Weissman C: Zur metastasierung maligner Tumoren in die Skelettperipherie. ROFO 129:621, 1978.
81. Gelberman RH, Stewart WR, Harrelson JM: Hand metastasis from melanoma. A case study. Clin Orthop 136:264, 1978.

82. Edelstyn GA, Gillespie PJ, Grebbell FS: The radiological demonstration of osseous metastases. Experimental observations. Clin Radiol *18*:158, 1967.

83. Lehrer HZ, Maxfield WS, Nice CM: The periosteal ''sunburst'' pattern in metastatic bone tumors. AJR *108*:154, 1970.

84. Wyche LD, de Santos LA: Spiculated periosteal reaction in metastatic disease resembling osteosarcoma. Orthopedics *1*:215, 1978.

85. Libson E, Bloom RA, Halperin I: Periosteal ''sunburst'' pattern due to a prostatic metastasis. Diagn Imaging *50*:146, 1981.

86. Vilar J, Lezana AH, Pedrosa CS: Spiculated periosteal reaction in metastatic lesions of bone. Skel Radiol *3*:230, 1979.

87. Dorn W III, Gladden P, Rankin EA: Regression of a renal-cell metastatic osseous lesion following treatment. J Bone Joint Surg [Am] *57*:869, 1975.

88. Bowers TA, Murray JA, Charnsangavej C, et al: Bone metastasis from renal carcinoma. The preoperative use of transcatheter arterial occlusion. J Bone Joint Surg [Am] *64*:749, 1982.

89. Golimbu C, Firooznia H, Rafii M: Hepatocellular carcinoma with skeletal metastasis. Radiology *154*:617, 1985.

90. Gelman M: Case report 25. Skel Radiol *1*:241, 1977.

91. Franck JL, Lhez JM, Arlet J: Une metastase osseuse exuberante d'origine prostatique. J Radiol *63*:209, 1982.

92. Resnik CS, Garver P, Resnick D: Bony expansion in skeletal metastasis from carcinoma of the prostate as seen by bone scintigraphy. South Med J *77*:1331, 1984.

93. Legier JF, Tauber LN: Solitary metastasis of occult prostatic carcinoma simulating osteogenic sarcoma. Cancer *22*:168, 1968.

94. Seife B: Osseous metastases from carcinoma of the large bowel. AJR *119*:414, 1973.

95. Caluori D, Gallo P: Case report of heterotopic bone formation in metastatic carcinoma of the colon. Tumori *65*:345, 1979.

96. Obley DL, Slasky BS, Peel RL, et al: Bone-forming gastric metastases in muscle-computed tomographic demonstration. J Comput Tomogr *7*:129, 1983.

97. Rosenbaum LH, Nicholas JJ, Slasky BS, et al: Malignant myositis ossificans: Occult gastric carcinoma presenting as an acute rheumatic disorder. Ann Rheum Dis *43*:95, 1984.

98. Chinn D, Genant HK, Quivey JM, et al: Heterotopic-bone formation in metastatic tumor from transitional-cell carcinoma of the urinary bladder. A case report. J Bone Joint Surg [Am] *58*:881, 1976.

99. Evison G, Pizey N, Roylance J: Bone formation associated with osseous metastases from bladder carcinoma. Clin Radiol *32*:303, 1981.

100. Patel S, Moso CJ: Ossification in metastases from carcinoma of the breast. JAMA *198*:1309, 1966.

101. Bettendorf U, Remmele W, Laaff H: Bone formation by cancer metastases. Case report and review of literature. Virchows Arch Pathol Anat Histol *369*:359, 1976.

102. Chalmers J, Gray DH, Rush J: Observations on the introduction of bone in soft tissues. J Bone Joint Surg [Br] *57*:36, 1974.

103. An T, Grathwohl M, Frable WJ: Breast carcinoma with osseous metaplasia: An electron microscopic study. Am J Clin Pathol *81*:127, 1984.

104. Huggins CB, McCarroll HR, Blocksom BH Jr: Experiments on the theory of osteogenesis. Arch Surg *32*:915, 1936.

105. Huggins CB: The formation of bone under the influence of epithelium of the urinary tract. Arch Surg *22*:377, 1931.

106. Clain A: Secondary malignant disease of bone. Br J Cancer *19*:15, 1965.

107. Bremmer RA, Jelliffe AM: The management of pathological fractures of the major long bones from metastatic cancer. J Bone Joint Surg [Br] *40*:652, 1958.

108. Gainor BJ, Buchert P: Fracture healing in metastatic bone disease. Clin Orthop *178*:297, 1983.

109. Altman H: Intramedullary nailing for pathological impending and actual fractures of long bones. Bull Hosp Joint Dis *13*:239, 1952.

110. Beals RK, Lawton GD, Snell WE: Prophylactic internal fixation of the femur in metastatic breast cancer. Cancer *28*:1350, 1971.

111. Parrish FF, Murray JA: Surgical treatment for secondary neoplastic fractures. J Bone Joint Surg [Am] *52*:665, 1970.

112. Fidler MW: Prophylactic internal fixation of secondary neoplastic deposits in long bones. Br Med J *1*:341, 1973.

113. Fidler MW: Incidence of fracture through metastases in long bones. Acta Orthop Scand *52*:623, 1981.

114. Koskinen EVS, Nieminen RA: Surgical treatment of metastatic pathological fracture of major long bones. Acta Orthop Scand *44*:539, 1973.

115. Heisterberg L, Johansen TS: Treatment of pathologic fractures. Acta Orthop Scand *50*:787, 1979.

116. Harrington KD, Sim FH, Enis JE, et al: Methylmethacrylate as an adjunct in the internal fixation of pathological fractures. J Bone Joint Surg [Am] *54*:1665, 1972.

117. Bonarigo BC, Rubin P: Nonunion of pathologic fracture after radiation therapy. Radiology *88*:889, 1967.

118. Rosen IW, Nadel HI: Button sequestrum of the skull. Radiology *92*:969, 1969.

119. Wells PO: Button sequestrum of eosinophilic granuloma of the skull. Radiology *67*:746, 1956.

120. Tirona JP: Roentgenological and pathological aspects of tuberculosis of the skull. AJR *72*:762, 1954.

121. Sholkoff SD, Mainzer F: Button sequestrum revisited. Radiology *100*:649, 1971.

122. Satin R, Usher MS, Goldenberg M: More causes of button sequestrum. J Can Assoc Radiol *27*:288, 1976.

123. Holthusen W, Lassrich MA, Steiner C: Epidermoids and dermoids of calvarian bones in early childhood: Their behavior in the growing skull. Pediatr Radiol *13*:189, 1983.

124. Keats TE, Holt JF: The calvarial ''doughnut lesion'': A previously undescribed entity. AJR *105*:314, 1969.

125. Royen PM, Ozonoff MB: Multiple calvarial ''doughnut lesions.'' A case report. AJR *121*:121, 1974.

126. Bartlett JM, Kishore PRS: Familial ''doughnut'' lesions of the skull. A benign hereditary dysplasia. Radiology *119*:385, 1976.

127. Thomas D, Hoeffel JC: L'acunes craniennes multiples d'orgine veineuse chez l'adulte. A propos de 14 observations. Ann Radiol *24*:226, 1981.

128. Branan R, Wilson CB: Arachnoid granulations simulating osteolytic lesions of the calvarium. AJR *127*:523, 1976.

129. Kirkwood JR, Margolis MT, Newton TH: Prostatic metastasis to the base of the skull simulating meningioma en plaque. AJR *112*:774, 1971.

130. Belanger WG, Dyke C: Roentgen diagnosis of malignant nasopharyngeal tumors. AJR *50*:9, 1943.

131. Potter GD: Sclerosis of base of skull as a manifestation of nasopharyngeal carcinoma. Radiology *94*:35, 1970.

132. Unger JD, Chiang LC, Unger GF: Apparent reformation of the base of the skull following radiotherapy for nasopharyngeal carcinoma. Radiology *126*:779, 1978.

133. Kendall B: Invasion of facial bone by basal meningioma. Br J Radiol *46*:237, 1973.

134. Tsai FY, Lisella RS, Lee KF, et al: Osteosclerosis of base of skull as a manifestation of tumor invasion. AJR *124*:256, 1975.

135. Leeds N, Seaman WB: Fibrous dysplasia of the skull and its differential diagnosis: Clinical and roentgenographic study of 46 cases. Radiology *78*:570, 1962.

136. Raycroft JF, Hockman RP, Southwick WO: Metastatic tumors involving the cervical vertebrae: Surgical palliation. J Bone Joint Surg [Am] *60*:763, 1978.

137. Boland PJ, Lane JM, Sundaresan N: Metastatic disease of the spine. Clin Orthop *169*:95, 1982.

138. Barron KD, Hirano A, Araki S, et al: Experience with metastatic neoplasms involving the spinal cord. Neurology *9*:91, 1959.

139. Shibasaki K, Harper CG, Bedbrook GM, et al: Vertebral metastases and spinal cord compression. Paraplegia *21*:47, 1983.

140. Fornasier VL, Czitrom AA: Collapsed vertebrae. A review of 659 autopsies. Clin Orthop *131*:261, 1978.

141. Ogden JA, Ogden DA: Skeletal metastasis: The effect on the immature skeleton. Skel Radiol *9*:73, 1982.

142. Deutsch A, Resnick D: Eccentric cortical metastases to the skeleton from bronchogenic carcinoma. Radiology *137*:49, 1980.

143. Bertin KC, Horstman J, Coleman SS: Isolated fracture of the lesser trochanter in adults: An initial manifestation of metastatic malignant disease. J Bone Joint Surg [Am] *66*:770, 1984.

144. Martini N, Huvos AG, Smith J, et al: Primary malignant tumors of the sternum. Surg Gynecol Obstet *138*:391, 1974.

145. Geha AS, Bernatz PE, Woolner LB: Bronchogenic carcinoma involving the thoracic wall: Surgical treatment and prognostic significance. J Thorac Cardiovasc Surg *54*:394, 1967.

146. Grillo HC, Greenberg JJ, Wilkins EW: Resection of bronchogenic carcinoma involving thoracic wall. J Thorac Cardiovasc Surg *51*:417, 1966.

147. de Gautard R, Dussault RG, Chahlaoui J, et al: Contribution of CT in thoracic bony lesions. J Can Assoc Radiol *32*:39, 1981.

148. Lally JF, Cossrow JI, Dalinka MK: Odontoid fractures in metastatic breast carcinoma. AJR *128*:817, 1977.

149. Goldschmidt RA, Resnik CS, Mills AS: Case report 266. Skel Radiol *11*:213, 1984.

150. Greenspan A, Klein MJ, Lewis MM: Case report 272. Skel Radiol *11*:297, 1984.

151. Greenspan A, Klein MJ, Lewis MM: Case report 284. Skel Radiol *12*:146, 1984.

152. Deutsch A, Resnick D, Niwayama G: Case report 145. Skel Radiol *6*:144, 1981.

153. Norman A, Greenspan A, Steiner G: Case report 173. Skel Radiol *7*:155, 1981.

154. Peavy PW, Rogers JV Jr, Clements JL Jr, et al: Unusual osteoblastic metastases from carcinoid tumors. Radiology *107*:327, 1973.

155. Greco MA, Waldo ED: Bronchial carcinoid tumors and bone metastases. NY State J Med *75*:102, 1975.

156. Manoli RS, Barthelemy CR: Osteolytic and osteoblastic metastases due to carcinoid tumors. Clin Nucl Med *5*:102, 1980.

157. Johnson DG, Osborne D, Bossen DH: Case report 185. Skel Radiol *7*:293, 1982.

158. Saitoh H: Distant metastasis of renal adenocarcinoma. Cancer *48*:1487, 1981.

159. Forbes GS, McLeod RA, Hattery RR: Radiographic manifestations of bone metastases from renal carcinoma. AJR *129*:61, 1977.

160. Aggarwal ND, Mittal RL, Bhalla R: Delayed solitary metastasis to the radius of renal-cell carcinoma. J Bone Joint Surg [Am] *54*:1314, 1972.

161. Neugut AI, Casper ES, Godwin A, Smith J: Osteoblastic metastases in renal cell carcinoma. Br J Radiol *54*:1002, 1981.

162. Marsden HB, Lawler W: Bone-metastasizing renal tumor of childhood. Br J Cancer *38*:437, 1978.

163. Eklof O, Mortensson W, Sandstedt B, et al: Bone metastases in Wilms' tumor: Occurrence and radiological appearance. Ann Radiol *27*:97, 1984.

164. Lamego CMB, Zerbini MCN: Bone-metastasizing primary renal tumors in children. Radiology 147:449, 1983.
165. Bertoni F: Case report 287. Skel Radiol 12:218, 1984.
166. McCook TA, Putman CE, Dale JK, et al: Medullary carcinoma of the thyroid: Radiographic features of a unique tumor. AJR 139:149, 1982.
167. Reyes J, Shimaoka K, Ghoorah J, et al: Osteoblastic metastases from medullary carcinoma of the thyroid. Br J Radiol 53:1003, 1980.
168. Goldman SM, Fajardo AA, Naraval RC, et al: Metastatic transitional cell carcinoma from the bladder: Radiographic manifestations. AJR 132:419, 1979.
169. Dunnick NR, Anderson T: Distant metastases to bone from bladder carcinoma: Report of three cases. AJR 132:469, 1979.
170. Mullin EM, Glenn JF, Paulson DF: Lesions of bone and bladder cancer. J Urol 113:45, 1975.
171. Jewett HJ, Strong GH: Infiltrating carcinoma of the bladder: Relation of depth of penetration of the bladder wall to incidence of local extension and metastases. J Urol 55:366, 1946.
172. Murray RO, Jacobson HG: The Radiology of Skeletal Disorders. 2nd Ed. Edinburgh, Churchill Livingstone, 1977, pp 584, 1090.
173. Stewart WR, Gelberman RH, Harrelson JM, et al: Skeletal metastases of melanoma. J Bone Joint Surg [Am] 60:645, 1978.
174. Steiner GM, MacDonald JS: Metastases to bone from malignant melanoma. Clin Radiol 23:52, 1972.
175. Fon GT, Wong WS, Gold RH, et al: Skeletal metastases of melanoma: Radiographic, scintigraphic, and clinical review. AJR 137:103, 1981.
176. Stanley P, Siegel SE, Isaacs H: Calcification in a paraspinal malignant melanoma in a child. AJR 129:143, 1977.
177. Blythe JG, Ptacek JJ, Buchsbaum HJ, Latourette HB: Bony metastases from carcinoma of cervix. Cancer 36:475, 1975.
178. Basson JS, Glaser MG: Bony metastasis in carcinoma of the uterine cervix. Clin Radiol 33:623, 1982.
179. Gelberman RH, Salamon PB, Huffer JM: Bone metastasis from carcinoma of the uterus. A case report. Clin Orthop 106:148, 1975.
180. Carstens SA, Resnick D: Diffuse sclerotic skeletal metastases as an initial feature of gastric carcinoma. Arch Intern Med 140:1666, 1980.
181. Baker LH, Vaitkevicius VK, Figiel SJ: Bony metastasis from adenocarcinoma of the colon. Am J Gastroenterol 62:139, 1974.
182. Joffe N, Antonioli DA: Osteoblastic bone metastases secondary to adenocarcinoma of the pancreas. Clin Radiol 29:41, 1978.
183. Cottin S, Caumon JP, Gibon M, et al: Metastases osseuses revelatrices d'hepatome. 13 cas. Rev Rhum Mal Osteoartic 48:347, 1981.
184. Pederson RT, Haidak DJ, Ferris RA, et al: Osteoblastic bone metastasis in Zollinger-Ellison syndrome. Radiology 118:63, 1976.
185. Khor TH, Tan BC, Chua EJ, et al: Distant metastases in nasopharyngeal carcinoma. Clin Radiol 29:27, 1978.
186. Debnam JW, Staple TW: Osseous metastases from cerebellar medulloblastoma. Radiology 107:363, 1973.
187. Courtney JV, Kelleher J, Radkowski MA: Skeletal metastases from medulloblastoma. Irish J Med Sci 148:189, 1979.
188. Damath HD Jr, Staple TW: Case report 212. Skel Radiol 9:64, 1982.
189. Das S, Dalby JE: Distant metastases from medulloblastoma. Acta Radiol Ther Phys Biol 16:117, 1977.
190. Booher KR Jr, Schmidtknecht TM: Cerebellar medulloblastoma with skeletal metastases. J Bone Joint Surg [Am] 59:684, 1977.
191. Kleinman GM, Hochberg FH, Richardson EP Jr: Systemic metastases from medulloblastoma: Report of two cases and review of the literature. Cancer 48:2296, 1981.
192. Gyepes MT, D'Anglio GJ: Extracranial metastases from central nervous system tumors in children and adolescents. Radiology 87:55, 1966.
193. Brutschin P, Culver GJ: Extracranial metastases from medulloblastomas. Radiology 107:359, 1973.
194. Schatzki SC, McIlmoyle G, Lowis S: Diffuse osteoblastic metastases from an intracranial glioma. AJR 128:321, 1977.
195. O'Connell DJ, Frank PH, Riddell RH: The metastases of meningioma—radiologic and pathologic features. Skel Radiol 3:30, 1978.
196. Jennings PG, Cook PL: Bony metastases from intracranial meningioma. Br J Radiol 56:421, 1983.
197. Punt J, Pritchard J, Pincott JR, et al: Neuroblastoma: A review of 21 cases presenting with spinal cord compression. Cancer 45:3095, 1980.
198. Roberts FF, Lee KR: Familial neuroblastoma presenting as multiple tumors. Radiology 116:133, 1975.
199. Merriam GR: Retinoblastoma: Analysis of 17 autopsies. Arch Ophthalmol 44:71, 1950.
200. Pullon PA, Cohen DM: Oral metastasis of retinoblastoma. Oral Surg 37:583, 1974.
201. Reed MH, Culham JAG: Skeletal metastases from retinoblastoma. J Can Assoc Radiol 26:249, 1975.
202. Brown DH: The urinary excretion of vanilmandelic (VMA) acid and homovanillic acid (HVA) in children with retinoblastoma. Am J Ophthalmol 62:239, 1966.
203. Loughran CF: Bone metastasis from squamous-cell carcinoma of the larynx. Clin Radiol 34:447, 1983.
204. Dubois PJ, Orr DP, Meyers EN, et al: Undifferentiated parotid carcinoma with osteoblastic metastases. AJR 129:744, 1977.
205. Abedelwahab IF, Norman A: Osteoblastic metastasis of lymphoepithelioma simulating osteoid osteoma. A case history. Bull Hosp Joint Dis 41:63, 1981.

206. Scalley JR, Collins J: Thymoma metastatic to bone. Report of a case diagnosed by percutaneous biopsy. Radiology 96:423, 1970.
207. James RE, Baker HL Jr, Scanlon PW: The roentgenologic aspects of metastatic pheochromocytoma. AJR 115:783, 1972.
208. Coulson WF: A metastasizing carotid-body tumor. J Bone Joint Surg [Am] 52:355, 1970.
209. Villiaumey J, Amouroux J, Rotterdam M, Pointud P, Delporte M-P: Les metastases osseuses des chemodectomes du corpuscule carotidien. Sem Hop Paris 50:857, 1974.
210. Meals RA, Hungerford DS, Stevens MB: Malignant disease mimicking arthritis of the hip. JAMA 239:1070, 1978.
211. Kagan AR, Steckel RJ: Metastatic carcinoma presenting as shoulder arthritis. AJR 129:137, 1977.
212. Lagier R: Synovial reaction caused by adjacent malignant tumors: Anatomico-pathological study of three cases. J Rheumatol 4:65, 1977.
213. Bevan DA, Ehrlich GE, Gupta VP: Metastatic carcinoma simulating gout. JAMA 237:2746, 1977.
214. Shenberger KN, Morgan GJ Jr: Recurrent malignant melanoma presenting as monoarthritis. J Rheumatol 9:328, 1982.
215. Ritch PS, Hansen RM, Collier BD: Metastatic renal cell carcinoma presenting as shoulder arthritis. Cancer 51:968, 1983.
216. Gall EA, Bennett GA, Bauer W: Generalized hypertrophic osteoarthropathy. A pathologic study of seven cases. Am J Pathol 27:349, 1951.
217. Hindmarsh JR, Emslie-Smith D: Monocytic leukemia presenting as polyarthritis in an adult. Br Med J 1:593, 1953.
218. Bennett RM, Ginsberg MH, Thomsen S: Carcinomatous polyarthritis. The presenting symptom of an ovarian tumor and association with a platelet activating factor. Arthritis Rheum 19:953, 1976.
219. Moutsopolous HM, Fye KH, Pugay PI, et al: Monoarthric arthritis caused by metastatic breast carcinoma. Value of cytologic study of synovial fluid. JAMA 234:75, 1975.
220. Stoler B, Staple TW: Metastases to the patella. Radiology 93:853, 1969.
221. Gall EP, Didizian NA, Park Y: Acute monoarticular arthritis following patellar metastasis. A manifestation of carcinoma of the lung. JAMA 229:188, 1974.
222. Benedek TG: Lysis of the patella due to metastatic carcinoma. Arthritis Rheum 8:560, 1965.
223. Weinblatt ME, Karp GI: Monoarticular arthritis: Early manifestation of a rhabdomyosarcoma. J Rheumatol 8:685, 1981.
224. Kaklamanis Ph, Yataganas X, Meletis J, et al: Carcinomatous monoarthritis. Clin Rheumatol 3:81, 1984.
225. Speerstra F, Boerbooms AMTh, van de Putte LBA, et al: Arthritis caused by metastatic melanoma. Arthritis Rheum 25:223, 1982.
226. Philipson JD, Birkhead R, Phillips PE: Arthritis of the elbow caused by metastatic bronchogenic carcinoma. Clin Exp Rheumatol 1:165, 1983.
227. Rozboril MB, Good AE, Zarbo RJ, et al: Sternoclavicular joint arthritis: An unusual presentation of metastatic carcinoma. J Rheumatol 10:499, 1983.
228. Naib ZM: Cytology of synovial fluids. Acta Cytol 17:299, 1973.
229. Meisels A, Berebichez M: Exfoliative cytology in orthopedics. Can Med Assoc J 84:957, 1961.
230. Goldenberg DL, Kelley W, Gibbons RB: Metastatic adenocarcinoma of synovium presenting as an acute arthritis. Diagnosis by closed synovial biopsy. Arthritis Rheum 18:107, 1975.
231. Fam AG, Kolin A, Lewis AJ: Metastatic carcinomatous arthritis and carcinoma of the lung. A report of two cases diagnosed by synovial fluid cytology. J Rheumatol 7:98, 1980.
232. Fam AG, Cross EG: Hypertrophic osteoarthropathy, phalangeal and synovial metastases associated with bronchogenic carcinoma. J Rheumatol 6:680, 1979.
233. Murray GC, Persellin RH: Metastatic carcinoma presenting as monarticular arthritis: A case report and review of the literature. Arthritis Rheum 23:95, 1980.
234. Spilberg I, Meyer GJ: The arthritis of leukemia. Arthritis Rheum 15:630, 1972.
235. Firooznia H, Pinto RS, Lin JP, et al: Chordoma: Radiologic evaluation of 20 cases. AJR 127:797, 1976.
236. Resnick D, Niwayama G: Intravertebral disk herniations: Cartilaginous (Schmorl's) nodes. Radiology 126:57, 1978.
237. Hubbard DD, Gunn DR: Secondary carcinoma of the spine with destruction of the intervertebral disk. Clin Orthop 88:86, 1972.
238. Resnick D, Niwayama G: Intervertebral disc abnormalities associated with vertebral metastases: Observations in patients and cadavers with prostatic cancer. Invest Radiol 13:182, 1978.
239. Schmorl G, Junghanns H: The Human Spine in Health and Disease. 2nd Ed. Translated by EF Besemann. New York, Grune & Stratton, 1971, p 141.
240. Hilton RC, Ball J, Benn RT: Vertebral end-plate lesions (Schmorl's nodes) in the dorsolumbar spine. Ann Rheum Dis 35:127, 1976.
241. Kuettner KE, Pauli BU: Resistance of cartilage to invasion. In L Weiss, HA Gilbert (Eds): Bone Metastasis. Boston, GK Hall, 1981, p 131.
242. Calabro JJ: Cancer and arthritis. Arthritis Rheum 10:553, 1967.
243. Holling HE: Pulmonary hypertrophic osteoarthropathy. Ann Intern Med 66:232, 1967.
244. MacKenzie AH, Scherbel AL: Connective tissue syndromes associated with carcinoma. Geriatrics 18:745, 1963.
245. Lansbury J: Collagen disease complicating malignancy. Ann Rheum Dis 12:301, 1953.
246. Simon RD Jr, Ford LE: Rheumatoid-like arthritis associated with a colonic carcinoma. Arch Intern Med 140:698, 1980.

247. Caldwell DS: Musculoskeletal syndromes associated with malignancy. Semin Arthritis Rheum 10:198, 1981.
248. Litwin SD, Allen JC, Kunkel HG: Disappearance of the clinical and serological manifestations of rheumatoid arthritis following thoracotomy for lung tumor (Abstr). Arthritis Rheum 9:865, 1966.
249. Lee JC, Yamauchi H, Hopper J Jr: The association of cancer and the nephrotic syndrome. Ann Intern Med 64:41, 1966.
250. Wybran J, Fudenberg HH: Thymus-derived rosette forming cells in various human disease states: Cancer, lymphoma, bacterial and viral infections, and other disease. J Clin Invest 52:1026, 1973.
251. Friou GJ: Current knowledge and concepts of the relationship of malignancy, autoimmunity, and immunologic disease. Ann NY Acad Sci 230:23, 1974.
252. Awerbuch MS, Brooks PM: Role of immune complexes in hypertrophic osteoarthropathy and nonmetastatic polyarthritis. Ann Rheum Dis 40:470, 1981.
253. Bradley JD, Pinals RS: Carcinoma polyarthritis: Role of immune complexes in pathogenesis. J Rheumatol 10:826, 1983.
254. Douglas GW, Levin RH, Sokoloff L: Infectious arthritis complicating neoplastic disease. N Engl J Med 270:299, 1964.
255. Keusch GT: Opportunistic infection in colon carcinoma. Am J Clin Nutr 27:1481, 1974.
256. Lyon LJ, Nevins MA: Carcinoma of the colon presenting as pyogenic arthritis. JAMA 241:2060, 1979.
257. Williams RC Jr: Dermatomyositis and malignancy: A review of the literature. Ann Intern Med 50:1174, 1959.
258. Curtis AC, Blaylock HC, Harrell ER Jr: Malignant lesions associated with dermatomyositis. JAMA 150:844, 1952.
259. Talal N, Bunim JJ: The development of malignant lymphoma in the course of Sjögren's syndrome. Am J Med 36:529, 1964.
260. Pagani JJ, Libshitz HI: Imaging bone metastases. Radiol Clin North Am 20:545, 1982.
261. Libshitz HI, Hortobagyi GN: Radiographic evaluation of therapeutic response in bony metastases of breast cancer. Skel Radiol 7:159, 1981.
262. Hortobagyi GN, Libshitz HI, Seabold JE: Osseous metastases of breast cancer. Clinical, biochemical, radiographic, and scintigraphic evaluation of response to therapy. Cancer. 53:577, 1984.
263. Barry WF Jr, Wells SA Jr, Cox CE, et al: Clinical and radiographic correlations in breast cancer patients with osseous metastases. Skel Radiol 6:27, 1981.
264. Pollen JJ, Reznek RH, Talner LB: Lysis of osteoblastic lesions in prostatic cancer: A sign of progression. AJR 142:1175, 1984.
265. Shortliffe LD, Freiha FS: Resolution of bony metastases after bilateral orchiectomy for carcinoma of prostate. Urology 17:353, 1981.
266. Pollen JJ, Shlaer WJ: Osteoblastic response to successful treatment of metastatic cancer of the prostate. AJR 132:927, 1979.
267. Merrick MV: Bone scans or skeletal surveys? Lancet 2:382, 1973.
268. Galasko CSB: Mechanism of uptake of bone imaging isotopes by skeletal metastases. Clin Nucl Med 12:565, 1980.
269. Shafer RB, Edeburn GF: Can the three-phase bone scan differentiate osteomyelitis from metabolic or metastatic bone disease? Clin Nucl Med 9:373, 1984.
270. Goergen TG, Alazraki NP, Halpern SE, et al: "Cold" bone lesions: A newly recognized phenomenon of bone imaging. J Nucl Med 15:1120, 1973.
271. Sy WM, Westring DW, Weinberger G: "Cold" lesions on bone imaging. J Nucl Med 16:1013, 1975.
272. Vieras F, Herzberg DL: Focal decreased skeletal uptake secondary to metastatic disease. Radiology 118:121, 1976.
273. Kagan AR, Steckel RJ: Lytic spine lesion and cold bone scan. AJR 136:129, 1981.
274. Witherspoon LR, Blonde L, Shuler SE, et al: Bone scan patterns of patients with diffuse metastatic carcinoma of the axial skeleton. J Nucl Med 17:253, 1976.
275. Constable AR, Cranage RW: Recognition of the superscan in prostatic bone scintigraphy. Br J Radiol 54:122, 1981.
276. Fukuda T, Inoue Y, Ochi H, et al: Abnormally high diffuse activity on bone scintigram. The importance of exposure time for its recognition. Eur J Nucl Med 7:275, 1982.
277. Corcoran RJ, Thrall JH, Kyle RW, et al: Solitary abnormalities in bone scans of patients with extraosseous malignancies. Radiology 121:663, 1976.
278. Sy WM, Mittal AK: Bone scan in chronic dialysis patients with evidence of secondary hyperparathyroidism and renal osteodystrophy. Br J Radiol 48:878, 1975.
279. Singh BN, Spies SM, Mehta SP, et al: Unusual bone scan presentation in osteomalacia: Symmetrical uptake—a suggestive sign. Clin Nucl Med 3:292, 1978.
280. Sostre S, Handler HL: Bony lesions in systemic mastocytosis: scintigraphic evaluation. Arch Dermatol 113:1245, 1977.
281. Bledin AG, Kim EE, Haynie TP: Bone scintigraphic findings related to unilateral mastectomy. Eur J Nucl Med 7:500, 1982.
282. Harbert JC, George FH, Kerner ML: Differentiation of rib fractures from metastases by bone scanning. Clin Nucl Med 6:359, 1981.
283. Hellman RS, Wilson MA: Discordance of sclerosing skeletal secondaries between sequential scintigraphy and radiographs. Clin Nucl Med 7:97, 1982.
284. Hardy JG, Kulatilake AE, Wastie ML: An index for monitoring bone metastases from carcinoma of the prostate. Br J Radiol 53:869, 1980.
285. Levenson RM, Sauerbrunn BJL, Bates HR, et al: Comparative value of bone scintigraphy and radiography in monitoring tumor response in systemically treated prostatic carcinoma. Radiology 146:513, 1983.
286. Condon BR, Buchanan R, Garvie NW, et al: Assessment of progression of secondary bone lesions following cancer of the breast or prostate using serial radionuclide imaging. Br J Radiol 54:18, 1981.
287. Rossleigh MA, Lovegrove FTA, Reynolds PM, et al: Serial bone scans in the assessment of response to therapy in advanced breast carcinoma. Clin Nucl Med 7:397, 1982.
288. DeLuca SA, Castronovo FP, Rhea JT: The effects of chemotherapy on bony metastases as measured by quantitative skeletal imaging. Clin Nucl Med 8:11, 1983.
289. McNeil BJ: Value of bone scanning in neoplastic disease. Semin Nucl Med 14:277, 1984.
290. Bitran JD, Bekerman C, Desser RK: The predictive value of serial bone scans in assessing response to chemotherapy in advanced breast cancer. Cancer 45:1562, 1980.
291. Pollen JJ, Witztum KF, Ashburn WL: The flare phenomenon on radionuclide bone scan in metastatic prostate cancer. AJR 142:773, 1984.
292. Collins JD, Bassett L, Main GD, et al: Percutaneous biopsy following positive bone scans. Radiology 132:439, 1979.
293. Harbin WP: Metastatic disease and the nonspecific bone scan: Value of spinal computed tomography. Radiology 145:105, 1982.
294. Hardy DC, Murphy WA, Gilula LA: Computed tomography in planning percutaneous bone biopsy. Radiology 134:447, 1980.
295. Braunstein EM, Kuhns LR: Computed tomographic demonstration of spinal metastases. Spine 8:912, 1983.
296. Redmond J III, Spring DB, Munderloh SH, et al: Spinal computed tomography scanning in the evaluation of metastatic disease. Cancer 54:253, 1984.
297. Hermann G, Rose JS, Strauss L: Tumor infiltration of the bone marrow: Comparative study using computed tomography. Skel Radiol 11:17, 1984.
298. Helms CA, Cann CE, Brunelle FO, et al: Detection of bone-marrow metastases using quantitative computed tomography. Radiology 140:745, 1981.
299. Pennes DR, Glazer GM, Wimbish KJ, et al: Chest wall invasion by lung cancer: Limitations of CT evaluation. AJR 144:507, 1985.
300. Zimmer WD, Berquist TH, McLeod RA, et al: Bone tumors: Magnetic resonance imaging versus computed tomography. Radiology 155:709, 1985.
301. Ramsey RG, Zacharias CE: MR imaging of the spine after radiation therapy: Easily recognizable effects. AJR 144:1131, 1985.
302. Simon MA, Karluk MB: Skeletal metastases of unknown origin. Diagnostic strategy for orthopedic surgeons. Clin Orthop 166:96, 1982.
303. Nystrom JS, Weiner JM, Heffelfinger-Juttner J, et al: Metastatic and histologic presentation in unknown primary cancer. Semin Oncol 4:53, 1977.
304. Steckel RJ, Kagan AR: Diagnostic persistence in working up metastatic cancer with an unknown primary site. Radiology 134:367, 1980.
305. Hebert J, Couser J, Seligson D: Closed medullary biopsy for disseminated malignancy. Clin Orthop 163:214, 1982.
306. Singer FR, Sharp CF Jr, Rude RK: Pathogenesis of hypercalcemia in malignancy. Mineral Electrol Metab 2:161, 1979.
307. Sharp CF Jr, Rude RK, Terry R, et al: Abnormal bone and parathyroid histology in carcinoma patients with pseudohyperparathyroidism. Cancer 49:1449, 1982.
308. Jung A, Schneider P, Millet R, et al: Hypercalcemia and parathyroid hyperplasia associated with renal adenocarcinoma. Postgrad Med J 52:106, 1976.
309. Smallridge RC, Wray HL, Schaaf M: Hypocalcemia with osteoblastic metastases in a patient with prostate carcinoma. A cause of secondary hyperparathyroidism. Am J Med 71:184, 1981.
310. Ludwig GD: Hypocalcemia and hypophosphatemia accompanying osteoblastic metastases: Studies of calcium and phosphate metabolism and parathyroid function. Ann Intern Med 56:676, 1962.
311. Lyles KW, Berry WR, Haussler M, et al: Hypophosphatemic osteomalacia: Association with prostatic carcinoma. Ann Intern Med 93:275, 1980.
312. Charhon S, Rouillat M, Bouvier M, et al: Osteomalacie vitaminosensible au cours des metastases osseuses condensantes prostatiques. A propos de deux cas. Rev Rhum Mal Osteoartic 48:469, 1981.
313. Franck JL, Bouteiller G, Fauchier C, et al: Profil biologique et histologique d'ostemalacie dans l'osteose condensante prostatique. A propos de 4 observations. Rev Rhum Mal Osteoartic 49:81, 1982.
314. Kabadi UM: Osteomalacia associated with prostatic cancer and osteoblastic metastases. Urology 21:65, 1983.
315. Weidner N, Bar RS, Weiss D, et al: Neoplastic pathology of oncogenic osteomalacia/rickets. Cancer 55:1691, 1985.
316. Gebhardt MC, Lippiello L, Bringhurst FR, et al: Prostaglandin E_2 synthesis by human primary and metastatic bone tumors in culture. Clin Orthop 196:300, 1985.
317. Sharp CF Jr: Humoral hypercalcemia of malignancy. The role of parathyroid hormone. NY State J Med 85:235, 1985.
318. Brushan B, Prasad J, Kaul V, et al: Osteoblastic metastases from thyroid carcinoma. Br J Radiol 58:563, 1985.
319. Garcia JF: Rapid regional osteolysis from pancreatic carcinoma. J Can Assoc Radiol 36:150, 1985.
320. Okazaki N, Yoshino M, Yoshida T, et al: Bone metastasis in hepatocellular carcinoma. Cancer 55:1991, 1985.
321. Leeson MC, Makley JT, Carter JR: Metastatic skeletal disease in the pediatric population. J Pediatr Orthop 5:261, 1985.
322. Amorosa JK, Weintraub S, Amorosa LF, et al: Sacral destruction: Foraminal lines revisited. AJR 145:773, 1985.
323. Manishen WJ, Sivananthan K, Orr FW: Resorbing bone stimulates tumor cell growth. A role for the host microenvironment in bone metastasis. Am J Pathol 123:39, 1986.

324. Leeson MC, Makley JT, Carter JR: Metastatic skeletal disease distal to the elbow and knee. Clin Orthop 206:94, 1986.

325. Healy JH, Turnbull ADM, Miedema B, et al: Acrometastases. J Bone Joint Surg [Am] 68:743, 1986.

326. Kuhlman JE, Fishman EK, Leichner PK, et al: Skeletal metastases from hepatoma: Frequency, distribution, and radiographic features. Radiology 160:175, 1986.

327. Keene JS, Sellinger DS, McBeath AA, et al: Metastatic breast cancer in the femur. A search for the lesion at risk of fracture. Clin Orthop 203:282, 1986.

328. Sartoris DJ, Clopton P, Nemcek A, et al: Vertebral-body collapse in focal and diffuse disease: Patterns of pathologic processes. Radiology 160:479, 1986.

329. Kagan AR, Steckel RJ, Bassett LW, et al: Radiologic contributions to cancer management. AJR 147:305, 1986.

330. Amin R: Regression of osteoblastic metastases from carcinoma of the prostate following therapy with tamoxifen. Br J Radiol 59:703, 1986.

331. Gold RH, Bassett LW: Radionuclide evaluation of skeletal metastases: Practical considerations. Skel Radiol 15:1, 1986.

332. Fink-Bennett D, Johnson J: Stippled ribs: A potential pitfall in bone scan interpretation. J Nucl Med 27:216, 1986.

333. Reiser M, Rupp N, Biehl Th, et al: MR in the diagnosis of bone tumours. Eur J Radiol 5:1, 1985.

334. Daffner RH, Lupetin AR, Dash N, et al: MRI in the detection of malignant infiltration of bone marrow. AJR 146:353, 1986.

335. Galasko CSB: Skeletal metastases. Clin Orthop 210:18, 1986.

336. Harrington KD: Metastatic disease of the spine. J Bone Joint Surg [Am] 68:1110, 1986.

337. Barnwell SL, Edwards MSB: Spinal intramedullary spread of medulloblastoma. Case report. J Neurosurg 65:253, 1986.

338. Vigorita VJ, Vitale A, Sclafani S, et al: Case report 403. Skel Radiol 15:680, 1986.

339. Lynn MD, Braunstein EM, Wahl RL, et al: Bone metastases in pheochromocytoma: Comparative studies of efficacy of imaging. Radiology 160:701, 1986.

340. Mink JH, Weitz I, Kagen AR, et al: Bone scan-positive and radiograph- and CT-negative vertebral lesion in a woman with locally advanced breast cancer. AJR 148:341, 1987.

341. Colson F, Tebib J, Bocquet B, et al: Ostéomalacie transitoire au cours du traitement hormonal des métastases ostéocondensantes prostatiques. Semin Hop Paris 62:2645, 1986.

342. Sim FH: Diagnosis and Management of Metastatic Bone Disease. A multidisciplinary Approach. Raven Press, New York, 1988.

343. Post MJD, Quencer RM, Green BA, et al: Intramedullary spinal cord metastases, mainly of nonneurogenic origin. AJR 148: 1015, 1987.

344. Krol G, Sze G, Malkin M, et al: MR of cranial and spinal meningeal carcinomatosis: Comparison with CT and myelography. AJR 151:583, 1988.

345. Frassica FJ, Sim FH: Pathophysiology. In FH Sim (Ed): Diagnosis and Management of Metastatic Bone Disease. A Multidisciplinary Approach. New York, Raven Press, 1988, p.7.

346. Aoki J, Yamamoto I, Hino M, et al: Osteoclast-mediated osteolysis in bone metastasis from renal cell carcinoma. Cancer 62:98, 1988.

347. Scher HI, Yagoda A: Bone metastases: Pathogenesis, treatment, and rationale for use of resorption inhibitors. Amer J Med 82:6, 1987.

348. Palmer E, Henrikson B, McKusick K, et al: Pain as an indicator of bone metastasis. Acta Radiolog 29:445, 1988.

349. Sim FH, Frassica FJ, Edmonson JH: Clinical and laboratory findings. In FH Sim (Ed): Diagnosis and Management of Metastatic Bone Disease. A Multidisciplinary Approach. New York, Raven Press, 1988, p. 25.

350. Kawamura H, Ogata K, Miura H, et al: Patellar metastases. A report of two cases. Intern Orthop (SICOT) 17:57, 1993.

351. Pazzaglia UE, Barbieri D, Cherubino P: Solitary metastasis of the patella as the first manifestation of lung cancer. Intern Orthop (SICOT) 13:75, 1989.

352. Libson E, Bloom RA, Husband JE, et al: Metastatic tumours of bones of the hand and foot. A comparative review and report of 43 additional cases. Skel Radiol 16:387, 1987.

353. Hattrup SJ, Amadio PC, Sim FH, et al: Metastatic tumors of the foot and ankle. Foot Ankle 8:243, 1988.

354. Amadio PC, Lombardi RM: Metastatic tumors of the hand. J Hand Surg [Am] 12:311, 1987.

355. Kerin R: The hand in metastatic disease. J Hand Surg [Am] 12:77, 1987.

356. Kolstad K, Högstorp H: Gastric carcinoma metastasis to a knee with a newly inserted prosthesis. A case report. Acta Orthop Scand 61:369, 1990.

357. Haller J, André MP, Resnick D, et al: Detection of thoracolumbar vertebral body destruction with lateral spine radiography. Part I: Investigation in cadavers. Invest Radiol 25:517, 1990.

358. Haller J, André MP, Resnick D, et al: Detection of thoracolumbar vertebral body destruction with lateral spine radiography. Part II: Clinical investigation with computed tomography. Invest Radiol 25:523, 1990.

359. Coerkamp EG, Kroon HM: Cortical bone metastases. Radiology 169:525, 1988.

360. Greenspan A, Norman A: Osteolytic cortical destruction: an unusual pattern of skeletal metastases. Skel Radiol 17:402, 1988.

361. Wendling D, Guidet M: Métastases osseuses pseudosarcomateuses. A propos de quatre observations. Sem Hôp Paris 65:5, 1989.

362. Bloom RA, Libson E, Husband JE, et al: The periosteal sunburst reaction to bone metastases. A literature review and report of 20 additional cases. Skel Radiol 16:629, 1987.

363. Toussirot E, Lafforgue P, Tonolli I, et al: Muscular metastasis as the first manifestation of malignancy: Distinctive features in three cases. Rev Rhum [Engl] 60:135, 1993.

364. Sridhar KS, Rao RK, Kunhardt B: Skeletal muscle metastases from lung cancer. Cancer 59:1530, 1987.

365. Menck H, Schulze S, Larsen E: Metastasis size in pathologic femoral fractures. Acta Orthop Scand 59:151, 1988.

366. Hipp JA, McBroom RJ, Cheal EJ, et al: Structural consequences of endosteal metastatic lesions in long bones. J Orthop Res 7:828, 1989.

367. McBroom RJ, Cheal EJ, Hayes WC: Strength reductions from metastatic cortical defects in long bones. J Orthop Res 6:369, 1988.

368. Leggon RE, Lindsey RW, Panjabi MM: Strength reduction and the effects of treatment of long bones with diaphyseal defects involving 50% of the cortex. J Orthop Res 6:540, 1988.

369. Habermann ET, Lopez RA: Metastatic disease of bone and treatment of pathologic fractures. Orthop Clin North Am 20:469, 1989.

370. Wong DA, Fornasier VL, MacNab I: Spinal metastases: The obvious, the occult, and the imposters. Spine 15:1, 1990.

371. Yochum TR, Sellers LT, Oppenheimer DA, et al: The sclerotic pedicle—how many causes are there? Skel Radiol 19:411, 1990.

372. Algra PR, Heimans JJ, Valk J, et al: Do metastases in vertebrae begin in the body or the pedicles? Imaging study in 45 patients. AJR 158:1275, 1992.

373. Asdourian PL, Weidenbaum M, DeWald RL, et al: The pattern of vertebral involvement in metastatic vertebral breast cancer. Clin Orthop 250:164, 1990.

374. Mirels H: Metastatic disease in long bones. A proposed scoring system for diagnosing impending pathologic fractures. Clin Orthop 249:256, 1989.

375. Phillips CD, Pope TL Jr, Jones JE, et al: Nontraumatic avulsion of the lesser trochanter: a pathognomonic sign of metastatic disease? Skel Radiol 17:106, 1988.

376. Turan I, Sjöden GOJ, Kalén A: Ovarian carcinoma metastasis to the little finger. A case report. Acta Orthop Scand 61:185, 1990.

377. Sherry MM, Greco FA, Johnson DH, et al: Metastatic breast cancer confined to the skeletal system. An indolent disease. Amer J Med 81:381, 1986.

378. Kamby C, Vejborg I, Daugaard S, et al: Clinical and radiologic characteristics of bone metastases in breast cancer. Cancer 60:2524, 1987.

379. Powell JM: Metastatic carcinoid of bone. Report of two cases and review of the literature. Clin Orthop 230:266, 1988.

380. Silverman JM: Case report 659. Skel Radiol 20:149, 1991.

381. Roblot P, Azais I, Alcalay M, et al: Une métastase hypertrophiante au cours d'un cancer de la prostate. Sem Hôp Paris 65:357, 1989.

382. Patten RM, Shuman WP, Teefey S: Metastasis from malignant melanoma to the axial skeleton: A CT study of frequency and appearance. AJR 155:109, 1990.

383. Motzkin NE, Rock MG, Wold LE, et al: Malignant melanoma metastatic to bone. Orthop 15:657, 1992.

384. Sanzari R, Paton P, Boutet O, et al: Métastases osseuses pseudo-sarcomateuses des cancers recto-sigmoïdo-coliques. Sem Hôp Paris 68:1369, 1992.

385. Reed JD, Fishman EK, Kuhlman JE, et al: Case report 535. Skel Radiol 18:161, 1989.

386. Vieco PT, Azouz EM, Hoeffel J-C: Metastasis to bone in medulloblastoma. A report of five cases. Skel Radiol 18:445, 1989.

387. Olson EN, Tien RD, Chamberlain MC: Osseous metastasis in medulloblastoma: MRI findings in an unusual case. Clin Imag 15:286, 1991.

388. Pelissou I, Roullet B, Vidal J, et al: Métastases extra-névraxiques d'un medulloblastome de l'adulte. Sem Hôp Paris 64:1045, 1988.

389. Algra PR, Postma T, Van Groeningen CJ, et al: MR imaging of skeletal metastases from medulloblastoma. Skel Radiol 21:425, 1992.

390. Jacobs JJ, Rosenberg AE: Extracranial skeletal metastasis from a pinealoblastoma. A case report and review of the literature. Clin Orthop 247:256, 1989.

391. Resnik CS, Young JWR, Aisner SC, et al: Case report 618. Skel Radiol 19:371, 1990.

392. David R, Eftenkhari F, Lamki N, et al: The many faces of neuroblastoma. RadioGraphics 9:859, 1989.

393. Dietrich RB, Kangarloo H, Lenarsky C, et al: Neuroblastoma: The role of MR imaging. AJR 148:937, 1987.

394. Chaloupka JC: Primary neuroblastoma of a vertebra: An unusual location for a variant of primitive neuroectodermal tumor of bone. AJR 159:1130, 1992.

395. Jaffe R, Santamaria M, Yunis EJ, et al: The neuroectodermal tumor of bone. Am J Surg Pathol 8:885, 1984.

396. Araki N, Uchida A, Kimura T, et al: Involvement of the retinoblastoma gene in primary osteosarcomas and other bone and soft-tissue tumors. Clin Orthop 270:271, 1991.

397. Zammit-Maempel I, Johnson RJ, Gattamaneni HR: Late presentation of bone metastases in phaeochromocytoma. Brit J Radiol 64:369, 1991.

398. Glassman AH, Kean JR, Martino JD, et al: Subtrochanteric pathologic fracture of both femora secondary to malignant pheochromocytoma. A case report. J Bone Joint Surg [Am] 72:1554, 1990.

399. Lynn MD, Braunstein EM, Shapiro B: Pheochromocytoma presenting as musculoskeletal pain from bone metastases. Skeletal Radiol 16:552, 1987.

400. Parnell AP, Dick DJ: Extradural metastases from paraganglionomas. Report of two cases. Clin Radiol 39:65, 1988.

401. Khurana JS, Kattapuram SV, Ehara S, et al: Case report 577. Skel Radiol 18:565, 1989.

402. Hermann G, Moss D, Norton KI, et al: Case report 450. Skel Radiol 16:657, 1987.

403. Moran C, Braunstein EM, Ulbright T, et al: Case report 689. Skel Radiol 20:465, 1991.

404. Jungreis CA, Sekhar LN, Martinez AJ, et al: Cardiac myxoma metastatic to the temporal bone. Radiology 170:244, 1989.
405. McLennan MK: Case report 657. Skel Radiol 20:141, 1991.
406. Ribalta T, Shannon RL, Ro JY, et al: Case report 645. Skel Radiol 19:616, 1990.
407. Meltzer CC, Fishman EK, Scott WW Jr: Computed tomography appearance of bone metastases of leiomyosarcoma. Skel Radiol 21:445, 1992.
408. Grober A, Goldberg I, Rotem A: Malignant eccrine poroma with metastatic involvement of the long bones. Clin Orthop 223:303, 1987.
409. Gerster J-C, Jaquier E, Ribaux C: Nonspecific inflammatory monoarthritis in the vicinity of bony metastases. J Rheumatol 14:844, 1987.
410. Benhamou CL, Tourliere D, Brigant S, et al: Synovial metastasis of an adenocarcinoma presenting as a shoulder monoarthritis. J Rheumatol 15:1031, 1988.
411. Schwarzer AC, Fryer J, Preston SJ, et al: Metastatic adenosquamous carcinoma presenting as an acute ankle monoarthritis, with a review of the literature. J Orthop Rheumatol 3:175, 1990.
412. Lario BA, Lopez JA, Santos JT, et al: Chronic metastatic arthritis as the first symptom of lung adenocarcinoma. Scand J Rheumatol 18:169, 1989.
413. Johnson JJ, Leonard-Segal A, Nashel DJ: Jaccoud's-type arthropathy: An association with malignancy. J Rheumatol 16:1278, 1989.
414. O'Keefe D, Gholkar A: Metastatic adenocarcinoma of the paraspinal muscles. Brit J Radiol 61:849, 1988.
415. Pauli B, Schwartz DE, Thoner EJM, et al: Tumor invasion and host extracellular matrix. Cancer Metab Review 2:129, 1983.
416. Hazeltine M, Duranceau L, Gariepy G: Presentation of breast carcinoma as Volkmann's contracture due to skeletal muscle metastases. J Rheumatol 17:1097, 1990.
417. Munk PL, Gock S, Gee R, et al: Case report 708. Skel Radiol 21:56, 1992.
418. Turosian M, Botet J, Paglia M: Colon carcinoma metastatic to the thigh, an unusual site of metastasis: Report of a case. Dis Colon Rectum 30:805, 1987.
419. Buerger LC, Montelone PN: Leukemic lymphomatous infiltration of skeletal muscle. Cancer 19:1416, 1966.
420. Pearson CM: Incidence and type of pathological alterations observed in muscle in a routine autopsy survey. Neurology 9:757, 1959.
421. Twining P, Williams MR, Morris AH, et al: The use of the pelvic radiograph alone to assess therapeutic response in bone metastases from breast cancer. Clin Radiol 39:583, 1988.
422. Tumeh SS, Beadle B, Kaplan WD: Clinical significance of solitary rib lesions in patients with extraskeletal malignancy. J Nucl Med 26:1140, 1985.
423. Massie JD, Sebes JI: The headless bone scan: an uncommon manifestation of metastatic superscan in carcinoma of the prostate. Skel Radiol 17:111, 1988.
424. Frank JA, Ling A, Patronas NJ, et al: Detection of malignant bone tumors: MR imaging vs scintigraphy. AJR 155:1043, 1990.
425. Jacobson AF, Cronin EB, Stomper PC, et al: Bone scans with one or two new abnormalities in cancer patients with no known metastases: Frequency and serial scintigraphic behavior of benign and malignant lesions. Radiology 175:229, 1990.
426. Kwai AH, Stomper PC, Kaplan WD: Clinical significance of isolated scintigraphic sternal lesions in patients with breast cancer. J Nucl Med 29:324, 1988.
427. Merrick MV: Bone scintigraphy—an update. Clin Radiol 40:231, 1989.
428. Colman LK, Porter BA, Redmond J III, et al: Early diagnosis of spinal metastases by CT and MR studies. J Comput Assist Tomogr 12:423, 1988.
429. Reinbold W-D, Wannenmacher M, Hodapp N, et al: Osteodensitometry of vertebral metastases after radiotherapy using quantitative computed tomography. Skel Radiol 18:517, 1989.
430. Rafii M, Firoozinia H, Golimbu C, et al: CT of skeletal metastasis. Semin Ultrasound, CT, MR 7:371, 1986.
431. Abdelwahab IF, Miller TT, Hermann G, et al: Transarticular invasion of joints by bone tumors: hypothesis. Skel Radiol 20:279, 1991.
432. Yasuma T, Yamauchi Y, Arai K, et al: Histopathologic study on tumor infiltration into the intervertebral disc. Spine 14:1245, 1989.
433. Ricci C, Cova M, Kang YS, et al: Normal age-related patterns of cellular and fatty bone marrow distribution in the axial skeleton: MR imaging study. Radiology 177:83, 1990.
434. Dawson KL, Moore SG, Rowland JM: Age-related marrow changes in the pelvis: MR and anatomic findings. Radiology 183:47, 1992.
435. Vogler JB III, Murphy WA: Bone marrow imaging. Radiology 168:679, 1988.
436. Smoker WRK, Godersky JC, Knutzon RK, et al: The role of MR imaging in evaluating metastatic spinal disease. AJR 149:1241, 1987.
437. Godersky JC, Smoker WRK, Knutzon R: Use of magnetic resonance imaging in the evaluation of metastatic spinal disease. Neurosurg 21:676, 1987.
438. Carmody RF, Yang PJ, Seeley GW, et al: Spinal cord compression due to metastatic disease: Diagnosis with MR imaging versus myelography. Radiology 173:225, 1989.
439. Williams MP, Cherryman GR, Husband JE: Magnetic resonance imaging in suspected metastatic spinal cord compression. Clin Radiol 40:286, 1989.
440. Kamholtz R, Sze G: MRI of spinal metastases. MRI Decisions, Nov/Dec 1990, p 2.
441. Algra PR, Bloem JL, Tissing H, et al: Detection of vertebral metastases: Comparison between MR imaging and bone scintigraphy. RadioGraphics 11:219, 1991.
442. Smolarz K, Jungehülsing M, Krug B, et al: Kernspintomographie des knochenmarks bei Karzinompatienten mit einer solitären Mehranreicherung im Skelettszintigramm. Nucl Med 29:269, 1990.
443. Kattapuram SV, Khurana JS, Scott JA, et al: Negative scintigraphy with positive magnetic resonance imaging in bone metastases. Skel Radiol 19:113, 1990.
444. Ruzal-Shapiro C, Berdon WE, Cohen MD, et al: MR imaging of diffuse bone marrow replacement in pediatric patients with cancer. Radiology 181:587, 1991.
445. Sze G, Krol G, Zimmerman RD, et al: Malignant extradural spinal tumors: MR imaging with Gd-DTPA. Radiology 167:217, 1988.
446. Stimac GK, Porter BA, Olson DO, et al: Gadolinium-DTPA–enhanced MR imaging of spinal neoplasms: Preliminary investigation and comparison with unenhanced spin-echo and STIR sequences. AJR 151:1185, 1988.
447. Baker LL, Goodman SB, Perkash I, et al: Benign versus pathologic compression fractures of vertebral bodies: Assessment with conventional spin-echo, chemical-shift, and STIR MR imaging. Radiology 174:495, 1990.
448. Yuh WTC, Zachar CK, Barloon TJ, et al: Vertebral compression fractures: distinction between benign and malignant causes with MR imaging. Radiology 172:215, 1989.
449. Barloon TJ, Yuh WTC, Yang CTC, et al: Spinal subarachnoid tumor seeding from intracranial metastasis: MR findings. J Comput Assist Tomogr 11:242, 1987.
450. Sze G: MRI of tumor metastases to the leptomeninges. MRI Decisions, Jan/Feb 1988, p. 2.
451. Sze G, Abramson A, Krol G, et al: Gadolinium-DTPA in the evaluation of intradural extramedullary spinal disease. AJR 150:911, 1988.
452. Lowe GM, Ramsey RG: MRI of spinal meningeal carcinomatosis. MRI Decisions, May/June 1992, p 24.
453. Lim V, Sobel DF, Zyloff J: Spinal cord pial metastases: MR imaging with gadopentetate dimeglumine. AJNR 11:975, 1990.
454. Paako E, Patronas NJ, Schellinger D: Meningeal Gd-DTPA enhancement in patients with malignancies. J Comput Assist Tomogr 14:542, 1990.
455. Grem JL, Burgess J, Trump DL: Clinical features and natural history of intramedullary spinal cord metastasis. Cancer 56:2305, 1985.
456. Sze G, Krol G, Zimmerman RD, et al: Intramedullary disease of the spine: Diagnosis using gadolinium-DTPA–enhanced MR imaging. AJR 151:1193, 1988.
457. Sze G, Bravo S, Krol G: Spinal lesions: Quantitative and qualitative temporal evolution of gadopentetate dimeglumine enhancement in MR imaging. Radiology 170:849, 1989.
458. Reijnierse M, Bloem JL, Doornbos J, et al: The signal intensity of the normal odontoid process (dens) displayed on magnetic resonance images. Skel Radiol 21:519, 1992.
459. Deutsch AL, Mink JH, Rosenfeld EP, et al: Incidental detection of hematopoietic hyperplasia on routine knee MR imaging. AJR 152:333, 1989.
460. Shellock FG, Morris E, Deutsch AL, et al: Hematopoietic bone marrow hyperplasia: High prevalence on MR images of the knee in asymptomatic marathon runners. AJR 158:335, 1992.
461. Nottebaert M, Exner GU, von Hochstetter AR, et al: Metastatic bone disease from occult carcinoma: a profile. Intern Orthop (SICOT) 13:119, 1989.
462. Le Chevalier T, Cvitkovie E, Caille P, et al: Early metastatic cancer of unknown primary origin at presentation. A clinical study of 302 consecutive autopsied patients. Arch Int Med 148:2035, 1988.
463. Pritchard DJ, Berquist TH: Role of biopsy. In FH Sim, (Ed): Diagnosis and Management of Metastatic Bone Disease. A Multidisciplinary Approach. Edited by New York, Raven Press, 1988, p. 69.
464. North CA, Zinreich ES, Christensen WN, et al: Multiple spinal metastases from paraganglioma. Cancer 66:2224, 1990.
465. Vanel D, Lacombe M-J, Couanet D, et al: Musculoskeletal tumors: Follow-up with MR imaging after treatment with surgery and radiation therapy. Radiology 164:243, 1987.
466. Nuovo MA, Dorfman HD, Sun C-CJ, et al: Tumor-induced osteomalacia and rickets. Amer J Surg Path 13:588, 1989.
467. Feldman F: Skeletal manifestations of ectopic and inappropriate endocrine and metabolic syndromes. Radiol Clin North Am 29:119, 1991.
468. Garrett IR: Bone destruction in cancer. Semin Oncol 20:4, 1993.
469. Shapeero LG, Couanet D, Vanel D, et al: Bone metastases as the presenting manifestation of rhabdomyosarcoma in childhood. Skel Radiol 22:433, 1993.
470. Rougraff BT, Kneisl JS, Simon MA: Skeletal metastases of unknown origin. A prospective study of a diagnostic strategy. J Bone Joint Surg [Am] 75:1276, 1993.
471. Mirowitz SA, Apicella P, Reinus WR, et al: MR imaging of bone marrow lesions: Relative conspicuousness on T1-weighted, fat-suppressed T2-weighted, and STIR images. AJR 162:215, 1994.
472. Georgy BA, Hesselink JR: MR imaging of the spine: Recent advances in pulse sequences and special techniques. AJR 161:923, 1994.
473. Schweitzer ME, Levine C, Mitchell DG, et al: Bull's eyes and halos: Useful MR discriminators of osseous metastasis. Radiology 188:249, 1993.
474. Sugimura H, Kisanuki A, Tamura S, et al: Magnetic resonance imaging of bone marrow changes after irradiation. Invest Radiol 29:35, 1994.

Congenital Diseases

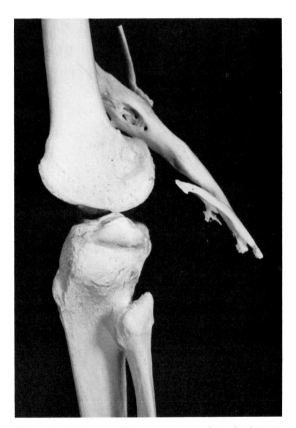

Fibrodysplasia ossificans progressiva: An irregular osseous sheet extends from the posterior surface of the femur across the back of the knee, and there is bony ankylosis of the proximal tibiofibular articulation. (From Resnick D: Skel Radiol *10*:131, 1983).

86

Developmental Dysplasia of the Hip

David J. Sartoris, M.D.

Developmental dysplasia of the hip (DDH) is a disease with extremely variable morphologic patterns. Although detection of DDH at birth by appropriate neonatal clinical and imaging examinations and immediate inception of treatment are desirable, the diagnosis is missed in many children, who subsequently come to medical attention for evaluation and treatment at several months to years of age.[1-3] At any stage of initial diagnosis, regardless of age, the primary goal is to delineate the specific pathologic morphology to direct the most appropriate treatment.

Subluxation and dislocation of the developing hip represent arbitrary definitions of static stages within a spectrum of dynamic morphologic alterations that often are of insidious onset and subtle in initial clinical and radiographic presentation. External factors, whether antenatal or postnatal, may have a significant role in the progressive deformation that inexorably occurs if the condition is not recognized clinically and radiographically.[4] Such factors may be breech presentation, anteversion of the femur, and contrac-

tures of the hip joint.[5, 6] During the neonatal period, when prompt diagnosis should be accomplished, routine radiography of the chondro-osseous hip has significant limitations, and imaging techniques capable of demonstrating unmineralized tissue frequently are required.

ETIOLOGY

The cause and pathogenesis of DDH are controversial and not completely understood. Although commonly used terminology implies that the dislocation occurs prenatally, most dislocations probably occur after birth. The factors predisposing to this situation, however, unquestionably are present in utero. The complex of musculoligamentous, capsular, cartilaginous, and osseous alterations that follow the dislocation are thought to be secondary effects and not causative. The alternative terms infantile dislocation, congenital dysplasia or displacement, and instability of the hip thus have been applied to the condition.[7]

Some investigators contend that instability, partial dislocation (subluxation), and complete dislocation exist as a continuum, with one form passing to another under appropriate conditions, whereas other researchers maintain that subluxation and dislocation are discrete fixed entities. Pathophysiologically, abnormal laxity rather than structural abnormality is most likely responsible for DDH, a hypothesis supported by an animal model of the disease (Fig. 86–1).[8] Increased laxity of the hip and other joints is seen in many patients with DDH as well as in otherwise normal members of their families. During the initial several days after birth, normal newborn infants may exhibit up to 6 mm of posterior femoral displacement on stress sonograms.[9] This may be secondary to the hormonal effect induced by maternal estrogen that is not completely inactivated by the immature fetal liver.

Although in the great majority of cases no other family members besides the patient have the disease, heritable factors are important.[10] The risk for normal parents of a child with DDH to have another affected child is about 6 per cent; if one parent also is affected, the risk increases to 36 per cent.[11] The risk to a patient's own children is estimated to be 12 per cent.

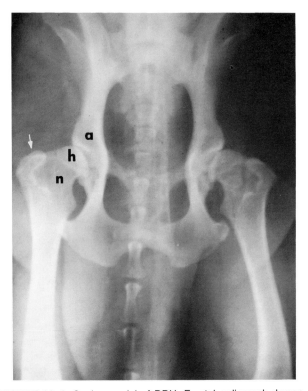

FIGURE 86–1. Canine model of DDH. Frontal radiograph demonstrates bilateral and symmetric abnormalities, including deformity of the femoral heads *(h)*, short and broad femoral necks *(n)*, greater trochanteric overgrowth (arrow), shallow acetabula *(a)*, and secondary degenerative joint disease.

The etiologic role of anatomic variation in the acetabulum or femoral neck is controversial. The acetabulum tends to become shallower and the femoral head more hemispherical during fetal life, a situation that could promote dislocation, and the parents of children with DDH are found to have diminished acetabular coverage. Of great importance is the role that the usually intrauterine position of hip flexion plays in maintaining proper position of the femoral head.[12] Both extreme flexion with knee extension (assumed with some breech positions) and sudden extension during birth tend to promote femoral head dislocation. The hyperflexion of breech presentation leads also to shortening and contracture of the iliopsoas muscle, which tends to perpetuate femoral displacement. DDH occurs in approximately 30 per cent of infants with breech presentation.[13] Associated abnormalities related to abnormal mechanical forces in utero include deformities of the lower extremity (equinovarus, metatarsus varus) and torticollis.[14]

Prenatal and postnatal pathologic patterns of the hip can be classified into three major groups (Fig. 86–2).[15] Type 1 is the most common group and corresponds to the dislocatable, unstable hip. Anatomic alterations include a slight increase in femoral anteversion and mild marginal abnormalities in the acetabular cartilage with early labral eversion. Type 2 includes the partially dislocated or subluxed hip, characterized by loss of femoral head sphericity, increased femoral anteversion, early labral eversion with hypertrophy, and a shallow acetabulum. In type 3, accentuated flattening of the femoral head and acetabulum occur, with inward growth and hypertrophy of the labrum (so-called limbus formation). Conventional radiography is relatively insensitive to these changes until acetabular ossification is advanced.

The concept of the dislocatable or unstable (type 1) hip is important clinically. Such instability is estimated to occur in from 0.25 to 0.85 per cent of all newborn infants. More than 60 per cent of these hips, however, will become stable when reexamined by Ortolani or Barlow maneuvers within 1 week of birth, and 88 per cent are stable by the age of 2 months. Thus, the vast majority of hips noted to be dislocatable at birth will not be dislocated persistently. As it is not possible to predict which of these will become stable spontaneously, all are treated conventionally to prevent established dislocation.

Although most dislocations occur during the first 2 weeks after birth, occasionally a dislocation will occur up to 1 year of age in patients documented to be normal previously. This is particularly true among infants with either a positive family history of DDH, breech presentation, or a persistent hip click on clinical examination.[16] Evidence also exists that rare late initial dislocations occur during childhood.

EPIDEMIOLOGY

Neonatal clinical examination will identify between 10 and 20 unstable hips per 1000 live births.[17] Female infants are affected by hip dislocation approximately eight times more frequently than male infants. Among affected infants, breech deliveries are six times more frequent than vertex presentations. DDH is significantly more common among white than among black newborn infants, and infants treated in a neonatal intensive care unit are at higher risk.[13]

Nearly two thirds of infants with hip instability are first-born, suggesting that the maternal uterus and abdominal wall in a primigravida are more confining and thus perpetuate abnormal stresses on the developing hip joint. The position of the fetus within the uterus and the relationship between the two legs may account for the 11:1:4 ratio of left to right to bilateral hip involvement.[18]

The prevalence of DDH in children with infantile idiopathic scoliosis has been shown to be 6.4 per cent, approximately 10 times its frequency in the general population. A female predominance exists in both disorders, and plagiocephaly may be an associated malformation when the conditions coexist. In patients with unilateral hip dislocation, the concavity of the thoracic scoliosis is on the contralateral side.[19] Occult spinal dysraphism also has been described in association with DDH.[38]

CLINICAL DETECTION

The most reliable methods for diagnosing DDH in the neonatal period are clinical: the Ortolani and Barlow maneuvers.[21] The Ortolani test assesses proximal femoral reduction into the acetabulum by progressive abduction of the hip. The Barlow test is the reverse; the proximal portion of the femur is displaced by progressive adduction. Despite routine application of these tests, which are positive for only a few days after birth, a 0.1 to 0.2 per cent prevalence of late diagnosis exists among infants found to be normal in the neonatal period.[22–26] Experienced examiners are required for accurate early clinical diagnosis of DDH.[27–29] It

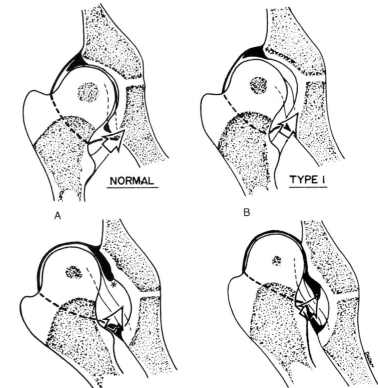

FIGURE 86–2. Schematic diagram of hip dysplasia patterns (arrows, course of iliopsoas tendon).

A Normal. The acetabular labrum *(L)* is in an everted position.

B Type 1. Positionally unstable or subluxatable hip. The pliable labrum may be deformed slightly.

C Type 2. Subluxated hip, with eversion of the fibrocartilaginous labrum, which may exhibit some inversion (asterisk). This type of hip subluxation may be reduced relatively easily in flexion.

D Type 3. Dislocated hip, with inversion and hypertrophy of the labrum, which presents an impediment to reduction.

(Courtesy of J. Ogden, M.D., Tampa, Florida.)

has been suggested that repeated clinical examination actually may increase hip instability.[30]

Primary anterior developmental dislocation of the hip can be diagnosed in infancy as an entity distinct from the more common posterior dislocation. Anterior dislocations are characterized by a fullness in the femoral triangle, external rotation at rest, marked limitation of abduction, severe pelvic tilt, and marked limb shortening. Conservative treatment with adduction splinting and closed reduction is recommended, although most patients also require derotational osteotomy for correction of femoral anteversion.[31]

During the first year, certain clinical findings become more obvious in the child with undiagnosed DDH. Anatomically, the surrounding soft tissues and chondro-osseous components gradually adapt to the abnormal relationship between the femoral head and the acetabulum. Reduction of the femoral head becomes progressively more difficult, and results of the Ortolani and Barlow tests become negative. Major muscle groups become shortened and contracted; adductor muscle tightness becomes increasingly apparent.

Subluxation or dislocation of the hip may be discovered months or years after multiple previous physical examinations with normal results. In such cases, an increased acetabular index may allow the femoral head to migrate laterally and become a delayed dislocation. The delayed subluxed or dislocated hip has been described as a condition that may be unrelated to neonatal hip instability.[32] Positive family history is a stronger predictor of late-presenting DDH than is breech presentation.[33–35]

DIAGNOSTIC IMAGING EVALUATION

Selection of appropriate imaging techniques in patients with DDH depends on age and differs for diagnostic versus management situations. Ultrasonography generally is preferred over conventional radiography among children under 1 year of age. Contrast arthrography and CT are indicated for preoperative planning. MR imaging also is a useful method, but its specific role remains to be completely established.[36]

Conventional Radiography

Neonatal Period. If the hip is unstable or has dislocated postnatally, conventional radiography in neutral and frog-leg projections will be unrevealing. Both of these positions may reduce a dislocatable hip and result in an erroneous impression of normality. The pelvis similarly will be normal as no secondary alterations in the osseous acetabulum will have occurred.

Radiologic confirmation of dislocation is not mandatory prior to initiation of treatment in clinically positive cases. A positive radiograph can, however, be obtained by applying a dislocating Ortolani or Barlow maneuver during the exposure (Fig. 86–3A). A dislocation-promoting position also has been described in which the legs are abducted to at least 45 degrees with simultaneous forced internal rotation. A line drawn along the axis of the femoral shaft in a nondislocated hip will pass through the upper edge of the acetabulum and cross the midline at the lumbosacral junc-

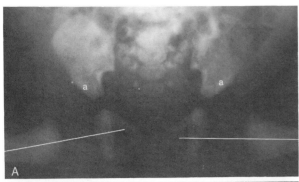

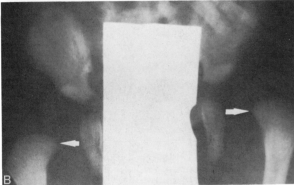

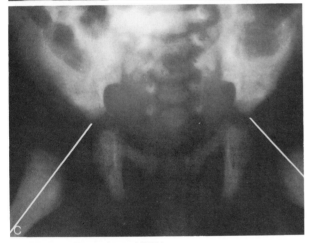

FIGURE 86-3. Bilateral type I DDH.

A On a radiograph with the hips in an Ortolani position, absence of femoral head ossification and shallow acetabula (a) are evident, as is symmetric malalignment. White lines indicate femoral shaft axes.

B Lateralization of both femora (arrows) is demonstrated with the joints in neutral position.

C On an abduction-internal rotation (von Rosen) view, alignment is normal (femoral shaft axes indicated by white lines passing symmetrically through the acetabula), indicating bilateral reduction.

tion. In a dislocated hip, this line will intersect the antero-superior iliac spine and traverse the midline in the lumbar region. The abduction-internal rotation position on occasion can lead to spontaneous hip reduction and a false-negative finding (Fig. 86-3B, C). Assessment of the relationship of the femoral head to the acetabulum in the neonate is complicated by the fact that the ossification center is not yet visible; hence its position must be inferred from the orientation of the femoral metaphysis (Fig. 86-4).[37] The femoral shaft should be located below a horizontal line drawn through the Y synchondroses, and the apex of the metaph-

ysis should lie medial to the edge of the acetabulum. The cartilaginous femoral epiphysis is slightly larger than the neck segment on which it rests. Hence, if a circle with diameter equivalent to the width of the femoral metaphysis is drawn on the shaft, the position of the epiphysis relative to the acetabulum can be estimated. Fat planes along the labrum and the edge of the joint capsule also help to delineate the position of the cartilaginous epiphysis.[38]

Childhood Period. Secondary capsular, ligamentous, muscular, and cartilaginous changes occur soon after persistent dislocation has been established. These abnormalities are extremely important to therapeutic decision making and prognosis but are occult radiologically. Early positive conventional radiographic findings imply that substantial cartilage and soft tissue deformation already has occurred. The earliest time at which the radiologic changes of a typical dislocated hip on a single radiograph can be recognized reliably is approximately 6 weeks of age.

As the child grows, the adaptive changes of the hip joint and femur become more evident on the routine radiograph. The characteristic findings include (1) proximal and lateral migration of the femoral neck adjacent to the ilium, (2) a shallow, incompletely developed acetabulum (acetabular dysplasia), (3) development of a false acetabulum, and (4) delayed ossification of the femoral ossific nucleus (Figs. 86-4 and 86-5).[39] Several radiologic lines have been described to distinguish between the normal and the dislocated hip (Fig. 86-6). The lines are drawn on an anteroposterior view of the pelvis and hips. Accurate positioning is critical; the hips must be extended, with the lower extremities aligned normally and in neutral rotation. Abnormal position can alter the diagnostic value of the lines considerably.[40]

The radiologic lines that have been found to be the most reliable and helpful in the diagnosis of DDH are summarized as follows:

1. The acetabular index or angle (Fig. 86-7) is a measurement of the apparent slope of the acetabular roof, which averages 27.5 degrees in newborn infants. The upper limit of normal is 30 degrees; a measurement greater than this strongly suggests acetabular dysplasia.

2. Lateral migration of the femoral head is measured by using the horizontal line of Hilgenreiner (through the triradiate cartilage) and its intersection with Perkin's line (a vertical line drawn downward from the lateral rim of the acetabulum). The intersection of these two lines divides the hip joint into quadrants. The femoral ossific nucleus, if present, or medial peak of the femoral metaphysis is within the inner lower quadrant if the hip is normal, but it is in the upper outer quadrant if the hip is dislocated.

3. Proximal migration of the femur is measured by observing the shortening of the vertical distance from the femoral ossific nucleus or the femoral metaphysis to Hilgenreiner's line.

4. Shenton's line is drawn between the medial border of the neck of the femur and the superior border of the obturator foramen. In the normal hip this line is an even, continuous arc, whereas in a dislocated hip with proximal displacement of the femoral head, it is broken and interrupted (Fig. 86-8).

These lines are helpful in the child with unilateral dislocation, when the abnormal side can be compared to the

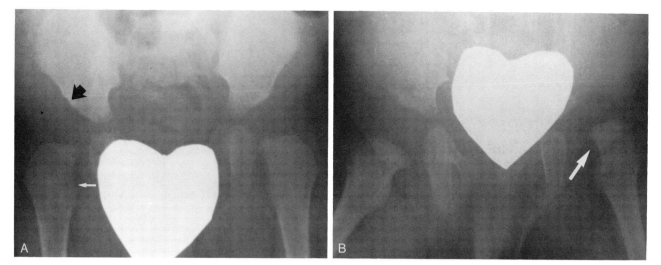

FIGURE 86–4. Types I and II DDH.

A Type I. The right femur is slightly lateralized (white arrow), in association with subtle flattening of the lateral acetabular margin (black arrow).

B Type II. In another patient, the left femur is displaced superolaterally (arrow).

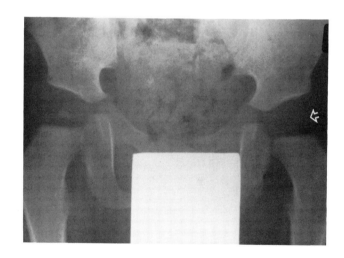

FIGURE 86–5. Type I DDH. Delayed development of the left femoral head ossification center (arrow) is evident by comparison with the normal right side.

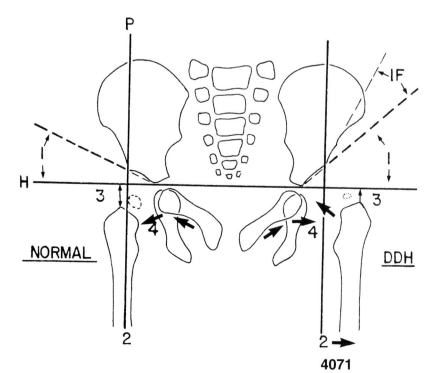

FIGURE 86–6. Radiographic indications of DDH (left side is abnormal). *I,* Acetabular index; *IF,* additional index of false acetabulum; *2,* lateral migration; *H,* Hilgenreiner's line; *P,* Perkin's line; *3,* superior migration; *4,* Shenton's line. (Courtesy of J. Ogden, M.D., Tampa, Florida.)

4071

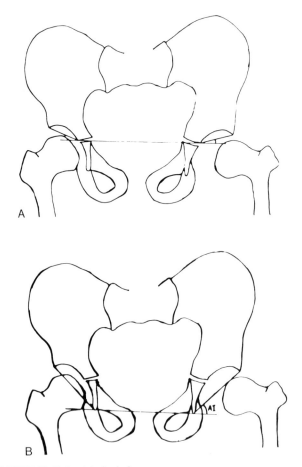

FIGURE 86–7. Acetabular index.

A Pediatric. The pediatric index is used when the triradiate cartilage clearly is open. It is defined as the angle that lies between a line connecting the superolateral margin of each triradiate cartilage (Y line) and a line drawn from the most superolateral ossified edge of the acetabulum to the superolateral margin of the triradiate cartilage.

B Adult. The angle that lies between a line connecting the teardrops on the inferior margin of the acetabula (Hilgenreiner's line) and a line drawn from the most superolateral ossified edge of the acetabulum to the teardrop constitutes the adult acetabular index (AI). (Courtesy of David S. Marcus, M.D., Tucson, Arizona.)

normal side, but they are of limited value in the child with bilaterally dislocated hips. It is important to recognize that the acetabular index may be normal despite significant dysplasia of the hip. Many of the changes associated with an increased acetabular index do not occur until the postnatal phase, when the hip gradually loses its intrauterine flexion contracture. Continued pressure from the femoral head eventually induces osteoclastic resorption and delayed endochondral bone formation at the lateral margin of the acetabular roof. The angle of acetabular acclivity relative to the pelvic baseline is variable; normally, at birth, it ranges from 18 to 36 degrees, and it decreases by 5 degrees during the ensuing 6 months. Measurement of this angle thus is of limited value (except for longitudinal follow-up of an individual patient) unless it is increased markedly.[41] Documenting the position of the femoral head relative to the acetabulum and characterizing the osseous acetabular margin are more important.

Several additional measurements have been developed (Fig. 86–9). The normal acetabulum has a slight central

concavity and a distinct lateral edge. Absence of either of these findings and persistent accentuated obliquity of the acetabular margin indicate abnormal femoral-acetabular relationships. Abnormal sclerosis of the outer aspect of the acetabulum is an associated finding. If these acetabular alterations are observed in a newborn infant, prenatal dislocation is assumed to be present.

Recently, conventional radiographic screening of the hip at 4 months of age has been described as a useful adjunct to neonatal screening among infants at high risk for DDH. Among a series of 357 patients with either positive family history, breech presentation, or persistent hip click on physical examination, 46 were found to have abnormal followup radiographs. Acetabular dysplasia predominated over subluxation in these children, 12 of whom required specific treatment.[42]

With appropriate early treatment, many of the radiographic abnormalities in DDH diminish or disappear completely. Ossification of a dislocated femoral head epiphysis generally lags behind that of the contralateral normal side, and disparity in size can persist for 6 to 12 months. Sequential radiographic examinations generally are performed at the time of clinical evaluation or cast change. The intervals between radiographic examinations should be as long as possible, and gonadal shielding is mandatory in both sexes.[43] If the condition is not treated, the dysplastic alterations will progress to a degree and then stabilize (Fig. 86–10). With persistent subluxation and associated instability, severe secondary degenerative abnormalities may occur at a young age and progress into adulthood (Fig. 86–11).[44] In untreated type III dysplasia, progressive changes will create a false acetabulum (Figs. 86–12 and 86–13).

Conventional Tomography

When visualization of the hip is impaired by a heavy cast, conventional tomography may be helpful. Restricting the arc of tube excursion or use of a book cassette can limit radiation exposure to an acceptable level, but in general conventional tomography should not be performed unless

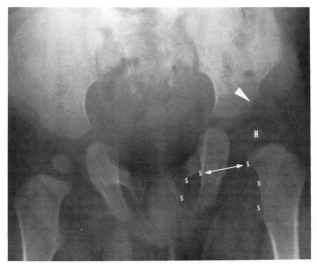

FIGURE 86–8. Type I DDH. The left femur is displaced superiorly and has a relatively small secondary ossification center (H) in association with a slightly shallow acetabulum (arrowhead). Shenton's line (S) is disrupted (white double-headed arrow).

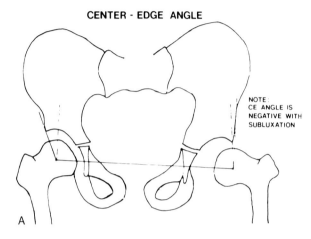

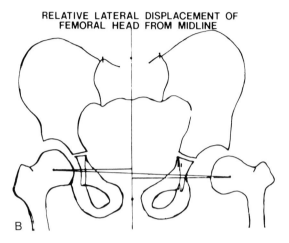

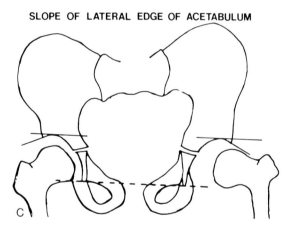

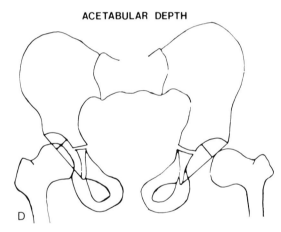

FIGURE 86–9. Additional measurements performed on conventional radiographs in DDH. In each illustration, the left hip is dysplastic.

A Center-edge (CE) angle. This angle lies between a line drawn from the center of the femoral head perpendicular to the line connecting the center of rotation of each femoral head and a line drawn from the center of the head to the superolateral ossified edge of the acetabulum. In a dislocated hip in which the center of the femoral head lies lateral to the superolateral ossified edge of the acetabulum, the CE angle will have a negative value.

B Relative lateral displacement of femoral head from midline. The pelvic midline is formed by a line connecting the point that lies equidistant between the superolateral margin on each side of the sacrum and the point that lies directly in the middle of the symphysis pubis. The lateral displacement of each femoral head is indicated by the length of a line drawn perpendicular to the midline from the center of the head.

C Slope of the lateral edge of the acetabulum. The angle formed between a line that is parallel to Hilgenreiner's line and tangent to the roof of the acetabulum and a line that is parallel to the lateral edge of the acetabulum is termed the slope. The normal acetabulum has a slope of the lateral edge that is defined as positive.

D Acetabular depth. The greatest perpendicular distance between the medial articular surface of the acetabulum and a line drawn from the teardrop to the most superolateral ossified edge of the acetabulum is the acetabular depth. (Courtesy of David S. Marcus, M.D., Tucson, Arizona.)

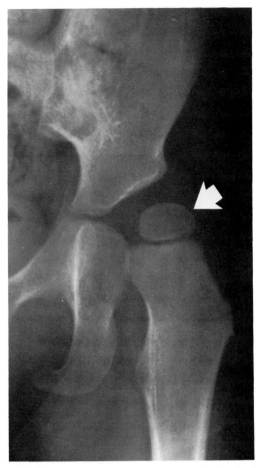

FIGURE 86–10. Untreated type I DDH. The acetabulum is shallow in association with aspherical deformity and lateral uncovering (arrow) of the femoral head.

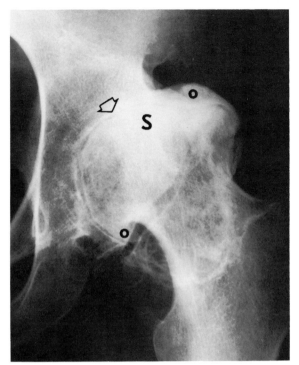

FIGURE 86–11. Degenerative joint disease secondary to untreated DDH. Deformity of the left femoral head and acetabulum is associated with superimposed joint space narrowing (arrow), subchondral sclerosis (S), osteophytosis (O), and lateralization of the femur.

absolutely necessary. This technique will demonstrate the femoral and acetabular margins more clearly.

Contrast Arthrography

Positive contrast arthrography is not indicated in the typical case of readily reducible neonatal hip instability, but it should be performed if concentric reduction is questionable or difficult to maintain. This procedure is indicated strongly when dislocation is discovered late or when sequential radiographic examinations do not document satisfactory therapeutic response. Arthrography is a useful adjunct to closed or open reduction of an infant hip and is beneficial for preoperative planning of acetabular reconstruction.[45] The method can be combined with CT, an approach that is particularly valuable for depicting posterior acetabular anatomy.[46]

Arthrography, which should be undertaken only after 2 to 3 weeks of traction to loosen soft tissue contracture, is done under a general anesthetic that will allow muscle relaxation and a proper assessment of reducibility. After sterile preparation of the skin, a narrow (20 gauge) spinal needle is introduced into the hip joint under fluoroscopic control. A trial injection ascertains whether the hip capsule is penetrated satisfactorily. A small amount of contrast material (1 to 2 ml) then is injected, again using fluoroscopy to determine satisfactory filling of the joint. The contrast

material should be dilute, as too dense a contrast medium (as well as too large a volume) will obscure the femoral head. The needle is removed and the hip is manipulated under fluoroscopy to determine reducibility and appropriate positions that maintain reduction. Spot films (anteroposterior views) then are taken in the following positions: (1) extension–external rotation, (2) extension–neutral rotation, (3) extension–internal rotation, (4) abduction–neutral rotation, (5) abduction–internal rotation, (6) abduction–flexion, (7) adduction, (8) adduction-push, and (9) adduction-pull. An inferomedial approach to this procedure has been described.[47]

On arthrographic images, the subluxed femoral head lies

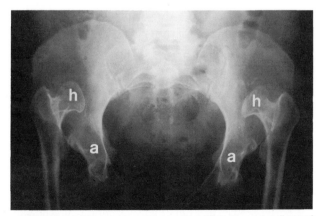

FIGURE 86–12. Bilateral type 3 untreated DDH. Frontal radiograph reveals symmetric acetabular hypoplasia (a) and abnormal articulation of the dysplastic femoral heads (h) with the iliac wings posteriorly.

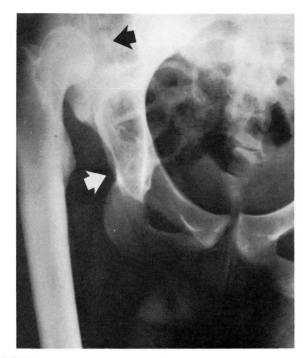

FIGURE 86–13. Untreated type III DDH in an adult. The right femur is hypoplastic and markedly displaced superolaterally, articulating with the iliac wing via a pseudoacetabulum (black arrow). The true acetabulum (white arrow) is underdeveloped.

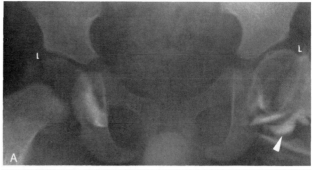

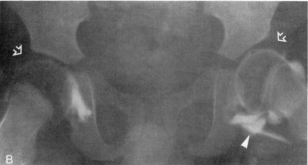

FIGURE 86–14. Arthrography in type I DDH. In both the neutral **(A)** and the abducted **(B)** positions, the left acetabular labrum (L, arrow) remains in a completely everted configuration, similar to that (L, arrow) of the contralateral normal hip. The joint capsule is more redundant on the left (arrowheads).

lateral to and below the margin of the labrum. The labrum may be displaced superiorly by the femoral head during stress maneuvers, but the head always remains below or lateral to its undersurface. The labrum may be elevated and flattened against the pelvis. Generally the joint capsule is loose, and the articular cavity is more capacious than normal (Fig. 86–14). Although reduction of the femoral head is easy, maintenance frequently is difficult. The femoral head often lies in normal position and displaces only with lateral stress. Pooling of contrast material then is observed medial to the lateralized femoral epiphysis.

In complete dislocation, the femoral head lies superior and lateral to the margin of the acetabular labrum (Fig. 86–15). As the femoral head migrates proximally on the ilium, the capsule is pushed ahead, stretching out and narrowing behind the femoral head. The iliopsoas tendon compresses the isthmus of the capsule as the tendon passes toward its insertion on the lesser trochanter. The capsule is adherent to the labrum, and these fused structures (termed the limbus) are interposed between the femoral epiphysis and the acetabulum. The portion of the capsule lying medial to the head is constricted in the form of an isthmus, resulting in a figure-of-eight capsular configuration. The ligamentum teres femoris frequently is thickened but occasionally is elongated and attenuated. The intra-acetabular capsular space is constricted and contains hyperplastic synovial fat, manifested as filling defects at its base. The limbus frequently is folded on itself (inverted) and lies within the acetabulum, with loss of the characteristic "rose thorn" appearance of the normal labrum. The capsular isthmus, interposed limbus, and tight iliopsoas muscle impede complete reduction, although the impression of the last-mentioned structure on the contrast medium–filled capsule ("hourglass" configuration) generally is not identifiable.

The hypertrophied intracapsular soft tissues or ligamentum teres femoris also may prevent complete medial seating of the femoral epiphysis.

The type 3 dislocation is not reducible, even when capsular laxity has been induced by preliminary traction. Arthrography overcomes the potential for a false impression of reduction on conventional radiographs owing to compression of the infolded labrum and capsule by the femoral head in this situation.

Ultrasonography

The initial application of ultrasonography to the diagnosis of DDH employed a static B-mode scanning unit and emphasized the assessment of acetabular morphology, an

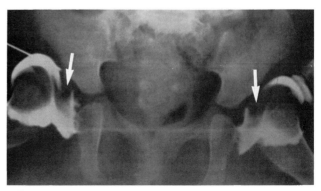

FIGURE 86–15. Arthrography in bilateral type III DDH. The acetabular labra (arrows) are totally inverted, effectively blocking reduction of the superolaterally displaced femoral heads. The ossified acetabula are shallow, and the joint capsules are capacious.

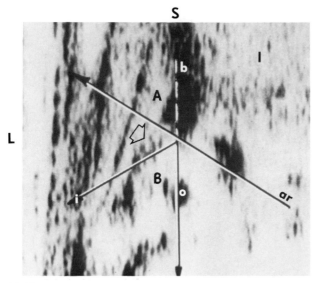

FIGURE 86–16. Normal hip sonogram, neutral coronal view. Graf alpha **(A)** and beta **(B)** angles are determined from bone and soft tissue landmarks. With dysplasia, alpha angle decreases and beta angle increases. *b,* Baseline; *i,* inclination line; *ar,* acetabular roof line; *arrow,* labrum; *o,* femoral head ossification center; *I,* ilium; *L,* lateral; *S,* superior.

approach that remains widely used in Europe (Fig. 86–16).[48–51] The reproducibility and tendency toward overdiagnosis associated with this method have been criticized.[52] Real-time systems have more recently provided increasingly accurate images of the infant hip as well as valuable information concerning function.[53–56] The advantages to this method include the following: (1) ultrasonography provides detailed depiction of the cartilaginous femoral head and its relationship to the bony and cartilaginous acetabulum; (2) patients in spica casts, Pavlik harnesses, and braces can be evaluated to ensure concentric reduction; (3) hip motion can be studied dynamically, documenting subluxation, dislocation, and reduction as they occur; and (4) exposure to ionizing radiation and sedation are avoided.[57–60] In addition, studies can be repeated as necessary for diagnosis and follow-up during treatment. Sonographic guidance of infant hip reduction under anesthesia also has been described.[61]

Technical Aspects

In most instances a lateral scanning approach is used to image the infant hip. Two body planes are used in this approach, the transverse plane, which produces a transaxial image of the hip and pelvis, and the longitudinal plane, at right angles to the transverse plane, which results in a coronal image. The infant may be placed supine, on its side, or prone, and the hip may be either flexed, with or without abduction, or extended. This scanning approach is well suited to evaluating infants in Pavlik harnesses, Ilfeld and other braces, and spica casts that have been windowed.

In all studies, a high frequency linear array transducer is recommended to provide the most detailed anatomic information. Sector scans may be used alternatively and frequently are necessary when scanning an infant in a spica cast. A transducer with a small scan head is necessary when using a window in the spica cast or the perineal opening at the groin. Scans in the longitudinal (coronal) and transverse (transaxial) planes are obtained with and without stress. The

following procedures for examination of the infant hip have been suggested: (1) a transverse neutral scan with the hip extended; (2) a transverse flexion scan of the hip with and without stress; and (3) a coronal (longitudinal) flexion scan with and without stress.[62]

When imaging an infant in a Pavlik harness, the hips are maintained in flexion throughout the sonographic examination. To stress an infant hip, the Barlow procedure is performed while using the lateral scanning approach. Movement of the femoral head laterally and posteriorly away from the center of the acetabulum is documented. Conversely, an Ortolani maneuver to reduce a subluxed or dislocated hip may be attempted.

Other methods for scanning the hip besides this technique and dynamic sonography using the lateral approach have been devised but at present have limited application. To use the anterior supine approach, the transducer is positioned over the groin in alignment with the long axis of the slightly abducted hip and proximal portion of the femur. This approach is employed with infants in spica casts in whom the degree of instability is such that windowing the molded cast over the femoral head is contraindicated. The perineal opening provides access to the groin. The femur is followed proximally to the rounded cartilaginous head, which is seated within the acetabulum. The ischium, which composes the posterior portion of the acetabulum, is seen immediately beneath the cartilaginous head. The cartilaginous labrum may be identified hugging the anterior contour of the femoral head within the acetabulum. A similar scanning technique that images the hip joint, proximal femoral metaphysis, and iliofemoral ligament in a sagittal plane is useful for determining the presence or absence of joint effusion.[63]

Normal Anatomy

The anatomy of the infant hip is easily and consistently demonstrated using a lateral scanning approach with real-time ultrasonography. The femoral head (composed of hyaline cartilage) is identified readily within the cup of the bony and cartilaginous acetabulum. The greater trochanter, also composed of hyaline cartilage, is contiguous with the inferior lateral margin of the femoral head. The joint capsule closely follows the contour of the cartilaginous head, attaching to the acetabulum just above the labrum. The labrum, also composed of hyaline cartilage with a fibrocartilaginous tip, forms the perimeter of the acetabular cup.[64–66] In normal term and preterm infants, the acetabular margin has been shown to grow and ossify more rapidly than the femoral head.[67]

The sonographic appearance of the infant hip on transverse (transaxial plane) and longitudinal (coronal plane) scans is characteristic.[68] The sound beam passes through the gluteal muscle and outlines the cartilaginous femoral head within the cup of the acetabulum. On the transaxial scan, the posterior bony acetabulum is formed by the ischium and the anterior margin by the pubis. Centrally located at the base of the acetabulum is the triradiate cartilage, an important landmark in sonographic hip imaging. Sound waves pass through the triradiate cartilage at the base of the acetabulum, producing a vertical echogenic line, whereas the bony acetabulum blocks passage of sound. The femoral head should be centered over the triradiate cartilage.

At right angles to the transaxial scan is the longitudinal

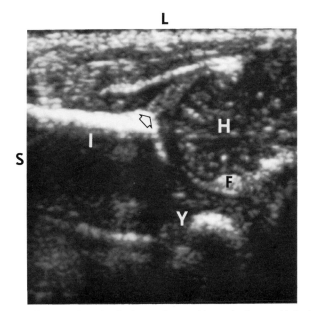

FIGURE 86–17. Longitudinal scan (coronal image) of normal infant hip. Ilium *(I)*, hyaline cartilage of acetabular labrum (arrow) with echogenic fibrocartilaginous tip, and cartilaginous femoral head *(H)* are shown. *Y,* Sound transmission through triradiate cartilage; *F,* fovea centralis; *L,* lateral; *S,* superior.

scan, representing the coronal plane. The bony ilium is visualized readily cephalad to the cartilaginous femoral head and forms the cup of the acetabulum. Triradiate cartilage sound transmission is seen at the base of the acetabular cup. The inferoposterior aspect of the acetabular cup on coronal images is the ischium.

Coronal Image (Fig. 86–17). The coronal scan of a normal infant hip reveals the femoral head as a discrete, spherical, homogeneous sphere of low echogenicity centered over the triradiate cartilage. The labrum is seen as an elongated triangle of hyaline cartilage with the fibrocartilaginous tip being more echogenic. The sound beam first penetrates the gluteal muscle lateral to the hip. Immediately beneath this structure lies the joint capsule, which follows closely the contour of the cartilaginous femoral head. When scanning in the coronal plane, the site of the greatest diameter of the femoral head is sought. In normal infants, at least half of the cartilaginous head should lie within the cup of the acetabulum. Subtle adjustment of transducer angulation allows identification of the deepest part of the acetabulum, which should contain the femoral head in its greatest diameter. The greater trochanter often is identified as it merges with the proximal femoral epiphysis. The bony metaphysis frequently is seen as a bright linear structure that blocks sound transmission at its junction with the cartilaginous head and greater trochanter.

To quantify the degree of subluxation, cursors may be used to quantitate both the diameter of the femoral head and the distance from the lateral margin to the base of the acetabulum (Fig. 86–18). Such measurements permit a containment ratio or percentage to be estimated. A midcoronal scan showing the greatest depth of the acetabular cup and largest diameter of the femoral head is necessary for accurate evaluation. Rotation of the transducer out of the true midcoronal plane either posteriorly or anteriorly may lead to underestimation of acetabular depth. Scans obtained an-

terior to the midcoronal plane may be recognized by the lateral flare of the bony ilium above the acetabulum. Conversely, images posterior to the midcoronal plane are characterized by a concave appearance to the ilium, due to the normal gluteal fossa of the posterior ilium.

Transaxial Image (Figs. 86–19 and 86–20). The transverse plane provides transaxial images of the hip. Once again, the femoral head appears as a moderately echogenic spherical mass cupped within the acetabulum. The sound transmission zone of the triradiate cartilage is seen at the base of the acetabulum between the pubic bone anteriorly and ischium posteriorly. The appearance of the femoral head centered over the triradiate cartilage has been likened to a lollipop: the femoral head constitutes the round candy, with the sound transmission through the triradiate cartilage comprising the lollipop stick. The posterior aspect of the bony acetabulum continues into a well-defined cartilaginous labrum, terminated by its small echogenic tip of fibrocartilage. Vascular pulsation at the ligamentum teres may be seen at the posterior base of the acetabulum. The ligamentum teres inserts into the fovea centralis, a small elliptical echogenic focus at the surface of the femoral head, best seen on transaxial images.

Sonographic Appearance of Specific Abnormalities

Ossification. Sonography identifies early bone formation within the cartilaginous head as a small central echogenic focus, well before radiographic demonstration of the ossification center.[69] As the secondary center grows, the resultant acoustic shadowing may obscure important anatomic landmarks such as the triradiate cartilage (Fig. 86–21). Therefore, sonography of the infant hip becomes less reliable after the age of approximately 12 months. Although older children may be imaged accurately with ultrasonography,

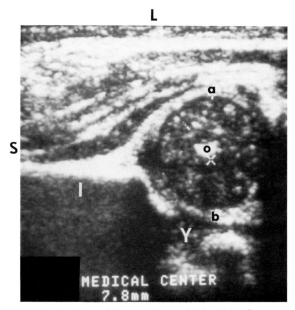

FIGURE 86–18. Coronal image of normal infant hip. Cursors are used to assess containment of femoral head within the acetabulum. *a-b* distance = diameter of cartilaginous head. The portion of the cartilaginous head within acetabulum is indicated by distance *x-b*. The ratio between these measurements estimates containment. *I,* Ilium; *Y,* triradiate cartilage; *o,* ossification center of femoral head; *L,* lateral; *S,* superior.

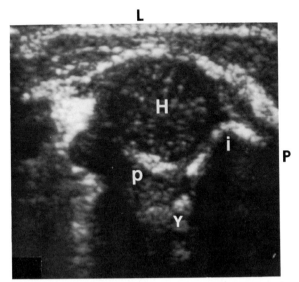

FIGURE 86–19. Transaxial scan of normal left hip. Cartilaginous femoral head *(H)*, pubis *(p,* representing anterior acetabulum), ischium *(i,* representing posterior acetabulum) and sound transmission through triradiate cartilage *(Y)* at the base of the acetabulum are shown ("lollipop" appearance). *L,* lateral; *P,* posterior.

the success of the procedure depends on the degree of ossification about the hip.

Growing evidence exists that sonographic demonstration of early ossification actually reflects collateral vascularization of the capital femoral epiphysis. This phenomenon precedes the appearance of the ossific center on radiography. The infant hip is particularly vulnerable to ischemic necrosis prior to the development of a collateral blood supply. Sonographic identification of early echogenic foci within the femoral head may signify the end of this vulnerable period and aid the orthopedic surgeon in treatment planning, particularly the timing of surgical reduction when indicated.[70]

Subluxation, Dislocation, and Dysplasia. In addition to allowing accurate imaging of the cartilaginous and bony components of the infant hip, real-time ultrasonography provides dynamic information about the position and stability of the femoral head with respect to the acetabulum. Just as the clinical diagnosis of DDH relies on the detection of hip instability using the Barlow and Ortolani maneuvers, the real-time sonographic evaluation of the hip should include dynamic techniques to elicit and record hip instability.[71] Motion and stability of the hip are evaluated on both transverse and longitudinal scans. While being scanned, the flexed hip may be abducted and adducted during the application of gentle stress. The sonographer may perform a push-pull movement in the anterior to posterior direction or "piston" the hip posteriorly to create stress. This is a provocative maneuver similar to the Barlow test, designed to reproduce subluxation or dislocation. Conversely, reduction of a subluxed or dislocated hip may be attempted with gentle flexion and abduction. While these maneuvers are being performed, hip position can be documented by video recording or by selected static images.

In the transverse plane with the hip flexed, gentle force is exerted on the femur in an attempt to displace the cartilaginous head posteriorly (Fig. 86–22). Although no movement should occur in the absence of DDH, normal infants may demonstrate sufficient capsular laxity to permit minor degrees of posterior subluxation during the first week of life.[72] This phenomenon should resolve within the first month after birth.

The normal range of hip instability in newborn infants has been determined quantitatively.[73] During the initial few days of life, normal hips may subluxate by 4 to 6 mm. Capsular laxity usually diminishes significantly during the first 2 days of life and should no longer be present by 2 to 4 weeks after birth. Depending on the degree of subluxation, the femoral head will move posteriorly and laterally away from the base of the acetabulum and the triradiate cartilage with stress. Scans in the longitudinal or coronal plane during this maneuver with the transducer centered posterior to the midcoronal plane demonstrate the maximum femoral head diameter overlying the posterior lip of the acetabulum (Fig. 86–23). Gentle push-pull movement induces return of the femoral head to the center of the acetabulum and, during stress, its reappearance at the posterior margin of the acetabular cup.

To measure excursion of the femoral head on transaxial scans during a piston or stress maneuver, two images are obtained. Prior to applying stress, the center of the cartilaginous head should be centered over the base of the acetabulum at the triradiate cartilage. When stress is applied, the subluxatable or dislocatable hip will move posteriorly. The linear distance between the center of the posteriorly displaced femoral head and the base of the acetabulum at the triradiate cartilage thus may be calculated (Fig. 86–24). In addition to moving posteriorly, the cartilaginous head also moves laterally, resulting in a gap between its margin and the acetabular base (Fig. 86–25).

Useful information may be obtained by attempting to reposition a subluxed or dislocated hip. Depending on the duration and degree of abnormality, an improvement in position may be demonstrated sonographically. A frankly dislocated hip is observed to lie superior, lateral, and posterior to the acetabulum on coronal or longitudinal scans (Fig. 86–26). Images through the greatest diameter of the cartilaginous head may falsely suggest a small acetabulum.

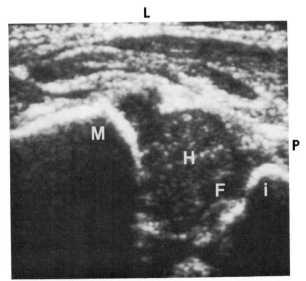

FIGURE 86–20. Transaxial scan of normal left hip. *M,* Bony femoral metaphysis distal to physis; *F,* fovea centralis of cartilaginous head *(H),* representing insertion of ligamentum teres; *i,* ischium; *L,* lateral; *P,* posterior.

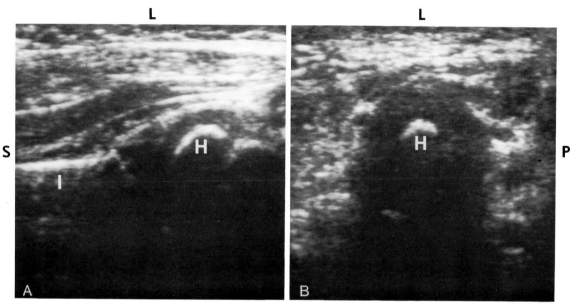

FIGURE 86–21. Coronal **(A)** and transaxial **(B)** scans of normal infant hip at 12 months of age. Ilium *(I)* and echogenic margin of capital femoral ossification center *(H)* are evident. Acoustic shadowing obscures base of acetabulum. *L,* Lateral; *P,* posterior; *S,* superior.

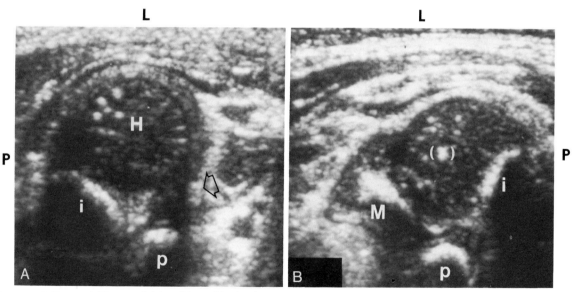

FIGURE 86–22. A, Transaxial image of right subluxatable hip after stress. The femoral head *(H)* has subluxated posteriorly and laterally with respect to acetabulum. **B,** Contralateral normal left hip for comparison. More advanced maturation of the femoral head ossific nucleus (parentheses) is evident. *i,* Ischium; *p,* pubis; arrow, echogenicity within acetabular fossa; *L,* lateral; *P,* posterior; *M,* femoral metaphysis.

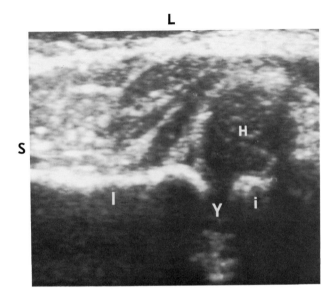

FIGURE 86–23. Longitudinal scan posterior to midcoronal plane. Subluxated femoral head *(H)* lies at the posterior margin of the acetabulum. *I,* Ilium; *i,* ischium; *Y,* triradiate cartilage; *L,* lateral; *S,* superior.

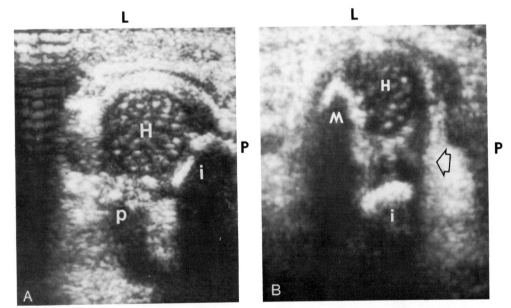

FIGURE 86–24. A, Transaxial scan of unstable left hip. The femoral head *(H)*, ischium *(i)*, and pubis *(p)* maintain normal relationship prior to stress. **B,** Same hip after posteriorly directed stress. The femoral head is displaced laterally and posteriorly (arrow) with respect to the ischium. Excursion can be measured using appropriate landmarks. *M,* Femoral metaphysis; *L,* lateral; *P,* posterior.

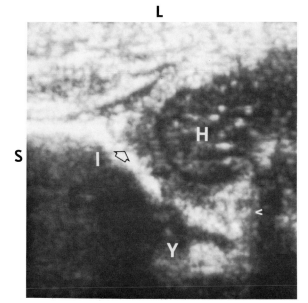

FIGURE 86–25. Coronal image of subluxatable right hip. The femoral head *(H)*, ilium *(I)*, triradiate cartilage *(Y)*, echogenic dysplastic acetabular labrum (arrow), and echogenic fibrofatty pulvinar (arrowhead) within the acetabular fossa are evident. *L,* Lateral; *S,* superior.

The acetabular labrum becomes echogenic, poorly defined, and frequently infolded, at times with a portion of the joint capsule. This labral interposition between the femoral head and acetabulum prevents closed reduction. Fibrofatty tissue or the pulvinar is identified as echogenic material within the cup of the acetabulum. A thickened, elongated ligamentum teres also may be identified (Fig. 86–28).

Acetabular dysplasia, which results from hip instability and is an anticipated consequence of untreated subluxation or dislocation, is evaluated optimally in the coronal plane.[74] This phenomenon will never be observed by ultrasonography in newborn infants with normally located and stable hips. The sonographic features of dysplasia include (1) present or past untreated hip instability; (2) a thick echogenic acetabular labrum; (3) a thick joint capsule; (4) a shallow acetabulum with rounding of the superior margin; and (5) occasional demonstration of a pulvinar and thickened ligamentum teres.

The acetabular labrum becomes echogenic secondary to metaplasia of hyaline cartilage to fibrocartilage. Changes in the contour of the superior margin of the acetabulum are similar to the radiographic appearance of acetabular dysplasia. Normal growth of the acetabulum is altered, resulting in loss of the well-defined angular margin of its superior aspect. The acetabular portion of the ilium is flattened and poorly defined.

Gentle flexion and abduction while scanning may demonstrate partial or complete reduction of the dislocation, which is useful for treatment planning. The same maneuver also demonstrates the dynamics of a dislocatable hip in the transaxial plane.

In long-standing unreducible dislocation, additional abnormalities may be identified with ultrasonography (Fig. 86–27). The cartilaginous head is situated posterior, lateral, and, frequently, superior to the acetabulum. Consequently, visualization of the acetabulum may be obscured partially by the bony metaphysis of the dislocated femur. The normally thin joint capsule becomes thickened and echogenic.

Reliability and Utility

Correlation of sonographic results with clinical findings, other available imaging studies, and long-term patient follow-up has demonstrated high sensitivity and specificity for dynamic ultrasonography of the neonatal hip.[75, 76] In one series, 23 per cent of patients with abnormal sonograms exhibited no clinical signs of DDH.[77] In addition to screening for the presence or absence of hip instability, real-time sonography has been shown to be beneficial for follow-up of infants undergoing treatment for DDH. Among patients managed with the Pavlik harness, optimal timing of follow-

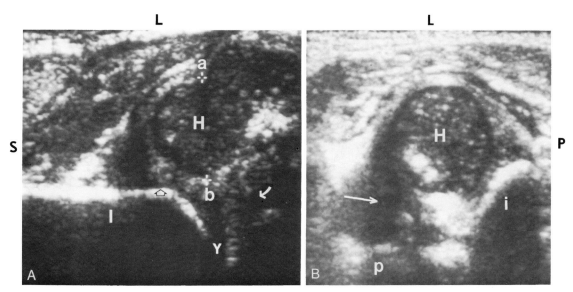

FIGURE 86–26. A, Coronal image of dislocated femoral head *(H)* lying lateral, superior, and posterior to the acetabulum. Black arrow indicates partially infolded acetabular labrum, whereas white arrow denotes fibrofatty pulvinar within the acetabular fossa. Gluteal muscles and joint capsule are stretched laterally. **B,** Transaxial image of the same left hip. The femoral head is dislocated laterally and posteriorly with respect to acetabulum. *a-b* distance, Cursor measurement of femoral head diameter; *L,* lateral; *S,* superior; *I,* ilium; *Y,* triradiate cartilage; *i,* ischium; *p,* pubis; arrow, pulvinar; *P,* posterior.

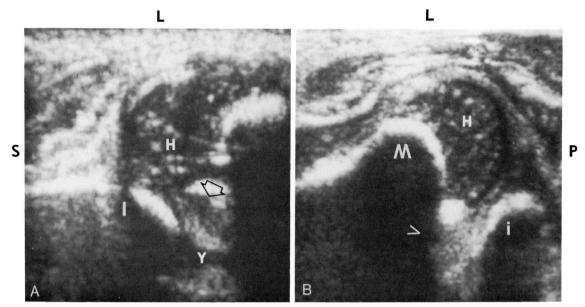

FIGURE 86–27. A, Coronal image of long-standing dislocation. The femoral head *(H)* is situated posterior, superior, and lateral to the acetabulum. The gluteal muscles are displaced laterally, and the joint capsule is echogenic and thick. The poorly defined, echogenic labrum is infolded (arrow), preventing reduction. **B,** Transaxial image of the same dislocated hip. The posterior acetabulum (represented by the ischium, *i*), the femoral head *(H)*, and the femoral metaphysis *(M)* are evident. The dislocated femoral head is held laterally by echogenic fibrofatty pulvinar (arrowhead). *I,* Ilium; *Y,* triradiate cartilage; *L,* lateral; *P,* posterior.

up scans is determined by consultation with the orthopedic surgeon. The average length of time for treatment with this device varies, but a period of 6 months followed by weaning generally is recommended, after which time a radiograph may be obtained.[78] The entire ultrasonographic examination, including gentle stress maneuvers, should be performed with the flexed hip in the harness. Documentation of stable concentric reduction in the Pavlik harness constitutes reassuring and valuable information for the orthopedic surgeon. Conversely, if ultrasonography documents persistent dislocation despite harness therapy, modification of the treatment plan is indicated.[79] Infants treated

by closed or open reduction and spica cast also may be examined sonographically. In collaboration with the sonographer, the orthopedic surgeon cuts a window in the cast posteriorly to provide access for the transducer. Dynamic evaluation of the hip obviously is not possible in a spica cast. The patient should not be moved from the prone position on the sonographic examination table until the window is replaced and plaster applied. As an alternative to windowing the cast, the hip may be imaged by ultrasonography from the anterior or groin aspect using the perineal opening of the spica cast.[80] Some investigators prefer CT or MR imaging for the evaluation of patients with casts.

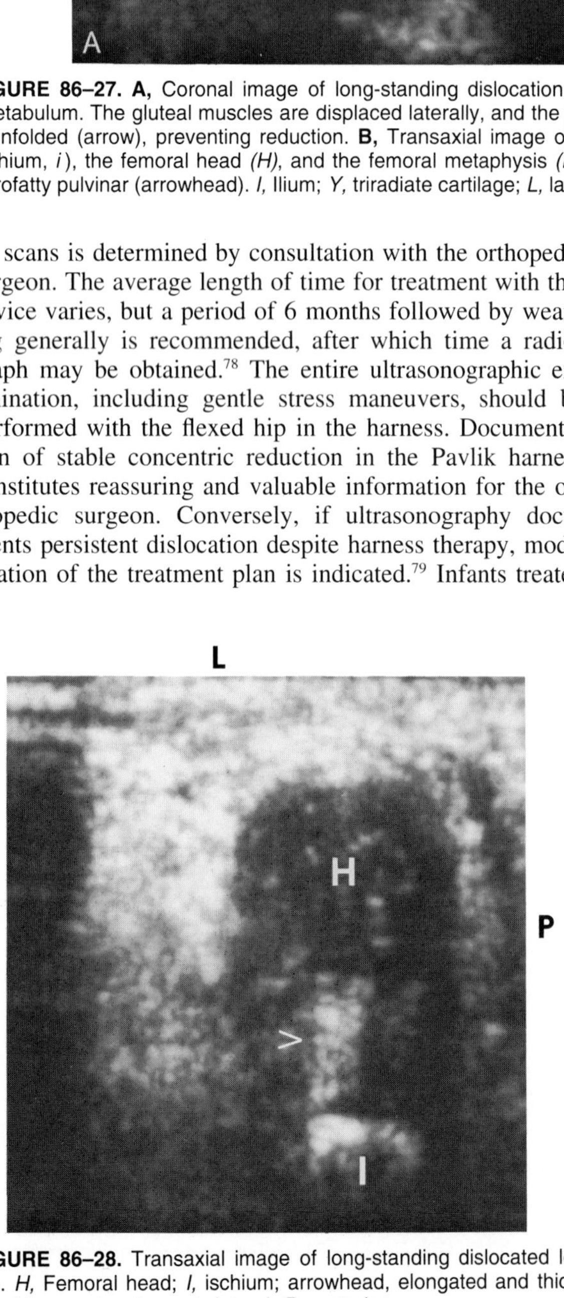

Several studies have addressed the value of ultrasonography versus clinical screening alone for the identification of hip instability among infants at risk for DDH, with encouraging results.[81–84] No late instances of DDH have occurred in infants subjected to prior sonographic screening. Unfortunately, the overall prevalence of late presenting DDH has not been altered significantly by neonatal hip sonography. The exact role of sonographic screening is not yet clear, but it may be required if late presentation of DDH is to be eliminated completely.

The value of real-time ultrasonography in diagnosis and follow-up of DDH is well established, and this method currently should be considered the imaging method of choice for documenting the condition objectively and monitoring the effectiveness of treatment.

Real-time ultrasonography of the infant's hip provides an accurate image of anatomic relationships as well as valuable information concerning function.[85–87] The technique allows clear imaging of the cartilaginous femoral head and permits accurate assessment of its size, shape, and symmetry.[88] The dynamic relationship of the cartilaginous head to the acetabulum is defined clearly, and instability, subluxation, and dislocation can be demonstrated quantitatively.[89] In the coronal plane, the edge of the acetabulum normally covers the femoral head over an arc of 55 to 57 degrees.[90, 91]

FIGURE 86–28. Transaxial image of long-standing dislocated left hip. *H,* Femoral head; *I,* ischium; arrowhead, elongated and thickened ligamentum teres; *L,* lateral; *P,* posterior.

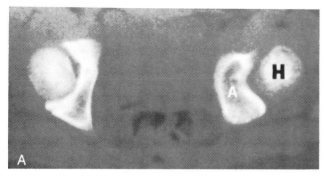
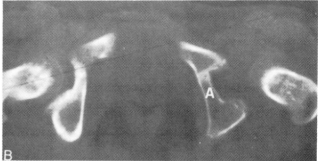

FIGURE 86–29. CT scan of untreated type II DDH. Sequential scans depict altered acetabular morphology *(A)* and deformity of the femoral head *(H)* on the left. The dysplastic femur is displaced superolaterally compared with the normal right femur. (From Sartoris DJ, Ogden JA. *In* D Resnick (Ed): Bone and Joint Imaging. Philadelphia, WB Saunders Company, 1989.)

The size, shape, and position of the hip can be monitored with the infant in a spica cast, brace, or harness. Real-time ultrasonography has been employed successfully for screening of high-risk babies to determine hip position, and it offers an alternative method for evaluating acetabular development.[92, 93]

A sonographic technique for evaluating the ossification center of the infant's hip allows the ossific nucleus to be identified before it can be visualized radiographically. Delay in ossification associated with pathologic conditions of the hip also can be recognized. Proper assessment of the size of the ossific nucleus requires scanning in orthogonal planes.[94] Acoustic shadowing causes the growing ossification center to appear curved and may make the medial acetabulum and triradiate cartilage difficult to identify.

Sonographic hip evaluation usually ceases to be reliable in children over 1 year of age, and it does not reduce the incidence of late cases.[95] In addition, direct quantitative measurements by this technique are subject to inter- and intraobserver variations and may yield false-negative results if stress is not applied.[96]

Computed Tomography

CT usually can provide accurate documentation of the adequacy of a reduction in DDH (Fig. 86–29).[97–99] It should supplement other diagnostic imaging examinations when the status of a reduction is in question because the patient is wearing a plaster cast (Fig. 86–30). CT provides a clear image of the reduction in the transverse plane, so that anterior or posterior subluxation of the femoral head can be detected readily with as few as one slice.[100, 101] Pulvinar hypertrophy, contracture of the iliopsoas tendon, and intra-articular osteocartilaginous bodies preventing relocation also can be demonstrated.[102, 103]

CT allows direct measurement of acetabular anteversion, which previously had not been possible with noninvasive studies in the living patient.[104] Acetabular anteversion is increased on the dislocated side as a result of excessive angulation of the anterior and posterior columns into the sagittal plane, and it returns to normal as treatment progresses.[105] Radiation exposure is less than that for conventional tomography and can be minimized by reducing tube current and number of slices.[106] The method also is applied readily in postoperative patients with spica casts.[107] CT, particularly with three-dimensional analysis, is extremely

useful in characterizing the abnormal acetabular morphology of untreated and postoperative DDH (Fig. 86–31).[108–111]

Magnetic Resonance Imaging

MR imaging offers great promise in the evaluation of DDH (Fig. 86–32), owing to its excellent depiction of unmineralized tissues, including cartilage, its direct multiplanar imaging capabilities, its lack of need for ionizing radiation, and its high sensitivity in the early detection of ischemic necrosis of bone.[112, 113] Three-dimensional image reconstruction of data derived by MR imaging also can be accomplished using sophisticated software and hardware.[114]

MR imaging is capable of depicting accurately the most important determinants of stability in the neonatal hip (Fig. 86–33).[115–117] These include femoral head shape, acetabular shape, position of the labrum, invagination of the joint capsule by the iliopsoas tendon, degree of femoral and acetabular anteversion, and position of the transverse acetabular ligament (Fig. 86–34).[118, 119] Femoral anteversion can be measured using MR imaging by obtaining an additional transaxial image through the femoral condyles, as has been described previously with CT (Fig. 86–35).[120] Addi-

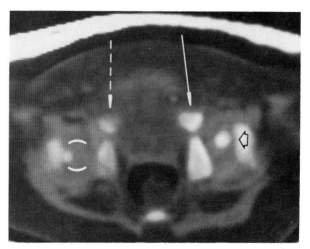

FIGURE 86–30. CT scan in unilateral DDH. With the patient in a plaster cast, delayed ossification and posterior displacement of the right femoral head (parentheses) are evident (compare with the normal left side, black arrow). The right acetabulum is underdeveloped and osteopenic (dashed arrow) in comparison to the normal left side (solid arrow).

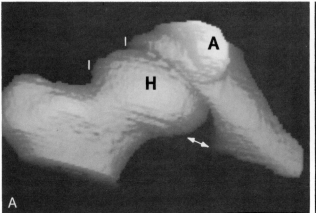
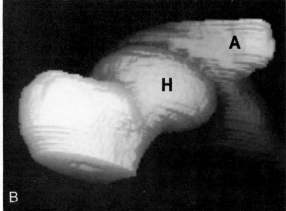

FIGURE 86–31. Three-dimensional CT scan in untreated DDH. Anterior **(A)** and right anterior oblique **(B)** images reveal an aspherical femoral head *(H)* with diminished lateral coverage (vertical lines), as well as femoral-acetabular *(A)* incongruence (double-headed arrow).

tional structures, including the ligamentum teres, the fat pad within the acetabular fossa, and various portions of the joint capsule, also are demonstrated by MR imaging.[115] The technique is performed readily through cast material and is the preferred method for early detection of ischemic necrosis in the developing proximal femoral epiphysis, a recognized complication of operative reduction in severe DDH.

Appropriate selection of pulse sequence, repetition time, echo time, section thickness, matrix size, field of view, and surface coil parameters (type, size, position) is critical for optimal resolution of the small anatomic structures in the neonatal hip. T1-weighted spin echo MR images provide adequate contrast between bone, cartilage, ligaments, and adjacent soft tissues. Coronal images are optimal for depicting the clinically important structures of the acetabular roof, including the labrum. Transaxial images are best suited for demonstrating the anterior and posterior structures of the joint. Routine use of both planes permits exact determination of the spatial relationship between the acetabulum and femoral head.[121, 122]

The application of rapid scanning techniques, such as gradient echo and fast spin echo imaging, allows the acquisition of scans in multiple hip positions within a reasonable time period, which partially overcomes the difficulty in obtaining dynamic images with MR imaging in young children (Figs. 86–36 and 86–37). Among the disadvantages of MR imaging, as compared to ultrasonography, are the greater cost and the need for sedation. Consequently, MR imaging should not be used for initial diagnosis or evaluation of routine DDH, but rather it should be reserved for complicated cases in which initial treatment has been unsuccessful.[115]

TREATMENT

Early (preferably neonatal) diagnosis and reduction of DDH is directed toward reestablishing normal chondroosseous development of the hip.[123, 124] When instability or frank dislocation has been detected clinically using the Ortolani or Barlow maneuver, the infant generally is placed in a flexion-abduction-external rotation apparatus such as the Pavlik harness, von Rosen splint, or Frejka pillow.[125–127] However, some investigators treat only dislocations; unsta-

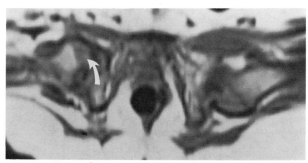

FIGURE 86–32. MR imaging in type I DDH. On a transaxial T1-weighted (TR/TE, 600/20) MR image with the hips in an abducted position, absence of marrow signal within the right femoral head (arrow) indicates delayed development of its secondary ossification center.

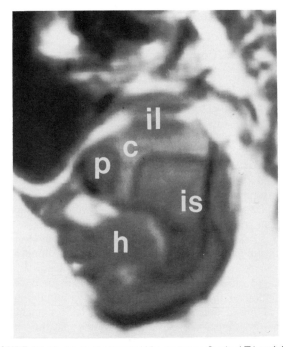

FIGURE 86–33. Normal neonatal hip anatomy. Sagittal T1-weighted (TR/TE, 600/20) MR image demonstrates osteocartilaginous structures including the ilium *(il)*, ischium *(is)*, pubic bone *(p)*, triradiate cartilage *(c)*, and femoral head *(h)*.

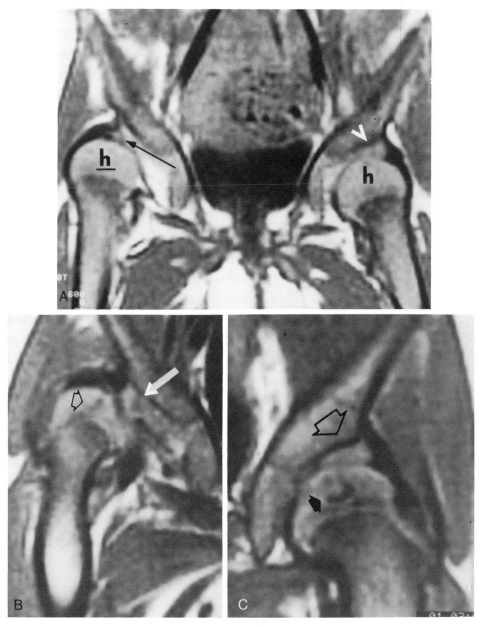

FIGURE 86–34. MR imaging in type 2 DDH.

  A Coronal T1-weighted (TR/TE, 600/25) spin echo MR image reveals superolateral subluxation of the right femoral head *(h)* when compared to the normal left side. Deformity of the right acetabular labrum (arrow) is evident in comparison to the normal left side (arrowhead).

  B At a slightly different level, a similar coronal MR image (TR/TE, 600/25) shows an underdeveloped secondary ossification center for the femoral head (black arrow). The acetabular labrum is both flattened and inverted partially (white arrow).

  C In a coronal T1-weighted (TR/TE, 600/25) spin echo MR image, the normal left hip is shown for comparison (solid arrow, femoral head ossification center; open arrow, acetabular labrum).

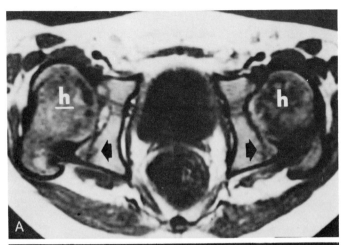

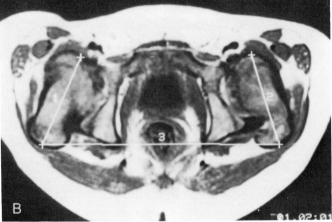

FIGURE 86–35. MR imaging in type 1 DDH.

A Transaxial T1-weighted (TR/TE, 800/25) spin echo MR image demonstrates an aspherical and deformed osteocartilaginous femoral head *(h)* on the right (compare with the normal left side). The posterior acetabular labra (arrows) are symmetric and positioned normally.

B The degree of femoral anteversion on the two sides is compared using quantitative software on a T1-weighted (TR/TE, 800/25) spin echo MR image through the femoral necks.

FIGURE 86–36. MR imaging in bilateral DDH. Transaxial gradient echo image (TR/TE, 100/25; flip angle, 40 degrees) reveals posterior dislocation of both femoral heads *(H)*. *c,* Triradiate cartilage. (Courtesy of A. Poznanski, M.D., Chicago, Illinois.)

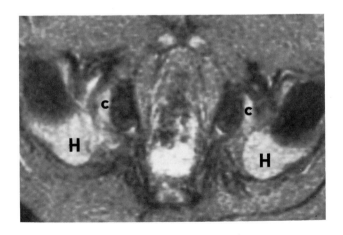

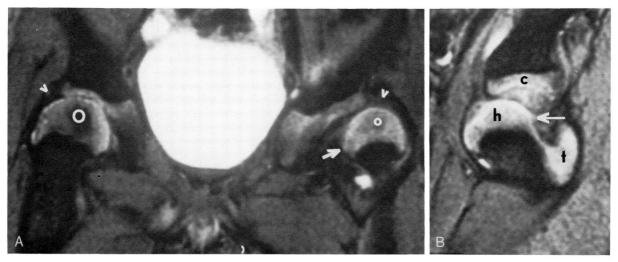

FIGURE 86–37. Gradient echo MR imaging in DDH.
A Coronal image (TR/TE, 100/25) reveals lateral subluxation of the left femur (arrow), the secondary ossification center of which is delayed in development *(O>o)*. Both acetabular labra are in the normal everted position (arrowheads).
B Sagittal image (TE/TE, 100/25) demonstrates mild anterior subluxation of the femoral head (arrow). Note the continuity between the cartilaginous femoral head *(h)* and the greater trochanter *(T)*. *c,* Triradiate cartilage.

ble hips they merely observe.[128] Treatment of DDH with the Pavlik harness requires frequent clinical and radiographic examination with the patient out of the device so that failure of reduction or adductor relaxation can be recognized and corrected promptly.[129] Scandinavian authors have reported better results with the von Rosen splint than with the Frejka pillow.[130] Regardless of the device used, sequential clinical and radiographic examinations subsequently document that satisfactory acetabular-femoral relationships are achieved in most patients.[131, 132]

In the minority of conservative treatment failures, arthrography is indicated, possibly followed by surgical intervention for achievement of complete anatomic reduction. Open reduction using the Ludloff approach is aimed at securing concentric relocation well before weight-bearing begins.[133] Congruent reductions accomplished before the age of 4 years lead to normal hip relationships in over 95 per cent of patients.[134] Late complications may result if a falsely reduced femoral head is pressed against an infolded labrum and capsule.[135] However, continuous pressure in a harness or cast may induce displacement or atrophy of obstructing structures and lead to normal femoral head seating.[136]

Unilateral DDH may be associated with abduction contracture of the contralateral hip, resulting in pelvic tilt, which directs the abnormal femoral head superolaterally and contributes to the development of acetabular dysplasia. In such cases, treatment of the dysplastic hip should include abduction splinting and stretching exercises of the contralateral hip.[137]

A large number of surgical procedures on the pelvis or femur have been designed for late salvage in cases of persistent acetabular maldevelopment and hip instability.[138, 139] The common goals of such intervention are the provision of improved acetabular coverage, enhanced femoral head-acetabular congruence, decreased pressure loading of the femoral head, and increased efficiency of the hip musculature.[140] These objectives can be achieved by many methods, of which the most commonly used include femoral varus

osteotomy, pelvic (Salter) or acetabular (Steel) rotation, increase in acetabular depth (Pemberton), or medialization of the femoral head (Chiari) (Fig. 86–38).[141–145] Although the hip-shelf procedure has been described as a safe, reliable, and conservative approach to the management of acetabular dysplasia, long-term results have been unfavorable and hence other stabilizing procedures currently are preferred.[146, 147] Similarly, the medial approach to open reduction of DDH may be less desirable because of the greater potential for direct arterial injury with secondary ischemic necrosis.[148, 149]

The innominate (Salter) osteotomy is the most frequently performed late surgical procedure. Indicated for persistent subluxation with mild to moderate acetabular dysplasia but a concentrically reduced hip, it reorients the acetabulum without changing its size or shape.[150, 151] The osteotomy is performed in a horizontal plane across the pelvis, just above the acetabulum. All three pelvic components are rotated forward and laterally as a unit using the pubic symphysis as a hinge axis. A bone block is used to maintain the open wedge. Postoperative radiographs demonstrate marked asymmetry between the two iliac wings and obturator foramina. Owing to pelvic flexibility, this disparity becomes progressively less pronounced with time. Quantitative assessment of femoral head size has been performed on conventional radiographs after this procedure. Long-term follow-up has revealed that innominate osteotomy does not cause overgrowth of the femoral head, although open reduction results in mild coxa magna.[152]

The circumacetabular (Pemberton) osteotomy is a means of reducing acetabular size and increasing articular congruence in patients with moderate to severe DDH. A pericapsular osteotomy is performed around the periphery of the acetabulum, the margin of which is displaced inferiorly, wrapped around the femoral head, and held in position by a bone block. The osteotomy is hinged at the pelvic Y synchondrosis and thus cannot be used after early adolescence, when the flexibility of the synchondrosis diminishes. Both the Salter and the Pemberton procedures increase

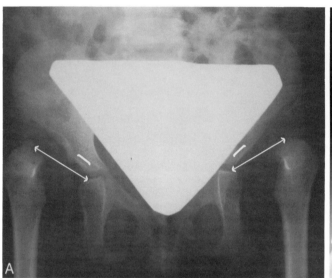

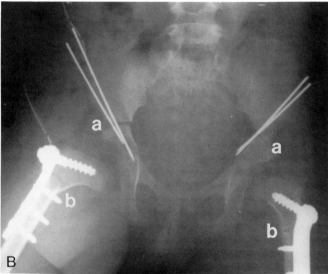

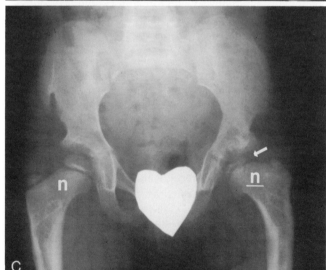

FIGURE 86–38. Bilateral pelvic and proximal femoral osteotomies in the management of DDH.

A Preoperative frontal radiograph reveals bilateral and symmetric dislocation (type 3) of the femoral heads (double-headed arrows) with shallow and underdeveloped acetabula (brackets).

B Frontal radiograph in immediate postoperative period demonstrates supra-acetabular *(a)* and subtrochanteric *(b)* varus osteotomy sites with internal fixation hardware and improved femoral-acetabular congruence.

C After hardware removal, an acceptable result has been achieved on the right side *(n)*, although the left femoral neck is short and broad *(n)*. Flattening and increased density of the left femoral head (arrow) indicate the development of ischemic necrosis as a complication.

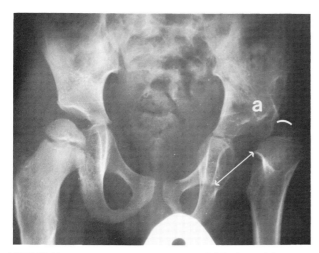

FIGURE 86–39. Recurrent unilateral type 2 DDH after pelvic osteotomy. Frontal radiograph demonstrates lateral subluxation (double-headed arrow) and rotation of the left femur, which articulates with the lateral edge of the deformed acetabulum *(a)*. Severely delayed ossification of the left femoral head (bracket) is evident.

pressure on the femoral head, predisposing to ischemic necrosis as a complication (Fig. 86–38).

The median displacement pelvic (Chiari) osteotomy medializes the femoral head and provides greater femoral head coverage by enlarging the acetabulum.[153–156] The biomechanical effect of medial weight-bearing transfer is to unload the femoral head and increase the efficiency of the abductor musculature. The angle of osteotomy is 10 to 20 degrees relative to the plane of the upper acetabular margin, and the lower segment is displaced medially by approximately half its width. A false radiographic impression of adequate medial shift can be produced by rotation as opposed to displacement. When performed bilaterally, this procedure may lead to significant pelvic narrowing with possible obstetric complications in women who later have children.

Eventually in untreated or unsuccessfully treated cases,

pain and disability secondary to residual deformity (Figs. 86–39 and 86–40) or osteoarthritis probably will necessitate reconstructive surgery or hip replacement at some time during adult life, although frequently not until the fifth or sixth decade.[157, 158] This is important to consider before embarking on any treatment when a child—particularly one who is over 1 year of age—has a unilateral or bilateral dislocation.

Complications

Inferior (obturator) dislocation of the hip resulting from excessive hip flexion has been described as a complication of Pavlik harness therapy for DDH.[159, 160] This phenomenon also can occur after treatment with spica cast immobilization, and it may require open reduction for management.[161]

Ischemic necrosis of the femoral head occurs in DDH only after treatment and can thus be considered an iatrogenic complication; it may lead to severe radiographic changes and a painful, dysfunctional hip in early adult life.[162–165] Among a large series of patients with DDH-associated ischemic necrosis, long-term follow-up has revealed an 80 per cent prevalence of secondary osteoarthritis by age 42 years.[166] Total hip arthroplasty ultimately may be required in some patients.[167] The reported frequency of ischemic necrosis in early-treated DDH has ranged from less than 1 per cent to as high as 12 per cent, and the condition can occur in the contralateral normal hip, particularly when both hips are immobilized.[28, 168–170] A dynamic canine model of DDH has been used to investigate the influence of hip position on femoral head vascularity.[171] Lack of preoperative traction and rigid immobilization in extreme positions of abduction may be causative factors, although the importance of the former is controversial.[172–176] Fortunately, modern therapeutic methods have decreased the prevalence of ischemic necrosis in DDH significantly.[177, 178]

Vascular occlusion may occur in vessels along the femoral neck or in the endochondral circulation. Identification of early ischemic necrosis is difficult by conventional radiography. Ossification of the cartilaginous head ensues

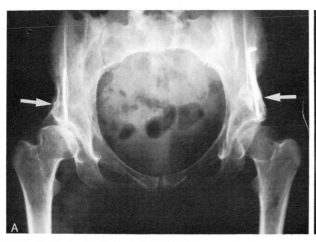
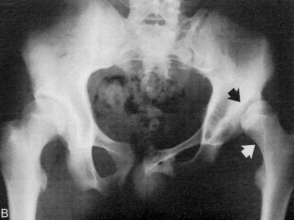

FIGURE 86–40. Surgically treated DDH (Salter procedure).
   A Healed iliac osteomy sites (arrows) and retained pins are noted on both sides, in association with deformity and slight lateralization of both femoral heads.
   B In a patient with type II dysplasia, the left femoral head is small, deformed, and displaced superolaterally (white arrow), and the left acetabulum is shallow (black arrow) with underdevelopment of the left hemipelvis, related in part to previous surgery. The right hip also is mildly dysplastic (type I).

soon after reduction and may be manifested as several granular foci rather than as a single homogeneous center. This phenomenon may represent early ischemic necrosis or a transient growth disturbance that does not result in significant late deformity.[179]

Failure of appearance or growth of the femoral ossification center during an interval of approximately 1 year after reduction is good evidence of necrosis. Characteristic manifestations of the process, such as broadening of the femoral neck, also may occur during this time or become evident later. Additional radiographic abnormalities may include irregular physeal margins, metaphyseal cysts, and the "sagging rope" sign, a U-shaped line projecting over the femoral neck that represents either the edge of the malpositioned femoral head or a reactive osseous ridge.[180]

Ischemic necrosis complicating the treatment of DDH has been classified into four radiographic patterns, early recognition of which can serve as a guide to subsequent therapy.[181] The type I pattern involves temporary fragmentation of the capital femoral ossific nucleus. Patients with this pattern have transient ischemia with early recovery and do not manifest significant growth disturbances requiring surgical treatment. The type II pattern is characterized by radiographic abnormalities localized to the lateral portions of the epiphysis, physis, and metaphysis. More extensive ischemia involving the entire proximal portion of the femur occurs in type III, resulting in premature physeal closure, femoral neck shortening, femoral head deformities, and trochanteric overgrowth. Patients with the second and third patterns are more likely to develop incomplete femoral head coverage and limb-length discrepancy requiring surgical intervention. The type IV pattern involves localized abnormalities of the medial epiphyseal ossification center and medial metaphysis, sometimes resulting in coxa magna with femoral neck shortening. Patients with the type IV pattern occasionally develop limb-length discrepancies, but surgery rarely is required.[182]

Premature fusion of the lateral growth plate with secondary external rotation of the femoral head may result from occlusion of the posterosuperior epiphyseal artery or immobilization-induced physeal compression.[183] Associated findings include shortening of the femoral neck and leg length discrepancy. Premature closure of the medial physis may induce coxa magna with mild shortening of the femoral neck. Generalized growth plate injury occurs with compromise of the medial circumflex artery, resulting in severe femoral neck shortening, leg-length discrepancy, and deformity of the femoral head.[179]

Three factors have been shown to correlate with the development of coxa magna after operative treatment of DDH. These include operation at a younger age, open reduction, and femoral osteotomy; the condition also may occur subsequent to type I ischemic necrosis. Coxa magna is not associated with an abnormal acetabular index or center-edge (CE) angle and should not be misinterpreted as hip subluxation or inadequate reduction. Satisfactory function can be anticipated in the setting of coxa magna provided that concentric, congruous reduction is obtained and sufficient acetabular growth potential exists for remodeling.[184]

The pattern of growth recovery lines in the femoral neck may be predictive of angular deformity or generalized growth impairment.[185] After treatment of DDH, such lines

normally occur parallel to the open growth plates, with the line-physis distance of the femoral neck being twice that of the greater trochanter owing to their differential growth rates. Nonparallelism or relative narrowing of the femoral neck line-physis distance is predictive of future angulation or shortening.[185, 186]

Relative trochanteric overgrowth also is a secondary phenomenon resulting from the unbalanced growth rates of the femoral neck and greater trochanteric physes.[187] This may result in alteration or reversal of the normal relationship between the superior margins of the femoral head and greater trochanter, manifested quantitatively as a decreased or negative articular-trochanteric distance. Inefficient abduction and functional coxa vara despite a normal neck-shaft angle are important biomechanical consequences. Management of this situation includes early trochanteric epiphysiodesis or inferior trochanteric displacement at an older age.[188, 189]

Acetabular dysplasia associated with DDH may persist or worsen in the setting of ischemic necrosis, owing to residual subluxation and lateral pressure from the deformed femoral head. Excision of the limbus as part of open reduction during infancy also may contribute to deficiency of the lateral acetabular margin in this situation.[190]

In the older child with initial late reduction, the radiographic appearance is that of Legg-Calvé-Perthes disease. The sequelae, however, generally are more severe; femoral neck shortening and epiphyseal deformity occur with much higher frequency. Incomplete epiphyseal necrosis is more difficult to recognize radiographically and can occur despite preliminary traction, gentle reduction, and avoidance of extreme immobilization positions. In a review of older children with DDH treated by limbus excision and derotation osteotomy, premature onset of degenerative arthritis was found to be the most important sign of poor long-term prognosis. This complication may occur despite apparent satisfactory reduction of the dislocated hip.[191]

In the setting of ischemic necrosis after closed reduction of developmental hip dislocation, lateral and proximal migration of the femoral head predisposes to premature degenerative joint disease in adulthood. Radiographic abnormalities in such patients include loss of femoral head sphericity with medial irregularity, lateral and proximal subluxation of the femur, and acetabular dysplasia.[166] Developmental coxa vara also has been described as a rare late complication of treated DDH. Vascular impairment with diminished medial growth plate activity may be responsible.

DIFFERENTIAL DIAGNOSIS

Incomplete Femoral Head Coverage. Inadequate acetabular coverage of the ossified femoral head epiphysis can be observed in a variety of conditions other than DDH. Lateral uncovering occurs in situations in which the acetabulum is developmentally small or the femoral head is enlarged (as in ischemic necrosis). Femoral neck valgus and anteversion tend to rotate the femoral head outward and contribute to poor coverage. The cause of deficient acetabular coverage may be evident on conventional radiographs (as in the pelvic tilt of cerebral palsy), although stress maneuvers or arthrography often is required for correct analysis.[180]

Inflammatory Disease. Hip subluxation, manifested as

lateralization of the femoral metaphysis, occurs in pyogenic arthritis of infancy. Soft tissue swelling and thigh flexion increase the density of the hip region and provide an important clue to the correct radiologic diagnosis. Associated growth plate dissolution and epiphyseal slip are best demonstrated by contrast arthrography.[180]

Neuromuscular Disease. Superior and lateral displacement of the femoral head is common in patients with meningomyelocele and may occur during infancy. The acetabulum may be shallow owing to prenatal onset of the disease, and evidence of spinal dysraphism should be present on pelvic radiographs (Fig. 86–41). The hip subluxation of cerebral palsy and other spastic conditions rarely develops during infancy and is associated with severe femoral anteversion and neck-shaft valgus.[180]

Traumatic Epiphyseal Slip. Traumatic epiphyseal slip may occur in the setting of infant abuse or birth trauma. If the epiphyseal ossification center is not yet mineralized, lateral shift of the femoral shaft can be misinterpreted as DDH rather than a shearing fracture.[180]

Congenital Coxa Vara. Congenital coxa vara without femoral shortening is extremely rare and can be distinguished from DDH by clinical examination and arthrography during the neonatal period.[180]

Abnormal Joint Laxity. Articular hypermobility is a feature of a variety of conditions other than DDH. Familial joint laxity probably is inherited as an autosomal dominant trait, and most affected persons do not have significant orthopedic problems. Hypotonia and joint laxity occur in Down's syndrome, and recurrent hip dislocation can be observed.[192] Cutaneous and articular hyperlaxity with inconstant spherical subcutaneous calcifications are part of the generalized connective tissue derangement seen in the Ehlers-Danlos syndrome.

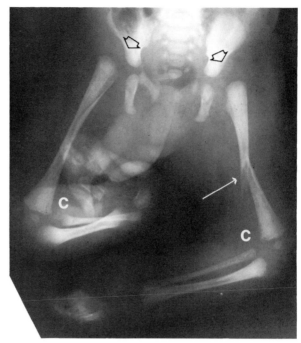

FIGURE 86–42. DDH associated with arthrogryposis multiplex congenita. Frontal radiograph reveals type 2 subluxation of both hips (arrowheads), bilateral lower extremity flexion contractures *(C)*, and a fracture of the left femoral shaft (white arrow).

In Larsen's syndrome, early joint laxity leads to multiple dislocations (particularly in the hips, elbows, and knees). Other typical features include flat facies with a saddle nose deformity and a distinctive juxtacalcaneal ossification center.

Within the group of children with arthrogryposis multiplex congenita, recurrent dislocation of many joints or only mild hyperextensibility of the metacarpophalangeal, elbow, or knee joints may be observed. When hip dislocation occurs in this disease, reduction is achieved readily but is difficult to maintain on cessation of immobilization. Conventional radiography reveals marked lateral femoral subluxation with relatively normal acetabula (Fig. 86–42). Arthrography demonstrates prominent redundant and lax capsular structures within which the femoral heads can be moved readily. When factors external to the hip joint per se are present, particularly neuromuscular diseases such as meningomyelocele and arthrogryposis multiplex congenita, the term ''teratologic hip'' often is applied.[180]

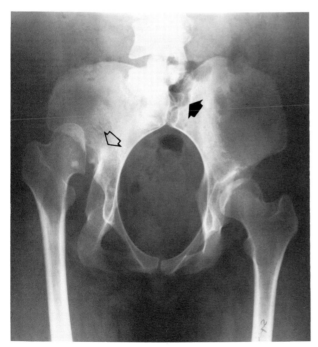

FIGURE 86–41. DDH associated with caudal regression syndrome. Frontal radiograph of the pelvis reveals sacral agenesis with hypoplasia of L5 (solid arrow) and type 3 dislocation of the right hip (open arrow).

SUMMARY

Developmental deformity of both sides of the hip joint (dysplasia) may be present at birth or become apparent months to years later. Early diagnosis and treatment are crucial in preventing severe long-term structural abnormalities. Three patterns of subluxation or dislocation are seen. Diagnostic methods include the Ortolani and Barlow maneuvers in newborn infants and analysis of radiologic lines drawn on anteroposterior views of the hip and pelvis. Conventional tomography, contrast arthrography, ultrasonography, CT, and MR imaging also are valuable for the evaluation of this disease.

References

1. Davies SJM, Walker G: Problems in the early recognition of hip dysplasia. J Bone Joint Surg [Br] 66:474, 1984.
2. Mackenzie IG, Wilson JG: Problems encountered in the early diagnosis and management of congenital dislocation of the hip. J Bone Joint Surg [Br] 63:38, 1981.
3. Williamson DM, Glover SD, Benson MK: Congenital dislocation of the hip presenting after the age of three years: A long-term review. J Bone Joint Surg [Br] 71:745, 1989.
4. Sherlock DA, Gibson PH, Benson MKD: Congenital subluxation of the hip: A long-term review. J Bone Joint Surg [Br] 67:390, 1985.
5. Ogden JA: Dynamic pathobiology of congenital hip dysplasia. In MO Tachdjian (Ed): Congenital Hip Disease. New York, Churchill Livingstone, 1982, pp 93–144.
6. Ogden JA: Development and growth of the hip. In JF Katz, RS Siffert (Eds): Management of Hip Disorders in Children. Philadelphia, JB Lippincott, 1983, pp 6–32.
7. Klisic PJ: Congenital dislocation of the hip—a misleading term: Brief report. J Bone Joint Surg [Br] 71:136, 1989.
8. Parker MD, Clark RL, Cuttino JT Jr, et al: Streptococcal antigen-induced dislocation and dysplasia of the hip in newborn rats: Radiologic and histologic evaluation of a model of congenital dislocation of the hip. Invest Radiol 24:604, 1989.
9. Keller MS, Weltin GG, Rattner Z, et al: Normal instability of the hip in the neonate: US standards. Radiology 169:733, 1988.
10. Hoaglund FT, Healey JH: Osteoarthrosis and congenital dysplasia of the hip in family members of children who have congenital dysplasia of the hip. J Bone Joint Surg [Am] 72:1510, 1990.
11. Lingg G, Torklus D, Nebel G: Hip dysplasia and congenital hip dislocation: A roentgenometric study in 110 families. Radiologe 21:538, 1981.
12. Good C, Walker G: The hip in the moulded baby syndrome. J Bone Joint Surg [Br] 66:491, 1984.
13. Westin GW, Ilfeld FW, Makin M, et al: Developmental hip dislocation. Contemp Orthop 16:17, 1988.
14. Hensinger RN: Congenital dislocation of the hip: Treatment in infancy to walking age. Orthop Clin North Am 18:597, 1987.
15. Walker JM: Morphological variants in the human fetal hip joint: Their significance in congenital hip disease. J Bone Joint Surg [Am] 62:1073, 1980.
16. Dwyer NS: Congenital dislocation of the hip: To screen or not to screen. Arch Dis Child 62:635, 1987.
17. Dunn PM: Screening for the detection of congenital dislocation of the hip. Arch Dis Child 61:921, 1986.
18. Bolton-Maggs BG, Crabtree SD: The opposite hip in congenital dislocation of the hip. J Bone Joint Surg [Br] 65:279, 1983.
19. Hooper G: Congenital dislocation of the hip in infantile idiopathic scoliosis. J Bone Joint Surg [Br] 62:447, 1980.
20. Wilkinson JA, Sedgwick EM: Occult spinal dysraphism in established congenital dislocation of the hip. J Bone Joint Surg [Br] 70:744, 1988.
21. Summers BN, Turner A, Wynn-Jones CH: Presentation of congenital hip dysplasia. J Bone Joint Surg [Br] 70:63, 1988.
22. Macnicol MF: Results of a 25-year screening programme for neonatal hip instability. J Bone Joint Surg [Br] 72:1057, 1990.
23. Yngve D, Gross R: Late diagnosis of hip dislocation in infants. J Pediatr Orthop 10:777, 1990.
24. Burger BJ, Burger JD, Bos CFA, et al: Neonatal screening and staggered early treatment for congenital dislocation or dysplasia of the hip. Lancet 336:1549, 1990.
25. Catford JC, Bennet GC, Wilkinson JA: Congenital hip dislocation: An increasing and still uncontrolled disability? Br Med J 285:1527, 1982.
26. Morrissy RT, Cowie GH: Congenital dislocation of the hip: Early detection and prevention of late complications. Clin Orthop 222:79, 1987.
27. Krikler SJ, Dwyer NSP: Comparison of results of two approaches to hip screening in infants. J Bone Joint Surg [Br] 74:701, 1992.
28. Poul J, Bajerova J, Sommernitz M, et al: Early diagnosis of congenital dislocation of the hip. J Bone Joint Surg [Br] 74:695, 1992.
29. Bernard AA, O'Hara JN, Bazin S, et al: An improved screening system for the early detection of congenital dislocation of the hip. J Pediatr Orthop 7:277, 1987.
30. Moore FH: Examining infants' hips—can it do harm? J Bone Joint Surg [Br] 71:4, 1989.
31. McCarroll HR, McCarroll HR Jr: Primary anterior congenital dislocation of the hip in infancy. J Bone Joint Surg [Am] 62:554, 1980.
32. Ilfeld FW, Westin GW, Makin M: Missed or developmental dislocation of the hip. Clin Orthop 203:276, 1986.
33. Bjerkreim I, Johansen J: Late diagnosed congenital dislocation of the hip. Acta Orthop Scand 58:504, 1987.
34. Dunn PM, Evans RE, Thearle MJ, et al: Congenital dislocation of the hip: Early and late diagnosis and management compared. Arch Dis Child 60:407, 1985.
35. Palmen K: Prevention of congenital dislocation of the hip: The Swedish experience of neonatal treatment of hip joint instability. Acta Orthop Scand 55(Suppl 208):1, 1984.
36. Sartoris DJ, Ogden JA: Congenital dysplasia of the hip. In D Resnick: Bone and Joint Imaging. Philadelphia, WB Saunders Company, 1989, p 1000.

37. Stewart RJ, Patterson CC, Mollan RAB: Ossification of the normal femoral capital epiphysis. J Bone Joint Surg [Br] 68:653, 1986.
38. Bertol P, Macnicol MF, Mitchell GP: Radiographic features of neonatal congenital dislocation of the hip. J Bone Joint Surg [Br] 64:176, 1982.
39. Ozonoff MB: The radiological assessment of congenital dislocation of the hip. Curr Orthop 1:258, 1987.
40. Rab GT: Preoperative roentgenographic evaluation for osteotomies about the hip in children. J Bone Joint Surg [Am] 63:306, 1981.
41. Broughton NS, Brougham DI, Cole WG, et al: Reliability of radiological measurements in the assessment of the child's hip. J Bone Joint Surg [Br] 71:6, 1989.
42. Garvey M, Donoghue VB, Gorman WA, et al: Radiographic screening at four months of infants at risk for congenital hip dislocation. J Bone Joint Surg [Br] 74:704, 1992.
43. Faure C, Schmit P, Salvat D: Cost-benefit evaluation of systematic radiological diagnosis of congenital dislocated hip. Pediatr Radiol 14:407, 1984.
44. Weinstein SL: Natural history of congenital hip dislocation (CDH) and hip dysplasia. Clin Orthop 225:62, 1987.
45. Drummond DS, O'Donnell J, Breed A, et al: Arthrography in the evaluation of congenital dislocation of the hip. Clin Orthop 243:148, 1989.
46. Harcke HT: Imaging in congenital dislocation and dysplasia of the hip. Clin Orthop 281:22, 1992.
47. Strife JL, Towbin R, Crawford A: Hip arthrography in infants and children: The inferomedial approach. Radiology 152:536, 1984.
48. Graf R, Schuler P: Sonography of the Infant Hip: An Atlas. Weinhein, Germany, VCH Verlagsgesellschaft MBH, 1986.
49. Scott ST: Infant hip ultrasound. Clin Radiol 40:551, 1989.
50. Zieger M, Hilpert S, Schulz RD: Ultrasonography of the infant hip. I. Basic principles. Pediatr Radiol 16:483, 1986.
51. Graf R: Ultrasonography of the infantile hip. In RC Sanders, MC Hill (Eds): Ultrasound Annual 1985. New York, Raven Press, 1985, p 177.
52. Harcke HT, Kumar SJ: The role of ultrasound in the diagnosis and management of congenital dislocation and dysplasia of the hip. J Bone Joint Surg [Am] 73:622, 1991.
53. Emerson DS, Brown DL, Mabie BC: Prenatal sonographic diagnosis of hip dislocation. J Ultrasound Med 7:687, 1988.
54. Boal DKB, Schwenker EP: The infant hip: Assessment with real-time US. Radiology 157:667, 1985.
55. Berman L, Catterall A, Meire HB: Ultrasound of the hip: A review of the applications of a new technique. Br J Radiol 59:13, 1986.
56. Novick G, Ghelman B, Schneider M: Sonography of the neonatal and infant hip. AJR 141:639, 1983.
57. Clarke NMP, Harcke HT, McHugh P, et al: Real-time ultrasound in the diagnosis of congenital dislocation and dysplasia of the hip. J Bone Joint Surg [Br] 67:406, 1985.
58. Clarke MNP: Sonographic clarification of the problems of neonatal hip instability. J Pediatr Orthop 6:527, 1986.
59. Keller MS, Chawla HS: Sonographic delineation of the neonatal acetabular labrum. J Ultrasound Med 4:501, 1985.
60. Keller MS, Chawla HS, Weiss AA: Real-time sonography of infant hip dislocation. RadioGraphics 6:447, 1986.
61. Keller MS, Weiss AA: Sonographic guidance for infant hip reduction under anesthesia. Pediatr Radiol 18:174, 1988.
62. Harcke HT, Grisson LE: Sonographic evaluation of the infant hip. Semin Ultrasound CT MR 7:331, 1986.
63. Miralles M, Gonzalez G, Pulpeiro JR, et al: Sonography of the painful hip in children: 500 consecutive cases. AJR 152:579, 1989.
64. Nichols GW, Schwenker EP, Boal DKB: Correlation of anatomy and ultrasonographic images in the infant hip: An experimental cadaver study. J Pediatr Orthop 6:410, 1986.
65. Harcke HT, Clarke NMP, Lee MS, et al: Examination of the infant hip with real-time ultrasonography. J Ultrasound Med 3:131, 1984.
66. Yousefzadeh DK, Ramilo HL: Normal hip in children: Correlation of US with anatomic and cryomicrotome sections. Radiology 165:647, 1987.
67. Zieger M, Hilpert S: Ultrasonography of the infant hip. IV. Normal development in the newborn and preterm neonate. Pediatr Radiol 17:470, 1987.
68. Novick GS: Sonography in pediatric hip disorders. Radiol Clin North Am 26:29, 1988.
69. Harcke HT, Lee MS, Sinning L, et al: Ossification center of the infant hip: Sonographic and radiographic correlation. AJR 7:317, 1986.
70. Boal DKB, Schwenker EP: Assessment of congenital hip dislocation with real-time ultrasound: A pictorial essay. Clin Imaging 15:77, 1991.
71. Berman L, Hollingdale J: The ultrasound appearance of positive hip instability tests. Clin Radiol 38:117, 1987.
72. Sosnierz A, Karel M, Maj S, et al: Ultrasound appearance of the hip joint in newborns during the first week of life. J Clin Ultrasound 19:271, 1991.
73. Keller MS, Weltin GG, Rattner Z, et al: Normal instability of the hip in the neonates: US standards. Radiology 169:733, 1988.
74. Morin C, Harcke HT, MacEwen GD: The infant hip: Real-time US assessment of acetabular development. Radiology 157:673, 1985.
75. Zieger M: Ultrasonography of the infant hip. II. Validity of the method. Pediatr Radiol 16:488, 1986.
76. Berman L, Klenerman L: Ultrasound screening for hip abnormalities: Preliminary findings in 1001 neonates. Br Med J 293:719, 1986.

77. Zieger M, Schulz RD: Ultrasonography of the infant hip. III. Clinical application. Pediatr Radiol *17*:226, 1987.
78. Polaneur PA, Harcke HT, Bowen JR: Effective use of ultrasound in the management of congenital dislocation and/or dysplasia of the hip. Clin Orthop *252*:176, 1990.
79. Grissom LE, Harcke HT, Kumar SJ, et al: Ultrasound evaluation of hip position in the Pavlik harness. J Ultrasound Med *7*:1, 1988.
80. Dahlstrom H, Oberg L, Friberg S: Sonography in congenital dislocation of the hip. Acta Orthop Scand *57*:402, 1986.
81. Langer R: Ultrasonic investigation of the hip in newborns in the diagnosis of congenital hip dislocation: Classification and results of a screening program. Skel Radiol *16*:275, 1987.
82. Tredwell SJ: Economic evaluation of neonatal screening for congenital dislocation of the hip. J Pediatr Orthop *10*:327, 1990.
83. Hadlow V: Neonatal screening for congenital dislocation of the hip: A prospective 21-year survey. J Bone Joint Surg [Br] *70*:740, 1988.
84. Fulton MJ, Barer ML: Screening for congenital dislocation of the hip: An economic appraisal. Can Med Assoc J *130*:1149, 1984.
85. Bialik V, Reuveni A, Pery M, et al: Utrasonography in developmental displacement of the hip: A critical analysis of our results. J Pediatr Orthop *9*:154, 1989.
86. Bick U, Muller-Leisse C, Troger J: Ultrasonography of the hip in preterm neonates. Pediatr Radiol *20*:331, 1990.
87. Graf R: The diagnosis of congenital hip-joint dislocation by the ultrasonic compound treatment. Arch Orthop Trauma Surg *97*:117, 1980.
88. Gardiner HM, Clarke NMP, Dunn PM: A sonographic study of the morphology of the preterm neonatal hip. J Pediatr Orthop *10*:663, 1990.
89. Graf R: Classification of hip joint dysplasia by means of sonography. Arch Orthop Trauma Surg *102*:248, 1984.
90. Terjesen T, Bredland T, Berg V: Ultrasound for hip assessment in the newborn. J Bone Joint Surg [Br] *71*:767, 1989.
91. Terjesen T, Runden T, Tangerud A: Ultrasonography and radiography of the hip in infants. Acta Orthop Scand *60*:651, 1989.
92. Jones DA, Powell N: Ultrasound and neonatal hip screening: A prospective study of "high risk" babies. J Bone Joint Surg [Br] *72*:457, 1990.
93. Tonnis D, Storch K, Ulbrich HJ: Results of newborn screening for CDH with and without sonography and correlation of risk factors. J Pediatr Orthop *10*:145, 1990.
94. Harcke HT, Grissom LE: Performing dynamic sonography of the infant hip. AJR *155*:837, 1990.
95. Clarke NMP, Clegg J, Al-Chalabi AN: Ultrasound screening of the hips at risk for CDH: Failure to reduce the incidence of late cases. J Bone Joint Surg [Br] *71*:9, 1989.
96. Engesaeter LB, Wilson DJ, Nag D, et al: Ultrasound and congenital dislocation of the hip: The importance of dynamic assessment. J Bone Joint Surg [Br] *72*:197, 1990.
97. Edelson JG, Hirsch M, Weinberg H, et al: Congenital dislocation of the hip and computerised axial tomography. J Bone Joint Surg [Br] *66*:472, 1984.
98. Helms CA, Goodman PC, Jeffrey RB Jr: Use of computed tomography in congenital dislocation of the hip. J Comput Assist Tomogr *7*:363, 1983.
99. Peterson HA, Klassen RA, Hoffman AD: The use of computerised tomography in dislocation of the hip and femoral neck anteversion in children. J Bone Joint Surg [Br] *63*:198, 1981.
100. Hernandez RJ: Concentric reduction of the dislocated hip: Computed tomographic evaluation. Radiology *150*:266, 1984.
101. Hernandez J, Poznanski AK: CT evaluation of pediatric hip disorders. Orthop Clin North Am *16*:513, 1985.
102. Hernandez RJ, Tachdjian MO, Dias LS: Hip CT in congenital dislocation: Appearance of tight iliopsoas tendon and pulvinar hypertrophy. AJR *139*:335, 1982.
103. Simons GW, Flatley TJ, Sty JR, et al: Intra-articular osteocartilaginous obstruction to reduction of congenital dislocation of the hip: Report of three cases. J Bone Joint Surg [Am] *70*:760, 1988.
104. Browning WH, Rosenkrantz H: Computed tomography in congenital hip dislocation: The role of acetabular anteversion. J Bone Joint Surg [Am] *64*:27, 1982.
105. Gugenheim JJ, Gerson LP, Sadler C, et al: Pathological morphology of the acetabulum in paralytic and congenital hip instability. J Pediatr Orthop *2*:397, 1982.
106. Guyer B, Smith DS, Cady RB, et al: Dosimetry of computerized tomography in the evaluation of hip dysplasia. Skel Radiol *12*:123, 1984.
107. Toby EB, Koman LA, Bechtold RE, et al: Postoperative computed tomographic evaluation of congenital hip dislocation. J Pediatr Orthop *7*:667, 1987.
108. Lang P, Genant HK, Steiger P, et al: Three-dimensional digital displays in congenital dislocation of the hip: Preliminary experience. J Pediatr Orthop *9*:532, 1989.
109. Lee DY, Choi IH, Lee CK, et al: Assessment of complex hip deformity using three-dimensional CT image. J Pediatr Orthop *11*:13, 1991.
110. Lafferty CM, Sartoris DJ, Tyson R, et al: Acetabular alterations in untreated congenital dysplasia of the hip: Computed tomography with multiplanar reformation and three-dimensional analysis. J Comput Assist Tomogr *10*:84, 1986.
111. Azuma H, Taneda H, Igarashi H, et al: Preoperative and postoperative assessment of rotational acetabular osteotomy for dysplastic hips in children by three-dimensional surface reconstruction computed tomography imaging. J Pediatr Orthop *10*:33, 1990.
112. Bos CFA, Bloem JL: Treatment of dislocation of the hip, detected in early childhood, based on magnetic resonance imaging. J Bone Joint Surg *71*:1523, 1989.
113. Bos CFA, Bloem JL, Obermann WR, et al: Magnetic resonance imaging in congenital dislocation of the hip. J Bone Joint Surg [Br] *70*:174, 1988.
114. Lang P, Steiger P, Genant HK, et al: Three-dimensional CT and MR imaging in congenital dislocation of the hip: Clinical and technical considerations. J Comput Assist Tomogr *12*:459, 1988.
115. Johnson ND, Wood BP, Jackman KV: Complex infantile and congenital hip dislocation: Assessment with MR imaging. Radiology *168*:151, 1989.
116. Toby BE, Koman LA, Bechtold RE: Magnetic resonance imaging of pediatric hip disease. J Pediatr Orthop *5*:665, 1985.
117. Fisher R, O'Brien TS, Davis KM: Magnetic resonance imaging in congenital dysplasia of the hip. J Pediatr Orthop *11*:617, 1991.
118. Hughes JR: Intrinsic obstructive factors in congenital dislocation of the hip: The role of arthrography. *In* MO Tachdjian (Ed): Congenital Dislocation of the Hip. New York, Churchill Livingstone, 1982, p 227.
119. Tachdjian MO: Treatment after walking age. *In* MO Tachdjian (Ed): Congenital Dislocation of the Hip. New York, Churchill Livingstone, 1982, p 344.
120. Hernandez RJ: Evaluation of congenital hip dysplasia and tibial torsion by computed tomography. J Comput Tomogr *7*:101, 1983.
121. Krasny R, Prescher A, Botschek A, et al: MR-anatomy of infant hips: Comparison to anatomical preparations. Pediatr Radiol *21*:211, 1991.
122. Johnson ND, Wood BP, Noh KS, et al: MR imaging anatomy of the infant hip. AJR *153*:127, 1989.
123. McKibbin B, Freedman L, Howard C, et al: The management of congenital dislocation of the hip in the newborn. J Bone Joint Surg [Br] *70*:423, 1988.
124. Schoenecker PL, Strecker WB: Congenital dislocation of the hip in children: Comparison of the effects of femoral shortening and of skeletal traction in treatment. J Bone Joint Surg [Am] *66*:21, 1984.
125. Bradley J, Wetherill M, Benson MKD: Splintage for congenital dislocation of the hip: Is it safe and reliable? J Bone Joint Surg [Br] *69*:257, 1987.
126. Elsworth C, Walker G: The safety of the Denis Browne abduction harness in congenital dislocation of the hip. J Bone Joint Surg [Br] *68*:275, 1986.
127. Iwasaki K: Treatment of congenital dislocation of the hip by the Pavlik harness: Mechanism of reduction and usage. J Bone Joint Surg [Am] *65*:760, 1983.
128. Gardiner HM, Dunn PM: Controlled trial of immediate splinting versus ultrasonographic surveillance in congenitally dislocatable hips. Lancet *336*:1553, 1990.
129. Mubarak S, Garfin S, Vance R, et al: Pitfalls in the use of the Pavlik harness for treatment of congenital dysplasia, subluxation, and dislocation of the hip. J Bone Joint Surg [Am] *63*:1239, 1981.
130. Heikkila E, Ryoppy S: Treatment of congenital dislocation of the hip after neonatal diagnosis. Acta Orthop Scand *55*:130, 1984.
131. Brougham DI, Broughton NS, Cole WG, et al: The predictability of acetabular development after closed reduction for congenital dislocation of the hip. J Bone Joint Surg [Br] *70*:733, 1988.
132. Race C, Herring JA: Congenital dislocation of the hip: An evaluation of closed reduction. J Pediatr Orthop *3*:166, 1983.
133. O'Hara JN, Bernard AA, Dwyer NS: Early results of medial approach open reduction in congenital dislocation of the hip: Use before walking age. J Pediatr Orthop *8*:288, 1988.
134. Zionts LE, MacEwen GD: Treatment of congenital dislocation of the hip in children between the ages of one and three years. J Bone Joint Surg [Am] *68*:829, 1986.
135. Renshaw TS: Inadequate reduction of congenital dislocation of the hip. J Bone Joint Surg [Am] *63*:1114, 1981.
136. Dahlstrom H, Friberg S, Oberg L: Stabilisation and development of the hip after closed reduction of late CDH. J Bone Joint Surg [Br] *72*:186, 1990.
137. Green NE, Griffin PP: Hip dysplasia associated with abduction contracture of the contralateral hip. J Bone Joint Surg [Am] *64*:1273, 1982.
138. Berkeley ME, Dickson JH, Cain TE, et al: Surgical therapy for congenital dislocation of the hips in patients who are twelve to thirty-six months old. J Bone Joint Surg [Am] *66*:412, 1984.
139. Perlik PC, Westin GW, Marafioti RL: A combination pelvic osteotomy for acetabular dysplasia in children. J Bone Joint Surg [Am] *67*:842, 1985.
140. Heikkila E, Ryoppy S, Louhimo I: The management of primary acetabular dysplasia: Its association with habitual side-lying. J Bone Joint Surg [Br] *67*:25, 1985.
141. Blockley NJ: Derotation osteotomy in the management of congenital dislocation of the hip. J Bone Joint Surg [Br] *66*:485, 1984.
142. Kasser JR, Bowen JR, MacEwen GD: Varus derotation osteotomy in the treatment of persistent dysplasia in congenital dislocation of the hip. J Bone Joint Surg [Am] *67*:195, 1985.
143. Marafioti RL, Westin GW: Factors influencing the results of acetabuloplasty in children. J Bone Joint Surg [Am] *62*:765, 1980.
144. Ninomiya S, Tagawa H: Rotational acetabular osteotomy for the dysplastic hip. J Bone Joint Surg [Am] *66*:430, 1984.
145. Williamson DM, Benson MKD: Late femoral osteotomy in congenital dislocation of the hip. J Bone Joint Surg [Br] *70*:614, 1988.
146. White RE, Sherman FC: The hip-shelf procedure: A long-term evaluation. J Bone Joint Surg [Am] *62*:928, 1980.
147. Summers BN, Turner A, Wynn-Jones CH: The shelf operation in the management of late presentation of congenital hip dysplasia. J Bone Joint Surg [Br] *70*:63, 1988.

148. Kalamchi A, Schmidt TL, MacEwen GD: Congenital dislocation of the hip: Open reduction by the medial approach. Clin Orthop *169*:127, 1982.

149. Powell EN, Gerratana FJ, Gage JR: Open reduction for congenital hip dislocation: The risk of avascular necrosis with three different approaches. J Pediatr Orthop *6*:127, 1986.

150. Barrett WP, Staheli LT, Chew DE: The effectiveness of the Salter innominate osteotomy in the treatment of congenital dislocation of the hip. J Bone Joint Surg [Am] *68*:79, 1986.

151. Fixsen JA: Anterior and posterior displacement of the hip after innominate osteotomy. J Bone Joint Surg [Br] *69*:361, 1987.

152. O'Brien T, Salter RB: Femoral head size in congenital dislocation of the hip. J Pediatr Orthop *5*:299, 1985.

153. Calvert PT, August AC, Albert JC, et al: The Chiari pelvic osteotomy: A review of the long-term results. J Bone Joint Surg [Br] *69*:551, 1987.

154. Hogh J, Macnicol MF: The Chiari pelvic osteotomy: A long-term review of clinical and radiographic results. J Bone Joint Surg [Br] *69*:365, 1987.

155. Malefijt MC, Hoogland T, Nielsen HKL: Chiari osteotomy in the treatment of congenital dislocation and subluxation of the hip. J Bone Joint Surg [Am] *64*:996, 1982.

156. Rejholec M, Stryhal F, Rybka V, et al: Chiari osteotomy of the pelvis: A long-term study. J Pediatr Orthop *10*:21, 1990.

157. Fairbank JCT, Howell P, Nockler I, et al: Relationship of pain to the radiological anatomy of the hip joints in adults treated for congenital dislocation of the hip as infants: A long-term follow-up of patients treated by three models. J Pediatr Orthop *6*:539, 1986.

158. Harley JM, Wilkinson JA: Hip replacement for adults with unreduced congenital dislocation: A new surgical technique. J Bone Joint Surg [Br] *69*:752, 1987.

159. Rombouts JJ, Kaelin A: Inferior (obturator) dislocation of the hip in neonates: A complication of treatment by the Pavlik harness. J Bone Joint Surg [Br] *74*:708, 1992.

160. Langkamer VG, Clarke NM, Witherow P. Complications of splintage in congenital dislocation of the hip. Arch Dis Child *66*:1322, 1991.

161. Mendez AA, Keret D, MacEwen GD: Obturator dislocation as a complication of closed reduction of the congenitally dislocated hip: A report of two cases. J Pediatr Orthop *10*:265, 1990.

162. Kalamchi A, MacEwen GD: Avascular necrosis following treatment of congenital dislocation of the hip. J Bone Joint Surg [Am] *62*:876, 1980.

163. Pool RD, Foster BK, Paterson DC: Avascular necrosis in congenital hip dislocation: The significance of splintage. J Bone Joint Surg [Br] *68*:427, 1986.

164. Suzuki S, Yamamuro T: Avascular necrosis in patients treated with the Pavlik harness for congenital dislocation of the hip. J Bone Joint Surg [Am] *72*:1048, 1990.

165. Robinson HJ Jr, Shannon MA: Avascular necrosis in congenital hip dysplasia: The effect of treatment. J Pediatr Orthop *9*:293, 1989.

166. Cooperman DR, Wallensten R, Stulberg SD: Post-reduction avascular necrosis in congenital dislocation of the hip. Long-term follow-up study of 25 patients. J Bone Joint Surg [Am] *62*:247, 1980.

167. McQueary FG, Johnston RC: Coxarthrosis after congenital dysplasia: Treatment by total hip arthroplasty without acetabular bone grafting. J Bone Joint Surg [Am] *70*:1140, 1988.

168. Wechsler RJ, Schwartz AM: Ischemic necrosis of the contralateral hip as a possible complication of untreated congenital hip dislocation. Skel Radiol *6*:279, 1981.

169. Smith MG: The results of neonatal treatment of congenital hip dislocation: A personal series. J Pediatr Orthop *4*:311, 1984.

170. Tredwell SJ, Davis LA: Prospective study of congenital dislocation of the hip. J Pediatr Orthop *9*:386, 1989.

171. Schoenecker PL, Lesker PA, Ogata K: A dynamic canine model of experimental hip dysplasia: Gross and histological pathology, and the effect of position of immobilization on capital femoral epiphyseal blood flow. J Bone Joint Surg [Am] *66*:1281, 1984.

172. Brougham DI, Broughton NS, Cole WG, et al: Avascular necrosis following closed reduction of congenital dislocation of the hip: Review of influencing factors and long-term follow-up. J Bone Joint Surg [Br] *72*:557, 1990.

173. Kahle WK, Anderson MB, Alpert J, et al: The value of preliminary traction in the treatment of congenital dislocation of the hip. J Bone Joint Surg [Am] *72*:1043, 1990.

174. Buchanan JR, Greer RB, Cotler JM: Management strategy for prevention of avascular necrosis during treatment of congenital dislocation of the hip. J Bone Joint Surg [Am] *63*:140, 1981.

175. Thomas IH, Dunin AJ, Cole WG, et al: Avascular necrosis after open reduction for congenital dislocation of the hip: Analysis of causative factors and natural history. J Pediatr Orthop *9*:525, 1989.

176. Fish DN, Herzenberg JE, Hensinger RN: Current practice in use of pre-reduction traction for congenital dislocation of the hip. J Pediatr Orthop *11*:149, 1991.

177. Bennett JT, MacEwen GD: Congenital dislocation of the hip: Recent advances and current problems. Clin Orthop *247*:15, 1989.

178. Gregosiewicz A, Wosko I: Risk factors of avascular necrosis in the treatment of congenital dislocation of the hip. J Pediatr Orthop *8*:17, 1988.

179. Thomas CL, Gage JR, Ogden JA: Treatment concepts for proximal femoral ischemic necrosis complicating congenital hip disease. J Bone Joint Surg [Am] *64*:817, 1982.

180. Ozonoff MB: Pediatric Orthopedic Radiology. 2nd Ed. Philadelphia, WB Saunders Company, 1992, p 164.

181. Carey TP, Guidera KG, Ogden JA: Manifestations of ischemic necrosis complicating developmental hip dysplasia. Clin Orthop *281*:11, 1992.

182. Thomas CL, Gage JR, Ogden JA: Treatment concepts for proximal femoral ischemic necrosis complicating congenital hip disease. J Bone Joint Surg [Am] *64*:817, 1982.

183. Campbell P, Tarlow SD: Lateral tethering of the proximal femoral physis complicating the treatment of congenital hip dysplasia. J Pediatr Orthop *10*:6, 1990.

184. Gamble JG, Mochizuki C, Bleck EE, et al: Coxa magna following surgical treatment of congenital hip dislocation. J Pediatr Orthop *5*:528, 1985.

185. O'Brien T: Growth-disturbance lines in congenital dislocation of the hip. J Bone Joint Surg [Am] *67*:626, 1985.

186. O'Brien T, Millis MB, Griffin PP: The early identification and classification of growth disturbances of the proximal end of the femur. J Bone Joint Surg [Am] *68*:970, 1986.

187. Iwersen LJ, Kalen V, Eberle C: Relative trochanteric overgrowth after ischemic necrosis in congenital dislocation of the hip. J Pediatr Orthop *9*:381, 1989.

188. Fernbach SK, Poznanski AK, Kelikian AS, et al: Greater trochanteric overgrowth: Development and surgical correction. Radiology *154*:661, 1985.

189. Gage JR, Cary JM: The effects of trochanteric epiphyseodesis on growth of the proximal end of the femur following necrosis of the capital femoral epiphysis. J Bone Joint Surg [Am] *62*:785, 1980.

190. O'Hara JN: Congenital dislocation of the hip: Acetabular deficiency in adolescence (absence of the lateral acetabular epiphysis) after limbectomy in infancy. J Pediatr Orthop *9*:640, 1989.

191. Gibson PH, Benson MKD: Congenital dislocation of the hip: Review at maturity of 147 hips treated by excision of the limbus and derotation osteotomy. J Bone Joint Surg [Br] *64*:169, 1982.

192. Bennet GC, Rang M, Roye DP, et al: Dislocation of the hip in trisomy 21. J Bone Joint Surg [Br] *64*:289, 1982.

87

Heritable Diseases of Connective Tissue, Epiphyseal Dysplasias, and Related Conditions

Amy Beth Goldman, M.D.

This chapter describes a group of disorders, many of which are associated with precocious osteoarthritis.

Marfan's syndrome, homocystinuria, the Ehlers-Danlos syndrome, and osteogenesis imperfecta all are inherited disorders of connective tissue. In varying degrees they involve the skin, ligaments, tendons, eyes, cardiovascular system, or skeleton. The joints of the extremities are not primarily affected by the connective tissue abnormalities. Incongruity resulting from the skeletal abnormalities and repetitive subclinical trauma resulting from ligamentous laxity, however, combine to produce precocious osteoarthritis. Myositis (fibrodysplasia) ossificans progressiva also is a primary disorder of connective tissues. It affects the joints of the extremities by causing peripheral ossification, the reverse of the other disorders in this category. Fibrogenesis imperfecta ossium and pseudoxanthoma elasticum do not result in joint changes but are included in this category because of possible similarities in pathogenesis.

The epiphyseal dysplasias are a heterogeneous group of inherited diseases, all of which result in abnormalities of the epiphyseal ends of the bones. Alterations in the contours of the articular surfaces result in incongruity and eventually in premature degeneration of the hyaline cartilage. Degenerative joint disease or degenerative disc disease frequently is the clinical complaint that brings these patients to medical attention.

Macrodystrophia lipomatosa and the Klippel-Trenaunay-Weber syndrome are two of the causes of congenital macrodactyly. The digital enlargement may be accompanied by articular changes. In macrodystrophia lipomatosa, secondary degenerative changes are dramatic and render the involved digit useless. In the Klippel-Trenaunay-Weber syndrome, the articular changes result from an associated bleeding diathesis.

MARFAN'S SYNDROME

Marfan's syndrome is a familial disorder of connective tissue that involves primarily the eye, the skeleton, and the cardiovascular system. It usually is an inherited autosomal dominant disorder with complete penetrance but variable expression.[1–5] Phenotypic heterogeneity varies from family to family and even within families.[2, 3, 6] Fifteen per cent of cases are sporadic.[1, 3, 7] The prevalence in the population is estimated to be 4 to 6 per 100,000 live births.[1, 5]

This syndrome was first described by Marfan in 1896. He emphasized the "spider-like" digits in a 5 year old patient and called the disorder "dolichostenomelia."[8] His original patient, however, no longer fits the definition of the disease owing to the associated joint contractures he had; in retrospect, the patient probably suffered from another familial disorder, which today is known as congenital contractural arachnodactyly.[7, 9, 10]

Pathology and Pathophysiology

The extreme phenotypic heterogeneity of Marfan's syndrome complicates clinical diagnosis based exclusively on the major physical findings (ectopia lentis, aortic root dilation or dissection, dural ectasia and dolichostenomelia).[2, 3, 6, 7, 10] This is particularly significant in cases in which there is no family history of the disorder. The highly variable clinical expression also has led to speculation that "mutations at different loci produce the same set of clinical manifestations in different families."[2]

Genetic linkage analysis studies have documented that one or more mutations in a locus (15q15–15q21) of the long arm of chromosome 15 (designated MFS1) result in Marfan's syndrome,[2, 5, 6] in both familial and sporadic cases.[6] Investigators also have identified the gene encoding fibrillin to be in the same locus on chromosome 15.[3, 5, 6, 11] Fibrillin is a large glycoprotein (350 kilodaltons) that is a component of elastin fibrils and linked to several smaller proteins.[6, 11] These fibrils are found in the periosteum, suspensory ligaments, and the tunica media of the aorta.[6] Immunohistochemical and biologic studies using monoclonal antibodies to fibrillin have shown a variety of abnormalities in families afflicted with Marfan's syndrome, including abnormal secretion, decreased synthesis, and abnormal extracellular assembly.[3, 11] The results suggest that any mutations that affect the structure of this glycoprotein have an adverse effect.[11]

Therefore, Marfan's syndrome results from mutations within the fibrillin gene on chromosome 15.[2, 3, 6, 11] Genetic analysis already has had practical clinical value in determining whether other disorders with similar phenotypic features are or are not a subset of Marfan's syndrome.[6] Patients with congenital contractural arachnodactyly (a milder syndrome without ocular findings) have shown no linkage to the fibrillin gene on chromosome 15 (negative lod scores) but have shown a positive linkage to the fibrillin gene on chromosome 5.[3, 6] Therefore, Marfan's syndrome and congenital arachnodactyly are genetically unrelated. Similarly, patients with isolated mitral prolapse and isolated anuloaortic ectasia have consistently negative lod scores for fibrillin gene 15.[6] However, cases with isolated ectopia lentis are genetically related to cases with Marfan's syndrome, despite the absence of musculoskeletal and vascular abnormalities.[3, 6] In the near future, genetic markers will provide an accurate means of prenatal or postnatal diagnosis of Marfan's syndrome despite its extreme phenotypic heterogeneity.

Pathologic changes in the tunica media of the aorta are part of the characteristic findings of Marfan's syndrome.[12–16] Accumulation of collagenous and mucoid material and fragmentation of elastic fibers predispose these patients to aortic dissection and rupture. The changes are most prominent in the ascending aorta, and early dilation of the proximal portion frequently results in incompetence of the aortic valve and dilation of the coronary sinuses.[13–16] Medial necrosis of the main pulmonary artery segment also has been described.

In addition to the abnormalities of the great vessels, fibromyxomatous changes may occur in the anulus, leaflets, and chordae tendineae of the aortic and mitral valves. They result in left-sided cardiac insufficiency related to the "floppy valve" syndrome.[17, 18]

The bilateral ectopia lentis that occurs in a majority of patients with Marfan's syndrome is related to changes in the suspensory ligaments of the lens.[13, 14, 18–20]

The precise cause and pathologic features of the skeletal changes have yet to be elucidated.

Clinical Findings

No sexual or racial predisposition is seen in Marfan's syndrome.[5, 13, 21, 22] Patients characteristically are tall and thin (greater than the 95th percentile by age and sex).[4] The limbs are disproportionately elongated in relation to the trunk (Fig. 87–1A), and arm span can exceed height.[1, 14, 19, 23] The lower extremities are affected more severely than the trunk or upper extremities. The increased length of the extremities is most exaggerated distally, particularly in the hands and feet.[13, 19, 20, 24] This gives the patient the typical appearance of arachnodactyly (Fig. 87–1B). Chest deformities (pectus carinatum or excavatum) and scoliosis (Fig. 87–1A) accentuate the limb-trunk discrepancy.[1, 13, 14, 19, 20, 24] Absence of normal subcutaneous fat and muscle atrophy also contribute to the appearance of abnormally long extremities. The skull typically is dolichocephalic, the face elongated, the jaw prominent, and the palate high and arched.[1, 13, 21, 24] Manifestations of ligamentous laxity, including angular deformities of the joints, pes planus, and scoliosis, frequently are evident.[25] Blue sclerae and poor dentition sometimes are present. Intelligence is normal.

It is unusual for the phenotypic findings of Marfan's syndrome to be apparent in infants.[7] In these infants, recognizable features include a peculiar facies characterized by large deep-set eyes (enophthalmus), malar hypoplasia, and micrognathia—an appearance referred to as the "worried look."[7] In these neonates, the disorder most often results from a sporadic mutation (only three of a series of 22 affected infants had a family history), and severe cardiac involvement is typical.[7, 26] Echocardiography can confirm the clinical impression by demonstrating a "cloverleaf" dilation of the sinuses of Valsalva.[7] These infantile cases are being treated with beta-blockade in an effort to reduce the morbidity of the disease.[7]

The most common ocular abnormalities are bilateral ectopia lentis and myopia, but strabismus and retinal detachments also may be present.[3, 11, 13, 14, 18–20] Cataracts occur late in the course of the disease and are secondary to the lens detachments.

The cardiac abnormalities are responsible for the shortened life expectancy of patients with Marfan's syndrome.[3, 27] The mean age at death is 28 years.[22] Cystic medial necrosis of the aorta or pulmonary artery occurs in a majority of patients and predisposes to dissection and rupture. Aortic and mitral valve insufficiency may result from the aortic dilation, from a "floppy valve" syndrome, or from both. Septal defects and sinus of Valsava aneurysms also are associated with Marfan's syndrome.

Difficulty in establishing the diagnosis of Marfan's syndrome is due to (1) variable expression; (2) the clinical findings that increase with age and, therefore, may not be apparent in the first years of life; and (3) the nonspecific nature of the "marfanoid phenotype."[7, 19, 28, 29] Indeed, in a series of 20 children with long fingers and myopia, three had other disorders (neurofibromatosis, Apert's syndrome, and premature craniosynostosis).[26] The diagnosis should be suspected by the clinician if at least two of the three systems are affected (ocular, cardiovascular, skeletal) and if

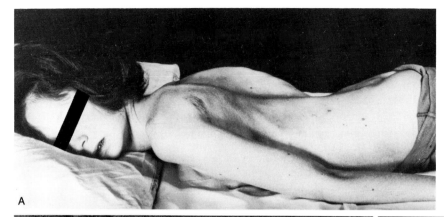

FIGURE 87–1. Marfan's syndrome: Adolescent girl. **A,** A prone view demonstrates disproportionately long arms and a thoracic kyphoscoliosis. **B,** The digits of the hands are elongated, and the thumb protrudes beyond the clenched fist **(C).**

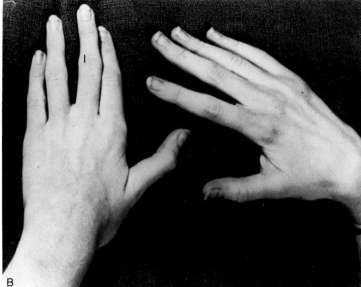

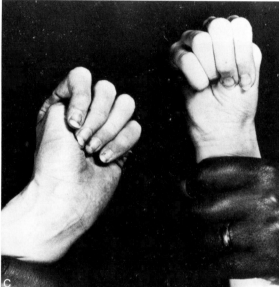

there is a family history of the disease.[1, 29, 30] In one orthopedic series, reported by Robins and coworkers, bilateral dislocation of the lens occurred in 57 per cent of cases, arachnodactyly in 89 per cent of cases, and aortic murmurs in 62 per cent of cases.[19] Ectopia lentis is the most reliable of the clinical changes but does not occur in all patients with Marfan's syndrome and has a mean age of onset of 2.7 years.[7] Identification of genetic markers is providing an accurate method of diagnosis in the majority of patients with Marfan's syndrome.[5]

The literature is replete with clinical and radiographic tests designed to identify the marfanoid phenotype. However, these tests may be negative in patients with documented Marfan's syndrome and falsely positive in patients with marfanoid phenotype but without ocular or cardiac changes.[31] The first of these tests is the "thumb sign" described by Steinberg,[20] in which the protrusion of the thumb beyond the confines of a clenched fist is used to reflect the narrow palm and long thumb that characterize arachnodactyly (Fig. 87–1C). The second test is the segmental measurement reported by Keech and associates.[29] The distance from the pubic symphysis to the floor and the distance from the top of the head to the floor are measured and a ratio is calculated. In normal adults, this ratio is less than 0.85. In patients with Marfan's syndrome and doli-

chostenomelia, the ratio is increased.[1, 29, 32] Skeletal proportions vary with age, and a table is necessary[33] to calculate the segmental index in children. The third test is the metacarpal index described by Parrish,[34] which is based on the lengths of the second through fifth metacarpal bones and is measured on radiographs of the hand (Figs. 87–2 and 87–3). The lengths of the metacarpal bones then are divided by the respective width of each diaphysis, and ratios are obtained. The four ratios are then averaged. In normal men, the metacarpal index is less than 8.8; in normal women, it is less than 9.4. The ratio is increased in patients with Marfan's syndrome.[13, 31, 33, 34] As in the clinical tests, application of the metacarpal index may result in false-positive and false-negative examinations.[31]

Radiographic Findings

The diagnosis of Marfan's syndrome usually is made after the child has begun to walk. Recently, ultrasonographic studies have attempted to identify mitral prolapse or aortic root dilation in the young child (less than 4 years of age)[7, 35] or abnormal segmental ratios in utero.[36] These studies as yet have identified only severely affected persons, however.[35, 36]

In the older child or adult with Marfan's syndrome,

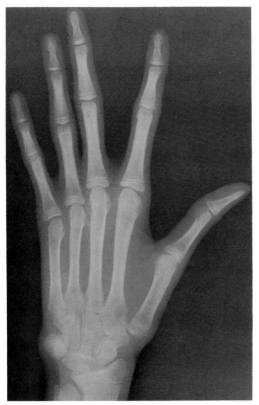

FIGURE 87-2. Marfan's syndrome. Posteroanterior view of the hand demonstrates absence of subcutaneous fat, elongation of phalanges and metacarpal bones, and normal bone density.

radiographs of the hands and feet demonstrate arachnodactyly with elongation of both the metacarpal bones and the phalanges (see Figs. 87–2 and 87–3). Frequently a 90 degree flexion deformity is present in one or both fifth digits of the hands (Fig. 87–3),[4] and a disproportionate elongation of the first digit of the foot may be seen. Bone age is normal or advanced. Other deformities in the hands and feet include hallux valgus, hammer toes, clubfeet, and calcaneal enthesophytes. Pes planus deformities and, rarely, carpal instability associated with perilunate dislocation result from ligamentous laxity.[19, 20, 28, 37, 38]

The extremities of patients with Marfan's syndrome demonstrate a marked diminution of soft tissue related to both muscular atrophy and sparse subcutaneous fat (Figs. 87–2 and 87–3).[4, 7] The long bones are slender and gracile. Osteoporosis is not present. Limb length discrepancies can occur. An increased frequency of slipped capital femoral epiphyses is seen.[4] Joints are hypermobile, predisposing to deformities (genu recurvatum, patella alta), dislocations (patellae, hips, clavicles, mandible), and joint instability.[38, 39] The hyperlaxity also is responsible for abnormal joint mechanics, repetitive subclinical trauma, and premature degenerative joint disease.[4]

Scoliosis occurs in 40 to 60 per cent of patients with Marfan's syndrome, further exaggerating the dolichostenomelia.[40] The curve pattern is similar to that of idiopathic scoliosis with a major thoracic curve convex to the right. Also, as in idiopathic scoliosis, an increased frequency of spondylolysis and spondylolisthesis occurs[1, 41, 42] (Fig. 87–4). The scoliosis of Marfan's syndrome, however, begins

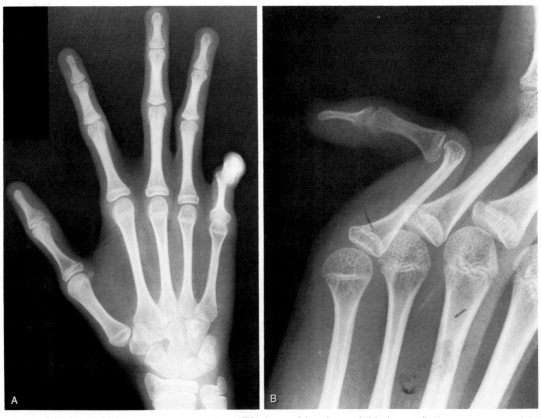

FIGURE 87-3. Marfan's syndrome. Frontal **(A)** and oblique **(B)** views of hand reveal 90 degree flexion contracture of fifth digit and arachnodactyly.

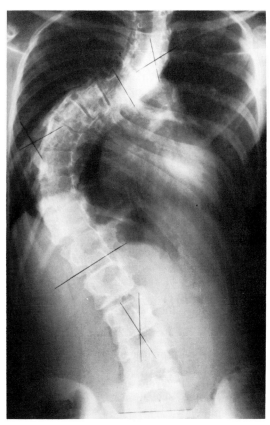

FIGURE 87–4. Marfan's syndrome: Scoliosis. The radiographic appearance is indistinguishable from that of idiopathic scoliosis.

earlier than the idiopathic form and does not exhibit the female predominance of the idiopathic type. It progresses more rapidly in young patients.[4, 10] The thoracic scoliosis often is accompanied by a lordotic deformity and may be painful.[4, 10] Treatment often is difficult, as the patient with Marfan's syndrome tends to be resistant to bracing, and surgery is associated with an increased frequency of complications, including pseudarthrosis.[42] Posterior scalloping of the vertebral bodies has been reported and is attributed to dural ectasia. An increased frequency of Scheuermann's disease likewise is seen.

Other spinal manifestations of Marfan's syndrome have been recognized, particularly since the advent of CT combined with metrizamide myelography and MR imaging.[43]

Sacral anomalies, characterized by focal widening of both the central canal and neural foramina, with or without a soft tissue mass (meningocele), are seen in older patients with Marfan's syndrome.[4, 22, 44, 45] Sixty-three per cent of patients in a clinical series reported by Pyeritz and coworkers[44] had dural ectasia observed on CT or MR imaging studies performed primarily for evaluation of the aorta. Of the two types of examinations, MR imaging appears superior to CT in allowing identification of spinal changes because of lower radiation dose.[46] Imaging studies demonstrate widening of the interpediculate distance (the side-to-side diameter of the spinal canal) and scalloping of the posterior aspects of one or more vertebral bodies (indicating an increase in the anteroposterior diameter of the canal). The mildest cases are limited to L5 and the sacrum and are associated with thinning of the pedicles and lamina and with foraminal expansion.[22, 44] Severely affected patients

have complete or almost complete absence of the pedicles accompanied by anterior or posterior sacral meningoceles.[22, 44] The severity of the spinal changes does not correlate with the severity of the ocular or aortic abnormalities.[44] The sacral anomalies of Marfan's syndrome are attributed to localized weakening of the dura, subjecting the vertebrae to transient increases in pressure created by the cerebrospinal fluid pulsations.[22] The sacrum is at greatest risk because in the upright position the arachnoid pressure is highest in the distal end of the spinal column. The majority of these lumbar or sacral anomalies are incidental findings. Neuralgia secondary to pressure on sacral roots has been reported[22, 44] but is unusual. Even more uncommon are headaches associated with bowel movements.[22] If an anterior meningocele is large, it may produce genitourinary or gynecologic complaints or be mistaken for a neoplasm.[22] The differential diagnosis of focal widening of the spinal canal with intraspinal or protruding meningoceles includes neurofibromatosis, Ehlers-Danlos syndrome, or increased intrathecal pressure resulting from surgery or trauma.

A rare but serious complication is atlantoaxial subluxation due to ligament laxity about the apophyseal joints of C1-C2 and resulting in compression of the medulla and cerebellar tonsils.[47]

Protrusio acetabuli deformities, associated with a decreased range of motion, have been described in Marfan's syndrome as well as in other collagen disorders, such as the Ehlers-Danlos syndrome.[1, 4, 10, 32] The cause of this finding is unclear but may relate to weakened acetabular bone.[32] Chest deformities associated with Marfan's syndrome include asymmetry with pectus excavatum or carinatum resulting from elongation of the ribs.[4, 7] Cystic disease of the lung has been observed. In the skull, findings include a longer, thicker, and, most significantly, taller osseous configuration than in normal persons.[21] Also noted are frontal bossing, a high-arched palate with dental crowding, and enlargement of the frontal sinuses.[4, 22]

The radiographic differential diagnosis includes other syndromes associated with marfanoid skeletal changes. Homocystinuria, a congenital disorder of methionine metabolism, is characterized by arachnodactyly, scoliosis, sternal deformities, and ligamentous laxity. Patients are mentally retarded, however, and in addition the skeleton is osteoporotic, the vascular changes involve fibrosis of both the media and the intima of the vessels, and arterial or venous thromboembolic phenomena occur.[1] Congenital contractural arachnodactyly, another inherited disorder of connective tissue, also is characterized by long, thin limbs, scoliosis, and dolichostenomelia.[12, 48–51] The absence of eye and cardiac changes and the presence of joint contractures and deformed ears can distinguish the two entities. Slowly progressive myopathies, particularly nemaline myopathy, constitute another differential possibility. Muscle biopsies and electromyographic studies in these patients are positive for primary abnormalities of the muscle fibers, however. Type I multiple endocrine neoplasia syndrome (parathyroid and pituitary tumors) and type IIb multiple endocrine neoplasia syndrome (mucosal neuromas, pheochromocytoma, medullary carcinoma of the thyroid) also are associated with marfanoid features,[52–54] as is the Ehlers-Danlos syndrome.[55] With these diseases, clinical history and genetic studies are necessary to establish the correct diagnosis. Lastly, Stickler's syndrome, a hereditary connective tissue disorder affecting ocular, skeletal, and orofacial structures, can be associated with marfanoid features. Its distinctive orofacial changes, however, establish the diagnosis.[1]

HOMOCYSTINURIA

The term homocystinuria encompasses a group of disorders characterized by inborn errors in methionine metabolism and excessive homocysteine in body fluids.[14, 56-59] Three different autosomal recessive genetic enzymatic defects that lead to disturbances in homocysteine homeostasis have been described.[56, 58-62] All three result in neurologic, ocular, and skeletal abnormalities as well as in premature occlusive vascular disease.[14, 56, 57, 62, 63] The best known of these entities is the syndrome associated with a deficiency in the enzyme cystathionine beta-synthase.[59, 60-62, 64] It is classified by McKusick[12] as a secondary disorder of the fibrous component of connective tissue and is grouped with Menkes' kinky hair syndrome, a disorder characterized by copper deficiency. Investigators have demonstrated that patients with homocystinuria have increased excretion of metals (copper, iron, manganese, lead, zinc, mercury) but also have increased levels of these substances in hair and plasma.[59] The mutations producing homocystinuria have been difficult to isolate owing to both allelic and genic heterogeneity.[58, 62]

The syndrome of homocystinuria was first described in 1962 by two separate groups of investigators.[65, 66] In 1964, Gibson and collaborators[116] identified the association of thromboembolic phenomena with marfanoid skeletal features, which led to the reclassification of many patients with so-called Marfan's syndrome. Homocystinuria also is referred to as cystathionine beta-synthase deficiency or hyperhomocysteinemia.[58]

Pathology and Pathophysiology

The heterogeneous biochemical phenotype, referred to as homocystinuria, can result from (1) abnormalities in the transsulfuration pathway responsible for the conversion of methionine to homocysteine and then to cystathionine and cystine or (2) defective remethylation of homocysteine into methionine.[58, 61, 62]

The enzyme cystathionine beta-synthase catalyzes the conversion of homocysteine to cystathionine.[57, 64, 67] A deficiency in this substance interferes with transsulfuration, creating a metabolic block in the conversion of homocysteine,[58, 61, 62] and cystathionine levels are decreased in the brain, skin, and liver.[64, 67-69] The second result is an abnormal accumulation of the substance that precedes the defective enzyme (i.e., homocysteine). The latter product of methionine metabolism accumulates in the tissues and may undergo methylation back to methionine or oxidation to disulfite homocystine.[64] Homocysteine, homocystine, and methionine accumulate in the plasma, and excessive homocysteine is excreted in the urine.[68]

Vitamin B_6 (pyridoxine) is a coenzyme in two steps of the methionine metabolic pathway. In some cases of homocystinuria, the clinical and chemical abnormalities can be altered by massive doses of this vitamin.[56, 63, 67, 68, 70, 71] The patients who respond to vitamin B_6 tend to have some cystathionine synthetase activity detectable in the skin or liver prior to treatment, whereas those who do not respond tend to have a more severe enzymatic deficit.[67, 68] It has been postulated that the variable clinical response to vitamin B_6 is an indication of genetic heterogeneity even among patients with cystathionine beta-sythetase deficiency.[62] However, it still is unknown why some patients are biochemically sensitive to pyridoxine (B_6) and others are resistant.[61, 63, 72] Other therapeutic measures that have been advocated include low methionine diets supplemented with cystine.[14, 58, 62, 63, 73]

Disorders of methionine metabolism also result from two types of enzymatic deficiencies in the remethylation pathway.[61] A deficiency in 5,10-methylenetetrahydrofolate reductase interferes with remethylation of homocysteine into methionine.[61] The patients with this inborn error of metabolism have low or normal serum methionine levels and moderate homocysteinemia.[61] A second extremely heterogeneous type of homocystinuria results from defective remethylation owing to abnormalities in the metabolism of the cofactor methylcobalamin.[61, 74, 75] The latter enzymatic defects interfere with the reduction of vitamin $B_{12}(Co^{3+})$ to $B_{12}(Co^{2+})$. Patients with absence of 5′-deoxyadenosylcobalamin and methylcobalamin (CblC and CblD) have low serum levels of methionine and homocystinuria as well as methylmalonic aciduria.[61, 74, 75] Phenotypic heterogeneity is present even within this group.[74] Type C usually is severe and occurs in neonates. Type D is milder and can develop later in life.[74] Patients with an isolated defect in the enzyme methylcobalamin (CblE, CblG) have low serum levels of methionine and homocystinuria but no methylmalonic aciduria.[61, 75] Patients with abnormal cobalamin metabolism manifest a megaloblastic anemia as well as ocular, skeletal, and severe neurologic abnormalities.[61, 75]

Experimental evidence, reported by Francis and coworkers,[76] Grieco,[77] Hurwitz and associates,[78] and Kang and Trelstad,[79] indicates that homocystinuria is associated with a defect in collagen synthesis. Studies of skin collagen have demonstrated an abnormal increase in the soluble component and an abnormal decrease in polymeric collagen.[79]

Arterial and venous thromboses complicate the course of homocystinuria. Several investigators have attributed this phenomenon to an increase in platelet "stickiness."[14, 66, 80, 81] The abnormal aggregation of platelets was reported by some investigators to result from changes in the vessel walls and from the presence of unstable collagen.[57, 60, 80, 81] Results of studies performed using ^{111}In-labeled platelets have not supported this hypothesis, however.[80] The cause of vascular damage and premature occlusive disease remains disputed, and other postulated mechanisms include induced activation of factor V by homocystine,[61] reduced antithrombin III levels,[61] and decreased platelet survival.[62] As in Marfan's syndrome, cystic medial necrosis and fragmentation of elastic fibers are found in the aortas of patients with homocystinuria.[66, 69] Unlike Marfan's syndrome, however, similar changes occur in the media of all elastic arteries and are uniquely accompanied by the presence of patchy intimal pads or ridges.[66] In addition, despite thinning of the media, aortic dissections are not a characteristic feature of homocystinuria as they are in Marfan's syndrome.[57] The thromboembolic phenomena are the most common cause of death in patients with homocystinuria.[58, 60, 61, 80] The type of treatment necessary to prevent these catastrophic events remains controversial.[82] Mortality at 30 years of age is 23 per cent in untreated or vitamin D–resistant patients.[62]

It is 4 per cent in patients responsive to high doses of vitamin D.[62]

Mental retardation, seizures, and even schizophrenia occur as a result of cystathionine beta-synthase deficiency.[64, 73] Approximately 30 per cent of 47 patients in one reported series had abnormally low intelligence.[69] Cystathionine, a major free amino acid in the brain, is decreased in amount. However, the exact cause of the central nervous system abnormalities is not yet known. Investigations are complicated by the coexisting changes of venous and arterial thromboses and by the peripheral neuropathy that may result from high dose pyridoxine therapy.[63, 71] Infants with homocystinuria resulting from defective cobalamin metabolism can be microcephalic and have cerebral atrophy and general hypotonia.[75] These abnormalities are reversible, if treated early, with cobalamin.[75]

The most characteristic ocular abnormality of homocystinuria is bilateral dislocation of the lens.[14, 60, 62, 71, 72] Described pathologic findings include thickening of the basement membrane of the ciliary body and atrophy of nonpigmented epithelium.[69]

Other pathologic abnormalities reported in patients with homocystinuria include fatty changes in the liver and electron microscopic abnormalities in the hepatocytes.[66–68] Muscle disturbances with changes in the electromyogram also have been described.[78]

Clinical Findings

The most frequent form of homocystinuria results from a defect in the enzyme cystathionine beta-synthase; the clinical manifestations of this form of disease are discussed first and in greatest detail here.[59–62] This disorder occurs most commonly in northern Europeans from Sweden, Germany, Holland, England, Ireland, and Scotland.[57] Estimated frequency varies from one in 24,000 to one in 260,000 population.[61]

Patients appear normal at birth and during infancy, the sole clinical finding being irritability.[65, 72] Even in infants, however, the urine does contain increased levels of homocystine[64] and, as in adults, the cyanide nitroprusside test produces a red-purple color.[12, 69] Enzyme assays for cystathionine beta-synthase and for detection of hyperhomocysteinuria are most sensitive after a methionine overload.[58] Antenatal diagnosis also is possible using recent techniques. Cystathionine beta-synthase activity can be measured in cultured amniotic cells.[83] The level of enzymatic activity can be measured in fibroblasts[83, 84] or even more accurately in fetal lymphocytes stimulated by phytohemagglutinin.[83] In the future, it may be possible to sample fetal blood directly using fetoscopy.[83]

In early childhood, motor development slows or even regresses.[85] Patients with homocystinuria tend to have thin skin with large pores and prominent venous markings.[69, 85] Striae occur over the buttocks and shoulders.[57] A malar flush is frequently present and "cigarette paper" scars occur with minor trauma. Livedo reticularis can be present over the extensor surfaces of the extremities or the buttocks.[85] Hair is thin and sparse.[85] Hair color is abnormal, possibly related to decreased activity of tyrosine (a copper containing enzyme).[59] A high, arched palate ("gothic" palate) and poor dentition both are characteristic of this disorder.[69, 86]

The most frequent physical finding is bilateral lens dislocations, which may be present at birth, but which are not obvious until 3 to 10 years of age.[14, 56, 72, 85] Ectopia lentis is present in 90 per cent of untreated patients at 10 years of age and most often is bilateral. The eye changes occur in only 55 per cent of treated vitamin D–responsive cases.[72] Other, less frequent eye abnormalities include cataracts, optic atrophy, microphthalmus, and congenital glaucoma.

The degree of mental retardation varies and may be modified by therapy.[56, 59, 60, 64, 72] The retardation is milder in pyridoxine-responsive patients.[60–62, 71] Epileptic seizures and vascular accidents also produce symptoms referable to the central nervous system.[56]

Spontaneous venous and arterial thromboses complicate the clinical course of homocystinuria and frequently are life-threatening. Although it is the main cause of morbidity, vascular thrombosis rarely is the presenting abnormality.[60] Common sites of arterial clotting are the intermediate-sized vessels, including the coronary, renal, and carotid arteries and the other major branches of the aorta.[14, 56, 57] Venous thromboses frequently involve the mesenteric vessels, the vena cava, the iliac vessels, and the pulmonary veins. Surgery may precipitate a major vascular accident.[14]

Interest has been expressed in identifying persons who are heterozygous for cystathionine beta-synthase deficiency.[58, 61] Investigators postulate that persons with this deficiency suffer from accelerated atherosclerosis, resulting in peripheral vascular and cerebrovascular disease ("homocysteine theory of atherosclerosis").[58, 61] The estimated frequency of this gene in the population of Ireland is 1 in 200.[58, 61] Documentation is difficult because the laboratory values of heterozygotic persons overlap those of normal persons.[58] A deficit of one enzyme that is less than complete can produce only a minor change in homocysteine concentrations, owing to heterogeneity of the synthase locus and encoding controls of homocysteine flux.[58] False-positive laboratory values can result in cases of acquired disorders of homocysteine homeostasis (e.g., renal failure, high protein intake).[61]

Twenty-five[56] to 60[14] per cent of patients with homocystinuria have skeletal abnormalities that resemble those of Marfan's syndrome.[60, 72] Patients are tall, with disproportionately long extremities, a "duck-like" or "Chaplin-like" gait, scoliosis, pectus excavatum, and joint laxity.[14, 61, 64, 78, 85, 86] Several clinical findings differentiate these two entities, however. First, mental retardation, the malar flush, and vascular thromboses are not found in Marfan's syndrome. Second, although both entities are characterized by bilateral lens dislocations, this sign can be detected in infancy in patients with homocystinuria. Third, the lens tends to dislocate downward in cases of homocytinuria and upward in Marfan's syndrome.[72] Fourth, in Marfan's syndrome, contractures occur only in the fifth digits of the hands, whereas in homocystinuria, contractures occur in multiple digits as well as in the elbows and knees.[14] Fifth, the primary life-endangering vascular changes in Marfan's syndrome are related to the aorta and its origin, as opposed to homocystinuria, in which sudden death more frequently is the result of thromboembolic phenomena or rupture of medium-sized vessels.[64] Lastly, unlike Marfan's syndrome, positive and specific laboratory findings are present in homocystinuria.[14] The plasma levels of homocysteine, homocystine, and methionine all are elevated, and the urine contains abnormal amounts of homocysteine, which, like cystine, gives a positive result on the nitroprusside test. Cystine and homocysteine can be differentiated by paper electrophoresis.[57] Liver and skin biopsies are necessary for a specific enzymatic diagnosis.[66]

The syndromes associated with defective remethylation pathway differ somewhat from the "classic" cases related to cystathionine beta-synthase deficiency and defective transsulfuration. Patients with absence of 5,10-methylene-tetrahydrofolate reductase have microcephaly and seizures in addition to ocular and vascular abnormalities.[61] The vascular changes tend not to be associated with clinical findings.[61] Patients with disorders of cobalamin metabolism exhibit failure to thrive, microcephaly, cerebral atrophy, and megaloblastic anemia.[61, 74, 75] These findings respond to treatment with cobalamin. Homocystinuria related to impaired synthesis of cobalamin has an extremely variable phenotypic expression. Types CblC and CblD are associated with presence of both methylmalonic acid and homocystine in the urine. Types CblE and CblG are accompanied by homocystinuria only.[61, 75]

Radiographic Findings

No radiographic abnormalities are present at birth in this disorder.[64] Skeletal changes occur gradually during childhood and do not appear to correlate with the severity of the enzymatic defect or with its response to vitamin B_6.

The skull can show a variety of changes, including enlargement of the sinuses,[14, 64, 69] widening of the diploic space,[56] extensive dural calcification,[56] or prognathism.[69] These changes may be present in any combination.[14, 64, 69, 72, 85] MR imaging studies of treated patients with homocystinuria reveal focal areas of gliosis in the white matter and diffuse cortical atrophy.[71] In one study, only one in seven patients revealed changes clearly related to cerebral infarction.[71] Therefore, homocysteic acid may produce neuronal damage directly.[71]

Examination of the spine early in childhood can reveal generalized osteoporosis and scoliosis (Fig. 87–5).[14, 64, 69, 72, 85] The vertebral bodies have an increased anteroposterior diameter and may be biconcave in shape.[14, 57] Compression fractures are frequent.[56, 85] Posterior scalloping of the vertebral bodies[86] and premature degenerative disc disease have also been described.[14, 87]

Changes in the extremities include dolichostenomelia, osteoporosis, and multiple growth recovery lines (Fig. 87–6).[56–58, 60, 64, 69, 72] Frequently seen deformities include flattening of the epiphyses (especially about the knees and hips), broad metaphyses (Fig. 87–6), and varus deformities of the humeri.[14, 69] A characteristic stippled appearance can occur in the growth plates of the distal radii and ulnae, which contain punctate areas of ossification.[14, 56, 69] Joint findings are variable. Abnormal laxity may be present and result in genu valgum deformities and patella alta (Fig. 87–6).[14, 64, 85] Coexisting with laxity of some joints, however, are flexion contractures of others, particularly in the digits, the elbows, and the knees.[14, 85] Bowing of the upper extremities and hemiatrophy have been reported in isolated cases.[56]

Characteristic changes in the hands include arachnodactyly (Fig. 87–7) and carpal deformities.[14, 56, 69, 72] Bone age may be normal, accelerated, or retarded.[69]

The nonosseous radiographic abnormalities of homocys-

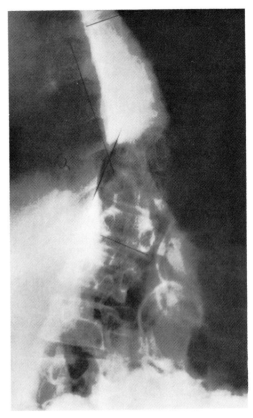

FIGURE 87–5. Homocystinuria. Scoliosis and osteoporosis are seen in the spine of a patient with homocystinuria.

tinuria include venous calcifications and an increased frequency of medullary sponge kidney.[56, 69]

The major radiographic differential diagnosis of homocystinuria involves Marfan's syndrome. The presence of osteoporosis, metaphyseal flaring, and multiple contractures should distinguish the radiographic appearance of dolichostenomelia in a patient with homocystinuria from that in a patient with Marfan's syndrome.[14, 56, 64]

EHLERS-DANLOS SYNDROME

The Ehlers-Danlos syndrome is a familial disorder of connective tissue that is characterized by hyperelasticity and fragility of the skin, hyperlaxity of the joints, and a bleeding diathesis.[88–91] The eye, gastrointestinal tract, bronchopulmonary tree, genitourinary system, and cardiovascular system also may be affected by this primary defect in mesenchyme.[92, 93]

The Ehlers-Danlos syndrome is not a single homogeneous disorder but a group of 11 syndromes that are associated with abnormal connective tissue; these syndromes vary genetically and biochemically but share the same complex of clinical abnormalities (Table 87–1).[94–96] It now is apparent that the clinical entity that is labeled the Ehlers-Danlos syndrome can result from genetic mutations of the procollagen genes (types IV and VII),[95, 97–106] enzymatic defects in posttranslational modification of fibrillar collagen (types IV and IX),[96, 105–110] or as yet unknown factors (Table 87–1). In addition, the syndrome in nearly 50 per cent of patients cannot be classified precisely,[96, 111, 112] and some types of syndrome have overlapping features.[111, 113] To further com-

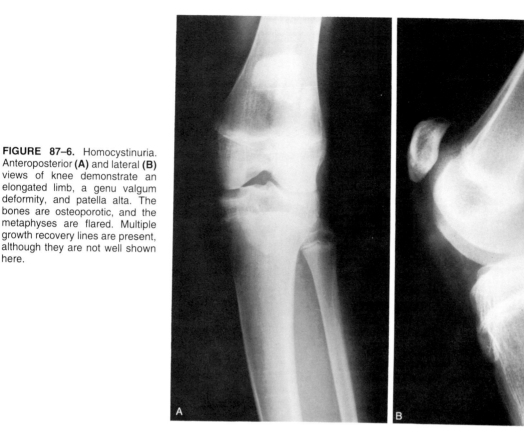

FIGURE 87–6. Homocystinuria. Anteroposterior **(A)** and lateral **(B)** views of knee demonstrate an elongated limb, a genu valgum deformity, and patella alta. The bones are osteoporotic, and the metaphyses are flared. Multiple growth recovery lines are present, although they are not well shown here.

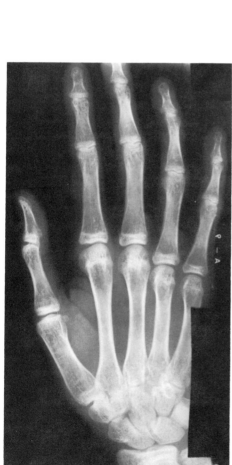

FIGURE 87–7. Homocystinuria. Frontal view of the hand reveals arachnodactyly and osteoporosis.

plicate the definition of Ehlers-Danlos syndrome, various authorities indicate that two of the 11 syndromes (IX, XI) should be reclassified under other disease categories: specifically, the type IX syndrome may be a disorder of copper transport and the type XI syndrome may represent a disorder of isolated joint instability.[96, 109]

The first efforts at organizing the spectrum of cases in the Ehlers-Danlos syndrome were published by Beighton and coworkers[89] and McKusick.[12] These classifications were based on the predominant mode of inheritance, the degree to which the three basic clinical findings were manifested, and any additional unique clinical abnormalities.[12, 89] More recent classification systems still are based on the severity of these same three phenotypic criteria (skin hyperelasticity, joint hypermobility, and skin fragility and bruising), and on the presence of additional unique clinical findings (Table 87–1).[94–98, 100, 103, 105, 108, 109]

Types I through IV are the most common forms of the Ehlers-Danlos syndrome.[95, 96] Type I, or the "gravis" form, is the classic form of this disorder and is characterized by dramatic hyperextensible skin, severe joint hypermobility, and easy bruisability (Table 87–1).[94–96] Type II, or the "mitis" form, is a milder syndrome than type I, with minimal cutaneous and joint manifestations; skin fragility is absent.[94, 96, 105] Type III is characterized by the predominance of severe joint hypermobility that results in slow physical development, poor coordination, and dislocations of small (temporomandibular, digital) and large (shoulders, knees, hips) joints.[96] Forty per cent of patients with the "benign hypermobility" syndrome require wheelchairs.[96] Types I,

TABLE 87–1. Classification of Ehlers-Danlos Syndrome

Type	Name	Pattern of Inheritance	Biochemical or Genetic Effect	Presence and Severity of the Three Basic Clinical Criteria	Additional Clinical Findings
I	Gravis	Autosomal dominant; rarely sporadic	Unknown	"Velvety" skin; severe laxity Severe joint hypermobility Bruisability	"Cigarette paper" scars Molluscoid tumors
II	Mitis	Autosomal dominant	Unknown	Mild skin laxity Mild joint hypermobility Absent skin fragility	Mitral prolapse Lumbar platyspondyly Papyraceous scars
III	Benign hypermobility	Autosomal dominant	Unknown	Mild skin laxity Severe joint hypermobility (40% wheelchair bound)	Joint dislocations
IV	Ecchymotic Acrogeric	Autosomal dominant Less frequent: autosomal recessive	Mutation in triple helical coding region of type III procollagen gene (COL3A1)	Easy bruisability of skin	Rupture of small and medium-sized vessels Acrogeria (aging of hands and feet) Rupture of hollow organs "Madonna" facies Blue sclerae Poor life expectancy
V	X-linked	X-linked recessive	Lysyl oxidase deficiency	Severe skin laxity Mild joint hypermobility Mild bruising	
VI	Ocular Scoliotic	Autosomal recessive	Collagen lysyl hydroxylase deficiency	Skin laxity Joint hypermobility Mild bruising	Ocular globe fragility Angioid steaking "Marfanoid" features Hypotonia during infancy Severe kyphoscoliosis
VII	Congenital arthrocholasys	Dominant or recessive	a. mutation in COLIA1 gene b. mutation in COLIA2 gene c. deficiency in procollagen N proteinase	Severe joint hypermobility Severe skin bruisability	Joint dislocations; developmental dysplasia of the hip Blue sclerae Micrognathia Criss-cross pattern on hands and soles Redundant skin folds
VIII	Periodontal form	Autosomal dominant	Unknown	Mild joint hypermobility Mild skin bruisability	Pretibial skin lesion Hyperpigmented scars Periodontitis with tooth loss
*IX	Occipital horn syndrome	X-linked recessive	?Disorder of copper metabolism	Skin hyperextensibility Joint hypermobility	Bony protuberance on occiput Poor extension of knees and elbows
X	Platelet dysfunction	Autosomal recessive	Abnormal fibronectin with abnormal platelet aggregation	Skin bruisability	Petechiae
*XI	Familial articular instability	Autosomal dominant	Unknown	Severe joint hypermobility	

*Beighton and coworkers[109] and Ainsworth and colleagues[96] exclude types IX and XI as forms of Ehlers-Danlos syndrome. Sarra-Carbonell and Jimenez,[94] Hamada and colleagues,[113] Hartsfield and Kousseff,[111] and Gamble and associates[121] still include types IX and XI as expressions of Ehlers-Danlos syndrome.

II, and III are associated with an autosomal dominant mode of inheritance (Table 87–1).[12, 89, 114] Type IV is the most serious form of the disease and has a decreased life expectancy related to spontaneous rupture of small or medium-sized vessels or rupture of hollow organs.[93, 96, 99–103, 115] Septal defects and insufficiency of the aortic and tricuspid valves further complicate the clinical course.[96] Type IV is referred to as the acrogeric type of Ehlers-Danlos syndrome because affected persons give the appearance of premature aging as a result of numerous skin folds in the face and extremities as well as prominent varicose veins (Table 87–1).[98–100, 102, 115] This type also is labeled the arterial form of Ehlers-Danlos syndrome because of vascular rupture and aneurysm formation. Autosominal dominant inheritance is commoner than autosomal recessive inheritance, although both types have been reported in families with type IV. Type V (an X-linked recessive form) is characterized by dramatic skin stretching. Type VI (autosomal recessive) is dominated by a variety of ocular abnormalities, including ocular fragility, angioid streaking, myopia, glaucoma, retinal detachment, and microcornea.[96, 105, 107, 114, 115] Type VI also can be associated with severe kyphoscoliosis, rheumatologic symptoms, and marfanoid features.[106, 107] Type VII

(autosomal dominant or recessive) is associated with short stature, severe joint hypermobility, and dislocations. It is characterized by abnormal skin collagen that occurs in sheets rather than fibrils (hieroglyphs), resulting in abnormal scarring, easy bruisability, redundant skin folds, and skin hyperextensibility.[98, 104–106] One of the three forms of type VII (type VIIC) resembles a disease of domestic animals (cattle, sheep, and Himalayan cats) referred to as dermatosparaxis.[106] Type VIII (autosomal dominant) is a rare syndrome associated with periodontal disease that results in loss of teeth and the surrounding alveolar bone by the second or third decade of life.[96, 117–120] Type VIII also is associated with pretibial skin lesions that resemble necrobiosis lipoidica diabeticorum.[111] Skin fragility and hypermobility are mild.[115] Type X (autosomal recessive) is associated with both skin bruisability and petechiae owing to platelet dysfunction. In 1986, the 7th Annual International Congress of Human Genetics sponsored a workshop to clarify and classify heritable disorders of connective tissue.[109] This committee removed types IX and XI from inclusion with the Ehlers-Danlos syndrome.[109]

Type IX (X-linked recessive) is associated with abnormalities in copper metabolism, relating it to the fatal childhood disease Menkes' syndrome (steely hair or kinky hair syndrome).[118, 120, 122] Clinically, patients with this disorder have skin fragility, hypermobile joints, skeletal abnormalities, spontaneous ruptures of visceral organs, and hernias.[118, 122] In addition, this disorder is associated with renal abnormalities (bladder diverticula, ureteral obstruction), chronic diarrhea, generalized dilation or tortuosity of vessels, and specific skeletal changes found in no other form of the Ehlers-Danlos syndrome (occipital "horns," deformed clavicles, bowed shafts of long bones). Previously, some of these patients were classified as having the X-linked recessive type of cutis laxa.[120] The nomenclature committee of the International Congress of Human Genetics reclassified this entity for the second time and included it with disorders of copper metabolism.[109] However, subsequent publications[94, 111, 113, 121] still included it as a form of Ehlers-Danlos syndrome. The type XI (autosomal dominant) syndrome is associated with severe joint laxity and absence of skin changes. Beighton and associates have reclassified it as a familial syndrome of articular instability.[109]

Despite efforts to bring order to a disease as heterogeneous as the Ehlers-Danlos syndrome, within each clinical type, heterogeneity is seen, not only in the clinical manifestations but also in the genetic or biochemical defects.[123]

The Ehlers-Danlos syndrome also has been referred to as cutis hyperelastica and dermatorrhexia.[124] The first documented case is attributed to Van Meeker, a Dutch surgeon, in 1682.[91, 119, 12] The skin fragility and hyperlaxity later were described in the German literature by Ehlers in 1901 and in the French literature by Danlos in 1906.[119]

Pathology and Pathophysiology

The skin of patients with the Ehlers-Danlos syndrome is abnormally thin and demonstrates a decrease in tensile strength.[91] The hair follicles and sebaceous glands are normal.[126] Various histologic studies of skin structure have described the elastic fiber content of the dermis to be increased,[126, 127] decreased,[124] and normal.[90, 91] It now is generally accepted, however, that the Ehlers-Danlos syndrome is primarily a disorder of collagen synthesis.[76, 89–91, 118, 128] Microscopic and ultrastructural studies have reported abnormal organization and interweaving of collagen bundles and abnormal shortening of the collagen chains.[90–92, 128]

At least 12 different types of collagen coded by a minimum of 20 genes have now been identified.[98] The major fibrillar kinds are types I, II, and III.[80] To date, abnormalities of types I, II, and III have been related to specific disease entities.[104, 105, 111, 112, 117]

The fibrillar collagens are triple helices composed of chains of approximately 1000 amino acids. Type I collagen is found in skin, bone, sclerae, tendons, ligaments, and vessel walls.[97, 98] It is a heterotrimer composed of two α1(I) chains and one α2(I) chain.[106] COLIA1 gene (locus in chromosome 17) encodes the proα1(I) chains and COLIA2 gene (locus in chromosome 7) encodes the proα2(I) chain.[95, 104, 105, 112, 129–131] Type III collagen is a component of skin, vessel walls, and walls of the hollow visceral organs.[97] It is a homotrimer composed of three identical chains. COL3A1 gene (locus on chromosome 2) encodes the proα(III) chain.[95, 104, 105, 112, 129] The procollagen molecules (proα1[I], proα2[I], proα[III]) are assembled within the rough endoplasmic reticulum of the cell. Each chain has an amino-

propeptide terminal (N-terminal) end and a globular (C-terminal) carboxyl terminal end.[97, 110, 131, 132] The terminals function in assembly and secretion.[97] Folding begins at the C-terminal ends of the chains.[98, 106, 131, 132] In both type I and type III collagen, glycine occurs in every third position in the helix[98, 132] and is part of a triplex (i.e., glycine-x-y, in which x is usually proline and y is hydroxyproline or lysine).[131, 132] During assembly of the procollagen molecules, progressive hydroxylation of the prolyl and lysyl residues occurs.[131, 132] This is a complex process and, to date, 11 posttranslational enzymes have been identified.[129] The glycine-x-y is repeated, and hydroxylation (modification of the chains) is crucial for stability and coherence.[96, 98] The completed triple helices, composed of procollagen chains, are secreted by the cell. Proteinases (proteolytic enzymes) then cleave off both the N- and the C-terminals of all chains to form the mature smaller, fibrillar collagen chains.[97, 98, 110, 131, 132]

Mature fibrillar collagen has two types of cross-links: (1) reducible by sodium borohydride and (2) nonreducible or "hard" cross-links (thought to result from condensation of two reducible cross-links).[13, 23, 25, 76, 133, 134] The nonreducible type of cross-links is more frequent in fibrillar collagen type II found in cartilage, vitreous humor, and nucleus pulposus.[13, 23, 25, 76, 98, 133, 134] Cultured fibroblasts synthesize large amounts of type I and type III collagen.[97] Cells can be obtained from punch biopsies of the dermis[97] and from chorionic villi, allowing for prenatal diagnosis of mutations in collagens type I and III.[98] DNA analysis for mutated collagen in patients suspected of having Ehlers-Danlos syndrome types IV and VII can be complicated by parental mosaicism.[97] Both phenotypes can result from heterogeneous mutations (i.e., point mutations, small and large deletions, substitutions, insertions, or regulatory mutations).[97, 98]

Type IV Ehlers-Danlos syndrome is related to a heterogeneous group of mutations that result in structural defects of procollagen III.[25, 95–98, 100–102, 113, 115, 118, 135] The abnormalities usually affect the triple helical coding region of the COL3A1 gene.[100, 103] Different mutation sites can lead to the same expression.[98, 100, 101] Families with the type IV syndrome can have autosomal dominant or autosomal recessive patterns of inheritance, but the dominant mode is more frequent.[100] Biochemical, genetic, and ultrastructural studies have revealed decreased synthesis of procollagen III,[94] abnormal nascent proteins resulting in decreased fibroblast secretion of procollagen III (decreased 10 to 80 per cent),[25, 100, 102, 103, 118, 123, 135] and destabilization of the collagen III triple helix.[100, 101, 103] Type III collagen occurs in walls of blood vessels (70 per cent of arterial collagen), skin (35 per cent of skin collagen), pleura, peritoneum, and the linings of hollow viscera (uterus, bladder, gastrointestinal tract).[98] Therefore, these tissues are affected most severely in type IV Ehlers-Danlos syndrome (ecchymotic or arterial form). Skin and arteries are elastin-rich but depleted of collagen.[98] The thickness of the dermis is diminished by 75 per cent.[115, 123] Pope and colleagues,[115] Lewkonia and Pope,[123] and Byers and coworkers[117] have theorized that type III collagen serves as a scaffold for type I collagen. Life expectancy is decreased in patients with type IV Ehlers-Danlos syndrome owing to aneurysm formation or spontaneous rupture of medium-sized vessels.[93, 96, 100, 103] Patients also can suffer from ruptured viscera (e.g., uterine rupture during pregnancy).[93]

Type VII Ehlers-Danlos syndrome encompasses a group of heterogeneous mutations that alter the structure of type I collagen, resulting in a deficiency or defect of procollagen N-proteinase.[95, 98, 104–106] Type VII is subdivided into three heritable disorders, either dominant or recessive, associated with the same phenotype: short stature, extreme joint hyperlaxity predisposing to dislocations, a criss-cross skin pattern on palms and soles, mild skin bruisability, and redundant skin folds and abnormal scars.[104–106] Type VIIA is related to a mutation in the COL1A1 gene resulting in changes in procollagen α1(I), and type VIIB is related to a mutation in the COL1A2 gene, resulting in changes in procollagen α2(I).[104–106] To date, six different mutations have been identified (five proα1[I] and one proα2[I]). However, all of these result in abnormal splicing or deletion of sequences encoded on exon 6, which is the domain of the cleavage site for N-proteinase and lysine (a component of collagen cross-links).[104–106] The abnormal procollagen peptidase cleavage results in abnormal processing of the N-terminal propeptide and 5′ end of proα1(I) and proα2(I), with failure to form a normal smaller collagen molecule.[84, 95, 98, 99, 105, 118] DNA studies in the type VIIC disorder (those cases that most closely resemble the domestic animal disorder dermatosparaxis) led to the postulate that the condition may result from mutations that alter the processing of the N-propeptide, possibly owing to a deficiency in procollagen N-proteinase. In type VII Ehlers-Danlos syndrome, the genetic or enzymatic changes result in abnormal fibril assembly, leading to production of sheets of skin collagen that resemble hieroglyphs.[106] Osteogenesis imperfecta is another heritable disorder related to mutations of type I collagen. Type VII Ehlers-Danlos patients can have blue sclerae[106] a frequent finding in osteogenesis imperfecta, and cases with overlap of the two syndromes have been reported.[98]

DNA studies of patients with types I and II Ehlers-Danlos syndrome (the commonest forms) reveal negative lod scores of COL1A1, COL1A2, and COL3A1.[95, 112] No evidence of a specific genetic defect has been identified. Electron microscopic studies have demonstrated abnormal dermal fibrils.

Types V and VI Ehlers-Danlos syndrome result from posttranslational enzyme defects in collagen synthesis.[97] In type V Ehlers-Danlos syndrome, studies have detected a decrease in the enzyme lysyl oxidase in some but not all cases.[96, 114, 118] Three variants of type VI Ehlers-Danlos syndrome exist.[96, 106, 107] Pinnell and collaborators[136] identified a decrease in the enzyme lysyl hydroxylase and in the hydroxylysine content of type I collagen. Hydroxylysine is necessary for the synthesis of stable collagen cross-links,[114, 117, 118] and a decrease in these stable cross-links has been associated with the Ehlers-Danlos syndrome since the studies of Jansen in 1955.[96, 107, 128] Type I collagen is the most severely affected. In other cases, families with similar clinical findings and classified as having type VI Ehlers-Danlos syndrome have shown a decrease in the lysyl hydroxylase content in fibroblast cultures but normal hydroxylysine content in skin.[96] In a third group of patients with this phenotype, the content of both lysyl hydroxylase and hydroxylysine appeared normal.[96] Patients with type IX syndrome (a phenotype that in the future may be excluded from the Ehlers-Danlos syndrome), like those with Menkes' syndrome, have a primary defect in copper metabolism that

results in a secondary defect in collagen formation.[118] In these cases, the mutation affects both the enzyme lysyl oxidase and intracellular copper transportation.[122] Specifically, lysyl oxidase converts newly synthesized collagen into its insoluble form and initiates the cross-linking of collagen and elastin.[118, 120, 122] Lysyl oxidase is a copper-dependent enzyme. In its absence serum copper and ceruloplasmin levels are decreased while skin levels of copper rise.[118, 122] Type X Ehlers-Danlos syndrome is associated with both easy bruisability of skin and failure of normal platelet aggregation.[96] Investigators have attributed the platelet changes to an abnormality of fibronectin.[96]

The mesenchymal defect in the various types of Ehlers-Danlos syndrome involves the joint capsules, the ligaments, and the paravertebral supporting tissues. No primary osseous abnormality has been reported in clinical studies of this syndrome. Immunofluorescent investigations, however, have shown a defect in tetracycline uptake, substantiating the theory of a primary abnormality in collagen production.[88, 91]

The molluscoid fibrous tumors, found predominantly on the pressure points of the body, are composed of proliferating connective tissue and degenerated fat.[90, 137] The vasculature is increased. Subcutaneous spherules of necrotic fat also are found in the skin and are thought to be related to subclinical trauma.[90, 137, 138]

The bleeding diathesis associated with the Ehlers-Danlos syndrome is ascribed to abnormalities in the vessel walls as well as to defects in the supporting perivascular tissues that result in failure of tamponade.[80, 90–92] Abnormal platelets and coagulation defects also have been reported in patients with type X Ehlers-Danlos syndrome.[89, 91, 96]

Clinical Findings

The diagnosis of Ehlers-Danlos syndrome continues to rest on the clinical triad of skin fragility, hyperelasticity of joints, and vascular fragility.[94–96, 113, 119] Molluscoid tumors on pressure points and subcutaneous nodules that form at sites of fatty degeneration also are considered diagnostic criteria. Clinical expression is extremely variable, however; the Ehlers-Danlos syndrome can represent a life-threatening disease or a mild disorder of mesenchymal tissues.[114]

The Ehlers-Danlos syndrome occurs most frequently in Caucasians of European origin.[96, 127] The disorder usually comes to medical attention during childhood (1 to 4 years of age),[90, 113] but some infants do have the "floppy baby" syndrome (types VI and VII).[88, 105–107, 139] A male predominance is seen,[96] and many of the patients are tall. Unlike cases of Marfan's syndrome and homocystinuria, dolichostenomelia can be present or absent,[12, 127] although families whose members have features of both Ehlers-Danlos and Marfan's syndromes have been reported.[55, 76] Typical facial characteristics in the Ehlers-Danlos syndrome include lop ears, redundant skin folds around the eyes, poor dentition, and a high, arched palate.[90, 91, 124, 127] As in osteogenesis imperfecta, blue sclerae may be seen (Table 87–1). Hypertelorism or "owl eyes" occur, particularly in types IV and IX.[79, 82] Mental retardation is not present. Patients affected with the Ehlers-Danlos syndrome walk with a characteristic gait that results from hyperextension of the hips to compensate for genu recurvatum deformities.[88] The gait disturbance

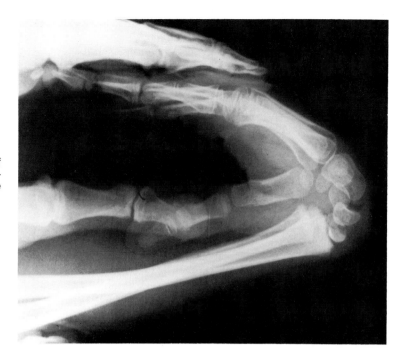

FIGURE 87–8. Ehlers-Danlos syndrome. Lateral view of the wrist shows a vacuum phenomenon in the lunate-capitate joint secondary to joint laxity. The patient is able to touch the forearm with the thumb.

is exacerbated by the presence of pes planus deformities and may be mistaken for tabes dorsalis.[91, 127]

The skin is velvety, thin, and hyperelastic. It can be raised in high folds and, unlike cases of cutis laxa, it retracts spontaneously. However, with advancing age and a concomitant decrease in the hyperelasticity of the skin, the folds become permanent and the skin lax. The skin also is easily bruised and tends to split with minor trauma. Scars are large and are covered by thin skin. The appearance of these scars has been compared to "cigarette paper."[91, 92, 137] Repeated hemorrhage results in a purple discoloration to the pretibial areas. Three types of skin nodules complicate the changes of the Ehlers-Danlos syndrome: molluscoid tumors occur at pressure points,[89, 91, 127] spherules of fat necrosis occur in the subcutaneous tissues, and subcutaneous hematomas are seen.[88, 90, 91, 124] All three can produce calcified masses. Skin ulcerations also occur in these patients.[70]

The passive and active hypermobility of joints in the Ehlers-Danlos syndrome has provided many a circus with an "India rubber man." Patients are able to (1) touch their thumbs to their forearms (Fig. 87–8), (2) passively dorsiflex their fifth fingers beyond 90 degrees, (3) hyperextend their elbows beyond 10 degrees, and (4) hyperextend their knees beyond 10 degrees (recurvatum).[88, 91, 140] Some patients also can touch the tip of the nose with the tongue.[91] Spontaneous dislocations are frequent, particularly in types I and VII, and correlate with the degree of laxity[88] (Table 87–1). Patients frequently are able to reduce these dislocations themselves.[86] Ligamentous as well as capsular laxity is present and results in kyphoscoliosis, pes planus, and inguinal and hiatal hernias. The ligamentous and capsular laxity is exacerbated by pregnancy and decreases with advancing age. Ligamentous laxity and recurrent dislocations lead to premature degenerative joint disease. Older patients complain of stiffness of hands, knees, and shoulders.[88] Treatment of articular symptoms resulting from either primary hypermo-bility or secondary degenerative changes consists of conservative measures, including splinting, rest, aspirin, and non-steroidal anti-inflammatory agents.[114]

The fragility of the vessel walls and lack of tamponade can result in bleeding from the gastrointestinal tract, the bronchopulmonary tree, or the gums.[91, 92] Such bleeding is most severe in the type IV (associated with abnormalities of type III collagen) and type X (associated with platelet abnormalities) syndromes (Table 87–1). Dissecting aneurysms of the aorta and spontaneous ruptures of the large vessels may occur and frequently result in death. Raynaud's phenomenon also has been reported in association with Ehlers-Danlos syndrome.[88, 90, 91, 141] The cause of acro-osteolysis in Ehlers-Danlos patients is unproved.[123] It has been theorized that a defect in perivascular connective tissue results in poor support of peripheral vessels and nerves, which, in turn, results in alterations of blood flow.[88]

Ocular abnormalities involve the cornea, sclera, fundus, and suspensory mechanism of the lens. Reported changes include strabismus, ectopia lentis, and retinal detachments.[91, 114] Type VI is the "ocular" type of Ehlers-Danlos syndrome (Table 87–1). Unlike Marfan's syndrome and homocystinuria, the presence of ectopia lentis is less consistent.[127]

Muscular weakness and easy fatigability also are features of the Ehlers-Danlos syndrome. Infants may be hypotonic, and older children frequently complain of muscle cramps.[91, 141, 142]

Visceral manifestations are most severe in type IV Ehlers-Danlos syndrome. These include segmental ectasia of the alimentary canal and respiratory tract. Spontaneous ruptures of bowel, uterus, and bronchi have been reported (Table 87–1). Cardiac abnormalities, including "floppy" mitral and tricuspid valves, also can occur, most frequently in patients with the type IV syndrome.

Surgery is poorly tolerated owing to a combination of bleeding problems and dehiscence.[90–92] Wounds, both iatrogenic and traumatic, gape in a "fish-mouth" fashion.[90, 96, 124, 126]

Radiographic Findings

Calcification of fatty spherules produces multiple subcutaneous dense lesions that are visible on radiographs.[91, 137, 143] They occur primarily in the forearms, shins, and extensor surfaces of the extremities and measure 2 to 8 mm in diameter. These calcifications usually have a dense rim and resemble phleboliths. Rarely the calcification is lamellated.[138] Other soft tissue calcifications occur in molluscoid lesions,[27] scars or hematomas,[91, 124] and areas of myositis ossificans.[84] An increased frequency of heterotopic ossification is seen in patients with the Ehlers-Danlos syndrome. Such ossification occurs primarily adjacent to the hips, extending from the inferior iliac spines to the greater trochanters. The cause of myositis ossificans in the Ehlers-Danlos syndrome and the reason for its predilection for the hips are unknown. The most widely accepted theory relates the heterotopic bone formation to poor support of vascular structures or friability of the vessel walls themselves, or both.[138]

Joint findings include persistent effusions or hemarthroses and occur in 20 per cent of patients with Ehlers-Danlos syndrome (Fig. 87–9).[88, 90, 91, 96, 140] Pain increases with age.[96] In one series, 16 of 42 patients over 40 years of age had osteoarthrosis.[96] The most common sites of joint involvement are the knee and ankle.[96] The fluid is thought to result from ligamentous and capsular laxity, which, in turn, produces repetitive subclinical trauma.[114, 140] Olecranon and prepatellar bursitis results from a similar process (Fig. 87–9). Particularly during childhood, these findings can initially be misinterpreted as the early manifestations of a rheumatologic disorder, and in young patients, the Ehlers-Danlos syndrome should be included in the differential diagnosis of pauciarticular arthritides.[114] The joint spaces may widen with minor stress (Fig. 87–8). Anteroposterior radiographs obtained with the patient standing can demonstrate varus deformities with widening of the lateral compartment.[140] Lateral knee films obtained with the joint in extension can show varying degrees of recurvatum (Figs. 87–9 and 87–10).

Dislocations and subluxations frequently complicate the clinical course (Figs. 87–9 to 87–11). The most frequent sites of dislocation are the digits, the glenohumeral joints, the patellofemoral joints, the temporomandibular joints, the radial heads, and the sternoclavicular and acromioclavicular joints.[88, 90, 91, 143] Digital dislocations often are recurrent.[121] Patients with the Ehlers-Danlos syndrome also can have midcarpal instability with capitate-scaphoid malalignment.[121] An increased frequency of congenital hip dislocations occurs most commonly in types I, II, V, VII, and IX (Fig. 87–11).[88, 91, 108, 144] Precocious osteoarthritis, occurring in the third and fourth decades of life, is the sequela of the repetitive minor trauma associated with capsular laxity and of the repetitive major trauma associated with dislocations.[88, 114] The prevalence of degenerative changes correlates with the severity of the laxity. Eventually contractures can occur and, combined with the degenerative cartilage changes, replace the primary joint laxity with secondary joint stiffness.[114, 123] The carpometacarpal joint of the thumb is particularly vulnerable; in a review of 24 children with Ehlers-Danlos syndrome (mean age, 15.9 years), 66 per cent of these joints were subluxated, 29 per cent were dislocated, and 16 per cent had stigmata of degenerative arthritis.[121]

Ligamentous laxity also results in pes planus deformities (Fig. 87–12) and abnormalities of the axial skeleton. The thorax can be asymmetric, with pectus carinatum (Fig. 87–

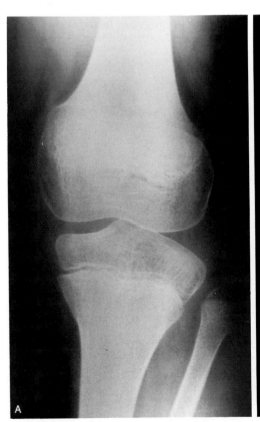
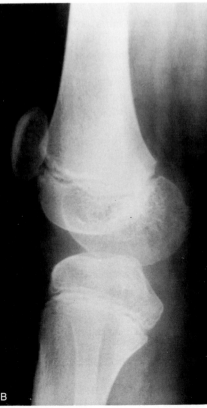

FIGURE 87–9. Ehlers-Danlos syndrome. Anteroposterior **(A)** and lateral **(B)** views of the knee reveal effusion and genu recurvatum deformity. Present but not well shown is soft tissue prominence in the region of the prepatellar bursa. The fibular head is malformed and does not articulate with the proximal portion of the tibia.

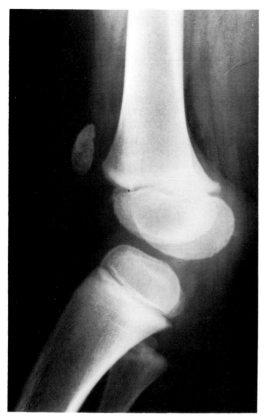

FIGURE 87–10. Ehlers-Danlos syndrome. Lateral view of the knee shows fibular head dislocation and genu recurvatum deformity.

13) and prominence of the costochondral junctions. The upper ribs may slant sharply downward (Fig. 87–13), giving the cervical spine an elongated appearance. Platyspondyly isolated to the lumbar spine has been observed.[145] Unlike cases of Scheuermann's disease or discitis, the vertebrae endplates remain smooth in patients with Ehlers-Danlos syndrome.[145] A kyphoscoliosis frequently is present at the thoracolumbar junction (Fig. 87–13)[126, 143, 446] and in older patients is associated with anterior wedging of the vertebrae. Rarely, a thoracic lordosis or "straight back" syndrome has been observed instead of a kyphosis.[88] In contrast to idiopathic scoliosis, abnormal spinal curvature may be present at birth (types I, II, VI).[107] Severe spondylolysis and spondylolisthesis have been reported in association with the scoliosis of Ehlers-Danlos syndrome (Fig. 87–14).[123, 141, 143] As in neurofibromatosis, posterior scalloping of the vertebral bodies (secondary to dural ectasia) has been reported.[87] If an associated Raynaud's disease is present, acro-osteolysis may be seen. This finding, particularly in patients who also have joint effusions, can further confuse the diagnosis and lead to an initial workup for a rheumatologic rather than a collagen disorder.[114, 123]

The radiographs also can demonstrate congenital anomalies associated with the Ehlers-Danlos syndrome, including arachnodactyly, triphalangeal thumbs, radioulnar synostoses, clubfeet, supernumerary teeth, delayed cranial ossification with large fontanelles and wide sagittal and metopic sutures, micrognathia, elongation of the ulnar styloid process, a short fifth proximal phalanx, and posterior radial head dislocations.[88, 106, 107, 137, 143] Imaging studies in patients with type VI Ehlers-Danlos syndrome (ecchymotic form) may reveal aneurysms, areas of liver necrosis, and other findings (e.g., diverticula of the colon or bladder, saccular dilations of the hepatic duct).[93] These patients can undergo spontaneous rupture of the large intestine, the uterus, or arterial aneurysms.

The radiographic differential diagnosis of joint laxity includes Marfan's syndrome, Larsen's syndrome, cachexia, Down's syndrome, and neuromuscular disorders.[91] A syndrome consisting of recurrent dislocations, an increased frequency of congenital hip dislocation, and a family history of ligamentous laxity also has been described and is not an

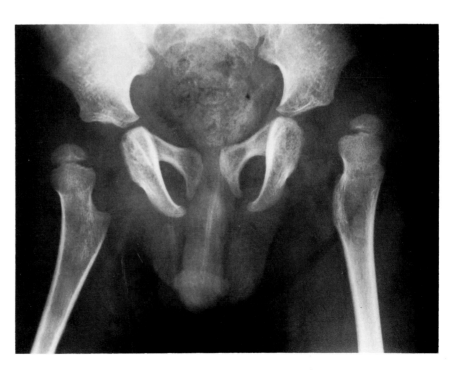

FIGURE 87–11. Ehlers-Danlos syndrome: Bilateral hip dislocations.

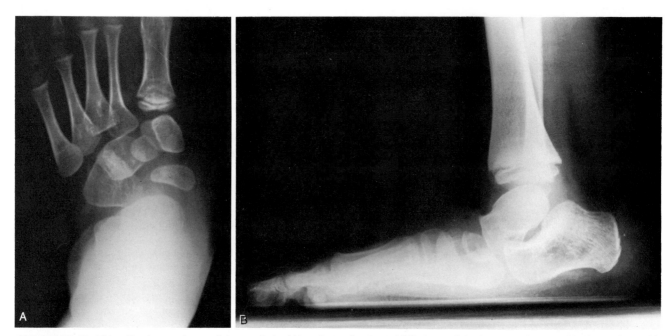

FIGURE 87–12. Ehlers-Danlos syndrome. Anteroposterior **(A)** and standing lateral **(B)** views of the foot reveal severe hindfoot valgus with pes planus deformity.

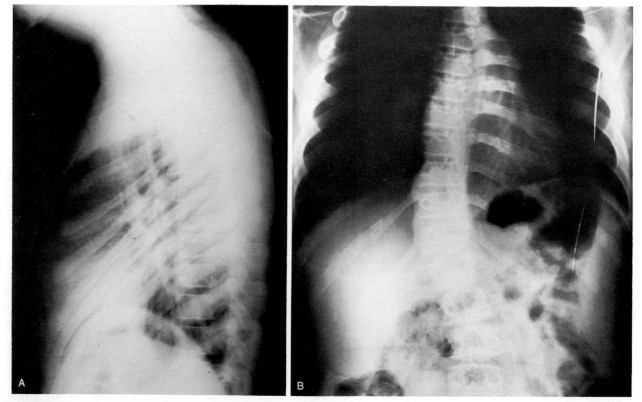

FIGURE 87–13. Ehlers-Danlos syndrome. Axial deformities include pectus carinatum **(A)**, thoracolumbar scoliosis **(A, B)**, and an exaggerated downward slant to the ribs **(B)**.

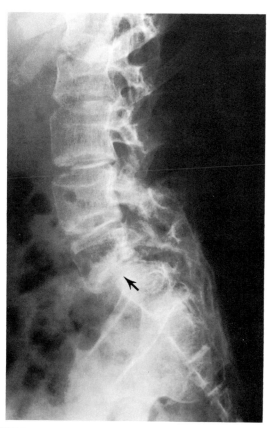

FIGURE 87–14. Ehlers-Danlos syndrome. Lateral view of the lumbar spine shows a spondylolysis and spondylolisthesis (arrow).

uncommon entity.[144, 146, 147] In this disorder, however, referred to as familial joint laxity, neither skin changes (fragility or masses) nor bleeding tendency are seen.[91, 114, 144, 146, 147]

The soft tissue calcifications of the Ehlers-Danlos syndrome may be mistaken for cysticercosis, vascular tumors, phleboliths, or collagen diseases. Their predilection for the lower extremities and their location in the subcutaneous tissues in the Ehlers-Danlos syndrome should help in establishing the correct diagnosis.

Type IX Ehlers-Danlos syndrome, unlike the other clinical categories, is associated with unique skeletal abnormalities, including horn-shaped excrescences on the occipital bone of the skull and deformed clavicles.[120] The shafts of the long bones are osteopenic and bowed and have wavy, thin cortices.[120] The location of these osseous changes corresponds to sites of membranous bone formation, and it has been suggested that they result from defective collagen within Sharpey's fibers of the periosteum. Other, less specific skeletal changes reported in patients with type IX Ehlers-Danlos syndrome are clinodactyly, micrognathia, and hypertelorism associated with flat orbits.[120]

OSTEOGENESIS IMPERFECTA

Osteogenesis imperfecta is an inherited disorder of connective tissue that affects the skeleton, ligaments, skin, sclerae, and dentin.[130, 148–155] The majority of patients have been proved to have mutations in one of the two genetic loci that encode type I collagen (COL1A1 and COL1A2).[97, 129, 131, 132, 154, 156] The resultant genetic disorder can be expressed by either abnormal synthesis (quantity) or abnormal structure (quality) of procollagen I (Table 87–2).[97, 155, 157, 158] Eighty-five per cent of genotypes are heterozygous for an autosomal dominant mutation.[154]

The four major clinical criteria are (1) osteoporosis with abnormal fragility of the skeleton, (2) blue sclerae, (3) dentinogenesis imperfecta, and (4) premature otosclerosis.[159, 160] The presence of two of these abnormalities confirms the diagnosis. Other features are ligamentous laxity, episodic diaphoresis with abnormal temperature regulation, easy bruisability, constipation, hyperplastic scars, premature vascular calcifications, and inappropriate euphoria.[148, 159, 161–164]

Osteogenesis imperfecta classically has been subclassified, on the basis of the severity of the skeletal findings, into two syndromes: the congenita form, which has a high infant mortality rate, and the tarda form, which is associated with a normal life expectancy. The terms tarda and congenita have largely been replaced in the Sillence classification,[165, 166] which is based on a combination of clinical, radiographic, and genetic factors.[98, 110, 130–132, 167, 168] The exact relationship between the nature of the mutations and the phenotype still remains to be investigated and, thus, the classification of osteogenesis imperfecta continues to be modified.[148, 152, 158, 159, 161, 164, 169, 170]

Sillence and coworkers[171] have offered a classification that divides osteogenesis imperfecta into four groups or types.

Type I is both the most common and the mildest phenotype of the disease.[165, 166] It is estimated to occur in 1 of 30,000 births.[170, 171] Osseous fragility results in an increased number of fractures but not dwarfing or bowing deformities. Patients either are of normal height or 2 to 3 standard deviations below the mean; they suffer presenile hearing loss and have sclerae that remain blue throughout life (Table 87–2).[165] Type I is subdivided into two groups depending on the presence (type IB) or absence (type IA) of dentinogenesis imperfecta (gray teeth). In most families with type I osteogenesis imperfecta, the genetic abnormality is poorly understood.[131, 132, 155, 172–174] The mode of transmission is autosomal dominant. Fibroblast cultures reveal a decrease in the quantity of type I collagen, but the molecules that are produced are normal structurally. DNA studies suggest the presence of a null allele (no deletions or rearrangements) in the COL1A1 locus but a failure to produce mRNA.[118, 173–175] Other, rarer modes of genetic transmission with known structural abnormalities in the type I collagen loci (COL1A1 and COL1A2) also are associated with the type I phenotype (Table 87–2).[131, 132, 158, 173, 174]

Type II is the lethal form of osteogenesis imperfecta. Severe osseous fragility results in dwarfing and fractures that occur in utero. The calvarium is very poorly mineralized. Infants with type II disease tend to have small, triangular faces, hypertelorism, small beaked noses, and, consistently, blue sclerae.[165, 170, 171] Type II has three recognizable subtypes: type A (telescoped long bones, beaded ribs), type B (lethal before or at birth), and type C (thin nodular ribs). Death usually occurs around the time of birth and is related to respiratory complications (Table 87–2).[176] Because infants with this lethal phenotype are born to phenotypically normal parents, earlier studies had concluded that the pattern of inheritance is autosomal recessive.[166] More recently investigators have demonstrated that most cases of type II osteogenesis imperfecta either result from a new dominant

TABLE 87–2. Sillence Clinical Classification and Genetic Mutations in Osteogenesis Imperfecta*

Type	Osseous Fragility	Sclerae	Presenile Hearing Loss	Dentinogenesis Imperfecta	Commonest Mode of Inheritance and Defect	Rarer Modes of Inheritance	Additional Clinical Observations
IA	+ Height normal to short (2 or 3 standard deviations less than normal)	Blue	+	−	Autosomal dominant resulting in null allele (no deletion or rearrangement but failure to produce mRNA) in the COLIA1 gene; 50 per cent sporadic	Autosomal dominant substitution for glycine residue in C-terminal telopeptide of proα1(I)	Joint hyperlaxity Premature arcus senilis Progressive kyphoscoliosis (can lead to loss of height postmenopausally)
IB	+ Height normal to short (2 or 3 standard deviations less than normal)	Blue	+	+		Autosomal dominant substitution or deletion in proα2(I)	
II	+ + + + Dwarfed "Crumpled" long bones Beaded ribs Severely affected	Blue	−	−	Autosomal dominant substitution for glycyl residues in triple helical domain of proα1(I) or proα2(I) (often point mutation) Sporadic or parental mosaicism	Autosomal dominant rearrangements in COLIA1 or COLIA2 genes Autosomal dominant deletions in triple helical domain of COLIA1 or COLIA2 genes Autosomal recessive deletion	Death usually perinatal and due to respiratory complications Small nose, "triangular" facies
III	+ + + Dwarfism—variable but progressive Limbs bowed	White (may be blue at birth but clear with age)	−	−	Autosomal dominant point mutations in COLIA1 or COLIA2 genes	Autosomal recessive frame-shift in COLIA2 gene that prevents incorporation of proα2(I) chains	Wormian bones in calvarium High childhood mortality due to thoracic deformity Shortest affected persons are more than 10 standard deviations below mean for age Progressive kyphosis
IV	+ → + + +	White	+	−	Autosomal dominant point mutation in COL1A2 or, less commonly, COL1A1 gene	Autosomal dominant exon-skipping mutations on COL1A2 gene	

*Based on data from references 131, 132, 158, 165.

point mutation in one of the two encoding genes for collagen I (COL1A1 or COL1A2) or occur as an autosomal dominant trait when one parent is genetically mosaic (only a percentage of germ cells contain the mutant gene).[131, 132, 158, 174, 177, 447] Several rare additional modes of transmission have been identified in families with this lethal phenotype (Table 87–2).

Type III is a rare phenotype of osteogenesis imperfecta, and in over two thirds of cases fractures are present at birth.[170, 171, 178] Osseous fragility is severe and, if patients with type III survive, they exhibit the most dramatic dwarfing among osteogenesis imperfecta cases (10 standard deviations below the mean).[165] The osseous fragility is progressive, with increasing bowing of long bones (Table 87–2). Kyphoscoliosis and thoracic deformities also are progressive, and the mortality rate is high in the third decade of life owing to pulmonary complications.[110, 165] Infants with type III disease may have blue sclerae at birth, but the sclerae become white or gray in adulthood. Type III usually is transmitted as an autosomal dominant trait with a point mutation in either of the two collagen I genetic loci.[110, 131, 132, 165] Rare families exist that exhibit type III disease, a recessive mode of transmission, and a "frame-shift" mutation in the COL1A2 locus.[131, 172]

Type IV osteogenesis imperfecta has the most variable osseous findings, and patients can range in height from normal to severely dwarfed.[165] Some patients with dwarfism are born with blue sclerae that become white with advanc-

ing age. Presenile deafness occurs in some type IV pedigrees.[110, 165] Inheritance is autosomal dominant, and the disorder most often is the result of a point mutation in one of the two collagen I loci.[131] Rare families with type IV phenotype have exon skipping mutations in the COL1A2 collagen I locus (Table 87–2).[131]

Even among these four types, considerable genetic, biochemical, and clinical variability is seen.[170, 179, 180] In addition, some patients simply defy classification.[98, 170, 179, 180] The use of sophisticated new techniques (i.e., identification of polymorphic markers within or close to the two encoding genes for collagen I, applied to skin biopsy and chorionic biopsy specimens) will add to or alter the Sillence classification.[98, 110, 156, 158, 181, 182]

Other names used in reference to osteogenesis imperfecta include Vrolik disease, van der Hoeve syndrome, osteopsathyrosis fetalis, and trias fragilis ossium.[170, 183] The first person described with symptoms that resemble severe osteogenesis imperfecta was a legendary Danish prince, Ivar Benlos.[183] This man was variously described as "boneless" or "legless" and was small enough to be carried into battle on a shield.[183] In the medical literature, the first description of the familial occurrence of fragile bones is attributed to Ekman, a Swedish military surgeon in 1788.[183] It was the Dutch anatomist Vrolik who, in 1849, coined the term osteogenesis imperfecta. He applied it only to dead neonates, however. Criteria other than fragile bones were recognized later. Spurway, in 1896, and Eddows, in 1900, noted the association of skeletal abnormalities and blue sclerae.[183] Adair-Dighton, in 1912, and van der Hoeve, in 1917, described a third major feature—premature hearing loss.[183] Although ligamentous laxity was observed by Velpeau as early as 1847, it was not until Bauer's research, in 1940, that osteogenesis imperfecta was attributed to a generalized defect in mesenchyme.[183] Bauer supported his hypothesis by identifying other features of the disease that involved tissues such as skin, cartilage, and blood vessels.[183]

Pathology and Pathophysiology

Osteogenesis imperfecta is an inherited connective tissue syndrome associated clinically with bone fragility and ligamentous laxity and genetically and biochemically with defects in fibrillar type I collagen synthesis (quantative or qualitative, or both).[130, 155, 175, 184, 185] Type I collagen composes 90 per cent of the organic matrix of bone.[186] As stated earlier, types I, II, and III are the fibrillar forms of collagen and make up the bulk of the extracellular component of connective tissues (e.g., skin, bones, tendons, ligaments, cartilage).[118, 187] DNA linkage studies have identified two diseases associated with defects of the encoding genes for type I collagen: osteogenesis imperfecta and type VII Ehlers-Danlos syndrome (Table 87–1).[97, 98, 131, 182]

The clinical defects in osteogenesis imperfecta involve tissues with high type I collagen content (e.g., bones, ligaments, tendons, fasciae, sclerae, and teeth).[118] In all forms of the disease, studies of cultured fibroblasts reveal a decrease in the amount of type I collagen and, therefore, a decrease in the ratio of type I to type III collagen.[118, 158, 170, 179, 184, 187] Using DNA linkage studies and newly identified genetic markers, the relationship between the Sillence phenotypes and the precise mutant locus are still being investigated (Table 87–2).[110, 129, 156, 158, 182] Several general observations have been made. First, osteogenesis imperfecta is a highly heterogeneous disease. Variability of expression occurs in the same pedigree, and each family studied with a particular phenotype may have a different mutation, although in the same limited number of loci.[156, 158, 188] Second, similar mutations can lead to different phenotypes.[132] Third, most families with type I disease have a quantitative defect in type I collagen, but those molecules that are produced are structurally normal.[76, 118, 131, 132, 166, 172, 173, 185] Types II, III, and IV and rare pedigrees of type I osteogenesis imperfecta have both a decrease in the synthesis of type I collagen and a type I collagen that is abnormal in quality. Those families with normal proα(I) chains tend to have a mild form of the disease, whereas in those families with abnormal molecules, the disease ranges from mild to lethal.[131, 155] Fourth, the triple helical domain of type I procollagen (amino acids 103 to 212) appears to be the site of the majority of point mutations.[131, 169, 188–190] Glycine can be replaced by arginine or serine; such substitutions result in a range of phenotypes.[131] Fifth, the position rather than the size of the mutation is related to the severity of the phenotypic manifestations.[98, 132, 173, 189] Those mutations that affect the C-terminal ends of the type I procollagen molecules produce a more severe phenotypic picture than those occurring closer to the N-terminal ends of the chains.[98, 131, 189] Sixth, a single point mutation in the triple helical domain of COL1A1 or COL1A2 can result in a severe degree of osteogenesis imperfecta.[188, 190, 191] Several factors amplify

the deleterious effects of a point mutation. For example, (1) if glycine is replaced by a "bulkier" amino acid (arginine or cysteine), a "kink" is produced in the molecule that delays assembly and allows for modification (overhydroxylation or overglycosylation) of the procollagen chains that, in turn, results in abnormal fibrils; (2) point mutation can affect the processing of the N-propeptides with persistence of the N-terminal; and (3) abnormal procollagen within a cell can result in degradation of the normal procollagen molecules produced by the same cell, a process called "procollagen suicide."[97, 157, 172, 191] Further, in cases of osteogenesis imperfecta, the presence of type III collagen has been detected in skeletal tissue.[118, 157, 170, 187] Type III collagen is not normally found in bone. In addition, biochemical studies reveal that the presence of abnormal glycosaminoglycan function can alter the aggregation of procollagen chains and exacerbate a primary defect in collagen cross-links.[192]

The pathologic and histologic changes in the osseous tissue in osteogenesis imperfecta are characterized by a primary defect in extracellular bone matrix.[193] Periosteal bone formation is decreased, which disturbs the normal circumferential growth of the bones.[110, 152, 194] Osteoblastic activity is slowed,[159, 164] and fetal bone is not replaced by normal lamellar bone,[76, 152, 161, 162, 165, 195] which leaves the cortex thinned and weakened mechanically. In the severe forms, osseous tissue can be devoid of normal trabeculae, whereas in the milder forms, a lamellar pattern predominates.[194] Even in cases that are not severely affected, however, histomorphometry with double tetracycline labeling demonstrates small areas of immature woven bone, a decrease in trabecular bone volume, and lamellae that are thinner than normal.[193, 196, 197] Osteoid seams can be prominent[193] or small.[197] Immature collagen in the matrix also results in granular material between the lamellae.[76, 160, 161, 170, 193]

The number of osteoblasts and osteocytes, per unit matrix, actually is increased.[131, 165, 170, 195, 198] Therefore, the decrease of bone synthesis per individual osteoblast is partly compensated for by an increase in the number of cells.[196, 199] Most investigators report an increase in the rate of bone turnover at the cellular level, which is postulated to be the result of a compensatory mechanism.[152, 163, 164, 170, 197] The osteocytes are large, oval, and arranged inhomogeneously.[193] They are surrounded by primitive woven bone, as opposed to mature lamellar bone.[193]

Electron microscopic studies of tissues from patients with various phenotypes of osteogenesis imperfecta have revealed alterations in the ultrastructure of the collagen fibrils, which have a smaller diameter than normal.[177, 184, 192] This observation can be related to one or more factors, including the abnormal presence of type III collagen in bone (type III is narrower than type I), restriction of fiber growth owing to the failure to cleave the terminal ends of the procollagen molecule, and, most likely, the increase in hydroxylysine content of procollagen in osteogenesis imperfecta (the amount of hydroxylysine is inversely proportional to the diameter of the fibril).[118, 184, 187] The functional significance of these narrow fibrils is unknown.[184] Other electron microscopic investigations have revealed dilation of the endoplasmic reticulum of skin and cartilage cells.[193]

Abnormalities of the cartilage growth plate have been reported, but their origin remains controversial. Spencer,[200] in 1962, observed an increase in the mucopolysaccharide content of the physis. Bullough and Davidson[201] published an autopsy study of a patient with the lethal form that revealed replacement of the growth plate by irregular islands of cartilage surrounded by thin rinds of spongy bone. Reports by Sillence[165] and Sanguinetti and colleagues[202] confirmed the presence of "cartilage nodules" in the region of the growth plates in the immature skeleton. It is uncertain whether these alterations represent a primary growth disturbance or whether they are secondary to trauma within the adjacent supporting bone, which is insufficiently stiff to supply support to the cartilage columns.[170, 203]

Bone, skin, and dentin share similar extracellular matrix, and therefore predictably defects described in fibroblast cultures and bone also occur in the teeth.[204] Immature collagen and abnormal granular calcifications have been observed in the pulp of the teeth,[159, 162, 164] just as in the skeleton.[193] Abnormalities of glycosaminoglycans have been identified,[193] and the dentin lacks the tubular structure of normal dentin. The enamel itself is normal, but it fractures and separates from the deficient dentin. No correlation exists between the severity of the dental changes and the number of fractures.[204]

The sclerae are thin and, as in other connective tissues, contain abnormal collagen. The blue translucency results from the brown choroid shining through the abnormal outer layer.[110, 164] Electron microscopic findings in the cornea include vacuolization of fibroblasts, thin collagen fibrils, dilated rough endoplasmic reticulum, and granular material between the lamellae—changes also observed in the skeleton and skin.[170]

The exact reason for premature otosclerosis in osteogenesis imperfecta is unknown.[149, 159, 164] Described pathologic abnormalities are related to (1) attenuation or discontinuity of the stapes crura or (2) thickening and softening of the stapes foot plates, which are inadequately fixed to the oval window.[110, 205-207] The tympanic membrane has been characterized as "transparent" and variously described as either bluish in some cases or rosy in others.[205] Sensory hearing loss also can complicate osteogenesis imperfecta, and it is thought to result from membrane distortion or perilymphatic hemorrhage.[205, 207] Abnormal external pinnae (lop ears, macrotia, notching of the helix) can occur with or without hearing loss.[205, 206]

A disturbance of the ATPase mechanism is thought to be related to abnormal temperature regulation[161, 164] and to defective platelet aggregation.[161] Abnormally large platelets have been described.[161]

Clinical Findings

Osteogenesis imperfecta occurs in all races. Some series report an equal sex distribution,[164] whereas others have observed a slight female predominance.[149, 160, 208] The severe forms (10 per cent) have high intrauterine and infant mortality rates owing to respiratory complications resulting from thoracic deformities or intracerebral hemorrhage.[110, 162] The age at which the diagnosis is established depends on the pattern of inheritance,[171] the severity of the clinical expression, and presence or absence of a known family history. Most cases are diagnosed at birth or, with the use of ultrasonography, in utero.[159, 209-211] Prenatal ultrasonography serves two purposes.[98, 129, 156, 158, 181, 190] First, the ultrasonograms allow identification of severely affected em-

bryos (those with Sillence types II, III, and occasionally IV syndromes), usually by 15 to 34 weeks of gestation.[110] Second, the study can serve as a guide to accurate biopsy of the chorionic villi.[110] Chorionic biopsy usually is reserved for members in families with a known history of osteogenesis imperfecta or for those mothers in whom an ultrasonographic examination has revealed a fetus with short stature and shortened, bowed extremities.[181]

Facial characteristics include temporal bulging, flattening of the features, micrognathia, and hypertelorism. These facial changes are observed most commonly in severely affected persons (Sillence types II and III) and create the impression of a small, triangular face.[212] Blue sclerae occur in over 90 per cent of cases,[159, 213] and intensity of the hue can vary with the patient's emotional status. A small ring of sclera surrounding the cornea can retain a normal white color and is called a "Saturn's ring" or arcus senilis.[164] Abnormal dentition with opalescent blue-gray or brown teeth is termed dentinogenesis imperfecta.[204, 206, 212] It is not as frequent a clinical finding as blue sclerae, but it is highly specific for osteogenesis imperfecta. Dental changes have even been found at autopsies of neonates with the lethal forms.[204] Dental changes are most consistent in the Sillence types IB and IVB syndromes (Table 87–2).[130] Permanent teeth usually are less discolored than deciduous teeth.[130] Even when the teeth appear normal, the dentin may be thin and poorly canalized.[97, 110]

Growth retardation occurs in most cases,[152, 214] and severely affected persons are dwarfed, with short, bowed long bones (Fig. 87–15).[97, 110] No abnormality in growth hormone is detectable, however.[168] The short stature is related to microscopic defects in collagen synthesis, the gross fracture deformities, telescoping fractures,[170] and fragmentation of the physeal plate.[203] Growth disturbances have been detected in utero.[210, 211, 214] The limbs are more involved than the trunk, and the lower extremities are more shortened than the upper extremities (Fig. 87–15).[159, 164, 208, 215] Skeletal

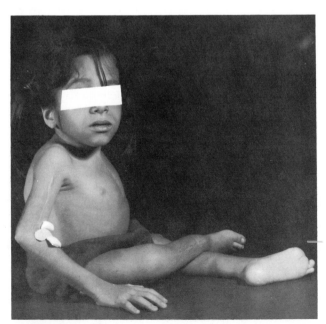

FIGURE 87–15. Osteogenesis imperfecta: Sillence type III. The limbs are disproportionately short and all four extremities are bowed. Thoracic deformities also are present.

deformities include kyphoscoliosis and bowing of the long bones, which exacerbates the limb-trunk discrepancy.[180] The spinal deformities can result in pain, paresthesias, difficulty in ambulating, and, in severe congenita-type cases, respiratory failure or paraplegia.[180, 216–218]

Multiple fractures, resulting from normal daily activities or minor trauma, are the predominant clinical finding in osteogenesis imperfecta. In severe congenita-type, the fractures occur even in the protected environment of the uterus.[159, 162, 219] The frequency of the pathologic fractures appears to decrease after puberty owing to either hormonal factors or the patient's increased awareness of the condition.[220] In both male and female patients, the frequency of fractures peaks in childhood and decreases in adolescence.[220] In women, however, renewed exacerbation occurs after menopause, probably as a result of the superimposition of postmenopausal osteoporosis on the preexisting collagen defect.[220] An alteration in the approach to fracture treatment in osteogenesis imperfecta using gentle physiotherapy, preferably in a pool, is recommended over complete immobilization to avoid aggravating the bone loss that characterizes the disease itself.[221] The Sillence classification system,[165] although useful in genetic counseling, has not proved consistent as a predictor of the therapeutic benefits of independent ambulation versus wheelchair usage.[167, 222]

Otosclerosis can occur prior to the age of 40 years.[159, 162, 164, 205, 207] Nerve conduction deafness occurs in 10 per cent of cases with associated vertigo and tinnitus.[205, 207]

As in other hereditary disorders of collagen synthesis, the clinical abnormalities of osteogenesis imperfecta include thin skin, a tendency to form hyperplastic scars, premature vascular calcifications, joint laxity, a high frequency of hernias, and platelet abnormalities.[149, 159, 162–164, 180, 212] Ligamentous laxity also can result in hypermobile joints, but no increase has been reported in the prevalence of dislocations.[110] Bleeding likewise results from capillary fragility, as it does in Ehlers-Danlos syndromes, but it tends to be less severe in osteogenesis imperfecta.[110, 180, 194]

The central nervous system similarly can be affected. Basilar impression effectively decreases the volume of the posterior fossa.[223, 224] In osteogenesis imperfecta, basilar impression is associated with platybasia or the "tam-o'-shanter" skull.[224] This complication, although partly related to fractures, does not correlate with the general severity of the disease, and, indeed, more instances have been reported in patients with the tarda forms than in those with the congenita forms. It is, therefore, postulated that this cranial finding is another example of the variety of defects that can occur in the collagen DNA sequence. Once present, basilar impression can interfere with the flow of cerebrospinal fluid (hydrocephalus), disturb cerebellar function, and result in compression of the brain stem (long tract signs, compression of the lower cranial nerves).[224] An increased frequency of pituitary deficiency has been attributed to intracranial hemorrhage at the time of birth.[164] A fragile calvarium, platelet abnormalities, and the connective tissue defect all may contribute to damage to the hypothalamopituitary axis.[164] The causes of hyperthermia and inappropriate euphoria are unknown.[161] Excessive sweating, noted predominantly in children, is thought to be related to heat loss through the abnormally thin dermis.[193]

Drug therapy for patients with osteogenesis imperfecta remains controversial.[110] Various studies have examined the efficacy of therapy with vitamin D and fluoride, calcitonin, and gonadal hormones.[110] Androgen and estrogen receptors have been demonstrated in bone cells, but the feared side effect of hormonal therapy is premature closure of the growth plates.[110]

Radiographic Findings

The most characteristic radiographic finding of osteogenesis imperfecta is a diffuse decrease in osseous density (Figs. 87–16 to 87–18), which involves equally the axial and appendicular portions of the skeleton.[164, 206, 208, 213, 225–228] The degree of osteopenia is highly variable, however, and at the mildest end of the spectrum, patients can appear to have normal bone density on plain films.[221] By definition, the decrease in osseous density is classified as a form of hereditary osteoporosis, because the primary abnormality involves synthesis of collagen matrix. In osteogenesis imperfecta, however, the primary defect in matrix is accompanied by a secondary alteration in mineralization, and although there is no disproportion of the mineral to matrix ratio, disordered alignment and binding of the mineral salts within the matrix is seen.[180, 193] Therefore, the radiographic changes are not exclusively those of osteoporosis. Often a rapid loss of bone mass occurs in middle-aged persons.[110]

On the basis of the radiographic appearance of the extremities, Fairbank[208] has subclassified patients with osteogenesis imperfecta into three groups. The first category encompasses those cases with thin, gracile bones (Fig. 87–16). This is the most common expression of the disease and

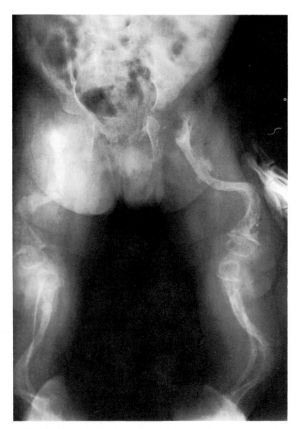

FIGURE 87–16. Osteogenesis imperfecta. Anteroposterior view of pelvis and lower extremities reveals a decrease in osseous density associated with thin, gracile long bones. Multiple fractures in various stages of healing are present. The long bones are bowed.

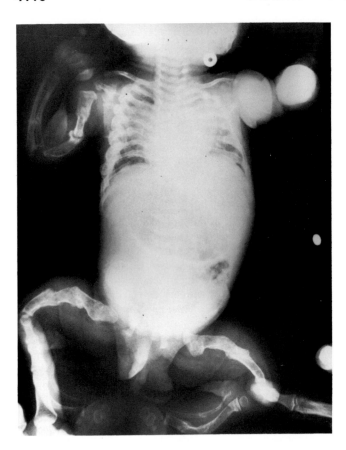

FIGURE 87–17. Osteogenesis imperfecta. Anteroposterior view of the skeleton shows a decrease in osseous density associated with short, thick bones and telescoping fractures. Both the upper and the lower extremities are bowed. Fractures are seen in all long bones and ribs.

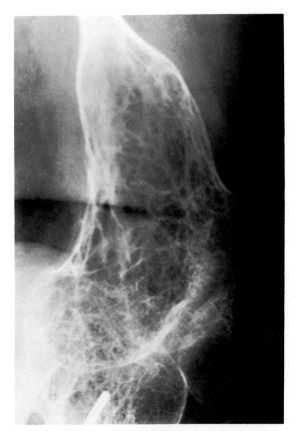

FIGURE 87–18. Osteogenesis imperfecta. Lateral view of knee demonstrates the rare cystic type of disease. The metaphyses are flared and honeycombed by thick, coarse trabeculae.

includes most of the patients in type I or mildly affected patients with type IV. The second group includes the patients with short, thick limbs (Fig. 87–17). This type of radiographic appearance occurs in patients with Sillence types II and III disease and, as with congenital bowing of the extremities, it usually is associated with severe micromelia (Fig. 87–17) and a poor prognosis. Third, and least frequent, is a group of cases with cystic changes in the extremities (Fig. 87–18). These occur in severely affected persons,[160] and the radiographic findings in this category are characterized by flared metaphyses, which are hyperlucent and traversed by a honeycomb of coarse trabeculae (Fig. 87–18). Bauze and collaborators[160] have associated the cystic appearance with abnormalities in stress patterns that, in turn, result in altered modeling of bone. As with the genetic categories, the radiographic classification is descriptive. Indeed, during periods of active growth, a patient may show change from one appearance to another.[130, 229] Patients with types II and III who survive infancy often undergo change from the thick limb type to the cystic or gracile type.[229] Considerable variation also exists within each category, as the radiographic appearance reflects a dynamic balance between the microscopic abnormalities and the gross fracture deformities. The cortices of the long bones may be either abnormally thin (Figs. 87–16 to 87–18) or abnormally thick (Fig. 87–19).[215, 221] The metaphyses may be flared (Fig. 87–18) or undermodeled (Fig. 87–16), and the shafts can be straight (Fig. 87–19) or bowed (Figs. 87–16 and 87–17). In an effort to better correlate the radiographic findings and the prognosis of the disease, Hanscom and associates have proposed a newer classification system,

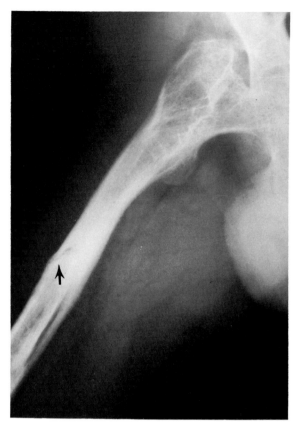

FIGURE 87–19. Osteogenesis imperfecta. Oblique view of the femur shows characteristic transverse fracture (arrow). Although the general density of the bone is decreased, the cortices are thickened as a result of previous trauma and bowing deformities.

which requires further investigation. Published in 1992, the results remain to be confirmed.[230]

The fractures that complicate the course of osteogenesis imperfecta occur most frequently in the lower extremities and usually are transverse (Fig. 87–19). Avulsion injuries also are common and result from normal muscle pull. Micromelia and bowing deformities are the sequelae of multiple telescoping fractures, which begin to occur during gestation (Fig. 87–17).[164, 226] Skull fractures are uncommon.[110, 130] Fracture healing usually is normal,[110] but tumoral callus (Fig. 87–20)[164, 227, 228, 231] and pseudarthroses (Fig. 87–21) may occur.[164] The tumoral callus of osteogenesis imperfecta is an unusual but important finding owing

to its ability to mimic an osteosarcoma.[180, 232] The femur is the most common anatomic site, but the abnormality may occur in multiple bones.[233] Hyperplastic callus can follow either trauma or surgical rodding. It is associated with a low grade fever, swelling, and pain and tenderness to palpation. Hyperplastic callus is observed most often in the Sillence types III and IV (white sclera) syndromes and in male patients.[130, 185] Collagen studies reveal overmodification (excessive hydroxylation or glycosylation) similar to that found in studies of skin fibroblasts.[185] No familial tendency to hyperplastic callus is present, however.[130, 185] In some cases, laboratory studies reveal a mild increase in the erythrocyte sedimentation rate or serum alkaline phosphatase levels (causing further confusion with tumors).

In children with severe osteogenesis imperfecta, the metaphyses or epiphyses of the long bones may contain multiple scalloped radiolucent areas with sclerotic margins (Fig. 87–22). The latter appearance is referred to as "popcorn calcifications," and it is thought to result from the traumatic fragmentation of the cartilage growth plate.[168, 203] Displaced epiphyseal separations are unusual.[110]

The joints of the extremities are affected by two separate processes, both of which lead to premature degenerative joint disease. First, fracture deformities distort the articular surfaces and result in incongruity (Fig. 87–23). The incongruity eventually leads to premature degeneration of the articular surfaces. Second, ligamentous and capsular laxity produces repetitive minor trauma, which also results in damage to the hyaline cartilage (Figs. 87–24 and 87–25).

Laxity is most prominent in groups I and III of Sillence and colleagues.[171] Tendon ruptures and recurrent sprains also can affect the joints.[130]

Since 1959, use of the Sofield procedure,[234] multiple osteotomies, and intramedullary rodding has changed the course of this disease. The intramedullary rods both correct the bowing deformities and protect the limb from further fractures.[221, 235] Correction of bowing deformities has increased the probability of ambulation, particularly in patients with the congenita forms.[235] Greater weight-bearing stress is placed on the joints, and intra-articular protrusion of the rods is possible, which may increase the prevalence of joint changes.[222] Modifications of Sofield and Millar's original procedure[234] include (1) percutaneous placement of rods combined with osteoclasis in very young patients[235] and (2) extensible rods (e.g., Bailey-Dubow[236]), which expand as the patient grows and obviate reoperation every 2 years.[222, 234, 236] With nonextensible rods, the bone can an-

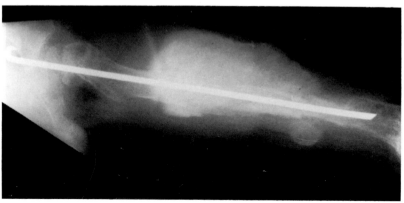

FIGURE 87–20. Osteogenesis imperfecta. Tumoral callus formation around Sofield osteotomies is seen.

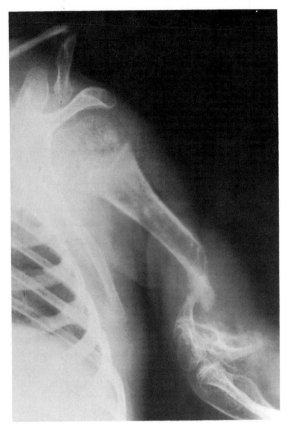

FIGURE 87–21. Osteogenesis imperfecta. Pseudarthroses of the humerus and clavicle complicate fractures.

gulate or fracture below the metal, or the rod can migrate through the cortex as growth occurs (Fig. 87–26).[221, 222, 236] Use of expanding rods is associated with more technical complications, however.[221, 222] Some investigators have advocated careful physiotherapy, beginning in infancy, in an effort to increase bone strength and to decrease the fracture rate.[167]

Radiographs of the skull demonstrate enlargement of the frontal and mastoid sinuses and wormian bones (Fig. 87–27).[130, 159, 164, 223, 227] These bones are defined as small, irregular intrasutural fragments that result from ununited portions of the primary ossification centers of the adjacent membranous bones.[180] To be considered a sign of abnormal ossification, as opposed to a normal variant, at least 10 fragments should be present, preferably arranged in a mosaic rather than in a linear fashion.[223] The presence of wormian bones probably is the sequela of abnormal skull development. Platybasia, with or without basilar impression, is a frequent deformity in osteogenesis imperfecta.[110, 159, 164, 223, 224] In this disease, it results from invagination of the occipital condyles with medial impingement on the foramen magnum.[224] CT of the skull can demonstrate hydrocephalus with ventricular enlargement. Very rarely, thickening and not thinning of the calvarium has been observed in cases of severe osteogenesis imperfecta and has been considered analogous to hyperplastic callus in the long bones.[232] In patients with premature otosclerosis, CT studies can reveal thickening of the stapes footplate, stapedial-crural fractures, failed fixation of the footplate, obliteration of the oval window, and flattening of the cochlea.[110] In patients with den-

tinogenesis imperfecta, dental radiographs demonstrate a decrease in the junction between the crown and roots and, prior to eruption, either absent or enlarged pulp chambers.[204]

The spine studies show flattening of the vertebral bodies, which are either biconcave or wedge-shaped anteriorly (Fig. 87–28).[159, 164] Cervical spine fractures (e.g., hangman's fracture) are an unusual complication.[237]

Severe kyphoscoliosis (Fig. 87–29) occurs in approximately 40 per cent of patients with osteogenesis imperfecta,[218] occurs in all four types of the disease, and results from a combination of ligamentous laxity, osteoporosis, posttraumatic damage to the vertebral growth plates, and osseous compression fractures.[3, 130, 159, 217, 220] Unlike idiopathic scoliosis, the spinal curves of osteogenesis imperfecta begin at an earlier age (less than 5 years), are not necessarily in an S shape compensatory configuration, and continue to progress at the same rate both before and after puberty.[216–218] In addition, the spinal changes are painful and interfere with sitting and ambulation.[3, 130] The multiple thoracic deformities, including fractured, beaded ribs, pectus carinatum, and kyphoscoliosis, contribute to compromised respiratory function.[153, 217, 218] Bracing not only is ineffective in halting the progress of the curves but also may exacerbate the pulmonary problems.[216, 217] Surgical stabilization also is a problem, owing to multiple technical difficulties. The vertebral arches are insufficiently rigid to sustain standard Harrington rods, and the hooks can result

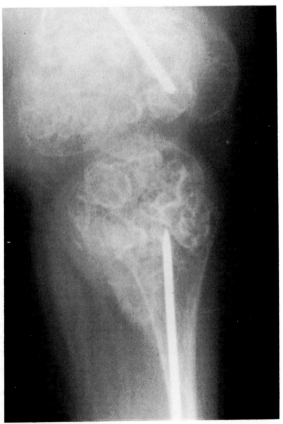

FIGURE 87–22. Osteogenesis imperfecta. Oblique view of the knee shows popcorn calcifications. These lucent areas with sclerotic margins are associated with absence of a normal horizontal growth plate and severe growth retardation. Sofield procedures have been performed.

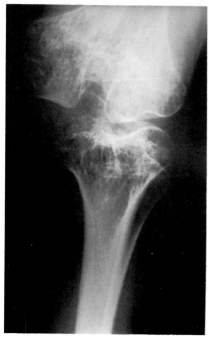

FIGURE 87–23. Osteogenesis imperfecta. Posttraumatic deformities result in irregularity of the articular surfaces of the knee. The opposite side was involved similarly.

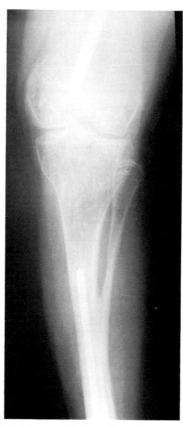

FIGURE 87–24. Osteogenesis imperfecta. Anteroposterior view of the knee reveals genu valgum.

in fractures. Despite difficulties in treatment, surgery is sometimes unavoidable because of the danger of paraplegia[180] or in patients in whom the severe axial deformity is interfering with sitting or respiration.

The pelvis is narrowed and frequently is triradiate in shape (Fig. 87–30), and compression fractures can be present.[221] Protrusion deformities of the acetabula (Figs. 87–30 and 87–31) and shepherd's crook deformities of the femora may be present. Premature vascular calcifications can be seen in the soft tissues.[159, 164]

In pregnant women with the disease, ultrasonography currently is being used in the detection of fetuses with severe osteogenesis imperfecta.[210, 211] The earliest reported cases were identified at 15 weeks of gestation.[102, 176, 229] It is not possible to differentiate among patients with the type II, type III, and severe type IV syndromes on the bases of

ultrasonograms alone.[229] Munoz and associates have described three major diagnostic criteria based on the results of the sonographic examination of the fetus.[176] First, multiple fractures result in discontinuity, "crumpling," or a "wrinkled" appearance of the long bones.[176] Second, severe demineralization of the calvarium is associated with excellent visualization of the intracranial contents. Third, shortening of the femur of more than three standard deviations below the mean value of the femoral length for gestional age is observed.[176] Other sonographic findings associated with fetal osteogenesis imperfecta are platyspondyly,

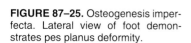

FIGURE 87–25. Osteogenesis imperfecta. Lateral view of foot demonstrates pes planus deformity.

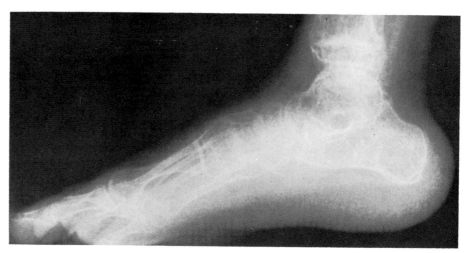

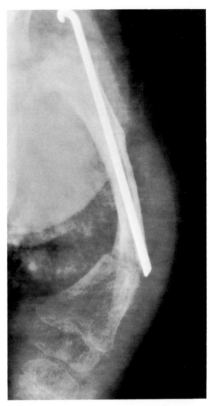

FIGURE 87–26. Osteogenesis imperfecta. Anteroposterior view of the femur shows two complications of nonexpandable rodding: fracture distal to the metal rod and erosion through the cortex.

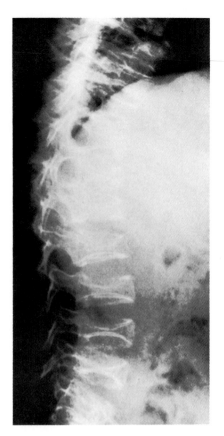

FIGURE 87–28. Osteogenesis imperfecta. Lateral view of the spine shows both biconcave vertebrae and vertebrae with anterior wedge deformities.

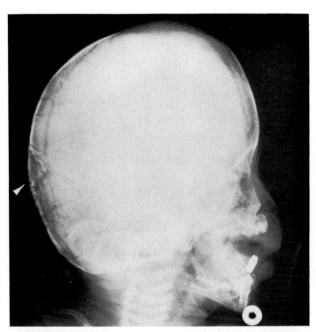

FIGURE 87–27. Osteogenesis imperfecta. Lateral view of the skull shows decreased osseous density, thinning of both tables, and multiple wormian bones (arrowhead).

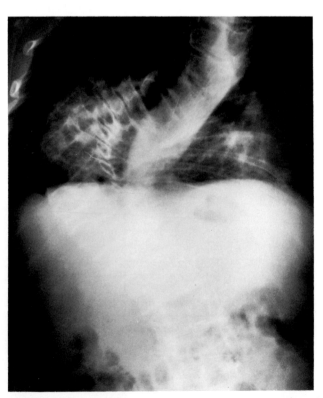

FIGURE 87–29. Osteogenesis imperfecta. Anteroposterior view of the spine reveals severe kyphoscoliosis, decreased osseous density, and flattening of the vertebral bodies.

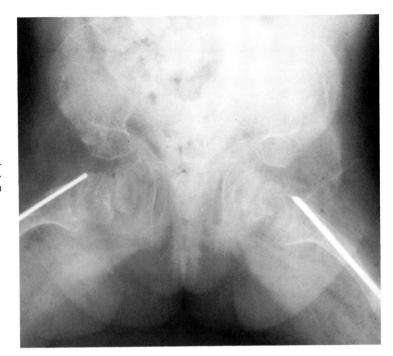

FIGURE 87–30. Osteogenesis imperfecta. Anteroposterior view of the pelvis shows a triradiate shape and protrusio acetabuli deformities. Sofield procedures have been performed in the femora.

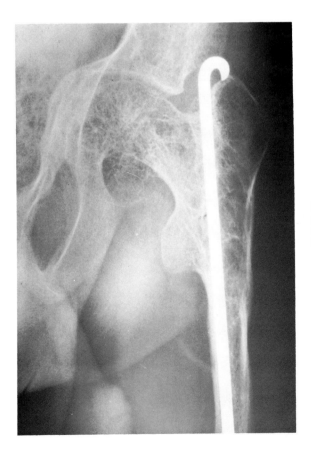

FIGURE 87–31. Osteogenesis imperfecta. Anteroposterior view of the hip demonstrates a protrusio acetabuli deformity and a coxa vara deformity. Owing to the severe varus deformity, the greater trochanter is higher than the femoral head (shepherd's crook deformity).

thick or thin "beaded" ribs, small thoracic circumference, and wormian bones.[176, 181, 238] Serial scans are important because changes may not be visible on the first examination, and sonographic studies are of help in determining prognosis and in planning for the type of delivery.[181] The differential diagnosis of severe (types II and III) osteogenesis imperfecta in utero includes thanotophoric dysplasia, thoracic asphyxiating dystrophy, camptomelic dwarfism, and hypophosphatasia.[130, 176, 238]

The differential diagnosis of osteogenesis imperfecta in infancy includes other entities with multiple fractures, such as the child abuse syndrome, congenital indifference to pain, scurvy, and Menke's kinky hair syndrome.[130] The relatively normal bone density at uninvolved sites and the absence of eye or dental abnormalities should distinguish these latter disorders from fragilitas ossium. Other differential diagnostic possibilities are diseases that produce a generalized decrease in osseous density. Hypophosphatasia is associated with lucent bones and bowing deformities of the extremities, but the metaphyseal changes of rickets also are present, distinguishing it from osteogenesis imperfecta. The radiographic findings of idiopathic juvenile osteoporosis and Cushing's disease may be indistinguishable from those of osteogenesis imperfecta, and in these instances clinical correlation is necessary.

MYOSITIS (FIBRODYSPLASIA) OSSIFICANS PROGRESSIVA

Myositis ossificans progressiva is a hereditary disorder of connective tissue characterized by symmetric congenital anomalies of the great toes and thumbs, progressive heterotopic chondrogeneses, and heterotopic ossification of striated muscles, tendons, ligaments, fasciae, aponeuroses, and occasionally skin.[239–245] The pattern of inheritance remains unknown. McKusick,[240] however, theorized that it is an autosomal dominant trait with a wide range of expressivity. The rare occurrence of this disease and the low reproduction rate in involved patients make the pattern of inheritance difficult to document.[246, 247] Indeed, most reported cases are the result of spontaneous mutations.[243, 244, 246–249] These sporadic cases correlate with advanced paternal age.[240, 247–249] No specific chromosomal defect has been identified,[245, 250] and no increase in the frequency of specific histocompatibility antigens is seen relative to that in the normal population.[251]

This syndrome was first described in 1692 by Patin, who reported the case of a young woman who in his words "turned to wood." It was Münchmeyer who reported the first series of cases, and this disorder often is referred to as Münchmeyer's disease. It also is called fibrogenesis ossificans progressiva or fibrodysplasia ossificans progressiva.

Pathology and Pathophysiology

The cause of myositis ossificans progressiva is unknown. It is classified as a hereditary disorder on the basis of two pieces of evidence. First, at least six sets of homozygous twins with the disease have been recorded.[245, 250, 252, 253] Second, a high association with congenital digital anomalies exists. Seventy-five to 90 per cent of patients with myositis ossificans progressiva and 5 per cent of their families have bilateral microdactyly of the first toes, often associated with synostosis of the phalanges (Figs. 87–32 and 87–33).[242] The nature of the association between the digital anomalies and the heterotopic ossification remains ob-

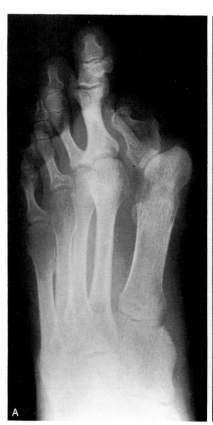
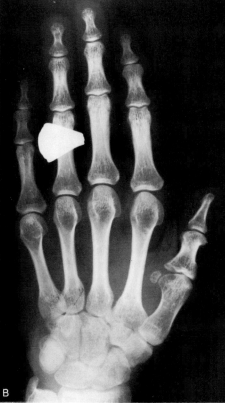

FIGURE 87–32. Myositis ossificans progressiva. Frontal views of the foot **(A)** and hand **(B)** demonstrate microdactyly of the first digits with hypoplasia and fusion of the phalanges.

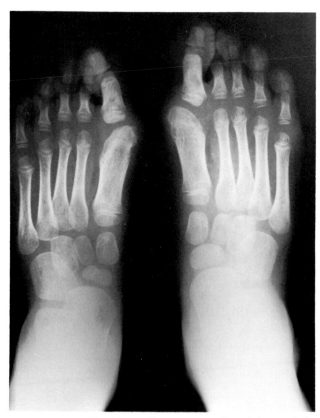

FIGURE 87–33. Myositis ossificans progressiva. Anteroposterior view of both feet shows the characteristic congenital anomalies of the first digits.

scure.[254] Embryologically, the critical time for the formation of the hands and feet is the 43rd and 44th days of gestation.[244, 249] The great toes are the last to form.[244]

Blood chemistry values, serum alkaline phosphatase concentrations, renal function, and parathyroid hormone levels all are within normal limits.[250, 252, 255] Calcium kinetic studies, using radioactive tracers, have indicated only the expected increase in the rates of bone deposition and bone resorption, with a disproportionate increase in deposition.[252] Even the target tissue is uncertain. The prevailing theory, supported by McKusick,[240] Kalukas and Adams,[241] and Smith,[245] postulates that the disease affects primarily the interstitial tissues and that muscle damage occurs secondary to pressure atrophy. Involvement of skin, tendons, and ligaments, which contain no muscle fibers, the detectable localized increase in alkaline phosphatase levels, and elevated urinary levels of collagen metabolites (hydroxyproline and hydroxylysine) support the concept of a fibrous defect.[241, 245, 246] It is known that the function of fibroblast cells can be modified by the environment and that the interaction of fibroblasts and collagen is mediated by cell surface proteins.[247] Fibroblast studies of skin collagen reveal reduced stability.[245] One theoretical possibility is that myositis ossificans progressiva is related to an abnormality in factors that regulate or increase the ability of fibroblast-like cells to modulate and acquire osteoblastic activity. It also has been proposed that the soft tissue changes are related to ectopic periosteal material. The abnormal deposition of calcium salts has been attributed either to absence of a circulating inhibitor[252] or to a primary defect in the collagen

itself.[240] Kaplan and associates[244] relate this disorder to a group of morphogenic proteins referred to as transforming growth factors. This family of proteins is capable of inducing endochondral ossification in vivo.[244] Changes in acid mucopolysaccharides (type, level of sulfation, degree of polymerization) can alter crystallization of inorganic salts.[256] Some investigators remain convinced, however, that the mesenchymal defect is primarily in the muscles themselves. Electromyographic studies, performed on unossified areas, have revealed abnormalities consistent with a myopathy.[245, 255, 257] Histochemical studies have demonstrated variability in muscle fiber size and a decrease in ATPase activity, which predates ossification.[245, 255, 257] Thus, the location of the metabolic error is still to be determined. Nerve conduction studies and sensitivity to parathyroid hormone are normal.[245]

The pathologic abnormalities that characterize the individual lesions are similar but not identical to those of myositis ossificans circumscripta.[252] The earliest histologic changes are edema and rapidly proliferating fibroblasts and myofibroblasts in a loose mucoid backround.[242, 245] The involved muscle fibrils reveal variations in diameter, loss of striations, flocculation of the sarcolemma proteins, a decrease in the number of nuclei, and hyaline degeneration of cytoplasm.[245, 252] Mesenchymal proliferation then results in the formation of multifocal interconnecting nodules composed of spindle cells and basophilic collagen, which, unlike normal collagen, is capable of accepting the deposition of calcium salts.[239, 241, 242, 247, 252] Gradually, the nodules coalesce to form large masses, the lesions become less cellular, the muscle fibers decrease in diameter, and the abnormal tissue is transformed into membranous bone.[247] Various stages of bone formation are present simultaneously,[247] and in some areas cartilage formation precedes ossification.[241] In myositis ossificans progressiva, the first spicules of bone can appear in the center of the nodules,[242, 247] which is the opposite of the peripheral pattern of ossification (the zonal phenomenon) that is characteristic of myositis ossificans circumscripta.[258] Eventually, the entire muscle or muscle group is replaced by columns or plates of lamellar bone, which, like normal bone, contain hematopoietic elements and adipose tissue (Fig. 87–34).[247, 252] These muscles are structurally and chemically identical to normal bone except for the persistence of a few intact fibers within the osseous mass.[241]

Clinical Findings

Myositis ossificans progressiva is a rare disease. By 1982, only 600 cases had been described in the literature.[245, 259, 260] The disorder has been variously reported to occur equally in both sexes[250, 252] or to occur more commonly in men.[261] Although the onset of symptoms usually is in the first decade of life, ossification rarely is present at birth.[252, 260] The mean age of onset is 3 years.[260] A few unusual cases have been reported with soft tissue changes in the neonatal period.[240, 247, 252] The most frequent presenting symptom is torticollis resulting from a painful, doughy mass within the sternocleidomastoid muscle.[243, 245, 252, 253, 257, 259, 260, 262] The initial clinical manifestations may simulate those of trauma, a tumor in the sternocleidomastoid muscle, or infection (e.g., mumps).[245]

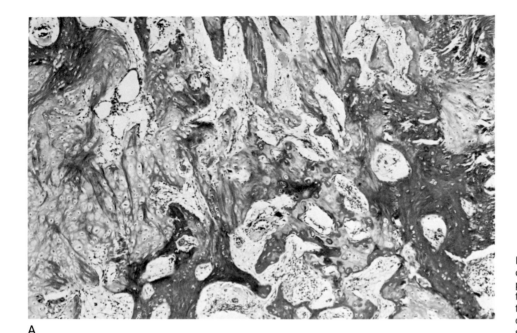

A

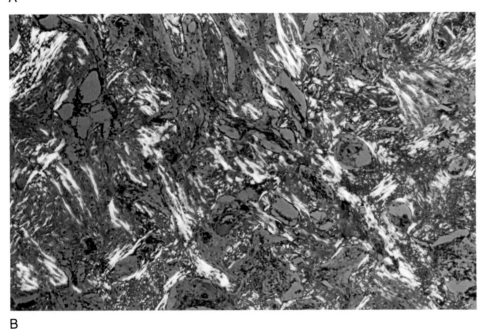

B

FIGURE 87–34. Myositis ossificans progressiva. An irregular piece of new bone was removed from the soft tissues surrounding the hip of a patient with myositis ossificans progressiva. Microscopic sections with unpolarized **(A)** and polarized **(B)** light show irregular collagen fibers and sheets of lamellar bone. Islands of woven bone also are present.

The disease usually progresses from the shoulder girdle to the upper arms, spine, and pelvis (Fig. 87–35).[241, 252, 253, 255] The distal portions of the extremities are involved late in the course of the disease. Diagnostic difficulty may be accentuated owing to failure to note the digital anomalies in the patient or parents.[245] Both CT scanning and MR imaging may be useful diagnostically as a supplement to plain films.[242, 243, 263]

Ossification proceeds from a cranial to caudal direction, from dorsal to ventral, and from axial to appendicular sites.[244] The heart, diaphragm, larynx, tongue, and sphincters are spared, as are all smooth muscle structures.[239–241, 253, 261] The natural history of myositis ossificans progressiva is one of erratic remissions and exacerbations.[252, 255, 261] The most rapid progression occurs during the second decade of life, but exacerbation of the disease continues throughout

life.[244, 260] In rare cases, there are long periods of disease inactivity.[245] Quiescent periods may last for years, or the course may be relentless.[264] A new episode of ossification frequently is precipitated by minor trauma, injections, or surgery,[242, 245, 260] but the injury is not the primary problem and determines only the site of new ossification.[241, 250, 252, 253] As an area becomes involved, the first symptoms are heat, edema, and a painful mass,[252, 265] a clinical appearance consistent with inflammation despite the pathologic changes that reveal no inflammation of the affected muscle.[245] The local changes may be accompanied by fever and an increase in the erythrocyte sedimentation rate.[239–241, 243, 257, 262, 264, 266] The pain decreases gradually while stiffness increases.[245] The mass slowly hardens as new bone formation progresses and contractures develop.[250, 252] The patient's trunk and head move together as a unit.[245] Joint ankylosis occurs as the

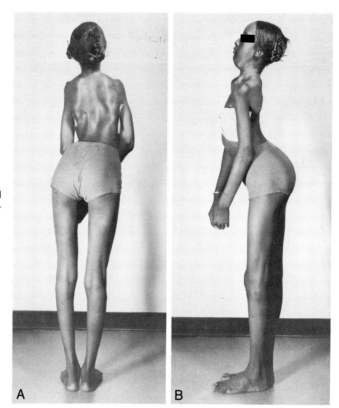

FIGURE 87–35. Myositis ossificans progressiva. Posterior **(A)** and lateral **(B)** views of an adolescent girl with myositis ossificans progressiva show the shoulder girdle and spine to be most affected.

result of ossification of the surrounding soft tissues, not as the result of primary synovial or cartilaginous abnormalities. Fusion of the hips usually is present by the third decade of life, leaving the patient wheelchair bound.[260, 267] Involvement of the temporomandibular joints limits nutrition.[262]

Simple surgical removal of the ectopic bone does little to restore motion.[250] Indeed, the initial lesion recurs with additional ossification in the scar tissue.[250, 259, 268] Operative intervention or even biopsy has been blamed for accelerating the disease process.[246, 259, 268] In recent years, surgical therapy has been combined with pre- and postoperative treatment with disodium etidronate (EHDP) in an effort to prevent recurrence or exacerbation of the disease.[245, 268, 269] EHDP is known to inhibit hydroxyapatite crystal formation and, theoretically, the areas of myositis ossificans are more sensitive to the inhibitory action of the medication than normal bone, owing to their high rate of bone turnover.[268] Several caveats relate to this treatment regimen, however. First, biopsies after surgery and EHDP therapy have shown some degree of recurrence of the lesion, although the new lesion has been incompletely mineralized.[259, 268] Second, excessive doses of EHDP do affect the normal skeleton and result in a decreased mineral to matrix ratio (i.e., osteomalacia).[246, 268, 270] Third, the natural course of the disease is one of remissions and recurrences, making evaluation of a therapeutic response difficult.[246]

Conductive hearing loss is another common complication of myositis ossificans progressiva.[245, 246, 260, 265] Whether such deafness is related to ossification of the stapedius muscle or represents an associated genetic defect is unknown.[265, 267] Nerve deafness, although rare, also has been reported.[260, 267]

Other clinical findings observed in this disease include premature baldness, particularly in female patients, abnormal teeth, hypogonadism, oily skin, and mental retardation.[245, 260, 267] As with hearing loss, these findings may be the result of primary genetic defects or result from malnutrition.

Early death is inevitable and may be secondary to respiratory failure with constriction of the chest wall and, in many cases, pneumonia,[241, 255, 261] or it may result from starvation with ossification of the masseter muscles.[253, 257, 259]

Radiographic Findings

Digital abnormalities are present at birth, are symmetric, and, in the vast majority of cases, precede the soft tissue ossification.[252, 257] The most common type of abnormality is a hallux valgus deformity associated with microdactyly of the first toes, with hypoplasia or synostosis of the phalanges, or both (Figs. 87–32 and 87–33).[241, 245, 252, 253, 260] The proximal phalanges of the great toes have an abnormal contour (broad and square) and are often fused to the distal phalanges.[249] The first metatarsals also are abnormal, and changes range from rounding of the distal articular surface to a hypoplastic cylindric ossification center with no epiphysis.[249] Connor and Evans[267] have subdivided the great toe anomalies of myositis ossificans progressiva into four categories: (1) shortened digit, a single fused phalanx, and lateral angulation at the first metatarsophalangeal joint, (2) normal length with fusion anomalies, (3) normal until heterotopic ossification supervenes and results in stiffness, and (4) other patterns of anomalies. Patients have been reported with hypoplasia of all toes[260] or total absence of the first digit.[252] In addition to anomalies of the great toes, in 44 per

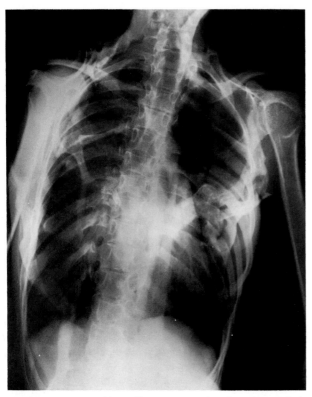

FIGURE 87–36. Myositis ossificans progressiva. An anteroposterior view of the thorax shows the early distribution of soft tissue ossification: shoulders, neck, and cervical spine.

87–37) or a plate of new bone with a "dotted veil" pattern outlining the fascial planes of the back or mandible.[241, 253] Pseudarthroses can occur within these masses of bone, particularly in the columns that surround the shoulder girdle.[259] These lucent areas are attributed to minor trauma.[259] The zonal phenomenon, a characteristic feature of myositis ossificans circumscripta,[258] is not present in progressiva cases. Involvement of the insertions of fasciae, ligaments, and tendons produces "pseudoexostoses" (not true osteochondromas) (Fig. 87–38), which arise from the metaphyses of the long bones, the occiput, and the calcaneus.[240, 259] Unlike a true osteochondroma, no cortical continuity of the outgrowth with the adjacent bone is present. Sesamoid bones that may fuse to the digits are another cause of "exostoses."[257, 271] Joint ankylosis (Fig. 87–39) results from ossification of the surrounding soft tissue structures, as opposed to a primary articular abnormality.[250, 262, 271] Ossification surrounding the hips limits ambulation. Ossification in the tissues adjacent to the temporomandibular joints is a serious clinical problem affecting nutrition. On radiographs, the soft tissue changes can be accompanied by abnormally shaped mandibular condyles.[262] Rarely, the shafts of the long bones become tethered while metaphyseal growth continues and the femoral or humeral heads literally are levered out of the joints, resulting in dislocations. As in other causes of hip dysplasia, the acetabular roofs become shallow and the femoral heads eventually fuse to pseudoacetabula.

CT scans are capable of identifying peripheral mineral-

cent of reviewed cases the middle phalanx of the fifth digit was small, and in childhood it had an accessory epiphysis.[249, 259] Similar abnormalities to those described in the feet frequently involve the hands (59 per cent of cases) (Fig. 87–32B).[241, 257, 260, 265] If the thumbs are involved, the anomalies are less severe than in the toes, and the most common finding is short first metacarpal bones.[249] As in the feet, small middle phalanges can be observed in the fifth digits with clinodactyly.[260] In no reported patient have abnormal thumbs been present in the absence of abnormal great toes. No correlation has been found between the digital anomalies and either the age at onset or the severity of ossification.

Other congenital anomalies of the skeleton associated with myositis ossificans progressiva are hallux valgus deformities (Fig. 87–32A),[175] broad femoral necks,[253, 260, 262, 267] bilateral thickening of the medial cortices of the tibiae,[259] an abnormal carrying angle at the elbow,[259] and an increased frequency of spina bifida.[241] In children, enlargement of the epiphyses has been observed.[259] The cause is unknown and can represent either another genetically determined anomaly or a secondary growth disturbance.[259]

After the onset of symptoms, the radiographic findings in the individual locations are similar to those of the traumatic form of myositis ossificans. The first radiographic finding is a soft tissue mass. The lesion gradually shrinks in size and ossifies. Mineralization often is evident in 3 to 4 weeks, earlier than in cases of traumatic heterotopic bone formation.[242, 260] The final appearance of the lesion may be that of a cylindric column of solid new bone replacing the entire muscle of the neck or extremities (Figs. 87–36 and

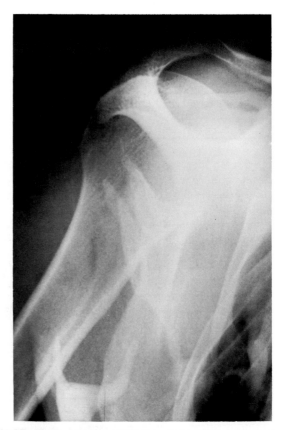

FIGURE 87–37. Myositis ossificans progressiva. Anteroposterior view of the shoulder demonstrates columns of mature bone replacing the normal soft tissue structures.

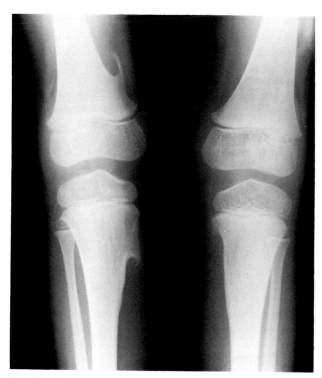

FIGURE 87–38. Myositis ossificans progressiva. Ossification of ligamentous insertions results in metaphyseal "exostoses."

ization and central low attenuation in cases of immature myositis ossificans circumscripta, prior to their appearance on plain films.[263] In 1986, Reinig and coworkers reported a series of 12 cases of myositis ossificans progressiva studied by CT.[243] The CT scans not only identified the presence of early heterotopic bone but also demonstrated a pattern of diffuse swelling of the musculofascial planes that could suggest the correct diagnosis even prior to visible mineralization. In this series,[243] cases that were studied in the first

8 weeks revealed extensive edema between the muscles on one or both sides of the neck. The edema extended beyond the clinically palpable mass.[243] The muscle or muscle bundles primarily involved by the disease also are edematous and can either be swollen or atrophied.[243] Mineralization is identifiable as early as 4 weeks after the onset of swelling and appears as small scattered flattened dense areas. The earliest mineralization occurs adjacent to or encircling the affected muscle, an appearance that supports the theory that the target of heterotopic ossification is fibrous tissue.[243] In more mature lesions, the muscle is entirely encircled by calcification or ossification, and the attenuation values of the muscle become abnormal (both increased and decreased).[243] In long-standing cases, all imaging methods demonstrate that the muscle tissue is replaced by mature bone.

A single published case report of an early unossified lesion in a patient with myositis ossificans progressiva included a description of the MR findings.[242] As in cases of early traumatic myositis ossificans circumscripta, in T1-weighted spin echo MR images, the palpable muscle mass has the same signal intensity as normal muscle but it displaces the surrounding soft tissue planes.[242, 263, 272] As in cases of early traumatic myositis ossificans, on T2-weighted spin echo images, the lesion is well defined, contains inhomogeneous areas of intermediate and high signal intensity, and is surrounded by an edema pattern.[263, 272] The high signal intensity on the T2-weighted images is postulated to result from hypercellularity.[242] A repeat MR study in this patient with myositis ossificans progressiva was performed 1 year after the first study.[242] The soft tissue mass had decreased in size, its signal intensity on T2-weighted spin echo MR images had decreased, and, on all sequences, small areas of low signal intensity crossed the mass (ossification or dense fibrous tissue or hemosiderin). MR imaging evaluation of both the progressiva and circumscripta forms of heterotopic bone is complicated by two factors. First, in

FIGURE 87–39. Myositis ossificans progressiva. Anteroposterior view of the hip shows joint ankylosis resulting from ossification of periarticular soft tissues (arrowhead).

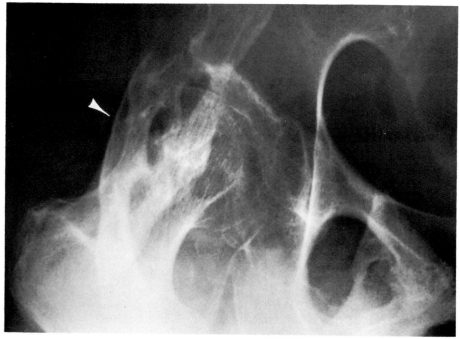

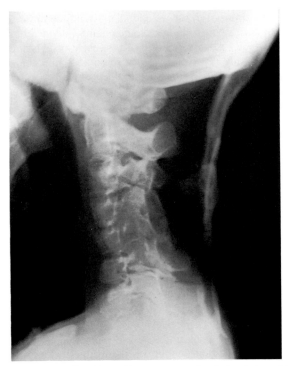

FIGURE 87–40. Myositis ossificans progressiva. Lateral view of the cervical spine reveals ossification of the soft tissues and secondary fusion of the apophyseal joints.

early lesions, surrounding edema can obscure the edge of the mass.[242, 263] Second, early areas of mineralization that result in small areas of low signal intensity may be recognized only in retrospect.[263]

Abnormalities in the spine occur as a result of loss of motion.[262] In the majority of cases, ossification of the soft tissues (interspinous ligament, supraspinous ligament, ligamentum nuchae, paraspinal muscles)[271] is followed by fusion of the posterior elements (laminae, spinous processes, apophyseal joints) (Figs. 87–40 and 87–41),[239, 241, 255, 271, 273] and finally, in adult patients, fusion of the vertebral bodies (Fig. 87–42).[271, 273] Secondary to the soft tissue ossification and the loss of motion of the posterior elements, the intervertebral discs become hypoplastic and calcified, and the anterior aspects of the vertebral bodies flatten.[271] The findings can mimic the appearance of ankylosing spondylitis. In the cervical spine, the canal appears wide and the pedicles are elongated.[259, 262, 267, 273] These findings result from the small size of the vertebral bodies (particularly in their anteroposterior diameters), which stopped growing when motion ceased.[259, 262, 267, 273] The spinous processes of the cervical spine become short and broad (Fig. 87–40).[262] In the thoracic and lumbar regions, so-called "dog vertebrae," which are higher than they are wide, occur as a result of limited weight-bearing.[259] Scoliotic deformities frequently are present.[259, 271] Ossification in the paraspinal soft tissues may or may not be visible.[259, 271, 274] The curves usually are mild, but severe deformities can occur, with ossification in the concavity producing a "bow-string" effect in the lumbar spine.[274] Thickman and colleagues[259] also have reported an increased frequency of spinal stenosis with a decrease in the width of the lumbar spinal canal associated with a decrease in the interpediculate distance.[259] The anteroposterior diameter of the lumbar canal was noted to remain

normal.[259] The sacroiliac joints, like other articulations, can become fused owing to extensive soft tissue ossification.[271]

In patients being treated with EHDP, coexisting radiographic changes of osteomalacia and pathologic fractures have been reported.[246, 267, 270]

The radiographic differential diagnosis includes the causes of metastatic calcifications (e.g., idiopathic calcinosis universalis, dermatomyositis, idiopathic tumoral calcinosis, and disorders of calcium metabolism). In all of these conditions, however, the dense lesions remain calcific and do not mature into trabecular bone. Systemic diseases related to multicentric areas of myositis circumscripta, including tetany, paraplegia, and burns, can mimic myositis ossificans progressiva on radiographs. The distribution of the ossified lesions is different, however; for example, in tetanus the lesions occur on extensor surfaces, in paraplegia ossification occurs adjacent to pressure points, and in burns ankylosis is found symmetrically about the elbows. In addition, the clinical history establishes the correct diagnosis clearly. In the cervical spine, other causes of fusion of the posterior elements (Klippel-Feil syndrome, Still's disease, ankylosing spondylitis) can resemble myositis ossificans progressiva.[259, 271, 273] The presence of soft tissue ossification and digital anomalies in cases of myositis ossificans progressiva greatly simplifies interpretation, however. During the initial stage of the disease, when the patient has an isolated tender soft tissue mass on the neck, face, or shoulder, the differential diagnosis is most difficult, and the swelling may be mistaken for a primary soft tissue tumor.[246, 262] Radiographs may show no mineralization or an

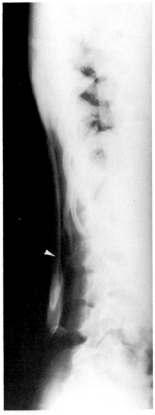

FIGURE 87–41. Myositis ossificans progressiva. Lateral view of the thoracic and lumbar spine shows a plate of bone resulting from involvement of the paraspinal ligaments (arrowhead).

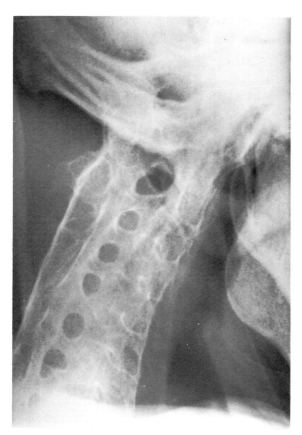

FIGURE 87–42. Myositis ossificans progressiva. Lateral view of the cervical spine shows the late changes of the disease with fusion of the soft tissues, apophyseal joints, and vertebral bodies.

The clinical expressions of pseudoxanthoma elasticum are protean, owing to genetic heterogeneity.[266, 277–281] Three autosomal recessive and two autosomal dominant pedigrees have been identified (Table 87–3).[266, 279] The autosomal recessive type I families have all three typical clinical manifestations: skin lesions in flexion folds, occlusive disease of medium-sized vessels, and angioid streaking. The autosomal recessive type II phenotype is characterized by severe generalized skin lesions but absence of ocular and vascular abnormalities. Autosomal dominant type I families suffer severe ocular changes with retinal degeneration and blindness, usually by 30 years of age. Typical skin lesions in a flexural distribution and occlusive vascular disease also are present. The autosomal dominant type II patients have minimal skin, ocular, and vascular abnormalities but have additional findings, including blue sclerae, hypermobile joints, and marfanoid features. The third type of autosomal recessive expression is the most recently described form of pseudoxanthoma elasticum and was identified in families in Belgium and South Africa.[266, 279] These pedigrees have revealed frequent consanguinity among members, and the syndrome is characterized by severe ocular changes and early blindness. The skin and vascular manifestations are mild (Table 87–3).

McKusick[277] attributes the first pathologic description of this disorder to Darier, who reported a case in 1896 and who coined the term pseudoxanthoma elasticum. Other names used in reference to this entity are elastorrhexis and the Grönblad-Strandberg syndrome, named for the authors who first recognized the association between the ocular and dermatologic findings.

insufficient amount of mineralization to determine its nature. Biopsy can add to the confusion as the histologic sections may suggest a fibrosarcoma or extraosseous osteosarcoma.[246, 247] At this stage, diagnosis rests on a good physical examination that identifies the digital anomalies.

PSEUDOXANTHOMA ELASTICUM

Pseudoxanthoma elasticum is an inherited disorder characterized by a defect in elastic fibers that involves the skin, eyes, and cardiovascular system.[275–277] The exact nature of the abnormality is unknown, but the elastic fibers have a tendency to calcify.

Pathology and Pathophysiology

The skin lesions of pseudoxanthoma elasticum are secondary to progressive mineralization of the elastin component of individual fibers.[280, 281] Skin biopsies of patients with pseudoxanthoma elasticum demonstrate rodlike or granular material occupying the deep and middle layers of the corium.[277, 282] The material shows staining properties similar to those of elastic fibers[277, 283–285] and is calcified or ossified.[276, 277, 283] The inorganic deposits consist of apatite $(CaPO_4)$.[281] Calcification of the "wooly" fragmented elastic fibers[286] and of the amorphous granular deposits of elastin[285] is an early and consistent finding. The epidermis is normal. On unstained sections examined with the fluorescent microscope, the upper one third of the dermis shows smooth

TABLE 87–3. Genetic and Phenotypic Classification of Pseudoxanthoma Elasticum

Type	Pattern of Inheritance	Skin Lesions	Ocular Findings	Other
I	Autosomal recessive	Peau d'orange, flexurally distributed	Retinal degeneration	Atherosclerosis
II	Autosomal recessive	Peau d'orange, generalized	—	—
I	Autosomal dominant	Peau d'orange, flexurally distributed	Severe retinal degeneration and early blindness	Atherosclerosis, often coronary
II	Autosomal dominant	Mild or absent	Mild retinal degeneration	Blue sclerae "Marfanoid" features Hyperextensible joints Mild vascular disease
III	Autosomal recessive*	Peau d'orange, mild and unusual distribution	Retinal degeneration	Mild arthrosclerosis

*Has been described in Belgium and in Afrikaner families.[266, 279]

discrete fibers that emit a normal light yellow-green autofluorescence.[284] In the lower two thirds of the dermis, the fibers emit an abnormal bright green autofluorescence.[284] Electron microscopic studies of biopsy material from skin lesions reveal no mineralization external to the elastic fibers.[287] The mineralization proceeds centrifugally from the center of the fiber. Fine granules progress to spicules that in turn are replaced by a broad mantle surrounding the abnormal fibers.[281, 287] In addition, electron microscopic studies of clinically normal but vulnerable skin sites show similar changes in the elastin moiety.[281] Identical studies of the skin of apparently normal children in afflicted families reveal similar findings.[281] Adjacent to areas of calcified elastin are abnormally thickened, "flower-like" collagen fibers and a marked increase in ground substance (similar to collagen changes in Ehlers-Danlos syndrome and osteogenesis imperfecta).[281, 287] The abnormal mineralization of the elastic fibers has variously been attributed to an increase in acid mucopolysaccharides that have been sulfated,[282] to polyionic deposits (possibly glycoproteins),[285] and to a copper deficiency that results in the production of abnormal elastin.[288]

The ocular changes are characterized by angioid streaks, which represent the fissuring and scarring of the membrane beneath the retina.[280, 282, 289] They are thought to be related either to sclerosis of the choroidal arteries or to tears of the lamina elastica of Bruch's membrane.[276, 277, 282, 289]

Narrowing and occlusion of the large muscular arteries of the extremities, viscera, and central nervous system also are findings of pseudoxanthoma elasticum. The pathologic changes include fragmentation of the external elastic membrane, thinning of the intima, and fibrous proliferation in the media. The vascular calcifications of pseudoxanthoma elasticum occur most frequently in the femoral arteries, involve the media of the vessel wall, and are uniform in distribution.[282] In atherosclerosis, the calcifications more often are intimal and are distributed in plaques.[282] The vascular stage of clotting also is abnormal.[290]

Ultrastructural studies of the endocardium reveal that some elastic fibers are heavily calcified.[277, 283] White areas of thickening affect the endocardium of the atria and ventricles.[282]

Clinical Findings

Pseudoxanthoma elasticum occurs in all races, and there is a slight female predominance.[277, 291] Skin abnormalities usually become apparent in the second decade of life, although a wide range in the age of onset is seen.[276, 277, 292] No correlation is found between the extent of skin lesions and the severity of the ocular changes (Table 87–3).[279] Changes in the skin involve primarily those areas that are subjected to mechanical wear and tear (flexion folds), such as the neck, the face, the axillary and inguinal folds, the cubital areas, and the periumbilical region.[277, 281, 282, 293, 294] Also affected are the heart, the soft palate, and the mucosae of the mouth, gastrointestinal tract, and vagina.[281] The earliest clinical findings are accentuation of the normal skin lines and cosmetic changes related to the neck or face. Particularly prominent are the nasolabial folds, and rubbing or stretching the skin makes the lesions more evident.[277, 292] Later, the skin becomes thickened, redundant, deeply grooved, and hyperextensible.[286] The normal compliance of

the skin is increased.[285] The most characteristic clinical feature is the yellow papules that occur between the thickened folds. These raised, abnormally colored areas give the skin a "pebbly" texture or a peau d'orange appearance.[277, 282, 286, 293] Hyperkeratotic lesions also have been observed on the abdominal wall, similar to those described in other connective tissue diseases (e.g., Marfan's syndrome, Ehlers-Danlos syndrome, osteogenesis imperfecta).[277]

The angioid streaks that characterize the ocular findings of pseudoxanthoma elasticum also begin in the second decade of life.[277] They appear as gray, red, or brown streaks radiating from the disc, which eventually involve the maculae and decrease central visual acuity.[276, 277, 289] Angioid streaks also occur in Paget's disease, sickle cell anemia, and the Ehlers-Danlos syndrome.[276, 282, 289, 294] Chorioretinitis, a more severe threat to vision, is a second ocular abnormality that may occur in pseudoxanthoma elasticum.[276, 277]

Involvement of the muscular arteries usually occurs in the third decade of life but in some instances begins in childhood.[291] Physical examination reveals weakening or even absence of the peripheral pulses.[277] The vascular changes may result in life-threatening complications. Resultant symptoms include intermittent claudication in both the upper and lower extremities, coronary insufficiency, abdominal angina, hypertension, and bleeding from almost every organ.[277, 282, 291] The gastrointestinal tract is the most frequent location of hemorrhage; indeed, severe gastrointestinal bleeding in a child should suggest the possibility of pseudoxanthoma elasticum.[277] Angiographic studies in patients with pseudoxanthoma elasticum and gastric hemorrhage reveal angiomatous malformations, aneurysmal dilation of some vessels, and narrowing and occlusion of medium-sized visceral arteries.[280] Other sites of hemorrhage include the subarachnoid space, the retina, the genitourinary tract, and the nasal passages. Pregnancy has been reported to be a precipitating factor.[277] Petechiae occur, but excessive bleeding from superficial lacerations is not a problem in this disorder. Cardiac changes result from a combination of hypertension, coronary artery disease, and endocardial abnormalities.[283] The early age at the onset of symptoms, plus the upper extremity involvement, differentiates these patients from those with atherosclerosis.[291] High serum cholesterol and serum triglyceride levels have been reported in patients with pseudoxanthoma elasticum.[276] Valvular abnormalities are unusual, but an increased frequency of mitral valve prolapse has been reported, relating pseudoxanthoma elasticum to other heritable disorders of connective tissue (Marfan's syndrome, Ehlers-Danlos syndrome).[295]

Psychiatric disturbances are another complication of this disease.[276]

Radiographic Findings

Radiographs of the skull frequently demonstrate premature calcification of the falx, the tentorium, the choroid plexus, and the petroclinoid ligaments.[277] Thickening of the calvarium and the base of the skull also has been reported.[296] Films of the extremities may demonstrate a variety of calcifications. Most typically, abnormal lesions with fibrillar linear calcifications are observed in the middle and deep layers of the dermis, the site of the pathologic abnormalities.[275] Calcifications also occur (1) within tendons and ligaments, (2) around the metacarpophalangeal joints, the hip joints, or the elbow joints, and (3) within both large peripheral veins and arteries.[280] Angiography of the extremities demonstrates localized occlusion and narrowing of large arteries (resembling fibromuscular dysplasia) as well as the formation of localized aneurysms and arteriovenous malformations.[296] Resorption of the tufts of the distal phalanges may result from the vascular changes.[277] Osseous abnormalities, including osteoporosis, bowing, metaphyseal ectasia, and abnormal lucent areas, also have been reported in association with four cases of pseudoxanthoma elasticum.[296] It is difficult to understand, however, why other such cases have not been recognized in large clinical series. It is possible that these osseous changes may represent only a coincidental dysplasia.

Four cases of pseudoxanthoma elasticum with punctate pulmonary opacities have been reported in the medical literature.[277, 280, 288] Both large nodules and miliary dense areas have been evident.[280] Whether these dense areas represent hemosiderin deposits related to hemorrhage or are a response to changes in the elastic fibers of the lung is unknown.[288]

Ultrasonography may allow identification of this disease in utero.[297] Increased echogenicity is identified in the corticomedullary junction of the kidneys secondary to calcification of the interlobar and arcuate arteries.[297]

The radiographic differential diagnosis includes other entities with both soft tissue and vascular calcification. Both renal disease and collagen vascular disease can produce calcifications in soft tissues as well as erosion of the distal tufts of the phalanges. In these two disorders, however, articular and osseous abnormalities coexist that should differentiate them from pseudoxanthoma elasticum. The Ehlers-Danlos syndrome and parasitic disorders also can produce soft tissue calcifications, but their distribution differs from that of pseudoxanthoma elasticum.

FIBROGENESIS IMPERFECTA OSSIUM

Fibrogenesis imperfecta ossium is a rare disorder of collagen synthesis.[298–301] The cause is unknown, and changes are limited to the skeleton. The entity was first described by Baker and Turnbull in 1950.[302]

Pathology and Pathophysiology

The characteristic pathologic abnormality of this disorder is the presence of abnormal collagen in the lamellar bones.[299–301] Unlike normal collagen, the fibrils are not birefringent when viewed with the polarizing microscope.[298, 299, 301, 303, 304] Reticulum stains show a decrease in the number of collagen fibrils.[305] The collagen defect, in turn, results in incomplete mineralization of the bone and in wide osteoid seams.[298, 301, 304] Therefore, although this disease is a form of osteoporosis (abnormal matrix), its pathologic and radiologic findings can resemble superficially those of osteomalacia (abnormal mineralization).

Gross specimens demonstrate that the normal trabecular architecture is replaced by wide, white, opaque columns of calcified tissue.[298, 299, 304] These irregular masses of abnormal tissue are oriented along lines of stress, roughly parallel to the replaced normal trabeculae.[298, 304] In some areas, the marrow space is severely compromised by the abnormal bone.[304] Histologic studies of biopsy specimens initially

reveal a layer of fiber-deficient bone covering the normal lamellar bone.[299] As the disease progresses, the rind of abnormal bone becomes thicker and the proportion of normal bone to abnormal bone decreases.[298, 299] On hematoxylin and eosin stained sections, the wide osteoid seams appear paler than those in osteomalacia.[304] Calcification is present in both the broad eosinophilic seams and in the abnormal bone.[298, 304] Indeed, the calcium content of the abnormal bone actually is increased because the collagen matrix is not as compact as that of normal bone, leaving room for enhanced mineral deposition.[298] Electron microscopic studies of the skeletal tissue in fibrogenesis imperfecta ossium reveal thin, randomly distributed collagen fibrils.[306] Similar pathologic changes to those described in bone also have been noted in the calcified zone of articular cartilage.[298] There are no reports of radiographically apparent joint changes associated with this disease, however. The collagen of tissue other than bone and calcified cartilage is normal.[304] In patients with fibrogenesis imperfecta ossium, the solubility of skin collagen is normal whereas that of osseous matrix is increased. A genetically determined defect in the amino acid sequence of collagen or procollagen has not been identified in this rare disorder. Clinical observations, including the late onset of symptoms (average age, 49 years)[307] and complaints isolated to the skeletal system, militate against a heritable disorder and favor an acquired one.

Clinical Findings

Fibrogenesis imperfecta ossium is an extremely rare disorder, with approximately 12 confirmed cases in the literature.[305–307] This disorder appears late in adult life.[299, 303, 304] The onset of symptoms is heralded by spontaneous fractures.[303, 305] Changes are rapidly progressive, with eventual debilitation of the patient owing to the severe bone and joint pain.[298, 301, 305] Serum calcium and phosphorus levels are normal.[300, 301, 304] Elevation of the serum alkaline phosphatase level may be present, however.[300, 304] The most characteristic laboratory abnormality is the excessive fecal excretion of calcium, with levels approaching those of hyperparathyroidism.[300] To date, results of studies of both renal function and gastrointestinal absorption have been normal.[304] Changes in the bone marrow distribution also have been reported,[301] and in some instances, monoclonal spikes have been noted on serum electrophoresis.[307] In one of the latter cases the patient had iliac crest biopsy findings suggestive of myeloma coexisting with the changes of fibrogenesis imperfecta ossium.[307] The diagnosis is suggested on the basis of the radiographic changes and confirmed by collagen studies of biopsy material.[298] Treatment of this disease with vitamin D_2 remains controversial, with conflicting reports of good versus poor symptomatic relief.[298, 304, 305]

Radiographic Findings

The radiographic changes in fibrogenesis imperfecta ossium are found in the entire skeleton, with relative sparing of the skull.[303] Autopsy studies confirm that abnormal bone matrix is present in the calvarium, as well as in other portions of the skeleton, but the changes are less advanced.[298] Two radiographic patterns have been described in association with this rare disorder.[307] First, and most typical, is the so-called fishnet appearance.[305, 307] A decrease in osseous density and in the number of trabeculae occurs but those that remain are coarse and dense.[298, 300, 303, 304] The thick, abnormal trabeculae still follow the lines of stress.[298, 299, 304] The cortices are replaced by a network of abnormal trabeculae,[300] but the size and contour of the bones remain normal.[303–305] The vertebral endplates are dense, mimicking the rugger-jersey spine of renal osteodystrophy.[304, 305] The skull may show widening of the vault and homogeneous sclerosis of the base.[305] The second, less common appearance of fibrogenesis imperfecta ossium is that of a generalized increase in osseous density with obliteration of the trabecular architecture.[307] Both radiographic patterns (fishnet and sclerotic) can coexist in the same patient,[305, 307] and both are most marked in the axial skeleton or around joints.[300, 305]

Multiple fracture deformities or pathologic fractures usually are present. In addition, pseudoexostoses of dense callus-like bone form around the axial skeleton and are thought to be the result of local trauma.[307] Extensive calcification of ligamentous and tendinous insertions as well as diffuse periosteal new bone formation has been described,[304] but whether these findings are the result of fibrogenesis imperfecta ossium itself or of the vitamin D_2 therapy is uncertain.[307]

A single reported isotopic bone scan demonstrated markedly augmented uptake of bone-seeking radionuclide in the axial skeleton, rivaling the intensity of uptake in Paget's disease.[307]

The radiographic differential diagnosis includes advanced osteitis fibrosa cystica (hyperparathyroidism), Paget's disease, fluorosis, and atypical axial osteomalacia. Atypical axial osteomalacia is rare and produces radiographic changes almost identical to those of fibrogenesis imperfecta ossium.[308] The principal differences are the abnormal collagen, which is found in fibrogenesis imperfecta ossium but not in the atypical form of osteomalacia,[303] and the distribution of the radiographic changes. In fibrogenesis imperfecta ossium, the skeletal changes are generalized. In atypical axial osteomalacia, the changes occur only in the central skeleton.[308]

MULTIPLE EPIPHYSEAL DYSPLASIAS

Spranger[309] has defined the term multiple epiphyseal dysplasia as "a group of heterogeneous disorders characterized by defective or excessive bone formation in the secondary ossification centers of the tubular bones and sometimes vertebrae." Unlike the mucopolysaccharidoses and hypothyroidism, which both are characterized by irregular ossification of articular surfaces, the epiphyseal dysplasias theoretically result from a heterogeneous group of mutations that lead to the formation of an abnormal cartilaginous anlage that, in turn, produces an epiphyseal center unable to tolerate normal cyclic loading.[310, 311] Therefore, these disorders are grouped together and are subclassified on the basis of morphologic and phenotypic changes. Rubin[312] has divided the epiphyseal dysplasias into two large categories: the spondyloepiphyseal dysplasias (with universal platyspondyly or beaking) and multiple epiphyseal dysplasias (with minimal or no spinal changes). The category of multiple epiphyseal dysplasias is far from homogeneous and contains isolated epiphyseal dysplasias, epiphyseal dysplasias associated with ocular, auditory, or endocrine abnormalities, and those which combine the findings of epiphyseal and metaphyseal dysostoses.[313–315] The problem of understanding epiphyseal dysplasias is further exacerbated by the multiple classifications and definitions used in various publications.[316, 317] For this textbook, the entity referred to as dysplasia epiphysealis multiplex (multiple epiphyseal dysplasia tarda) is considered to be the prototype of the epiphyseal dysplasias. At the end of this section, chondrodystrophia calcificans (multiple epiphyseal dysplasia congenita) and Meyer's dysplasia are discussed in brief.

In 1937, Ribbing[318] published a description of a multiple epiphyseal dysplasia with mild osseous abnormalities and with an autosomal dominant mode of inheritance. Ten years later, Fairbank[319] reported similar, but more severe, osseous changes in 20 additional cases and coined the term dysplasia epiphysealis multiplex. Since these original reports, this disease has been shown to be a classic example of genetic heterogeneity.[311, 316, 320–323] Most affected families have an inheritance pattern consistent with an autosomal dominant gene with high penetrance.[309, 311, 314, 317, 322–328] Cases of spontaneous mutation and pedigrees with autosomal recessive inheritance also have been reported, however.[311, 320, 321, 329, 330] Other terms used in reference to this entity are Fairbank-Ribbing disease, multiple epiphyseal dysplasia tarda, and dysplasia polyepiphysaire.[317] The "pseudoachondroplastic" type of epiphyseal dysplasia is a designation that has been applied to severely affected patients who are dwarfed.[309, 312, 326] The name pseudoachondroplasia has been applied to a variety of other entities, however,[331] and incorrectly implies a similarity between the epiphyseal dysplasias and such entities as achondroplasia or achondrogenesis.

Pathology and Pathophysiology

The primary defect in dysplasia epiphysealis multiplex appears to involve the epiphyseal chondrocyte.[317, 324, 332, 333] On gross specimens, the growth plate is found to be widened and to have an irregular metaphyseal margin. Tongues of cartilage extend into the osseous metaphysis, and the peripheral trabeculae are irregular. Histologic specimens of the growth plate demonstrate a decrease in the number of chondrocytes in all zones, invasion of vessels into the cartilage, and loss of the normal columnar arrangement of the chondrocytes.[332–334] Excessive matrix as well as areas of degeneration and cleft formation are observed.[320, 333, 334] Bars of calcified fibrous tissue extend from the epiphysis to the metaphysis. The collagen within the growth plate is normal but with decreased mucopolysaccharide content, specifically of galactosamine. This finding is thought to be related to a defect in chondroitin sulfate.[333] The result of these abnormalities is delayed and disorderly ossification of the epiphyseal ends of the bones. The midportion of the secondary ossification centers contains woven bone, and the peripheries are irregular in contour.[324] However, the morphologic abnormalities of the growth plate are not pathognomonic.[335] Joint incongruity inevitably leads to angular deformities (varus or valgus) and to secondary degenerative joint disease (Fig. 87–43).[324, 335]

Considerable progress has been made in establishing that most spondyloepiphyseal and spondyloepimetaphyseal dysplasias result from a variety of mutations in the type II collagen locus (COL2A1) of chromosome 12.[323, 336–345] The

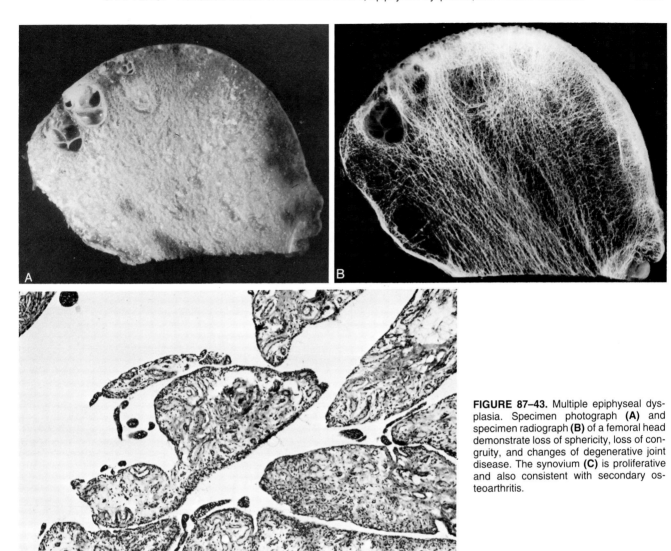

FIGURE 87–43. Multiple epiphyseal dysplasia. Specimen photograph **(A)** and specimen radiograph **(B)** of a femoral head demonstrate loss of sphericity, loss of congruity, and changes of degenerative joint disease. The synovium **(C)** is proliferative and also consistent with secondary osteoarthritis.

spondyloepiphyseal dysplasias are a heterogeneous group of disorders characterized by irregular epiphyses, universal platyspondyly, kyphoscoliosis, cervical instability (Fig. 87–44), ocular abnormalities (myopia, retinal detachment), and oral manifestations (cleft palate).[336, 338–340, 346] At one end of the phenotypic spectrum, spondyloepiphyseal dysplasia can result in severe dwarfing and be recognized at birth.[339–342, 346] At the opposite end of the spectrum are a group of disorders referred to as "chondrodysplasias."[323, 347] The chondrodysplasias come to medical attention when precocious secondary osteoarthritis occurs owing to incongruity of the articular surfaces.[339, 341, 342, 345, 346] The spinal and genetic changes are found, in retrospect, after the onset of joint pain.

Type II collagen is found in hyaline cartilage (95 per cent of resting cartilage collagen), in nucleus pulposus, and in the vitreous of the eye—all sites that are affected in spondyloepiphyseal dysplasias.[340, 344] Resting hyaline cartilage also contains small amounts of types IX and XI collagen, whereas active growth plates contain type X collagen.[337, 342] Type II collagen forms a network in which the

spaces are filled by hydrated proteoglycans.[342] The interaction between the four types of collagen (II, IX, X, XI), proteoglycans, and hyaluronic acid is still incompletely understood.[337] Type II collagen is a homotrimer with a triple helix composed of three identical chains encoded by gene COL2A1.[337, 341] Linkage studies have demonstrated that the majority of autosomal dominant types of spondyloepiphyseal dysplasia, achondrogenesis, hypochondrogenesis, Stickler's syndrome and Kniest's syndrome result from mutation in the type II collagen gene.[337, 339–341, 343, 344, 348, 349] Heterogeneity of position is seen as well as a variety of different types of mutations that produce the spondyloepiphyseal dysplasia phenotype.[336–340, 343] It is difficult to maintain human chondrocytes in culture; therefore, biologic material is limited.[338] However, electrophoretic mobility studies have demonstrated that type II collagen specimens from most families with spondyloepiphyseal dysplasia demonstrate slower mobility than those from normal controls.[336, 345] The inference is that the abnormal type II collagen has a higher molecular weight than that of normal

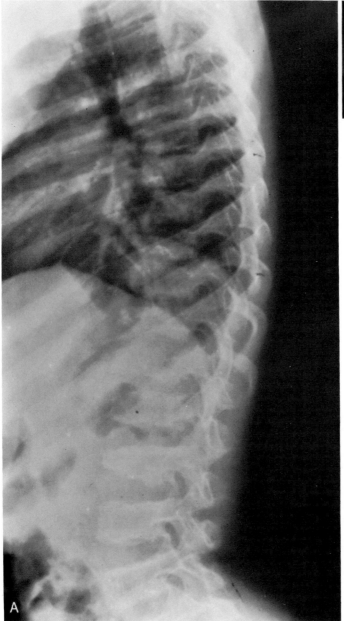

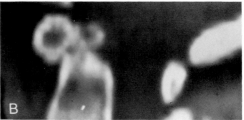

FIGURE 87–44. Spondyloepiphyseal dysplasia.

A A lateral projection of the thoracolumbar spine demonstrates universal platyspondyly and irregular endplates.

B A sagittal reformatted CT scan of the atlantoaxial junction shows a hypoplastic unfused odontoid process.

controls owing to a delay in the formation of the triple helix that, in turn, results in overmodification.[336, 345] As in diseases related to type I collagen overmodification (osteogenesis imperfecta and Ehlers-Danlos syndrome type VII), the closer the mutation is to the C-terminus, the more severe the phenotypic expression.[336, 338] However, rare pedigrees of autosomal dominant spondyloepiphyseal dysplasia, recessive forms of spondyloepiphyseal dysplasia, and the multiple epiphyseal dysplasias do not result from primary mutations of the type II collagen gene (negative lod scores with genetic markers of the COL2A1 gene).[337–341, 343, 345, 348] The inherited cartilaginous defects in such disorders remain unknown. With further investigation, the nosology of the epiphyseal dysplasias may be changed and clarified, on the basis of further biochemical, histochemical, and DNA linkage studies.

Clinical Findings

Dysplasia epiphysealis multiplex affects both sexes equally,[317, 319, 324, 332] intelligence is normal,[320, 329, 330] and osseous involvement is bilateral and symmetric.[311] Considerable variation exists in the severity of the disease among families and even among members of the same family.[316, 324, 330, 350] This group of conditions is characterized by disturbance of two or more paired epiphyses,[310, 311] irregular epiphyseal growth, minimal irregularity of the vertebral endplates, particularly at the thoracolumbar junction, and absence of features suggesting other diseases.[311, 322, 323, 328] The most frequent sites of involvement are the hips, knees, shoulders, ankles, and wrists.[328] In the absence of dwarfism, the patient usually first manifests the disease early in childhood, and common presenting complaints include articular pain,[309, 324, 334] gait disturbances, and difficulty in running and climbing stairs. The last-mentioned complaints result from a combination of restricted motion of the incongruous joints and secondary varus or valgus deformities. In milder cases, symptoms may not occur until adulthood, when secondary degenerative joint disease supervenes, usually in the large joints of the lower extremity.[311, 351]

Physical examination reveals short stature, but only in severe cases is dwarfism present. The growth disturbance may lead to symmetric shortening of the skeleton, if the spine is involved (Fig. 87–45),[326] or to micromelia if only the limbs are affected.[322] The hands and feet have a characteristic stubby appearance. In normal persons, when the arms are placed alongside the body, the fingertips usually reach the level of the greater trochanters; in dysplasia epiphysealis multiplex, the fingertips extend to the midthigh owing to a decreased limb length that affects predominantly the lower segment of the body.[328, 332, 335] A waddling gait is common and associated deformities include coxa vara, genu valgum, genu varum, or tibiotalar slants. Muscular development is normal.[329, 330] In adolescent and young adult patients, precocious degenerative joint disease leads to stiffness and decreased range of motion.[322, 328] Affected members in a single family tend to have the same distribution of involved epiphyses and the same susceptibility to secondary osteoarthritis.[310, 322, 328, 335] The elbows and knees are incapable of full extension.[311, 335, 339] Hematologic and urinary studies are normal. The diagnosis of multiple epiphyseal dysplasia is established on the basis of the positive radiographic findings in combination with the absence of biochemical abnormalities.[320, 327] The identification of fami-

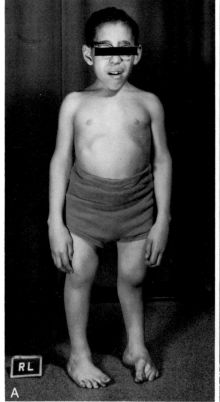
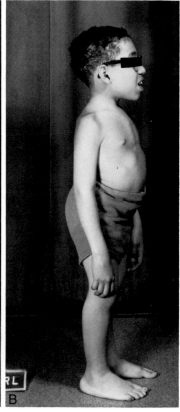

FIGURE 87–45. Multiple epiphyseal dysplasia. Frontal **(A)** and lateral **(B)** views of patient with this disease reveal short stature, protuberant joints, and scoliosis.

lies with autosomal dominant spondyloepiphyseal dysplasia is based on a combination of phenotopic features, electrophoretic studies of type II collagen, and genetic linkage studies.[336–341, 343, 346]

Radiographic Findings

Radiographic abnormalities appear in the second or third year of life and are most marked in the hips, knees, wrists, and ankles. Peripheral weight-bearing and non–weight-bearing joints can be affected.[339, 346] The number of joints affected and the degree of severity vary even among members of the same family.[316, 324, 330, 350] Osseous involvement is always bilaterally symmetric.

In young children, the epiphyseal centers of the long bones are late in appearing and slow in mineralizing, and when they begin to ossify they are irregularly fragmented (Figs. 87–46 to 87–48). The epiphyses frequently ossify from multiple centers and have a mulberry-like appearance (Fig. 87–46)[327, 332] or the central ossific nucleus can be surrounded by ''specks'' of calcification.[328] The secondary centers may be either small (Figs. 87–46 to 87–48) or flattened, with poor congruity or containment (Fig. 87–49).[310] Rarely, the ends of the bones may be enlarged and mushroom-shaped (Fig. 87–50). In one study, sequential radiographs revealed progressive flattening of the femoral capital epiphyses, postulated to be the result of cyclic loading.[311] Severe irregularity of the epiphyses however, does not correlate with the severity of dwarfing.[328]

In older children, slipped epiphyses complicate the coxa vara deformities (Fig. 87–51).[352] The decrease in the neck-shaft angle rotates the growth plate into a more vertical alignment than normal and, in turn, increases the shear stress on the cartilage. The widening of the growth plate and the disordered columnar arrangement of chondrocytes that occur in this disease also predispose to epiphyseal separations.[333] Incongruity and angular deformities, particularly of the knee and hip joints,[317, 334] result in premature

osteoarthritis.[310, 346] Articular symptoms (pain, limitation of motion, effusions, and contractures) occasionally occur as early as the first decade (Figs. 87–51 and 87–52).[334, 339, 341, 346] Arthrography frequently is necessary to determine the cause of joint pain in young patients with multiple epiphyseal dysplasia, as delayed ossification of the secondary centers prevents accurate plain film diagnosis of slipped epiphyses, degenerative arthritis, or intra-articular bodies (Figs. 87–51 to 87–53).[352] Fusion of epiphyseal centers also is delayed, and, in the knees or elbows, a fragmented piece of the secondary center remains ununited and forms an intra-articular body (Fig. 87–53).[320, 328]

In adolescents, apparent improvement in the radiographic appearance has been reported to occur as the result of puberty.[320, 327, 334] The smoother appearance of the ends of the bones is simply the result of the completion of skeletal growth and the fusion of the multiple centers of ossification, however. If an arthrogram is performed on a child with multiple epiphyseal dysplasia, the radiolucent cartilage surfaces always look ''better'' than the multiple ossific nuclei within them (Fig. 87–52). Even after puberty, the affected articular surfaces of the long bones remain irregular and abnormal in shape (Figs. 87–53 to 87–55). The femoral heads and femoral condyles are flattened (Figs. 87–53 and 87–55).[320, 330] The proximal end of the tibia is square instead of biconcave (Fig. 87–56).[320] The talar articular surface also is flat.[320, 332] Differential growth rates within the same physeal plate result in wedge-shaped epiphyses and eventually angular deformities of the articular surfaces. Common abnormalities include coxa vara (Figs. 87–46 and 87–51),[324, 327] genu valgum (Fig. 87–56),[333] genu varum (Fig. 87–57),[333] tibiotalar slant (Fig. 87–58),[332] and V-shaped deformities of the wrist (Fig. 87–59).[324] An unusual growth disturbance associated with multiple epiphyseal dysplasia is hypoplastic irregular ''double patellae'' (Fig. 87–60).[320, 353] On the lateral and Merchant projections, two crescent-shaped ossification centers are observed one inside the other.[320, 353] This anomaly has not been described in other

Text continued on page 4142

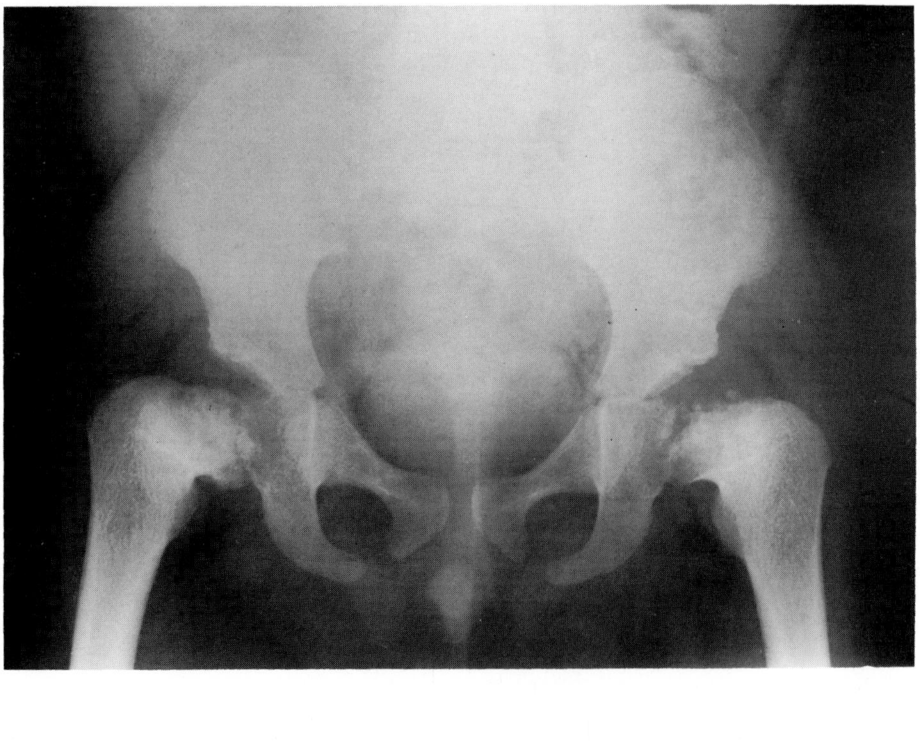

FIGURE 87–46. Multiple epiphyseal dysplasia. Anteroposterior view of the pelvis shows irregular femoral epiphyses and multiple epiphyseal ossification centers. Bilateral coxa vara deformities are present. Mild irregularity of the metaphyses also is noted, and the acetabula show minimal irregularities.

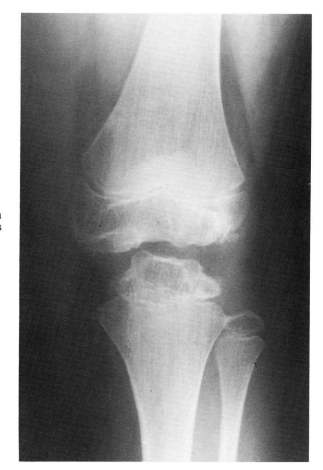

FIGURE 87–47. Multiple epiphyseal dysplasia. Anteroposterior view of a knee demonstrates flattening of condyles and irregularity of the contours of the epiphyses.

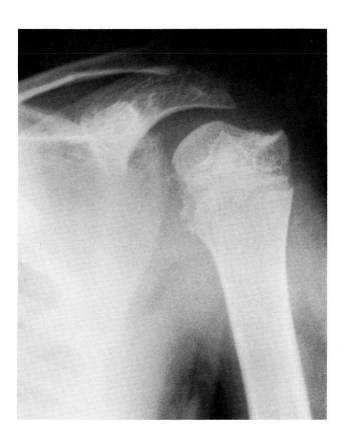

FIGURE 87–48. Multiple epiphyseal dysplasia. Anteroposterior view of a shoulder reveals an irregular contour and abnormal shape to the humeral head.

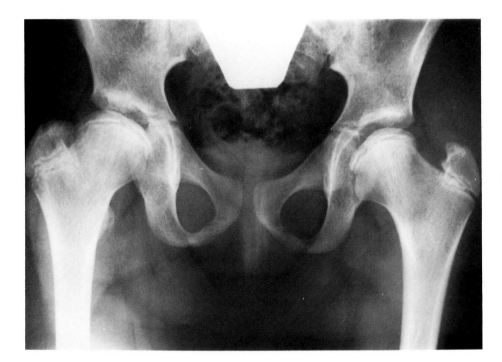

FIGURE 87–49. Multiple epiphyseal dysplasia. Anteroposterior view of both hips shows flattening of the femoral heads and irregularity of the acetabular margins.

FIGURE 87–50. Multiple epiphyseal dysplasia. Anteroposterior view of the hip shows enlargement of the epiphyses. Premature degenerative joint disease is present.

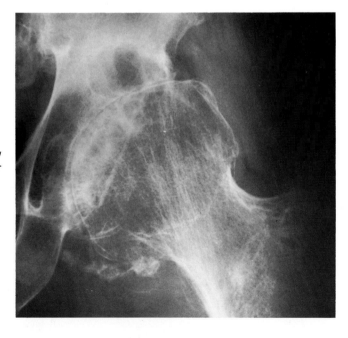

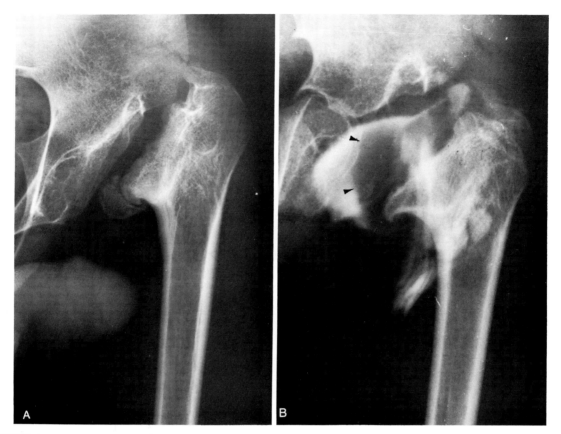

FIGURE 87-51. Multiple epiphyseal dysplasia.
A Anteroposterior view of hip shows small irregular femoral head and marked coxa vara deformity.
B The arthrogram reveals displacement of the cartilaginous femoral head (arrowheads) associated with a slipped epiphysis.

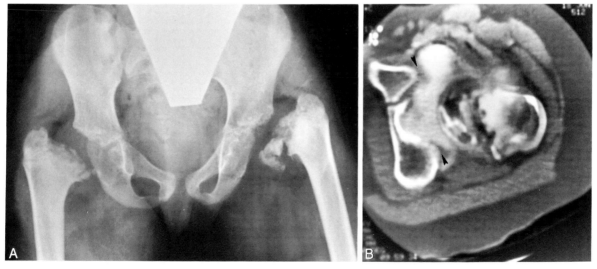

FIGURE 87-52. Multiple epiphyseal dysplasia. Anteroposterior **(A)** view of the pelvis shows small, irregular epiphyses, delayed ossification of the femoral heads (right greater than left), and severe coxa vara deformities. CT scan **(B)** obtained after an arthrogram of the left hip reveals (1) a relatively normal-sized cartilaginous femoral head and (2) severe incongruity of the hip with excessive pooling of contrast material in the medial joint space. The poor fit between the cartilaginous head and acetabulum predisposes to precocious degenerative joint disease; even this 8 year old patient demonstrates irregularity of the cartilaginous surface of the acetabulum (arrowheads).

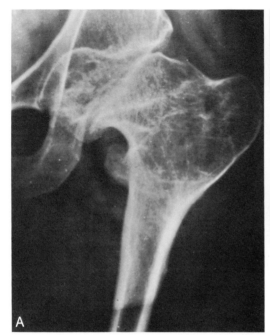

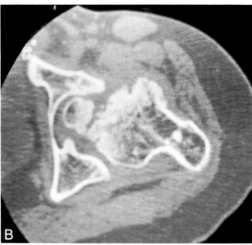

FIGURE 87–53. Multiple epiphyseal dysplasia. Anteroposterior **(A)** view of the left hip reveals a lucent line persisting between the femoral head and neck in this skeletally mature patient. CT scan **(B)** demonstrates one large and several small ununited fragments that have failed to fuse with the rest of the femoral head.

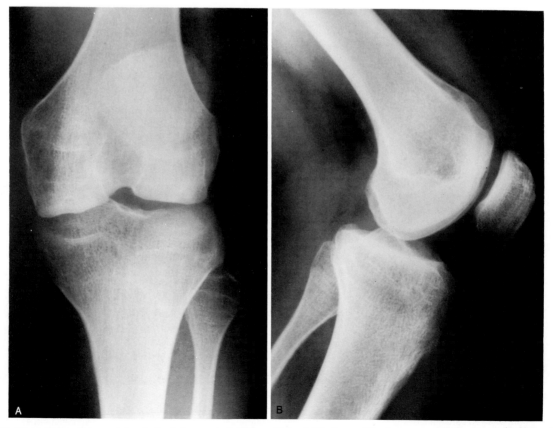

FIGURE 87–54. Multiple epiphyseal dysplasia. Anteroposterior **(A)** and lateral **(B)** views of the knee reveal flattening of the femoral condyles and irregularities of the articular surfaces.

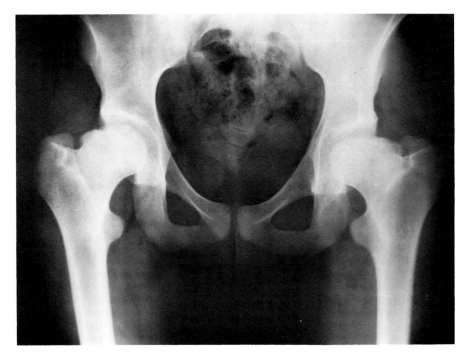

FIGURE 87–55. Multiple epiphyseal dysplasia. Anteroposterior view of the pelvis demonstrates flattening and irregularity of the surfaces of the femoral heads.

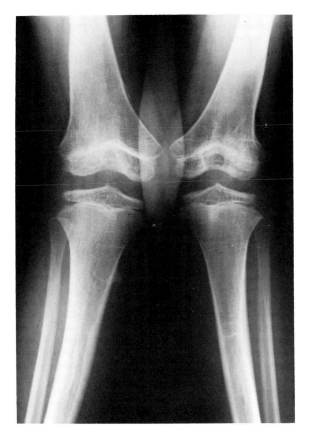

FIGURE 87–56. Multiple epiphyseal dysplasia. Anteroposterior standing view of the knees shows irregular flattened epiphyses and genu valgum deformities.

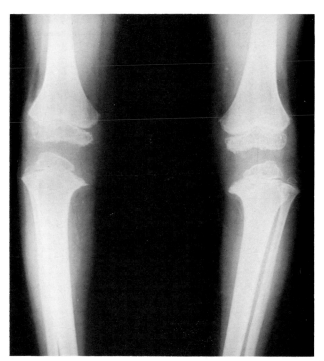

FIGURE 87–57. Multiple epiphyseal dysplasia. Anteroposterior standing view of the knees shows genu varum deformity and beaking of proximal tibial metaphyses. Epiphyses show characteristic irregularities of ossification.

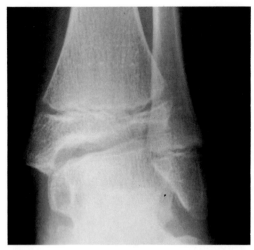

FIGURE 87–58. Multiple epiphyseal dysplasia. Anteroposterior view of the ankle demonstrates tibiotalar slant with a wedge-shaped distal tibial epiphysis.

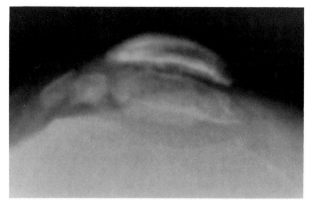

FIGURE 87–60. Multiple epiphyseal dysplasia. Merchant's view of the knee, revealing hypoplastic crescent-shaped "double patellae."

dysplasias and results in chronic subluxations and dislocations.[353]

In most cases of multiple epiphyseal dysplasia, changes of secondary degenerative joint disease are present before the third or fourth decade of life (Fig. 87–61).[310] Cartilage changes result from a combination of joint incongruity produced by the abnormal shape of the articular surfaces and abnormal weight-bearing forces resulting from the malalignment of the joint surfaces. In some cases, mild flaring and irregularity of the metaphyses may be seen (Fig. 87–46). In children, fraying and irregular mineralization also may be present. The metaphyseal changes are particularly noticeable in the metacarpal and metatarsal bones (Fig. 87–

62). If, however, gross metaphyseal changes are present, the diagnosis should be changed to metaepiphyseal or epimetaphyseal dysplasia.

The hands and feet of patients with dysplasia epiphysealis multiplex demonstrate small, broad phalanges, sometimes with irregularity of both epiphyseal and nonepiphyseal ends of the bones (Figs. 87–59 and 87–62). Fusion anomalies or hypoplasia of the carpal bones also occurs in association with this disorder.[313, 316, 326] Bone age is delayed.[322, 328, 351]

The spine is affected in two thirds of patients, and the radiographic changes are similar to those of Scheuermann's disease (Fig. 87–63). The frequency of spinal involvement does not correlate with the severity of the peripheral changes.[350] The vertebral abnormalities associated with this entity include irregularity of the anterior aspects of the vertebral endplates, anterior wedging of the vertebral bodies, mild platyspondyly, and scoliosis. These changes usually are localized to the midthoracic spine. In one series of 18 patients with multiple epiphyseal dysplasia, the odontoid process was absent in six, although neurologic complications were rare.[354]

Maroteaux[317] has based his classification of multiple epiphyseal dysplasia on the distribution (spine versus extremities) of the epiphyseal changes. Type I affects primarily the limbs, including the hands and feet. Little or no axial involvement is seen. Type II has a central distribution, with abnormalities involving the spine and large joints but sparing the distal portions of the extremities. Type III is a conglomerate of localized dysplasias.[316, 317] In all cases, the skull and thorax are spared.[326]

The radiographic differential diagnosis includes other causes of irregular articular surfaces, such as juvenile inflammatory arthritis,[339, 341, 346] osteonecrosis,[311] cretinism, the mucopolysaccharidoses,[323, 344, 349] and other dysplasias. Still's disease may produce abnormalities of the epiphyses; however, the osseous changes are not always symmetric and are accompanied by effusions and juxta-articular osteoporosis. In 10 per cent of cases, Legg-Calvé-Perthes disease is bilateral. The radiographic changes are not symmetric and are limited to the hips, however.[331] In addition, early changes of osteonecrosis are isolated to the superolateral aspect of the epiphysis, whereas epiphyseal dysplasias involve the entire articular surface.[310] Cretinism also is associated with epiphyseal irregularities, but in addition patients have retardation of bone age, generalized osteoporosis,

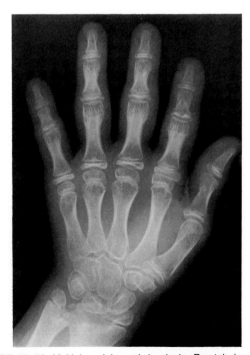

FIGURE 87–59. Multiple epiphyseal dysplasia. Frontal view of the hand shows the characteristic stubby phalanges and a V-shaped deformity of the wrist. The epiphyses of the radius and ulna have an abnormal wedge shape.

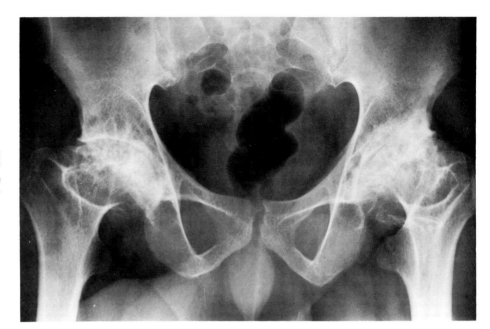

FIGURE 87–61. Multiple epiphyseal dysplasia. Anteroposterior view of hips shows secondary degenerative changes complicating the epiphyseal dysplasia.

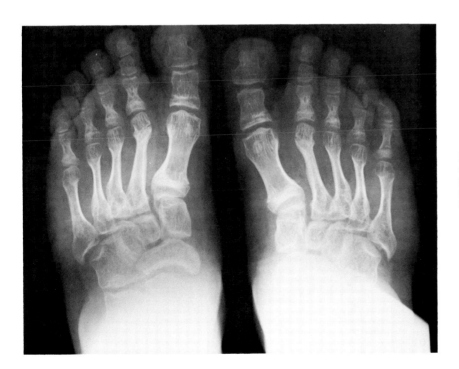

FIGURE 87–62. Multiple epiphyseal dysplasia. Anteroposterior view of feet shows epiphyseal irregularity, forefoot adductus deformities, and stubby phalanges. Mild flaring of the metaphyses also is present.

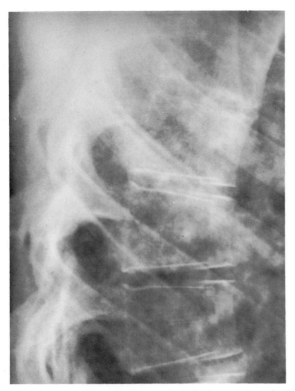

FIGURE 87–63. Multiple epiphyseal dysplasia. Lateral view of spine shows the mild changes that are associated with epiphyseal dysplasias. The vertebral bodies and intervertebral discs are wedge-shaped and minor irregularities of the vertebral endplates are present.

wormian bones, and broad femoral necks. The radiographic findings of spondyloepiphyseal dysplasias and the mucopolysaccharidoses are characterized by more severe spinal changes than those noted in epiphysealis dysplasia multiplex.[320, 326, 330] Beaking of the vertebral bodies and universal platyspondyly differentiate the former entities from the latter, but radiographic differentiation is not always clear-cut. However, unlike multiple epiphyseal dysplasias, the vast majority of autosomal dominant and X-linked spondyloepiphyseal and spondyloepimetaphyseal dysplasias are the result of mutations at type II collagen (COL2A1 gene) and,

in conjunction with radiographs of the spine, can be diagnosed on the basis of results of genetic linkage studies.[336, 338–340, 342, 343, 346] Dysplasias exist that combine epiphyseal and metaphyseal abnormalities.[315] In general, these problem syndromes are grouped together under the name metaepiphyseal dysplasia or epimetaphyseal dysplasia.[315]

Chondrodysplasia Punctata

Chondrodysplasia punctata is a form of multiple epiphyseal dysplasia that is characterized by calcification of unossified cartilaginous epiphyseal centers during the first year of life (Fig. 87–64).[309, 354]

To date, five types of primary chondrodysplasia punctata have been recognized (Table 87–4).[323, 355] They share varying degrees of short-limbed dwarfism, joint contractures, ichthyosiform skin lesions, and cataracts. The categories were established in 1986 by an international group working on constitutional diseases of bone.[323] The types were based on phenotype, mode of inheritance, and, in groups II and III, gene localization.

The first type is the rhizomelic form, which follows an autosomal recessive pattern of inheritance and is characterized by symmetric limb involvement; this form is lethal early in childhood.[214, 324, 347, 354–358] Most patients die of respiratory tract infections.[359] Patients with the type I form have severe psychomotor retardation, seizures, and delayed growth.[354] Physical examination reveals characteristic facies (bulbous nasal tip), sensorineural deafness, symmetric cataracts, microcephaly, and the characteristic ichthyosiform skin lesion.[323, 355] Laboratory studies demonstrate that rhizomelic chondrodysplasia punctata, like Zellweger's syndrome, is an inherited peroxisomal disorder.[354, 358] In rhizomelic infants, a deficiency of an enzyme, dihydroxyacetone-phosphate acetyltransferase, results in decreased hepatic peroxisomes and decreased plasmalogen synthesis in both fibroblasts and red blood cells.[354, 358] Patients also exhibit abnormal accumulation of phytanic acid in plasma and liver.[347] In rhizomelic chondrodysplasia punctata, unlike Zellweger's syndrome, other peroxisomal functions, including levels of long-chain fatty acids and bile, are normal.[354, 358] Prenatal diagnosis of both entities now is possible by biochemical analysis of cultured amniotic cells or chorionic trophoblasts.[354, 358]

TABLE 87–4. Genetic, Clinical, and Radiographic Classification of Primary Chondrodysplasia Punctata*

Type	Mode of Inheritance	Genetic Defect	Midface	Psychomotor Retardation	Prognosis	Limb Shortening	Other
1. Rhizomelic	Autosomal recessive	Peroxisomal enzyme defect	"Bulbous" nasal tip	Severe (rare cases survive)	Lethal	Rhizomelic Symmetric Joint contractures	Ichthyosiform lesions Cataracts—symmetric Microcephaly Sensorineural deafness
2. X-linked dominant Conradi-Hunermann	X-linked dominant	Mutation in short arm of X chromosome	Nasal hypoplasia with bifid tip	Mild	Males—lethal; females—normal survival	Asymmetric Joint contractures	"Blotchy" skin lesions Vertebral body clefts Asymmetric cataracts
3. X-linked recessive Curry-type	X-linked recessive	Mutation in short arm of X chromosome	Nasal hypoplasia	Mild	Normal survival	Symmetric Telebrachydactyly	Severe ichthyosiform lesions
4. Sheffield type†	?X-linked recessive	Unknown	Flat nose	+	Normal survival	Mild Symmetric Mesomelic	
5. Tibia-metacarpal type	Unknown	Unknown	Hypoplasia of entire midface	Normal	Normal survival	Symmetric Mesomelic	

*Based on data from references 323, 355, 361, 363.
†Same as warfarin embryopathy.

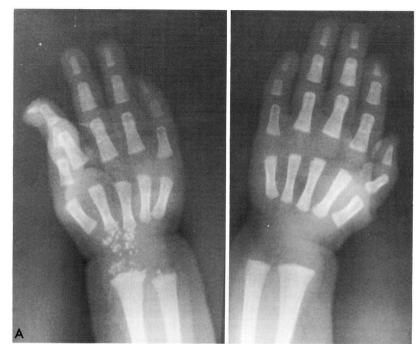

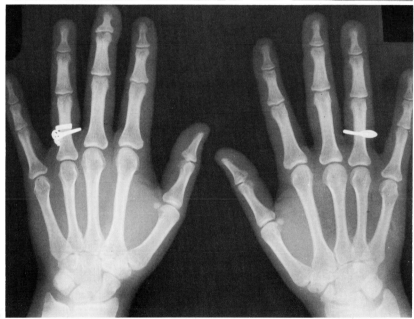

FIGURE 87–64. Chondrodysplasia punctata.
A Posteroanterior views of hands obtained at birth demonstrate asymmetric stippling of cartilage epiphyses.
B Posteroanterior view of the hands at 13 years of age demonstrates almost normal ossification. Only the carpal scaphoid remains abnormal.

The second form of chondrodysplasia punctata is the X-linked dominant form that includes cases previously classified as Conradi-Hünermann syndrome (Fig. 87–64).[358, 360] This variety is consistent with normal life expectancy in women but is lethal in men (Table 87–4).[323, 355, 358] The mutation has been mapped to chromosome Xq 27-28 (short arm of the X chromosome).[361–363] Limb shortening is asymmetric and associated with joint contractures.[354] Cataract formation also is asymmetric, and skin lesions may be either ichthyosiform or "blotchy" and "lyonized." Coronal clefts in the vertebral bodies of the thoracic and lumbar spine are reported in both rhizomelic[356] and X-linked dominant types.[354]

The third category, or Curry type, of chondrodysplasia

punctata (Table 87–4) has an X-linked recessive mode of inheritance; the mutation has been mapped to chromosome Xp-22.3 (short arm of the X chromosome), and the phenotype may be the result of either deletions or translocations.[354, 361–363] Female carriers apparently may be normal but often are short in stature (although not dwarfed); they do have a high rate of spontaneous abortions of male fetuses.[362] The ichthyosiform skin lesions are severe and generalized. Hypoplastic distal phalanges are present on radiographs.[364]

The fourth form, or Sheffield type, is thought to have an X-linked recessive mode of inheritance because of the disproportionately high number of afflicted male infants (66 per cent).[323, 355] This phenotype is associated with mild sym-

1. Zellweger's syndrome: lethal, autosomal recessive, peroxisomal defect as in primary rhizomelic form

2. Embryopathies: warfarin, phenytoin, alcohol

3. Rubella infection

4. Vitamin K epoxide reductase deficiency

5. Trisomies 18 and 21

6. Multiple epiphyseal dysplasia (in rare pedigrees)

metric limb shortening, mental retardation, and a flat nose (Table 87–4). Warfarin embryopathy most closely resembles the Sheffield phenotype (Table 87–5).[323, 355, 365–369]

The fifth form of chondrodysplasia punctata is the tibiametacarpal phenotype. The mode of inheritance and site of genetic mutation are unknown. Limb shortening is symmetric and mesomelic (Table 87–4).[355] This phenotype is associated with hypoplasia of the entire midface.

In addition to the five recognized primary phenotypes of chondrodysplasia punctata, many other syndromes can be associated with localized or generalized stippling of the cartilage anlagen. The secondary causes (Table 87–5) include (1) Zellweger's syndrome (Fig. 87–65), (2) embryopathies related to maternal use of warfarin, phenytoin, or alcohol, (3) rubella infection, (4) trisomies 18 and 21, (5) vitamin K reductase deficiency, and (6) some pedigrees of multiple epiphyseal dysplasia.[355]

Described pathologic findings in the epiphyseal centers in chondrodysplasia punctata include mucoid degeneration, cyst formation, and calcification.[309, 370, 371] Calcifications, although present at birth, are resorbed during the first year of life, but during growth the epiphyses ossify in an irregular

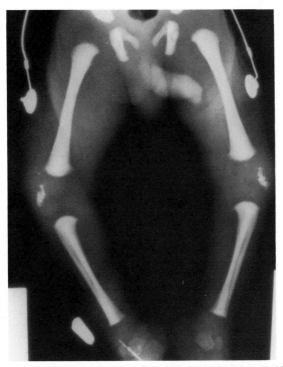

FIGURE 87–65. Zellweger's syndrome. View of the lower extremities of a newborn infant reveals chondrodysplasia punctata, limited to the patellae.

fashion. The abnormalities preceding cartilage degeneration are unknown. Studies performed on beagle puppies, which develop a form of chondrodysplasia punctata,[370, 372] suggest a three-stage process, however. In the animals, the first pathologic findings are areas of abnormal matrix with large amounts of free chondroitin sulfate.[372] During the second stage, abnormal matrix coalesces with liquefaction and cyst formation. In the third stage, calcification occurs both in the contents of the cyst and in the surrounding abnormal cartilage.

The clinical findings include short stature with disproportionate shortening of the extremities and scoliosis.[309, 357, 365, 367, 373] In the X-linked dominant form, limb changes are asymmetric and spine deformities are severe (Fig. 87–66).[309, 359, 371] Midface anomalies are present and usually affect the nose. Cataracts form with a high frequency in the first months of life, and optic atrophy also is frequent.[359, 364, 371] Other findings include mental retardation, cardiac anomalies, recurrent infections (particularly pulmonary), fibrous joint contractures, alopecia, and ichthyosiform rashes.[209, 356, 371, 373] In the X-linked recessive form, children have small distal phalanges.[364]

The radiographic changes differ in the more common phenotypes. In the milder X-linked dominant and recessive pedigrees, radiographs obtained in the first year of life demonstrate punctate or stippled calcifications at the ends of the long bones (Fig. 87–64), at the ends of the short tubular bones, in the vertebral endplates, in the cartilage rings of the trachea, and in the cartilage structures of the pharynx.[309, 354, 360] The calcifications have been described as "spattered paint" or "cluster of pearls."[359] The extent of calcification does not correlate with the overall prognosis, but does correlate with the severity of the skeletal deformities.[360] In rare instances, the tracheal ring calcifications have resulted in clinically significant tracheal stenosis. The punctate calcifications decrease with age, and the stippled cartilage calcifications usually are replaced by bone within 2 years.[347, 354, 374]

Radiographic changes occurring later in life are variable. In some cases, the ossified skeleton is normal. More frequently, however, the early cartilage changes result in a diffuse asymmetric epiphyseal dysplasia (Fig. 87–66).[309, 356, 357] The late epiphyseal changes are not specific for chondrodysplasia punctata.[357] The asymmetric limb involvement, brachydactyly, and scoliotic deformity of this syndrome should suggest the correct diagnosis and initiate a search for skin, eye, or facial stigmata in the patient or family members.[357, 375] The metaphyses and shafts of the long bones usually are normal. However, an appearance in the tibia resembling infantile Blount's disease can be observed.[374] A kyphoscoliosis frequently results from the irregular shape of the vertebral bodies (Fig. 87–66C).[309, 375, 376] Segmentation anomalies also are present frequently. Rare instances of chondrodysplasia punctata complicated by a hypoplastic unfused odontoid[377] or spinal cord anomalies[378] have been reported.

In the severe autosomal recessive form of chondrodysplasia punctata, the stippled calcifications occur primarily in the hips and shoulders.[356] Shortening of the extremities is symmetric and more severe proximally than distally.[209] Ossification of epiphyses is delayed.[347] The metaphyses are flared, and the shafts of the long bones are bowed. The vertebral bodies show a characteristic coronal cleft, which results from failure of the normal ossification centers to

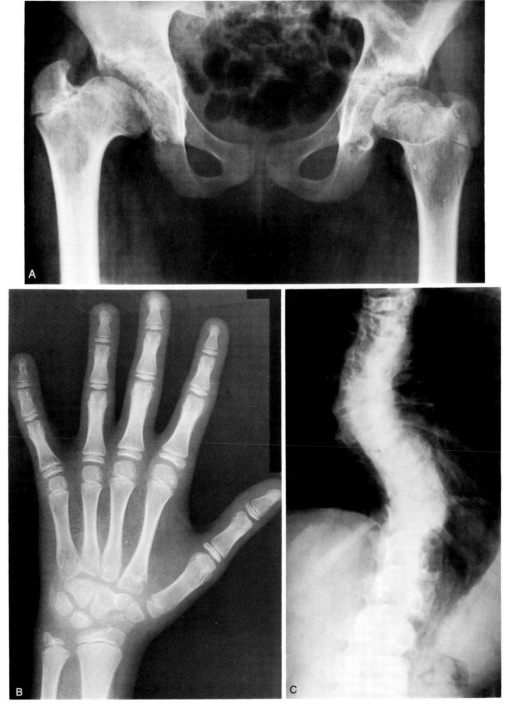

FIGURE 87–66. Chondrodysplasia punctata.
  A Anteroposterior view of hips shows epiphyseal dysplasia resulting from the Conradi-Hünermann syndrome.
  B Patient's wrist has suffered delayed ossification and residual stippling of the scaphoid, which has not yet ossified.
  C Anteroposterior view of spine reveals severe scoliotic deformity.

fuse. If the patient survives infancy, radiographs show irregularity of the cartilaginous growth plate and abnormal contours of the secondary ossification centers.

The radiographic differential diagnosis of chondrodysplasia punctata includes other causes of "stippled epiphyses" (Table 87–5). Prenatal ultrasonography is capable of establishing a diagnosis of chondrodysplasia punctata (short-limbed dwarfism with stippled epiphyses, splayed metaphyses, disproportionate rhizomelic or mesomelic segmental shortening, and, in some cases, vertebral clefts).[354, 379] However, information regarding the family history and past medical history is necessary to allow differentiation between primary and secondary causes of epiphyseal stippling (Tables 87–4 and 87–5).

Meyer's Dysplasia

The cause of Meyer's dysplasia is unknown. It represents either a mild localized epiphyseal dysplasia limited to the femoral capital epiphyses[380, 381] or a normal variant of ossification.[382] Patients and family members are not at risk for developing a diffuse epiphyseal dysplasia. The nature of the pathologic changes is unknown. Most cases are discovered as an incidental finding on hip or pelvic radiographs that are obtained for other reasons.[383] This disorder is more common in men than in women.[383] Occasionally patients complain of mild pain and a limp.[381] The most serious problem encountered is the risk of misdiagnosing the condition as Legg-Calvé-Perthes disease. Radiographic studies reveal delayed ossification of the femoral heads, which appear at approximately 2 years of age instead of at 6 months.[380–382] Bone age is retarded, and the delay is more severe than that reported in Legg-Calvé-Perthes disease.[381] In unilateral cases, the diagnosis can be suspected prior to ossification because the cartilaginous femoral head is smaller on the affected side.[383] Furthermore, the abnormal side shows a 30 to 50 per cent decrease in the distance between the femoral metaphysis and Hilgenreiner's line when compared to the normal side.[383] As the femoral capital epiphyses begin to ossify, granular foci or multiple irregular centers develop with an abnormal flattened appearance (Fig. 87–67). As growth continues, serial radiographic studies reveal consolidation of the granular ossific nuclei and a return to the normal hemispheric shape of the femoral heads.[381] Unlike osteonecrosis, the changes are bilaterally symmetric in 50 per cent of cases, no predilection for the superior aspect of the femoral heads is seen, the density of the epiphyses is not increased, and the children usually are

younger (Fig. 87–67).[383] If serial films are available, they are extremely useful as children with Meyer's dysplasia initially have abnormal proximal femora and show improvement with age. Minimal flattening of the articular surface may persist, but by 5 years of age the granular foci in the affected epiphysis have fused and the radiographs are nearly normal (Fig. 87–68). Children with Legg-Calvé-Perthes disease initially have normal femoral heads that become more deformed as the disease progresses.[381] Lastly, in children with Meyer's dysplasia, all three phases of the radionuclide bone scan (blood flow, blood pool, static) are normal, and the signal intensity of the multiple foci in the femoral head is normal on all MR imaging sequences.[383] These imaging methods allow definitive exclusion of an ischemic process such as Legg-Calvé-Perthes disease.

MACRODYSTROPHIA LIPOMATOSA

Macrodystrophia lipomatosa is a rare form of localized gigantism characterized by a congenital and progressive overgrowth of all the mesenchymal elements of a digit, with a disproportionate increase in the fibroadipose tissue.[384–387] Rarely it involves portions of an entire extremity.[388–390] In the latter instances, it usually affects the lateral aspect of the upper extremity and the medial aspect of the lower extremity.[390, 391] It is classified as a developmental anomaly and is not hereditary.[387]

In 1967, Barsky[384] defined true macrodactyly as "a rare congenital malformation characterized by an increase in the size of all elements or structures of a digit or digits." By this definition, only 56 reported cases and seven of his own patients could be said to have true macrodactyly. The total, by 1985, had reached only 76 documented cases.[389, 392] According to Kelikian,[385] it was Feriz, in 1925, who coined the term macrodystrophia lipomatosa, referring only to localized gigantism in the lower extremity. In 1966, Ranawat and coworkers[393] accepted macrodystrophia lipomatosa as a term applicable to gigantism in the upper extremity.

Dramatic proliferation of fatty tissue associated with localized gigantism has been described in the literature under many titles, including partial acromegaly, macrosomia, elephantiasis, megalodactyly, dactylomegaly, macrodactyly macroceir, and club finger.

Pathology and Pathophysiology

The cause of macrodystrophia lipomatosa remains obscure, and theories include lipomatous degeneration,[385] dis-

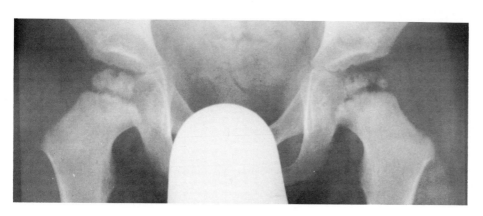

FIGURE 87–67. Meyer's dysplasia in a 2 year old boy. Anteroposterior view of the pelvis demonstrates irregular ossification of both femoral heads. The irregularity involves the entire epiphysis, and the changes are symmetric. The femoral heads are of normal density.

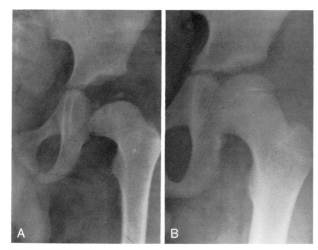

FIGURE 87–68. Meyer's dysplasia.
A Anteroposterior view of the left hip of a 2 year old child shows multiple ossification centers for the femoral capital epiphysis. The density of the ossific nucleus is normal. The opposite hip was involved similarly.
B Repeat anteroposterior view at 6 years of age reveals an almost normal femoral head with only slight residual flattening.

turbed fetal circulation,[394] an error in segmentation,[394] the trophic influence of a tumefied nerve,[385] and the in utero disturbance of a growth-limiting factor.[384] Gupta[391] suggested that an in utero insult occurs at the apex of the limb bud. Several other authors postulated that macrodystrophia lipomatosa is an expression of neurofibromatosis.[395–397] The evidence supporting this theory includes (1) the favored distribution in the hand, corresponding to the territory of the median nerve,[394, 397] (2) the pathologic similarities, including neural enlargement,[394, 397] (3) the predominant involvement of those mesenchymal elements that are under neural control,[394] and (4) the observation that macrodactyly occurs in patients with documented neurofibromatosis.[395, 398]

The evidence against the association of macrodystrophia lipomatosa and neurofibromatosis is based on (1) the lack of neurocutaneous or other systemic abnormalities in patients with macrodystrophica lipomatosa,[384, 385, 387] (2) the absence of an increased frequency of localized gigantism or other anomalies in family members, in contrast to neurofibromatosis, which is clearly hereditary,[387] (3) the neural enlargement, which is not present in all cases and which is the result of fibrosis of the sheath, not neural tumefaction,[394] (4) the disproportionate increase in adipose tissue,[384, 385] and (5) the difference in the radiographic appearance. On the basis of the latter evidence, most investigators[384, 385, 387, 399–401] postulate that in the absence of the cutaneous findings of neurofibromatosis, isolated congenital macrodactyly is an independent pathologic process.

The most dramatic pathologic finding is the increase in adipose tissue, interspersed in a fine mesh of fibrous tissue, which involves the bone marrow, periosteum, muscles, nerve sheaths, and subcutaneous tissues (Fig. 87–69).[385, 394, 397, 398] Neural enlargement and irregularity may be prominent, most frequently involving the median nerve in the hand and the plantar nerve in the foot.[384, 388, 389, 391, 394, 397] On microscopic sections, the increase in size of the nerve is noted to be due to infiltration of the sheath by fibroadipose tissue,[394] not to an increase in the number of axons.[399] The phalanges are enlarged by both endosteal and periosteal

deposition of bone.[385] The periosteum is studded with nodules approximately 1 mm in diameter that consist of chondroblasts and osteoblasts and that become larger and more numerous toward the distal ends of the phalanges.[395] This probably accounts for the predominantly distal enlargement of the osseous structures.

A pathologic study of 26 cases with macrodactyly has emphasized the coexistence of an entity termed fibrolipomatous hamartoma of nerve and macrodactyly of one or more digits.[392] In a series of 26 patients with fibrofatty enlargement of a nerve, seven had overgrowth of the digits supplied by that nerve. The 26 subjects all had localized neural enlargement due to excessive mature fat that probably was of nerve sheath origin. The affected nerves also were surrounded by epineural and perineural fibrosis. Most cases in this series were first manifested by symptoms of compression neuropathy, including carpal tunnel syndrome. Only those patients with abnormalities of the median nerve or pedal nerves had associated macrodactyly. The cause-and-effect relationship between the hamartomatous changes of nerve sheath origin and macrodystrophia lipomatosa remains unclear. The predilection for involvement of the median nerve in both entities also is unexplained. On the basis of this research,[392, 401, 402] a new synonym has been added for macrodystrophia lipomatosa—specifically, ''nerve territory oriented macrodactyly.''

Clinical Findings

The localized gigantism associated with macrodystrophia lipomatosa is recognizable at birth.[384, 385, 387] There is no known sexual predilection. The rate of accelerated growth varies from patient to patient and even from digit to digit.[385] Involvement almost always is unilateral, although one or more adjacent digits in the same extremity may be enlarged (Figs. 87–69 and 87–70). The lower extremity is involved more commonly than the upper extremity. The second and third digits are the favored sites in both upper (the distribution of the median nerve) and lower extremities (Figs. 87–69 and 87–70).[385, 391, 394, 397, 398, 403] The fifth digit is the least likely to be affected.[404] Only a single published report of a case has appeared in which the macrodactyly corresponded to the distribution of the ulnar nerve with enlargement isolated to the fourth and fifth fingers.[404] The usual reason for seeking surgical correction is cosmetic.[387] Mechanical problems are not encountered until adolescence, when secondary degenerative joint disease reduces function and large osteophytes result in compression of the neurovascular structures.[384, 391, 394, 404] Rarely, the patient has carpal tunnel syndrome as a presenting feature.[392, 393]

The affected part is increased in both length and girth.[391, 400] The skin is thickened, pale, and glossy.[385, 387, 398] Growth of the digit ceases at puberty.[404]

Radiographic Findings

Radiographs of patients with macrodystrophia lipomatosa demonstrate abnormalities in both soft tissues and osseous structures (Figs. 87–69 and 87–70).[401] The soft tissue overgrowth is most marked at the distal end of the digit and along its volar aspect in the distribution of the median and plantar nerves.[387–389, 391, 401] Volar overgrowth produces dorsal deviation of the affected parts (Figs. 87–69 and 87–70).

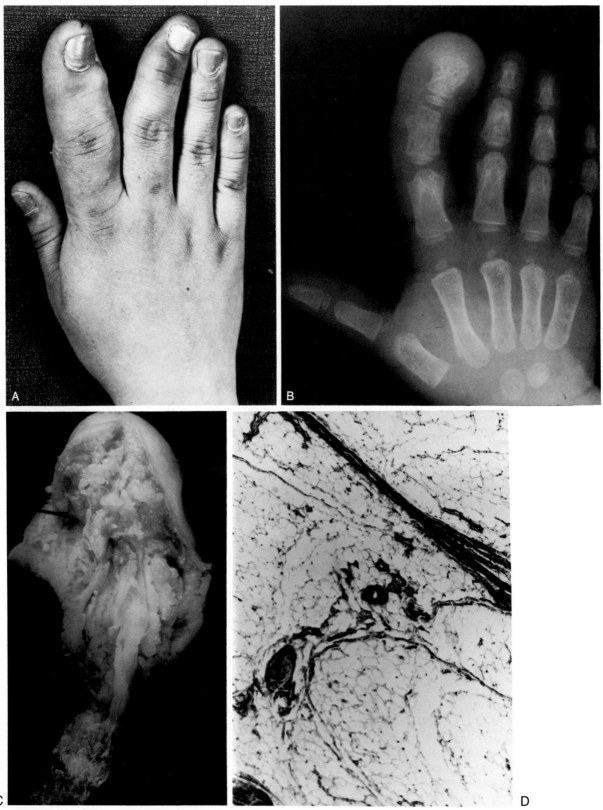

FIGURE 87–69. Macrodystrophia lipomatosa.

A Clinical appearance of involvement of the second and third digits of the hand.

B Posteroanterior radiograph shows osseous and soft tissue enlargement, affecting predominantly the distal end of the second digit, and splaying of the ends of the phalanges.

C,D Gross specimen **(C)** and section of specimen **(D)** show bulk of digit to be composed of fat. Enlarged nerve is seen in gross specimen. (From Goldman AB, Kaye JJ: AJR *128*:101, 1977. Copyright 1977, American Roentgen Ray Society.)

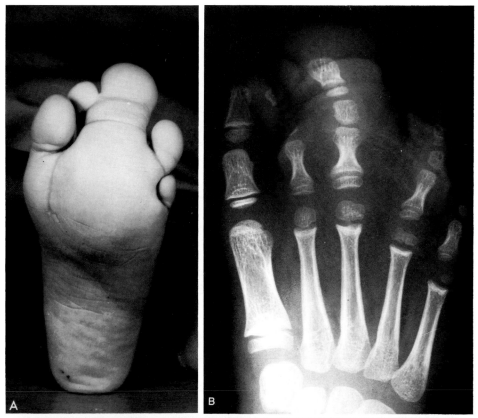

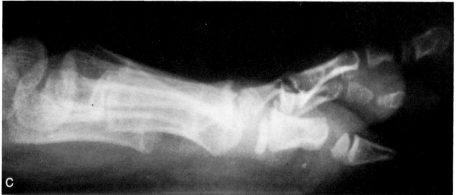

FIGURE 87–70. Macrodystrophia lipomatosa.

A Clinical appearance of involvement of the second and third digits of foot with soft tissue syndactyly.

B,C Anteroposterior **(B)** and lateral **(C)** radiographs demonstrate soft tissue and osseous overgrowth with predominant involvement of the distal ends of the digits and the volar surface of the foot. Soft tissue lucent areas are apparent.

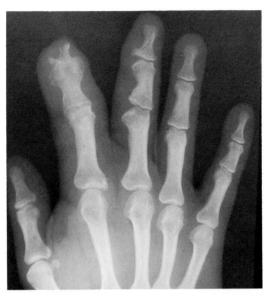

FIGURE 87–71. Macrodystrophia lipomatosa. Adult patient with involvement of second and third digits of hand. Radiograph demonstrates osseous overgrowth and exuberant secondary degenerative joint disease.

Small lucent areas reflecting overgrowth of fat usually are detectable within the soft tissues. The phalanges are long, broad, and often splayed at their distal ends.[387] The trabeculae are normal.[391] The distal phalanx or phalanges have a mushroom shape.[391] If more than one digit is involved, the digits are always adjacent to one another. Rare bilateral cases have been observed.[404]

Two subtypes of macrodystrophia lipomatosa have been described.[392, 393] First are the so-called static cases, in which growth of the enlarged digit or digits progresses at the same rate as growth of the normal digits.[404] Second are the progressive cases, in which the enlarged digit or digits grow at a more rapid rate than the rest of the extremity.[387, 404] The progressive type is more likely to affect the proximal bones (metacarpal and metatarsal bones) than is the static group, but in both the changes are more severe at the distal ends of the digits.[404] The articular surfaces may slant, and, late in childhood, severe secondary degenerative joint disease supervenes (Figs. 87–71 and 87–72).[385, 394, 398] The osteophytes and reactive new bone are disproportionately large in relation to the joint space narrowing, which may be the result of the periosteal nodules associated with overgrowth (Fig. 87–71).[401] A high frequency of associated local anomalies is seen, including syndactyly (Fig. 87–70) and polydactyly. Clinodactyly is present almost invariably, as a result of the side-to-side variations in the accelerated rate of growth (Figs. 87–69 to 87–71).[401]

CT scanning in a patient with macrodystrophia lipomatosa showed the presence of large linear radiolucent bands of fat within the affected muscle.[388] MR imaging in a patient with involvement of the arm revealed an increase in subcutaneous fat in one aspect of the extremity with displacement of adjacent muscle bundles.[389] Fibrous strands and a thickened median nerve accompanied the excessive adipose tissue.[389] The excessive fat had the same signal intensity as normal subcutaneous fat and was not well marginated, as in patients with lipomas.

The radiographic differential diagnosis of localized gigantism includes both acquired and congenital disorders.

On the basis of the history, the acquired causes (dactylitis secondary to infection, trauma, infarction, or Still's disease, osteoid osteoma, melorheostosis)[386, 405–408] can be eliminated from the differential diagnosis of macrodystrophia lipomatosa. The majority of congenital causes also can be excluded. Hyperemia, secondary to tumorous overgrowth of hemangiomatous and lymphangiomatous elements, produces soft tissue hypertrophy and symmetric overgrowth of the bones.[386, 405] The Klippel-Trenaunay-Weber syndrome has obvious cutaneous abnormalities.[386, 393, 409] The absence of enchondromas eliminates the possibility of Ollier's disease.[387, 396] Furthermore, CT scanning and MR imaging in patients with macrodystrophia lipomatosa allow identification of a disproportionate amount of normal mature fat.[388] In Klippel-Trenaunay-Weber syndrome, these studies reveal varicose veins or capillary hemangiomas in the skin.[389] In lymphedema, abnormal signal intensity is seen in the muscles characterized by a relative decrease in signal intensity on T1-weighted spin echo images when compared to normal muscle and a relative increase in signal intensity on T2-weighted spin echo images when compared to subcutaneous fat.[389]

The most difficult differential diagnosis on radiographs, as on pathologic examination, involves neurofibromatosis (Fig. 87–73). Macrodactyly in patients with von Recklinghausen's disease is the result of plexiform neurofibromas (with hemangiomatous and lymphangiomatous elements), combined with a mesodermal dysplasia.[410, 411] Several radiographic findings can help to differentiate macrodystrophia lipomatosa from neurofibromatosis, however. First, the distribution of localized gigantism in neurofibromatosis is not identical to that of macrodystrophia lipomatosa. In neurofibromatosis, unlike macrodystrophia lipomatosa, the enlarged digits may be bilateral, involvement of one extremity does not necessarily involve contiguous digits, and the dis-

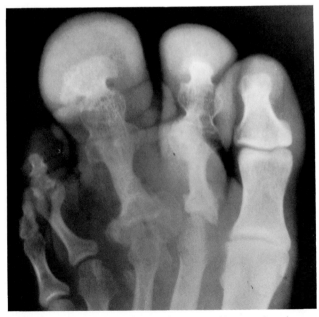

FIGURE 87–72. Macrodystrophia lipomatosa with secondary degenerative arthritis. A frontal view of the forefoot demonstrates overgrowth of the second and third digits, abnormal radiolucent areas in the soft tissues, and a mushroom shape of the third distal phalanx. Large osteophytes arise from the slanting articular surfaces of the third metatarsophalangeal joint.

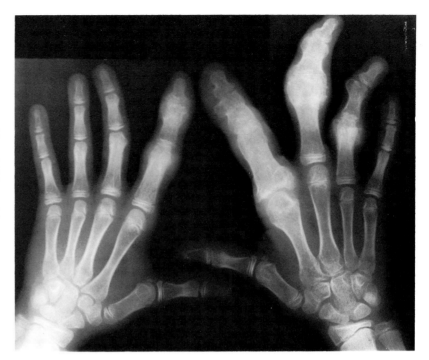

FIGURE 87–73. Neurofibromatosis. Bilateral macrodactyly can be evident in this disease. In addition, digital overgrowth is not most severe in the distal phalanges, premature fusion of the growth plates has occurred, and the cortices of the affected phalanges are dense and wavy. (From Goldman AB, Kaye JJ: AJR, *128*:101, 1977. Copyright 1977, American Roentgen Ray Society.)

tal phalanges are not the most severely affected (Fig. 87–73).[401] Second, the hemangiomatous elements of the plexiform neurofibroma can produce premature fusion of the growth plates.[410] Growth in a digit involved by macrodystrophia lipomatosa ceases with puberty. Third, the enlarged osseous structures in neurofibromatosis may have a wavy cortex and an elongated, sinuous appearance (Fig. 87–73).[410, 411] The latter deformity is related to the periosteal abnormalities in neurofibromatosis. Fourth, the observation of soft tissue lucent areas has not been reported in patients with macrodactyly who have the neurocutaneous manifestations of neurofibromatosis. Last, if necessary, MR imaging can be performed, demonstrating neurofibromas as localized areas of increased signal intensity contiguous to neural structures.[389]

KLIPPEL-TRENAUNAY-WEBER SYNDROME

The Klippel-Trenaunay-Weber syndrome is characterized by a clinical triad that includes unilateral cutaneous capillary hemangiomas, varicose veins, and local gigantism with both soft tissue and osseous overgrowth (Fig. 87–74).[412–418] Although not included in the three major clinical criteria of this disease, arteriovenous malformations often are present and are responsible for major complications.[419] Lymphatic anomalies also are associated with this disorder, which also is referred to as angio-osteohypertrophy syndrome.[420]

The cause of the Klippel-Trenaunay-Weber syndrome is unknown.[421] To date, four families with more than one affected member have been reported.[418, 422, 423] In addition, in a series of 26 cases of Klippel-Trenaunay-Weber syndrome,[422] 25 per cent of families had members with osseous abnormalities of the digits but without nevi or venous distention.[422] In another series of 86 patients, four families had first and second degree members with cutaneous nevi flammei or angiomatous nevi.[423] One family had a member with hemihypertrophy but no vascular abnormalities.[423] These

studies suggest that the disease in most affected patients results from spontaneous mutations but that osseous or vascular lesions (but not the full-blown syndrome) may be inherited.[422, 423]

The association of limb hypertrophy and port-wine hemangiomas was reported independently by Klippel and Trenaunay in 1900[424] and by Parke-Weber in 1907.[425] The latter author, in a later publication, described additional cases with associated arteriovenous malformations. Some investigators[413, 426] prefer to split the syndrome into two forms: those without arteriovenous malformations (Klippel-Trenaunay syndrome) and those with arteriovenous malformations (Parke-Weber syndrome), but most authors consider them a single entity under the term Klippel-Trenaunay-Weber syndrome.[417, 419, 427] Other names used in reference to this disease are angio-osteohypertrophy, acro-osteochondral hypertrophy, partial hypertrophy with angioectasia, congenital angioectatic hypertrophy, and nevus varicosis osteohypertrophicus.[417, 428, 429]

Pathology and Pathophysiology

Most investigators attribute the Klippel-Trenaunay-Weber syndrome to a disturbance in embryogenesis.[418, 427, 430] Persistence of embryonic microscopic arteriovenous communications within the limb bud has been proposed in the pathophysiology of this disorder and would explain its three major clinical abnormalities.[420] The insult probably occurs between the third and the sixth week of gestation.[418, 422] Disagreement exists concerning the target tissue, and theories of pathogenesis include (1) a disturbance at the time of vascular differentiation, with invasion of the limb bud, and (2) injury to the sympathetic ganglia or intermediate lateral tract, with secondary loss of the vascular control mechanisms.[418, 428] In one reported case, Klippel-Trenaunay-Weber syndrome was associated with maternal abuse of butabarbital.[431] The syndrome is associ-

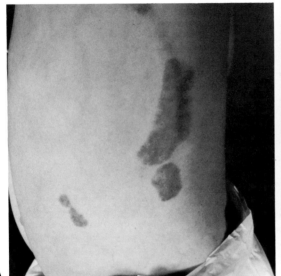

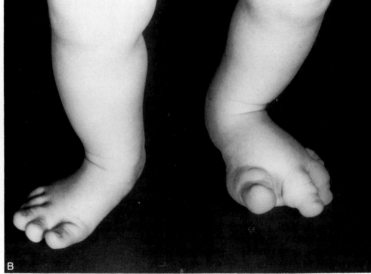

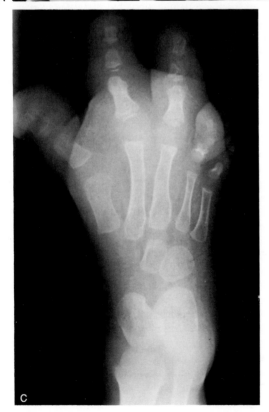

FIGURE 87–74. Klippel-Trenaunay-Weber syndrome.
  A Photograph of abdomen shows unilateral cutaneous hemangiomas and prominent venous markings.
  B View of legs demonstrates overgrowth of one extremity.
  C Anteroposterior view of the foot reveals both osseous and soft tissue overgrowth.

ated with a variety of vascular abnormalities, including superficial blue and pigmented hemangiomas, varicose veins, arteriovenous fistulae, lymphangiomas, and absence of the deep venous system.[416, 417, 432] Skin biopsies of affected limbs have revealed scattered groups of thin-walled vessels and increased collagen proliferation.[429, 433] The arteriovenous malformations, if present, provide a low resistance pathway for the cardiac output.[416, 434] They dilate progressively with age and can result in both local and systemic complications (bleeding, high output failure). A high frequency of spinal arteriovenous fistulae has been observed, and Djindjian and coworkers[435] have suggested that these are traceable to the embryogenesis of the vascular supplies of the spine and skin, which originate from the paired dorsolateral arteries.

Superficial varicose veins and edema result from agenesis, atresia, or compression of the deep venous system.[436] Lymphatic malformations are also related to the deficient deep veins.[436] The venous abnormalities can result in stasis ulcers or thrombophlebitis.[420]

The osseous and soft tissue overgrowth that characterizes the Klippel-Trenaunay-Weber syndrome occurs in the same area as the vascular malformations (Fig. 87–74).[426] No specific primary osseous abnormalities seem to occur, and local gigantism is attributed to the abnormal vascular supply.[412, 415, 416, 418, 419, 425] Brooksaler,[428] on the basis of studies of animal models, has suggested that the osseous overgrowth is related to paralysis of the normal vasoconstrictor mechanism. Lindenauer[413, 426] observed that in patients with arteriovenous malformations, the augmented rate of blood flow may be a primary factor contributing to excessive growth. Barek and colleagues[419] attributed the gigantism to a combination of excessive arterial perfusion and an increase in venous capacity.

Clinical Findings

The Klippel-Trenaunay-Weber syndrome has no sex predilection.[419, 437] It usually is unilateral and most frequently affects the lower extremities (Fig. 87–74). The vascular anomalies may occur in the upper extremity, in two ipsilateral extremities, in the face, or in the trunk.[427–429] Hemihypertrophy, bilateral involvement, and crossed forms are rare, however.[422]

The diagnosis can be established at any time between birth and adulthood.[418] In one clinical series, the average age at which the patient sought medical attention was 13.2 years.[413] The most frequent chief complaint is related to the varicosities. Progression ceases during the second or third decade of life.[419]

The port-wine cutaneous hemangiomas (nevus flammeus) represent the earliest clinical finding (Fig. 87–74).[296, 415, 419, 426, 427, 437] They may be present at birth or appear in the first months of life.[415] The color of the skin lesions varies from bright orange to dark purple to faint pink.[413, 426, 436] The lesions stop abruptly at the midline[413, 426] and are more apparent when the patient is standing (Fig. 87–74A).[297] Associated with the cutaneous hemangiomas are increased skin temperature, altered sweating, hair loss, and dyskeratosis.[414, 418, 429] Extension of the hemangiomatous lesions into the pelvis is common, as is involvement of the viscera, with resultant organomegaly.[418, 419] Involvement of

the face may result in alterations of lacrimation and salivation.[428]

Varicose veins become obvious when the child begins to walk (Fig. 87–74).[415, 418, 419, 426–428] They vary in size from slightly dilated to finger thickness.[415] Ulcerations, thrombophlebitis, and edema further complicate the venous changes.[418, 419, 432] Pulmonary varices also can occur in association with this syndrome.[414, 427] The related lymphangiectasia has been reported to result in chyluria or a chylothorax.[436]

Localized gigantism develops early in childhood and may involve all or only a part of an extremity (Fig. 87–74).[416, 418, 427, 430] The hypertrophy affects both the length and girth of the extremity.[420] Periods of rapid growth alternate with periods of no change.[415, 428] The rate of growth is unpredictable,[438] and the limb disparity may either improve or worsen as the patient matures.[418] The prepubertal growth spurt and pregnancy are periods of greatest risk for a sudden exacerbation.[418] If the upper extremity is involved, a carpal tunnel syndrome may result from the combination of tissue hypertrophy and augmented blood supply.[427] Facial involvement usually affects the mandible and maxilla, with unilateral exophthalmos[414] and premature eruption of permanent teeth.[427, 428]

Arteriovenous malformations, often associated with aneurysmal dilation of vessels, create both local and systemic complications.[418, 434] Their presence and size to a great extent determine the overall prognosis.[418, 419, 434] In the extremities, vascular fistulae may produce intermittent claudication or high output congestive heart failure.[414, 416, 434] Physical examination may reveal thrills, bruits, or pulsatile masses.[426] Visceral vascular malformations have been reported in the colon, producing hematochezia and ulcerations.[418, 432, 436, 439] In the bladder, they result in hematuria,[418, 440] and in the spinal canal they create subarachnoid hemorrhages.[435] Central nervous system involvement may lead to seizures, mental retardation, migraine headaches, macro- or microcephaly, hemangiomas, fistulas, bifrontal varices, ischemic infarcts, aplasia of the internal carotid arteries, malformations of the arterial circle of Willis, and optic nerve anomalies.[421]

Owing to the extensive nature of the angiodysplasia, cosmetic surgery, radiation therapy, and soft tissue reduction procedures are of questionable value.[418, 419, 432] Therapy usually is limited to elevation of the limb and use of compression stockings. In severe cases, when there are numerous arteriovenous fistulae and high output failure, amputation may be necessary.[416, 419] Transcatheter embolization holds some promise in treating urinary or gastrointestinal bleeding, but experience is limited.[419]

Formes frustes of the Klippel-Trenaunay-Weber syndrome also have been described and are subclassified into neviforme, osteohypertrophic, and avaricose types.[428] Angio-osteohypertrophy also may occur in combination with the bleeding diathesis of the Kasabach-Merritt syndrome[439] or with Sturge-Weber syndrome.[421]

Radiographic Findings

The gigantism associated with the Klippel-Trenaunay-Weber syndrome may affect an entire extremity or only the distal digits.[419, 430] The enlargement involves all layers of the soft tissues as well as osseous structures.[418, 419] Both the length and the girth of the affected part are increased (Fig. 87–74).[413, 418, 419, 426, 436] In one series,[438] the average limb length discrepancy was 5.4 cm. Radionuclide bone scans have demonstrated an increase in the rate of bone turnover at the growth plates and rapid augmented uptake in the soft tissue during blood flow and blood pool phases of the study.[416, 420] The phalanges, metatarsals, and metacarpals all are increased in size (Fig. 87–74) and may demonstrate cortical thickening.[415, 433] The limb with the angiomatous anomalies rarely is shorter than the normal limb.[426, 427] The coarse ''sunburst'' trabeculae, characteristic of the intraosseous hemangioma, have been observed in isolated bones (skull, hand).[431, 432] Congenital osseous abnormalities are frequent and include syndactyly, polydactyly, and congenital hip dislocations.[415, 427, 428] A scoliotic deformity may be present as a result of leg length discrepancies.[415, 418, 428, 433] Calcified phleboliths can be observed in the soft tissues.

Venograms obtained from patients with the Klippel-Trenaunay-Weber syndrome have demonstrated a variety of abnormalities.[412, 413, 418, 419, 436] The deep venous system can be totally absent or demonstrate areas of agenesis, atresia, or extreme obstruction owing to fibrous bands or arteries.[412, 413, 418, 419, 436, 438] The perforators are incompetent.[418] The superficial veins are dilated and valveless.[419] A network of abnormal superficial veins provides the major pathway for venous return from the affected extremity.[419] The femoral and popliteal veins are involved more frequently than the deep calf veins. Phleboliths within the varicosities produce multiple soft tissue calcifications. If present, arteriovenous malformations usually are small and numerous.[419] Arteriographic findings are variable. In some cases, the arterial phase is normal. In other patients, the presence of arteriovenous malformations is reflected indirectly by early venous drainage or hypertrophy of feeding vessels. In still others, the vascular malformations are of sufficient size to be visualized directly by use of a contrast agent.[419, 442] Arteriovenous malformations also produce skeletal changes, including multiple lytic lesions.[416, 442] Those involving the viscera may be detected on plain films by the presence of a fixed collection of phleboliths.[439] Unlike phleboliths that occur in normal adults, these dense structures are found in children and are located in atypical sites.[439, 443] Barium studies performed on patients with colonic hemangiomas have revealed thickened folds secondary to varices, extrinsic compression by a soft tissue mass, infiltration of the bowel wall, and secondary mucosal ulcerations.[439, 443]

Lung nodules can be hamartomas or pulmonary varices.[414, 419, 427]

If coexisting changes of the Kasabach-Merritt syndrome are present, joint findings occur and resemble those of hemophilia.[439]

Ultrasonographic examination has identified stigmata of the Klippel-Trenaunay-Weber syndrome in utero[444]—specifically, echolucent areas corresponding to cutaneous hemangiomas and lymphangiomas. After birth, sonography and CT scanning have proved useful in identifying those patients with visceral involvement who are at risk for bleeding complications.[443] As in the embryo, the hemangiomas are sonolucent,[443, 444] but in children, punctate hyperechoic foci also are present, possibly corresponding to phleboliths. CT scanning, after the administration of oral and intravenous contrast material, reveals areas of low density in the

pelvis, abdominal cavity, and affected viscera. Calcifications are apparent where clusters of phleboliths occur and the normal structures are displaced by the vascular lesions. CT, like barium enema examinations, can demonstrate thickening of the wall of the colon associated with luminal compromise in the rectosigmoid, reflecting vascular lesions and varices.

MR imaging studies of the cranium after intravenous administration of gadolinium compounds reveal enhancement of signal intensity in the choroid plexus and leptomeninges and cerebral atrophy.[421]

The major radiographic differential diagnoses involve Maffucci's syndrome, macrodystrophia lipomatosa, and neurofibromatosis.[445] Maffucci's syndrome, like the Klippel-Trenaunay-Weber syndrome, does exhibit both soft tissue and osseous enlargement, soft tissue phleboliths, and brachydactyly. However, unlike the Klippel-Trenaunay-Weber syndrome, osseous enchondromas or cartilaginous ''organ-pipe'' deformities are present, whereas soft tissue varicosities are absent. Macrodystrophia lipomatosa is distinguishable from the Klippel-Trenaunay-Weber syndrome because overgrowth is limited to the digits, enlargement is most dramatic around the distal phalanges, and the soft tissue overgrowth is accompanied by lucent areas representing fat deposits.[401] Neurofibromatosis is the most difficult problem in differential diagnosis.[445] Gigantism in this systemic disorder usually is associated with plexiform neurofibromas—soft tissue lesions that combine hemangiomatous and lymphangiomatous elements with the neural tumors. In neurofibromatosis, however, either the patient or the family members have the two classic stigmata of this hereditary disease (café-au-lait spots or subcutaneous neurofibromas). In addition, unlike the Klippel-Trenaunay-Weber syndrome, in neurofibromatosis the limb overgrowth is associated with an osseous dysplasia, and the bones are grossly deformed, often with sinuous, irregular cortices.

SUMMARY

Certain disorders of connective tissue that can lead to significant radiologic alterations have been discussed. Included in this discussion are diseases of connective tissue synthesis and disorders of epiphyses. The radiographic changes are diverse, ranging from joint incongruity with secondary degeneration to soft tissue calcification or ossification with or without osseous overgrowth. Although clinical and laboratory features exist in some of these diseases that provide important clues to the correct diagnosis, an awareness of the radiographic alterations allows early and appropriate assessment in cases in which the diagnosis may be more obscure.

References

1. Fast A, Otremsky Y, Pollack D, Floman Y: Protrusio acetabuli in Marfan's syndrome. Report of two cases. J Rheumatol 11:549, 1984.
2. Kainulainen K, Pulkkinen L, Savolainen A, et al: Location on chromosome 15 of the gene defect causing Marfan syndrome. N Engl J Med 323:935, 1990.
3. Tsipouras P: Marfan syndrome: A mystery solved. J Med Genet 29:73, 1992.
4. Magid D, Pyeritz RE, Fishman EK: Musculoskeletal manifestations of the Marfan syndrome: radiologic features. AJR 155:99, 1990.
5. Sararazi M, Tsipouras P, Del Mastro R, et al: A linkage map of 10 loci flanking the Marfan syndrome locus on 15q: Results of an international consortium study. J Med Genet 2:75, 1992.
6. Tsipouras P, Del Mastro R, Sarafaraz M, et al: The International Marfan Syndrome Collective Study. Genetic linkage of the Marfan syndrome, ectopia

lentis, and congenital contractural arachnodactyly to the fibrillin genes on chromosomes 15 and 5. N Engl J Med *326*:905, 1992.

7. Morse RP, Rockenmacher S, Pyeritz RE, et al: Diagnosis and management of infantile Marfan syndrome. Pediatrics *86*:888, 1990.

8. Marfan AB: Un cas de déformation congénitale des quatre membres, trés prononcée aux extrémitiés caracterisée par d'allongement des os avec un certain degré d'amincissement. Bull Mém Soc Méd Hôp Paris, 3rd Series, *13*:220, 1896.

9. Langenskiold A: Congenital contractural arachnodactyly. Report of a case and of an operation for knee contracture. J Bone Joint Surg [Br] *67*:44, 1985.

10. Joseph KN, Kane HA, Milner RS, et al: Orthopedic aspects of the Marfan phenotype. Clin Orthop *277*:251, 1992.

11. Milewicz DM, Pyeritz RT, Crawford ES, et al: Marfan syndrome: Defective synthesis, secretion, and extracellular matrix formation of fibrillin by cultured dermal fibroblasts. J Clin Invest *89*:79, 1992.

12. McKusick VA: The classification of heritable disorders of connective tissue. Birth Defects *11*:1, 1975.

13. McKusick VA: Heritable Disorders of Connective Tissue. 4th Ed. St Louis, CV Mosby Co, 1972, p 61.

14. Brenton DP, Dow CJ: Homocystinuria and Marfan's syndrome. A comparison. J Bone Joint Surg [Br] *54*:277, 1972.

15. Baer RW, Taussig HB, Oppenheimer FH: Congenital aneurysmal dilatation of aorta associated with arachnodactyly. Bull Johns Hopkins Hosp *72*:309, 1943.

16. Murdoch JL, Walker BA, Halpern BL, Kuzma LW, McKusick VA: Life expectancy and causes of death in Marfan syndrome. N Engl J Med *286*:804, 1972.

17. Case records of the Massachusetts General Hospital. N Engl J Med *277*:92, 1967.

18. Papaioannou AC, Matsaniotis N, Cantez T, Durst MD: Marfan syndrome. Onset and development of cardiovascular lesions in Marfan syndrome. Angiology *21*:580, 1970.

19. Robins PR, Moe JH, Winter RB: Scoliosis in Marfan's syndrome. Its characteristics and results of treatment in thirty-five patients. J Bone Joint Surg [Am] *57*:358, 1975.

20. Steinberg I: A simple screening test for the Marfan syndrome. Am J Roentgenol *97*:118, 1966.

21. Beals RK, Mason L: The Marfan skull. Radiology *140*:723, 1981.

22. Arroyo JF, Garcia JF: Case report 582. Skel Radiology *18*:614, 1989.

23. Hirst AE, Gore I: Marfan's syndrome: A review. Prog Cardiovasc Dis *16*:187, 1973.

24. Stinson HK, Cruess RL: Marfan's syndrome with marked limb-length discrepancy. A case report. J Bone Joint Surg [Am] *49*:735, 1967.

25. Pyeritz RE, McKusick VA: Basic defects in the Marfan syndrome. N Engl J Med *305*:1011, 1981.

26. Tayel S, Kurczynski TW, Levine M, et al: Marfanoid children. Etiology, heterogeneity and cardiac findings. Am J Dis Child *145*:90, 1991.

27. Phornphutkeil C, Rosenthal A, Nadas AS: Cardiac manifestations of Marfan syndrome in infancy and childhood. Circulation *47*:587, 1973.

28. McKusick VA: More speculation on Marfan syndrome. J Pediatr *80*:530, 1972.

29. Keech MR, Wendt VE, Reed RC, Bistue AR, Bianchi FA: Family studies of the Marfan syndrome. J Chronic Dis *19*:57, 1966.

30. Lee JD: Marfan syndrome. JAMA *218*:597, 1961.

31. Joseph KN: The metacarpal index—obsolete in Marfan syndrome. Skel Radiol *21*:371, 1992.

32. Wenger DR, Ditkoff TJ, Herring JA, Mauldin DM: Protrusio acetabuli in Marfan's syndrome. Clin Orthop Rel Res *147*:134, 1980.

33. Joseph MC, Meadow SR: The metacarpal index of infants. Arch Dis Child *44*:515, 1969.

34. Parrish JG: Heritable disorders of connective tissue. Proc R Soc Med *53*:515, 1960.

35. Sisk HE, Zahka KG, Pyeritz RE: The Marfan syndrome early in childhood: Analysis of 15 patients at less than 4 years of age. Am J Cardiol *52*:353, 1983.

36. Konigsberg M, Factor S, Cho S, Herskowitz A, Nitowski H, Morecki R: Fetal Marfan syndrome: Prenatal ultrasound diagnosis with pathological confirmation of skeletal and aortic lesions. Prenat Diagn *1*:241, 1981.

37. Heldrich FJ Jr, Wright CE: Marfan's syndrome. Diagnosis in the neonate. Am J Dis Child *114*:419, 1967.

38. Pennes DR, Braunstein EM, Shiraz KK: Carpal ligamentous laxity with bilateral perilunate dislocation in Marfan syndrome. Skel Radiol *13*:62, 1985.

39. Walker BA, Beighton PH, Murdock JL: The marfanoid hypermobility syndrome. Ann Intern Med *71*:349, 1969.

40. Amis J, Herring JA: Iatrogenic kyphosis: A complication of Harrington instrumentation in Marfan's syndrome. J Bone Joint Surg [Am] *66*:460, 1984.

41. Ogden JA, Southwick WO: Contraposed curve patterns in monozygotic twins. Clin Orthop Rel Res *116*:35, 1976.

42. Winter RB: Severe spondylolisthesis in Marfan's syndrome: Report of two cases. J Pediatr Orthop *2*:51, 1982.

43. Fishman EK, Zinreich J, Kumar AJ, Rosenbaum AE, Seigelman SS: Sacral abnormalities in Marfan syndrome. J Comput Assist Tomogr *7*:851, 1983.

44. Pyeritz RE, Fishman EK, Bernhardt BA, et al: Dural ectasia is a common feature of the Marfan syndrome. Am J Hum Genet *43*:726, 1988.

45. Harkens KL, El-Khoury GY: Intrasacral meningocoele in a patient with Marfan syndrome. Spine *15*:610, 1990.

46. Soulen RL, Fishman EK, Pyeritz RE, et al: Marfan syndrome: Evaluation with MR imaging versus CT. Radiology *165*:697, 1987.

47. Levander B, Mellström A, Grepe A: Atlantoaxial instability in Marfan's syndrome. Diagnosis and treatment. Neuroradiology *21*:43, 1981.

48. Bjerkreim I, Skogland LB, Trygstad O: Congenital contractural arachnodactyly. Acta Orthop Scand *47*:250, 1976.

49. Epstein CJ, Graham CB, Hodgkin WE, Hecht F, Motulsky AG: Hereditary dysplasia of bone with kyphoscoliosis, contractures and abnormally shaped ears. J Pediatr *73*:379, 1968.

50. Ghosh S: Marfan syndrome or variant. J Pediatr *74*:840, 1969.

51. MacLeod PM, Fraser C: Congenital contractural arachnodactyly. A heritable disorder of connective tissue distinct from Marfan syndrome. Am J Dis Child *126*:810, 1973.

52. Manning GS, Stevens KA, Stock JL: Multiple endocrine neoplasia, type I. Association with marfanoid habitus, optic atrophy and other abnormalities. Arch Intern Med *143*:2315, 1983.

53. Forsman PJ, Jenkins ME: Medullary carcinoma of the thyroid with Marfan-like habitus. Pediatrics *52*:188, 1973.

54. Gutjahr P, Spranger J: Thyroidectomy in type IIb multiple-endocrine-neoplasia syndrome. Lancet *1*:1149, 1977.

55. Goodman RM, Wooley CF, Frazier RL, Covault L: Ehlers-Danlos syndrome occurring together with the Marfan syndrome. N Engl J Med *273*:514, 1965.

56. Brill PW, Mitty JA, Gaull GE: Homocystinuria due to cystathionine synthetase deficiency: Clinical-roentgenologic correlations. Am J Roentgenol *121*:45, 1974.

57. Schimke RN, McKusick VA, Pollack AD: Homocystinuria simulating the Marfan syndrome. Trans Assoc Am Physicians *78*:60, 1965.

58. McGill JJ, Mettler G, Rosenblatt DS, et al: Detection of heterozygotes for recessive alleles. Homocyst(e)inemia: Paradigm of pitfalls in phenotypes. Am J Med Genet *36*:45, 1990.

59. Yoshida Y, Nakana A, Hamada R, et al: Patients with homocystinuria: High metal concentrations in hair, blood and urine. Acta Neurol Scand *86*:490, 1992.

60. Cochran FB, Sweetman L, Schmidt K, et al: Pyridoxine unresponsive homocystinuria with an unusual clinical course. Am J Med Genet *35*:519, 1990.

61. Skovby F: Introduction. Inborn errors of metabolism causing homocysteinemia and related vascular involvement. Haemostasis *19*(Suppl 1):1, 1989.

62. Mudd SH, Skovby F, Levy HL, et al: The natural history of homocystinuria due to cystathionine β-synthase deficiency. Am J Hum Genet *37*:1, 1985.

63. Mpofu C, Alani SM, Whitehouse C, et al: No sensory neuropathy during pyridoxine treatment in homocystinuria. Arch Dis Child *66*:1081, 1991.

64. Smith SW: Roentgen findings in homocystinuria. Am J Roentgenol *100*:147, 1967.

65. Carson NAJ, Dent CE, Field CMB, Gaull GE: Homocystinuria: Clinical and pathological review of ten cases. J Pediatr *66*:565, 1965.

66. Gerittsen T, Waisman HA: Homocystinuria, an error in metabolism of methionine. Pediatrics *33*:413, 1964.

67. Gaull G, Sturman JA, Schaffner F: Homocystinuria due to cystathionine synthase deficiency: Enzymatic and ultrastructural studies. J Pediatr *84*:381, 1974.

68. Gaull GE: Homocystinuria, vitamin B_6 and folate: Metabolic interrelationships and clinical significance. J Pediatr *81*:1014, 1972.

69. McKusick VA: Heritable Disorders of Connective Tissue. 4th Ed. St Louis, CV Mosby Co, 1972, p 224.

70. Maddocks JJ, MacLochlan J: Application of new fluorescent thiol reagent to diagnosis of homocystinuria. Lancet *2*:1043, 1991.

71. Ludolph AC, Ullrich K, Bick U, et al: Functional and morphological deficits in late treated patients with homocystinuria: A clinical, electrophysiologic and MRI study. Acta Neurol Scand *83*:161, 1991.

72. Cacciari E, Salardi S: Clinical and laboratory features of homocystinuria. Haemostasis *19* (Suppl 1):10, 1989.

73. London Letter: Can Med Assoc J *99*:1013, 1968.

74. Ribes A, Briones P, Vilaseca MA, et al: Methylmalonic aciduria with homocystinuria: Biochemical studies, treatment and clinical course of a cbl-C patient. Eur J Pediatr *149*:412, 1990.

75. Watkins D, Rosenblatt DS: Functional methionine synthase deficiency (cbiE and CblG): Clinical and biochemical heterogeneity. Am J Med Genet *34*:427, 1989.

76. Francis MJO, Smith R: Polymeric collagen of skin in osteogenesis imperfecta, homocystinuria, and Ehlers-Danlos and Marfan syndromes. Birth Defects *11*:15, 1975.

77. Grieco AJ: Homocystinuria: Pathogenic mechanisms. Am J Med Sci *273*:120, 1977.

78. Hurwitz LJ, Chopra JS, Carson NAJ: Electromyographic evidence of a muscle lesion in homocystinuria. Acta Paediatr Scand *57*:401, 1968.

79. Kang AH, Trelstad RL: A collagen defect in homocystinuria. J Clin Invest *52*:2571, 1973.

80. Davis JW, Flournoy LD, Phillips PE: Amino acids and collagen-induced platelet aggregation. Lack of effect of three amino acids that are elevated in homocystinuria. Am J Dis Child *129*:1020, 1975.

81. Hill-Zobel RL, Pyeritz RE, Scheffel U, Malpica O, Engin S, Camargo EE, Abbott M, Guilarte TR, Hill J, McIntyre PA, Murphy EA, Tsan MF: Kinetics and distribution of ¹¹¹indium-labeled platelets in patients with homocystinuria. N Engl J Med *307*:781, 1982.

82. Shulman JD, Agarwal B, Mudd HS, Shulman NR: Pulmonary embolism in homocystinuria patient during treatment with dipyridamole and acetylsalicylic acid. N Engl J Med *299*:661, 1978.

83. Fensom AA, Benson PF, Crees MJ, Ellis M, Rodeck CH, Vaughan RW: Prenatal exclusion of homocystinuria (cystathionine-β-synthetase deficiency) by assay of phytohaemagglutinin-stimulated lymphocytes. Prenat Diagn *3*:127, 1983.

84. Fowler B, Borresen AL, Bowman N: Prenatal diagnosis of homocystinuria. Lancet 2:875, 1982.

85. Beals RK: Homocystinuria. A report of two cases and review of the literature. J Bone Joint Surg [Am] 51:1561, 1969.

86. Leonard MS: Homocystinuria: A differential diagnosis of Marfan syndrome. Oral Surg 36:214, 1973.

87. Mitchell GE, Lourie H, Berne AS: The various causes of scalloped vertebrae with notes on their pathogenesis. Radiology 89:67, 1967.

88. Beighton P, Horan F: Orthopaedic aspects of the Ehlers-Danlos syndrome. J Bone Joint Surg [Br] 51:444, 1969.

89. Beighton P, Trice A, Lord T, Dickson E: Variants of Ehlers-Danlos syndrome. Clinical, biochemical, haematological and chromosomal features of 100 patients. Ann Rheum Dis 28:251, 1969.

90. Svane S: Ehlers-Danlos syndrome. A case with some skeletal changes. Acta Orthop Scand 37:49, 1966.

91. McKusick VA: Heritable Disorders of Connective Tissue. 4th Ed. St. Louis, CV Mosby Co, 1972, p 292.

92. Rybka FJ, O'Hara ET: The surgical significance of Ehlers-Danlos syndrome. Am J Surg 113:431, 1967.

93. Schippers E, Dittler HJ: Multiple hollow organ dysplasia in Ehlers-Danlos syndrome. J Pediatr Surg 24:1181, 1989.

94. Sarra-Carbonell S, Jimenez SA: Ehlers-Danlos syndrome associated with acute pancreatitis. J Rheum 16:1390, 1989.

95. Sokolov BP, Prytkov AN, Tromp G, et al: Exclusion of COL1A1, COL1A2 and COL3A1 genes as candidate genes for Ehlers-Danlos syndrome type I in one large family. Hum Genet 88:125, 1991.

96. Ainsworth SR, Aulicino PL: A survey of patients with Ehlers-Danlos syndrome. Clin Orthop 286:250, 1993.

97. Cohn DH, Byers PH: Clinical screening for collagen defects in connective tissue diseases. Clin Perinatol 17:793, 1990.

98. Pope FM, Daw CM, Narcisi P, et al: Prenatal diagnosis and prevention of inherited abnormalities with collagen. J Inher Metab Dis 12(Suppl 1):135, 1989.

99. Richards AJ, Ward PN, Narcisi P, et al: A single base mutation in the gene for type III collagen (COL3A1) converts glycine 847 to glutamic acid in a family with Ehlers-Danlos syndrome type IV. An unaffected family member is mosaic for the mutation. Hum Genet 89:414, 1992.

100. Superti-Furga A, Steinmann B, Ramirez F, et al: Molecular defects of type III procollagen in Ehlers-Danlos syndrome type IV. Hum Genet 82:104, 1989.

101. Richards AJ, Lloyd JC, Narcisi P, et al: A 27-bp deletion from one allele of the type III collagen gene (COL3A1) in a large family with Ehlers-Danlos syndrome type IV. Hum Genet 89:325, 1992.

102. Kontusaari S, Tromp SG, Kuivaniemi H, et al: Substitution of aspartate for glycine 1018 in the type III procollagen (COL3A1) gene causes type IV Ehlers-Danlos syndrome: The mutated allele is present in most leukocytes of the asymptomatic mosaic mother. Am J Hum Genet 51:497, 1992.

103. Lee B, D'Alesso M, Vissing H, et al: Characterization of large deletion associated with a polymorphic block of repeated dinucleotides in type III procollagen gene (COL3A1) of a patient with Ehlers-Danlos syndrome type IV. Am J Hum Genet 48:511, 1991.

104. Vasan NS, Kuivaniemi H, Vogel BE, et al: A mutation in the proα2(I) gene (COL1A2) for type I procollagen in Ehlers-Danlos syndrome type VII: Evidence suggesting that skipping of exon 6 in RNA splicing may be a common cause of phenotype. J Hum Genet 48:305, 1991.

105. Pope FM, Nicholls AC, Palan A, et al: Clinical features of an affected father and daughter with Ehlers-Danlos syndrome type VIIIB. Br J Dermatol 126:77, 1992.

106. Wertelecki W, Smith LT, Byers PH: Initial observation of human dermatosparaxis: Ehlers-Danlos syndrome type VIIC. J Pediatr 121:558, 1992.

107. Wenstrup RJ, Murad S, Pinnell SR: Ehlers-Danlos syndrome type VI: Clinical manifestations of collagen lysyl hydroxylase deficiency. J Pediatr 115:405, 1989.

108. Horton WA, Collins DL, DeSmet AA, et al: Familial joint instability syndrome. Am J Med Genet 6:221, 1980.

109. Beighton P, dePaepe AV, Danks D, et al: International nosology of heritable disorders of connective tissue, Berlin, 1986. Am J Med Genet 29:581, 1988.

110. Gertner JM, Root L: Osteogenesis imperfecta. Orthop Clin North Am 21:151, 1990.

111. Hartsfield JK, Kousseff BG: Phenotypic overlap of Ehlers-Danlos syndrome types IV and VIII. Am J Med Genet 37:465, 1990.

112. Wordsworth BP, Ogilvie DJ, Sykes BC: Segregation analysis of the structural genes of the major fibrillar collagens provides further evidence of molecular heterogeneity in type II Ehlers-Danlos syndrome. Br J Rheumatol 30:173, 1991.

113. Hamada S, Hiroshima K, Oshita S, et al: Ehlers-Danlos syndrome with soft tissue contractures. J Bone Joint Surg [Br] 74:902, 1992.

114. Osborn TG, Lichtenstein JR, Moore TL, Weiss T, Zuckner J: Ehlers-Danlos syndrome presenting as rheumatic manifestations in the child. J Rheumatol 8:79, 1981.

115. Pope FM, Jones PM, Wells RS, Lawrence D: Ehlers-Danlos syndrome IV (acrogeria): New autosomal dominant and recessive types. J R Soc Med 73:180, 1980.

116. Gibson JB, Carson MDJ, Neill DW: Pathological findings in homocystinuria. J Clin Pathol 17:427, 1964.

117. Byers PH, Barsh GS, Holbrook KA: Molecular mechanisms of connective tissue abnormalities in the Ehlers-Danlos syndrome. Coll Relat Res 5:475, 1981.

118. Prockop DJ, Kivirikko KI: Heritable diseases of collagen. N Engl J Med 311:376, 1984.

119. Kornberg M, Aulicino PL: Hand and wrist problems in patients with Ehlers-Danlos syndrome. J Hand Surg 10:193, 1985.

120. Sartoris DJ, Luzzatti L, Weaver DD, MacFarlane JD, Hollister DW, Parker BR: Type IX Ehlers-Danlos syndrome. A new varient with pathognomonic radiologic features. Radiology 152:665, 1984.

121. Gamble JG, Mochizuki C, Rinsky LA: Trapeziometacarpal abnormalities in Ehlers-Danlos syndrome. J Hand Surg 14:89, 1989.

122. Kuivaniemi H, Peltonen L, Palotie A, Kaitila I, Kivirikko KI: Abnormal copper metabolism and deficient lysyl oxidase activity in a heritable connective tissue disorder. J Clin Invest 69:730, 1982.

123. Lewkonia RM, Pope FM: Joint contractures and acroosteolysis in Ehlers-Danlos syndrome type IV. J Rheumatol 12:140, 1985.

124. Brown A, Stock VF: Dermatorrhexis: Report of a case. Am J Dis Child 54:956, 1967.

125. Pearl W, Spicer M: Ehlers-Danlos syndrome. South Med J 74:80, 1981.

126. Freeman JT: Ehlers-Danlos syndrome. Am J Dis Child 79:1049, 1950.

127. Coventry MB: Some skeletal changes in the Ehlers-Danlos syndrome. A report of two cases. J Bone Joint Surg [Am] 43:855, 1961.

128. Jansen LH: The structure of the connective tissue, an explanation of the symptoms of the Ehlers-Danlos syndrome. Dermatologica 110:108, 1955.

129. Tsipouras P, Myers JC, Ramirez F, et al: Restriction fragment length polymorphism associated with the proα2(I) gene of human type I procollagen. Application to a family with an autosomal dominant form of osteogenesis imperfecta. J Clin Invest 72:1262, 1983.

130. Stoltz MR, Dietrich SL, Marshall GJ: Osteogenesis imperfecta perspectives. Clin Orthop 242:120, 1989.

131. Byers PH: Brittle bones—fragile molecules: Disorders of collagen gene structure and expression. Trends Genet 6:293, 1990.

132. Byers PH, Steiner RD: Osteogenesis imperfecta. Annu Rev Med 43:269, 1992.

133. Bacchus H: A quantitative abnormality in serum mucoproteins in the Marfan syndrome. Am J Med 25:744, 1958.

134. Boucek RJ, Noble NL, Gunja-Smith Z, Butler WT: The Marfan syndrome: A deficiency in chemically stable collagen cross-links. N Engl J Med 305:988, 1981.

135. Stolle CA, Pyeritz RE, Myers JC, Prockop DJ: Synthesis of an altered type III procollagen in patients with Type IV Ehlers-Danlos syndrome. J Biol Chem 260:1937, 1985.

136. Pinnell SR, Krane SM, Kenzora JE, Glimcher MJ: A heritable disorder of connective tissue. Hydroxylysine-deficient collagen disease. N Engl J Med 286:1013, 1972.

137. Holt JF: The Ehlers-Danlos syndrome. Am J Roentgenol 55:420, 1946.

138. Katz I, Stuner K: Ehlers-Danlos syndrome with ectopic bone formation. Radiology 65:352, 1955.

139. Badelon O, Bensahel H, Csukonyi Z, et al: Congenital dislocation of the hip in Ehlers-Danlos syndrome. Clin Orthop 255:138, 1990.

140. Sutro CJ: Hypermobility of bones due to "overlengthened" capsular and ligamentous tissue. A case for recurrent intra-articular effusions. Surgery 21:67, 1947.

141. Newton TH, Carpenter ME: The Ehlers-Danlos syndrome with acroosteolysis. Br J Radiol 32:739, 1959.

142. Kirk JA, Ansell BM, Bywaters EGL: The hypermobility syndrome—musculoskeletal complaints associated with generalized joint hypermobility. Ann Rheum Dis 26:419, 1967.

143. Beighton P, Thomas ML: The radiology of Ehlers-Danlos syndrome. Clin Radiol 20:354, 1969.

144. Carter C, Wilkinson T: Persistent joint laxity and congenital dislocation of the hip. J Bone Joint Surg [Br] 46:40, 1964.

145. Koslowski K, Padilla C, Sillence D: Lumbar platyspondyly—characteristic sign of Ehlers-Danlos syndrome. Skel Radiol 20:589, 1991.

146. Carter C, Sweetran R: Familial joint laxity and recurrent dislocation of the patella. J Bone Joint Surg [Br] 40:664, 1958.

147. Carter C, Sweetran R: Recurrent dislocation of the patella and of the shoulder. Their association with familial joint laxity. J Bone Joint Surg [Br] 42:721, 1960.

148. Haebara H, Yamasaki Y, Kyogoku M: An autopsy case of osteogenesis imperfecta congenita—histochemical and electron microscopical studies. Acta Pathol Jpn 19:377, 1967.

149. Ibsen KH: Distinct varieties of osteogenesis imperfecta. Clin Orthop Rel Res 50:279, 1967.

150. Sykes B, Francis MJO, Smith R: Altered relation of two collagen types in osteogenesis imperfecta. N Engl J Med 296:1200, 1977.

151. Fugi K, Tanzer ML: Osteogenesis imperfecta: Biochemical studies of bone collagen. Clin Orthop Rel Res 124:271, 1977.

152. King JD, Bobechko WP: Osteogenesis imperfecta. An orthopedic description and surgical review. J Bone Joint Surg [Br] 53:72, 1971.

153. Versfeld GA, Beighton PH, Katz K, et al: Costovertebral anomalies in osteogenesis imperfecta. J Bone Joint Surg [Br] 67:602, 1985.

154. Cohn DH, Byers PH: Cysteine in triple helical domain of proα2(I) chain of type I collagen in nonlethal forms of osteogenesis imperfecta. Hum Genet 87:167, 1991.

155. Edwards MS, Graham JM Jr: Studies of type I collagen in osteogenesis imperfecta. J Pediatr 117:67, 1990.

156. Lynch JR, Ogilvie D, Priestly L, et al: Prenatal diagnosis of osteogenesis

imperfecta by identification of concordant collagen I allele. J Med Genet 28:145, 1991.

157. Tenni R, Valli M, Rossi A, et al: Possible role of overglycosylation in type I collagen triple helical domain in the molecular pathogenesis of osteogenesis imperfecta. Am J Med Genet 45:252, 1993.

158. Sykes B, Ogilvie D, Wordsworth P, et al: Consistent linkage of dominantly inherited osteogenesis imperfecta to type I collagen loci: COL1A1 and COL1A2. Am J Hum Genet 46:293, 1990.

159. Falvo KA, Root L, Bullough PG: Osteogenesis imperfecta: Clinical evaluation and management. J Bone Joint Surg [Am] 56:783, 1974.

160. Bauze RJ, Smith R, Francis MJO: A new look at osteogenesis imperfecta. J Bone Joint Surg [Br] 57:2, 1975.

161. Solomons CC, Millar EA: Osteogenesis imperfecta—new perspectives. Clin Orthop Rel Res 96:299, 1973.

162. Falvo KA, Bullough PG: Osteogenesis imperfecta: A histometric analysis. J Bone Joint Surg [Am] 55:275, 1973.

163. Castells S: New approaches to treatment of osteogenesis imperfecta. Clin Orthop Rel Res 93:239, 1973.

164. McKusick VA: Heritable Disorders of Connective Tissue. 4th Ed. St Louis, CV Mosby Co, 1972, p 399.

165. Sillence D: Osteogenesis imperfecta: An expanding panorama of variants. Clin Orthop 159:11, 1981.

166. Sillence DO, Senn A, Danks DM: Genetic heterogeneity in osteogenesis imperfecta. J Med Genet 16:101, 1979.

167. Gerber LH, Binder H, Weintrob J, et al: Rehabilitation of children and infants with osteogenesis imperfecta. A program for ambulation. Clin Orthop 251:254, 1990.

168. Vetter U, Pontz B, Zauner E, et al: Osteogenesis imperfecta: A clinical study of the first ten years of life. Calcif Tissue Int 50:36, 1992.

169. Starman BJ, Eyre E, Charbonneau H, et al: Osteogenesis imperfecta. The position of substitution for glycine by cysteine in triple helical domain of the proα1(I) chains of type I collagen determines the clinical phenotype. J Clin Invest 84:1206, 1989.

170. Sillence D: Osteogenesis imperfecta: An expanding panorama of variants. Clin Orthop Rel Res 159:11, 1981.

171. Sillence DO, Senn A, Danks DM: Genetic heterogeneity in osteogenesis imperfecta. J Med Genet 16:101, 1979.

172. Willing MC, Cohn DH, Byers PH: Frameshift mutation near 3' end of COL1A1 gene of type I collagen predicts an elongated proα1(I) chain and results in osteogenesis imperfecta type I. J Clin Invest 85:282, 1990.

173. Wenstrup RJ, Willing MC, Starman BJ, et al: Distinct biochemical phenotypes predict clinical severity in nonlethal varients of osteogenesis imperfecta. Am J Hum Genet 46:975, 1990.

174. Willing MC, Pruchno CJ, Atkinson M, et al: Osteogenesis imperfecta type I is commonly due to a COL1A1 null allele of type I collagen. Am J Hum Genet 51:508, 1992.

175. Barash GS, David KE, Byers PH: Type 1 osteogenesis imperfecta: A nonfunctional allele for pro alpha 1(I) chains of type 1 procollagen. Proc Natl Acad Sci USA 79:3938, 1982.

176. Munoz C, Filly RA, Golbus MS: Osteogenesis imperfecta type II: Prenatal sonographic diagnosis. Radiology 174:181, 1990.

177. Stoss H, Freisinger P: Collagen fibrils of osteoid in osteogenesis imperfecta: Morphometrical analysis of fibril diameter. Am J Med Genet 45:257, 1993.

178. Paterson CR, McAllison S, Miller R: Osteogenesis imperfecta with dominant inheritance and normal sclera. J Bone Joint Surg [Br] 65:35, 1983.

179. Byers PH, Bonadio JF, Steinmann B: Osteogenesis imperfecta: Update and perspective. Am J Med Genet 17:429, 1984.

180. Beighton P, Spranger J, Versveld G: Skeletal complications in osteogenesis imperfecta. S Afr Med J 64:565, 1983.

181. Thompson EM: Non-invasive prenatal diagnosis of osteogenesis imperfecta. Am J Med Genet 45:201, 1993.

182. Sykes B: Linkage analysis in dominantly inherited osteogenesis imperfecta. Am J Med Genet 45:212, 1993.

183. Weil VH: Osteogenesis imperfecta: historical background. Clin Orthop Rel Res 159:7, 1981.

184. Jones CJP, Cummings C, Ball J, Beighton P: Collagen defect of bone in osteogenesis imperfecta (type I). An electron microscopic study. Clin Orthop Rel Res 183:208, 1984.

185. Brenner RE, Vetter U, Nerlich A, et al: Biochemical analysis of callus tissue in osteogenesis imperfecta type IV. Evidence for transient overmodification in collagen types I and III. J Clin Invest 84:915, 1989.

186. Vetter U, Fisher LW, Mintz KP, et al: Osteogenesis imperfecta: Changes in noncollagenous proteins in bone. J Bone Miner Res 6:501, 1990.

187. Eyre DR: Concepts in collagen biochemistry: Evidence that collagenopathies underlie osteogenesis imperfecta. Clin Orthop Rel Res 159:97, 1981.

188. Superti-Furga A, Pistone F, Romano C, et al: Clinical variability of osteogenesis imperfecta linked to COL1A2 and associated with a structural defect in type I collagen molecule. J Med Genet 26:358, 1989.

189. Bachinger HP, Morris NP, Davis JM: Thermal stability and folding of the collagen triple helix and effects of mutations in osteogenesis imperfecta on the triple helix of type I collagen. Am J Med Genet 45:152, 1993.

190. Pruchno CJ, Cohn DH, Wallis GA, et al: Osteogenesis imperfecta due to recurrent point mutations at GpG dinucleotides in COL1A1 gene of type I collagen. Hum Genet 87:33, 1991.

191. Prockop DJ, Constantinou CD, Dombrowski KE, et al: Type I procollagen: The gene-protein system that harbors most of the mutations causing osteogenesis

imperfecta and probably more common heritable disorders of connective tissue. Am J Med Genet 34:60, 1989.

192. Brown DM: Biochemical abnormalities in osteogenesis imperfecta. Clin Orthop Rel Res 159:95, 1981.

193. Bullough PG, Davidson D, Lorenzo JC: The morbid anatomy of the skeleton in osteogenesis imperfecta. Clin Orthop Rel Res 159:42, 1981.

194. Ramser JR, Villanueva AR, Pirok D, Frost HM: Tetracycline-based measurement of bone dynamics in 3 women with osteogenesis imperfecta. Clin Orthop Rel Res 49:151, 1966.

195. Doty SB, Mathews RS: Electron microscope and histochemical investigation of osteogenesis imperfecta tarda. Clin Orthop Rel Res 80:191, 1971.

196. Deak SB, Nicholls A, Pope FM, Prockop DJ: The molecular defect in a nonlethal variant of osteogenesis imperfecta. Synthesis of proα2 (I) chains which are not incorporated into trimers of procollagen. J Biol Chem 258:15192, 1983.

197. Baron R, Gertner JM, Lang R, Vignery A: Increased bone turnover with decreased bone formation by osteoblasts in children with osteogenesis imperfecta tarda. Pediatr Res 17:204, 1983.

198. Engfeldt B, Engstrom A, Zetterstorm R: Bio-physical studies of bone tissue in osteogenesis imperfecta. J Bone Joint Surg [Br] 36:654, 1954.

199. Ste-Marie LG, Charhon SA, Edouard C, Chapuy MC, Meunier PJ: Iliac bone histomorphometry in adults and children with osteogenesis imperfecta. J Clin Pathol 37:1081, 1984.

200. Spencer AT: A histochemical study of long bones in osteogenesis imperfecta. J Pathol Bacteriol 83:423, 1962.

201. Bullough PG, Davidson D: The morphology of the growth plate in osteogenesis imperfecta. (Abstr) Clin Orthop Rel Res 116:259, 1976.

202. Sanguinetti C, Greco F, DePalma L, et al: Morphologic changes in growth-plate cartilage in osteogenesis imperfecta. J Bone Joint Surg [Br] 72:475, 1990.

203. Goldman AB, Davidson D, Pavlov H, Bullough PG: "Popcorn calcifications." A prognostic sign of osteogenesis imperfecta. Radiology 136:351, 1980.

204. Levin LS: The dentition in osteogenesis imperfecta syndromes. Clin Orthop Rel Res 159:64, 1981.

205. Bergstrom L: Fragile bones and fragile ears. Clin Orthop Rel Res 159:58, 1981.

206. Smith R, Francis MJO, Houghton CR: The Brittle Bone Book. London, Butterworths, 1983.

207. Tabor E, Curtin HD, Hirsch BE, et al: Osteogenesis imperfecta tarda: Appearance of the temporal bones at CT. Radiology 175:181, 1990.

208. Fairbank T: Atlas of General Affectations of the Skeleton. Edinburgh, E & S Livingstone, 1951.

209. Bailey JA: Forms of dwarfism recognized at birth. Clin Orthop Rel Res 76:150, 1971.

210. Aylsworth AS, Seeds JW, Guildford WB, Burns CB, Washburn DB: Prenatal diagnosis of a severe deforming type of osteogenesis imperfecta. Am J Med Genet 19:707, 1984.

211. Milson I, Matteson L-A, Dahlen-Nilsson I: Antenatal diagnosis of osteogenesis imperfecta by real time ultrasound: Two case reports. Br J Radiol 55:310, 1982.

212. Wynne-Davies R, Gormley J: Clinical and genetic patterns in osteogenesis imperfecta. Clin Orthop Rel Res 159:26, 1981.

213. Caffee J: Pediatric X-Ray Diagnosis. 6th Ed. Chicago, Year Book Medical Publishers, 1973, pp 54, 1037.

214. Elias S, Simpson JL, Griffin LP: Intrauterine growth retardation in osteogenesis imperfecta. JAMA 239:23, 1978.

215. Wright PG, Gernsetter SL, Greenblatt RB: Therapeutic acceleration of bone age in osteogenesis imperfecta. A case report. J Bone Joint Surg [Br] 36:654, 1954.

216. Gitelis S, Whiffen J, DeWald RL: The treatment of severe scoliosis in osteogenesis imperfecta. Case report. Clin Orthop Rel Res 175:56, 1983.

217. Norimatsu H, Mayuzumi T, Takahashi H: The development of spinal deformities in osteogenesis imperfecta. Clin Orthop Rel Res 162:20, 1982.

218. Yong-Hing K, MacEwen GD: Scoliosis with osteogenesis imperfecta. Results of treatment. J Bone Joint Surg [Br] 64:36, 1982.

219. Falvo KA, Root L: Osteogenesis imperfecta tarda. J Hosp Special Surg 1:44, 1975.

220. Patterson CR, McAllison S, Stellman JL: Osteogenesis imperfecta after menopause. N Engl J Med 310:1694, 1984.

221. Root L: The treatment of osteogenesis imperfecta. Orthop Clin North Am 15:775, 1984.

222. Porat S, Heller E, Seidman DS, et al: Functional results of operation in osteogenesis imperfecta: Elongating and nonelongating rods. J Pediatr Orthop 11:200, 1991.

223. Cremin B, Goodman H, Spranger J, Beighton P: Wormian bones in osteogenesis imperfecta and other diseases. Skel Radiol 8:35, 1982.

224. Pozo JL, Crockard HA, Ransford AO: Basilar impression in osteogenesis imperfecta. A report of three cases in one family. J Bone Joint Surg [Br] 66:233, 1984.

225. Brailsford JF: The Radiology of Bones and Joints. Baltimore, Williams & Wilkins Co, 1948, p 547.

226. Edeiken J, Hodes PJ: Roentgen Diagnosis of Diseases of Bone. 2nd Ed. Baltimore, Williams & Wilkins Co, 1973, p 145.

227. Greenfield GB: Radiology of Bone Disease. Philadelphia, JB Lippincott Co, 1979, p 209.

228. Currano G, Brooksaler F: Osteogenesis imperfecta. In HJ Kaufman (Ed): Intrinsic Disease of Bones. Progress in Pediatric Radiology, Vol 4. Basel, S Karger, 1973, p 346.

229. Pendola F, Borrone C, Filocamo M, et al: Radiological "metamorphosis" in a

patient with severe congenital osteogenesis imperfecta. Eur J Pediat *149*:403, 1990.

230. Hanscom DA, Winter RB, Lutter L, et al: Osteogenesis imperfecta. Radiographic classification, natural history and treatment of spinal deformity. J Bone Joint Surg [Am] *74*:598, 1992.

231. Laurent LE, Salenius P: Hyperplastic callus formation in osteogenesis imperfecta. Report of a case simulating sarcoma. Acta Orthop Scand *38*:280, 1967.

232. Campbell JB: Case report 217. Skel Radiol *9*:141, 1982.

233. McCall RE, Bax JA: Hyperplastic callus formation in osteogenesis imperfecta. Pediatr Orthop *4*:361, 1984.

234. Sofield HA, Millar EA: Fragmentation realignment and intramedullary rod fixation of deformities of the long bones in children. A ten year appraisal. J Bone Joint Surg [Am] *41*:1371, 1959.

235. Middleton RWD: Closed intramedullary rodding for osteogenesis imperfecta. J Bone Joint Surg [Br] *66*:652, 1984.

236. Lang-Stevenson AI, Sharrard WJW: Intramedullary rodding with Bailey-Dubow extensible rods in osteogenesis imperfecta. An interim report of results and complications. J Bone Joint Surg [Br] *66*:227, 1984.

237. Rush GA, Burke SW: Hangman's fracture in a patient with osteogenesis imperfecta. Case report. J Bone Joint Surg [Am] *66*:778, 1984.

238. Constantine G, McCormack J, Mchugo J, et al: Prenatal diagnosis of severe osteogenesis imperfecta. Prenat Diagn *11*:103, 1991.

239. Simpson AJ, Friedman S: Myositis ossificans progressiva. Mt Sinai J Med *38*:416, 1971.

240. McKusick VA: Fibrodysplasia ossificans progressiva. *In* Heritable Disorders of Connective Tissue. 4th Ed. St Louis, CV Mosby Co, 1972, p 687.

241. Kalukas BA, Adams RD: Disease of Muscle. 4th Ed. Philadelphia, Harper & Row, 1985, p 659.

242. Caron KH, Dipietro MA, Aisen AM, et al: MR imaging of early fibrodysplasia ossificans progressiva. J Comput Assist Tomogr *14*:318, 1990.

243. Reinig JW, Hill SC, Fang M, et al: Fibrodysplasia ossificans progressiva. Radiology *159*:153, 1986.

244. Kaplan FS, Tabas JA, Zasloff MA: Fibrodysplasia ossificans progressiva: A clue from the fly. Calif Tissue Int *47*:117, 1990.

245. Smith R: Myositis ossificans progressiva: A review of current problems. Arthritis Rheum *4*:369, 1975.

246. Rogers JG, Geho WB: Fibrodysplasia ossificans progressiva. A survey of forty-two cases. J Bone Joint Surg [Am] *61*:709, 1979.

247. Cramer SF, Ruehl A, Mandel MA: Fibrodysplasia ossificans progressiva. Cancer *48*:1016, 1981.

248. Rogers JG, Chase GA: Paternal age effect on fibrodysplasia ossificans progressiva. J Med Genet *16*:147, 1979.

249. McKusick VA, Pyeritz RE: The hand and foot malformations in fibrodysplasia ossificans progressiva. Johns Hopkins Med J *147*:73, 1980.

250. Letts RM: Myositis ossificans progressiva. A report of two cases with chromosome studies. Can Med Assoc J *99*:856, 1976.

251. Connor JM, Woodrow JC, Evans DAP: Histocompatibility antigens in patients with ectopic ossification due to fibrodysplasia ossificans progressiva. Ann Rheum Dis *41*:646, 1982.

252. Ludwak L: Myositis ossificans progressiva. Mineral, metabolic, and radioactive calcium studies of the effects of hormones. Am J Med *37*:269, 1964.

253. Illingworth RS: Myositis ossificans progressiva (Münchmeyer's disease). Brief review with report of 2 cases treated with corticosteroids and observed for 16 years. Arch Dis Child *46*:264, 1971.

254. Letts RM: Myositis ossificans progressiva. Can Med Assoc J *100*:133, 1969.

255. Smith DM, Zerman W, Johnston CC, Deiss WP: Myositis ossificans progressiva. Case report with metabolic and histochemical studies. Metabolism *15*:521, 1966.

256. Blumenkrantz N, Asboe-Hansen G: Fibrodysplasia ossificans progressiva. Biochemical changes in blood serum, urine, skin, bone and ectopic ossification. Scand J Rheum *7*:85, 1978.

257. Fletcher E, Moss MS: Myositis ossificans progressiva. Ann Rheum Dis *24*:267, 1965.

258. Ackerman LV: Extraosseous localized non-neoplastic bone and cartilage formation (so-called myositis ossificans). Clinical and pathological confusion with malignant neoplasms. J Bone Joint Surg [Am] *40*:279, 1958.

259. Thickman D, Bonakdar-pour A, Clancy M, Van Orden J, Steel H: Fibrodysplasia ossificans progressiva. Am J Roentgenol *139*:935, 1982.

260. Connor JM, Evans DAP: Fibrodysplasia ossificans progressiva. The clinical features and natural history of 34 patients. J Bone Joint Surg [Br] *64*:76, 1982.

261. Gwinn JL: Radiological case of the month. Progressive myositis ossificans. Am J Dis Child *116*:655, 1968.

262. Cremin B, Connor M, Beighton P: The radiological spectrum of fibrodysplasia ossificans progressiva. Clin Radiol *33*:499, 1982.

263. Kransdorf MJ, Meis JM, Jelinek JS: Myositis ossificans: MR appearance with radiologic-pathologic correlation. AJR *157*:1243, 1991.

264. Seibert JJ, Morrissy RT, Fuller J, Young LW: Radiological case of the month. Am J Dis Child *137*:77, 1983.

265. Ludman H, Hamilton EBD, Eade AWT: Deafness in myositis ossificans progressiva. J Laryngol *82*:57, 1968.

266. Viljoen D: Pseudoxanthoma elasticum (Gronblad-Strandberg syndrome). J Med Genet *25*:488, 1988.

267. Connor JM, Evans DAP: Fibrodysplasia ossificans progressiva. The clinical features and natural history of 34 patients. J Bone Joint Surg [Br] *64*:76, 1982.

268. Russell RGG, Smith R, Bishop MC, Price DA: Treatment of myositis ossificans progressiva with diphosphonate. Lancet *1*:10, 1972.

269. Holmsen H, Ljunghall S, Hierson T: Myositis ossificans progressiva. Clinical and metabolical observations in a case treated with diphosphonate (EHDP) and surgical removal of ectopic bone. Acta Orthop Scand *50*:33, 1976.

270. Hall JG, Schaller JG, Worsham NG, Horning MR, Staheli LT: Fibrodysplasia ossificans progressiva (myositis ossificans progressiva) treatment with disodium etidronate (letter). J Pediatr *94*:679, 1979.

271. Resnick D: Case report 240. Skel Radiol *10*:131, 1983.

272. Ehara S, Nakosato T, Tamakawa Y, et al: MRI of myositis ossificans circumscripta. Clin Imaging *15*:130, 1991.

273. Connor JM, Smith R: The cervical spine in fibrodysplasia ossificans progressiva. Br J Radiol *55*:492, 1982.

274. Ferdinand R, Stefanelli A: Myositis ossificans progressiva associated with severe scoliosis. Clin Orthop Rel Res *139*:49, 1979.

275. Najjar SS, Farah FS, Kurban AK, Melhem RE, Khatchadouria AK: Tumoral calcinosis and pseudoxanthoma elasticum. J Pediatr *72*:243, 1968.

276. Alinder I, Boström H: Clinical studies on a Swedish material of pseudoxanthoma elasticum. Acta Med Scand *191*:273, 1972.

277. McKusick VA: Heritable Disorders of Connective Tissue. 4th Ed. St Louis, CV Mosby Co, 1972, p 475.

278. Pope FM: Two types of autosomal recessive pseudoxanthoma elasticum. Arch Dermatol *110*:209, 1974.

279. De Palpe A, Viljoen D, Matton M, et al: Pseudoxanthoma elasticum: Similar autosomal recessive subtype in Belgian and Afrikaner families. Am J Med Genet *38*:16, 1991.

280. Belli A, Cawthorne S: Visceral angiographic findings in pseudoxanthoma elasticum. Br J Radiol *61*:368, 1988.

281. Hausser I, Anton-Lamprecht I: Early preclinical diagnosis of dominant pseudoxanthoma elasticum by specific ultrastructural changes of dermal elastic and collagen tissue in a family at risk. Hum Genet *87*:693, 1991.

282. Shevick M: Pseudoxanthoma elasticum. Angiology *122*:629, 1971.

283. Akhtar M, Brody H: Elastic tissue in pseudoxanthoma elasticum. Ultrastructural study of endocardial lesions. Arch Pathol *99*:667, 1975.

284. Fellner MJ, Chen AS, McCabe JB: Pseudoxanthoma elasticum. Arch Dermatol *114*:288, 1978.

285. Sandberg LB, Soskel NT, Leslie JG: Elastin structure, biosynthesis, and relation to disease states. N Engl J Med *304*:566, 1981.

286. Eng AM: Pseudoxanthoma elasticum in hyperphosphatasia. Arch Dermatol *111*:271, 1975.

287. Walker ER, Frederickson RG, Mayes MD: The mineralization of elastic fibers and alterations of extracellular matrix in pseudoxanthoma elasticum: Ultrastructure, immunocytochemistry and x-ray analysis. Arch Dermatol *125*:70, 1989.

288. Mamtora H, Cope V: Pulmonary opacities in pseudoxanthoma elasticum: Report of two cases. Br J Radiol *54*:65, 1981.

289. Hogan JF, Heaton CL: Angioid streaks and systemic disease. Br J Dermatol *89*:411, 1973.

290. Cocco AE, Grayer DI, Walker BA, Martyn LJ: The stomach in pseudoxanthoma elasticum. JAMA *210*:2381, 1972.

291. Schachner L, Young D: Pseudoxanthoma elasticum with severe cardiovascular disease in a child. Am J Dis Child *127*:571, 1974.

292. Judd KP: Hyperelasticity syndromes. Cutis *33*:494, 1984.

293. Engelman MW, Fliegelman MT: Pseudoxanthoma elasticum. Cutis *21*:837, 1978.

294. Mehta HK: Grönblad-Strandberg syndrome. Proc R Soc Med *61*:548, 1968.

295. Lebwohl MG, Distefano D, Prioleau PG, Uram M, Yannuzzi LA, Fleishmajer R: Pseudoxanthoma elasticum and mitral valve prolapse. N Engl J Med *307*:229, 1982.

296. Prick JJG, Thijssen HDM: Radiodiagnostic signs in pseudoxanthoma elasticum generalisatum (dysgenesis elastofibrillaris mineralisans). Clin Radiol *28*:549, 1977.

297. Suarez MJ, Garcia JB, Orense M, et al: Sonographic aspects of pseudoxanthoma elasticum. Pediatr Radiol *21*:538, 1991.

298. Baker SL: Fibrogenesis imperfecta ossium. J Bone Joint Surg [Br] *34*:378, 1956.

299. Baker SL, Dent CE, Freidman M, Watson L: Fibrogenesis imperfecta ossium. J Bone Joint Surg [Br] *48*:804, 1966.

300. Golding FC: Fibrogenesis imperfecta. J Bone Joint Surg [Br] *50*:619, 1968.

301. Golde D, Greipp P, Sanzenbacher L, Gralnick HR: Hematologic abnormalities in fibrogenesis imperfecta ossium. J Bone Joint Surg [Am] *53*:365, 1971.

302. Baker SL, Turnbull HM: Two cases of a hitherto undescibed disease characterized by a gross defect in collagen matrix. J Pathol Bacteriol *62*:132, 1950.

303. Murray RO, Jacobson JG: The Radiology of Skeletal Disorders. 2nd Ed. Edinburgh, Churchill Livingstone, 1977, p 1170.

304. Swan CHJ, Shah K, Brewer DB, Cooke WT: Fibrogenesis imperfecta ossium. Q J Med *178*:233, 1976.

305. Byers PD, Stamp TCK, Stoker DJ: Case report 296. Skel Radiol *13*:77, 1985.

306. Stamp TCB, Byers PD, Ali SY, Jenkin MV, Willoughby JMT: Fibrogenesis imperfecta ossium: Remission with melphalan. Lancet *1*:582, 1985.

307. Stoddart PGP, Wickremaratchi T, Watt I: Fibrogenesis imperfecta ossium. Br J Radiol *57*:744, 1984.

308. Frost HM, Frame B, Ormond RS, Hunter RB: Atypical axial osteomalacia. A report of three cases. Clin Orthop Rel Res *23*:283, 1962.

309. Spranger J: The epiphyseal dysplasias. Clin Orthop Rel Res *114*:46, 1976.

310. Trebel NJ, Jensen FO, Bankier A, et al: Development of the hip in multiple epiphysical dysplasia. Natural history and susceptibility to osteoarthritis. J Bone Joint Surg [Br] 72:1061, 1990.

311. Bassett GS: Orthopaedic aspects of skeletal dysplasias. Instr Course Lect 39:381, 1990.

312. Rubin P: Dynamic Classification of Bone Dysplasias. Chicago, Year Book Medical Publishers, 1964, p 120.

313. Pfeiffer RA, Jünemann G, Polster J, Bauer H: Epiphyseal dysplasia of the femoral head, severe myopia and perceptive hearing loss in three brothers. Clin Genet 4:141, 1973.

314. Wolcott ED, Rallison ML: Infancy-onset diabetes mellitus and multiple epiphyseal dysplasia. J Pediatr 80:292, 1972.

315. Koslowski K, Budzinska A: Combined metaphyseal and epiphyseal dystosis. Report of two cases—one in which metaphyseal changes predominate, and a second one in which epiphyseal changes are more marked. Am J Roentgenol 97:21, 1966.

316. Lie SO, Siggers DC, Dorst JP, Kopits SE: Unusual multiple epiphyseal dysplasia. Birth Defects 10:165, 1974.

317. Maroteaux P: Epiphyseal dysplasia, multiple. In D Bergsma (Ed): Birth Defects Compendium. New York, National Foundation, March of Dimes, Alan R Liss Inc, 1979, p 409.

318. Ribbing S: Studien über hereditäre, multiple Epiphysenstörungen. Acta Radiol Suppl 34:1, 1937.

319. Fairbank T: Dysplasia epiphysialis multiplex. Br J Surg 34:225, 1947.

320. Mansoor IA: Dysplasia epiphysealis multiplex. Clin Orthop Rel Res 72:287, 1970.

321. Juberg RC: Hereditary and multiple epiphyseal dysplasia. JAMA 237:2600, 1977.

322. Villarreal T, Carnevale A, Mayén DG, et al: Anthropometric studies in five children and their mothers with a severe form of multiple epiphyseal dysplasia. Am J Med Genet 42:415, 1992.

323. Beighton P, Giedon A, Gorlin R, et al: International classification of osteochondrodysplasias. Eur J Pediatr 151:407, 1992.

324. Hoefnagel D, Sycamore LK, Russel SW, Bucknall WE: Hereditary multiple epiphyseal dysplasia. Ann Hum Genet 30:201, 1967.

325. Koslowski K, Lipska E: Hereditary dysplasia epiphysealis multiplex. Clin Radiol 18:330, 1967.

326. Felman AH: Multiple epiphyseal dysplasia. Three cases with unusual vertebral anomalies. Radiology 93:119, 1969.

327. Mena HR, Pearson EO: Multiple epiphyseal dysplasia. JAMA 236:2629, 1976.

328. Versteylen RJ, Zwemmer A, Lorié CAM, et al: Multiple epiphyseal dysplasia complicated by severe osteochondritis dissecans of the knee. Incidence in two families. Skel Radiology 17:401, 1988.

329. Gamboa I, Lisker R: Multiple epiphyseal dysplasia tarda. A family with autosomal recessive inheritance. Clin Genet 6:15, 1974.

330. Juberg RC, Holt JF: Inheritance of multiple epiphyseal dysplasia tarda. Am J Hum Genet 20:549, 1968.

331. Crossan JF, Wynne-Davies R, Fulford GE: Bilateral failure of the capital femoral epiphyses: Bilateral Perthes' disease, multiple epiphyseal dysplasia, pseudoachondroplasia, spondyloepiphyseal dysplasia, congenita and tarda. J Pediatr Orthop 3:297, 1983.

332. Berg PK: Dysplasia epiphysialis multiplex. Am J Roentgenol 97:31, 1966.

333. Hunt DD, Ponseti IV, Pedrine-Mille A, Pedrini V: Multiple epiphyseal dysplasia in two siblings. J Bone Joint Surg [Am] 49:1611, 1967.

334. Pattrone NA, Kredich DW: Arthritis in children with multiple epiphyseal dysplasia. J Rheumatol 12:1, 1985.

335. Shapiro F: Epiphyseal disorders. N Engl J Med 317:1702, 1987.

336. Murray LW, Bautista J, James PL, et al: Type II collagen defects in chondrodysplasias. Spondyloepiphyseal dysplasias. Am J Hum Genet 45:5, 1989.

337. Byers PH: Molecular heterogeneity in chondrodysplasias. Am J Hum Genet 45:1, 1989.

338. Lee B, Vissing H, Ramirez F, et al: Identification of molecular defect in a family with spondyloepiphyseal dysplasia. Science 244:978, 1989.

339. Knowlton RG, Katzenstein PL, Moskowitz RW, et al: Genetic linkage of a polymorphism in the type II procollagen gene (COL2A1) to primary osteoarthritis associated with mild chondrodystrophy. N Engl J Med 322:526, 1990.

340. Anderson IJ, Goldberg RB, Marion RW, et al: Spondyloepiphyseal dysplasia congenita: Genetic linkage to type II collagen (COL2A1). Am J Hum Genet 48:896, 1990.

341. Sher C, Ramesar R, Martell R, et al: Mild spondyloepiphyseal dysplasia (Namaqualand type): genetic linkage to type II collagen gene (COL2A1). Am J Hum Genet 48:518, 1991.

342. Eyre DR, Weis MA, Moskowitz RW: Cartilage expression of a type II collagen mutation in an inherited form of osteoarthritis associated with a mild chondrodysplasia. J Clin Invest 87:357, 1991.

343. Ramesar R, Beighton P: Spondyloepiphyseal dysplasia in Cape Town family: linkage with gene for type II collagen (COL2A1). Am J Med Genet 43:833, 1992.

344. Temple JK: Stickler's syndrome. J Med Genet 26:119, 1989.

345. Anderson IJ, Tsipouras P, Sher C, et al: Spondyloepiphyseal dysplasia, mild autosomal dominant type is not due to primary defects in type II collagen. Am J Med Genet 37:272, 1990.

346. Robinson D, Tuder M, Halperin N, et al: Spondyloepiphyseal dysplasia associated with progressive arthropathy. Acta Orthop Trauma Surg 108:397, 1989.

347. Poulos A, Sheffield L, Sharp P, et al: Rhizomelic chondrodysplasia punctata: Clinical, pathologic, and biochemical findings in two patients. J Pediatr 113:685, 1988.

348. Oestreich AE, Prenger EC: MR demonstrates megaepiphyses of the hips in Kniest dysplasia of the young child. Pediatr Radiol 22:302, 1992.

349. Schantz K, Anderson PE Jr, Justesen P: Spondyloepiphyseal dysplasia tarda. Report of a family with autosomal dominant transmission. Acta Orthop Scand 59:716, 1988.

350. Hulvey JT, Keats T: Multiple epiphyseal dysplasia. A contribution to the problem of spinal involvement. Am J Roentgenol 106:170, 1969.

351. Ingram RR: Early diagnosis of multiple epiphyseal dysplasia. J Pediatr Orthop 12:241, 1992.

352. Goldman AB: Procedures in Skeletal Radiology. Orlando, Florida, Grune and Stratton, 1984, p 15.

353. Dahners LE, Francisco WD, Halleran WJ: Findings of arthrotomy in a case of double layered patellae associated with multiple epiphyseal dysplasia. J Pediatr Orthop 2:67, 1982.

354. Wardinski TD, Pagon RA, Powell BR, et al: Rhizomelic chondrodysplasia punctata and survival beyond one year: A review of the literature and five case reports. Clin Genet 38:84, 1990.

354a. Wynne-Davies R: Instability of the upper cervical spine. Skeletal dysplasia group. Arch Dis Child 64:283, 1989.

355. Wulfsberg EA, Curtis J, Jayne CH: Chondrodysplasia punctata: A boy with X-linked recessive chondrodysplasia punctata due to an inherited X-Y translocation with a current classification of these disorders. Am J Med Genet 43:823, 1992.

356. Mason RC, Kozlowski K: Chondrodysplasia punctata. A report of 10 cases. Radiology 109:145, 1973.

357. Silengo MC, Luzzatti L, Silverman FN: Clinical and genetic aspects of Conradi-Hünermann disease. A report of three familial cases and review of the literature. J Pediatr 97:911, 1980.

358. Hoefler G, Hoefler S, Watkins PA, et al: Biochemical abnormalities in rhizomelic chondrodysplasia punctata. J Pediatr 112:726, 1988.

359. Heselson NG, Cremin BJ, Beighton P: Lethal chondrodysplasia punctata. Clin Radiol 29:679, 1978.

360. Lawrence JJ, Schlesinger AE, Kozlowski K, et al: Unusual radiographic manifestations of chondrodysplasia punctata. Skel Radiology 18:15, 1989.

361. Agematsu K, Koike K, Morosawa H, et al: Chondrodysplasia punctata with X;Y translocation. Hum Genet 80:105, 1988.

362. Wohrle D, Gotthold B, Schulz W, et al: Heterozygous expression of X-linked chondrodysplasia punctata. Complex chromosome aberration including deletion of MIC2 and STS. Hum Genet 86:215, 1990.

363. Petit C, Melki J, Levilliers J, et al: An interstitial deletion in Xp 22.3 in a family with X-linked recessive chondrodysplasia punctata and short stature. Hum Genet 85:247, 1990.

364. Curry CJR, Magenis RE, Brown M, et al: Inherited chondrodysplasia punctata due to deletion of terminal short arm of an X chromosome. N Engl J Med 311:1010, 1984.

365. Shaul WL, Emery J, Hall JG: Chondrodysplasia punctata and maternal warfarin use during pregnancy. Am J Dis Child 129:360, 1975.

366. Warkany J: A warfarin embryopathy? Am J Dis Child 129:287, 1975.

367. Whitfield MF: Chondrodysplasia punctata after warfarin early in pregnancy. Case report and summary of the literature. Arch Dis Child 55:139, 1980.

368. Happle R: X-linked dominant chondrodysplasia punctata. Review of the literature and report of a case. Hum Genet 53:65, 1979.

369. Manzke H, Chrisophers E, Wiederman HR: Dominant sex-linked inherited chondrodysplasia punctata: A distinct type of chondrodysplasia punctata. Clin Genet 17:97, 1979.

370. Rasmussen PG, Reimann I: Multiple epiphyseal dysplasia with special reference to histologic findings. Acta Pathol Microbiol Scand 81:381, 1973.

371. Sugarman GI: Chondrodysplasia punctata (rhizomelic type): Case report and pathologic findings. Birth Defects 10:399, 1974.

372. Rasmussen PG: Multiple epiphyseal dysplasia. Two morphological and histochemical investigations of cartilage matrix, particularly in the precalcification stage. Acta Pathol Microbiol Scand 83:493, 1975.

373. Gwinn JL, Lee FA: Radiological case of the month. Am J Dis Child 129:287, 1975.

374. Ikegawa S, Nagano A, Nakamura K: Chondrodysplasia punctata mimicking Blount's disease. A case report. Acta Orthop Scand 61:580, 1990.

375. Wenger DR, Ezaki M: Bilateral femoral head collapse in an adolescent with brachydactyly (multiple epiphyseal dysplasia tarda type 1 c). Pediatr Orthop 1:267, 1981.

376. Herring JA: Rapidly progressive scoliosis in multiple epiphyseal dysplasia. J Bone Joint Surg [Am] 50:703, 1976.

377. Bethem D, Falls C: Os odontoideum in chondrodysplasia calcificans congenita. A case report. J Bone Joint Surg [Am] 64:1385, 1982.

378. Curless RG: Dominant chondrodysplasia punctata with neurologic symptoms. Neurology 33:1095, 1983.

379. Spirt BA, Oliphant M, Gottlieb RH, et al: Prenatal sonographic evaluation of short-limbed dwarfism: An algorithmic approach. RadioGraphics 10:217, 1990.

380. Meyer J: Dysplasia epiphysealis capitis femoris. A clinico-radiological syndrome and its relationship to Legg-Calvé-Perthes' disease. Acta Orthop Scand 34:183, 1964.

381. Harrison S: Dysplasia epiphysealis capitis femoris. Clin Orthop Rel Res 80:118, 1971.

382. Brower AC: The osteochondroses. Orthop Clin North Am *14*:99, 1983.
383. Khermosh O, Wientroub S: Dysplasia epiphysealis capitis femoris. Meyer's dysplasia. J Bone Joint Surg [Br] *73*:621, 1991.
384. Barsky AJ: Macrodactyly. J Bone Joint Surg [Am] *49*:1255, 1967.
385. Kelikian H: Macrodactyly. *In* Congenital Deformities of the Hand and Forearm. Philadelphia, WB Saunders Co, 1974, p 610.
386. Posnanski AK: The Hand in Radiologic Diagnosis. Philadelphia, WB Saunders Co, 1974, pp 193, 328, 416.
387. Moran B, Butler F, Colville J: X-ray diagnosis of macrodystrophia lipomatosa. Br J Radiol *57*:523, 1984.
388. Jain R, Sawhney S, Berry M: CT diagnosis of macrodystrophia lipomatosa. A case report. Acta Radiol *33*:554, 1992.
389. Blacksin B, Barnes FJ, Lyons MM: MR diagnosis of macrodystrophia lipomatosa. AJR *158*:1295, 1992.
390. Viola RW, Kahn A, Pottenger LA: Case Report. Paraxial macrodystrophia lipomatosa of the medial right lower limb. J Pediatr Orthop *11*:671, 1991.
391. Gupta SK, Sharma OP, Sharma SV, et al: Macrodystrophia lipomatosa: Radiographic observations. Br J Radiol *65*:769, 1992.
392. Silverman TA, Enzinoer FM: Fibrolipomatous hamartoma of nerve. A clinicopathologic analysis of 26 cases. Am J Surg Pathol *9*:7, 1985.
393. Ranawat CS, Arora MM, Singh RG: Macrodystrophia lipomatosa with carpal tunnel syndrome. A case report. J Bone Joint Surg [Am] *50*:1242, 1968.
394. Littler JW, Cramer LM, Smith JW: Symposium on Reconstructive Hand Surgery. St Louis, CV Mosby Co, 1974, p 218.
395. Moore BH: Macrodactylism and associated peripheral nerve changes associated with congenital deformities. J Bone Joint Surg *26*:282, 1944.
396. Inglis K: Local gigantism (a manifestation of neurofibromatosis): Its relation to general gigantism and to acromegaly. Illustrating the influence of intrinsic factors in disease when development of the body is abnormal. Am J Pathol *26*:1059, 1950.
397. Tuli SM, Khanna NN, Sinha GP: Congenital macrodactyly. Br J Plast Surg *22*:237, 1969.
398. Thorne FL, Posch JL, Mladick RA: Megalodactyly. Plast Reconstr Surg *41*:232, 1968.
399. Minkowitz S, Minkowitz F: A morphological study of macrodactylism. A case report. J Pathol Bacteriol *90*:323, 1965.
400. Ben-Bassat M, Casper J, Kaplan I, Laron Z: Congenital macrodactyly. A case report with three-year follow-up. J Bone Joint Surg [Br] *48*:359, 1966.
401. Goldman AB, Kaye JJ: Macrodystrophia lipomatosa: Radiographic diagnosis. Am J Roentgenol *128*:101, 1977.
402. Kelikian H: Congenital Deformities of the Hand and Forearm. Philadelphia, WB Saunders Co, 1974, p 610.
403. Herring JA: Macrodactyly. Pediatr Orthop *4*:503, 1984.
404. Stern PJ, Nyquist SR: Macrodactyly in ulnar nerve distribution associated with cubital tunnel syndrome. J Hand Surg *7*:569, 1982.
405. Cockshott WP: Dactylitis and growth disorders. Br J Radiol *36*:19, 1963.
406. Rosborough D: Osteoid osteoma. Report of a lesion in the terminal phalanx of a finger. J Bone Joint Surg [Br] *48*:485, 1966.
407. McCarthy DM, Dorr CA, Mackintosh CE: Unilateral localized gigantism of the extremities with lipomatosis, arthropathy, and psoriasis. J Bone Joint Surg [Br] *51*:348, 1969.
408. Bloem JJ, Donner R: Hyperplasia of palmar plates and macrodactyly in a young child. J Bone Joint Surg [Br] *63*:114, 1981.
409. Johnson EW, Ghormley RK, Dockerty MB: Hemangiomas of the extremities. Surg Gynecol Obstet *102*:531, 1956.
410. Meszaros WT, Guzzo F, Schorsch H: Neurofibromatosis. Am J Roentgenol *98*:557, 1966.
411. Pitt MJ, Mosher JF, Edeiken J: Abnormal periosteum and bone in neurofibromatosis. Radiology *103*:143, 1972.
412. Gamsu G: The Klippel-Trenaunay syndrome. A case report. J Can Assoc Radiol *21*:287, 1970.
413. Lindenauer SM: Congenital arteriovenous fistula and the Klippel-Trenaunay syndrome. Ann Surg *174*:248, 1971.
414. Belovic B, Nethercott J, Donsky HJ: An unusual variant of Klippel-Trenaunay-Weber syndrome. Can Med Assoc J *111*:439, 1974.
415. Gellis SS, Feingold M: Picture of the month. Klippel-Trenaunay-Weber syndrome (angioosteohypertrophy). Am J Dis Child *128*:213, 1974.
416. Letts RM: Orthopaedic treatment of hemangiomatous hypertrophy of the lower extremity. J Bone Joint Surg [Am] *59*:777, 1977.
417. MacPherson RI, Letts RM: Skeletal disease associated with angiomatosis. J Can Assoc Radiol *29*:90, 1978.

418. You CK, Rees J, Gillis DA, Steeves J: Klippel-Trenaunay syndrome: A review. Can J Surg *26*:399, 1983.
419. Barek L, Ledor S, Ledor K: The Klippel-Trenaunay syndrome: A case report and review of the literature. Mt Sinai J Med *49*:66, 1982.
420. Snow RD, Lecklitner ML: Musculoskeletal findings in Klippel-Trenaunay syndrome. Clin Nucl Med *16*:928, 1991.
421. Williams DW III, Elster AD: Cranial CT and MR in Klippel-Trenaunay-Weber syndrome. AJNR *13*:291, 1992.
422. McGrory BJ, Amadio PC, Dobyns JH, et al: Anomalies of the fingers and toes associated with Klippel-Trenaunay syndrome. J Bone Joint Surg [Am] *73*:153, 1991.
423. Aelvoet GE, Jorens PG, Roelen LM: Genetic aspects of the Klippel-Trenaunay syndrome. Br J Dermatol *126*:603, 1992.
424. Klippel M, Trenaunay P: Du naevus variqueux ostéohypertrophique. Arch Gen Med *3*:641, 1900.
425. Parke-Weber F: Angioma formation in connection with hypertrophy of the limbs and hemihypertrophy. Br J Dermatol *19*:231, 1907.
426. Lindenauer SM: The Klippel-Trenaunay syndrome: Varicosity, hypertrophy and hemangioma with no arteriovenous fistula. Ann Surg *162*:303, 1965.
427. Owens DW, Garcia E, Pierce RR, Castrow FF II: Klippel-Trenaunay-Weber syndrome with pulmonary vein varicosity. Arch Dermatol *108*:111, 1973.
428. Brooksaler F: The angioosteohypertrophy syndrome, Klippel-Trenaunay-Weber syndrome. Am J Dis Child *112*:161, 1966.
429. Inui M, Chiba R, Shike S: An autopsy case of Klippel-Trenaunay-Weber disease. Acta Pathol Jpn *19*:251, 1969.
430. Moynahan JA: Nevoid hypertrophy of the lower limbs, with gigantism of digits (Klippel-Trenaunay-Weber syndrome). Proc R Soc Med *54*:695, 1961.
431. Baar AJ: Klippel-Trenaunay's syndrome in connection with a possible teratogenic effect of butobarbital. Dermatologica *154*:314, 1977.
432. Baskerville PA, Ackroyd JS, Thomas ML, Browse NL: The Klippel-Trenaunay syndrome: Clinical, radiological and haemodynamic features and management. Br J Surg *72*:232, 1985.
433. Harper PS, Horton WA: Klippel-Trenaunay-Weber syndrome. Birth Defects *78*:315, 1971.
434. Gwinn DL, Lee FA: Radiologic case of the month. Am J Dis Child *131*:89, 1977.
435. Djindjian M, Djindjian R, Hurth M, Rey A, Houdart R: Spinal cord arteriovenous malformations and Klippel-Trenaunay-Weber syndrome. Surg Neurol *8*:229, 1977.
436. Seville M: Klippel and Trenaunay's syndrome. 768 operated cases. Ann Surg *201*:365, 1985.
437. Sehgal VN, Aggarwal SP, Gupta RC: Klippel-Trenaunay-Parke-Weber syndrome. Derm Int *7*:212, 1968.
438. McCullough CJ, Kenwright J: The prognosis in congenital lower limb hypertrophy. Acta Orthop Scand *50*:307, 1979.
439. Ghahremani GG, Kangarloo H, Volberg F, Meyers MA: Diffuse cavernous hemangioma of the colon in the Klippel-Trenaunay syndrome. Radiology *118*:637, 1976.
440. Hall BD: Bladder hemangiomas in Klippel-Trenaunay-Weber syndrome. N Engl J Med *285*:1032, 1971.
441. Johnson JF: Hemangiomatous calvarial trabecular pattern in newborns. Am J Neuroradiol *2*:48, 1981.
442. Ekerot L, Jonsson K, Eiken O, Cederholm C: Hemangioma of the lunate (Klippel-Trenaunay syndrome). Case report. Scand J Plast Surg *15*:153, 1981.
443. Jafri SZH, Bree RL, Glazer GM, Francis IR, Schwab RE: Computed tomography and ultrasound findings in Klippel-Trenaunay syndrome. J Comput Assist Tomogr *7*:457, 1983.
444. Hatjis CG, Philip AG, Anderson GG, Mann LI: The in utero ultrasonographic appearance of Klippel-Trenaunay-Weber syndrome. Am J Obstet Gynecol *139*:972, 1981.
445. Pear J, Viljoen D, Beighton P: Limb overgrowth—clinical observations and nosological considerations. S Afr J Med *64*:905, 1983.
446. Nerlich AG, Brenner RE, Wiest I, et al: Immunohistochemical localization of interstitial collagens in bone tissue from patients with various forms of osteogenesis imperfecta. Am J Med Genet *45*:258, 1993.
447. Cohn DH, Starman BJ, Blumberg B, et al: Recurrence of lethal osteogenesis imperfecta due to parental mosaicism for a dominant mutation in a human type I collagen gene (COL1A1). Am J Hum Genet *45*:591, 1990.

88

Osteochondrodysplasias, Dysostoses, Chromosomal Aberrations, Mucopolysaccharidoses, and Mucolipidoses

William H. McAlister, M.D., and
Thomas E. Herman, M.D.

Osteochondrodysplasias
  Achondroplasia Group
    Thanatophoric Dysplasia
    Classic (Heterozygous) Achondroplasia
    Homozygous Achondroplasia
    Hypochondroplasia
  Achondrogenesis Group
  Spondyloepiphyseal Dysplasia Congenita Group
    Hypochondrogenesis
    Spondyloepiphyseal Dysplasia Congenita
  Metatropic Dysplasia Group
    Fibrochondrogenesis
    Metatropic Dysplasia
  Short Rib Dysplasia Group
    Short Rib Syndromes (With or Without Polydactyly)
    Asphyxiating Thoracic Dysplasia (Jeune's Syndrome)
    Ellis–van Creveld Dysplasia (Chondroectodermal
      Dysplasia)
  Atelosteogenesis and Diastrophic Dysplasia Group
    Atelosteogenesis Dysplasias
    Otopalatodigital Syndrome
    Diatrophic Dysplasia
  Kniest and Stickler Dysplasia Group
    Dyssegmental Dysplasia
    Kniest's Dysplasia
    Otospondylomegaepiphyseal Dysplasia
    Stickler's Dysplasia
  Other Spondyloepimetaphyseal Dysplasias
    X-Linked Spondyloepiphyseal Dysplasia Tarda
    Spondyloepimetaphyseal Dysplasia
    Progressive Pseudorheumatoid Chondrodysplasia
    Dyggve-Melchior-Clausen Dysplasia
    Wolcott-Rallison Dysplasia
    Pseudoachondroplasia
    Myotonic Chondrodysplasia (Catel-Schwartz-Jampel
      Dysplasia)

Spondylometaphyseal Dysplasias
    Spondylometaphyseal Dysplasia, Multiple Types
    Spondyloenchondroplasia
  Multiple Epiphyseal Dysplasias
  Chondrodysplasia Punctata (Stippled Epiphyses) Group
  Metaphyseal Dysplasias
    Jansen Type
    Schmid Type
    McKusick Type
    Schwachman-Diamond Type
    Adenosine Deaminase Deficiency
    Metaphyseal Anadysplasia
  Brachyrachia (Short Spine Dysplasia)
    Brachyolmia
  Mesomelic Dysplasias
    Dyschondrosteosis
    Nievergelt Type
    Langer Type
    Robinow Type
  Acromelic and Acromesomelic Dysplasias
    Acromesomelic Dysplasia
    Trichorhinophalangeal Dysplasia
    Saldino-Mainzer Dysplasia
    Pseudohypoparathyroidism
  Dysplasias with Significant (but not Exclusive) Membranous
    Bone Involvement
    Cleidocranial Dysplasia
    Osteodysplasty (Melnick-Needles Syndrome)
  Bent-Bone Dysplasia Group
    Campomelic Dysplasia
    Kyphomelic Dysplasia
  Multiple Dislocations with Dysplasia
    Larsen's Syndrome
    Desbuquois' Syndrome
    Spondyloepimetaphyseal Dysplasia with Joint Laxity
  Osteodysplastic Primordial Dwarfism Group

Dysplasias with Decreased Bone Density
  Menkes' Syndrome
Dysplasias with Defective Mineralization
Dysplasias with Increased Bone Density
  Osteopetrosis, Multiple Types
  Dysosteosclerosis
  Pyknodysostosis
  Osteosclerosis, Stanescu Type
  Axial Osteosclerosis
  Osteopoikilosis, Melorheostosis, Osteopathia Striata
  Diphyseal Dysplasia (Camurati-Engelmann Disease)
  Craniodiaphyseal Dysplasia
  Lenz-Majewski Dysplasia
  Craniometaphyseal Dysplasia, Wormian Bone Type
  Endosteal Hyperostosis
  Pachydermoperiostosis
  Frontometaphyseal Dysplasia
  Craniometaphyseal Dysplasia
  Pyle's Dysplasia
  Osteoectasia with Hyperphosphatasia
  Oculodento-osseous Dysplasia (Oculodentodigital Syndrome)
  Familial Infantile Cortical Hyperostosis (Caffey's Disease)
Disorganized Development of Cartilaginous and Fibrous Components of the Skeleton
  Dysplasia Epiphysealis Hemimelica
  Multiple Cartilaginous Exostoses
  Enchondromatosis (Ollier's Disease)
  Enchondromatosis with Hemangiomas (Maffucci's Syndrome)
  Metachondromatosis
  Osteoglophonic Dysplasia
  Fibrous Dysplasia and Myofibromatosis
Miscellaneous
  Tubular Stenosis (Kenny-Caffey Syndrome)
  Parastremmatic Dysplasia
  Occipital Horn Syndrome
Dysostoses
  Craniosynostosis
  Craniofacial Dysostosis (Crouzon's Syndrome)
  Acrocephalosyndactyly
    Apert's Syndrome
    Saethre-Chotzen Acrocephalosyndactyly
    Pfeiffer's Syndrome
    Jackson-Weiss Syndrome
  Acrocephalopolysyndactyly
  Other Craniosynostosis Syndromes
    Baller-Gerold Syndrome
    Antley-Bixler Syndrome
    Trigonencephaly Syndromes
    Cephalopolysyndactyly (Greig's Syndrome)
    Mandibulofacial Dysostosis (Treacher Collins Syndrome)
    Acrofacial Dysostosis, Preaxial (Nager's Syndrome)
    Acrofacial Dysostosis, Postaxial (Miller's Syndrome)
    Oculoauriculovertebral Dysplasia (Goldenhar's Syndrome)
    Hemifacial Microsomia
    Oculomandibulofacial Syndrome (Hallermann-Streiff-François Syndrome)
Chromosomal Aberrations
  4p − Syndrome (Wolf-Hirschhorn Syndrome)
  5p − Syndrome
  Trisomy 8 Syndrome
  Trisomy 9p Syndrome
  Trisomy 13 Syndrome
  Trisomy 18 Syndrome
  Trisomy 21 (Down's Syndrome)
  Monosomy 21 Syndrome
  Turner's Syndrome
  Kleinfelter's Syndrome
Mucopolysaccharidoses (MPS) and Related Disorders
  MPS I-H (Hurler's Syndrome)
  MPS I-S (Scheie's Syndrome)
  MPS I-H-S
  MPS II (Hunter's Syndrome)
  MPS III (Sanfilippo's Syndrome)

MPS IV (Morquio's and Related Syndromes)
MPS VI (Maroteaux-Lamy Syndrome)
MPS VII (Sly's Syndrome)
Aspartylglucosaminuria
Mannosidosis
Fucosidosis
GM₁ Gangliosidosis
Mucolipidoses
  Mucolipidosis I (Sialidosis)
  Mucolipidosis II (I-Cell Disease)
  Mucolipidosis III (Pseudo-Hurler's Polydystrophy)

A modified version of the international classification of osteochondrodysplasias published in 1992 is used in this chapter.[1] The approach to the skeletal dysplasias taken here is based primarily on radiographic findings with the addition of pertinent clinical data, including inheritance patterns. Space limitations do not permit detailed histochemical and histopathologic analyses of each disorder. Certain conditions, such as fibrous dysplasia, osteogenesis imperfecta, idiopathic juvenile osteoporosis, epiphyseal dysplasias, osteopoikilosis, osteopathia striata, and melorheostosis, are discussed in other chapters. The interested reader is referred to some excellent general references[2-11] and to those cited in this chapter in the discussion of each condition.

OSTEOCHONDRODYSPLASIAS

Achrondroplasia Group

Thanatophoric Dysplasia. Since its original description in 1967, thanatophoric, or "death bearing" dysplasia, has become a well-recognized clinical and pathologic entity.[12] Affected children usually are stillborn or die shortly after birth owing to hypoplastic lungs; however, occasional survival into infancy occurs. Polyhydramnios and poor fetal activity are common; the diagnosis has been made in utero by sonography.[13] The fetus or infant has marked short-limbed dwarfism, a large head with frontal bossing, and a depressed nasal bridge. Numerous skin folds are present. The anteroposterior diameter of the chest is narrow, and the child has a relatively long trunk.

Radiographic findings include marked shortening of the long tubular bones in a rhizomelic pattern of distribution, with metaphyseal flaring and osseous bowing and widening (Fig. 88–1A).[14, 15] The bowed femora resemble telephone receivers. Pronounced flattening of the vertebral bodies with more constriction of their midportions and wide intervertebral disc spaces are evident (Fig. 88–1B). Because the neural arches are better developed than the vertebral bodies, the appearance of each vertebra on frontal radiographs resembles an inverted U or H. Narrowing of the spinal canal is most marked in the lumbar region. The thorax is slender owing to short ribs with flared anterior ends. Small, rectangular iliac bones, small sacroiliac notches, and short and wide pubic and ischial bones are seen. The phalanges are short, relatively broad, and cupped (Fig. 88–1C). The base of the skull is short and the foramen magnum is small. Autopsies have demonstrated that the narrowed foramen magnum can indent the cervical cord. A variety of extraskeletal malformations have been described, including a dysplastic temporal cortex and basal ganglia,[16] megalo-

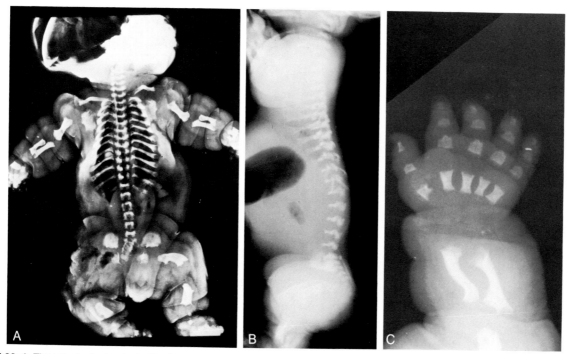

FIGURE 88–1. Thanatophoric dysplasia. Radiographs from three patients are shown.
A Findings include short tubular bones with flared metaphyses, squared iliac bones, and short ribs.
B The vertebral bodies are markedly flattened with wide disc spaces.
C The tubular bones of the hands are markedly shortened but relatively broad. Bowing and metaphyseal flaring are evident in the bones of the forearm.

cephaly, polymicrogyria, heart defects, and some degree of hydronephrosis.

The histopathologic features consist of disorganized endochondral bone formation with lack of ordered rows of cartilage cells and hypertrophy of chondrocytes.[17] The basic pathogenetic mechanism may be persistence of abnormal fetal mesenchyme, which appears to be transformed into the severely abnormal bone and cartilage.[18] Fibrous bands continuous with the periosteum or perichondrium extend into the growth zone.[19] A cloverleaf skull and hemangiomatosis of the occipital bone have been seen in association with thanatophoric dysplasia.[20–22] Cases of thanatophoric dysplasia have been subclassified into those with and without cloverleaf skull.

The pattern of inheritance of this condition is unclear, but a dominant new mutation still is the most likely cause.[23] The radiographic findings cannot be distinguished from those of some patients with homozygous achondroplasia.

Certain cases of platyspondylodysplastic lethal neonatal short-limbed dwarfism have been classified as thanatophoric variants, such as Torrance, San Diego, and Luton types. These are separate entities, however, and are rare.

Classic (Heterozygous) Achondroplasia. Classic achondroplasia, a relatively common type of dwarfism of autosomal dominant inheritance, is evident at birth and is compatible with a long life span. Clinical manifestations include short limbs, especially of the proximal portions (rhizomelic micromelia), a large head with a prominent forehead and a depressed nasal bridge, thoracolumbar kyphosis in infancy, and exaggerated lumbar lordosis with prominent buttocks in children and adults.[24] The hands are stubby and trident, and often elbow motion is limited. Because of the constricted basicranium, foramen magnum, and spinal canal, persons with achondroplasia at any age may develop compression of the spinal cord, lower brain stem, cauda equina, and nerve roots. This compression by the foramen magnum can be associated with serious neurologic problems,[25] and such compression can cause apnea and sudden death.[26–31] Degenerative changes of the spine, herniated intervertebral discs, and exaggerated spinal curvatures, especially kyphosis, compromise the already narrow spinal canal.[31] Modest increases in height can be seen with recombinant human growth hormone.[32]

Radiographic findings include a cranium that is large compared with the size of the face, with defective growth of the base of the skull, resulting in a pinched appearance (Fig. 88–2). The foramen magnum is small and is well shown by CT scanning.[25] MR imaging of the craniocervical junction, cranium, and brain shows narrowing of the subarachnoid space at the level of the foramen magnum.[33] Some patients demonstrate compressive deformities of the cervicomedullary junction, hydrocephalus, stretching of the optic nerves and pituitary stalk, and bifrontal widening of the subarachnoid space.[33] The interpediculate distances of the lower lumbar vertebrae, which normally increase on proceeding distally, remain the same at all levels or decrease in the lower lumbar region (Fig. 88–3). In the lateral projection of the spine, the pedicles are short, the backs of the vertebral bodies often are concave, and the spinal canal is small (Fig. 88–4). Growth failure occurs at the neurocentral synchondrosis. The vertebral bodies are flattened and appear bullet-shaped in infancy and early childhood. The iliac bones are squared with small sacrosciatic notches and flat acetabular angles (Fig. 88–5). Shortening of the tubular bones, especially the proximal ones, and metaphyseal flaring are seen (Fig. 88–6). The proximal femora are rounded with a lucent appearance in infancy. The fibula is disproportionately long (Fig. 88–6). A V-shaped configuration of

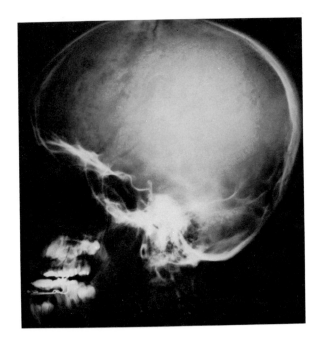

FIGURE 88–2. Heterozygous achondroplasia: Skull. Note the pinched base of the skull.

FIGURE 88–3. Heterozygous achondroplasia: Spine.

A The interpediculate distances in the lumbar vertebrae narrow distally. The iliac bones are squared, the sacrosciatic notches are small, and the ischial bones are shortened.

B A myelogram in an older child reveals marked spinal stenosis.

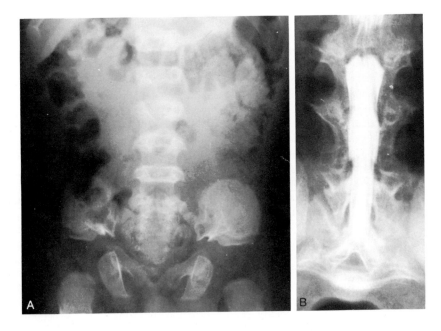

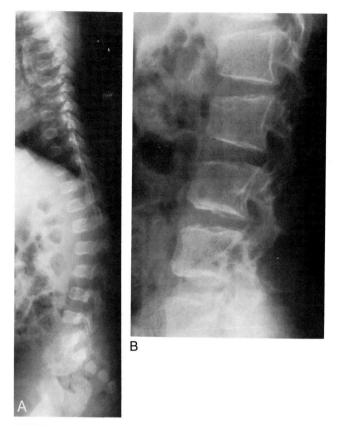

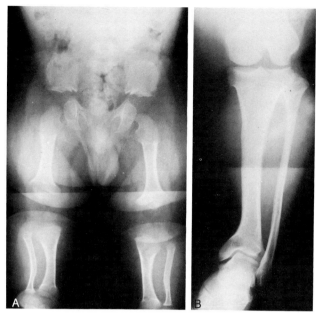

FIGURE 88–6. Heterozygous achondroplasia: Lower extremities.

A Newborn. Rhizomelic shortening of the tubular bones with metaphyseal flaring and medial slanting of distal femoral metaphyses are seen.

B Adult. A V-shaped configuration of the distal femoral epiphysis and a disproportionately long fibula, with resultant inversion of the foot, are present.

FIGURE 88–4. Heterozygous achondroplasia: Lateral spine.

A Four month old child. Bullet-shaped vertebral bodies with diminished heights and wide disc spaces are seen.

B In an older child, the vertebral bodies have a posterior concavity, diminished heights, anterior wedging, and short pedicles, and the spinal canal is small.

flared. The lung volumes are decreased and intrathoracic narrowing may lead to airway compression (Fig. 88–8).[34, 35]

The skeletal abnormalities of achondroplasia are the result of a generalized defect in the process of endochondral

the distal femoral growth plate may be seen. Shortening of the tubular bones in the hands and feet is evident, with the proximal and middle phalanges having the greatest degree of shortening as well as of widening (Fig. 88–7). The ribs also are shortened, and the anteroposterior diameter of the chest is decreased. The anterior ends of the ribs may be

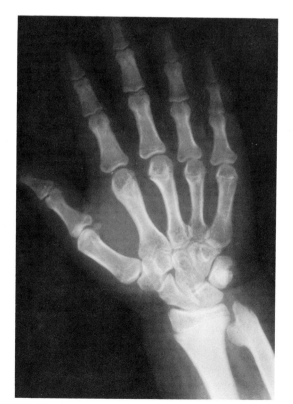

FIGURE 88–7. Heterozygous achondroplasia: Hand. The tubular bones are shortened. The distal portion of the ulna is deformed, with a prominent styloid process, and the metaphysis of the radius appears flared.

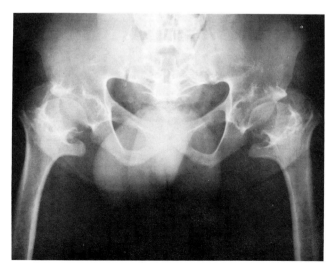

FIGURE 88–5. Heterozygous achondroplasia: Pelvis. In this adult patient, findings include spinal stenosis, lack of flaring of the iliac wings (which have rounded corners), and short femoral necks.

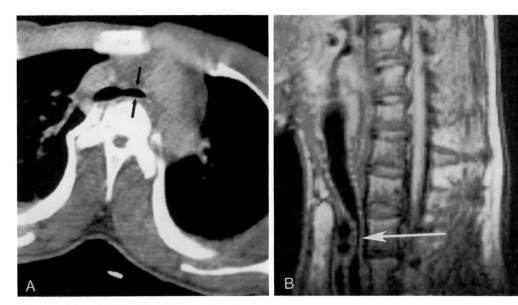

FIGURE 88–8. Heterozygous achondroplasia: Thorax and neck.

A Transaxial CT scan of chest. The bifurcation of the trachea is compressed (arrows). The posterior aspects of the ribs are posteriorly directed with the vertebral bodies situated in an anterior position.

B Sagittal T$_1$-weighted spin echo MR image of neck and thoracic inlet. Marked tracheal narrowing (arrow) is seen at the level of the great vessels in the superior mediastinum. The trachea is constricted between the sternum anteriorly and the vertebral bodies posteriorly. The innominate artery and left brachiocephalic vein are anterior to the trachea. The spinal canal is narrowed.

bone formation. Although the histologic features of endochondral bone formation may be altered only slightly, the rate of such formation appears to be depressed.

Homozygous Achondroplasia. Homozygous achondroplasia is an extremely rare type of congenital short-limbed dwarfism that is lethal; an affected infant dies within the first days or weeks of life.[36] The condition results when both parents have achondroplasia. Characteristic clinical features of the disease include a large cranium, depressed nasal bridge, and limb shortening in an infant with respiratory distress. The radiographs outline changes that are more severe than those in classic (heterozygous) achondroplasia; indeed, they may be indistinguishable from those of thanatophoric dysplasia (Fig. 88–9).

The abnormalities in endochondral bone formation that are observed in homozygous achondroplasia are far more prominent than in heterozygous achondroplasia and more closely resemble those in thanatophoric dysplasia.[37, 38, 39]

Hypochondroplasia. Hypochondroplasia, an autosomal dominant disorder, first becomes manifest in childhood with clinical and radiologic findings that are similar to but less severe than those of achondroplasia (Figs. 88–10 to 88–12).[40–45] Small stature, increased lumbar lordosis, bowlegs, and limited elbow extension may be noted on clinical evaluation. Radiographic findings include narrowing of the interpediculate distances distally and exaggerated posterior concavity of vertebral bodies in the lumbar region, mild platyspondyly, small spinal canals, shortening of the tubular bones, and a short, broad femoral neck. Mild metaphyseal flaring occurs. The iliac bones are shortened with flattened acetabular roofs and small sciatic notches. The fibulae may be slightly long and the distal ends of the ulnae are short with prominent ulnar styloid processes. The skull is not affected significantly, although macrocephaly, shortening of the base, and smallness of the foramen magnum can be seen.[44] Mild radiographic findings can be seen at birth. The

condition has been seen but not diagnosed on prenatal sonograms.[46]

An achondroplasia-hypochondroplasia complex has been described with radiographic findings quite different from those of either of these two conditions in a child born of a mother with hypochondroplasia and a father with achondroplasia.[47] An autosomal recessive condition also exists that resembles hypochondroplasia but is associated with more dramatic shortening of the humerus, the absence of tibial and ulnar shortening, and normal interpediculate distances.[48]

Achondrogenesis Group

Achondrogenesis. Achondrogenesis, a type of dwarfism of neonates, is characterized by a disproportionately large head, short trunk, protuberant abdomen, severe micromelia, and hydrops.[49] The disease has been reported in twins, is considered to be of autosomal recessive inheritance, and commonly is associated with polyhydramnios.[50] Achondrogenesis has been classified into two varieties: type I and type II.[51] Radiographic findings common to both types include severe lack of ossification of the vertebral bodies (especially caudally); small deformed iliac bones; absent or poor ossification of pubic and ischial bones, calcaneus, and talus; tubular bones that are strikingly short and malformed with wide, cupped ends; and short ribs with cupped and flared ends. Type I is subdivided into IA (Houston-Harris) with rib fractures and IB (Fraccaro) without rib fractures. Neonates with type IB may have more extensive skull ossification but shorter limbs and no fibular ossification.[52] Some degree of ischial ossification occurs in persons with type IA. In the type I syndrome, more severe shortening and bowing of the tubular bones are seen, with some widening (rectangular bones) and metaphyseal spur formation, and poorer ossification of the vertebral bodies and skull (Fig. 88–13A). Type II (Langer-Saldino) or hypochondro-

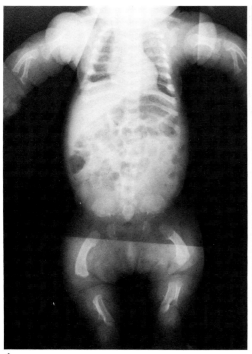

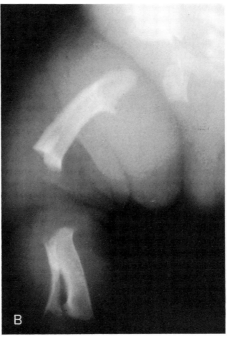

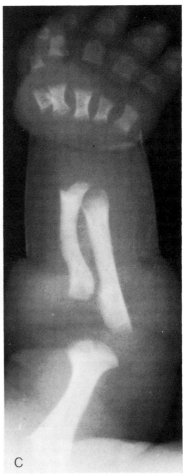

A

FIGURE 88–9. Homozygous achondroplasia.

A In this newborn infant, the changes are more severe than those seen in heterozygous achondroplasia but less severe than those in thanatophoric dysplasia.

B,C In a second newborn infant, the tubular bones show severe shortening, bowing, widening, and metaphyseal flaring, and the iliac bone has a square configuration. These findings cannot be distinguished from those of thanatophoric dysplasia.

C

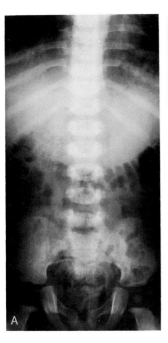

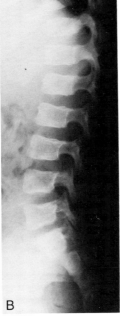

FIGURE 88–10. Hypochondroplasia: Spine.

A In the lumbar spine of a 7 month old child, the increase in interpediculate distances that normally is seen in the lower lumbar spine is not present. Shortening of the iliac bones and small sacrosciatic notches are evident.

B In an 8 year old patient, posterior concavity of the vertebral bodies and slight narrowing of the spinal canal are observed.

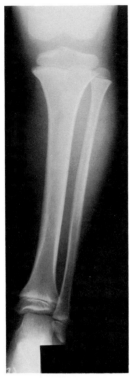

FIGURE 88–11. Hypochondroplasia: Long tubular bones. Although both bones are decreased in length, the fibula is long with respect to the tibia.

genesis represents the severe end of the spondyloepiphyseal dysplasia congenita group. Patients with the more severe type II form are distinguished from those with type I on the basis of iliac bone features: in the type II form, the iliac bones have a crescent-shaped inner border that is smoother,

longer, and less deformed (Fig. 88–13B). In addition the skull is better ossified, the changes in the tubular bones are less severe, and less rib shortening is found.

Additional classification schemes for achondrogenesis have been developed. After a review of 79 cases, Whitley and Gorlin proposed the existence of four types of disease ranging from classic achondrogenesis type I to a milder type IV or hypochondrogenesis.[53] A wide spectrum of bone changes, from mild to severe, occurs in Type II (Langer-Saldino).[54] Collagen type II, shown to be abnormal in severe cases, may be normal in mild cases.[55] Antenatal diagnosis of achondrogenesis has been made by sonography.[56, 57]

Spondyloepiphyseal Dysplasia Congenita Group

Hypochondrogenesis. Hypochondrogenesis is believed to represent type II achondrogenesis (Langer-Saldino), and patients may survive for months[58]; its histopathologic features are identical to those of achondrogenesis. Hypochondrogenesis is part of a spectrum that includes spondyloepiphyseal dysplasia congenita with milder clinical and radiographic findings. Affected patients have a large head, depressed nasal bridge, micromelia, and short neck and trunk. The radiographic appearance includes short but well-developed tubular bones, metaphyseal flaring with mild irregularity, delayed epiphyseal ossification, relatively long fibulae, absence of rib fractures, modestly developed iliac bones with poor pubic bone development and flat acetabula, small flattened or oval vertebral bodies, and defective skull ossification behind the foramen magnum (Figs. 88–13B and

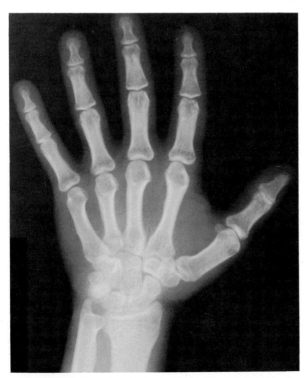

FIGURE 88–12. Hypochondroplasia: Hand. The tubular bones are short and the ulnar styloid process is long.

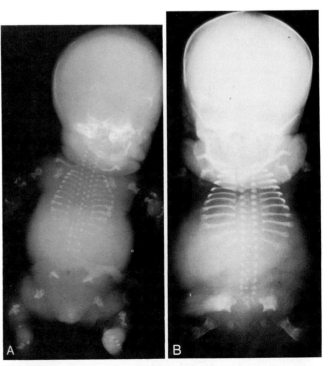

FIGURE 88–13. Achondrogenesis.

A Type 1A (Houston-Harris). The vertebrae are poorly ossified. The tubular bones are short, bowed, and deformed, with wide cupped ends and metaphyseal osteophytes. Small deformed iliac bones and short ribs with fractures and cupped ends also are seen.

B Type II (Langer-Saldino). The ribs are short, the vertebral bodies are poorly ossified, the tubular bones are short with mushroom-stem femora, and the iliac bones have a crescent-shaped inner border.

88–14).[59] In the more severe cases the long tubular bones have been described as resembling mushroom stems. Hypochondrogenesis probably is of autosomal recessive inheritance.

Spondyloepiphyseal Dysplasia Congenita. This short-trunk dwarfism is distinguished by mild shortening of the limbs, flat face, cleft palate, short neck, increased anteroposterior chest diameter, and joint restriction.[60] During growth, progressive kyphoscoliosis, dorsal kyphosis, or lumbar lordosis occurs. The hands and feet often are normal except for the presence of equinovarus deformity. Important additional features include myopia and retinal detachment, which can lead to blindness, and atlantoaxial instability, which can result in spinal cord compression that can be shown nicely by MR imaging. Although the pattern of inheritance usually is autosomal dominant, an autosomal recessive form of the disorder also is probable. A lethal form of the disease exists called hypochondrogenesis or achondrogenesis type II (discussed previously). Respiratory complications may be severe.[61]

Radiographic findings include a decreased height of the vertebral bodies and, in infancy, pear-shaped vertebrae (Fig. 88–15A)[60] related to the lack of development of the posterior portion of the vertebral bodies. In childhood, anterior wedging, irregularity, and generalized flattening of the vertebral bodies occur, with the appearance of kyphoscoliosis and lumbar lordosis. The interpediculate distances in the lower lumbar vertebrae may be narrowed. Hypoplasia of the odontoid process can be associated with atlantoaxial dislocation (Fig. 88–15B). Typical radiographic findings in the pelvis include a marked delay in the ossification of the pubic bones and proximal portion of the femora (Fig. 88–16A). The femoral heads often ossify from multiple centers, and a progressive coxa vara develops, with premature os-

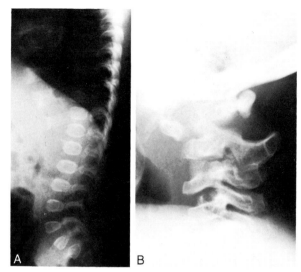

FIGURE 88–15. Spondyloepiphyseal dysplasia congenita.
A Decreased height of the vertebral bodies is seen, with pear-shaped vertebrae noted in the thoracic and lower lumbar regions.
B Hypoplasia of the odontoid process has resulted in atlantoaxial instability. The vertebral bodies are flat.

teoarthritis. Prominent shortening of the femoral necks may be evident, with small femoral heads that appear well below the level of the greater trochanters (Fig. 88–16B). The chest is broad and bell-shaped and has a decreased vertical height. The scapulae are short and squared. Flaring of the ends of the ribs anteriorly, pectus carinatum, and delay in sternal ossification are present. The long tubular bones have delayed epiphyseal ossification. The epiphyses are irregular and metaphyses show variable irregularity and flaring (Fig. 88–16A). Genu valgum or genu varum may be seen. The proximal carpal and tarsal bones may be small, with delayed ossification (Fig. 88–17). The calcaneus and talus may not be ossified at birth.

This condition exhibits considerable genetic heterogeneity, including lethal variants (Fig. 88–18).[61a, 62] The histopathologic features are characteristic.[63] Heterozygous mutations of type II collagen have been found.[64]

Metatropic Dysplasia Group

Fibrochondrogenesis. Fibrochondrogenesis, a fatal dwarfism appearing in neonates, probably is of autosomal recessive inheritance and is distinguished by posteriorly flattened, pear-shaped thoracic and lumbar vertebral bodies containing coronal fissures; short limbs with markedly flared, slightly irregular metaphyses; short and thin ribs with cupped ends; long, thin clavicles; small scapulae; iliac bones that are decreased in size and have rounded lateral borders; small sacrosciatic notches; and typical morphologic changes in the growth plate (Fig. 88–19).[65, 66]

Metatropic Dysplasia. Metatropic dysplasia is characterized by short extremities and a normal or elongated trunk at birth, and by a short trunk with kyphoscoliosis later in life. The term metatropic means ''changing'' and was selected by Maroteaux to stress the evolving stages of the disease. At birth, the ends of the long tubular bones are prominent, and joint movement is limited. In infancy, the thorax appears to be long and narrow, and a small soft tissue fold resembling a tail may be present over the sacrum. The hands and feet initially are long and slender but

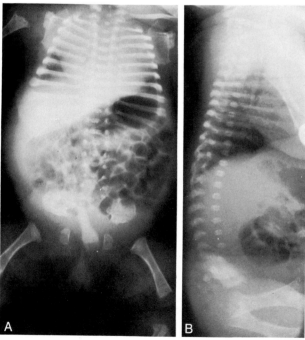

FIGURE 88–14. Hypochondrogenesis. Frontal **(A)** and lateral **(B)** radiographs show that the ribs, vertebral bodies, and pelvic and tubular bones are affected less severely than in achondrogenesis, type I.

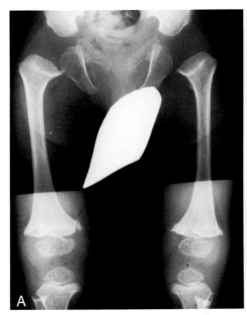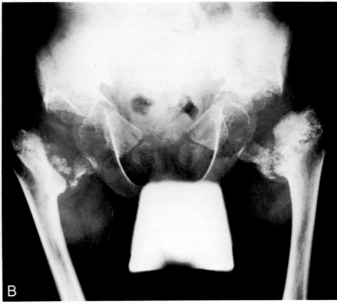

FIGURE 88–16. Spondyloepiphyseal dysplasia congenita.

A In a 2 year old patient, delayed ossification of the pubic bones and proximal portion of the femora is evident. The iliac bones are small, and metaphyseal irregularity is seen in the bones about the knees.

B In another patient (11 years old), the femoral heads are small and inferiorly placed, and the femoral necks and pubic bones are poorly developed.

become relatively shortened later in life. The patient may have progressive (and, sometimes, marked) kyphoscoliosis, with severe anterior bowing of the sternum.

The radiographic findings are dramatic. The tubular bones of the extremities are short and have marked metaphyseal widening, which resembles the appearance of a trumpet or dumbbell (Fig. 88–20).[67, 67a] The trochanters are particularly large, especially the lesser trochanter, and the appearance simulates that of a battle-axe, especially in infancy. The fibula may be relatively long. The epiphyses are delayed in appearance and are small, flat, and deformed. The vertebral bodies are rectangular or diamond-shaped in infancy and reduced markedly in height, and the intervertebral disc spaces appear large. Although the vertebral bodies increase in size, they remain flat, irregular, and wedged anteriorly (Fig. 88–21). The neural arches are fairly well developed. Atlantoaxial instability may be present, with abnormal development of the odontoid process and resultant neurologic deficits (Fig. 88–22).[68] The pelvis is characterized by shortened ilia with curved lateral margins, flat acetabular roofs, and small sacrosciatic and lateral iliac notches (Fig. 88–23). The Y-shaped triradiate cartilage is wide. In infancy the thorax is elongated and has a decreased anteroposterior diameter as a consequence of the short ribs, which exhibit flared anterior ends; the development of kyphoscoliosis and sternal protrusion during childhood leads to the deformed appearance of the thorax. The tubular bones of the hands and feet have metaphyseal expansion and delayed and irregular epiphyseal ossification (Fig. 88–

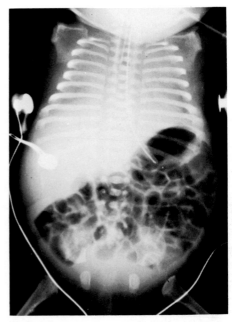

FIGURE 88–18. Spondyloepiphyseal dysplasia congenita. This severely affected newborn infant has a bell-shaped thorax, flattening of the vertebral bodies, defective pubic ossification, small scapulae, and hyaline membrane disease.

FIGURE 88–17. Spondyloepiphyseal dysplasia congenita. Note small and deformed carpal bones.

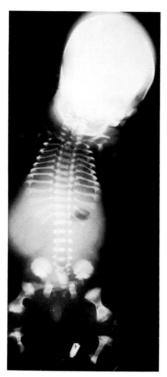

FIGURE 88–19. Fibrochondrogenesis. The vertebrae are flattened, the tubular bones are shortened, with flared metaphyses, and the ribs are short and thin, with cupped ends. The iliac wings are round, with narrow sacrosciatic notches. (Courtesy of H. Taybi, M.D., Oakland, California.)

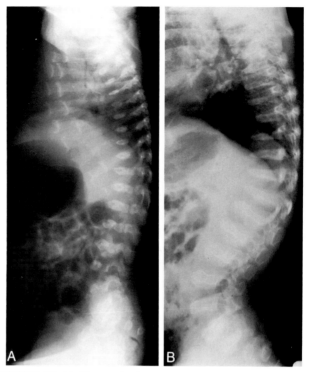

FIGURE 88–21. Metatropic dysplasia. Lateral radiographs of the spine in the newborn period **(A)** and at the age of 14 months **(B)** show marked vertebral flattening and anterior wedging. The initially present coronal cleft vertebrae, especially at the fourth lumbar level, have undergone further ossification.

24). The carpal and tarsal bones also are irregular with delayed ossification.

The inheritance of this condition is uncertain, but three genetic patterns appear to exist: (1) a nonlethal type with autosomal recessive inheritance, (2) a nonlethal autosomal dominant type, and (3) a lethal type with probable autosomal recessive inheritance (Fig. 88–25).[68–70] Although considerable heterogeneity occurs in this disorder, its separation into variant forms has been questioned.[71]

Short Rib Dysplasia Group

Multiple syndromes are characterized by a narrow thorax with short ribs, micromelia, and frequent polydactyly. Early death occurs from pulmonary hypoplasia. Four types of short rib–polydactyly syndromes are discussed here, and

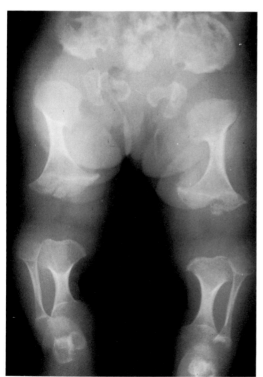

FIGURE 88–20. Metatropic dysplasia. In this newborn infant, the bones are shortened, with marked metaphyseal flaring and large femoral trochanters. The iliac bones are short, with curved lateral margins and small sacrosciatic notches.

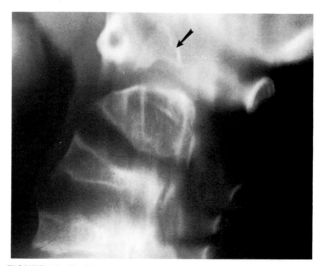

FIGURE 88–22. Metatropic dysplasia. A conventional tomogram of the upper cervical spine in a 7 year old patient demonstrates a small and deformed, separate odontoid process (arrow) and flattened vertebral bodies.

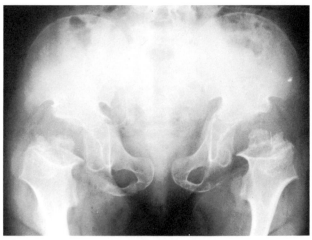

FIGURE 88–23. Metatropic dysplasia. Note the "battle axe" appearance of the iliac bones, with small sacrosciatic notches, deformed capital femoral epiphyses, and broad femoral necks.

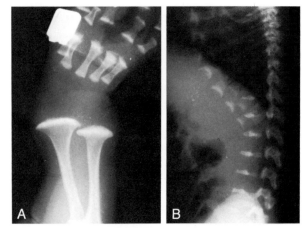

FIGURE 88–25. Metatropic dysplasia. The more lethal form of the disease is associated with marked metaphyseal flaring of the radius and ulna **(A)** and marked vertebral body flattening **(B).**

each has probable autosomal recessive inheritance. Also included are asphyxiating thoracic dystrophy and Ellis–van-Creveld dysplasia.

Short Rib–Polydactyly Syndrome, Type I (Saldino-Noonan). Newborn infants with this condition appear hydropic and have extreme limb shortening, postaxial polydactyly, and a narrow thorax.[72, 73] The polydactyly occasionally is preaxial. Radiographic features include severely shortened ribs that are horizontal, small scapulae, and deformed clavicles (Fig. 88–26). The tubular bones are extremely short, have irregular ends, and sometimes are pointed (Fig. 88–26). The femora may lack corticomedullary differentiation and the fibulae may be absent. The fingers are short, with phalangeal ossification that is either absent, round, or irregular. Similar changes occur in the metacarpal bones. The vertebral bodies are distorted, flattened or squared, and irregular; coronal clefts may be pres-

ent (Fig. 88–26B) The iliac bones are small, with flat acetabular roofs that have medial and lateral spurs and short sacroiliac notches. Dolichocephaly and a small mandible are seen. Multiple anomalies of the respiratory, cardiac, genital, and gastrointestinal tracts may be evident. The diagnosis has been established in utero by sonography or fetoscopy.[74, 75]

Short Rib–Polydactyly Syndrome, Type II (Majewski). In the type II variety, in addition to severe rib reduction and polydactyly, affected patients have hydrops, a small flat nose, low-set ears, and cleft lip or cleft palate.[76] In comparison to the type I syndrome, radiographic findings in the type II syndrome include rounded but not irregular metaphyses of the long tubular bones. The tibia can be disproportionately short and have an oval appearance. The spine and pelvis are involved only mildly. The proximal femoral epiphyses may be ossified at birth. The mandible is small, but the skull reveals minor ossification abnormalities. Multiple cardiovascular, gastrointestinal, genital, and brain anomalies have been reported, as have a hypoplastic epiglottis and renal cysts.[77] Microscopic changes have some similarities to those of the Ellis–van Creveld syndrome.[78]

Short Rib–Polydactyly Syndrome, Type III (Verma-Naumoff). In this syndrome in addition to the narrow thorax, short ribs, and short and squared scapulae and iliac bones, the vertebrae bodies are increased in size with prominent vascular channels.[79, 80] The tubular bones are better formed and have characteristic metaphyseal spurs, especially in the femora (Fig. 88–27).[79, 80] The base of the skull is short, and the frontal bone is prominent. Multiple congenital anomalies are found in other organ systems. Distinguishing between the type I and the type III syndromes sometimes is difficult, as both may be part of a spectrum of the same disease process, although type III has milder changes, including better-formed tubular bones with metaphyseal spurs, and better-formed fibulae and ribs.[81]

Short Rib–Polydactyly Syndrome, Type IV (Breemer). Type IV has similarities to type II except for the presence of mild platyspondyly, smaller iliac wings, bowing of tubular bones, and a tibia longer than the fibula.[82]

Asphyxiating Thoracic Dysplasia (Jeune's Syndrome). Initial reports of this autosomal recessive condition described infants with constricted chests and mild shorten-

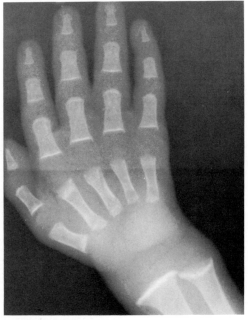

FIGURE 88–24. Metatropic dysplasia. Metaphyseal expansion and a delay in ossification of the epiphyses and carpal bones are seen.

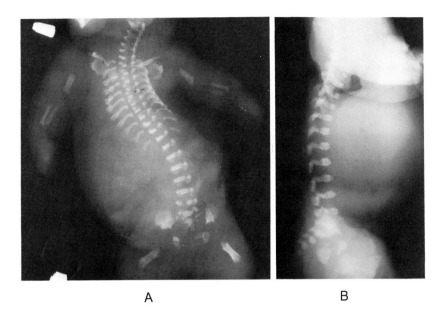

FIGURE 88–26. Short rib–polydactyly syndrome, type I (Saldino-Noonan). Radiographs **(A,B)** in two different infants are shown. The ribs are severely shortened, the scapulae are small, the tubular bones are short with irregular ends, the iliac bones have a squared configuration with medial and lateral excrescences, and the vertebral bodies are slightly flattened and irregular.

A   B

ing of the extremities who died from pulmonary hypoplasia. Later reports included patients with less severe respiratory symptoms,[83–85] although the patients who survive to childhood generally succumb to progressive renal disease.[86] Prenatal sonographic diagnosis of this disorder has occurred on the basis of an appropriate family history, a flat thorax, and shortened extremities.[87, 88]

The striking radiographic features are a narrow thorax and short, horizontally oriented ribs with wide, irregular

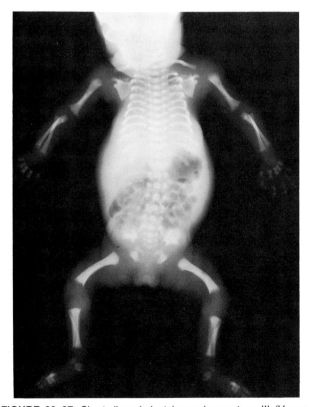

FIGURE 88–27. Short rib–polydactyly syndrome, type III (Verma-Naumoff). The ribs are extremely short, the tubular bones are better formed than in the type I syndrome, and metaphyseal outgrowths are evident. The iliac bones are squared, with inferior acetabular excrescences. The spine shows only mild changes.

costochondral junctions (Fig. 88–28). The clavicles may have a high, handle-bar appearance. The neonatal pelvic findings, similar to those in chondroectodermal dysplasia, are short iliac, pubic, and ischial bones, with the lateral borders of the ilia being rounded. The acetabular roofs are flat, with downward spikelike projections at the medial, lateral, and, sometimes, central aspects of the acetabular roofs, the so-called triradiate or trident acetabulum (Fig. 88–29). Premature ossification of the proximal femoral epiphyses occurs in a majority of patients. The sacrosciatic notches are small. The pelvis becomes normal with age, but the proximal femoral metaphyses may become progressively irregular. The long tubular bones are slightly shortened, with minimal metaphyseal flaring. Prominent findings in the hand may be evident (Fig. 88–30). Infants have mild digital shortening, especially in the distal phalanges, and inconstant polydactyly. Later, the epiphyses become cone-shaped and fuse prematurely, producing further shortening of the middle and distal phalanges. Similar findings are present in the feet. The skull and spine are normal.

Asphyxiating thoracic dystrophy has many radiographic and histopathologic features that are similar to those of

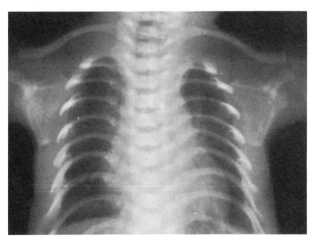

FIGURE 88–28. Asphyxiating thoracic dysplasia: Chest. Note the short ribs and handle-bar appearance of the clavicles.

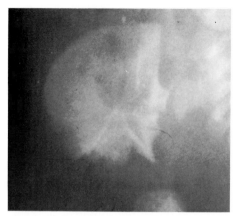

FIGURE 88–29. Asphyxiating thoracic dystrophy: Pelvis. Observe the three downward-projecting acetabular spikes.

chondroectodermal dysplasia,[89] but it differs from the latter disorder in being characterized by shorter ribs, a higher prevalence of progessive renal disease, hepatic fibrosis, less prominent nail changes, and less frequent polydactyly, especially in the hands. In addition, it is not associated with congenital heart disease or changes in the proximal portion of the tibia.

Ellis–van Creveld Dysplasia (Chondroectodermal Dysplasia). The Ellis–van Creveld dysplasia, a short-limbed dwarfism, is characterized by ectodermal dysplasia, polydactyly, and congenital heart disease.[90–96] The condition is inherited as an autosomal recessive trait and is evident at birth. Short stature, distal shortening of limbs, polydactyly, absent or hypoplastic fingernails or toenails, dysplastic teeth, upper lip abnormalities, and, less commonly, cardiac defects (atrial septal defect or a single atrium) are clinical features of the disease. In addition, renal abnormalities and hydrocephalus have been noted in some persons. Some radiographic features resemble those of familial asphyxiating thoracic dystrophy and include an elongated chest, shortened ribs with anterior osseous expansion, small sacrosciatic notches, hypoplastic ilia, a trident pelvis, and premature ossification of the proximal femoral epiphyses. In addition some patients have shortening of the tubular bones (especially the phalanges), polydactyly (especially in the

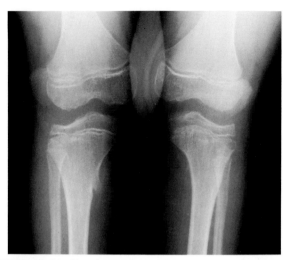

FIGURE 88–31. Chondroectodermal dysplasia. The tubular bones are shortened, with metaphyseal flaring. The lateral portion of the proximal tibial epiphyses is poorly developed. A medial diaphyseal excrescence is present on the tibia, and the patellae are dislocated.

hands), carpal fusion, an extra carpal bone, cone-shaped epiphyses, enlargement of the proximal end of the ulna and distal end of the radius (drumstick appearance), and anterior dislocation of the radial heads. A wider but hypoplastic lateral aspect of the proximal end of the tibia, medial tibial diaphyseal exostoses, genu valgum, and fibular shortening are typical (Figs. 88–31 to 88–33). The skull and spine usually are normal. Histopathologic findings in fetuses are dissimilar from those of larger infants and older children.[97]

Death in childhood is common owing to cardiac and pulmonary complications.

Atelosteogenesis and Diastrophic Dysplasia Group

Atelosteogenesis Dysplasias. Maroteaux and associates derived the term atelosteogenesis from the Greek word *atelas,* meaning ''incomplete.''[98] At least three types of this lethal short-limbed dwarfism occur. The patients exhibit dislocated large joints, clubfeet, bowed legs, midface hypoplasia, micrognathia, flat nasal bridge, and cleft palate. The radiographic features include incomplete ossification of the vertebrae, which, in addition, have coronal or sagittal clefts, and hypoplasia of the upper thoracic vertebral bodies and cervical kyphosis (Fig. 88–34).[99] The ribs may be hy-

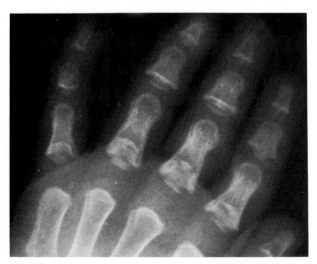

FIGURE 88–30. Asphyxiating thoracic dystrophy: Hand. Cone-shaped epiphyses and short phalanges are present.

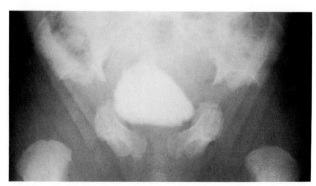

FIGURE 88–32. Chondroectodermal dysplasia. In this newborn infant, note the three downward-projecting acetabular spikes. Contrast material is present in the bladder.

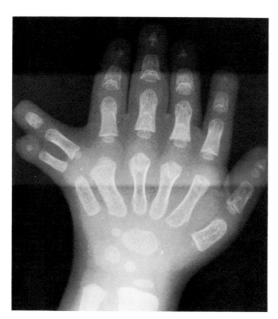

FIGURE 88–33. Chondroectodermal dysplasia. Postaxial polydactyly and shortening of the tubular bones (especially the distal phalanges, which appear as linear streaks) are apparent. Cone-shaped epiphyses are best seen in the middle phalanges. The capitate and hamate are fused, and an extra carpal ossicle appears lateral to the hamate.

poplastic. The humeri and femora are club-shaped and are narrowed distally (Fig. 88–34). The humeri and fibulae may be absent or hypoplastic. Other long tubular bones may be shortened or bowed. Some short tubular bones, especially

the proximal phalanges, are unossified. The distal phalanges may be better ossified than other bones of the hands and feet. The bones of the hands and feet can show considerable dysplastic-hypoplastic changes.[100] The pubic bones may have poor ossification or additional ossification centers.[101]

Patients with type III syndrome may survive past the newborn period. In type I, the distal phalanges are well ossified, short and wide. The other short tubular bones are unossified or hypoplastic. In type II, all the tubular bones of the hands are ossified but dysplastic. The second or third metacarpal bone, or both, may be larger than the other tubular bones. The fibula may be small but is ossified. Fewer vertebral abnormalities are present than in type I. In type III, the metacarpals are short but ossified more evenly. The proximal phalanges may have a tombstone shape.[102]

Otopalatodigital Syndrome. Two types of otopalatodigital syndrome are discussed, with the more common type I having milder findings. The type II variety overlaps with atelosteogenesis. Type II syndrome is associated with a characteristic facies, hearing defects, and digital abnormalities in the hands and feet resembling those of a tree frog, with short first digits and broad terminal phalanges.[103] The "prize fighter" facial appearance results from a prominent brow with widely spaced eyes, a broad nose, and lateral slanting of the eyes. Cleft palate is seen frequently. The inheritance pattern includes both X-linked and autosomal recessive types, with more severe involvement in boys.[104] The recessive form is associated with growth retardation and a number of minor clinical and radiologic features.[105] An association with omphaloceles is seen.[106]

The most characteristic radiographic findings found in

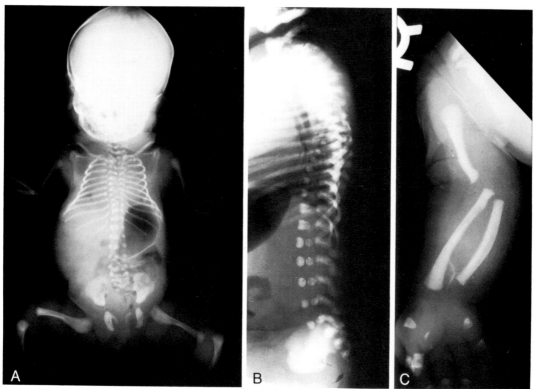

FIGURE 88–34. Atelosteogenesis dysplasias.
A Club-shaped humeri and femora, short limbs, dislocated elbows and left knee, and hypoplasia of the upper thoracic vertebrae are present. The fibulae are absent.
B Coronal cleft vertebrae are well shown.
C The humerus is club-shaped, with a hooklike distal end. The elbow is dislocated, and ossification in the hand is retarded.
(Courtesy of R. Lachman, M.D., Los Angeles, California.)

type I are in the hands and feet, consisting of shortening of the first digits and broad distal phalanges (Fig. 88–35).[107] Pseudoepiphyses and widening of the metacarpal and metatarsal bones, and short first digits, especially in the feet, may be evident. Abnormalities of the carpal bones are frequent, with a transversely oriented capitate, carpal fusions, and accessory ossicles. Similar anomalies occur in the tarsal bones. The bones of the extremities can demonstrate a lack of normal tubulation and mild bowing. Coxa valga deformity may be apparent. Radial head dislocation and underdevelopment of the proximal portion of the radius also may be seen.

The skull findings include a prominent supraorbital ridge with a thick frontal bone, absence of the frontal sinuses, a vertical clivus, prominent posterior parietal and occipital regions, and small wormian bones in the lambdoid sutures. The mastoids are poorly aerated. The chest may show pectus excavatum. Failure of ossification is seen in the vertebral bodies and the neural arches in the upper portion of the cervical spine and in some of the spinous processes. The lumbosacral canal can be widened (Fig. 88–36). Osteosclerosis is seen occasionally.[108] As mentioned earlier, features of the otopalatodigital syndrome type II overlap those of atelosteogenesis type I.[102] Death occurs in most infants with the type II syndrome due to respiratory complications. The type II patient has bowed long bones, large wavy scapulae, wavy thin ribs, long hooked clavicles, and hand and foot abnormalities.[109]

Diastrophic Dysplasia. Lamy and Maroteaux used the term diastrophic, which means ''twisted'' or ''crooked,'' to emphasize the twisted extremities and vertebral column that are found in this autosomal recessive disorder, which is characterized by short stature, progressive scoliosis and kyphosis, clubfeet, multiple contractures and dislocations, and distinctive abnormalities of the hands, feet, and ears.[110] In addition to short and broad hands and feet, the thumbs and great toes are held in a hitchhiker's position. The ear lobes are deformed from cystic masses appearing in the first few

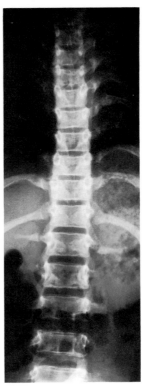

FIGURE 88–36. Otopalatodigital syndrome. Note interpediculate widening with failure of ossification in the neural arches in the lower thoracic and lumbar regions.

months of life. A cleft palate is common. Although the prognosis is good, respiratory complications resulting from tracheal collapse can cause death in infancy. A wide variability of expression is seen in this disorder, with some patients having mild symptoms. The condition may be seen in patients with E trisomy mosaicism.[111] Pseudodiastrophic dysplasia is a separate condition with platyspondyly, proximal interphalangeal joint dislocations, clubfeet that respond to therapy, and the absence of enlarged cystic ears.[112]

Radiographic findings of diastrophic dysplasia include marked shortening of the tubular bones with metaphyseal widening and rounding (Fig 88–37).[113] The epiphyses are delayed in appearance, especially the proximal femoral epiphysis, and are flattened and deformed (Fig. 88–38). Flattening is particularly marked in the outer portion of the distal femoral epiphysis. The tibial ossification center in infancy is located medially. Disproportionate shortening of the ulna and the fibula occurs. The radial heads may be dislocated. The bones of the hands and feet are small, especially the first metacarpal, which may be round or oval (Fig. 88–37). The epiphyses in the hands may be irregular, distorted, and wide. The carpal bones may ossify prematurely (Fig. 88–37), appear deformed, or reveal accessory ossification centers. The feet show similar findings in addition to equinovarus deformity. The most common finding in the foot is hindfoot valgus deformity and metatarsus adductus.[114] Narrowing of the joint spaces may be marked, especially in the hips and elbows, with late degenerative changes. Femora may have broad intertrochanteric regions with short femoral necks (Fig. 88–38). Scoliosis sometimes is evident at or soon after birth and tends to be progressive and rigid. The cervical vertebrae may reveal defective development, which can lead to kyphosis, spinal instability,

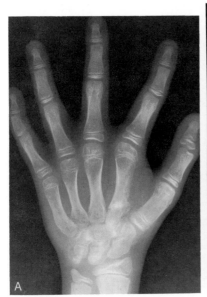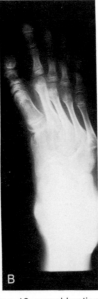

FIGURE 88–35. Otopalatodigital syndrome. In a 12 year old patient, findings include osseous shortening, especially in the first digits, a proximally pointed pseudoepiphysis of the second metacarpal bone, carpal deformities, epiphyseal flattening, and tarsal fusions.

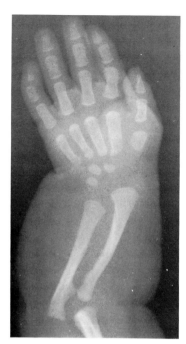

FIGURE 88–37. Diastrophic dysplasia. The tubular bones of the forearm are shortened, especially the distal portion of the ulna, and bowing of the distal portion of the radius is seen. Premature carpal ossification, a rounded first metacarpal bone, and clinodactyly of the fifth digit also are present.

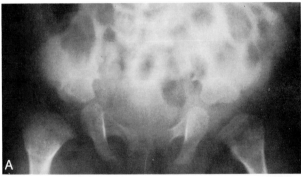

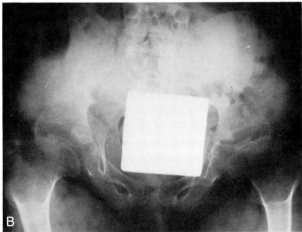

FIGURE 88–38. Diastrophic dysplasia.
A In this newborn infant, the hip joints are narrow, the femoral necks are short, and the intertrochanteric regions of the femur are broad.
B These findings persist 5 years later. Small, flat femoral epiphyses now are present.

spinal cord compression, and death.[115, 116] Slight narrowing of the interpediculate distances is seen distally in the lumbar spine. Calcification of the pinna of the ear and airway cartilages sometimes is seen.

Kniest and Stickler Dysplasia Group

Dyssegmental Dysplasia. Dyssegmental dysplasia, a neonatal condition characterized by short curved limbs, narrow thorax, short neck, and limitation of joint motion, has been confused with Kniest's dysplasia.[117] Two forms exist: the lethal Silverman-Handmaker type (Fig. 88–39) and the less severe Rolland-Desbuquois type.[118, 119] A variety of other findings include hydrocephalus, hydronephrosis, cleft palate, and inguinal hernias. The condition is considered to be of autosomal recessive inheritance.

Radiographically, the spine is characterized by marked variation in the size, width, and shape of the vertebral bodies; coronal clefts; sagittal clefts; vertebral wedging; and the absence of normal widening of the interpediculate distances in the lower lumbar spine (Fig. 88–39). Anisospondyly is the term given to these abnormal vertebral bodies, which do not correspond in shape to normal vertebrae.[120] The long tubular bones are short and wide and reveal metaphyseal widening, cupping, angular deformities, and even pseudofractures. Epiphyseal ossification is delayed, whereas ossification of the carpal bones may not be delayed. The short tubular bones are short and thick. The first metatarsal bone may be enlarged. The thorax is small with flared, irregular rib ends. Hypoplasia of the scapula can be present. The iliac bones are decreased in height and have rounded lateral contours and small sacrosciatic notches; the pubic and ischial bones are broad and short. The midface and mandible may be hypoplastic. The spine changes are more severe in the Silverman-Handmaker type and seen more easily on both the frontal and lateral radiographs of the spine.

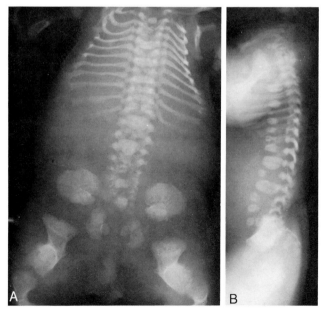

FIGURE 88–39. Dyssegmental dysplasia. The vertebrae vary in size and demonstrate faulty segmentation and coronal clefts. The tubular bones are short and have wide ends and angular deformities. The iliac bones also are short, with rounded lateral margins. (Courtesy of A. Poznanski, M.D., Chicago, Illinois.)

The abnormalities in this syndrome may relate to a defect in the early embryonic process of segmentation. A genetically determined fault in collagen development may have occurred.[121] The diagnosis has been made prenatally.[122]

Kniest's Dysplasia. The clinical findings in Kniest's dysplasia include a short trunk, prominent joints (especially the knees), and flattened face with a depressed nasal bridge. Ocular abnormalities (particularly myopia and retinal detachments), stiff joints, deafness, inguinal hernias, hip dislocation, delayed ambulation, cleft palate, and clubfeet occur. Marked dorsal kyphosis or kyphoscoliosis and lumbar lordosis develop. This disease has been associated with a severe form of the Pierre Robin syndrome and external hydrocephalus.[123] It is believed to be of autosomal dominant inheritance.

Radiographic findings include shortening of the tubular bones, with flaring of the ends, including both the metaphyses and the epiphyses.[124] Epiphyseal development is delayed, especially in the proximal portion of the femora (Fig. 88–40A). MR imaging has shown small ossified femoral heads surrounded by large cartilaginous femoral heads.[125] The epiphyses may be flattened and irregular, although those about the knees may become somewhat large as the child grows. The changes are progressive. Irregularity occurs on both sides of the growth plate. The epiphyses of the hand are fragmented, flattened, and squared. Swelling about the interphalangeal joints may be associated with periarticular osseous enlargement similar to Heberden's and Bouchard's nodes. The carpal bones are small and irregular, and the adjacent joint spaces may be narrowed (Fig. 88–40B). The spine demonstrates generalized osseous flattening with anterior tapering of the vertebral bodies (Fig. 88–41). Some vertebral endplate irregularity may be present. Coronal clefts, usually in the lumbar spine, often are apparent in infants. Kyphoscoliosis develops. The odontoid may be enlarged. In addition to marked delay in ossification of the femoral capital epiphyses and pubic bones, pelvic abnormalities include broad and short femoral necks, marked coxa vara, and hip contractures. The iliac bones are decreased in vertical height, rounded, and underdeveloped inferiorly.

Histologic evaluation reveals friable cartilage with irregularity in both cellular size and matrix staining. The combination of hypertrophic cartilage cells and surrounding loose matrix containing large holes resembles Swiss cheese.[126, 127] A basic defect in type II collagen has been proposed as the abnormality in this syndrome.[128]

Otospondylomegaepiphyseal Dysplasia. By introducing four new cases and reviewing two previously reported cases, Giedion and collaborators, in 1982, defined a syndrome consisting of deafness, extremity shortening, enlarged knees and elbows, back pain, and prominent proximal interphalangeal joints in the hands.[129] Presumably it is inherited as an autosomal recessive trait. Radiographically enlarged epiphyses are evident, especially in the knees, after infancy. The lower thoracic spine contains vertebral bodies that are flattened. Coronal cleft vertebrae may be seen in the very young. The odontoid process may be enlarged. The soft tissues of the fingers may be increased, and the carpal and tarsal bones as well as the epiphyses of the metacarpal and metatarsal bones are large. The iliac wings may be square.

McAlister and coworkers described a patient in whom enlarged epiphyses, osteoporosis, wrinkly skin, and an aged appearance were seen (Fig. 88–42).[130] Silverman and Reiley reported eight patients with megaepiphyses, defective vertebral and pelvic ossification, and metaphyseal dysplasia.[131]

Stickler's Dysplasia. In 1965, Stickler and coworkers described a kindred having eye problems and swollen joints.[132] The predominant ophthalmic features of this autosomal dominant disease, also called arthro-ophthalmopathy, are severe myopia, retinal detachment, vitreoretinal degeneration, and blindness. Enlargement, swelling, and redness of joints, particularly the knees, ankles, and wrists, are noted in childhood. The face may reveal a depressed nasal bridge, cleft palate, and small mandible. The Pierre Robin syndrome is seen frequently in infants. Neurosensory hearing loss is common.[133] Radiographic features (which often are the most helpful clue to the diagnosis)[134] include flattening of the epiphyses and joint space narrowing. Underdevelopment of the lateral portion of the distal tibial epiphysis is especially characteristic (Fig. 88–43A). Premature degen-

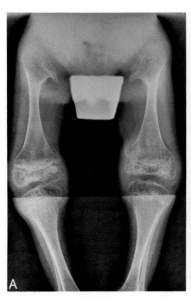
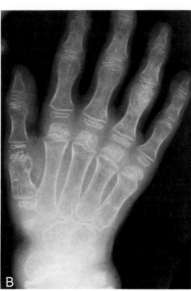

FIGURE 88–40. Kniest's dysplasia.

  A In the lower extremities, observe metaphyseal expansion and irregular epiphyseal ossification. Note the delay in appearance of ossification in the capital femoral epiphyses.

  B In the hand, osteopenia, prominence about the joints, irregular carpal bones, and epiphyseal irregularity and flattening are seen.

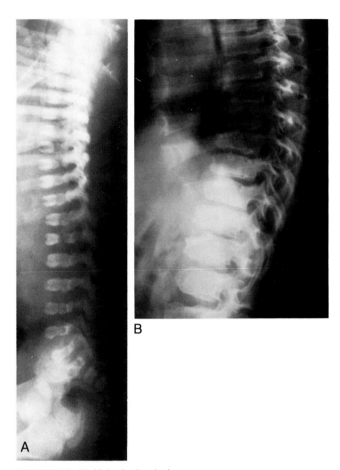

FIGURE 88–41. Kniest's dysplasia.
  A Newborn. Some vertebral flattening with anterior tapering and coronal cleft vertebrae are shown.
  B Child. Note vertebral flattening and irregularity.

erative joint disease is noted in adults. The metacarpal bones of the hands can be broad, with adjacent joint space narrowing, accessory ossicles, and clinodactyly of the fifth digit (Fig. 88–43B). Also noted are relative metaphyseal expansion, wide femoral necks, coxa valga, and hypoplasia of the iliac wings. Underdevelopment of the anterior por-

tion of the maxilla is common.[135] Mild alterations in a few of the vertebral endplates resemble those seen in Scheuermann's disease (Fig. 88–43C). Mutations in type II collagen may be responsible for Stickler's syndrome.[136]

Other Spondyloepimetaphyseal Dysplasias

X-Linked Spondyloepiphyseal Dysplasia Tarda. The X-linked recessive condition occurs only in male subjects and generally becomes evident between the ages of 5 and 10 years because of impaired spinal growth.[137] In addition, autosomal dominant and autosomal recessive forms occur.[138] Complaints of back and hip pain are common, particularly in adults. The extremities and face are normal. Radiographic findings in the spine predominate in the lumbar area and are quite characteristic, consisting of vertebral bodies that have a hump-shaped area of dense bone on the central and posterior portions of the endplates (Fig. 88–44). The disc spaces appear narrow posteriorly and wide anteriorly. The odontoid process may be deformed. Degenerative spinal changes develop in early adulthood.[139] The bones in the pelvis and the femoral necks may appear slightly small. Coxa vara may be present. The chest has a relative increase in its anteroposterior diameter. Mild flattening of the epiphyses occurs about the major joints, especially the hips and the shoulders. Osteoarthritis, particularly in the hips, eventually can become disabling.[140] Affected persons may have thoracic disc herniation.[141]

Spondyloepimetaphyseal Dysplasia. Spondyloepimetaphyseal dysplasia encompasses a heterogeneous group of conditions that are characterized by involvement of the spine, epiphyses, and metaphyses, resulting in osseous shortening and deformities. These conditions are to be distinguished from others that may affect similar portions of the skeleton, such as metatropic dysplasia and pseudoachondroplasia. Kozlowski, in 1974, described the micromelic type of spondyloepimetaphyseal dysplasia, presumed to be of autosomal recessive inheritance, with greatest shortening in the proximal portion of the limbs, relatively long hands and feet, and genu valgum.[142] Affected patients had scoliosis, increased lordosis, facial flattening, and hypertelorism. Another variety, the Irapa type (named after

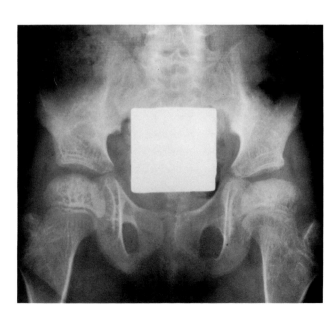

FIGURE 88–42. Macroepiphyseal dysplasia with osteoporosis, wrinkled skin, and aged appearance. This 5 year old child has osteoporosis and markedly enlarged femoral capital epiphyses.

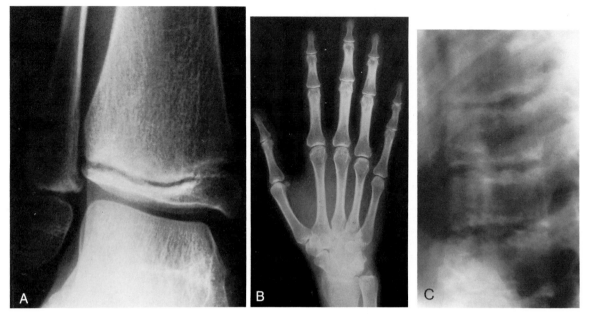

FIGURE 88–43. Arthro-ophthalmopathy (Stickler's dysplasia).
  A The distal tibial epiphysis is underdeveloped, most marked in its lateral portion, producing a talar slant in this 7 year old child.
  B Observe mild joint space narrowing in the hand and wrist.
  C A radiograph of the spine reveals narrowing of the intervertebral discs and endplate irregularity, simulating the appearance of Scheuermann's disease.

the Indians of the Irapa tribe of Venezuela, in whom the disease was evident), is characterized by shortening of the tubular bones, epimetaphyseal dysplasia, platyspondyly, osteopenia, abnormal carpal bones, a decreased size of the pelvic bones, coxa vara, and premature degenerative joint disease.[143] Other types include that associated with joint laxity, cone epiphyses, severe platyspondyly, and hypotrichosis.[144]

In 1982, Anderson and collaborators[145] reviewed 14 patients with a unique form of spondyloepimetaphyseal dysplasia, the Strudwick type (Fig. 88–45).[146] Considerable heterogeneity may exist in this latter condition. In the neonatal period, the radiographic findings of this form of spondyloepimetaphyseal dysplasia resemble those of spondyloepiphyseal dysplasia congenita, with delayed epiphyseal ossification and flattened epiphyses. The failure of epiphys-

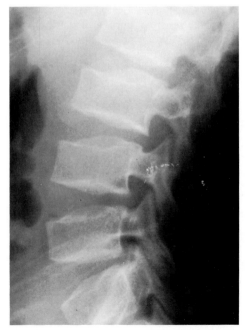

FIGURE 88–44. Spondyloepiphyseal dysplasia tarda, X-linked recessive syndrome. The characteristic osseous "humps" are evident in the central and posterior portions of the vertebral endplates. The disc spaces are narrow posteriorly and wide anteriorly.

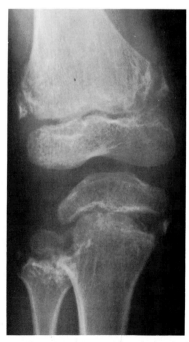

FIGURE 88–45. Spondyloepimetaphyseal dysplasia (Strudwick type). Flattened epiphyses and irregularly ossified metaphyses are evident.

eal ossification is especially marked in the proximal portion of the femora. The metaphyses develop a mottled appearance, with both sclerotic and lucent areas (Fig. 88–45). The fibula may be more involved than the tibia and the ulna more than the radius. The irregularity of the metaphyses that develops during infancy distinguishes this condition from spondyloepiphyseal dysplasia congenita.[147] Findings in the pelvis and hips include coxa vara, which may be severe, small sacrosciatic notches, delayed ossification of the pubic bones, and prominent proximal regions of the femora. The vertebral bodies may be pear-shaped, with posterior hypoplasia, findings best observed in the lumbar spine. The ribs reveal anterior flaring. Spinal cord compression can result from hypoplasia of the odontoid process and atlantoaxial instability.

A number of other related conditions exist that are difficult to classify but some have typical radiographic changes, such as found in opsismodysplasia, a condition with severe platyspondyly, tubular bone shortening, metaphyseal cupping, and marked delay in epiphyseal ossification.[148]

Progressive Pseudorheumatoid Chondrodysplasia. This autosomal recessive condition is characterized by progressive arthropathy and platyspondyly.[149, 150] Between the ages of 3 and 8 years, pain, swelling, and stiffness develop about multiple joints, particularly in the hands. The disease can start in early infancy, however.[151] The symptoms are similar to those of rheumatoid arthritis, but synovitis is absent. Progressive joint disease and contractures occur that are crippling to the patients. Short stature results from spinal abnormalities that include generalized flattening of the vertebrae with occasional kyphosis or scoliosis (Fig. 88–46A). Defective ossification can be evident in the anterior portions of the vertebral bodies.[149] Elsewhere, generalized epiphyseal irregularity and flattening of varying degree occur.[152] Enlargement of the epiphyses and metaphyses in the bones of the hands, particularly those about the proximal interphalangeal joints, is evident, and subsequent joint space narrowing is seen. Periarticular osteoporosis is common. The femoral necks are short, and the proximal femoral epiphyses are large. Eventually, epiphyseal flattening and secondary osteoarthritis become apparent (Fig. 88–46B).[153]

Dyggve-Melchior-Clausen Dysplasia. Dyggve, Melchior, and Clausen first described a dysplasia in three dwarfed and mentally retarded siblings; however, mental retardation is not uniformly present in this syndrome.[154] Affected persons have a short trunk, a protruding sternum, lumbar lordosis, genu valgum, a waddling gait, and a small head. Joint mobility is decreased.

Radiographic findings in the spine include flattened vertebral bodies that are pointed anteriorly[155, 156] and commonly contain notchlike defects that lead to a ''camel hump'' appearance (Fig. 88–47A). Scoliosis or kyphosis and increased lumbar lordosis are evident. A hypoplastic odontoid process may result in atlantoaxial instability. The iliac bones are short and broad with lacelike borders. Indeed, this lacelike appearance of the iliac crests is one of the more characteristic components of the disease (Fig. 88–47B). Patients show a relative increase in the transverse diameter of the pelvic inlet. The ischial bones are widened, shortened, and somewhat irregular. Ossification in the femoral heads is delayed. The acetabula become progressively dysplastic as a consequence of hip dislocations. In younger patients, the proximal femoral growth plate may be oriented horizontally, with a prominent medial projection and irregular metaphyses. In the hand, the tubular bones may be shortened (especially in the first digit); in addition pseudoepiphyses may be present in the proximal portion of the second metacarpal bone, and the proximal and middle phalanges can have cone-shaped epiphyses. During their development, the carpal bones may be small and irregular. In the thorax, anterior bowing of the sternum, a decreased size of the scapula, and widened anterior ends of the ribs are seen.

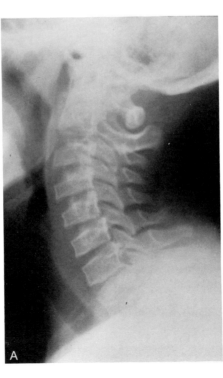
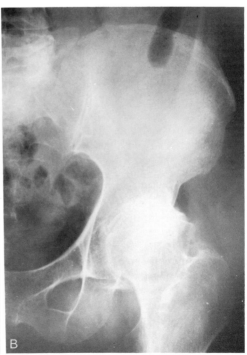

FIGURE 88–46. Progressive pseudorheumatoid chondrodysplasia.

A In this 13 year old patient, flattening of the vertebral bodies is evident.

B In a 30 year old woman, marked narrowing of the joint space of the hip is accompanied by bone sclerosis and osteophytosis.

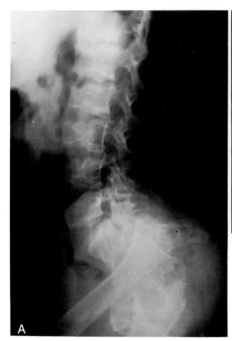

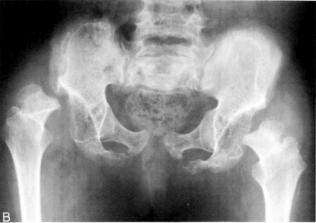

FIGURE 88–47. Dyggve-Melchior-Clausen dysplasia.
A The lumbar vertebral bodies show superior and inferior defects in the endplates, producing a "camel hump" appearance.
B The lacelike iliac crests are well seen in an 11 year old child. The right hip is dislocated; on the left side, subluxation of the femoral head is evident.

The long tubular bones contain flattened epiphyses with adjacent joint space narrowing. Additionally, metaphyseal defects are seen in childhood.

Histopathologic and histochemical studies on biopsy specimens have been described.[157, 158] This syndrome is considered to be an autosomal recessive disease, although reports also have documented an X-linked recessive inheritance pattern.[159]

Wolcott-Rallison Dysplasia. Wolcott-Rallison dysplasia is a mild spondyloepiphyseal dysplasia with an onset of diabetes mellitus in infancy.[160] The epiphyseal development is delayed and the proximal femoral epiphysis may become reabsorbed, with hip dislocation. The platyspondyly is mild.

Pseudoachondroplasia. In 1959, Maroteaux and Lamy described a type of dwarfism that resembled achondroplasia, with short stature becoming apparent after the age of 2 years. In pseudoachondroplasia, the head is normal and the hands and feet are shorter than those seen in true achondroplasia.[161] The legs may be bowed, and the gait is waddling.

Radiographic findings become apparent in late infancy and are modified throughout childhood.[162] Initially, the epiphyses are small and flattened (Fig. 88–48A). The metaphyses are wide, with dense, mushroom-shaped provisional zones of calcification (Fig. 88–48A). In the adult, the tubular bones are short and expanded at their ends (Fig. 88–48B). The epiphyses remain abnormal, and premature degenerative arthritis develops as the metaphyseal irregularity resolves. A long fibula may be seen. The vertebral bodies initially are oval or biconvex, with central tongue-like anterior projections (Fig. 88–49A); later they become wedged or flattened, but the vertebral bodies can have a more normal appearance in adulthood. About one half of patients have some vertebral endplate irregularity in childhood. Mild to moderate scoliosis with lumbar lordosis is common; atlantoaxial instability and odontoid hypoplasia also may be present. In early childhood, small capital femoral epiphyses and delayed development of the pubic bones and ischia are seen. The widening and delayed development

of the triradiate cartilage is characteristic. The inferior border of the ilium has a sloping acetabular angle and a spiked appearance (Fig. 88–49B). The iliac wings may be slightly underdeveloped. As the patient grows, the pelvis becomes more normal in appearance, although coxa vara and deformity of the femoral heads persist. The hands and feet have short, wide tubular bones with irregular epiphyses. Proxi-

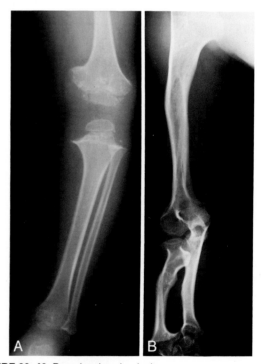

FIGURE 88–48. Pseudoachondroplasia.
A Note the small epiphyses and metaphyseal flaring in a 5 year old child.
B In an adult, the bones of the upper extremity are short, especially those in the forearm, and reveal metaphyseal flaring.

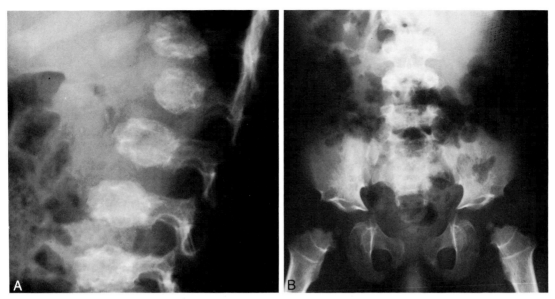

FIGURE 88–49. Pseudoachondroplasia.
  A In a 5 year old child, the vertebral bodies are rounded, with anterior tongues. Note hypoplasia of the first lumbar vertebra.
  B Typical pelvic findings include tiny capital femoral epiphyses, sloping acetabular roofs with medial and lateral osseous spikes, and a delay in pubic ossification.

mal pointing of the metacarpal bones may resolve by older childhood. The carpal bones initially are delayed in appearance and irregular but become more normal in appearance in adulthood. The distal portions of the radius and ulna can be angled toward one another. The posterior end of the ribs is cupped in childhood and the lower angle of the scapula is slow to develop.

On the basis of histologic studies, pseudoachondroplasia has been assumed to be a generalized cartilage disorder related to abnormalities of proteoglycans.[163] Although this condition has been separated into various types, the delineations are not complete because of the inability to differentiate clearly among apparent autosomal dominant and recessive forms.[164, 165] Wynn-Davies and coworkers suggested that both forms be subdivided into mild and severe.[166]

Myotonic Chondrodysplasia (Catel-Schwartz-Jampel Dysplasia). Myotonic chondrodysplasia, an autosomal recessive condition, is characterized by short stature, myotonia, immobile or masklike facies, blepharophimosis, joint contracture, kyphosis, and pectus carinatum. Precise further classification of this condition is unclear, although some patients have evidence of an immune deficiency.[167] Radiographic findings include changes in the capital femoral epiphyses consisting of delayed ossification, osseous irregularity and flattening, premature degenerative changes, coxa vara or coxa valga, and a triangular deformity of the pelvis with flared iliac wings.[168] Diffuse platyspondyly, coronal cleft vertebrae, kyphosis or kyphoscoliosis, and basilar invagination also have been noted (Fig. 88–50). With the exception of the hips, the epiphyseal and metaphyseal changes in the tubular bones are mild, although tibial bowing can be present. One 16 year old patient developed a Brown-Sequard syndrome secondary to stenosis in the cervical spine.[169]

Spondylometaphyseal Dysplasias

This poorly defined and complex group of diseases is characterized by abnormalities in the vertebrae and metaphyses of tubular bones. Considerable heterogeneity can be found in the clinical and radiographic appearances.[170–172] Maroteaux and Spranger tried to clarify the situation by subdividing the disorder into three subgroups on the basis of the appearance of the femoral necks and into a distinctive Kozlowski type.[173] A modified version of their classification is given here.

1. Kozlowski type
2. Severe coxa vara
   a. Mild vertebral abnormalities
      1. Discrete metaphyseal change (Sutcliffe)
      2. More severe metaphyseal changes (corner fracture type)

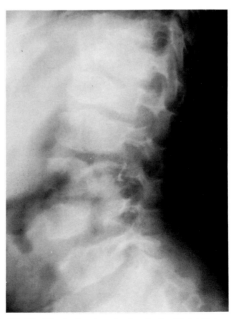

FIGURE 88–50. Myotonic chondrodysplasia (Catel-Schwartz-Jampel dysplasia). Diffuse vertebral flattening and residual coronal cleft vertebrae are seen.

b. Round vertebral bodies

c. Flattened vertebral bodies with tonguelike deformity

3. Moderate changes of the femoral neck

a. Slight vertebral body irregularity, short tubular bones of the hands with irregular metaphyses

b. Generalized platyspondyly

4. Discrete metaphyseal changes of the femoral neck

a. Squared vertebral bodies with irregular contours

b. Moderately flattened and long vertebral bodies (in the lateral projection)

c. Trapezoidal aspect of the vertebral bodies

The most common type of spondylometaphyseal dysplasia, described by Kozlowski in 1967, is accompanied by a short stature, kyphosis and scoliosis, diminutive hands and feet, bowing of the bones, and, in the lower extremities, joint limitation and gait disturbance. It is an autosomal dominant disorder.[170] Radiographically, the vertebral bodies are flattened appreciably and can be deformed further with spinal curvatures (Fig. 88–51A). The pedicles are located medially. Irregular metaphyses are most marked in the proximal portion of the femora, where coxa vara also is evident (Fig. 88–51B); the metaphyseal disease can improve with immobilization techniques, including bracing.[174] The ilia are shortened in their craniocaudal dimension, and the sacrosciatic notches are small. Some irregularity occurs in the horizontally oriented acetabular roofs (Fig. 88–51B). Flattening and irregularity in the epiphyses usually are mild, although premature degenerative changes are noted in the joints. The carpal and tarsal bones reveal markedly retarded skeletal maturation.

Patients with the corner fracture type have severe coxa vara, small triangular bone fragments (corner fracture appearance) at the periphery of the metaphyses adjacent to the growth plate, lower thoracic and upper lumbar exaggerated endplate convexity, and some anterior vertebral wedging.[175]

Spondyloenchondroplasia. Schorr and coworkers[176] described two brothers with enchondromatous-like changes in the long tubular bones, platyspondyly, and irregular vertebral endplates. Radiolucent islands in the posterior portions of the vertebral bodies and metaphyseal lucent and sclerotic streaks extending into the shafts of the bones of the extremities were evident. Changes were more obvious in the fibulae and ulnae than in the tibiae or radii.[177] Basal ganglia calcifications may be seen. The inheritance pattern of this syndrome probably is autosomal recessive.

Multiple Epiphyseal Dysplasias

This condition is discussed in Chapter 87.

Chondrodysplasia Punctata (Stippled Epiphyses) Group

A great deal of confusion has surrounded the disorder chondrodysplasia punctata owing to the variability of its clinical findings and to the number of disorders associated with stippled epiphyses, a hallmark of this condition. The separation of this disorder into at least four types has lessened the confusion.

Chondrodysplasia Punctata, Rhizomelic Type. This autosomal recessive disorder is the most clearly recognizable one and is characterized by marked rhizomelic shortening of the extremities, a flat face, a depressed nasal bridge, microcephaly, lymphedema of the cheeks, psychomotor retardation, cataracts, and joint contractures.[178] The skin may be thick, scaly, and dry. Most infants die from failure to thrive or from recurrent infections.

Radiographic findings include severe, symmetric rhizo-

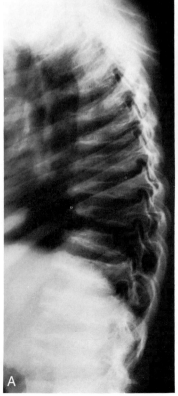
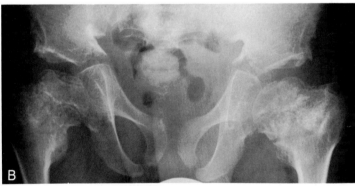

FIGURE 88–51. Spondylometaphyseal dysplasia, Kozlowski type.

A Marked flattening of the vertebral bodies with anterior wedging in the thoracic spine is seen.

B In the pelvis, shortened femoral necks, metaphyseal and epiphyseal irregularities, flat broad acetabula, and narrow sacrosciatic notches are evident.

melic shortening of the tubular bones, with metaphyseal splaying and abundant stippled calcification in the ends of the long bones (Fig. 88–52A). Epiphyseal ossification is delayed. Calcifications are seen adjacent to the spine, especially in the cervical and sacral regions, and adjacent to the pubic, ischial, tarsal, and carpal bones, patellae, and ribs. The respiratory airway can be narrowed by abnormal calcification in the laryngeal and tracheal cartilages. Lateral radiographs of the spine show anterior and posterior ossification centers separated by a lucent band. This so-called coronal cleft appearance appears to be due to an overproduction of cartilage in the zone between the dorsal and central ossification centers of the vertebral body (Fig. 88–52B).[179] The vertebral bodies are irregular, and kyphoscoliosis may develop. The iliac wings lack normal flaring. The stippling tends to resolve, especially in the patients who survive beyond infancy, and the bones become more osteopenic.

The most striking histologic changes are seen in the growth plates of the long bones, where maturation of cartilage cells is disturbed and a lack of the normal columnar arrangement of chondrocytes is evident.[180] Similar but less severe changes have been seen in the Conradi-Hünermann form (see subsequent discussion). An inborn error of peroxisome metabolism similar to that seen in the Zellweger syndrome has been found in this rhizomelic type of chondrodysplasia punctata, although radiographically the Zellweger syndrome resembles the Conradi-Hünermann form of chondrodysplasia punctata more closely. The diagnosis of the rhizomelic type of disease has been made prenatally by biochemical analysis.[181]

Chondrodysplasia Punctata, Conradi-Hünermann or Conradi's Type.[182, 183] This form is autosomal dominant in

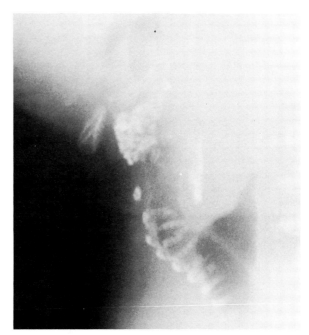

FIGURE 88–53. Chondrodysplasia punctata: Conradi-Hünermann form. The laryngeal and tracheal cartilages are irregularly calcified.

its inheritance pattern and affects girls more often than boys. It may be apparent at birth, owing to facial characteristics that include a flattened nasal tip with a deep nasal bridge and a prominent forehead. Some degree of limb shortening occurs in a majority of patients but may be asymmetric. Limitation of articular motion and joint contractures are common. Other findings include "squareness" and deformity of the hands, clubfeet, dislocated hips, genu valgum, kyphoscoliosis, and short stature. Cataracts are far less common than in the rhizomelic form of the disease. Other ocular anomalies include glaucoma, corneal clouding, and microphthalmia. Cutaneous manifestations of the disease are present in approximately 20 per cent of patients; these include cutaneous thickening and scaling, an orange peel appearance of the skin, sparse eyebrows and eyelashes, and alopecia. Congenital cardiac malformations are found in approximately 10 per cent of the patients.

Radiographic findings consist of calcific deposits in and around epiphyses and other cartilaginous areas, such as the trachea (Fig. 88–53). These calcifications often resolve by early childhood.[184] Areas that commonly are involved include the acetabulum, proximal portion of the femur, patella, spine, and carpal and tarsal bones (Fig. 88–54). Shortening of the long tubular bones in a unilateral or bilateral distribution is seen. The metaphyseal regions appear normal. In addition to stippling, the spine may show scoliosis, which may be partly attributable to limb shortening. Coronal cleft vertebrae are infrequent. In more severe cases, epiphyseal dysplasia and early degenerative changes often are evident.

Lawrence and coworkers described five atypical findings that may be seen in this condition, namely, an absent long bone, unilateral stippling, thick cone-shaped epiphyses in the distal phalanges, severe bowing of long tubular bones, and shortening of a single digit.[185]

Chondrodysplasia Punctata, X-Linked Recessive Type. Curry and associates reported two families in which an

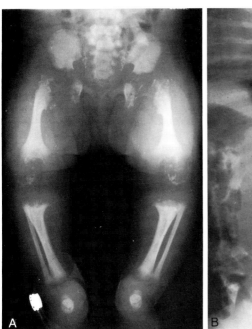
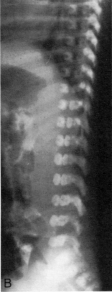

FIGURE 88–52. Chondrodysplasia punctata: Autosomal recessive rhizomelic form.

A The lower extremities reveal rhizomelic shortening, stippled calcifications, particularly about the hips and knees, and metaphyseal flaring.

B Coronal cleft vertebrae are shown.

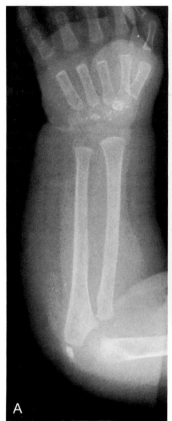

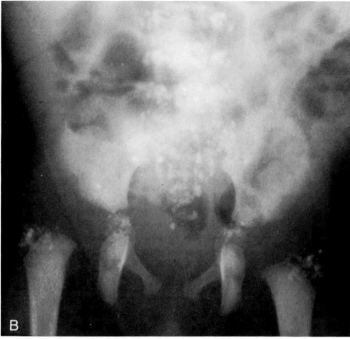

FIGURE 88–54. Chondrodysplasia punctata: Conradi-Hünermann form.

A Calcifications are seen about the elbow and wrist. Otherwise, the bones appear relatively normal.

B In a newborn infant, abundant calcifications are evident in the spine, acetabula, and proximal portion of the femora.

inherited deletion of the short arm of the X chromosome was evident in four boys who had features resembling most closely those of the Conradi-Hünermann form.[186] The patients were mentally retarded, had symmetrically distributed epiphyseal stippling in infancy (Fig. 88–55), and had distal phalangeal hypoplasia. Female carriers either had broad wrists, short arms, and decreased carpal angles or were normal.

The condition is characterized by the stippled calcifica-

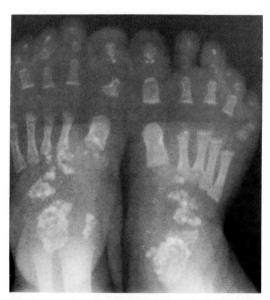

FIGURE 88–55. Chondrodysplasia punctata: X-linked recessive form. In this newborn infant, multiple calcifications, particularly about the tarsal bones, are accompanied by phalangeal deformities.

tions and skin lesions of ichthyosis in early infancy; later, atrophic skin changes occur.[187] Scoliosis or kyphoscoliosis, asymmetric shortening of the tubular bones, short stature, and joint dislocations also are seen. Murine models of this disorder exist,[188] and the disease has been associated with chromosomal abnormalities.[189] An X-linked dominant form may exist.

Chondrodysplasia Punctata, Tibia-Metacarpal Type. The features of this form include midface hypoplasia, depressed nasal bridge, small mandible, and short neck and limbs.[190] Radiographic findings include shortening of the metacarpal bones, especially the fourth, with calcific stippling. The tibiae are short with relatively long fibulae. The distal ends of the ulnae are hypoplastic, with proximal dislocation and bowing of the radii. The distal ends of the phalanges, humeri, and femora also may be shortened. Tarsal stippling is seen. The vertebrae show deficient ossification in the cervical spine, coronal clefts, and stippling of the sacrum in infancy.[190]

Epiphyseal stippling also can be found in infants born to mothers taking warfarin sodium or phenytoin and in patients with the fetal alcohol syndrome, chromosomal abnormalities, prenatal rubella infection, the CHILD syndrome, and Zellweger's syndrome. The last-mentioned disorder is characterized by manifestations that include craniofacial dysmorphism, profound hypotonia, dysgenesis of the brain, renal cortical cysts, and soft tissue calcifications, especially about the patella and hip.

Metaphyseal Dysplasias

This term applies to a number of conditions in which the greatest involvement occurs in the metaphyses, which are flared and irregular; the epiphyses and diaphyses also may be abnormal, however. The spine is normal or involved minimally. The Jansen, Schmid, McKusick, and Schwachman-Diamond syndromes, adenosine deaminase deficiency, and metaphyseal anadysplasia are discussed here. Less common forms, such as those described by Vaandrager, Spahr, Koslowski, Pena, Wiedemann, Spranger, Jequier, and Kaitila, and the metaphyseal dysplasias associated with hereditary lymphopenic agammaglobulinemia and cone epiphyses, are not discussed here.[191, 192]

Metaphyseal Dysplasia, Jansen Type. The Jansen type is a rare but severe disorder characterized by marked dwarfism, swelling of the joints, and bowed forearms and legs.[193] The face has typical features: frontonasal hyperplasia, hypertelorism, and a receding chin. The inheritance pattern is autosomal dominant. Radiographic findings depend on the patient's age. In infancy marked irregularity of the metaphyses, widening of the growth plates, diffuse osteopenia, and mild bowing of long tubular bones are seen. The metaphyseal changes also are apparent in the short tubular bones. In this age group, permeative radiolucent areas are seen throughout the long bones. Subperiosteal bone resorption and fractures have led to diagnostic confusion with hyperparathyroidism, a clinical dilemma that is compounded in some patients by the presence of hypercalcemia. In childhood, the metaphyses become cupped, with wide zones of irregular calcification that eventually disappear as the growth plate closes in adults. The resultant bones are shortened and bowed and have metaphyseal flaring (Fig. 88–56).[194] The phalanges of the hand are more affected than the metacarpal bones. The skull is osteopenic, with basilar and supraorbital ridge sclerosis, underdevelopment of the mastoid air cells and sinuses, and mandibular hypoplasia.[195] The spine shows minimal platyspondyly. The anterior ends of the ribs are flared. Ozonoff reported a patient who died at the age of 6 years with cor pulmonale secondary to

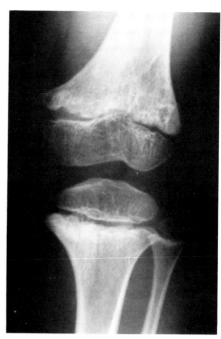

FIGURE 88–57. Metaphyseal dysplasia: Schmid type. In a 5 year old child, the tubular bones are short, and V-shaped metaphyseal irregularities are present, best observed in the femur.

progressive rib involvement, at the same time that the changes in the long bones were improving.[196]

Metaphyseal Dysplasia, Schmid Type. The inheritance of the Schmid type is autosomal dominant. Patients have short stature of variable severity and bowed legs; the disorder usually becomes manifest after infancy.[197] Radiographically metaphyseal irregularity, flaring, and growth plate widening are present and most obvious about the knees and hips (Fig. 88–57). Proximal femoral metaphyseal involvement with resultant coxa vara beginning after the third year of life is common.[198] The anterior ends of the ribs are flared, but the spine and hands are not involved. After physeal closure, osseous shortening and deformities remain. Histologically, nonspecific disorganization of the cartilage in the growth plate and retardation of endochondral bone formation are seen.[199] The abnormalities in this condition may be confused with the skeletal changes of child abuse.[200]

Metaphyseal Dysplasia, McKusick Type. The McKusick type was first described in 1964 by McKusick and collaborators in the Amish.[201] Of autosomal recessive inheritance, it often is termed cartilage-hair hypoplasia. The patients are of normal intelligence and are very short, with fine, light-colored hair, small hands, bowed legs, and joint laxity. The rate of congenital megacolon is increased. Complex immune deficiencies are seen with a resultant increase in the frequency of infections (some of which may be fatal) and malignant tumors.[202, 203] Radiographic findings include minimal epiphyseal flattening and an irregular provisional zone of calcification, with metaphyseal cupping and flaring (Fig. 88–58).[204] Discrete round or cystic metaphyseal irregularities are interspersed with normal-appearing provisional zones of calcification. Metaphyseal abnormalities are most prominent in the lower extremities and, when severe, are associated with a shorter stature.[205] The fibula is relatively long and contributes to the foot deformities seen in some persons. Subluxation or dislocation of the radial head oc-

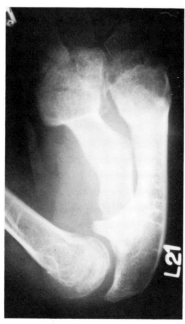

FIGURE 88–56. Metaphyseal dysplasia: Jansen type. Marked shortening, bowing, and metaphyseal expansion of the bones in the forearm are seen in an 11 year old patient.

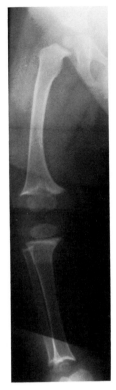

FIGURE 88–58. Metaphyseal dysplasia: McKusick type. In a 9 month old child the tubular bones are short, and V-shaped metaphyseal irregularities are present, best observed in the femur.

casionally is present. The bones in the hands and feet are small, and the carpal bones appear irregular. The vertebral bodies are small. Additional vertebral abnormalities include atlantoaxial subluxation with odontoid hypoplasia,[206] mild endplate abnormalities believed to represent Schmorl's nodes, mild scoliosis, and accentuated lumbar lordosis. Flaring and lucent regions in the anterior end of the ribs, a short sternum, and pectus carinatum also may be evident.

Metaphyseal Dysplasia, Schwachman-Diamond Type. The Schwachman-Diamond type of metaphyseal dysplasia is associated with exocrine pancreatic insufficiency and cyclic neutropenia and is characterized by anemia, leuko-

penia, neutropenia, thrombocytopenia, failure to thrive, growth retardation, ectodermal dysplasia, recurrent pulmonary infections, and malabsorption related to the pancreatic disease.[207] Diarrhea is almost always present. The osseous abnormalities, although not uniformly evident, consist of metaphyseal alterations that are found more frequently in the lower extremities than in the upper extremities. The provisional zone of calcification can be widened and radiolucent, and sclerotic areas may be present in the metaphysis (Fig. 88–59A).[208] Abnormal metaphyseal areas are located adjacent to normal-appearing ones. Coxa vara or a slipped capital femoral epiphysis may result. The fifth finger may be short, and skeletal maturation is delayed.[209] Osteopenia is frequent and probably secondary to the gastrointestinal disease. Spine changes similar to those of Scheuermann's disease are common.[210] Shortened ribs with flared and irregular anterior ends may result in a clinically small thoracic cage, but this is not a prominent feature of the disease.[211] Fatty replacement in the pancreas can be shown nicely by CT scanning (Fig. 88–59B).[207]

Adenosine Deaminase Deficiency. This disorder is associated with severe combined immunodeficiency, flared and cupped anterior ends of the ribs, and flared metaphyses.[212] The bone changes can be reversed with bone marrow transplantation.

Metaphyseal Anadysplasia. In this disorder, minimal growth impairment and metaphyseal irregularities that occur in infancy and improve in childhood are seen.[213]

Brachyrachia (Short Spine Dysplasia)

Brachyolmia. A mild trunk dwarfism, brachyolmia encompasses a heterogeneous group of conditions that are characterized by generalized platyspondyly with minimal involvement of the limbs. Four types have been proposed and all have platyspondyly without significant radiographic findings in the extremities. The Hoback type is associated with modestly flattened vertebral bodies, irregular endplates, and extension of the lateral margins of the vertebral bodies (Fig. 88–60); the Toledo type is accompanied by corneal opacities and precocious ossification of costal cartilage; the Maroteaux type is characterized by rounding of the anterior and posterior margins of the vertebral borders

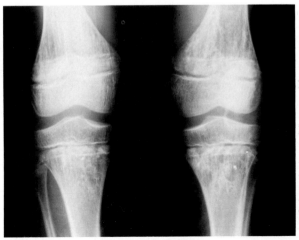
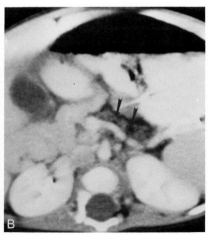

FIGURE 88–59. Metaphyseal chondrodysplasia with exocrine pancreatic insufficiency and neutropenia (Schwachman-Diamond syndrome).
  A Multiple sclerotic and radiolucent areas are observed in the metaphyses about the knees.
  B CT scan of the abdomen shows fatty replacement of the pancreas (arrows).

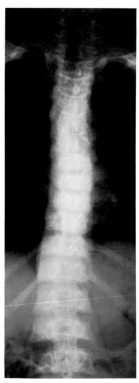

FIGURE 88–60. Brachyolmia. This 14 year old patient has platyspondyly. Note that the vertebral bodies project laterally beyond the pedicles.

with less elongation in the lateral view and less lateral extension in the frontal view; and the dominant inheritance type is associated with the most severe spinal changes.[214] All but the last type are autosomal recessive conditions. Histopathologic changes are present in the growth plates in the recessive forms of the disease.[215]

Mesomelic Dysplasias

The term "mesomelic" indicates that limb shortening results primarily from changes in the forearms and lower legs. Only four types are discussed here. These varieties of dwarfism are associated with a normal life span and an inheritance pattern that usually is autosomal dominant.

Dyschondrosteosis. This common condition also is called the Léri-Weill syndrome and is characterized by a mild mesomelic type of limb shortening with a Madelung's deformity of the forearm.[216, 217] The inheritance pattern is autosomal dominant, and the disease expresses itself more frequently and severely in female patients.[218] Radiographic findings include a shortened radius that is bowed dorsally and laterally and a distal segment of the ulna that often is subluxed or dislocated dorsally (Fig. 88–61).[219] The distal portion of the radius is underdeveloped and tilts in an ulnar and volar direction. This lack of development of the distal radial epiphysis with premature fusion of the medial side of the physis is the most characteristic finding in dyschondrosteosis. The carpal bones fit into the resulting V-shaped deformity of the radius and ulna. The distance between the radius and the ulna is increased, and the radial head may be flattened and dislocated. A lesser degree of shortening of the tibia and the fibula is seen, and a medial spicule of bone may project from the proximal portion of the tibia. When accompanied by tibia varum, a relatively long fibula can distort the shape of the ankle mortise, and surgical management may be required.[217] Coxa valga also can occur, and the tubular bones in the hands and feet may be shortened.

Nievergelt Type. This is the most severe form of mesomelic dysplasia.[218] Mesomelic shortening is accompanied by bone protuberances in the lower legs. Foot and hand deformities, limitation of joint motion, and genu valgum may be seen. Radiographic findings include marked hypoplasia of the bones in the forearms and lower legs, with a rhomboid or triangular shape of the tibia. Although both of the bones are dysplastic, the fibula is longer than the tibia, and the growth plates may be slanted, especially in the tibia. Proximal radioulnar synostosis with adjacent elbow dislocation and fusion of the carpal and tarsal bones can be seen. The fibula may be absent.[219]

Langer Type. The limb shortening in the Langer type is

FIGURE 88–61. Dyschondrosteosis.
A In this 5 year old girl, a radiograph shows separation of the radius and ulna and underdevelopment of the medial aspect of the radius. The carpal bones fit into the V-shaped deformity of the wrist.
B In the mother of the child in **A,** a classic V-shaped deformity of the radiocarpal joint is present.

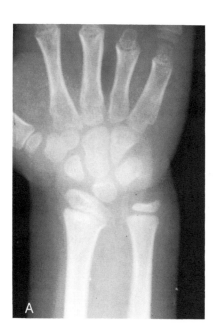

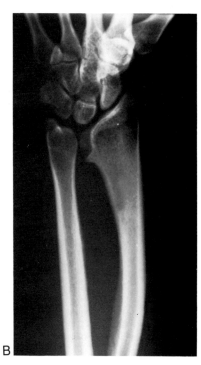

not as great as that found in the Nievergelt type. The mandible may be hypoplastic. Radiographically, the radius is short, with dorsolateral bowing, and it appears wide relative to its length (Fig. 88–62).[220, 221] The distal end of the radius slopes forward toward the ulna. Hypoplasia of the ulna is greatest in its distal portion. The carpal angles are decreased, and the hands reveal ulnar deviation. A short and wide tibia with metaphyseal flaring is characteristic. The fibula is hypoplastic, with absence or hypoplasia of its proximal portion. The epiphysis of the tibia ossifies late and fuses prematurely with the metaphysis. This condition is believed to be inherited as an autosomal recessive trait, but it also may be autosomal dominant.[220, 222]

Robinow Type. The Robinow type is accompanied by milder mesomelic shortening, especially in the upper limbs. Affected patients have a characteristic face, described as "fetal,"[223, 224] a prominent forehead with hypertelorism, a small upturned nose, and a small jaw. Multiple other reported abnormalities include genital hypoplasia and growth delay. Radiographic findings include shortening of the bones in the forearms and lower legs, with dislocation of the radial heads. The distal part of the ulna is severely hypoplastic. A cleft may be present in the distal phalanx of the thumb. Clinodactyly involving the fifth finger can be seen. Vertebral anomalies, particularly hemivertebrae, are common.

Other types of mesomelic dwarfism also occur,[225] including the Werner type that is accompanied by absent or extremely hypoplastic tibiae, polydactyly, and absence of thumb. Congenital heart disorders and Hirschsprung's disease may be associated with the Werner type of mesomelic dysplasia.[226]

Acromelic and Acromesomelic Dysplasias

Acromesomelic Dysplasia. Acromesomelic dysplasia, a short-limbed type of dwarfism of autosomal recessive in-

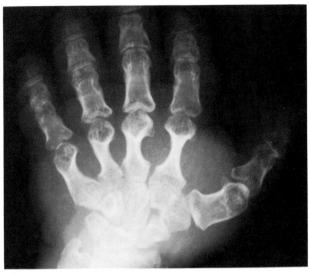

FIGURE 88–63. Acromesomelic dysplasia. This 26 year old patient has marked shortening and widening of the tubular bones.

heritance, was described in 1971 and is characterized by primary involvement of the forearms, hands, legs, and feet. The limb shortening, which becomes more apparent with age, is greater in the upper extremities.[227, 228] Lower thoracic kyphosis and increased lumbar lordosis may be observed. Radiographic findings include shortening of the midportion of the tubular bones, bowing of the radius, and dislocation of the radial head. The ulna often is shorter than the radius or the fibula. Widening of the short tubular bones is most marked in the proximal and middle phalanges (Fig. 88–63). Mild playtyspondyly and localized vertebral hypoplasia are seen in the thoracolumbar area and can lead to kyphosis.[229] The basilar part of the ilia is relatively hypoplastic. Hydrocephalus may be present.[230]

The markedly shortened bones in the hands, feet, and forearms and the changes in the spine allow separation of acromesomelic dysplasia from other mesomelic dysplasias and from pseudohypoparathyroidism. It is uncertain whether the Maroteaux and Campailla-Martinelli forms of this dysplasia truly are distinct disorders. Acromelic dysplasia is characterized by mild facial anomalies, growth retardation, mild shortening of the tubular bones, and widening of the proximal and middle phalanges. The proximal portions of the second, third, fourth, and fifth metacarpal bones are pointed.[231] Geleophysic dysplasia patients have a happy expression on their faces. Small hands and feet result from shortened tubular bones. Short stature and progressive valvular cardiac disease also are seen.[232]

Trichorhinophalangeal Dysplasia, Type I. Trichorhinophalangeal dysplasia consists of two types. The clinical features of the type I, autosomal dominant disorder include scalp hair that is sparse and slow to grow, a large pear-shaped nose, deformity of the proximal interphalangeal joints similar to that in rheumatoid arthritis, short stature, and joint laxity.[233–235] The most characteristic radiographic findings occur in the hands; cone-shaped epiphyses, producing a U-shaped pattern, and osseous shortening are present, particularly in the middle phalanges (Fig. 88–64A). Ivory epiphyses are common in the distal phalanges. The proximal femoral capital epiphyses are small and often have changes resembling those occurring in Legg-Calvé-Perthes

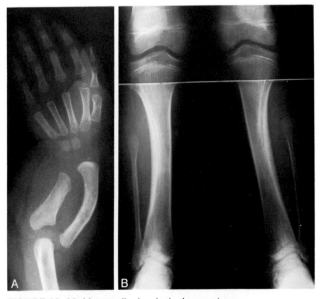

FIGURE 88–62. Mesomelic dysplasia: Langer type.

A In a 2 year old child, observe marked hypoplasia of the distal portion of the ulna and radial bowing.

B In a 5 year old patient, hypoplastic fibulae, tibial shortening with metaphyseal flaring, and talar slanting are seen.

(**B,** Courtesy of A. Oestreich, M.D., Cincinnati, Ohio.)

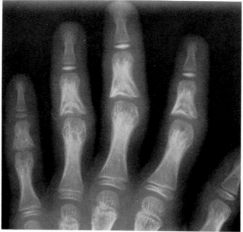
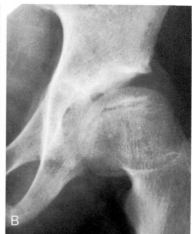

FIGURE 88–64. Trichorhinophalangeal dysplasia, type I.

A In a 10 year old child, the proximal interphalangeal joints are swollen; cone-shaped epiphyses, producing a U-shaped pattern, and ivory epiphyses (in the distal phalanges) are seen.

B A radiograph of the pelvis in a teen-ager shows a wide, flattened left femoral head.

disease (Fig. 88–64B). Coxa magna and degenerative joint disease may result and, later in life, patients may have articular symptoms and signs in the hips, elbows, fingers, and thoracic spine. Pectus carinatum, mild scoliosis, and kyphosis also can be seen.[236]

Trichorhinophalangeal Dysplasia, Type II. The type II (Giedion-Langer) disorder also is called acrodysplasia with exostoses and is associated with clinical findings that are similar to those of type I. Some features in the face, hands, and other locations are different, however, such as mental retardation and multiple exostoses.[237, 238] Such exostoses have not been reported in trichorhinophalangeal dysplasia type I.[238, 239] The mode of inheritance of the type II disorder is believed to be autosomal dominant, and a deletion of the long arm of chromosome 8 may be present.[239] The type II form is far more common in male subjects. The exostoses develop between the first and fifth years of life and increase until skeletal maturity.[240] They often will distort and expand a bone and do not resemble the bone outgrowths seen in multiple cartilaginous exostoses (Fig. 88–65). In addition to exostoses, radiographic findings include cone-shaped

epiphyses in the thumb and other digits of the hand, with resultant U-shaped deformities (Fig. 88–65B), and changes in the hips similar to those of Legg-Calvé-Perthes disease.[241] Additional features include a short fibula, tibiofibular synostosis, a wide femoral neck, segmentation errors in the spine, asymmetric limb growth, foot deformities, and microcephaly.

Saldino-Mainzer Dysplasia. The Saldino-Mainzer syndrome also is called acrodysplasia with retinitis pigmentosa and nephropathy and consists of cone-shaped epiphyses in the hands (Fig. 88–66), uremia, retinitis pigmentosa, cerebellar ataxia, and renal disease characterized by functional defects in the distal tubules and collecting ducts and manifested by a failure to concentrate and acidify the urine. The renal findings are those of nephronophthisis. The capital femoral epiphyses often are poorly developed. Other diseases with cone-shaped epiphyses of the hands that can be associated with renal disease are discussed by Mainzer and associates[242] and by Giedion.[243]

Pseudohypoparathyroidism. This condition is discussed in Chapter 57.

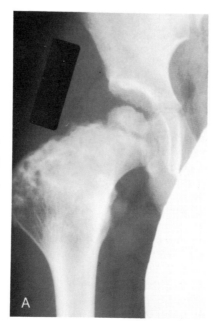
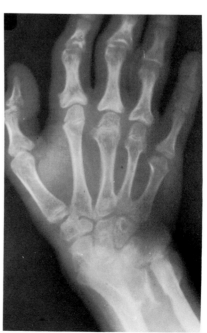

FIGURE 88–65. Trichorhinophalangeal dysplasia, type II (Giedion-Langer syndrome).

A The pelvis shows exostoses with expansion of the proximal portion of the femur.

B The hands in another patient show exostoses and cone-shaped epiphyses.

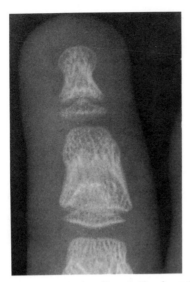

FIGURE 88–66. Acrodysplasia with retinitis pigmentosa and nephropathy (Saldino-Mainzer syndrome). Cone-shaped epiphyses in a finger are evident in a 7 year old child.

Dysplasias with Significant (but not Exclusive) Membranous Bone Involvement

Cleidocranial Dysplasia. Cleidocranial dysplasia, an autosomal dominant disorder with high penetrance, has a wide range of clinical manifestations.[244] Mild shortening of stature may be seen. The head is large and brachycephalic, with a small face and bossing of the frontal and parietal bones. The sutures are wide, and their closure is delayed. Oral findings include a high-arched palate with delayed eruption of poorly formed[245] and supernumerary teeth (Fig. 88–67). The shoulders may droop, and the patient may have an increased range of motion of the glenohumeral joint. Hearing loss is not uncommon owing to abnormalities of the ossicles.[246] Genu valgum and short fingers can be seen. A narrow thorax may lead to respiratory distress in infancy.

Radiographic findings include poor ossification of the skull with wide sutures and multiple wormian bones, most marked in the lambdoid sutures (Fig. 88–67).[247] Parietal bone ossification may be absent at birth. In adults, the frontal bone often is thickened.[248] The foramen magnum may be large and deformed, the basal angle of the skull may be increased, and basilar impression often is evident (Fig. 88–67). Caudal bulging of the occipital bone may be present. The paranasal sinuses and mastoids are not well developed. The mandible may be broad, with persistence of its synchondrosis. Although total clavicular absence is uncommon, any portion of the clavicle may be absent; the middle or outer portion is affected most commonly (Fig. 88–68). The scapula is hypoplastic, with a small glenoid cavity, and the thorax may be bell-shaped, especially in patients with more severe clavicular abnormalities. Pelvic alterations occur frequently and consist of a delay in ossification of the pubic bones, a wide symphysis pubis, and narrow iliac wings (Fig. 88–69). Although coxa valga deformity is more frequent, unilateral or bilateral coxa vara deformity may develop and lead to disturbances of gait (Fig. 88–69A). Mild diaphyseal narrowing and expanded metaphyses of the tubular bones may be evident. The spinal changes consist primarily of spina bifida occulta, which is most marked in the cervical and upper thoracic spine, but some patients have multiple vertebral ossification centers, wedged vertebrae with scoliosis, or defects in the pars interarticularis in the lumbar spine. The findings in the hand include small tapered distal phalanges, slightly small middle phalanges, pseudoepiphyses in the metacarpal bones, somewhat large phalangeal epiphyses (especially in the distal phalanges), cone-shaped epiphyses, and retarded ossification of the carpal bones (Fig. 88–70). Multiple anomalies also have been seen in a hereditary condition resembling cleidocranial dysplasia. These anomalies include severe micrognathia, absence of the thumbs, and lack of distal phalangeal ossification.[249]

Osteodysplasty (Melnick-Needles Syndrome). Osteodysplasty was first reported by Melnick and Needles in 1966.[250] The clinical appearance of affected patients is more or less characteristic. Typically, the face is small, with large ears, protruding eyes, micrognathia, and malaligned teeth; the upper portions of the arms are short, and the thorax is narrow. Bowing of the extremities and scoliosis may be present. The inheritance pattern of the disorder is autosomal dominant, and it probably is lethal in male subjects[251, 252]; osteodysplasty is seen only in female patients. Radiographically, the cortex of the tubular bone is irregular, with an undulating contour and multiple constrictions of the medullary cavities (Fig. 88–71).[253] Lateral bowing of the tibia is typical. A ribbon-like appearance and cortical irregularity of the ribs are present. The normal curvature of the clavicle is accentuated, and cortical irregularity and wide medial ends of this bone may occur. Pectus excavatum also may be seen. The scapulae are small and deformed. The thin iliac wings are flared, with constriction of the bases of the ilia and sharply concave sacrosciatic notches; the pubic and ischial bones are narrow. Coxa valga, long femoral necks, and subtrochanteric narrowing are seen. The changes in the hands are mild, although dysplasia of the distal phalanges can occur. Sclerosis appears in the base of the skull and mastoid bones, and the anterior portion of the cranial fossa is small. Closure of the anterior fontanelle is delayed. The mandible is thin and small, with an obtuse angle and hypoplastic coronoid processes.[254, 255] In the spine the vertebral bodies show an increased height and anterior concavity; in the lumbar region, the spinal canal may be enlarged and the laminae appear thinned. Scoliosis or kyphoscoliosis can occur. Extraskeletal findings include ureterovesical obstruction and cardiac enlargement secondary to pulmonary hypertension.[253] Although the precise pathogenesis of this syndrome is unknown, an aberration of collagen synthesis may be present.[256]

Bent-Bone Dysplasia Group

Campomelic Dysplasia. Campomelic (meaning bent limbs) dysplasia describes an entity distinct from a number of other conditions that are accompanied by bending of the extremities.[257, 258] Affected newborn infants have a large head and a short trunk and short limbs. The anterolateral bowing of the limbs is most marked in the legs. Dimples may be present over the area of bowing in the tibia. Clubfeet, joint contractures, bowing of the bones in the forearm, small hands, and a short neck are seen. The calvarium is large, with a small facies, depressed nasal root, low-set ears, small jaw, and cleft palate. The disease prob-

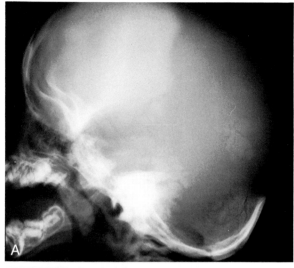 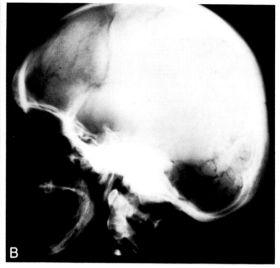

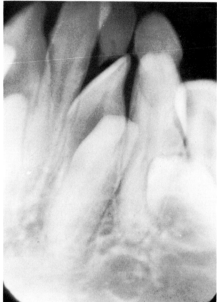

FIGURE 88–67. Cleidocranial dysplasia.

A A skull radiograph in a 15 month old patient demonstrates wide sutures, poor ossification of the parietal bone, and multiple wormian bones.

B In an adult, inferior bulging of the occipital bone, wormian bones in the lambdoid suture, and segmental thickening in the supraorbital portion of the frontal bone are evident.

C Jaw. Delayed dental eruption and supernumerary teeth are shown.

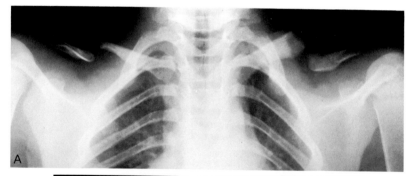

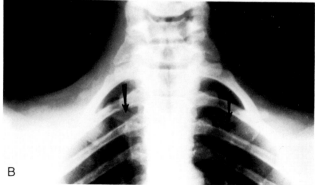

FIGURE 88–68. Cleidocranial dysplasia.

A In an 8 year old patient, note clavicular defects at the junction of the outer and middle thirds of the bone.

B In this adult, tiny residual clavicles are evident (arrows).

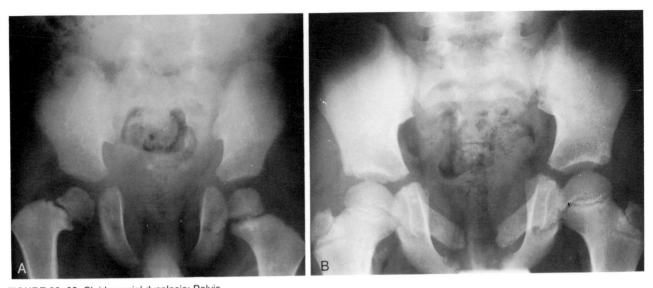

FIGURE 88–69. Cleidocranial dysplasia: Pelvis.
A A radiograph in a 5 year old child shows no ossification of pubic bones and the development of idiopathic coxa vara of the right femur.
B In an 8 year old child, incomplete ossification of the pubic bones and narrow iliac wings are evident.

ably is of autosomal recessive inheritance and usually is fatal in infancy, although long-term survival is reported. The diagnosis has been made in utero.[259]

Radiographic findings, which are most marked in the extremities, consist of anterolateral angulation of the femora, slightly above the middle third of the diaphysis (Fig. 88–72). Tibial bowing occurs primarily in an anterior direction at the junction of the middle and distal thirds of the bone. The cortex is markedly thin at the convexity of the curve. The fibula is hypoplastic. The long tubular bones of the upper extremities are slightly shortened and minimally angulated. Patients have small hands, with shortening especially of the middle and distal phalanges and clinodactyly of the fifth digit. The chest is bell-shaped and has a decreased anteroposterior diameter; other features are thin, wavy ribs, slender clavicles, and a narrow tracheal caliber resulting from defective tracheobronchial cartilage. The scapula is small, and often only 11 pairs of ribs are found. Typical findings in the pelvis include the absence of the ala of the sacrum, narrow iliac bones, acetabular hypoplasia, poor pubic ossification, and widely separated, short ischial bones. The hips frequently are dislocated. Delayed ossification occurs in the epiphyses about the knees, in the talus, and in the sternum. Vertebral anomalies—especially hypo-

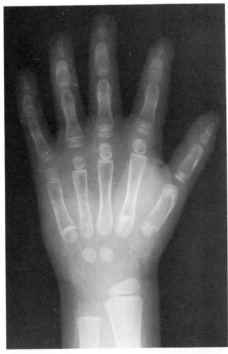

FIGURE 88–70. Cleidocranial dysplasia. The phalangeal epiphyses are large, and the distal phalanges and carpal bones are small. Pseudoepiphyses in the metacarpal bones and hypoplasia of the distal portion of the ulna are seen.

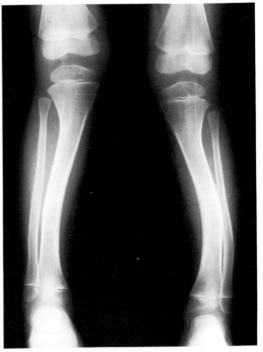

FIGURE 88–71. Osteodysplasty (Melnick-Needles syndrome). Note the characteristic lateral bowing of the tibiae.

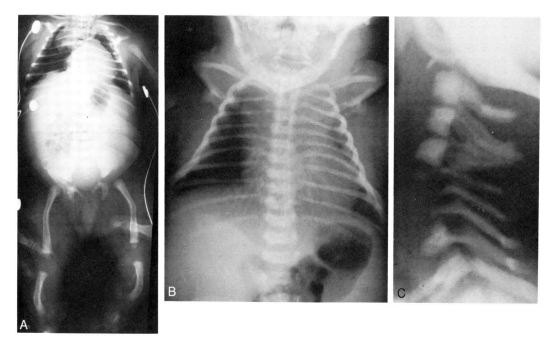

FIGURE 88–72. Campomelic dysplasia.
  A In the lower extremity, the tubular bones reveal anterolateral bowing. The iliac bones, scapulae, fibulae, and lungs are hypoplastic, and the hips are dislocated. The 11 pairs of ribs and the clavicles are thin, and the pedicles of the thoracic spine are hypoplastic.
  B In another patient, hypoplasia of the vertebrae and scapulae and thin ribs are seen.
  C Dysplastic lower cervical vertebrae are present in this patient.

plasia of the upper thoracic pedicles and lower cervical vertebrae with narrow interpediculate distances—and hypoplasia of the cervical vertebrae are characteristic (Fig. 88–72B,C). The thoracic spine, scapulae, and pelvic abnormalities and the clinical findings can occur in cases without limb bowing.[260] Abnormal spinal curvature is common.[261] The most characteristic radiographic findings are the curved femora and tibiae, small scapulae, hypoplastic pedicles of the thoracic spine, and hypoplasia in the cervical spine. These characteristic abnormalities serve to separate campomelic dysplasia from other conditions with curved bones.[262]

A variety of abnormalities of internal organs are seen in campomelic dysplasia, including pulmonary hypoplasia, hydronephrosis, hydroureters, congenital heart disease, absence of the olfactory bulbs and tracts, and hydrocephalus. Some boys with campomelic dysplasia and gonadal dysgenesis lack the H-Y antigen.

Kyphomelic Dysplasia. Kyphomelic dysplasia is characterized by short, broad, bent femora with metaphyseal flaring and irregularity (Fig. 88–73). Dimples can be found over the apex of the bowed femora. Mild platyspondyly, shortening and bowing of other long tubular bones (especially the humeri), and short flared ribs are additional findings.[263]

Multiple Dislocations with Dysplasia

Larsen's Syndrome. In 1950, Larsen and collaborators described six patients with multiple dislocations, clubfeet, and a characteristic clinical appearance consisting of a recessed midface, widely spaced eyes, and a depressed nasal bridge.[264] Larsen's syndrome is a generalized disorder of connective tissue and collagen. Additional findings include a cleft palate, broad thumbs, and spinal involvement that may lead to progressive neurologic impairment. Laryngomalacia, tracheomalacia, or tracheal stenosis may be seen.

Radiographs show dislocations, usually of major joints such as the knees, hips, and elbows (Fig. 88–74).[265, 266] The ends of the bones are distorted (Fig. 88–74B). Multiple ossification centers may be seen after dislocation of the elbow.[267] The carpal and tarsal bones may be supernumerary or possess an abnormal shape (Fig. 88–75), and the calcaneus typically ossifies from two separate centers (Fig. 88–76). The tubular bones of the hands and feet may be broad and shortened, and pseudoepiphyses in the metacarpal and metatarsal bones often are present (Fig. 88–75). Abnormalities of the vertebral bodies, particularly in the cervical spine, consist of errors in segmentation or flattening, and these can be associated with kyphosis or kyphoscoliosis (Fig. 88–77). Encroachment on the subdural space at the apex of the kyphosis has been documented.[268] Radiographs of the skull demonstrate hypertelorism, a small jaw, and brachycephaly.

Both autosomal dominant and autosomal recessive transmission patterns have been reported.[269] Because the dislocations are difficult to treat, the patients may develop considerable disability and secondary degenerative changes. Many extraskeletal abnormalities have been reported in this syndrome, including dilation of the aortic root, other cardiac malformations, and tortuosity and dilation of the cranial and abdominal arteries.[270–272]

Desbuquois' Syndrome. Desbuquois' syndrome is characterized by short stature, multiple dislocations, osteopenia, and characteristic findings about the hips, including large and pointed lesser trochanters with a "monkey wrench" appearance of the femoral necks.[273] Extra ossification centers are present in the hands.

Spondyloepimetaphyseal Dysplasia with Joint Laxity. In 1980 Beighton and Kozlowski reported seven children with short-limbed dwarfism who also had a severe progressive high dorsal kyphoscoliosis, joint hypermobility, short

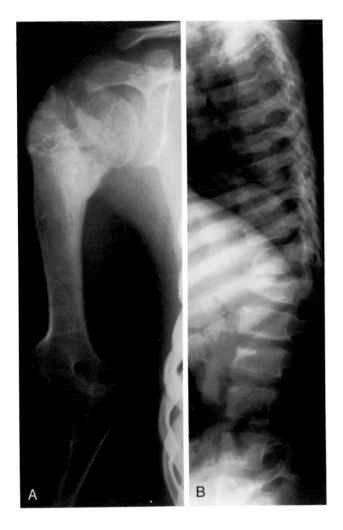

FIGURE 88–73. Kyphomelic dysplasia.
  A The right humerus in a 4 year old child shows bowing and metaphyseal irregularity.
  B In the same patient, the spine shows platyspondyly, with marked changes between T11 and T12.

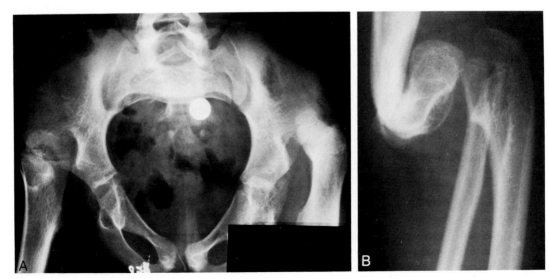

FIGURE 88–74. Larsen's syndrome.
  A Bilateral dislocations of the hip are seen.
  B A dislocation of the elbow with considerable osseous deformity is evident.

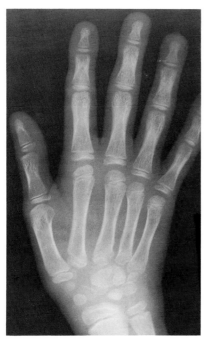

FIGURE 88–75. Larsen's syndrome. Multiple small carpal bones, metacarpal pseudoepiphyses, and some degree of epiphyseal flattening are seen.

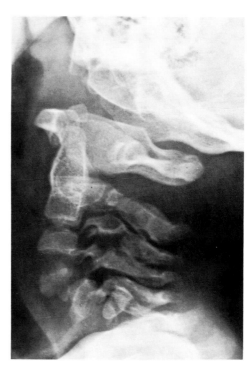

FIGURE 88–77. Larsen's syndrome. Dysplastic vertebrae are seen in the cervical spine.

nonrigid thumbs, an oval face with protuberant eyes, a cleft palate, and normal mentation.[274] The condition is inherited as an autosomal recessive trait.[275] Radiographic findings include generalized osteoporosis and vertebral bodies that are flattened or oval and irregular. Epiphyseal development is delayed. The metaphyses are wide and contain cystic areas. The radius characteristically is short and bowed and the elbows are dislocated. Genu valgum and clubfeet are common. The tubular bones of the hands and feet are shortened but the distal phalanges are widened. The iliac wings are large and flared, with small hypoplastic iliac bodies, and

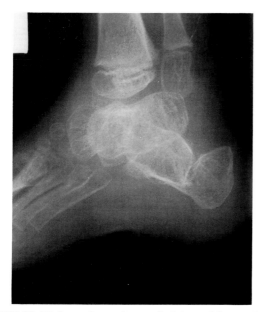

FIGURE 88–76. Larsen's syndrome. A deformed foot and partial fusion of two ossification centers in the os calcis are present.

the acetabula are underdeveloped. The proximal femoral epiphyses are flattened, irregular, and small. The hips often dislocate. Patients have short femoral necks and coxa valga. The thorax is asymmetric owing to rib deformities associated with thoracic kyphoscoliosis. Progressive kyphoscoliosis can lead to spinal cord and nerve root compression, paraplegia, and severe cardiorespiratory failure.

Osteodysplastic Primordial Dwarfism Group

Osteodysplastic Primordial Dwarfism. The type I and type II forms of this disease can be differentiated by their radiographic features. Patients with the type I form have bowed and shortened humeri and femora. The pelvis is dysplastic inferiorly. Patients with the type II form have shortening of the legs and forearms with medial bowing of the radii, shortening of the ulnae, and coxa vara (Fig. 88–78A). The distal and proximal femoral epiphyses align themselves with a central indentation of the adjacent metaphyses (Fig. 88–78B).[276] Severe prenatal and postnatal delay in growth is evident.

Dysplasias with Decreased Bone Density

Osteogenesis imperfecta, homocystinuria, and idiopathic juvenile osteoporosis are discussed in other portions of this book.

Menkes' Syndrome. Menkes' syndrome (or Menkes' kinky hair syndrome) is an X-linked disorder leading to defective copper absorption from the intestine. The typical patient is a male infant with sparse, light, kinky hair, profound failure to thrive, and progressive degeneration of the central nervous system. Serum levels of copper and ceruloplasmin are decreased. Radiographic findings, which include osteopenia and metaphyseal spurs, have been confused with changes in the child abuse syndrome and rickets (Fig. 88–79). Periosteal new bone formation is common,

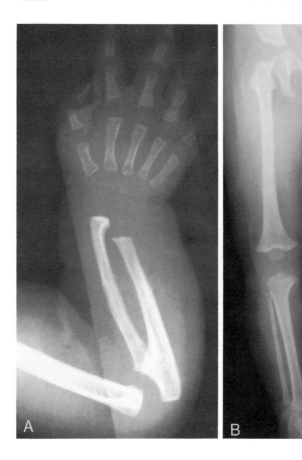

FIGURE 88–78. Osteodysplastic primordial dwarfism, type II.

A The radius is elongated and bowed toward the ulna.

B A triangular shape of the distal femoral epiphyses (which fit into a central femoral notch) is evident. The metaphyses flare slightly. The fibulae are shorter than the tibiae.

and wormian bones are identified in the lambdoid sutures. Thin tubular bones, a wooly appearance of certain ossification centers, flaring of the ends of the ribs, a small mandible, and scalloping of the posterior surface of the vertebral bodies are other radiographic features.[277] Dramatic changes occur in the blood vessels, particularly in the brain, presumably secondary to fragmentation of the elastic layer that results in tortuosity of the cerebral and systemic vasculature.[278] Bladder diverticula,[279] dilation of portions of the urinary tract, and emphysema have been seen in this condition. CT scanning and MR imaging of the brain show cerebral atrophy, infarctions, subdural fluid, and markedly tortuous vessels.[280]

Dysplasias with Defective Mineralization

Hypophosphatasia, rickets, and neonatal hyperparathyroidism are discussed in Chapters 53 and 57.

Dysplasias with Increased Bone Density

Osteopetrosis. Osteopetrosis is a complex disease of at least four different types that have very distinct clinical, radiologic, and histopathologic features.

Osteopetrosis, Precocious Type. The precocious type is an autosomal recessive form, also called the lethal form, but this designation is misleading because some patients survive for a number of years. Clinical abnormalities include failure to thrive, hepatosplenomegaly, and cranial nerve dysfunction, especially blindness[281] and deafness. The head may be large owing to hydrocephalus. The obliteration of the marrow cavity by abnormal bone leads to anemia and thrombocytopenia and predisposes to recurrent infections with early death in most patients.

The radiographic findings are characterized by generalized osteosclerosis. Tubular bones show a failure of differentiation between the cortex and the medullary cavity (Figs. 88–80 and 88–81). Modeling in these bones is defective and, in some instances, leads to a clublike appearance (Fig. 88–81). Infants may exhibit a rickets-like configuration in the ends of the bones, with mottled, radiolucent areas related to the presence of an excessive number of hyper-

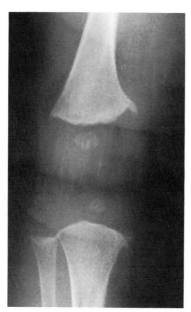

FIGURE 88–79. Menkes' kinky hair syndrome. Observe metaphyseal excrescences in the femur and tibia in a 3 month old infant.

trophic, degenerating chondrocytes (Fig. 88–81).[282] Longitudinal striations, observed occasionally, are believed to correspond to sites of blood vessels that are surrounded by connective tissue; more frequently seen transverse striations are due to alternating areas of mature bone and intensely sclerotic and disorganized osseous tissue (Figs. 88–80*B* and 88–81*C*). The presence of a "bone within bone" (or an endobone) appearance is an unusual but characteristic finding. According to Engfeld and associates,[283] the miniature central bones are a core of more primitive, coarsely fibrillar and cellular osseous tissue separated from the surrounding cortex by nonsclerotic bone or a rudimentary medullary cavity. Periostitis may be seen, particularly in infants, and fractures, which generally heal, are common.

MR imaging shows the marrow stores to be located in the skull base and ends of the long tubular bones in children under 1 year of age. Between 3 and 5 years of age, marrow stores are shifted to the diaphyses of the long tubular bones and the calvarium. In the long bones, the sites of the greatest accumulation of marrow correspond to areas of decreased opacity on radiographs.[284]

The entire skull is involved, but the cartilaginous portion at its base is the cranial site that is affected most frequently and severely (Fig. 88–82*A*). The cranial foramina are small. A detailed study using CT scanning and MR imaging by Elster and associates showed macrocephaly, a thick calvarium with dense inner and outer tables, and broadened diploic spaces with poorly defined borders.[285] Later a hair-

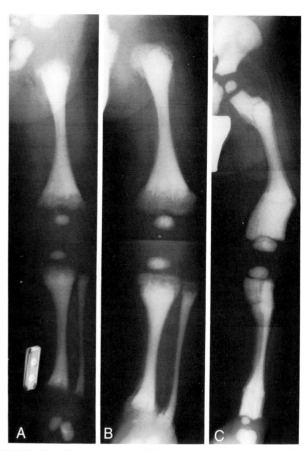

FIGURE 88–81. Osteopetrosis: Precocious or autosomal recessive lethal type. Radiographs of the same patient at 4 months **(A)**, 8 months **(B)**, and 24 months **(C)** of age. Initially, osteosclerosis, radiolucent areas in the metaphyses, and wide physes are evident. Subsequently, the radiolucent regions disappear and are replaced by increasing metaphyseal expansion and pathologic fractures.

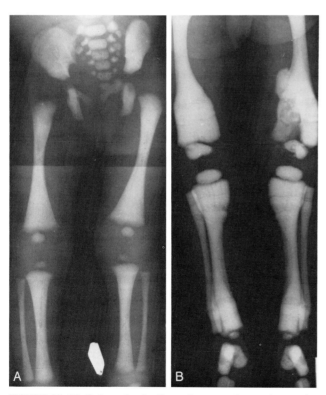

FIGURE 88–80. Osteopetrosis: Precocious or autosomal recessive lethal type.

A In a newborn infant, diffuse osteosclerosis and slight metaphyseal expansion of the tubular bones are evident.

B In a second patient, 16 months of age, marked osteosclerosis and bone expansion are seen. Note the transverse and horizontal radiolucent lines in the metaphyses and a pathologic fracture in the left femur.

on-end appearance may develop. The skull base has appreciable marrow activity (as shown with MR imaging) despite sclerotic bones.[284] The teeth may be malformed and the mandible may contain a dense endobone corresponding to a condylar cartilage center.[285] The mastoid regions and paranasal sinuses are poorly developed. Osteomyelitis of the mandible or maxilla may be seen. The internal acoustic meatus may be narrowed or the canal through which the facial nerve passes may be stenotic. In the spine, the vertebral bodies tend to be uniformly radiodense, with a prominent anterior vascular notch (Fig. 88–82*B*). As the child matures, exaggeration of the sclerosis occurs in the vertebral endplates. The brain can exhibit delayed myelination, white matter disease, calcification in the basal ganglia and deep portions of the cerebrum, atrophy, hydrocephalus, and optic nerve atrophy.[286]

The histopathologic and biochemical features of this syndrome have been studied extensively.[282, 287–291] Primary parenchymal disease in the brain with cytoplastic storage in the neurons has been documented.[292] Clinical improvement has been reported after bone marrow transplantation,[293] and treatment with high dose calcitriol may be of use in those infants in whom the osteoclasts lack ruffled borders.[294]

Osteopetrosis, Delayed Type. The delayed type, an autosomal dominant variety of osteopetrosis, was originally described by the German radiologist Albers-Schönberg. Af-

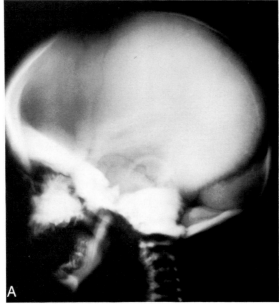
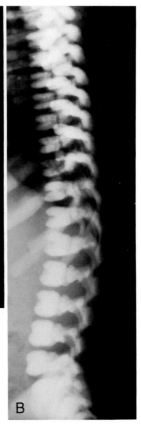

FIGURE 88–82. Osteopetrosis: Precocious or autosomal recessive lethal type.

A Diffuse osteosclerosis of the skull, most marked at the base, is present.

B Diffuse vertebral sclerosis and accentuation of the anterior vascular notches are evident.

fected persons may be relatively asymptomatic. The disease may be detected because of a pathologic fracture, problems after tooth extraction, mild anemia, or cranial nerve palsies.[295-298] The radiographic findings are similar to but less severe than those in the autosomal recessive form of the disease (Fig. 88–83A). The bones are diffusely osteosclerotic, with defective tubulation and a thickened cortex. The vertebral endplates become accentuated, especially with advancing age (Fig. 88–83B). A ''bone within bone'' appearance or radiolucent bands in the ends of the diaphyses are sometimes seen (Fig. 88–84).

Osteopetrosis, Intermediate Recessive Type. Beighton and associates[298] have described a milder, recessive form of osteopetrosis that is distinct from both the more severe, recessive form of the disease that is seen in infants and the less severe, autosomal dominant form. Affected patients often are of short stature, with pathologic fractures, anemia, and hepatomegaly (Fig. 88–85).[299] The radiographic findings are characterized by diffuse bone sclerosis, especially in the base of the skull, interference with normal bone modeling, a ''bone within bone'' appearance, and retained primary and impacted permanent teeth. The facial bones also are involved. Ischemic necrosis of the femoral head has been reported in this form of the disease.[300]

Osteopetrosis with Tubular Acidosis. The variety with tubular acidosis, also called ''marble brain'' disease or Sly's disease, was reported initially in 1972 and consists of osteopetrosis, renal tubular acidosis, and cerebral calcifications.[301] The inheritance pattern is autosomal recessive, and the clinical course is compatible with long survival. Many of the patients, however, are mentally retarded. A deficiency in carbonic anhydrase has been identified in some affected persons.[302] Typical clinical findings include a fail-

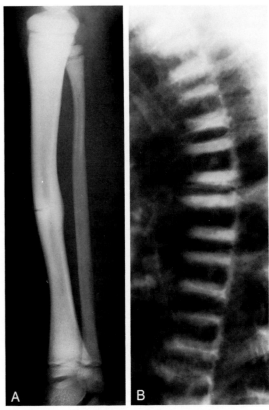

FIGURE 88–83. Osteopetrosis: Delayed or autosomal dominant type.

A Osteosclerosis, cortical thickening, and an incomplete fracture are evident.

B Osteosclerosis in the superior and inferior portions of the vertebral bodies has produced a ''sandwich'' appearance.

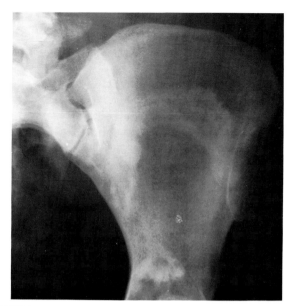

FIGURE 88–84. Osteopetrosis: Delayed or autosomal dominant type. The "bone within bone" appearance is seen in the ilium of an adult patient.

ure to thrive, symptoms related to renal tubular acidosis, muscle weakness, and hypotonia.[303, 304]

Radiographic findings are detected throughout the skeleton and include osteosclerosis, obliteration of the medullary cavity, and pathologic fractures (Figs. 88–86 and 88–87). An unusual aspect of this disease is the occurrence of progressive improvement in the radiographic abnormalities, a

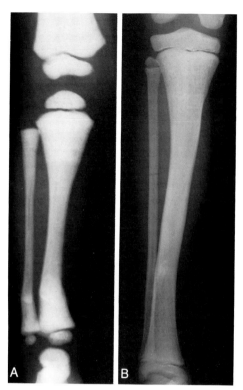

FIGURE 88–86. Osteopetrosis: Recessive type with tubular acidosis (in a patient with carbonic anhydrase II deficiency).

A At the age of 2 years, diffuse osteosclerosis, a failure of normal bone modeling, and fractures of the tibia and fibula are present.

B At 10 years of age, osteosclerosis is less prominent, osseous bowing is evident, and a new fracture of the fibula has developed.

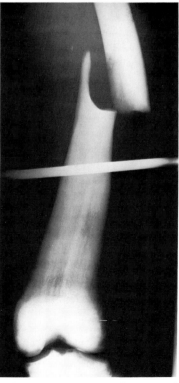

FIGURE 88–85. Osteopetrosis: Intermediate recessive type. In an 18 year old patient, a pathologic fracture of the femur followed modest trauma. Diffuse osteosclerosis and failure of normal bone modeling are seen.

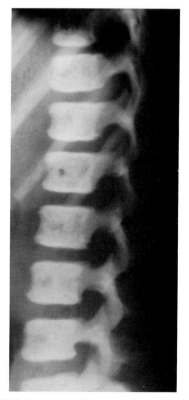

FIGURE 88–87. Osteopetrosis: Recessive type with tubular acidosis (in a patient with carbonic anhydrase II deficiency). Diffuse osteosclerosis is observed in the spine.

finding that is more characteristic of this syndrome than of other forms of osteopetrosis (Fig. 88–86). Although intracranial calcification can be detected on routine radiographs, it is best shown by CT scanning.[305] This calcification can be located anywhere in the brain, but generally it is found in the basal ganglia and periventricular areas (Fig. 88–88).

Dysosteosclerosis. Dysosteosclerosis is an autosomal recessive disorder manifested in early childhood as small stature, dental anomalies, increased bone fragility, and, occasionally neurologic abnormalities, including nerve palsies.[306, 307] Although thickening and sclerosis of the cranial vault, base of the skull, ribs, clavicles, and tubular bones may resemble the findings in osteopetrosis, the presence of platyspondyly with irregular vertebral endplates and expanded dense metadiaphyseal segments of long bones containing even denser transverse lines and a less dense diaphyseal segment allows recognition of this syndrome (Fig. 88–89). There may be absorption of the phalangeal tufts.

Pyknodysostosis. The syndrome of pyknodysostosis consists of osteosclerosis, short stature, frontal and occipital bossing, a small face with receding chin, short broad hands, and hypoplasia of the nails. This disorder is of autosomal recessive inheritance and often is accompanied by multiple fractures. The painter Toulouse-Lautrec is believed to have had this syndrome. Radiographic findings include generalized and uniform osteosclerosis (Fig. 88–90).[308, 309] In the tubular bones, metaphyseal modeling is only mildly abnormal, and the medullary cavities may be narrowed. The bones of the hands and feet are short, with hypoplasia or osteolysis of the distal phalanges, which may become progressively more severe (a characteristic aspect of the disease) (Fig. 88–90A). In the skull, a marked delay in the closure of the sutures is evident (Fig. 88–90B), and the

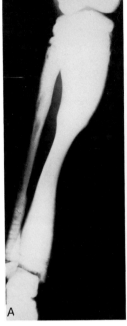
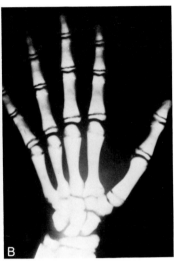

FIGURE 88–89. Dysosteosclerosis.
  A Note failure of normal tubulation and osteosclerosis with several radiolucent transverse zones.
  B Similar findings are present in the hand.
  (Courtesy of R. Lachman, M.D., Los Angeles, California.)

anterior fontanelle may remain open, even in adults. Wormian bones are common, especially in the lambdoid sutures. A thick and sclerotic skull base and a thin vault without diploic markings represent additional cranial manifestations of the disease. The mastoids are poorly developed, the orbits are radiodense, the mandible is hypoplastic without normal angulation, the maxilla is small, and the teeth are malformed, malpositioned, and hypoplastic.[310] A long uvula in combination with diminutive facial bones may obstruct the nasopharynx, leading to hypoventilation during sleep, cor pulmonale, and hepatic failure.[311, 312] The vertebral bodies are sclerotic, and errors in vertebral segmentation may be present in the upper portion of the cervical spine. Spondylolisthesis of the lower lumbar vertebrae also is seen. The acromial ends of the clavicles may be resorbed.

Osteosclerosis, Stanescu Type. The Stanescu type, a rare, autosomal dominant disease, is characterized by short stature, brachycephaly, brachydactyly, a small jaw, and cortical thickening of the long bones.[313] Shortening is more prominent in the upper extremities than in the lower extremities. The skull is small and brachycephalic, with poor development of the sinuses and mastoids. The spine may be osteosclerotic and the short tubular bones (with the exception of the distal phalanges) are decreased in length.

Axial Osteosclerosis

Osteomesopyknosis. Clinical manifestations of osteomesopyknosis typically begin in the second decade of life and consist of back pain and discomfort.[314] Radiographs reveal patchy areas of osteosclerosis in the vertebral endplates, osseous pelvis, and proximal femora (Fig. 88–91). In the femora, cystic changes also may be evident. The skull, hands and feet, and remaining tubular bones are normal.

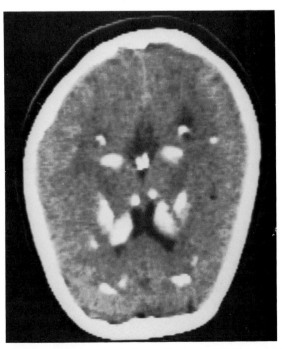

FIGURE 88–88. Osteopetrosis: Recessive type with tubular acidosis (in a patient with carbonic anhydrase II deficiency). Diffuse intracranial calcifications, particularly in the basal ganglia and periventricular areas, are seen.

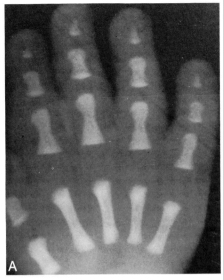
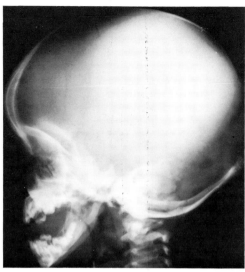

FIGURE 88–90. Pyknodysostosis.
A In a newborn infant, diffuse osteosclerosis with hypoplasia of the distal phalanges is present.
B In a 4 month old child, wide sutures and basal sclerosis represent the significant cranial abnormalities. The mandible is hypoplastic.

An autosomal dominant pattern of inheritance appears most likely.[315]

Central Osteosclerosis with Ectodermal Dysplasia. This condition is characterized by ichthyosis, brittle hair, impaired intelligence, decreased fertility, and short stature (IBIDS).[316] Osteosclerosis is present predominantly in the skull, spine, ribs, clavicles, pelvis, and proximal portions of the long tubular bones (Fig. 88–92). The tubular bones in the limbs are osteopenic (Fig. 88–92C). This condition may be a form of trichothiodystrophy.

Axial Osteosclerosis with Bamboo Hair. The condition, which also is called Netherton syndrome, may be associated with central osteosclerosis and congenital ichthyosiform erythroderma (bamboo hair).[316, 317]

Osteopoikilosis, Melorheostosis, Osteopathia Striata. These conditions are discussed in Chapter 93.

Diaphyseal Dysplasia (Camurati-Engelmann Disease). Camurati-Englemann disease is a generalized, bilaterally symmetric dysplasia of bone that is characterized by cortical thickening, narrowing of the medullary cavity, and a sclerotic and expanded diaphyseal segment that results from periosteal and endosteal bone formation.[318–323] The epiphyses are spared. Diaphyseal dysplasia is an autosomal dominant disorder with considerable variability of expression and occasionally complete lack of penetrance. In some patients the presenting symptoms initially appear in the first decade of life, whereas in others the disease is discovered in the second, third, or fourth decade of life. A reduction of muscle mass and subcutaneous fat, muscular weakness, abnormal gait, bone enlargement, and leg pain may be evident. Occasionally, the erythrocyte sedimentation rate is elevated. Characteristic radiographic features include cortical thickening and sclerosis of the diaphyses of the tubular bones (Fig. 88–93). The osteosclerosis is irregular and inhomogeneous, and endosteal involvement is greater than periosteal involvement.[324] In order of decreasing frequency, the tibia, femur, humerus, ulna, radius, and bones of the hands and feet are affected. In addition, the fibula, clavicle, ribs, and pelvis can be involved. A symmetric distribution is typical but not present uniformly. Sclerosis of the base of the skull is common. The sclerosis in the vertebrae is greatest in the posterior portion of the vertebral bodies and neural arches.[324]

The course of this disease is variable. Progressive findings are common, but spontaneous improvement in adolescence also has been recognized. Increased intracranial pressure and encroachment on cranial nerves can lead to significant complications in some patients.

Craniodiaphyseal Dysplasia. Craniodiaphyseal dysplasia, an autosomal recessive disorder, is characterized by early deformity of the face that is caused by marked sclerosis and thickening of the skull, including the mandible.[325, 326] The head is large, the nasal bridge is flat-

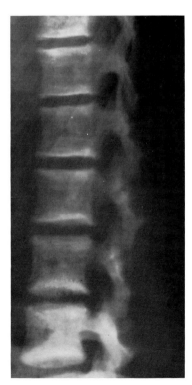

FIGURE 88–91. Osteomesopyknosis. In this teenage patient, patchy areas of osteosclerosis are observed in the spine.

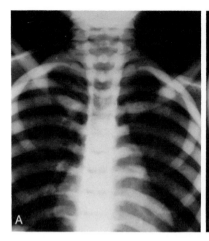
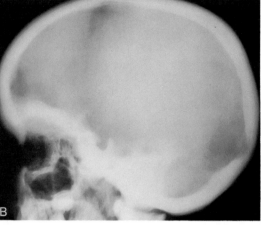
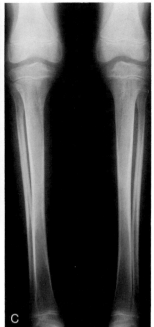

FIGURE 88–92. Central osteosclerosis with ectodermal dysplasia.
A The chest shows osteosclerosis of the spine, ribs, and clavicles.
B The skull shows marked sclerosis.
C Osteopenia without sclerosis is evident in the long tubular bones.

tened, and the forehead is wide and high. Hypertrophy of bone also causes nasal and lacrimal obstruction and cranial nerve palsies. The patient is of short stature and may be mentally retarded. Radiographically, at birth, massive and progressive hyperostosis in the skull and facial bones leads to obliteration of the paranasal sinuses.[327] Involvement of the long and short tubular bones varies in severity, although

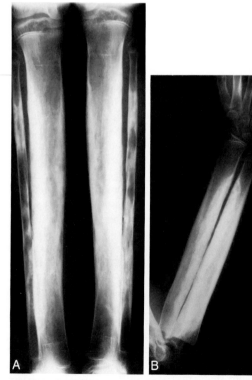

FIGURE 88–93. Diaphyseal dysplasia (Camurati-Engelmann disease). The tubular bones are wide, with thickened cortices and narrowed medullary canals. Mottled areas of rarefaction are present, best observed in the fibulae.

cortical thickening and a lack of normal modeling are typical. Varying degrees of osseous expansion and sclerosis are seen. The ribs, clavicles, and ilia are widened and sclerotic, whereas changes in the spine are milder and predominate in the vertebral arches.[328]

Lenz-Majewski Dysplasia. Lenz-Majewski dysplasia probably is of autosomal dominant inheritance and is characterized by a large head, loose skin, large ears, failure to thrive, and mental retardation. Radiographically, closure of the anterior fontanelle is delayed and thickening and sclerosis of the skull, especially the base, orbital rims, and facial bones is seen.[329] The metaphyses of the tubular bones are flared, and the diaphyses are short and sclerotic. Similar findings can be noted in the hands and feet. The middle phalanges are short. The rib cage, vertebrae, and central portions of the iliac and ischial bones are sclerotic.

Craniometadiaphyseal Dysplasia, Wormian Bone Type. This uncommon, probably autosomal recessive condition is associated with a thin superior part of the cranium and multiple wormian bones. Later, minimal sclerosis of the skull base may be seen. The long bones are wide with normal metaphyseal flaring. The short tubular bones also are wide, without diaphyseal constriction, and the clavicles and ribs are broad.[330]

Endosteal Hyperostosis. Although the terminology that has been used to describe the group of diseases termed endosteal hyperostosis is inconstant and a definitive classification system has yet to be proposed, three types of hyperostosis are considered appropriately here: an autosomal recessive type that occurs in childhood (Van Buchem's type), a more severe autosomal recessive syndrome (sclerosteosis), and an autosomal dominant type appearing in late childhood (Worth's type).

Van Buchem's Type. Symptoms and signs occur at an earlier age in Van Buchem's syndrome than in the autosomal dominant form of the disease and are characterized by more severe enlargement of the mandible and more frequent cranial nerve involvement, including facial nerve palsy and deafness.[331-333] Affected patients also have a prominent forehead and widened nasal bridge, and serum levels of alkaline phosphatase may be elevated. Unlike the case with sclerosteosis, stature is normal. Radiographic findings are similar to but more severe than those in the dominant form of the disease (Fig. 88–94). Specific abnormalities include periosteal excrescences in the tubular bones, osteosclerotic and enlarged ribs and clavicles, and increased radiodensity of the spine, particularly prominent in the spinous processes.

Sclerosteosis. The autosomal recessive form was first delineated by Truswell in 1958, and the designation "sclerosteosis" was introduced by Hansen in 1967.[334-336] This disorder usually becomes evident in infancy or early childhood. Clinical findings are excessive height and weight, peculiar facies with a broad, flat nasal bridge, ocular hypertelorism, mandibular prominence, deafness, facial palsy, cutaneous or bony syndactyly of the second and third fingers, absent or dysplastic nails, and radial deviation of the terminal phalanges. In adults, headaches due to elevation of intracranial pressure have been described.

Radiographs show a progressive marked hyperostosis of the skull and mandible.[339] The vertebral endplates and pedicles and the bones of the pelvis are sclerotic. The long bones are enlarged, with cortical hyperostosis, moderate alteration of the bone contours, and lack of normal diaphyseal constriction. Pathologic fractures do not occur.

Worth's Type. Worth's syndrome, an autosomal dominant form of endosteal hyperostosis, may be detected incidentally on radiographs obtained for unrelated reasons; however, asymmetric enlargement of portions of the face, particularly the jaw,[338] and the presence of a palatal mass (torus palatinus) are important clinical signs. Radiographic

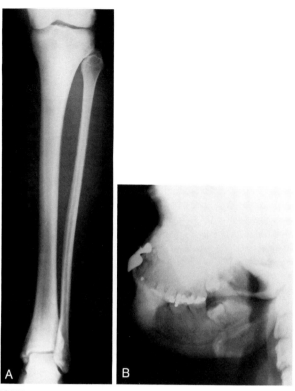

FIGURE 88–95. Endosteal hyperostosis: Autosomal dominant syndrome (Worth's syndrome).
A In an adult, endosteal thickening of the cortices has led to encroachment on the medullary canals.
B Mandibular findings include osteosclerosis, loss of the normal antegonial notch, coarse trabeculation, and a prominent mandibular canal.

findings include endosteal thickening in the cortex of the tubular bones with encroachment on the medullary cavity (Fig. 88–95A).[339] The bones are not expanded, and abnormal modeling is absent. In the skull, osteosclerosis begins in the base and subsequently involves the facial bones, especially the mandible. The latter bone lacks the normal antegonial notch, and the mandibular canal may be prominent (Fig. 88–95B). In the spine the sclerosis is most evident in the spinous processes. The ribs and osseous pelvis are affected only mildly. Unlike the recessive form of the disease, in Worth's type the serum levels of alkaline phosphatase are normal, the basilar foramina are not affected, cranial nerve involvement is rare, and the clinical course is benign.[340, 341]

Pachydermoperiostosis. The clinical and radiologic features of pachydermoperiostosis,[338-341] which resemble, in part, those of secondary hypertrophic osteoarthropathy (Fig. 88–96), are discussed in Chapter 93.

Frontometaphyseal Dysplasia. Frontometaphyseal dysplasia initially was described by Gorlin and Cohen in 1969[342] and encompasses cranial hyperostosis, abnormal tubulation of cylindrical bone, and additional skeletal and extraskeletal abnormalities.[343-346] Clinical manifestations include childhood onset, prominent hornlike supraorbital ridges, micrognathia, defective dentition, a wide nasal bridge, a high-arched palate, hearing loss, visual disturbances, a short trunk with long extremities, elongated fingers with ulnar deviation of the hands, genu valgum, decreased joint mobility, and contractures. The initial

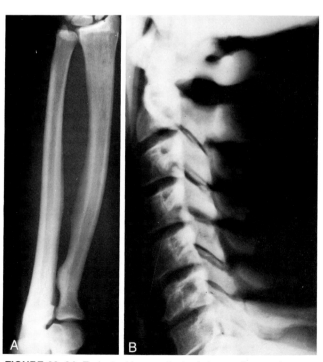

FIGURE 88–94. Endosteal hyperostosis: Autosomal recessive syndrome (Van Buchem's syndrome).
A Note diffuse osteosclerosis and cortical thickening.
B Osteosclerosis is especially marked in the neural arches and spinous processes.

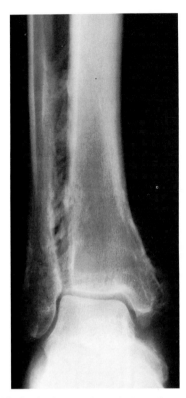

FIGURE 88–96. Pachydermoperiostosis. Irregular periosteal bone formation is characteristic of this disorder.

manifestations usually are related to the craniofacial abnormalities. An X-linked recessive inheritance is likely.

Radiographic features consist of a prominent supraorbital ridge, calvarial hyperostosis, absent frontal sinuses, antegonial notching of the mandibular body, hypoplasia of the angle and condylar process of the mandible, dental malformations, accentuated flaring of the iliac wings, metaphyseal splaying in the tubular bones, tibial and fibular waviness and bowing, genu valgum, tibia recurvatum, and elongation and widening of the metacarpal bones and phalanges (Fig. 88–97). Rib contours can be irregular. The ischial bones can be wide, and coxa valga may be present. In older patients, progressive erosion and fusion of the carpal and tarsal bones have been noted, which may simulate the findings in juvenile chronic arthritis or various osteolytic syndromes.

Although the exact relationship of frontometaphyseal dysplasia to other craniotubular disorders is not clear, the presence of prominent cranial abnormalities allows its differentiation from Pyle's dysplasia. The features of frontometaphyseal dysplasia resemble those of craniometaphyseal dysplasia, although it has been suggested that facial and occipital bone involvement and a normal pelvic contour in the craniometaphyseal variety allow separation of the two disorders.

Craniometaphyseal Dysplasia. The basic features of craniometaphyseal dysplasia in both its autosomal dominant and its recessive forms are facial deformity, cranial hyperostosis, and failure of normal modeling of tubular bones.[347–349] The recessive forms of the disease are accompanied by more severe facial involvement, which, in some cases, leads to striking abnormalities consisting of a broad mass at the base of the nose and hypertelorism. In fact, nasal obstruc-

tion due to bone proliferation causes many of these patients to be mouth-breathers. Dental malocclusion and facial paralysis often occur. Deafness results, in part, from foraminal constriction with encroachment on the auditory nerve and from direct involvement of the ossicles in the inner ear (Fig. 88–98). Similar osseous proliferation leads to optic nerve atrophy and compression of the brain stem. Although some patients are mentally retarded and have hydrocephalus and leukoencephalopathy, their life span usually is within normal limits.

Radiographically, progressive sclerosis of the base of the skull and about the cranial sutures, obliteration of the paranasal sinuses, and loss of the lamina dura about the teeth are seen.[350] In infancy, osteosclerosis in the diaphysis of the tubular bones, similar to that observed in diaphyseal dysplasia, is evident; subsequently it disappears, being replaced by a severe modeling defect manifested as metaphyseal expansion, cortical thinning, and club-shaped epiphyses (Fig. 88–98). The spine rarely is affected, although the ribs and the medial aspect of the clavicles can be widened. Intense uptake of the pharmaceutical agent can be seen on radionuclide bone scans in the skull and diaphyses of the tubular bones.[351]

Pyle's Dysplasia. Pyle's (or metaphyseal) dysplasia is a rare disorder that demonstrates either recessive or dominant transmission; it becomes manifest at a variable age with mild clinical symptoms and signs, including joint pain, muscular weakness, scoliosis, genu valgum, dental malocclusion, and bone fragility.[352–355] The radiographic abnormalities are striking (Fig. 88–99). Marked expansion of the metaphyseal segments of tubular bones leads to an Erlenmeyer flask appearance, especially in the distal portion of the femur and proximal portions of the tibia and fibula. Changes in the upper extremity are similar but less extensive. In both locations, a relatively abrupt transition occurs between the cylindrical and flared portions of the bone. Minor alterations in the skull include supraorbital prominence, an obtuse angle of the jaw, and mild sclerosis of the cranial vault. The bones of the pelvis, medial portions of the clavicles, and sternal ends of the ribs are expanded.

Osteoectasia with Hyperphosphatasia. This disorder, which also is known as juvenile Paget's disease, chronic osteopathy with hyperphosphatasia, and hereditary hyperphosphatasia, is a rare condition of infancy and childhood characterized by generalized cortical thickening of bones and chronic sustained elevation of serum levels of alkaline phosphatase.[356–359] It was first described by Bakwin and Elger in 1956[360] and is detected in early life because of an abnormal modeling of bones that leads to marked skeletal deformity. An autosomal recessive inheritance seems to exist, with considerable variability of expression. Involvement may be severe or mild, and clinical variation is evident even in a single family. Overproduction of bone and bone collagen by osteocytes and failure of primitive fibrous bone to mature into compact lamellar or haversian bone are present with increased bone turnover. Affected children have a small stature, large skull, fusiform swelling and bowing of the tubular bones, and a tendency toward fracture. They may exhibit severely limited motion and are unable to walk, crawl, or sit up. Laboratory abnormalities, in addition to elevated serum levels of alkaline phosphatase, include increased serum levels of acid phosphatase, uric acid, and leucine aminopeptidase and increased urinary lev-

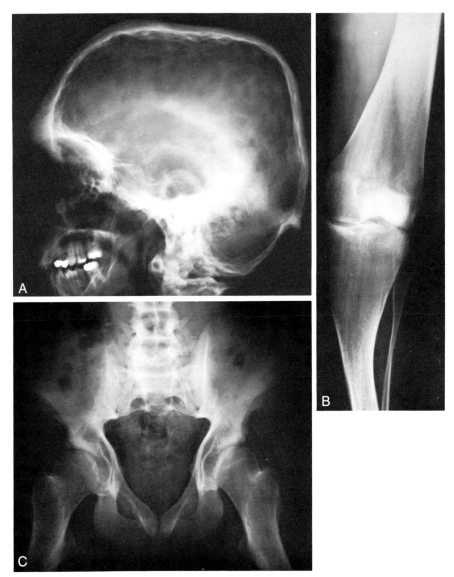

FIGURE 88–97. Frontometaphyseal dysplasia.
A Marked thickening of the supraorbital ridges is evident.
B The long tubular bones reveal metaphyseal splaying.
C Flaring of the iliac wings, wide ischial bones and femoral necks, and coxa valga are evident.
(Courtesy of L. Langer, M.D., Minneapolis, Minnesota.)

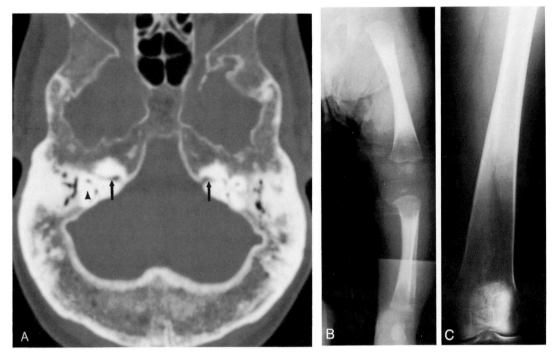

FIGURE 88–98. Craniometaphyseal dysplasia.
A CT scan of the temporal bones shows a thick diploic space, narrow internal auditory canals (arrows), and sclerotic otic capsules (arrowhead).
B,C Radiographs of the leg in a 2 month old child **(B)** and her mother **(C)** show the changing appearance of the radiographic abnormalities. The dominant finding in the child is diaphyseal osteosclerosis and that in the mother is metaphyseal expansion.

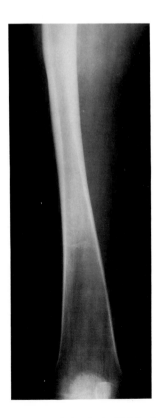

FIGURE 88–99. Metaphyseal dysplasia (Pyle's dysplasia). The femur has an "Erlenmeyer flask" appearance.

els of peptide-bound hydroxyproline. On radiographic analysis, virtually every bone is seen to be affected (Fig. 88–100). Marked calvarial thickening with wide diploic spaces and uneven mottled mineralization of the skull are seen. The tubular bones are bowed and widened. The cortex is thick with coarse trabeculae. The lack of a discrete cortical shadow is noteworthy. The medullary cavity usually is widened but can be narrowed. Vertebral body flattening and protrusio acetabuli are seen. By the second or third decade of life, most patients are severely deformed and incapacitated. Much recent attention has been directed toward the use of thyrocalcitonin or pamidronate in the treatment of this disease.[361]

Oculodento-osseous Dysplasia (Oculodentodigital Syndrome). Affected patients have a typical facies consisting of microphthalmia, a thin nose with narrow nostrils, a large jaw, and hypoplasia of the enamel of the teeth.[362] They also may have syndactyly or clinodactyly, sparse hair (especially about the eyes), and glaucoma. The clinical expressions of this disease vary greatly and, although the condition is presumed to be an autosomal dominant one, other patterns of inheritance also are possible.[363]

Radiographs of the skull reveal osteosclerosis, especially in the basal area, and enlargement of the mandible (Fig. 88–101A). Calcification may be observed on radiographs of the orbits and basal ganglia, although it is detected more easily with CT scanning.[364] The tubular bones show metaphyseal widening and cortical thickening (Fig. 88–101B). Similar widening occurs in the ribs and in the medial as-

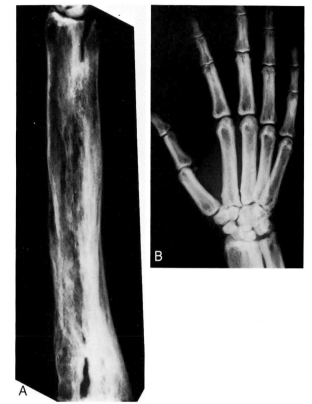

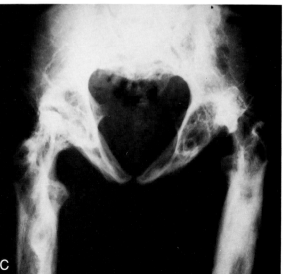

FIGURE 88–100. Hereditary hyperphosphatasia.

  A Cortical thickening in the radius and ulna is associated with loss of definition between the cortex and the medullary bone.

  B Similar findings are present in the hand.

  C In the pelvis, a pagetoid appearance is evident. Subluxation of the left femoral head is present.

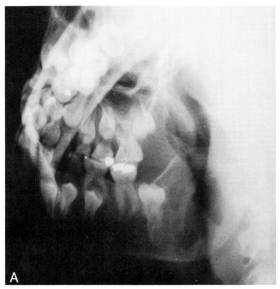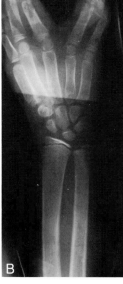

FIGURE 88–101. Oculodento-osseous dysplasia.

A The mandible is expanded in an 11 year old child.

B In the upper extremity, failure of normal tubulation of the bones is noted. Soft tissue syndactyly between the second and third digits and the fourth and fifth digits can be seen.

pects of the clavicles. Mild vertebral flattening in the thoracic spine, syndactyly, absent or osseous fusion of the phalanges, clinodactyly, and bony abnormalities of the inner ear are additional radiographic findings.

Familial Infantile Cortical Hyperostosis (Caffey's Disease). This condition is discussed in Chapter 93.

Disorganized Development of Cartilaginous and Fibrous Components of the Skeleton

Dysplasia Epiphysealis Hemimelica. Dysplasia epiphysealis hemimelica, also known as Trevor's disease or tarsoepiphyseal aclasis, is characterized by asymmetric cartilaginous overgrowth (histologically identical to that of an osteochondroma) in one or more epiphyses or a tarsal or carpal bone.[365, 366] A painless, bony swelling or deformity about a joint, usually in the lower extremities and especially adjacent to the ankle or knee, becomes evident, typically when the patient is 2 to 14 years of age, although occasionally it may appear in infancy.[367] Boys are affected more commonly than girls, and the clinical manifestations are variable, leading to the recognition of localized, classic, and generalized forms of the disease.[368, 369]

Characteristic radiographic features include the early appearance and excessive growth of the involved epiphysis, with a resultant irregularly calcified or partially calcified mass projecting from the epiphysis or a tarsal or carpal bone (Fig. 88–102). Although the irregular mass initially may appear distinct from the surrounding bone, eventually it fuses with the adjacent epiphysis. In fact, an entire epiphysis may be involved. When the malformation involves the epiphyses on one side of the body, it may be associated with hemihypertrophy. Spinal abnormalities, including scoliosis, may occur. Although the masses usually cease growing at the time of skeletal maturity, on rare occasions growth may recur in adulthood. Joint dysfunction or deformity may require surgical intervention. MR imaging and CT scanning are useful in determining a plane of separation between the mass and the remaining normal epiphysis (Fig. 88–103).[370, 371] Although it has been seen in several members of a single family, this disorder generally is accepted as nongenetic in origin.[372]

Multiple Cartilaginous Exostoses. The true frequency of this autosomal dominant condition, also called diaphyseal aclasis, is unknown, but it is a common disease, characterized by cartilage-capped exostoses that usually arise near the diaphyseal side of the physeal line.[373] The patients, usually boys, develop painless lumps near the ends of the long tubular bones and have mild shortness of stature.

The radiographic appearance and size of the exostoses are extremely variable and, in part, depend on their site of origin (Fig. 88–104).[374] They arise in the metaphyseal side of the growth plate, and the apex of the exostosis points away from the epiphysis. The origin can be in an epiphysis, however, as often occurs in the hands. Associated metaphyseal expansion and deformity are evident adjacent to the base of the exostosis, except when the lesions are small. Of great importance, growth of the osteochondromas can be apparent as long as endochondral ossification is proceeding in the adjacent physis but should cease when this normal ossification halts with closure of the growth plate.

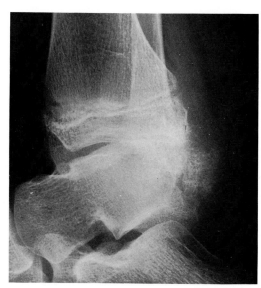

FIGURE 88–102. Dysplasia epiphysealis hemimelica. Note a bony mass arising from the posterior surface of the talus.

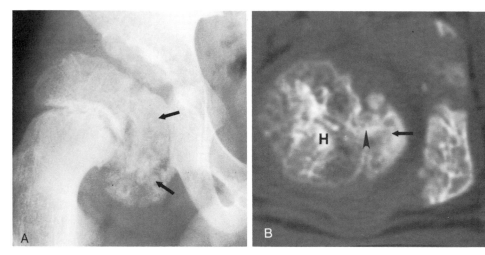

FIGURE 88–103. Dysplasia epiphysealis hemimelica. A radiograph **(A)** and transaxial CT scan **(B)** show a partially calcified mass separate from (arrows) and connected to (arrowhead) the right femoral epiphyses (H).

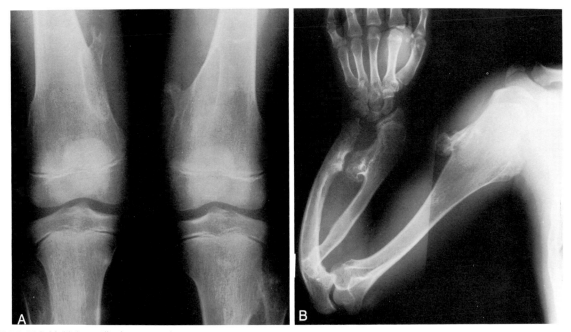

FIGURE 88–104. Multiple cartilaginous exostoses.
  A Observe multiple exostoses arising from expanded metaphyses.
  B Similar exostoses are seen in association with metaphyseal expansion, shortening, and bowing of bones. The radial head is dislocated.

With regard to abnormalities at specific sites, the bones of the forearm frequently are deformed with ulnar angulation of the distal articular surface of the radius, bowing of the radius, ulnar shift of the carpus, shortening of the ulna, and dislocation of the radial head (Fig. 88–104B).[376] The fibula also may be shortened, with lateral obliquity of the ankle joint. Although the ends of the long tubular bones are involved most frequently, the ribs, scapula, and iliac bone often are affected. Vertebral involvement, although uncommon, can lead to spinal cord and nerve root compression. Small lesions in the metaphyseal region of the phalanges or the metacarpal bones may lead to V-shaped physeal lines.[376]

Complications related to the osteochondromas are interference with growth, compression of surrounding structures, including vessels,[377] nerves, and tendons, and malignant transformation. Although the frequency of malignant conversion of an osteochondroma to a chondrosarcoma is unknown, reported estimates are as high as 25 per cent. Gordon and collaborators[378] believed that a more realistic estimate of this frequency is 3 per cent. The radiographic diagnosis of malignant transformation is difficult prior to closure of the physis because the configuration of the cartilaginous cap is variable and can simulate the appearance of a malignant tumor. The findings that suggest malignant transformation are continued growth of the osteochondroma after cessation of normal growth, a changing appearance of calcifications in the cartilage cap, an irregular outline of the osteochondroma, evidence of bone destruction at the base of the exostosis, and angiographic findings that include an increased number of blood vessels adjacent to the osteochondroma with early venous filling and displacement of the surrounding structures.[378] CT scanning, MR imaging, and bone scintigraphy represent additional techniques that may be used to help diagnose malignant transformation of an osteochondroma.

Enchondromatosis (Ollier's Disease). Ollier's disease, a nonhereditary condition, is characterized by multiple enchondromas distributed throughout the tubular and flat bones of the body. The presenting clinical manifestations are masses that increase in size as the child grows, asymmetric limb shortening, and either genu varum or genu valgum deformity.[379] The femur and tibia are affected most commonly.[380] Radiographically, the lesions are seen clearly in infancy and consist of radiolucent masses that can be either round, triangular, or linear (Figs. 88–105 and 88–106). The tubular bones may exhibit considerable expansion, especially in the hands. Pathologic fractures may occur. Focal areas of calcification may appear within the mass. Cartilaginous areas that extend from the physis can lead to considerable interference with growth, resulting in osseous shortening and deformity. Angular deformities are most common in the distal portion of the femur and are associated with nonuniform metaphyseal involvement.[380] In the pelvis, V-shaped radiolucent areas appear in the iliac crest.

The enchondromas typically stabilize or even regress in adulthood. Malignant transformation to chondrosarcoma may occur in up to 25 per cent of the patients by the age of 40 years.[381] One patient developed four primary chondrosarcomas over an 11 year period.[382] Other malignant tumors do occur. Spranger and associates have described six types of enchondromatosis, including one characterized by severe

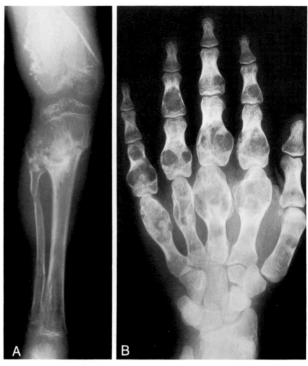

FIGURE 88–105. Enchondromatosis (Ollier's disease).
 A Radiolucent masses of varying shapes are present, containing calcifications that are best demonstrated in the femur and fibula.
 B Multiple expanded radiolucent lesions are evident.

involvement of the hands and feet, mild platyspondyly, and deformity of the skull.[383]

Enchondromatosis with Hemangiomas (Maffucci's Syndrome). Maffucci's syndrome represents the combina-

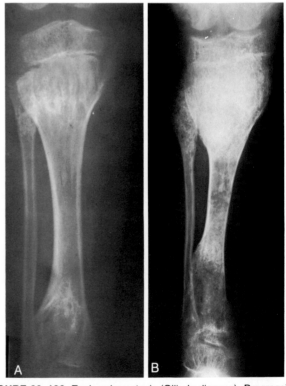

FIGURE 88–106. Enchondromatosis (Ollier's disease). Progressive changes are noted in a child between the ages of 2 years **(A)** and 12 years **(B).**

tion of enchondromatosis and soft tissue hemangiomas.[384] The hemangiomas are detected at birth or shortly thereafter and are of variable size and number. They can produce large masses and distortion of bone growth, including scoliosis.[385] The distribution of the hemangiomas does not correlate with that of the enchondromas. Hemangiomas may occur in other organs, including those of the gastrointestinal tract. Hemangiomas in the head and neck may distort the trachea and produce dysphagia or epistaxis.[386] CT scanning and MR imaging are useful in the evaluation of the nature, extent, and vascularity of the soft tissue and bony lesions.[387]

The radiographic features in Maffucci's syndrome are similar to those of Ollier's disease with the addition of phleboliths and soft tissue masses (Fig. 88–107). Involvement of the hands and feet is frequent and severe. A higher frequency of malignant transformation of the enchondromas is seen in Maffucci's syndrome than in Ollier's disease.[387–389]

Metachondromatosis. Metachondromatosis, an autosomal dominant condition, is characterized by multiple cartilaginous exostoses and enchondromas with prominent marginal calcifications.[390, 391] The principal sites of the exostoses are the hands and feet (Fig. 88–108), although the entire skeleton, including the spine, may be affected. In contrast to typical cartilaginous exostoses, the exostoses in this syndrome point toward the growth plate, are small, and may decrease in size or resolve completely. The enchondromas are seen in the iliac crests and the metaphyses of the tubular bones, and appear as irregular, calcified lesions.[392, 393] Extrarticular calcification and ossification are common. Failure of skeletal growth and distortion of limbs are uncommon.

Osteoglophonic Dysplasia. Osteoglophonic dysplasia, a severe form of rhizomelic dwarfism, is characterized by facial deformities, including a flat bridge of the nose, frontal bossing, hypertelorism, and enlargement of the jaw.[394] Radiographic findings include craniostenosis, prognathism, cystic lesions in the jaws, mild platyspondyly, multiple metaphyseal radiolucent areas that are most frequent in the distal portions of the femora, and epiphyseal alterations.[395]

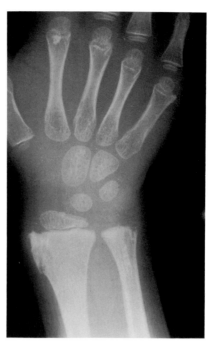

FIGURE 88–108. Metachondromatosis. Exostoses (best seen in the fifth metacarpal bone and radius) and cartilaginous streaks in the distal end of the radius and ulna are present.

The term osteoglophonic refers to the hollowed-out appearance in the metaphyses. The carpal and tarsal bones are small and deformed, and cone-shaped epiphyses occur in the bones of the hands. The hands and feet are short and broad.

Fibrous Dysplasia and Myofibromatosis. These disorders are discussed in Chapters 84, 92, and 95.

Miscellaneous

Tubular Stenosis (Kenny-Caffey Syndrome). Kenny-Caffey syndrome is characterized by a short stature, transient hypocalcemia that may lead to tetany, delayed closure of the anterior fontanelle, widening of the cranial sutures, and stenosis of the medullary canal in multiple bones.[396, 397] The hypocalcemia is a consequence of hypoparathyroidism and resolves with increasing age.[398] The syndrome probably is of dominant inheritance[399] and may be associated with deficiency of the growth hormone. Ocular findings are myopia, hyperopia, and microphthalmia.[400] Radiographs show thinning of the shafts of the long and short tubular bones with a narrow medullary canal (Fig. 88–109). The cortex is thickened, and the metaphyses are flared. Tracheobronchomegaly has been reported.[401]

Parastremmatic Dysplasia. The name for this severe form of dwarfism, which may be of autosomal dominant inheritance, is derived from the Greek words for "distorted limb." Prominent, asymmetric changes occur in the lower limbs, including a twisting type of deformity, progressive kyphoscoliosis, and multiple joint contractures. The hands and feet are short and stubby. Radiographic features include markedly irregular ossification of the epiphyses and metaphyses ("flocky bone" appearance) (Fig. 88–110).[404] The tubular bones are short, have expanded ends, and are osteopenic and grossly deformed. The vertebral bodies are flat, with irregularly ossified endplates. Scoliosis or kyphoscoli-

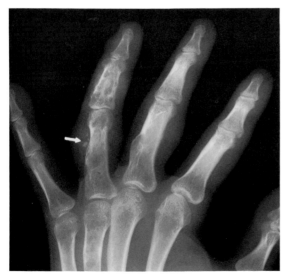

FIGURE 88–107. Enchondromatosis with hemangiomas (Maffucci's syndrome). In addition to multiple enchondromas, phleboliths with calcification are evident in the proximal portion of the fourth digit (arrow).

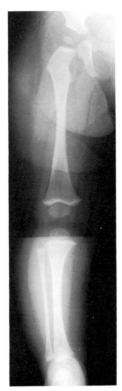

FIGURE 88–109. Tubular stenosis (Kenny-Caffey syndrome). The marked tubular stenosis is evident in the bones of the lower extremities in a 9 month old child.

osis can be severe.[403] The pelvic bones are small, with ilia that have irregular, lacy borders (Fig. 88–110B). Femoral neck ossification is defective, and the femoral heads are small and frequently dislocated. The ends of the ribs are cupped. The carpal and tarsal bones are irregular in both contour and structure.

Occipital Horn Syndrome. Occipital horn syndrome is a rare disease of copper metabolism associated with an unusual skeletal dysplasia that also is referred to as Ehlers-Danlos syndrome, type IX.[404] This X-linked recessive condition is characterized by parasagittal bony exostoses (or horns) arising from the occipital bone (Fig. 88–111A).[405] Other skeletal findings include unusual boxlike deformities

of the bones about the elbow with radial head dislocation (Fig. 88–111B), abnormal hammer-shaped lateral portions of the clavicles (Fig. 88–111C), and abnormal hips and pelvis.[406] Tortuous vessels and obstructive uropathy also are seen. Serum levels of copper and ceruloplasmin are depressed, as are serum levels of lysyloxidase, a copper-dependent enzyme required for the formation of collagen and elastin cross-links.[407]

DYSOSTOSES

Craniosynostosis

The term craniosynostosis implies premature fusion of one or more of the calvarial sutures. These sutures are not true growth centers but rather respond to the stimulus provided by the expanding intracranial contents by laying down new bone.[408] Restraint of the fetal head may be one of the factors leading to isolated closure of a suture.[409] Premature closure of a suture results in local cessation of growth and distortion of the calvarial configuration. Accurate radiographic interpretation should be directed toward the identification of the affected sutures rather than toward the use of specific but, sometimes, confusing terminology that describes the abnormal shape of the skull. The affected suture can be identified by a straight rather than a serrated radiolucent line, osseous proliferation at the suture line, or frank osseous fusion. As a supplement to conventional radiography, CT scanning may be used to delineate any associated abnormalities of the face and central nervous system.[410] Occasionally, bone scintigraphy also can be useful.[411]

Isolated closure of the sagittal suture is the pattern of craniosynostosis that is encountered most commonly, accounting for more than 50 per cent of cases. Closure of the sagittal suture results in an increased anteroposterior diameter of the skull and a decreased biparietal diameter (Fig. 88–112A,B). Synostosis of both coronal sutures produces a skull that is short in its anteroposterior diameter, often with a decrease in the depth of the orbits and maxillary hypoplasia (Fig. 88–112C). Unilateral closure of a coronal suture produces flattening of the orbit on the involved side, best seen on the submentovertical projection of the skull; on the

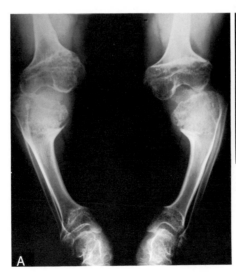

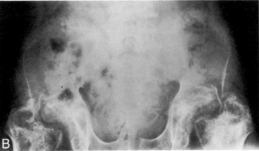

FIGURE 88–110. Parastremmatic dysplasia. The epiphyses are poorly developed, the ilia have lacy margins, and a "flocky bone" appearance about the knees and hips is seen. (Courtesy of E. Miller, M.D., Chicago, Illinois.)

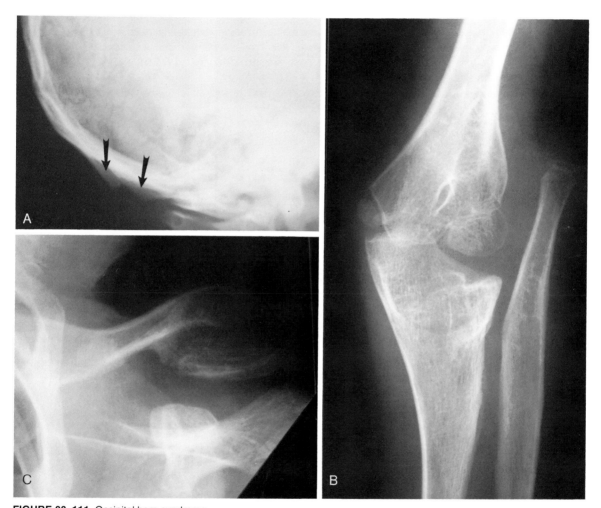

FIGURE 88–111. Occipital horn syndrome.
A The small occipital horns (arrows) are seen in the midline posterior to the foramen magnum.
B A boxlike deformity of the proximal portion of the ulna and a dislocated radial head can be noted.
C The outer region of the clavicle has a hammer-shaped appearance.

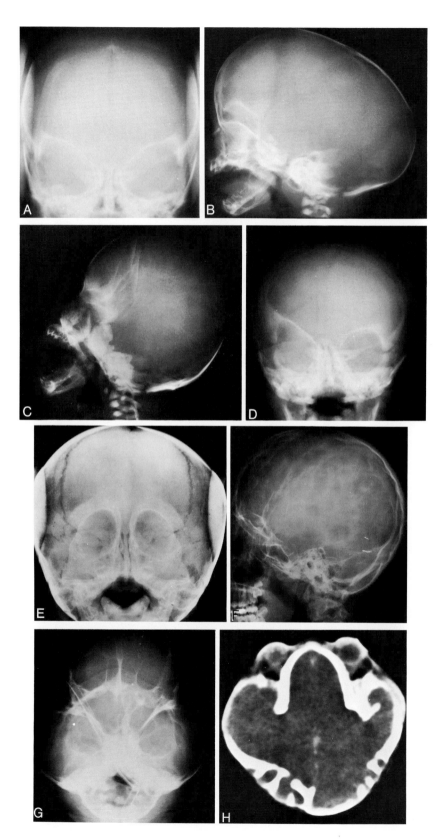

FIGURE 88–112. Craniosynostosis.

A, B Closure of the sagittal suture. Dolichocephaly has occurred.

C Closure of both coronal sutures. The skull is brachycephalic, with a small anterior fossa and a hypoplastic maxilla.

D Closure of one coronal suture. Note the harlequin-shaped right orbit.

E Closure of the metopic suture. Hypotelorism and a triangular-shaped forehead are observed.

F Closure of all sutures. The skull is brachycephalic, with prominent digital markings.

G,H Kleeblattschädel skull. Note osseous scalloping and a trilobed appearance of the cranial vault. The brain projects into the multiple bone channels.

frontal projection, a classic harlequin-shaped orbit is identified (Fig. 88–112D). Unilateral closure of the lambdoid suture leads to flattening of one side of the back of the head, or plagiocephaly. An isolated metopic synostosis creates a triangular forehead with hypotelorism (Fig. 88–112E). In cases of closure of multiple sutures, the skull is variable in shape, although generally it is brachycephalic, and digital markings in the cranium are quite prominent (Fig. 88–112F). The Kleeblattschädel, or clover-leaf skull configuration, also is associated with premature synostosis of multiple sutures (Fig. 88–112G,H). It frequently is accompanied by hypoplasia of the midportion of the face, hydrocephalus, and mental retardation. CT examinations, especially with three-dimensional reconstructions, are useful in surgical planning (Fig. 88–113). Thanatophoric dwarfism, the Pfeiffer syndrome, limb anomalies, and unclassified bone dysplasias can be found in association with Kleeblattschädel.

Craniosynostoses can be further classified into primary and secondary types. Primary closure sometimes occurs as an isolated phenomenon or in conjunction with other malformation syndromes. Secondary synostoses are evident in rickets, hypophosphatasia, thyroid disorders, and hypercalcemia, and they may follow surgical decompression of the intracranial contents. Certain patients with craniosynostosis have characteristic abnormalities of the limbs, and the specific combination of findings forms the basis of some common and recognizable syndromes.

Craniofacial Dysostosis (Crouzon's Syndrome)

Crouzon's syndrome is characterized by craniosynostosis, exophthalmos, and midface retrusion.[412] It has an auto-

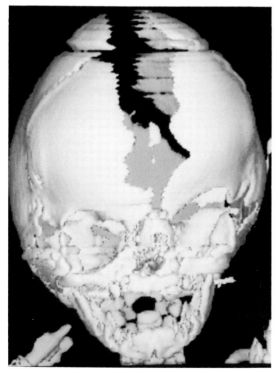

FIGURE 88–113. Apert's syndrome. A three dimensional reconstruction of CT data of the cranium in a newborn infant shows that the coronal suture is solidly closed and the sagittal suture is open.

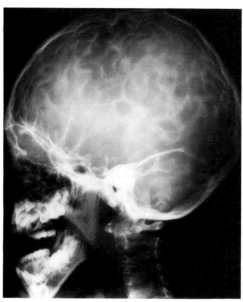

FIGURE 88–114. Craniofacial dysostosis (Crouzon's syndrome). The skull is brachycephalic, and slight maxillary hypoplasia is evident. Abnormal osseous fusion in the cervical spine also was present.

somal dominant mode of transmission, but its expressivity is variable. The skull usually is brachycephalic, with fusion of the coronal and sagittal sutures (Fig. 88–114). In addition, fusion of the lambdoid suture has been reported in 80 per cent of patients.[412] Such craniosynostoses usually are evident by the age of 3 years. Other findings include prominent digital markings in the skull in over 90 per cent of the cases, calcification in the stylohyoid ligament, and deviation of the nasal septum. The maxilla is hypoplastic, and, in combination with sutural closure, influences the degree of exophthalmos that will occur. The prognathic appearance of the mandible also is related, in large part, to the hypoplastic maxilla. Hypertelorism is common and hydrocephalus may occur. Although the absence of significant abnormalities of the hands and feet helps to distinguish Crouzon's syndrome from other disorders accompanied by craniosynostosis, careful analysis will reveal minor alterations in these locations.[413] Spinal anomalies are seen in approximately one third of the patients and usually consist of fusions between the second and third cervical vertebrae (Fig. 88–114). Subluxation of the radial head and ankylosis of the elbows also may occur. Cor pulmonale, related to obstruction of the nasopharyngeal airway, is a recognized complication of this disease.[414]

Acrocephalosyndactyly

Acrocephalosyndactyly encompasses a number of disorders, not all clearly distinct.

Apert's Syndrome. Apert's syndrome is an autosomal dominant condition with sutural closure, midface hypoplasia, and symmetric syndactyly of the hands and feet involving, at a minimum, the second, third, and fourth digits.[415] The abnormality of cranial sutures that occurs in Apert's syndrome may better be regarded as sutural agenesis than as premature closure of a normal suture. The characteristic skull findings at birth are a closed coronal sutural area and an extensive midline calvarial defect from the glabella to the posterior fontanelle, often producing a wide metopic suture area (Fig. 88–112C,D). The calvarium is thin and undermineralized. During the first 4 years of life, islands of ossification occur in the midline defect, coalesce, and ultimately close the sagittal suture area (Fig. 88–115A).[416] Three general patterns of brachycephaly occur: excessively high brachycephaly, excessively wide brachycephaly, and brachycephaly with frontal keel.[417] Facial abnormalities include small orbits with resultant ocular proptosis, a hypoplastic and retropositioned maxilla, and a small nasopharynx[417] (Fig. 88–112C). CT scanning with three-dimensional reconstruction has proved to be valuable in the operative management of patients with Apert's syndrome.[418] Hand abnormalities include a short deviated thumb, complex osteocartilaginous syndactyly of the distal phalanges in the second, third, and fourth digits, and simple syndactyly of the fourth and fifth digits. Three patterns of hand anomalies occur; these sometimes are referred to as spade hand, mitten hand, and rosebud hand[419] (Fig. 88–115B,C). Foot anomalies include complete simple syndactyly (but without complex osteocartilaginous syndactyly), a triangular first proximal phalanx, and progressive osseous fusion of tarsal and metatarsal bones[419] (Fig. 88–115C).

Cerebral abnormalities are common and include hydrocephalus, agenesis of the corpus callosum, septal agenesis, septo-optic dysplasia, megencephaly, gyral abnormalities, encephalocele, hypoplasia of white matter, and heterotopic gray matter.[420, 421]

Osseous fusions also may be evident in other joints of the extremities, and the limbs may be short.[422, 423] In addition, subluxation of the glenohumeral joint, irregularities of the glenoid region, and progressive fusion of the vertebrae, particularly in the cervical spine, may be evident.[424, 425] Cervical spine fusion is common and almost always involves C5-C6, in contrast to the C2-C3 fusion usually seen in Crouzon's syndrome.[426]

Saethre-Chotzen Acrocephalosyndactyly. Saethre-Chotzen syndrome is characterized by craniosynostosis, low frontal hairline, ptosis, brachydactyly, and cutaneous syndactyly of the fingers and the second and third toes. Saethre-Chotzen syndrome is relatively common but of variable, often mild, expression.[427] Brachycephaly relates to craniosynostosis, although some members of a single family may have malformations of the extremities without craniosynostosis.[428] Additional osseous abnormalities include a bifid distal phalanx in the great toe, brachydactyly, coxa valga, small iliac bones, and hypoplasia of the clavicle.[429] Cranial abnormalities are variable.[430] The posterior portion of the base of the skull usually is short and oriented vertically, and the sella turcica is abnormally low in position. The length of the mandibular ramus is reduced.

Pfeiffer's Syndrome. Pfeiffer's syndrome, an autosomal dominant condition, is characterized by craniosynostosis, broad thumbs and toes, variable maxillary retrusion, and partial soft tissue syndactyly. The cranial and extracranial findings are variable, but premature closure of the coronal sutures is typical.[431, 432] Three clinical subtypes of Pfeiffer's syndrome occur. Type I is classic Pfeiffer's syndrome, associated with normal intelligence and a good prognosis. Type II is manifested by cloverleaf skull, severe proptosis, and ankylosis of the elbows. Type III is manifested by the absence of cloverleaf skull but the presence of elbow ankylosis and a high morbidity in infancy.[433] A hallux valgus deformity with a triangular shape of the proximal phalanx in the great toe and an enlarged first metatarsal bone (Fig. 88–116) are common. In the hands and feet, cutaneous syndactyly of the second and third digits and shortening of the middle phalanges often are present. The thumb is broad and deformed, with frequent fusion of the interphalangeal joints. Symphalangism of other digits, carpal and tarsal fusions, and accessory epiphyses are among some of the additional malformations in the hands and feet. Cervical spine fusion, cone-shaped epiphyses, and hypoplasia of the bones about the elbow are encountered.[434]

Jackson-Weiss Syndrome. Jackson-Weiss syndrome, an autosomal dominant condition characterized by midface hypoplasia, craniosynostosis, and anomalies of the feet (but usually with normal hands), is uncommon.[435] A tremendous variety of anomalies of the feet have been observed, ranging from abnormalities of the great toe identical to those seen in Pfeiffer's syndrome to more extensive synostosis, as seen in Apert's syndrome. The facial appearance in pa-

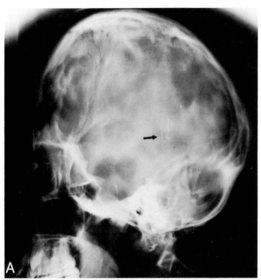
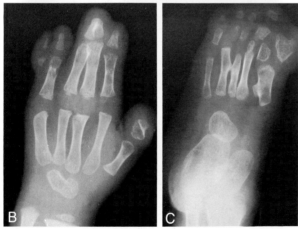

FIGURE 88–115. Acrocephalosyndactyly—Apert's syndrome.

A Findings in the skull include brachycephaly, a hypoplastic anterior fossa, a prominent sella turcica, and choroid calcifications (arrow). Abnormalities in the cervical spine also are present in this adult.

B In the hand of a child, symphalangism, osseous and soft tissue syndactyly, phalangeal deformity in the thumb, polydactyly, and carpal fusion are seen.

C Similar abnormalities are observed in the foot.

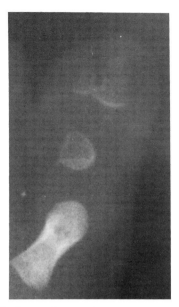

FIGURE 88–116. Acrocephalosyndactyly—Pfeiffer's syndrome. The first toe is broad, with a triangular proximal phalanx and a bifid distal phalanx.

tients with the Jackson-Weiss syndrome has been likened to that in patients with Crouzon's syndrome, but marked proptosis is absent.

Acrocephalopolysyndactyly

The basic features of the acrocephalopolysyndactyly syndromes are craniosynostosis and polysyndactyly. The best known of these disorders is *Carpenter's syndrome,* of autosomal recessive inheritance. Acrocephaly, obesity, hypogonadism, abdominal hernias, and congenital heart disease[436] are among its many associated abnormalities. Mental retardation may be present but its occurrence is not invariable.[437] Radiographic findings include a relatively late closure of the coronal suture and a variety of abnormalities in the hands and feet. The tubular bones of the hands, particularly the middle phalanges and metacarpal bones,[438] are shortened, and syndactyly commonly occurs between the third and fourth digits (Fig. 88–117A). The proximal phalanx of the thumb often is broad or duplicated. A ''tongue-like'' appearance may be seen on the radial aspect of the epiphysis of the proximal phalanx of the second finger. In the foot, preaxial polydactyly with duplication of the first

or second toe, soft tissue syndactyly (Fig. 88–117B), and a short and broad first metatarsal bone are typical alterations. Coxa valga, flared iliac wings, genu valgum, and spinal anomalies also can be seen. Two other syndromes of acrocephalopolysyndactyly should be noted. Patients with *Noack's syndrome* exhibit enlarged thumbs and duplication of the great toes. *Sakati's syndrome* is characterized by craniosynostosis, polysyndactyly, shortened tibiae and fibulae, and bowed femora. Goodman's syndrome and Summit's syndrome now are considered variants of Carpenter's syndrome in which the patients have normal intelligence (Summit's syndrome) or clinobrachydactyly (Goodman's syndrome).[439]

Other Craniosynostosis Syndromes

Baller-Gerold Syndrome. The Baller-Gerold syndrome is an autosomal recessive craniosynostosis syndrome associated with radial hypoplasia. No typical pattern of sutural closure is seen; plagiocephaly, turricephaly, and trigonencephaly all have been described.[440] Radial anomalies often are asymmetric, including bilateral radial hypoplasia and asymmetric thumbs and first metacarpal bones. Anal anomalies, particularly imperforate anus, with associated genitourinary anomalies are seen in over one third of patients.[441, 442]

Antley-Bixler Syndrome. The Antley-Bixler syndrome is a craniosynostosis syndrome associated with radiohumeral synostosis, choanal stenosis, and femoral bowing. The inheritance probably is autosomal recessive.[443, 444] Craniosynostosis is most frequent in the skull base but also involves coronal, lambdoid, and metopic sutures. Fractures of the femur at the point of maximum bowing may be present at birth.

Trigonencephaly Syndromes. Trigonencephaly denotes a triangular head with a prominent keel-shaped forehead usually attributed to metopic synostosis, although some controversy exists as to whether the synostosis is primary or secondary.[445] Ethmoid hypoplasia and orbital hypotelorism also are important features. Trigonencephaly may be inherited as an autosomal dominant condition without other abnormalities. Trigonencephaly occurs as an occasional manifestation in several syndromes, including Baller-Gerold and Saethre-Chotzen syndromes. However, it is a phenotypic feature of the Opitz C syndrome and several other rare conditions. Opitz C syndrome is an autosomal recessive condition associated with limb anomalies, particularly

FIGURE 88–117. Acrocephalopolysyndactyly (Carpenter's syndrome).

A Hand. Soft tissue syndactyly involves the third and fourth digits. The middle phalanges of the fingers are either absent or hypoplastic, and the proximal phalanx of the thumb is hypoplastic.

B Foot. Soft tissue syndactyly with preaxial polydactyly and some phalangeal deformities are seen. The first metatarsal bone is short and broad.

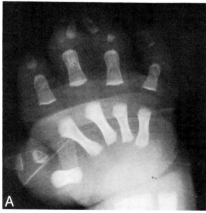
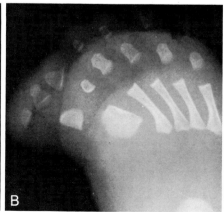

polysyndactyly, high-arched palate, multiple oral frenula, and psychomotor retardation.[446] Cardiac anomalies, especially septal and atrioventricular canal defects, are common.

Cephalopolysyndactyly (Greig's Syndrome). Greig's syndrome is characterized by both preaxial (in the feet) and postaxial (in the hands) polydactyly,[447] syndactyly, a large head, and minor craniofacial abnormalities[448, 449] (Fig. 88–118). Hypertelorism no longer is considered a necessary part of this syndrome, nor is there evidence of craniosynostosis or mental retardation. The forehead often is high and prominent, with a broad nasal bridge and epicanthal folds.

The features of the acrocallosal syndrome resemble those of Greig's syndrome but include, in addition, severe mental retardation, hypotonia, and absence of the corpus callosum.[449]

Mandibulofacial Dysostosis (Treacher Collins Syndrome). Patients with Treacher Collins syndrome, an autosomal dominant disorder, have characteristic clinical features consisting of an antimongoloid slant to the eyes, flat cheekbones, small mandible, dysplastic ears, deafness, coloboma, and deficient lashes in the lower eyelids. Radiographic findings include marked hypoplasia of the zygomatic arches, the maxilla, and the paranasal sinuses. The orbits are egg-shaped, and the mandible is hypoplastic, with a broad concave curve on the lower border of the body (Fig. 88–119). It appears that this basic shape of the mandible is established in utero and is maintained throughout postnatal development.[450] The coronoid process may be broad, and the condylar process is small. The external auditory canal sometimes is absent, and a poorly formed middle portion of the ear contains abnormal ossicles.[451, 452] Narrowing of the upper portion of the airway is related to facial involvement, and this may lead to sleep apnea, which has been improved by mandibular surgery.[453] Occasionally, vertebral anomalies and malformations in the extremities also are observed.

Acrofacial Dysostosis, Preaxial (Nager's Syndrome). The facial characteristics of Nager's syndrome, an autosomal recessive disorder, are similar to those of mandibulo-

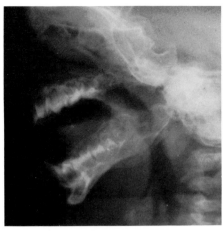

FIGURE 88–119. Mandibulofacial dysostosis (Treacher Collins syndrome). Note the hypoplastic mandible with a broad, concave curve in its lower aspect.

facial dysostosis.[454] In addition, this syndrome is associated with preaxial reduction abnormalities in the upper limbs.[455] Both the thumb and the radius may be absent (Fig. 88–120). Syndactyly in the feet also may be observed. More severe abnormalities have been encountered in several patients.

Acrofacial Dysostosis, Postaxial (Miller's Syndrome). Miller's syndrome probably is an autosomal dominant condition with facial features similar to those of the Treacher Collins syndrome but with aplasia or hypoplasia of the fifth digits in both the hands and the feet and accessory nip-

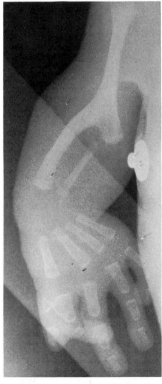

FIGURE 88–120. Acrofacial dysostosis (Nager's syndrome). In a 1 month old infant, osseous fusion of the ulna and the humerus, a hypoplastic radius, four rather than five metacarpal bones, radial deviation of the hand, and an additional two phalanges with soft tissue syndactyly on the ulnar side of the hand are evident.

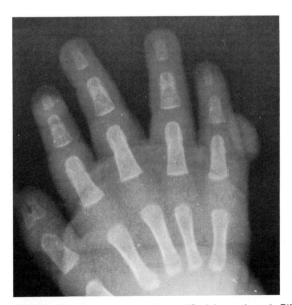

FIGURE 88–118. Cephalopolysyndactyly (Greig's syndrome). Bifid distal phalanx of the thumb and polydactyly are seen.

ples.[456] The radius and ulna often are short and radioulnar synostosis is common.[457]

Oculoauriculovertebral Dysplasia (Goldenhar's Syndrome). Goldenhar's syndrome is a malformation spectrum of ocular, auricular, and skeletal defects of unknown cause and often of discordant manifestations in monozygotic twins.[459] Although some cases are of autosomal dominant inheritance, probably significant etiologic heterogeneity exists.[458, 459] Its dominant features are hypoplasia of the face (usually unilateral), abnormalities of the ear (consisting of preauricular tags or pits and deformity or absence of pinna), and eye anomalies (including epibulbar dermoids, lipodermoids or lipomas, and colobomas of the upper lids). Radiographic findings confirm the presence of hypoplasia of the mandible, maxilla, and mastoids.[460] The external auditory canals and ossicles in the ear reveal varying degrees of hypoplasia or may be absent altogether.[460] Similarly, the zygoma and the temporomandibular joints are hypoplastic. Common vertebral abnormalities include osseous fusion, hemivertebrae, supernumerary vertebrae, and an elongated odontoid process; scoliosis and rib involvement also may be associated (Fig. 88–121). A variety of other abnormalities occur, including hypoplasia of the radius, absent digits, renal anomalies, imperforate anus, congenital heart disease, bronchopulmonary malformations,[461] cranial defects, hydrocephalus, and lipoma of the corpus callosum.[462, 463]

Hemifacial Microsomia. The characteristic features of the disease are unilateral abnormalities of the ear and hypoplasia involving one side of the face.[464] Macrostomia and malformation of the mandibular ramus and condylar process also are present. Although much variablity occurs in the manifestations in this syndrome,[465] many similarities with oculoauriculovertebral dysplasia exist, and the two conditions are not always clearly separable. In most instances, hemifacial microsomia occurs sporadically, but the condi-

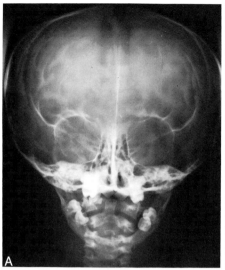
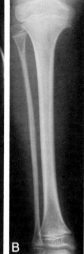

FIGURE 88–122. Oculomandibulofacial syndrome (Hallermann-Streiff-François syndrome).
 A Findings include bulging of the parietal bones, prominent digital markings, and a hypoplastic mandible.
 B The tubular bones are narrowed.

tion may have an autosomal dominant or autosomal recessive inheritance.[466]

Oculomandibulofacial Syndrome (Hallermann-Streiff-François Syndrome). Oculomandibulofacial syndrome consists of craniofacial malformations, ocular and dental abnormalities, and a proportionate dwarfism that may be severe.[467] The face and mandible are small, and the nose is narrow and beaklike. Frontal bossing is noted, and the patient has a diminished amount of hair and skin atrophy. Ocular findings include microphthalmia and cataracts. The teeth may be malformed and have a variety of other abnormalities. Deficiency of humoral immunity and hypoparathyroidism have been observed.[468]

Radiographs show a small mandible with primary involvement of its ascending ramus.[469] Hypoplasia or aplasia of the temporomandibular joints and hypoplasia of the maxilla may be present. The shape of the skull varies, but it often is brachycephalic, with frontal and parietal bossing (Fig. 88–122A). The long tubular bones, ribs, and clavicles are thin (Fig. 88–122B). Additional findings include flattening of the vertebral bodies, dislocations of joints, calcification of the falx cerebri, winged scapulae, syndactyly, metacarpal shortening, and osteoporosis.[470]

CHROMOSOMAL ABERRATIONS

Chromosomal abnormalities tend to result from genetic imbalances and involve either autosomal or sex chromosomes. Many are lethal, owing to the severe defects in normal morphogenesis they cause. They can be classified as trisomies (in which three rather than the normal pair of chromosomes are present), translocations (in which part of a chromosome becomes transposed to another chromosome), and deletions (in which a portion of a chromosome is absent). Only the more common chromosomal abnormalities are summarized here.

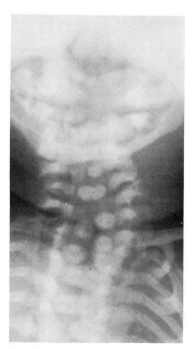

FIGURE 88–121. Oculoauriculovertebral dysostosis (Goldenhar's syndrome). Multiple developmental errors are noted in the cervical and upper thoracic regions of the spine.

4p− Syndrome (Wolf-Hirschhorn Syndrome)

Patients with deletion of the short arm of chromosome 4 reveal mental and growth retardation, seizures, eye deformities, cleft lip and cleft palate, hypoplastic dermal ridges, and nonspecific skeletal alterations, including dolicocephaly with severe microretrognathia producing a Greek-helmet craniofacial profile, hypertelorism, foot deformities, hypoplastic ilia, thin posterior ribs, and vertebral abnormalities.[471, 472] Poor ossification of the pubis, sacral alae, and cervical spine may be prominent radiographic findings (Fig. 88–123). Renal anomalies are frequent, especially severe renal hypoplasia with oligonephronia.[471]

5p− Syndrome

Deletion of the short arm of chromosome 5 results in a well-known syndrome named after the characteristic cry made by affected patients (cat cry or cri du chat syndrome). Mental retardation is severe, growth is slow, and microcephaly, a round face, hypertelorism, epicanthal folds, and an antimongoloid slant of the palpebral fissures are seen. Nonspecific radiographic features include microcephaly, hypertelorism, abnormal development of long bones (perhaps due to muscular hypotonia), scoliosis, shortening of some of the metacarpal bones, and small iliac wings.[473]

Trisomy 8 Syndrome

Patients with trisomy 8 syndrome have a large skull with a prominent bulging forehead, hypotelorism, a broad shallow nose, thick lips, a small mandible, and a short neck.[474] The trunk appears somewhat long and narrow, and multiple joint contractures and clubfeet are seen. Mental retardation is mild. Radiographically generalized osteopenia, multiple joint subluxations or dislocations, hypoplastic iliac bones with loss of the lateral wings, small patellae, coxa valga, and metaphyseal flaring in the tubular bones are seen.[475] Skeletal maturation is delayed. Multiple anomalies in the spine include extra vertebrae, spina bifida, hemivertebrae, and other errors of vertebral segmentation. The interpediculate distances in the lumbar spine often are narrow. The clavicles can be sclerotic, the scapulae are small, and Sprengel's deformity sometimes is present. Accessory and nar-

row ribs are common, and pectus excavatum and abnormal sternal ossification may be found. Cardiac and renal anomalies, including cystic nephroblastomas, also can occur.[476]

San Luis Valley recombinant (SLVR) chromosome 8 is a chromosomal anomaly found in the Hispanic population of the southwest portion of the United States. Hypertelorism, clinodactyly, and small patellae occur. Interestingly there is a 93 per cent incidence of congenital heart disease with a 55 per cent incidence of conotruncal abnormalities.[477]

Trisomy 9p Syndrome

Trisomy 9p is associated with growth disturbance and mental retardation, hypertelorism, a large nose, cup-shaped ears, kyphoscoliosis, small hands and feet with short digits, clinodactyly, syndactyly, hypoplastic terminal phalanges and nails, and characteristic dermatoglyphic patterns.[478–480] Radiographic findings are evident in the feet, hands, and pelvis during the period of physeal growth and include retardation of osseous maturation, pseudoepiphyses, and delayed ossification of the pubic bones.

Trisomy 13 Syndrome

Trisomy 13 syndrome is a clearly defined chromosomal disorder first noted in 1960 by Patau and associates[481] and subsequently described by other investigators.[482–485] Affected infants have severe anomalies, with mental retardation, seizures, and apnea. A small skull, arhinencephaly, holoprosencephaly (occurring in 66 per cent of patients),[486] abnormal eyes and ears, cleft lip, cleft palate, cutaneous hemangiomas, flexion deformities of fingers, congenital heart disease, and renal cystic disease are evident.[486] The most common skeletal alterations are polydactyly, syndactyly, asymmetry of the thorax, prominence of the calcaneus, midline craniofacial anomalies, small first ribs, and rocker-bottom feet (Fig. 88–124).

Trisomy 18 Syndrome

The increased age of mothers of infants with trisomy 18 is similar to that which is noted in Down's syndrome.

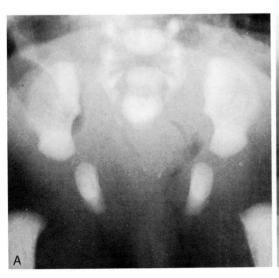
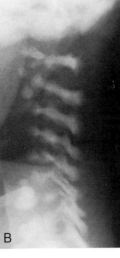

FIGURE 88–123. 4p− syndrome (Wolf-Hirschhorn syndrome).

A In a newborn infant, poor ossification of the pubic bones, hypoplastic ilia, and poor sacral ossification are seen.

B Dysplastic cervical vertebrae also are evident.

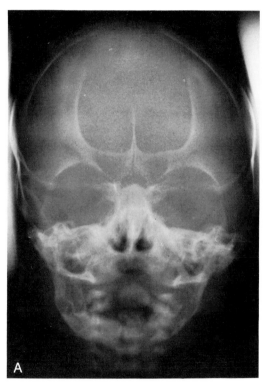

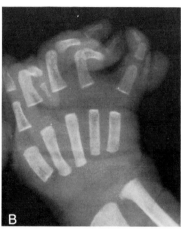

FIGURE 88–124. Trisomy 13 syndrome.

A In a newborn infant, observe hypotelorism, a cleft palate, skull defects, and microcrania.

B Flexion contractures and postaxial polydactyly also are evident.

Affected infants are of low birth weight and possess a narrow head, prominent occiput, malformed ears, micrognathia, high-arched palate, finger deformities, hypertonicity, and hernias.[487-490] Cardiac anomalies (especially ventricular septal defect), omphalocele (10 to 20 per cent of patients), and renal anomalies (especially horseshoe-shaped kidneys) are frequent features of this syndrome.[491, 492] Radiographs of the hand reveal adduction of the thumb, superimposition of the second and third fingers, and hypoplasia of the first metacarpal bone. Rocker-bottom feet, metatarsus varus, a shortened first toe, hypoplastic terminal phalanges of the toes, hypoplasia of ribs, clavicles, and sternum, and pelvic deformities complete the radiographic picture (Fig. 88–125). Cerebral anomalies include cerebellar hypoplasia and large choroid plexus cysts.[492]

Trisomy 21 (Down's Syndrome)

In 1959, Lejeune and coworkers[493] observed that patients with certain phenotypic characteristics of Down's syndrome had 47 chromosomes. Ninety to 95 per cent of persons with this syndrome possess the extra chromosome designated number 21. Patients with this syndrome are identified at birth by the ocular abnormalities (which include oblique palpebral fissures, epicanthal folds, cataracts, Brushfield spots, nystagmus, and strabismus), hypotonia, brachycephaly, mental retardation, and large tongue. Developmental hip dysplasia is evident in approximately 40 per cent of infants. Gastrointestinal abnormalities, including duodenal atresia,[494] Hirschsprung's disease,[495] and tracheoesophageal and anorectal anomalies,[496] are well recognized. Pulmonary hypertension[497] occurs with high frequency, probably secondary to pulmonary, tracheal, and nasopharyngeal anomalies.[498, 499]

Radiographs of the pelvis reveal flared iliac wings and flattened acetabular roofs (Fig. 88–126),[500-504] findings that may persist into adulthood.[500] Hypoplasia of the middle

phalanx of the fifth finger with clinodactyly, short and irregular metacarpal bones, accessory epiphyses, an extra manubrial ossification center, cuboid vertebral bodies, 11 pairs of ribs, microcephaly, a high-arched and short palate, delayed sutural closure, and sinus hypoplasia may be identified. These abnormalities vary in prevalence, related in part to whether the patients have trisomy 21 or chromosomal translocation and mosaicism.[505]

Atlanto-occipital[506] and atlantoaxial instability[503] can be associated with neurologic deficits (Fig. 88–126C). The exact mechanism for the neurologic findings is not certain, although a high degree of ligamentous laxity, with cord compression, is suspected.[507, 508] Additional factors that are responsible for atlantoaxial instability may include trauma, pharyngeal infection, osseous abnormalities of the odontoid process, and hypoplastic posterior arch of the atlas.[509] This instability generally is not symptomatic and may decrease with increasing age of the patient.

Monosomy 21 Syndrome

Monosomy 21 syndrome has features that resemble those of arthrogryposis multiplex congenita, including joint contractures, dislocations, and kyphoscoliosis. The patient has severe growth retardation and a typical facial appearance consisting of a broad nose, an antimongoloid slant of the palpebral fissures, a carplike mouth, large and low-set ears, and a small mandible. Osseous syndactyly, vertebral malformations, a short and broad thorax, a narrow pelvis, flexed fingers, and poor pubic ossification as well as other inconstant skeletal malformations may be present.[510, 511]

Turner's Syndrome

Turner's syndrome occurs in persons with female phenotype and a 45, XO chromosome complement. As many as 99.9 per cent of fetuses with this chromosomal comple-

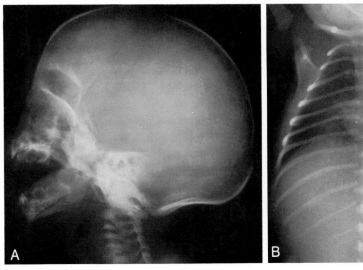
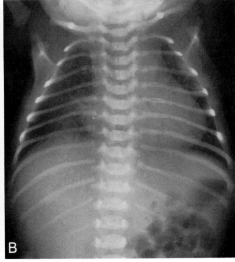

FIGURE 88–125. Trisomy 18 syndrome.
A The skull is elongated, with a prominent occiput and hypoplastic mandible.
B The clavicles and ribs are thin. Cardiac abnormalities are present.

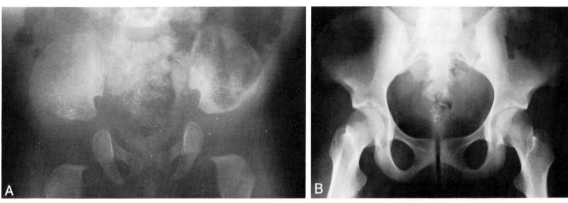

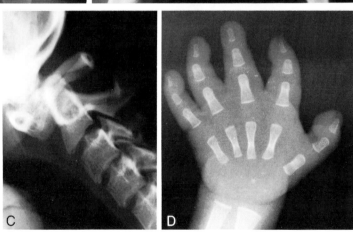

FIGURE 88–126. Trisomy 21 (Down's syndrome).

A In a newborn infant, observe flared iliac wings with resultant decreased acetabular and iliac angles.

B In an adult, the iliac wings remain flared.

C Note considerable atlantoaxial subluxation.

D Hypoplasia of the middle phalanx of the fifth digit and clinodactyly are present.

ment are aborted spontaneously in the first trimester of pregnancy. Mosaicism is more frequent in live-born infants with Turner's syndrome. In fact, some chromosomally normal cells in the fetus or placenta may be necessary for survival.[512, 513] In the newborn infant, edema of the hands and feet may be evident, and large edematous masses about the neck, which can even be detected in utero,[514] occur. Secondary sex characteristics do not appear, primary amenorrhea is frequent, and the ovaries are small and streak-like.[515] Clinical manifestations include lymphedema of the lower extremities, loose skin about the neck, congenital anomalies of the heart, great vessels,[516] and kidneys, short stature, and laterally displaced nipples on a shieldlike chest.

Many radiographic abnormalities may be evident in this syndrome[517–520] (Fig. 88–127). Osteoporosis is present except in the very young and may be related to an estrogen deficiency occurring early in life.[521] The decreased bone density is most pronounced in the spine, carpus, and tarsus. Although skeletal maturation may appear to proceed normally, epiphyseal fusion is delayed and may not occur until the third decade of life. Shortening of the metacarpal bones, especially the fourth, and of the metatarsal bones can be

evident. Drumstick phalanges have been observed. Although a decrease in the carpal angle has been noted in this syndrome, it is not common.[522] Deformity of the knees with flattening of the medial tibial plateau, beaking or exostoses of the medial and proximal portions of the tibia, and enlargement of the medial femoral condyle are observed. Cubitus valgus, thin clavicles and ribs, vertebral body irregularities, and abnormalities of the odontoid process and atlas also have been described. With regard to the skull and face, brachycephaly, small facial bones, mandibular prominence, enlarged sinuses, and calcification in the petroclinoid ligaments have been observed. Extraskeletal findings include hyperplasia or neoplasms of the pituitary gland,[523] coarctation of the aorta, hemangiomas, intestinal telangiectasia, inflammatory bowel disease,[524] renal anomalies (e.g., malrotation and horseshoe kidneys), and a variety of other tumors.[525]

Klinefelter's Syndrome

Klinefelter's syndrome usually results from the presence of two or more X chromosomes and a Y chromosome,

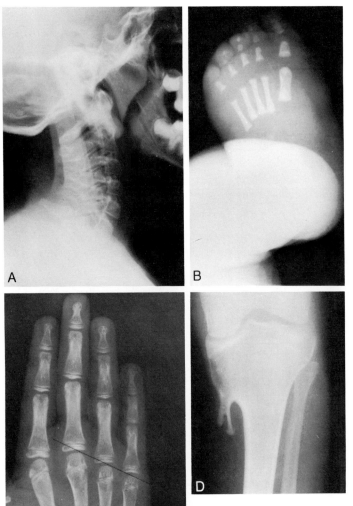

FIGURE 88–127. Turner's syndrome.

A In an 8 year old patient, soft tissue abnormality, related to webbing of the neck, projects over the posterior portion of the vertebrae. Osteopenia is evident.

B In a newborn infant, note soft tissue edema.

C The fourth metacarpal bone is relatively short, and the phalanges are relatively long, with a drumstick configuration.

D Findings include an exostosis projecting from the medial aspect of the tibia and prominence of the medial femoral condyle.

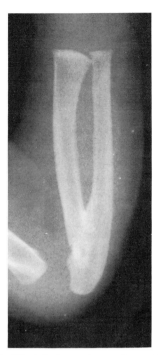

FIGURE 88–128. Klinefelter's syndrome. In a child with an XXY chromosomal pattern, radioulnar synostosis is observed.

although a number of variant chromosomal patterns also are recognized, such as XXYY.[526–528] Muscular weakness, mental retardation, delayed puberty, azoospermia, and infertility are frequent. A variety of nonspecific radiographic changes have been outlined, including metacarpal shortening, clinodactyly, accessory epiphyses, a flattened ulnar styloid process, pointed phalangeal tufts, radioulnar synostosis, and retarded bone age (Fig. 88–128).

MUCOPOLYSACCHARIDOSES (MPS) AND RELATED DISORDERS

The term mucopolysaccharidosis (MPS) was first used in 1952 by Brante[529] in a description of the histologic findings in patients with gargoylism, which included swollen collagen tissues filled with water-soluble material. The same material was discovered in other sites and organs. Later studies indicated extensive amounts of certain mucopolysaccharides in the urine of affected patients.[530] In the ensuing years, the detection of different chemical substances in the urine of patients with similar varieties of dwarfism led to the delineation of closely related but distinct disorders. Currently, the MPS are classified into various types, and additional diseases are recognized, some of which are mucolipidoses, which demonstrate similar clinical and radiologic findings (Table 88–1). Common to the MPS and mucolipidoses are certain clinical and radiographic characteristics; the radiographic abnormalities are designated dysostosis multiplex and are described in the following paragraph.

The skull usually is large and dolichocephalic, with premature closure of the sagittal suture (Fig. 88–129). The mastoids and paranasal sinuses are poorly developed. Commonly, an elongated J-shaped sella turcica (Fig. 88–129), prominent adenoids, malformed teeth, flattened mandibular condyles, a large tongue, and a thick diploic space are seen. Central nervous system changes are discussed later in the

section dealing with Hurler's syndrome. In the spine, there is defective development of the anterosuperior portion of the vertebral bodies at the thoracolumbar junction with gibbus formation owing to the presence of hook-shaped vertebrae (Fig. 88–130). The vertebral bodies are oval, slightly diminished in height, or flattened (Fig. 88–131). In the pelvis, the superior acetabular region is underdeveloped, resulting in a widened acetabular roof and wide acetabular angle (Fig. 88–132). Coxa valga is frequent, and the femoral heads are delayed in development and become dysplastic. In the chest, the ribs are widened but taper near their vertebral margins (Fig. 88–132). The clavicles are thick, short, and widened. The changes in the long tubular bones are greater in the upper extremities than in the lower extremities, with diaphyseal and metaphyseal expansion, delay in epiphyseal ossification, and cortical thinning (Fig. 88–133A). Constriction of the humeral and femoral necks with resultant varus deformities may occur (Fig. 88–133B). In the hand, diffuse osteopenia, cortical thinning, and proximal tapering of the second to fifth metacarpal bones (Fig. 88–134) are observed. The proximal and middle phalanges are short and wide, and the terminal phalanges are hypoplastic. The carpal bones are small and deformed. Similar but less dramatic changes also occur in the phalanges of the foot and metatarsal and tarsal bones. The distal portions of the radius and ulna taper, thus altering the carpal angle. In addition, cardiomegaly and hepatosplenomegaly, flexion contractures, and umbilical and inguinal hernias may be seen.

A more precise diagnosis requires clinical information, including the pattern of genetic transmission, and biochemical data, including the pattern of increased urinary excretion of acid mucopolysaccharides. Three clinical-genetic syndromes due to alpha-L-iduronidase deficiency now are recognized: MPS I-H (Hurler's syndrome), MPS I-S (Scheie's syndrome), and MPS I-H-S (a distinct intermediate syndrome). Hurler's syndrome is the most severe variety.

MPS I-H (Hurler's Syndrome)

Hurler's syndrome, an autosomal recessive disorder, becomes manifest in the first few years of life.[531] Patients reveal distinctive facies, mental retardation, deafness, dwarfism, corneal opacities, hepatosplenomegaly, cardiomegaly, and cardiac murmurs. Laboratory analysis indicates increased urinary excretion of dermatan sulfate and heparan sulfate, abnormal mucopolysaccharide accumulation in the bone marrow and peripheral leukocytes, and low or absent activity of alpha-L-iduronidase in various tissues. Radiographs reveal macrocephaly, craniostenosis, a J-shaped sella turcica, widening of the anterior portion of the ribs, ovoid vertebral bodies with hypoplasia of vertebrae about the thoracolumbar junction resulting in kyphosis, atlantoaxial subluxation,[532] hypoplasia and stenosis of the bases of the ilia with pseudoenlargement of the acetabulum and coxa valga, shortening and widening of the shafts of the long tubular bones, pointing of the proximal portions of the metacarpal bones, and osteoporosis (Figs. 88–129, 88–130, 88–133, and 88–134). Mental retardation and skeletal deformities may be progressive, leading to considerable disability. Death usually occurs in the first decade of life from heart failure or respiratory complications.[533] Severe involve-

TABLE 88–1. Mucopolysaccharidoses, Mucolipidoses, and Other Conditions with Dysostosis Multiplex

Designation	Eponym or Synonym	Enzyme Deficient	Clinical Features
Mucopolysaccharidoses (MPS):			
MPS I-H	Hurler's syndrome	Alpha-L-iduronidase	Early clouding of cornea, mental retardation, heart disease, coarse facial features
MPS I-S	Scheie's syndrome	Alpha-L-iduronidase	Late onset, stiff joints, cloudy cornea, aortic valve disease, intelligence unaffected, mild facial dysmorphism
MPS I-H-S	Hurler-Scheie syndrome	Alpha-L-iduronidase	Intermediate between Hurler's and Scheie's syndromes
MPS II	Hunter's syndrome	Iduronate-2-sulfatase	Severe: Diagnosed early, mental retardation, death in second decade
			Mild: Survival into adulthood with little intellectual impairment
MPS III	Sanfilippo's syndrome (Types A, B, C, D)	IIIA Heparan N-sulfatase	Severe mental retardation, very mild skeletal and somatic features
		IIIB alpha-N-acetyl glucosaminidase	
		IIIC Acetyl CoA: a-Glucosaminide-N-acetyl transferase	
		III N-acetyl glucosamine-6-sulfate sulfatase	
MPS IV	Morquio's syndrome (Types A and B)	IVA: Galactosamine-6-sulfate sulfatase	Severe dwarfism, short trunk and neck, knock-knees, corneal changes (seen with slit lamp), intelligence unaffected
MPS VI	Maroteaux-Lamy syndrome	N-acetylgalactosamine-4-sulfatase	Dwarfism, coarse facial features, corneal clouding, normal intelligence
MPS VII	Sly syndrome	Beta-glucuronidase	Hepatosplenomegaly, variable mental retardation
Other Conditions:			
Aspartyl-glucosaminuria		Aspartyl glucosaminidase	Intellectual deterioration, coarse features
Alpha-beta-mannosidosis		Alpha-beta-mannosidase	Variable, mental retardation
Fucosidosis		Alpha-fucosidase	Upper respiratory infections, developmental delay
GM$_1$ gangliosidosis (several forms)	GM$_1$ gangliosidosis	Beta-galactosidase	Severe to mild somatic features, onset in infancy
Mucolipidoses (ML):			
ML I (sialidosis)	Lipomucopolysaccharidosis	N-acetyl-neuraminidase	Mild somatic features, progressive neuromuscular symptoms
ML II	I-cell disease	UDP-N-acetyl-glucosaminyl-phosphotransferase	Exaggerated somatic features, marked gingival hyperplasia
ML III	Pseudo-Hurler's polydystrophy	UDP-N-acetyl-glucosaminyl-phosphotransferase	Variable somatic features, stiff joints, corneal clouding, short stature

From Blighton, P (ed): Heritable Disorders of Connective Tissue 5th ed. St. Louis, CV Mosby, 1993.

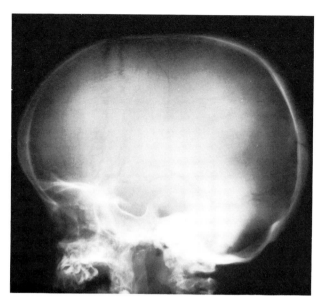

FIGURE 88–129. Dysostosis multiplex (MPS I, Hurler's syndrome). The skull is large, the mastoids are poorly developed, and the sella turcica is J-shaped.

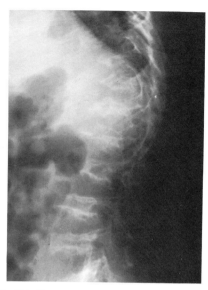

FIGURE 88–131. Dysostosis multiplex (MPS IV, Morquio's syndrome). The vertebral bodies are flattened and possess anterior tongues of bone.

ment of the thoracic and abdominal aorta in Hurler's syndrome leading to coarctations and occlusions of costal and lumbar arteries may be common, being manifested clinically as hypertension.[534] Coronary artery disease occurs.[535] Airway obstruction is a common problem resulting from various causes, including mucopolysaccharide infiltration of the larynx and trachea, a high epiglottis, adenoid enlargement, an abnormal cervical spine, and abnormal chest motion and configuration.[536, 537]

With regard to other imaging techniques, CT scanning of the brain may reveal hydrocephalus that can be progressive, enlargement of the interhemispheric fissures and cortical sulci, and symmetric areas of low attenuation in the white matter.[538] MR imaging reveals delayed or deficient myeli-

nation in the brain that can improve after bone marrow transplantation, diminished gray-white matter differentiation, and cystic changes in the periventricular and supraventricular white matter with frequent involvement of the corpus callosum and basal ganglia.[539]

MPS I-S (Scheie's Syndrome)

An autosomal recessive disorder, MPS I-S is characterized by deficiency of alpha-L-iduronidase and is manifested primarily as peripheral clouding of the cornea, normal men-

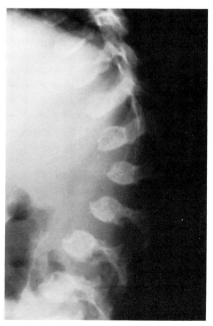

FIGURE 88–130. Dysostosis multiplex (MPS I, Hurler's syndrome). Note the hook-shaped vertebrae and a gibbus deformity at the thoracolumbar junction.

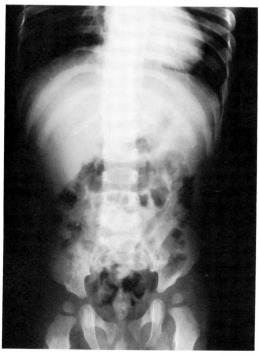

FIGURE 88–132. Dysostosis multiplex (MPS II, Hunter's syndrome). Underdevelopment of the superior acetabular region, wide femoral necks, coxa valga deformity, and wide ribs with posterior tapering are seen.

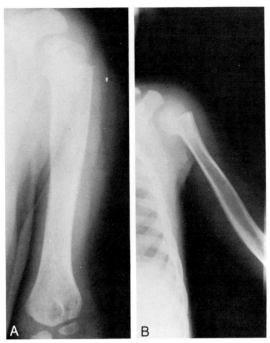

FIGURE 88–133. Dysostosis multiplex (MPS I, Hurler's syndrome). Radiographs of the upper extremity in a patient aged 18 months **(A)** and 4 years **(B)** show initial osseous expansion and subsequent osseous constriction in the proximal portion of the humerus.

tality, normal or slightly reduced stature, stiff joints, hirsutism, flexion of the hands, and aortic regurgitation.[540] Airway obstruction may lead to apnea during sleep and require operative intervention.[541] Increased excretion of dermatan sulfate and heparan sulfate is seen. Radiographs demonstrate proximal tapering of the metacarpal bones, widening of the ribs, and mild alterations of the spine and skull.[542] An arthropathy in adult patients with Scheie's syndrome has been described. Periarticular cysts have been seen in the hands, wrists, and hips.[543, 544]

MPS I-H-S

MPS I-H-S is intermediate between MPS I-H and MPS I-S in its clinical and radiologic severity as a result of the presence of different allelic mutations at the alpha-L-iduronidase locus.[545, 546] Myelography may reveal spinal cord compression, especially in the cervical region, related to thickening of the dura.[547]

MPS II (Hunter's Syndrome)

Hunter's syndrome, an X-linked recessive disorder, is differentiated from MPS I by its occurrence only in male subjects, mild mental retardation, absence of corneal clouding, less significant hearing impairment, and a relatively benign clinical course. However, in addition to a mild form, a severe form of the disease does exist.[548–552] The latter form, often fatal in the second decade of life, is accompanied by mental retardation and more marked radiographic and clinical features. The milder form is associated with normal intelligence and less dramatic radiographic abnormalities, although osteoarthritis of the hip may occur (Figs. 88–132 and 88–135).[552] Survival into middle age or beyond is not infrequent, although serious problems involving the heart or lungs can develop, leading to the patient's death.

MPS III (Sanfilippo's Syndrome)

Sanfilippo's syndrome encompasses a group of diseases that result from deficiencies of lysosomal enzymes involved in the degradation of heparan sulfate. These diseases have

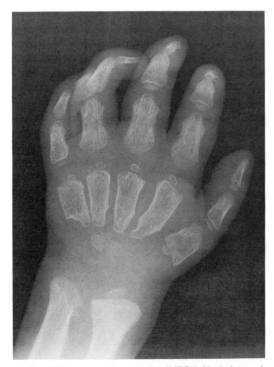

FIGURE 88–134. Dysostosis multiplex (MPS I, Hurler's syndrome). Osteopenia, pointing of the proximal portion of the metacarpal bones, widening of the proximal and middle phalanges, small carpal bones, and a V-shaped deformity of the distal portion of the radius and ulna are evident.

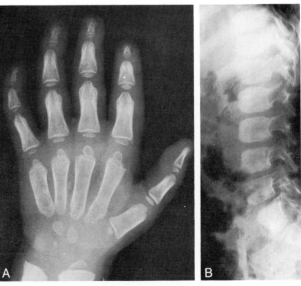

FIGURE 88–135. MPS II (Hunter's syndrome).
A The changes of dysostosis multiplex are mild, with phalangeal widening, metacarpal pointing, and a delay in carpal ossification.
B The vertebral bodies are slightly rounded and have an accentuated posterior concavity.

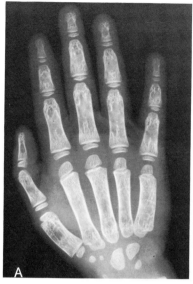
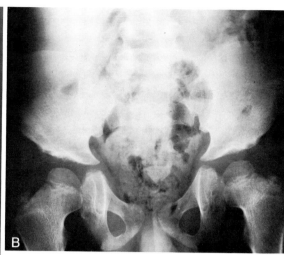

FIGURE 88–136. MPS III (Sanfilippo's syndrome).
A Osteopenia and mild changes of dysostosis multiplex are seen.
B Mild flaring of the iliac bones with underdevelopment of their supra-acetabular portion and slight widening of the femoral necks are evident.

been designated as types A, B, C, and D, depending on the nature of the specific deficiency.[553, 554] The different types are similar clinically,[553–555] although type A generally is more severe. Abnormal facial features, limitation of joint mobility, hepatosplenomegaly, and mental retardation usually become evident after the age of 2 or 3 years. Radiographic findings of dysostosis multiplex are relatively mild (Fig. 88–136); the skull is thick and the mastoids are underdeveloped. In the spine, a mild gibbus deformity and oval vertebral bodies with occasional small anterior osteophytes are evident. A leading cause of death is pneumonia. Central nervous system changes are similar to those evident in Hurler's syndrome.

MPS IV (Morquio's and Related Syndromes)

MPS IV includes a type A or Morquio's syndrome, related to a deficiency of galactosamine-6-sulfate sulfatase, and a type B syndrome, due to a deficiency of beta-galactosidase.[556] Clinical findings in these syndromes are highly variable[557] but typically include severe dwarfism, spinal

shortening and kyphoscoliosis, anterior bulging of the sternum, joint laxity, prominence of the lower face, hypoplasia of the enamel in the deciduous and secondary teeth, a short neck, exaggerated lumbar lordosis, and flat feet. Corneal clouding and deafness also occur. Normal intelligence and a variable life span are additional features.

The abnormalities on spinal radiographs are most helpful in the accurate diagnosis of MPS IV. In early infancy, the vertebral bodies are slightly rounded, with a small anterior beak.[558] With subsequent growth, a central tongue or projection appears, protruding from the anterior surface of the vertebral bodies. In adulthood, the vertebrae are flat and rectangular, with irregular margins (Figs. 88–131 and 88–137A). Instability may lead to upper spinal cord damage during anesthesia (Fig. 88–137B).

The anteroposterior diameter of the chest is increased, with a decrease in its vertical height. Anterior bowing of the prematurely fused sternum is associated with short, wide ribs with bulbous ends. Cardiac enlargement occurs as the result of aortic valvular involvement. In the pelvis, increased obliquity in the lateral aspect of the acetabular

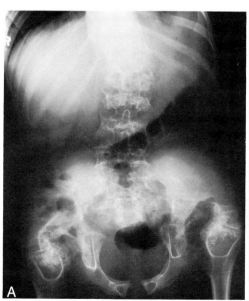
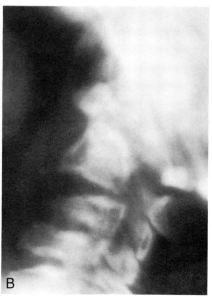

FIGURE 88–137. MPS IV (Morquio's syndrome).
A In a 10 year old patient, marked platyspondyly, flared iliac wings, and severe changes about the hips are evident.
B A lateral conventional tomogram of the cervical spine shows odontoid hypoplasia and narrowing of the spinal canal.

roofs and considerable flaring of the iliac wings are observed. Coxa valga deformity and progressive dysplasia of the capital femoral epiphysis also are seen (Fig. 88–137A).[559] Additional findings include flattening and deformity of the mandibular condyles, mild expansion of the metacarpal bones with pointed proximal ends, small and irregular carpal bones, and slanting of the distal articular surfaces of the radius and ulna. The long tubular bones exhibit diminished growth, metaphyseal flaring, and epiphyseal deformity.

MPS VI (Maroteaux-Lamy Syndrome)

Maroteaux-Lamy syndrome, which is an autosomal recessive disorder, is characterized by short stature that usually becomes evident at about 2 years of age in association with lumbar kyphosis, sternal protrusion, knock knees, abnormal facies, hepatosplenomegaly, and joint contractures.[560, 561] A spectrum of abnormalities that range from mild to severe is seen. Corneal opacification and normal intelligence are additional clinical findings. Radiographs reveal macrocephaly, an enlarged sella turcica, ilial hypoplasia, flared iliac crests, dysplasia of capital femoral epiphyses, constriction of the proximal femoral and humeral necks, coxa valga, biconvexity of vertebral endplates, hypoplasia of the anterior aspects of the upper lumbar vertebrae and odontoid process, deformities of the long tubular bones, narrowing of the ribs near their vertebral ends, widening of the medial aspects of the clavicles, and shortening, widening, and proximal tapering of metacarpal bones (Fig. 88–138). Cardiac disease develops in adolescence and adulthood as a severe cardiomyopathy that includes endocardial fibroelastosis or valvular heart involvement.[562]

MPS VII (Sly's Syndrome)

Sly and collaborators in 1973 described MPS VII in an infant with short stature, mental retardation, beta-glucuronidase deficiency, and radiographic findings typical of the MPS.[563] At least three forms of the disorder are recognized on the basis of clinical criteria: a fatal neonatal form; an infantile form with an early onset and with features and clinical course similar to that of Hurler's syndrome; and a much milder juvenile form with later clinical onset.[564, 565] Ischemic necrosis of the proximal femoral epiphysis and spinal abnormalities are the dominant radiographic changes (Fig. 88–139). The changes of dysostoses multiplex are most pronounced and progressive in the infantile form.

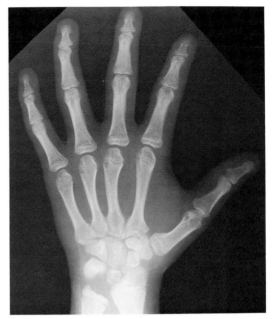

FIGURE 88–138. MPS VI (Maroteaux-Lamy syndrome). In a 13 year old patient, note minimal flexion contractures of the fingers and deformity of the distal portion of the radius and ulna.

Aspartylglucosaminuria

Patients with aspartylglucosaminuria are mentally retarded, with facial features resembling those in Hurler's syndrome, dorsal kyphosis, and abnormal urinary excretion of aspartylglucosamine.[566] Radiographic findings are mild, with osteopenia, a small skull with a thickened diploic portion, hypoplastic vertebrae in the thoracolumbar region, and osteoporosis.

Mannosidosis

Mannosidosis is a storage disorder associated with a deficiency of the enzyme alpha-D-mannosidase in the liver. This deficiency results in the intracellular accumulation and excessive urinary excretion of mannose-containing oligosaccharides. Radiographs reveal calvarial thickening, flattening and deformity of vertebral bodies, ilial hypoplasia, and mild expansion of the tubular bones of the hand.[567, 568] Infantile and juvenile types occur, with the former being associated with severe radiographic changes, mental deterioration, and death in childhood. The juvenile type is accom-

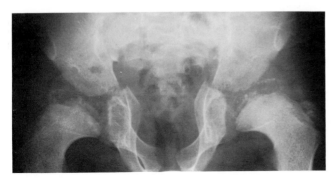

FIGURE 88–139. MPS VII (Sly's syndrome). In this 8 year old patient, obvious flattening and fragmentation of the capital femoral epiphyses are seen.

panied by milder clinical and radiographic changes of dysostosis multiplex.

Fucosidosis

Fucosidosis is a lysosomal storage disorder that leads to psychomotor deterioration and even death. The majority of patients are of Italian descent.[569] A deficiency of alpha-fucosidase enzyme allows abnormal accumulation of fucosyl components in the lysosomes.

Three patterns of this autosomal recessive disease have been described. In the type I disorder, clinical onset occurs in the first few months of life, with rapid psychomotor deterioration and early death. In the type II disorder, the symptoms and signs commence in the second year of life and relate to progressive cerebral degeneration. A later onset of the disease with slower progression characterizes the type III syndrome. In the various types the radiographic abnormalities of dysostosis multiplex are mild.[570, 571] Some reviews suggest that the different types of the disease are part of a continuous clinical spectrum of severity.[569]

GM₁ Gangliosidosis

GM₁ gangliosidosis, an autosomal recessive disease, relates to beta-galactosidase deficiency. The clinical findings include progressive cerebral degeneration, visceromegaly, features resembling those of Hurler's syndrome, and dysostosis multiplex.[572] The condition has three forms: infantile, juvenile, and adult.[573] The infantile form of the disease is characterized by severe neurologic disability, hepatosplenomegaly, blindness, seizures, cherry-red maculae, and early death. Neonatal edema is common, and some infants may have frank ascites. Radiographic findings are dramatic, as the tubular bones are short, expanded, and osteopenic, with metaphyseal irregularity and periosteal cloaking (Fig. 88–140). Fractures are common. An underdeveloped supra-acetabular portion of the ilium and flaring of the iliac wings

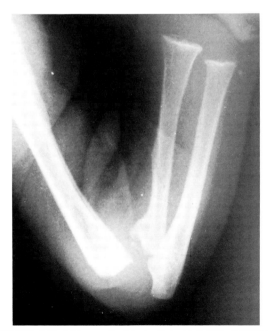

FIGURE 88–140. GM₁ gangliosidosis. Note periostitis, particularly in the humerus and the radius.

are evident. The vertebral bodies are hypoplastic. In one report, excessive accumulation of hyaline cartilage occurred in a notched defect in the lumbar vertebrae at the site of a gibbus deformity.[574] The juvenile form of the disease has a later onset, a slower course, and milder clinical and radiographic findings.[573] The adult type of the disease has a wide range of clinical and radiographic features.[575]

Mucolipidoses

The mucolipidoses are a group of disorders that clinically and radiographically resemble Hurler's syndrome, with the absence of abnormal mucopolysacchariduria and the presence of prominent accumulations of complex lipids. Four types exist, but type IV is not associated with skeletal manifestations.

Mucolipidosis I (Sialidosis)

Mucolipidosis I, also called sialidosis, is a lysosomal storage disease that results from a deficiency of *N*-acetyl neuraminidase.[576] Considerable phenotypic diversity is seen. Typically, affected patients possess physical features similar to those of Hurler's syndrome, a neurodegenerative process affecting the white and gray matter in the brain, cherry-red macular changes, and hepatosplenomegaly. Radiographs reveal a thick skull, a small sella turcica, slender tubular bones, severe thoracolumbar scoliosis, and dislocations of the hip and other joints.[577] Additional findings include a bifid calcaneus, premature fusion of the metopic suture, and hypoplasia of the odontoid process.[578]

Mucolipidosis II (I-Cell Disease)

At several months of age, the clinical and radiologic features of I-cell disease or Leroy's syndrome, an autosomal recessive disorder, simulate those of Hurler's syndrome (Fig. 88–141) but with normal levels of glycosaminoglycan excretion.[579–581] Abnormal fibroblast inclusion bodies characterize this disorder.[582]

In the neonatal period the radiographic abnormalities include osteoporosis, periosteal bony deposition in the long tubular bones, metaphyseal irregularity, cortical destruction, fractures, ovoid vertebral bodies, gibbus deformity at the thoracolumbar junction, narrow supra-acetabular regions, elongated ischial bones, and short phalanges. In later infancy and childhood, severe changes of dysostosis multiplex are seen. The hips may be dislocated. The prognosis in this condition is poor, and many patients die in early childhood as a result of cardiac or respiratory failure. The histologic findings of the bone lesions in neonates are similar to those of rickets and hyperparathyroidism.[583, 585] Radiographically, the condition may be confused with neonatal hyperparathyroidism.

Mucolipidosis III (Pseudo-Hurler's Polydystrophy)

Mucolipidosis III, an autosomal recessive disorder, is characterized by mucopolysaccharides in the fibroblasts, viscera, and mesenchymal tissue, normal urinary excretion of mucopolysaccharides, dwarfism, restricted joint mobility, peculiar facies, corneal opacification, and mild or moderate mental retardation.[585–587] Radiographic abnormalities simulate those in MPS I and MPS II and are of variable severity (Fig. 88–142). Clawhands, flattening of the femoral epiph-

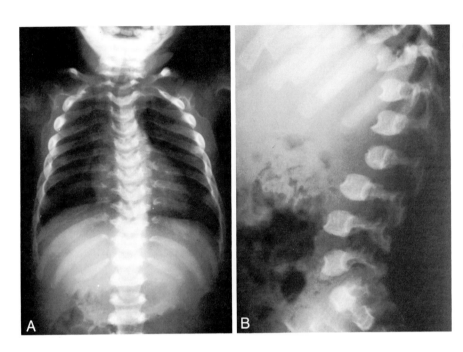

FIGURE 88–141. Mucolipidosis II (I-cell disease). Findings include widening of the ribs, deformed scapulae, varus deformity of the humeri, and hook- and hourglass-shaped vertebrae.

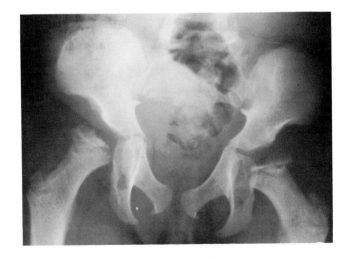

FIGURE 88–142. Mucolipidosis III. In a 9 year old child, note narrow supra-acetabular portions of the iliac bones, small irregular femoral heads, coxa valga, and tapering of the ischial bones.

yses, platyspondyly, and flaring of the iliac wings can be seen.

References

1. Spranger JW: International classification of osteochondrodysplasias. Eur J Pediatr 151:407, 1992.
2. Spranger JW, Langer LO Jr, Wiedemann H-R: Bone Dysplasias. An Atlas of Constitutional Disorders of Skeletal Development. Philadelphia, WB Saunders Company, 1974.
3. Silverman FN: Caffey's Pediatric X-Ray Diagnosis: An Integrated Imaging Approach. Chicago, Year Book Medical Publishers, 1985.
4. Kozlowski K, Beighton P: Gamut Index of Skeletal Dysplasias. New York, Springer-Verlag, 1984.
5. Taybi H, Lachman R: Radiology of Syndromes, Metabolic Disorders and Skeletal Dysplasias. 3rd Ed. Chicago, Year Book Medical Publishers, 1990.
6. Wynne-Davies R, Hall CM, Apley AG: Atlas of Skeletal Dysplasias. New York, Churchill Livingstone, 1985.
7. Rimoin DL, Lachman RS: Genetic Disorders of the Osseous Skeleton. In P Beighton (Ed): McKusick's Heritable Disorders of Connective Tissue. 5th ed. St. Louis, CV Mosby, 1993, pp 557–689.
8. Gorlin RJ, Cohen MM, Levin LS: Syndromes of the Head and Neck. 3rd Ed. New York, Oxford University Press, 1990.
9. Wiedemann, HR, Kunze J, Grosse FR, et al: Atlas of Clinical Syndromes. 3rd Ed. St. Louis, Mosby–Year Book, 1992.
10. Poznanski AK: The Hand in Radiologic Diagnosis. 2nd Ed. Philadelphia, WB Saunders Company, 1984.
11. Beighton P, Cremin BJ: Sclerosing Bone Dysplasias. New York, Springer-Verlag, 1980.
12. Maroteaux P, Lamy M, Robert JM: Le nanisme thanatophore. Presse Med 75:2519, 1967.
13. Burrows PE, Stannard MW, Pearrow JK, et al: Early antenatal sonographic recognition of thanatophoric dysplasia with cloverleaf skull deformity. AJR 143:841, 1984.
14. McAlister WH: Thanatophoric dwarfism. Semin Roentgenol 8:158, 1973.
15. Kaufman RL, Rimoin DL, McAlister WH, et al: Thanatophoric dwarfism. Am J Dis Child 120:53, 1970.
16. Wongmongkolrit T, Bush M, Roessmann U: Neuropathological findings in thanatophoric dysplasia. Arch Pathol Lab Med 107:132, 1983.
17. Rimoin DL, McAlister WH, Saldino RM, et al: Histologic appearances of some types of congenital dwarfism. In H Kaufman (Ed): Intrinsic Diseases of Bones. Progress in Pediatric Radiology, Vol 4. Basel, S Karger, 1973, p 68.
18. Ornoy A, Adomian GE, Burgeson RE, et al: The role of mesenchyme-like tissue in the pathogenesis of thanatophoric dysplasia. Am J Med Genet 21:613, 1985.
19. Sundkvist L: Thanatophoric dysplasia. Acta Pathol Microbiol Immunol Scand, Sect A, 91:335, 1983.
20. Isaacson G, Blakemore KJ, Chervenak FA: Thanatophoric dysplasia with cloverleaf skull. Am J Dis Child 137:896, 1983.
21. Kremens B, Kemperdick H, Borchard F, et al: Thanatophoric dysplasia with cloverleaf skull. Case report and review of the literature. Eur J Pediatr 139:298, 1982.
22. Langer LO, Yang SS, Hall JG, et al: Thantophoric dysplasia and cloverleaf skull. Am J Med Genet 3(Suppl):167, 1987.
23. Serville F, Carles D, Maroteaux P: Thanatophoric dysplasia of identical twins. Am J Med Genet 17:703, 1984.
24. Langer LO, Baumann PA, Gorlin RJ: Achondroplasia. AJR 100:12, 1967.
25. Hecht JT, Nelson FW, Butler IJ, et al: Computerized tomography of the foramen magnum: Achondroplastic values compared to normal standards. Am J Med Genet 20:355, 1985.
26. Pauli RM, Scott CI, Wassman ER, et al: Apnea and sudden unexpected death in infants with achondroplasia. J Pediatr 104:342, 1984.
27. Fremion AS, Garg BP, Kalsbeck J: Apnea as the sole manifestation of cord compression in achondroplasia. J Pediatr 104:398, 1984.
28. Stokes DC, Phillips JA, Leonard CO, et al: Respiratory complications of achondroplasia. J Pediatr 102:534, 1983.
29. Pierre-Kahn A, Hirsch JF, Renier D, et al: Hydrocephalus and achondroplasia. A study of 25 observations. Child's Brain 7:205, 1980.
30. Hall JG, Horton W, Kelly T, et al: Head growth in achondroplasia: Use of ultrasound studies. Am J Med Genet 13:105, 1982.
31. Wynne-Davis R, Walsh WK, Gormley J: Achondroplasia and hypochondroplasia: Clinical variation and spinal stenosis. J Bone Joint Surg [Br] 63:458, 1981.
32. Horton WAH, Hecht JT, Hood OJ, et al: Growth hormone therapy in achondroplasia. Am J Med Genet 42:667, 1992.
33. Kao SCS, Wazin MH, Smith WL, et al: MR imaging of the craniovertebral junction, cranium, and brain in children with achondroplasia. AJR 153:565, 1989.
34. Stokes DC, Wohl ME, Wise RA, et al: The lungs and airways in achondroplasia. Chest 98:145, 1990.
35. Herman TE, Siegel MJ, McAlister WH: Chest wall deformity and respiratory distress in a 17-year-old patient with achondroplasia: CT and MRI evaluation. Pediatr Radiol 22:233, 1992.
36. Pauli RM, Conroy MM, Langer LO, et al: Homozygous achondroplasia with survival beyond infancy. Am J Med Genet 16:459, 1983.
37. Stanescu R, Stanescu V, Maroteaux P: Homozygous achondroplasia: Morphologic and biochemical study of cartilage. Am J Med Genet 37:412, 1990.
38. Rimoin DL, Hughes GN, Kaufman RL, et al: Endochondral ossification in achondroplastic dwarfism. N Engl J Med 283:728, 1970.
39. Aterman K, Welch JP, Taylor PG: Presumed homozygous achondroplasia. A review and report of a further case. Pathol Res Pract 178:27, 1983.
40. Glascow JFT, Nevin NC, Thomas PS: Hypochondroplasia. Arch Dis Child 53:868, 1978.
41. Hall BD, Spranger J: Hypochondroplasia: Clinical and radiological aspects in 39 cases. Radiology 133:95, 1979.
42. Bridges NA, Hindmarsh PC, Brook CGD: Growth of children with hypochondroplasis treated with growth hormone for up to three years. Horm Res 36(Suppl 1):56, 1991.
43. Heselson NG, Cremin BJ, Beighton P: Radiographic manifestations of hypochondroplasia. Clin Radiol 30:79, 1979.
44. Oberklaid F, Danks DM, Jensen F, et al: Achondroplasia and hypochondroplasia. J Med Genet 16:140, 1979.
45. Dominguez R, Young LW, Stelle MW, et al: Multiple exostotic hypochondroplasia: Syndrome of combined hypochondroplasia and multiple exostoses. Pediatr Radiol 14:356, 1984.
46. Jones SM, Robinson LK, Sperrazza R: Prenatal diagnosis of skeletal dysplasia identified postnatally as hypochondroplasia. Am J Med Genet 36:404, 1990.
47. Sommer A, Young-Wee T, Frye T: Anchondroplasia-hypochondroplasia complex. Am J Med Genet 26:949, 1987.
48. Desch LW, Horton WA: An autosomal recessive bone dysplasia syndrome resembling hypochondroplasia. Pediatrics 75:786, 1985.
49. Houston CS, Awen CF, Kent HP: Fatal neonatal dwarfism. J Can Assoc Radiol 23:45, 1972.
50. Anderson PE Jr: Achondrogenesis Type II in twins. Br J Radiol 54:61, 1981.
51. Chen H, Liu CT, Yang SS: Achondrogenesis. A review with special consideration of Type II (Langer-Saldino). Am J Med Genet 10:379, 1971.
52. van der Harten HJ, Brons JTJ, Dijkstra PF, et al: Achondrogenesis-hypochondrogenesis: The spectrum of chondrogenesis imperfecta. A radiological, ultrasonographic, and histopathologic study of 23 cases. Pediatr Pathol 8:571, 1988.
53. Whitley CB, Gorlin RJ: Achondrogenesis: New nosology with evidence of genetic heterogeneity. Radiology 148:693, 1983.
54. Borochowitz, Z, Ornoy A, Lachman R, et al: Achondrogenesis II-hypochondrogenesis: Variability versus heterogeneity. Am J Med Genet 24:273, 1986.
55. Batge B, Nerlich A, Brenner R, et al: Collagen type II in Langer-Saldino achondrogenesis: Absence of major abnormalities in a less severe case. Acta Paediatr 81:158, 1992.
56. Mohony BS, Filly RA, Cooperberg PL: Antenatal sonographic diagnosis of achondrogenesis. J Ultrasound Med 3:333, 1984.
57. Benacerraf B, Osathanondh R, Bieber FR: Achondrogenesis type I: Ultrasound diagnosis in utero. J Clin Ultrasound 12:357, 1984.
58. Maroteaux P, Stanescu V, Stanescu R: Hypochondrogenesis. Eur J Pediatr 141:14, 1983.
59. Hendrickx G, Hoefsloot F, Kramer P, et al: Hypochondrogenesis; an additional case. Eur J Pediatr 140:278, 1983.
60. Spranger JW, Langer LO: Spondyloepiphyseal dysplasia congenita. Radiology 94:313, 1970.
61. Harding CO, Green CG, Perloff WH, et al: Respiratory complications in children with spondyloepiphyseal dysplasia congenita. Pediatr Pulmonol 9:49, 1990.
61a. Macpherson RI, Wood BP: Spondyloepiphyseal dysplasia congenita. A cause of lethal neonatal dwarfism. Pediatr Radiol 9:217, 1980.
62. Harrod ME, Friedman JM, Currarino G, et al: Genetic heterogeneity in spondyloepiphyseal dysplasia congenita. Am J Med Genet 18:311, 1984.
63. Engfeldt B, Bolme P, Eklof O, et al: Congenital spondyloepiphyseal dysplasia. Morphological and biochemical examination of skeletal tissue in an unusual case of this disorder. Pediatr Radiol 14:118, 1984.
64. Cole WG, Hall RK, Rogers JG: The clinical features of spondyloepiphyseal dysplasia congenita resulting from the substitution of glycine 997 by serine in the α (II) chain of type II collagen. J Med Genet 30:27, 1993.
65. Whitley B, Langer LO, Ophoven J, et al: Fibrochondrogenesis: Lethal, autosomal recessive chondrodysplasia with distinctive cartilage histopathology. Am J Med Genet 19:265, 1984.
66. Eteson DJ, Adomian GE, Ornoy A, et al: Fibrochondrogenesis: Radiologic and histologic studies. Am J Med Genet 19:277, 1984.
67. Batge B, Nerlich A, Brenner R, et al: Collagen type II in Langer-Saldino achondrogenesis: Absence of major abnormalities in a less severe case. Acta Paediatr 81:158, 1992.
67a. McAlister WH: Metatropic dwarfism. Semin Roentgenol 8:154, 1973.
68. Beck M, Roubicek M, Rogers JG, et al: Heterogeneity of metatropic dysplasia. Eur J Pediatr 140:231, 1983.
69. Perri G: A severe form of metatropic dwarfism. Pediatr Radiol 7:183, 1978.
70. Shanske AL, Baden M, Fernando M, et al: A possible lethal variant of metatropic dwarfism. Birth Defects 18:135, 1982.
71. Kozlowski K, Morris L, Reinwein H, et al: Metatropic dwarfism and its variants: Report of six cases. Aust Radiol 20:367, 1976.
72. Saldino RM, Noonan CD: Severe thoracic dystrophy with striking micromelia, abnormal osseous development including the spine and multiple visceral anomalies. AJR 114:257, 1972.
73. Kaibara N, Eguchi M, Shibata K, et al: Short rib–polydactyly syndrome Type I, Saldino-Noonan. Eur J Pediatr 133:63, 1980.

74. Johnson VP, Petersen LP, Holzwarth DR, et al: Midtrimester prenatal diagnosis of short-limb dwarfism (Saldino-Noonan syndrome). Birth Defects *18*:133, 1982.

75. Toftager-Larsen K, Benzie RJ: Fetoscopy in prenatal diagnosis of the Majewski and the Saldino-Noonan types of the short rib–polydactyly syndromes. Clin Genet *26*:56, 1984.

76. Walley VM, Coates CF, Gilbert JJ, et al: Brief clinical report: Short rib–polydactyly syndrome, Majewski type. Am J Med Genet *14*:445, 1983.

77. Chen H, Yang SS, Gonzalez E, et al: Short rib–polydactyly syndrome, Majewski type. Am J Med Genet *7*:215, 1980.

78. Bergstrom K, Gusafson K-H, Jorulf H, et al: A case of Majewski syndrome with pathoanatomic examination. Skel Radiol *4*:134, 1979.

79. Naumoff P, Young LW, Mazer J, et al: Short rib–polydactyly syndrome Type 3. Radiology *122*:443, 1977.

80. Yang SS, Lin C-S, Al Saadi A, et al: Short rib–polydactyly syndrome, type 3 with chondrocytic inclusions: Report of a case and review of the literature. Am J Med Genet *7*:205, 1980.

81. Sillence DO: Non-Majewski short rib–polydactyly syndrome. Am J Med Genet *7*:223, 1980.

82. Lungarotti MS, Martello C, Marinelli I, et al: Lethal short rib syndrome of the Beemer type without polydactyly. Pediatr Radiol *23*:325, 1993.

83. Langer LO Jr: Thoracic-pelvic-phalangeal dystrophy. Asphyxiating thoracic dystrophy of the newborn, infantile thoracic dystrophy. Radiology *91*:447, 1968.

84. Koslowski K, Masel J: Asphyxiating thoracic dystrophy without respiratory disease. Report of two cases of the latent form. Pediatr Radiol *5*:30, 1976.

85. Cortina H, Beltran J, Olague R, et al: The wide spectrum of the asphyxiating thoracic dysplasia. Pediatr Radiol *8*:93, 1979.

86. Shah KJ: Renal lesion in Jeune's syndrome. Br J Radiol *53*:432, 1980.

87. Lipson M, Waskey J, Rice J, et al: Prenatal diagnosis of asphyxiating thoracic dysplasia. Am J Med Genet *18*:273, 1984.

88. Schinzel A, Savoldelli G, Briner J, et al: Prenatal sonographic diagnosis of Jeune syndrome. Radiology *154*:777, 1985.

89. Oberklaid F, Danks DM, Mayne V, et al: Asphyxiating thoracic dysplasia. Arch Dis Child *52*:758, 1977.

90. McKusick FA, Egeland JA, Eldridge R, et al: Dwarfism in the Amish I. The Ellis–van Cleveld syndrome. Bull Johns Hopkins Hosp *115*:306, 1964.

91. Da Silva EO, Janovitz D, De Albuquerque SC: Ellis–van Creveld syndrome: Report of 15 cases in an inbred kindred. J Med Genet *17*:349, 1980.

92. Muller LM, Cremin BJ: Ultrasonic demonstration of fetal skeletal dysplasia. S Afr Med J *67*:222, 1985.

93. Bui T-H, Marsk L, Eklof O: Prenatal diagnosis of chondroectodermal dysplasia with fetoscopy. Prenat Diagn *4*:155, 1984.

94. Taylor GA, Jordan CE, Dorst SK, et al: Polycarpaly and other abnormalities of the wrist in chondroectodermal dysplasia: The Ellis–van Creveld syndrome. Radiology *151*:393, 1984.

95. Jequier S, Dunbar JS: The Ellis–van Creveld syndrome. *In* H Kaufman (Ed): Intrinsic Diseases of Bones. Progress in Radiology, Vol 4. Basel, S Karger, 1973, p 167.

96. Rosemberg S, Carneiro PC, Zerbini MCN, et al: Brief clinical report: Chondroectodermal dysplasia (Ellis–van Creveld) with anomalies of CNS and urinary tract. Am J Med Genet *15*:291, 1983.

97. Qureshi F, Jacques SM, Evans MI, et al: Skeletal histopathology in fetuses with chondroectodermal dysplasia (Ellis–van Creveld Syndrome). Am J Genet *45*:471, 1993.

98. Maroteaux P, Spranger J, Stanescu V, et al: Atelosteogenesis. Am J Genet *31*:15, 1982.

99. Kozlowski K, Tsuruta T, Kameda Y, et al: New forms of neonatal death dwarfism: Report of three cases. Pediatr Radiol *10*:155, 1981.

100. Sillence DO, Kozlowski K, Rogers JG, et al: Atelosteogenesis: Evidence for heterogeneity. Pediatr Radiol *17*:112, 1987.

101. Nores JA, Rotmensch S, Romero R, et al: Atelosteogenesis type II: Sonographic and radiological correlation. Prenatal Diagn *12*:74, 1992.

102. Stern HJ, Graham JM, Lachman RS, et al: Atelosteogenesis type III: A distinct skeletal dysplasia with features overlapping atelosteogenesis and oto-palato-digital syndrome type II. Am J Med Genet *36*:183, 1990.

103. Langer LO: The roentgenographic features of oto-palato-digital (OPD) syndrome. AJR *100*:63, 1967.

104. Gall JC Jr, Stern AM, Poznanski AK, et al: Oto-palato-digital syndrome. Am J Hum Genet *124*:24, 1972.

105. Fitch N, Jequier S, Gorlin R: The oto-palato-digital syndrome, proposed Type II. Am J Med Genet *15*:655, 1983.

106. Young K, Barth CK, Moore C, et al: Otopalatodigital syndrome type II associated with omphalocele: Report of three cases. Am J Med Genet *45*:481, 1993.

107. Poznanski AK, MacPherson RI, Gorlin RJ, et al: The hand in the oto-palato-digital syndrome. Ann Radiol *16*:203, 1973.

108. Kozlowski K, Turner J, Scougall J, et al: Oto-palato-digital syndrome with severe x-ray changes in two half brothers. Pediatr Radiol *6*:97, 1977.

109. Gendall PW, Kozlowski K: Oto-palato-digital syndrome Type II. Pediatr Radiol *22*:267, 1992.

110. Langer LO: Diastrophic dwarfism in early infancy. AJR *93*:399, 1965.

111. Holmgren G, Jagell S, Lagerkvist B, et al: A pair of siblings with diastrophic dysplasia and E trisomy mosaicism. Hum Hered *34*:266, 1984.

112. Eteson DJ, Beluffi G, Burgio GR, et al: Pseudodiastrophic dysplasia: A distinct newborn skeletal dysplasia. J Pediatr *109*:635, 1986.

113. Lachman R, Sillence D, Rimoin D, et al: Diastrophic dysplasia: The death of a variant. Radiology *140*:79, 1981.

114. Ryoppy S, Poussa M, Merikanto J, et al: Foot deformities in diastrophic dysplasia. J Bone Joint Surg [Br] *74*:441, 1992.

115. Bethen D, Winter RB, Lutter L: Disorders of the spine in diastrophic dwarfism. J Bone Joint Surg [Am] *62*:529, 1980.

116. Poussa M, Merikanto J, Ryoppy S, et al: The spine in diastrophic dysplasia. Spine *16*:881, 1991.

117. Handmaker SD, Campbell JA, Robinson LD, et al: Dyssegmental dwarfism: A new syndrome of lethal dwarfism. Birth Defects *13*:79, 1977.

118. Fasanelli S, Kozlowski K, Reiter S, et al: Dyssegmental dysplasia (report of two cases with a review of the literature). Skel Radiol *14*:173, 1985.

119. Aleck KA, Grix A, Clericuzio C, et al: Dyssegmental dysplasias: Clinical, radiographic, and morphologic evidence of heterogeneity. Am J Med Genet *27*:295, 1987.

120. Gruhn JG, Gorlin RJ, Langer LO: Dyssegmental dwarfism: A lethal and anisospondylic camptomicromelic dwarfism. Am J Dis Child *132*:382, 1978.

121. Svejcar J: Biochemical abormalities in connective tissue of osteodysplasty of Melnick-Needles and dyssegmental dwarfism. Clin Genet *23*:369, 1983.

122. Anderson PE Jr, Hauge M, Bang J: Dyssegmental dysplasia in siblings: Prenatal ultrasonic diagnosis. Skel Rad *17*:29, 1988.

123. Silengo MC, Davi GF, Bianco R, et al: Kniest disease with Pierre Robin and hydrocephalus. Pediatr Radiol *13*:106, 1983.

124. Lachman RS, Rimoin DL, Hollister DW, et al: The Kniest syndrome. AJR *123*:805, 1975.

125. Oestreich AE, Prenger EC: MR demonstrates cartilaginous megaepiphyses of the hips in Kniest dysplasia of the young child. Pediatr Radiol *22*:302, 1992.

126. Rimoin DL. Hollister DW, Siggers DC, et al: Clinical, radiographic, histologic and ultrastructure definition of the Kniest syndrome. Pediatr Res *7*:348, 1973.

127. Chen H, Yang SS, Gonzales E: Kniest dysplasia: Neonatal death with necroscopy. Am J Med Genet *6*:171, 1980.

128. Poole AR, Rosenberg L, Murray L, et al: Kniest dysplasia: A probable type II collagen defect. Pathol Immunopathol Res *7*:95, 1988.

129. Giedion A, Brandner M, Lecannellier J, et al: Oto-spondylo-mega-epiphyseal dysplasia (OSMED). Helv Paediatr Acta *37*:361, 1982.

130. McAlister WH, Coe JD, Whyte MP: Macroepiphyseal dysplasia with symptomatic osteoporosis, wrinkled skin, and aged appearance. A presumed autosomal recessive condition. Skel Radiol *15*:47, 1986.

131. Silverman FN, Reiley MA: Spondylo-megaepiphyseal-metaphyseal dysplasia: A new bone dysplasia resembling cleidocranial dysplasia. Radiology *156*:365, 1985.

132. Stickler GB, Belau PG, Farrell FJ, et al: Hereditary progressive arthro-ophthalmopathy. Mayo Clin Proc *40*:433, 1965.

133. Liberfarb RM, Hirose T, Holmes LB: The Wagner-Stickler syndrome: A study of 22 families. J Pediatr *99*:394, 1981.

134. Schreiner RL, McAlister WH, Marshall RE: Stickler syndrome in a pedigree of Pierre Robin syndrome. Am J Dis Child *126*:86, 1973.

135. Hall JG, Herrod H: The Stickler syndrome presenting as a dominantly inheritance, cleft palate and blindness. J Med Genet *12*:397, 1975.

136. Ahmad NN, McDonald-McGinn DM, Zackai EH, et al: A second mutation in the type II procollagen gene (COL2A1) causing stickler syndrome (arthro-ophthalmopathy) is also a premature termination codon. Am J Hum Genet *52*:39, 1993.

137. Langer LO: Spondyloepiphysial dysplasia tarda, hereditary chondrodysplasia with characteristic vertebral configuration in the adult. Radiology *82*:833, 1964.

138. Schantz K, Andersen PE Jr, Justesen P: Spondyloepiphyseal dysplasia tarda: Report of a family with autosomal dominant transmission. Acta Orthop Scan *59*:716, 1993.

139. Poker N, Finby N, Archibald RM: Spondylolepiphysial dysplasia tarda: Four cases in childhood and adolescence, and some considerations regarding platyspondyly. Radiology *85*:474, 1965.

140. Kozlowski K, Masel J: Spondyloepiphysial dysplasia tarda (report of 7 cases). Australas Radiol *27*:285, 1983.

141. Ikegawa S, Nakamura K, Hoshino Y, et al: Thoracic disc herniation in spondyloepiphyseal dysplasia. Acta Orthop Scand *64*:105, 1993.

142. Kozlowski K: Micromelic type of spondylo-meta-epiphyseal dysplasia. Pediatr Radiol *2*:61, 1974.

143. Hernandez A, Ramirez ML, Nazara Z, et al: Autosomal recessive spondylo-epimetaphyseal dysplasia (Irapa type) in a Mexican family: Delineation of the syndrome. Am J Med Genet *5*:179, 1980.

144. Whyte MP, Petersen DJ, McAlister WH: Hypotrichosis with spondyloepimetaphyseal dysplasia in three generations: A new autosomal dominant syndrome. Am J Med Genet *36*:288, 1990.

145. Anderson CE, Sillence DO, Lachman RS, et al: Spondylo-meta-epiphyseal dysplasia. Strudwick Type. Am J Med Genet *13*:243, 1983.

146. Kousseff BG, Nichols P: Autosomal recessive spondylo-meta-epiphyseal dysplasia, type Strudwick. Am J Med Genet *17*:547, 1984.

147. Shebib SM, Chudley AE, Reed MH: Spondylometepiphyseal dysplasia congenita, Strudwick Type. Pediatr Radiol *21*:298, 1991.

148. Maroteaux P, Stanescu V, Stanescu R, et al: Opsismodysplasia: A new type of chondrodysplasia with predominant involvement of the bones and the hand and the vertebrae. Am J Med Genet *19*:171, 1984.

149. Spranger J, Albert C, Schilling F, et al: Progressive pseudorheumatoid arthritis of childhood (PPAC). A hereditary disorder simulating rheumatid arthritis. Eur J Pediatr *140*:34, 1983.

150. Al-Awada SA, Farag TI, Naguib K, et al: Spondyloepiphyseal dysplasia tarda with progressive arthropathy. J Med Genet *21*:193, 1984.

151. Lewkonia RM, Bech-Hansen NT: Spondyloepiphyseal dysplasia tarda simulating juvenile arthritis: Clinical and molecular genetic observations. Clin Exp Rheum *10*:411, 1992.

152. Kaibara N, Takagishi K, Katsuki I, et al: Spondyloepiphyseal dysplasia tarda with progressive arthropathy. Skel Radiol *10*:13, 1983.

153. Wynne-Davies R, Hall C, Ansell BM: Spondyloepiphyseal dysplasia tarda with progressive arthropathy. A ''new'' disorder of autosomal recessive inheritance. J Bone Joint Surg [Br] *64*:44, 1982.

154. Dyggve HV, Melchoir JC, Clausen J: Morquio-Ullrich's disease. An inborn error of metabolism? Arch Dis Child *37*:525, 1962.

155. Kaufman RL, Rimoin DL, McAlister WH: The Dyggve-Melchior-Clausen syndrome. Birth Defects *7*:144, 1971.

156. Spranger J, Maroteaux P, DerKaloustian VM: The Dyggve-Melchior-Clausen Syndrome. Radiology *114*:415, 1975.

157. Horton WA, Scott CI: Dyggve-Melchior-Clausen syndrome. A histochemical study of the growth plate. J Bone Joint Surg [Am] *64*:408, 1982.

158. Rimoin DL, Hollister DW, Lachman RS, et al: Histologic studies in the chondrodystrophies. Birth Defects *10*:274, 1974.

159. Yunis E, Fontalvo J, Quintero L: X-linked Dyggve-Melchior-Clausen syndrome. Clin Genet *18*:284, 1980.

160. Stob H, Pesch HJ, Pontz B, et al: Wolcott-Rallison syndrome: Diabetes mellitus and spondyloepiphyseal dysplasia. Eur J Pediatr *138*:120, 1982.

161. Horton WA, Hall JG, Scott CI, et al: Growth curves for height for diastrophic dysplasia, spondyloepiphyseal dysplasia congenita, and pseudoachondroplasia. Am J Dis Child *136*:316, 1982.

162. Heselsonn GL, Beighton P: Pseudoachondroplasia: Report of 13 cases. Br J Radiol *50*:473, 1977.

163. Pedrini-Mille A, Maynard JA, Pedrino VA: Pseudoachondroplasia: Biochemical and histochemical studies of cartilage. J Bone Joint Surg [Am] *66*:1408, 1984.

164. Maroteaux P, Stanescu R, Stanescu V, et al: The mild form of pseudoachondroplasia. Identity of the morphologic and biochemical alterations of growth cartilage with those of typical pseudoachondroplasia. Eur J Pediatr *133*:227, 1980.

165. Dennis NR, Renton P: The severe recessive form of pseudoachondroplastic dysplasia. Pediatr Radiol *3*:169, 1975.

166. Wynne-Davies R, Hall CM, Young ID: Pseudoachondroplasia: Clinical diagnosis at different ages and comparison of autosomal dominant and recessive types. A review of 32 patients (26 kindreds). J Med Genet *23*:425, 1986.

167. Pavone L: Immunologic abnormalities in Schwartz-Jampel syndrome. J Pediatr *98*:512, 1981.

168. Horan F, Beighton P: Orthopedic aspects of Schwartz syndrome. J Bone Joint Surg [Am] *57*:542, 1975.

169. Smith DL, Shoumaker R, Shuman R: Compressive myelopathy in the Schwartz-Jampel syndrome. Ann Neurol *9*:497, 1981.

170. Kozlowski K: Spondylometaphyseal dysplasia. Prog Pediatr Radiol *4*:299, 1973.

171. Thomas PS, Nevin NC: Spondylometaphyseal dysplasia. AJR *128*:89, 1977.

172. Lachman RS, Zonana J, Khajavi A, et al: Spondylometaphyseal dysplasia. Clinical, radiologic and pathologic correlations. Ann Radiol *22*:125, 1979.

173. Maroteaux P, Spranger J: The spondylometaphyseal dysplasias. A tentative classification. Pediatr Radiol *21*:293, 1991.

174. Kim GS, McAlister WH, Whyte MP: Intermittent radiographic changes of rickets without detector trabecular bone mineralization in a case of spondylometaphyseal dysplasia. Bone *7*:1, 1986.

175. Langer LO Jr, Brill PW, Ozonoff MB, et al: Spondylometaphyseal dysplasia, corner fracture type: A heritable condition associated with coxa vara. Radiology *175*:761, 1990.

176. Schorr S, Legum C, Ochshorn M: Spondyloenchondroplasia: Enchondromatomosis with severe platyspondyly in two brothers. Radiology *118*:133, 1976.

177. Frydman M, Bar-Ziv, J, Preminger-Shapiro R, et al: Possible heterogeneity in spondyloenchondroplasia: Quadriparesis, basal ganglia calcifications, and chondrocyte inclusions. Am J Med Genet *36*:279, 1990.

178. Spranger JW, Opitz JM, Bidder U: Heterogeneity of chondrodysplasia punctata. Humangenetik *11*:190, 1971.

179. Wells TR, Landing BH, Bostwick FH: Studies of vertebral coronal cleft in rhizomelic chondrodysplasia punctata. Pediatr Pathol *12*:593, 1992.

180. Gilbert EF, Opitz JM, Spranger JW, et al: Chondrodysplasia punctata—rhizomelic form. Eur J Pediatr *123*:89, 1976.

181. Schutgen RBH, Wanders RJA, Nijenhues HA, et al: Rhizomelic chondrodysplasia punctata. Prenatal diagnosis by biochemical analyses. Int Pediatr *8*:45, 1993.

182. Sheffield LJ, Danks DM, Mayne V, et al: Chondrodysplasia punctata—23 cases of a mild and relatively common variety. J Pediatr *89*:916, 1976.

183. Silengo MC, Luzzatti L, Silverman FN: Clinical and genetic aspects of Conradi-Hünermann disease. J Pediatr *97*:911, 1980.

184. Theander G, Pettersson H: Calcification in chondrodysplasia punctata. Relation to ossification and skeletal growth. Acta Radiol (Diagn) *19*:205, 1978.

185. Lawrence JJ, Schlesinger AE, Kozlowski K, et al: Unusual radiographic manifestations of the chondrodysplasia punctata. Skel Radiol *18*:15, 1989.

186. Curry CJR, Magenis RE, Brown M, et al: Inherited chondrodysplasia punctata due to a deletion of the terminal short arm of an X chromosome. N Engl J Med *311*:1010, 1984.

187. Manzke H, Christophers E, Wiedemann HR: Dominant sex-linked inherited

188. chondrodysplasia punctata: A distinct type of chondrodysplasia punctata. Clin Genet *17*:97, 1980.

188. Happle R, Phillips RJS, Roessner A, et al: Homologous genes for X-linked chondroplasia punctata in man and mouse. Hum Genet *63*:24, 1983.

189. Hunter AGW, Rimoin DL, Koch UM, et al: Chondrodysplasia punctata in an infant with duplication 16p due to a 7;16 translocation. Am J Med Genet *21*:581, 1985.

190. Rittler M, Menger H, Spranger J: Chondrodysplasia punctata, tibia-metacarpal (MT) type. Am J Med Genet *37*:200, 1990.

191. Jequier S, Bellini F, Mackenzie DA: Metaphyseal chondrodysplasia with ectodermal dysplasia. Skel Radiol *7*:107, 1981.

192. Kaitila II, Halttunen P, Snellman O, et al: A new form of metaphyseal chondrodysplasia in two sibs: Surgical treatment of tracheobronchial malacia and scoliosis. Am J Med Genet *11*:415, 1982.

193. Nazara Z, Hernandez A, Corona-Rivera E, et al: Further clinical and radiological features in metaphyseal chondrodysplasia Jansen type. Radiology *140*:697, 1981.

194. Charrow J, Poznanski AK: The Jansen Type of metaphyseal chondrodysplasia: Confirmation of dominant inheritance and review of the radiographic manifestations in the newborn and adult. Am J Med Genet *18*:321, 1984.

195. Holthausen W, Holt JF, Stoeckenius M: The skull and metaphyseal chondrodysplasia type Jansen. Pediatr Radiol *3*:137, 1975.

196. Ozonoff MB: Asphyxiating thoracic dysplasia as a complication of metaphyseal chondrodysplasia (Jansen type). Birth Defects *10*:72, 1974.

197. Pavone L, Mollica F, Giovanni S, et al: Metaphyseal chondrodysplasia Schmid type. Am J Dis Child *134*:699, 1980.

198. Lachman RS, Rimoin DL, Spranger J: Metaphyseal chondrodysplasia, Schmid type. Clinical and radiographic delineation with a review of the literature. Pediatr Radiol *18*:93, 1988.

199. Wasylenko MJ, Wedge JH, Houston CS: Metaphyseal chondrodysplasia, Schmid type. A defect in ultrastructure metabolism: Case report. J Bone Joint Surg [Am] *62*:660, 1980.

200. Kleinman P: Schmid-like metaphyseal chondrodysplasia simulating child abuse. AJR *156*:576, 1991.

201. McKusick VA, Eldridge R, Hostetler JA, et al: Dwarfism in the Amish. II. Cartilage-hair hypoplasia. Bull Johns Hopkins Hosp *116*:285, 1965.

202. Pierce GF, Palmar SH: Lymphocyte dysfunction and cartilage-hair hypoplasia. II. Evidence of a cell cycle specific deficit in T-cell growth. Clin Exp Immunol *50*:621, 1982.

203. Makitie O, Kaitila I: Cartilage-hair hypoplasia—clinical manifestations in 108 Finnish patients. Eur J Pediatr *152*:211, 1993.

204. McAlister WH: Metaphyseal chondroplasia, type McKusick. Semin Roentgenol *8*:222, 1973.

205. Makitie O, Marttinen E, Kaitila I: Skeletal growth in cartilage-hair hypoplasia. A study of 82 patients. Pediatr Radiol *22*:434, 1992.

206. Ray HC, Dorst JP: Cartilage-hair hypoplasia. In H Kaufman (Ed): Intrinsic Diseases of Bones. Progress in Pediatric Radiology, Vol 4. Basel, S Karger, 1973, p 270.

207. Robberecht E, Nachtegaele P, Van Rattinghe R, et al: Pancreatic lipomatosis in the Schwachman-Diamond syndrome. Identification by sonography and CT-SCAN. Pediatr Radiol *15*:348, 1985.

208. McClennan TW, Steinbach HL: Schwachman's syndrome—a broad spectrum of bony abnormality. Radiology *112*:167, 1974.

209. Stanley P, Sutcliffe J: Metaphyseal chondrodysplasia with dwarfism, pancreatic insufficiency and neutropenia. Pediatr Radiol *1*:119, 1973.

210. Aggett PJ, Cavanagh NPC, Matthew DJ, et al: Schwachman's syndrome. Arch Dis Child *55*:331, 1980.

211. Michels VV, Donovan GK: Schwachman syndrome: Unusual presentation as asphyxiating thoracic dystrophy. Birth Defects *18*:129, 1982.

212. Chakravarti VS, Borns P, Lobell J, et al: Chondroosseous dysplasia in severe combined immunodeficiency due to adenosine deaminase deficiency (chondroosseous dysplasia in ADA deficiency SCID). Pediatr Radiol *21*:447, 1991.

213. Maroteaux P, Verloes A, Stanescu V, et al: Metaphyseal anadysplasia: A metaphyseal dysplasia of early onset with radiological regression and benign course. Am J Med Genet *39*:4, 1991.

214. Shohat M, Lachman R, Gruber HE, et al: Brachyolmia: Radiographic and genetic evidence of heterogeneity. Am J Med Genet *33*:209, 1989.

215. Horton WA, Langer LO, Collins DL, et al: Brachyolmia, recessive type (Hobaek): A clinical, radiographic, and histologic study. Am J Med Genet *16*:201, 1983.

216. Langer LO: Dyschondrosteosis of the inheritable bone dysplasia with characteristic roentgenographic features. AJR *95*:178, 1965.

217. Dawe C, Wynne-Davies R, Fulford GE: Clinical variation in dyschondrosteosis. A report of 13 individuals in 8 families. J Bone Joint Surg [Br] *64*:377, 1982.

218. Linchenstein JR, Sindaramn M, Burdge R: Sex influence expression of Madelung's deformity in a family with dyschondrosteosis. J Med Genet *17*:41, 1980.

219. Mohan V, Shrivastava K, Bhushan B, et al: Dyschondrosteosis. Australas Radiol *28*:39, 1984.

220. Langer LO: Mesomelic dwarfism of hypoplastic ulna, fibula, mandible type. Radiology *89*:654, 1967.

221. Kaitila II, Liessti JT, Rimoin DL: Mesomelic skeletal dysplasia. Clin Orthop *114*:94, 1976.

222. Espiritu C, Chen H, Woolley PV: Mesomelic dwarfism as the homozygous expression of dyschondrosteosis. Am J Dis Child *129*:375, 1975.

223. Wadlington WB, Tucker VL, Schimke RN: Mesomelic dwarfism with hemiver-

tebrae and small genitalia (the Robinow syndrome). Am J Dis Child 126:202, 1973.

224. Petit P, Fryns JP, Goddeeris P, et al: The Robinow syndrome. Ann Genet 23:221, 1980.
225. Sandomenico C, Sandomenico ML: Mesomelic dysplasia with "normal and relative long fibula," slight micrognathia and brachymetatarsals (IV-V) in a six-year-old girl. Pediatr Radiol 13:47, 1983.
226. Hall CM: Werner's mesomelic dysplasia with ventricular septal defect and Hirschsprung's disease. Pediatr Radiol 10:247, 1981.
227. Langer LO Jr, Garrett RT: Acromesomelic dysplasia. Radiology 137:349, 1980.
228. Borrelli P, Fasanelli S, Marini R: Acromesomelic dwarfism in a child with an interesting family history. Pediatr Radiol 13:165, 1983.
229. Hall CM, Stoker DJ, Robinson DC, et al: Acromesomelic dwarfism. Br J Radiol 53:999, 1980.
230. Fernandez del Moral R, Santolaya Jimenez JM, Rodriguez Gonzalez JI, et al: Report of a case: Acromesomelic dysplasia. Radiologic, clinical, and pathological study. Am J Med Genet 33:415, 1989.
231. Maroteaux P, Stanescu R, Stanescu V, et al: Acromicric dysplasia. Am J Med Genet 24:447, 1986.
232. Spranger J, Gilbert EF, Arya S, et al: Geleophysic dysplasia. Am J Med Genet 19:487, 1984.
233. Giedion A, Burdea M, Fruchter Z, et al: Autosomal-dominant transmission of trichorhinophalangeal syndrome: Report of four unrelated families, review of 60 cases. Helv Paediatr Acta 28:249, 1973.
234. Felman AH, Frias JL: The trichorhinophalangeal syndrome: Study of 16 patients in one family. AJR 129:631, 1977.
235. Ferrandez A, Remirez J, Saenz P, et al: The trichorhinophalangeal syndrome. Report of 4 familial cases belonging to 4 generations. Helv Paediat Acta 35:559, 1980.
236. Hornsby VPL, Pratt AE: The tricho-rhino-phalangeal syndrome. Clin Radiol 35:243, 1984.
237. Giedion A, Kesztler R, Muggiasca F: The widened spectrum multicartilaginous exostosis (MCE). Pediatr Radiol 3:93, 1975.
238. Buhler EM, Malik NJ: The tricho-rhino-phalangeal syndrome(s): Chromosome 8 long arm deletion: Is there a shortest region of overlap between reported cases? TRP I and TRP II syndromes: Are they separate entities? Am J Genet 19:113, 1984.
239. Langer LO Jr, Krassikoff N, Laxova R, et al: The tricho-rhino-phalangeal syndrome with exostoses (or Langer-Giedion syndrome): Four additional patients without mental retardation and review of the literature. Am J Med Genet 19:81, 1984.
240. Bauermeister S, Letts M: The orthopaedic manifestations of the Langer-Giedion syndrome. Orthop Rev 21:31, 1992.
241. Kozlowski K, Harrington G, Barylak A, et al: Multiple exostosis–mental retardation syndrome (Ale-Calo or MEMR syndrome). Description of 2 childhood cases. Clin Pediatr 16:219, 1977.
242. Mainzer F, Saldino RM, Ozonoff MB, et al: Familial nephropathy associated with retinitis pigmentosa, cerebellar ataxia, and skeletal abnormalities. Am J Med 49:556, 1970.
243. Giedion A: Phalangeal cone shaped epiphysis of the hands (PhCSEH) and chronic renal disease—the conorenal syndromes. Pediatr Radiol 8:32, 1979.
244. Chitayat D, Hodgkinson KA, Azouz EM: Intrafamilial variability in cleidocranial dysplasia: A three generation family. Am J Med Genet 42:298, 1992.
245. Monasky GE, Winkler S, Icenhower JB, et al: Cleidocranial dysostosis. Two case reports. NY State Dent J 49:236, 1983.
246. Hawkins HB, Shapiro R, Petrillo CJ: The association of cleidocranial dysostosis with hearing loss. AJR 125:944, 1975.
247. Tan KL, Tan LKA: Cleidocranial dysostosis in infancy. Pediatr Radiol 11:114, 1981.
248. Jarvis JL, Keats TE: Cleidocranial dysostosis. The review of 40 cases. AJR 121:5, 1974.
249. Yunis E, Varon H: Cleidocranial dysostosis, severe micrognathism, bilateral absence of thumbs and first metatarsal bone, and distal aphalangia. Am J Dis Child 134:649, 1980.
250. Melnick JC, Needles CF: An undiagnosed bone dysplasia. A two family study of four generations and three generations. AJR 97:39, 1966.
251. Gorlin RJ, Knier J: X-linked or dominant, lethal in the male, inheritance of Melnick-Needles (osteodysplasty) syndrome? A reappraisal. Am J Med Genet 13:465, 1982.
252. Oeyen P, Holmes LB, Trelstad RL, et al: Omphalocele and multiple severe congenital anomalies associated with osteodysplasia (Melnick-Needles syndrome). Am J Med Genet 13:453, 1982.
253. Klint RV, Agustsson NH, McAlister WH: Melnick-Needles osteodysplasia associated with pulmonary hypertension, obstructive uropathy, and marrow hypoplasia. Pediatr Radiol 6:49, 1977.
254. Leonard MS, Gorlin RJ: The nature of the mandibular lesion in Melnick-Needles syndrome. Radiology 150:844, 1984.
255. Eggli K, Giudici M, Ramer J, et al: Melnick-Needles syndrome. Four new cases. Pediatr Radiol 22:257, 1992.
256. Svejcar J: Biochemical abnormalities in connective tissue of osteodysplasia of Melnick-Needles and dyssegmental dwarfism. Clin Genet 23:369, 1983.
257. Hall BD, Spranger JW: Campomelic dysplasia. Am J Dis Child 134:285, 1980.
258. Kozlowski K, Butzler HO, Galatius-Jensen F, et al: Syndromes of congenital bowing of the long bones. Pediatr Radiol 7:40, 1978.
259. Balcar I, Bieber FR: Sonographic and radiologic findings in campomelic dysplasia. AJR 141:481, 1983.

260. Macpherson RI, Skinner SA, Donnenfeld AE: Acampomelic campomelic dysplasia. Pediatr Radiol 20:90, 1989.
261. Coscia MF, Bassett GS, Bowen JR, et al: Spinal abnormalities in campomelic dysplasia. J Pediat Orthop 9:6, 1989.
262. Houston CS, Opitz JM, Spranger JW, et al: The campomelic syndrome: Review, report of 17 cases, and follow-up on the currently 17-year-old boy first reported by Maroteaux et al in 1971. Am J Med Genet 15:3, 1983.
263. Viljoen D, Beighten P: Kyphomelic dysplasia. Dysmorph Clin Genet 1:136, 1988.
264. Larsen LJ, Schottstaedt ER, Boist FC: Multiple congenital dislocations associated with a characteristic facial deformity. J Pediatr 37:574, 1950.
265. McAlister WH: Larsen's syndrome. Semin Roentgenol 8:246, 1973.
266. Kozlowski KA, Robertson F, Middleton R: Radiographic findings in Larsen syndrome. Australas Radiol 18:336, 1974.
267. Houston CS, Reed MH, Desautels JEL: Separating Larsen syndrome from the "arthrogryposis basket." J Can Assoc Radiol 32:206, 1981.
268. Micheli LJ, Hall JE, Watts HG: Spinal instability in Larsen's syndrome. Report of 3 cases. J Bone Joint Surg [Am] 58:562, 1976.
269. Trigueros AP, Vazquez JL, DeMiguel CF: Larsen's syndrome: Report of three cases in the family, mother and two offsprings. Acta Orthop Scand 49:582, 1978.
270. Swensson RE, Linnebur AC, Paster SB: Striking aortic root dilatation in a patient with Larsen syndrome. J Pediatr 86:914, 1975.
271. Strisciuglio P, Sebastio G, Andria G, et al: Severe cardiac anomalies in sibs with Larsen syndrome. J Med Genet 20:422, 1983.
272. Rasooly R, Gomori JM, BenEzra D: Arterial tortuosity and dilatation in Larsen syndrome. Neuroradiology 30:258, 1988.
273. LeMerrer M, Young ID, Stanescu V, et al: Desbuquois syndrome. Eur J Pediatr 150:793, 1991.
274. Beighton P, Kozlowski K: Spondylo-epimetaphyseal dysplasia with joint laxity and severe progressive kyphoscoliosis. Skel Radiol 5:205, 1980.
275. Beighton P, Gericke G, Kozlowski K, et al: The manifestation and natural history of spondylo-epi-metaphyseal dysplasia and joint laxity. Clin Genet 26:308, 1984.
276. Herman TE, Mendelsohn NJ, Dowton SB, et al: Microcephalic osteodysplastic primordial dwarfism, type II. A report of a case with characteristic skeletal features. Pediatr Radiol 21:602, 1991.
277. Kozlowski K, McCrossin R: Early osseous abnormalities in Menkes' kinky hair syndrome. Pediatr Radiol 8:191, 1980.
278. Farrelly C, Stringer DA, Daneman A, et al: CT manifestations in Menkes' kinky hair syndrome (trichopoliodystrophy). J Can Assoc Radiol 35:406, 1984.
279. Harcke HT, Capitanio MA, Grover WD, et al: Bladder diverticulum in Menkes' syndrome. Radiology 124:459, 1977.
280. Menkes JH: Kinky hair disease: Twenty five years later. Brain Dev 10:77, 1988.
281. Hoyt CS, Billson FA: Visual loss in osteopetrosis. Am J Dis Child 133:955, 1979.
282. Bonucci E, Sartori E, Spina M: Osteopetrosis fetalis. Report on a case, with special reference to ultrastructure. Virchows Arch Pathol Anat 368:109, 1975.
283. Engfeld B, Fajers CM, Lodin H, et al: Studies of osteopetrosis. Roentgenological and pathologic-anatomical investigations on some of the bone changes. Acta Pediatr 49:391, 1960.
284. Elster AD, Theros EG, Key LL, et al: Autosomal recessive osteopetrosis: Bone marrow imaging. Radiology 182:507, 1992.
285. Elster AD, Theros EG, Key IL, et al: Cranial imaging in autosomal recessive osteopetrosis. Part I. Facial bones and calvarium. Radiology 183:129, 1992.
286. Elster AD, Theros EG, Key IL, et al: Cranial imaging in autosomal recessive osteopetrosis. Part II. Skull base and brain. Radiology 183:137, 1992.
287. Shapiro F, Glimcher MJ, Holtrop ME, et al: Human osteopetrosis. A histological, ultrastructural, and biochemical study. J Bone Joint Surg [Am] 62:384, 1980.
288. Teitelbaum SL, Coccia PF, Brown DM, et al: Malignant osteopetrosis: A disease of abnormal osteoclast proliferation. Metab Bone Dis Rel Res 3:99, 1981.
289. Milgram JW, Jasty M: Osteopetrosis. A morphological study of twenty-one cases. J Bone Joint Surg [Am] 64:912, 1982.
290. Marks CR, Seifert MF, Marks SC III: Osteoclast populations in congenital osteopetrosis: Additional evidence of heterogeneity. Metab Bone Dis Rel Res 5:259, 1984.
291. Milhaud G, Labat M-L, Litwin I, et al: Osteopetro-rickets: A new congenital bone disorder, Metab Bone Dis Rel Res 3:91, 1981.
292. Ambler MW, Trice J, Grauerholz J, et al: Infantile osteopetrosis and neuronal storage disease. Neurology 33:437, 1983.
293. Coccia PF, Krivit W, Cervenka J, et al: Successful bone marrow transplantation for infantile malignant osteopetrosis. N Engl J Med 302:701, 1980.
294. Blazar BR, Fallon MD, Teitelbaum SL, et al: Calcitriol for congenital osteopetrosis. N Engl J Med 311:55, 1984.
295. Hinkel CL, Beiler D: Osteopetrosis in adults. AJR 74:46, 1955.
296. Johnson CC Jr, Lavy N, Lord T, et al: Osteopetrosis. A clinical genetic, metabolic and morphologic study of the dominantly inherited benign type. Medicine 47:149, 1968.
297. Fish RM: Osteopetrosis in trauma. J Emerg Med 1:125, 1983.
298. Beighton P, Hamersma H, Cremin BJ: Osteopetrosis in South Africa. The benign, lethal and intermediate forms. S Afr Med J 55:659, 1979.
299. Kahler SG, Burns JA, Aylsworth AS: A mild autosomal recessive form of osteopetrosis. Am J Genet 17:451, 1984.

300. Kivara N, Katsuki I, Hotokebuchi T, et al: Intermediate form of osteopetrosis with recessive inheritance. Skel Radiol 9:47, 1982.
301. Sly WS, Lang R, Avioli L, et al: Recessive osteopetrosis. A new clinical phenotype. Am J Hum Genet 24:34, 1972.
302. Sly WS, Whyte MP, Sundaram V, et al: Carbonic anhydase II deficiency in twelve families with autosomal recessive syndrome of osteopetrosis and renal tubular acidosis and cerebral calcification. N Engl J Med 313:139, 1985.
303. Whyte MP, Murphy WA, Fallon MD, et al: Osteopetrosis renal tubular acidosis and basal ganglia calcification in three sisters. Am J Med 69:74, 1980.
304. Bergman H, Brown J, Rodgers A, et al: Osteopetrosis with combined proximal and distal renal tubular acidosis. Am J Kidney Dis 2:357, 1982.
305. Cummings WA, Ohlsson A: Intracranial calcification in children with osteopetrosis caused by carbonic anhydrase II deficiency. Radiology 157:325, 1985.
306. Houston CS, Gerrard JW, Ives EJ: Dysosteosclerosis. AJR 130:988, 1978.
307. Leisti J, Kaitila I, Lachman RS, et al: Dysosteosclerosis. Birth Defects 11:349, 1975.
308. Canalis D, Reardon GE, Baron R: Dynamic bone morphometric and studies on the effects of serum on bone metabolism in vitro in a case of pycnodysostosis. Metab Bone Dis Rel Res 2:99, 1980.
309. Elmore SM: Pycnodysostosis. A review. J Bone Joint Surg [Am] 49:153, 1967.
310. Zachariades N, Koundouris I: Maxillofacial symptoms in two patients with pyknodysostosis. J Oral Maxillofac Surg 42:819, 1984.
311. Yousefzadeh DK, Agha AS, Reinertson J: Radiographic studies of upper airway obstruction with cor pulmonale in a patient with pycnodysostosis. Pediatr Radiol 8:45, 1979.
312. Aronson DC, Heymans HSA, Bijlmer RPGM: Cor pulmonale and acute liver necrosis, due to upper airway obstruction as part of pycnodysostosis. Eur J Pediatr 141:251, 1984.
313. Dipierri JE, Guzman JD: A second family with autosomal dominant osteosclerosis—type Stanescu. Am J Med Genet 18:13, 1984.
314. Proschek R, Labelle H, Bard C, et al: Osteomesopyknosis. J Bone Joint Surg [Am] 67:652, 1985.
315. Renowden SA, Cole T, Hall M: Osteomesopyknosis: A benign familial disorder of bone. Clin Radiol 46:46, 1992.
316. Civitelli R, McAlister WH, Teitelbaum SL, et al: Central osteosclerosis with ectodermal dysplasia: Clinical laboratory, radiologic, and histopathologic characterization with review of the literature. J Bone Miner Res 4:863, 1989.
317. Porter PS, Starke JC: Netherton's syndrome. Arch Dis Child 43:319, 1968.
318. Girdany BR, Sane F, Graham CB: Engelmann's disease. In H Kaufman (Ed): Intrinsic Diseases of Bones. Progress in Pediatric Radiology, Vol 4. Basel, S Karger, 1973, p 414.
319. Crisp AJ, Brenton DP: Engelmann's disease of bone—a systemic disorder? Ann Rheum Dis 41:183, 1982.
320. Naveh Y, Kaftori JK, Alan V, et al: Progressive diaphyseal dysplasia: Genetics and clinical and radiographic manifestations. Pediatrics 74:399, 1984.
321. Kumar B, Murphy WA, Whyte MP: Progressive diaphyseal dysplasia (Engelmann disease): Scintigraphic-radiographic-clinical correlations. Radiology 140:87, 1981.
322. Minford M, Hardy GH, Forsythe WI, et al: Engelmann's disease and effects of cortical steroids. Case report. J Bone joint Surg [Br] 63:597, 1981.
323. Wirth CR, Kay J, Bourke J: Diaphyseal dysplasia (Engelmann's syndrome). A case report demonstrating a deficiency in cortical Haversian system formation. Clin Orthop 171:186, 1982.
324. Kaftori JK, Kleinhaus U, Naveh Y: Progressive diaphyseal dysplasia (Camurati-Engelmann): Radiographic follow-up and CT findings. Radiology 164:777, 1987.
325. Tucker AS, Klein L, Anthony GL: Craniodiaphyseal dysplasia. Evolution of a five year period. Skel Radiol 1:47, 1976.
326. MacPherson RI: Craniodiaphyseal dysplasia, a disease or group of diseases. J Can Assoc Radiol 25:22, 1974.
327. Kaitila I, Stewart RE, Landow E, et al: Craniodiaphyseal dysplasia. Birth Defects 11:359, 1975.
328. Brueton LA, Winter RM. Craniodiaphyseal dysplasia. J Med Genet 27:701, 1990.
329. Gorlin RJ, Whitley CB: Lenz-Majewski syndrome. Radiology 149:129, 1983.
330. Langer LO Jr, Brill PW, Afshani E: Radiographic features of craniometadiaphyseal dysplasia, wormian bone type. Skel Radiol 20:37, 1991.
331. Eastman JR, Bixler D: Generalized cortical hyperostosis (Van Buchem's disease): Nosological considerations. Radiology 125:297, 1977.
332. Jacobs P: Van Buchem's disease. Postgrad Med 53:479, 1977.
333. Dixon JM, Cull RE, Gamble P: Two cases of Van Buchem's disease. J Neurol Neurosurg Psychiatry 45:913, 1982.
334. Cremin BJ: Sclerosteosis in children. Pediatr Radiol 8:173, 1979.
335. Beighton P, Hamersma H: Sclerosteosis in South Africa. S Afr Med J 55:783, 1979.
336. Stein SA, Witkop C, Hill S, et al: Sclerosteosis. Neurogenic and pathophysiologic analysis of American kinship. Neurology 33:267, 1983.
337. Beighton P: Sclerosteosis. J Med Genet 25:200, 1988.
338. Rimoin DL: Pachydermoperiostitis (idiopathic clubbing and periostitis). Genetic and physiologic considerations. N Engl J Med 272:923, 1965.
339. Currarino G, Tierney RC, Giesel RJ, et al: Familial idiopathic osteoarthropathy. AJR 84:633, 1961.
340. Cremin BJ: Familial idiopathic osteoarthropathy of children: A case report and progress. Br J Radiol 43:568, 1970.
341. Irie T, Takahashi M, Kaneko M: Case report 546. Skel Radiol 18:310, 1989.
342. Gorlin RJ, Cohen MM Jr: Frontometaphyseal dysplasia: A new syndrome. Am J Dis Child 118:487, 1969.
343. Beighton P, Hamersma H: Frontometaphyseal dysplasia: An autosomal dominant or X-linked? J Med Genet 17:53, 1980.
344. Gorlin RJ, Winter RB: Frontometaphyseal dysplasia—evidence of X-linked inheritance. Am J Med Genet 5:81, 1980.
345. Fitzsimmons JS, Fitzsimmons EM, Barrow M, et al: Frontometaphyseal dysplasia. Further delineation of the clinical syndrome. Clin Genet 22:195, 1982.
346. Jend-Rossnann I, Jend HH, Ringe JD, et al: Frontometaphyseal dysplasia: Symptoms and possible mode of inheritance. J Oral Maxillofac Surg 42:743, 1984.
347. Carnevale A, Grether P, Del Castillo V, et al: Autosomal dominant craniometaphyseal dysplasia. The clinical variability. Clin Genet 23:17, 1983.
348. Penchaszadeh VB, Gutierrez ER, Figueroa E: Autosomal recessive craniometaphyseal dysplasia. Am J Med Genet 5:43, 1980.
349. Beighton P, Hamersma A, Turan F: Craniometaphyseal dysplasia—variability of expression within a large family. Clin Genet 15:252, 1979.
350. Bricker SL, Langlais RP, Van Dis ML: Dominant craniometaphyseal dysplasia. Literature review and case report. Dentomaxillofac Radiol 12:95, 1983.
351. Ramseyer LTH, Leonard JC, Stacy TM: Bone scan findings in craniometaphyseal dysplasia. Clinical Nuc Med 18:137, 1993.
352. Gorlin RJ, Koszalk MS, Spranger J: Pyle's disease (familial metaphyseal dysplasia). A presentation of 2 cases and argument for its separation from craniometaphyseal dysplasia. J Bone Joint Surg [Am] 52:347, 1970.
353. Shibuya H, Suzuki S, Okuyama T, Yukawa Y: The radiological appearances of familial metaphyseal dysplasia. Clin Radiol 33:439, 1982.
354. Heselson NG, Raad MS, Hamersma H, et al: Radiologic manifestations of metaphyseal dysplasia (Pyle's disease). Br J Radiol 52:431, 1979.
355. Beighton P: Pyle disease (metaphyseal dysplasia). J Med Genet 24:321, 1987.
356. Caffey J: Familial hyperphosphatemia with ateliosis and hypermetabolism of growing membranous bone. Prog Pediatr Radiol 4:438, 1973.
357. Iancu TC, Almagor G, Friedman E, et al: Chronic familial hyperphosphatasemia. Radiology 129:669, 1978.
358. Whalen JP, Horwith M, Krook L, et al: Calcitonin treatment in hereditary bone dysplasia with hyperphosphatasemia. A radiographic and histologic study of bone. AJR 129:29, 1977.
359. Dunn V, Condon VR, Rallison ML: Familial hyperphosphatasemia. Diagnosis in early infancy and response to human thyrocalcitonin therapy. AJR 132:541, 1979.
360. Bakwin H, Elger MS: Fragile bones with macrocranium. J Pediatr 49:558, 1956.
361. Spindler A, Berman A, Mautalen C, et al: Chronic idiopathic hyperphosphatasia. Report of a case treated with pamidronate and a review of the literature. J Rheumatol 19:642, 1992.
362. Reisner SH, Kott E, Bornstein B, et al: Oculo-dento-digital dysplasia. Am J Dis Child 118:600, 1969.
363. Patton MA, Laurence KM: Three new cases of oculodentodigital (ODD) syndrome: Development of the facial phenotype. J Med Genet 22:386, 1985.
364. Beighton P, Hamersma H, Raad M: Oculodento-osseous dysplasia: Heterogeneity or variable expression? Clin Genet 16:169, 1979.
365. Carlson DH, Wilkinson RH: Variability of unilateral epiphyseal dysplasia (dysplasia epiphysialis hemimelica). Radiology 133:369, 1969.
366. Lamesch AJ: Dysplasia epiphysealis hemimelica of the carpal bones. Report of a case and review of the literature. J Bone Joint Surg [Am] 65:398, 1983.
367. Wiedemann HR, Mann M, vonKreudenstein PS: Dysplasia epiphysealis hemimelica—Trevor disease. Severe manifestations in a child. Eur J Pediatr 136:311, 1981.
368. Azour EM, Slomic AM, Marton D, et al: The variable manifestations of dysplasia epiphysealis hemimelica. Pediatr Radiol 15:44, 1985.
369. Cruz-Condi R, Amaya S, Valdivia P, et al: Dysplasia epiphysealis hemimelica. J Pediatr Orthop 4:625, 1984.
370. Keret D, Spatz DK, Caro PA, et al: Dysplasia epiphysealis hemimelica: Diagnosis and treatment. J Pediatr Orthop 12:365, 1992.
371. Gerscovich EO, Greenspan A: Computed tomography in the diagnosis of dysplasia epiphysealis hemimelica. J Can Assoc Radiol 40:313, 1989.
372. Connor JM, Horan FT, Beighton P: Dysplasia epiphysialis hemimelica. A clinical and genetic study. J Bone Joint Surg [Br] 65:350, 1983.
373. Crandell BF, Field LL, Sparkes RS, et al: Hereditary multiple exostoses. Report of a family. Clin Orthop 190:217, 1984.
374. Shapiro F, Simon S, Glimcher MJ: Hereditary multiple exostoses: Anthropometric, roentgenologic and clinical aspects. J Bone Joint Surg [Am] 61:815, 1979.
375. Burgess RC, Cates H: Deformities of the forearm in patients who have multiple cartilaginous exostosis. J Bone Joint Surg [Am] 75:13, 1993.
376. Shupe JL, Leone NC, Gardner EJ, et al: Hereditary multiple exostoses. Hereditary multiple exostoses in horses. Am J Pathol 104:285, 1981.
377. deMatos AN, Mendonca JM, Pereira MC: Hereditary multiple exostoses. A rare cause of arterial insufficiency. Angiology 34:362, 1983.
378. Gordon SL, Buchanan JR, Ladda RL: Hereditary multiple exostosis. Report of a kindred. J Med Genet 18:428, 1981.
379. Mainzer F, Minagi H, Steinbach HL: The variable manifestation of multiple enchondromatosis. Radiology 99:377, 1971.
380. Shapiro F: Ollier's disease. An assessment of angular deformity, shortening, and pathological fracture in twenty-one patients. J Bone Joint Surg [Am] 64:95, 1982.

381. Schwartz HS, Zimmerman NB, Simon MA, et al: The malignant potential of enchondromatosis. J Bone Joint Surg [Am] 69:269, 1987.

382. Cannon SR, Sweetnam DR: Multiple chondrosarcomas in dyschondroplasia (Ollier's disease). Cancer 55:836, 1985.

383. Spranger J, Kemperdieck H, Bakowski H, et al: Two peculiar types of enchondromatosis. Pediatr Radiol 7:215, 1978.

384. McAlister WH: Enchondromatosis with hemangioma. Semin Roentgenol 8:230, 1973.

385. Niechajev IA, Hansson LI: Maffucci's syndrome. Case report. Scand J Plast Reconstr Surg 16:215, 1982.

386. Lowell SH, Mathoy RH: Head and neck manifestations of Maffucci's syndrome. Arch Otolaryngol 105:427, 1979.

387. Collins PS, Han W, Williams LR, et al: Maffucci's syndrome (hemangiomatosis osteolytica): A report of four cases. J Vasc Surg 16:364, 1992.

388. Kessler HB, Recht MP, Dalinka MK: Vascular anomalies in association with osteodystrophies—a spectrum. Skel Radiol 10:95, 1983.

389. Lewis RJ, Kotchan AS: The Maffucci's syndrome: Functional and neoplastic significance. J Bone Joint Surg [Am] 55:1465, 1973.

390. Beals RK: Metachondromatosis. Clin Orthop 169:167, 1982.

391. McAlister WH, Cacciarelli AA, Gilula LA: Roentgen rounds #89. Orthop Rev 16:71, 1987.

392. Kennedy LA: Metachondromatosis. Radiology 148:117, 1983.

393. Lachman RS, Cohen A, Hollister D, et al: Metachondromatosis. Birth Defects 10:171, 1974.

394. Beighton P, Cremin BJ, Kozlowski K: Osteoglophonic dwarfism. Pediatr Radiol 10:46, 1980.

395. Beighton P: Osteoglophonic dysplasia. J Med Genet 26:572, 1989.

396. Frech RS, McAlister WH: Medullary stenosis of the tubular bones with associated hypercalcemic convulsions and short stature. Radiology 91:45, 1968.

397. Caffey J: Congenital stenosis of the medullary spaces and tubular bones and calvaria in two proportionate dwarfs—mother and son; coupled with transient hypercalcemic tetany. AJR 100:1, 1967.

398. Lee WK, Vargas A, Barnes J, et al: The Kenny-Caffey syndrome. Growth retardation and hypercalcemia in a young boy. Am J Med Genet 14:773, 1983.

399. Majewski F, Rosendahl W, Ranke M, et al: The Kenny syndrome, a rare type of growth deficiency with tubular stenosis, transient hypoparathyroidism and anomalies. Eur J Pediatr 136:21, 1981.

400. Abdel-Al YK, Auger LT, El-Gharbawy F: Kenny-Caffey syndrome. Case report and literature review. Clin Pediatr 28:175, 1989.

401. Sane AC, Effmann EL, Brown SD: Tracheobronchiomegaly. The Mounier-Kuhn syndrome in a patient with the Kenny-Caffey syndrome. Chest 102:618, 1992.

402. Langer LO, Petersen D, Spranger JW: An unusual bone dysplasia: Parastremmatic dwarfism. AJR 110:550, 1970.

403. Horan F, Beighton P: Parastremmatic dwarfism. J Bone Joint Surg [Br] 58:343, 1976.

404. Herman TE, McAlister WH, Boniface A, et al: Occipital horn syndrome. Additional radiographic findings in two new cases. Pediatr Radiol 22:363, 1992.

405. Sartoris DJ, Resnick D: The horn: A pathognomonic feature in pediatric bone dysplasias. Aust Paediatr J 23:347, 1987.

406. Sartoris DJ, Luzzatti L, Weaver DD, et al: Type 1X Ehlers-Danlos syndrome. Radiology 152:665, 1984.

407. Kuivaniemi H, Peltonen L, Kivirikko KI: Type IX Ehlers-Danlos syndrome and Menkes syndrome: The decrease in lysyl oxidase activity is associated with a corresponding deficiency in the enzyme protein. Am J Hum Genet 37:798, 1985.

408. Marsh JL, Vannier MW: Comprehensive Care for Craniofacial Deformities. St. Louis, CV Mosby, 1985.

409. Graham JM Jr: Craniostenosis: A new approach to management. Pediatr Ann 10:258, 1981.

410. Pilgram TK, Vannier MW, Hildebolt CF, et al: Craniosynostosis: Imaging quality, confidence, and correctness in diagnosis. Radiology 173:675, 1989.

411. Gellad FE, Haney PJ, Sun JCC, et al: Imaging modalities of craniosynostosis with surgical and pathological correlation. Pediatr Radiol 15:285, 1985.

412. Kreiborg S: Crouzon syndrome. A clinical and roentgencephalometric study. Scand J Plast Reconstr Surg (Suppl) 18:1, 1981.

413. Kaler SG, Bixler D, Yu P: Radiographic hand abnormalities in fifteen cases of Crouzon syndrome. J Craniofac Genet Dev Biol 2:205, 1982.

414. Dawn N, Sigger DC: Cor pulmonale and Crouzon's disease. Arch Dis Child 46:394, 1971.

415. Cohen MM, Kreiborg S: Visceral anomalies in the Apert syndrome. Am J Med Genet 45:758, 1993.

416. Kreiborg S, Cohen MM: Characteristics of the infant Apert skull and its subsequent development. J Craniofacial Genet Dev Biol 10:399, 1990.

417. Marsh JL, Galic M, Vannier MW: The craniofacial anatomy of Apert syndrome. Clin Plast Surg 18:237, 1991.

418. Vannier MW, Hildebolt C, Marsh JL: Craniosynostosis: Diagnostic value of 3-D CT reconstruction. Radiology 173:669, 1989.

419. Upton J: Classification and pathology anatomy of limb anomalies. Apert syndrome. Clin Plast Surg 18:321, 1991.

420. Cohen MM, Kreiborg S: Agenesis of the corpus callosum: Its associated anomalies and syndromes with special reference to Apert syndrome. Neurosurg Clin North Am 2:565, 1991.

421. Teng RJ, Wang PJ, Wang TS, et al: Apert syndrome associated with septo-optic dysplasia. Pediatr Neurol 5:384, 1989.

422. Yonenobu K, Tada K, Tsuyuguchi Y: Apert's syndrome—a report of five cases. Hand 14:317, 1982.

423. Green SM: Pathologic anatomy of the hands in Apert's syndrome. J Hand Surg 7:450, 1982.

424. Beligere N, Harris V, Pruzansky S: Progressive bone dysplasia in Apert syndrome. Radiology 139:593, 1981.

425. Schauerte EW, St Aubin PM: Progressive synostosis in Apert's syndrome (acrocephalosyndactyly) with description of roentgenographic changes in the feet. AJR 97:67, 1966.

426. Kreiborg S, Barr M, Cohen MM: Cervical spine in the Apert syndrome. Am J Med Genet 43:704, 1992.

427. Cristofori G, Filippi G: Saethre-Chotzen syndrome with trigonencephaly. Am J Med Genet 44:611, 1992.

428. Friedman JM, Hanson JW, Graham CB, et al: Saethre-Chotzen syndrome. A broad and variable pattern of skeletal malformations. J Pediatr 91:929, 1977.

429. Kopysz Z, Stanska N, Ryzko J, et al: The Saethre-Chotzen syndrome with partial bifid of the distal phalanges of the great toes. Observations of three cases in one family. Hum Genet 56:195, 1980.

430. Evans CA, Christiansen RL: Cephalic malformations in Saethre-Chotzen syndrome. Acrocephalosyndactyly type II. Radiology 121:399, 1976.

431. Baraitser M, Bowen-Bravery M, Saldana-Garcia P: Pitfalls in genetic counseling in Pfeiffer syndrome. J Med Genet 17:250, 1980.

432. Sanchez JM, DeNegrotti TC: Variable expression of Pfeiffer syndrome. J Med Genet 18:73, 1981.

433. Cohen MM: Pfeiffer syndrome update, clinical subtypes and guidelines for differential diagnosis. Am J Med Genet 45:300, 1993.

434. Saldino RM, Steinbach HL, Epstein CJ: Familial acrocephalosyndactyly (Pfeiffer syndrome). AJR 116:609, 1972.

435. Jackson C, Weiss L, Reynolds WA, et al: Craniosynostosis, midfacial hypoplasia, and foot abnormalities: An autosomal dominant phenotype in a large Amish kindred. J Pediatr 88:963, 1976.

436. Frias JL, Felman AH, Rosenbloom AL, et al: Normal intelligence in two children with Carpenter's syndrome. Am J Med Genet 2:191, 1978.

437. Robinson LK, Jameds HE, Mubarak SJ, et al: Carpenter syndrome: Natural history and clinical spectrum. Am J Med Genet 20:461, 1985.

438. Kaler SG, Bixler D, Yu P: Metacarpophalangeal pattern profile in ACPS Type II (Carpenter syndrome). J Craniofac Genet Dev Biol 1:373, 1981.

439. Gershoni-Baruch R: Carpenter syndrome: Marked variability of expression to include the Summitt and Goodman syndromes. Am J Med Genet 35:236, 1990.

440. Mandergem LV, Verloes A, Lejeune L, et al: The Baller-Gerold syndrome. J Med Genet 29:266, 1992.

441. Dallapiccola B, Zalente L, Mingorelli R, et al: Baller-Gerold syndrome: Case report and clinical and radiological review. Am J Med Genet 42:365, 1992.

442. Lin AE, McPherson E, Nwokoro MA, et al: Further delineation of the Baller-Gerold syndrome. Am J Med Genet 45:519, 1993.

443. Jacobsen RL, Dignan PSJ, Miiodovnik M, et al: Antley-Bixler syndrome. J Ultrasound Med 11:161, 1992.

444. Escobar LF, Bixler D, Sadove M, et al: Antley-Bixler syndrome from a prognostic perspective. Am J Med Genet 29:829, 1988.

445. Zanini SA, Paglioli E, Viterbo F, et al: Trigonencephaly. J Craniofac Surg 3:85, 1992.

446. Schaap C, Schrander-Stumpel CT, Fryns JP: Opitz-C syndrome: On the nosology of mental retardation and trigonocephaly. Genet Counseling 3:209, 1992.

447. Gollop TR, Fontes LR: The Greig cephalopolysyndactyly syndrome: Report of a family and review of the literature. Am J Med Genet 22:59, 1985.

448. Duncan PA, Greig L, Klein RM: Cephalosyndactyly syndrome. Am J Dis Child 133:818, 1979.

449. Chudley AE, Houston CS: The Greig encephalopolysyndactyly syndrome in a Canadian family. Am J Med Genet 13:269, 1982.

450. Behrent RG: The continuity of mandibular form in mandibulofacial dysostosis. J Dent Res 61:1240, 1982.

451. Lloyd GAS, Phelps PD: Radiology of the ear in mandibulo-facial dysostosis—Treacher-Collins syndrome. Acta Radiol 20:233, 1979.

452. Mafee MF, Schild JA, Kumar A, et al: Radiographic features of the ear-related developmental anomalies in patients with mandibulofacial dysostosis. Int J Pediatr Otorhinolaryngol 7:229, 1984.

453. Johnson C, Taussig LM, Koopmann C, et al: Obstructive sleep apnea in Treacher-Collins syndrome. Cleft Palate 17:103, 1980.

454. Bowen AD, Harley F: Mandibulofacial dysostosis with limb malformations (Nager acrofacial dysostosis). Birth Defects 10:109, 1974.

455. Krauss CM, Hassell LA, Gang DL: Brief clinical report: Anomalies in an infant with Nager acrofacial dysostosis. Am J Med Genet 21:761, 1985.

456. Ogelvi-Stuart AL, Parsons AC: Miller syndrome (postaxial acrofacial dysostoses): Further evidence for autosomal recessive inheritance and expansion of the phenotype. J Med Genet 28:695, 1991.

457. Miller M, Fineman R, Smith DW: Postaxial acrofacial dysostosis syndrome. J Pediatr 95:970, 1979.

458. Setzer E, Ruiz-Castaneda N, Severn C, et al: Etiologic heterogeneity in the oculo-auriculo-vertebral syndrome. J Pediatr 98:88, 1981.

459. Schrander-Stumpel CTRM, Die Smulders CEM, Hennekam RCM, et al: Oculoauriculovertebral spectrum and cerebral anomalies. J Med Genet 29:326, 1992.

460. Rees DO, Collum LMT, Bowen DI: Radiologic aspects of oculo-auriculo-vertebral dysplasia. Br J Radiol 45:15, 1972.

461. Bowen AD, Parry WH: Bronchopulmonary foregut malformation in Goldenhar anomalad. AJR 134:186, 1980.

462. Pauli RM, Jung JH, McPherson EW: Goldenhar association and cranial defects. Am J Med Genet 15:177, 1983.

463. Beltinger C, Saule H: Imaging of lipoma of the corpus callosum and intracranial dermoids in the Goldenhar syndrome. Pediatr Radiol 18:72, 1988.

464. Gorlin RJ, Pindborg JJ, Cohen MM Jr: Syndromes of the Head and Neck. 2nd Ed. New York, McGraw-Hill Book Company, 1976.

465. Rollnick BR, Kaye CI: Hemifacial microsomia and variants: Pedigree data. Am J Med Genet 15:233, 1983.

466. Burch U: Genetic aspects of hemifacial microsomia. Hum Genet 64:291, 1983.

467. Steel RW, Bass JW: Hallerman-Streiff syndrome. Clinical and prognostic consideration. Am J Dis Child 120:462, 1970.

468. Chanddra RK, Joglekar S, Antonio Z: Deficiency of humoral immunity in hypoparathyroidism associated with the Hallermann-Streiff syndrome. J Pediatr 93:892, 1978.

469. Kurlander GJ, Lavy NW, Campbell JA: Roentgen differentiation of oculodento-digital in the Hallermann-Streiff syndrome in infancy. Radiology 86:77, 1966.

470. Dinwiddie R, Gewitz M, Taylor JFN: Cardiac defects in Hallermann-Streiff syndrome. J Pediatr 92:77, 1978.

471. Magill HI, Shackelford GD, McAlister WH, et al: 4p− (Wolf-Hirschhorn) syndrome. AJR 135:283, 1980.

472. Tachdjian G, Fondacci C, Tapia S, et al: The Wolf-Hirschhorn syndrome in fetuses. Clin Genet 42:281, 1992.

473. James AE, Adkins L, Feingold M, et al: The cri-du-chat syndrome. Radiology 92:50, 1969.

474. Breg WR, Steele MW, Miller OJ, et al: The cri du chat syndrome in adolescents and adults: Clinical findings in 13 older patients with partial deletion of the short arm of chromosome No. 5 (5p−). J Pediatr 77:782, 1970.

475. Riccardi VM: Trisomy 8: An international study of 70 patients. Birth Defects 13:171, 1977.

476. Silengo MC, Davi CF, Franceschini P: Radiological features of trisomy 8. Pediatr Radiol 8:116, 1979.

477. Gelb B, Towbin JA, McCabe RB, et al: San Luis Valley recombinant chromosome 8 and tetralogy of Fallot: A review of chromosome 8 anomalies and congenital heart disease. Am J Med Genet 4:471, 1991.

478. Pilling DW, Levick RK: Radiologic abnormalities associated with anomalies of the 9th chromosome. Pediatr Radiol 6:215, 1978.

479. Schinzel A: Trisomy 9p, a chromosomal aberration with distinct radiologic findings. Radiology 130:125, 1979.

480. Wilson GN, Raj AN, Baker D: The phenotypic and cytogenetic spectrum of partial trisomy 9. Am J Med Genet 20:277, 1985.

481. Patau K, Smith DW, Therman E, et al: Multiple congenital anomalies caused by an extra autosome. Lancet 1:790, 1960.

482. James AE, Belcourt CL, Atkins L, et al: Trisomy 13–15. Radiology 92:44, 1969.

483. Scarbough PR, Finley WH, Finley SC: A review of trisomies 21, 18, and 13. Ala J Med Sci 19:174, 1982.

484. Cabin HS, Lester LA, Roberts WC: Congenital heart disease with trisomy 13: Use of the echocardiogram in delineating the location of a left to right shunt. Am Heart J 100:563, 1980.

485. Franceschini P, Fabris C, Bogetti G, et al: First rib hypoplasia in Patau's disease. Pediatr Radiol 2:65, 1974.

486. Moerman P, Fryns JP, van der Steen K, et al: The pathology of trisomy 13 syndrome, a study of 12 cases. Human Genetics 80:341, 1988.

487. James AE, Belcourt CL, Atkins L, et al: Trisomy 18. Radiology 92:37, 1969.

488. Christianson AL, Nelson MM: Four cases of trisomy 18 syndrome with limb reduction malformations. J Med Genet 21:293, 1984.

489. Moerman P, Fryns JP, Goddeeris P, et al: Spectrum of clinical and autopsy findings in trisomy 18 syndrome. J Genet Hum 30:17, 1982.

490. Robinson MG, McCorquodale MM: Trisomy 18 and neurogenic neoplasia. J Pediatr 99:428, 1981.

491. Kinoshita M, Nakamura Y, Nakano R, et al: Thirty-one autopsy cases of trisomy 18: Clinical features and pathologic findings. Pediatr Pathol 9:445, 1989.

492. Nyberg DA, Kramer D, Resta RG, et al: Prenatal sonographic findings of trisomy 18: Review of 47 cases. J Ultrasound Med 2:103, 1993.

493. Lejeune J, Gautier M, Turpin R: Etude des chromosomes somatiques de neuf enfants mongoliens. C R Acad Sci 248:1721, 1959.

494. Smith GV, Teele RL: Delayed diagnosis of duodenal obstruction in Down's syndrome. AJR 134:937, 1980.

495. Ryan ET, Ecker JL, Christakis NA, et al: Hirschsprung's disease: Associated abnormalities and demography. J Pediatr Surg 27:76, 1992.

496. Torfs CP, Bateson TF, Curry CJR: Anorectal and esophageal anomalies with Down syndrome. Am J Med Genet 44:847, 1992.

497. Laughlin GM, Wynne JW, Victorica BE: Sleep apnea as a possible cause of pulmonary hypertension in Down's syndrome. J Pediatr 98:435, 1981.

498. Aboussouan LS, O'Donovan PB, Moodie DS, et al: Hypoplastic trachea in Down's syndrome. Am Rev Respir Dis 147:72, 1993.

499. Cooney TP, Thurlbeck WM: Pulmonary hypoplasia in Down's syndrome. N Engl J Med 307:1170, 1982.

500. Roberts GM, Starey N, Harper P, et al: Radiology of the pelvis and hips in adults with Down's syndrome. Clin Radiol 31:475, 1980.

501. Austin JHM, Preger L, Siris E, et al: Short hard palate in newborn: Roentgen sign of mongolism. Radiology 92:775, 1969.

502. Ieshima A, Kisa T, Yoshino K, et al: A morphometric CT study of Down's syndrome showing small posterior fossa and calcification of basal ganglia. Neuroradiology 26:493, 1984.

503. Hungerford GD, Akkaraju V, Rawe SE, et al: Atlanto-occipital and atlanto-axial dislocations with spine cord compression in Down's syndrome: A case report and review of the literature. Br J Radiol 54:758, 1981.

504. Currarino G, Swanson GE: A developmental variant of ossification in manubrium sterni in mongolism. Radiology 82:916, 1964.

505. Willich E, Fuhr U, Kroll W: Skeletal manifestations in Down's syndrome. Correlation between roentgenologic and cytogenetic findings. Ann Radiol 18:355, 1975.

506. Stein SM, Kirchner SG, Horev G, et al: Atlanto-occipital subluxation in Down syndrome. Pediatr Radiol 21:121, 1991.

507. Tishler JM, Martel W: Dislocation of the atlas in mongolism. A preliminary report. Radiology 84:904, 1965.

508. Martel W, Tishler JM: Observations on the spine in mongoloidism. AJR 97:630, 1966.

509. Martich V, Ben-Ami T, Yousefzadeh DK, et al: Hypoplastic posterior arch of C-1 in children with Down syndrome: A double jeopardy. Radiology 183:125, 1992.

510. Houston CS, Chudley A: Separating monosomy-21 from the "arthrogryposis basket." J Can Assoc Radiol 32:220, 1981.

511. Herva R, Koivisto M, Seppanen U: 21-Monosomy in a liveborn male infant. Eur J Pediatr 140:57, 1983.

512. Hall JG, Gilchrist DM: Turner syndrome and its variants. Pediatr Clin North Am 37:1421, 1990.

513. Lippe B: Turner syndrome. Endocrinol Metab Clin North Am 20:121, 1991.

514. Robinow M, Spisso K, Buschi AJ, et al: Turner's syndrome. Sonography showing fetal hydrops simulating hydramnios. AJR 135:846, 1980.

515. Lester PD, McAlister WH: Pneumopelvigraphy in childhood. AJR 131:607, 1978.

516. Herman TE, Kusner DC, Cleveland RH: Premature sternal fusion in gonadal dysgenesis with coarctation. Pediatr Radiol 15:350, 1985.

517. Baker DH, Berdon WE, Morishima A, et al: Turner syndrome and pseudo-Turner's syndrome. AJR 100:40, 1967.

518. Kosowicz J: The roentgen appearance of the hand and wrist in gonadal dysgenesis. AJR 93:354, 1965.

519. Cleveland RH, Done S, Correia JA, et al: Small carpal bone surface area, a characteristic of Turner's syndrome. Pediatr Radiol 15:168, 1985.

520. Rzymski K, Kosowicz J: The skull and gonadal dysgenesis and roentgenometric study. Clin Radiol 26:379, 1975.

521. Brown DM, Jowsey J, Bradford DS: Osteoporosis in ovarian dysgenesis. J Pediatr 84:816, 1974.

522. Poznanski AK, Garn SM, Shaw HA: The carpal angle in the congenital malformation syndromes. Ann Radiol 19:141, 1976.

523. Nishi Y, Sakano T, Hyodo S, et al: Pituitary abnormalities detected by high resolution computed tomography with thin slices in primary hypothyroidism and Turner syndrome. Eur J Pediatr 142:25, 1984.

524. Arulananthan K, Kramer MS, Gryboski JD: The association of inflammatory bowel disease in X-chromosomal abnormalities. Pediatrics 66:63, 1980.

525. Ochi H, Takeuchi J, Sandberg AA: Multiple cancers in a Turner's syndrome with 45,X/46,XXp − /46,XX/47,XXX karyotype. Cancer Genet Cytogenet 16:335, 1985.

526. Ohsawa T, Furuse M, Kikuchi Y, et al: Roentgenographic manifestation of Kleinfelter syndrome. AJR 112:78, 1971.

527. Kosowicz J, Rzymski K: Radiologic features of the skull in Kleinfelter's syndrome and male hypogonadism. Clin Radiol 26:371, 1975.

528. Houston CS: Roentgen findings in XXXXY chromosomal anomaly. J Can Assoc Radiol 18:258, 1967.

529. Brante G: Gargoylism: A mucopolysaccharidosis. Scand J Clin Lab Invest 4:43, 1952.

530. Dorfman A, Lorincz AE: Occurrence of urinary acid mucopolysaccharides in the Hurler syndrome. Proc Natl Acad Sci 43:443, 1957.

531. Hurler G: Uber einen Typ multipler Abartungen, vorwiegend am Skelettsystem. Z Kinderheilkd 24:220, 1919.

532. Thomas SL, Childress MH, Quinton B: Hypoplasia of the odontoid with atlanto-axial subluxation in Hurler's syndrome. Pediatr Radiol 15:353, 1985.

533. Peters ME, Arya S, Langer LO, et al: Narrow trachea in mucopolysaccharidoses. Pediatr Radiol 15:225, 1985.

534. Taylor DB, Blaser SI, Burrows PE, et al: Arteriopathy and coarctation of the abdominal aorta in children with mucopolysaccharidosis: Imaging findings. AJR 157:819, 1991.

535. Braunlin EA, Hunter DW, Krivit W, et al: Evaluation of coronary artery disease in the Hurler syndrome by angiography. Am J Cardiol 69:1489, 1992.

536. Myer CM: Airway obstruction in Hurler's syndrome—radiographic features. Int J Pediatr Otorhinolaryngol 22:91, 1991.

537. Bredenkamp JK, Smith ME, Dudley JP, et al: Otolaryngologic manifestations of the mucopolysaccharidoses. Ann Otol Rhinol Laryngol 101:472, 1992.

538. Watts RWE, Spellacy E, Kendall BE, et al: Computed tomography studies on patients with mucopolysaccharidosis. Neuroradiology 21:9, 1981.

539. Murata R, Nakajima S, Tanaka A, et al: MR imaging of the brain in patients with mucopolysaccharidosis. AJNR 10:1165, 1989.

540. Stevenson RE, Howell RR, McKusick VA, et al: The iduronidase-deficient mucopolysaccharidoses: Clinical and roentgenographic features. Pediatrics 57:111, 1976.

541. Perks WH, Cooper RA, Bradbury S, et al: Sleep apnea in Scheie syndrome. Thorax 35:85, 1980.

542. Lamon MJ, Trojak JE, Abbott MH: Bone cysts in mucopolysaccharide I-S Scheie syndrome. Johns Hopkins Med J 146:73, 1980.

543. Hamilton E, Pitt P: Articular manifestations of Scheie's syndrome. Ann Rheum Dis 51:542, 1992.

544. Lamon JM, Trojak JE, Abbott MH: Bone cysts in mucopolysaccharidosis IS (Scheie syndrome). Johns Hopkins Med J 146:71, 1980.

545. Kaibara N, Katsuki I, Hotokebuchi T, et al: Hurler-Scheie phenotype with parental consanguinity: Report of additional case supporting the concept of genetic heterogeneity. Clin Orthop 175:233, 1983.

546. Roubicek M, Gehler J, Spranger J: The clinical spectrum of alpha-L-iduronidase deficiency. Am J Med Genet 20:471, 1985.

547. Sostrin RD, Hasso AN, Peterson DI, et al: Myelographic features in mucopolysaccharidosis—a new sign. Radiology 125:421, 1977.

548. Young ID, Harper PS, Newcombe RG, et al: A clinical and genetic study of Hunter's syndrome. II. Differences between mild and severe forms. J Med Genet 19:408, 1982.

549. Young ID, Harper PS: The natural history of the severe form of Hunter's syndrome. A study based on 52 cases. Dev Med Child Neurol 4:481, 1983.

550. Grossman H, Dorst JP: Mucopolysaccharidosis and mucolipidosis. In H Kaufman (Ed): Intrinsic Diseases of the Bone Progress in Pediatric Radiology, Vol 4. Basel, S Karger, 1973, p 395.

551. Archer IM, Kingston HM, Harper PS: Prenatal diagnosis of Hunter syndrome. Prenat Diagn 4:195, 1984.

552. Zlotogora J, Bach G: Heterozygote detection in Hunter syndrome. Am J Med Genet 17:661, 1984.

553. Van de Kamp JJP, Niermeijer MF, Von Figura K, et al: Genetic heterogeneity and clinical variability in the Sanfilippo syndrome, types A, B, and C. Clin Genet 20:152, 1981.

554. Coppa GV, Giorgi PL, Felici L, et al: Clinical heterogeneity in Sanfilippo disease (mucopolysaccharidosis III) type D: Presentation of two new cases. Eur J Pediatr 140:130, 1983.

555. Andria G, Di Natale P, Del Gieidice E, et al: Sanfilippo B syndrome (MPS): Mild and severe forms in the same sibling. Clin Genet 15:500, 1979.

556. Holzgrave W, Grobe H, von Figura K, et al: Morquio syndrome. Clinical findings of 11 patients with MPS IV-A and 2 patients with MPS IV-B. Hum Genet 57:360, 1981.

557. van Gemund JJ, Giesberts NAH, Eerdmans RF, et al: Morquio-B disease, spondyloepiphyseal dysplasia associated with acid β-galactosidase deficiency. Report of three cases in one family. Hum Genet 64:50, 1983.

558. Grossman H, Dorst JP: Mucopolysaccharidosis and mucolipidosis. In H Kaufman (Ed): Intrinsic Diseases of Bones. Progress in Pediatric Radiology, Vol 4. Basel, S Karger, 1973, p 495.

559. Hecht JT, Scott CI, Smith TK, et al: Mild manifestations of the Morquio syndrome. Am J Med Genet 18:369, 1984.

560. Wald SL, Schmidek HH: Compressive myelopathy associated with type IV mucopolysaccharidosis (Maroteaux-Lamy syndrome). J Neurol 14:83, 1984.

561. Krivit W, Pierpont ME, Ayaz KL, et al: Bone-marrow transplantation in Maroteaux-Lamy syndrome (mucopolysaccharidosis type VI biochemical and clinical status 24 months after transplantation). N Engl J Med 311:1606, 1984.

562. Hayflick S, Rowe S, Kavanaugh-McHugh A, et al: Acute infantile cardiomyopathy as a presenting feature of mucopolysaccharidosis VI. J Pediatr 120:269, 1992.

563. Sly WS, Quinton BA, McAlister WH, et al: Beta glucuronidase deficiency: Report of clinical, radiologic, and biochemical features of a new mucopolysaccharidosis. J Pediatr 82:249, 1973.

564. Gitzelman R, Wiesmann UN, Spycher MA, et al: Unusually mild course of beta glucuronidase deficiency in two brothers (mucopolysaccharidosis VII). Helv Paediatr Acta 33:413, 1978.

565. Hoyme HE, Jones KL, Higginbottom MC, et al: Presentation of mucopolysaccharidosis VII (beta glucuronidase deficiency in infancy). J Med Genet 18:237, 1981.

566. Gehler J, Sewell AC, Becker C, et al: Clinical and biochemical evaluation of aspartyl-glucosaminuria as observed on two members of an Italian family. Helv Pediatr Acta 36:179, 1981.

567. Spranger J, Gehler J, Cantz M: The radiographic features of mannosidosis. Radiology 119:401, 1976.

568. Mitchell ML, Erickson RP, Schmid D, et al: Mannosidosis of two brothers with different disease severity. Clin Genet 20:191, 1981.

569. Willems PJ, Gatti R, Darby JK, et al: Fucosidosis revisited: A review of 77 patients. Am J Med Genet 38:111, 1991.

570. Brill PW, Beratis NJ, Kousseff BG, et al: Roentgenographic findings in fucosidosis Type II. AJR 124:75, 1975.

571. Lee FL, Donnell GN, Gwinn JL: Radiographic features of fucosidosis. Pediatr Radiol 5:204, 1977.

572. O'Brien JS: Generalized gangliosidosis. In JB Stanbury, et al (Eds): Metabolic Basis of Inherited Disease. 4th Ed. New York, McGraw-Hill Book Company, 1982.

573. Farrell DF, Och U: GM-I gangliosidosis phenotypic variation in a single family. Ann Neurol 9:225, 1981.

574. Rabinowitz JC, Sacher M: Gangliosidosis (GM-I)—a re-evaluation of vertebral deformity. AJR 121:155, 1974.

575. Rosenberg H, Frewen TC, Li MD, et al: Cardiac involvement in diseases characterized by beta-galactosidase deficiency. J Pediatr 106:77, 1985.

576. Spranger J, Gehler J, Cantz M: Mucolipidosis I—a sialidosis. Am J Med Genet 1:21, 1977.

577. Staalman CR, Bakker HD: Mucopilidosis. Skel Radiol 12:153, 1984.

578. Kelly TE, Vartosheski L, Harris DJ, et al: Mucolipidosis I (acid neuraminidase deficiency). Am J Dis Child 135:703, 1981.

579. Lemaitre L, Remy J, Farriaux JP, et al: Radiologic signs of mucolipidosis II or I-cell disease. Pediatr Radiol 7:97, 1978.

580. Babcock DS, Bove KE, Hug G, et al: Fetal mucolipidosis II (I-cell disease): Radiologic and pathologic correlation. Pediatr Radiol 16:32, 1986.

581. Patriquin HB, Kaplan P, Kind HP, et al: Neonatal mucolipidosis II (I-cell disease): Clinical and radiologic features in three cases. AJR 129:37, 1977.

582. Brown WJ, Farquhar MG: Accumulation of coated vesicles bearing mannose-6-phosphate receptors for lysosomal enzymes in the Golgi region of I-cell fibroblasts. Proc Natl Acad Sci USA 81:5135, 1984.

583. Pazzaglia UE, Beluffi G, Danesino C, et al: Neonatal mucolipidosis II. The spontaneous evolution of early bone lesions and the effect of vitamin D treatment. Pediatr Radiol 20:80, 1989.

584. Pazzaglia UE, Beluffi G, Campbell JB, et al: Mucolipidosis II: Correlation between radiological features and histopathology of the bones. Pediatr Radiol 19:406, 1989.

585. Herd JK, Dvorak AD, Wiltse HE, et al: Mucolipidosis type III. Elevated serum and urine enzyme activities. Am J Dis Child 33:1181, 1978.

586. Nolte K, Spranger J: Early skeletal changes in mucolipidosis III. Ann Radiol 19:151, 1976.

587. Melhem R, Dorst JP, Scott CI, et al: Roentgen findings in mucolipidosis III (pseudo-Hurler's polydystrophy). Radiology 106:153, 1973.

89

Spinal Anomalies and Curvatures

M. B. Ozonoff, M.D.

This chapter discusses various spinal anomalies and abnormal curvatures. Although the discussion is brief, emphasis is placed on some important structural abnormalities of the vertebral body or arch, or both, and of the craniovertebral junction and sacrum. Also summarized are disorders leading to open or closed (occult) spinal dysraphism and the causes and characteristics of congenital scoliosis, kyphosis, and lordosis, and of other varieties of scoliosis, both idiopathic and that related to other conditions or syndromes.

CONGENITAL ANOMALIES OF THE SPINE

Structural Abnormalities

Many congenital vertebral anomalies are of such minor degree and resolve so quickly, as a result of skeletal growth and maturation, that properly they are considered normal developmental variants; a typical example of this would be the transient coronal cleft vertebra of infancy.[1, 2] Other defects are remnants of previous embryologic states that have failed to evolve completely but nevertheless have little or no clinical importance (e.g., nonfusion of the lumbar or sacral neural arches). Nevertheless, many, such as myelomeningocele, are of major structural and clinical significance.

Some anomalies are restricted to skeletal structures, either isolated at one or two levels or part of larger complexes. Other abnormalities are associated with neural tube defects (myelomeningocele, diastematomyelia, and congenital intraspinal tumors). Additionally, the skeletal and neural anomalies may be part of a multisystem abnormality, such as the VATER (vertebral, anorectal, tracheal, esophageal, renal/rectal) complex[3-5] and numerous dysplasias and syndromes. The term "dysraphism" refers to a failure of midline fusion and development and often is used synonymously with any congenital anomaly of the spine, even if no fusional abnormality is present.

Structural spinal abnormalities can be classified generally into those resulting from nondevelopment, from nonfusion, or from nonsegmentation of embryologic structures.[6] Detailed analysis has confirmed the visible spatial disorientation, but no abnormal histologic patterns have been found to explain the findings.

Anomalies of the Vertebral Body. The vertebral body develops originally from paired chondral centers and, at a later stage, from a single ossification focus that is separated transiently by the notochordal remnant into anterior and posterior centers. Total aplasia can be explained by failure of development of the mesoderm in the involved segment. Lack of development of one of the paired chondral centers produces a lateral hemivertebra, whereas if the failure occurs at the ossification stage, anterior agenesis will result in a posterior hemivertebra.

Hemivertebrae may vary in size, and the contralateral segment at the same level may be completely absent or hypoplastic (Fig. 89–1). The pedicle on the side of the hemivertebra may be normal or enlarged, and its counterpart at the same level may be either absent or hypoplastic. The same may be true with respect to the ribs, with the hypoplastic or aplastic side of the vertebra rarely possessing a rib. The hemivertebra may exist in place of a normal vertebra, or it may be a supernumerary structure, often slightly displaced from the main axis of the spinal column.

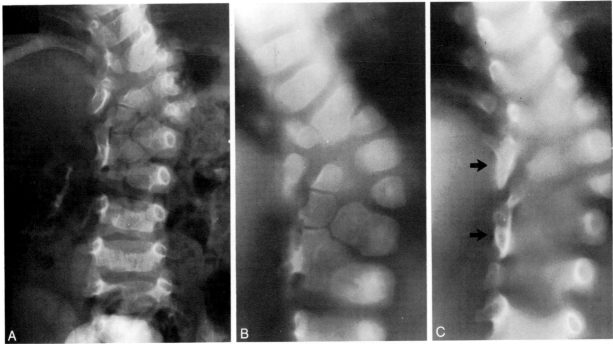

FIGURE 89–1. Congenital scoliosis. A left thoracolumbar scoliosis is associated with right upper lumbar pediculate bars and multiple supernumerary hemivertebrae on the left.

   A Abnormalities of the vertebral body are difficult to differentiate from those of the neural arch on this routine frontal radiograph.

   B Multidirectional planar tomography at the level of the vertebral bodies reveals multiple hemivertebrae with several centers fused with each other.

   C Multidirectional planar tomography at a more posterior level demonstrates normal pedicles on the left and pediculate-laminar bars on the right (arrows).

   (From Theros EG, Harris JH Jr [Eds]: American College of Radiology Bone Syllabus IV. Chicago, American College of Radiology, 1989.)

In many cases, the anomaly that is present in the vertebral body is associated with fusion or segmentation defects in the neural arch.

The vertebral body occasionally is constricted centrally, most probably after incomplete fusion of the two chondral centers, with hypoplasia where they join (butterfly vertebra). Two or more vertebral somites also may be subject to nonsegmentation, in which case a block vertebra is formed. The intervertebral discs may be completely absent or may be represented by rudimentary, irregularly calcified structures. Often a waistlike constriction of the fused structure is found at the level of the intervertebral disc (causing an hourglass appearance), and the total height of the block vertebra usually is less than expected from the number of segments that are involved. In the cervical spine, this congenital anomaly may be difficult to differentiate from abnormalities caused by juvenile chronic arthritis. In an analysis of adult cervical spines with vertebral fusion, 13 per cent were believed to be congenital.[7]

Anomalies of the Vertebral Arch. The same anomalies of formation, segmentation, and maturation may affect the neural arches. Each neural arch develops from a separate chondrification (and subsequently an ossification) center; these paired arches normally unite in the midline by the age of 2 years but frequently remain open at the L5 or S1 spinal level, or both; less commonly, they may remain open at the T11 or T12 spinal level.[8–10] The frequency of such nonfusion is so high that it must be considered a normal variant rather than an abnormality, and many of these apparent vertebral "splits" in fact are composed of cartilage and fibrous tissue. The use of the term "spina bifida occulta" for these minor failures of fusion is to be strongly discouraged as the term implies significant clinical abnormalities, which generally are not present. The term "spina bifida," if it is to be used at all, should be restricted to those instances of severe dysraphism with neurologic consequences.

Abnormalities of the neural arch (including the pedicles, which originate from the same developmental centers) include total absence, underdevelopment with wide osseous separation, and failure of segmentation (Fig. 89–2). In addition, rare anomalies of the spine have been reported, including absent lumbosacral facets,[11] a double spinal canal,[12] and duplication of the spine.[13, 14]

When pediculate aplasia occurs, it is most common in the cervical and lumbar regions. Although usually it is asymptomatic when present in the thoracic and lumbar segments, neck pain and neurologic symptoms reportedly were present in two thirds of patients with cervical involvement.[15–19] In a small series of patients, nearly 50 per cent also had genitourinary abnormalities.[20]

The outline of the pedicle on the involved side is absent and the opposite pedicle at the same level frequently is hyperplastic, although this finding is less common in children than in adults.[20, 21] Hypoplasia of the ipsilateral superior articular facet may be present as well as abnormality of the inferior facet of the vertebra above. The spinous process at the affected level frequently tilts toward the abnormal

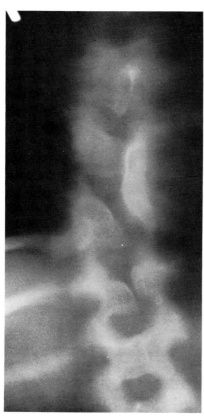

FIGURE 89–2. Congenital scoliosis. Multidirectional planar tomography in this 4 year old girl demonstrates both nonfused neural arches and fusion of laminae at adjacent levels.

side, and the transverse process may be more anterior than usual.[22–24] Facet, laminar, or spinous process fusion may be an associated finding.

The use of CT scanning in the evaluation of these abnormalities has shown that in some instances the pedicle actually may not be absent but may be only very hypoplastic and oriented more coronally, thus explaining its apparent absence on plain films; frequently an associated retroisthmic laminar defect is present.[25]

Failure of segmentation leads to linkage and fusion of adjacent laminae or pedicles, termed congenital vertebral bars.[26] Although these abnormalities can occur bilaterally, usually they are unilateral and important clinically, owing to their restrictive effect on growth on the side on which they lie. Radiographically, pediculate bars appear as a discrete osseous line encircling the pedicles at two or more vertebral levels (Fig. 89–1C).

Laminar fusions are difficult to delineate on plain films and are best shown with planar tomography. They often are associated with vertebral body fusion or hemivertebrae. In younger children, such fusions may be cartilaginous and thus not demonstrable radiologically; serial examinations may show the functional effect produced by unilateral tethering before the bony fusion is demonstrated.

Klippel-Feil Syndrome. The Klippel-Feil syndrome originally was described as a major fusion abnormality in which the cervical and upper thoracic vertebrae were merged into one bony mass, associated with webbing of the neck and a low hairline.[27] Subsequently, the term Klippel-Feil syndrome has been used as a designation for any type

and degree of congenital fusion in the cervical spine, whether or not the clinical triad is present. In fact, in fewer than one half of reported cases was the full syndrome present.[28, 29]

Owing to the blocklike fusions, abnormal degrees of motion may exist at the unfused levels, at times with impingement on neural structures (Fig. 89–3).

The Klippel-Feil syndrome and its associated abnormalities (scoliosis, undescended scapula, and renal abnormalities)[30–32] are discussed more fully in Chapter 90.

Craniovertebral Junction Abnormalities. The craniovertebral junction, like the thoracolumbar and lumbosacral junctions, is a developmentally unstable transitional region in which congenital anomalies are common.[33–42] Embryologically, the cranial half of the first sclerotome is incorporated into the occipital condyles, and only the tip of the odontoid process (dens) retains a contribution from this segment. The caudal half of this sclerotome forms the anterior, lateral, and posterior masses and arches of the atlas. The dens is formed mainly from the second cervical sclerotome. Incomplete incorporation or failure of segmentation leads to a spectrum of fusional anomalies and accessory structures in this area.[43] Many of these are minor and asymptomatic, but some are of significant clinical importance, even if symptoms and signs have not yet developed.[44]

The length of the normal odontoid process in the adult is 16 to 18 mm, and this length is positively correlated with the height of the centrum and the diameter of the spinal canal.[45] The size of the ossified structure obviously is less in a child; owing to the large amount of cartilage in childhood, the atlantoaxial space, which is considered to be abnormal if it is more than 3 mm wide in an adult, normally can be as great as 5 mm in a child.[46, 47] A sagittal cleft is seen in the odontoid process in infancy but usually the cleft fuses by the second year of life.[48, 49]

Many abnormalities of this region have been described.[50] These include agenesis of the odontoid process and its base or of the odontoid process alone, incomplete formation of the apex of the dens, os odontoideum, and nonfusion of the apical apophysis of the dens (ossiculum terminale). Abnormalities at other levels in the cervical spine are seen in two thirds of patients.[51]

In odontoid aplasia, no extension of the dens above the body of the axis is present. Odontoid aplasia (or hypoplasia) may be an isolated congenital anomaly, or it may be associated with the mucopolysaccharidoses and other syndromes. Reports also document the dissolution of a previously ossified odontoid process after trauma.[52, 53]

The os odontoideum is a well-defined ossicle that lies at the tip of the odontoid process and is about one half the size of a normal dens.[54, 55] There is strong evidence that this also is an acquired rather than a congenital lesion, as it has been shown to be present after trauma when the odontoid process had previously been normal.[54, 56] Hypertrophy of the anterior arch of C1, indicating a long-standing process, may help distinguish os odontoideum from an acute fracture.[57]

Occipitalization (assimilation) of the atlas is a normal variant that is asymptomatic in most cases. Typically, the anterior arch of the atlas is fused to the skull base, and other portions of the ring of the atlas reveal similar fusion in many cases. As many as one half of patients with occipitalization of the atlas also have vertebral fusion at the C2-

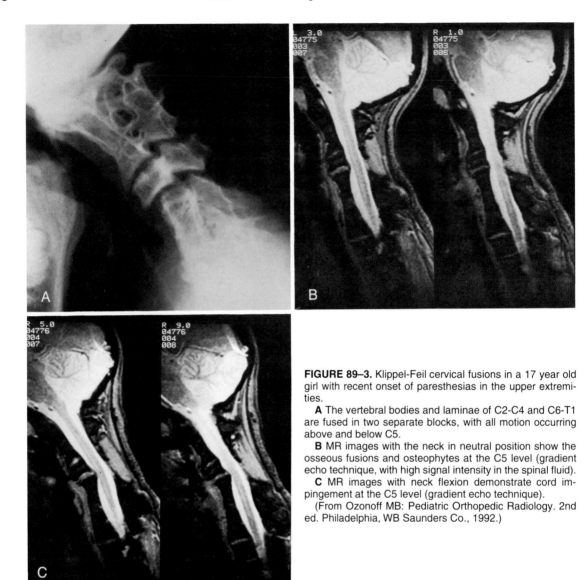

FIGURE 89–3. Klippel-Feil cervical fusions in a 17 year old girl with recent onset of paresthesias in the upper extremities.

A The vertebral bodies and laminae of C2-C4 and C6-T1 are fused in two separate blocks, with all motion occurring above and below C5.

B MR images with the neck in neutral position show the osseous fusions and osteophytes at the C5 level (gradient echo technique, with high signal intensity in the spinal fluid).

C MR images with neck flexion demonstrate cord impingement at the C5 level (gradient echo technique).

(From Ozonoff MB: Pediatric Orthopedic Radiology. 2nd ed. Philadelphia, WB Saunders Co., 1992.)

C3 spinal level. Although the odontoid process is high, directly beneath the foramen magnum, platybasia and basilar impression are uncommon. Fusion of the anterior arch of the atlas to the dens also has been reported as a rare phenomenon.[58]

The evaluation of high cervical anomalies by standard radiography is hampered by the complexity of the structures at this level and their radiologic superimposition. CT scanning with two-dimensional or three-dimensional reconstruction often is needed to delineate the abnormality; MR imaging will help in determining the vulnerability of adjacent neural structures.

Sacral Agenesis. Sacral agenesis is a well-known spinal anomaly with characteristic clinical findings.[59-61] In about one third of patients, the entire sacrum is absent; in the remainder, one or more sacral segments are present, but in some not only the sacrum but also the lumbar or even the lower thoracic column may be absent.[62, 63] Focal lumbar agenesis with an intact sacrum has been described in the 13q− deletion syndrome,[64] but this is a very rare occurrence. Many patients with sacral agenesis will have an associated meningomyelocele and gastrointestinal or genitourinary abnormalities.[3, 65, 66] Diabetes mellitus is present in 19 per cent of mothers of these patients, and sacral agenesis occurs in 0.1 to 0.2 per cent of all infants of diabetic mothers. This anomaly occurs to a significant extent as part of the VATER and VACTERL (vertebral, anorectal, cardiac, tracheal, esophageal, renal, limb) complexes.[67] Flexion contractures of the hips and knees and hip dislocation commonly are present.[59] Severe neurologic abnormalities frequently are encountered. Partial sacral agenesis may take the form of complete absence of one or more distal sacral segments or a paraxial defect with unilateral aplasia or hypoplasia, through which an anterior sacral meningocele may protrude.[68-70]

Several radiologic patterns are seen. With complete sacral (or lumbosacral) agenesis, the ilia may be fused in the midline (Fig. 89–4) or may articulate with each other below the terminal vertebral segment. In other cases, the ilia will articulate with the lowest vertebral body rather than with each other. With partial sacral agenesis, the remaining segments are placed in their usual position between the iliac wings (Fig. 89–5). Scoliosis occurs in more than one half of patients, and many of them have spine anomalies above

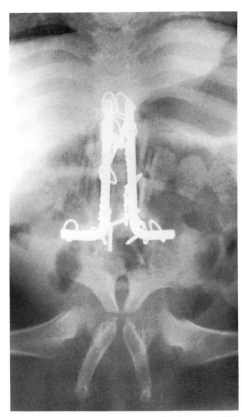

FIGURE 89–4. Lumbar and sacral agenesis. Segmental fusion with Luque rods has been used to stabilize the lower thoracic spine and pelvis. The ilia are fused in the midline. The lower pelvis and acetabula are dysplastic.

the level of the sacrum (hemivertebra, pediculate bar, diastematomyelia, or idiopathic scoliosis).[71]

The imaging workup should include flexion and extension radiographs to determine vertebral and pelvic stability.[71] Dural sac stenosis (with the subarachnoid space ending above the level of the defect) and a low conus medullaris with tethering and arachnoid adhesions may be present.[72] MR imaging will detect these and other neural anomalies. Renal sonography or urography and cystography are essential, as these patients have bladder dysfunction and, frequently, upper urinary tract abnormalities (Fig. 89–5).[73] Anterior sacral meningocele is best evaluated with CT scanning and MR imaging.

Spinal Dysraphism Complexes

Dysraphism represents a failure of midline fusion that encompasses not only structural vertebral defects but also associated abnormalities of embryonic tissue in those organ systems developing at the same time as the neural tube, including the neurologic, gastrointestinal, and genitourinary systems. Dysraphic abnormalities are described as open (uncovered) or closed (covered or occult) lesions. Open defects, such as myelomeningocele, usually are obvious clinically at birth.[74] Closed or occult lesions may have a cutaneous marker such as a nevus, hairy patch, hemangioma, or lipoma that signals the possible presence of an underlying abnormality; in most of these cases, obvious vertebral anomalies are evident radiologically, but occasionally the spine is normal. Diagnostic evaluation of open

dysraphism or detection of occult dysraphism may involve the complete imaging armamentarium (plain radiography, conventional tomography, CT scanning, sonography, and MR imaging) to fully delineate these complex lesions.[75-85]

Myelomeningocele. Myelomeningocele, an example of open spinal dysraphism, is evident clinically at birth. The origin of this anomaly is not completely settled, with one theory relating it to spinal cord rupture after fetal hydrocephalus and hydromyelia.[86] That portion of the spinal cord which is proximal to the obvious neural abnormality often is intrinsically abnormal (e.g., diplomyelia and hydrosyringomyelia).[87]

Plain film radiography usually is sufficient as a preoperative guide but often is deferred until emergency surgery has been performed. The radiologic landmark indicating the highest level of abnormality is that point at which the spinal architecture is visibly distorted. In the infant, however, this frequently is difficult to determine. The point at which widening of the interpediculate distance and vertebral body occurs usually is taken as the superior limit of the anomaly, but the upper extent of the lesion predicted radiologically may not correlate with the functional neurologic level.

The expanding neural and meningeal mass causes reorientation of the laminae from an oblique to a sagittal or even coronal plane (Figs. 89–6 to 89–8). The pedicles are

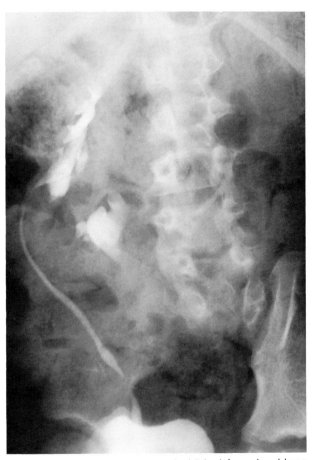

FIGURE 89–5. Partial sacral agenesis. L5 is deformed and hypoplastic, and there are two pedicles at the S1 level with a rudimentary left S2 pedicle fused to that above. The sacrum is absent below this level. The hypoplastic upper portion of the sacrum articulates with the ilia. The intravenous urogram demonstrates crossed fused ectopia of the left kidney.

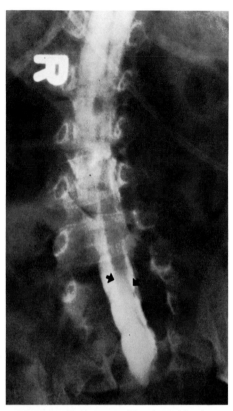

FIGURE 89–6. Myelomeningocele. The dysraphic abnormalities include a widened interpediculate distance at the L3 spinal level and distally. The myelogram demonstrates tethering of the spinal cord (arrows) in the sacral area.

pushed laterally and displaced from a sagittal to a more coronal plane, and the transverse processes are rearranged similarly. Many of these changes are difficult to visualize with routine radiography, and CT scanning, with or without the administration of contrast agents, or MR imaging is necessary to show the vertebral and neural abnormalities (Fig. 89–7C).[88–91]

Vertebral hypoplasia, hemivertebra, laminar and pediculate fusion, diastematomyelia, and lipoma all may be associated with the myelomeningocele. Congenital abnormalities of the spine also may be present above the level of the neural defect. Although no abnormality of spinal curvature is seen initially in about one third of patients, scoliosis is present at an early age in one half of all patients[74] and in 80 per cent of those more than 10 years of age; kyphosis is present in about one fifth of patients.[92] The scoliotic curvature at the level of the spinal defect frequently is progressive, but scoliosis often develops also well above the level of the neurologic and spinal defects. This has been related to persistent and progressive hydromyelia[93] and frequently is halted by ventricular shunting.[94–96]

The status of the urinary tract should be evaluated at standard intervals with cystography, urography, and ultrasonography. MR imaging may be helpful in symptomatic patients needing surgical revision of the closure area in the spine later in childhood; cord tethering at the site of original repair is seen in more than one half of patients (Fig. 89–7).[89, 91, 97] Aortic hypoplasia with branching anomalies may interfere with anterior surgical intervention.[98]

Anterior sacral meningoceles are rarer than the typical posterior protrusions. They usually are associated with a unilateral, scimitar-like hemisacral osseous defect and a mass protruding through the defect that may be detectable on barium studies of the rectum[68, 69] or on CT scanning. Accompanying gastrointestinal or genitourinary anomalies also are common.

Occult Spinal Dysraphism. Dysraphic changes in systems derived from the primitive germ layers but covered with skin have been termed occult, closed, or covered spinal dysraphism. The basic pathogenic processes are identical to those causing open lesions: failure of midline fusion; duplication (diplomyelia, diastematomyelia); overgrowth of normal tissues (lipoma, dermoid); herniation of one germ layer through another (neurenteric cyst)[99]; and abnormalities due to differences in the growth patterns of neural and skeletal structures or abnormal fixation (tethered cord). Among the numerous solitary or combined lesions that may occur are abnormal or supernumerary nerve roots, dural and arachnoid adhesions, spinal cord angiomas and hamartomas, and failure of differentiation of the conus.[100–102]

Occult dysraphism is twice as common in girls as in boys, whereas open lesions are seen with equal frequency in the two sexes. Approximately one half of these abnormalities have cutaneous markers[103]; additional clinical manifestations include leg length and motor power discrepancy, pes cavus and other foot deformities, gait abnormality, and neurogenic bladder.

Radiologic evaluation generally will reveal structural vertebral defects, although 15 per cent of patients may have no radiographic abnormalities. Neural arch anomalies are common, and more than two levels usually are involved. Interpediculate widening and enlargement of the spinal canal often are present, and the vertebral bodies may be deformed or scalloped. An associated mediastinal mass may be present. MR imaging studies are necessary to delineate the neural defect associated with the structural skeletal abnormalities.[104–106]

The most common occult spinal dysraphic lesions are diastematomyelia, low conus (tethered filum), and congenital intraspinal tumors (lipomas and dermoids).

Diastematomyelia refers to a congenital longitudinal diastasis in the spinal cord, leading to two parts that usually are of unequal size.[107–109] Although an osseous spur may be present between the two parts of the spinal cord, approximately one half of patients with this anomaly have no true septum.[110]

It is doubtful that traction on such a spur, if present, is the cause of the symptoms in diastematomyelia, as the cord reaches its final level in relation to the spine in the first few months of life and symptoms characteristically occur much later.[106] In addition, the septum often is not at the upper end of the split in the cord, and resection of it rarely leads to regression of neurologic manifestations.[111]

Diastematomyelia occurs in 15 per cent of all patients with congenital scoliosis[111, 112] and is two times more common in girls than in boys. Skin changes are noted in about 80 per cent of patients, are similar to those described in other types of occult spinal dysraphism, and do not correspond in distribution to the level of any septum or spur. The latter is most common at the L1 to L4 spinal segment, with an abnormal osseous structure visible in about 75 per cent of cases (Fig. 89–8). CT scanning has revealed that only 50 per cent of spurs are recognized easily on plain

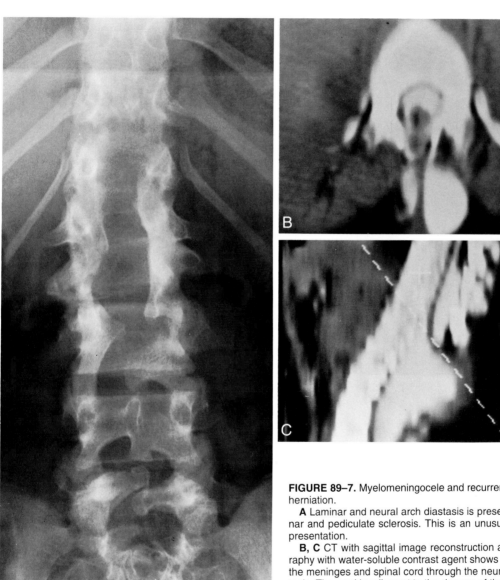

FIGURE 89–7. Myelomeningocele and recurrent meningeal herniation.

A Laminar and neural arch diastasis is present with laminar and pediculate sclerosis. This is an unusual radiologic presentation.

B, C CT with sagittal image reconstruction after myelography with water-soluble contrast agent shows herniation of the meninges and spinal cord through the neural arch diastasis. The cord is adherent to the dorsum of the sac.

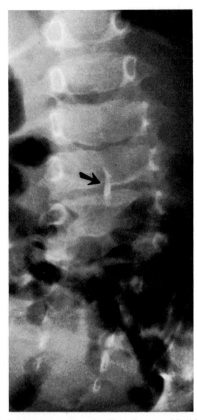

FIGURE 89–8. Diastematomyelia. This 2 year old girl with myelo-meningocele has a well-defined bony spicule projecting over the third lumbar vertebra (arrow). Associated dysraphic changes include widened interpediculate distances, asymmetric development of the lower vertebral bodies, and undeveloped sacral neural arches.

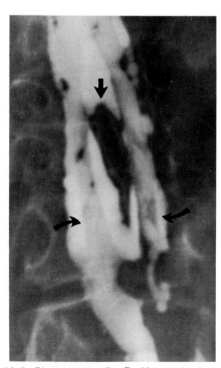

FIGURE 89–9. Diastematomyelia. Positive contrast myelography demonstrates two separate spinal cords (curved lower arrows) and a bony mound in the intramedullary space (upper straight arrow). (From Ozonoff MB: Pediatric Orthopedic Radiology. Philadelphia, WB Saunders Co, 1979.)

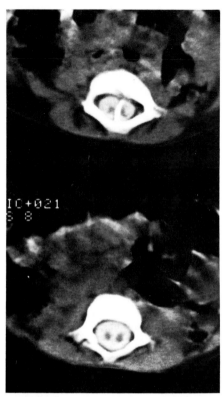

FIGURE 89–10. Diastematomyelia. CT scanning with water-soluble intrathecal contrast material shows the two separate spinal cords and an osseous septum separating them. (Same patient as in Figure 89–8.)

films, but many can be seen in retrospect once their level has been identified with CT scanning.[113, 114] Such scanning also is useful in the identification of moundlike osseous abnormalities and can demonstrate nonosseous septa when intrathecal contrast material is employed. When a bony septum is present, it frequently extends from the neural arch forward, not necessarily being fused anteriorly to the vertebral body. When unilateral laminar fusion is present, the spur extends from the side of fusion.

The most common radiologic finding in diastematomyelia is an intersegmental laminar fusion associated with a defect in the neural arch at the same level or at an adjacent level.[115] An increased interpediculate distance and scoliosis[116] are present in about two thirds of patients.[110] In fewer than 10 per cent of patients, the spine is completely normal.

Myelography alone or combined with CT scanning using positive contrast material or MR imaging[117] will show the perimedullary space surrounding the normal and the divided portions of the spinal cord (Fig. 89–9).[118] Within the intermedullary space lying between the divided cord, a thin fibrous, cartilaginous, or bony septum or a large mound of deformed bone may be found. The length of the divided cord averages five vertebral segments,[116] but it may be as long as 15 vertebrae. Transaxial CT and MR images demonstrate that the two portions of the spinal cord are unequal in size (Fig. 89–10).[114]

Meningoceles, dermoids, neurenteric cysts, or hamartomas may coexist with diastematomyelia.

The low conus (tethered conus, tight filum terminale, cord traction) syndrome is believed by many investigators to represent another manifestation of occult spinal dysraphism.[119] Intraspinal dermoids, lipomas, congenital bands, and myelomeningoceles (Fig. 89–6) all may cause tethering of the conus, but in many cases of such tethering no associated lesions are found.[111, 119] Whether the conus medullaris actually is prevented from accomplishing its normal ascent from a lower lumbar to an upper lumbar level during development owing to adhesions, or whether this low position is a sign of spinal cord maldevelopment, is debated.[100] The conus medullaris is considered abnormally low when it lies below the L2-L3 spinal level at the age of 2 months.[106] Its precise position can be determined with ultrasonography in infants 6 months of age or younger[120] or with MR imaging.[121] The low position of the conus causes the nerve roots to emerge more horizontally than usual. The dural sac usually is increased in volume. The filum terminale may be thickened, often owing to fatty infiltration; a diameter exceeding 2 mm is considered abnormal.[106]

Congenital intraspinal tumors are associated with identical vertebral changes, cutaneous manifestations, and clinical symptoms as other forms of occult spinal dysraphism. Of these congenital tumors, dermoids, and lipomas constitute a large proportion. Lipomas may be intramedullary, intradural, or extradural in location and frequently are associated with open dysraphism in the form of lipomeningocele.[122–125] Characteristic congenital iliac anomalies also may occur.[126, 127] Enterogenous cysts within the spinal canal have been described.[128]

Vertebral scalloping at the level of an intraspinal tumor is frequent.[123] The conus may be low, and extradural abnormalities are seen, consisting of smooth compression or dural adhesions or bands causing plication, with a sharply defined abnormality or an irregular deformity. Cross-sectional imaging studies are particularly useful in the evaluation of an extradural lipoma or lipomeningocele.[88]

SPINAL CURVATURES

Scoliosis (Greek: curvature, crookedness) refers to lateral spinal curvature in the coronal plane. Scoliosis may be caused by congenital architectural imbalance or growth asymmetry; neoplastic, traumatic, or infectious damage; radiation; reflexive splinting due to nerve irritation; bone dysplasias; or asymmetric neuromuscular control.[129] The great majority of cases, however, are of unknown cause (idiopathic scoliosis) and have an onset during childhood rather than being present at birth.

Imaging Techniques in Evaluating Scoliosis

After clinical examination of the patient, including visual analysis of the spinal curvature with the patient standing and bending forward, plain film radiography should be employed. Although moiré screen and other projectional techniques have been used by some investigators, they may not be more helpful than simple visual evaluation.[130] The initial radiologic examination should be a limited one, obtained to confirm the existence of an abnormal spinal curvature, estimate its magnitude and location, and detect any congenital anomalies. The entire spine is examined in the erect position with the patient standing without shoes. If a lateral film is needed to evaluate accompanying kyphosis, it should be obtained with the patient standing with his or her forearms

resting on a stand so that they are completely horizontal, relieving the upper torso of this weight and avoiding a forward or backward lean. Gonadal shielding is used in all patients and, in girls, should cover the lower one half of the pelvic inlet. In very young patients, films accomplished with the patient erect may be misleading as a result of poor balance, and a supine film may be all that can be obtained; in such cases it should be realized that the true curvature will be reduced when the patient is supine.[131]

The cumulative radiation exposure resulting from multiple serial examinations has been predicted to increase the relative risk of the development of breast cancer by 1.35 per cent.[132] Therefore, every attempt should be made to reduce radiation exposure to the lowest level feasible.[133] Dose reduction techniques that include the use of posteroanterior radiographs,[134, 135] lead acrylic filters,[136] high speed screen-film combinations, added filtration in the tube collimator, and breast shielding will lower the thyroid dose to one twentieth of that expected if these techniques were not used; the breast exposure will be reduced even further.[137, 138] Gradient screens also have been employed to reduce radiation exposure and enhance visualization.[139]

Posteroanterior rather than anteroposterior views are recommended for routine use, with the main advantage being reduction of radiation to the breast.[138, 139] Although visualization of the upper endplates of the vertebrae is slightly poorer in kyphotic patients, and edge sharpness is minimally decreased owing to magnification, visualization of the sacroiliac joints is better.[138, 139]

The long film format described earlier does not show specific areas in good detail and, if there is a question of a lesion or congenital anomaly, supine spot films are indicated.[140] If surgery is contemplated or if the need for orthotic (bracing) treatment is not certain, supine bending films may be helpful to determine whether the curve is structural and to what degree it is correctable. The interval chosen between radiographic examinations depends on the age of the child and the degree of spinal curvature. Rapid progression may occur during the adolescent growth spurt, and examinations during this period may need to be spaced more closely. It should be noted that measurement uncertainty in the range of 3 or 4 degrees, compared with a theoretical maximum progression rate of 1 degree per month, suggests that radiography repeated at intervals of less than 3 or 4 months may not be reliable.

Specialized imaging techniques are helpful in certain situations.[141–144] Segmented field radiography has been suggested as a means to eliminate total spine radiation.[145] Digital radiography[146] also will lower radiation exposure but has a greater interobserver error. An axial projection of the flexed spine using tangential radiography is feasible to evaluate neural arch defects in infants,[147] although CT scanning is now the standard. Whereas thermography has shown differential temperature patterns on the two sides of the spine in patients with scoliosis,[148] it is of dubious clinical value. Bone scintigraphy is valuable in confirming the presence of osteoid osteomas, osteoblastomas, or other irritative foci[149]; it also is helpful for detecting pseudarthroses after surgery.[150]

MR imaging and ultrasonography represent additional techniques that may be employed.[103, 120, 151–155] Specifically, ultrasonography can evaluate the contents of the spinal canal in normal infants under 6 months of age and in older children if there is an open neural arch or previous laminectomy.[103, 120, 151, 152] Fetal ultrasonography likewise may reveal congenital anomalies of the spine.[153]

Myelography is not indicated in patients with idiopathic scoliosis; its role in the evaluation of congenital scoliosis was always somewhat controversial[6, 111, 156], and it has been supplanted by MR imaging. Although MR imaging is of undoubted value in the evaluation of congenital scoliosis, its utilization in the workup of idiopathic scoliosis is controversial. MR imaging has found a high incidence of abnormality in patients with pain, weakness, and abnormal neurologic findings and a remarkable association of otherwise idiopathic left thoracic and thoracolumbar curves with hydrosyringomyelia.[157]

Maturity may be estimated roughly from the degree of development of the iliac crest apophyses.[158] If a more reliable evaluation of maturity is needed, bone age analysis of the hand and wrist is indicated. Although disparity in maturity is known to occur between different body parts, the magnitude of difference probably is not clinically significant.

Evaluation of the genitourinary tract in patients with congenital scoliosis is indicated. This can be accomplished by screening ultrasonography followed by intravenous urography when indicated.

Radiologic Analysis of Scoliosis

On a frontal radiograph, the normal child's spine is straight, without curvature in the coronal plane. On a lateral radiograph, the newborn infant has a relatively straight spine but develops thoracic kyphosis and lumbar lordosis as he or she adopts an erect position. The median T5 to T12 thoracic kyphosis in normal older children is 27 degrees (ninetieth percentile, 40 degrees). The median L1 to L5 lumbar lordosis is normally 40 degrees (ninetieth percentile, 54 degrees).[159] It should be noted that the lumbar lordosis is measured between L1 and L5, not to the superior surface of the sacrum. Because the angle between the lower border of L5 and the upper border of S1 varies from 5 to 21 degrees, an increase in apparent lumbar lordosis would occur if measurements were calculated from the top of the sacrum.

According to the standardized terminology adopted by the Scoliosis Research Society,[112, 160] the scoliotic curvature should be identified as nonstructural (flexible, with correction to linear alignment with lateral bending) or structural (curvature not completely corrected with lateral bending), with associated architectural asymmetry common. Although attempts to label the spinal curvatures as primary or secondary usually are speculative, the curvature above or below the level of the major structural curve usually is considered to be compensatory, allowing the patient's head to be returned to its usual relationship over the midline of the sacrum. These compensatory curves generally are nonstructural and will be corrected with lateral bending, although, when present for a long period of time, a permanent structural alteration related to asymmetric growth may develop.

The first task in the radiologic analysis of scoliosis is the identification of the vertebrae at either end of the curvature (the end vertebrae). The most laterally displaced and rotated vertebra is designated the apical vertebra and will be located between these two terminal vertebrae. The degree of

rotation and displacement from the midline of the vertebrae above and below the apical vertebra will diminish progressively until the end vertebrae are reached, at which point the spine will straighten or a second curve in the opposite direction will be detected. The intervertebral disc adjacent to each end vertebra will be maximally wedged. The psoas margin on the concave side of a lumbar curve often is absent.[161]

The curvature is measured by constructing lines along the superior endplate of the highest vertebra and along the inferior endplate of the lowest vertebra (Fig. 89–11). If these landmarks are indistinct, the tops or bottoms of the pedicles can be used as alternative selections. In the case of mild or moderate curvatures, lines drawn perpendicular to these endplate lines will ease the task of measuring the angle of scoliosis. This method (Cobb's method) often will give a misleadingly high value for the degree of scoliosis owing to the presence of wedging of the end vertebrae.[162, 163] The Cobb method also may miscalculate the degree of correction after treatment. Despite these and other drawbacks,[164–167] this method is the standard means of description; an alternative technique described by Ferguson (in which lines connecting the centers of the end and apical vertebrae are measured) is no longer recommended for the analysis of scoliosis.

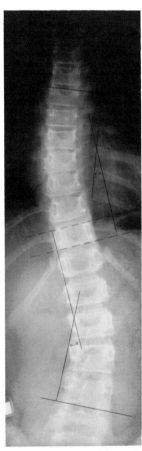

FIGURE 89–11. Measurement of idiopathic scoliosis (Cobb method). This 10 year old girl has a T4-T11 right spinal curvature of 20 degrees and a T11-L4 left scoliosis of 27 degrees. Note that T11 is included in both curve measurements. Minimal rotation occurs in the thoracic region and essentially none in the lumbar segment. (From Ozonoff MB: Pediatric Orthopedic Radiology. 2nd ed. Philadelphia, WB Saunders Co., 1992.)

A slight discrepancy (of approximately 2 degrees) occurs in measurements of scoliotic curves derived from postero-anterior radiographs and those derived from anteroposterior radiographs,[138, 139] with the degree of curvature being somewhat greater in the former situation.[138] This difference in measurement has very little influence on the clinical evaluation of the patient. Furthermore, variability in the measured degree of curvature occurs as an intraobserver error when such measurements are derived without comparison to previous examinations. Differences in the measurements of spinal curvature in the range of 4 degrees occur when several observers measure the same film.[168–170] Measurement error is increased when digital radiography is employed, owing to the small size of the image.[146]

Rotation of the spine is greatest at the level of the apical vertebra but is quite variable from one patient to another. Scoliotic curves of the same magnitude in two patients may appear to have different degrees of vertebral rotation. In general, curves of less than 40 degrees are more rotated proportionately than larger ones.[162, 171] Although it formerly was believed that spinal rotation always was toward the convexity and limited to the extent of curvature, this pattern actually is found in less than a majority of cases.[172] Such rotation extends past the limits of the curvature in 22 per cent of patients and may occur in some patients in the absence of scoliosis.

Normally, pedicles are placed symmetrically with respect to the vertebral edges; when spinal rotation occurs, the pedicle will move inward from the edge of the body; the degree of rotation can be calculated by various methods.[173–175] Vertebral rotation also can be analyzed by sonography[176] or CT scanning and seems to correlate with the magnitude of the curvature but not with its length or position. Computer analysis also can be used to define the degree of spinal curvature on the routine radiographs.[177, 178]

Kyphosis and lordosis are measured in the same manner by constructing lines along the vertebral endplates on the lateral radiograph. In severe scoliosis, the normal patterns of kyphosis and lordosis are diminished and the lateral profile of the spine is straightened.[179]

Evaluation of the skeletal maturity is a helpful clinical tool as most mild or moderate spinal curvatures will no longer progress after the cessation of growth. Exceptions to this rule occur, and many severe spinal curvatures will increase throughout the life of the patient.[180] Skeletal maturity can be determined by analysis of the development of the apophysis of the iliac crest. Risser[181] reported that most curves will not increase after the appearance of complete ossification of the iliac apophysis (which occurs at an average age of 15 years 3 months in girls and about 6 months later in boys).[182, 183] The validity of this observation has been questioned, and, in some patients, complete fusion of the iliac apophysis rather than its total ossification seems to correlate better with cessation of progression of the spinal curvature. In cases in which the exact definition of skeletal maturity is required, it is best to obtain a bone age by standard methods.

Congenital Scoliosis

Scoliosis initiated and perpetuated by a congenital anomaly of the spine is termed congenital scoliosis. The spinal angulation is caused by both an architectural imbalance and the presence of differing growth potentials in the two sides of the spine.[6, 184] Congenital scoliosis may be caused by failure of formation (wedge vertebra or hemivertebra), partial duplication (supernumerary hemivertebra), failure of segmentation (unilateral block vertebra, pediculate bar, neural arch fusion), or a combination of these lesions.[6, 185–188] Several different abnormalities may exist in the same portion of the spine, or anomalies may be present at different spinal levels. The thoracolumbar region is affected most commonly.[184]

Progression of congenital scoliosis is seen in about 75 per cent of patients, the poorest prognosis occurring in the association of a unilateral bar and a contralateral hemivertebra; the abnormal growth potential caused by the hemivertebra and the tethering effect of the bar will act in concert to cause progressive spinal angulation. Associated rib abnormalities are common, although synostosis of ribs that occurs at a distance from the spine does not contribute significantly to the progression of a scoliotic curve.

The radiologic evaluation of congenital scoliosis should include erect radiographs of the entire spine and detailed supine spot and oblique radiographs of any area of abnormality detected during initial workup. In the young child, an axial projection occasionally can be obtained by flexing the spine and angling the beam in a tangential fashion; the normal neural arch cleft has been reported to curve medially, but it will curve laterally in dysraphic states.[147] Conventional tomography or CT is especially helpful in detecting laminar fusion and in defining abnormalities when anomalies of both the centrum and the neural arch are present (Fig. 89–1).

Ultrasonography of the intraspinal contents in congenital scoliosis and dysraphism is feasible prenatally,[153, 189] in the young infant, and in those infants with large osseous defects.[103, 152, 153] MR imaging demonstrates well the status of the neural contents of the spine and probably is indicated if surgery is contemplated.[190, 191] CT scanning, with or without myelography,[97, 192–197] is indicated when simpler measures fail to reveal the information needed for surgical revision of osseous structures.

Examination of the genitourinary tract is indicated in all patients with congenital anomalies of the spine.[65, 198–200] Investigations have shown that associated genitourinary tract abnormalities, especially unilateral renal agenesis, horseshoe kidneys, and renal duplications and ectopia, are frequent and unrelated to the level, side, or severity of the spinal changes. Other abnormalities associated with congenital scoliosis include congenital heart disease, undescended scapulae, and thumb anomalies.

Patients with congenital scoliosis should be followed carefully for evidence of progression of the spinal curvature.[185–187, 201] Surgical fusion should be reserved for those situations in which an unacceptable degree of curvature is predicted; it should be delayed as long as possible and restricted to the smallest area of the spine that is feasible to effect the desired result. As any segment of the spine that is fused will not grow further, extensive fusion in a young child will result in a markedly reduced spinal length. In the thoracic spine, this may result in unacceptable growth restriction and respiratory problems.

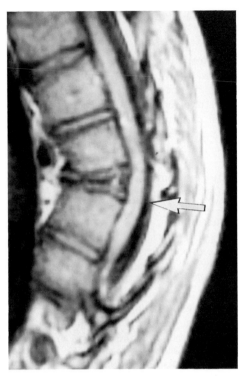

FIGURE 89–12. Congenital kyphosis associated with a posterior hemivertebra in a 15 year old girl. A sagittal T1-weighted (TR/TE, 550/20) spin echo MR image demonstrates the spinal cord (arrow) to be displaced anteriorly, curving around the point of kyphosis. (From Ozonoff MB: Pediatric Orthopedic Radiology. 2nd ed. Philadelphia, WB Saunders Co., 1992.)

Congenital Kyphosis and Lordosis

Congenital lordosis is uncommon and usually is limited to the thoracic region, where growth inhibition will lead to a severe restrictive thoracic dysplasia. The lordosis is caused by fusion of the posterior neural elements and continued anterior vertebral growth. Synostosis of the posterior portion of the ribs also may add to the growth inhibition and is a common finding in the hyperlordosis of spondylocostal and spondylothoracic dysplasia.[202] Congenital lordosis and hyperextension also have been reported as a rare finding secondary to intrauterine positional deformations.[203]

Congenital kyphosis is much more frequent than congenital lordosis and is related to agenesis or underdevelopment of the anterior portion of the vertebral centrum, resulting in a posterior hemivertebra (Fig. 89–12); less commonly, it is related to failure of segmentation anteriorly with a congenital bar formed between the vertebral bodies (Fig. 89–13).[6, 204] (This congenital situation must be distinguished from a developmental anterior fusion, which takes place in childhood, termed progressive noninfectious anterior vertebral body fusion. This fusion eventually will resemble a congenital bar[205] [Fig. 89–14].) As with congenital scoliosis, genitourinary abnormalities are common. Some patients with congenital kyphosis also will have Klippel-Feil fusional anomalies in the cervical spine. Congenital kyphosis is common in myelomeningocele, diastrophic dwarfism, and certain other dysplasias.[206, 207]

The thoracolumbar spine is the area that is involved most typically. The vertebral body may be deficient laterally as well as anteriorly, and associated scoliosis may be evident.

Anterior subluxation of the spine above the level of the anomaly may lead to displacement of the hypoplastic vertebral body into the neural canal,[208] causing thecal deformity (Fig. 89–12). Paraplegia is a potential complication both before and during surgery.[209]

Idiopathic Scoliosis

The frequency of idiopathic scoliosis in the normal population depends on the magnitude of the curvature being described. Kane[210] estimated that scoliosis equal to or greater than 10 degrees was present in 25 of 1000 persons and scoliosis greater than 20 degrees was present in 5 of 1000 persons; another study described a scoliosis of more than 10 degrees in 2 to 3 per cent of adolescents.[211] The frequency of scoliosis of more than 25 degrees has been documented as 1.5 per 1000 persons in the United States, 4 per 1000 persons in the United Kingdom, and 3 per 1000 persons in Sweden. DeSmet[112] has reviewed the prevalence, progression, sex distribution, and pattern of idiopathic scoliosis.

Mandatory visual screening of school populations has been instituted in many areas of the world.[212] One clinical study[213] showed a 13.6 per cent prevalence of scoliosis in seventh and eighth grade students, but another showed that only 3 per cent of children required follow-up radiographic analysis, and only 1 per cent of such children had scoliosis of greater than 5 degrees.[214] On the basis of the foregoing facts, the economic and radiation costs of school screening, with detection of many small nonsignificant curves ("schooliosis")[211, 215] have been subjected to serious scru-

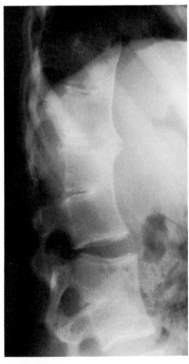

FIGURE 89–13. Congenital kyphosis secondary to anterior vertebral nonsegmentation. The congenital fusion is incomplete, with rudimentary posterior discs evident at several levels. Increased motion at the complete disc spaces has caused hypertrophic bone formation. (From Theros EG, Harris JH Jr [Eds]: American College of Radiology Bone Syllabus IV. Chicago, American College of Radiology, 1989.)

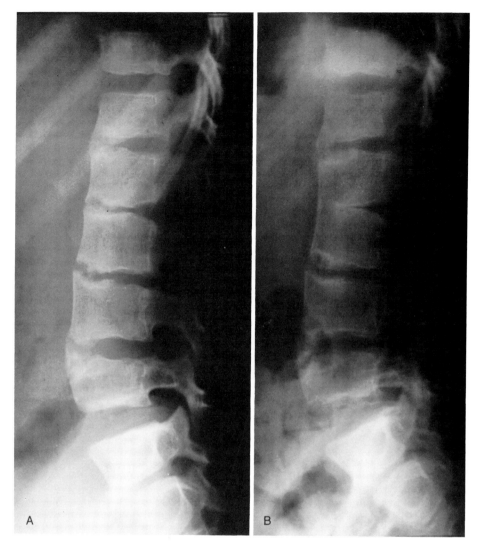

FIGURE 89–14. Progressive noninfectious anterior vertebral body fusion syndrome simulating anterior bar formation.

A At the age of 6 years, anterior disc narrowing with localized endplate irregularity has occurred.

B Two years later, fusion has occurred at L1-L2.

(From Ozonoff MB: Pediatric Orthopedic Radiology. 2nd ed. Philadelphia, WB Saunders Co., 1992.)

tiny, as the value of such studies in predicting progressive curvature is limited.[216–219]

The demography and epidemiology of idiopathic scoliosis are variable.[220] One half of patients with idiopathic scoliosis in Europe are first seen at an age younger than 8 years, whereas only 8 per cent of similar cases in the United States are detected by that age. Scoliosis seems to be more common in taller and heavier persons[221, 222] and in those with decreased skeletal maturation. Adolescent scoliosis is four to eight times more common in girls than in boys, but there is evidence that its frequency in the two sexes is more nearly equal at younger ages; for unknown reasons, the spinal curvatures in girls are more progressive and clinically significant.

Idiopathic scoliosis is evident in as many as 16 per cent of patients with congenital heart disease.[223–225] It also is more common in patients with Scheuermann's deformity,[226] spondylolisthesis,[227] and amelic or phocomelic states[228, 229] and in a large number of other syndromes and mesenchymal disorders.[230–232]

The ability to predict which curves will progress and which will regress or remain stable obviously is of great clinical importance. The reported frequency of progression of the spinal curvature has varied from 5 per cent to 79 per cent.[233, 234] Sixty per cent of curvatures in rapidly growing prepubertal children will progress[234, 235]; 10 to 22 per cent of curves will improve, especially those that initially are less than 15 degrees in older children. Curvatures less than 30 degrees generally will not progress after the child is mature, but severe curvatures (50 to 75 degrees) will continue to increase at the rate of about 1 degree per year in adults. Marked tilting and lateral subluxation of vertebral bodies occur in older patients with severe idiopathic scoliosis[236] (Fig. 89–15). This situation must be differentiated from the scoliosis of elderly patients due to degenerative disc disease and facet disease not related to idiopathic adolescent disease: 70 per cent of older patients (50 to 84 years) have been reported to have scoliosis, with 30 per cent having curvatures of more than 10 degrees.[237, 238] The frequency of low back pain in these older patients was the same as that in the general population, even though lateral subluxation and degenerative changes were frequent.[239] Cardiorespiratory function definitely is decreased in those with scoliosis of greater than 65 degrees, however.

Investigations of neurologic and endocrine status, labyrinthine sensitivity, postural equilibrium reactions, muscular fiber properties, and growth rates and patterns in various portions of the spine[240] have been performed, but the cause

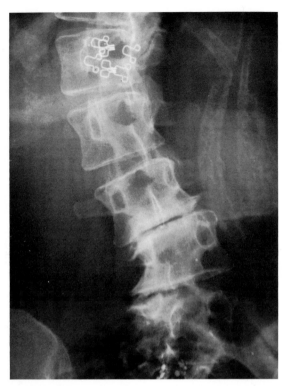

FIGURE 89–15. Idiopathic adolescent scoliosis. The residual effect of this condition is shown in a 43 year old woman. Disc space narrowing, osteophyte formation, vertebral sclerosis, and lateral vertebral subluxation are present.

or causes of idiopathic scoliosis remain elusive.[241] One third of first-degree relatives of patients with idiopathic scoliosis have spinal curvatures of 10 degrees or greater. If both parents have idiopathic scoliosis, the possibility of its occurrence in their children is increased by a factor of 50. Although there is some evidence for a dominant, X-linked inheritance pattern with incomplete penetrance and variable expressivity,[241] most studies tend to favor a multifactorial inheritance pattern.[242, 243]

Clinical Patterns. Idiopathic scoliosis has been divided into three groups (infantile, juvenile, adolescent) on the basis of age of the patient at the time the condition is recognized.

Infantile scoliosis is detected before the age of 4 years.[244–248] It has a striking geographic distribution; for example, it is more common in the United Kingdom and rare in the United States. Resolution of the spinal curvature occurs in 74 per cent of cases of infantile scoliosis; scoliotic curves that are greater than 50 degrees are the ones that usually progress. Associated plagiocephaly has been noted in 86 per cent of affected infants, with the skull depression invariably located on the convex side of the curve. As the cranial flattening and the scoliosis both develop in the first 6 months of life and rarely are present at birth, both deformities are believed to result from plastic deformation of bone in infants who were wrapped tightly and placed obliquely supine in their cribs. With the increased use of prone positioning for these children, the frequency of infantile scoliosis has diminished markedly.[249]

Juvenile scoliosis is that which is recognized between the ages of 4 and 10 years.[250] About 13 per cent of all cases of scoliosis are discovered in this age period, but, because many of the abnormal curvatures found later in life had their inception at a young age, the establishment of juvenile scoliosis as a separate category is of doubtful validity.[251] In distinction to adolescent scoliosis, boys are affected predominantly when the diagnosis is established prior to the age of 6 years; between the ages of 7 and 10 years, girls are affected principally.[250] Juvenile scoliosis almost invariably progresses with growth.

Adolescent scoliosis is detected between the ages of 10 years and the time of skeletal maturity and is by far the most common type of idiopathic scoliosis in the United States. The ratio of affected girls to boys ranges between 4 to 1 and 8 to 1.

Evolution and Treatment of Idiopathic Scoliosis. As a general rule, spinal curvatures of less than 25 degrees are not treated actively unless they occur in preadolescent children and show evidence of rapid progression. With more severe curvature, thoracolumbar orthotic braces are used with pressure pads placed over those ribs leading to the apical vertebrae.[235] High thoracic curves occasionally require the use of a brace with supports extending into the cervical area.

The purpose of bracing is to restrict the degree of spinal curvature to that which was encountered when treatment was instituted. The braces are removed when spinal growth has been completed. Electrical stimulation of the muscles on the convex side of the scoliotic curve in an attempt to cause spinal straightening has been the subject of much interest, with conflicting results. One study has shown reduction or stabilization of the curvature in 85 per cent of patients,[251, 252] but other investigations have had much less favorable results.

Surgical treatment is based on the induction of an osseous spinal fusion achieved with implanted bone graft after excisional decortication and facet fusion. Hardware implants are used to stabilize the fusion length until a mature continuous fusion has occurred. These instruments vary from two point distraction (Harrington rods and hooks) to segmental corrections with a variety of rods, hooks, sublaminar wires, and cross-links (Luque, Cotrel-Dubousset, Texas Scottish Rite Hospital, Wisconsin, Dwyer, Isola, and other systems).[253–265]

Complications of spinal fusion include breakage of wires or rods, loosening and migration of hooks,[266] spondylolysis,[267] pseudarthrosis, bronchial compression by the fusion mass,[268] dislocation above the fusion site after trauma to the long lever arm of the ankylosed spine,[269] gastric volvulus, aortic aneurysm, and retroperitoneal fibrosis. Superior mesenteric artery compression can be caused by either the straightening of the spine after surgery[270] or the pressure of a cast.[271–273] Rod breakage cannot occur without spinal motion, and the presence of metal failure indicates a pseudarthrosis,[274] although an actual fracture line may not be evident on routine radiographs and the break may subsequently have healed; only 68 per cent of confirmed pseudarthroses were visible on routine radiography[275] (Fig. 89–16). Oblique radiologic projections may define an abnormal radiolucent line clearly at the site of fusion, often with sclerosis or spurring of the osseous edges[276] (Fig. 89–17). Small gaps in bone continuity and poorly defined radiolucent areas are common in the fusion mass during the healing process and may make the diagnosis of a pseudarthrosis difficult. In such cases, bone scintigraphy is useful,[277, 278]

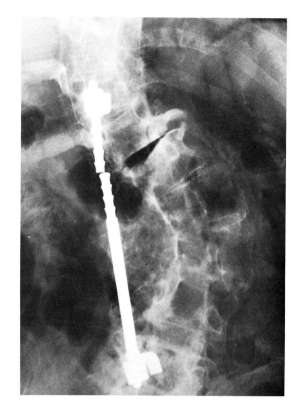

FIGURE 89–16. Broken Harrington rod after spinal fusion. Gas is present in the T12-L1 intervertebral disc with lateral subluxation, osteophytosis, and bone sclerosis. Although no pseudarthrosis is evident on this film, the presence of the broken rod and evidence of vertebral motion indicate that a zone of incomplete fusion or pseudarthrosis must be present.

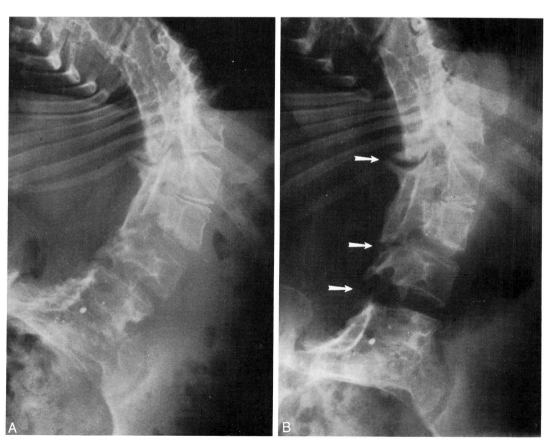

FIGURE 89–17. Congenital scoliosis with previous surgical fusion.
   A Osteophytes and a radiolucent cleft across the fusion mass are seen at T12-L1, and the fusion is incomplete at L3-L4.
   B Traction demonstrates right-sided diastasis at multiple levels (arrows).

demonstrating a localized region of increased radionuclide activity in the area of abnormal motion and bone formation. Owing to the accumulation of the radiopharmaceutical agent that normally may occur in the first 6 months after spinal surgery, scintigraphic abnormalities are easier to detect 1 year or more after the surgical procedure.[150]

Neuromuscular Scoliosis

Asymmetric innervation or unbalanced muscular function may lead to scoliosis.[279] Gravitational forces also may cause or worsen spinal curvature when muscle power is diminished. The typical neuromuscular curvature is a long, C-shaped scoliosis extending from the upper thoracic region to the pelvis. Pelvic obliquity is characteristic. In some instances, however, neuromuscular scoliosis may be indistinguishable from idiopathic scoliosis.

Cerebral palsy is the most common cause of neuromuscular scoliosis.[280–283] Scoliosis is more common and marked in those patients with severe neurologic disability and is uncommon in the presence of mild dysfunction. Spinal curvature is most frequent in patients with spastic quadriplegia, may be severe, and is closely correlated with mental and motor retardation, especially lack of ambulation.[284, 285] Pelvic obliquity and hip dislocation are other typical features in patients with spastic quadriplegia (Fig. 89–18).

Scoliosis is common in diseases of the spinal cord. It is seen in as many as 70 per cent of patients with syringomyelia[94] and may occur before neurologic symptoms have developed.[286] MR imaging will assist in the differentiation of syringomyelia and spinal cord tumors, which also may lead to scoliosis.[286–293]

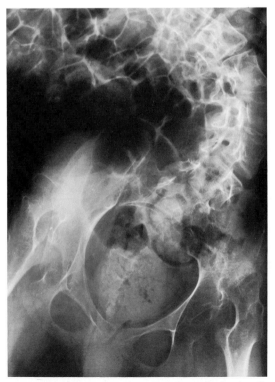

FIGURE 89–18. Neuromuscular scoliosis in cerebral palsy. Severe left lumbar scoliosis with marked rotation is present. The pelvis is oblique, with bilateral hip dislocations. (From Theros EG, Harris JH Jr [Eds]: American College of Radiology Bone Syllabus IV. Chicago, American College of Radiology, 1989.)

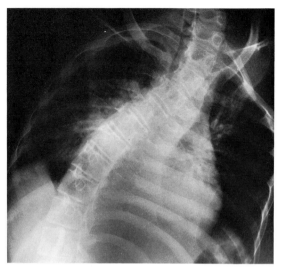

FIGURE 89–19. Scoliosis in Duchenne muscular dystrophy. Cardiomegaly and pulmonary vascular congestion also are present.

Abnormal curvatures occurring after traumatic paraplegia or quadriplegia also are common.[294, 295] If the injury occurs before the adolescent growth spurt, over 90 per cent of patients will have progressive scoliosis and two thirds will have abnormal kyphosis.[296] An injury occurring after this age is less likely to lead to scoliosis, although kyphosis is common after laminectomy.[297] All quadriplegic patients who have been injured prior to 14 years of age may be expected to develop scoliosis, kyphoscoliosis, or lordoscoliosis.[298]

Scoliosis developing after poliomyelitis is no longer a common occurrence[299]; the paralysis seems to trigger the scoliosis but does not in itself cause a pattern correlated with muscle asymmetry.[300] In spinal muscular atrophy, scoliosis occurs in more than 60 per cent of patients and usually develops between the ages of 3 and 6 years.[301, 302] Spinal curvature also is common in many other neurologic conditions. It is seen in as many as 80 per cent of patients with Friedreich's ataxia and actually may involve almost all patients who live long enough.[303] The curvature progresses after maturity and is not correlated with muscular weakness.[304, 305] Pelvic obliquity usually is not present. Scoliosis also has been described in epilepsia partialis continua[306] and torsional dystonia[307] and is frequent in familial dysautonomia, hypertrophic interstitial polyneuritis, and peroneal muscular atrophy.

Scoliosis is of variable onset and severity in different types of muscular dystrophy.[308] In the Duchenne type,[309, 310] scoliosis usually does not develop until the child is older than 10 years and confined to a wheelchair.[311, 312] Sixty to 95 per cent of such patients develop scoliosis, often after asymmetric hip contracture with pelvic obliquity; the curvature is aggravated by gravity in these very weak persons.[313, 314] The terminal event in many of these patients is cardiomyopathy and circulatory failure (Fig. 89–19).

Scoliosis Associated with or Secondary to Other Conditions

Although most cases of scoliosis are idiopathic, others occur as part of many different syndromes or are associated

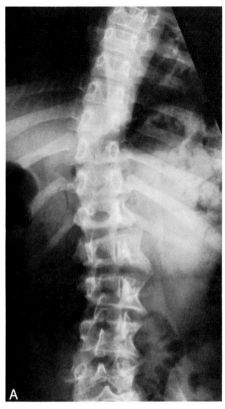
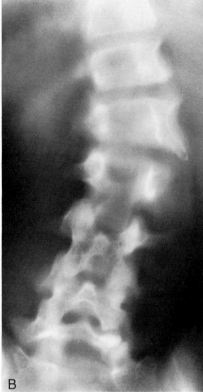
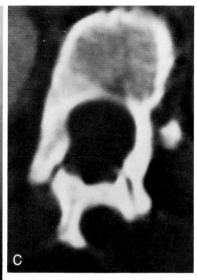

FIGURE 89–20. Neurofibromatosis.

  A Scoliosis is associated with asymmetric development of the lumbar vertebral bodies, lateral vertebral scalloping, and coarse trabeculae.

  B Planar tomography demonstrates vertebral body and pediculate dysplasia and sclerosis.

  C Pediculate sclerosis and elongation are confirmed with CT scanning.

with systemic disease, regional irritative foci, or fibromuscular change adjacent to or remote from the spine.

Abnormalities of spinal curvature may be associated with pathologic changes in osseous and collagen structure. In idiopathic juvenile osteoporosis, progressive scoliosis and kyphosis are difficult to treat surgically prior to adolescence, owing to osseous weakening and progressive bending of the fusion mass.[315, 316] Similar therapeutic failures have been observed in osteogenesis imperfecta.[317]

The scoliosis of neurofibromatosis[318–320] classically has been described as one with sharp angulation and associated kyphosis but, in reality, many abnormal spinal curvatures in this disease resemble those of idiopathic scoliosis. When abrupt angulation of the spine, kyphosis, and adjacent rib dysplasia are evident, however, the radiologic diagnosis of neurofibromatosis is ensured. Associated findings may include a paravertebral soft tissue mass, deformed transverse processes, enlarged vertebral foramina, marked rotation of the spinal curvature, and a coarsened and sclerotic trabecular pattern[321–327] (Fig. 89–20). MR imaging studies will delineate abnormal neural elements, often in the form of extensive plexiform paravertebral masses, not recognizable on routine radiography or CT scanning.[328–331]

Tumors in the vertebrae or adjacent ribs may be associated with scoliosis, presumably on an irritative basis.[332] In this situation, osteoid osteomas or osteoblastomas[333–343] generally are located on the concave side of the spinal curvature at its apex (Fig. 89–21). These curvatures generally are nonstructural in type but will become structural if present during a prolonged period of growth.[333–336] Intense uptake of bone-seeking radionuclide agents occurs in these tumors.[344]

Scoliosis occurring after a fracture of the transverse process of the vertebra is convex to the side of the injury, rather than concave to this side, as it would be if it were due to splinting and irritation. It is believed to result from ineffective quadratus lumborum function.[345]

Scoliosis is seen in about 10 per cent of patients with intraspinal tumors.[346] In over 50 per cent of such cases, radiologic changes are seen in the pedicles, spinal canal, or paravertebral area.[292]

The spinal curvature that results from significant leg length discrepancy[347, 348] is convex to the side of the shorter leg, characteristically involves the lumbar or thoracolumbar region, and is a functional rather than a structural scoliosis. In time, however, the curvature may become structural through long-term contractural changes or growth,[348] and some asymmetry of lateral flexion of the spine may remain after leg length equalization.[347] Scoliosis with sacral tilt also may be due to pelvic asymmetry rather than leg length discrepancy and will not progress.[212]

Scoliosis may be caused by adjacent soft tissue changes. Although rare, it may occur in retroperitoneal fibrosis, either idiopathic or secondary to trauma,[349] and it has been reported after thoracotomy or empyema[350–352] and congenital pulmonary aplasia.[353]

Radiation therapy employed in the treatment of malignant tumors of the kidney, thorax, or retroperitoneum will cause both clinical and radiologic spinal deformity.[112, 351, 354–358] Although the abnormal curvature is most severe when only a portion of the spine is included in the radiation field, it nevertheless can result even when the entire spine is irradiated. Scoliosis has been reported in 70 per cent of patients receiving radiation therapy and chemotherapy for

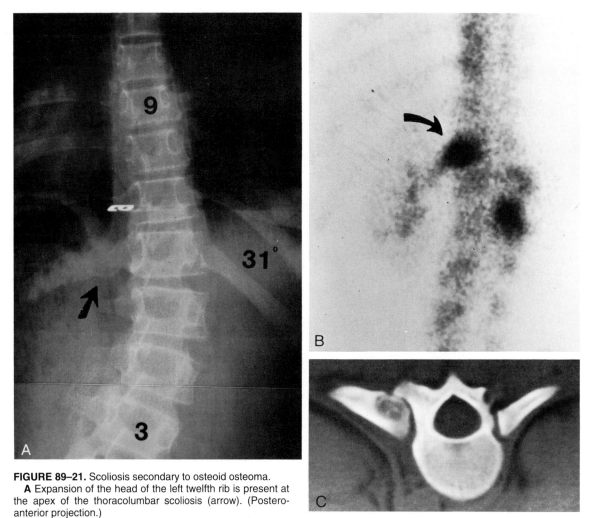

FIGURE 89–21. Scoliosis secondary to osteoid osteoma.
A Expansion of the head of the left twelfth rib is present at the apex of the thoracolumbar scoliosis (arrow). (Postero-anterior projection.)
B A technetium bone scan shows intense uptake of the radionuclide in the left twelfth rib (arrow).
C CT scanning demonstrates expansion and sclerosis of the proximal portion of the left twelfth rib. A central nidus is present. (The orientation of the CT scan has been reversed to correspond with that of the other images.)

Wilms' tumor and in 76 per cent of 5 year survivors after treatment for neuroblastoma.[354] The spinal changes are most marked with radiation levels over 3000 cGy (rad), and the curvature is accentuated if there has been a laminectomy or if the patient is paraplegic.[354]

The abnormalities after radiation therapy are caused by damage to blood vessels and soft tissues adjacent to the spine as well as to osteocytes, chondroblasts, and vascular structures in bone; the resulting damage not only is immediate but also affects future skeletal growth. Growth recovery lines may produce a bone-within-bone appearance. Unilateral vertebral body wedging caused by asymmetric growth on the two sides of the spine is common, as are vertebral contour irregularities and anterior vertebral wedging (Fig. 89–22). Decreased axial growth also may be expected, both in the spine and in adjacent irradiated structures, such as the ilia. Osteochondromas occasionally may develop within the radiation field.[359–361]

Scoliosis is common with upper limb deficiency, with an overall prevalence of 16 per cent. All patients with bilateral upper limb amelia would be predicted to develop scoliosis, with less frequent involvement in children with unilateral amelia or those with radial or ulnar hemimelia or phoco-melia.[228, 229, 362] Scoliosis has been reported in cystic fibrosis[363] and in Scheuermann's deformity.[226, 364]

Scoliosis in Bone Dysplasias and Generalized Syndromes

Scoliosis (or kyphosis) is a common feature of many bone dysplasias and syndromes.[207, 365, 366] A specific diagnosis may not be possible on the basis of spinal deformity alone, although structural features in the individual vertebrae occasionally are distinctive. This is especially true in achondroplasia, in which the abnormal growth patterns lead to pediculate shortening and premature fusion of the neurocentral synchondroses.[367] The spinal canal thus is reduced in size, and the stenosis may be exacerbated by laminar thickening and bulging of the intervertebral discs.[368–370] Thoracolumbar vertebral wedging and kyphosis are seen in 30 per cent of older patients with achondroplasia[371] and may be accentuated in infants who are carried with the spine in persistent flexion.[372]

Scoliosis also is seen in spondyloepiphyseal dysplasia congenita, spondylometaphyseal dysplasia,[373] diastrophic dwarfism, metatropic dwarfism, chondrodysplasia punctata,

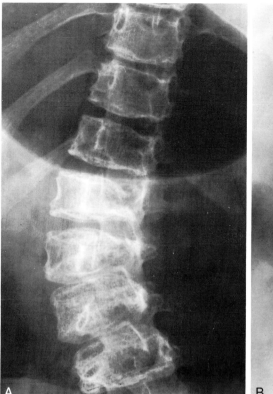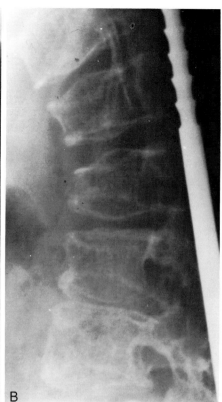

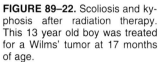
FIGURE 89–22. Scoliosis and kyphosis after radiation therapy. This 13 year old boy was treated for a Wilms' tumor at 17 months of age.

A Abnormal bone formation and asymmetric growth have produced vertebral body wedging and a coarsened trabecular pattern.

B Also note the inhibited anterior vertebral growth with resultant kyphosis.

(From Theros EG, Harris JH Jr [Eds]: American College of Radiology Bone Syllabus IV. Chicago, American College of Radiology, 1989.)

and the mucopolysaccharidoses.[206, 207] The scoliosis in diastrophic dwarfism is rapidly progressive, and the spine soon becomes rigid and severely rotated.[206] In spondylocostal and spondylothoracic dysplasias,[374–376] multiple congenital anomalies of the spine are present, including block vertebrae, hemivertebrae, neural arch clefts, atlantoaxial hypoplasia, and craniovertebral anomalies. Rib fusions, bifurcations, and variations in size and thickness are evident.[202]

In arthrogryposis, the frequency of scoliosis is about 30 per cent.[377] In the rigid spine syndrome, restricted spinal flexion and extension are associated with diminished muscle bulk and power[378]; some affected patients will develop scoliosis.[379] Scoliosis also is a component of many rare syndromes and constitutional disorders,[365] including maple syrup urine disease,[380] cerebral gigantism, spondyloepiphyseal dysplasia tarda,[381] and the Laurence-Moon-Biedl, Larsen, Melnick-Needles,[382] Fragile X,[383] Marfan,[384] Ehlers-Danlos, Cornelia deLange, and Down syndromes. Almost all patients with the Prader-Willi syndrome[385, 386] will develop scoliosis, most with structural curves greater than 10 degrees.[385, 387]

SUMMARY

A great variety of congenital and developmental anomalies may become evident in the spine, and causes and patterns of abnormal spinal curvature also are varied. Accurate diagnosis of these alterations relies on careful clinical evaluation supplemented with imaging examinations that include routine radiography, conventional tomography, CT scanning, ultrasonography, and MR imaging.

References

1. Cohen J, Currarino G, Neuhauser EBD: A significant variant in the ossification centers of the vertebral bodies. AJR 76:469, 1956.
2. Wollin DG, Elliott MB: Coronal cleft vertebrae and persistent notochordal derivatives of infancy. J Can Assoc Radiol 12:78, 1961.
3. Beals RK, Rolfe B: VATER association: A unifying concept of multiple anomalies. J Bone Joint Surg [Am] 71:948, 1989.
4. Lawhon SM, MacEwen GD, Bunnell WP: Orthopaedic aspects of the VATER association. J Bone Joint Surg [Am] 68:424, 1986.
5. Weaver DD, Mapstone CL, Yu P: The VATER association: Analysis of 46 patients. Am J Dis Child 140:225, 1986.
6. Winter RB, Lonstein JE, Leonard AS, et al: Congenital Deformities of the Spine. New York, Thieme-Stratton Inc. 1983.
7. Brown MW, Templeton AW, Hodges FJ III: The incidence of acquired and congenital fusions in the cervical spine. AJR 92:1255, 1964.
8. Cowell MJ, Cowell HR: The incidence of spina bifida occulta in idiopathic scoliosis. Clin Orthop 118:116, 1976.
9. Sutow WW, Pryde AW: Incidence of spina bifida occulta in relation to age. Am J Dis Child 91:211, 1956.
10. Hollinshead WH: Anatomy of the spine: Points of interest to orthopaedic surgeons. J Bone Joint Surg [Am] 47:209, 1965.
11. Arcomano JP, Spyros K: Congenital absence of the lumbosacral articular processes. Skel Radiol 8:133, 1982.
12. McKay DW, Nason SS: Congenital duplication of the spinal canal. A case report. Spine 5:390, 1980.
13. Kelly A, Towbin R, Kaufman R, et al: Spine duplication. Spine 10:15, 1985.
14. Kelly A, Towbin R, Kaufman R, et al: Spine duplication. Spine 10:15, 1985.
15. Schwartz AM, Wechsler RJ, Landy MD, et al: Posterior arch defects of the cervical spine. Skel Radiol 8:135, 1982.
16. Bardsley JL, Hanelin LG: The unilateral hypoplastic lumbar pedicle. Radiology 101:315, 1971.
17. Morin ME, Palacios E: The aplastic hypoplastic lumbar pedicle. AJR 122:639, 1974.
18. Oestreich A, Young LW: The absent cervical pedicle syndrome: A case in childhood. AJR 107:505, 1969.
19. Tomsick TA, Lebowitz ME, Campbell C: The congenital absence of pedicles in the thoracic spine. Report of two cases. Radiology 111:587, 1974.
20. Yousefzadeh DK, El-Khoury GY, Lupetin AR: Congenital aplastic-hypoplastic lumbar pedicle in infants and young children. Skel Radiol 7:259, 1982.
21. Yochum TR, Sellars LT, Oppenheimer DA, et al: The sclerotic pedicle—how many causes are there? Skel Radiol 19:411, 1990.

22. Stelling CB: Anomalous attachment of the transverse process to the vertebral body: An accessory finding in congenital absence of a lumbar pedicle. Skel Radiol 6:47, 1981.
23. Polly DW Jr, Mason DE: Congenital absence of a lumbar pedicle presenting as back pain in children. J Pediatr Orthop 11:214, 1991.
24. Wiener MD, Martinez S, Forsberg DA: Congenital absence of a cervical spinal pedicle: Clinical and radiologic findings. AJR 155:1037, 1990.
25. Wortzman G, Steinhardt MI: Congenitally absent lumbar pedicle: A reappraisal. Radiology 152:713, 1984.
26. MacEwen GD, Conway JJ, Millet WT: Congenital scoliosis with a unilateral bar. Radiology 90:711, 1968.
27. Klippel M, Feil A: Un cas d'absence des vertèbres cervicales. Avec cage thoracique remontant jusqu'à la base du crâne (cage thoracique cervicale). Nouv Iconogr Salpêtrière 25:223, 1912 (cited in Clin Orthop 109:3, 1975).
28. Hensinger RN, Lang JE, MacEwen GD: Klippel-Feil syndrome. A constellation of associated anomalies. J Bone Joint Surg [Am] 56:1246, 1974.
29. Hall JE, Simmons ED, Danlychuk K, et al: Instability of the cervical spine and neurological involvement in Klippel-Feil syndrome: A case report. J Bone Joint Surg [Am] 72:460, 1990.
30. Winter RB, Moe JH, Lonstein JE: The incidence of Klippel-Feil syndrome in patients with congenital scoliosis and kyphosis. Spine 9:363, 1984.
31. Moore WB, Mathews TJ, Rabinowitz R: Genitourinary anomalies associated with Klippel-Feil syndrome. J Bone Joint Surg [Am] 57:355, 1975.
32. Ramsey J, Bliznak J: Klippel-Feil syndrome with renal agenesis and other anomalies. AJR 113:460, 1971.
33. Lombardi G: The occipital vertebra. AJR 86:260, 1961.
34. McRae DL: Bony abnormalities in the region of the foramen magnum: Correlation of the anatomic and neurologic findings. Acta Radiol 40:335, 1953.
35. McRae DL, Barnum AS: Occipitalization of the atlas. AJR 70:23, 1953.
36. McRae DL: Craniovertebral junction. In TH Newton, DG Potts (Eds): Radiology of the Skull and Brain. St Louis, CV Mosby, 1971, p 260.
37. Sauvegrain J, Mareschal J-L: Malformations de la charnière craniocervicale chez l'enfant. Ann Radiol 15:263, 1972.
38. Shapiro R, Robinson F: Anomalies of the craniovertebral border. AJR 127:281, 1976.
39. El Gammal T, Brooks BS: Anatomy of the craniovertebral junction. In JM Taveras, JT Ferrucci (Eds): Radiology. Diagnosis—Imaging—Intervention. Vol 3. Philadelphia, JB Lippincott, 1986.
40. El Gammal T, Brooks BS: Radiologic evaluation of the craniovertebral junction. In JM Taveras, JT Ferrucci (Eds): Radiology. Diagnosis—Imaging—Intervention. Vol 3. Philadelphia, JB Lippincott, 1986.
41. Ogden JA, Murphy MJ, Southwick WO, et al: Radiology of postnatal development: XIII. C-1–C-2 interrelationships. Skel Radiol 15:433, 1968.
42. Schweitzer ME, Hodler J, Cervilla V, et al: Craniovertebral junction: Normal anatomy with MR correlation. AJR 158:1087, 1992.
43. Motateanu M, Gudinchet F, Sarraj H, et al: Case report 665. Congenital absence of posterior arch of atlas. Skel Radiol 20:231, 1991.
44. McClellan R, El Gammal T, Willing S, et al: Persistent infantile odontoid process: A variant of abnormal atlantoaxial segmentation. AJR 158:1305, 1992.
45. McManners T: Odontoid hypoplasia. Br J Radiol 56:907, 1983.
46. Bohrer SP, Klein A, Martin W III: "V" shaped predens space. Skel Radiol 14:111, 1985.
47. Locke GR, Gardner JI, Van Epps EF: Atlas-dens interval (ADI) in children. AJR 97:135, 1966.
48. Ogden JA: Radiology of postnatal skeletal development. XI. The first cervical vertebra. Skel Radiol 12:12, 1984.
49. Harwood-Nash DC: Computed tomography of the craniocervical junction in children. Ann Radiol 27:235, 1984.
50. Dawson EG, Smith L: Atlanto-axial subluxation in children due to vertebral anomalies. J Bone Joint Surg [Am] 61:582, 1979.
51. Hibri NS, El-Khoury GY, Menezes AH, et al: Gas and metrizamide myelography in abnormalities of the craniovertebral junction. Skel Radiol 6:85, 1981.
52. Fielding JW: Disappearance of the central portion of the odontoid process. A case report. J Bone Joint Surg [Am] 47:1228, 1965.
53. Freiberger RH, Wilson PD Jr, Nicholas JA: Acquired absence of the odontoid process. A case report. J Bone Joint Surg [Am] 47:1231, 1965.
54. Fielding JW, Hensinger RN, Hawkins RJ: Os odontoideum. J Bone Joint Surg [Am] 62:376, 1980.
55. Schuler TC, Kurz L, Thompson DE, et al: Natural history of os odontoideum. J Pediatr Orthop 11:222, 1991.
56. Thomason M, Young JWR: Case Report 261. Os odontoideum. Skel Radiol 11:144, 1984.
57. Holt RG, Helms CA, Munk PL, et al: Hypertrophy of C-1 anterior arch: Useful sign to distinguish os odontoideum from acute dens fracture. Radiology 173:207, 1989.
58. Olbrantz K, Bohrer SP: Fusion of the anterior arch of the atlas and dens. Skel Radiol 12:21, 1984.
59. Banta JV, Nichols O: Sacral agenesis. J Bone Joint Surg [Am] 51:693, 1969.
60. Passarge E, Lenz W: Syndrome of caudal regression in infants of diabetic mothers: Observations of further cases. Pediatrics 37:672, 1966.
61. Guidera KJ, Raney E, Ogden JA, et al: Caudal regression: A review of seven cases, including the mermaid syndrome. J Pediatr Orthop 11:743, 1991.
62. Frantz CH, Aitken GT: Complete absence of the lumbar spine and sacrum. J Bone Joint Surg [Am] 49:1531, 1967.
63. Mongeau M, LeClaire R: Complete agenesis of the lumbosacral spine. J Bone Joint Surg [Am] 54:161, 1972.
64. Grace E, Drennan J, Colver D, et al: The 13q-deletion syndrome. J Med Genet 8:351, 1971.
65. Fernbach SK: Urethral abnormalities in male neonates with VATER association. AJR 156:137, 1991.
66. Loder RT, Dayioglu MM: Association of congenital vertebral malformations with bladder and cloacal exstrophy. J Pediatr Orthop 10:389, 1990.
67. Azouz EM, Slomic A: Radiographic gradation of lumbosacral dysgenesis. J Can Assoc Radiol 30:90, 1979.
68. De Klerk DJJ, McCusker I, Loubser JS: Anterior sacral meningoceles. S Afr Med J 54:361, 1978.
69. Sumner TE, Crowe JE, Phelps CR II, et al: Occult anterior sacral meningocele. Am J Dis Child 134:385, 1980.
70. Anderson FM, Burke BL: Anterior sacral meningocele. A presentation of three cases. JAMA 237:39, 1977.
71. Renshaw TS: Sacral agenesis: A classification and review of twenty-three cases. J Bone Joint Surg [Am] 60:373, 1978.
72. Brooks BS, El Gammal T, Hartlage P, et al: Myelography of sacral agenesis. AJNR 2:319, 1981.
73. White RI, Klauber GT: Sacral agenesis. Analysis of 22 cases. Urology 8:521, 1976.
74. Piggott H: The natural history of scoliosis in myelodysplasia. J Bone Joint Surg [Br] 62:54, 1980.
75. Altman NR, Altman DH: MR imaging of spinal dysraphism. AJNR 8:533, 1987.
76. Bale JF Jr, Bell WE, Dunn V, et al: Magnetic resonance imaging of the spine in children. Arch Neurol 43:1253, 1991.
77. Barkovitch AJ, Edwards MSB, Cogen PH: MR evaluation of spinal dermal sinus tracts in children. AJR 156:791, 1991.
78. Barkovitch AJ, Naidich TP: Congenital anomalies of the spine. In AJ Barkovitch (Ed): Pediatric Neuroimaging. New York, Raven Press, 1990.
79. Caro PA, Marks HG, Keret D, et al: Intraspinal epidermoid tumors in children: Problems in recognition and imaging techniques for diagnosis. J Pediatr Orthop 11:288, 1991.
80. Davis PC, Hoffman JC Jr, Ball TI, et al: Spinal abnormalities in pediatric patients: MR imaging findings compared with clinical, myelographic, and surgical findings. Radiology 166:679, 1988.
81. Philips WA, Hensinger RN, Kling TF Jr: Management of scoliosis due to syringomyelia in childhood and adolescence. J Pediatr Orthop 10:351, 1990.
82. Walker HS, Lufkin RB, Dietrich RB, et al: Magnetic resonance imaging of the pediatric spine. RadioGraphics 7:1129, 1987.
83. Zieger M, Dörr U: Pediatric spinal sonography: I. Anatomy and examination technique. Pediatr Radiol 18:9, 1988.
84. Schumacher R, Kroll B, Schwarz M, et al: M-mode sonography of the caudal spinal cord in patients with meningomyelocele. Radiology 184:263, 1992.
85. Szalay EA, Roach JW, Smith H, et al: Magnetic resonance imaging of the spinal cord in spinal dysraphisms. J Pediatr Orthop 7:541, 1987.
86. Gardner WJ: Hydrodynamic mechanism of syringomyelia: Its relationship to myelocele. J Neurol Neurosurg Psychiatry 28:247, 1965.
87. Donaldson WF: Neural spinal dysraphism (myelomeningocele, etc.). In J Hardy (Ed): Spinal Deformity in Neurological and Muscular Disorders. St Louis, CV Mosby, 1974, p 140.
88. Naidich TP, McLone DG, Mutluer S: A new understanding of dorsal dysraphism with lipoma (lipomyeloschisis): Radiologic evaluation and surgical correction. AJNR 4:103, 1983.
89. Just M, Schwarz M, Ludwig B, et al: Cerebral and spinal MR findings in patients with post-repair myelomeningocele. Pediatr Radiol 20:262, 1990.
90. Kramer PPG, Scheers IM: Round anterior margin of lumbar vertebral bodies in children with a meningomyelocele. Pediatr Radiol 17:263, 1987.
91. Nelson MD Jr, Bracchi M, Naidich TP, et al: The natural history of repaired myelomeningocele. RadioGraphics 8:695, 1988.
92. Barson AJ: Radiological studies of spina bifida cystica. The phenomenon of congenital lumbar kyphosis. Br J Radiol 38:294, 1965.
93. Samuelsson L, Bergström K, Thuomas K-Å, et al: MR imaging of syringohydromyelia and Chiari malformations in myelomeningocele patients with scoliosis. AJNR 8:539, 1987.
94. Hall P, Lindseth R, Campbell R, et al: Scoliosis and hydrocephalus in myelocele patients: The effect of ventricular shunting. J Neurosurg 50:174, 1979.
95. Hall PV, Campbell RL, Kalsbeck JE: Meningomyelocele and progressive hydromyelia. Progressive paresis in myelodysplasia. J Neurosurg 43:457, 1975.
96. Hall PV, Lindseth RE, Campbell RL, et al: Myelodysplasia and developmental scoliosis. A manifestation of syringomyelia. Spine 1:48, 1976.
97. Heinz ER, Rosenbaum AE, Scarff TB, et al: Tethered spinal cord following meningomyelocele repair. Radiology 131:153, 1979.
98. Loder RT, Shapiro P, Towbin R, et al: Aortic anatomy in children with myelomeningocele and congenital lumbar kyphosis. J Pediatr Orthop 11:31, 1991.
99. Neuhauser EBD, Harris GBC, Berrett A: Roentgenographic features of neurenteric cysts. AJR 79:235, 1958.
100. Burrows FGO: Some aspects of occult spinal dysraphism: A study of 90 cases. Br J Radiol 41:496, 1968.
101. James CCM, Lassman LP: Spinal dysraphism. The diagnosis and treatment of progressive lesions in spina bifida occulta. J Bone Joint Surg [Br] 44:828, 1962.
102. Gillespie R, Faithfull DK, Roth A, et al: Intraspinal anomalies in congenital scoliosis. Clin Orthop 93:103, 1973.
103. Scheible W, James HE, Leopold GR, et al: Occult spinal dysraphism in infants: Screening with high-resolution real-time ultrasound. Radiology 146:743, 1983.

104. Roos RAC, Vielvoye GJ, Voormolen JHC, et al: Magnetic resonance imaging in occult spinal dysraphism. Pediatr Radiol 16:412, 1986.
105. Scatliff JG, Kendall BE, Kingsley DPE, et al: Closed spinal dysraphism: Analysis of clinical, radiological, and surgical findings in 104 consecutive patients. AJR 152:1049, 1989.
106. Wilson DA, Prince JR: MR imaging determination of the location of the normal conus medullaris throughout childhood. AJR 152:1029, 1989.
107. McClelland RR, Marsh DG: Double diastematomyelia. Radiology 123:378, 1977.
108. Till K: Spinal dysraphism. A study of congenital malformations of the lower back. J Bone Joint Surg [Br] 51:415, 1969.
109. Winter RB, Haven JJ, Moe JH, et al: Diastematomyelia and congenital spine deformities. J Bone Joint Surg 56:27, 1974.
110. Kennedy PR: New data on diastematomyelia. J Neurosurg 51:355, 1979.
111. McMaster MJ: Occult intraspinal anomalies and congenital scoliosis. J Bone Joint Surg [Am] 66:588, 1984.
112. De Smet AA: Radiology of Spinal Curvature. St Louis, CV Mosby, 1985.
113. Hood RW, Riseborough EJ, Nehme A-M, et al: Diastematomyelia and structural spinal deformities. J Bone Joint Surg [Am] 62:520, 1980.
114. Arredondo F, Haughton VM, Hemmy DC, et al: The computed tomographic appearance of the spinal cord in diastematomyelia. Radiology 13:685, 1980.
115. Hilal SK, Marton D, Pollack E: Diastematomyelia in children. Radiographic study of 34 cases. Radiology 112:609, 1974.
116. Keim HA, Greene AF: Diastematomyelia and scoliosis. J Bone Joint Surg [Am] 55:1425, 1973.
117. Castillo M: MRI of diastematomyelia. MRI Decisions, Sept/Oct, p 12, 1991.
118. Scatliff JH, Till K, Hoare RD: Incomplete, false, and true diastematomyelia. Radiological evaluation by air myelography and tomography. Radiology 116:349, 1975.
119. Kaplan JO, Quencer RM: The occult tethered conus syndrome in the adult. Radiology 137:387, 1980.
120. Raghavendra BN, Epstein FJ, Pinto RS, et al: The tethered spinal cord: Diagnosis by high-resolution real-time ultrasound. Radiology 149:123, 1983.
121. Raghavan N, Barkovich AJ, Edwards M, et al: MR imaging in the tethered spinal cord syndrome. AJR 152:843, 1989.
122. Ammerman BJ, Henry JM, DeGirolami V, et al: Intradural lipomas of the spinal cord: A clinicopathological correlation. J Neurosurg 44:331, 1976.
123. Gold LHA, Kieffer SA, Peterson HO: Lipomatous invasion of the spinal cord associated with spinal dysraphism: Myelographic evaluation. AJR 107:479, 1969.
124. Taviere V, Brunelle F, Baraton J, et al: MRI study of lumbosacral lipoma in children. Pediatr Radiol 19:316, 1989.
125. Wippold FJ, Citrin C, Barkovich AJ, et al: Evaluation of MR in spinal dysraphism with lipoma: Comparison with metrizamide computed tomography. Pediatr Radiol 17:184, 1987.
126. Sauer JM, Ozonoff MB: Congenital bone anomalies associated with lipomas. Skel Radiol 13:276, 1985.
127. Theander G: Malformation of the iliac bone associated with intraspinal abnormalities. Pediatr Radiol 3:235, 1975.
128. Holmes GL, Trader S, Ignatiadis P: Intraspinal enterogenous cysts. A case report and review of pediatric cases in the literature. Am J Dis Child 132:906, 1978.
129. Herman R, Mixon J, Fisher A, Malulucci R, et al: Idiopathic scoliosis and the central nervous system: A motor control problem. Spine 10:1, 1985.
130. Adair IV, Van Wijk MC, Armstrong GWD: Moiré topography in scoliosis screening. Clin Orthop 129:165, 1977.
131. Torell G, Nachemson A, Haderspeck-Grib K, et al: Standing and supine Cobb measures in girls with idiopathic scoliosis. Spine 10:425, 1985.
132. De Smet AA, Fritz SL, Asher MA: A method for minimizing the radiation exposure from scoliosis radiographs. J Bone Joint Surg [Am] 63:156, 1981.
133. Dutkowsky JP, Shearer D, Schepps B: Radiation exposure to patients receiving routine scoliosis radiography measured at depth in an anthropomorphic phantom. J Pediatr Orthop 10:532, 1990.
134. Schock CC, Brenton L, Agarwal KK: The effect of PA versus AP X-rays on the apparent scoliotic angle. Orthop Trans 4:32, 1980.
135. DeSmet AA, Goin JE, Asher MA, et al: A clinical study of the differences between the scoliotic angle measured on posteroanterior and anteroposterior radiographs. J Bone Joint Surg [Am] 64:489, 1982.
136. Gray JE, Stears JG, Frank ED: Shaped, lead-loaded acrylic filters for patient exposure reduction and image-quality improvement. Radiology 146:825, 1983.
137. Gray JE, Hoffman AD, Peterson HA: Reduction of radiation exposure during radiography for scoliosis. J Bone Joint Surg [Am] 65:5, 1983.
138. Bhatnagar JP, Gorson RO, Krohmer JS: X-ray doses to patients undergoing full-spine radiographic examination. Radiology 138:231, 1981.
139. Ritter EM, Wright CE, Fritz SL, et al: Use of a gradient intensifying screen for scoliosis radiography. Radiology 135:230, 1980.
140. Libson E, Bloom RA, Dinari G, et al: Oblique lumbar spine radiographs: Importance in young patients. Radiology 151:89, 1984.
141. Howell FR, Dickson RA: The deformity of idiopathic scoliosis made visible by computer graphics. J Bone Joint Surg [Br] 71:399, 1989.
142. Singer KP, Jones TJ, Breidahl PD: A comparison of radiographic and computer-assisted measurements of thoracic and thoracolumbar sagittal curvature. Skel Radiol 19:21, 1990.
143. Drerup B, Hierholzer E: Evaluation of frontal radiographs of scoliotic spines. Part I. Measurement of position and orientation of vertebrae and assessment of clinical shape parameters. J Biomech 25:1357, 1992.
144. Drerup B, Hierholzer E: Evaluation of frontal radiographs of scoliotic spines. Part II. Relations between lateral deviation, lateral tilt and axial rotation of vertebrae. J Biomech 25:1443, 1992.
145. Daniel WW, Barnes GT, Nasca RJ, et al: Segmented-field radiography in scoliosis. AJR 144:325, 1985.
146. Harcke HT, Mandell GA, Lee MS, et al: Evaluating scoliosis with digital radiographic techniques. Abstract, Society for Pediatric Radiology, Boston, April 20, 1985.
147. Shackelford GD, MacAllister WH: Axial radiography of the spine: A projection for evaluation of the neural arches in children. Radiology 3:798, 1979.
148. Cooke ED, Carter LM, Pilcher MF: Identifying scoliosis in the adolescent with thermography: A preliminary study. Clin Orthop 148:172, 1980.
149. Papanicolaou N, Treves S: Bone scintigraphy in the preoperative evaluation of osteoid osteoma and osteoblastoma of the spine. Ann Radiol 27:104, 1984.
150. McMaster MJ, Merrick MV: The scintigraphic assessment of the scoliotic spine after fusion. J Bone Joint Surg [Br] 62:65, 1980.
151. Knake JE, Gabrielsen TO, Chandler WF, et al: Real-time sonography during spinal surgery. Radiology 151:461, 1984.
152. Miller JH, Reid BS, Kemberling CR: Utilization of ultrasound in the evaluation of spinal dysraphism in children. Radiology 143:737, 1982.
153. Abrams SL, Filly RA: Congenital vertebral malformations: Prenatal diagnosis using ultrasonography. Radiology 155:762, 1985.
154. Nokes SR, Murtagh RF, Jones JD III, et al: Childhood scoliosis: MR imaging. Radiology 164:791, 1987.
155. Winter RB: Prevalence of spinal canal or cord abnormalities in idiopathic, congenital, and neuromuscular scoliosis (Abst). J Pediatr Orthop 12:680, 1992.
156. Gryspeerdt GL: Myelographic assessment of occult forms of spinal dysraphism. Acta Radiol 1:702, 1963.
157. Barnes PD, Brody JD, Jaramillo D, et al: Atypical idiopathic scoliosis: MR imaging evaluation. Radiology 186:247, 1993.
158. Scoles PV, Salvagno R, Villalba K, et al: Relationship of iliac crest maturation to skeletal and chronologic age. J Pediatr Orthop 8:639, 1988.
159. Propst-Proctor SL, Bleck EE: Radiographic determination of lordosis and kyphosis in normal and scoliotic children. J Pediatr Orthop 3:344, 1983.
160. A glossary of scoliosis terms. Spine 1:57, 1976.
161. Williams SM, Harned RK, Hultman SA, et al: The psoas sign: A reevaluation. RadioGraphics 5:525, 1985.
162. Aaro S, Dahlborn M: Estimation of vertebral rotation and the spinal and rib cage deformity in scoliosis by computer tomography. Spine 6:460, 1981.
163. Jeffries BF, Tarlton M, De Smet AA, et al: Computerized measurement and analysis of scoliosis. A more accurate representation of the shape of the curve. Radiology 134:381, 1980.
164. George K, Rippstein J: A comparative study of the two popular methods of measuring scoliotic deformity of the spine. J Bone Joint Surg [Am] 43:809, 1961.
165. Sevastikoglou JA, Berquist E: Evaluation of the reliability of radiological methods for registration of scoliosis. Acta Orthop Scand 40:608, 1969.
166. Deacon P, Flood BM, Dickson RA: Idiopathic scoliosis in three dimensions. A radiographic and morphometric analysis. J Bone Joint Surg [Br] 66:509, 1984.
167. Morrissy RT, Goldsmith GS, Hall EC, et al: Measurement of the Cobb angle on radiographs of patients who have scoliosis: Evaluation of intrinsic error. J Bone Joint Surg [Am]. 72:320, 1990.
168. Oda M, Rauh S, Gregory PB, et al: The significance of roentgenographic measurement in scoliosis. J Pediatr Orthop 2:378, 1982.
169. Gross C, Gross M, Kuschner S: Error analysis of scoliosis curvature measurement. Bull Hosp Joint Dis 43:171, 1983.
170. Carman DL, Browne RH, Birch JG: Measurement of scoliosis and kyphosis radiographs: Intraobserver and interobserver variation. J Bone Joint Surg [Am] 72:328, 1990.
171. Aaro S, Dahlborn M: The longitudinal axis rotation of the apical vertebra, the vertebral, spinal and rib cage deformity in idiopathic scoliosis studied by computer tomography. Spine 6:567, 1981.
172. Armstrong GWD, Livermore NB III, Suzuki N, et al: Nonstandard vertebral rotation in scoliosis screening patients. Its prevalence and relation to the clinical deformity. Spine 7:50, 1982.
173. Mehta MH: Radiographic estimation of vertebral body rotation in scoliosis. J Bone Joint Surg [Br] 55:513, 1973.
174. Nash CL Jr, Moe JH: A study of vertebral rotation. J Bone Joint Surg [Am] 51:223, 1969.
175. Benson DR, Schultz AB, DeWald RL: Roentgenographic evaluation of vertebral rotation. J Bone Joint Surg [Am] 58:1125, 1976.
176. Suzuki S, Yamamuro T, Shikata J, et al: Ultrasound measurement of vertebral rotation in idiopathic scoliosis. J Bone Joint Surg [Br] 71:252, 1989.
177. De Smet AA, Tarlton MA, Cook LT, et al: A radiographic method for three-dimensional analysis of spinal configuration. Radiology 137:343, 1980.
178. De Smet AA, Tarlton MA, Cook LT, et al: The top view for analysis of scoliosis progression. Radiology 147:369, 1983.
179. Raso VJ, Russell GG, Hill DL, et al: Thoracic lordosis in idiopathic scoliosis. J Pediatr Orthop 11:599, 1991.
180. Collis DK, Ponseti IV: Long-term follow-up of patients with idiopathic scoliosis not treated surgically. J Bone Joint Surg [Am] 51:425, 1969.
181. Risser JC: Scoliosis: Past and present. J Bone Joint Surg [Am] 46:167, 1964.
182. Urbaniak JR, Schaefer WW, Stelling FH III: Iliac apophyses. Prognostic value in idiopathic scoliosis. Clin Orthop 116:80, 1976.
183. Biondi J, Weiner DS, Bethem D, et al: Correlation of Risser sign and bone age determination in adolescent idiopathic scoliosis. J Pediatr Orthop 5:697, 1985.

184. McMaster MJ, Ohtsuka K: The natural history of congenital scoliosis. A study of two hundred and fifty-one patients. J Bone Joint Surg [Am] *64*:1128, 1982.

185. Nasca RJ, Stelling FH III, Steel HA: Progression of congenital scoliosis due to hemivertebrae and hemivertebrae with bars. J Bone Joint Surg [Am] *57*:456, 1975.

186. Winter RB, Moe JH, Eilers VE: Congenital scoliosis. A study of 234 patients treated and untreated. Part I. Natural history. J Bone Joint Surg [Am] *50*:1, 1968.

187. Winter RB: Congenital scoliosis. Clin Orthop *93*:75, 1973.

188. Jaffray D, O'Brien JP: A true anterior thoracic meningocele associated with a congenital kyphoscoliosis. J Pediatr Orthop *5*:717, 1985.

189. Birnholz JC: Fetal lumbar spine: Measuring axial growth with US. Radiology *158*:805, 1986.

190. Bradford DS, Heithoff KB, Cohen M: Instraspinal abnormalities and congenital spine deformities: A radiographic and MRI study. J Pediatr Orthop *11*:36, 1991.

191. Privett GW Jr: MRI of congenital anomalies of the spine. MRI Decisions *4*:24, 1990.

192. Pettersson H, Harwood-Nash DCF, Fitz CR, et al: Conventional metrizamide myelography (MM) and computed tomographic metrizamide myelography (CTMM) in scoliosis. A comparative study. Radiology *142*:111, 1982.

193. Resjö IM, Harwood-Nash DC, Fitz CR, et al: Normal cord in infants and children examined with computed tomographic metrizamide myelography. Radiology *130*:691, 1979.

194. Hirschfelder H: Computerized tomography: A new dimension in the assessment of scoliosis. Electromedica *51*:132, 1983.

195. Pettersson H, Harwood-Nash DCF: CT and Myelography of the Spine and Cord. Techniques, Anatomy and Pathology in Children. New York. Springer-Verlag, 1982.

196. Resjö IM, Harwood-Nash DC, Fitz CR, et al: Computed tomographic metriza-mide myelography in spinal dysraphism in infants and children. J Comput Assist Tomogr *2*:549, 1978.

197. Johnson S, Nayanar VV, Jones RFC: Metrizamide myelography in spinal dys-raphism. Australas Radiol *24*:161, 1980.

198. MacEwen GD, Winter RB, Hardy JH: Evaluation of kidney anomalies in congenital scoliosis. J Bone Joint Surg [Am] *54*:1451, 1972.

199. Vitki RJ, Cass AS, Winter RB: Anomalies of the genitourinary tract associated with congenital scoliosis and congenital kyphosis. J Urol *108*:655, 1972.

200. Schey WL: Vertebral malformations and associated somaticoviscieral abnormal-ities. Clin Radiol *27*:341, 1976.

201. Winter RB, Moe JH, Wang JF: Congenital kyphosis. Its natural history and treatment as observed in a study of one hundred and thirty patients. J Bone Joint Surg [Am] *55*:223, 1973.

202. Franceschini P, Grassi E, Fabris C, et al: The autosomal recessive form of spondylocostal dysostosis. Radiology *112*:673, 1974.

203. Ezaki M, Herring JA: Congenital hyperextension of the lumbar spine. A case report. J Bone Joint Surg [Am] *63*:1177, 1981.

204. Beals RK: Familial vertebral hypoplasia and kyphosis. J Bone Joint Surg [Am] *51*:190, 1969.

205. Smith JRG, Martin IR, Shaw DG, et al: Progressive noninfectious anterior vertebral fusion. Skel Radiol *15*:599, 1986.

206. Bethem D, Winter RB, Lutter L, et al: Spinal disorders of dwarfism. Review of the literature and report of eighty cases. J Bone Joint Surg [Am] *63*:1412, 1981.

207. Bethem D, Winter RB, Lutter L: Disorders of the spine in diastrophic dwarfism. A discussion of nine patients and review of the literature. J Bone Joint Surg [Am] *62*:529, 1980.

208. Lorenzo RL, Hungerford GD, Blumenthal BI, et al: Congenital kyphosis and subluxation of the thoracolumbar spine due to vertebral aplasia. Skel Radiol *10*:255, 1983.

209. Winter RB, Moe JH, Lonstein JE: The surgical treatment of congenital kypho-sis. A review of 94 patients age 5 years or older, with 2 years or more follow-up in 77 patients. Spine *10*:224, 1985.

210. Kane WJ: Scoliosis prevalence: A call for a statement of terms. Clin Orthop *126*:43, 1977.

211. Renshaw TS: Screening school children for scoliosis. Clin Orthop *229*:26, 1988.

212. Dickson RA, Stamper P, Sharp A-M, et al: School screening for scoliosis: Cohort study of clinical course. Br Med J *281*:265, 1980.

213. Brooks HL, Azen SP, Gerberg E, et al: Scoliosis: A prospective epidemiologi-cal study. J Bone Joint Surg [Am] *57*:968, 1975.

214. Lonstein JE, Bjorklund S, Wanninger MH, et al: Voluntary school screening for scoliosis in Minnesota. J Bone Joint Surg [Am] *64*:481, 1982.

215. Dvoonch VM, Siegler AH, Cloppas CC, et al: The epidemiology of "school-iosis." J Pediatr Orthop *10*:206, 1990.

216. Lonstein JE: Adolescent idiopathic scoliosis: Screening and diagnosis. Am Acad Orthop Surgeons Instructional Course Lectures *38*:105, 1989.

217. US Preventive Services Task Force: Screening for adolescent idiopathic sco-liosis. Review article. JAMA *269*:2667, 1993.

218. US Preventive Services Task Force: Screening for adolescent idiopathic sco-liosis. Policy statement. JAMA *269*:2664, 1993.

219. Sox HC Jr, Woolf SH: Evidence-based practice guidelines from the US Preven-tive Services Task Force. JAMA *269*:2678, 1993.

220. Weinstein SL: Adolescent idiopathic scoliosis: Prevalence and natural history. Am Acad Orthop Surgeons Instructional Course Lecture *38*:115, 1989.

221. Archer IA, Dickson RA: Stature and idiopathic scoliosis. A prospective study. J Bone Joint Surg [Br] *67*:185, 1985.

222. Nordwall A, Willner S: A study of skeletal age and height in girls with idiopathic scoliosis. Clin Orthop *110*:6, 1975.

223. Reckles LN, Peterson HA, Bianco AJ Jr, et al: The association of scoliosis and congenital heart defects. J Bone Joint Surg [Am] *57*:449, 1975.

224. Roth A, Rosenthal A, Hall JE, et al: Scoliosis and congenital heart disease. Clin Orthop *93*:95, 1973.

225. Farley FA, Phillips WA, Herzenberg JE, et al: Natural history of scoliosis in congenital heart disease. J Pediatr Orthop *11*:42, 1991.

226. Deacon P, Berkin CR, Dickson RA: Combined idiopathic kyphosis and sco-liosis. An analysis of the lateral spinal curvatures associated with Scheuer-mann's disease. J Bone Joint Surg [Br] *67*:189, 1985.

227. McPhee IB, O'Brien JP: Scoliosis in symptomatic spondylolisthesis. J Bone Joint Surg [Br] *62*:155, 1980.

228. Powers TA, Haher TR, Devlin VJ, et al: Abnormalities of the spine in relation to congenital upper limb deficiencies. J Pediatr Orthop *3*:471, 1983.

229. Herring JA, Goldberg MJ: Instructional case. Amelia and scoliosis. J Pediatr Orthop *5*:605, 1985.

230. Beals RK: Nosologic and genetic aspects of scoliosis. Clin Orthop *93*:23, 1973.

231. McAlister WH, Shackelford GD: Classification of spinal curvatures. Radiol Clin North Am *13*:93, 1975.

232. McAlister WH, Shackelford GD: Measurement of spinal curvatures. Radiol Clin North Am *13*:113, 1975.

233. Lonstein JE, Carlson JM: The prediction of curve progression in untreated idiopathic scoliosis during growth. J Bone Joint Surg [Am] *66*:1061, 1984.

234. Perdriolle R, Vidal J: Thoracic idiopathic scoliosis curve. Evolution and prog-nosis. Spine *10*:785, 1985.

235. Nash CL: Current concepts review. Scoliosis bracing. J Bone Joint Surg [Am] *62*:848, 1980.

236. Weinstein SL, Ponseti IV: Curve progression in idiopathic scoliosis. J Bone Joint Surg [Am] *65*:447, 1983.

237. Robin GC, Span Y, Steinberg R, et al: Scoliosis in the elderly. A follow-up study. Spine *7*:365, 1982.

238. Gillespie T III, Gillespy T Jr, Revak CS: Progressive senile scoliosis: Seven cases of increasing spinal curves in elderly patients. Skel Radiol *13*:280, 1985.

239. Richter DE, Nash CL Jr, Moskowitz RW, et al: Idiopathic adolescent sco-liosis—a prototype of degenerative joint disease. The relation of biomechanic factors to osteophyte formation. Clin Orthop *193*:221, 1985.

240. Dickson RA, Lawton JO, Archer IA, et al: The pathogenesis of idiopathic scoliosis. Biplanar spinal asymmetry. J Bone Joint Surg [Br] *66*:8, 1984.

241. Nachemson AL, Sahlstrand T: Etiologic factors in adolescent idiopathic sco-liosis. Spine *2*:176, 1977.

242. Riseborough EJ, Wynne-Davies R: A genetic survey of idiopathic scoliosis in Boston, Massachusetts. J Bone Joint Surg [Am] *55*:974, 1973.

243. Wynne-Davies R: Familial (idiopathic) scoliosis. A family survey. J Bone Joint Surg [Br] *50*:24, 1968.

244. Ferreira JH, James JIP: Progressive and resolving infantile idiopathic scoliosis. The differential diagnosis. J Bone Joint Surg [Br] *54*:648, 1972.

245. James JIP, Lloyd-Roberts GC, Pilcher MF: Infantile structural scoliosis. J Bone Joint Surg [Br] *41*:719, 1959.

246. Lloyd-Roberts GC, Pilcher MF: Structural idiopathic scoliosis in infancy. A study of the natural history of 100 patients. J Bone Joint Surg [Br] *47*:520, 1965.

247. Mehta MH: The rib-vertebra angle in the early diagnosis between resolving and progressive infantile scoliosis. J Bone Joint Surg [Br] *54*:230, 1972.

248. Wynne-Davies R: Infantile idiopathic scoliosis. Causative factors, particularly in the first six months of life. J Bone Joint Surg [Br] *57*:138, 1975.

249. McMaster MJ: Infantile idiopathic scoliosis: Can it be prevented? J Bone Joint Surg [Br] *65*:612, 1983.

250. Figueiredo UM, James JIP: Juvenile idiopathic scoliosis. J Bone Joint Surg [Br] *63*:61, 1981.

251. Dickson RA: Conservative treatment for idiopathic scoliosis. J Bone Joint Surg [Br] *67*:176, 1985.

252. Brown JC, Axelgaard J, Howson DC: Multicenter trial of a noninvasive stimu-lation method for idiopathic scoliosis. A summary of early treatment results. Spine *9*:382, 1984.

253. Aaro S, Dahlborn M: The effect of Harrington instrumentation on the longitu-dinal axis rotation of the apical vertebra and on the spinal and rib-cage defor-mity in idiopathic scoliosis studied by computer-tomography. Spine *7*:456, 1982.

254. Luque ER: The correction of postural curves of the spine. Spine *7*:270, 1982.

255. Luque ER: Current concepts review. The anatomic basis and development of segmental spinal instrumentation. Spine *7*:256, 1982.

256. Thompson GH, Wilber RG, Shaffer JW, et al: Segmental spinal instrumentation in idiopathic scoliosis. A preliminary report. Spine *10*:623, 1985.

257. Edgar MA, Mehta MH: Long-term follow-up of fused and unfused idiopathic scoliosis. J Bone Joint Surg [Br] *70*:712, 1988.

258. Engler GL: Preoperative and intraoperative considerations in adolescent idio-pathic scoliosis. Am Acad Orthop Surgeons Instructional Course Lecture *38*:137, 1989.

259. Fitch RD, Turi M, Bowman BE, et al: Comparison of Cotrel-Dubousset and Harrington rod instrumentations in idiopathic scoliosis. J Pediatr Orthop *10*:44, 1990.

260. Herndon WA, Sullivan JA, Gruel CR, et al: A comparison of Wisconsin instrumentation and Cotrel-Dubousset instrumentation. J Pediatr Orthop *13*:615, 1993.

261. McCall RE, Bronson W: Criteria for selective fusion in idiopathic scoliosis using Cotrel-Dubousset instrumentation. J Pediatr Orthop 12:475, 1992.

262. Slone RM, MacMillan M, Montgomery WJ, et al: Spinal fixation. Part 2. Fixation techniques and hardware for the thoracic and lumbosacral spine. RadioGraphics 13:521, 1993.

263. Kostuik JP: Current concepts review. Operative treatment of idiopathic scoliosis. J Bone Joint Surg [Am] 72:1108, 1990.

264. Renshaw TS, Solga PM, Drennan JC, et al: Studies of an L-rod sublaminar wire spinal fusion. J Pediatr Orthop 11:226, 1991.

265. Tolo VT: Surgical treatment of adolescent idiopathic scoliosis. Am Acad Orthop Surgeons Instructional Course Lecture 38:143, 1989.

266. Slone RM, MacMillan M, Montgomery WJ: Spinal fixation. Part 3. Complications of spinal instrumentation. RadioGraphics 13:797, 1993.

267. Friedman RJ, Micheli LJ: Acquired spondylolisthesis following scoliosis surgery. A case report. Clin Orthop 190:132, 1984.

268. Karoll M, Hernandez RJ, Wessel HU: Computed tomography diagnosis of bronchial compression by the spine after surgical correction of scoliosis. Pediatr Radiol 14:335, 1984.

269. Drennan JC, King EW: Cervical dislocation following fusion of the upper thoracic spine for scoliosis. J Bone Joint Surg [Am] 60:1003, 1978.

270. Amy BW, Priebe CJ Jr, King A: Superior mesenteric artery syndrome associated with scoliosis treated by a modified Ladd procedure. J Pediatr Orthop 5:361, 1985.

271. Griffiths GJ, Whitehouse GH: Radiological features of vascular compression of the duodenum occurring as a complication of the treatment of scoliosis. Clin Radiol 29:77, 1978.

272. Berk RN, Coulson DB: The body cast syndrome. Radiology 94:303, 1970.

273. Evarts CM, Winter RB, Hall JE: Vascular compression of the duodenum associated with the treatment of scoliosis. Review of the literature and report of eighteen cases. J Bone Joint Surg [Am] 53:431, 1971.

274. McMaster MJ, James JIP: Pseudarthrosis after spinal fusion for scoliosis. J Bone Joint Surg [Br] 58:305, 1976.

275. Lauerman WC, Bradford DS, Transfeldt EE, et al: Management of pseudarthrosis after arthrodesis of the spine for idiopathic scoliosis. J Bone Joint Surg [Am] 73:222, 1991.

276. Risser JC, Iqbal QM, Nagata K, et al: Roentgenographic detection of preventable occult pseudarthrosis in the treatment of scoliosis. Clin Orthop 107:171, 1975.

277. Slizofski WJ, Collier BD, Flatley TJ, et al: Painful pseudarthrosis following lumbar spinal fusion: Detection by combined SPECT and planar bone scintigraphy. Skel Radiol 16:136, 1987.

278. Hannon KM, Wetta WJ: Failure of technetium bone scanning to detect pseudarthroses in spinal fusion for scoliosis. Clin Orthop 123:42, 1977.

279. Hensinger RN, McEwen GD: Spinal deformity associated with heritable neurological conditions: Spinal muscular atrophy, Friedreich's ataxia, familial dysautonomia, and Charcot-Marie-Tooth disease. J Bone Joint Surg [Am] 58:13, 1976.

280. Balmer GA, MacEwen GD: The incidence and treatment of scoliosis in cerebral palsy. J Bone Joint Surg [Br] 52:134, 1970.

281. Gersoff WK, Renshaw TS: The treatment of scoliosis in cerebral palsy by posterior spinal fusion with Luque-rod segmental instrumentation. J Bone Joint Surg [Am] 70:41, 1988.

282. Thometz JG, Simon SR: Progression of scoliosis after skeletal maturity in institutionalized adults who have cerebral palsy. J Bone Joint Surg [Am] 70:1290, 1987.

283. Guidera KJ, Borrelli J Jr, Raney E, et al: Orthopaedic manifestations of Rett syndrome. J Pediatr Orthop 11:204, 1991.

284. Madigan RR, Wallace SL: Scoliosis in the institutionalized cerebral palsy population. Spine 6:583, 1981.

285. Lonstein JE, Akbarnia BA: Operative treatment of spinal deformities in patients with cerebral palsy or mental retardation. An analysis of one hundred and seven cases. J Bone Joint Surg [Am] 65:43, 1983.

286. Baker AS, Dove J: Progressive scoliosis as the first presenting sign of syringomyelia. Report of a case. J Bone Joint Surg [Br] 65:472, 1983.

287. Resjö IM, Harwood-Nash DC, Fitz CR, et al: Computed tomographic metrizamide myelography in syringohydromyelia. Radiology 131:405, 1979.

288. Kan S, Fox AJ, Viñuela F, et al: Spinal cord size in syringomyelia: Change with position on metrizamide myelography. Radiology 146:409, 1983.

289. Citron N, Edgar MA, Sheehy J, et al: Intramedullary spinal cord tumours presenting as scoliosis. J Bone Joint Surg [Br] 66:513, 1984.

290. Evans GA, Drennan JC, Russman BS: Functional classification and orthopaedic management of spinal muscular atrophy. J Bone Joint Surg [Br] 63:516, 1981.

291. Williams B: Orthopaedic features in the presentation of syringomyelia. J Bone Joint Surg [Br] 61:314, 1979.

292. DeSousa AL, Kalsbeck JE, Mealey J Jr, et al: Intraspinal tumors in children. A review of 81 cases. J Neurosurg 51:437, 1979.

293. Huebert HT, MacKinnon WB: Syringomyelia and scoliosis. J Bone Joint Surg [Br] 51:338, 1969.

294. Dearolf WW II, Betz RR, Vogel LC, et al: Scoliosis in pediatric spinal cord-injured patients. J Pediatr Orthop 10:214, 1990.

295. Hackney DB: Denominators of spinal cord injury. Radiology 177:18, 1990.

296. Mayfield JK, Erkkila JC, Winter RB: Spine deformity subsequent to acquired childhood spinal cord injury. J Bone Joint Surg [Am] 63:1401, 1981.

297. Lancourt JE, Dickson JH, Carter RE: Paralytic spinal deformity following traumatic spinal-cord injury in children and adolescents. J Bone Joint Surg [Am] 63:47, 1981.

298. Brown JC, Swank SM, Matta J, et al: Late spinal deformity in quadriplegic children and adolescents. J Pediatr Orthop 4:456, 1984.

299. Pavon SJ, Manning C: Posterior spinal fusion for scoliosis due to anterior poliomyelitis. J Bone Joint Surg [Br] 52:420, 1970.

300. Duval-Beaupère G, Lespargot A, Grossiord A: Scoliosis and trunk muscles. J Pediatr Orthop 4:195, 1984.

301. Schwentker EP, Gibson DA: Orthopaedic aspects of spinal muscular atrophy. J Bone Joint Surg [Am] 58:32, 1976.

302. Riddick MF, Winter RB, Lutter LD: Spinal deformities in patients with spinal muscle atrophy. A review of 36 patients. Spine 7:476, 1982.

303. Labelle H, Tohme S, Duhaime M, et al: Natural history of scoliosis in Friedreich's ataxia. J Bone Joint Surg [Am] 68:564, 1986.

304. Cady RB, Bobechko WP: Incidence, natural history, and treatment of scoliosis in Friedreich's ataxia. J Pediatr Orthop 4:673, 1984.

305. Daher YH, Lonstein JE, Winter RB, et al: Spinal deformities in patients with Friedreich ataxia: A review of 19 patients. J Pediatr Orthop 5:553, 1985.

306. Winter RB, Kriel RL: Scoliosis due to epilepsia partialis continua. J Pediatr Orthop 5:94, 1985.

307. Stantiski CJ, Micheli LJ, Hall JE: The correction of spinal deformity in idiopathic torsional dystonias. J Bone Joint Surg [Am] 65:980, 1983.

308. Daher YH, Lonstein JE, Winter RB, et al: Spinal deformities in patients with muscular dystrophy other than Duchenne: A review of 11 patients having surgical treatment. Spine 10:614, 1985.

309. Siegel IM: Scoliosis in muscular dystrophy. Some comments about diagnosis, observations on prognosis, and suggestions for therapy. Clin Orthop 93:235, 1973.

310. Wilkins KE, Gibson DA: The patterns of spinal deformity in Duchenne muscular dystrophy. J Bone Joint Surg [Am] 58:24, 1976.

311. Smith AD, Koreska J, Moseley CF: Progression of scoliosis in Duchenne muscular dystrophy. J Bone Joint Surg [Am] 71:1066, 1989.

312. Oda T, Shimizu N, Yonenobu K, et al: Longitudinal study of spinal deformity in Duchenne muscular dystrophy. J Pediatr Orthop 13:478, 1993.

313. Hsu JD: The natural history of spine curvature progression in the nonambulatory Duchenne muscular dystrophy patient. Spine 7:771, 1983.

314. Daher YH, Lonstein JE, Winter RB, et al: Spinal deformities in patients with muscular dystrophy other than Duchenne. A review of 11 patients having surgical treatment. Spine 10:614, 1985.

315. Bartal E, Gage JR: Idiopathic juvenile osteoporosis and scoliosis. J Pediatr Orthop 2:295, 1982.

316. Jones ET, Hensinger RN: Spinal deformity in idiopathic juvenile osteoporosis. Spine 6:1, 1981.

317. Yong-Hing K, MacEwen GD: Scoliosis associated with osteogenesis imperfecta. Results of treatment. J Bone Joint Surg [Br] 64:36, 1982.

318. Chaglassian JH, Riseborough EJ, Hall JE: Neurofibromatous scoliosis. Natural history and results of treatment in thirty-seven cases. J Bone Joint Surg [Am] 58:695, 1976.

319. Curtis BH, Fisher RL, Butterfield WL, et al: Neurofibromatosis with paraplegia. Report of eight cases. J Bone Joint Surg [Am] 51:843, 1969.

320. Scott JC: Scoliosis and neurofibromatosis. J Bone Joint Surg [Br] 47:240, 1965.

321. Hsu LCS, Lee PC, Leong JCY: Dystrophic spinal deformities in neurofibromatosis. Treatment by anterior and posterior fusion. J Bone Joint Surg [Br] 66:495, 1984.

322. Winter RB, Moe JH, Bradford DS, et al: Spine deformity in neurofibromatosis. A review of one hundred and two patients. J Bone Joint Surg [Am] 61:677, 1979.

323. Sirois JL III, Drennan JC: Dystrophic spinal deformity in neurofibromatosis. J Pediatr Orthop 10:522, 1990.

324. Calvert PT, Edgar MA, Webb PJ: Scoliosis in neurofibromatosis: The natural history with and without operation. J Bone Joint Surg [Br] 71:246, 1989.

325. Crawford AH Jr, Bagamery N: Osseous manifestations of neurofibromatosis in childhood. J Pediatr Radiol 6:72, 1986.

326. Stone JF, Bridwell KH, Shackelford GD, et al: Dural ectasia associated with spontaneous dislocation of the upper part of the thoracic spine in neurofibromatosis: A case report and review of the literature. J Bone Joint Surg [Am] 69:1079, 1987.

327. Akbarnia BA, Gabriel KR, Beckman E, et al: Prevalence of scoliosis in neurofibromatosis (abstract). J Pediatr Orthop 13:278, 1993.

328. Burk DL Jr, Brunberg JA, Kanal E, et al: Spinal and paraspinal neurofibromatosis: Surface coil MR imaging at 1.5 T. Radiology 162:797, 1987.

329. Mirowitz SA, Sartor K, Gado M: High-intensity basal ganglia lesions on T1-weighted MR images in neurofibromatosis. AJR 154:369, 1990.

330. Stull MA, Moser RP Jr, Kransdorf MJ, et al: Magnetic resonance appearance of peripheral nerve sheath tumors. Skel Radiol 20:9, 1991.

331. Shu HH, Mirowitz SA, Wippold FJ II: Neurofibromatosis: MR imaging findings involving the head and spine. AJR 160:159, 1993.

332. Fabris D, Candiotto S, Mammano S, et al: Antalgic scoliosis due to nonosteogenic fibroma of the L1 neural arch: Report of a case. J Pediatr Orthop 6:103, 1986.

333. Fabris D, Trainiti G, Di Comun M, et al: Scoliosis due to rib osteoblastoma: Report of two cases. J Pediatr Orthop 3:370, 1983.

334. Ransford AO, Pozo JL, Hutton PAN, et al: The behavior pattern of the scoliosis associated with osteoid osteoma or osteoblastoma of the spine. J Bone Joint Surg [Br] 66:16, 1984.

335. Kehl DK, Alonso JE, Lovell WW: Scoliosis secondary to an osteoid-osteoma of the rib. A case report. J Bone Joint Surg [Am] 65:701, 1983.

336. Kirwan EO, Hutton PAN, Ransford AO: Osteoid osteoma and benign osteo-

blastoma of the spine. Clinical presentation and treatment. J Bone Joint Surg [Br] 66:21, 1984.

337. Freiberger RH: Osteoid osteoma of the spine. A cause of backache and scoliosis in children and young adults. Radiology 75:232, 1960.

338. Keim HA, Reina EG: Osteoid-osteoma as a cause of scoliosis. J Bone Joint Surg [Am] 57:159, 1975.

339. MacLellen DI, Wilson FC Jr: Osteoid osteoma of the spine. A review of the literature and report of six new cases. J Bone Joint Surg [Am] 49:111, 1967.

340. McLeod RA, Dahlin DC, Beabout JW: The spectrum of osteoblastoma. AJR 126:321, 1976.

341. Pochaczevsky R, Yen YM, Sherman RS: The roentgen appearance of benign osteoblastoma. Radiology 75:429, 1960.

342. Von Ronnen JR: Case report 4: Osteoblastoma spinous process of C-2. Skel Radiol 1:61, 1976.

343. Azouz EM, Kozlowski K, Marton D, et al: Osteoid osteoma and osteoblastoma of the spine in children. Report of 22 cases with brief literature review. Pediatr Radiol 16:25, 1986.

344. Winter PF, Johnson PM, Hilal DK, et al: Scintigraphic detection of osteoid osteoma. Radiology 122:177, 1977.

345. Gilsanz V, Miranda J, Cleveland R, et al: Scoliosis secondary to fractures of the transverse processes of lumbar vertebrae. Radiology 134:627, 1980.

346. Tachdjian MO, Matson DD: Orthopaedic aspects of intraspinal tumors in infants and children. J Bone Joint Surg [Am] 47:223, 1965.

347. Papaioannou T, Stokes I, Kenwright J: Scoliosis associated with limb-length inequality. J Bone Joint Surg [Am] 64:59, 1982.

348. Giles LGF, Taylor JR: Lumbar spine structural changes associated with leg length inequality. Spine 7:159, 1982.

349. Letts M: Scoliosis in children secondary to retroperitoneal fibrosis. Report of two cases. J Bone Joint Surg [Am] 64:1363, 1982.

350. Durning RP, Scoles PV, Fox OD: Scoliosis after thoracotomy in tracheoesophageal fistula patients. A follow-up study. J Bone Joint Surg [Am] 62:1156, 1980.

351. Kinsella JP, Brasch RD, Ablin AA: Unilateral hypoplasia of the hemithorax causing ''pseudoscoliosis'' after lung irradiation in a child with Wilm's tumor. Pediatr Radiol 15:340, 1985.

352. DeRosa GP: Progressive scoliosis following chest wall resection in children. Spine 10:618, 1985.

353. Meehan PL, Lovell WW, Ahn JI: Congenital absence of the lung. J Pediatr Orthop 5:708, 1985.

354. Mayfield JK, Riseborough EJ, Jaffe N, et al: Spinal deformity in children treated for neuroblastoma. The effect of radiation and other forms of treatment. J Bone Joint Surg [Am] 63:183, 1981.

355. Neuhauser EBD, Wittenborg MH, Berman CZ, et al: Irradiation effects of roentgen therapy on the growing spine. Radiology 59:637, 1952.

356. Riseborough EJ, Grabias SL, Burton RI, et al: Skeletal alterations following irradiation for Wilm's tumor. With particular reference to scoliosis and kyphosis. J Bone Joint Surg [Am] 58:526, 1976.

357. Rubin P, Duthie RB, Young L: The significance of scoliosis in postirradiated Wilm's tumor and neuroblastoma. Radiology 79:539, 1962.

358. Vaeth JM, Levitt SH, Jones MD, et al: Effects of radiation therapy in survivors of Wilm's tumor. Radiology 79:560, 1962.

359. Katzman H, Waugh T, Berdon W: Skeletal changes following irradiation of childhood tumors. J Bone Joint Surg [Am] 51:825, 1969.

360. Libshitz HI, Cohen MA: Radiation-induced osteochondromas. Radiology 142:643, 1982.

361. DeSimone DP, Abdelwahab IF, Kenan S, et al: Case report 785: Radiation-induced osteochondroma of the ilium. Skel Radiol 22:289, 1993.

362. Makely JT, Heiple KG: Scoliosis associated with congenital deficiencies of the upper extremity. J Bone Joint Surg [Am] 52:279, 1970.

363. Paling MR, Spasovsky-Chernick M: Scoliosis in cystic fibrosis—an appraisal. Skel Radiol 8:63, 1982.

364. Mau H: Die Differentialdiagnose der beginnenden Skoliose beim M. Scheuermann gegenüber der idiopathischen Skoliose. Z Orthop 120:58, 1982.

365. Beneux J, Rigault P, Pouliquen JC, et al: Scolioses et cypho-scolioses des maladies constitutionnelles rares. Ann Chir Infant 18:261, 1977.

366. Taybi H, Lachman RS: Radiology of Syndromes, Metabolic Disorders, and Skeletal Dysplasias. 3rd Ed. Chicago, Year Book Medical Publishers, 1990.

367. Kao SCS, Waziri MH, Smith WL, et al: MR imaging of the craniovertebral junction, cranium, and brain in children with achondroplasia. AJR 153:565, 1989.

368. Suss RA, Udvarhelyi GB, Wang H, et al: Myelography in achondroplasia: Value of a lateral C1-2 puncture and non-ionic, water-soluble contrast medium. Radiology 149:159, 1983.

369. Morgan DF, Young RF: Spinal neurological complications of achondroplasia. J Neurosurg 52:463, 1980.

370. Lutter LD, Langer LO: Neurological symptoms in achondroplastic dwarfs—surgical treatment. J Bone Joint Surg [Am] 59:87, 1977.

371. DuVoisin RC, Yahr MD: Compressive spinal cord and root syndromes in achondroplastic dwarfs. Neurology 12:202, 1962.

372. Beighton P, Bathfield CA: Gibbal achondroplasia. J Bone Joint Surg [Br] 63:328, 1981.

373. Winter RB, Bloom B-A: Case report: Spine deformity in spondylometaphyseal dysplasia. J Pediatr Orthop 10:535, 1990.

374. Moseley JE, Bonforte RJ: Spondylothoracic dysplasia—a syndrome of congenital anomalies. AJR 106:166, 1969.

375. Pochaczevsky R, Ratner H, Perles D, et al: Spondylothoracic dysplasia. Radiology 98:53, 1971.

376. Fogarty EE, Beatty T, Dowling F: Spondylocostal dysplasia in identical twins. J Pediatr Orthop 5:720, 1985.

377. Drummond DS, MacKenzie DA: Scoliosis in arthrogryposis multiplex congenita. Spine 2:146, 1978.

378. Colver AF, Steer CR, Godman MJ, et al: Rigid spine syndrome and fatal cardiomyopathy. Arch Dis Child 56:148, 1981.

379. Daher YH, Lonstein JE, Winter RB, et al: Spinal deformities in patients with arthrogryposis. A review of 16 patients. Spine 10:609, 1985.

380. Herndon WA: Case report. Scoliosis and maple syrup urine disease. J Pediatr Orthop 4:126, 1984.

381. Kozlowski K, Masel J: Spondylo-epiphysealis dysplasia tarda (report of 7 cases). Australas Radiol 27:285, 1983.

382. Bartolozzi P, Calabrese C, Falcini F, et al: Case report. Melnick-Needles syndrome: Osteodysplasty with kyphoscoliosis. J Pediatr Orthop 3:387, 1983.

383. Davids JR, Hagerman RJ, Eilert RE: Orthopaedic aspects of fragile-X syndrome. J Bone Joint Surg [Am] 72:889, 1990.

384. Magid D, Pyeritz RE, Fishman EK: Musculoskeletal manifestations of the Marfan syndrome: Radiologic features. AJR 155:99, 1990.

385. Gurd AR, Thompson TR: Case report. Scoliosis in Prader-Willi syndrome. J Pediatr Orthop 1:317, 1981.

386. Rees D, Jones MW, Owen R, et al: Scoliosis surgery in the Prader-Willi syndrome. J Bone Joint Surg [Br] 71:685, 1989.

387. Holm VV, Laurnen EL: Prader-Willi syndrome and scoliosis. Dev Med Child Neurol 23:192, 1981.

90

Additional Congenital or Heritable Anomalies and Syndromes

Donald Resnick, M.D.

In the preceding chapters, important congenital and inherited disorders, including diseases of collagen and developing epiphyses, many of the bone dysplasias, and aberrations of spinal development, are discussed. In the following pages, additional congenital or heritable anomalies and syndromes are outlined that may lead to significant abnormalities in the growing skeleton and that, in some cases, may produce clinical and radiologic alterations that simulate those of certain acquired conditions. The discussion of each entity is brief, and the interested reader should consult standard available textbooks for more detailed analysis.[1–5, 171]

TERMINOLOGY

The separation of skeletal anomalies and skeletal variations is not accomplished uniformly with ease. An *anomaly* represents a marked deviation from normal standards, especially as a result of a congenital or hereditary defect, whereas a *variation* indicates a modification of some characteristics that are considered normal (variant of normal) or typical of a disease (variant of a disease). In some ways, then, the designation of a particular finding (or findings) as a skeletal anomaly or, alternatively, as a skeletal variation is arbitrary and accomplished on the basis of the presence and severity of accompanying clinical manifestations. Anomalies can be classified further as *deformations* (representing the normal response of a tissue to unusual mechanical forces), *malformations* (representing a primary problem in the morphogenesis of a tissue), and *disruptions* (occurring as a breakdown of a previously normal tissue).[172]

In Chapter 2, some of the sources of diagnostic errors are described that may be encountered during the radiographic evaluation of musculoskeletal symptoms and signs. These errors generally are related to misdiagnosis occurring when the appearance of entirely normal structures, modified by overlying shadows created by gas or soft tissues, is interpreted as abnormal; when anatomic rarefactions, irregularities, depressions, or proliferations of bone are regarded as evidence of disease; or when slight modifications in osseous anatomy (e.g., normal variations) are judged to be significant. Although the present chapter is concerned principally with more extensive alterations in anatomy (e.g., anomalies), a few additional comments regarding normal and variant radiographic findings are appropriate here.

AREAS OF NORMAL AND ANOMALOUS TRABECULAR DIMINUTION OR PROMINENCE

Although the precise factors that govern the development and ultimate form of the human skeleton are complex and not entirely understood, it is inevitable that concepts of engineering and mechanics have been used to analyze osseous structure. The composition of bone, consisting of a tubelike outer surface, or cortex, with ridges and other areas of thickening and an inner latticework of trabecular bone, appears well suited to the application of the tensile and compressive forces with which it must deal. It has been suggested that the internal or trabecular architecture of bone

coincides with routes of stress. Although this theory is not accepted fully, there can be little argument that trabeculae are not distributed uniformly in the human skeleton but rather are more prominent and numerous in certain regions and sparse or absent in others. The radiographic consequence of this inhomogeneity of trabecular structure is the appearance of radiolucent areas that are entirely normal yet easily misinterpreted as evidence of disease. The size and shape of such zones of trabecular diminution are somewhat variable but their locations are remarkably constant. Important examples include the normal areas of rarefaction in the femoral neck (Ward's triangle), the body of the calcaneus, and the proximal portion of the humerus adjacent to the greater tuberosity[194, 195] (Fig. 90–1). Alternatively, prominent trabeculae normally are encountered at many different sites, of which the distal portion of the humerus deserves emphasis (Fig. 90–2).

The external surface of bone is not uniformly smooth but, rather, possesses normal sites of elevation, depression, and irregularity. At joints, condyles (shaped like a knuckle), trochleae (with grooves simulating those of a pulley), fac-

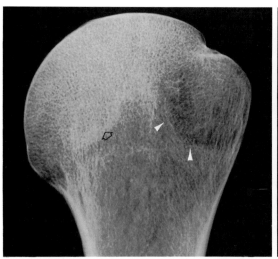

A

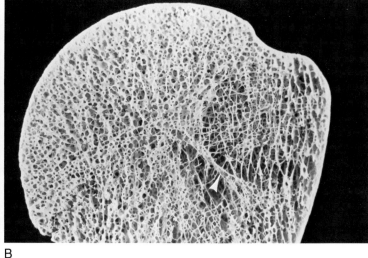

B

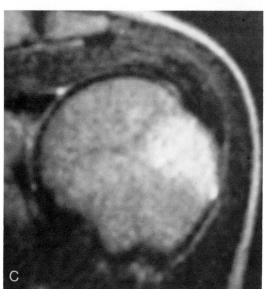

C

FIGURE 90–1. Normal sites of trabecular diminution. Proximal portion of the humerus.

A, B The area of rarefaction adjacent to the greater tuberosity is termed a humeral pseudocyst and is a normal finding. The curvilinear inferior margin (arrowheads) represents a distinct band of trabeculae that separate the relatively porous region laterally and the more compact spongiosa medially. A fusion line, marking the site of closure of a portion of the physis, is faintly visible (arrow). (From Resnick D, Cone RO III: Radiology *150*:27, 1984.)

C In a patient, a coronal oblique T2-weighted (TR/TE, 2000/80) spin echo MR image reveals that the humeral pseudocyst contains sparse trabeculae and fatty marrow whose signal intensity is greater than that in other portions of the proximal end of the humerus. (Courtesy of M. Stull, M.D., Washington, D.C.)

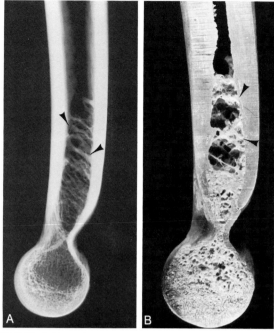

FIGURE 90–2. Normal sites of trabecular prominence. Distal portion of the humerus. As shown in this sagittal section, prominent trabeculae normally exist in this region (arrowheads). On frontal radiographs, they lead to a V-shaped radiodense area.

ets, or foveae are evident. Along with areas of osseous irregularity that occur at regions of tendon and ligament attachments, these normal sites of bone protuberances or excrescences may lead to diagnostic difficulty during the interpretation of the radiographs. Important examples of such sites include the linea aspera in the posterior surface of the middle third of the femur (Fig. 90–3), which serves as the insertion of strong adductor and extensor muscles[173, 174]; the soleal line on the posterior surface of the proximal third of the tibia, to which attaches the strong fascia that covers the popliteus and the soleus[175]; and the deltoid tuberosity in the lateral surface of the midportion of the humerus.

Although accompanying radiographic findings at these regions may be misinterpreted as evidence of periostitis or hyperostosis, the propensity for error is far less than that occurring with cystic areas and cortical irregularities in the posterior aspect of the distal part of the femur at the site of attachment of tendinous fibers of the adductor magnus muscle. A variety of terms have been applied to these latter lesions, including fibrous cortical defects; subperiosteal, periosteal, and cortical defects; subperiosteal, periosteal, and cortical desmoids; and (benign) metaphyseal and avulsive cortical irregularities.[176–190] Although some early reports grouped together cystic and proliferative lesions of the distal posterior femoral metaphysis and, in fact, considered them to represent a single entity observed in different stages of development and healing,[181, 190] subsequent investigators have stressed the different clinical and radiographic features of the typical cystic cortical lesion and the proliferative cortical irregularity. The former lesion is considered a fibrous cortical defect, predominating in children and young adolescents and appearing as a cortical lucency or excavation. It occurs lateral to the medial supracondylar ridge of the femur, analogous to cortical defects at other

skeletal sites. The proliferative cortical lesion may be observed in slightly older patients, occurs along the medial supracondylar ridge, and appears as cortical spiculation or irregularity that may simulate neoplasm.

The proximity of the extensor tendon of the adductor magnus muscle to the site of the typical femoral proliferative lesion is consistent with a traumatic pathogenesis (Fig. 90–4). Although histologic studies fail to document aponeurotic, muscular, or tendinous fibers at the precise site of the lesion, the observed pathologic aberrations, although not specific, appear to represent a response to stress. Proliferation of fibrous and osteoid tissue and periosteum, osteoclastic activity, local hemorrhage, bony spicules, and a soft tissue mass could result from a traumatic insult to the periosteum. Strengthening of the bone and firm adherence of the periosteum that occur with maturity could explain the relative infrequency of the changes in adults. The presence of this lesion in physically active adolescents and of an exaggerated abnormality in extremely athletic persons[187] (Fig. 90–5) also supports a traumatic pathogenesis. There are no histologic data that indicate a neoplastic or infectious cause.

In studies of cadavers[191] and patients,[192] a second area of rarefaction has been identified lateral to the medial supracondylar line and adductor tubercle, approximately 1 cm above the superior limit of the medial condyle (Fig. 90–6). This location corresponds to the osseous site of attachment of the medial head of the gastrocnemius muscle and is lateral to the site of the attachment of the tendon of the

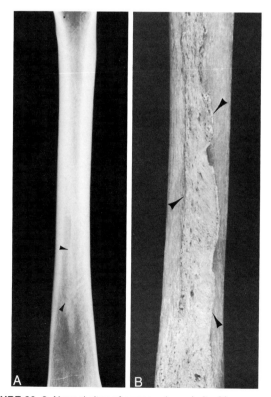

FIGURE 90–3. Normal sites of osseous irregularity: Linea aspera in the femur. The linear radiodense region (arrowheads) in the frontal radiograph **(A)** represents the site of the linea aspera, which is an elevated and irregular normal bone protuberance (arrowheads) in the posterior, middiaphyseal region of the femur, as shown in the specimen photograph **(B)**.

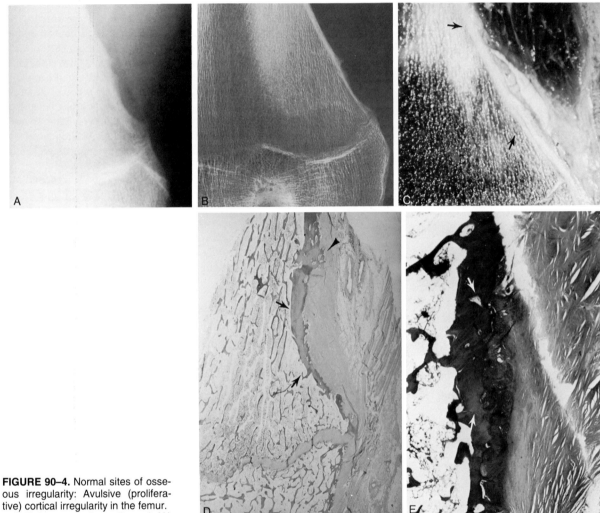

FIGURE 90–4. Normal sites of osseous irregularity: Avulsive (proliferative) cortical irregularity in the femur.

A, B A preoperative radiograph **(A)**
and specimen radiograph **(B)** delineate the characteristics of this lesion. Observe the normal cortical thickening and small periosteal
excrescences extending into the soft tissue. The spongiosa is entirely normal, and a soft tissue mass is not apparent.

C A photograph of a coronal section demonstrates cortical thickening and irregularity (arrows). No tendinous fibers are identified at
the site of the lesion.

D, E Low **(D)** and high power **(E)** photomicrographs delineate a shallow cortical defect with an irregular cortical base (arrows) and
persistent thickening with new bone formation (arrowhead). Fibrous connective tissue is seen within the lesion, composed of uniform
spindle-shaped cells with eosinophilic fibrillar cytoplasm. Osteoclastic activity is evident.

(From Resnick D, Greenway G: Radiology *143*:345, 1982.)

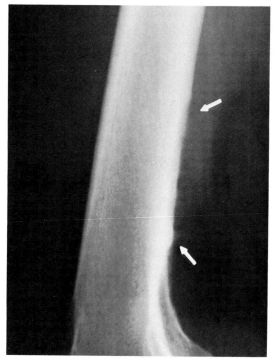

FIGURE 90–5. Normal sites of osseous irregularity: Avulsive (proliferative) cortical irregularity in the femur. This 24 year old woman was engaged in many athletic activities, including gymnastics. She had a 2 week history of knee pain. Conservative therapy was instituted with clinical improvement occurring within the next 4 to 6 weeks. Extensive cortical irregularity along the posteromedial aspect of the distal end of the femur is seen (between arrows). Observe excavation of the cortex and thick horizontal strands of new bone extending into the soft tissues. (From Resnick D, Greenway G: Radiology *143*:345, 1982.)

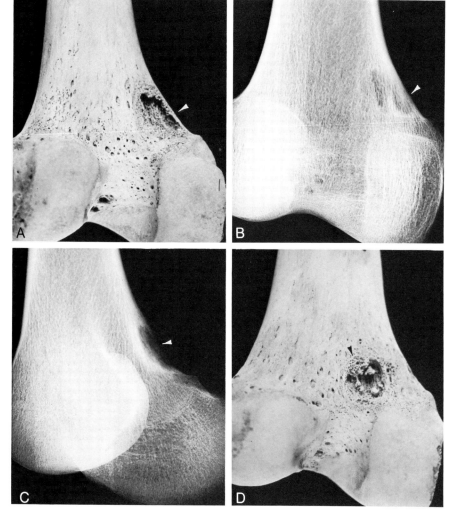

FIGURE 90–6. Normal sites of osseous irregularity: Excavation in the femur.

A–C A photograph of the posterior surface **(A)** of the distal portion of the femur and accompanying frontal **(B)** and oblique **(C)** radiographs reveal the typical location and configuration of the distal femoral cortical excavation (arrowheads), measuring 1.2 × 1.9 cm. Note its intracortical location and well-circumscribed appearance. No associated periostitis is seen.

D A photograph of the posterior surface of the distal portion of the femur demonstrates a similar cortical excavation (arrowhead), measuring approximately 1.4 cm in diameter. Observe the bony spicules at the base of the lesion.

(From Resnick D, Greenway G: Radiology *143*:345, 1982.)

adductor magnus muscle. The circular or oval lesions are variable in size, although they may be larger than 2 cm in diameter. The osseous floor of the lesion commonly is irregular, with several protruding bone spicules. The precise pathogenesis of this distal femoral cortical excavation is not clear, although a stress-related phenomenon appears most likely: The site of the abnormality corresponds to the area of attachment of the medial head of the gastrocnemius muscle; the presence of small osseous irregularities at the base of the lesion could be the result of traction on muscle fibers; and the cystlike appearance evident on gross pathologic and radiologic examination could represent focal osteoporosis owing to the hyperemia provoked by the traumatic insult. Radiolucent lesions have been described at osseous sites of insertion of other muscles.[193]

SKELETAL CANALS, APERTURES, AND FORAMINA

A channel that extends through a bone is termed a foramen or, when large, an aperture. When the channel is oriented obliquely and, therefore, is of considerable length, it is referred to as a canal. Nutrient canals, through which pass the nutrient arteries, extend in an oblique fashion from one or more foramina on the osseous surface (Fig. 90–7). In the long tubular bones of the extremities, the nutrient canals typically point away from the dominant growing end

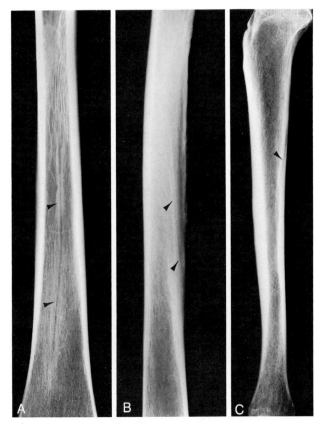

FIGURE 90–7. Normal nutrient canals.
A, B Femur. A frontal **(A)** and lateral **(B)** radiograph of two different femoral specimens indicate the position and configuration of the normal nutrient canal (arrowheads), which pierces the posterior cortex and extends proximally. It may simulate a fracture.
C Tibia. The nutrient canal (arrowhead) extends through the posterior cortex of the bone in a proximal to distal direction.

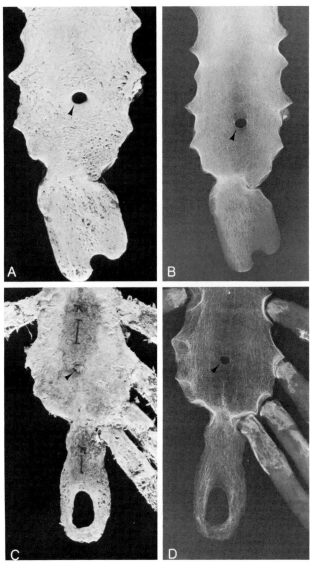

FIGURE 90–8. Sternal foramina. Specimen photographs **(A, C)** and radiographs **(B, D)** of two examples are given (arrowheads). Note their location in the lower portion of the sternal body and their oval configuration. Bifid xiphoid processes also are apparent and, in one case **(C, D)**, have led to a second foramen in the distal portion of the sternum.

of the bone, a fact that forms the basis of the mnemonic phrase ''To the elbow I go, from the knee I flee.'' Resulting radiolucent channels rarely lead to diagnostic difficulty, although, on occasion, they resemble a fracture line. Numerous and sometimes prominent nutrient foramina are encountered in several sites, of which those in the distal portion of the femur should be emphasized. In flat bones such as the scapula and ilium, nutrient canals create linear or branching radiolucent areas that, although distinctive, can produce diagnostic uncertainty during routine radiography or even CT scanning.[196, 424]

Sites of osseous thinning or true foramina are common in bones containing thin plates, or laminae, such as the parietal and occipital bones of the skull,[197–200] the sternum,[201–204] and the scapula.[205] Foramina of the sternum usually are single, oval to circular, and located in the lower portion of the sternal body (Fig. 90–8). Scapular foramina occur at the superior border of the bone at its junction with

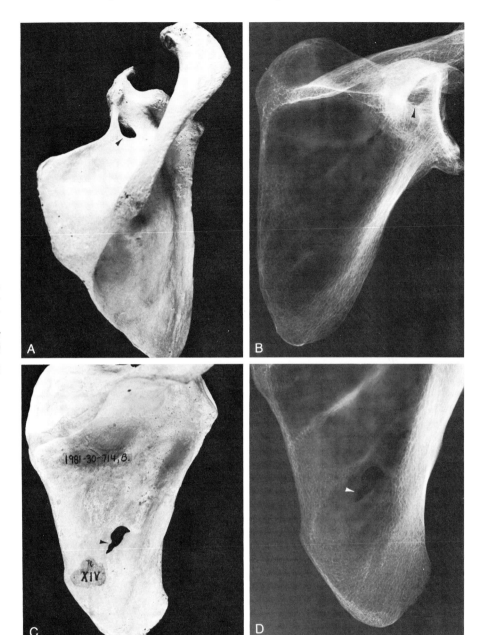

FIGURE 90–9. Scapular foramina.

A, B Foramen adjacent to the coracoid process. This foramen (arrowheads) relates to ossification of the superior transverse ligament.

C, D Foramen within the scapular body. A typical example (arrowheads) is shown.

(From Pate D, et al: Skel Radiol *14*:270, 1985.)

the coracoid process and are attributable to ossification of the superior transverse ligament, in the body of the bone inferior to the scapular spine, in the superior fossa as a clasplike defect, and at the superomedial border above the scapular spine (Fig. 90–9). These should be differentiated from scapular thinning, which most typically is evident in the body of the bone and results in large radiolucent areas of variable shape (Fig. 90–10).

Another commonly encountered aperture, designated a herniation pit, is seen in the anterior surface of the femoral neck.[425] Ingrowth of fibrous and cartilaginous elements occurs through a perforation in the cortex in a roughened reaction area of sclerotic bone, resulting in unilateral or bilateral, small, rounded radiolucent areas in the anterolateral aspect of the femoral neck.[425, 426] Although the lucent regions generally are stable, they may enlarge in persons of all ages, perhaps related to changing mechanics such as the pressure and abrasive effect of the overlying hip capsule

and anterior muscles.[427] Such enlargement, which may occur rapidly,[427] is evident more frequently in patients with a history of athletic physical activity.[425, 427] Bone scintigraphy, although typically negative in persons with herniation pits, occasionally may be positive with increased accumulation of the radiopharmaceutical agent.[427, 428] MR imaging generally shows a focus of low signal intensity on T1-weighted spin echo MR images and high signal intensity, consistent with that of fluid, on T2-weighted spin echo images.[427, 429]

ACCESSORY OSSIFICATION CENTERS AND FRAGMENTED SESAMOID BONES

Although the appearance of more than one center of ossification during the development of an epiphysis can be a manifestation of disease (as in the epiphyseal dysgenesis that accompanies hypothyroidism), such centers frequently are encountered in asymptomatic children and adolescents

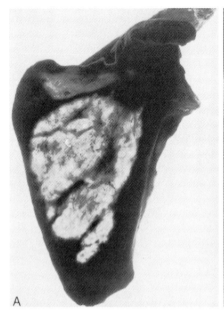
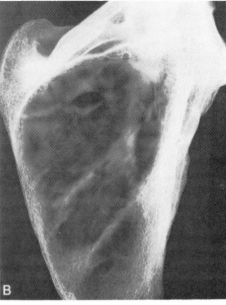

FIGURE 90–10. Scapular thinning. These areas of normal osseous thinning produce large radiolucent regions of varying shape. (From Pate D, et al: Skel Radiol *14*:270, 1985.)

and, as such, generally are regarded as a variation of normal. Accessory ossicles also are seen, especially in the hands, wrist, and feet (see later discussion) but also elsewhere such as the sternum (episternal ossicles)[459]; these occur in approximately 1 per cent of normal persons.[17] Multiple centers of epiphyseal ossification and accessory ossicles should be differentiated from sesamoid bones, such as the patella and fabella, which usually are embedded in tendons in close relation to a joint or occur at sites of tendinous angulation about an osseous surface.

Although, in the past, emphasis has been given to the differentiation of accessory ossicles or ossification centers from fractures, the possibility that some of these ossific foci are acquired after injury and that they may be associated with significant clinical manifestations has led to a recent, renewed interest in these ''normal variations.''[409] The os trigonum near the posterior surface of the talus,[430, 431] the os vesalianum adjacent to the cuboid and base of the fifth metatarsal,[206] the os intermetatarsale between the bases of the first and second metatarsals, and the os supratrochleare dorsale in the olecranon fossa[207] are examples of accessory ossicles that reportedly have been accompanied by pain (Fig. 90–11). Although many ossicles may have clinical significance, several deserve emphasis.

1. *Accessory navicular bone (os tibiale externum or naviculare secundarium).* Two distinct types of accessory navicular bone have been described: A separate ossicle may occur as a sesamoid bone in the posterior tibial tendon (type I); and an accessory ossification center may appear in the tubercle of the navicular bone (type II)[208, 417] (Figs. 90–12 and 90–13). Type I ossicles account for approximately 30 per cent of cases, generally are well defined, are round or oval, measure 2 to 6 mm in diameter, and are situated up to 5 mm medial and posterior to the medial aspect of the navicular. Type II accessory ossification centers represent approximately 70 per cent of cases, are triangular or heart-shaped, measure 9 to 12 mm in size, and are located within 1 to 2 mm from the medial and posterior aspect of the

navicular.[208] An anomaly termed a cornuate navicular involves the medial aspect of the navicular bone and is related to the presence of an osseous bridge connecting an accessory bone with the medial aspect of the navicular.

Of these three patterns, it is the type II ossification center and the cornuate navicular that have been associated with clinical manifestations, particularly pain, which usually becomes evident in the second decade of life. Increased accumulation of a bone-seeking radionuclide during scintigraphy represents a sensitive (but not entirely specific) finding of a painful accessory navicular bone.[545] Histologic analysis has revealed inflammatory chondro-osseous changes compatible with chronic stress-related injury.[208, 432]

With regard to the sesamoid bone that characterizes the type I anomaly, a relationship with pes planus, due to the abnormal insertion of the tibialis posterior tendon into the accessory ossicle, has been proposed but is unproved.[209, 210]

2. *Carpal boss (os styloideum).* A commonly occurring bony protuberance on the dorsum of the wrist at the base of the second and third metacarpals adjacent to the capitate and trapezoid bones is termed a carpal boss or carpe bossu[211–214, 433, 434] (see Chapter 39). It relates to either an osteophyte or an accessory ossification center, the os styloideum. Although generally asymptomatic or associated only with a lump or bump, the carpal boss occasionally can lead to pain and limitation of hand motion owing to an overlying ganglion, bursitis, osteoarthritis, or slippage of an extensor tendon.[214] Radiographs obtained with 30 degrees of supination and ulnar deviation of the wrist demonstrate the osteophyte or os styloideum to good advantage[214] and may be supplemented with bone scintigraphy (Fig. 90–14), conventional tomography, or CT scanning.

3. *Bipartite and dorsal defect of the patella.* The occurrence of multiple ossification centers in a sesamoid bone, of which the bipartite patella is the best example, has long been regarded as a normal variation with little or no clinical significance. Ogden and collaborators[215] and others[216, 409, 552] have challenged this concept, emphasizing that local pain may accompany this patellar variation and, further, that

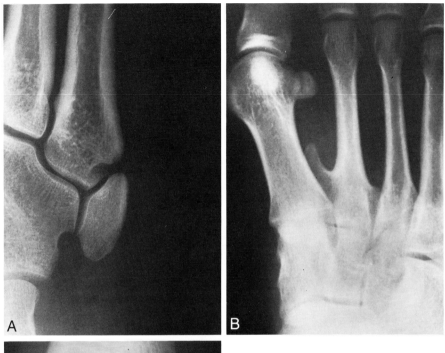

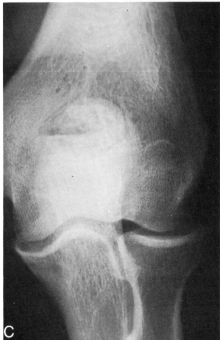

FIGURE 90–11. Accessory ossicles.
   A Os vesalianum.
   B Os intermetatarsale.
   C Os supratrochleare posterius (dorsale).

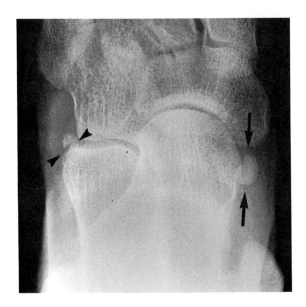

FIGURE 90–12. Accessory navicular bone: Type I (sesamoid bone in the tibialis posterior tendon). In this 22 year old woman with pain over the lateral aspect of the foot after a fall, an anteroposterior radiograph of the foot shows a fracture of the anterolateral margin of the calcaneus (arrowheads). A well-defined oval ossicle (arrows) is noted adjacent to the posteromedial margin of the navicular bone. (From Lawson JP, et al: Skel Radiol *12*:250, 1984.)

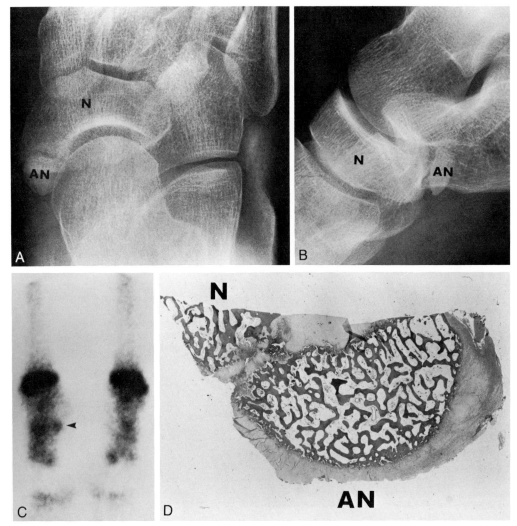

FIGURE 90–13. Accessory navicular bone: Type II (accessory ossification center in the tubercle of the navicular bone). This 12 year old girl developed progressive pain over the medial aspect of the foot, which was aggravated by gymnastics and skiing.

A, B Anteroposterior **(A)** and lateral **(B)** radiographs demonstrate the triangular, accessory navicular bone (AN) adjacent to the medial and posterior margin of the navicular (N).

C A bone scan shows increased accumulation of the radiopharmaceutical agent in the region of this accessory bone (arrowhead).

D A low power photomicrograph of the specimen after surgical excision shows the accessory navicular bone (AN), intervening cartilage, and a portion of the true navicular bone (N). At higher power (not shown) the histologic findings, which included proliferating vascular mesenchymal tissue and cartilage and osteoblastic activity, were consistent with chronic trauma.

(From Lawson JP, et al: Skel Radiol *12*:250, 1984.)

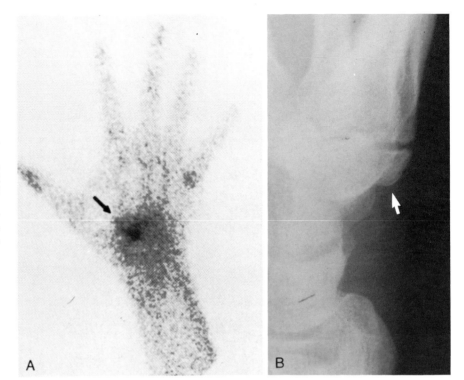

FIGURE 90–14. Carpal boss (os styloideum).

A Increased accumulation of a bone-seeking radionuclide (arrow) is evident at the site of the carpal boss, at the base of the second and third metacarpal bones.

B In a different patient, a typical os styloideum (arrow) is seen. (Courtesy of J. Spaeth, M.D., Albuquerque, New Mexico, and G. Greenway, M.D., Dallas, Texas.)

histologic analysis suggests the presence of a chronic chondro-osseous tensile failure of the bone in skeletally immature persons, similar to that occurring in Osgood-Schlatter and Sinding-Larsen-Johansson lesions. The bipartite patella usually, but not invariably, is bilateral in distribution. The predilection for the superolateral aspect of the bone (Fig. 90–15), with rare exceptions, remains the radiographic hallmark of the finding, usually allowing differentiation from

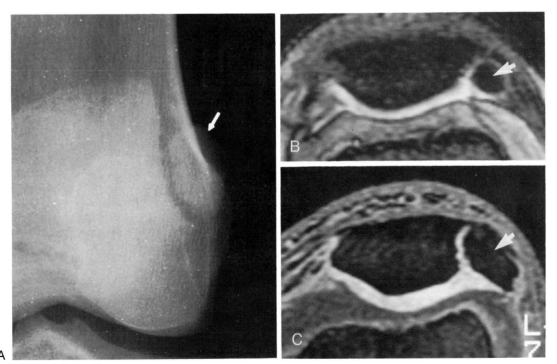

FIGURE 90–15. Bipartite patella.

A Localization to the superolateral aspect of the patella (arrow) is the most characteristic radiographic finding.

B In a transaxial gradient echo (MPGR) MR image (TR/TE, 500/17; flip angle, 20 degrees) obtained with chemical presaturation of fat (ChemSat), the separate ossification center (arrow) in the superolateral aspect of the patella is evident. Cartilage with high signal intensity is seen between the ossicle and remaining portion of the patella and on the posterior articular surface of the bone.

C In a different patient, a transaxial gradient echo (spoiled gradient recalled acquisition in the steady state—SPGR) MR image (TR/TE, 58/10; flip angle, 60 degrees) obtained with volumetric acquisition and chemical presaturation of fat (ChemSat), resulting in a section thickness of 1.5 mm, shows a larger ossicle (arrow) in the superolateral portion of the patella. The cartilage again reveals high signal intensity. The accompanying joint effusion is of low signal intensity. (Courtesy of M. Recht, M.D., Cleveland, Ohio.)

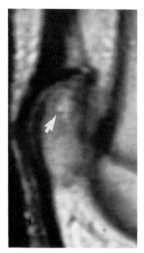

FIGURE 90–16. Dorsal defect of the patella.
A sagittal T2-weighted (TR/TE, 2000/60) spin echo MR image shows a subchondral lesion (arrow) with high signal intensity in the superior portion of the patella. The lesion was of low signal intensity on T1-weighted images (not shown).

acute fractures and anomalies[217] of the patella. Rarely, other forms of partition of the patella, either in the sagittal[435] or coronal[436] plane, are encountered.

The dorsal defect of the patella initially was believed to be a variation in normal ossification of the bone,[437, 438] perhaps related to bipartite patellae, and occurring in 0.3 to 1 per cent of persons,[439, 440] either unilaterally or bilaterally.[441–443] More recently, a traumatic pathogenesis related to traction occurring in the insertion site of the vastus lateralis muscle has been emphasized.[440] In common with a bipartite patella, the dorsal defect occurs in the superolateral aspect of the bone (Fig. 90–16), and the two conditions may coexist in the same person.[440] Histologically, the dorsal defect is characterized by the presence of nonspecific fibrous components with or without areas of bone necrosis. Although patients with this finding generally are asymptomatic, local pain and tenderness may be present.

The radiographic characteristics of the dorsal defect of the patella include a well-circumscribed lesion in the superolateral portion of the bone, adjacent to the articular cartilage. CT confirms the typical location of the defect and may demonstrate fissuring of the adjacent superficial, or external, surface of the bone. This latter feature is compatible with a relationship between the dorsal defect and bipartite patella, perhaps representing stages of the same process. MR imaging reveals some variability in the signal intensity characteristics of the dorsal patellar defect: On T1-weighted spin echo MR images, the lesion may be inhomogeneous with signal that is isointense or slightly hyperintense to that of articular cartilage, or that, in some areas, is hypointense to that of articular cartilage; on gradient echo images, the signal intensity of the lesion generally is equal to or greater than that of the cartilage.[444] Although, in general, the articular cartilage adjacent to the dorsal defect is intact, this is not uniformly the case.[546]

Healing of the dorsal defect of the patella may occur spontaneously or after surgical intervention. New bone initially develops at the margins of the lesion and proceeds centrally.[440] Dorsal defects rarely are observed after the third decade of life.

4. *Os trigonum.* The normal ossification process of the body of the talus progresses posteriorly. A separate ossification center in the posterior border of the talar body may occur, however, appearing between the ages of 8 and 10 years in girls and 11 and 13 years in boys.[445] This center usually fuses with the remainder of the bone within a year of its appearance.[445] If it persists after skeletal maturation, it is designated an os trigonum.[430, 431]

Historically, an os trigonum generally has been regarded as an insignificant developmental variation,[431] although, rarely, it has been described as a fracture.[446] It more frequently is bilateral than unilateral and has been reported to occur in 1 to 25 per cent of adults.[431, 447, 448]

A specific syndrome, the os trigonum or talar compression syndrome, has been associated with a persistent and often large os trigonum[447, 449] (Fig. 90–17) (see Chapter 70). This syndrome relates to compression of the posterior structures of the ankle during repeated plantar flexion of the foot and is seen most typically in ballet dancers.[449] In this foot position, the os trigonum is caught between the posterior edge of the tibia above and the calcaneus below, resulting in localized pain and tenderness. The injury may affect the bone itself or the synchondrosis that exists between the talus and the os trigonum.[431] Scintigraphy using bone-seeking radionuclides can be used to further diagnose the condition, and removal of the accessory ossification center generally is curative.[449]

5. *Os subtibiale and os subfibulare.* Accessory ossicles are encountered beneath the medial malleolus (os subtibiale) and lateral malleolus (os subfibulare) in asymptomatic

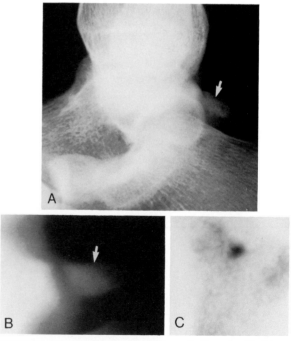

FIGURE 90–17. Os trigonum syndrome. A 16 year old girl complained of pain and tenderness in the posterior region of the ankle. Routine radiography **(A)** and conventional tomography **(B)** reveal a prominent os trigonum (arrows) with an irregular gap between it and the posterior margin of the talus. Bone scintigraphy **(C)**, accomplished in the lateral projection, shows uptake of the radionuclide in the area of the os trigonum. Surgery confirmed the presence of fibrous tissue between the talus and the os trigonum, and symptoms disappeared after excision of the latter. (Courtesy of G. Greenway, M.D., Dallas, Texas.)

children. Although these ossicles generally have been regarded as variations in ossification, there is evidence to suggest that at least those on the lateral side of the ankle are of traumatic pathogenesis. Ogden and Lee[450] found that irregularities of ossification of the medial malleolus were far more frequent than those of the lateral malleolus and more commonly were bilateral. Furthermore, pain, although associated with both medial and lateral ossicles, was more characteristic of the lateral ossicles. Griffiths and Menelaus[451] observed symptomatic lateral ossicles of the ankle in three children, all of whom had suffered recurrent ankle sprains and responded clinically to surgical excision of the ossicle with reconstruction of the fibular collateral ligament. Berg[452] confirmed similar findings in four adults with both symptomatic ankle instability and an associated os subfibulare; operative exploration in each patient revealed that the ossicle represented a nonunion of an avulsion fracture at the site of attachment of the anterior talofibular ligament.

Although ossicles about the medial and lateral malleoli occasionally may represent variations in ossification,[453] it appears likely that most, especially those on the lateral aspect of the ankle, are traumatic in origin.

6. *Ossicles about the elbow.* Separate ossicles commonly are seen in and about the elbow. Typical sites of involvement are the regions of the olecranon fossa and the coronoid fossa. Ossicles in the olecranon fossa have been designated os supratrochleare posterius[454, 455] (Fig. 90–11*C*), and those in the coronoid fossa, the os supratrochleare anterius or fabella cubiti.[456, 457] Although these ossicles have been regarded as normal variations, injuries to the elbow are common and may result in free intra-articular osseous bodies that eventually lodge in the fossae in the anterior and posterior surfaces of the distal end of the humerus. Therefore, it is probable that many of the accessory ossicles about the elbow in reality have resulted from injury.[458]

7. *Os acromiale.* A persistent ossification center at the free end of the acromion occurs in as many as 15 per cent of persons. Typically, this center fuses with the acromion before the person reaches 25 years of age; a separate site of ossification after this age is designated an os acromiale (Fig. 90–18). The os acromiale is variable in size and most commonly is triangular in shape. It usually forms a synchondrosis with the acromion and may articulate also with the clavicle. Pain and a higher prevalence of the shoulder impingement syndrome and tears of the rotator cuff have been associated with an os acromiale (see Chapter 70). Its appearance simulates that of a fracture of the acromion.

SKELETAL APLASIA AND HYPOPLASIA

An entire bone or a portion thereof may fail to form in the normal fashion, producing a variety of congenital deficiencies.[218] These have been studied extensively and classified by Frantz and O'Rahilly[6] and later by other investigators.[7, 8] Initially, in 1961,[6] deficiencies were subdivided into two basic types: terminal deficiencies, in which all skeletal elements were absent distally along a designated axis; and intercalary deficiencies, in which parts ordinarily interposed between the proximal and distal aspects of the remaining limb were absent. Each of these two types was further divided into transverse and longitudinal varieties on the basis of whether the absent bone(s) extended across the width of a limb or ran parallel to the long axis of the limb.[8] This schema subsequently was changed in 1966,[7] at which time the general term meromelia was used to describe all partial absences. The four major categories that had been described previously—terminal, intercalary, transverse, and longitudinal—were retained, and a new category, central defects, was added. In 1974, an international classification system was formulated.[9, 10] In it, all limb deficiencies were classified as transverse or longitudinal. The transverse category encompassed those congenital anomalies that previously had been described as terminal transverse deficiencies, and the longitudinal category consisted of all of the remaining deficiencies.

Of the major tubular bones, aplasia or hypoplasia most typically affects the fibula, radius, femur, ulna, and humerus in order of descending frequency.

Fibular Aplasia and Hypoplasia

The severity of this most common osseous deficiency is variable.[11–15, 219, 460] Congenital absence or severe hypoplasia of the fibula can be combined with ventral and medial bowing of the companion tibia, a skin dimple at the apex of the bow, an equinovalgus foot, absence of one or two of the lateral rays of the foot, tarsal aplasia or fusion, and retarded development or shortening of the ipsilateral femur (Fig. 90–19). Milder varieties of fibular hypoplasia also may be more difficult to recognize. Distal or proximal deficiencies can be seen; distal fibular hypoplasia may be associated with a valgus deformity of the ankle, whereas proximal fibular hypoplasia can be accompanied by valgus knee deformity and instability at the proximal tibiofibular articulation.[16]

Radial and Ulnar Aplasia and Hypoplasia

Radial anomalies may include total or partial aplasia or hypoplasia (Fig. 90–20). Bilateral abnormalities are common and may be combined with hypoplasia or absence of the thumb or radial carpal bones. Such radial lesions can be

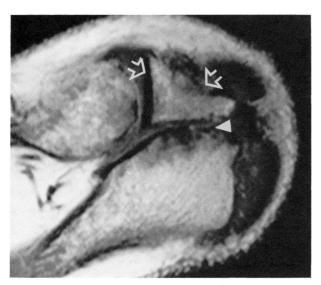

FIGURE 90–18. Os acromiale. A transaxial proton density weighted (TR/TE, 1000/20) spin echo MR image shows a triangular os acromiale (arrows) articulating with the clavicle and, in an irregular fashion (arrowhead), with the acromion. (Courtesy of S. Eilenberg, M.D., San Diego, California.)

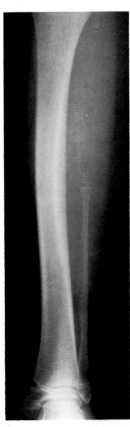
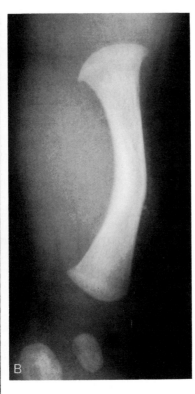

FIGURE 90–19. Hypoplasia and aplasia: Fibula.
  A Note severe hypoplasia of the fibula with medial bowing of the midshaft of the tibia.
  B In a different patient, a 1 month old infant, aplasia of the fibula is accompanied by medial bowing of the tibia.
  (**B,** Courtesy of H. S. Kang, M.D., Seoul, Korea.)

A

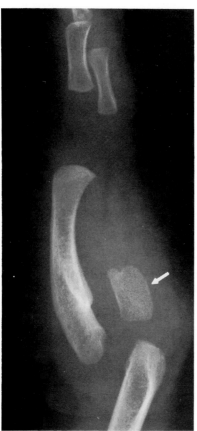

FIGURE 90–20. Hypoplasia: Radius. Severe hypoplasia of the radius (arrow) is associated with a deformed ulna and absence of some bones in the hand and the wrist.

associated with systemic disorders in some cases. These include the VATER syndrome (Fig. 90–21); cardiac abnormalities, including ventricular septal defect, atrial septal defect, pulmonary artery atresia, and patent ductus arteriosus; and thrombocytopenia with absent radius (TAR syndrome)[17–20, 411, 461] (Fig. 90–22). With regard to the VATER syndrome, major components are vertebral anomalies, anal atresia, tracheoesophageal fistula with or without esophageal atresia, radial dysplasia, renal anomalies including aplasia, and congenital heart disease. Other, less constant components include the Klippel-Feil syndrome, Sprengel deformity, hemifacial microsomia, the Goldenhar triad (epibulbar dermoids, preauricular appendages, and vertebral abnormalities), and genital anomalies.[461]

Deficiency of the ulna is less frequent and severe than that of the radius. Three types of deformity are recognized: hypoplasia, partial aplasia, and total aplasia.[21] Ulnar deviation of the hand occurs, suggesting that a tethering effect exists in which a radiographically invisible fibrocartilaginous band attaches distally to the distal radial epiphysis, the ulnar side of the carpus, or both, extending from the proximal ulnar primary ossification center. Resection of this band may reduce the angular growth deformities, although this surgical procedure is not recommended uniformly.[220]

Proximal Femoral Focal Deficiency (PFFD)

Proximal femoral focal deficiency is the term applied to a spectrum of conditions characterized by partial absence and shortening of the proximal portion of the femur.[22–26, 221–223] Additional designations for this congenital but not inherited disorder are dysgenesis of the proximal femur, congenital

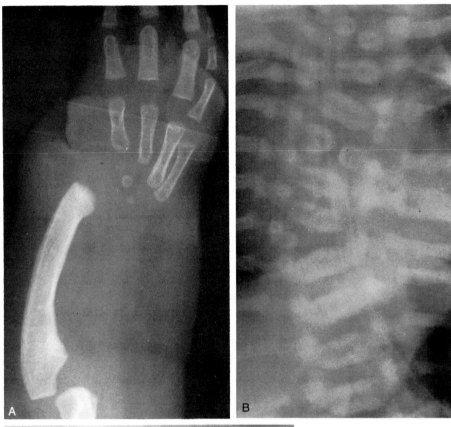

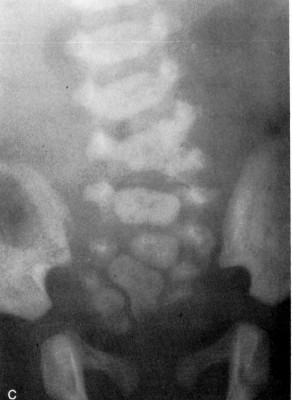

FIGURE 90–21. Vertebral-anal-tracheal-esophageal-radial-renal (VATER) syndrome. This 2½ year old child demonstrates radial aplasia, absence of the thumb, and severe spinal anomalies. Additional abnormalities included a tracheoesophageal fistula and renal and anal anomalies.

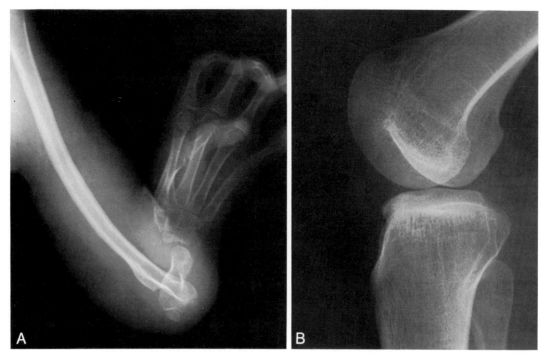

FIGURE 90–22. Thrombocytopenia with absent radius (TAR syndrome).
A In this child, absence of the radius and deformity of the forearm are evident.
B Absence of the patella also is seen.

short femur, congenital hypoplasia of the upper femur, and femoral hypoplasia with coxa vara. PFFD is distinguished from total femoral agenesis and coxa vara without shortening of the femoral shaft.[224] Although some cases of PFFD are associated with other skeletal defects, including aplasia of the cruciate ligaments of the knee,[225] this disorder usually is an isolated occurrence, appearing in a unilateral fashion in 90 per cent of patients. A variety of classification systems have been suggested on the basis of presence and location of the femoral head and neck[23, 222, 223] (Table 90–1) (Figs. 90–23 and 90–24). The designation of a specific type of PFFD in an individual patient may require both radiography and arthrography.[463] The role of MR imaging in the classification of the disorder is promising but not entirely clear.[463]

Radiographs of a newborn infant demonstrate a short femur that is displaced superiorly, posteriorly, and laterally to the iliac crest. The distal end of the femur usually is normal. Ossification of the femoral capital epiphysis invariably is delayed. After the second year of life, affected children reveal either dysgenesis or absence of subtrochanteric ossification, the severity of the abnormalities varying with the type of PFFD that is present. At skeletal maturity, changes include subtrochanteric varus deformity or pseudarthrosis, a large unossified gap between the femoral capital epiphysis and dysplastic shaft, or ossification of only the distal femoral epiphysis.[22] Secondary abnormalities of the pelvis and acetabulum are common, correlating with the degree of femoral head deformity or hypoplasia. The major differential diagnosis of the radiographic findings is developmental coxa vara, in which familial and bilateral characteristics may be seen and in which abnormalities are less

TABLE 90–1. Classification of Proximal Femoral Focal Deficiency

Class	Head of Femur	Acetabulum	Femoral Segment	Relationship Among Components of Femur and Acetabulum at Skeletal Maturity
A	Present	Adequate	Short	Bony connection between components of femur; head in acetabulum; subtrochanteric varus, often with pseudarthrosis
B	Present	Adequate or moderately dysplastic	Short; usually proximal bony tuft	No osseous connection between head and shaft; head in acetabulum
C	Absent or represented by ossicle	Severely dysplastic	Short; usually proximally tapered	May be osseous connection between shaft and proximal ossicle; no osseous connection between femur and acetabulum
D	Absent	Absent; obturator foramen enlarged; pelvis squared in bilateral cases	Short, deformed	

(From Levinson ED, Ozonoff MB, Royers PM: Proximal femoral focal deficiency [PFFD]. Radiology 125:197, 1977.)

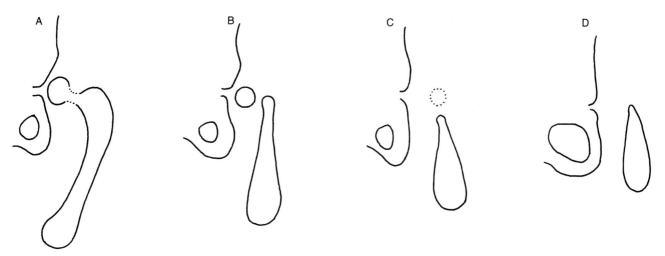

FIGURE 90–23. Proximal femoral focal deficiency (PFFD): Classification system. Classes A to D are described. In all classes, the femoral shaft is very short. Dashed lines indicate structures that will (Class A) or may (Class C) ossify at a later date. (After Levinson ED, et al: Radiology 125:197, 1977.)

severe, delayed in appearance, progressive, and related to a true decrease in the neck-shaft angle as opposed to the subtrochanteric varus that appears in PFFD.

The cause of this disorder is obscure. It has been suggested that the condition arises from a cellular nutritional disturbance at the time of cell division (4 to 6 weeks after ovulation).[27] The occurrence of some cases of PFFD in children of diabetic mothers and the production of similar osseous defects in chick embryos by the injection of insulin suggest that an abnormality of carbohydrate metabolism may be important in this malformation.[22, 23, 28] Additional possible pathogeneses include vascular damage to mesenchymal tissue in the upper portion of the femur, mechanical injury,[23, 29] or a genetic defect.[221] Histopathologic study of the physes has revealed altered proliferation and maturation of chondrocytes, manifested in every zone of the growth plate, and the lack of normal preparation of matrix by the hypertrophic cells.[462]

Skeletal Aplasia and Hypoplasia About the Knee

Although distal femoral focal deficiency is rare and generally is accompanied by dysgenesis of a variable portion of the proximal end of the femur, it has been observed as an isolated phenomenon or in combination with agenesis of the tibia.[226, 227] Congenital deficiency or absence of the tibia (Fig. 90–25) usually is associated with fibular hypoplasia and hemimelia, although it has been described in children with an intact fibula.[228, 464] Four categories of tibial deficiency are recognized: In type 1, the tibia is completely absent and the distal end of the femur is hypoplastic, or a rudimentary tibia articulates with the distal end of a relatively normal femur; in type 2, the proximal end of the tibia is well developed, and the distal end of the tibia is absent; in type 3, the tibia is represented by an amorphous segment of bone, which is present more distally than proximally; and in type 4, the proximal end of the tibia is normal, and the distal end is shortened, with a congenital diastasis of the ankle joint.[465] In addition to alterations of the adjacent fibula, abnormalities that may accompany deficiencies of

the tibia include flexion contracture of the knee, inversion and adduction of the foot, femoral hypoplasia, diastasis of the tibiofibular syndesmosis, and anomalies of the hand.[228] Congenital absence of the cruciate ligaments also may be encountered in patients with osseous dysplasias about the knee.[229, 418]

Hypoplasia (Dysplasia) of the Glenoid Neck of the Scapula

This entity also is termed glenoid hypoplasia and dentated glenoid anomaly[230–236, 466–468] (Fig. 90–26). Men and women are affected with about equal frequency. Although the age at which the diagnosis is established varies, most patients have been evaluated in the third to seventh decades of life. Children and adolescents also may be discovered to have this abnormality, however.[236] Shoulder pain and limitation of motion frequently are evident[553]; less commonly, the condition may be discovered as an incidental finding. Severe glenohumeral joint instability is infrequent or rare. In one series, however, 25 per cent of affected patients had multidirectional instability of this joint.[553] A family history of similar abnormalities has been apparent in some of the reported patients, suggesting that the changes may represent a hereditary trait, possibly due to a dominant gene with low penetrance.[230]

Radiography reveals abnormalities that usually are confined to the shoulder. Bilateral and relatively symmetric changes predominate, consisting of dysplasia of the scapular neck and irregularity of the glenoid surface. A dentate or notched articular surface becomes apparent[234] (Fig. 90–27A). Additional findings may include hypoplasia of the humeral head and neck, varus deformity of the proximal portion of the humerus, and enlargement and bowing of the acromion and the clavicle. The glenohumeral joint appears widened, especially inferiorly. Premature development of osteoarthritis at this site may occur.

Arthrography or computed arthrotomography of the glenohumeral joint reveals smooth, concentric articular surfaces with thick cartilage covering the glenoid cavity, particularly on its inferior aspect.[230, 235, 469, 470] A channel-like

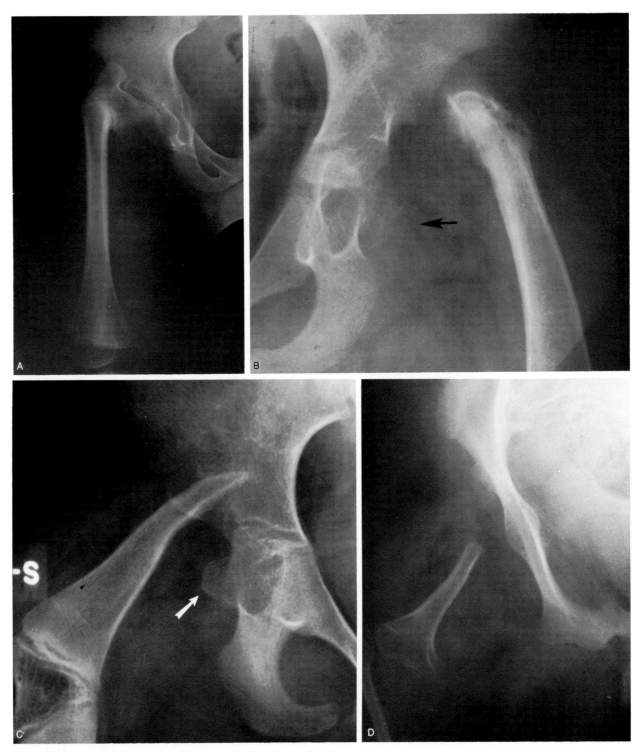

FIGURE 90–24. Proximal femoral focal deficiency (PFFD): Types of involvement.

  A Class A. The short right femoral shaft, continuity of head and shaft, femoroacetabular articulation, and subtrochanteric varus alignment are characteristic.

  B Class B. The left femoral shaft is short. The femoral head (arrow) is seated in the acetabulum, but there is no bony continuity between head and shaft.

  C Class C. The right femoral shaft is short, tapered, and elevated. No femoral head is evident. The dysplastic acetabulum contains a bony protuberance (arrow), which, on other views, represented a part of the acetabulum. A right knee fusion had previously been performed.

  D Class D. Complete absence of the acetabulum and femoral head is apparent. Note the changes in the knee.

  (**A–C,** From Levinson ED, et al: Radiology *125*:197, 1977.)

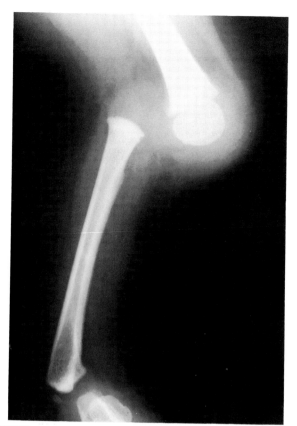

FIGURE 90–25. Aplasia: Tibia. In this 11 month old girl, a type 1 tibial deficiency is evident with malalignment of the femur and hypertrophied fibula. (Courtesy of H. S. Kang, M.D., Seoul, Korea.)

collection of contrast material has been observed at the apparent site of the thickened glenoid cartilage[235] (Fig. 90–27B). The precise cause of this peculiar arthrographic abnormality is unclear. Such an appearance can result from a developmental splitting or acquired ulceration of the articular cartilage or glenoid labrum. The observation of such channels in symptomatic patients suggests also that the cartilaginous abnormalities relate to injury associated with subluxations of the humeral head[470] (Fig. 90–27C). Pathologic data, however, are lacking.

The radiographic abnormalities associated with dysplasia of the neck of the scapula are virtually diagnostic. The absence of alterations in other epiphyses eliminates the diagnosis of multiple epiphyseal dysplasia. Similarly, the lack of significant anomalies at other skeletal sites in almost all reported cases of this disorder allows its differentiation from various other skeletal dysplasias. In a few reports of dysplasia of the scapular neck, however, the presence of additional anomalies has been noted, including spina bifida, hemivertebrae, cervical ribs, and webbing of the axillae. Other disorders, such as occupational trauma, ischemic necrosis of bone, osteochondritis dissecans, hemophilia, pigmented villonodular synovitis, ochronosis, and Sprengel's deformity, are not realistic diagnostic choices.

An injury to the brachial plexus occurring at birth can lead to an upper arm type of paralysis (Erb's paralysis) with subsequent radiographic abnormalities about the shoulder that might resemble dysplasia of the scapular neck. Clinical findings in Erb's paralysis ensure accurate diagnosis in most cases. In the newborn infant and young child, these include an arm that is held at the patient's side with the extremity rotated internally and the forearm pronated, soft tissue atrophy, retardation of epiphyseal ossification in the proximal portion of the humerus, and elevation and outward rotation of the scapula. In the older child, adolescent, and adult, the scapula continues to be elevated and rotated externally, the acromion and coracoid process may be elongated, and the clavicle may be hypoplastic.

The precise cause and pathogenesis of glenoid hypoplasia are unknown. It is possible that the precartilage destined to ossify and become the inferior segment of the glenoid fails to develop[232, 470]; however, the stimulus for this lack of normal development remains obscure. The radiographic abnormalities resemble those seen in developmental dysplasia of the hip, but a meaningful association of the two conditions has not been established.

Sacrococcygeal Agenesis (Caudal Regression Syndrome)

This well-known anomaly, which also is discussed in Chapter 89, leads to absence of one or more segments of the sacrum, which may be combined with aplasia of the lower thoracic and upper lumbar spine[30–33, 237–241] (Fig. 90–28). Approximately 20 per cent of persons with this syndrome are the children of diabetic mothers. Associated abnormalities include neurogenic bladder and serious urologic problems, hip dislocations, flexion contractures of the knees and hips, and foot deformities. Radiographic findings vary with the severity of the anomaly. Complete sacral agenesis is combined with deformed ilia that may articulate with each other or with the lowest vertebral body or that fuse in the midline. When combined with complete fusion of the lower extremities, the sacral agenesis has been referred to as the mermaid syndrome.[471] Partial agenesis may lead to a deformed and sickle-shaped sacrum through which an anterior meningocele may protrude. Central sacral defects may be combined with hereditary presacral teratoma.[34]

The detection of associated skeletal and visceral abnor-

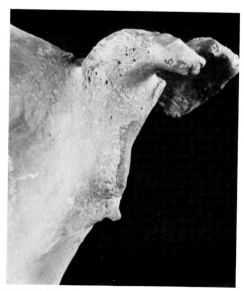

FIGURE 90–26. Hypoplasia (dysplasia) of the glenoid neck of the scapula. A photograph of the scapula reveals an irregular, dentate, or notched articular surface and hypoplasia of the glenoid neck.

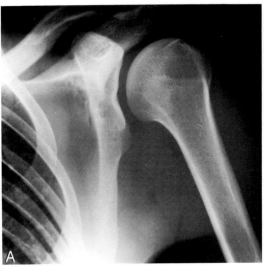

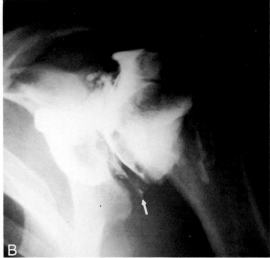

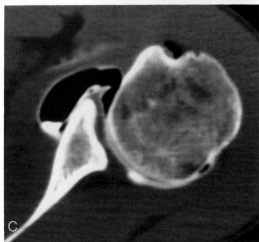

FIGURE 90–27. Hypoplasia (dysplasia) of the glenoid neck of the scapula.

A Hypoplasia of the scapular neck, an irregular notched glenoid articular surface, and widening of the lower portion of the joint space are evident. The opposite side was affected similarly.

B Arthrography of the glenohumeral joint in a different patient shows a channel-like collection of contrast material inferiorly (arrow).

(**A, B,** From Resnick D, et al: AJR *139*:387, 1982. Copyright 1982, American Roentgen Ray Society.)

C In a third patient, computed arthrotomography shows posterior subluxation of the humeral head and redundancy of the anterior portion of the joint capsule. The findings are compatible with multidirectional instability.

(**C,** Courtesy of G. Greenway, M.D., Dallas, Texas.)

malities requires myelography,[241] urography, cystography, MR imaging,[471] and contrast studies of the gastrointestinal tract in addition to plain film radiography.[35, 36]

SKELETAL HYPERPLASIA

Congenital enlargement may involve a single bone, a portion of a limb, or the entire limb. In some instances, one half of the body can be affected. Soft tissue hypertrophy generally accompanies the osseous abnormality. Although they are idiopathic in a large number of cases, similar changes can be evident in a wide variety of disorders, including neurofibromatosis, lipomatosis, the Proteus syndrome, hemangiomatosis, lymphangiomatosis, arteriovenous malformations, endocrine disorders, cerebral gigantism, Wilms' tumor, and neoplasms of the adrenal glands.[37–39] Localized osseous overgrowth can be noted in macrodystrophia lipomatosa and in response to hyperemia in articular and inflammatory disorders, such as hemophilia, juvenile chronic arthritis, and osteomyelitis.

MALSEGMENTATIONS AND FUSIONS

Errors in segmentation frequently are inherited and result in osseous fusion of neighboring bones, such as the radius

and ulna. Bony ankylosis also can occur between longitudinally arranged bones, as in the digits of the hand and the foot. On the opposite side of the spectrum, hypersegmentation and duplication anomalies exist. In both of these situations, radiographs are particularly helpful, outlining the presence and characteristics of the malformation.

Hyperphalangism and Polydactyly

Extra phalanges in humans virtually are confined to the thumb (Fig. 90–29). The triphalangeal thumb is a rare familial disorder[40, 41, 242] that leads to a small or large ossicle in the abnormal digit. Although the anomaly can occur as an isolated finding, it also may be associated with other anomalies, including polydactyly, duplications, and absent bones, and with certain syndromes, including Holt-Oram syndrome, trisomy 13–15, and Blackfan-Diamond anemia.[42] Accessory phalanges should be differentiated from pseudoepiphyses of the digits that may accompany certain syndromes, such as cleidocranial dysostosis and hypothyroidism.

Polydactyly, representing an increased number of digits, can appear in the hand or the foot (Fig. 90–30). Polydactyly is more common in blacks than in whites, and the presence and pattern of its inheritance depend on the type of anomaly

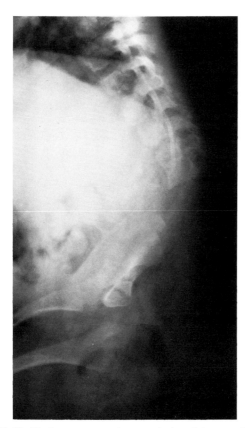

FIGURE 90–28. Sacrococcygeal agenesis (caudal regression syndrome). In this child of a diabetic mother, observe absence of much of the lumbar spine and all of the sacrum. Deformity of the ilia is evident.

that is evident. In the foot, the fifth digit usually is involved.[472] Its appearance on the radial side of the hand (including the thumb)[243] is termed preaxial polydactyly, and its existence on the ulnar side of the hand is known as postaxial polydactyly. Preaxial polydactyly may be associated with acrocephalosyndactyly, brachydactyly B, acropectorovertebral dysplasia, Fanconi's syndrome, Holt-Oram syndrome, and other conditions; postaxial polydactyly can appear in chondroectodermal dysplasia (Ellis–van Creveld syndrome), Laurence-Moon-Biedl syndrome, trisomy 13, asphyxiating thoracic dystrophy, Goltz's focal dermal hypoplasia, and other diseases.[42]

An unusual condition that may or may not be associated with polydactyly is termed the longitudinally bracketed epiphysis, or the delta phalanx.[244–246] Occurring in the hand or the foot with predominant involvement of the first ray, the delta phalanx leads to a trapezoid-shaped, diaphyseal-metaphyseal unit with alterations in physeal configuration. Phalangeal, metacarpal, or metatarsal localization is possible, and bilateral or unilateral distributions are encountered. In addition to polydactyly, the delta phalanx has been associated with clinodactyly, extra phalanges, and a variety of congenital syndromes.

Syndactyly

Syndactyly, a common anomaly, relates to a lack of differentiation between two or more digits.[43] It may be subdivided into cases with either soft tissue or osseous

involvement and classified into partial (involving the proximal segments of a digit) and complete (involving the entire digit) types (Fig. 90–31). Other classification systems also are used.[42] Most cases are inherited, although some appear in a sporadic fashion. Men are affected more commonly than women. A large number of syndromes have been associated with syndactyly.[42] Included in this list is Poland's syndrome, in which syndactyly occurs and the pectoral muscles are absent.[44, 247, 248] It has been suggested that Poland's syndrome is present in approximately 10 per cent of patients with syndactyly[473] (Fig. 90–32). Additional anomalies in this nonhereditary syndrome are hypoplasia of the hand, nipple, clavicle, sternum, or ribs, pectus excavatum, pectus carinatum, elevated scapulae, carpal coalition,[249] abnormalities of tendons,[247] hemivertebrae, and scoliosis. Also reported are dextrocardia; herniation of the lung; shortening of the humerus, radius, or ulna; radioulnar synostosis; and agenesis of the nails.[473] A possible association of Poland's syndrome with leukemia has been noted.[45, 46] A similar association with lymphoma, thrombocytopenia, and spherocytosis has been indicated.[473]

Symphalangism

Symphalangism represents a fusion of one phalanx to another within the same digit, presumably resulting from a failure of differentiation of the intervening articulation.[47, 48] This usually is inherited as a dominant trait. On radiographs in the infant, the anomaly may be difficult to recognize owing to the "invisible" nature of the cartilaginous tissue. Hypoplasia of the joint and an adjacent abnormal epiphysis

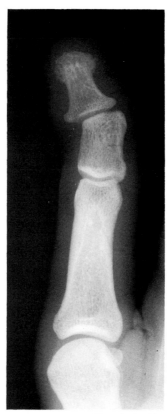

FIGURE 90–29. Hyperphalangism: Thumb. In this patient with the Holt-Oram syndrome, observe three separate phalanges in the thumb.

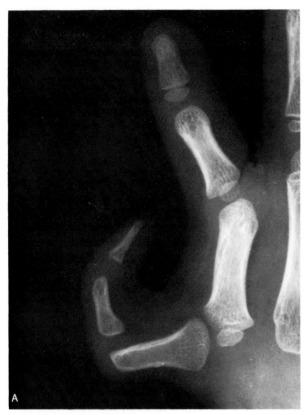
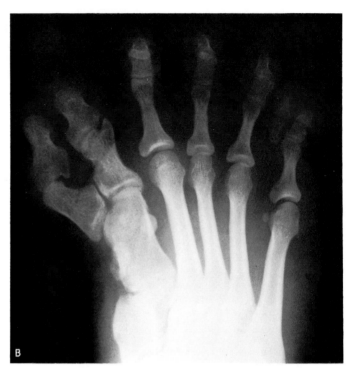

FIGURE 90–30. Polydactyly.
  A Hand: Preaxial polydactyly has resulted in an extra digit adjacent to the thumb.
  B Foot: Observe the extra digit medial to the great toe, which is associated with deformity of the adjacent phalanges, metatarsals, and tarsal bones. Also note extra phalanges in the fifth toe.

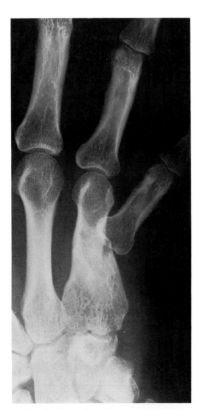

FIGURE 90–31. Syndactyly. A partial osseous fusion involves the fourth and fifth metacarpal bones. Note the ulnar displacement of the fifth finger. (Courtesy of C. Robinson, M.D., San Francisco, California.)

represent radiographic clues even at this early age, however. Typical sites of involvement include the proximal interphalangeal joints of the fingers and the distal interphalangeal joints of the toes, with predilection for the ulnar side of the hand.[42] The thumb rarely is affected. Additional abnormalities may include shortening and flattening of the metacarpals, carpal and tarsal fusions,[49] and osteoarthritis of adjacent joints.[474] Associated syndromes include diastrophic dwarfism, Bell's brachydactyly types A and C, popliteal pterygium syndrome, and certain acrocephalosyndactyly syndromes.[42]

It is important to differentiate this anomaly from acquired intra-articular fusions accompanying various arthritides, including juvenile chronic arthritis and psoriatic arthritis. With congenital symphalangism, the proximal and middle phalanges may be joined by a smooth osseous contour, although a slight expansion of the bony margin may be encountered at the level of the affected joint. Furthermore, a small lucent cleft at the site of fusion and hypoplasia of distal phalanges and metacarpal heads are helpful signs.

Carpal Fusion (Coalition)

Carpal fusion or coalition is a relatively common abnormality that may occur as an isolated phenomenon or as part of a generalized congenital malformation syndrome. As a rule, isolated fusions involve bones in the same carpal row (proximal or distal), whereas syndrome-related fusions may affect bones in different rows (proximal and distal).[42, 50]

The most common site of the isolated fusion is between

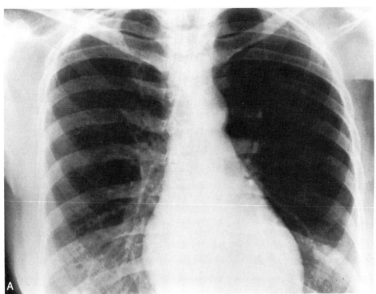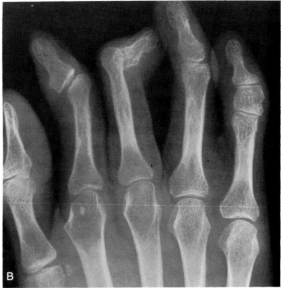

FIGURE 90–32. Poland's syndrome.
   A Note the absence of the left pectoral muscles, creating increased lucency of the left hemithorax. Elevation of the scapula and deformity of the ribs are also seen.
   B The involved hand reveals aplasia (second, third, and fourth digits) and hypoplasia (fifth digit) of the middle phalanges, partial soft tissue syndactyly between the fourth and fifth fingers and between the second and third fingers, and osseous deformities.

the triquetrum and the lunate bones; in this location the fusion occurs in 0.1 to 1.6 per cent of the general population, more frequently in men and in blacks,[51] and has little or no clinical significance[52] (Fig. 90–33). The fusion is bilateral in approximately 60 per cent of cases.[478] Widening of the scapholunate interosseous space is a frequent finding in cases of lunotriquetral fusion, although the scapholunate interosseous ligament generally is intact. Less common isolated coalitions that may be encountered include capitate-hamate fusion,[53] trapezium-trapezoid fusion, and pisiform-hamate fusion.[54, 475] In fact, isolated fusions have been described in almost all possible combinations[55, 250] including those affecting more than two bones.[251] The presence and exact location of coalition are not always easy to identify on radiographic examination. This difficulty relates to the partial or incomplete nature of the ankylosis in some cases, the need for multiple projections owing to the obliquity of the osseous surfaces of the normal carpal bones, and the requirement that congenital and acquired coalition must be differentiated. In most cases, symptoms and signs are entirely lacking, although pain has been observed in some cases,[252] especially in association with partial coalitions and cystic changes in the adjacent bones,[419, 476, 477] and a definite risk of fracture exists in the presence of a fused carpus.[56, 57]

Massive carpal fusion usually is associated with other anomalies. Similarly, fusion between bones of the proximal and distal carpal rows or between the carpal bones and radius or ulna generally is associated with additional malformations. The associated alterations may include tarsal coalition or one of a variety of congenital syndromes, such as acrocephalosyndactyly syndrome, arthrogryposis, diastrophic dwarfism, Ellis–van Creveld syndrome, hand-foot-uterus syndrome, Holt-Oram syndrome, otopalatodigital syndrome, Turner's syndrome, or symphalangism.[42] Many such carpal fusions are familial.

The anomaly develops from a failure of segmentation of

the primitive cartilaginous canals and absence of joint formation.[53, 58] The osseous centers of the involved carpus coalesce at variable ages, usually between 6 and 15 years of age (Fig. 90–34). On radiographs, continuous trabeculae can be traced from one bone to the next, although a small notch or cleft may remain at the site of coalition. Discrete intraosseous cysts adjacent to the area of coalition sometimes are seen. The changes usually can be differentiated from acquired ankylosis that may accompany infection, certain arthritides, such as juvenile chronic arthritis and rheumatoid arthritis, trauma, and surgery.

Accessory Carpal Bones

A number of extra ossification centers may appear in the wrist adjacent to the eight normal carpal bones. These have been well described by Poznanski.[42] Although they produce no symptoms or signs, they must be differentiated from small fracture fragments (Fig. 90–35). In addition, certain ossicles are associated with specific malformation syndromes. Accessory bones in the distal carpal row can accompany diastrophic dwarfism, Ellis–van Creveld syndrome, Larson's syndrome, otopalatodigital syndrome, and brachydactyly A-1. The os centrale or remnant of a central row of carpal bones can be an isolated finding,[479] although it also is noted in the hand-foot-uterus syndrome, Holt-Oram syndrome, otopalatodigital syndrome, and Larsen's syndrome.

Radioulnar Synostosis

A common site of osseous fusion in the tubular bones of the extremities is between the proximal portions of the radius and ulna[59] (Fig. 90–36). Two distinct types have been recognized: proximal or true radioulnar synostosis, in which the radius and ulna are fused smoothly at their prox-

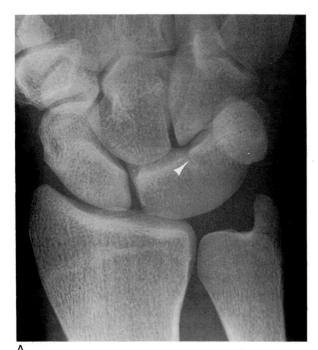

A

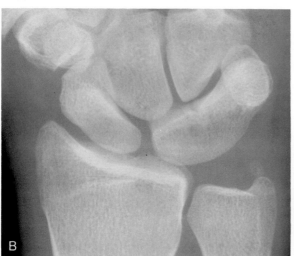

B

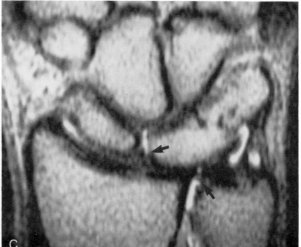

C

FIGURE 90–33. Carpal fusion (coalition).

A Note the bony fusion between the lunate and the triquetrum with a small cleft (arrowhead) at the site of ankylosis.

B, C In a second case, a solid lunotriquetral coalition is associated with a widened scapholunate interosseous space **(B).** A coronal T2-weighted (TR/TE, 1000/80) spin echo MR image **(C)** shows fluid of high signal intensity (arrows) that outlines defects in the scapholunate interosseous ligament and triangular fibrocartilage. Usually, in such cases, the scapholunate interosseous ligament is intact.

FIGURE 90–34. Carpal fusion (coalition). Radiographs obtained over an 18 month period show progressive lunotriquetral coalition. In **A,** an abnormal alignment of the two bones is visible when the patient was 9 years of age; in **B,** partial bone ankylosis is apparent.

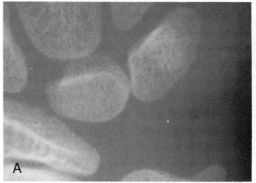

A

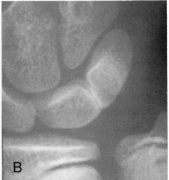

B

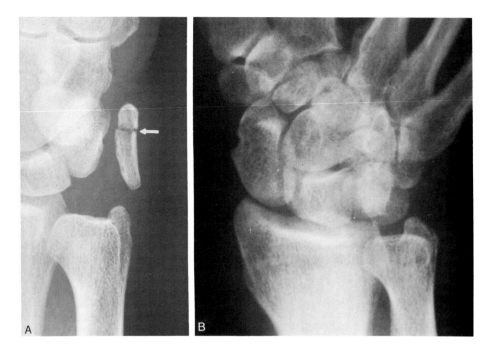

FIGURE 90–35. Accessory carpal bones.

A An extra area of ossification containing a fracture (arrow) is evident in an otherwise normal wrist.

B In this dramatic example, more than 12 carpal bones are present.

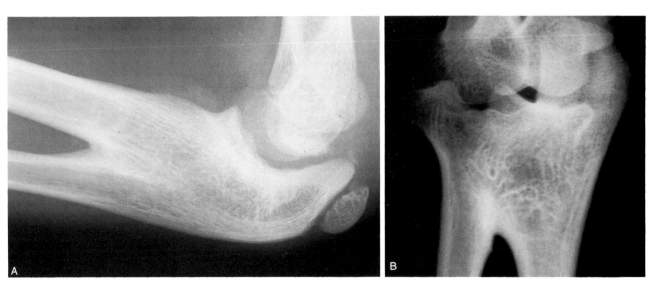

FIGURE 90–36. Radioulnar synostosis.

A In this patient, note smooth osseous fusion of the proximal segments of the radius and the ulna.

B In a different patient, fusion has occurred just distal to the proximal border of the radius, and a congenital dislocation of the radial head is seen.

imal borders for a distance of about 2 to 6 cm; and a second variety, in which fusion just distal to the proximal radial epiphysis is associated with congenital dislocation of the radial head.[60] In both types, interference with normal forearm supination is seen. Other descriptions of radioulnar synostosis indicate additional radiographic types of this anomaly[253] or a spectrum of involvement that can range from fibrous to complete bone fusion. The condition is bilateral in approximately 60 per cent of patients, affecting men and women equally or showing a slight male predominance.[253] Sporadically occurring examples appear more often than familial cases. Radioulnar synostosis is regarded as an anomaly of longitudinal segmentation in which, instead of the formation of the superior radioulnar joint space, the interzonal mesenchyme persists, undergoing chondrification and ossification.

Additional anomalies that may accompany radioulnar synostosis are clubbed feet, developmental dysplasia of the hip, knee anomalies, hypoplasia of the thumb, carpal fusion, symphalangism, and Madelung's deformity. Radioulnar synostosis also may appear as part of arthrogryposis, multiple hereditary exostoses, acrocephalopolysyndactyly, acrocephalosyndactyly, Holt-Oram syndrome, mandibulofacial dysostosis, Nievergelt-Pearlman syndrome, Klinefelter's syndrome, and other chromosomal aberrations, including those with excessive X chromosomes (XXXXY, XXXY, or XXYY).[60, 61, 254] Furthermore, such synostosis can be acquired when osseous proliferation of one or both bones appears in the course of infection or infantile cortical hyperostosis.

The diagnosis of congenital radioulnar synostosis is not difficult when the ossified bridge has formed, appearing as a bar that eventually may engulf the radial head. Prior to such ossification, the continuous cartilaginous tissue extending between the proximal portions of the radius and ulna is invisible radiographically, although abnormal traction or tethering can produce secondary changes in the adjacent osseous tissue. Lateral bowing of the distal end of the radius may accompany this synostosis.

Synostosis of Other Long Tubular Bones

Additional patterns of synostosis in the long tubular bones are less frequent than that between the radius and ulna and include humeroulnar[255] and tibiofibular synostoses.[256] Of interest, bifurcations of long tubular bones also have been described.[257]

Tarsal Fusion (Coalition)

Tarsal coalition represents an abnormal fusion of one or more of the tarsalia. The union may be fibrous, cartilaginous, or osseous and can be congenital (developmental) or acquired in response to infection, trauma, articular disorders, or surgery.[482]

Congenital, or developmental, tarsal coalition is of unknown cause. It appears to arise on the basis of a failure of differentiation and segmentation of the primitive mesenchyme that results in lack of formation of intervening joints, a theory that gains support from the identification of such anomalies in the fetus.[62] Although in 1896, Pfitzner[63] proposed that tarsal coalitions were caused by the gradual incorporation of accessory ossicles into adjacent tarsal

bones, a suggestion that was supported at least in part by later investigators,[64–67] the observation of tarsal fusion in fetuses discounts such a proposal. In some cases, a familial history of identical abnormalities is obtained.[68–70] In fact, Leonard[71] reported that 39 per cent of 98 first-degree relatives of 31 patients with peroneal spastic flatfoot and partial coalition had some type of fusion, although the presence and degree of symptoms and signs and the pattern of ankylosis varied among some patients and relatives. He suggested that the disorder was of autosomal dominant inheritance with genetic variability of expression. It appears that familial factors indeed are important in some cases, particularly those with massive tarsal fusions.

The condition dates from antiquity, cases having been found in pre-Columbian Indian skeletons.[72] Despite an early description of peroneal spastic flatfoot by Sir Robert Jones in 1897,[73] it was not until 1921 that a relationship of this clinical entity and tarsal coalition was documented.[64] This association now is well recognized,[65, 74] although it is not uniform in all cases of peroneal spastic flatfoot; other conditions, such as juvenile chronic arthritis, tuberculosis, osteoarthritis, and fracture can cause a similar clinical problem. Typically, symptoms and signs of tarsal coalition appear in the second or third decade of life; an earlier age of onset is rare, perhaps owing to the fact that the fusion is fibrous or cartilaginous in the young child or adolescent, and only with the appearance of ossification do pain and restricted motion become evident. After minor trauma or unusual activity, the affected person complains of vague pain in the foot, aggravated by prolonged standing or athletic endeavor.[75] Limited subtalar motion, pes planus, and shortening with persistent or intermittent spasm of the peroneal muscles are seen on physical examination. The rigid foot may be held in a valgus attitude, although anterior tibial spasm can lead to varus deformity.[76, 77] Coalition also can be manifested as a cavus foot[78, 79] or as an incidental finding in an asymptomatic person.

Isolated partial coalitions can be classified according to the bones that are affected; calcaneonavicular, talocalcaneal, talonavicular, and calcaneocuboid fusions, in order of decreasing frequency, can be detected. Tarsal fusions accompanying multiple malformation syndromes may have "atypical" patterns or may involve the entire tarsus.[80] In the otopalatodigital syndrome and the hand-foot-uterus syndrome, coalition among the cuneiforms and metatarsal bases may be encountered.[81, 82] Tarsal fusions also may accompany hereditary symphalangism,[48, 83] arthrogryposis,[84] acrocephalosyndactyly (Apert's syndrome),[85] and many other disorders.[1, 2] Identification of the nature and extent of a coalition frequently requires routine radiography that in some instances can be supplemented with special views, conventional tomography, CT scanning, MR imaging, scintigraphy, and even arthrography.[75, 86–88, 258–261, 412]

Calcaneonavicular Coalition. This type of coalition is one of the most frequent,[262–265] is sometimes bilateral,[266] and can be asymptomatic or associated with rigid flatfoot.[413] In general, symptoms and signs are less severe than those accompanying talocalcaneal coalitions, and "secondary" radiographic abnormalities may be less marked. Coalition is identified optimally on a 45 degree medial-oblique view of the foot and, in fact, may be completely overlooked on anteroposterior and lateral projections[89] (Fig. 90–37). The diagnosis is simplified by the presence of a solid bony bar

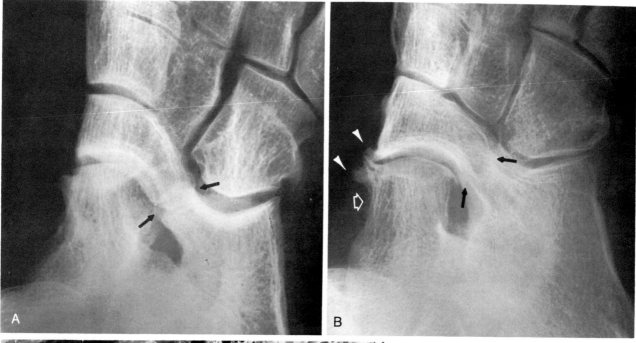

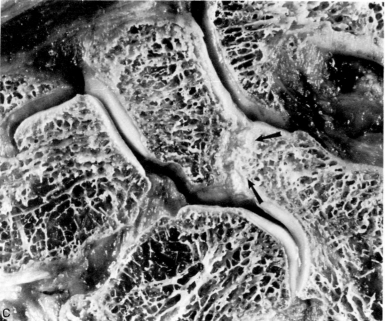

FIGURE 90–37. Calcaneonavicular tarsal coalition.

A Observe the approximation of the osseous surfaces of the calcaneus and navicular bone (arrows) on the medial oblique view. Mild abnormalities are apparent at the calcaneocuboid joint.

B In this patient, a complete osseous coalition (solid arrows) is evident on the medial oblique view. Observe the bony excrescences at the talonavicular joint space (arrowheads) and hypoplasia of the distal aspect of the talus (open arrow).

C A photograph of a sagittal section of a cadaveric foot reveals evidence of a fibrous ankylosis between calcaneus and navicular bone (arrows). A partial joint space can be identified.

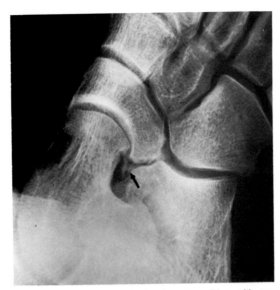

FIGURE 90–38. Calcaneonavicular tarsal coalition with possible fracture. After an episode of trauma, this patient developed severe pain and swelling of the midfoot. An incomplete calcaneonavicular bar is associated with osseous fragmentation (arrow). This finding may represent a fibrous or cartilaginous coalition alone or one that has fractured. A bone scan (not shown) revealed intense uptake of the radiopharmaceutical agent in the midfoot. (Courtesy of P. Kaplan, M.D., Charlottesville, Virginia.)

extending between the calcaneus and the navicular bone but is more difficult in cases of cartilaginous or fibrous coalition. Normally, a joint does not exist between the two bones; a close approximation of their bony contours, especially if adjacent eburnation or sclerosis is evident, should raise the possibility of a nonosseous coalition. Elongation of the anterosuperior portion of the calcaneus also suggests the diagnosis, and such elongation, when viewed on the lateral radiograph, has been designated the "anteater nose" sign.[480] Bony fusion may be identified between the ages of

8 and 12 years. A secondary radiographic sign of calcaneonavicular coalition is hypoplasia of the head of the talus.[90] Talar "beaking" is uncommon and, when present, may be the result of an associated talocalcaneal fusion. Rarely, a fracture of the abnormal calcaneonavicular osseous bridge is identified[265] (Fig. 90–38).

Although other diagnostic techniques such as scintigraphy, CT, and MR imaging have been used to evaluate patients with this common type of coalition,[258, 481] generally they are not required (Figs. 90–39 and 90–40).

Talocalcaneal Coalition. The talocalcaneal fusion represents the other common type of tarsal coalition. Almost all such fusions occur at the middle facet, between the talus and sustentaculum tali (Figs. 90–41 and 90–42); ankylosis of the posterior subtalar joint or of the anterior facets is far less frequent (Fig. 90–43). The condition is more common in boys than in girls and is bilateral in 20 to 25 per cent of patients. Cartilaginous, fibrous, or bony bridges may be identified, although radiographic evaluation often requires special views in addition to standard anteroposterior and lateral projections. A penetrated axial radiograph (Harris-Beath view) obtained with varying degrees of beam angulation, oblique radiographs, and anterior and lateral conventional tomograms may be necessary. These techniques may identify the actual site of osseous fusion, although closely apposed and irregular bony articular surfaces can indicate the presence of bridging fibrous or cartilaginous tissue.[483] Cartilaginous coalitions usually are associated with marked narrowing of the joint, whereas fibrous coalitions, which typically involve the most posterior part of the sustentaculum tali, may lead only to subtle diminution of the interosseous space,[483] although hypoplasia of the sustentaculum tali also may be apparent.[484] In both fibrous and cartilaginous coalitions, CT alone, arthrography alone, or CT and arthrography together may be helpful. Contrast medium introduced into the talonavicular space of this joint will fail to flow beneath the anterior aspect of the talus and over the sustentaculum tali owing to the abnormal tissue elements[91] (see Chapter 13).

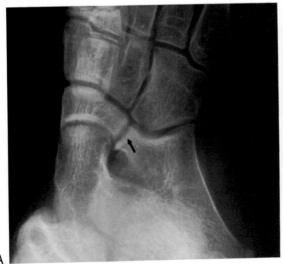
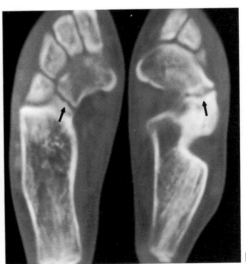

FIGURE 90–39. Calcaneonavicular tarsal coalition.
A An oblique radiograph shows an incomplete osseous bar (arrow) extending between the calcaneus and the navicular bone. Similar abnormalities were evident on the opposite side.
B A transverse CT scan confirms the presence of bilateral calcaneonavicular coalitions (arrows).
(Courtesy of G. Greenway, M.D., Dallas, Texas.)

FIGURE 90–40. Calcaneonavicular tarsal coalition.

A A sagittal T1-weighted (TR/TE, 400/20) spin echo MR image reveals a nonosseous coalition (arrow) between the calcaneus and navicular bones. Its signal characteristics are compatible with the presence of fibrocartilaginous tissue.

B A sagittal gradient echo (MPGR) image (TR/TE, 500/20; flip angle, 25 degrees) also shows the coalition (arrow) and confirms the cartilaginous nature of the abnormal union.

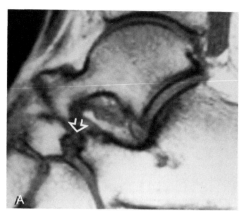
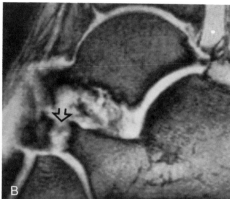

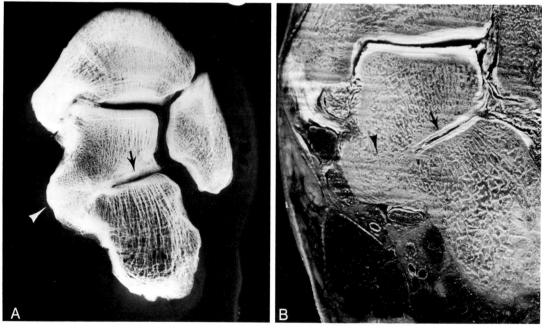

FIGURE 90–41. Talocalcaneal tarsal coalition: Middle facets. A radiograph **(A)** and photograph **(B)** of a coronal section of the hindfoot reveal a complete osseous bridge (arrowheads) involving the middle facets of the talus and the calcaneus. Note the relatively normal posterior subtalar joint (arrows) and ankle.

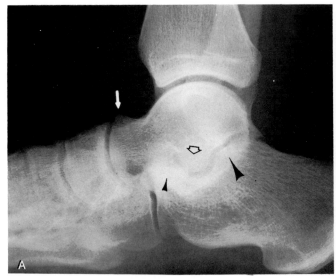
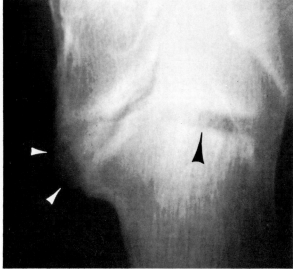

FIGURE 90–42. Talocalcaneal tarsal coalition: Middle facets.

A A lateral radiograph reveals talar beaking (solid arrow), broadening of the lateral process of the talus (open arrow), narrowing of the posterior subtalar joint (large arrowhead), and nonvisualization of the space between the sustentaculum tali and talus (middle subtalar joint) (small arrowhead).

B In a different patient, a Harris-Beath view outlines partial bony ankylosis (small arrowheads) between the sustentaculum tali and talus. Note the intact posterior subtalar joint (large arrowhead).

Fortunately, a number of secondary radiographic signs have been described in association with talocalcaneal coalition.[75, 86] These include the following:

1. Talar beaking. Dorsal subluxation of the navicular bone produced by subtalar rigidity leads to elevation of the periosteum below the talonavicular ligament with subperiosteal proliferation and the production of a beak or excrescence at the dorsal surface of the talar head adjacent to the talonavicular space, best identified on lateral projections (Fig. 90–44). A similar but less constant outgrowth occurs on the adjacent navicular bone. This "beak," which rarely may fracture after an acute injury or chronic stress,[547] should be differentiated from a normal talar ridge on the dorsum of the bone[267] and, when present, is not pathognomonic of talocalcaneal coalition; it may be identified in other conditions associated with abnormal motion at the talonavicular space, such as rheumatoid arthritis. A similar beak may be identified in diffuse idiopathic skeletal hyperostosis[267] and acromegaly. Osseous excrescences at the talonavicular space or on the dorsal aspect of the proximal navicular bone related to osteoarthritis of the midfoot and

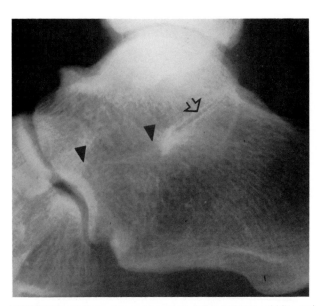
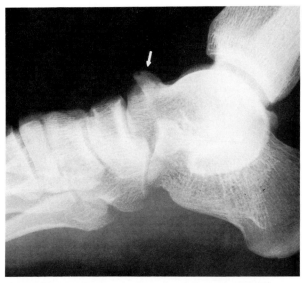

FIGURE 90–43. Talocalcaneal tarsal coalition: Anterior, middle, and posterior facets. Observe bony ankylosis of the anterior and middle facets (arrowheads) and incomplete ankylosis of the posterior facets (arrow). (Courtesy of S. Moreland, M.D., San Diego, California.)

FIGURE 90–44. Talocalcaneal tarsal coalition: Talar beak. In a patient with a talocalcaneal coalition involving the middle facets, observe a large osseous excrescence (arrow) on the dorsal surface of the talus. (Reprinted from Sartoris DJ, Resnick D: Arthritis Rheum *28*:331, 1985. Copyright 1985. Used by permission of the American Rheumatism Association.)

ankle (respectively) are differentiated easily from the talar beak of talocalcaneal coalition.

2. Broadening of the lateral process of the talus. Broadening or rounding of this process (Fig. 90–42) is identified easily when comparison views of the opposite (uninvolved) foot are part of the radiographic examination. It is present in 40 to 60 per cent of patients, may occur in the absence of a talar beak, and apparently is related to a valgus angulation of the calcaneus.

3. Narrowing of the posterior subtalar joint. This finding can be evident in as many as 50 to 60 per cent of patients with or without additional secondary signs of coalition and represents degenerative arthritis or a nontangential position of the articular surface due to calcaneal eversion.

4. Concave undersurface of the talar neck and asymmetry of the talocalcaneonavicular joint. Comparison views

are helpful in the detection of this sign, although care must be taken to ensure that similar projections are available on both sides.

5. Failure of visualization of the "middle" subtalar joint. The inability to identify this joint on lateral views is a useful finding but is one that is difficult to apply in some cases because of a faulty position of the foot.[268]

6. Ball-and-socket ankle joint. A rounded, convex appearance of the proximal talar articular surface and a concomitant concave appearance of the distal end of the tibia may accompany talocalcaneal coalition, presumably owing to an adaptation of the ankle joint to provide the inversion and eversion function that is restricted at the talocalcaneal articulations[92–95, 269, 420] (Fig. 90–45). This change also may accompany other congenital anomalies, including short extremities, absence or fusion of rays, genu valgum defor-

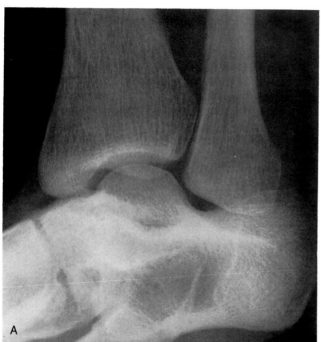

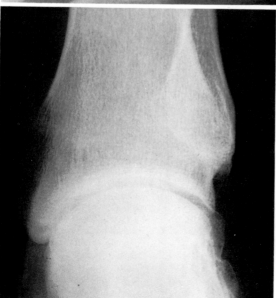

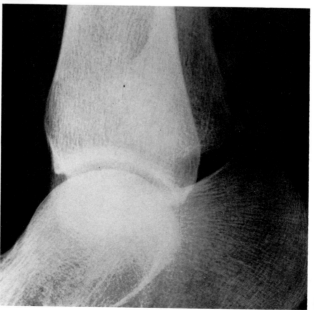

FIGURE 90–45. Tarsal coalition with ball-and-socket ankle joint (congenital coalition).

A An oblique radiograph outlines bony coalition among most of the tarsal bones, including the talocalcaneal joints. Note the ball-and-socket appearance of the ankle with associated deformity of the distal end of the fibula.

B, C In a different patient, talocalcaneal coalition again is associated with a ball-and-socket ankle joint and with a shortened fibula.

(**B, C,** Courtesy of F. Brahme, M.D., San Diego, California.)

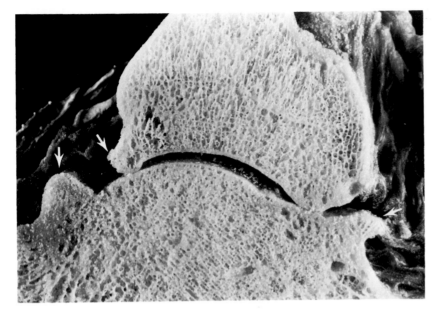

FIGURE 90–46. Tarsal coalition with ball-and-socket ankle joint (acquired coalition). A surgical fusion of the talocalcaneal joints can be associated with deformity of the ankle. The degree of deformity is greater in those cases in which ankylosis occurs at a young age. In this case, a photograph of a sagittal section of the ankle of a cadaver indicates rounding of the talar surface and osteophytes (arrows).

mity, and hypoplasia or aplasia of the fibula.[269, 485, 486] Ball-and-socket ankle joints also may result from acquired disorders of the midfoot, although the degree and smoothness of the deformity are less in the acquired conditions (Fig. 90–46). Secondary osteoarthritis later may appear in a ball-and-socket ankle joint.[486]

Although direct visualization of the bone bridge or identification of one or more of these secondary signs ensures accurate radiographic diagnosis of talocalcaneal coalition in many instances, the importance of bone scintigraphy as a screening examination[260, 261] and of CT as a definitive examination[258–260, 412, 481, 487–491] should be understood. With regard to scintigraphy, abnormal uptake of the bone-seeking

radionuclide occurs about the subtalar joints and in the dorsum of the foot; with regard to CT scanning, a coronal scanning plane, with or without slight angulation of the x-ray beam, appears to be best, and the technique allows assessment of both feet at the same time (Figs. 90–47 and 90–48). Plantar plane images as well as those obtained in a modified sagittal plane also may be useful.[489] The technique can be applied successfully to the assessment of fibrous and cartilaginous coalitions.[483, 484]

Talonavicular Coalition. This is an uncommon type of coalition that may reveal an autosomal dominant[96, 97] or recessive[98] hereditary transmission and an association with anomalies of the little finger.[97] Patients may be asymptomatic or may have pain[492] or peroneal spasm.[264, 270] The

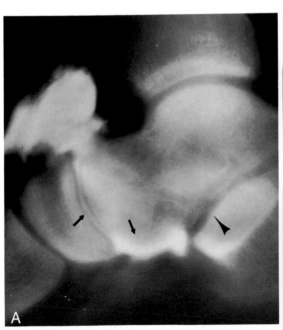
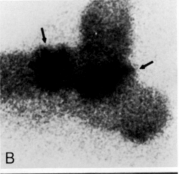
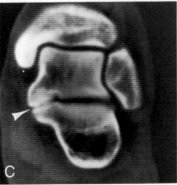

FIGURE 90–47. Talocalcaneal tarsal coalition: Use of arthrography, scintigraphy, and CT. This 24 year old man developed pain that intensified with recreational parachuting.

A Arthrography of the anterior talocalcaneonavicular joint followed by conventional tomography indicates opacification of the talonavicular space and anterior talocalcaneal space (arrows) but absence of contrast material in the area of the middle facets (arrowhead). Incidentally noted is extravasation of the contrast agent into the dorsal soft tissue.

B Bone scintigraphy shows accumulation of the radionuclide about the anterior and posterior subtalar joints (arrows).

C A direct coronal CT scan shows a fibrous or cartilaginous coalition (arrowhead) in the area of the middle facets. The normal interosseous space in this region is narrowed with adjacent bone sclerosis.

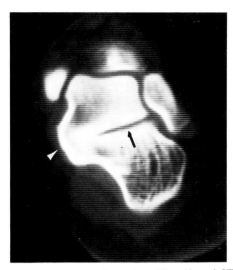

FIGURE 90–48. Talocalcaneal tarsal coalition: Use of CT. A solid bone union (arrowhead) in the region of the middle facets is well documented on a direct coronal CT scan. The posterior subtalar joint is slightly narrowed (arrow).

onset of symptoms generally occurs at the age of 5 years, although children younger than this may report vague pain and discomfort during physical activity. Limitation of subtalar motion and a bone protuberance at the level of the navicular bone may be apparent on physical examination. Radiography usually outlines the osseous bridge, and little difficulty in diagnosis is encountered (Fig. 90–49).

Other Coalitions. Calcaneocuboid coalitions are very rare, are readily identified on radiographs, and may be asymptomatic or associated with peroneal spasm.[99–101] A bilateral or unilateral distribution can be seen, and other anomalies may coexist. Isolated examples of cubonavicular and naviculocuneiform coalitions have been reported.[102–105, 271, 493] An association of naviculocuneiform coalition and Köhler's disease of the tarsal navicular bone has been suggested[104, 494] but is unproved.

Rib Anomalies

Accessory *cervical ribs* may develop in a unilateral or bilateral distribution at the level of the seventh and, rarely, the sixth cervical vertebrae (Fig. 90–50). Their size is variable, and in some instances elongated transverse processes arising from the vertebrae simulate true cervical ribs. The scalenus anticus syndrome is a recognized complication of this anomaly.

Intrathoracic ribs usually are supernumerary and are extremely rare.[272–275] These ribs are unilateral, are more common on the right side, and usually, but not invariably,[273] are unassociated with additional skeletal anomalies. Although generally they are asymptomatic and are discovered as an incidental finding during chest radiography, intrathoracic ribs may have a fibrous, diaphragmatic attachment, which can cause a restrictive ventilatory defect.[272] The anomalous rib usually arises from the posteroinferior margin of another rib or directly from a vertebral body.[272] The midthoracic region typically is affected.[273] Radiographs allow accurate identification of the intrathoracic rib, which appears as an opaque region overlying the inner part of the lung field in the frontal projection of the chest or is located posteriorly in the lateral projection (Fig. 90–51). CT can be used to analyze the anomaly further,[274] revealing in some cases a lung-based opaque region containing intrathoracic fat,[495] but it rarely is required.

Pelvic ribs also are rare, being asymptomatic and discovered on radiographic examinations performed for nonrelated reasons.[276–282, 496, 548] These ribs may arise as single or multiple radiodense areas, adjacent to the upper portion of the lumbar spine, ilium, acetabulum, sacrum, or coccyx (Fig. 90–52), and they possess a bony, cartilaginous, or ligamentous site of attachment. Their size, shape, and configuration are extremely variable, and they course in a horizontal, oblique, or vertical direction. The osseous nature of the anomaly is apparent radiographically owing to the presence of a cortex and internal trabeculation. Jointlike gaps in the ossified structure sometimes are seen. Major differential diagnostic possibilities include posttraumatic hetero-

FIGURE 90–49. Talonavicular tarsal coalition. Bony fusion of the talus and the navicular bone is evident. Deformity of the apposing surfaces of talus and calcaneus also is apparent.

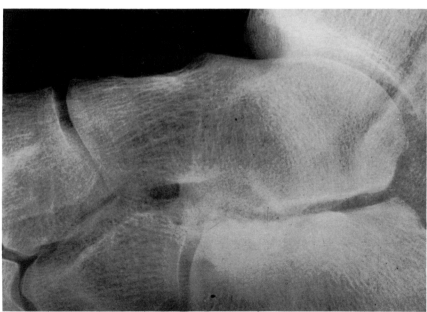

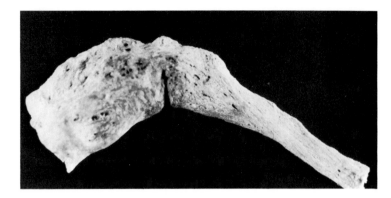

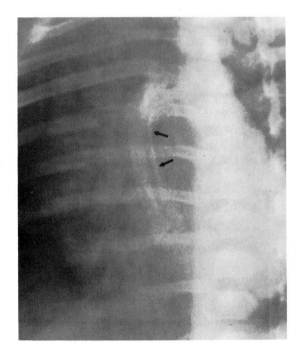

FIGURE 90–50. Cervical rib. Observe the accessory rib arising from the transverse process of the seventh cervical vertebra.

FIGURE 90–51. Intrathoracic rib. The supernumerary rib (arrows) arises from the posteroinferior margin of another rib and is projected over the inner portion of the lung field in this frontal radiographic projection. (Courtesy of S. Hilton, M.D., San Diego, California.)

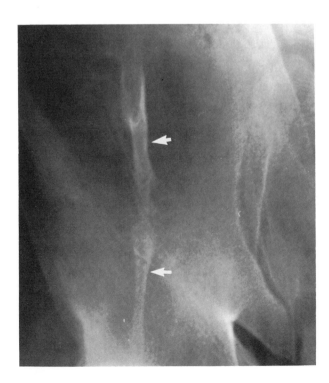

FIGURE 90–52. Pelvic rib. An example is shown (arrows).

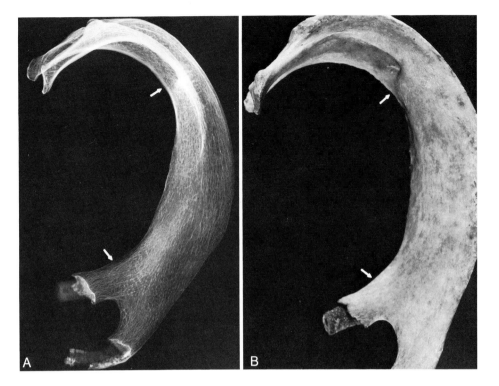

FIGURE 90–53. Synostosis of the ribs. Solid bone (between arrows) unites the middle segment of two upper thoracic ribs. They are separate posteriorly and bifurcate into separate structures again anteriorly.

topic ossification, neurologic injury or a burn with soft tissue ossification, osteochondroma, hemophilia, and ligamentous ossification related to diffuse idiopathic skeletal hyperostosis or fluorosis.

Synostosis involving ribs may occur either as an isolated phenomenon, usually affecting the first and second ribs, or in association with abnormalities of spinal segmentation (Fig. 90–53). *Bifurcation* of the sternal end of the ribs is relatively common and usually is without clinical significance. Either anomaly, however, may represent a manifestation of an underlying disorder, such as the basal cell nevus syndrome (Gorlin's syndrome).

Klippel-Feil Syndrome

The term Klippel-Feil deformity is applied loosely to many types of congenital fusions of the cervical vertebrae; however, the original syndrome, as described by Klippel and Feil in 1912,[106, 107] consisted of a triad of signs: a short neck, a low posterior hairline, and a limitation of movement of the neck. These easily recognized clinical manifestations are present at birth, yet the relatively minor nature of the affliction may delay the patient's coming to medical attention until the second or third decade of life. At this time, in addition to the physical signs noted previously, neurologic abnormalities may be present. As applied currently, the designation of the Klippel-Feil syndrome indicates a congenital fusion of two or more cervical vertebrae; the classic triad is not apparent in more than 50 per cent of patients.

The reported frequency of congenital cervical vertebral fusion has varied considerably. Some investigators regard the finding as being exceedingly rare,[108] whereas others report its occurrence in nearly 0.5 per cent of spinal radiographs.[109] Men and women are affected with approximately equal frequency. The level and extent of cervical involvement are not constant. In most cases, fusion begins at the occiput and the first cervical vertebra, at the first and second cervical vertebrae, or at the second and third cervical vertebrae[110] (Fig. 90–54). With involvement of the upper cervical region, the segment of the second and third vertebrae represents a typical distal location of the fusion; with involvement of the lower cervical region, it is the segment between the sixth and seventh vertebrae that generally denotes the distal extent of disease. The joints of the second and third and of the fifth and sixth cervical vertebrae are altered most frequently. Occasionally, cases involve upper thoracic vertebrae as well, usually ending at the fourth and fifth thoracic levels. These findings are not constant, nor is the fusion solid throughout its extent. In some instances, one or more intervening levels may not be affected. This allows for some degree of motion in involved spinal segments and, in some cases, cervical instability with neurologic involvement.[497]

Patients with Klippel-Feil syndrome or related deformity usually do not reveal evidence of a familial history of disease; exceptions to this rule occur, as evidenced by several reports.[111, 112] On clinical examination, the patient has a short neck, which, when the syndrome is severe, may create the illusion that the head is resting directly on the thorax. Restriction of motion may be marked, particularly that of lateral motion rather than flexion and extension.[498, 499] Torticollis can be present in some cases. Neurologic abnormalities are variable and may include spasticity, hyperreflexia, pain, muscle atrophy, oculomotor disturbances, pyramidal tract findings, paralysis, anesthesia, and paresthesia. In the presence of high cervical fusions, neurologic findings tend to be more prominent and appear earlier in the course of the disease. Such findings also may develop acutely after minor injury.[283]

Many associated malformations have been described.[110]

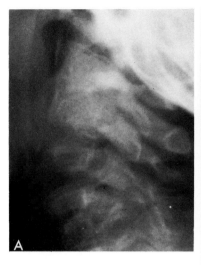
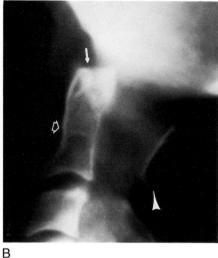
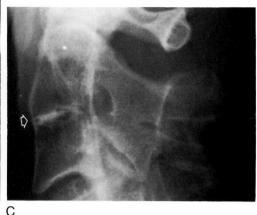

FIGURE 90–54. Klippel-Feil syndrome.

A Observe bony fusion of the atlas and the axis with deformity of the base of the skull. Both the vertebral bodies and the posterior elements are involved.

B In a different patient, conventional tomography indicates osseous fusion of cervical vertebrae. Note the incorporation of the odontoid process into the anterior arch of the atlas (solid arrow), the narrowed "waist" of the fused vertebral bodies (open arrow), and ankylosis of the posterior elements (arrowhead).

C In a third patient, fusion of the second and third cervical vertebrae is seen. Note the ankylosis of the posterior elements and the atrophic intervertebral disc containing calcification (open arrow).

1. Sprengel's deformity. Unilateral or bilateral elevation of the scapula is present in approximately 20 to 25 per cent of cases, especially in those with high and extensive cervical fusions (Fig. 90–55). It may be associated with an omovertebral bone connecting the scapula and vertebrae. This bone, which is present in approximately 30 to 40 per cent of cases of fixed elevated scapula, is not always ossified.[284] It may consist of osseous, cartilaginous, or fibrous tissue, and the connection between scapula and omovertebral element may be cartilaginous, bony, or fibrous[285] or be a true joint. The connection usually is at the middle to lower portion of the vertebral border of the scapula.[286, 287] Rarely, a similar bone connects the vertebrae and ribs[288] or scapula and clavicle (omoclavicular bone).[500] Alterations of the adjacent clavicle may be evident.

2. Cervical ribs. Anomalous ribs are evident in approximately 10 to 15 per cent of cases, most frequently in women.

3. Webbed neck (pterygium colli). Webbing of the soft tissues on each side may accentuate the shortness of the neck and may involve the skin, muscles, and fascia. Reports of cervical spinal fusions and webbed necks in patients with Turner's syndrome also have appeared.[113]

4. Hemivertebrae. A hemivertebrae is present in approximately 15 to 20 per cent of cases and can lead to scoliosis.

5. Spina bifida. Anterior or posterior spina bifida is frequent in patients with cervical fusions. The abnormalities may be apparent in one or more levels in the cervical or thoracic regions.

6. Other anomalies. Kyphosis, scoliosis, spinal stenosis, fused, absent, or deformed ribs, basilar impression, cranial asymmetry, congenital defects of the brain or spinal cord, deformed dens, cleft palate, supernumerary lobes of the lung, patent foramen ovale, interventricular septal defect, renal anomalies, and enteric cysts or duplications represent some of the additional malformations that may be apparent.[114–116, 289, 549]

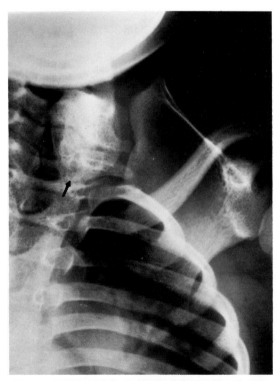

FIGURE 90–55. Klippel-Feil syndrome with Sprengel's deformity. Note the elevated position of the scapula, an omovertebral bone (arrow), and cervical spinal abnormalities.

On radiographs, the fusion may be partial or complete and may affect the vertebral bodies, the pedicles, the laminae, or the spinous processes (Fig. 90–54). Initially detected changes may progress in severity and extent on serial radiographs.[118, 290] With fusion of the vertebral bodies, small atrophic intervertebral discs may be apparent, which can contain calcification. The anteroposterior diameter of the vertebral bodies at the level of an affected discovertebral junction may be smaller than that at the superior and inferior limits of the vertebrae adjacent to uninvolved discs, forming the basis for the wasp-waist sign.[554] The resulting trapezoidal shape of the vertebral body is very suggestive of a congenital fusion or at least of one that has occurred at an early age, as it is related to the interference with normal growth at the site of fusion; continued growth at the unaffected aspects of the vertebrae then produces the altered vertebral shape that is characteristic of the condition.

The Klippel-Feil deformity apparently results from an insult to the developing fetus, preventing normal embryogenesis. Oxygen deprivation in rabbits during the 9th to 11th days of gestation, a period corresponding to the 25th day of gestation in humans, can lead to vertebral anomalies in the offspring.[116] Gardner and Collins[117] have postulated that overdistention of the neural tube in embryonal life is a common factor in the pathogenesis of the Klippel-Feil syndrome, syringomyelia, diastematomyelia, meningomyelocele, and the Arnold-Chiari syndrome, although this theory may be an oversimplification of the processes leading to varied spinal malformations.[110] Additional factors, such as hereditary effects and chromosomal abnormalities, have yet to be fully explored.

The radiographic features of a congenital fusion of cervical vertebral bodies must be distinguished from those in acquired cases of ankylosis (Fig. 90–56). Although this is not always possible, the following signs are helpful in the diagnosis of Klippel-Feil syndrome and related anomalies: trapezoidal shape of vertebral bodies with intervening atrophic intervertebral discs, irregularity of the intervertebral foramina, and fusion of both the anterior (vertebral bodies and intervertebral discs) and posterior (pedicles, laminae, spinous processes) columns of the spine. Application of these criteria in the evaluation of spinal radiographs may allow differentiation of congenital fusion from other processes, particularly juvenile chronic arthritis, yet a review of some of the earlier reports of Klippel-Feil syndrome indicates that cases of juvenile chronic arthritis were included in the analyses. Although it is the clinical history that is most helpful in differentiating between these two conditions, the radiographic findings of juvenile chronic arthritis do not include ankylosis of adjacent spinous processes. Furthermore, in this articular disease, abnormalities of other skeletal sites are apparent, and an elevated position of the scapula is not seen. In ankylosing spondylitis, ankylosis of vertebral bodies and apophyseal joints is noted, but the vertebrae and intervertebral discs are not diminutive. Differentiation of congenital cervical fusion from tuberculosis and traumatic and surgical changes usually is not difficult.

Congenital Block Vertebrae

Congenital synostosis of vertebrae in the thoracic and lumbar spine also may be encountered, again related to a derangement of embryologic development (Fig. 90–57). The anomaly usually is limited in extent, affecting two adjacent vertebrae, and commonly is asymptomatic, being discovered on radiographs obtained for other reasons. The

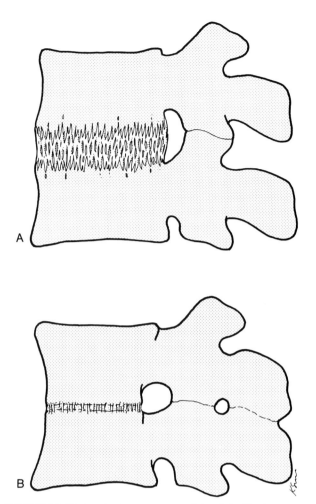

FIGURE 90–56. Acquired versus congenital vertebral fusion.
  A Acquired ankylosis. Note the absence of constriction at the level of the intervertebral disc and the absence of posterior element fusion.
  B Congenital ankylosis. A constricted appearance at the level of the intervertebral disc has produced a trapezoidal shape of the bony mass. The posterior elements also are ankylosed, and the intervertebral disc is atrophic.

fusion typically affects the vertebral bodies, although the posterior elements also can be incorporated into an ossified mass. The intervening intervertebral disc is atrophic and calcified or completely obliterated. Partial fusion of one side of the vertebrae can lead to scoliosis or other abnormalities of spinal curvature. The same radiographic guidelines noted in the discussion of the Klippel-Feil syndrome apply to the recognition of congenital fusion of thoracic and lumbar vertebrae.

ARTICULAR ABNORMALITIES

Madelung's Deformity

In 1878, Madelung[119] described a painful wrist deformity in a young woman that he considered to be the result of an overloading of a joint that already was predisposed to malformation. Subsequently, Madelung's deformity has attracted the attention of numerous investigators.[120–125] The primary deformity is a bowing of the distal end of the radius. Typically, the radial bowing occurs in a volar direction while the ulna continues to grow in a straight fashion.

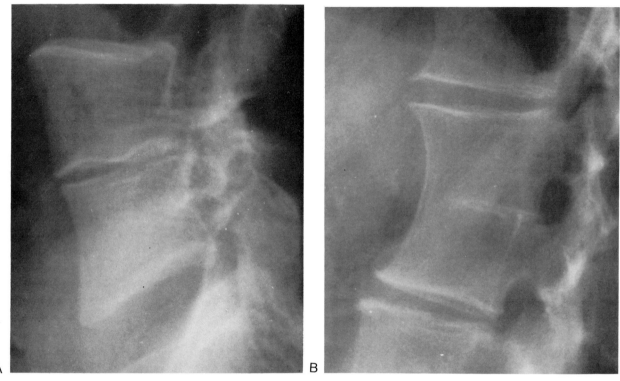

A   B

FIGURE 90–57. Congenital block vertebrae: Lumbar spine.

A Note incomplete fusion between the fourth and fifth lumbar vertebral bodies. The intervertebral disc is atrophic and the anteroposterior width of the vertebral bodies at the site of fusion is less than at the uninvolved portions of the bodies, creating a trapezoidal vertebral shape.

B In this more exaggerated example, note the concave anterior vertebral surface and atrophic intervertebral disc containing minimal calcification. Observe the degenerative changes (osteophytes and bone sclerosis) at the adjacent discal levels.

The curvature and growth disturbance of the radius result in its being shorter than the ulna. Thus, the ulna is relatively long in comparison to its osseous neighbor, and the carpal angle, formed by the intersection of two lines (the first tangent to the proximal surfaces of the scaphoid and the lunate bones, the second tangent to the proximal margins of the triquetrum and the lunate bones), which normally is 130 to 137 degrees, is decreased[126, 127] (Table 90–2). In recent years, numerous radiographic alterations have been reported in Madelung's deformity[124] (Fig. 90–58).

1. Radial abnormalities. Dorsal and ulnar curvature, decreased length, triangularization of the distal radial epiphysis with unequal growth of the epiphysis, premature fusion of the medial half of the radial epiphysis, a localized area of lucency along the ulnar border of the radius, osteophy-

TABLE 90–2. Syndromes Associated with Abnormality of the Carpal Angle

Decreased	Increased
Madelung's deformity	Arthrogryposis
Dyschondrosteosis	Diastrophic dwarfism
Turner's syndrome	Epiphyseal dysplasias
Morquio's syndrome	Frontometaphyseal dysplasia
Hurler's syndrome	Otopalatodigital syndrome
	Pfeiffer's syndrome
	Spondyloepiphyseal dysplasia
	Trisomy 21

(From Poznanski AK: The Hand in Radiologic Diagnosis. Philadelphia, WB Saunders Co, 1974, p 140.)

tosis along the inferior ulnar portion of the radius, and ulnar and volar angulation of the distal radial articular surface have been reported.

2. Ulnar abnormalities. Dorsal subluxation, enlargement and distortion of the ulnar head, and changes in length have been observed.

3. Carpal abnormalities. Wedging of the carpus between the deformed radius and protruding ulna, triangular configuration with the lunate at the apex, and arched curvature in the lateral projection as a direct continuation of the arch of posterior bowing of the radial epiphysis have occurred.

Much confusion has existed regarding the cause of this deformity. Some of this confusion was stimulated by the report in 1929 by Léri and Weill[128] in which a case of hereditary dwarfism was characterized by a wrist alteration that appeared identical to Madelung's deformity. In addition, the forearms and the lower legs were shorter than the proximal and distal parts of the extremities. This mesomelic variety of dwarfism has become known as dyschondrosteosis, and additional reports of this disease have confirmed the constant and prominent role that Madelung's deformity assumes in its radiographic features.[501] Considerable debate has occurred regarding the relationship of dyschondrosteosis and Madelung's deformity. At the extremes are the opinions that the two are not related[129] and that they are identical syndromes.[130] It appears that this wrist deformity is frequent in patients with dyschondrosteosis but that it also is evident as an isolated phenomenon without associated dwarfism. Whether this latter pattern represents a

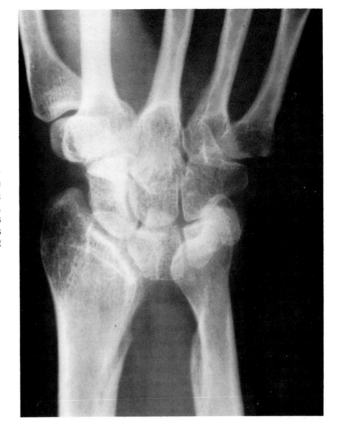

FIGURE 90–58. Madelung's deformity. Abnormalities include increased width between the distal portions of the radius and ulna, an ulna that is relatively long compared to the length of the radius, a decreased carpal angle, triangularization of the distal radial epiphysis, osseous excrescences on apposing metaphyseal regions of radius and ulna, distortion of the ulnar head, and wedging of the carpus between the deformed radius and protruding ulna, with the lunate at the apex of the wedge.

forme fruste of dyschondrosteosis cannot be ascertained with certainty. Golding and Blackburne[129] believe that isolated Madelung's deformity is not heritable and is restricted to women, whereas dyschondrosteosis is confined to men. This opinion is not accepted uniformly, and, in fact, reports of familial cases of isolated Madelung's deformity have appeared.[291]

Madelung's deformity has been classified into several types, including posttraumatic (due to extension injuries to the radial epiphysis), dysplastic (due to dyschondrosteosis and multiple hereditary exostoses) (Fig. 90–59), genetic (in association with Turner's syndrome), and idiopathic.[125] This classification system is complicated by the fact that the wrist abnormality in some of these conditions is not a typical Madelung's deformity but rather is a "reverse" deformity in which the distal end of the radius is tilted dorsally, the carpus is shifted dorsally, and the distal end of the ulna appears to be dislocated anteriorly.[502]

The isolated variety of Madelung's deformity is more commonly bilateral than unilateral, is asymmetric in severity, and, if not restricted to women, is at least three to five times more common in female patients. Clinical manifestations usually become evident in the adolescent or young adult, in whom visible deformity, pain, fatigue, and limited range of motion, especially dorsal extension, ulnar deviation, and supination, are noted. The carpal tunnel syndrome may be evident.[503] After several years of progressive symptoms and signs, the findings may become stationary, and the pain actually may decrease, although in some cases, surgical intervention is required. Rarely, spontaneous rupture of extensor tendons may be evident.[131]

Congenital Subluxation and Hyperextension of the Knee

Congenital subluxation and hyperextension of the knee is a rare congenital deformity, occurring approximately one fortieth to one eightieth as frequently as developmental dysplasia of the hip, in which the tibia and femur are abnormally related.[132–135, 504–507] Blacks are affected more commonly than whites. A definite female preponderance is seen, with a reported ratio of approximately 3 to 1. Hereditary factors appear to be important in some cases as judged by a familial history of the deformity[136, 137] and its occurrence in twins[292]; associated congenital deformities include dislocation of the hip, foot abnormalities, and dislocation of the elbow, in order of decreasing frequency.[138] Other factors that may be important in the cause of this condition include abnormal fetal position during pregnancy,[139] breech delivery,[505] perinatal injury, neuromuscular imbalance,[293] quadriceps contracture,[140, 507] and absence or hypoplasia of the cruciate ligaments.[138] The last two findings may be the result of, rather than the cause of, the knee malposition.

The severity of the deformity is variable[141] (Fig. 90–60). Hyperextension can occur without tibial malposition, tibial subluxation or dislocation can appear without hyperextension, or both hyperextension and subluxation or dislocation may occur together (Fig. 90–61); habitual anterior subluxation of the tibia on the femur during extension of the knee[508] may represent a very mild form of this deformity. At birth, an affected infant frequently reveals a hyperextended knee or knees with limited flexion capabilities and anterior transverse skin folds or creases at the point of

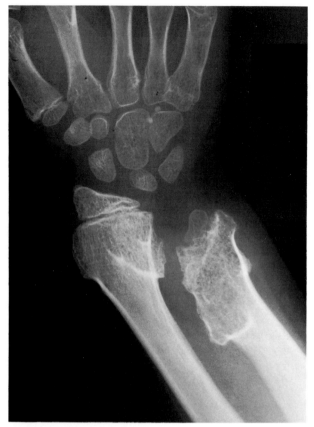

FIGURE 90–59. Wrist deformity in multiple hereditary exostoses. Observe broad-based exostoses of the radius and ulna with metaphyseal widening. The ulna is relatively short compared to the radius. The distal radial epiphysis is triangular in shape.

tibial epiphysis and obliteration of the suprapatellar pouch secondary to local fibrous adherence to the quadriceps muscle. Surgical observations confirm the presence of ablation of the suprapatellar pouch and also reveal quadriceps fibrosis, anterior dislocation of the hamstring tendons, dysplasia of the articular surfaces of the femur and tibia, and elongation and attenuation of the anterior cruciate ligament.[505]

This condition should be distinguished from genu recurvatum due to ligament laxity, acquired quadriceps contracture, and traumatic changes.

Congenital Dislocation of the Radial Head

Although it is a rare condition, congenital dislocation of the radial head represents the most common anomaly of the elbow region. It may occur as an isolated phenomenon or in association with other congenital abnormalities, particularly those of the hand.[294, 295, 509] In some instances, a familial history of the anomaly, suggesting an autosomal recessive inheritance pattern, is evident.[296] Clinical findings usually appear in infancy or childhood and include a decrease in elbow motion.[294] Radiographic abnormalities include a relatively short ulna or long radius, hypoplasia or aplasia of the capitulum, a partially defective trochlea, prominence of the ulnar epicondyle, a dome-shaped radial head with an elongated radial neck, and grooving of the distal portion of the humerus.[295] Unilateral or bilateral involvement is seen, and progressive subluxation or dislocation of the radial head usually proceeds in a posterior direction.

Diagnostic difficulty is encountered in the differentiation of congenital versus traumatic dislocation of the radial head, and, in fact, the former surprisingly may be encountered during attempted surgical reduction of a dislocation that was considered traumatic in origin.[297] As congenital dislocation of the radial head may produce minor symptoms and signs, it is expected that some patients with this disorder will be evaluated only after a significant injury to the elbow, increasing the likelihood of diagnostic error. In these instances, the radiographic abnormalities indicated previously show that malpositioning of the radial head is of long

hyperextension. Radiographs confirm the anterior position of the proximal portion of the tibia with respect to the distal end of the femur and, possibly, lateral subluxation and valgus deformity of the knee. Anterior tibial bowing and patellar hypoplasia also may be seen. Arthrography can delineate flattening of the chondral surface in the posterior

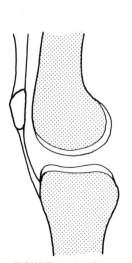
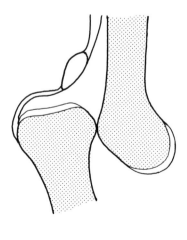
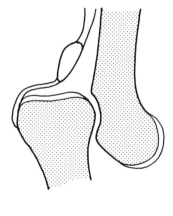

FIGURE 90–60. Congenital subluxation and hyperextension of the knee. Variable patterns can be encountered. Mild subluxation or frank dislocation with anterior femoral erosion may be seen.

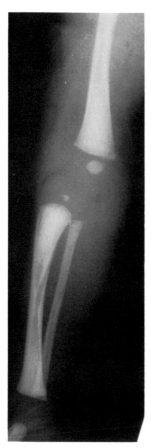

FIGURE 90–61. Congenital subluxation of the knee. In a 2 day old infant, note anterior displacement of the tibia and fibula with respect to the femur.

duration but may not allow differentiation between traumatic or congenital alterations.

Infantile Coxa Vara

Normally, the angle of intersection of the axis of the femoral neck with that of the femoral shaft varies with age but is approximately 150 degrees at birth and 120 to 130 degrees in the adult. The relative valgus position in the infant's femur is due to an increased growth of the medial portion of the cartilage plate in the prenatal period. With an acceleration of growth in the lateral portion of the plate in the child, a more varus position becomes apparent.

The term coxa vara indicates a neck-shaft angle that is less than 120 degrees despite the variation of normal values that occurs in different age groups. Coxa vara may accompany various processes, including PFFD, osteogenesis imperfecta, renal osteodystrophy, rickets, and fibrous dysplasia.[142] Infantile or developmental coxa vara is a designation of a proximal femoral deformity that usually becomes apparent in the first few years of life, especially the age at which the child first walks. Boys and girls are affected with approximately equal frequency, and the condition is unilateral in 60 to 75 per cent of cases.[298] Clinically, the affected child has a painless lurching gait or, in the case of bilateral involvement, a ''duck-waddle'' gait.[143–148] Limited joint motion also is seen. Additional features include a short stature and excessive lumbar lordosis.

Radiographs reveal a decrease in the femoral shaft–neck angle and a medially located triangular piece of bone in the neck adjacent to the head that is bounded by two radiolucent bands traversing the neck and forming an inverted V. The growth plate itself is widened, and its alignment is more vertical than normal. With further growth, the varus deformity frequently progresses, probably related to the forces of weight-bearing (Fig. 90–62). The triangular piece of bone may merge with the shaft, remodeling thickens the medial cortex of the femoral neck, the greater trochanter enlarges, and secondary degenerative joint disease can appear. MR imaging reveals a widened growth plate with expansion of cartilage mediodistally between the capital femoral epiphysis and metaphysis.[510] Histologically, the growth plate is composed of irregularly distributed germinal cartilage cells with abundant matrix.[510]

The precise cause of this condition has not been delineated. A familial occurrence of the deformity is noted in some cases, suggesting a genetic cause or predisposition.[148–152] Additional mechanisms that have been proposed in infantile coxa vara are a juvenile osteochondrosis similar to Legg-Calvé-Perthes disease,[143] pathologic ossification of the femoral neck, embryonic interference with blood supply to the proximal portion of the femur,[153] and trauma.[154] Experimentally, coxa vara can be produced by inducing growth arrest in the capital femoral epiphysis.[155]

The differential diagnosis of infantile coxa vara includes PFFD, slipped capital femoral epiphysis, septic arthritis and osteomyelitis, rickets, and fibrous dysplasia.[299]

Primary Protrusion of the Acetabulum

Acetabular protrusion refers to intrapelvic displacement of the medial wall of the acetabulum. It may be evident in many articular and nonarticular disorders, including rheumatoid arthritis, ankylosing spondylitis, septic arthritis, de-

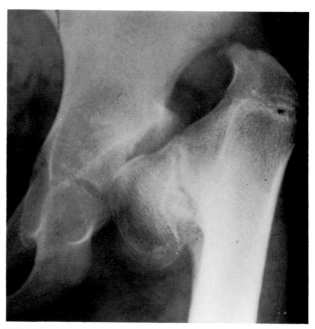

FIGURE 90–62. Infantile coxa vara. Note the severe varus deformity of the proximal portion of the femur, the vertically located and irregular growth plate, thickening of the medial cortex of the femoral neck, a prominent greater trochanter, and acetabular flattening.

generative joint disease, osteomalacia, Paget's disease, sickle cell anemia, neoplasm, and trauma, and as an effect of irradiation. Protrusio acetabuli also can appear in the absence of any recognizable cause, and, in such a case, it is termed primary acetabular protrusion. The primary variety was recognized first by Otto in 1824[156] and sometimes is referred to as Otto pelvis.

The cause of primary acetabular protrusion is unknown. A failure of ossification[157, 158] or premature fusion[159] of the Y cartilage has been offered as a possible etiologic factor. Alexander[160] suggested that the deep acetabulum was unrelated to any pathologic process in the joint, the adjacent bone, or the Y cartilage but instead was a direct consequence of normal stress on the Y cartilage; under normal circumstances, the protrusion was reversible owing to the diminishing stresses after the age of 8 years, but under abnormal circumstances, a failure of correction of the protrusion resulted in its persistence into adult life. This investigator noted that acetabular protrusion was more common in the female sex and in association with premature fusion of the Y cartilage and coxa vara. He also noted persistent beaking of the Y cartilage as a feature in young children that was associated with acetabular protrusion in the adult. Thus, according to Alexander, the deformity was the direct result of a failure of normal acetabular remodeling. A familial nature of the disorder was emphasized first by Rechtman in 1936[161] and subsequently was confirmed in numerous reports.[162–164]

Primary acetabular protrusion usually affects both hips and is much more frequent in women than in men. Hooper and Jones[165] divided patients with the disorder into three subgroups: a juvenile group, in which boys and girls were affected in equal numbers, a family history was frequent, and symptoms and signs occurred in adolescence, progressed rapidly, and became incapacitating; a middle-aged group, in which symptoms and signs appeared later in life and in which osteoarthritis was not uncommon; and an elderly group, in which osteoarthritis was invariable. These investigators noted that the deformity was aggravated during periods of rapid hormone flux, namely at puberty and at or after menopause.

The predictive value of beaking of the Y cartilage of the acetabular region may be somewhat limited. Such a change is not infrequent in the developing skeleton, probably as a result of medial displacement of the Y synchondrosis due to normal weight-bearing, and is reversible in most persons. Marked beaking combined with abnormal varus angulation of the femoral neck or premature fusion of the Y cartilage is a more alarming finding that may be accompanied later by protrusion of the acetabulum. Such protrusion is confirmed readily on radiographic examination, although appropriate criteria that differ in the male and female patient must be applied (see Chapter 22).

With progressive protrusion deformity, the femoral head assumes an intrapelvic location, and the joint space may be normal, narrowed, or obliterated. Pathologic examination confirms the existence of fibrocartilaginous replacement and osteophytosis of the femoral head.[164]

Acetabular deformity in mild cases of primary protrusion must be distinguished from normal variations in acetabular depth. The radiographic diagnosis of abnormal protrusion based on the mere "crossing" of the acetabular line and ilioischial line is inadequate; rather, an abnormal situation exists in the adult pelvis when the distance between the medially located acetabular line and the laterally located ilioischial line is 6 mm or more in women and 3 mm or more in men (Fig. 90–63). With the onset of joint degeneration and narrowing in primary acetabular protrusion, the findings must be distinguished from those of other articular disorders of the hip. The joint space loss in idiopathic acetabular protrusion usually results in axial or medial migration of the femoral head with respect to the acetabulum. In osteoarthritis alone, superior or, less commonly, medial migration of the femoral head is typical. Axial migration of the femoral head is seen in rheumatoid arthritis, ankylosing spondylitis, chondrolysis, chondral atrophy due to immobilization, and calcium pyrophosphate dihydrate crystal deposition disease, but other radiographic features ensure ac-

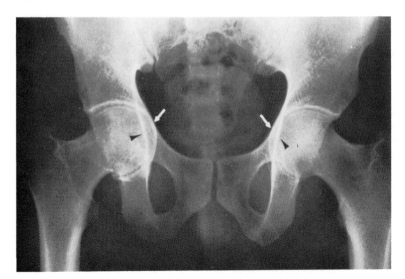

FIGURE 90–63. Primary protrusion of the acetabulum. This 30 year old man reveals bilateral acetabular protrusion with concentric loss of joint space. Note that the acetabular line (arrows) is located medial to the ilioischial line (arrowheads) by a considerable distance.

curate diagnosis of most of these conditions. It should be noted, however, that idiopathic acetabular protrusion and idiopathic chondrolysis share many clinical and radiologic features, and differentiation between them may be difficult.[300]

Joint Hypermobility Syndrome

Joint hypermobility syndrome, which also is referred to as congenital laxity of ligaments, indicates hypermobility of joints that is independent of inflammatory conditions, neurologic disorders, diseases of connective tissue (including the Ehlers-Danlos syndrome), and other congenital disorders.[421] Its occurrence as an isolated phenomenon has been documented,[301–303] although such documentation requires the application of strict diagnostic criteria of joint laxity[304, 305] and knowledge of ethnic, age-related, and sex-related differences in articular mobility.[306] For example, such mobility normally is more pronounced in women than in men, in younger than in older persons, and in blacks and Native Americans than in whites of the same age and sex.[307, 308, 513, 517] Furthermore, some types of motion can become more exaggerated owing to prolonged occupational or recreational (e.g., ballet dancing) activities,[309] and, in fact, such activities can lead to changes in joint alignment (e.g., axial radial rotation of the ulnar digits in pianists).[310]

The syndrome of joint hypermobility may be familial, related to the presence of a dominant gene. Although the condition may be entirely asymptomatic, clinical manifestations have been reported, ranging from minor articular discomfort, acute pain, or joint effusions to recurrent subluxations or dislocations of the patella, hip, elbow, or glenohumeral joint, idiopathic scoliosis, carpal tunnel syndrome and other neuropathies, temporomandibular joint dysfunction, or prolapse of the mitral valve.[301, 303, 304, 312, 313, 511, 512, 514–516] Foot abnormalities, including equinovarus and calcaneovalgus deformities, also have been associated with this syndrome,[314] as have osteoarthritis and chondrocalcinosis.[315]

Foot Deformities

Although a detailed discussion of the complexities of the deformed foot is well beyond the scope of this textbook, a brief summary of the major foot deformities is included here. The interested reader should consult the excellent radiographic reviews provided by Ozonoff,[166] Freiberger and colleagues,[167] and Ritchie and Keim,[168] from which many of the following observations are derived. Proper radiographic analysis requires both anteroposterior and lateral projections exposed during weight-bearing. The anteroposterior projection is obtained with the sagittal plane of the leg perpendicular to the film and with the knees together; the lateral view is exposed with the foot in maximal dorsiflexion, a technique that usually requires the use of a support beneath the plantar surface of the foot. The following terms are applied to the deformities.

Talipes: a long-established name for congenital deformities of the foot (for example, talipes equinovarus).
Pes: a name that should be restricted to acquired deformities of the foot (such as pes equinovarus).

Valgus: the bones distal to a specified joint are oriented in a plane away from the midline of the body.
Varus: the opposite of valgus, in which the bones distal to a specified joint are oriented in a plane toward the midline of the body.
Equinus: fixed plantar flexion of the hindfoot.
Calcaneus: fixed dorsiflexion of the hindfoot.
Cavus: a raised longitudinal arch of the foot.
Planus: a flattened longitudinal arch of the foot.
Adduction: displacement in a transverse plane toward the axis of the body.
Abduction: displacement in a transverse plane away from the axis of the body.

The normal alignment of the foot is inferred from the information obtained on anteroposterior and lateral radiographs using, in large part, the relationship of the talus and the calcaneus (Figs. 90–64 and 90–65). In the anteroposterior projection, a line through the long axis of the talus extended distally falls on, or close to, the medial border of the first metatarsal, and one through the long axis of the calcaneus falls at the base of the fourth metatarsal. The angle between the two lines, the talocalcaneal angle, averages approximately 35 degrees in the adult and is somewhat greater in the infant. The axes of the metatarsals are roughly parallel and fan out slightly in a distal direction. In the lateral projection, the foot can be dorsiflexed to such an extent that an angle between it and the lower leg is considerably less than 90 degrees. In neutral position, the long axis of the calcaneus extends dorsally from posterior to anterior, and the long axis of the talus is flexed in a plantar direction and is mildly angulated with the long axis of the first metatarsal bone. The talocalcaneal angle averages 35 degrees and is about equal to that noted on the anteroposterior view. The longitudinal axes of the metatarsals are approximately parallel, with the fifth metatarsal being most plantar, the others superimposed, and the first metatarsal being most dorsal in location.

The talus is used as the point of reference in the description of foot deformities. It generally is assumed that the talus is relatively fixed in relation to the lower leg, so that a change in the relationship of the talus and the calcaneus reflects a movement of the latter bone. The calcaneus can abduct, increasing the talocalcaneal angle, or adduct, decreasing the talocalcaneal angle.

In *hindfoot (heel) valgus* (Fig. 90–64), an anteroposterior projection reveals an increase in the talocalcaneal angle. An extended line through the longitudinal axis of the talus will fall medial to the first metatarsal, and the navicular and other tarsal bones will be displaced laterally to the talus. On the lateral projection, the talus will be tilted more vertically than normal, owing to the abduction of the calcaneus, which decreases the plantar support on the anterior portion of the talus. The long axis of the talus and that of the first metatarsal will angulate in a plantar direction.

In *hindfoot (heel) varus* (Fig. 90–64), on anteroposterior views the long axis of the talus falls lateral to the base of the first metatarsal owing to the adduction of the anterior end of the calcaneus. The talocalcaneal angle is decreased, and the talus and calcaneus are more parallel to each other than in the normal foot. The navicular bone is displaced medially. On the lateral view, the calcaneus and talus both are more horizontal and parallel with each other.

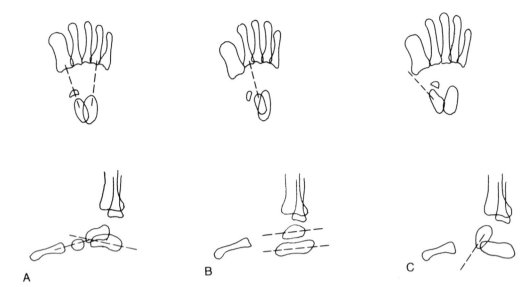

FIGURE 90–64. Foot: Normal and abnormal hindfoot and forefoot relationship.

A Normal. On an anteroposterior radiograph, the talar axis intersects or points slightly medial to the first metatarsal bone, and the navicular bone is situated directly opposite the head of the talus. The calcaneus points toward the fourth metatarsal bone, creating a talocalcaneal angle of approximately 35 degrees in the adult and somewhat greater in the infant. On a lateral radiograph, the anterior portion of the talus is mildly flexed in a plantar direction, and the calcaneus is slightly dorsiflexed. An extended line through the longitudinal axis of the talus is directed along the axis of the first metatarsal bone. The talocalcaneal angle is approximately 35 degrees.

B Hindfoot varus deformity. The anteroposterior radiograph reveals a decrease in the talocalcaneal angle as the two bones lie closely together and more parallel to each other. The navicular bone is displaced medially, and the talar axis points lateral to the first metatarsal base. In the lateral projection, the talus and the calcaneus are both more horizontal and parallel with each other.

C Hindfoot valgus deformity. On the anteroposterior radiograph, the talocalcaneal angle is increased, with the navicular bone and remaining tarsal bones being located lateral to the talus. The talar axial line passes medial to the first metatarsal bone. On the lateral radiograph, the talus is oriented more vertically, and the long axis of the talus and that of the first metatarsal bone angulate in a plantar direction.

(After Ozonoff MB: Pediatric Orthopedic Radiology. Philadelphia, WB Saunders Co, 1979.)

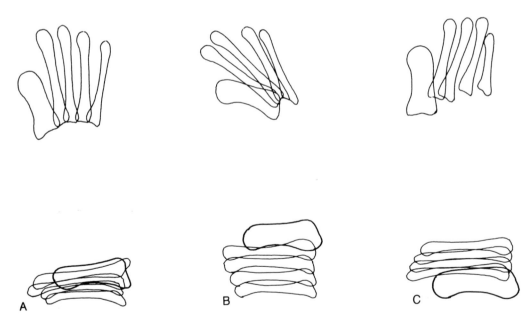

FIGURE 90–65. Foot: Normal and abnormal forefoot alignment.

A Normal. On the anteroposterior radiograph, the metatarsal bones converge proximally with overlapping at their bases. On the lateral projection, the fifth metatarsal bone is in the most plantar position, with the other metatarsals being superimposed.

B Forefoot varus deformity. On the frontal radiograph, the forefoot is narrowed, with increased convergence at the metatarsal bases, resulting in more overlap than normal. On the lateral radiograph, a ladder-like arrangement is seen, with the first metatarsal bone being most dorsal.

C Forefoot valgus deformity. The forefoot is broadened, with the metatarsal bones being more prominent than normal and with decreased overlap at the metatarsal bases. In the lateral projection, a ladder-like arrangement can be noted in some cases, with the first metatarsal bone being in the most plantar position.

(After Ozonoff MB: Pediatric Orthopedic Radiology. Philadelphia, WB Saunders Co, 1979.)

Hindfoot or heel valgus is present in flatfoot, metatarsus varus, congenital vertical talus, and certain congenital and neurologic deformities of the foot. Hindfoot or heel varus commonly is visible in talipes equinovarus and some paralytic deformities.

In *hindfoot equinus,* in the lateral projection, the calcaneus is flexed in a plantar direction so that the angle between the axes of the calcaneus and the tibia is greater than 90 degrees. This deformity accompanies talipes equinovarus and congenital vertical talus. Equinus of the entire foot is evident in various neuromuscular disorders. In *calcaneal hindfoot deformity,* in the lateral projection, the calcaneus is dorsiflexed abnormally so that its anterior end has a more superior position, and the bone possesses a boxlike appearance. Calcaneal positions of the calcaneus appear in association with cavus deformities of the foot.

The term *clubfoot* represents a condition associated with equinovarus foot deformity and hindfoot varus (Fig. 90–66). Thus, the anteroposterior radiograph reveals a decreased talocalcaneal angle, and the talus and calcaneus are roughly parallel. The forefoot is adducted and in varus alignment. On the lateral radiograph, an equinus heel and a plantar flexed forefoot are evident. Again, the axes of the talus and calcaneus are roughly parallel. The clubfoot deformity is relatively common, occurs more frequently in male children, and can be unilateral or bilateral.[316] Its exact

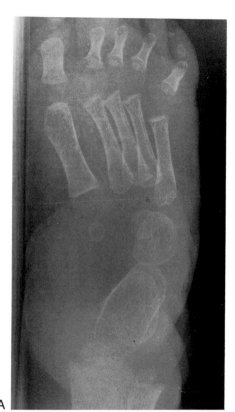

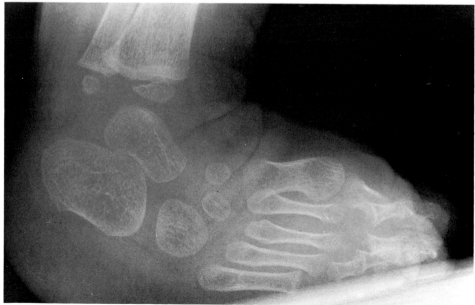

FIGURE 90–66. Clubfoot (equinovarus) deformity.

A Anteroposterior projection. The hindfoot is in marked varus position, with superimposition of the talar and calcaneal centers. A line drawn through the talus will pass far laterally to the first metatarsal bone. The navicular is not ossified, but its abnormal position can be inferred from the location of the first metatarsal base and the first cuneiform center. The forefoot is narrowed, with increased overlap of the metatarsal bases.

B Lateral projection. The talus and the calcaneus are more parallel than normal. The calcaneus is in equinus position, abnormally flexed in a plantar direction. Forefoot inversion with a ladder-like arrangement of the metatarsal bones is apparent.

(From Ozonoff MB: Pediatric Orthopedic Radiology. Philadelphia, WB Saunders Co, 1979.)

cause is not clear, although a considerable number of theories have been proposed: defective connective tissue with ligamentous laxity, muscular imbalance, intrauterine position deformity, central nervous system or vascular abnormality, and persistence of early normal fetal relationships.[166, 316–320] It seems probable that the precise cause of the clubfoot is complex and multifactorial. Anatomic studies in some cases have revealed a small talus containing a talar dome that is less convex than normal and a neck that is dislocated in a medial and plantar direction.[169] These changes result in an articular surface between the talus and the navicular bone that faces medially with the subtalar surface tilted in varus, equinus, and medial rotation.[166] The calcaneus may be diminished in size and displaced into varus, equinus, and internal rotation. This produces talonavicular and calcaneocuboid spaces that are located in a vertical line.[166] Anomalous tendon insertions and aberrations in fibular movement due to a posterolateral tether[320] also have been identified as significant anatomic features of the equinovarus foot deformity. In some instances, the ankle joint itself is abnormal, in the form of tibial hemimelia or tibiofibular diastasis.[321]

The accurate diagnosis of the clubfoot deformity relies on routine radiography, which may be supplemented with arthrography, conventional tomography, CT scanning, and arteriography,[322] and the diagnosis can be accomplished prenatally with ultrasonography.[323] The value of MR imaging in the analysis of this deformity is not clear, although the delineation of unossified cartilage with this technique is advantageous in the assessment of the infant's foot.

After inadequate or improper treatment of the clubfoot, certain deformities may remain. These include the rocker-bottom deformity, which is due to correction of the foot dorsiflexion before the equinus, and the flattop talus, which is due to flattening of the superior surface of the plantar flexed talus that is articulating with the tibia (Fig. 90–67). The navicular bone may appear truncated or wedged.[414]

A *congenital vertical talus* (congenital flatfoot with talo-navicular dislocation) can occur as an isolated condition or as part of a generalized malformation syndrome or disorder.[324] The condition occurs with approximately equal frequency in boys and girls and in a unilateral or bilateral distribution. It frequently is associated with arthrogryposis or myelomeningocele. On the anteroposterior radiograph, severe heel valgus and forefoot abduction result in an increased talocalcaneal angle with the talar axis lying medial to the first metatarsal bone. On the lateral radiograph, an equinus heel with plantar flexion of both the calcaneus and the talus is evident (Fig. 90–68). In fact, the talar axis is almost vertical in orientation, producing an increase in the talocalcaneal angle. The forefoot is dorsiflexed at the midtarsal level, resulting in a convex plantar surface of the foot, the rocker-bottom deformity. The navicular bone is dislocated dorsally, locking the talus into its plantar flexed position. With ossification of the navicular bone, the talonavicular dislocation becomes visible.

The *cavus foot deformity* is a frequent accompaniment of neurologic or muscular disorders, such as peroneal muscular atrophy, poliomyelitis, and meningomyelocele.[170] An abnormally high longitudinal arch of the foot is seen, as the calcaneus is dorsiflexed (calcaneus position) and the metatarsals are plantar flexed (Fig. 90–69).

The *flexible flatfoot deformity* is associated, on the anteroposterior view, with an increase in the talocalcaneal angle, heel valgus, and forefoot abduction. The midtarsal transverse arch is flattened, and the metatarsals are approximately parallel in their orientation. On the lateral projection, hindfoot valgus again is noted, with the talus in a more vertical attitude than normal (Fig. 90–70). The calcaneus and the metatarsals are aligned horizontally, and the plantar arch is flattened. Although the resulting radiographic picture may resemble superficially that seen in congenital vertical talus, the flexible flatfoot deformity is not associated with equinus, and the navicular bone retains its normal position with regard to the distal surface of the talus.

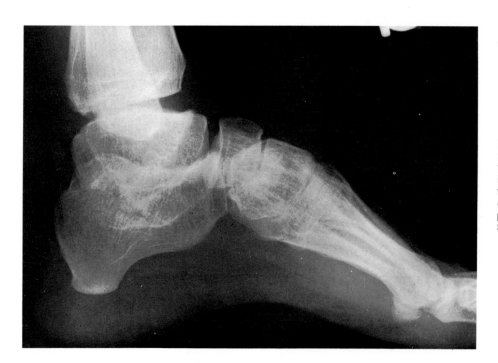

FIGURE 90–67. Corrected clubfoot (equinovarus) deformity with flat-topped talus. Note also the flattening of the articular surface of the tibia. A cavus arch is apparent. (From Ozonoff MB: Pediatric Orthopedic Radiology. Philadelphia, WB Saunders Co, 1979.)

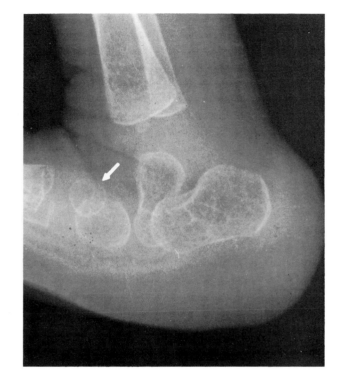

FIGURE 90–68. Congenital vertical talus. The talar axis is markedly vertical in orientation, and the calcaneus is in equinus position, producing an inferior convexity to the plantar surface of the foot. The navicular is unossified, but, because of the position of the ossified third cuneiform (arrow), it should be displaced dorsally, occupying the space between the cuneiform and the talus.

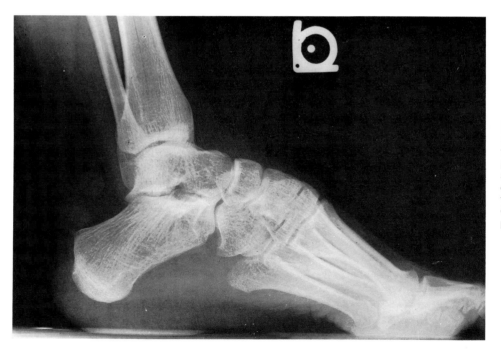

FIGURE 90–69. Cavus foot. After poliomyelitis, this 18 year old woman reveals an increased plantar arch with a calcaneus position of the os calcis and increased plantar flexion of the forefoot. (From Ozonoff MB: Pediatric Orthopedic Radiology. Philadelphia, WB Saunders Co, 1979.)

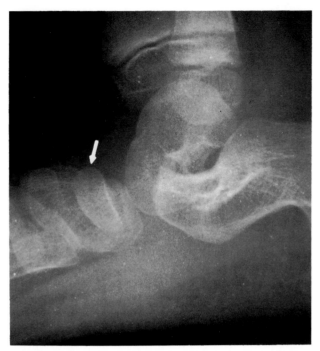

FIGURE 90–70. Flexible flatfoot (pronated foot). A lateral radiograph demonstrates an increased vertical position of the talus. The calcaneus and metatarsals are more horizontal than normal, flattening the plantar arch. Note the relatively normal position of the tarsal navicular (arrow). An anteroposterior view revealed hindfoot valgus deformity, with an increased talocalcaneal angle.

Metatarsus adductus and metatarsus varus is a common deformity of unknown cause (Fig. 90–71).[325] The forefoot is adducted and in varus alignment, with a concave medial border, convex lateral border, and high arch. The hindfoot is normal in mild cases and is in valgus alignment in severe cases. Dorsiflexion of the foot is normal or exaggerated.

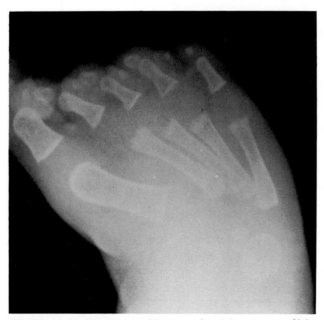

FIGURE 90–71. Metatarsus adductus and metatarsus varus. Note the adducted varus position of the forefoot, with a concave medial border and convex lateral border.

Some authors have classified patterns of forefoot adduction into several types based on the presence or absence of associated deformities of the midfoot and hindfoot; described categories included simple metatarsus adductus with adduction of the forefoot alone, complex metatarsus adductus with adduction of the forefoot combined with abnormal alignment of the midfoot, simple skewfoot deformity with adduction of the forefoot combined with a valgus position of the hindfoot, and complex skewfoot with adduction of the forefoot combined with abnormal alignment of the midfoot and a valgus position of the hindfoot.[518]

Peroneal spastic flatfoot is a deformity that is associated frequently with a tarsal coalition (discussed previously).

TORSION OF THE FEMUR AND TIBIA

Twisting of a tubular bone on its longitudinal axis is termed torsion. Torsional deformities of the human femur and tibia have received considerable attention as they have been linked to a variety of clinically significant conditions.[550] In femoral torsion, the lower or condylar portion of the bone represents the segment on which the proximal portion rotates on its longitudinal axis: in anteversion or antetorsion, the axis of the femoral neck is twisted in a forward or anterior direction with respect to the frontal or coronal plane of the femoral condyles; in retroversion or retrotorsion, this axis is rotated posteriorly or directed backward with reference to the coronal condylar plane.[326] In tibial torsion, the distal segment of the tibia is rotated toward either the medial malleolus (internal or medial tibial torsion) or the lateral malleolus (external or lateral tibial torsion).[326] The precise cause of these torsional deformities is not clear; potential factors include aberrations in the normal development of the limbs with persistence of fetal patterns of alignment, malposition of the limbs in early postnatal life, and genetic predispositions.

Internal femoral torsion or anteversion is an important finding in congenital dislocation of the hip, Legg-Calvé-Perthes disease, and neuromuscular disorders.[327] It also is observed as an isolated finding in children who otherwise appear to be normal and in whom internal femoral torsion generally is present at birth but becomes more apparent when the child begins to walk with a "toe-in" or pigeon-toed gait.[328] The inward rotation of the femur is accompanied by limitation of lateral rotation of the hips.[326] Compensatory findings include a valgus position of the hindfoot, adduction of the forefoot, and tibial torsion.[328] Although spontaneous correction of femoral anteversion is common, it is not expected if the torsional deformity persists beyond the age of 7 years,[326] and, therefore, it may require operative intervention in the older child.

A number of radiographic techniques have been employed to diagnose femoral anteversion and to assess its severity. These may require a series of frontal and lateral radiographs, axial projections, fluoroscopy, biplane radiography, specialized devices and frames for positioning the leg, and considerable expertise on the part of both the technician and the physician.[329–331, 519, 544] Although ultrasonography also has been used for this purpose,[332, 520, 551, 555] CT (or transaxial tomography[410]) appears better suited for the analysis of torsional deformities, allowing measurements of femoral torsion as well as acetabular torsion through the use of several transaxial scans.[333–336, 415, 422, 423, 521–523]

Internal or medial tibial torsion may occur as an isolated phenomenon or, more commonly, in association with congenital metatarsus varus or developmental genu varum deformity.[326] Accompanying femoral anteversion may be noted in some patients, but a relationship between the two conditions is not accepted uniformly.[524] The diagnosis may escape detection until the age of 1 year or beyond, becoming apparent when the child walks with a bowlegged or pigeon-toed gait. Spontaneous correction of this deformity is encountered, especially in those instances in which there is no family history of the abnormality.[326] *Abnormal external or lateral tibial torsion* may be congenital or acquired, the latter occurring principally in association with a contracture of the iliotibial band.[326]

The accurate diagnosis of tibial torsional malalignment requires knowledge of the changing patterns of tibial torsion that are encountered in normal infants and children[337, 338] and the use of routine radiography and CT scanning.[557]

MISCELLANEOUS SYNDROMES AND CONDITIONS

Osteo-onychodysostosis

Osteo-onychodysostosis, an autosomal dominant disorder, also is referred to as the nail-patella syndrome, hereditary osteo-onychodysplasia (HOOD), and Fong's syndrome.[342–349, 525] It is characterized by dysplastic fingernails, hypoplastic or absent patellae, additional bony deformities, particularly about the pelvis and elbows, iliac horns, widespread soft tissue changes, and renal dysplasia.[350] Proteinuria and, occasionally, hematuria may be present in infancy, although significant renal impairment usually is not evident until adulthood. Renal osteodystrophy[343] and death can result from the kidney disease. The exact nature of the renal changes is not clear; a characteristic abnormality of the glomerular basement membrane can be evident with electron microscopy, and an enzymatic defect in collagen metabolism may be the common link to the skeletal and renal lesions.[351–353, 359, 526]

Clinical manifestations can become evident in the child, adolescent, or adult but most frequently are seen in the second and third decades of life. Hypoplasia or splitting of fingernails, palpable absence of the patellae, presence of iliac protuberances, increased carrying angle of the elbow, abnormal pigmentation of the iris, and proteinuria may be recognized on initial clinical examination. Laboratory analysis can confirm the presence of more severe renal dysfunction.

The radiographic changes are highly characteristic and may allow accurate diagnosis even in the absence of clinical suspicion of the disease. Thus, in infancy, the demonstration of posterior iliac horns allows identification of this dysplasia.[349] Skeletal changes also are apparent in other regions of the body. In the knee, absence or hypoplasia of the fibula and patella, asymmetric development of the femoral condyles with hypoplasia of the lateral condyle and an apparent or true enlargement of the medial condyle, and a sloping tibial plateau with a prominent tibial tubercle are identified (Fig. 90–72).[527] These changes can lead to deformity, abnormal gait, patellar instability, and genu valgum. In the elbow, asymmetric development of the humeral con-

dyles, hypoplasia of the capitulum, and subluxation or dislocation of the radial head are the major changes (Fig. 90–73).[361]

Abnormalities of the pelvis consist of dysplasia of the iliac wings and the presence of iliac horns (Fig. 90–74). Iliac horns first were described by Kieser in 1939[354] and Fong in 1946.[355] Their association with nail, elbow, and knee dysplasia was recognized by Mino and coworkers in 1948.[356] Bilateral outgrowths from the posterior ilium, which occasionally are capped by an epiphysis, are virtually pathognomonic of osteo-onychodysostosis, although they are absent in a small percentage of cases. Unilateral iliac horns apparently can be unassociated with other skeletal abnormalities.[357]

Additional bony changes can be evident in the shoulder,[528] wrist, ankle, and subtalar joints, emphasizing the generalized nature of this dysplasia. Soft tissue alterations include flexion contractures of the hip, knee, elbow, fingers, and foot[362, 529]; web formation; and deltoid, triceps, and quadriceps hypoplasia.[344]

The basic defect is not known. Osteoporosis has been documented with histomorphologic techniques applied to bone in patients with this dysplasia.[360] An abnormality in the connective tissue due to an alteration of the enzymatic system of the ground substance has been suggested.[358] Other mechanisms also have been proposed and are summarized by Valdueza.[344]

Progeria

Progeria is a rare syndrome that was described by Hutchinson in 1886.[363] Infants appear normal at birth, and typical clinical manifestations become evident within the first few years of life. Dwarfism, alopecia, brown pigmentation of the trunk, atrophic skin, loss of subcutaneous fat, impaired extension at the hips and knees, a receding chin, a beaked nose, and exophthalmos are seen.[364] Radiographic findings include hypoplastic facial bones and mandible, delay in closure of cranial sutures, and coxa valga.[367] Acro-osteolysis of the terminal phalanges of the hands and feet and of the clavicles is a distinctive finding.[365, 366] Progressive dissolution of these bones and others, including the ribs and humerus, can lead to pathologic fractures that heal slowly and often progress to nonunion.[368] The pattern and degree of osteolysis may be reminiscent of that in hyperparathyroidism or massive osteolysis of Gorham in some cases. Another syndrome, acrogeria, resembles progeria and leads to premature aging of the skin.[530, 531] Additional features of this rare syndrome include female predominance, short stature, micrognathia, superficial venous distention, acro-osteolysis of terminal phalanges, delayed closure of cranial sutures, wormian bones, antegonial notching of the mandible, and linear, metaphyseal radiolucent regions.[532]

Arthrogryposis Multiplex Congenita

The term arthrogryposis is derived from two Greek words meaning curved joints,[369] an appropriate name for this disorder. The role of hereditary factors in arthrogryposis has long been disputed, and a precise mode of inheritance has not been documented.[370, 374] Numerous causes for the condition have been proposed,[375] including mechanical, neurologic,[371, 377] and infectious, but none has been substan-

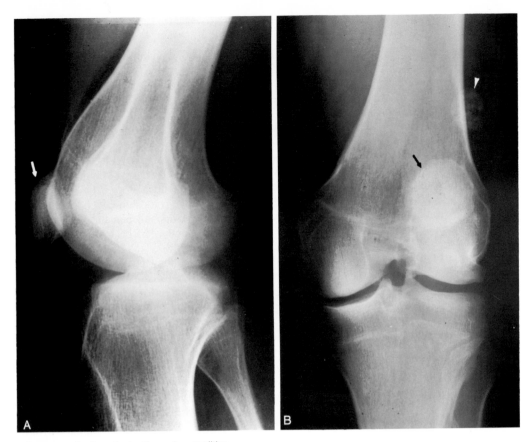

FIGURE 90–72. Osteo-onychodysostosis: Knee abnormalities.

A Observe the hypoplastic patella (arrow). (Courtesy of A. Goldman, M.D., New York, New York.)

B In a different patient, the patella is hypoplastic (arrow), the lateral condyle of the femur is relatively small in comparison to the medial condyle, and an intra-articular osseous body within the suprapatellar pouch (arrowhead) can be seen. (Courtesy of V. Vint, M.D., La Jolla, California.)

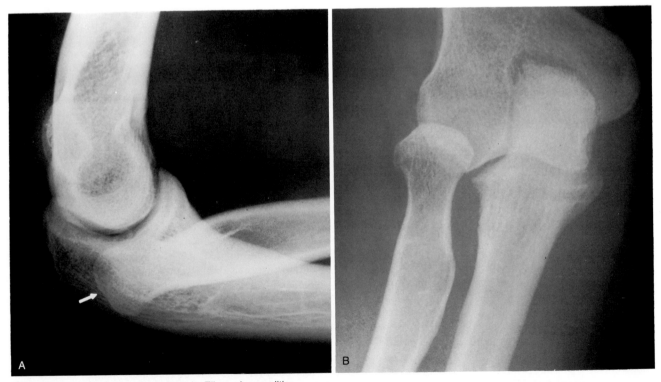

FIGURE 90–73. Osteo-onychodysostosis: Elbow abnormalities.

A The dislocation and deformity of the proximal portion of the radius (arrow) and irregularity of the humeral condyles can be seen. (Courtesy of A. Goldman, M.D., New York, New York.)

B In another patient, observe subluxation and deformity of the proximal part of the radius and hypoplasia of the distal lateral portion of the humerus.

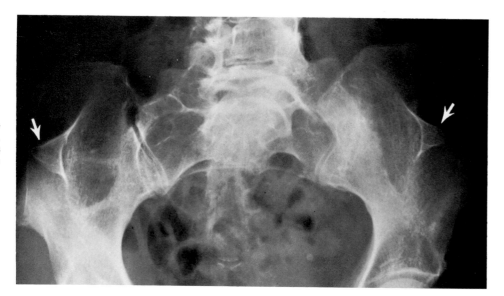

FIGURE 90–74. Osteo-onycho-dysostosis: Pelvic abnormalities. Bilateral posterior iliac outgrowths or horns can be identified (arrows).

tiated. At birth, affected infants display multiple and frequently symmetric joint contractures involving many of the peripheral joints, with limitation of both active and passive motion. A ''diamond deformity'' of the lower extremities is typical, with the hips abducted, flexed, and rotated externally and with the knees flexed. Sensation is intact.

Radiographic features include decreased muscle mass and contractures. Equinovarus deformity of the foot, talocalcaneal coalition,[376] clubhand in ulnar deviation, carpal fusion, and dislocation of the hips are frequent[372, 373] (Fig. 90–75). Additional abnormalities include patellar elongation and malposition, hemophilia-like changes of the distal portion of the femur and proximal end of the tibia, and fibular hypoplasia.[533] Fractures are not unusual, and scoliosis can be detected in many persons.[416] Multiple surgical procedures may be required, although a high rate of recurrence of deformities is apparent.

Werner's Syndrome

Werner's syndrome is named after the investigator who, in 1904, described four siblings with similar clinical findings: shortness of stature, premature aging, scleroderma-like skin changes, and cataracts.[378] Werner attributed the peculiar clinical abnormalities to a failure of ectoderm-derived cells. Since this original description, more than 100 cases have been documented, which are well summarized in the classic review by Epstein and collaborators.[379] Werner's syndrome is similar to but distinct from progeria. Its principal clinical manifestations include a symmetric retardation of growth with absence of the adolescent growth spurt, graying and loss of the hair, voice alterations, cataracts, skin ulcerations, and, in some cases, mild diabetes mellitus.[379] Additional changes are vascular and soft tissue calcifications, generalized osteoporosis, atrophy of muscle

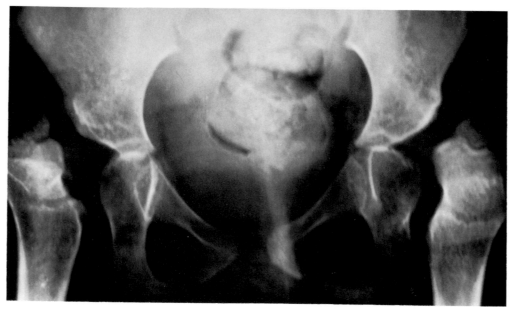

FIGURE 90–75. Arthrogryposis multiplex congenita. Note bilateral dislocations of the hip.

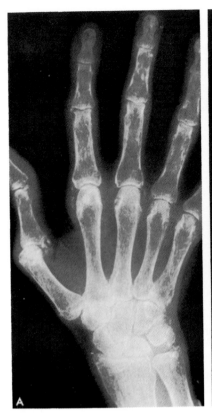
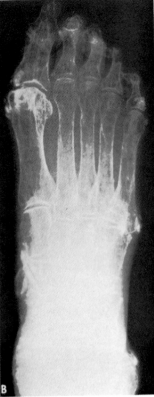

FIGURE 90–76. Werner's syndrome. Observe osteoporosis and soft tissue calcifications, most prominent in periarticular locations. (Courtesy of P. Major, M.D., Winnipeg, Manitoba, Canada.)

and fat, and hypogonadism with small genitalia and decreased libido and potency in men, and small breasts and menstrual abnormalities in women. Neoplasms, especially sarcomas (e.g., osteosarcoma, fibrosarcoma, leiomyosarcoma, melanoma) and meningiomas, may complicate the clinical picture in as many as 10 per cent of patients.[383, 534] The prognosis is guarded, as many patients succumb by the fourth or fifth decade of life to complications of cardiovascular involvement, including myocardial infarction and stroke. Genetic studies in Werner's syndrome reveal findings compatible with an autosomal recessive mode of inheritance.[384] Although it has been suggested that a defect in a single protein or enzyme could account for the findings, the exact nature of the disorder remains elusive.[379]

Radiographic evaluation reveals patchy or generalized osteoporosis.[380–382] Extensive arterial calcifications may be evident, particularly in the vessels of the extremities, coronary arteries, and aorta. Aortic and mitral valvular calcification also may be apparent in association with cardiac enlargement and congestive heart failure. Soft tissue calcification is observed in approximately one third of cases and predominates about bony protuberances, including the distal ends of the tibia and fibula, and areas about the knees, feet, and hands (Fig. 90–76). Soft tissue atrophy also may be apparent. Destructive osseous lesions related to osteomyelitis and septic arthritis and neurotrophic changes in the feet resembling the findings of diabetes mellitus can be evident.[380] Degenerative changes in the spine also have been described. Osteosclerosis of the phalanges, especially in the hand, has been evident in some cases (Fig. 90–77).[535, 536]

Clinically, Werner's syndrome resembles progeria, although cataracts, hyperkeratosis, skin ulcerations, and diabetes mellitus are not characteristics of progeria.[379] Werner's syndrome also bears some resemblance to Rothmund's syndrome, myotonic dystrophy, scleroderma, and the Cockayne syndrome. Radiographically, the findings are

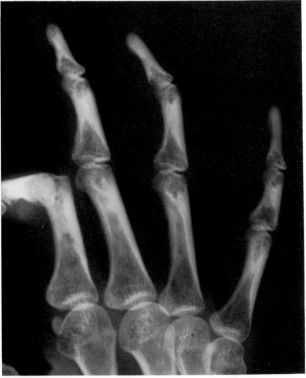

FIGURE 90–77. Werner's syndrome. Observe osteosclerosis and cortical thickening of all of the phalanges.

most reminiscent of those in collagen vascular disorders and hyperparathyroidism.

Congenital Pseudarthrosis

Congenital pseudarthrosis is an unusual condition associated with fracture followed by a nonunion. It is identified most typically in the tibia,[385–387, 537, 538] although pseudarthroses also may be seen in the fibula, femur, clavicle, humerus, ulna, radius, rib, and, rarely, other bones.[388–391, 403, 539–542] Its classification and pathogenesis have been the source of a great deal of confusion and debate.[404] In some patients, pseudarthroses are present at birth (true congenital pseudarthrosis), whereas in other patients, they develop in the first few years of life (infantile pseudarthrosis).[392] Rarely, pseudarthroses first develop in late childhood or adolescence.[556] Some affected persons may have stigmata of neurofibromatosis or fibrous dysplasia,[388] although others do not; the reported frequency of neurofibromatosis in cases of pseudarthrosis has varied considerably (0 to 70 per cent), in part related to the criteria used to substantiate the diagnosis of neurofibromatosis. Histologic evaluation of the affected site may reveal intraosseous tissue that appears to be representative of a neurofibroma or schwannoma, although ultrastructural characteristics may demonstrate subtle differences between the dense cellular tissue of a pseudarthrosis and the tissue of a neural tumor.[393] Thus, the precise relationships among congenital pseudarthrosis, neurofibromatosis, and fibrous dysplasia remain a mystery, although in some cases, pseudarthrosis can apparently represent a localized and isolated phenomenon.

It is the more common infantile variety of the disease as

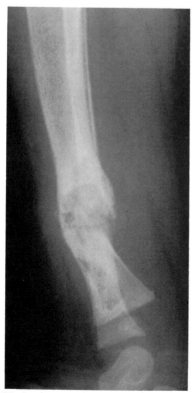

FIGURE 90–78. Congenital pseudarthrosis: Tibia. A fracture of the distal portion of the tibia is associated with bone resorption and angulation. (Courtesy of M. Pathria, M.D., San Diego, California.)

it appears in the tibia that has attracted the most attention in the literature. This lesion usually develops in the first or second year of life, although occasionally it may appear after this time and rarely may be delayed until the eighth to eleventh years of life. Unilateral changes predominate. Initially, anterior bowing of the lower half of the tibia is recognized with or without abnormality of the adjacent fibula. Rarely, the fibula is involved alone or initially.[539] At the apex of the tibial curve, sclerosis, narrowing of the medullary canal, and cystic abnormality may indicate impending fracture and pseudarthrosis. These early prefracture findings have been emphasized by Lloyd-Roberts and Shaw[394] and have been attributed to an abnormality of the primary cartilaginous anlage by some investigators. Badgley and collaborators[395] noted that the site of tibial angulation coincided with the location of the primary ossification center, suggesting that cartilaginous changes in this center could produce the typical osseous defect, a theory that was supported by histologic data derived from later clinical and laboratory investigations.[396–398] Although additional theories abound, including those that suggest that the tibial pseudarthrosis is related to trauma, amnionic bands, genetic aberration, vascular anomalies, and nutritional or metabolic disturbance, the possibility of a primary alteration in the cartilaginous anlage producing this lesion is attractive and possibly could explain the development of similar defects at other sites, such as the clavicle and proximal portion of the femur.[398] Once the fracture appears, the margins of the adjacent bone ends taper further (Figs. 90–78 and 90–79). The prognosis for ultimate union at the fracture site varies with the age of the patient (fractures developing before 2 years of age carry a poor prognosis), the pattern of radiographic abnormality (a cystic appearance may be associated with a better prognosis), and the type of therapy that is employed[388, 405, 406]; if a graft is applied, healing may be expected in approximately 25 to 35 per cent of patients.

Congenital pseudarthrosis of the bones of the forearm is rare. The radius and ulna are affected with nearly equal frequency (Fig. 90–80).[540] Involvement of both bones together is extremely rare, although reports of this phenomenon exist,[540] as do reports in which congenital pseudarthroses have involved bones in the forearm and lower leg together.[541] Pseudarthrosis of the radius or ulna generally is associated with neurofibromatosis. Any portion of either bone may be affected. Deformities appear in infancy or, rarely, at birth and may be discovered during evaluation after a traumatic insult.[540] Radiographic findings resemble those encountered in cases of pseudarthrosis of the tibia.

Congenital pseudarthrosis of the clavicle occurs almost exclusively on the right side of the body, although it may be bilateral in 10 per cent of cases.[391, 402, 542] Its occurrence on the left side[407] may be associated with dextrocardia, suggesting that the position of adjacent vascular structures such as the subclavian artery may be important in the pathogenesis of this osseous defect; the pulsation of a nearby artery located between the clavicle and first rib or cervical rib conceivably could produce bony resorption.[399] Cervical ribs occur with increased frequency in patients with congenital pseudarthrosis of the clavicle. Other theories emphasize the role of trauma, a defect in the primary ossification center of the clavicle, or a failure of coalescence of two centers of clavicular ossification.[400, 401] A familial occurrence of the disorder occasionally is noted. The lesion usu-

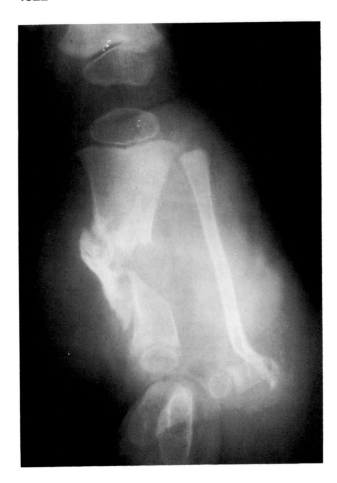

FIGURE 90–79. Congenital pseudarthrosis: Tibia and fibula. Fractures with pseudarthroses are observed in the middle third of the tibia and the lower third of the fibula. Some of the ends of the fractured bones are tapered. Considerable soft tissue swelling and hypertrophy are evident, although this child had no clinical evidence of neurofibromatosis.

FIGURE 90–80. Congenital pseudarthrosis: Radius. In this child with neurofibromatosis, observe resorption and tapering of the bone about the fracture site in the radius and bowing, osteosclerosis, and periostitis of the ulna. (Courtesy of M. Pathria, M.D., San Diego, California.)

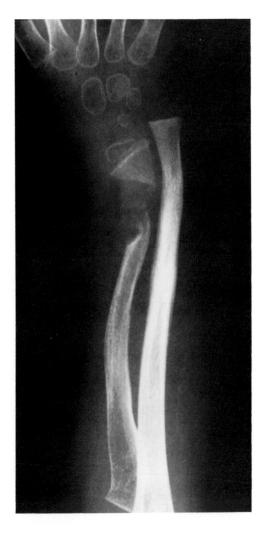

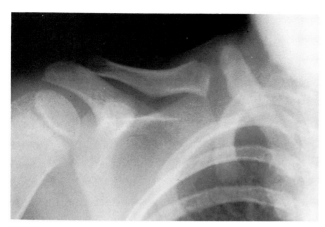

FIGURE 90–81. Congenital pseudarthrosis: Clavicle. This 4 year old girl had a prominent symptomatic mass over her right clavicle. Note the superior position of the medial end of the clavicle and the absence of visible callus. (From Schnall SB, et al: J Pediatr Orthop 8:316, 1988.)

ally is discovered within the first few months of life owing to the presence of a painless lump over the middle one third of the clavicle. On radiographs, the medial end of the clavicle is seen to be superior to the lateral end, osseous discontinuity is evident, and callus formation is absent (Fig. 90–81). It is the absence of pain and visible callus that usually allows differentiation from a posttraumatic pseudarthrosis.[408] A third disorder leading to similar clavicular changes is cleidocranial dysostosis. Another entity, designated the wavy clavicle, similarly occurs predominantly on the right side of the body, is seen in adults, and may have a vascular pathogenesis that is similar to that postulated for cases of congenital pseudarthrosis of the clavicle.[543] On pathologic examination of the clavicle in cases of congenital pseudarthrosis, fibrous tissue is found to separate the two cartilage-covered bone ends, and there is no evidence of neurofibromatosis or fibrous dysplasia.[401]

SUMMARY

A summary of some of the many congenital and inherited disorders of the skeleton has been undertaken. It is evident that these have varied clinical and radiologic manifestations. In some instances, radiographic features are entirely specific, whereas in others, they must be interpreted with knowledge of clinical abnormalities to arrive at a correct diagnosis.

References

1. Caffey JP: Pediatric X-ray Diagnosis. 7th ed. Chicago, Year Book Medical Publishers, 1978.
2. Spranger JW, Langer LO Jr, Wiedemann HR: Bone Dysplasias. An Atlas of Constitutional Disorders of Skeletal Development. Philadelphia, WB Saunders Co, 1974.
3. McKusick VA: Heritable Disorders of Connective Tissue. St Louis, CV Mosby Co, 1972.
4. Rubin P: Dynamic Classification of Bone Dysplasias. Chicago, Year Book Medical Publishers, 1964.
5. Bailey JA: Disproportionate Short Stature. Diagnosis and Management. Philadelphia, WB Saunders Co, 1973.
6. Frantz CH, O'Rahilly R: Congenital skeletal limb deficiencies. J Bone Joint Surg [Am] 43:1202, 1961.
7. Burtch RL, Fishman S, Kay HW: Nomenclature for congenital skeletal limb deficiencies, a revision of the Frantz and O'Rahilly classification. Artif Limbs 10:24, 1966.
8. Mital MA: Limb deficiencies: Classification and treatment. Orthop Clin North Am 7:457, 1976.
9. Kay HW: A proposed international terminology for the classification of congenital limb deficiencies. Interclinic Information Bull 13:1, 1974.
10. Kay HW: A proposed international terminology for the classification of congenital limb deficiencies. Orthot Prosth 28:33, 1974.
11. Coventry MB, Johnson EW Jr: Congenital absence of the fibula. J Bone Joint Surg [Am] 34:941, 1952.
12. Kruger LM, Talbott RD: Amputation and prosthesis as definitive treatment in congenital absence of the fibula. J Bone Joint Surg [Am] 43:625, 1961.
13. Achterman C, Kalamchi A: Congenital deficiency of the fibula. J Bone Joint Surg [Br] 61:133, 1979.
14. Jansen K, Andersen KS: Congenital absence of the fibula. Acta Orthop Scand 45:446, 1974.
15. Westin GW, Sakai DN, Wood WL: Congenital longitudinal deficiency of the fibula. Follow-up of treatment by Syme amputation. J Bone Joint Surg [Am] 58:492, 1976.
16. Ogden JA: Proximal fibular growth deformities. Skel Radiol 3:223, 1979.
17. Barnes JC, Smith WL: The VATER association. Radiology 126:445, 1978.
18. Simcha A: Congenital heart disease in radial clubbed hand syndrome. Arch Dis Child 46:345, 1971.
19. Hall JG, Levin J, Kuhn JP, et al: Thrombocytopenia with absent radius (TAR). Medicine 48:411, 1969.
20. Omenn GS, Figley MM, Graham CB, et al: Prospects for radiographic intrauterine diagnosis—the syndrome of thrombocytopenia with absent radii. N Engl J Med 288:777, 1973.
21. Ogden JA, Watson HK, Bohne W: Ulnar dysmelia. J Bone Joint Surg [Am] 58:467, 1976.
22. Goldman AB, Schneider R, Wilson PD Jr: Proximal focal femoral deficiency. J Can Assoc Radiol 29:101, 1978.
23. Levinson ED, Ozonoff MB, Royen PM: Proximal femoral focal deficiency (PFFD). Radiology 125:197, 1977.
24. Lange DR, Schoenecker PL, Baker CL: Proximal femoral focal deficiency: Treatment and classification in forty-two cases. Clin Orthop 135:15, 1978.
25. Panting AL, Williams PF: Proximal femoral focal deficiency. J Bone Joint Surg [Br] 60:46, 1978.
26. Fixsen JA, Lloyd-Roberts GC: The natural history and early treatment of proximal femoral dysplasia. J Bone Joint Surg [Br] 56:86, 1974.
27. Shands AR Jr, MacEwen GD: Congenital abnormalities of the femur. Acta Orthop Scand 32:307, 1962.
28. Pedersen LM, Tygstrup I, Pedersen J: Congenital malformations in newborn infants of diabetic women. Correlation with maternal diabetic vascular complications. Lancet 1:1124, 1964.
29. Holden CEA: Congenital shortening of one femur in one identical twin. Postgrad Med J 44:813, 1968.
30. Blumel J, Evans EB, Eggers GWN: Partial and complete agenesis or malformation of the sacrum and associated anomalies. J Bone Joint Surg [Am] 41:497, 1958.
31. Banta JV, Nichols O: Sacral agenesis. J Bone Joint Surg [Am] 51:693, 1969.
32. Passarge E, Lenz W: Syndrome of caudal regression in infants of diabetic mothers: Observations of further cases. Pediatrics 37:672, 1966.
33. Renshaw TS: Sacral agenesis: A classification and review of twenty-three cases. J Bone Joint Surg [Am] 60:373, 1978.
34. Hunt PT, Davidson KC, Ashcraft KW, et al: Radiography of hereditary presacral teratoma. Radiology 122:187, 1977.
35. Wilkinson RH, Strand RD: Congenital anomalies and normal variants. Semin Roentgenol 13:7, 1979.
36. Dounis E: Sacrococcygeal agenesis. A report of four new cases. Acta Orthop Scand 49:475, 1978.
37. Poznanski AK, Stephenson JM: Radiographic findings in hypothalamic acceleration of growth associated with cerebral atrophy and mental retardation (cerebral gigantism). Radiology 88:446, 1967.
38. Inglis K: Local gigantism (a manifestation of neurofibromatosis): Its relation to general gigantism and to acromegaly. Illustrating the incidence of intrinsic factors in disease when development of the body is abnormal. Am J Pathol 26:1059, 1950.
39. Barsky AJ: Macrodactyly. J Bone Joint Surg [Am] 49:1255, 1967.
40. Poznanski AK, Garn SM, Holt JF: The thumb in the congenital malformation syndromes. Radiology 100:115, 1971.
41. Swanson AB, Brown KS: Hereditary triphalangeal thumb. J Hered 53:259, 1962.
42. Poznanski AK: The Hand in Radiologic Diagnosis. Philadelphia, WB Saunders Co, 1974.
43. Warkany J: Congenital Malformations: Notes and Comments. Chicago, Year Book Medical Publishers, 1971.
44. Ireland DCR, Takayama N, Flatt AE: Poland's syndrome. A review of forty-three cases. J Bone Joint Surg [Am] 58:52, 1976.
45. Hoefnagel D, Rozycki A, Worster-Hill D, et al: Leukaemia and Poland's syndrome. Lancet 2:1038, 1972.
46. Mace JW, Kaplan JM, Schanberger JE, et al: Poland's syndrome: Report of seven cases and review of the literature. Clin Pediatr 11:98, 1972.
47. Elkington SG, Huntsman RG: The Talbot fingers: A study in symphalangism. Br Med J 1:407, 1967.
48. Strasberger AK, Hawkins MR, Eldridge R, et al: Symphalangism: Genetic and clinical aspects. Johns Hopkins Med J 117:108, 1965.

49. Harle TS, Stevenson JR: Hereditary symphalangism associated with carpal and tarsal fusions. Radiology 89:91, 1967.

50. Cope JR: Carpal coalition. Clin Radiol 25:261, 1974.

51. Garn SM, Frisancho AR, Poznanski AK, et al: Analysis of triquetral-lunate fusion. Am J Phys Anthropol 34:431, 1971.

52. Dean RFA, Jones PRM: Fusion of triquetral and lunate bones shown in several radiographs. Am J Phys Anthropol 17:279, 1959.

53. Cockshott WP: Carpal fusions. AJR 89:1260, 1963.

54. Cockshott WP: Pisiform hamate fusion. J Bone Joint Surg [Am] 51:778, 1969.

55. O'Rahilly R: A survey of carpal and tarsal anomalies. J Bone Joint Surg [Am] 35:626, 1953.

56. McGoey PF: Fracture-dislocation of fused triangular and lunate (congenital). Report of a case. J Bone Joint Surg 25:928, 1943.

57. Smitham JH: Some observations on certain congenital abnormalities of the hand in African natives. Br J Radiol 21:513, 1948.

58. McCredie J: Congenital fusion of bones: Radiology, embryology, and pathogenesis. Clin Radiol 26:47, 1975.

59. Green WT, Mital MA: Congenital radio-ulnar synostosis: Surgical treatment. J Bone Joint Surg [Am] 61:738, 1979.

60. Mital MA: Congenital radioulnar synostosis and congenital dislocation of the radial head. Orthop Clin North Am 7:375, 1976.

61. Davenport CB, Taylor HL, Nelson LA: Radio-ulnar synostosis. Arch Surg 8:705, 1924.

62. Harris BJ: Anomalous structures in the developing human foot. Anat Rec 121:399, 1955.

63. Pfitzner W: Die Variationen im Aufbau des Fussskelets. Morphol Arb 6:245, 1896.

64. Slomann HC: On coalition calcaneo-navicularis. J Orthop Surg 3:586, 1921.

65. Harris RI, Beath T: Etiology of peroneal spastic flat foot. J Bone Joint Surg [Br] 30:624, 1948.

66. Chambers CH: Congenital anomalies of the tarsal navicular with particular reference to calcaneo-navicular coalition. Br J Radiol 23:580, 1950.

67. Hark FW: Congenital anomalies of the tarsal bones. Clin Orthop 16:21, 1960.

68. Rothberg AS, Feldman JW, Schuster OF: Congenital fusion of astragalus and scaphoid: Bilateral, inherited. NY State Med J 35:29, 1935.

69. Webster FS, Roberts WM: Tarsal anomalies and peroneal spastic flatfoot. JAMA 146:1099, 1951.

70. Bersani FA, Samilson RL: Massive familial tarsal synostosis. J Bone Joint Surg [Am] 39:1187, 1957.

71. Leonard MA: The inheritance of tarsal coalition and its relationship to spastic flat foot. J Bone Joint Surg [Br] 56:520, 1974.

72. Heiple KG, Lovejoy CO: The antiquity of tarsal coalition. J Bone Joint Surg [Am] 51:979, 1969.

73. Jones Sir R: Peroneal spasm and its treatment. Report of a meeting of the Liverpool Medical Institution. Liverpool Med Chir J 17:442, 1897.

74. Badgley CE: Coalition of the calcaneus and the navicular. Arch Surg 15:75, 1927.

75. Conway JJ, Cowell HR: Tarsal coalition: Clinical significance and roentgenographic demonstration. Radiology 92:799, 1969.

76. Kendrick JI: Treatment of calcaneonavicular bar. JAMA 172:1242, 1960.

77. Simmons EH: Tibialis spastic varus foot with tarsal coalition. J Bone Joint Surg [Br] 47:533, 1965.

78. Schmidt F: Über eine symmetrische Synostosis calcaneo-navicularis bei gleichzeitigem Klumphohlfuss. Arch Orthop Unfallchir 30:289, 1931.

79. Lapidus PW: Spastic flat foot. J Bone Joint Surg 28:126, 1946.

80. Poznanski AK: Foot manifestations of the congenital malformation syndromes. Semin Roentgenol 5:354, 1970.

81. Poznanski AK, Stern AM, Gall JC Jr: Radiographic findings in the hand-foot-uterus syndrome (HFUS). Radiology 95:129, 1970.

82. Langer LO Jr: The roentgenographic features of the oto-palato-digital (OPD) syndrome. AJR 100:63, 1967.

83. Geelhoed GW, Neel JV, Davidson RT: Symphalangism and tarsal coalitions: A hereditary syndrome. A report on two families. J Bone Joint Surg [Br] 51:278, 1969.

84. Poznanski AK, LaRowe PC: Radiographic manifestations of the arthrogryposis syndrome. Radiology 95:353, 1970.

85. Schauerte EW, St. Aubin PM: Progressive synostosis in Apert's syndrome (acrocephalosyndactyly), with a description of roentgenographic changes in the feet. AJR 97:67, 1966.

86. Beckly DE, Anderson PW, Pedegana LR: The radiology of the subtalar joint with special reference to talo-calcaneal coalition. Clin Radiol 26:333, 1975.

87. Jack EA: Bone anomalies of the tarsus in relation to "peroneal spastic flat foot." J Bone Joint Surg [Br] 36:530, 1954.

88. Feist JH, Mankin JH: The tarsus. I. Basic relationships and motions in the adult and definition of optimal recumbent oblique projection. Radiology 79:250, 1962.

89. Herschel H, von Ronnen JR: The occurrence of calcaneonavicular synosteosis in pes valgus contractus. J Bone Joint Surg [Am] 32:280, 1950.

90. Braddock GTF: A prolonged follow-up of peroneal spastic flat foot. J Bone Joint Surg [Br] 43:734, 1961.

91. Kaye JJ, Ghelman B, Schneider R: Talocalcaneonavicular joint arthrography for sustentacular-talar tarsal coalitions. Radiology 115:730, 1975.

92. Brahme F: Upper talar enarthrosis. Acta Radiol 55:221, 1961.

93. Schrieber RR: Congenital and acquired ball-and-socket ankle joint. Radiology 84:940, 1965.

94. Lamb D: The ball and socket ankle joint—a congenital abnormality. J Bone Joint Surg [Br] 40:240, 1958.

95. Channon GM, Brotherton BJ: The ball and socket ankle joint. J Bone Joint Surg [Br] 61:85, 1979.

96. Boyd HB: Congenital talonavicular synostosis. J Bone Joint Surg 26:682, 1944.

97. Challis J: Hereditary transmission of talonavicular coalition in association with anomaly of the little finger. J Bone Joint Surg [Am] 56:1273, 1974.

98. Zeide MS, Wiesel SW, Terry RL: Talonavicular coalition. Clin Orthop 126:225, 1977.

99. Mahaffey HW: Bilateral congenital calcaneocuboid synostosis, a case report. J Bone Joint Surg 27:164, 1945.

100. Veneruso LC: Unilateral congenital calcaneocuboid synostosis with complete absence of a metatarsal and toe, a case report. J Bone Joint Surg 27:718, 1945.

101. Outland T, Murphy ID: Relation of tarsal anomalies to spastic and rigid flatfeet. Clin Orthop 1:217, 1953.

102. Waugh W: Partial cubo-navicular coalition as a cause of peroneal spastic flat foot. J Bone Joint Surg [Br] 39:520, 1957.

103. Lusby HLJ: Naviculo-cuneiform synostosis. J Bone Joint Surg [Br] 41:150, 1959.

104. Gregersen HN: Naviculocuneiform coalition. J Bone Joint Surg [Am] 59:128, 1977.

105. Del Sel JM, Grand NE: Cubo-navicular synostosis. A rare tarsal anomaly. J Bone Joint Surg [Br] 41:149, 1959.

106. Klippel MM, Feil A: Absence de colonne cervicale. Cage thoracique remontant jusqu'à la base du crâne. Presse Med 20:411, 1912.

107. Klippel M, Feil A: Anomalie de la colonne vertébrale par absence des vertébres cervicales; cage thoracique remontant jusqu'à la base du crâne. Bull Mem Soc Anat Paris 87:185, 1912.

108. Luftman II, Weintraub S: Klippel-Feil syndrome in a full term stillborn infant. NY State J Med 51:2035, 1951.

109. Shands AR Jr, Bundens WD: Congenital deformities of the spine. An analysis of the roentgenograms of 700 children. Bull Hosp Joint Dis 17:110, 1956.

110. Gray SW, Romaine CB, Skandalakis JE: Congenital fusion of the cervical vertebrae. Surg Gynecol Obstet 118:373, 1964.

111. Sicard JA, Lermoyez J: II. Formes frustes, évolutive, familiale du syndrome de Klippel-Feil. Rev Neurol Paris 39:71, 1923.

112. Masi A, Vichi GF: La sindrome di Klippel-Feil: Contributo statistics e clinico radiologico. Riv Clin Pediatr 65:22, 1960.

113. Haddad HM, Wilkins L: Congenital anomalies associated with gonadal aplasia, review of 55 cases. Pediatrics 23:885, 1959.

114. Hensinger RN, Lang JE, MacEwen GD: Klippel-Feil syndrome. A constellation of associated anomalies. J Bone Joint Surg [Am] 56:1246, 1974.

115. Ramsay J, Bliznak J: Klippel-Feil syndrome with renal agenesis and other anomalies. AJR 113:460, 1971.

116. Degenhardt KH, Kladetsky J: Malformaciones de la columna vertebrale y del esbozo de la corda dorsalis. Arch Pediatr 7:1, 1956.

117. Gardner WJ, Collins JS: Klippel-Feil syndrome. Syringomyelia, diastematomyelia and myelomeningocele—one disease? Arch Surg 83:638, 1961.

118. Fietti VG Jr, Fielding JW: The Klippel-Feil syndrome: Early roentgenographic appearance and progression of the deformity. J Bone Joint Surg [Am] 58:891, 1976.

119. Madelung OW: Die spontane Subluxation der Hand nach vorne. Verh Dtsch Ges Chir 7:259, 1878.

120. Anton JI, Reitz GB, Spiegel MB: Madelung's deformity. Ann Surg 108:411, 1938.

121. Felman AH, Kirkpatrick JA Jr: Madelung's deformity: Observations in 17 patients. Radiology 93:1037, 1969.

122. Nielsen JB: Madelung's deformity: A follow-up study of 26 cases and a review of the literature. Acta Orthop Scand 48:379, 1977.

123. Dannenburg M, Anton JI, Spiegel MB: Madelung's deformity. Consideration of its roentgenological diagnostic criteria. AJR 42:671, 1939.

124. Ranawat CS, DeFiore J, Straub LR: Madelung's deformity. An end-result study of surgical treatment. J Bone Joint Surg [Am] 57:772, 1975.

125. Henry A, Thorburn MJ: Madelung's deformity. A clinical and cytogenetic study. J Bone Joint Surg [Br] 49:66, 1967.

126. Kosowicz J: The carpal sign in gonadal dysgenesis. J Clin Endocrinol Metab 22:949, 1962.

127. Kosowicz J: The roentgen appearance of hand and wrist in gonadal dysgenesis. AJR 93:354, 1965.

128. Léri A, Weill J: Une affection congénitale et symétrique du développement osseux: La dyschondrostéose. Bull Mem Soc Hop Paris 53:1491, 1929.

129. Golding JSR, Blackburne JS: Madelung's disease of the wrist and dyschondrosteosis. J Bone Joint Surg [Br] 58:350, 1976.

130. Herdman RC, Langer LO, Good R: Dyschondrosteosis, the most common cause of Madelung's deformity. J Pediatr 68:432, 1966.

131. Goodwin DRA, Michels CH, Weissman SL: Spontaneous rupture of extensor tendons in Madelung's deformity. Hand 71:72, 1979.

132. Niebauer JJ, King DE: Congenital dislocation of the knee. J Bone Joint Surg [Am] 42:207, 1960.

133. Carlson DH, O'Connor J: Congenital dislocation of the knee. AJR 127:465, 1976.

134. Laurence M: Genu recurvatum congenitum. J Bone Joint Surg [Br] 49:121, 1967.

135. Curtis BH, Fisher RL: Congenital hyperextension with anterior subluxation of the knee. J Bone Joint Surg [Am] 51:255, 1969.

136. McFarlane AL: A report on four cases of congenital genu recurvatum occurring in one family. Br J Surg *34*:388, 1947.

137. Provenzano RW: Congenital dislocation of the knee. Report of a case. N Engl J Med *236*:360, 1947.

138. Katz MP, Grogono BJS, Soper KC: The etiology and treatment of congenital dislocation of the knee. J Bone Joint Surg [Br] *49*:112, 1967.

139. Shattock SG: Genu recurvatum in a foetus at term. Trans Pathol Soc Lond *42*:280, 1891.

140. Middleton DS: The pathology of congenital genu recurvatum. Br J Surg *22*:696, 1935.

141. Ahmadi B, Shahriaree H, Silver CM: Severe congenital genu recurvatum. Case report. J Bone Joint Surg [Am] *61*:622, 1979.

142. Calhoun JD, Pierret G: Infantile coxa vara. AJR *115*:561, 1972.

143. Babb FS, Ghormley RK, Chatterton CC: Congenital coxa vara. J Bone Joint Surg [Am] *31*:115, 1949.

144. Hark FW: Congenital coxa vara. Am J Surg *80*:305, 1950.

145. Johanning K: Coxa vara infantum. I. Clinical appearance and aetiological problems. Acta Orthop Scand *21*:273, 1951.

146. Zadek I: Congenital coxa vara. Arch Surg *30*:62, 1935.

147. Golding FC: Congenital coxa vara. J Bone Joint Surg [Br] *30*:161, 1948.

148. Fisher FL, Waskowitz WJ: Familial developmental coxa vara. Clin Orthop *86*:2, 1972.

149. Letts RM, Shokeir MHK: Mirror-image coxa vara in identical twins. J Bone Joint Surg [Am] *57*:117, 1975.

150. Almond HG: Familial infantile coxa vara. J Bone Joint Surg [Br] *38*:539, 1956.

151. Barrington-Ward LE: Double coxa vara with other deformities occurring in brother and sister. Lancet *1*:157, 1912.

152. Say B, Taysi K, Pirnar T, et al: Dominant congenital coxa vara. J Bone Joint Surg [Br] *56*:78, 1974.

153. Morgan JD, Somerville EW: Normal and abnormal growth at the upper end of the femur. J Bone Joint Surg [Br] *42*:264, 1960.

154. Magnusson R: Coxa vara infantum. Acta Orthop Scand *23*:284, 1953.

155. Compere EL, Garrison M, Fahey JJ: Deformities of the femur resulting from arrestment of growth of capital and greater trochanteric epiphysis. J Bone Joint Surg *22*:909, 1940.

156. Otto AW, Ein Becken: Mit hagelformig aus gedehnten pfannen. *In* Neue seltene Beobachtungen zur Anatomie, Physiologie, und Pathologie gehörig. Berlin, August Rücker, 1824.

157. Eppinger H: Pelvis-Chrobak: Coxarthrolisthesis-Becken (Festschir R Chrobak). Beitr Geb Gynakol *2*:176, 1903.

158. Golding FC: Protrusio acetabuli (central luxation). Br J Surg *22*:56, 1934.

159. Gilmour J: Adolescent deformities of the acetabulum and investigation into the nature of protrusio acetabuli. Br J Surg *26*:670, 1939.

160. Alexander C: The aetiology of primary protrusio acetabuli. Br J Radiol *38*:567, 1965.

161. Rechtman AM: Etiology of deep acetabulum and intrapelvic protrusion. Arch Surg *33*:122, 1936.

162. Macdonald D: Primary protrusio acetabuli. Report of an affected family. J Bone Joint Surg [Br] *53*:30, 1971.

163. Bilfield BS, Janecki CJ, Evarts CM: Primary protrusion of the acetabulum. Report of affected identical twins. Clin Orthop *94*:257, 1973.

164. D'Arcy K, Ansell BM, Bywaters EGL: A family with primary protrusio acetabuli. Ann Rheum Dis *37*:53, 1978.

165. Hooper JC, Jones EW: Primary protrusion of the acetabulum. J Bone Joint Surg [Br] *53*:23, 1971.

166. Ozonoff MB: Pediatric Orthopedic Radiology. Philadelphia, WB Saunders Co, 1979.

167. Freiberger RH, Hersh A, Harrison MO: Roentgen examination of the deformed foot. Semin Roentgenol *5*:341, 1970.

168. Ritchie GW, Keim HA: A radiographic analysis of major foot deformities. Can Med Assoc J *91*:840, 1964.

169. Settle GW: The anatomy of congenital talipes equinovarus: Sixteen dissected specimens. J Bone Joint Surg [Am] *45*:1341, 1963.

170. Brewerton DA, Sandifer PH, Sweetnam DR: ''Idiopathic'' pes cavus. An investigation into its etiology. Br Med J *2*:659, 1963.

171. Silverman FN: Caffey's Pediatric X-ray Diagnosis. An Integrated Imaging Approach. 8th Ed. Chicago, Year Book Medical Publishers, 1985.

172. Smith DW: Recognizable Patterns of Human Deformation. Identification and Management of Mechanical Effects on Morphogenesis. Philadelphia, WB Saunders Co, 1981.

173. Pitt MJ: Radiology of the femora linea aspera-pilaster complex: The track sign. Radiology *142*:66, 1982.

174. Rivoal A, Dal Soglio S, Viallet J-F, et al: Une ligne méconnue: La ligne après du fémur. J Radiol *61*:615, 1980.

175. Levine AH, Pais MJ, Berinson H, et al: The soleal line: A cause of tibial pseudoperiostitis. Radiology *119*:79, 1976.

176. Sontag LW, Pyle SI: The appearance and nature of cyst-like areas in the distal femoral metaphyses of children. AJR *46*:185, 1941.

177. Kimmelstiel P, Rapp IH: Cortical defect due to periosteal desmoids. Bull Hosp Joint Dis *12*:286, 1951.

178. Allen DH: A variation of diaphyseal development which simulates the roentgen appearance of primary neoplasms of bone. AJR *69*:940, 1953.

179. Simon H: Medial distal metaphyseal femoral irregularity in children. Radiology *90*:258, 1968.

180. Johnson LC, Genner BA III, Engh CA, et al: Cortical desmoids. J Bone Joint Surg [Am] *50*:828, 1968.

181. Brower AC, Culver JE Jr, Keats TE: Histologic nature of the cortical irregularity of the medial posterior distal femoral metaphysis in children. Radiology *99*:389, 1971.

182. Young DW, Nogrady MB, Dunbar JS, et al: Benign cortical irregularities in the distal femur of children. J Can Assoc Radiol *23*:107, 1972.

183. Bufkin WJ: The avulsive cortical irregularity. AJR *112*:487, 1971.

184. Barnes GR Jr, Gwinn JL: Distal irregularities of the femur simulating malignancy. AJR *122*:180, 1974.

185. Dunham WK, Marcus NW, Enneking WR, et al: Developmental defects of the distal femoral metaphysis. J Bone Joint Surg [Am] *62*:801, 1980.

186. Kreis WR, Hensinger RN: Irregularity of the distal femoral metaphysis simulating malignancy. Case report. J Bone Joint Surg [Am] *59*:38, 1977.

187. Kirkpatrick JA, Wilkinson RH. Case report 52. Skel Radiol *2*:189, 1978.

188. Caffey J, Silverman FN: Pediatric X-ray Diagnoses. 5th Ed. Chicago, Year Book Medical Publishers, 1967, p 777.

189. Kohler A, Zimmer EA: Borderlands of the Normal and Early Pathologic in Skeletal Roentgenology. 11th Ed. New York, Grune & Stratton, 1968, p 416.

190. Caffey J: On fibrous defects in cortical walls of growing tubular bones: Their radiologic appearance, structure, prevalence, natural course, and diagnostic significance. Adv Pediatr *7*:13, 1953.

191. Resnick D, Greenway G: Distal femoral cortical defects, irregularities, and excavations. A critical review of the literature with the addition of histologic and paleopathologic data. Radiology *143*:345, 1982.

192. Husson JL, Marquer Y, Jourdain R, et al: Anatomical relationship between the medial head of the gastrocnemius and the occurrence of a dystrophic bony lacuna. Anat Clin *6*:37, 1984.

193. Brower AC: Cortical defects of the humerus at the insertion of the pectoralis major. AJR *128*:677, 1977.

194. Resnick D, Cone RO III: The nature of humeral pseudocysts. Radiology *150*:27, 1984.

195. Helms CA: Pseudocysts of the humerus. AJR *131*:287, 1978.

196. Richardson ML, Montana MA: Nutrient canals of the ilium: A normal variant simulating disease on computed tomography. Skel Radiol *14*:117, 1985.

197. Lane B: Erosions of the skull. Radiol Clin North Am *12*:257, 1974.

198. Cederlund D-G, Andren L, Olivecrona H: Progressive bilateral thinning of the parietal bones. Skel Radiol *8*:29, 1982.

199. Haden MA, Keats TE: The anatomic basis for localized occipital thinning: A normal anatomic variant. Skel Radiol *8*:221, 1982.

200. Swischuk LE: The normal pediatric skull. Variations and artefacts. Radiol Clin North Am *10*:277, 1972.

201. Noonan CD: Congenital perforation of the sternum. Radiologe *3*:467, 1963.

202. Resnik CS, Brower AC: Midline circular defect of the sternum. Radiology *130*:657, 1979.

203. McCormick WF: Sternal foramina in man. Am J Forensic Med Pathol *2*:249, 1981.

204. Stark P: Midline sternal foramen: CT demonstration. J Comput Assist Tomogr *9*:489, 1985.

205. Pate D, Kursunoglu S, Resnick D, et al: Scapular foramina. Skel Radiol *14*:270, 1985.

206. Smith AD, Carter JR, Marcus RE: The os vesalianum: An unusual cause of lateral foot pain. A case report and review of the literature. Orthopedics *7*:86, 1984.

207. Obermann WR, Loose HWC: The os supratrochleare dorsale: A normal variant that may cause symptoms. AJR *141*:123, 1983.

208. Lawson JP, Ogden JA, Sella E, et al: The painful accessory navicular. Skel Radiol *12*:250, 1984.

209. Kidner FC: The prehallux (accessory scaphoid) in its relation to flatfoot. J Bone Joint Surg *11*:831, 1929.

210. Sullivan JA, Miller WA: The relationship of the accessory navicular to the development of the flat foot. Clin Orthop *144*:233, 1979.

211. Lamphier TA: Carpal bossing. Arch Surg *81*:1013, 1960.

212. Bassoe E, Bassoe HH: The styloid bone and carpe bossu disease. AJR *74*:886, 1955.

213. Carter RM: Carpal boss: Commonly overlooked deformity of the carpus. J Bone Joint Surg *23*:935, 1941.

214. Conway WF, Destouet JM, Gilula LA, et al: The carpal boss: An overview of radiographic evaluation. Radiology *156*:29, 1985.

215. Ogden JA, McCarthy SM, Jokl P: The painful bipartite patella. J Pediatr Orthop *2*:263, 1982.

216. Green WT Jr: Painful bipartite patellae. A report of three cases. Clin Orthop *110*:197, 1975.

217. Weinberg S: Case report 177. Skel Radiol *7*:223, 1981.

218. Lenz W: Genetics and limb deficiencies. Clin Orthop *148*:9, 1980.

219. Hootnick DR, Levinsohn EM, Packard DS Jr: Midline metatarsal dysplasia associated with absent fibula. Clin Orthop *150*:203, 1980.

220. Marcus NA, Omer GE Jr: Carpal deviation in congenital ulnar deficiency. J Bone Joint Surg [Am] *66*:1003, 1984.

221. Gupta DKS, Gupta SK: Familial bilateral proximal femoral focal deficiency. Report of a kindred. J Bone Joint Surg [Am] *66*:1470, 1984.

222. Kalamchi A, Cowell HR, Kim KI: Congenital deficiency of the femur. J Pediatr Orthop *5*:129, 1985.

223. Gillespie R, Torode IP: Classification and management of congenital abnormalities of the femur. J Bone Joint Surg [Br] *65*:557, 1983.

224. Hamanishi C: Congenital short femur. J Bone Joint Surg [Br] *62*:307, 1980.

225. Johansson E, Aparisi T: Missing cruciate ligament in congenital short femur. J Bone Joint Surg [Am] *65*:1109, 1983.

226. Tsou PM: Congenital distal femoral focal deficiency: Report of a unique case. Clin Orthop 162:99, 1982.

227. Gilsanz V: Distal focal femoral deficiency. Radiology 147:105, 1983.

228. Kalamchi A, Dawe RV: Congenital deficiency of the tibia. J Bone Joint Surg [Br] 67:581, 1985.

229. Thomas NP, Jackson AM, Aichroth PM: Congenital absence of the anterior cruciate ligament. A common component of knee dysplasia. J Bone Joint Surg [Br] 67:572, 1985.

230. Pettersson H: Bilateral dysplasia of the neck of the scapula and associated anomalies. Acta Radiol 22:81, 1981.

231. Triquet J, Trellu M, Trellu X, et al: Dysplasie monoepiphysaire de la cavité glenoid de l'omoplate. Arch Fr Pediatr 37:683, 1980.

232. Owen R: Bilateral glenoid hypoplasia. Report of five cases. J Bone Joint Surg [Br] 35:262, 1953.

233. McClure JG, Raney RB: Anomalies of the scapula. Clin Orthop 110:22, 1975.

234. Sutro CJ: Dentated articular surface of the glenoid—an anomaly. Bull Hosp Joint Dis 28:104, 1967.

235. Resnick D, Walter RD, Crudale AS: Bilateral dysplasia of the scapular neck. AJR 139:387, 1982.

236. Kozlowski K, Colavita N, Morris L, et al: Bilateral glenoid dysplasia. (Report of 8 cases.) Australas Radiol 29:174, 1985.

237. Abraham E: Sacral agenesis with associated anomalies (caudal regression syndrome): Autopsy case report. Clin Orthop 145:168, 1979.

238. Stanley JK, Owen R, Koff S: Congenital sacral anomalies. J Bone Joint Surg [Br] 61:401, 1979.

239. Helin I, Pettersson H, Alton D: Extensive spinal dysraphism and sacral agenesis without urologic disturbances. Acta Radiol (Diagn) 24:209, 1983.

240. Hotston S, Carty H: Lumbosacral agenesis: A report of three new cases and review of the literature. Br J Radiol 55:629, 1982.

241. Brooks BS, Gammal TE, Hartlage P, et al: Myelography of sacral agenesis. Am J Neuroradiol 2:319, 1981.

242. Wood VE: Congenital thumb deformities. Clin Orthop 195:7, 1985.

243. Tada K, Yonenobu K, Tsuyuguchi Y, et al: Duplication of the thumb. A retrospective review of two hundred and thirty-seven cases. J Bone Joint Surg [Am] 65:584, 1983.

244. Ogden JA, Light TR, Conlogue GJ: Correlative roentgenography and morphology of the longitudinal epiphyseal bracket. Skel Radiol 6:109, 1981.

245. Neil MJ, Conacher C: Bilateral delta phalanx of the proximal phalanges of the great toes. A report on an affected family. J Bone Joint Surg [Br] 66:77, 1984.

246. Theander G, Carstam N, Rausing A: Longitudinally bracketed diaphyses in young children. Radiologic histopathologic correlation. Acta Radiol (Diagn) 23:293, 1982.

247. Senrui H, Egawa T, Horiki A: Anatomical findings in the hands of patients with Poland's syndrome. Report of four cases. J Bone Joint Surg [Am] 64:1079, 1982.

248. Gausewitz SH, Meals RA, Setoguchi Y: Severe limb deficiency in Poland's syndrome. Clin Orthop 185:9, 1984.

249. Hadley MDM: Carpal coalition and Sprengel's shoulder in Poland's syndrome. J Hand Surg [Br] 10:253, 1985.

250. Smith-Hoefer E, Szabo RM: Isolated carpal synchondrosis of the scaphoid and trapezium. A case report. J Bone Joint Surg [Am] 67:318, 1985.

251. Carlson DH: Coalition of the carpal bones. Skel Radiol 7:125, 1981.

252. Simmons BP, McKenzie WD: Symptomatic carpal coalition. J Hand Surg [Am] 10:190, 1985.

253. Cleary JE, Omer GE Jr: Congenital proximal radio-ulnar synostosis. Natural history and functional assessment. J Bone Joint Surg [Am] 67:539, 1985.

254. Küsswetter W, Heisel A: Die radio-ulnare Synostose als Merkmal von Chromosomen-aberrationen. Z Orthop 119:10, 1981.

255. Jacobsen ST, Crawford AH: Humeroradial synostosis. J Pediatr Orthop 3:96, 1983.

256. Gamble JG: Proximal tibiofibular synostosis. J Pediatr Orthop 4:243, 1984.

257. Lenart G: Bifurcation of long tubular bones. Arch Orthop Trauma Surg 97:165, 1980.

258. Sarno RC, Carter BL, Bankoff MS, et al: Computed tomography in tarsal coalition. J Comput Assist Tomogr 8:1155, 1984.

259. Sartoris DJ, Resnick DL: Tarsal coalition. Arthritis Rheum 28:331, 1985.

260. Deutsch AL, Resnick D, Campbell G: Computed tomography and bone scintigraphy in the evaluation of tarsal coalition. Radiology 144:137, 1982.

261. Goldman AB, Pavlov H, Schneider R: Radionuclide bone scanning in subtalar coalitions: Differential considerations. AJR 138:427, 1982.

262. Stormont DM, Peterson HA: The relative incidence of tarsal coalition. Clin Orthop 181:28, 1983.

263. Mosier KM, Asher M: Tarsal coalitions and peroneal spastic flat foot. A review. J Bone Joint Surg [Am] 66:976, 1984.

264. Rosen JS: Tarsal coalitions: Rare or not. J Am Podiatry Assoc 74:572, 1984.

265. Richards RR, Evans JG, McGoey PF: Fracture of a calcaneonavicular bar: A complication of tarsal coalition. A case report. Clin Orthop 185:220, 1984.

266. Wheeler R, Guevera A, Bleck EE: Tarsal coalitions: A review of the literature and case report of bilateral dual calcaneonavicular and talocalcaneal coalitions. Clin Orthop 156:175, 1981.

267. Resnick D: Talar ridges, osteophytes, and beaks: A radiologic commentary. Radiology 151:329, 1984.

268. Shaffer HA Jr, Harrison RB: Tarsal pseudo-coalition—a positional artifact. J Can Assoc Radiol 31:236, 1980.

269. Pappas AM, Miller JT: Congenital ball-and-socket ankle joints and related lower-extremity malformations. J Bone Joint Surg [Am] 64:672, 1982.

270. Cowell HR, Elener V: Rigid painful flatfoot secondary to tarsal coalition. Clin Orthop 177:54, 1983.

271. Miki T, Yamamuro T, Iida H, et al: Naviculo-cuneiform coalition. A report of two cases. Clin Orthop 196:256, 1985.

272. Kelleher J, O'Connell DJ, MacMahon H: Intrathoracic rib: Radiographic features of two cases. Br J Radiol 52:181, 1979.

273. Thery Y, Spindler R, Mabille JP: Côtes surnuméraires intrathoraciques. Ann Radiol 19:669, 1976.

274. Stark P, Lawrence DD: Intrathoracic rib—CT features of a rare chest wall anomaly. Comput Radiol 8:365, 1984.

275. Friedrich M, Gerstenberg E, Goy W: Die intrathorakale rippe. ROFO 122:438, 1975.

276. Sullivan D, Cornwell WS: Pelvic rib. Report of a case. Radiology 110:355, 1974.

277. Greenspan A, Normal A: The pelvic digit. Bull Hosp J Dis 44:72, 1984.

278. Dunaway CL, Williams JP, Brogdon BG: Case report 222. Skel Radiol 9:212, 1983.

279. Greenspan A, Norman A: The "pelvic digit"—an unusual developmental anomaly. Skel Radiol 9:118, 1982.

280. Bohutova J, Kolar J, Vitovec J, et al: Accessory caudal axial and pelvic ribs. ROFO 133:641, 1980.

281. Lame EL: Case report 32. Skel Radiol 2:47, 1977.

282. Pais MJ, Levine A, Pais SO: Coccygeal ribs: Development and appearance in two cases. AJR 131:164, 1978.

283. Elster AD: Quadriplegia after minor trauma in the Klippel-Feil syndrome. A case report and review of the literature. J Bone Joint Surg [Am] 66:1473, 1984.

284. Ogden JA, Conlogue GJ, Phillips SB, et al: Sprengel's deformity. Radiology of the pathologic deformation. Skel Radiol 4:204, 1979.

285. Wilkinson JA, Campbell D: Scapular osteotome for Sprengel's deformity. J Bone Joint Surg [Br] 62:486, 1980.

286. Carson WG, Lovell WW, Whitesides TE Jr: Congenital elevation of the scapula. Surgical correction by the Woodward procedure. J Bone Joint Surg [Am] 63:1199, 1981.

287. Grogan DP, Stanley EA, Bobechko WP: The congenital undescended scapula. Surgical correction by the Woodward procedure. J Bone Joint Surg [Br] 65:598, 1983.

288. Goodwin CB, Simmons EH, Taylor I: Cervical vertebral-costal process (costovertebral bone)—a previously unreported anomaly. A case report. J Bone Joint Surg [Am] 66:1477, 1984.

289. Prusick VR, Samberg LC, Wesolowski DP: Klippel-Feil syndrome associated with spinal stenosis. A case report. J Bone Joint Surg [Am] 67:161, 1985.

290. Southwell RB, Reynolds AF, Badger VM, et al: Klippel-Feil syndrome with cervical cord compression resulting from cervical subluxation in association with an omo-vertebral bone. Spine 5:480, 1980.

291. Nixon JE: Bilateral Madelung's disease of the wrist: A familial condition? J R Soc Med 76:313, 1983.

292. Dungy C, Leupp M: Congenital hyperextension of the knees in twins. Clin Pediatr 23:169, 1984.

293. Jacobsen K, Vopalecky F: Congenital dislocation of the knee. Acta Orthop Scand 56:1, 1985.

294. Kelly DW: Congenital dislocation of the radial head: Spectrum and natural history. J Pediatr Orthop 1:295, 1981.

295. Mardam-Bey T, Ger E: Congenital radial head dislocation. J Hand Surg 4:316, 1979.

296. Cockshott WP, Omololu A: Familial posterior dislocation of both radial heads. J Bone Joint Surg [Br] 40:484, 1958.

297. McFarland B: Congenital dislocation of the head of the radius. Br J Surg 24:41, 1936.

298. Weinstein JN, Kuo KN, Millar EA: Congenital coxa vara. A retrospective review. J Pediatr Orthop 4:70, 1984.

299. Pavlov H, Goldman AB, Freiberger RH: Infantile coxa vara. Radiology 135:631, 1980.

300. Hughes AW: Idiopathic chondrolysis of the hip: A case report and review of the literature. Ann Rheum Dis 44:268, 1985.

301. Finsterbush A, Pogrund H: The hypermobility syndrome. Musculoskeletal complaints in 100 consecutive cases of generalized joint hypermobility. Clin Orthop 168:124, 1982.

302. Sutro CJ: Hypermobility of bone due to "overlengthened" capsular and ligamentous tissues: A cause for recurrent intra-articular effusions. Surgery 21:67, 1947.

303. Kirk JA, Ansell BM, Bywaters EGL: The hypermobility syndrome. Musculoskeletal complaints associated with generalized hypermobility. Ann Rheum Dis 26:414, 1967.

304. Carter C, Sweetnam R: Familial joint laxity and recurrent dislocation of the patella. J Bone Joint Surg [Br] 40:664, 1958.

305. MacNab I, MacNab L: Ligamentous laxity and scar formation. Clin Orthop 135:154, 1978.

306. Beighton P, Solomon L, Soskolne CL: Articular mobility in an African population. Ann Rheum Dis 32:413, 1973.

307. Ellis FE, Bundick WR: Cutaneous elasticity and hyperelasticity. Arch Dermatol 74:22, 1956.

308. Harris H, Joseph J: Variation in extension of the metacarpophalangeal and interphalangeal joints of the thumb. J Bone Joint Surg [Br] *31*:547, 1949.

309. Klemp P, Stevens JE, Isaacs S: A hypermobility study in ballet dancers. J Rheumatol *11*:692, 1984.

310. Bard CC, Sylvestre JJ, Dussault RG: Hand osteoarthropathy in pianists. J Can Assoc Radiol *35*:154, 1984.

311. Pitcher D, Grahame R: Mitral valve prolapse and joint hypermobility: Evidence for a systemic connective tissue abnormality? Ann Rheum Dis *41*:352, 1982.

312. Carter C, Sweetnam R: Recurrent dislocation of the patella and of the shoulder: Their association with familial joint laxity. J Bone Joint Surg [Br] *42*:721, 1960.

313. Wynne-Davies R: Acetabular dysplasia and familial joint laxity: Two etiological factors in congenital dislocation of the hip. J Bone Joint Surg [Br] *52*:704, 1970.

314. Wynne-Davies R: Family studies and the cause of congenital club foot (talipes equinovarus). J Bone Joint Surg [Br] *46*:445, 1964.

315. Bird HA, Tribe CR, Bacon PA: Joint hypermobility leading to osteoarthrosis and chondrocalcinosis. Ann Rheum Dis *37*:203, 1978.

316. Somppi E: Clubfoot. Review of the literature and an analysis of 135 treated clubfeet. Acta Orthop Scand (Suppl) *209*:7, 1984.

317. Ippolito E, Ponseti IV: Congenital club foot in human fetus. A histological study. J Bone Joint Surg [Am] *62*:8, 1980.

318. Atlas S, Menacho LCS, Ures S: Some new aspects in the pathology of clubfoot. Clin Orthop *149*:224, 1980.

319. Victoria-Diaz A, Victoria-Diaz J: Pathogenesis of idiopathic clubfoot. Clin Orthop *185*:14, 1984.

320. Scott WA, Hosking SW, Catterall A: Club foot. Observations on the surgical anatomy of dorsiflexion. J Bone Joint Surg [Br] *66*:71, 1984.

321. Gilsanz V, Teitelbaum G, Condon VR: Clubfoot deformity and tibiofibular diastasis. AJR *140*:759, 1983.

322. Greider TD, Siff SJ, Gerson P, et al: Arteriography in club foot. J Bone Joint Surg [Am] *64*:837, 1982.

323. Benacerraf BR, Frigoletto FD: Prenatal ultrasound diagnosis of clubfoot. Radiology *155*:211, 1985.

324. Jacobsen ST, Crawford AH: Congenital vertical talus. J Pediatr Orthop *3*:306, 1983.

325. Reimann I, Werner HH: The pathology of congenital metatarsus varus. A post-mortem study of a newborn infant. Acta Orthop Scand *54*:847, 1983.

326. Tachdjian MO: Pediatric Orthopedics. Philadelphia, WB Saunders Co, 1972, p 1442.

327. Fabry G, MacEwen GD, Shands AR Jr: Torsion of the femur. A follow-up study in normal and abnormal conditions. J Bone Joint Surg [Am] *55*:1726, 1973.

328. McSweeny A: A study of femoral torsion in children. J Bone Joint Surg [Br] *53*:90, 1971.

329. Ruby L, Mital MA, O'Connor J, et al: Anteversion of the femoral neck. Comparison of methods of measurement in patients. J Bone Joint Surg [Am] *61*:46, 1979.

330. Herrlin K, Ekelund L: Radiographic measurements of the femoral neck anteversion. Comparison of two simplified procedures. Acta Orthop Scand *54*:141, 1983.

331. Proubasta IR, Lluch AL, Roig JL, et al: A new method of measuring the femoral anteversion and neck-shaft angles. Clin Radiol *35*:323, 1984.

332. Moulton A, Upadhyay SS: A direct method of measuring femoral anteversion using ultrasound. J Bone Joint Surg [Br] *64*:469, 1982.

333. Visser JD, Jonkers A, Hillen B: Hip joint measurements with computerized tomography. J Pediatr Orthop *2*:143, 1982.

334. Weiner DS, Cook AJ, Hoyt WA Jr, et al: Computed tomography in the measurement of femoral anteversion. Orthopedics *1*:299, 1978.

335. Reikerås O, Bjerkreim I, Kolbenstvedt A: Anteversion of the acetabulum in patients with idiopathic anteversion of the femoral neck. Acta Orthop Scand *53*:847, 1982.

336. Hernandez RJ, Tachdjian MO, Poznanski AK, et al: CT determination of femoral torsion. AJR *137*:97, 1981.

337. Khermosh O, Lior G, Weissman SL: Tibial torsion in children. Clin Orthop *79*:25, 1971.

338. Staheli LT, Engel GM: Tibial torsion. A method of assessment and a survey of normal children. Clin Orthop *86*:183, 1972.

339. Jeno HH, Heller M, Dalek M, et al: Measurement of tibial torsion by computer tomography. Acta Radiol (Diagn) *22*:271, 1981.

340. Laasonen EM, Jokio P, Lindholm JS: Tibial torsion measured by computed tomography. Acta Radiol (Diagn) *25*:325, 1984.

341. Jakob RP, Haertel M, Stusi E: Tibial torsion calculated by computerised tomography and compared to other methods of measurement. J Bone Joint Surg [Br] *62*:238, 1980.

342. Turner JW: A hereditary arthrodysplasia associated with hereditary dystrophy of the nails. JAMA *100*:882, 1933.

343. Eisenberg KS, Potter DE, Bovill EG Jr: Osteo-onychodystrophy with nephropathy and renal osteodystrophy. A case report. J Bone Joint Surg [Am] *54*:1301, 1972.

344. Valdueza AF: The nail-patella syndrome. A report of 3 families. J Bone Joint Surg [Br] *55*:145, 1973.

345. Gilula LA, Kantor OS: Familial colon carcinoma in nail-patella syndrome. AJR *123*:783, 1975.

346. Preger L, Miller EH, Winfield JS, et al: Hereditary onycho-osteo-arthrodysplasia. AJR *100*:546, 1967.

347. Darlington D, Hawkins CF: Nail-patella syndrome with iliac horns and hereditary nephropathy. Necropsy report and anatomical dissection. J Bone Joint Surg [Br] *49*:164, 1967.

348. Palacios E: Hereditary osteo-onycho-dysplasia. The nail-patella syndrome. AJR *101*:842, 1967.

349. Williams HJ, Hoyer JR: Radiographic diagnosis of osteo-onychodysostosis in infancy. Radiology *109*:151, 1973.

350. Hawkins CF, Smith OE: Renal dysplasia in a family with multiple hereditary abnormalities including iliac horns. Lancet *1*:803, 1950.

351. Hoyer JR, Michael AF, Vernier RL: Renal disease in nail-patella syndrome: Clinical and morphologic studies. Kidney Int *2*:231, 1972.

352. Ben-Bassat M, Cohen L, Rosenfeld J: The glomerular basement membrane in the nail-patella syndrome. Arch Pathol *92*:350, 1971.

353. Uranga VM, Simmons RL, Hoyer SR, et al: Renal transplantation for the nail patella syndrome. Am J Surg *125*:777, 1973.

354. Kieser W: Die sog. Flughaut beim Menschen. Ihre Beziehung zum Status dysraphicus und ihre Erblichkeit. (Dargestellt an der Sippe Fr.) Z Menschl Vererb-u Konstitutionslehre *23*:594, 1939.

355. Fong EE: "Iliac horns" (symmetrical bilateral central posterior iliac processes). A case report. Radiology *47*:517, 1946.

356. Mino RA, Mino VH, Livingstone RG: Osseous dysplasia and dystrophy of the nails. Review of the literature and report of a case. AJR *60*:633, 1948.

357. Wasserman D: Unilateral iliac horn (central posterior iliac process). Case report. Radiology *120*:562, 1976.

358. Cosack G: Hereditäre Arthro-Osteo-Onycho-Dysplasie mit Beckenhörnern ("Turner-Kieser-Syndrom") in Verbindung mit Hyposiderämie. Z Kinderheilk *75*:449, 1954.

359. Neuhold A, Seidl G, Stummvoll H, et al: Nail-patella syndrom. Radiologe *22*:568, 1982.

360. Rossi JF, Kha Tu D, Baldet P, et al: Osteo-onycho-dysplasie hereditaire. Sem Hop Paris *59*:403, 1983.

361. Garces MA, Muraskas JK, Muraskas EK, Abdel-Hameed MF: Hereditary onycho-osteo-dysplasia (HOOD syndrome): A report of two cases. Skel Radiol *8*:55, 1982.

362. Hogh J, Macnivol MF: Foot deformities associated with onycho-osteo-dysplasia. Int Orthop (SICOT) *9*:135, 1985.

363. Hutchinson J: Congenital absence of hair and mammary glands: With atrophic condition of skin and its appendages in a boy whose mother had been almost wholly bald from alopecia areata from the age of six. Med Chir Trans *69*:473, 1886.

364. Margolin FR, Steinbach HL: Progeria. Hutchinson-Gilford syndrome. AJR *103*:173, 1968.

365. Franklyn PP: Progeria in siblings. Clin Radiol *27*:327, 1976.

366. Ozonoff MB, Clemett AR: Progressive osteolysis in progeria. AJR *100*:75, 1967.

367. Gamble JG: Hip disease in Hutchinson-Gilford progeria syndrome. J Pediatr Orthop *4*:585, 1984.

368. Moen C: Orthopaedic aspects of progeria. J Bone Joint Surg [Am] *64*:542, 1982.

369. Lewin P: Arthrogryposis multiplex congenita. J Bone Joint Surg *7*:630, 1925.

370. Friedlander HL, Westin GW, Wood WL Jr: Arthrogryposis multiplex congenita. A review of forty-five cases. J Bone Joint Surg [Am] *50*:89, 1968.

371. Brown LM, Robson MJ, Sharrard WJW: The pathophysiology of arthrogryposis multiplex congenita neurologica. J Bone Joint Surg [Br] *62*:291, 1980.

372. Poznanski AK, LaRowe PC: Radiographic manifestations of arthrogryposis syndrome. Radiology *95*:353, 1970.

373. Bléry M, Pannier S, Barre JL: Étude radiologique de l'arthrogrypose. À propos de 28 cas. J Radiol Electrol Med Nucl *58*:597, 1977.

374. Hall JG: Genetic aspects of arthrogryposis. Clin Orthop *194*:44, 1985.

375. Swinyard CA, Bleck EE: The etiology of arthrogryposis (multiple congenital contracture). Clin Orthop *194*:15, 1985.

376. Grant AD, Rose D, Lehman W: Talocalcaneal coalition in arthrogryposis multiplex congenita. Bull Hosp J Dis *42*:236, 1982.

377. Imamura M, Yamanaka N, Nakamura F, et al: Arthrogryposis multiplex congenita: An autopsy case of a fatal form. Hum Pathol *12*:699, 1981.

378. Werner O: Über kataract in verbindung mit sklerodermie. (Doctoral dissertation, Kiel University.) Kiel, Germany, Schmidt & Klaunig, 1904.

379. Epstein CJ, Martin GM, Schultze AL, et al: Werner's syndrome. A review of its symptomatology, natural history, pathologic features, genetics and relationship to the natural aging process. Medicine *45*:177, 1966.

380. Jacobson HG, Rifkin H, Zucker-Franklin D: Werner's syndrome: A clinical-roentgen entity. Radiology. *74*:373, 1960.

381. Rosen RS, Cuwini R, Cablentz D: Werner's syndrome. Br J Radiol *43*:193, 1970.

382. Herstone ST, Bower J: Werner's syndrome. AJR *51*:639, 1944.

382a. Magill HL, Shackelford GD, McAlister WH, et al: 4p–(Wolf-Hirschhorn) syndrome. AJR *135*:283, 1980.

383. Usui M, Ishii S, Yamawaki S, et al: The occurrence of soft tissue sarcomas in three siblings with Werner's syndrome. Cancer *54*:2580, 1984.

384. Goto M, Tanimoto K, Horiuchi Y, et al: Family analysis of Werner's syndrome: A survey of 42 Japanese families with a review of the literature. Clin Genet *19*:8, 1981.

385. Andersen KS: Congenital angulation of the lower leg and congenital pseudarthrosis of the tibia in Denmark. Acta Orthop Scand *43*:539, 1972.

386. Andersen KS: Radiological classification of congenital pseudarthrosis of the tibia. Acta Orthop Scand *44*:719, 1973.

387. Boyd HB, Sage FB: Congenital pseudarthrosis of the tibia. J Bone Joint Surg [Am] *40*:1245, 1958.

388. Brown GA, Osebold WR, Ponseti IV: Congenital pseudarthrosis of long bones. A clinical, radiographic, histologic, and ultrastructural study. Clin Orthop *128*:228, 1977.

389. Gibson DA, Carroll N: Congenital pseudarthrosis of the clavicle. J Bone Joint Surg [Br] *52*:629, 1970.

390. Owen R: Congenital pseudarthrosis of the clavicle. J Bone Joint Surg [Br] *52*:644, 1970.

391. Ahmadi B, Steel HH: Congenital pseudarthrosis of the clavicle. Clin Orthop *126*:130, 1977.

392. VanNes CP: Congenital pseudarthrosis of the leg. J Bone Joint Surg [Am] *48*:1467, 1966.

393. Briner J, Yunis E: Ultrastructure of congenital pseudarthrosis of the tibia. Arch Pathol *95*:97, 1973.

394. Lloyd-Roberts GC, Shaw NE: The prevention of pseudarthrosis in congenital kyphosis of the tibia. J Bone Joint Surg [Br] *51*:100, 1969.

395. Badgley CE, O'Connor J, Kudner DF: Congenital kyphoscoliotic tibia. J Bone Joint Surg [Am] *34*:349, 1952.

396. Duraiswami PK: Comparison of congenital defects induced in developing chickens by certain teratogenic agents with those caused by insulin. J Bone Joint Surg [Am] *37*:277, 1955.

397. Dunn AW, Aponte GE: Congenital bowing of the tibia and femur. J Bone Joint Surg [Am] *44*:737, 1962.

398. Newell RLM, Durbin FC: The aetiology of congenital angulation of tubular bones with constriction of the medullary canal and its relationship to congenital pseudarthrosis. J Bone Joint Surg [Br] *58*:444, 1976.

399. Lloyd-Roberts GC, Apley AG, Owen R: Reflection upon the etiology of congenital pseudarthrosis of the clavicle. J Bone Joint Surg [Br] *57*:24, 1975.

400. Wall JJ: Congenital pseudarthrosis of the clavicle. J Bone Joint Surg [Br] *52*:1003, 1970.

401. Manashil G, Laufer S: Congenital pseudarthrosis of the clavicle: Report of three cases. AJR *132*:678, 1979.

402. Quinlan WR, Brady PG, Regan BF: Congenital pseudarthrosis of the clavicle. Acta Orthop Scand *51*:489, 1980.

403. Ostrowski DM, Eilert RE, Waldstein G: Congenital pseudarthrosis of the ulna: A report of two cases and review of the literature. J Pediatr Orthop *5*:463, 1985.

404. Boyd HB: Pathology and natural history of congenital pseudarthrosis of the tibia. Clin Orthop *166*:5, 1982.

405. Murray HH, Lovell WW: Congenital pseudarthrosis of the tibia. A long-term follow-up study. Clin Orthop *166*:14, 1982.

406. Morrissy RT: Congenital pseudarthrosis of the tibia. Factors that affect results. Clin Orthop *166*:21, 1982.

407. March HC: Congenital pseudarthrosis of the clavicle. J Can Assoc Radiol *33*:35, 1982.

408. Freedman M, Gamble J, Lewis C: Intrauterine fracture simulating a unilateral clavicular pseudarthrosis. J Can Assoc Radiol *33*:37, 1982.

409. Lawson JP: Symptomatic radiographic variants in extremities. Radiology *157*:625, 1985.

410. Kushner DC, Cleveland RH, Ehrlich MG, et al: Low-dose transaxial tomography. An alternative to computed tomography for the evaluation of anteversion of the femur during childhood. Invest Radiol *20*:978, 1985.

411. Lawhon SM, MacEwen GD, Bunnell WP: Orthopaedic aspects of the VATER association. J Bone Joint Surg [Am] *68*:424, 1986.

412. Pineda C, Resnick D, Greenway G: Diagnosis of tarsal coalition with computed tomography. Clin Orthop *208*:282, 1986.

413. Inglis G, Buxton RA, Macnicol MF: Symptomatic calcaneonavicular bars. The results 20 years after surgical excision. J Bone Joint Surg [Br] *68*:128, 1986.

414. Miller JH, Bernstein SM: The roentgenographic appearance of the "corrected clubfoot." Foot Ankle *6*:177, 1986.

415. Jend H-H: Die computertomographische Antetorsionswinkelbestimmung. ROFO *144*:447, 1986.

416. Daher YH, Lonstein JE, Winter RB, et al: Spinal deformities in patients with arthrogryposis. A review of 16 patients. Spine *10*:609, 1985.

417. Sella EJ, Lawson JP, Ogden JA: The accessory navicular synchondrosis. Clin Orthop *209*:280, 1986.

418. Kaelin A, Hulin PH, Carlioz H: Congenital aplasia of the cruciate ligaments. A report of six cases. J Bone Joint Surg [Br] *68*:827, 1986.

419. Resnik CS, Grizzard JD, Simmons BP, et al: Incomplete carpal coalition. AJR *147*:301, 1986.

420. Takakura Y, Tamai S, Masuhara K: Genesis of the ball-and-socket ankle. J Bone Joint Surg [Br] *68*:834, 1986.

421. Child AH: Joint hypermobility syndrome: Inherited disorder of collagen synthesis. J Rheumatol *13*:239, 1986.

422. Gelberman RH, Cohen MS, Desai SS, et al: Femoral anteversion. A clinical assessment of idiopathic intoeing gait in children. J Bone Joint Surg [Br] *69*:75, 1987.

423. Mahboubi S, Horstmann H: Femoral torsion: CT measurement. Radiology *160*:843, 1986.

424. Moser RP, Wagner GN: Nutrient groove of the ilium, a subtle but important forensic radiographic marker in the identification of victims of severe trauma. Skel Radiol *19*:15, 1990.

425. Pitt MJ, Graham AR, Shipman JH, et al: Herniation pit of the femoral neck. AJR *138*:1115, 1982.

426. Angel JL: The reaction area of the femoral neck. Clin Orthop *32*:130, 1964.

427. Crabbe JP, Martel W, Matthews LS: Rapid growth of femoral herniation pit. AJR *159*:1038, 1992.

428. Thomason CB, Silverman ED, Walter RD, et al: Focal bone tracer uptake associated with a herniation pit of the femoral neck. Clin Nucl Med *8*:304, 1983.

429. Nokes SR, Vogler JB, Spritzer CE, et al: Herniation pits of the femoral neck: Appearance at MR imaging. Radiology *172*:231, 1989.

430. Mann RW, Owsley DW: Os trigonum. Variation of a common accessory ossicle of the talus. J Am Podiatr Assoc *80*:536, 1990.

431. Grogan DP, Walling AK, Ogden JA: Anatomy of the os trigonum. J Pediatr Orthop *10*:618, 1990.

432. Grogan DP, Gasser SI, Ogden JA: The painful accessory navicular: A clinical and histopathological study. Foot Ankle *10*:164, 1989.

433. Hultgren T, Lugnegård H: Carpal boss. Acta Orthop Scand *57*:547, 1986.

434. Keats TE: Normal variants of the hand and wrist. Hand Clinics *7*:153, 1991.

435. Hägglund G, Pettersson H: A case of bilateral duplication of the patella. Acta Orthop Scand *60*:725, 1989.

436. Gasco J, Del Pino JM, Gomar-Sancho F: Double patella. A case of duplication in the coronal plane. J Bone Joint Surg [Br] *69*:602, 1987.

437. Goergen TG, Resnick D, Greenway G, et al: Dorsal defect of the patella: A characteristic radiographic lesion. Radiology *130*:333, 1979.

438. Haswell DM, Berne AS, Graham CB: The dorsal defect of the patella. Pediatr Radiol *4*:238, 1976.

439. Johnson JF, Brogden BG: Dorsal defect of the patella: Incidence and distribution. AJR *139*:339, 1982.

440. van Holsbeeck M, Vandamme B, Marchal G, et al: Dorsal defect of the patella: concept of its origin and relationship with bipartite and multipartite patella. Skel Radiol *16*:304, 1987.

441. Owsley DW, Mann RW: Bilateral dorsal defect of the patella. AJR *154*:1347, 1990.

442. Hunter LY, Hensinger RN: Dorsal defect of the patella with cartilaginous involvement: A case report. Clin Orthop *143*:131, 1979.

443. Denham RH: Dorsal defect of the patella. J Bone Joint Surg [Am] *66*:116, 1984.

444. Ho VB, Kransdorf MJ, Jelinek JS, et al: Dorsal defect of the patella: MR features. J Comput Assist Tomogr *15*:474, 1991.

445. McDougall A: The os trigonum. J Bone Joint Surg [Br] *37*:257, 1955.

446. Shepherd FJ: A hitherto undescribed fracture of the astragalus. J Anat Physiol *17*:79, 1882.

447. Quirk R: Talar compression syndrome in dancers. Foot Ankle *3*:65, 1982.

448. Lapidus PW: A note on the fracture of the os trigonum. Bull Hosp Joint Dis *33*:150, 1972.

449. Brodsky AE, Khalil MA: Talar compression syndrome. Foot Ankle *7*:338, 1987.

450. Ogden JA, Lee J: Accessory ossification patterns and injuries of the malleoli. J Pediatr Orthop *10*:306, 1990.

451. Griffiths JD, Menelaus MB: Symptomatic ossicles of the lateral malleolus in children. J Bone Joint Surg [Br] *69*:317, 1987.

452. Berg EE: The symptomatic os subfibulare. Avulsion fracture of the fibula associated with recurrent instability of the ankle. J Bone Joint Surg [Am] *73*:1251, 1991.

453. Coral A: The radiology of skeletal elements in the subtibial region: Incidence and significance. Skel Radiol *16*:298, 1987.

454. Obermann WR, Loose HW: The os supratrochleare dorsale: A normal variant that may simulate disease. AJR *141*:123, 1983.

455. Canigiani G, Wickenhauser J, Czech W: Beitrag zur Osteochondritis dissecans in Foramen supratrochleare. ROFO *117*:66, 1972.

456. Schwarz GS: Bilateral antecubital ossicles (fabella cubiti) and other rare accessory bones of the elbow. Radiology *69*:730, 1957.

457. Gudmundsen TE, Østensen H: Accessory ossicles in the elbow. Acta Orthop Scand *58*:130, 1987.

458. Bassett LW, Mirra JM, Forrester DM, et al: Post-traumatic osteochondral "loose body" of the olecranon fossa. Radiology *141*:635, 1981.

459. Stark P, Watkins GE, Hildebrandt-Stark HE, et al: Episternal ossicles. Radiology *165*:143, 1987.

460. Maffulli N, Fixsen JA: Fibular hypoplasia with absent lateral rays of the foot. J Bone Joint Surg [Br] *73*:1002, 1991.

461. Beals RK, Rolfe B: VATER association. A unifying concept of multiple anomalies. J Bone Joint Surg [Am] *71*:948, 1989.

462. Boden SD, Fallon MD, Davidson R, et al: Proximal femoral focal deficiency. Evidence for a defect in proliferation and maturation of chondrocytes. J Bone Joint Surg [Am] *71*:1119, 1989.

463. Hillmann JS, Mesgarzadeh M, Revesz G, et al: Proximal femoral focal deficiency: Radiologic analysis of 49 cases. Radiology *165*:769, 1987.

464. Pattinson RC, Fixsen JA: Management and outcome in tibial dysplasia. J Bone Joint Surg [Br] *74*:893, 1992.

465. Schoenecker PL, Capelli M, Millar EA, et al: Congenital longitudinal deficiency of the tibia. J Bone Joint Surg [Am] *71*:278, 1989.

466. Lintner DM, Sebastianelli WJ, Hanks GA, et al: Glenoid dysplasia. A case report and review of the literature. Clin Orthop *283*:145, 1992.

467. Kozlowski K, Scougall J: Congenital bilateral glenoid hypoplasia: a report of four cases. Br J Radiol 60:705, 1987.

468. Borenstein ZCF, Mink J, Oppenheim W, et al: Case report 655. Skel Radiol 20:134, 1991.

469. Callaghan JJ, York JJ, McNeish LM, et al: Unusual anomaly of the scapula defined by arthroscopy and computed tomographic arthrography. Report of a case. J Bone Joint Surg [Am] 70:452, 1988.

470. Manns RA, Davies AM: Glenoid hypoplasia: Assessment by computed tomographic arthrography. Clin Radiol 43:316, 1991.

471. Guidera KJ, Raney E, Ogden JA, et al: Caudal regression: A review of seven cases, including the mermaid syndrome. J Pediatr Orthop 11:743, 1991.

472. Nogami H: Polydactyly and polysyndactyly of the fifth toe. Clin Orthop 204:261, 1986.

473. Lord MJ, Laurenzano KR, Hartmann RW Jr: Poland's syndrome. Clin Pediatr 29:606, 1990.

474. Krohn KD, Brandt KD, Braunstein E, et al: Hereditary symphalangism. Association with osteoarthritis. J Rheumatol 16:977, 1989.

475. Ganos DL, Imbriglia JE: Symptomatic congenital coalition of the pisiform and hamate. J Hand Surg [Am] 16:646, 1991.

476. Simmons BP, McKenzie WD: Symptomatic carpal coalition. J Hand Surg [Am] 10:190, 1985.

477. Gross SC, Watson K, Strickland JW, et al: Triquetral-lunate arthritis secondary to synostosis. J Hand Surg [Am] 14:95, 1989.

478. Knezevich S, Gottesman M: Symptomatic scapholunatotriquetral carpal coalition with fusion of the capitatometacarpal joint. Report of a case. Clin Orthop 251:153, 1990.

479. Gerscovich EO, Greenspan A: Case report 598. Skel Radiol 19:143, 1990.

480. Oestreich AE, Mize WA, Crawford AH, et al: The "anterior nose": A direct sign of calcaneonavicular coalition on the lateral radiograph. J Pediatr Orthop 7:709, 1987.

481. Warren MJ, Jeffree MA, Wilson DJ, et al: Computed tomography in suspected tarsal coalition. Examination of 26 cases. Acta Orthop Scand 61:554, 1990.

482. Bower BL, Keyser CK, Gilula LA: Rigid subtalar joint—a radiographic spectrum. Skel Radiol 17:583, 1988.

483. Kumar SJ, Guille JT, Lee MS, et al: Osseous and non-osseous coalition of the middle facet of the talocalcaneal joint. J Bone Joint Surg [Am] 74:529, 1992.

484. Lee MS, Harcke HT, Kumar SJ, et al: Subtalar joint coalition in children: New observations. Radiology 172:635, 1989.

485. Pistoia F, Ozonoff MB, Wintz P: Ball-and-socket ankle joint. Skel Radiol 16:447, 1987.

486. Dennis DA, Clayton ML, Ferlic DC: Osteoarthritis associated with a ball-and-socket ankle joint. A case report. Clin Orthop 215:196, 1987.

487. Scranton PE Jr: Treatment of symptomatic talocalcaneal coalition. J Bone Joint Surg [Am] 69:533, 1987.

488. Takakura Y, Sugimoto K, Tanaka Y, et al: Symptomatic talocalcaneal coalition. Its clinical significance and treatment. Clin Orthop 269:249, 1991.

489. Wechsler RJ, Karasick D, Schweitzer ME: Computed tomography of talocalcaneal coalition: Imaging techniques. Skel Radiol 21:353, 1992.

490. Herzenberg JE, Goldner JL, Martinez S, et al: Computerized tomography of talocalcaneal tarsal coalition: A clinical and anatomic study. Foot Ankle 6:273, 1986.

491. Percy EC, Mann DL: Tarsal coalition: A review of the literature and presentation of 13 cases. Foot Ankle 9:40, 1988.

492. Bonk JH, Tozzi MA: Congenital talonavicular synostosis. A review of the literature and a case report. J Am Podiatr Assoc 79:186, 1989.

493. Wiles S, Palladino SJ, Stavosky JW: Naviculocuneiform coalition. J Am Podiatr Assoc 78:355, 1988.

494. Ertel AN, O'Connell FD: Talonavicular coalition following avascular necrosis of the tarsal navicular. J Pediatr Orthop 4:482, 1984.

495. Hawass N-E-D, Bahakim H, Al-Boukai AA: Intrathoracic fat. A new CT feature of intrathoracic rib. Case report. Clin Imaging 15:31, 1991.

496. Nguyen VD, Matthes JD, Wunderlich CC: The pelvic digit: CT correlation and review of the literature. Comput Med Imaging Graphics 14:127, 1990.

497. Hall JE, Simmons ED, Danylchuk K, et al: Instability of the cervical spine and neurological involvement in Klippel-Feil syndrome. A case report. J Bone Joint Surg [Am] 72:460, 1990.

498. Hensinger RN: Congenital anomalies of the cervical spine. Clin Orthop 264:16, 1991.

499. O'Connor JF, Cranley WR, McCarten KM, et al: Radiographic manifestations of congenital anomalies of the spine. Radiol Clin North Am 29:407, 1991.

500. Mikawa Y, Watanabe R, Yamano Y: Omoclavicular bar in congenital elevation of the scapula. A new finding. Spine 16:376, 1991.

501. Fagg PS: Wrist pain in the Madelung's deformity of dyschondrosteosis. J Hand Surg [Br] 13:11, 1988.

502. Fagg PS: Reverse Madelung's deformity with nerve compression. J Hand Surg [Br] 13:23, 1988.

503. Luchetti R, Mingione A, Monteleone M, et al: Carpal tunnel syndrome in Madelung's deformity. J Hand Surg [Br] 13:19, 1988.

504. Bell MJ, Atkins RM, Sharrard WJW: Irreducible congenital dislocation of the knee. Aetiology and management. J Bone Joint Surg [Br] 69:403, 1987.

505. Johnson E, Audell R, Oppenheim WL: Congenital dislocation of the knee. J Pediatr Orthop 7:194, 1987.

506. Bensahel H, Dal Monte A, Hjelmstedt A, et al: Congenital dislocation of the knee. J Pediatr Orthop 9:174, 1989.

507. Ferris B, Aichroth P: The treatment of congenital knee dislocation. A review of nineteen knees. Clin Orthop 216:135, 1987.

508. Ferris BD, Jackson AM: Congenital snapping knee. Habitual anterior subluxation of the tibia in extension. J Bone Joint Surg [Br] 72:453, 1990.

509. Campbell CC, Waters PM, Emans JB: Excision of the radial head for congenital dislocation. J Bone Joint Surg [Am] 74:726, 1992.

510. Bos CFA, Sakkers RJB, Bloem JL, et al: Histological, biochemical, and MRI studies of the growth plate in congenital coxa vara. J Pediatr Orthop 9:660, 1989.

511. Arroyo IL, Brewer EJ, Giannini EH: Arthritis/arthralgia and hypermobility of the joints in schoolchildren. J Rheumatol 15:978, 1988.

512. March LM, Francis H, Webb J: Benign joint hypermobility with neuropathies: Documentation and mechanism of median, sciatic, and common peroneal nerve compression. Clin Rheumatol 7:35, 1988.

513. Silman AJ, Day SJ, Haskard DO: Factors associated with joint mobility in an adolescent population. Ann Rheum Dis 46:209, 1987.

514. Rovetta G, Bianchi G, Monteforte P: Syndrome du canal carpien dans l'hyperlaxité ligamentaire. Rev Rhum Mal Osteoartic 57:661, 1990.

515. Harinstein D, Buckingham RB, Braun T, et al: Systemic joint laxity (the hypermobile joint syndrome) is associated with temporomandibular joint dysfunction. Arthritis Rheum 31:1259, 1988.

516. Amir D, Frankl U, Pogrund H: Pulled elbow and hypermobility of joints. Clin Orthop 257:94, 1990.

517. Larsson L-G, Baum J, Mudholkar GS: Hypermobility features and differential incidence between the sexes. Arthritis Rheum 30:1426, 1987.

518. Berg EE: A reappraisal of metatarsus adductus and skewfoot. J Bone Joint Surg [Am] 68:1185, 1986.

519. Høiseth A, Reikerås O, Fønstelien E: Evaluation of three methods for measurement of femoral neck anteversion. Femoral neck anteversion, definition, measuring methods and errors. Acta Orthop 30:69, 1989.

520. Upadhyay SS, O'Neil T, Burwell RG, et al: A new method using ultrasound for measuring femoral anteversion (torsion): Technique and reliability. Br J Radiol 60:519, 1987.

521. Berman L, Mitchell R, Katz D: Ultrasound assessment of femoral anteversion. A comparison with computerised tomography. J Bone Joint Surg [Br] 69:268, 1987.

522. Lausten GS, Jørgensen F, Boesen J: Measurement of anteversion of the femoral neck. Ultrasound and computerised tomography compared. J Bone Joint Surg [Br] 71:237, 1989.

523. Murphy SB, Simon SR, Kijewski PK, et al: Femoral anteversion. J Bone Joint Surg [Am] 69:1169, 1987.

524. Reikerås O: Is there a relationship between femoral anteversion and leg torsion? Skel Radiol 20:409, 1991.

525. Guidera KJ, Satterwhite Y, Ogden JA, et al: Nail patella syndrome: A review of 44 orthopaedic patients. J Pediatr Orthop 11:737, 1991.

526. Croock AD, Kahaleh MB, Powers JM: Vasculitis and renal disease in nail-patella syndrome: Case report and literature review. Ann Rheum Dis 46:562, 1987.

527. Banskota AK, Mayo-Smith W, Rajbhandari S, et al: Case report 548. Skel Radiol 18:318, 1989.

528. Loomer RL: Shoulder girdle dysplasia associated with nail patella syndrome. A case report and literature review. Clin Orthop 238:112, 1989.

529. Fiedler BS, DeSmet AA, Kling TF Jr, et al: Foot deformity in hereditary onycho-osteodysplasia. J Can Assoc Radiol 38:305, 1987.

530. Gottron H: Familiare akrogerie. Arch Dermatol Syphilis 181:571, 1941.

531. Calvert HT: Acrogeria (Gottron type). Br J Dermatol 69:69, 1957.

532. Ho A, White SJ, Rasmussen JE: Skeletal abnormalities of acrogeria, a progeroid syndrome. Skel Radiol 16:463, 1987.

533. Guidera KJ, Kortright L, Barber V, et al: Radiographic changes in arthrogrypotic knees. Skel Radiol 20:193, 1991.

534. Khraishi M, Howard B, Little H: A patient with Werner's syndrome and osteosarcoma presenting as scleroderma. J Rheumatol 19:810, 1992.

535. Gaetani SA, Ferraris AM, D'Agosta A: Case report 485. Skel Radiol 17:298, 1988.

536. Goto M, Kindynis P, Resnick D, et al: Osteosclerosis of the phalanges in Werner's syndrome. Radiology 172:841, 1989.

537. Crossett LS, Beaty JH, Betz RR, et al: Congenital pseudarthrosis of the tibia. Long-term follow-up study. Clin Orthop 245:16, 1989.

538. McGinnis MR, Mullen JO: Congenital pseudarthrosis of the tibia associated with cleidocranial dysostosis and osteogenesis imperfecta. A case report. Clin Orthop 220:228, 1987.

539. Dal Monte A, Donzelli O, Sudanese A, et al: Congenital pseudarthrosis of the fibula. J Pediatr Orthop 7:14, 1987.

540. Bell DF: Congenital forearm pseudarthrosis: Report of six cases and review of the literature. J Pediatr Orthop 9:438, 1989.

541. Younge D, Arford C: Congenital pseudarthrosis of the forearm and fibula. A case report. Clin Orthop 265:277, 1991.

542. Schnall SB, King JD, Marrero G: Congenital pseudarthrosis of the clavicle: A review of the literature and surgical results of six cases. J Pediatr Orthop 8:316, 1988.

543. Levin B: The unilateral wavy clavicle. Skel Radiol 19:519, 1990.

544. Kane TJ, Henry G, Furry D: A simple roentgenographic measurement of femoral anteversion. A short note. J Bone Joint Surg [Am] 74:1540, 1992.

545. Romanowski CAJ, Barrington NA: The accessory navicular—an important cause of medial foot pain. Clin Radiol 46:261, 1992.

546. Sueyoshi Y, Shimozaki E, Matsumoto T, et al: Two cases of dorsal defect of the patella with arthroscopically visible cartilage surface perforations. J Arthrosc Rel Surg 9:164, 1993.

547. Resnik CS, Aiken MW, Kenzora JE: Case report 780. Skel Radiol 22:214, 1993.

548. Hoeffel C, Hoeffel JC, Got I: Bilateral pelvic digits. A case report and review of the literature. ROFO 158:275, 1993.

549. Ulmer JL, Elster AD, Ginsberg LE, et al: Klippel-Feil syndrome: CT and MR of acquired and congenital abnormalities of the cervical spine and cord. J Comput Assist Tomogr 17:215, 1993.

550. Staheli LT: Rotational problems in children. J Bone Joint Surg [Am] 75:939, 1993.

551. Terjesen T, Anda S, Rønningen H: Ultrasound examination for measurement of femoral anteversion in children. Skel Radiol 22:33, 1993.

552. Ogata K: Painful bipartite patella. A new approach to operative treatment. J Bone Joint Surg [Am] 76:573, 1994.

553. Wirth MA, Lyons FR, Rockwood CA Jr: Hypoplasia of the glenoid. A review of sixteen patients. J Bone Joint Surg 75:1175, 1993.

554. Nguyen VD, Tyrrel R: Klippel-Feil syndrome: Patterns of bony fusion and wasp-waist sign. Skeletal Radiol 22:519, 1993.

555. Hinderaker T, Uden A, Reikerås O: Direct ultrasonographic measurement of femoral anteversion in newborns. Skeletal Radiol 23:133, 1994.

556. Roach JW, Shindell R, Green NE: Late-onset pseudarthrosis of the dysplastic tibia. J Bone Joint Surg [Am] 75:1593, 1993.

557. Eckhoff DG, Johnson KK: Three-dimensional computed tomography reconstruction of tibial torsion. Clin Orthop Rel Res 302:42, 1994.

SECTION

XVIII

Miscellaneous Diseases

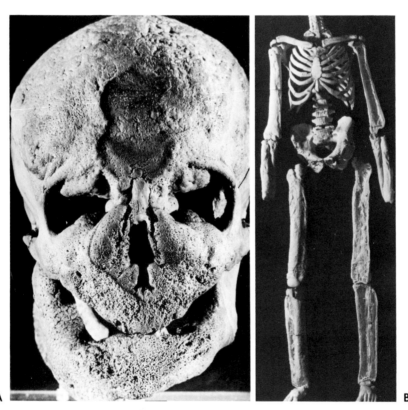

A Leontiasis ossea: Notice the massive deposition of bone involving the cranium and face. The paranasal sinuses are obliterated.
B Pachydermoperiostosis: Generalized hyperostosis is evident.
(**A, B,** from Ortner DJ, Putschar WGJ: Identification of Pathological Condition in Human Skeletal Remains. Washington, D.C., Smithsonian Institution Press, 1981.)

91

Sarcoidosis

Donald Resnick, M.D., and Gen Niwayama, M.D.

Sarcoidosis is a granulomatous disorder of unknown cause affecting multiple organ systems, especially in young adults, and leading principally to bilateral hilar adenopathy, pulmonary infiltrates, and skin or eye lesions.[1] The diagnosis of the disease is substantiated by a combination of clinical, radiologic, and histologic features, the last consisting predominantly of widespread, noncaseating epithelioid cell granulomas. The histologic appearance of the granulomas, although characteristic, is not diagnostic by itself, and accurate identification of sarcoidosis requires careful elimination of other conditions that may have similar histologic alterations. The course of the disease is variable, and it may be associated with significant musculoskeletal abnormalities.

ETIOLOGY AND PATHOGENESIS

Theories of the cause of this disorder abound, yet none has been confirmed. Many of its features, such as the disseminated distribution, the presence of granulomas that morphologically resemble those associated with infection, and the familial and geographic clustering, suggest that sarcoidosis is an infectious disorder.[2] *Mycobacterium tuberculosis* and other mycobacteria, fungi, and viruses have been offered as possible etiologic agents. Typical or atypi-

cal mycobacteria are not recovered consistently from the granulomatous lesions of sarcoidosis, however. Similarly, isolation of fungal or viral agents has not been accomplished.[3] Although elevation of antibody titers to viruses such as Epstein-Barr, herpes simplex, rubella, measles, and parainfluenza is recorded, the finding is not consistent, nor does it correlate with the clinical activity or stage of the disease.[2] Evidence has existed that an agent from human sarcoid tissue can be transmitted into the foot pads of mice much more consistently than from normal lymph node tissue; autoclaved or irradiated sarcoid tissue does not induce granuloma formation.[2]

The occasional reports of sarcoidosis occurring in families suggest that hereditary influences also may be important in the cause or pathogenesis of this disease[3]; the clinical and radiologic features of familial sarcoidosis generally are similar to those of sporadic sarcoidosis. No significant association between sarcoidosis and either serologically defined or lymphocyte-defined transplantation antigens has been demonstrated, however, although there may be a higher frequency of HLA-B8 in patients with early resolution of the disease and in those with erythema nodosum and polyarthralgias.[2]

Although immunologic abnormalities are well-recognized manifestations of the disease, they are not fully understood, they vary from one person to another, and they occur in patients with a variety of other disorders. The immune mechanisms influence the clinical symptoms and signs associated with the various forms of the disease, but the abnormal immune reactivity per se does not cause sarcoidosis.[2] With regard to pulmonary involvement in sarcoidosis, proliferation of activated T lymphocytes in the lung possibly is related to the release of interleukin-2.[115]

CLINICAL ABNORMALITIES

Sarcoidosis has a worldwide distribution (with its greatest incidence having been reported in Sweden) and by no means is rare in the United States, where the highest concentration of cases occurs in the Southeast. The disease affects men and women equally, although it is particularly common in women of childbearing age. It usually becomes apparent between 20 and 40 years of age. Approximately 70 per cent of patients with sarcoidosis are less than 40 years of age. Blacks are more frequently affected than whites; in the United States, the disease is ten times more common in black patients. Black women are affected about twice as often as black men, and, in general, the disease is more severe in blacks than whites. Sarcoidosis appears to be rare in Chinese persons.

The clinical manifestations are highly variable. In some patients, radiographic evidence of hilar adenopathy may appear in the absence of any symptoms and signs.[4] In others, an acute or chronic form of the disease becomes evident.[3] One form of acute disease, accompanied by erythema nodosum, polyarthritis, iritis, and fever, is designated Lofgren's syndrome. Pulmonary manifestations are frequent (as many as 90 per cent of patients eventually will have pulmonary abnormalities) and include cough, chest pain, and dyspnea. Ocular abnormalities, occurring in about 25 per cent of patients with the disease, include a granulomatous uveitis, iritis, and iridocyclitis. Discrete, agglomerated, reddish skin nodules that are flat or slightly raised are seen, which on histologic examination are found to consist of typical granulomas. Also, in acute sarcoidosis, erythema nodosum is common,[116] which, when combined with hilar adenopathy and arthralgia, indicates a favorable prognosis. Malaise, anorexia, weight loss, fever, hepatosplenomegaly, and lymphadenopathy also are detected in many cases. Additional findings relate to involvement of other organs, including those of the central or peripheral nervous system, the heart, and the musculoskeletal system. Enlargement of the salivary and lacrimal glands occurs in approximately 10 per cent of patients with sarcoidosis.

Laboratory analysis may indicate anemia, leukopenia, eosinophilia, a reduction in serum albumin concentration, and an elevation of serum globulin level. Hypercalcemia can be seen in approximately 25 per cent of cases, reflecting increased sensitivity to vitamin D and increased intestinal absorption of calcium. Recent studies indicate that alveolar macrophages and sarcoid granulomas are involved actively in the metabolism of vitamin D and apparently lead to the synthesis of 1,25-dihydroxyvitamin D, the cause of the hypercalcemia in sarcoidosis.[151–153] Hypercalcemia usually is mild and may be associated with normal or slightly elevated serum phosphate levels and hypercalciuria. The administration of cortisone reduces the hypercalcemia.[5]

In 60 to 80 per cent of patients with sarcoidosis, especially those with early disease and prominent adenopathy,[6] an intradermal injection of 0.2 ml of a 10 per cent saline suspension of sarcoid tissue produces a nodule containing noncaseating granulomas. This represents a positive Kveim test,[7] a reaction that is present in only 3 to 4 per cent of patients with other granulomatous disorders.[2] The general lack of availability of Kveim antigen and the occasional positivity of the test in other diseases such as regional enteritis[8] limit the usefulness of this reaction, however. Furthermore, as hypergammaglobulinemia and cutaneous anergy[9] represent nonspecific findings of sarcoidosis, a search for more diagnostic laboratory tests has been undertaken. The demonstration that circulating levels of angiotensin-converting enzyme (ACE) are elevated in approximately 80 per cent of patients with acute pulmonary sarcoidosis, perhaps related to increased synthesis of the enzyme by epithelioid cells in the granuloma, may indicate

that a more specific test for the disorder is available, although elevations of ACE also have been recorded in Gaucher's disease and leprosy.[10, 117, 118]

The natural course of sarcoidosis is extremely variable, although a favorable outcome is most typical. Radiographic evidence of pulmonary fibrosis, in general, indicates a poor prognosis, as does multiorgan involvement.

GENERAL PATHOLOGIC ABNORMALITIES

The accurate diagnosis of sarcoidosis is made on the basis of compatible clinical and radiologic findings, the presence of supporting laboratory data, such as a positive reaction to Kveim antigen, anergy, and elevated levels of serum gamma globulins, and the demonstration of typical noncaseating granulomas in the absence of other identifiable causes for such lesions. Although the histologic features of sarcoidosis are well known, it must be recognized that noncaseating granulomas can be evident in additional neoplastic and infectious disorders. The granuloma is composed of discrete hyperplastic tubercles consisting predominantly of epithelioid cells[11, 12] (Fig. 91–1). Additional cell types that are present are lymphocytes (typically, helper T lymphocytes), giant cells, and plasma cells. Caseation characteristically is absent. Granulomas can be apparent in almost any organ, including the bone marrow (in about 20 per cent of cases),[119] but most often are present in the lung, lymph nodes, liver, and spleen.[11] They can grow slowly or rapidly, but in many cases they remain relatively unchanged in both size and number. As they resolve, the granulomas frequently are replaced with fibrous elements. It is this fibrosis, in addition to the mechanical compression of the adjacent tissue by the granuloma itself, that accounts for the clinically apparent organ dysfunction in many systems of the body that characterizes sarcoidosis.[2]

MUSCULOSKELETAL ABNORMALITIES

Sarcoidosis can involve muscles, subcutaneous tissues, bones, and joints and results in prominent clinical, radiologic, and pathologic findings.

Muscle Involvement

Noncaseating granulomas are evident in skeletal muscle in 50 to 80 per cent of patients who have had sarcoidosis for less than 2 years, although their detection requires meticulous examination of ample specimens. Granulomatous involvement of muscular tissues in sarcoidosis can be symptomatic or, more commonly, asymptomatic. Pain, tenderness, and nodular swelling are typical clinical findings. Muscle contractures have been reported.[121] A true symmetric proximal sarcoid myopathy can occur with or without evidence of disease in other locations.[13, 120, 166] The myopathy, which can cause weakness, elevated muscle enzyme levels, and abnormal electromyograms, may respond favorably to corticosteroid treatment and is associated with noncaseating granulomatous, lymphocytic infiltration, and muscle necrosis and regeneration.

Reports of muscle involvement in sarcoidosis have emphasized that although symptomatic disease is relately rare in comparison to asymptomatic disease, several types of sarcoid muscle involvement may lead to symptoms:

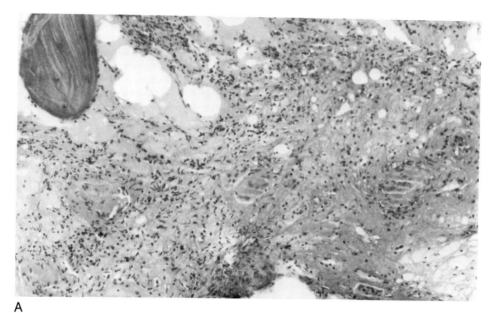

FIGURE 91–1. Sarcoidosis: Pathologic abnormalities.

A The bone marrow spaces are replaced by granulomatous lesions (180×). Epithelioid cells and multiple Langhans giant cells are observed.

B In this photomicrograph, note the epithelioid cells, multiple Langhans giant cells (arrowheads), lymphocytes, and fibroblasts. No caseation is present. Special stains and culture for acid-fast bacilli and fungi gave negative results (360×).

A

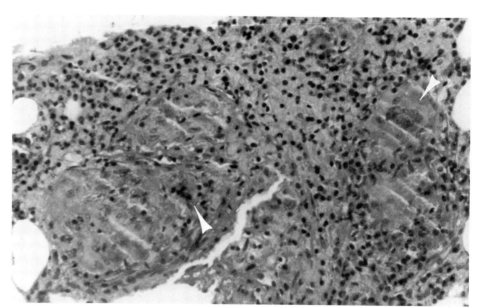

B

Chronic myopathy, the most common type, usually is accompanied by other manifestations of chronic sarcoidosis, is manifested as symmetric involvement typically of proximal muscle groups, is associated with muscle contractures, hypertrophy, or atrophy, and affects middle-aged and elderly patients, especially postmenopausal women; nodular myopathy is accompanied by small tender nodules in various musculotendinous junctions; and acute myositis, which is rare, leads to muscle tenderness, weakness, and myalgias, usually accompanied by acute polyarthritis or erythema nodosum.[167] Differentiation among these three types of symptomatic muscle disease can be accomplished through careful clinical and laboratory assessment and, perhaps, MR imaging (see later discussion).[168]

Subcutaneous Involvement

In addition to a variety of cutaneous manifestations of sarcoidosis and to erythema nodosum, subcutaneous nodules may be identified in approximately 5 per cent of patients with this disease. Such nodules usually are observed in men and women between the third and sixth decades of life; associated visceral involvement, particularly of the lungs, liver, and spleen, is not uncommon, although osseous lesions typically are absent.[169] As described by Kalb and associates,[169] subcutaneous nodules in sarcoidosis have an insidious onset; are painless, round, and mobile; are distributed in the extremities with fewer nodules in the trunk and face; and may increase in number over a period of weeks to months, thereafter becoming constant in number, ranging from 1 to 100. Histologically, these nodules generally are noncaseating, lying in the subcutaneous fat with or without extension into the dermis. The designation of Darier-Roussy sarcoidosis sometimes is applied to these and other lesions of the subcutaneous tissue. Radiographically, lobulated masses, sometimes in a periarticular distribution, are seen (Fig. 91–2). Subjacent erosion of bone may be evident,

TABLE 91–1. Frequency of Bone Lesions in Large Series of Sarcoidosis Patients from 10 Cities*

City	Number of Patients		Bone Lesions	
	With Sarcoidosis	Undergoing Skeletal Radiography	Number	Per Cent
London	537	475	19	4
New York	311	139	13	9
Paris	329	165	6	3.5
Los Angeles	150	60	3	4
Tokyo	282	282	5	2
Reading	425	425	5	1
Lisbon	89	89	12	13
Edinburgh	502	502	6	1.2
Novi Sad	285	225	25	11
Geneva	121	121	4	3
Total	3031	2483	98	5

*Used by permission from James DG, Neville E, Carstairs LS: Bone and joint sarcoidosis. Semin Arthritis Rheum 6:53–81, 1976.

although calcification generally is not apparent. Differential diagnostic considerations include gouty tophi, rheumatoid nodules, and xanthomas.

Osseous Involvement

Frequency. Clinical evidence of bone involvement in sarcoidosis was noted before the discovery of x-rays. Pronounced chronic swelling about affected fingers and toes in association with lupus pernio (Boeck's sarcoid) was recognized by Besnier in 1898[14] and described further by Kreibich in 1904.[15] Rieder in 1910[16] and Jüngling in 1928[17] noted radiographic findings in lupus pernio, although accurate differentiation of the sarcoid lesions from tuberculosis was not accomplished until later. Although innumerable reports of osseous involvement in sarcoidosis are now available that define its radiographic characteristics,[18–22, 122] there has been much disagreement about the frequency of skeletal involvement in the disease. In a review of reports of sarcoidosis throughout the world, the frequency of radiographic evidence of osseous involvement varied from 1 to 13 per cent, averaging 5 per cent[3] (Table 91–1). It is obvious that variations in these reports and others are related to differences in patient selection and method of examination. As many of the skeletal lesions of sarcoidosis are asymptomatic, an accurate appraisal of the frequency of osseous involvement in this disease would require complete skeletal surveys of patients with all forms of sarcoidosis, regardless of their clinical manifestations. Furthermore, as minor cystic bone changes in this disorder may resemble findings in normal persons,[23] an age- and sex-matched control population also must be evaluated. Because this type of comprehensive investigation has not been accomplished to date, the quoted figure of 5 per cent must be viewed with caution.

Osseous sarcoidosis rarely is detected in the absence of skin lesions,[24] although the skeletal abnormalities can be prominent even when cutaneous alterations are quite subtle. It has been estimated that 80 to 90 per cent of patients with sarcoidosis involving bone have radiographic evidence of pulmonary disease.[2] Bone changes in this disease, in the

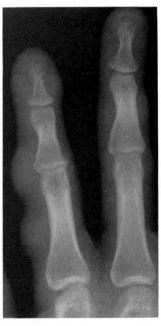

FIGURE 91–2. Sarcoidosis: Subcutaneous nodules. Observe prominent soft tissue nodules in the second and third digits, with acro-osteolysis of the terminal tufts.

absence of additional clinical or radiologic manifestations, are distinctly unusual.

Clinical Manifestations. Although bone changes often are entirely asymptomatic,[11, 18, 25, 26] clinical manifestations in some cases may be prominent. Soft tissue swelling and cutaneous lesions of the hands and, less typically, the feet can accompany osseous disease. These clinical findings frequently are symmetric and are most prominent over the proximal and middle phalanges of the digits. Less often, the areas of the metacarpals, metatarsals, terminal phalanges, wrists, and midfeet are affected.[12] Tenderness, stiffness, and restricted motion can be seen. Soft tissue swelling and deformity may be apparent also at other sites, including the nose,[27–29] face and sinuses,[30–34] skull, and extremities. Pathologic fractures of the ribs[123] or long or short tubular bones of the extremities[35, 131, 158, 159] and spinal cord compression[36–38, 124–127] due to sarcoidosis also can lead to prominent clinical manifestations.

Radiographic Manifestations. The radiographic manifestations of sarcoidosis vary with the region of the skeleton that is affected.[154] Certain specific patterns can be recognized, especially in the bones of the hand.

Osteoporosis producing generalized osteopenia, a decrease in cortical thickness, and striations of the cortex has been observed in sarcoidosis, perhaps related to granulomatous destruction and displacement of spongy trabeculae and perivascular infiltration of the haversian systems. A coarsened, reticulated, or lacework trabecular pattern becomes evident (Fig. 91–3). Localized rarefactions or cystic lesions may lead to a ''punched-out'' appearance that can simulate that which is encountered in a variety of benign or malignant processes. These cysts can be located centrally or eccentrically, may be sharply marginated, and may be round or ovoid, and frequently they are combined with alterations in the adjacent trabecular structure. At times, osseous destruction can appear rapidly, associated with a permeative pattern, cortical violation, and sequestration.

Remarkably, even in the presence of this aggressive dissolution of bone, periostitis, although reported,[170] is distinctly unusual.[171] Furthermore, osteosclerosis about these rarefactions is absent or mild.

Less typically, localized or generalized osteosclerosis is evident (Fig. 91–4), sometimes appearing long after the lung involvement in sarcoidosis has become arrested.[172] Nodular opacities can appear in the medullary cavities of the tubular bones of the hands and feet, or about the terminal phalanges (acro-osteosclerosis) (see discussion later in this chapter). In unusual circumstances, a widespread increase in skeletal radiodensity may be seen.[39–42, 172, 173] The latter osteosclerotic changes are most frequent in the spine, pelvis, skull, ribs, and proximal ends of the long bones; they can be diffuse or focal, resembling changes in Paget's disease, skeletal metastasis, lymphoma, myelofibrosis, mastocytosis, hemoglobinopathies, renal osteodystrophy, and fluorosis. Skeletal biopsy has revealed typical granulomas, confirming the diagnosis of sarcoidosis as the cause of the increased radiodensity.

Hands and Feet. The hand is the predominant site of skeletal sarcoidosis.[18–21, 43, 44, 109, 122, 128, 129, 155] Involvement of the wrist and foot is less frequent.[130] Unilateral or bilateral changes can be encountered, but close symmetry between lesions on the two sides of the body is unusual. In the hand, abnormalities are found in the middle and distal phalanges, and, less often, the proximal phalanges[163] and metacarpals. Several types of lesions are seen (Fig. 91–5). Diffuse trabecular alterations are especially characteristic, leading to a honeycomb or latticework configuration. More localized lytic lesions produce cystic defects that, as they heal, may become surrounded by a thin rim of sclerosis. These lesions can appear centrally in the spongiosa or eccentrically, leading to marginal scalloping of the bone. An entire phalanx can be affected in association with pathologic fracture, fragmentation, soft tissue swelling, and telescoping of a digit (Fig. 91–6). Periostitis is uncommon.

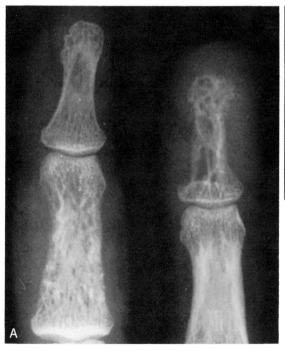

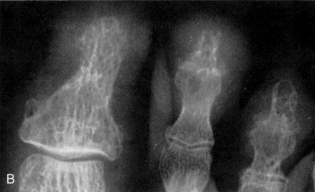

FIGURE 91–3. Sarcoidosis: Abnormal trabecular pattern. Observe the coarsened, reticulated, or lacework appearance of the trabeculae in the phalanges of the hand **(A)** and foot **(B)**. Soft tissue swelling is evident. (Courtesy of P. Stern, M.D., Covina, California.)

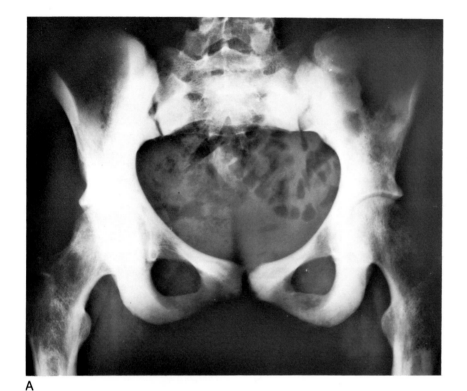

A

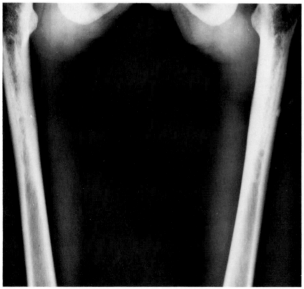

B

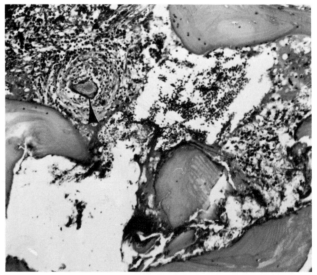

C

FIGURE 91–4. Sarcoidosis: Osteosclerosis. This 29 year old black woman had an established diagnosis of sarcoidosis of 13 years' duration with involvement of lungs, lymph nodes, and liver.

A In the pelvis, there is uniform increased bone density, especially in the iliac bones, ischii, and superior pubic rami.

B A "bone within bone" appearance in the femora is evident. Observe the increased density in the proximal two thirds of the bones.

C After an iliac crest biopsy a low power view reveals thickened, cancellous bone with a noncaseating granuloma containing a characteristic giant cell (arrowhead).

(From Bonakdarpour A, et al: *AJR 113*:646, 1971. Copyright 1971, American Roentgen Ray Society.)

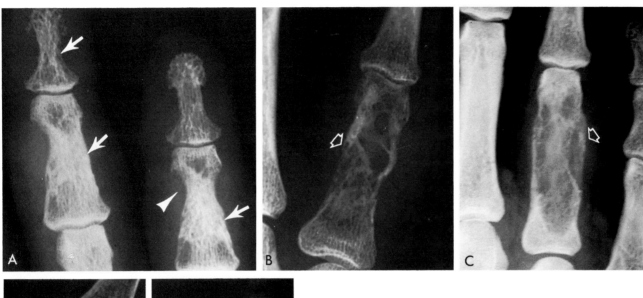

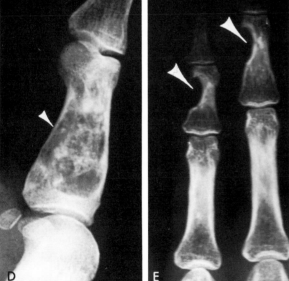

FIGURE 91–5. Sarcoidosis: Hand.

A–E A variety of radiographic changes can be seen. Trabecular alterations can produce a honeycomb or latticework configuration (solid arrows), more localized defects (open arrows), which may rarely calcify (small arrowhead), and marginal scalloping of bone (large arrowheads).

(**A,** Courtesy of A. Brower, M.D., Washington, D.C.; **B,** courtesy of M. Dalinka, M.D., Philadelphia, Pennsylvania.)

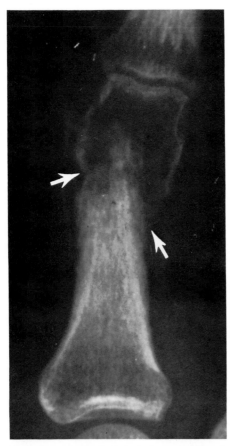

FIGURE 91–6. Sarcoidosis: Pathologic fracture. Note the fracture (arrows) that extends across an osteolytic lesion of the distal portion of a proximal phalanx. No periostitis is seen. (Courtesy of L. Rogers, M.D., Chicago, Illinois.)

The circumscribed areas need not be homogeneously lucent. Residual trabeculae or small nodular opaque areas can produce recognizable radiodense shadows. In some instances, calcification of the lesion may simulate the appearance of one or more enchondromas.

Acro-osteosclerosis has been reported as a sign of sarcoidosis of the hands (Fig. 91–7). This was emphasized by McBrine and Fisher in 1975[45] as well as by other investigators,[46, 47] although authors of earlier reports of the radiographic appearance in sarcoidosis had dismissed acro-osteosclerosis as an incidental finding.[18] The appearance is characterized by focal opaque areas, frequently of the terminal phalanges, and endosteal thickening. The finding is not specific, having been noted in scleroderma,[48] rheumatoid arthritis, systemic lupus erythematosus,[49] Hodgkin's disease, and hematologic disorders.[46] Its usefulness as a diagnostic sign of sarcoidosis is limited further by the appearance of one or more opaque nodules in phalanges of normal persons. Sclerosis of the digits has been observed in 31 per cent[47] and 54 per cent[45] of patients with sarcoidosis, however—statistics that underscore the fact that osteolysis should not be regarded as the sole skeletal manifestation of the disease.

Changes in the wrist can include cystic or marginal lucent shadows, whereas those in the feet parallel the findings in the hand, with a coarsened trabecular pattern, localized lesions, and opaque areas (see Fig. 91–3).

Long Tubular Bones. Examples of destructive lesions of the long tubular bones of the extremities are rare.[35, 50, 51, 171] Single or multiple lytic foci (Fig. 91–8) can lead to cortical erosion and violation, with pathologic fracture.[131] Although periostitis usually is not observed, hypertrophic osteoarthropathy, with widespread and prominent periosteal new bone formation, has been reported in association with systemic sarcoidosis.[174, 175]

Skull and Face. Calvarial destruction in sarcoidosis is unusual.[52–57, 122, 156, 157, 182] When present, such destruction may be asymptomatic and is characterized by single or multiple lytic lesions of varying size, usually without adjacent eburnation (Fig. 91–9A). These defects, which nearly always are associated with evidence of sarcoidosis elsewhere in the body, must be differentiated from eosinophilic granuloma, chronic infections, and tumors such as metastases, plasma cell myeloma, lymphoma, and meningioma.

Osseous destruction of the facial bones can reflect the presence of granulomatous lesions in adjacent structures, such as the nasal skin, paranasal sinuses, nasal mucosa, optic nerve and canal, and lacrimal sac. Nasal bone destruction (Fig. 91–9B) is especially characteristic,[27–29, 58, 59] although dissolution of the walls of the paranasal sinuses[32, 60, 61] and orbit[30, 34, 62, 132] and enlargement of one or both

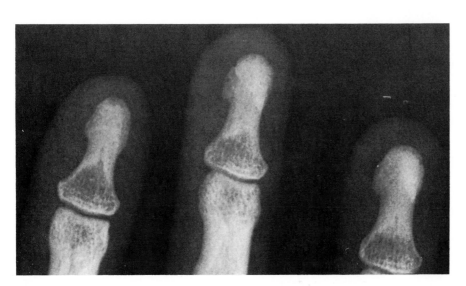

FIGURE 91–7. Sarcoidosis: Acro-osteosclerosis. Observe widespread sclerosis of the terminal aspects of the phalanges. This appearance is not specific.

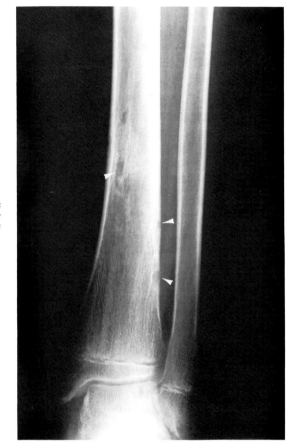

FIGURE 91–8. Sarcoidosis: Long tubular bones. Small, eccentric osteolytic lesions (arrowheads) in the tibia of a child are observed. They are sharply circumscribed, with minimal marginal sclerosis and no periostitis. (Courtesy of L. Cooperstein, M.D., Pittsburgh, Pennsylvania.)

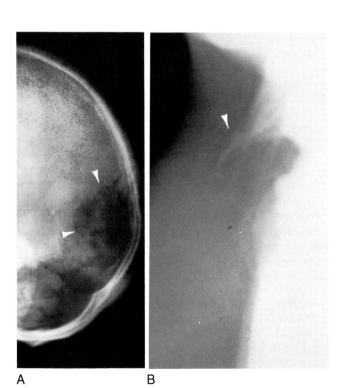

A   B

FIGURE 91–9. Sarcoidosis: Skull and face.
  A Observe an osteolytic lesion in the occipital region (arrowheads).
  B Soft tissue swelling and destruction of the nasal bones (arrowhead) are characteristic of the disease.

optic canals[63, 64] have been noted, simulating the changes associated with other granulomatous processes, such as leprosy or Wegener's granulomatosis.

Thorax. Rib involvement is infrequent; lesions may be entirely lytic, entirely sclerotic, or both lytic and sclerotic.[133] Pathologic fractures may occur.[123] Sternal abnormalities are rare.[160]

Pelvis. As in other sites, the innominate bones, when involved in sarcoidosis, may reveal a pattern of osteolysis, osteosclerosis, or a combination of the two.[176]

Spine and Spinal Cord. Although vertebral sarcoidosis is uncommon, postmortem[65, 66] and antemortem[67–72] studies have verified the localization of granulomas within vertebral marrow. Clinical findings include pain, tenderness, deformity, and neurologic dysfunction. On radiographs, bone lysis with marginal sclerosis can involve one or more contiguous or noncontiguous vertebral bodies, generally with preservation of the intervening intervertebral disc spaces.[67–74, 161, 177] Predilection for the lower thoracic and upper lumbar vertebrae is noted, although cervical involvement,[51, 72] including a pathologic fracture of the odontoid process,[57] has been recorded. Extension into the pedicles can be observed, although isolated involvement of the posterior elements of the spine apparently is rare. Paraspinal swelling also is evident in some cases (Fig. 91–10); occasionally, such swelling may accompany posterior lymphadenopathy without osseous involvement.[75] The radiographic appearance can simulate osteomyelitis, particularly when the in-

tervertebral disc space is narrowed,[178] or neoplasm. The involvement of multiple levels and the absence of intervertebral disc space narrowing in some cases are helpful clues to the correct diagnosis.

Spinal cord and cauda equina involvement in sarcoidosis is rare.[36–38, 76–81, 179, 183, 186] Such involvement can occur from intramedullary granulomas (a rare manifestation),[127] or granulomatous infiltration of the meninges or peripheral nerves.[124] Myelography or MR imaging (see later discussion) may reveal an intramedullary or intradural mass or evidence of arachnoiditis and meningeal thickening. Prominent neurologic findings usually are associated with other evidence of the disease.

Articular Involvement

Joint symptoms and signs appear in 10 to 35 per cent of patients with sarcoidosis, more frequently in women than in men.[6, 19, 22, 82–89, 111, 114, 134, 135] Two fundamental patterns of articular disease occur: acute polyarthritis and chronic polyarthritis (Fig. 91–11). Rarely, other patterns are seen.

Acute Polyarthritis. Peripheral symmetric polyarthralgia or polyarthritis affects small and medium-sized joints, especially the ankles, knees, elbows, wrists, and joints of the hands, appearing early in the course of the disease in association with erythema nodosum, hilar lymph node enlargement, fever, uveitis, and typical skin lesions. This pattern of joint disease, which is virtually identical to that in uncomplicated erythema nodosum,[134] leads to soft tissue swelling, joint effusion, pain, tenderness, limitation of motion, and stiffness, findings that disappear in 4 to 6 weeks. Radiographs generally reveal soft tissue swelling and, perhaps, osteoporosis. Sonographic findings are indicative of joint effusions, tenosynovitis, and subcutaneous inflammation,[180] and histologic examination of the synovial membrane confirms a nonspecific inflammatory response.[164] Laboratory analysis may indicate elevation of the erythrocyte sedimentation rate and C-reactive protein.

Chronic Polyarthritis. A second variety of joint disease, which occurs in cases of sarcoidosis that have persisted for months to years, is a chronic polyarthritis that subsides and recurs, and that eventually may lead to permanent disability and irreversible joint damage. On initial evaluation some of the patients who have chronic disease have had acute episodes of polyarthritis. A gradual transition ensues in which symptoms and signs wax and wane over a period of years. The joints most typically affected are the ankles, knees, shoulders, wrists, and small joints of the hands. Rarely, monoarticular arthritis rather than polyarticular arthritis is evident. Cutaneous and pulmonary alterations are frequent. Analysis of synovial fluid may indicate an elevated total protein level, with white blood cell counts in the range of 15,000 to 20,000 cells/cu mm and a predominance of lymphocytes.[2]

On radiographs, osseous sarcoidosis may or may not be present.[90, 91, 136–140] In those cases in which adjacent bony involvement is evident, articular destruction and collapse may occur secondary to extension of the osseous disease into the subchondral bone. Without such extension, radiologic changes related to the joint disease are unusual. Soft tissue swelling may be evident, in combination with periarticular osteoporosis. Mild diffuse joint space loss and

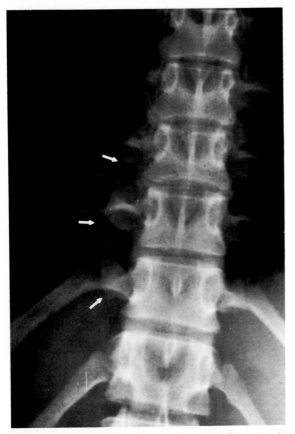

FIGURE 91–10. Sarcoidosis: Paraspinal swelling. Observe a large paraspinal mass (arrows) in the thoracic spine of this patient with sarcoidosis. Such a finding can accompany vertebral involvement or represent a manifestation of posterior lymphadenopathy.

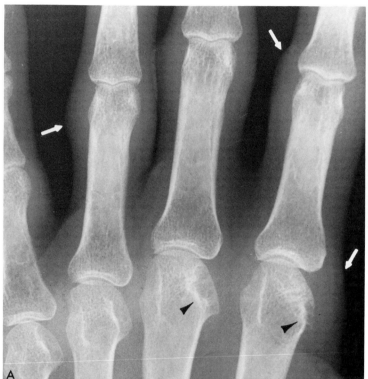

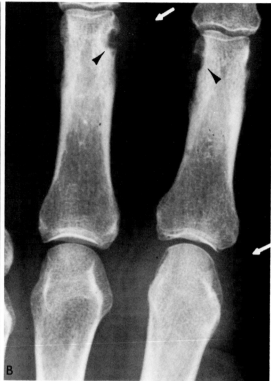

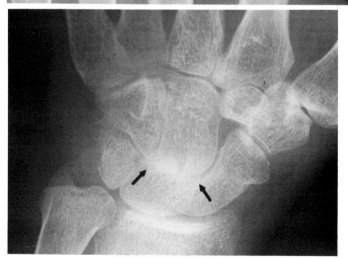

FIGURE 91–11. Sarcoidosis: Articular involvement (radiographic abnormalities).

A Observe soft tissue swelling of multiple proximal interphalangeal and metacarpophalangeal joints (arrows) with articular space narrowing and small osseous defects (arrowheads). The absence of obvious osseous sarcoid is unusual in patients with such joint alteration.

B In another patient, prominent soft tissue swelling is evident about the proximal interphalangeal and metacarpophalangeal joints (arrows), and osseous defects (arrowheads) again are seen.

C A radiograph in a 30 year old black woman with sarcoidosis shows soft tissue swelling and joint space narrowing (arrows), mainly confined to the midcarpal compartment of the wrist. Osteoporosis and marginal osseous erosions are not evident. The appearance is not diagnostic, resembling that in rheumatoid arthritis and other disorders.

eccentric and well-defined erosive alterations also can be noted (Fig. 91–12). Without detection of characteristic changes in periarticular osseous tissues, the radiographic findings related to the chronic polyarthritis of sarcoidosis are not diagnostic.

Histologic examination of the synovium in either situation can indicate the presence of noncaseating granulomas[91, 92, 141] (Fig. 91–13). These lesions are not specific, resembling the findings in tuberculosis, mycotic infections, berylliosis, and certain foreign body reactions,[93] although no fungi or acid-fast organisms are recovered from the granuloma.[92] An additional or isolated inflammatory component also is evident in some cases, characterized by infiltration of leukocytes and plasma cells, and proliferation of fibroblasts.[142] The synovial lining of tendon sheaths may be affected similarly.[165]

Other Patterns. Sarcoid arthritis occurring in children has been emphasized in several reports.[143–146] Although rare, articular abnormalities simulate those seen in some forms of juvenile chronic arthritis and usually are accompanied by both cutaneous and ocular involvement. Polyarticular disease predominates, with changes present in large and small joints of the extremities. Prominent but painless articular effusions and swelling of tendon sheaths are associated with boggy and thickened synovial membranes. Soft tissue enlargement and osteopenia are the characteristic radiographic abnormalities; rarely, cartilaginous and osseous destruction is apparent (Fig. 91–14).

Pelvic and spinal changes resembling those in ankylosing spondylitis or other seronegative spondyloarthropathies rarely are observed in sarcoidosis.[84, 94–98, 147, 177] Sacroiliac joint erosions, sclerosis, and bony ankylosis with or without spinal changes have been described, although the pathogenesis is unknown. Perlman and coworkers[99] noted a young black man with granulomatous disease of the vertebrae who developed quadriplegia after a fall. Destructive osseous spinal lesions were combined with anterior and lateral para-

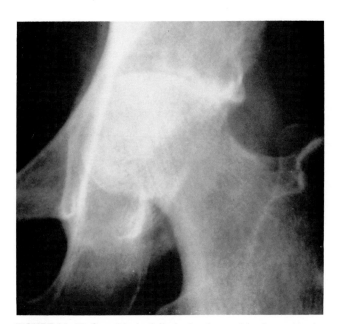

FIGURE 91–12. Sarcoidosis: Articular involvement (radiographic abnormalities). Concentric joint space loss occurred during a 4 month period in this 53 year old woman with sarcoidosis. (Courtesy of D. Sauser, M.D., Loma Linda, California.)

vertebral ossification in the cervical, thoracic, and lumbar regions, resembling changes in psoriasis or Reiter's syndrome. The sacroiliac joints were normal. The authors postulated that the bony outgrowths represented a reparative response to the extensive vertebral granulomatous process.

The occurrence of a Jaccoud-type arthropathy, with reducible, painless flexion deformities of the interphalangeal joints of the hand, has been identified in one patient with sarcoidosis.[181] Sarcoidosis also has been reported in association with psoriasis, hyperuricemia and pseudopodagra, eosinophilic fasciitis, rheumatoid arthritis, and elevation of serum rheumatoid factor.[2, 100–102, 148] Steroid therapy in patients with sarcoidosis can be complicated by osteonecrosis. The presence of this complication in patients with sarcoidosis not receiving such medication is extremely rare and may not be related to the disease process itself.

Rarely, sarcoidosis may be associated with large periosseous or periarticular soft tissue masses with or without calcification (see previous discussion).[112] An association of sarcoidosis and hyperparathyroidism also has been suggested.[113]

Other Diagnostic Techniques

Scintigraphy has been employed to delineate the extent of skeletal involvement in sarcoidosis.[103, 149] Abnormalities occurring after administration of ^{99m}Tc-pyrophosphate (Fig. 91–15) are more extensive than those depicted on corresponding radiographic studies and appear to relate to sites of histologically evident noncaseating granulomas. Further use of this sensitive diagnostic technique may lead to identification of bone involvement in a high percentage of patients with sarcoidosis.[110]

Gallium-67 citrate imaging is useful in defining the extent of sarcoid involvement of the skin, lungs, lymph nodes, spleen, salivary and lacrimal glands, and skeletal muscles.[150, 162, 187] With regard to muscle, abnormal accumulation of the radiotracer decreases or disappears after institution of corticosteroid therapy.[150]

MR imaging has been applied in a limited fashion to the analysis of osteoarticular and muscular manifestations of sarcoidosis.[168, 178] The signal intensity characteristics of intraosseous lesions in this disease are not unique. Typically, low signal intensity, similar to that of muscle, on T1-weighted spin echo images and high signal intensity on T2-weighted spin echo and most gradient echo images are observed (Fig. 91–16). With involvement of the spine, MR imaging findings resemble those of infective spondylitis; affected vertebral bodies and intervertebral discs show low signal intensity on the T1-weighted images, hyperintensity on T2-weighted images, and enhancement of signal intensity after the intravenous administration of a gadolinium chelate.[178, 184] Paraspinal extension of the disease process may be apparent (Fig. 91–17). Sarcoidosis of the spinal cord may lead to nodular lesions with signal hypointensity on T1-weighted images and with enhancement of signal intensity after intravenous administration of a gadolinium contrast agent.[179, 183] The spinal cord may appear swollen.

The MR imaging appearance of muscular sarcoidosis appears to depend on the type of involvement present (see previous discussion).[168, 185] Nodular myopathy is characterized by the presence of oval nodules consisting of a star-

FIGURE 91–13. Sarcoidosis: Articular involvement (pathologic abnormalities). A 51 year old black woman with sarcoidosis developed bilateral knee effusions and stiffness. Radiographs revealed lytic lesions of the subchondral bone in both femora. The photomicrograph of the synovium of one knee following biopsy reveals noncaseating granulomas and scattered chronic inflammatory cells (75×). Cultures for bacteria and fungi were negative. (From Bjarnason DJ, et al: J Bone Joint Surg [Am] 55:618, 1973.)

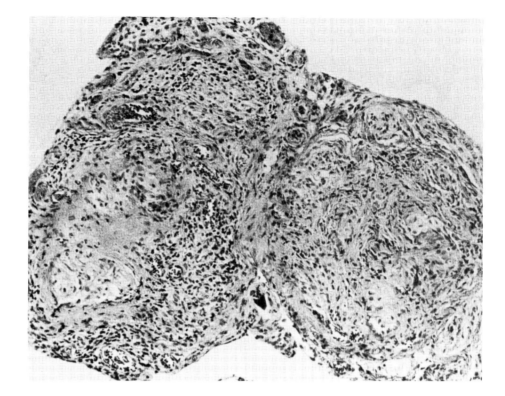

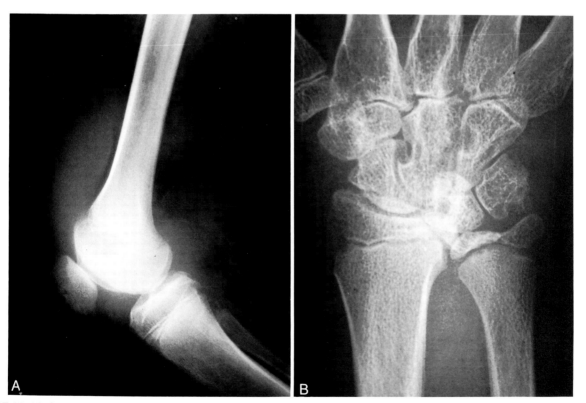

FIGURE 91–14. Childhood sarcoidosis. In this child, radiographic findings include osteopenia, a large effusion in the knee, and joint space narrowing and bone erosions throughout the wrist. (Courtesy of L. Cooperstein, M.D., Pittsburgh, Pennsylvania.)

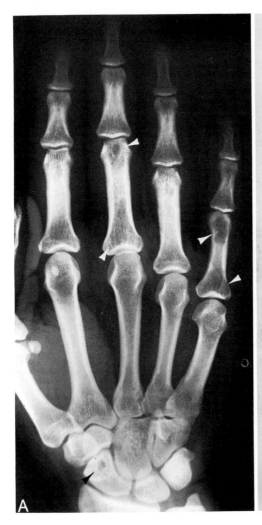

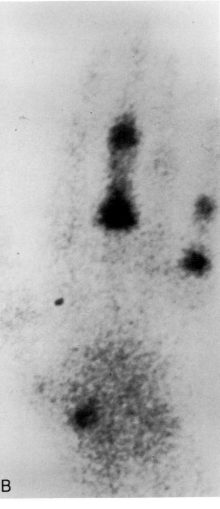

FIGURE 91–15. Sarcoidosis: Scintigraphic abnormalities.

A Observe areas of subtle bone destruction in the scaphoid and phalanges (arrowheads), characterized by poorly defined and well-defined osteolytic lesions.

B The bone scan shows abnormal accumulation of the radiotracer at these sites.

(Courtesy of V. Vint, M.D., San Diego, California.)

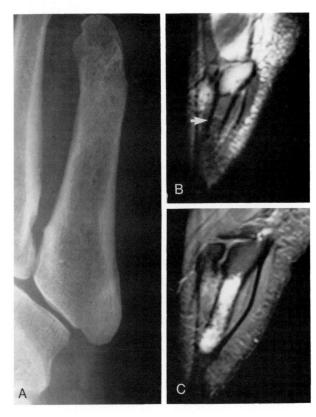

FIGURE 91–16. Sarcoidosis: MR imaging abnormalities. Bone involvement. This 54 year old woman had histologic evidence of sarcoidosis affecting the fifth metatarsal bone and other osseous sites.

A A radiograph shows bone expansion, osteopenia, and small radiolucent lesions confined to the fifth metatarsal bone.

B A sagittal T1-weighted (TR/TE, 600/16) spin echo MR image shows a well-defined lesion of low signal intensity in this bone (arrow).

C A similar image (TR/TE, 800/20) using chemical presaturation (ChemSat) of fat and intravenous administration of a gadolinium chelate reveals the hyperintense lesion.

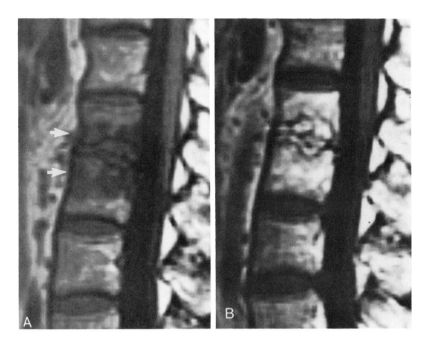

FIGURE 91–17. Sarcoidosis: MR imaging abnormalities. Spine involvement. In a 53 year old woman, sarcoid involvement of the upper lumbar spine led to routine radiographic abnormalities simulating those of infection.

A A sagittal T1-weighted (TR/TE, 600/20) spin echo MR image reveals low signal intensity in adjacent portions of the first and second lumbar vertebral bodies (arrows) and intervening disc.

B A gadolinium-enhanced T1-weighted (TR/TE, 600/20) spin echo MR image shows increased signal intensity in these vertebral bodies and disc.

(From Kenney CM, et al: J Comput Assist Tomogr *16*:660, 1992.)

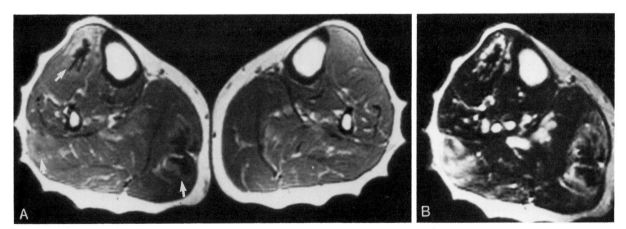

FIGURE 91–18. Sarcoidosis: MR imaging abnormalities. Muscular involvement. This 64 year old woman had nodular myopathy involving the right lower extremity.

A A transaxial T1-weighted (TR/TE, 550/30) spin echo MR image shows three oval nodules: two in the gastrocnemius muscle and one in the tibialis anterior muscle (arrows). In each lesion, a star-shaped area of low signal intensity is surrounded by a region of slightly higher signal intensity.

B A transaxial T2-weighted (TR/TE, 1800/100) spin echo MR image reveals high signal intensity in the peripheral portion of each lesion.

(From Otake S, et al: Radiology *176*:145, 1990.)

shaped area of low signal intensity surrounded by an area of high signal intensity on both T1- and T2-weighted spin echo images (Fig. 91–18); histopathologic correlation documents that such nodules contain a central fibrotic region surrounded by inflammatory granulomatous tissue.[168] The foci of inflammatory tissue may show enhancement of signal intensity after intravenous administration of a gadolinium compound.[185] Chronic sarcoid myopathy generally escapes detection on MR images.

Differential Diagnosis

The skeletal alterations in sarcoidosis are sufficiently characteristic in most cases to allow an accurate radiographic diagnosis. Occasionally, the trabecular and cystic changes in the hand may be confused with abnormalities in other disorders (Table 91–2). In *tuberous sclerosis*, cystlike foci in the phalanges and metacarpals usually are associated with a distinctive variety of periosteal proliferation, leading to nodular excrescences attached to the outer aspect of the bones (Fig. 91–19).[104] Adjacent eburnation frequently is evident, and periostitis of metatarsal shafts and intracranial calcification substantiate the correct diagnosis (see Chapter 92).

Fibrous dysplasia can produce monostotic or polyostotic abnormalities. A widened medullary space of phalanges and metacarpals with a diffuse ground-glass appearance is typical, commonly combined with focal areas of lucency or sclerosis and more widespread skeletal abnormalities[105] (Fig. 91–20) (see Chapter 92).

Enchondromas are benign tumors composed of cartilage that often are identified in the hands of asymptomatic persons. The tumor commonly produces a central rarefied area with or without calcification, and scalloping of the endosteal margin of the cortex.[106] Occasionally, enchondromas are eccentric or parosteal in location, producing an altered radiographic picture. Although the appearance of a lucent lesion containing calcification in sarcoidosis can simulate an enchondroma exactly, other skeletal findings ensure accurate diagnosis.

Enchondromatosis or *Ollier's disease* is a syndrome of multiple enchondromas that produce soft tissue swelling in one or more extremities.[107] This nonfamilial disorder is related to the persistence of cartilaginous islands in the metaphyses and diaphyses of tubular bones that can lead to disturbances in skeletal growth and deformity. Although the

TABLE 91–2. Multiple Cystlike Lesions of the Metacarpal Bones and Phalanges*

Sarcoidosis
Gout
Rheumatoid arthritis
Xanthomatosis
Tuberous sclerosis
Fibrous dysplasia
Enchondromatosis (Ollier's disease)
Tuberculosis
Fungal disease
Metastasis (r)
Plasma cell myeloma (r)
Hyperparathyroidism (r)
Basal cell nevus syndrome (r)
Hemangiomas (r)

*r = Rare manifestation of the disease.

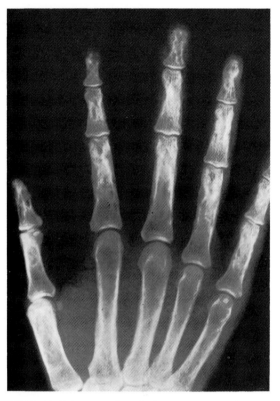

FIGURE 91–19. Tuberous sclerosis. In a 38 year old black woman, cystlike lesions of variable size are evident in the phalanges and metacarpal bones. Periosteal apposition of bone has led to broadening of the phalanges and an irregular and nodular surface, especially in the metacarpal bones. (Courtesy of G. Greenway, M.D., Dallas, Texas.)

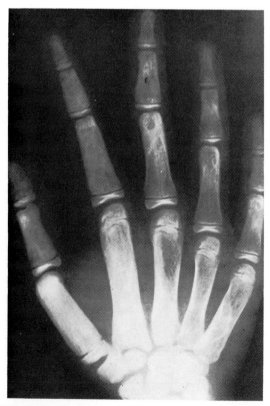

FIGURE 91–20. Fibrous dysplasia. In this child with polyostotic fibrous dysplasia, note the diffuse ground-glass appearance of the metacarpals and phalanges. Cortical thinning and osseous expansion are seen.

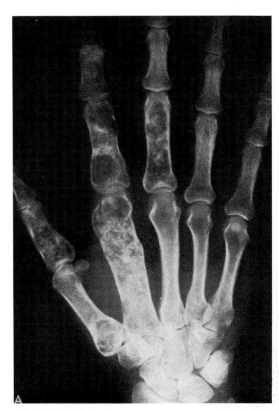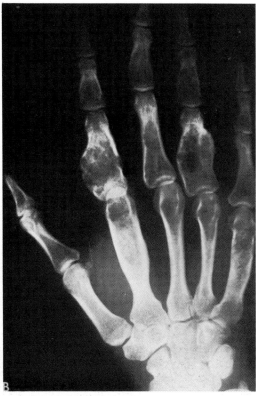

FIGURE 91–21. Enchondromatosis (Ollier's disease). In one patient **(A),** observe radiolucent foci containing calcification in the first, second, and third digits. Note endosteal scalloping, cortical diminution, and osseous expansion. The distal phalanx of the second finger had been removed surgically. In a second patient **(B),** lesions are present in the second, third, fourth, and fifth digits. They are associated with a coarsened trabecular pattern, endosteal scalloping, and localized osseous expansion.

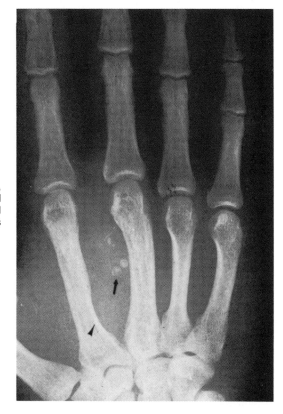

FIGURE 91–22. Hemangiomatosis. Observe a coarsened trabecular pattern, most evident in the middle phalanges and metacarpal bones of the second and third digits, and a soft tissue mass containing phleboliths (arrow), which has led to pressure erosion of the second metacarpal bone (arrowhead). The findings are diagnostic of osseous and soft tissue hemangiomatosis.

clinical findings can be mistaken for arthritis, the soft tissue prominences are hard. Furthermore, radiographs reveal multiple lucent and calcified lesions, although a more diffuse and bizarre appearance can be seen (Fig. 91–21). When enchondromatosis is combined with cavernous hemangiomas, *Maffucci's syndrome* is diagnosed.[108] Considerable malignant potential of the cartilaginous lesions exists in this latter syndrome, which is less striking in multiple enchondromatosis alone and rare in the solitary enchondroma. In all three of these disorders, the radiographic features easily are differentiated from those of sarcoidosis.

Multiple lucent lesions of phalanges, metacarpals, and metatarsals also can accompany tuberculosis and other granulomatous infections (see Chapter 66), hemangiomatosis (Fig. 91–22), xanthomatosis, fat necrosis, hyperparathyroidism, Gorlin's basal cell nevus syndrome, lipomatosis, plasma cell myeloma, and skeletal metastasis.

Nasal and facial bone destruction is encountered in sarcoidosis, syphilis, fungal and other infections, Wegener's granulomatosis, and neoplasms.

The articular findings in sarcoidosis are not specific. Acute arthritis with soft tissue swelling and osteoporosis is seen in numerous processes. Chronic changes with joint space narrowing and osseous destruction simulate alterations in many infections, particularly tuberculosis. The absence of periostitis in sarcoid skeletal lesions is a helpful sign.

SUMMARY

Skeletal abnormalities in sarcoidosis are encountered most frequently in the hand; in this location, a coarsened trabecular pattern, cystic and marginal bone defects, and sclerosis are virtually diagnostic. Although findings can be encountered in other skeletal sites, such as the skull, facial bones, spine, and long tubular bones, as well as various joints, these alterations usually are not specific. Thus, skull abnormalities can simulate eosinophilic granuloma and various neoplasms, spinal changes can mimic infection, and articular alterations can resemble rheumatoid arthritis, gout, and infectious arthritis.

References

1. Siltzbach LE (Ed): Seventh International Congress on Sarcoidosis and Other Granulomatous Disorders. Ann NY Acad Sci 278:1, 1976.
2. Stobo JD: Sarcoidosis. *In* AS Cohen (Ed): The Science and Practice of Clinical Medicine. Vol. 4. Rheumatology and Immunology. New York, Grune & Stratton, 1979, p 290.
3. James DG, Neville E, Carstairs LS: Bone and joint sarcoidosis. Semin Arthritis Rheum 6:53, 1976.
4. Bacharach T: Sarcoidosis. A clinical review of 111 cases. Am Rev Resp Dis 84:12, 1961.
5. Goetz AA: Effect of cortisone on hypercalcemia in sarcoidosis. Relief of gastrointestinal, dermatological, and renal symptoms with steroid therapy. JAMA 174:380, 1960.
6. Israel HL, Sones M: Selection of biopsy procedures for sarcoidosis diagnosis. Arch Intern Med 113:255, 1964.
7. Kveim A: En ny og spesifikk kutan-reaksjon ved Boecks sarcoid. Nord Med 9:169, 1941.
8. Mitchell DN, Cannon P, Dyer NH, et al: The Kveim test in Crohn's disease. Lancet 2:571, 1969.
9. Sulzberger MB: Sarcoid of Boeck (benign miliary lupoid) and tuberculin anergy. Am Rev Tuberc 28:734, 1933.
10. Lieberman J: Elevated serum angiotensin-converting-enzyme (ACE) levels in sarcoidosis. Am J Med 59:365, 1975.
11. Longcope WT, Freiman DG: A study of sarcoidosis based on a combined investigation of 160 cases including 30 autopsies from Johns Hopkins and Massachusetts General Hospitals. Medicine 31:1, 1952.
12. Jaffe HL: Metabolic Degenerative and Inflammatory Diseases of Bones and Joints. Philadelphia, Lea & Febiger, 1972, p 1004.
13. Talbot PS: Sarcoid myopathy. Br Med J 4:465, 1967.
14. Besnier E: Lupus pernio de la face. Ann Dermatol Syphilol 10:333, 1898.
15. Kreibich K: Über-Lupus pernio. Arch Dermatol Syphilol 7:3, 1904.
16. Rieder H: Über Kombination von chronischer Osteomyelitis (Spina ventosa) mit Lupus-Pernio. ROFO 15:125, 1910.
17. Jüngling O: Über Ostitis tuberculosa multiplex cystoides, Zugleich ein Beitrag zur Lehre von der Tuberkuliden des Knochens. Beitr Klin Chir 143:401, 1928.
18. Holt JF, Owens WI: The osseous lesions of sarcoidosis. Radiology 53:11, 1949.
19. Israel HL, Sones M: Sarcoidosis. Clinical observation on one hundred sixty cases. Arch Intern Med 102:766, 1958.
20. Stein GN, Israel HL, Sones M: A roentgenographic study of skeletal lesions in sarcoidosis. Arch Intern Med 97:532, 1956.
21. FitzGerald P, Meenan FOC: Sarcoidosis of the hands. J Bone Joint Surg [Br] 40:256, 1958.
22. Mayock RL, Bertrand P, Morrison CE, et al: Manifestations of sarcoidosis: Analysis of 145 patients with a review of 9 series selected from the literature. Am J Med 35:67, 1963.
23. Baltzer G, Behrend H, Behrend T, et al: Zur Häufigkeit zystischer Knochenveränderungen (Ostitis cystoides multiplex Jüngling) bei der Sarkoidose. Dtsch Med Wochenschr 95:1926, 1970.
24. James DG: Dermatological aspects of sarcoidosis. Q J Med 28:109, 1959.
25. Reisner D: Boeck's sarcoid and systemic sarcoidosis (Besnier-Boeck-Schaumann disease). A study of thirty-five cases. I. Clinical observations. Am Rev Tuberc 49:289, 1944.
26. Mather G: Calcium metabolism and bone changes in sarcoidosis. Br Med J 1:248, 1957.
27. Bridgman JF, Mistry PK: Sarcoidosis of the nose. Practitioner 208:393, 1972.
28. Fletcher R: Sarcoid of the nose. Arch Otolaryngol 39:470, 1949.
29. O'Brien P: Sarcoidosis of the nose. Br J Plast Surg 23:242, 1970.
30. Stein HA, Henderson JW: Sarcoidosis of the orbit. Survey of the literature and report of a case. Am J Ophthalmol 41:1054, 1956.
31. Neault RW, Riley FC: Report of a case of dacrocystitis secondary to Boeck's sarcoid. Am J Ophthalmol 70:1011, 1970.
32. Livingstone G: Sarcoidosis of maxillary antrum. J Laryngol Otol 70:426, 1956.
33. Fischer OE, Burton GG, Bryan WF: Sarcoidosis involving the lacrimal sac. Am Rev Respir Dis 103:708, 1971.
34. Bodian M, Lasky MA: Sarcoidosis of the orbit. Am J Ophthalmol 33:343, 1950.
35. Watson RC, Cahen I: Pathological fracture in long bone sarcoidosis. Report of a case. J Bone Joint Surg [Am] 55:613, 1973.
36. Nathan MPR, Chase PH, Elguezabel A, et al: Spinal cord sarcoidosis. NY State J Med 76:748, 1976.
37. Snyder R, Towfighi J, Gonatas NK: Sarcoidosis of the spinal cord. Case report. J Neurosurg 44:740, 1976.
38. Bernstein J, Rival J: Sarcoidosis of the spinal cord as the presenting manifestation of the disease. South Med J 71:1571, 1978.
39. Bonakdarpour A, Levy W, Aergerter EE: Osteosclerotic changes in sarcoidosis. AJR 113:646, 1971.
40. Lin S-R, Levy W, Go EB, et al: Unusual osteosclerotic changes in sarcoidosis simulating osteoblastic metastases. Radiology 106:311, 1973.
41. Young DA, Laman ML: Radiodense skeletal lesions in Boeck's sarcoid. AJR 114:553, 1972.
42. Smith J, Farr GH Jr: An unusual case of dense bones. Clin Bull Memorial Sloan-Kettering Cancer Center 7:40, 1977.
43. Knutsson F: Skeletal changes in sarcoidosis. Acta Radiol 51:429, 1959.
44. Centea A, Gherman E: Knochenveränderungen bei Sarkoidose. Z Orthop 111:321, 1973.
45. McBrine CS, Fisher MS: Acrosclerosis in sarcoidosis. Radiology 115:279, 1975.
46. Godin E, Capesius P, Kempf F: Acro-ostéosclérose au course de la maladie de Besnier-Boeck-Schaumann. J Radiol Electrol Med Nucl 58:115, 1977.
47. Pavlica P, Stasi G, Tonti R, et al: L'ostéosclérose phalangienne dans la sarcoïdose. J Radiol Electrol Med Nucl 58:603, 1977.
48. Edeikin L: Scleroderma with sclerodactylia. Report of 3 cases with roentgen findings. AJR 22:42, 1929.
49. Goodman N: The significance of terminal phalangeal osteosclerosis. Radiology 89:709, 1967.
50. Robert F: Les manifestations osseuses de la maladie de Besnier-Boeck-Schaumann (la maladie de Perthes-Jüngling). Sem Hôp Paris 25:2327, 1944.
51. Toomey F, Bautista A: Rare manifestations of sarcoidosis in children. Radiology 94:569, 1970.
52. Nielsen J: Recherches radiologiques sur les lésions des os et des poumons dans les sarcoïdes de Boeck. Bull Soc Fr Dermatol Syphiligr 41:1187, 1934.
53. Posner I: Sarcoidosis: Case report. J Pediatr 20:486, 1942.
54. Teirstein AS, Wolf BS, Siltzbach LE: Sarcoidosis of the skull. N Engl J Med 265:65, 1961.
55. Olsen TG: Sarcoidosis of the skull. Radiology 80:232, 1963.
56. Turner OA, Weiss SR: Sarcoidosis of the skull. Report of a case. AJR 105:322, 1969.
57. Zimmerman R, Leeds NE: Calvarial and vertebral sarcoidosis. Case report and review of the literature. Radiology 119:384, 1976.
58. Curtis GT: Sarcoidosis of the nasal bones. Br J Radiol 37:68, 1964.
59. Trachtenberg SB, Wilkinson EE, Jacobson G: Sarcoidosis of the nose and paranasal sinuses. Radiology 113:619, 1974.

60. Hoggins GS, Allan D: Sarcoidosis of the maxillary region. Oral Surg 28:623, 1969.
61. Bordley JE, Proctor DF: Destructive lesion in the paranasal sinuses associated with Boeck's sarcoid. Arch Otolaryngol 36:740, 1942.
62. Rider JA, Dodson JW: Sarcoidosis. Report of a case manifested by retrobulbar mass, proptosis, destruction of the orbit, and infiltration of the paranasal sinuses. Am J Ophthalmol 33:117, 1950.
63. Goodman SS, Margulies ME: Boeck's sarcoid simulating a brain tumor. Arch Neurol Psychiatry 81:419, 1959.
64. Anderson WB, Parker JJ, Sondheimer FK: Optic foramen enlargement caused by sarcoid granuloma. Radiology 86:319, 1966.
65. Nickerson DA: Boeck's sarcoid. Report of six cases in which autopsies were made. Arch Pathol 24:19, 1937.
66. Rubin EH, Pinner M: Sarcoidosis. One case report and literature review of autopsied cases. Am Rev Tuberc 49:146, 1944.
67. Rodman T, Funderburk EE Jr, Myerson RM: Sarcoidosis with vertebral involvement. Ann Intern Med 50:213, 1959.
68. Goodbar JE, Gilmer WS Jr, Carroll DS, et al: Vertebral sarcoidosis. JAMA 178:1162, 1961.
69. Zener JC, Alpert M, Klainer LM: Vertebral sarcoidosis. Arch Intern Med 111:696, 1963.
70. Berk RN, Brower TD: Vertebral sarcoidosis. Radiology 82:660, 1964.
71. Brodey PA, Pripstein S, Strange G, et al: Vertebral sarcoidosis. A case report and review of the literature. AJR 126:900, 1976.
72. Stump D, Spock A, Grossman H: Vertebral sarcoidosis in adolescents. Radiology 121:153, 1976.
73. Baldwin DM, Roberts JG, Croft HE: Vertebral sarcoidosis. A case report. J Bone Joint Surg [Am] 56:629, 1974.
74. Bloch S, Movson IJ, Seedat YK: Unusual skeletal manifestations in a case of sarcoidosis. Clin Radiol 19:226, 1968.
75. Schabel SI, Foote GA, McKee KA: Posterior lymphadenopathy in sarcoidosis. Radiology 129:591, 1978.
76. Wood EH, Bream CA: Spinal sarcoidosis. Radiology 73:226, 1959.
77. Banerjee T, Hunt WE: Spinal cord sarcoidosis. Case report. J Neurosurg 36:490, 1972.
78. Semins H, Nugent GR, Chou SM: Intramedullary spinal cord sarcoidosis. Case report. J Neurosurg 37:233, 1972.
79. Walker AG: Sarcoidosis of the brain and spinal cord. Postgrad Med J 37:431, 1961.
80. Moldover A: Sarcoidosis of the spinal cord. Report of a case with remission associated with cortisone therapy. Arch Intern Med 102:414, 1958.
81. Wiederholt WC, Siekert RG: Neurological manifestations of sarcoidosis. Neurology 15:1147, 1965.
82. Siltzbach LE, Duberstein JL: Arthritis in sarcoidosis. Clin Orthop 57:31, 1968.
83. Gumpel JM, Johns CJ, Shulman LE: The joint disease of sarcoidosis. Ann Rheum Dis 26:194, 1967.
84. Cabanel G, Jacquot F, Phelip X, et al: Les formes articulaires de la sarcoïdose. Sem Hôp Paris 49:3051, 1973.
85. Gayrard M, Bouteiller G, Durroux R, et al: Le rhumatisme sarcoïdosique. A propos de 2 observations. Rev Med Toul 14:543, 1978.
86. Kaplan H: Sarcoid arthritis: A review. Arch Intern Med 112:924, 1963.
87. Kitridou RC, Schumacher HR: Arthritis of acute sarcoidosis (Abstr). Arthritis Rheum 13:328, 1970.
88. Lebacq E, Ruelle M: Les manifestations articulaires de la sarcoïdose. Rev Rhum Mal Osteoartic 33:611, 1966.
89. Sèze S de, Caroit M, Leonetti P: Les manifestations articulaires de la sarcoïdose. Rev Rhum Mal Osteoartic 35:571, 1968.
90. Turek SL: Sarcoid disease of bone at the ankle joint. J Bone Joint Surg [Am] 35:465, 1953.
91. Bjarnason DF, Forrester DM, Swezey RL: Destructive arthritis of the large joints. A rare manifestation of sarcoidosis. J Bone Joint Surg [Am] 55:618, 1973.
92. Sokoloff L, Bunim JJ: Clinical and pathological studies of joint involvement in sarcoidosis. N Engl J Med 260:841, 1959.
93. Grier RS, Nash P, Freiman DG: Skin lesions in persons exposed to beryllium compounds. J Indust Hyg Toxicol 30:228, 1948.
94. Blanchon P, Paillas J, Lauriat H, et al: Localisations pelvirachidiennes et rachidiennes de la sarcoïdose de B.B.S. Ann Med Interne 127:843, 1976.
95. Deshayes P, Desseauve J, Hubert J, et al: Un cas de polyarthrite au cours d'une sarcoïdose. Un cas de spondylarthrite ankylosante au cours d'une sarcoïdose. Rev Rhum Mal Osteoartic 32:671, 1965.
96. Verstraetten JM, Bekaert J: Association de spondylite ankylosante et de sarcoïdose. Acta Tuberc Belg 42:149, 1951.
97. Martin E, Fallet GH: Pneumopathies chroniques et rhumatisme. Schweiz Med Wochenschr 83:776, 1953.
98. Brun J, Pozzetto H, Buffat JJ, et al: Sarcoïdose vertébrale et sacro-iliaque avec image de pseudo-abcès pottique. Guérison par corticothérapie. Presse Med 74:511, 1966.
99. Perlman SG, Damergis J, Witorsch P, et al: Vertebral sarcoidosis with paravertebral ossification. Arthritis Rheum 21:271, 1978.
100. Putkonen T, Virkkunen M, Wager O: Joint involvement in sarcoidosis with special reference to the coexistence of sarcoidosis and rheumatoid arthritis. Acta Rheum Scand 11:53, 1965.
101. Kaplan H, Klatskin G: Sarcoidosis, psoriasis, and gout: Syndrome or coincidence? Yale J Biol Med 32:335, 1960.
102. Loefgren S, Norberg R: Metabolic aspect of sarcoidosis. Acta Tuberc Scand Suppl 45:40, 1959.
103. Reginato AJ, Schiappaccasse V, Guzman L, et al: 99mTechnetium-pyrophosphate scintiphotography in bone sarcoidosis. J Rheumatol 3:426, 1976.
104. Holt JF, Dickerson WW: The osseous lesions of tuberous sclerosis. Radiology 58:1, 1952.
105. Pritchard JE: Fibrous dysplasia of the bones. Am J Med Sci 222:313, 1951.
106. Takigawa K: Chondroma of the bones of the hand. A review of 110 cases. J Bone Joint Surg [Am] 53:1591, 1971.
107. Mainzer F, Minagi H, Steinbach HL: The variable manifestations of multiple enchondromatosis. Radiology 99:377, 1971.
108. Andrén L, Dymling JF, Elner A, et al: Maffucci's syndrome. Report of 4 cases. Acta Chir Scand 126:397, 1963.
109. Forouzesh S, Fan PT, Bluestone R: Universal sarcoid dactylitis: A case report. Arthritis Rheum 22:1403, 1979.
110. Rohatgi PK: Radioisotope scanning in osseous sarcoidosis. AJR 134:189, 1980.
111. Prier A, Camus J-P: Les manifestations rhumatologiques de la sarcoïdose. Rev Méd 22:1109, 1980.
112. Schwartz JM: Sarcoid tumor of knee. NY State J Med 80:806, 1980.
113. Lavalard JF, Philippe JM, Preux MC, et al: Sarcoïdose hypercalcémique révélée par une biopsie osseuse. Ann Méd Interne 131:35, 1980.
114. Müller W, Wurum K: Rheumatische syndrome bei der Sarcoidose. Akt Rheumatol 5:39, 1980.
115. Pinkston P, Bitterman PB, Crystal RG: Spontaneous release of interleukin-2 by lung T lymphocytes in active pulmonary sarcoidosis. N Engl J Med 308:793, 1983.
116. Lewis JE: Sarcoidosis presenting as inflammatory nodose lesions of the legs. South Med J 73:1416, 1980.
117. Rohatgi PK, Ryan J, Lindeman P: Value of serial measurement of angiotensin converting enzyme in the management of sarcoidosis. Am J Med 70:44, 1981.
118. Rohrback MS, DeRemee RA: Pulmonary sarcoidosis and serum angiotensin converting enzyme. Mayo Clin Proc 57:64, 1982.
119. Bodem CR, Hamory BH, Taylor HM, et al: Granulomatous bone marrow disease. A review of the literature and clinicopathologic analysis of 58 cases. Medicine 62:372, 1983.
120. Itoh J, Akiguchi I, Midorikawa R, et al: Sarcoid myopathy with typical rash of dermatomyositis. Neurology 30:1118, 1980.
121. Cameron HU: Symmetrical muscle contractures in tumorous sarcoidosis. Report of a case. Clin Orthop 155:108, 1981.
122. Yaghmai I: Radiographic, angiographic and radionuclide manifestations of osseous sarcoidosis. RadioGraphics 3:375, 1983.
123. Guilford WB, Mentz WM, Kopelman HA, et al: Sarcoidosis presenting as a rib fracture. AJR 139:608, 1982.
124. Atkinson R, Ghelman B, Tsairis P, et al: Sarcoidosis presenting as cervical radiculopathy. A case report and literature review. Spine 7:412, 1982.
125. Martin CA, Murali R, Trasi SS: Spinal cord sarcoidosis. Case report. J Neurosurg 61:981, 1984.
126. Baum J, Solomon M, Alba A: Sarcoidosis as a cause of transverse myelitis: Case report. Paraplegia 19:167, 1981.
127. Hitchon PW, Haque AU, Olson JJ, et al: Sarcoidosis presenting as an intramedullary spinal cord mass. Neurosurgery 15:86, 1984.
128. Adler DD, Blane CE, Holt JF: Case report 220. Skel Radiol 9:205, 1983.
129. Lieberman J, Krauthammer M: Pseudoclubbing in a patient with sarcoidosis of the phalangeal bones. Arch Intern Med 143:1017, 1983.
130. Lovy MR, Hughes GRV: Sarcoidosis presenting as subacute polydactylitis. J Rheumatol 8:350, 1981.
131. Redman DS, McCarthy RE, Jimenez JF: Sarcoidosis in the long bones of a child. A case report and review of the literature. J Bone Joint Surg [Am] 65:1010, 1983.
132. Wolk RB: Sarcoidosis of the orbit with bone destruction. AJR 5:204, 1984.
133. Rockoff SD, Rohatgi PK: Unusual manifestations of thoracic sarcoidosis. AJR 144:513, 1985.
134. Fitzgerald AA, Davis P: Arthritis, hilar adenopathy, erythema nodosum complex. J Rheumatol 9:935, 1982.
135. Perruquet JL, Harrington TM, Davis DE, et al: Sarcoid arthritis in a North American Caucasian population. J Rheumatol 11:521, 1984.
136. Pitt P, Hamilton EBD, Innes EH, et al: Sarcoid dactylitis. Ann Rheum Dis 42:634, 1983.
137. Yasui N, Tsuyuguchi Y: Sarcoid disease of the wrist joint. Hand 15:246, 1983.
138. LeGoff P, Jaffres R, Schwarzberg C, et al: Arthrite chronique destructive du genou d'origine sarcoïdosique associée à des geodes des os longs. Rev Rhum Mal Osteoartic 49:647, 1982.
139. Feldman C: Chronic sarcoid arthritis. Rheumatol Rehabil 20:18, 1981.
140. Boyd RE, Andrews BS: Sarcoidosis presenting as cutaneous ulceration, subcutaneous nodules and chronic arthritis. J Rheumatol 8:311, 1981.
141. Scott DGI, Porto LOR, Lovell CR, et al: Chronic sarcoid synovitis in the Caucasian: An arthroscopic and histological study. Ann Rheum Dis 40:121, 1981.
142. Palmer DG, Schumacher HR: Synovitis with nonspecific histological changes in synovium with chronic sarcoidosis. Ann Rheum Dis 43:778, 1984.
143. Castellanos A, Galan E: Sarcoidosis (Besnier-Boeck-Schaumann's disease). Report of a case simulating Still's disease. Am J Dis Child 71:513, 1946.
144. North AF, Fink CW, Gibson WM, et al: Sarcoid arthritis in children. Am J Med 48:449, 1970.

145. Rosenberg AM, Yee EH, Mackenzie JW: Arthritis in childhood sarcoidosis. J Rheumatol *10*:987, 1983.

146. Thomas AL, Thomas CS, Dodge JA, et al: A case of sarcoid arthritis in a child. Ann Rheum Dis *42*:343, 1983.

147. Gerster JC, Chappuis PH: Association d'une sarcoidose aigue et d'une spondylarthrite ankylosante. Schweiz Rundsch Med Prax *70*:2356, 1981.

148. Cohen MD, Allen GL, Ginsburg WW: Eosinophilic fasciitis and sarcoidosis: A case report. J Rheumatol *10*:347, 1983.

149. Cinti DC, Hawkins HB, Slavin JD Jr: Radioisotope bone scanning in a case of sarcoidosis. Clin Nucl Med *10*:192, 1985.

150. Edan G, Bourguet P, Delaval P, et al: Gallium-67 imaging in muscular sarcoidosis. J Nucl Med *25*:776, 1984.

151. Adams JS, Sharma OP, Gacad MA, et al: Metabolism of 25-hydroxyvitamin D_3 by cultured pulmonary alveolar macrophages in sarcoidosis. J Clin Invest *72*:1856, 1983.

152. Mason R, Frankel T, Chan Y-L, et al: Vitamin D conversion by sarcoid lymph node homogenate. Ann Intern Med *100*:59, 1984.

153. Sharma OP: Hypercalcemia in sarcoidosis. The puzzle finally solved. Arch Intern Med *145*:626, 1985.

154. Sartoris DJ, Resnick D, Resnik C, et al: Musculoskeletal manifestations of sarcoidosis. Semin Roentgenol *20*:376, 1985.

155. Leibowitz MR, Essop AR, Schamroth CL, et al: Sarcoid dactylitis in black South African patients. Semin Arthritis Rheum *14*:232, 1985.

156. Koeger AC, Milleron B, Prier A, et al: Sarcoidose de la voute cranienne. A propos d'une observation. Sem Hôp Paris *61*:1577, 1985.

157. Madoule P, Ellrodt A, Chevrot A, et al: Case report 306. Skel Radiol *13*:304, 1985.

158. Terranova WA, Williams GS, Kuhlman TA, et al: Acute phalangeal fractures due to undiagnosed sarcoidosis. J Hand Surg [Am] *10*:902, 1985.

159. Lunn PG, McGlone R, Varian JPW: Sarcoidosis presenting with pathological fracture of a metacarpal. J Hand Surg [Br] *11*:137, 1986.

160. Oven TJ, Sones M, Morrissey WL: Lytic lesion of the sternum. Rare manifestation of sarcoidosis. Am J Med *80*:285, 1986.

161. Bundens DA, Rechtine GR: Sarcoidosis of the spine. Case report and literature review. Spine *11*:209, 1986.

162. Glickstein MF, Velchik MG: Gallium uptake in cutaneous sarcoidosis. Clin Nucl Med *11*:119, 1986.

163. Van Linthoudt D, Ott H: An unusual case of sarcoid dactylitis. Br J Rheumatol *25*:222, 1986.

164. Kremer JM: Histologic findings in siblings with acute sarcoid arthritis: Association with the B8, DR3 phenotype. J Rheumatol *13*:593, 1986.

165. Merle M, Bour C, Foucher G, et al: Sarcoid tenosynovitis in the hand. A case report and literature review. J Hand Surg [Br] *11*:281, 1986.

166. Wolfe SM, Pinals RS, Aelion JA, et al: Myopathy in sarcoidosis: Clinical and pathologic study of four cases and review of the literature. Semin Arthritis Rheum *16*:300, 1987.

167. Jamal MM, Cilursu AM, Hoffman EL: Sarcoidosis presenting as acute myositis. Report and review of literature. J Rheumatol *15*:1868, 1988.

168. Otake S, Banno T, Ohba S, et al: Muscular sarcoidosis: Findings at MR imaging. Radiology *176*:145, 1990.

169. Kalb RE, Epstein W, Grossman ME: Sarcoidosis with subcutaneous nodules. Am J Med *85*:731, 1988.

170. Lesser RS, Dadparvar S, Weiss AA, et al: Aggressive lesion in osseous sarcoidosis. J Rheumatol *15*:510, 1988.

171. Beasley EW III, Peterman SB, Hertzler GL: An unusual form of tibial sarcoidosis. AJR *149*:754, 1987.

172. Abdelwahab IF, Norman A: Osteosclerotic sarcoidosis. AJR *150*:161, 1988.

173. Hall FM, Shmerling RH, Aronson M, et al: Case report 705. Skel Radiol *21*:182, 1992.

174. Rahbar M, Sharma OP: Hypertrophic osteoarthropathy in sarcoidosis. Sarcoidosis *7*:125, 1990.

175. Alloway JA, Nashel DJ, Rohatgi FK: Sarcoidosis and hypertrophic osteoarthropathy. J Rheumatol *19*:180, 1992.

176. Resnik CS, Young JWR, Aisner SC, et al: Case report 594. Skel Radiol *19*:79, 1990.

177. Mijiyawa M, Fereres M, Deutsch JP, et al: Atteinte pelvirachidienne de la sarcoïdose. A propos d'une observation. Revue de la literature. Rev Rhum Mal Osteoartic *56*:529, 1989.

178. Kenney CM III, Goldstein SJ: MRI of sarcoid spondylodiskitis. J Comput Assist Tomogr *16*:660, 1992.

179. Morita H, Hayashi R, Tako K, et al: Spinal cord sarcoidosis: MRI findings in response to treatment. Eur Neurol *32*:126, 1992.

180. Kellner H, Späthling S, Herzer P: Ultrasound findings in Löfgren's syndrome: Is ankle swelling caused by arthritis, tenosynovitis, or periarthritis? J Rheumatol *19*:38, 1992.

181. Sukenik S, Hendler N, Yerushalmi B, et al: Jaccoud's-type arthropathy: An association with sarcoidosis. J Rheumatol *18*:915, 1991.

182. Maña J, Segarra MI, Casas R, et al: Multiple atypical bone involvement in sarcoidosis. J Rheumatol *20*:394, 1993.

183. Junger SS, Stern BJ, Levine SR, et al: Intramedullary spinal sarcoidosis: Clinical and magnetic resonance imaging characteristics. Neurology *43*:333, 1993.

184. Ginsberg LE, Williams DW III, Stanton C: MRI of vertebral sarcoidosis. J Comput Assist Tomogr *17*:158, 1993.

185. Otake S: Sarcoidosis involving skeletal muscle: Imaging findings and relative value of imaging procedures. AJR *162*:369, 1994.

186. Le Breton C, Ferroir J-P, Cadranel J, et al: Case report 825. Skeletal Radiol *23*:297. 1994.

187. Kobayashi H, Kotoura Y, Sakahara H, et al: Solitary muscle sarcoidosis: CT, MRI, and scintigraphic characteristics. Skeletal Radiol *23*:293, 1994.

92

Tuberous Sclerosis, Neurofibromatosis, and Fibrous Dysplasia

Frieda Feldman, M.D.

Tuberous sclerosis, neurofibromatosis, and polyostotic fibrous dysplasia involve multiple systems in multiple ways and may, therefore, be associated with a variety of seemingly unrelated radiographic stigmata. Often the physician's knowledge of these entities is fragmented and complicated by their diverse clinical presentations, which usually are seen and treated by physicians in a variety of specialties. Specialists, although readily recognizing the particular expression of the disease to which they are most attuned, often are unaware of its relationship to a larger mosaic, which is steadily assuming greater proportions as finer facets of these entities are appreciated.

Before discussing dissimilarities, it is important to note that tuberous sclerosis, neurofibromatosis, and fibrous dysplasia share certain common characteristics. Although they are grouped with the neuroectodermal and mesodermal dysplasias, all three germ layers may be involved in the development of each of these entities. Moreover, all have been associated with certain classic clinical triads, which are considered as aids in their identification. Although mutations do occur, in the majority of cases the three disorders are hereditary or familial diseases. Therefore, more detailed histories and examinations of patients and their relatives frequently reveal incomplete, unfamiliar, or atypical expressions of the classic syndromes. When recognized, these expressions have often served to reclassify many so-called sporadic cases as hereditary or familial.

TUBEROUS SCLEROSIS

General Features

Tuberous sclerosis or Bourneville's disease[1] (or "epiloia," which combines the words epilepsy and anoia—i.e., "mindless") is a disease of autosomal dominant inheritance. New mutations have been reported in 25 to 90 per cent of cases[2, 3] and prevalence has ranged from 1 per 10,000 to 1 per 200,000 births.[4, 5] It has no known geographic, ethnic, or gender predilection.

The disorder classically is characterized by a clinical triad of epileptic seizures, mental retardation, and skin lesions that have been regarded as hamartomas. Hamartomas may occur in many organs with a variety of clinical manifestations. Their recognition is of prime importance as the components of the classic triad may not appear simultaneously or may not appear at all, owing to occurrence of formes frustes. Furthermore, seizures, although observed in the first decade of life, are nonspecific, mental retardation is difficult to evaluate at birth, and skin lesions may be subtle or absent in early life.

Cutaneous, Cranial, and Ocular Abnormalities

Almost all patients have cutaneous stigmata, four of which (adenoma sebaceum, shagreen patches, periungual fibromas, and hypopigmented macules) are believed to be diagnostic. Adenoma sebaceum (Fig. 92–1) occurs in 80 to 90 per cent of cases but is present in only 13 per cent of patients during the first year of life. It usually appears between 2 and 5 years of age but often is not manifest until puberty or until pregnancy occurs.[3, 6] No correlation has been found between the extent of this skin lesion and the severity of other aspects of tuberous sclerosis.[7] Sensitivity to cold represents the only reported symptom of adenoma sebaceum. Shagreen skin, an anglicized name for ''peau chagrine,'' meaning ''skin like untanned leather,'' occurs in 20 to 50 per cent of cases with a similar time of onset as that of adenoma sebaceum.[8] The dull, red or tan, firm

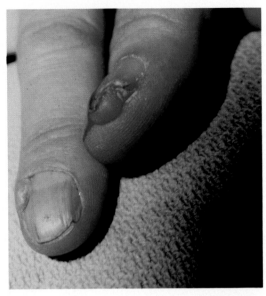

FIGURE 92–2. Tuberous sclerosis: Periungual fibromas. Such fibromas occur in about 20 per cent of patients and usually appear at puberty. They may be solitary or multiple and affect the toes as well as the fingers. (Courtesy of L. Shapiro, M.D., New York, New York.)

plaque has a wrinkled surface, protrudes slightly above the surrounding skin, favors the lumbar region of the trunk, and may be painful. Gingival and periungual fibromas (Fig. 92–2) predominate in female patients and usually appear at puberty. They are more common in the toes than in the fingers and are more prone to grow and recur after excision than are the other cutaneous lesions.[6, 7] Hypopigmented macules (leukoderma) may be noted at birth or in the neonatal period.[2, 8–10] Erroneously called vitiligo or depigmented nevi, the macules are not as milk-white in color as they are not completely lacking in melanin pigmentation, and they may be overlooked in fair-skinned patients. A Wood's ultraviolet lamp is helpful in enhancing their contrast with normal skin.[9] The macules are oval, lanceolate, or ash leaf-shaped, have irregular margins, reveal an average diameter of 1.3 cm, and are most frequent on the trunk and buttocks (Fig. 92–3). The presence of hypopigmented macules in infants makes the diagnosis of tuberous sclerosis probable, whereas their occurrence in conjunction with seizures makes it highly probable.[9] Café-au-lait spots and soft fibromas also are common. Recombinant research has identified a genetic defect in tuberous sclerosis on chromosome 11 near the gene for tyrosinase. This may explain the skin pigment abnormalities in 95 per cent of cases, as this enzyme is involved with melanin synthesis.[159, 160]

Lesions of the central nervous system are responsible for the epilepsy and mental retardation that constitute the remaining two components of the classic diagnostic triad. Of 71 Mayo Clinic patients with tuberous sclerosis, 93 per cent had seizures, 87 per cent had abnormal findings on electroencephalograms, and 38 per cent had average intelligence.[3, 6] Almost all patients who are mentally retarded have epileptic seizures. Routine skull films may show patchy areas of calvarial sclerosis due to hyperostosis of the inner table and prominent trabeculae in the diploic spaces (Fig. 92–4). Generalized thickening and increased density of both tables of the vault also may be noted. Evidence of raised intracranial pressure (i.e., sutural diastasis, sellar changes, in-

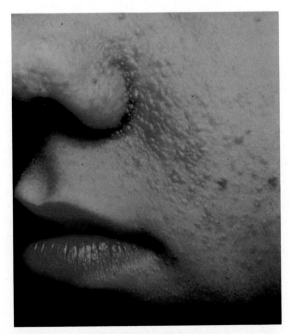

FIGURE 92–1. Tuberous sclerosis: Adenoma sebaceum. This 15 year old girl had had seizures since birth. These skin lesions usually develop in the first 5 years of life but most commonly occur after the onset of seizures. (Courtesy of L. Shapiro, M.D., New York, New York.)

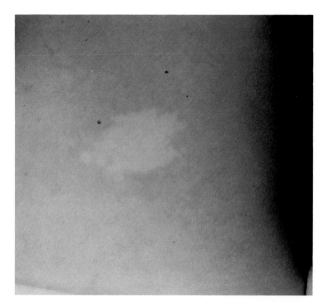

FIGURE 92–3. Tuberous sclerosis. The hypopigmented macule usually is oval or leaf-shaped with irregular margins, has an average diameter of 10 to 15 cm, and most commonly occurs on the abdomen and legs. (Courtesy of L. Shapiro, M.D., New York, New York.)

creased convolutional markings) and thinning adjacent to cortical tubers have been reported.[11]

Intracerebral calcifications occur in 50 to 80 per cent of cases (Fig. 92–4). They increase in frequency as the patient becomes older and commonly are undetectable on routine films of the very young. Skull radiographs in 45 children with tuberous sclerosis yielded 21 cases in which intracranial calcifications were evident.[12] Only three patients were less than 2 years old; one was 7 months of age. Frequency of the calcifications ranged from 14 per cent in infants under 1 year old to 60 per cent in those 10 to 14 years of age. Calcifications may be multiple, nodular, discrete, and

several millimeters in diameter. Occasional linear or single calcified conglomerates 2 to 3 cm in diameter may be noted (Fig. 92–5).

Brain lesions in tuberous sclerosis occur predominantly in three main loci: the ventricles, the white matter, and the cortex.[13, 14] The hamartomatous foci, which may or may not calcify, vary in size and number and may be found in the cerebrum, cerebellum, medulla, and spinal cord. Most lie adjacent to cerebrospinal fluid pathways and are either subependymal nodules or cortical tubers located about the ventricles and arising within the basal ganglia. The nodules usually are small and multiple, and they may produce a candle guttering effect on the ventricular surface, where they often are hemorrhagic, necrotic, and calcified (Fig. 92–5). Larger lesions near the foramen of Monro may be giant cell astrocytomas, which occur in 2 to 10 per cent of cases. They may be single or multiple and may result in obstructive hydrocephalus. Lesions of the third ventricle are less frequent.[15] Previously, identification depended on pneumoencephalography (Fig. 92–5) and ventriculography; however, CT with or without contrast enhancement can demonstrate lesions in the brain at an earlier stage, particularly if they are calcified (Fig. 92–6). They are detectable on CT scans in 50 per cent of patients by the age of 10 years.

Tuberous sclerosis literally means hard swellings (i.e., tuber is the Latin word for "swelling" and skleros is the Greek word for "hard"). Bourneville[1] first used the term tuber to describe the potato-like appearance of cortical lesions in the brain. Cortical tubers are present in almost all cases of tuberous sclerosis and involve any portion of the cortex. A direct correlation between the number of cortical tubers and the degree of mental retardation has been noted. The tubers often are barely visible on involved gyri, however, and are more easily palpated than visualized on the surface of the brain. MR imaging has demonstrated otherwise inapparent lesions (Fig. 92–7). The lesions of the central nervous system in tuberous sclerosis behave differ-

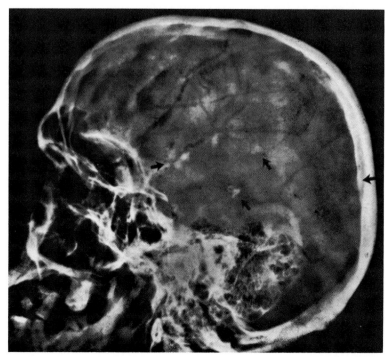

FIGURE 92–4. Tuberous sclerosis: Lateral view of the skull. Multiple intracerebral calcific deposits are noted, together with several scattered areas of calvarial sclerosis (arrows).

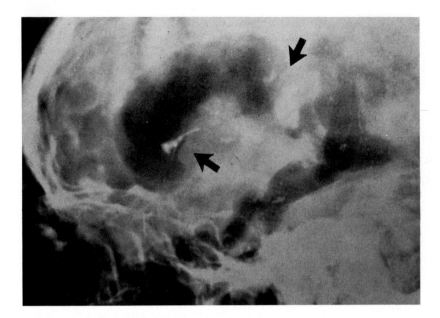

FIGURE 92–5. Tuberous sclerosis: Pneumoencephalogram. The multiple calcified paraventricular subependymal nodules or "tubers" are well outlined by air, so-called candle guttering (arrows).

ently on CT and MR imaging. Subependymal hamartomas do not show enhancement on CT despite the administration of intravenous contrast agents, whereas giant cell astrocytomas characteristically do. On MR imaging, subependymal nodules usually are isointense or hypointense relative to gray matter in T1-weighted spin echo MR images and hypointense relative to gray matter in T2-weighted spin echo images depending on their degree of calcification (Fig. 92–7B). Reversals of signal intensity patterns are noted again in neonates.[161–163] About 30 per cent of such nodules show enhancement of signal intensity after intravenous administration of gadopentetate dimeglumine (a gadolinium chelate), with one third showing serpentine flow voids in dilated tumor vessels, indicating their origin near vascular

germinal matrix.[161] However, an enhancing subependymal nodule near the foramen of Monro, if enlarging or associated with hydrocephalus (or both), suggests the presence of a subependymal giant cell astrocytoma. This type of astrocytoma differs from other cerebral astrocytomas owing to its benign biologic and pathologic features. It grows slowly, has no surrounding edema, and is noninvasive. Its recurrence rate is low after total surgical resection, and it rarely undergoes malignant degeneration.[161] In general, enhancement of lesion conspicuity after intravenous administration of contrast agents in MR images, unlike CT images, is not indicative of neoplastic transformation.

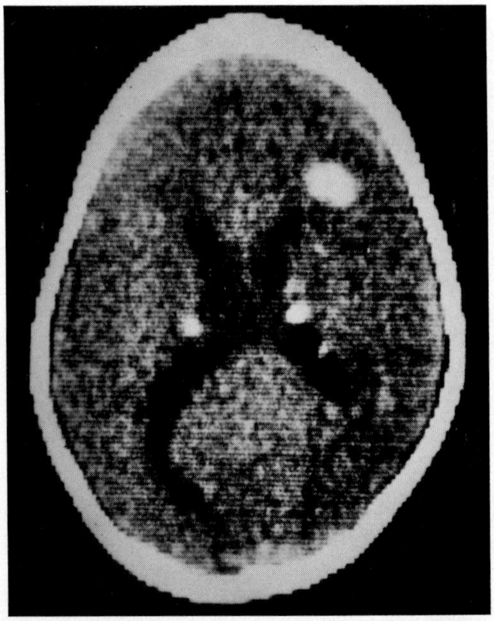

Calcified cortical tubers are detected with CT scanning by their high density. The majority of cortical tubers, however, are subtle, uncalcified subcortical masses of low density that go undetected on CT scans.[159] They are defined best in MR images. Cortical tubers are of low signal intensity on T1-weighted spin echo MR images and of high signal intensity on T2-weighted spin echo images, presumably owing to increased central free water in their loose stroma and to adjacent disordered myelination. In neonates, signal intensity patterns are reversed, with tubers appearing hyperintense in T1-weighted spin echo MR images and hypointense in T2-weighted spin echo images.[159] Again, high signal intensity in T2-weighted spin echo MR images does not imply malignant degeneration, which is rare in cortical tubers.

Heterotopic islets of neurons and glial cells in the white matter in 90 per cent of cases occur in direct proportion to the numbers of cortical tubers.[161] They appear wedge-shaped, tumefactive, linear, or striated[164]; are difficult to see in T1-weighted spin echo MR images in older patients; and are of high signal intensity in T2-weighted spin echo MR images, with zones of low signal intensity if calcified. Ten per cent of white matter lesions show homogeneous enhancement of signal intensity after intravenous administration of gadolinium-based contrast agents.

Ultrastructurally, the abnormal cells in tuberous sclerosis have features of both astrocytes and neurons. Whether they are cortical, ventricular, or in white matter, the lesions re-

FIGURE 92–6. Tuberous sclerosis: CT scanning. Transaxial CT scan of a 9 year old boy taken at the level of the ventricles shows numerous subependymal and intracerebral calcifications.

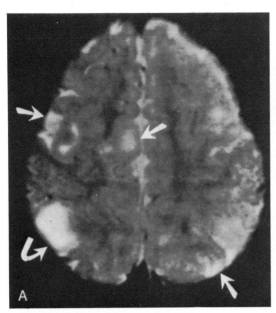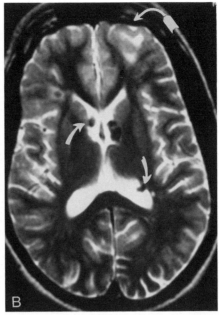

FIGURE 92–7. Tuberous sclerosis: MR imaging—brain.
  A This 22 month old girl had had leukodermia and seizures since she was 4 months old. CT showed only ventricular calcifications that were not detected with MR imaging. However, MR imaging clearly defines multiple tubers (arrows). Flat lesions (curved arrow) may fail to be appreciated grossly at surgery, although they are large and superficial. (Courtesy of J. Bello, M.D., New York, New York.)
  B A transaxial fast spin echo MR image (TR/TE, 3000/102) in a 22 year old man with seizures shows numerous calcified subependymal nodules of low signal intensity (small arrows) and a left frontal cortical tuber (large arrow). (Courtesy of R. Mosesson, M.D., New York City, New York.)

sult from disordered migration, differentiation, and maturation of embryonic cells. They are, therefore, dysplasias or hamartomas rather than true neoplasms. Distinction between nodules and tumors is made on the basis of whether or not the mass produces symptoms. Histologically, giant astrocytes in some lesions may resemble the giant cells of glioblastoma multiforme; however, a malignant astrocytoma or glioblastoma multiforme is so rare in association with tuberous sclerosis that the coexistence probably is coincidental. Unlike neurofibromatosis, tuberous sclerosis has limited potential for the development of malignant tumors. Hence, patients with tuberous sclerosis who show loss of control of epilepsy, disturbances in mentation in the context of previously normal intelligence, or hydrocephalus should undergo examination with CT, MR imaging, or both (Figs. 92–6 and 92–7). Early detection of operable lesions is desirable for effective therapy.

Appropriate intracranial calcification, combined with such dermatologic stigmata as white macules and a history of seizures, with or without mental deficiency, ensures the diagnosis of tuberous sclerosis. Ultrasonography has been able to identify cerebral nodules in utero (at 28 weeks' gestation), as confirmed by autopsy. Cranial ultrasonography in newborn infants affords excellent visualization of subependymal ventricular nodules. Peripheral lesions are more difficult to detect, with those that are solid having sonographic properties similar to those of the surrounding normal tissues.[16–18]

Ocular abnormalities are seen at birth in 52 per cent of cases and may be evident as early as 3 months' gestation. Although many lesions have been described, only retinal hamartomas (i.e., phakomas), characteristically seen at the posterior pole or in the juxtapapillary region, clearly are part of the syndrome. Exophytic, mulberry-like lesions are the most classic abnormality. Fluorescein angiography often is used to locate intensely vascular, flat, poorly circumscribed, and otherwise undetectable lesions. Hypopigmented spots in the iris analogous to the skin lesions also may occur. Calcified retinal hamartomas may be seen near the optic nerve head in CT scans.

Extracranial Skeletal Abnormalities

In addition to the skull, the remainder of the skeleton may be involved focally or diffusely with medullary or cortical cystlike radiolucent areas or dense sclerotic deposits.[19] Cortical lesions in the form of localized concretions or nodules, defects, and pits or depressions as well as irregular, subperiosteal new bone deposition that results in a thickened, undulating cortical contour most often involve the short tubular bones of the hands and feet[20, 21] (Figs. 92–8 and 92–9) and, occasionally, the long tubular bones. Sharply demarcated, rounded radiolucent lesions, identified macroscopically as nonspecific fibrous tissue, predominate in the distal phalanges of the hand, which also rarely may be eroded by subungual fibromas (Figs. 92–2 and 92–8).

The spine and pelvis are additional sites for medullary osteoblastic deposits ranging from a few millimeters to centimeters in diameter,[22] which may be discrete and round, ovoid, or flame-shaped (Figs. 92–10 and 92–11). The usually homogeneously dense intraosseous lesions occasionally have a mottled appearance. They do not expand the bone or transgress osseous contours. Unusual prior to puberty,[23, 24] these lesions occur as later, asymptomatic manifestations, which often are overlooked but may enlarge slowly over a period of years. An awareness of their association with tuberous sclerosis as well as correlation with other

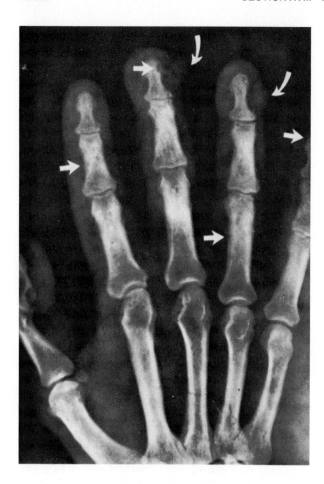

FIGURE 92–8. Tuberous sclerosis: Posteroanterior view of the hand. Numerous rounded intramedullary radiolucent lesions are seen in several phalanges of various digits, together with cortical pitting (straight arrows). Note neighboring periungual fibromas in the third and fourth digits (curved arrows).

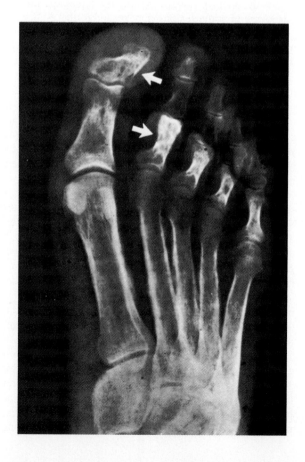

FIGURE 92–9. Tuberous sclerosis: Frontal view of the foot. A thickened, undulating cortex with well-defined external contours cloaks the first four metatarsal bones. Several small, rounded intramedullary radiolucent areas are seen in the distal phalanx of the first toe and the proximal phalanx of the second toe (arrows).

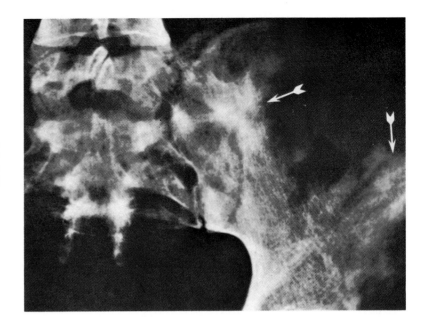

FIGURE 92–10. Tuberous sclerosis: Anteroposterior view of the left ilium. Irregular intramedullary osteosclerotic deposits are noted within both the ilium and the sacrum. Several are flame-shaped (arrows).

clinical data should eliminate their confusion with osteoblastic metastases.

The relationship between tuberous sclerosis and scoliosis has received little emphasis. In a series of 12 patients, six had scoliotic curves ranging from 12 degrees to 78 degrees with a mean value of 37 degrees.[25]

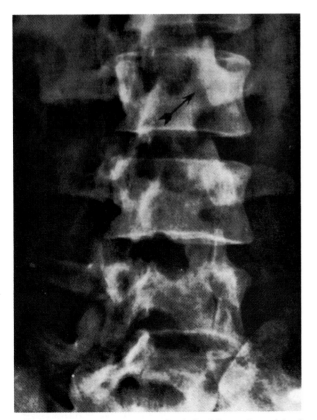

FIGURE 92–11. Tuberous sclerosis: Left oblique view of lumbar spine. The left pedicle and superior articular facet of a lumbar vertebra of a 32 year old man are homogeneously dense (arrow). This was an incidental finding on intravenous pyelography.

Visceral Abnormalities

The viscera and the skin, eyes, brain, and bones serve as silent sites of tumor-like formations; the kidneys, heart, gastrointestinal tract organs, liver, lungs, and spleen all may be involved. Lesions containing varying proportions of vascular, smooth muscle, fat, and fibrous tissue may variously be identified as angiomyomas, angiofibromas, or myolipomas depending on the predominant cellular elements; if histologic pleomorphism is present, they are termed sarcomas. These hamartomas, which rarely are noted in embryonic life[5] or in neonates, increase in frequency with age. New imaging techniques are assuming increasingly important roles in their earlier identification (Figs. 92–7 and 92–12).

Kidney. Approximately 50 per cent of patients with tuberous sclerosis have associated renal lesions, including cysts, angiomyolipomas, and aneurysms.[26, 27] The occurrence of aneurysms of the renal artery and, rarely, of the intracranial vessels in tuberous sclerosis suggests a common developmental arterial wall defect.[28] Coarctation of the aorta and renal artery stenosis also have been documented; hypertension, well recognized in neurofibromatosis, likewise may occur in tuberous sclerosis.[29] Renal angiomyolipomas or epithelial cysts, or both, have been noted in 42 to 100 per cent of cases. Conversely, 50 per cent of all renal angiomyolipomas occur in patients with tuberous sclerosis. They are circumscribed but not encapsulated and may bulge from the renal surface. Renal angiomyolipomas may be detected on routine radiographs owing to the presence of intraparenchymal radiolucent areas related to their high fat content and to contour irregularities and enlargement of the kidneys. CT or ultrasonography serves to delineate secondary pelvocaliceal distortion or displacement due to adjacent angiomyolipomas (Fig. 92–12). CT can be used effectively to differentiate the renal abnormalities of tuberous sclerosis from those of adult type polycystic kidney disease (Fig. 92–12B).[26, 27, 29]

Renal angiomyolipomas have been misinterpreted histologically owing to the characteristics of nuclear hyperchro-

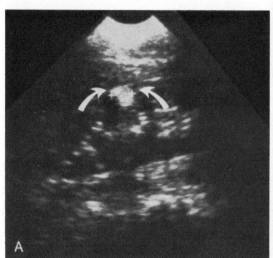
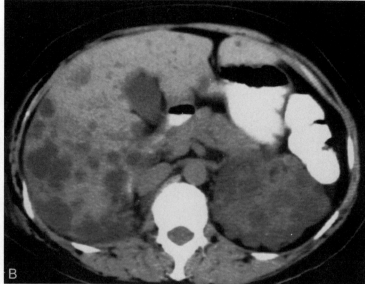

FIGURE 92–12. Tuberous sclerosis: Visceral abnormalities.

A Ultrasonogram of right kidney of a 20 year old woman. Rounded, hyperechoic masses representing angiomyolipomas (arrows) involve the cortices of both kidneys. Cardiac sonography revealed multiple rhabdomyomas within the right atrium and both ventricles.

B In a 49 year old woman with an acute abdomen and chest pains, an abdominal CT scan shows an enlarged liver and left kidney with multiple parenchymal cysts.

matism and mitoses in their dysplastic smooth muscle cells and to invasion of large vascular channels. Arteriography, although delineating increased and abnormal vasculature with tortuous vessels and contrast media "puddling," cannot distinguish definitively between renal neoplasms and angiomyolipomas.[230, 31]

Associated renal cysts usually are superficial and cortical in location. They have a distinctive, hyperplastic, eosinophilic epithelial lining, show no mitoses, and may protrude into lumina.[32] Occasionally cysts may replace the parenchyma extensively, so that hypertension and renal insufficiency, common sequelae of cystic kidneys per se, may be the earliest presenting signs of tuberous sclerosis. Although they may mimic certain types of polycystic renal disease on sonograms,[165] they may be differentiated from angiolipomas by their thin-walled, anechoic areas with posterior enhancement.[166, 167] Episodic flank pain and renal colic secondary to hemorrhage are occasional symptoms that may be evident in patients with renal carcinoma. When such symptoms occur bilaterally, tuberous sclerosis is favored, as more than 90 per cent of renal carcinomas are unilateral.

In a patient with epilepsy and "cystic" renal enlargement, tuberous sclerosis is a serious diagnostic consideration, whereas a combination of renal cysts and angiomyolipomas is now thought to be pathognomonic of this disease, requiring a detailed history and sonographic evaluation of family members. In infants with cystic renal disease and no family history of the disorder, tuberous sclerosis may be confirmed with a CT scan of the brain.

Heart. The coincident occurrence of tuberous sclerosis of the brain and rhabdomyoma of the heart was noted in von Recklinghausen's original description. This association is reported in 30 to 50 per cent of patients with tuberous sclerosis, although its true frequency may be higher, as many neonates with cardiac rhabdomyomas have not survived.[33, 34] Such rhabdomyomas have been demonstrated at autopsy in fetuses at 28 and 32 weeks' gestation. They

may reach several centimeters in diameter, rarely calcify, are well circumscribed but not encapsulated, occur in any cardiac chamber, and may arise in the myocardium or project from the endocardium or epicardium. Symptoms may be due to intraluminal obstruction by projecting tumors, obstruction of the valvular orifice, myocardial dysfunction, and disturbance of cardiac rhythm. Although lack of symptoms does not exclude the presence of a cardiac rhabdomyoma, most patients have circulatory difficulties leading to death in the first year of life. Although an irregular cardiac contour may be apparent on routine chest films, radiographs most commonly are normal or show nonspecific abnormalities. Ultrasonography should be used as a screening procedure in high risk cases.[34]

Congenital rhabdomyomas in tuberous sclerosis seldom show significant growth. Metastases have not been demonstrated convincingly, so that rather than true neoplasm, these lesions have been regarded as hamartomatous clusters of myocardial cells with disordered maturation and no disruption of organization beyond the cellular level.[35]

Lung and Pleura. Pulmonary lesions occur in approximately 1 per cent of patients with tuberous sclerosis, almost all of whom are female.[19, 36, 37] Pulmonary symptoms are of late onset, developing at an average age of 30 years and usually not before 20 years of age. Dyspnea, a presenting symptom in 58 per cent of cases, may be secondary to spontaneous pneumothorax, which occurs in 50 per cent of cases. Respiratory insufficiency, usually severe and progressive, also may be related to subpleural blebs or cor pulmonale.[19]

Although some patients have had a chylothorax, this is seen more commonly in lymphangiomyomatosis (66 per cent of cases). Some authors contend, however, that the latter condition represents an incomplete form of tuberous sclerosis with pulmonary involvement. Pleural complications are frequent in both entities; pneumothorax occurs in 50 per cent of cases in both diseases, together with progressive dyspnea and cor pulmonale[37]; pregnancy may exacerbate both diseases; and, in both, chest radiographs display thoracic distention and a uniform, diffuse, or basilar interstitial infiltration with a honeycomb pattern.[38, 39]

Grossly, the lung in tuberous sclerosis typically demonstrates two findings: (1) a honeycomb of cystic, spongelike spaces and multiple small fibroleiomyomatous nodules, some of which surround blood vessels, and (2) capillary angiomas. Thickened pulmonary arteries also have been noted. Long-term prognosis in patients with tuberous sclerosis and pulmonary involvement is poor, with an average survival of less than 10 years from the onset of symptoms. Treatment with progesterone, recently shown to be effective in pulmonary lymphangiomatosis, therefore has been advocated.[37]

Endocrine Abnormalities

The association of endocrine and metabolic abnormalities with tuberous sclerosis is not well known. Hepatic, splenic, thyroid, and pancreatic adenomas[15] and lipomyomas have been noted, as have pituitary, adrenal, and thyroid dysfunction and diabetes mellitus. Abnormalities in the size of the sella turcica are included among the reported skeletal defects.[40]

NEUROFIBROMATOSIS

General Features

Neurofibromatosis, like tuberous sclerosis, is a phakomatosis in which embryologically established defects may involve all three cell layers. Neurocutaneous abnormalities may, therefore, be accompanied by a wide range of lesions in multiple organ systems. Regional or limited involvement, shared characteristics, and a lack of specific diagnostic laboratory tests make knowledge of the varied clinical expressions of neurofibromatosis essential for diagnosis.

Neurofibromatosis, which has an estimated frequency of 1 in 3000 births, is one of humanity's most common genetic disorders. It is inherited as an autosomal dominant trait with no sex predilection.[41] The purported mutation rate of nearly 1 per 10,000 gametes per generation is greater than that for other common genetic disorders. At least 50 per cent of all index cases are thought to have resulted from mutations; this estimate has been challenged by computerized analyses, however, which revealed abnormal congenital dermatoglyphic patterns in the parents of many patients previously thought to have had spontaneous mutations.[42] Fathers over 35 years of age have had a twofold risk of producing a child with a new mutation, whereas maternal age has had no significant effect. Further analysis, however, reveals that factors other than advancing paternal age are important in explaining the relatively high mutation rate in this disease.[43] Additional factors, such as pregnancy and puberty, aggravate the manifestations of neurofibromatosis.

Initial reports by Tiresius[44] (1793), Smith[45] (1849), Virchow[46] (1863), and Payne[47] (1887) antedated von Recklinghausen's[48] report (1882), which first associated the neural and fibrous elements in neurofibromatosis. This disorder is thought by some investigators to be of multiple cell origin on the basis of studies using the X-linked glucose-6-phosphate dehydrogenase locus[49] and by other authors to more specifically represent a neurocristopathy.[43, 49–51] The National Institutes of Health Consensus Development Conference, on the basis of genetic and epidemiologic studies, has held neurofibromatosis to be a group of diseases with eight subtypes.[168] Diagnostic criteria for neurofibromatosis-1 and neurofibromatosis-2, which account for 99 per cent of cases, are summarized in Table 92–1.

Cutaneous and Ocular Abnormalities

Classically, prior to the development of the previously mentioned classification, neurofibromatosis was noted to consist of a clinical triad that includes cutaneous lesions, mental deficiency, and skeletal deformities. In addition to its characteristic skin tumors, which histologically are neurofibromas, plexiform neurofibromas, and schwannomas, café-au-lait spots are common (Fig. 92–13). Although the café-au-lait spots are not pathognomonic of neurofibromatosis, differences in their distribution, configuration, and number compared with those in tuberous sclerosis and fibrous dysplasia make them useful indicators of neurofibromatosis. Six or more macules 1.5 cm or more in diameter are unusual in tuberous sclerosis and have been considered reliable evidence of neurofibromatosis.[41] Placing undue emphasis on identifying a minimum of six café-au-lait spots, however, has led to underdiagnosis, overdiagnosis, and misdiagnosis of neurofibromatosis. Fewer than 1 per cent of normal children have more than two café-au-lait spots (Fig. 92–13). In neurofibromatosis, the spots are age related and not uniformly present at birth, but they tend to increase in number, size, and pigmentation until the middle of the third decade of life, when they may begin to fade.

The soft, flat, elevated or pedunculated, nipple-like lesions of molluscum fibrosum are another cutaneous lesion of neurofibromatosis (Fig. 92–14). Localized or diffuse plexiform neurofibromas of peripheral nerves also occur and may lead to elephantiasis neuromatosa, with massive enlargement of the skin, soft tissues, and underlying skeleton. The reason for such overgrowth is unknown. An in-

---

TABLE 92–1. Diagnostic Criteria for Neurofibromatosis-1 and Neurofibromatosis-2*

Criteria for Neurofibromatosis-1 (two or more of the following):

Six or more café-au-lait macules (diameter > 5 mm before puberty, > 15 mm after puberty)
Two or more neurofibromas (any type) or one plexiform neurofibroma
Inguinal or axillary freckling
Optic glioma
Two or more Lisch nodules (iris hamartomas)
Characteristic osseous lesions
  (sphenoid dysplasia, thinning of long bone cortices, with or without pseudarthrosis)
First degree relative with neurofibromatosis-1 (parent, sibling, or child)

Criteria for Neurofibromatosis-2 (one of the following):
Bilateral eighth nerve masses
Neurofibromatosis-2 in a first degree relative (parent, sibling, or child) and either a unilateral eighth nerve mass or two of the following:
  neurofibroma, meningioma, glioma, schwannoma, juvenile posterior capsular lenticular opacity

---

*Some patients, particularly children, if they do not have sufficient findings to meet these criteria, may require follow-up evaluations. Molecular genetics may permit a diagnosis in some patients.

(Modified from National Institutes of Health Consensus Development Conference: Arch Neurol 45: 575, 1988.)

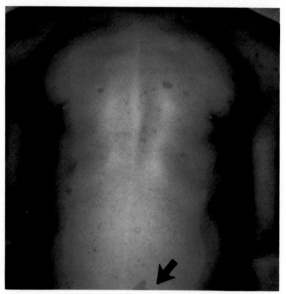

FIGURE 92–13. Neurofibromatosis in a 16 year old boy. Café-au-lait spots are scattered over the anterior chest and abdominal wall. They may vary in size from freckles to larger macules (arrow) with smooth edges. Any patient with six or more café-au-lait spots measuring 1.5 cm or more in diameter may be presumed to have neurofibromatosis.

crease in serum nerve growth factor has been noted in some patients.[52] This factor has had mixed success as a disease marker, however, because fibroblasts cultured from neurofibromas grow without nerve growth factor and without contact with neuronal elements from affected patients.[43, 51–53] Inherent defects in cells forming the lesions, rather than

anomalous nerve growth factor activity, may be important in the pathogenesis of the soft tissue and osseous overgrowth.[54] Foci of dermal hypoplasia made up of discrete, depressed, pale violaceous areas with poor vascular responses also have been noted in neurofibromatosis. They have been related to perineural cells that bar diffusion of pharmacologic agents.[55]

The iris or Lisch nodule is a common ocular manifestation. It varies in color from light tan to dark brown and in size from small spots detectable only with slit lamp biomicroscopy to large nodules readily apparent on direct examination. The nodules may be superficial or deep within the iris stroma and flat, like freckles, with indistinct borders, or dome-shaped, protruding from the iridic surface. They usually are bilateral, vary in number, and are most common after the age of 5 years. Their histogenesis is disputed. They have been thought to be neurofibromas arising from peripheral schwannian elements or melanocytic hamartomas of neural crest origin.

A patient of any age with the three stigmata of café-au-lait spots, neurofibromas, and iris nodules is considered to have neurofibromatosis. Other ocular manifestations, such as bilateral prominent corneal nerves, occur in this disease but are of lesser diagnostic significance.[56]

Osseous Abnormalities

Cranium. The orbit frequently displays a characteristic unilateral defect of the greater and lesser wings of the sphenoid bone (Fig. 92–15). Neurofibromatous tissue usually is not present in the vicinity of the defect, which has been attributed to an underlying mesodermal dysplasia or

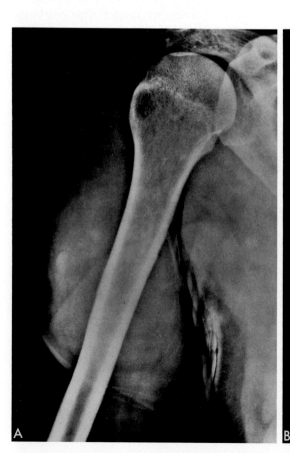

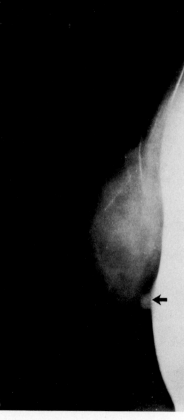

FIGURE 92–14. Neurofibromatosis in a 50 year old man: Fibroma molluscum.

A Anteroposterior view of the right arm. These soft tissue nodules or masses may be single or multiple and may grow under, be flush with, or be raised above skin level. Lesions also may be pedunculated.

B Tangential view of the right arm. Note second lesion with nipple-like configuration (arrow). These lesions have a tendency to invaginate on digital compression. Tumors involving nerves are designated neurofibromas or neurilemomas depending on their relationship with the nerve fibers. Diffuse neoplastic involvement of a nerve and its branches is termed a plexiform neuroma.

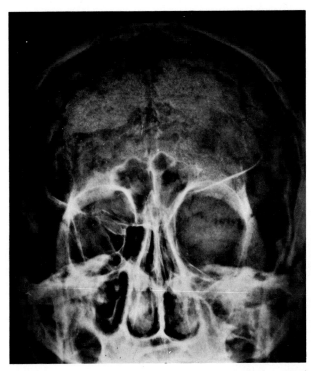

FIGURE 92–15. Neurofibromatosis: Patient with pulsating exophthalmos (posteroanterior view of the skull). The left orbit is enlarged and appears "empty" owing to loss of normal osseous landmarks that are present on the right. Note absence of both sphenoid wings and small ethmoid sinuses.

complete absence of bone. The deficient posterosuperior orbital wall may give rise to pulsating exophthalmos due to a temporal meningocele or temporal lobe herniation through the defect. Enophthalmos may occur rarely.[57–59] Another bony defect tends to occur on the left side of the skull in the lambdoid suture just posterior to the junction of the parietomastoid and occipitomastoid sutures (Fig. 92–16). Enlarged ipsilateral middle cranial fossae or orbital fissures, thickened superolateral orbital muscles with medial optic nerve displacement, an underdeveloped ipsilateral mastoid, and hypoplastic maxillary and ethmoid sinuses also are common.[59, 60] The mandible, maxilla, zygoma, and overlying soft tissues may be affected, with resultant facial deformity. CT scans or MR images help to distinguish skeletal abnormalities due to mesodermal dysplasia from those caused by neighboring neoplastic or dysplastic soft tissues.

Another sign of neurofibromatosis evident on routine films is aggregated granular calcifications in the area of the temporal lobe.[61] These calcifications are similar to those seen within the choroid plexus glomus; however, usually they spare the glomus, may be unilateral or bilateral, and appear to extend along the wall of the temporal horn choroid plexus.[61]

Spine. The spinal column is affected frequently.[62–64] In a population with neurofibromatosis, 60 per cent of patients will have some abnormality of the spine. Scoliosis (with or without kyphosis) is the most common spinal manifestation.[65] Scoliosis has two presenting patterns: One resembles an ordinary idiopathic spinal curve; the other is a dysplastic, sharply angulated, short segment kyphoscoliosis that commonly involves fewer than six middle or lower thoracic

vertebrae, may be rapidly progressive,[66] and is considered virtually diagnostic of neurofibromatosis (Figs. 92–17 and 92–18). The spinal deformity in neurofibromatosis is distinguished by the predominance of kyphosis over scoliosis. Rotation and lateral subluxation of vertebral bodies may be so severe that apical vertebrae face posterolaterally rather than anteriorly, in total misalignment with the remainder of the spine. Severe kyphoscoliosis and many of the other spinal abnormalities (vertebral body wedging and scalloping, pedicle erosion, foraminal enlargement, and penciling and spindling of transverse processes and ribs) (Figs. 92–19 to 92–24) have been attributed to a primary mesodermal dysplasia.

Surgical results have been poor. The marked vertebral malalignment makes anterior access for both grafting and use of instruments difficult and mechanically ineffective in preventing spinal progression. Local vascular anomalies and hypervascular neurofibromatous tissue may be associated with intraoperative and postoperative hemorrhage and cerebrospinal fluid fistulae.[67] The frequency of postoperative pseudarthroses ranges from 17 per cent in cases of idiopathic spinal curves to 64 per cent in patients with dysplastic spinal curves with more than 50 degrees of kyphosis.[68] Spondylolysis occurs less frequently than in the general population, however.[65]

Other Sites. In addition to the skull and spine, the ribs, pelvis, and long bones are sites of abnormal or deficient bone formation that reflect the basic mesodermal dysplasia (Figs. 92–24 to 92–27). Bowing, pathologic fracture, and pseudarthrosis of long bones occur, and callus formation and fracture healing may be defective (Figs. 92–26 and 92–

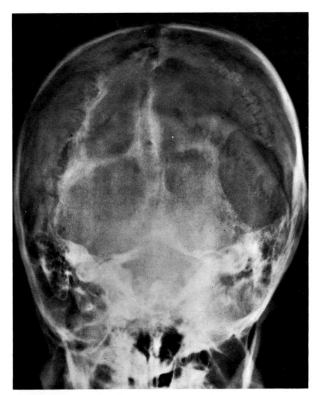

FIGURE 92–16. Neurofibromatosis: Posteroanterior (Towne) view of the skull. An oval calvarial defect involves the left lambdoid suture and extends toward the midline. This type of defect usually occurs on the left side.

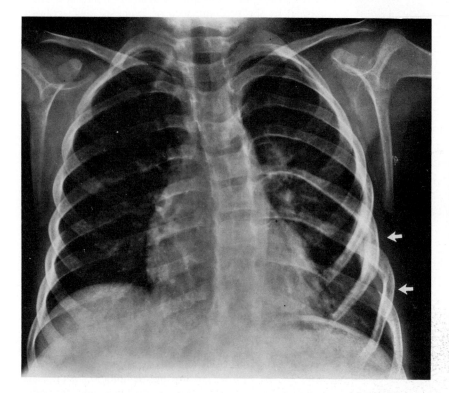

FIGURE 92–17. Neurofibromatosis: Postero-anterior view of the chest. A moderate degree of thoracic spine scoliosis is associated with widened interpediculate distances of the thoracic vertebrae and deformed, widely spaced, overconstricted, and irregularly contoured ribs on the left side (arrows).

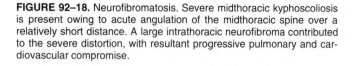

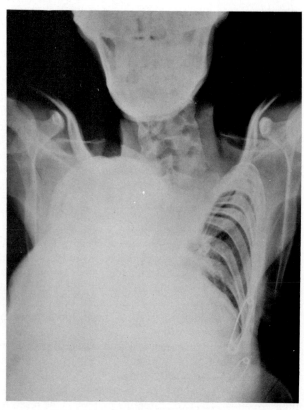

FIGURE 92–18. Neurofibromatosis. Severe midthoracic kyphoscoliosis is present owing to acute angulation of the midthoracic spine over a relatively short distance. A large intrathoracic neurofibroma contributed to the severe distortion, with resultant progressive pulmonary and cardiovascular compromise.

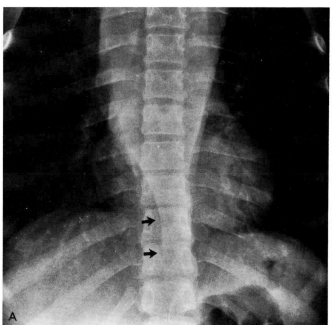

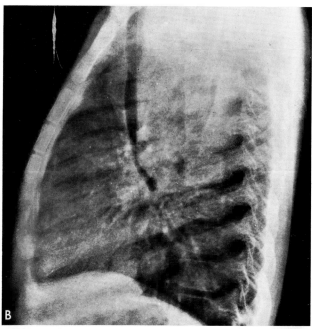

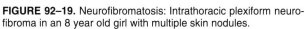

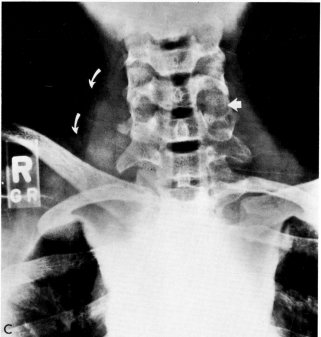

FIGURE 92–19. Neurofibromatosis: Intrathoracic plexiform neurofibroma in an 8 year old girl with multiple skin nodules.

A Posteroanterior view of the chest. The extensive triangular tumor was broadly based at both apices but descended to involve the entire mediastinum. Note the apex at the T10-T11 level (arrows) and slightly lobulated contours of the right side of the mass.

B Lateral view of the chest. The tumor impinged on the trachea and left main-stem bronchus. Note that the mass is entirely posterior to the trachea. At surgery extensive tumor mass was found to be fixed along the posterior gutter. The lungs were uninvolved. The vertebrae, foramina, and ribs appear normal.

C Anteroposterior view of the chest—apical lordotic view at 14 years of age. The tumor has grown proportionately. Enlarging neurofibroma at the base of the right side of the neck (curved arrows) necessitated readmission to the hospital. Note the markedly enlarged left cervical spine foramen (straight arrow).

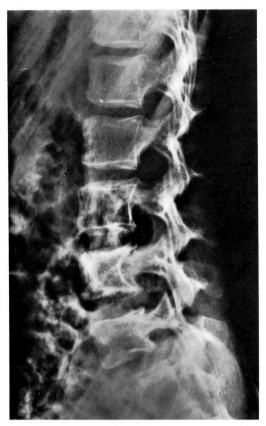

FIGURE 92–20. Neurofibromatosis. Marked posterior vertebral body scalloping is localized to the L3, L4, and L5 levels. There is no associated scoliosis and no change in the intervertebral disc spaces. Scalloping may result from the intrinsic dysplastic change within bone as well as from neighboring dural ectasia (see Fig. 92–22**B**) rather than from mechanical pressure exerted by a local neurofibroma.

27). The tibia is affected most commonly. Anterolateral bowing of this bone, usually evident in the first years of life, is particularly characteristic and may be accompanied by a gracile, abnormally formed, or hypoplastic fibula.

The occurrence of fracture and pseudarthrosis in neurofibromatosis has received a great deal of attention. When deformed or attenuated bones fracture in this disease, frequently they fail to reunite. Pseudarthroses ultimately may result, a finding that is most common in the tibia (Fig. 92–

26). Pseudarthroses in this bone (or others) usually are evident during childhood and may be the sole manifestation of neurofibromatosis. The failure of fracture healing may be accompanied by inhibition of growth in an adjacent physis, contributing to a significant loss in bone length. In paired bones, such as the radius and ulna or the tibia and fibula, deformity resulting from aberrations in normal growth leads to malalignment of joints, compromised function, and even dislocation (e.g., radial head).[69, 70]

The precise cause of defective fracture healing and pseudarthroses in neurofibromatosis is not clear. Callus formation appears to be defective rather than absent. Microscopically, the interrupted bone ends are embedded in a homogeneous fibrous matrix admixed with hyaline cartilage and fibrocartilage, occasionally resembling fibrous dysplasia. No evidence is seen of neural hypertrophy, osteomalacia, or impaired osteoblastic function at the site of pseudarthrosis. Electron microscopic studies of three cases of tibial pseudarthrosis have confirmed the absence of perineural or Schwann cells.[7] Such findings indicate that neural tissue within the bone is not essential in the pathogenesis of pseudarthrosis and have led to the belief that the primary causative factor may reside in the surrounding soft tissues. Removal of both bone and soft tissues has not proved to be beneficial therapeutically, however.

Pseudarthrosis, therefore, remains a difficult orthopedic problem, with many procedures having been advocated to improve alignment and stability. Various grafting techniques, including free vascularized bone grafts (with or without resection of the pseudarthrosis), osteotomies, intramedullary nails, and electric stimulation, all have had limited success in achieving adequate fixation or osteogenesis.[71] In addition, the older the patient, the less likely it is that union will be achieved.

Neural Tumors and Tumor-like Lesions

Spinal Nerves. Two important manifestations of neurofibromatosis are neurofibromas and, far more frequently, meningoceles. In fact, 70 to 80 per cent of all meningoceles occur in patients with neurofibromatosis, in whom they commonly are multiple and often (60 per cent) are asymptomatic. Radiographic differentiation of meningoceles and neurofibromas is difficult as both lesions may produce focal, posterior, paravertebral masses protruding laterally

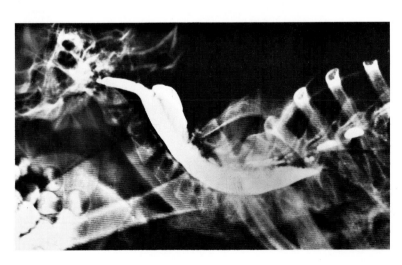

FIGURE 92–21. Neurofibromatosis. Prone cervical-thoracic myelogram demonstrates gross enlargement of the spinal canal with posterolateral dural ectasia.

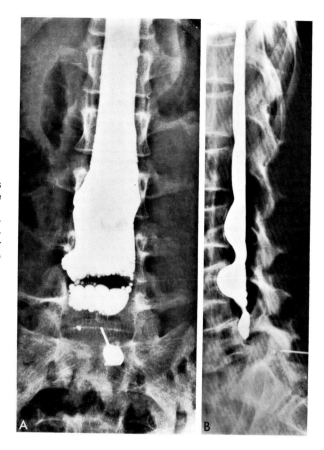

FIGURE 92–22. Neurofibromatosis: Lumbar myelogram.

A Posteroanterior view. The grossly enlarged subarachnoid space has uniform lateral boundaries outlined by the iophendylate column. Note widened interpediculate distances.

B Prone lateral view reveals evidence of localized pooling of the contrast medium at the L3, L4, and L5 levels owing to dural ectasia. Scalloping usually occurs earlier than interpediculate widening, as the trabecular bone of vertebral bodies offers less resistance to local pressure than the compact bone of the pedicles.

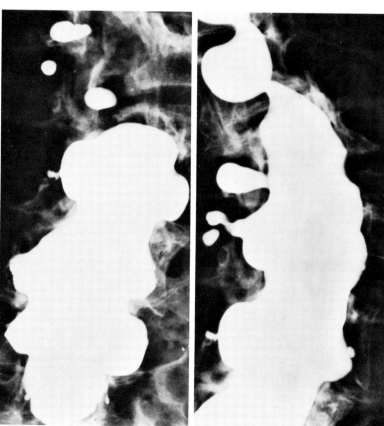

FIGURE 92–23. Neurofibromatosis: Lumbar myelogram. This patient had severe lumbar scoliosis and widespread vertebral body dysplasia. Note marked dural ectasia with involvement of multiple nerve root sleeves.

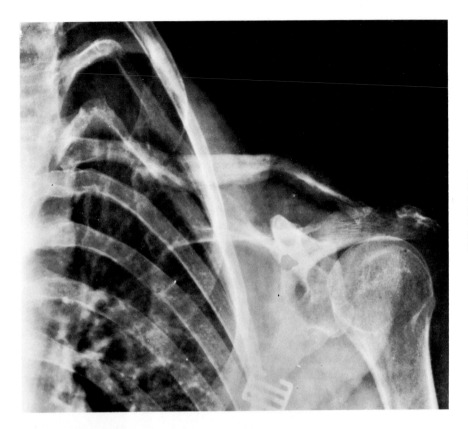

FIGURE 92–24. Neurofibromatosis: Left upper hemithorax. Typical appearing ribs are angulated and overconstricted. Some have wavy, undulating, ribbon-like configurations. The upper ribs are widely separated. A pseudarthrosis of the left clavicle is another associated abnormality.

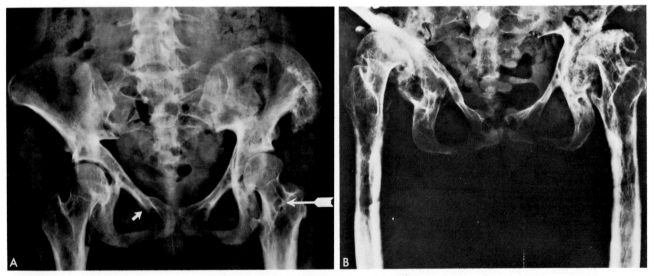

FIGURE 92–25. Neurofibromatosis: Anteroposterior view of the pelvis (13 year follow-up).

A Radiograph of 5/17/65. Marked pelvic asymmetry and hypertrophy accentuated by irregular mineralization and beaklike projections of the left inferior and superior iliac spines and proximal portion of the left femur are seen. Note the elongated and partially detached right lesser trochanter and deformed right pubis (small arrow) due to previously fractured dysplastic bone. The involved acetabula still have a cuplike configuration. Note associated spinal involvement, relatively enlarged, flattened femoral heads, and the rounded, sharply circumscribed radiolucent area in the left femoral neck (large arrow). Intraosseous defects that are considered as characteristically associated abnormalities and commonly attributed to intraosseous neurofibromas are controversial. Superficial cortical depressions when not radiographed in profile may simulate intraosseous lesions. They may, in fact, be due to incidental causes unrelated to the basic disease. There is particular disagreement among authorities who dispute the existence of intramedullary or intracortical nerve fibers. Some defects result from periosteal proliferations that have formed a shell of bone enclosing a previous subperiosteal hemorrhage or an originally external neurofibroma.

B Radiograph of 7/18/78. All deformities have progressed markedly. Severe bilateral acetabular distortion and thinning and overconstriction of the ischial and pubic bones have resulted in a triradiate pelvis. Note overgrowth, flattening, and cephalad subluxation of the femoral head. The left femoral neck defect appears relatively large. Larger, less well defined radiolucent lesions now involve the left pubis, ischium, and acetabulum, however. Intermittent fractures and osteomalacia had intervened.

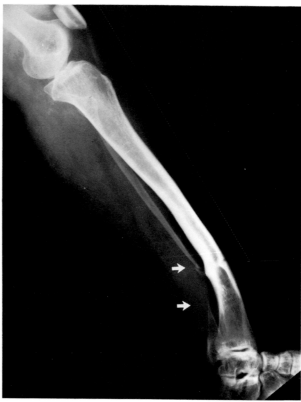

FIGURE 92–26. Neurofibromatosis: Lateral view of the tibia and fibula. Note pseudarthrosis at the most common site (i.e., junction of the middle and lower thirds of the tibia or fibula, or both, with attenuation and "penciling" of the neighboring fibular segments [arrows]), disuse osteoporosis distal to the pseudarthrosis, and secondary deformities of the talus and calcaneus. Anterior bowing of the leg is characteristic and usually is evident in the first years of life. Pseudarthrosis may develop spontaneously, after fracture, or after an osteotomy done to correct bowing.

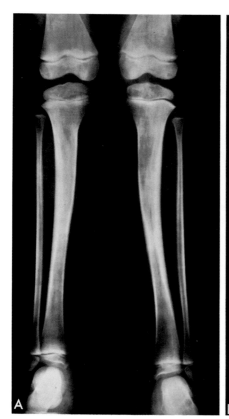

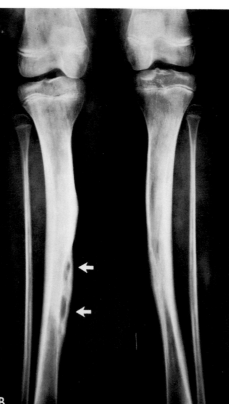

FIGURE 92–27. Neurofibromatosis: Anteroposterior view of tibiae and fibulae.

A Initial radiograph. Dysplastic changes in both lower legs include bilateral bowing, most marked on the left, overgrowth and increased leg length on the left, distal femoral modeling deformities resulting in Ehrlenmeyer flask configurations, and genu valgum.

B Radiograph obtained approximately 6 years later. Progression of the deformities in **A** has occurred, particularly along the medial aspect of right midtibial shaft. Cortical thickening and hypertrophy have resulted in the development of two intracortical radiolucent lesions (arrows). These cystlike, apparently intraosseous lesions may result from subperiosteal hemorrhage, with subsequent periosteal proliferation and repair, or from the incorporation or overgrowth of the periosteum around a previously external soft tissue lesion, such as a neurofibroma.

from enlarged neural foramina. Recognition of meningoceles is important, however, as their resection may result in the formation of cerebrospinal fluid fistulae. Their causation is not entirely certain, and factors such as bone dysplasia (leading to weakened vertebrae that are susceptible to the normal pulsatile pressure of the cerebrospinal fluid), meningeal dysplasia (leading to ectatic, pulsatile dural sacs that may erode bone), or both types of dysplasias (representing manifestations of the basic mesodermal dysplasia of the disease) may be important.

In the radiographic differentiation of meningoceles and neurofibromas, the presence of eccentric, unilateral spinal column scalloping has been said to favor the diagnosis of an adjacent nerve tumor (Fig. 92–19C), whereas central scalloping reputedly is more frequent with dural ectasia (Figs. 92–20 and 92–21). This distinction is not absolute, however. A paraspinal neuroma eventually may grow centripetally through intervertebral foramina into the spinal canal and assume a dumbbell or hourglass shape identical to that of a meningocele (Figs. 92–28 and 92–29). Focal, paravertebral nerve tumors, with or without intraspinal dumbbell segments, are in fact less frequent. In the mediastinum, however, neurofibromas commonly appear as larger, lobular, smoothly contoured masses extending from the thoracic inlet and lung apices to the hila on each side of the mediastinum, at sites corresponding to loci for the vagus nerves (Fig. 92–19). The presence of a scoliosis with the convex region directed toward the mass is a feature that favors the diagnosis of a meningocele.[60]

CT also may fail to distinguish meningoceles from neural tumors definitively. Metrizamide myelography, when combined with CT, often provides more detailed anatomic and pathologic information than either method alone (Figs. 92–29 and 92–30). Calcification within a paraspinal mass, best seen on CT scans, rules against the presence of a meningocele. Conversely, a posterior mediastinal lesion in a patient with neurofibromatosis, particularly one that is cystic, is most likely to be a meningocele. Pooled contrast material within an otherwise nonspecific mass of low density permits the specific diagnosis of meningocele and simultaneously defines the degree of spinal cord compromise (Fig. 92–29). MR imaging and ultrasonography have further aided in defining the size, shape, and extent of paraspinal and intraspinal lesions and their relation to neighboring vital structures, often additionally demonstrating asymptomatic and unsuspected coexisting lesions[72] (Figs. 92–29 and 92–30).

Peripheral neurofibromatosis (neurofibromatosis-1), in addition to having neurofibromas, shares other features with the central subtype (neurofibromatosis-2). For example, it may be associated with peripheral schwannomas. Moreover, spinal nerve lesions rarely may be complicated by neuropathic osteoarthropathy.[169–172] A similar mechanism led to the production of a neuropathic knee in a patient with an intraspinal lipoma that was described by Robinson and Sweeney.[170] Sartoris and Jones[171] reported another case of a 50 year old man with neurofibromatosis and presumptive axial neuropathic osteoarthropathy.

Because any nerves may be involved, including those of the sympathetic chain and intercostal regions, solid lesions in neurofibromatosis may occur in other than mediastinal or paraspinal locations. Intercostal neuromas may appear as extrapleural masses with or without erosion of adjacent ribs. Twisted, ribbon-like, notched, scalloped, or generally deformed and irregularly contoured ribs more frequently are due to dysplastic bone formation, however (Figs. 92–17 and 92–24). Whereas rib notching resembles the focal depressions usually seen in conjunction with coarctation of the aorta only superficially, coarctation may coexist in neurofibromatosis.[73]

Although many of these lesions are asymptomatic, despite being present at birth or at an early age, neurologic sequelae, including paraparesis and paraplegia, may complicate severe kyphoscoliosis, bony dysplasia, or coexistent central nervous system lesions. Kyphosis rather than scoliosis is believed to contribute more to the production of paraplegia in patients with neurofibromatosis. Biomechanical studies have shown that spinal flexion elongates the spinal canal and deforms the spinal cord, which thereby is subjected to excessive axial tension. Concomitant pulmonary and cardiovascular compromise may be evident and, in fact, may occur at an early or unrecognized stage of neurofibromatosis. Therefore, shortness of breath may constitute an early, seemingly unrelated symptom of the disease (Fig. 92–19).

Cranial Nerves. Tumors of cranial nerves are a recognized manifestation of neurofibromatosis (Fig. 92–31). In the new classification system (Table 92–1), neurofibromatosis-1 is referred to as peripheral neurofibromatosis or von Recklinghausen's disease. It is transmitted as an autosomal dominant trait in 50 per cent of cases and as a presumed spontaneous mutation of a genetic locus on chromosome 17 in the others. It is classified as a disease of astrocytes and nerves, per se, with glial tumors predominating.[159] Neurofi-

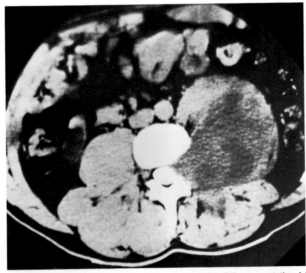

FIGURE 92–28. Neurofibromatosis: Transaxial CT scan at the L3 vertebral level. The patient was a 25 year old black man with known maternal neurofibromatosis, café-au-lait spots noted at age 13 years, back discomfort since age 18 years, and 6 weeks of progressive left flank pain radiating to the left thigh and knee. Routine films (not shown) revealed a poorly defined mass causing eccentric scalloping of the posterior portion of the vertebral body and superior portion of the L4 transverse process and lateral deviation of the left kidney. CT defines a large intradural mass with extradural extension engulfing the nerve root, eroding the posterolateral aspect of the L3 vertebral body and foramen, and involving the psoas and spinothalamic muscles down to the level of the pelvis. The mass, whose rim is enhanced irregularly after the injection of contrast material, represented a moderately cellular, focally necrotic, benign neurofibroma.

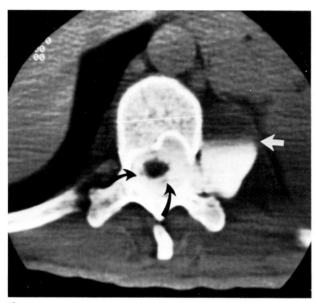

A

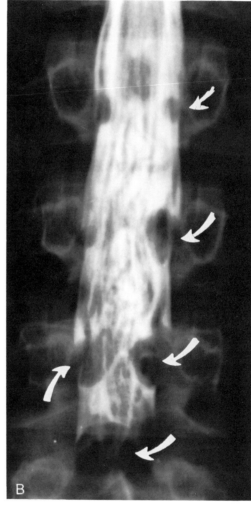

B

FIGURE 92–29. Neurofibromatosis: CT scanning and myelography.

A CT of the T10 level after metrizamide myelogram. A dumb-bell-shaped paravertebral mass on the left side, arising within the spinal canal, causes eccentric erosion of the left pedicle and posterior hemivertebra. Pooled contrast agent with a fluid level within the confines of the mass (white arrow) is indicative of a meningocele. Rounded radiolucent shadows represent intradural neurofibromas (black arrows).

B Metrizamide myelogram of a 24 year old man with lower extremity paresthesias shows multiple intrathecal neurofibromas (arrows).

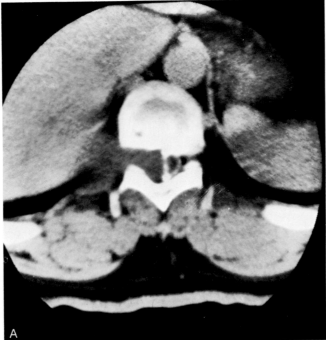

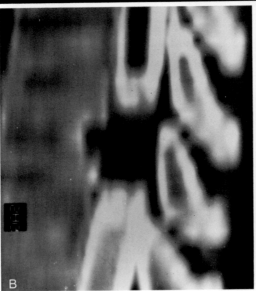

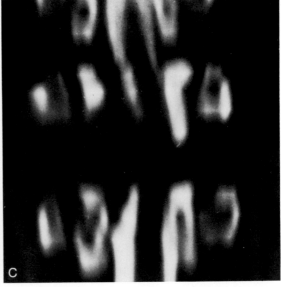

FIGURE 92–30. Neurofibromatosis: CT after metrizamide myelogram. The patient was a 32 year old man with an asymptomatic neurofibroma.

A A low density, right paravertebral mass, with a dumbbell-shaped component in the spinal canal, enlarges the neural foramen, flattens the right hemivertebra focally, and displaces the cord markedly to the left. Contrast agent fails to enter the substance of the mass, which has no discernible fluid level.

B, C Sagittal and coronal reconstructions of the CT data further define the marked spinal cord displacement and the focal, osseous defect in the vertebral body. Its sclerotic base indicates chronicity.

(Courtesy of G. Carson, M.D., New York, New York.)

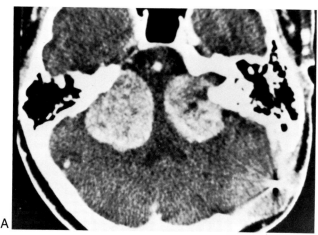

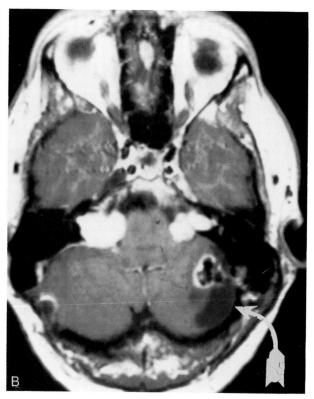

FIGURE 92–31. Neurofibromatosis: Acoustic nerve abnormalities.

A Bilateral acoustic schwannomas. CT with intravenous contrast agent from a 17 year old woman with a 1 year history of progressive hearing loss, greater on the right. Bilaterally enhancing masses project from both acoustic meati. A markedly enlarged left internal auditory canal is evident.

B In a second patient, a transaxial T1-weighted (TR/TE, 656/15) spin echo MR image obtained after the intravenous injection of a gadolinium compound shows schwannomas of both acoustic nerves with enhancement of signal intensity. Similar, but less dramatic, enhancement of a cerebellar cystic glioma (arrow) and enlarged tortuous optic nerves also are seen.

bromatosis-2, referred to as central neurofibromatosis, is transmitted as an autosomal dominant trait with nearly 100 per cent penetrance and is due to a defective locus on the long arm of chromosome 22.[173, 174] It is considered a disease of the covering membranes of the central nervous system, with schwannomas or neurinomas predominating. In neurofibromatosis-1, glial tumors predominate. Optic nerve gliomas represent the most common lesions of the central nervous system, with a reported prevalence of from 5 to 70 per cent.[173] Conversely, the reported prevalence of neurofibromatosis in those patients with optic gliomas has varied from 6 to 58 per cent.[159, 160] Retrobulbar and palpebral plexiform neurofibromas and retrograde extension to the cavernous sinus also are noted[75] (Figs. 92–32 to 92–34).

On MR images, optic nerve gliomas appear as enlarged nerves, usually of normal signal intensity; hypointense involved optic chiasms, tracts, and radiations may be hypointense or isointense to normal brain parenchyma in T1-weighted spin echo MR images and hyperintense to brain parenchyma in T2-weighted spin echo MR images.[174]

MR imaging is superior to CT scanning in allowing simultaneous assessment of all segments of the optic nerve (i.e., intraorbital, intracanalicular, and intracranial). MR imaging also is superior to CT scanning in the evaluation of other central glial cell tumors occurring in neurofibromatosis-1, such as ependymomas, glioblastomas, and astrocytomas of the brain stem, spinal cord, and basal ganglia.

In neurofibromatosis-2, schwannomas of the cranial (and spinal) nerves are the most common tumors, followed by meningiomas. They are composed of cells that form nerve sheaths without neoplastic involvement of the nerves themselves.[172] The frequently associated meningiomas often are multiple and predominate in the sphenoid ridge, intraventricular and presellar regions, falx, and optic nerve sheath. Fifty per cent of meningiomas occur in neurofibromatosis and, in this disease, meningiomas frequently recur.

Bilateral schwannomas usually become manifest in the third or fourth decade of life, but they may appear earlier in patients with unilateral lesions. The acoustic and trigeminal nerves are affected most often. Unilateral lesions typically arise from the vestibular portion of the eighth nerve and produce tinnitus and deafness owing to compression of the cochlear nerve; bilateral acoustic neurinomas tend initially to infiltrate and spread fibers of the cochlear nerve without compressing it, accounting for a delay in clinical manifestations.

CT has been effective in allowing detection of these lesions.[74] MR imaging, however, allows detection of schwannomas as well as of other associated and often unsuspected lesions. In MR images, schwannomas are hypointense or isointense relative to brain parenchyma in images obtained with a short repetition time (TR), are hyperintense in images obtained with a long TR, and show homogeneous enhancement of signal intensity after intravenous administration of gadopentetate dimeglumine. Necrotic or calcified lesions show heterogeneous signal intensity.[161, 176] In MR images, meningiomas often are multiple and coexist with acoustic schwannomas. They are hypointense or isointense to cerebral white matter in short TR images and isointense to hyperintense in long TR images. Detection of small or multiple meningiomas is improved after intravenous injection of a gadolinium-based contrast agent.

Segmental neurofibromatosis (type 5) is a rare form of the disease distinguished by schwannomas, neurofibromas,

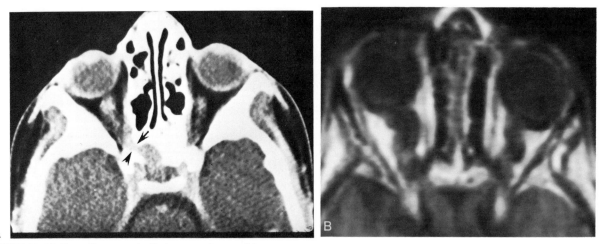

FIGURE 92–32. Neurofibromatosis: Optic nerve abnormalities.

   A CT of the skull. An opticochiasmatic glioma erodes the right optic foramen (arrows) to involve the right optic nerve. (Courtesy of J. Silver, M.D., New York, New York.)

   B In a different patient, a transaxial T1-weighted (TR/TE, 750/32) spin echo MR image shows large, tortuous optic nerves of low signal intensity.

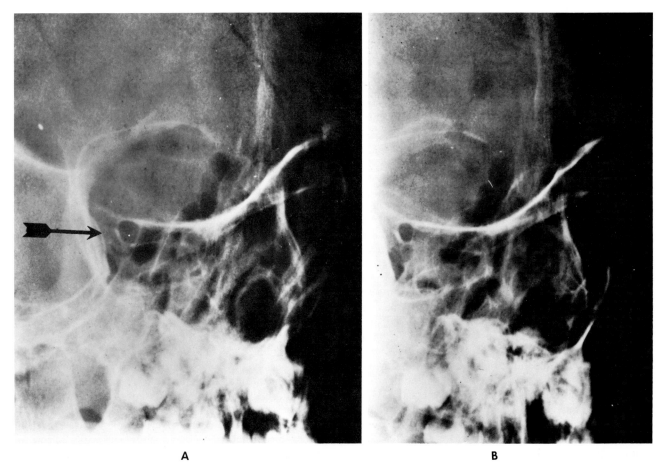

A   **B**

FIGURE 92–33. Neurofibromatosis: Optic foramina. A 4 year old boy has a normal right optic foramen **(B)** with concentric enlargement of the left owing to an optic nerve glioma (arrow) **(A).** Neurofibromas of the orbital nerve and meningiomas of the optic nerve sheath are other orbital lesions that may be encountered in association with neurofibromatosis.

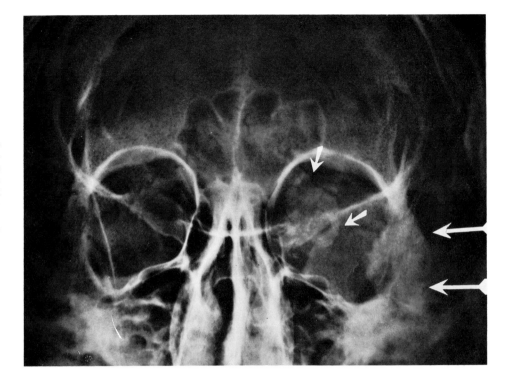

FIGURE 92–34. Neurofibromatosis with meningioma: Posteroanterior view of the skull. Note intraorbital calcification and sclerosis and expansion of the left lesser sphenoid wing, which was the site of a meningioma (small arrows). Note also the dysplastic zygoma (large arrows).

and café-au-lait spots with limited dermatomal distributions.[177] Occasional pain and pruritus are attributed to large numbers of mast cells in neurofibromas.

Benign as well as malignant central nervous system tumors account for much of the mortality in neurofibromatosis. Bilateral acoustic neurinomas, opticochiasmatic gliomas with optic nerve involvement, meningiomas, and astrocytomas may exist in various combinations. Furthermore, basilar impression, ventricular dilation, macrencephaly, and atlantoaxial dislocation all have been documented in neurofibromatosis.[13, 76, 77] As in other congenital mesenchymal disorders, such as Marfan's syndrome, atlantoaxial dislocation has been related to maldeveloped and flaccid supporting ligaments. Rarely, neurofibromas intervene between the odontoid process and anterior arch of the atlas, further contributing to atlantoaxial malalignment.[76]

Macrocranium (increased skull size) and macrencephaly (increased brain size) are associated with neurofibromatosis. Historically, macrocranium was a prominent feature in one of the earliest documented cases of neurofibromatosis; the large misshapen head of the so-called "elephant man" was repeatedly referred to by Treves,[78] yet it took a century for macrocranium and macrencephaly to be appreciated as frequent and significant clinical manifestations of the disease. Macrocranium was identified in 75 per cent of 24 children with neurofibromatosis in one reported series,[79] and in another, 70 per cent of 52 children with this disease had cranial capacities above the fiftieth percentile.[80] The frequency of this finding is lower in patients with tuberous sclerosis.

Idiopathic ventricular dilation, which may coexist with macrencephaly, has been noted in 32 to 45 per cent of cases of neurofibromatosis. Although it has been associated with intraventricular obstruction by central nervous system neurofibromas, disturbance of cerebrospinal fluid absorption, bone dysplasia, and subcortical atrophy, it may occur in their absence.

The causes of mental retardation in patients with neurofibromatosis are multiple. Changes in intelligence or mental status in those patients with initially mild mental deficiency should initiate a careful search for hydrocephalus, brain tumors, or cerebral ischemia resulting from vascular lesions. Abnormalities of intracranial arteries occur in approximately one third of patients with neurofibromatosis[81–83] and include narrowing or stenosis of dysplastic vascular channels and aneurysms. Small arterioles or major arteries, or both, may be affected.[77, 82]

Peripheral Nerves. Peripheral nerve tumors in neurofibromatosis most frequently involve neural supporting tissues. The two most common benign forms are solitary or multiple neurofibromas (Fig. 92–35) and neurilemomas (schwannomas) (Fig. 92–36). The latter are encapsulated lesions that lie on the surface of the nerve. They are more common than neurofibromas, which infiltrate involved nerves diffusely and incorporate all nerve elements (i.e., Schwann cells, nerve fibers, and fibroblasts). Tumors of nerves may, therefore, appear as focal fusiform enlargements or diffuse, multinodular, or coalescent sheetlike masses. Benign plexiform or cirsoid neurofibromas, observed only in neurofibromatosis, appear as bizarre soft tissue networks that interdigitate imperceptibly with adjacent fat and muscle, recur after resection, and have a potential for malignant degeneration. They are recognized most easily in massively enlarged extremities (e.g., elephantiasis neuromatosa), although the face, head, and trunk also may be involved. Such lesions may occur anywhere along the course of central or peripheral nerves or within deep or superficial tissues.

Tumors of the genitourinary tract may involve the genitalia (e.g., the scrotum, penis, clitoris, or vulva) or the retroperitoneum (e.g., kidney, ureter, or bladder). Extraperitoneal lesions occurring anterior to the sacrum often extend laterally along pelvic side walls and have attentuation coefficients on CT scans below those of muscles.[84] Although

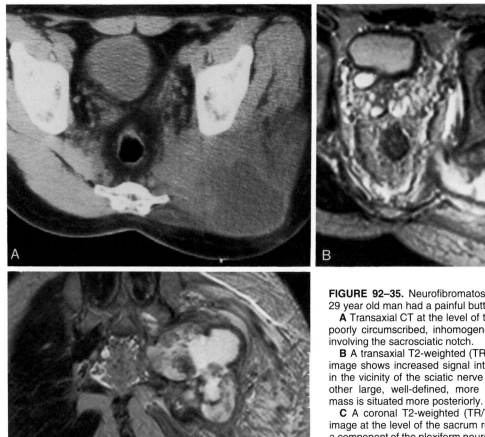

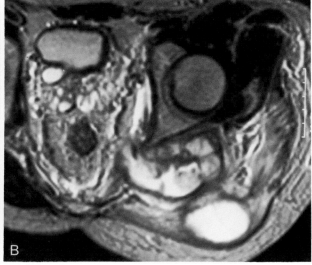

FIGURE 92–35. Neurofibromatosis: Plexiform neurofibroma. A 29 year old man had a painful buttock mass.

A Transaxial CT at the level of the acetabulum shows a large, poorly circumscribed, inhomogeneous, left-sided buttock mass involving the sacrosciatic notch.

B A transaxial T2-weighted (TR/TE, 3000/102) spin echo MR image shows increased signal intensity within rounded masses in the vicinity of the sciatic nerve and in adjacent muscles. Another large, well-defined, more homogeneously hyperintense mass is situated more posteriorly.

C A coronal T2-weighted (TR/TE, 3000/102) spin echo MR image at the level of the sacrum reveals centripetal extension of a component of the plexiform neurofibroma through the left sacral foramen.

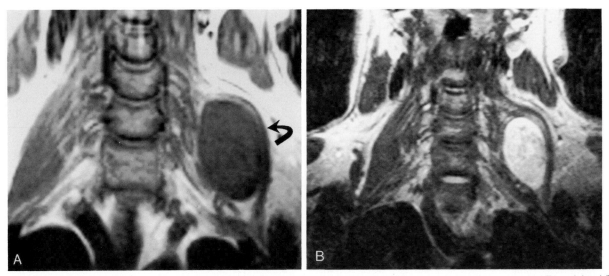

FIGURE 92–36. Neurofibromatosis: Schwannoma. In a 38 year old man with pain and paresthesias in the left arm, coronal T1-weighted (TR/TE, 633/20) **(A)** and T2-weighted (TR/TE, 1800/70) **(B)** spin echo MR images show a well circumscribed mass in the brachial plexus. It is of low signal intensity (arrow) in **A** and of high signal intensity in **B**.

overlap with lymphoid tissues exists, their neurogenic origin is suggested by a presacral location associated with sacral deformities, such as enlarged sacral nerve root foramina, and absent prevertebral or periaortic lymphadenopathy. It is important to note, however, that lymphoma itself has a higher rate of occurrence in neurofibromatosis.[85, 86]

Neurofibromas and leiomyomas are the most frequently encountered benign tumors of the gastrointestinal tract, so that their occurrence does not necessarily imply the presence of neurofibromatosis. Neurogenic neoplasms in this location usually arise from subserosal nerves and from Auerbach's plexus and the submucosal plexus. Resulting symptoms are variable in nature and severity. Anemia occurs in approximately 25 per cent of cases of neurofibromatosis. Malignant degeneration of neuromas in the gastrointestinal tract is no more common than in neuromas of other areas.[87–89]

CT and MR imaging are far more sensitive than routine radiography in the detection of tumors of peripheral nerves.[90] The findings lack specificity, however, making difficult the differentiation of neurofibromas and neurilemomas from each other, and from meningoceles, cysts, abscesses, metastases, and malignant degeneration.[36, 91] In general, both neurofibromas and neurilemomas have lower attenuation coefficients on CT than does muscle, a characteristic that has been ascribed to increased amounts of water and endoneurial myxoid matrix (Fig. 92–28). Some neurofibromas are isodense with muscle, however, possibly because of their increased collagen content, whereas schwannomas, which lack collagen, may display densities as low as 5 to 10 Hounsfield units.[36, 54] Criteria for benignity have required that neuromas appear as rounded, elliptical, smoothly marginated masses with homogeneously low attenuation coefficients and that neurofibrosarcomas appear as lesions with irregular contours with inhomogeneous central or peripheral zones of diminished density. Such gross morphologic characteristics have proved to be unreliable, however, as sarcomas may appear spherical and sharply marginated, whereas benign plexiform neurofibromas may be aggressive and invasive.[36, 90, 91] Low density zones also may be nonspecific and represent hemorrhage, necrosis, and cystic degeneration, whereas calcification and differences in attenuation between high and low density areas, as well as rim enhancement after intravenous instillation of contrast material, occur in both benign and malignant lesions.[36, 90, 91] Although the average values of 20 to 25 Hounsfield units in benign lesions have, with intravenous contrast material, been enhanced to 30 to 50 Hounsfield units, sarcomas also increased an average of 10 Hounsfield units or more after administration of the contrast agent. Size, too, is an inaccurate gauge of malignancy because benign nervous tissue overgrowths may encroach extensively on neighboring soft tissue planes. Recurrent benign tumors likewise cannot be distinguished reliably from new primary or metastatic lesions.[92]

Malignant Degeneration. Estimates of malignant degeneration of neurogenic tumors in patients with neurofibromatosis vary from 2 to 29 per cent, with 5 per cent representing an average estimate. As pain is an unreliable indicator, asymptomatic, new, or enlarging masses may be malignant. The hypothesis that trauma and surgery predispose to sarcomatous degeneration remains unsubstantiated. The prognosis in patients with such sarcomas is poor,[87, 93]

underscoring the need for early and accurate diagnosis. Diagnostic techniques involving ionizing radiation should be used with discretion in neurofibromatosis owing to the known occurrence of neurosarcomas at sites of previous irradiation.[94] Despite the existence of reports that indicate the effectiveness of gallium-67 scanning in the diagnosis of neural tumors[95] and a possible role for MR imaging in such diagnosis, biopsy may be required. Unfortunately, this invasive procedure is not without risk owing to the extreme vascularity of affected tissues. An abundance of vessels and local extension are characteristics of these tumors (even when benign) that defy surgical extirpation and often preclude operative intervention.

Although the vast majority of soft tissue sarcomas complicating neurofibromatosis are of nerve trunk origin and uniform composition (e.g., malignant schwannomas or neurofibrosarcomas), a second type of sarcoma showing pleomorphism, with or without demonstrable nerve trunk relationships, also may occur. The latter type, attributed to multipotential neurilemmal cells that produce fat, striated muscle, cartilage, and osteoid by metaplasia, accounts for the occasional rhabdomyosarcoma, liposarcoma, or osteosarcoma occurring in soft tissues in patients with this disease.[92] Primary intraosseous sarcomas, however, occur sporadically in neurofibromatosis and are of no predominant histologic type.[94] Only three of a series of 4774 malignant bone tumors occurred in patients with neurofibromatosis: two malignant fibrous histiocytomas of the tibia and one fibrosarcoma of the humerus.[93, 94] Review of another 65 cases of neurofibromatosis and malignant peripheral nerve sheath tumors yielded no associated non-neurogenic, primary malignant bone tumor.[93, 94] Primary neurogenic, intraosseous tumors are extremely rare, and their malignant counterparts (i.e., primary neurogenic sarcomas arising in bone) are even rarer.[96] Fawcett and Dahlin[96] found only seven intraosseous neurilemomas among 3987 primary bone tumors. Only one of these was in a patient who had neurofibromatosis.

Miscellaneous Abnormalities

Other Associated Neoplasms. Tumors other than those of neural supporting tissues occur much more frequently in patients with neurofibromatosis than in the general population. They include both lesions of neural crest origin (e.g., neuroblastoma, pheochromocytoma, medullary thyroid carcinoma, and melanoma) and lesions not clearly derived from the neural crest (e.g., Wilms' tumor, rhabdomyosarcoma, and leukemia). Juvenile chronic myelogenous and acute myelomonocytic leukemia, which account for fewer than 5 per cent of childhood leukemias, occur more commonly in neurofibromatosis. Therefore, this disorder is linked with leukemogenesis as well as with carcinogenesis. Common adult cancers of the breast, lung, colon, and prostate seem underreported in neurofibromatosis, however.[7, 43, 85, 86]

Aberrations in Growth of Limbs. Skeletal aberrations frequently associated with neurofibromatosis may be due to deficient or premature cessation of growth as well as to overgrowth of bones and soft tissues. These stigmata may appear separately or together and in various permutations and combinations.[97] Elephantoid soft tissue hypertrophy of an entire limb or part of a limb, such as gigantism of a finger, may exist with normal-appearing bony structures or with hypertrophied or underdeveloped osseous elements. The cause of these abnormalities is not clear, although hypervascularity or hemorrhage, or both, may be important.

Hemorrhage occurring in neurofibromatosis, which may be massive, recurrent, and fatal, is a commonly unappreciated associated finding.[98–101] Subperiosteal and soft tissue hemorrhage has been noted after comparatively minor insults. An inherent abnormality of the periosteum, which is a mesodermal derivative, or looseness in its adherence to the cortex has been incriminated. Large subperiosteal collections of fluid and blood may be related to the poor tamponade effect.

Cystic Lesions in Bone. Reports of so-called cystic bone lesions in neurofibromatosis have been a source of controversy, particularly as the term "cystic" has often been used descriptively when lesions have not been biopsied.[102] Two types of cysts, subperiosteal and intraosseous, have been noted. The subperiosteal form, described as caves, pits, or notches on cortical surfaces, has been attributed to mechanical pressure from adjacent neurogenic tissue[65, 98–101] and to focal hemorrhage from poorly adherent, dysplastic periosteum, which then proliferates over the lesion. Intraosseous cystic lesions have been ascribed to direct invasion of the periosteum, cortex, and haversian canals by neurofibromatous tissue. Most authorities believe bona fide intraosseous cystic lesions to be nonexistent or, at best, rare expressions of neurofibromatosis.

Jaffe considered that multiple nonossifying fibromas coexisting with brown skin patches might represent a forme fruste of neurofibromatosis.[103] Other investigators thought the nonossifying fibromas were present with increased frequency in neurofibromatosis.[102, 104] Most authors believe nonossifying fibromas to be a coincidental finding in this disorder, however. In one report 14 patients with neurofibromatosis were noted to have multiple radiolucent bone lesions about the knee. They were variously diagnosed as nonossifying fibromas, fibrous cortical defects, and intraosseous neurofibromas solely on the basis of their radiographic appearance. None was biopsied.[102]

Vascular Lesions. Vascular lesions are common in neurofibromatosis. Most have been asymptomatic. Arterial abnormalities, including thickened walls, stenoses, and aneurysms, may involve the genitourinary and gastrointestinal systems, spleen, endocrine glands, brain, heart, and great vessels. Abdominal and thoracic aortic coarctations have been described[105, 106] (Fig. 92–37). Rib notching may, therefore, result from aortic coarctation as well as directly from bone dysplasia. Coarctation, however, most often is associated with focal depressions along the undersurfaces of ribs, whereas longer, generalized, ribbon-like deformities are more typical of dysplasia. Congenital heart disease, including ventricular and atrial septal defects and pulmonary valvular stenoses, also have been noted.[60, 107] Another, less well appreciated vascular abnormality is stenosis or occlusion of arteries at the base of the brain.[108]

Microscopic patterns have varied depending on the size of the involved artery and have included internal hypertrophy, disorganized muscular and elastic fibers of the tunica media, and true aneurysm formation. Neurofibromatous changes may involve only the adventitia and may compromise arteries by extrinsic compression.

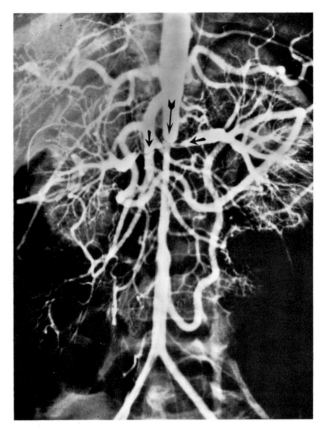

FIGURE 92–37. Neurofibromatosis: Abdominal aortogram in a 10 year old girl with neurofibromatosis and a 4 month history of hypertension. Severe coarctation of the abdominal aorta as well as bilateral renal artery stenoses with poststenotic dilations are defined (arrows). Both kidneys were normal in size and were perfused normally. Note rich collateral network. Concomitant stenoses or coarctation of the abdominal aorta occurs in approximately 25 per cent of patients with neurofibromatosis and renal artery stenosis.

Renal artery stenosis constitutes a common underlying cause of hypertension in neurofibromatosis[109, 110] (Fig. 92–37). Renal artery stenosis is the most likely cause of hypertension in a child with neurofibromatosis, whereas in an adult hypertensive patient, pheochromocytoma is the more common causative favor.[60, 111] Approximately 1 per cent of patients with neurofibromatosis have pheochromocytomas, but 5 to 25 per cent of patients with pheochromocytomas have neurofibromatosis. In addition to renovascular hypertension, the clinical manifestations of vasculopathy in neurofibromatosis include occlusive cerebrovascular disease, mesenteric artery insufficiency, congenital heart disease, major branch arterial stenoses, and coarctations and aneurysms.[83]

The histogenesis of arterial alterations is controversial. They have been believed to represent generalized proliferations of somatic soft tissues, true nerve tissue neoplasms within vessel walls, and altered fibroblasts and smooth muscle fibers resulting from mesodermal dysplasia.

Pulmonary Lesions. Kerley's B lines, cystic bullae, and interstitial honeycomb-patterned infiltrates reminiscent of the changes in tuberous sclerosis have been described in the lungs of patients with neurofibromatosis. Severe interstitial fibrosis, indistinguishable from fibrosing alveolitis, with alveolar destruction leading to bulla formation and obliteration of blood vessels, has been documented histologically.[3, 112] The pathogenesis of the pulmonary changes is uncertain.

Endocrine Abnormalities. Associated endocrine abnormalities include hyperparathyroidism, osteomalacia,[113] small bowel carcinoid tumors,[60] multiple endocrine adenomatosis, and Sipple's syndrome. Sipple's syndrome is a hereditary disorder consisting of medullary thyroid carcinoma, pheochromocytoma, and multiple mucosal neuromas involving the lips, tongue, eyes, or gastrointestinal tract.[114] It has overlapping features with neurofibromatosis (e.g., multiple neuromas, café-au-lait spots, and scoliosis), but cutaneous neurofibromas are not present. Precocious sexual development, which is linked more frequently with fibrous dysplasia, also has been reported.[115]

FIBROUS DYSPLASIA

General Features

Fibrous dysplasia is a skeletal developmental anomaly of bone-forming mesenchyme in which osteoblasts fail to undergo normal morphologic differentiation and maturation. It is of unknown cause and not hereditary, and it may affect one bone, a few bones, or many bones.[116] The polyostotic variety and rarely the monostotic type,[117] when associated with endocrine dysfunction—typically manifested by precocious female sexual development and cutaneous pigmentation—is known as the McCune-Albright syndrome.[118, 119]

The name fibrous dysplasia was coined by Lichtenstein in 1938[120] to describe a disorder of expanding fibro-osseous lesions that had variously been referred to as fibrous osteodystrophy, osteodystrophia fibrosa, and osteitis fibrosa disseminata. Previous efforts had been directed largely toward differentiating it from osteitis fibrosa cystica (i.e., hyperparathyroidism) or associating it with other endocrine dysfunctions. Moreover, because fibrous dysplasia, like neurofibromatosis, was associated with abnormalities of the skin, skeleton, central nervous system, and endocrine glands, some authorities suggested that they were, in fact, the same disease.[121, 122]

Cutaneous and Mucosal Abnormalities

Abnormal cutaneous pigmentation is the most common extraskeletal manifestation of fibrous dysplasia. Although occasionally it is associated with monostotic involvement, the pigmentation is evident in more than one half of persons with polyostotic disease and almost always is present in those with both multiple bone lesions and endocrine dysfunction. The pigmented macules or café-au-lait spots of fibrous dysplasia are related to increased amounts of melanin in the basal cells of the epidermis. They are not raised, and their texture is identical to that of adjacent normal cutaneous tissue. They may occur in isolation, but when multiple they tend to be arranged in a linear or segmental pattern near the midline of the body. Although frequently paralleling the distribution of skeletal lesions, they often overlie the regions of the lower lumbar spine, sacrum, buttocks, upper back, neck, and shoulders. Similar lesions may occur on the lips and oral mucosa.

Pigmentation may date from birth, but the initial appearance or enlargement of pigmented areas in childhood, or even after puberty, is not unusual. Pigmentation may, in fact, occasionally precede the development of skeletal or endocrine abnormalities. The café-au-lait spots of fibrous dysplasia, although brown and widely distributed as in neurofibromatosis, usually are fewer in number, contoured more irregularly, and darker in color. Differences in pattern and pigment granule content in the two diseases have been documented using histochemical dopa reactions.[66] Cutaneous lesions that further distinguish neurofibromatosis from fibrous dysplasia include white, freckle-shaped axillary macules, molluscum fibrosum, and plexiform neurofibromas.

Skeletal Abnormalities

Fibrous dysplasia may be associated with either solitary or multiple lesions in one or more bones. Approximately 70 to 80 per cent of cases are monostotic and 20 to 30 per cent are polyostotic; 2 to 3 per cent are associated with endocrinopathies. In the majority of cases one or only a few bones are involved, but virtually any bone may be affected.[123–128] Monostotic fibrous dysplasia is encountered most frequently in a rib, femur, tibia, gnathic bone, calvarium, and humerus, in order of decreasing frequency. Polyostotic fibrous dysplasia more frequently involves the skull and facial bones, pelvis, spine, and shoulder girdle. A noteworthy characteristic of skeletal distribution is the infrequent solitary involvement of the ilium, which usually is affected concomitantly with the femur. Conversely, however, solitary femoral involvement is not uncommon.[129] A ''ray'' pattern characterized by involvement of phalanges in one or more deformed digits also has been noted, but, as in the pelvis, it is unusual for the phalanges to be affected without other accompanying skeletal stigmata.

Polyostotic fibrous dysplasia may be unilateral or bilateral and may affect several bones of a single limb or both limbs, with or without axial skeletal involvement. Although it is said to favor one side,[116, 120] extensive polyostotic disease commonly is associated with generalized and bilateral, albeit asymmetric, involvement. Despite the designation, however, polyostotic fibrous dysplasia often is limited to a few osseous sites. In one series, only one fourth of patients had more than 50 per cent of the skeleton involved at the time of initial presentation. The severity and degree of osseous involvement, including gross deformities owing to bowing, angular and curvilinear distortion, fusiform expansion, and linear growth discrepancies, are significantly more marked in polyostotic disease than in monostotic disease. Polyostotic involvement also is correlated with a higher frequency of clinical symptoms. Pain in an extremity associated with a limp or spontaneous fracture, or both, often constitutes the initial symptom or symptom complex. In one series, 85 per cent of subjects with polyostotic fibrous dysplasia had sustained fractures, whereas 40 per cent had had three or more fractures.[130]

Monostotic lesions may be entirely asymptomatic for long periods until an obvious pathologic fracture (with or without an associated injury) or an occult stress fracture develops. Severe deformities are unusual in monostotic disease. Bowing ordinarily is slight, with skeletal abnormalities most commonly limited to focal bone expansion with cortical thinning or hypertrophy. Conversely, in polyostotic fibrous dysplasia, larger segments of the bone usually are affected. In fact, an entire bone may be involved, although its ends usually are spared. The more pronounced deformities in polyostotic fibrous dysplasia reflect the deposition of greater amounts of abnormal bone and fibrous tissue, both of which serve to compromise skeletal strength.

The ages of patients with monostotic disease have ranged from 10 to 70 years, but recognition is most frequent in the second and third decades of life. The age distribution is considerably younger in polyostotic fibrous dysplasia, as its more severe manifestations lead to earlier clinical and radiographic recognition. Two thirds of patients are symptomatic before the age of 10 years.[130] Such differences in degree, distribution, and presentation of skeletal abnormalities, as well as the absence of well-documented conversion from monostotic to polyostotic involvement, have led some authors to postulate that two independent forms of fibrous dysplasia exist.

The only significant laboratory abnormality associated with fibrous dysplasia has been an elevated serum alkaline phosphatase level, which occurred in one third of a series of 90 patients.[130] Such elevations, noted during periods of fracture healing or exacerbation of disease, however, also have been documented in the absence of fractures in both adults and children. Therefore, poor correlation exists between serum alkaline phosphatase levels and the extent of skeletal involvement.

Skull and Facial Bones. Involvement of the skull and lesions of the facial bones occur with nearly equal frequency and are noted in approximately 10 to 25 per cent of patients with monostotic fibrous dysplasia and in 50 per cent of those with polyostotic involvement (Figs. 92–38 and 92–39). Common loci include the frontal, sphenoid, maxillary, and ethmoid bones; the occipital and temporal bones are affected less commonly.[131] Although such lesions may be asymptomatic, progression often leads to clinically evident, albeit innocuous, asymmetry and deformity of the head and face as well as to a variety of neurologic complications.

Hypertelorism, displacement of the globe, exophthalmos, diplopia, and visual impairment, which may evolve gradually into blindness as a result of optic nerve compromise, are related to associated alterations in orbital and periorbital bones[131, 132] (Fig. 92–40). Distortion of the sphenoid wing and temporal bone similarly may lead to compromise of the internal auditory nerve with tinnitus, vestibular dysfunction, and hearing loss (Fig. 92–41), whereas involvement of the cribriform plate may produce hyposmia or anosmia.

Routine radiographs commonly reveal single or multiple, symmetric or asymmetric, radiolucent or sclerotic lesions in the skull or facial bones, or both. Profound and often extensive sclerosis tends to predominate in the skull and affects the base and sphenoid wings particularly, a stigma shared with Paget's disease. Concomitant involvement of the facial bones and prominence of the external occipital protuberance in fibrous dysplasia, however, are features that are less frequent in Paget's disease, neurofibromatosis, or meningioma. The maxilla and mandible, when involved in fibrous dysplasia, most commonly exhibit a mixed radiolucent and radiopaque pattern with frequent displacement of teeth and distortion of the nasal and sinus cavities.

Hazy radiolucent lesions, which generally are the most common manifestations of fibrous dysplasia at all sites, often are associated with widened diploic spaces and expansion in the skull and facial bones. The osseous expansion, which may be focal or widespread, almost always is in an outward direction. The outer table of the vault in fibrous dysplasia therefore invariably is convex, whereas both tables, although occasionally thinned, remain essentially intact rather than transgressed or destroyed, as frequently is the case in Paget's disease. CT is an excellent means of

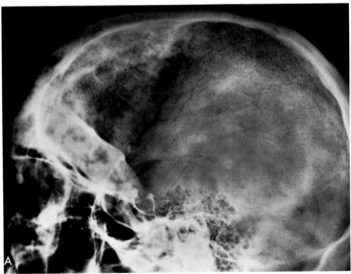
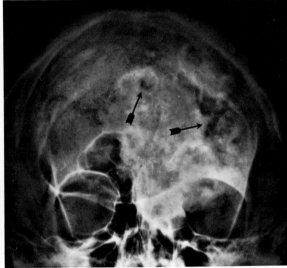

B

FIGURE 92–38. Fibrous dysplasia in a 22 year old man.
   A Lateral view of the skull.
   B Posteroanterior view of the skull. The frontal bone and anterior fossa are affected predominantly. The sphenoid and orbital portions of the frontal bone are involved markedly by the hyperostotic, sharply defined productive process, which also obliterates the left frontal and ethmoid sinuses partially. Several patchy, well-marginated radiolucent lesions (arrows) are evident within the area of sclerosis.

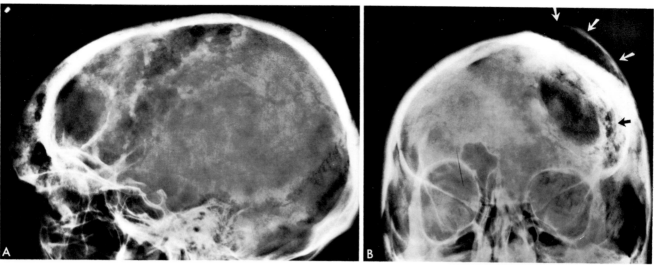

FIGURE 92–39. Fibrous dysplasia in a 30 year old woman.

A Lateral view. The frontal bone is involved by a mixed sclerotic and lytic process. The multiple irregular radiolucent areas all are bounded by sclerotic rims. Note the relative preservation of the inner table, with expansion of the outer frontal table.

B Posteroanterior view. The large ovoid radiolucent lesion in the left frontal bone is margined by a sclerotic rim or "rind." Faint, punctate radiodense areas within the confines of the lesion (black arrow) represent calcified osteoid. Note the marked expansion and attenuation of the outer table, which now is a thin bony shell (white arrows). Although the lesions of fibrous dysplasia tend to stabilize with adulthood, some may enlarge after puberty owing to "cystification" rather than malignant change.

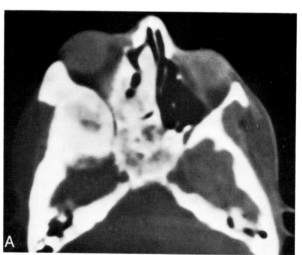

FIGURE 92–40. Fibrous dysplasia: CT of the skull.

A Transaxial CT of both orbits. Large, mottled, bony masses encroach on the right orbital contents, with resultant exophthalmos. The right nasal cavity and the ethmoid and sphenoid sinuses are obstructed and expanded by fibro-osseous masses. The thickened squamous portion of the temporal bone is convex externally.

B Coronal CT scan. This scan further defines the predominantly outward calvarial expansion (arrow) with an undisturbed inner table. The dappled, smoky appearance of the expanded bones rimming the right orbit and deforming the right maxilla and maxillary sinus results from their high fibrous and unmineralized osteoid content.

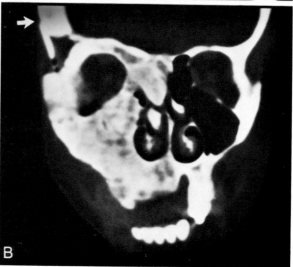

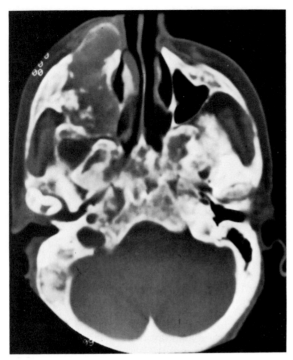

FIGURE 92–41. Fibrous dysplasia: Transaxial CT of the base of the skull. A hazy, homogeneous, partially calcified mass fills and expands the right maxillary and sphenoid sinuses. The entire skull base, including the sphenoid, petrous, and mastoid portions of the temporal bone, all foramina, and the external auditory canal are compromised. Deformities are predominantly right sided.

documenting this point of differential diagnosis as well as of defining the degree of craniofacial bone involvement and the occasional extracortical extensions of fibrous dysplasia.

Another radiographic pattern associated with fibrous dysplasia in the cranial vault is that of a varying sized but localized zone of relative radiolucency, which, when surrounded by a sclerotic rim, may take on a doughnut-shaped configuration. Another unusual but important association is the occasional marked hypervascularity of fibrous dysplasia in the skull; spontaneous, recurrent hemorrhage has been a well-documented complication corroborated by both angiographic[133–135] and scintigraphic studies.[136]

Spine. Involvement of the spine is infrequent in polyostotic fibrous dysplasia and rare in monostotic disease.[137] Radiographic characteristics, similar to those noted in sites affected more frequently, have included well-defined, expansile, radiolucent lesions with multiple internal septations or striations that have involved the vertebral body and, occasionally, the pedicles and vertebral arch. Rarely associated sequelae have included paraspinal soft tissue extension and vertebral collapse, which in turn may lead to angular deformity and spinal cord compression (Figs. 92–42 and 92–43).

Varying degrees of neurologic deficit, including paralysis, have been noted in association with vertebral compression or osseous expansion or, more rarely, with masses of fibrous tissue extending into the spinal canal. Myelography, CT, and MR imaging are superior to routine radiography in defining the extent of involvement of the vertebral column and compromise of the spinal cord.

Tubular Bones. Lesions in the long bones of the extremities usually are intramedullary and predominantly diaphy-

seal in location, with only occasional epiphyseal involvement. They may be eccentric or centrally placed and most often are radiolucent, with a hazy quality classically described as a "ground glass" appearance (Figs. 92–44 to 92–46). The lesions usually are well defined and frequently are bordered by a zone of reactive sclerosis or a thickened, hypertrophied neighboring cortex. Occasional endosteal scalloping or erosion may be accompanied by focal cortical thinning. The resultant locally expansile lesions contribute to the regionally bulging or undulating contours that are a characteristic radiographic feature of fibrous dysplasia. More extensive modeling deformities may appear as areas of fusiform expansion of a long segment of bone with gradual tapering at the junction of abnormal and normal bone. In all instances, however, external cortices invariably are smooth and intact unless fracture or infection has supervened. An internally loculated or trabeculated configuration and a focally calcified or ossified matrix contribute to radiographically appreciated intralesional opaque shadows (Fig. 92–46).

In polyostotic fibrous dysplasia, unilateral changes predominate, but bilateral, albeit asymmetric, alterations also are frequent.[116, 120] The major effect of fibrous dysplasia is to weaken the structural integrity of involved bone. Weight-bearing bones, in particular, become bowed with varying degrees of resultant deformity. Pronounced curvature of the femoral neck and proximal portion of the femoral shaft due

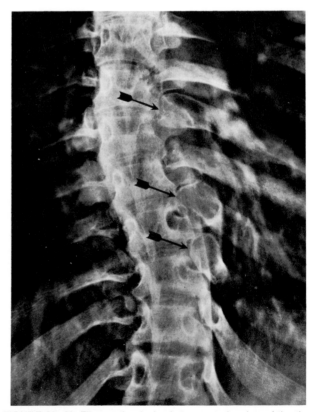

FIGURE 92–42. Fibrous dysplasia: Anteroposterior view of the thoracic spine in a 14 year old boy. The vertebral column is more likely to be involved in polyostotic than in monostotic fibrous dysplasia. The dysplastic bone per se, as well as multiple fractures owing to poorly tolerated mechanical stresses, results in both primary and secondary scolioses. Note several lucent expansile lesions involving the left posterior ribs at the costovertebral junctions (arrows).

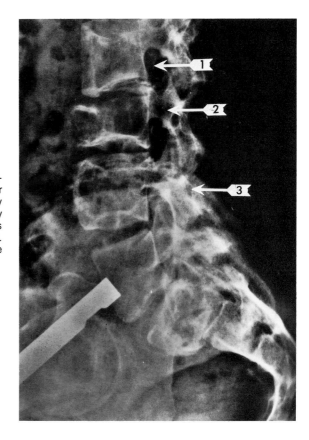

FIGURE 92–43. Fibrous dysplasia: Lateral view of the lumbar spine. Vertebral involvement may take the form of deformed vertebral bodies or posterior elements having a "ground glass" appearance (arrow 1) or clearer, purely radiolucent lesions having a "cystic" appearance. The latter most frequently contain a rubbery, fibrous tissue that does not weaken bone (arrow 3) as much as do actual cystic, fluid-filled cavities, which also have been noted. The last-mentioned cysts have been presumed to be related to hemorrhage or ischemia and are more prone to compression and collapse (arrow 2).

to an intrinsic femoral lesion commonly produces a severe coxa vara abnormality referred to as a "shepherd's crook" deformity, which is a characteristic stigma of the disease (Fig. 92–47). Overgrowth or undergrowth of bones and adjacent soft tissues also may occur and on radiographs may resemble superficially the changes in neurofibromatosis. Leg length discrepancies may, therefore, reflect abnormalities in shape, modeling, and linear growth as well as asymmetry secondary to fracture.

Fractures frequently follow minor injuries. They seldom are displaced, however, and generally heal within a normal time period with identifiable callus formation. Stress (insufficiency) fractures, although more difficult to detect with conventional radiographic techniques, also are encountered. Bone scintigraphy in such cases is characterized by increased accumulation of radiopharmaceutical agent at the fracture site. Owing to the intrinsic hypervascularity of fibrous dysplasia per se, however, and the fact that osteomyelitis and a variety of benign and malignant lesions show similar patterns of increased activity, radionuclide bone scanning remains nonspecific in the diagnosis of fibrous dysplasia or any of its complications, and the scintigraphic abnormalities must be correlated with other imaging data and with clinical findings.

The radiographic features of fibrous dysplasia in metacarpal and metatarsal bones and phalanges are similar to those encountered in the long tubular bones (Fig. 92–48). An entire short tubular bone occasionally may be involved with evidence of the typical "ground glass" appearance and either complete loss of modeling or mild expansion with or without cortical thinning.

Other Skeletal Sites. Among additional osseous sites, the ribs and innominate bones are affected most commonly, whereas the clavicle, scapula, sacrum, and carpal and tarsal bones are involved only occasionally. Of diagnostic importance, fibrous dysplasia is the most frequently occurring benign lesion of the rib cage, representing 30 per cent of primary benign chest wall lesions (Figs. 92–49 to 92–51). Rib involvement, although most often innocuous, may be associated with considerable osseous expansion and deformity as well as with extraosseous extension of dysplastic tissue. This last finding has been held responsible for disabling restrictive pulmonary involvement with accompanying hypoxia, pulmonary hypertension, and cardiac failure.[138] Unilateral, fusiform enlargement of one or more ribs is characteristic of fibrous dysplasia. This unilateral distribution, despite the presence of polyostotic involvement, serves as a means of distinction from other diseases, such as hyperparathyroidism and skeletal metastases, that characteristically are disseminated more widely throughout the skeleton.

Unilateral or asymmetric, bilateral involvement of the innominate bones is a frequent eventuality in polyostotic fibrous dysplasia, but it usually is associated with concomitant disease in the proximal portion of the femur (Fig. 92–52). Acetabular deformity, including protrusion, and a markedly distorted triradiate pelvis often are evident. When polyostotic fibrous dysplasia affects adjacent bones, pelvic involvement with accompanying acetabular protrusion may result in telescoping of the bones about the hip.

Other Imaging Techniques. CT scanning is extremely useful in defining accurately the full extent and nature of skeletal involvement in fibrous dysplasia, particularly in such complex anatomic areas as the spine, pelvis, and skull. It further demonstrates, often to better advantage than plain films, the characteristically expansile, well-defined osseous lesions of fibrous dysplasia as well as their hazy, amorphous contents and occasionally subtle mineral deposits.

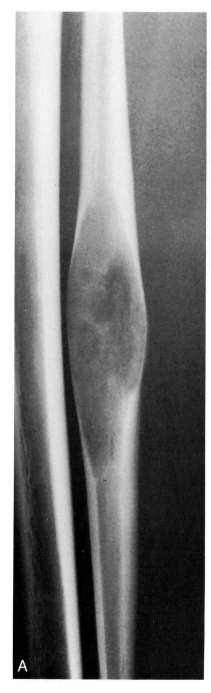

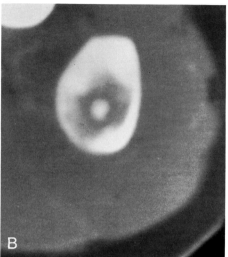

FIGURE 92–44. Fibrous dysplasia. In a 14 year old boy, a monostotic lesion in the diaphysis of the fibula **(A)** is centrally located, hazy in appearance, well marginated, and slightly expansile. Transaxial CT **(B)** confirms its central location, cortical thinning, and internal calcification. Excision of the lesion confirmed the preoperative diagnosis of fibrous dysplasia. (Courtesy of G. Greenway, M.D., Dallas, Texas.)

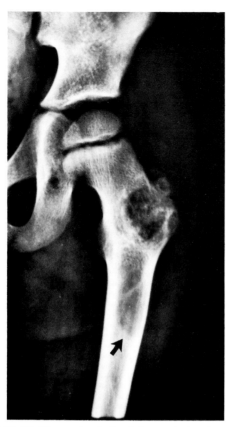

FIGURE 92–45. Fibrous dysplasia: Anteroposterior view of the femur. The hazy, irregularly contoured, but well-defined lesion typically is situated in the diametaphysis. Note the partially calcified osseous matrix and the sclerotic rim of the proximal portion of the lesion. Its lowermost extension has an entirely lucent bladelike configuration, which is not as well demarcated (arrow).

CT also permits a more objective evaluation of a bone lesion by means of measurements of attenuation coefficients. Usually in the range of 70 to 130 Hounsfield units, these coefficients may be further increased by intralesional calcification or ossification, whereas disorders such as osteomyelitis or eosinophilic granuloma more often display lower attenuation values, ranging from 20 to 40 Hounsfield units. CT is likewise indispensable for the accurate delineation of large lesions. Those associated with extraosseous soft tissue components are particularly significant as they

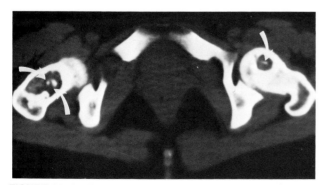

FIGURE 92–46. Fibrous dysplasia: Transaxial CT of the hips. The right femoral neck and left femoral head harbor sharply demarcated, radiolucent lesions with internal calcifications (arrows). The lesion on the right, bordered by a thick sclerotic rind, is associated with a shepherd's crook deformity.

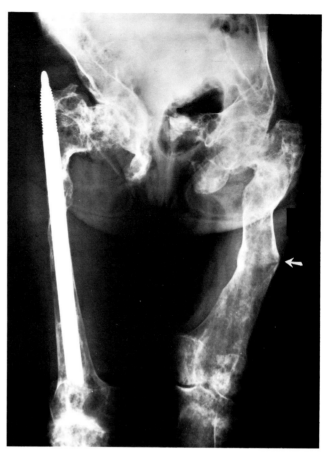

FIGURE 92–47. Fibrous dysplasia: Anteroposterior view of the pelvis and femora. Polyostotic involvement is seen in a 20 year old woman with McCune-Albright syndrome and a history of multiple fractures and surgical interventions. Note the severe pelvic distortion and bilateral proximal femoral varus deformities, the so-called shepherd's crook deformities. The femoral shafts are poorly modeled, with an intrinsic hazy, lucent appearance and little sclerosis or lesional calcification. The entire shafts, including the bone ends, are affected. There is an acute angulation at the site of a previously healed fracture (arrow).

may impinge on vital neighboring structures and occasionally are suspected erroneously of having undergone malignant transformation.

MR imaging also can be applied to the assessment of fibrous dysplasia. In common with CT, MR imaging allows analysis of the full extent of the process, both in spinal (Fig. 92–53) and in extraspinal sites. The signal intensity characteristics of fibrous dysplasia are variable. Although, typically, areas of involvement are of low signal intensity in T1-weighted spin echo MR images, low, intermediate (Fig. 92–54), or high (Fig. 92–55) signal intensity may be evident in T2-weighted spin echo MR images. In some cases, irregular regions of low signal intensity about an area of high signal intensity may be apparent in the T2-weighted spin echo images. The degree of enhancement of signal intensity after the intravenous administration of gadolinium-based contrast agents also is variable (Fig. 92–56).

Natural History. The prognosis in fibrous dysplasia generally depends on the extent and degree of initial skeletal involvement as well as on extraskeletal features. Monostotic involvement is not usually converted to polyostotic disease, and, in most instances, the size and number of

Text continued on page 4390

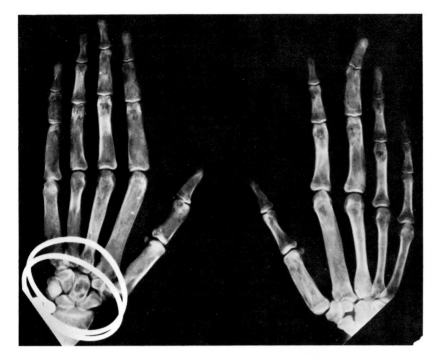

FIGURE 92–48. Fibrous dysplasia: Posteroanterior view of the hands. Expansion of the spongiosa, cortical thinning, and alteration of bone texture are common radiographic findings in affected tubular bones. This 16 year old girl had widespread failure of modeling with abnormal angulation and localized overgrowth of bones and soft tissues. Several metacarpal bones and phalanges have rectangular or fusiform shapes, with a loss of definition between medullary and cortical bone. The hazy or "ground glass" appearance is particularly uniform in the second metacarpal bones. Localized radiolucent lesions with endosteal scalloping and areas of medullary sclerosis also are seen in several phalanges.

FIGURE 92–49. Fibrous dysplasia: Anteroposterior view of the rib. This solitary, expansile, multilocular-appearing lesion with an intact cortex was an incidental finding on a chest film of a teen-age boy. The likeliest cause of such a focal rib lesion is fibrous dysplasia. Rib lesions more commonly are associated with prominent fibrous replacement of bone and therefore commonly are radiolucent.

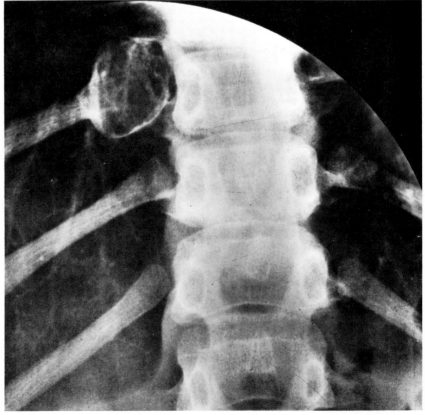

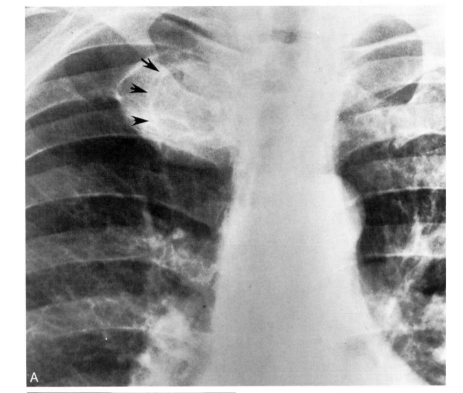

FIGURE 92–50. Fibrous dysplasia.

A Posteroanterior view of the chest in a 45 year old man. A hazy, expansile lesion with a sclerotic lateral margin and internal curvilinear calcifications (arrows) involves the posteromedial aspect of the right fourth rib at its costovertebral junction.

B Transaxial CT scan of the ribs. The lesion's amorphous, generally homogeneous internal architecture, medial calcific deposits, and thin rim of unmineralized matrix extending laterally beyond a circumferentially sclerotic rim (arrows) are defined.

C ^{99m}Tc-methylene diphosphonate bone scan. The lesion concentrates the radionuclide intensely.

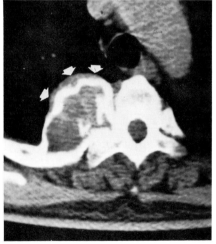

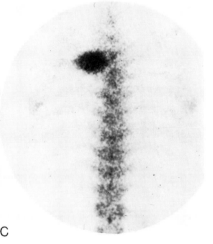

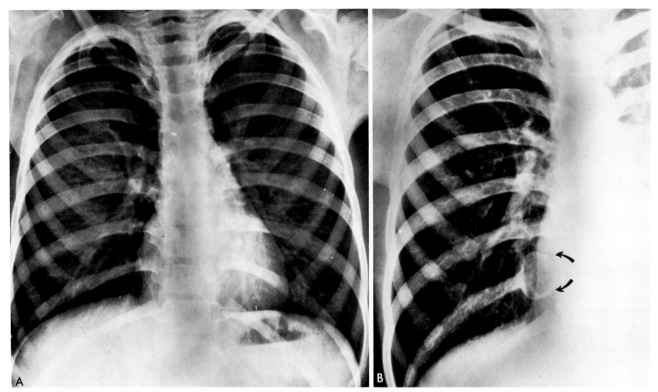

FIGURE 92–51. Fibrous dysplasia: De novo appearance in the rib of an asymptomatic patient.
   A Posteroanterior view of the chest. Note normal rib cage at 8 years of age.
   B Posteroanterior view of the chest obtained 5 years later. Note the expansile lesion of the right tenth rib, discovered as an incidental finding at 13 years of age. The lesion is hazy in appearance and sharply outlined by an attenuated but intact cortex (arrows).
   (Courtesy of W. B. Seaman, M.D., New York, New York.)

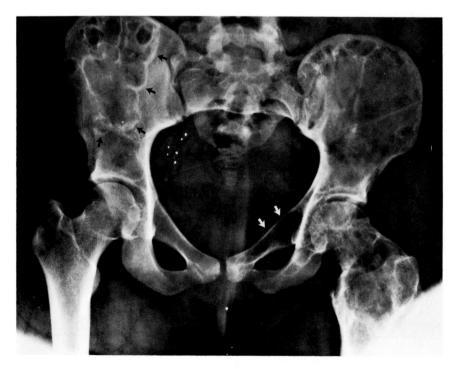

FIGURE 92–52. Fibrous dysplasia: Anteroposterior view of the pelvis in a 16 year old girl with polyostotic fibrous dysplasia and McCune-Albright syndrome. The dysplasia has resulted in a thickened, fore-shortened femoral neck and shaft held in varus position (a shepherd's crook deformity). Note the hazy, "ground glass" appearance of the involved left femur, with relative sparing of the femoral head. The left pubis and both ilia also are involved by radiographically typical lesions of fibrous dysplasia. The purely radiolucent pubic lesion is expansile and nonmineralized (white arrows). The central segments of the right iliac locus are hazy and smoky in appearance owing to a high proportion of osteoid and are well demarcated by an almost continuous curvilinear sclerotic rim (black arrows).

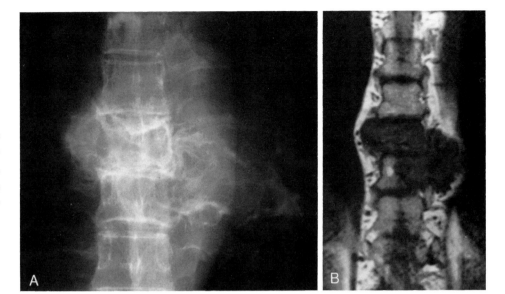

FIGURE 92–53. Fibrous dysplasia: MR imaging abnormalities.

A A routine radiograph shows osteolysis and bone expansion of two contiguous thoracic vertebrae and adjacent ribs.

B A coronal T1-weighted (TR/TE, 800/20) spin echo MR image reveals the extent of the process, which is of low signal intensity.

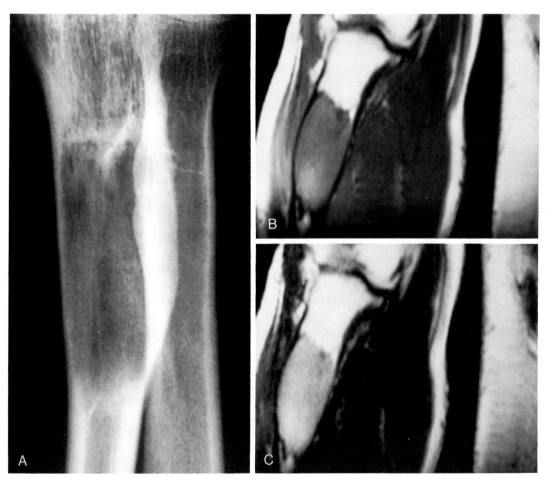

FIGURE 92–54. Fibrous dysplasia: MR imaging abnormalities.

A A routine radiograph shows a slightly expansile, osteolytic lesion in the proximal portion of the ulna.

B, C Coronal proton density (TR/TE, 1200/20) **(B)** and T2-weighted (TR/TE, 1200/70) **(C)** MR images reveal the expansile lesion. It is of low signal intensity in **B** and intermediate signal intensity in **C**.

(Courtesy of C. Sebrechts, M.D., San Diego, California.)

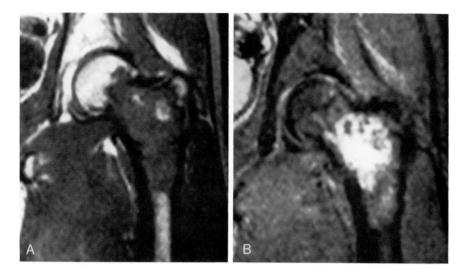

FIGURE 92–55. Fibrous dysplasia: MR imaging abnormalities. In this patient with a lesion in the proximal portion of the femur, a coronal T1-weighted (TR/TE, 786/30) spin echo MR image **(A)** reveals a lesion of inhomogeneous but mainly low signal intensity. The femoral head is not involved. A coronal T2-weighted (TR/TE, 2000/80) spin echo MR image **(B)** shows increased signal intensity in the lesion. Note peripheral nodular regions of low signal intensity.

skeletal lesions do not increase from those noted on the initial radiographic evaluation.[129] Exceptions to these rules have been documented occasionally, however, including extension of an existing lesion to another segment of an involved bone[139] or the appearance of new lesions in additional bones. Although both polyostotic and monostotic fibrous dysplasia generally become quiescent at puberty and remain so throughout the remainder of life, in some instances progressive deformity supervenes, particularly when extensive fibrous dysplasia occurs early in life. In such cases, fractures are common, deformity is severe, and ultimate prognosis is poor. Conversely, initially limited disease usually is associated with slow progression and a favorable prognosis independent of the age of onset.[130] Reac-

tivation of skeletal lesions in fibrous dysplasia also has been noted during the course of pregnancy and estrogen therapy.

Malignant Degeneration. Malignant transformation of skeletal lesions is a rare complication of fibrous dysplasia, with an estimated frequency ranging from 0.4 to 1 per cent in fewer than 50 reported cases.[140–144] Less than half of such cases occurred in patients with polyostotic fibrous dysplasia. In many presumed examples, prior radiation to involved bones has complicated accurate determination of spontaneous malignant degeneration.

In monostotic fibrous dysplasia, malignant transformation is noted most often in the skull and facial bones, whereas in polyostotic disease the femur and facial bones are affected most frequently. Osteosarcoma and fibrosar-

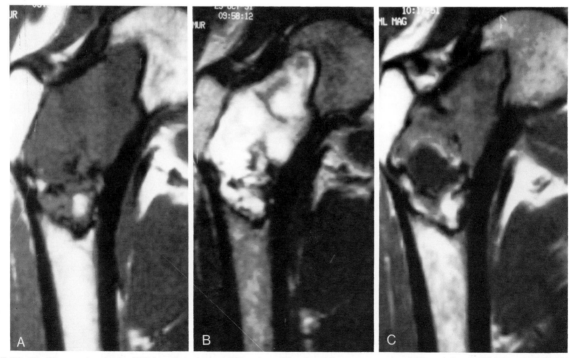

FIGURE 92–56. Fibrous dysplasia: MR imaging abnormalities. In a 50 year old woman, coronal T1-weighted (TR/TE, 500/15) **(A)** and T2-weighted (TR/TE, 2000/80) **(B)** spin echo MR images and a coronal T1-weighted (TR/TE, 500/15) image obtained after the intravenous administration of a gadolinium compound **(C)** are shown. The femoral lesion is of low signal intensity in **A** and inhomogeneous but predominantly of high signal intensity in **B**. Note irregular areas of low signal intensity within the lesion in **B**. Inhomogeneous enhancement of signal intensity is seen in **C**. (Courtesy of J. Kramer, M.D., Vienna, Austria.)

coma are the types of tumors that have been encountered most often. Although chondrosarcoma reputedly occurs less frequently, its recognition is particularly difficult in view of the intrinsic cartilaginous islands or nodules that frequently coexist with fibrous dysplasia and that may lead to an erroneous diagnosis of low-grade chondrosarcoma, particularly in cases with polyostotic disease. The significance of radiographic evidence of calcification in fibrous dysplasia (of the type associated with cartilage), rather than being indicative of potential malignancy, more often is prognostic of further deformity, particularly at the time of the adolescent growth spurt.

The elapsed time between the diagnosis of fibrous dysplasia and that of malignancy has been variable but is most often cited in years or even decades. Clinically, pain and swelling accompanied by such radiographic changes as poorly defined areas of osteolysis, cortical destruction, and soft tissue masses in the vicinity of disrupted cortices have been regarded as highly suggestive of malignant transformation.

Pathologic Abnormalities. The relatively radiolucent or radiopaque areas appreciated on radiographs, classically described as of milky or "ground glass" appearance, reflect the relative amounts of fibrous and osseous tissue in a specific lesion at a particular time. Trabeculae of woven bone, which may be well mineralized, although irregular in size and shape, are embedded haphazardly within a largely fibrous collagenous matrix and contribute to the overall generalized haziness of the characteristic lesion. Conversely, predominantly fibrous zones appear more radiolucent. Some lesions additionally exhibit focal, fluid-filled areas attributed to degeneration and cellular necrosis. If large enough, they appear markedly radiolucent, often simulating cystic lesions on radiographs.

Grossly, the masses of dysplastic tissue usually appear solid and are gritty or sandy to the touch. Microscopically, lesions are composed of varying sized, irregular ossicles of woven bone scattered throughout a fibrocellular matrix rich in alkaline phosphatase. The trabeculae characteristically are not rimmed by osteoblasts, an important feature in the histologic differentiation of fibrous dysplasia from ossifying fibroma (see Chapter 83).

Cartilage islands or nodules, which usually occupy only small segments of a lesion, occur in at least 10 per cent of cases but are less well known constituents of fibrous dysplasia.[145] Recognition of such cartilaginous foci, however, is of vital importance, because their degree of cellularity and nuclear atypia, particularly when calcified, may strongly suggest chondrosarcoma both radiologically and pathologically. The suggested sources of these foci have included callus formation secondary to fracture, cartilaginous rests, particularly near the growth plate, and coexisting enchondromatosis. Indeed, several cases of fibrous dysplasia with such benign cartilaginous inclusions have been reported under such designations as fibrocartilaginous dysplasia and fibrochondrodysplasia, which may lead to their being considered evidence of quasi-independent entities rather than minor constituents of the basic lesion of fibrous dysplasia itself.[143, 146, 147]

Endocrine Abnormalities

Fibrous dysplasia has no sexual predilection. The greater the number of polyostotic cases included in any review of

the disease, the greater the likelihood of a female bias. Its characteristically associated endocrinopathy, the McCune-Albright syndrome, predominates in girls and classically consists of polyostotic fibrous dysplasia, cutaneous pigmentation, and precocious sexual development. Not all patients with fibrous dysplasia characterized by polyostotic disease and cutaneous pigmentation, however, exhibit sexual precocity or endocrine disturbance. Furthermore, incomplete forms of the syndrome include sexual precocity and osseous lesions in the absence of cutaneous pigmentation.

Sexual precocity, rare in boys, occurs in 30 to 50 per cent of girls and is characterized by the early appearance of vaginal bleeding, breast development, and axillary and pubic hair. The gynecomastia associated with fibrous dysplasia in boys is of uncertain cause.[139, 148] The term sexual precocity or precocious pseudopuberty is preferred over that of precocious puberty[149, 150] because puberty implies mature gonadal function.[117, 122, 139, 148, 151, 152] In fact, there have been few documented instances of ovulation,[153] of circulating ovulatory luteinizing hormone, or of testicular biopsies yielding mature spermatozoa in patients with this syndrome. Precocious puberty has, therefore, not been substantiated adequately in many of the presumptive cases of McCune-Albright syndrome.[149, 150] In this syndrome, the possibility of increased sensitivity of target organs (i.e., gonads and breasts) to normal or minimally elevated prepubertal circulating pituitary hormones has been suggested. Premature vaginal bleeding has, therefore, been explained by early release of or ovarian hypersensitivity to follicle-stimulating hormone. Alternatively, another theory suggesting end-organ autonomy was postulated in a 6 month old girl whose vaginal bleeding ceased after removal of a functioning luteinized ovarian cyst.[151, 153] She also had Cushing's syndrome secondary to adrenal nodular hyperplasia. Biochemical evidence supported adrenal and gonadal autonomy and refuted hyperfunction mediated by the hypothalamic-pituitary axis.

Additional pluriglandular involvement has long been recognized in polyostotic fibrous dysplasia, including Cushing's disease, acromegaly, hyperthyroidism, hyperparathyroidism, and extrainsular hypothalamic diabetes mellitus.[125, 126, 149, 150, 154, 155] Albright, noting a variety of associated endocrinopathies, initially stressed end-organ sensitivity as a cause, whereas other authors subsequently maintained that hypersecretion of hypothalamic releasing hormones was responsible.[154] Such hypersecretion, however, generally has not been substantiated, neither in the hyperthyroidism with toxic nodular goiter that occurs in 5 to 30 per cent of cases[155] nor in many of the early reported cases of reputed acromegaly or Cushing's syndrome that have failed to satisfy modern endocrinologic criteria.[156] Some of these clinical diagnoses also must be regarded with caution because acromegalic facies, the exophthalmos of Graves' disease, and visual defects suggesting a pituitary tumor all may be mimicked by facial and skeletal involvement in fibrous dysplasia alone.

It is noteworthy that even in the absence of overt sexual precocity, apparent hormonal disturbances have been reflected in advanced skeletal maturation and accelerated linear growth, with or without subsequent premature closure of the physes. Such altered growth, particularly when predominantly unilateral in distribution, may lead to profound isolated deformities or marked, multicentric distortions in skeletal architecture that are, in themselves, classic hallmarks of polyostotic fibrous dysplasia.

Although pituitary nodularity and hyperplasia have been said to exist in fibrous dysplasia, frank tumors have not been documented consistently. The significance of demonstrations by CT and ultrasonography of presumed pituitary and ovarian structural abnormalities remains uncertain, because CT standards for endocrinologically normal subjects have yet to be established.[127] The observed "pituitary prominence" may, in fact, represent physiologic enlargement of the normal prepubertal gland. Discoveries of single and multiple adenomas in the pituitary, adrenal, thyroid, and parathyroid glands, however, in addition to hyperplasia of target organs, lend support to the thesis of glandular autonomy and strengthen the hypothesis of an existing variant of multiple endocrine adenomatosis.[125, 126]

Therefore, the association of endocrinopathies in fibrous dysplasia, with or without a concomitant McCune-Albright syndrome, has been explained by two major theories. One contends that congenital hypothalamic dysfunction with hypersecretion of releasing hormones results in increased stimulation of target organs.[154] The other theory postulates an underlying form of multiple endocrine neoplasia with autonomous function of involved endocrine glands.[126]

A new, third suggested unifying mechanism explaining the autonomous hyperfunction of multiple endocrine systems in the McCune-Albright syndrome has implicated a mutation in the alpha subunit of a Gs protein.[178–181] Such mutations have been found in isolated growth hormone–secreting pituitary tumors and in thyroid nodules,[182] both of which occur in the McCune-Albright syndrome. The mutation in Gs alpha (arginine-201) to either histidine or cysteine serves to attenuate Gs alpha GTPase activity and activates adenylate cyclase. The mutation has been found in virtually all affected tissues of patients with the McCune-Albright syndrome, including the ovary, testis, adrenal, pituitary, and thyroid glands, skin, and bones, and it is present in various degrees in different tissues of the same patient.[178–182] Somatic mosaicism of the Gs alpha gene also can account for the varying sites and degrees of involvement of different tissues in different patients, with some having gonadal involvement alone and others exhibiting severe multisystemic disease. Gs alpha activating mutations also occur in nonendocrine tissues and in the liver, gastrointestinal tract, and heart. In McCune-Albright syndrome they have been associated with chronic hepatitis, intestinal polyps, and cardiac arrhythmias.[181]

Sexual precocity in the McCune-Albright syndrome initially was thought erroneously to occur exclusively in girls. To date, about 100 cases have been described in girls,[178] and approximately 12 cases have been described in boys. Analysis of the Gs alpha gene in five testicular biopsies revealed the expected mutation in all cases.[180]

Other Abnormalities

Hypophosphatemic rickets and osteomalacia have been noted in patients with either monostotic or polyostotic fibrous dysplasia, both with and without the McCune-Albright syndrome.[157, 158] Clinical signs and symptoms, which have included skeletal pain, tenderness, and osseous deformity, have been documented in association with pertinent biochemical abnormalities. The findings are analogous to those seen when rickets and osteomalacia accompany neoplastic disorders of bone or soft tissue (see Chapter 53). In these instances, as well as in fibrous dysplasia, resection of the lesion may be followed by disappearance of the findings of rickets or osteomalacia. The synthesis of a phosphaturic hormone by a concomitant bone or soft tissue tumor or by benign fibrous lesions, such as fibrous dysplasia, has been one hypothesis developed to explain the associated metabolic disorder.

SUMMARY

In view of the many ramifications of all of these syndromes, prompt and proper identification of tuberous sclerosis, neurofibromatosis, and fibrous dysplasia cannot be overemphasized. The advantages that accrue from early recognition include not only the anticipation, prevention, and treatment of some of their associated disorders and complications but also the use of genetic planning where applicable.

Tuberous sclerosis represents a widespread aberration, which begins during embryonic life and which may involve all germ layers. Its classic clinical triad consists of epileptic seizures, mental retardation, and skin lesions.

Neurofibromatosis, previously characterized by a classic clinical triad consisting of cutaneous lesions, mental deficiency, and skeletal deformities, now has been reclassified into several subtypes. When stipulated components are present, or when patients with classic neurofibromatosis have a variety of other lesions in addition to the triad, diagnosis is not difficult. Less familiar lesions, however, although recognized individually, may not be recognized as "part and parcel" of the neurofibromatosis complex, particularly when they may constitute the patient's initial or major complaint.

Fibrous dysplasia is a disorder of heretofore unknown causation in which the skeleton represents a prominent target tissue. A variety of endocrine abnormalities, including the McCune-Albright syndrome, may accompany the osseous abnormalities. As in the other two disorders, accurate appraisal of both the osseous and the extraosseous components of fibrous dysplasia is mandatory.

Recognition of all facets of these three diseases, including their unusual manifestations, is important in view of rapid advances being made in basic laboratory and clinical imaging technology. New biomolecular techniques have prompted new classifications of many phakomatoses on the basis of underlying chromosomal abnormalities, such that insight into the category of disease into which a particular clinical manifestation belongs, whether suggested or confirmed by modern imaging methods, takes on new importance. This is particularly true of MR imaging, which now, in a noninvasive fashion, allows detection of numerous subtle central neurologic manifestations of several of the phakomatoses. Because of such detection, genetic counseling and prenatal testing are made more immediately effective to parents and siblings of affected children.[183] Moreover, new surgical and enzymatic therapies of metabolic, endocrine, and neurologic disorders associated with many of the phakomatoses require accurate recognition and categorization of presenting clinical manifestations before they can be applied. Tuberous sclerosis, neurofibromatosis, and fibrous dysplasia all are diseases that greatly benefit from modern imaging technology.

References

1. Bourneville DM: Contribution à l'étude de l'idiotie. Arch Neurol *1*:69, 1880.
2. Bunde S: The significance of a white macule on the skin of a child. Dev Med Child Neurol *12*:805, 1970.
3. Medley BE, McLeod RA, Houser OW: Tuberous sclerosis. Semin Roentgenol *11*:35, 1976.
4. Critchley M, Earl CJC: Tuberose sclerosis and allied conditions. Brain 55:311, 1932.
5. Thibault JH, Manuelidis EE: Tuberous sclerosis in a premature infant. Report of a case and review of the literature. Neurology 20:139, 1970.
6. Lagos JC, Holman CB, Gomez MR: Tuberous sclerosis: Neuroroentgenologic observations. AJR *104*:171, 1968.
7. Bender BL, Yunis EJ: The pathology of tuberous sclerosis. Pathol Annu *17*:339, 1982.
8. Hurwitz S, Braverman IM: White spots in tuberous sclerosis. J Pediatr 77:587, 1970.
9. Fitzpatrick TB, Szabó G, Hori Y, et al: White leaf-shaped macules: Earliest visible signs of tuberous sclerosis. Arch Dermatol 98:1, 1968.
10. Gold AP, Freeman JM: Depigmented nevi: The earliest sign of tuberous sclerosis. Pediatrics 35:1003, 1965.
11. Terada T, Nakai E, Moriwaki H, et al: Tuberous sclerosis with an atypical radiologic skull change: Case report. Neurosurgery *16*:804, 1985.
12. Fitz CR, Harwood-Nash DCF, Thompson JR: Neuroradiology of tuberous sclerosis in children. Radiology *110*:635, 1974.
13. Gardeur D, Palmiere A, Mashaly R: Cranial computed tomography in the phakomatoses. Neuroradiology 25:292, 1983.
14. Khangure MS: Intraventricular brain tumors associated with tuberous sclerosis: Clinical and radiographic characteristics. Australas Radiol 27:115, 1983.
15. Charlot-Charles J, Jones GW: Renal antiomyolipoma associated with tuberous sclerosis. Review of the literature. Urology *3*:465, 1974.
16. Frank LM, Chaves-Carballo E, Earley L: Early diagnosis of tuberous sclerosis by cranial ultrasonography. Arch Neurol *41*:1302, 1984.
17. Legge M, Sauerbrei E, Macdonald A: Intracranial tuberous sclerosis in infancy. Radiology *153*:667, 1984.
18. Wilson RD, Hall JG, McGillivray BC: Tuberous sclerosis: Case report and investigation of family members. J Can Med Assoc *132*:807, 1985.
19. Green GJ: The radiology of tuberose sclerosis. Clin Radiol *19*:135, 1968.
20. Brown B: The radiologic features of bone changes in tuberous sclerosis with a case report. J Can Assoc Radiol *12*:1, 1961.
21. Whitaker PH: Radiological manifestations in tuberose sclerosis. Br J Radiol *32*:152, 1959.
22. Komar NN, Gabrielsen TO, Holt JF: Roentgenographic appearance of lumbosacral spine and pelvis in tuberous sclerosis. Radiology 89:701, 1967.
23. Ashby DW, Ramage D: Lesions of the vertebrae and innominate bones in tuberous sclerosis. Br J Radiol *30*:274, 1957.
24. Nathanson N, Avnet NL: An unusual x-ray finding in tuberous sclerosis. Br J Radiol *39*:786, 1966.
25. Madigan RR, Wallace SL: Scoliosis associated with tuberous sclerosis. J Tenn Med Assoc 74:643, 1981.
26. Elkin M, Bernstein J: Cystic diseases of the kidney. Clin Radiol 20:65, 1969.
27. Mitnick JS, Bosniak MA, Hilton S, et al: Cystic renal disease in tuberous sclerosis. Radiology *147*:85, 1983.
28. Beal S, Delaney P: Tuberous sclerosis with intracranial aneurysms. Arch Neurol *40*:826, 1983.
29. Flynn PM, Robinson MB, Stapleton FB, et al: Coarctation of the aorta and renal artery stenosis in tuberous sclerosis. Pediatr Radiol *14*:337, 1984.
30. Hamburger RJ, Clark JE, Moran JJ, et al: Symptomatic benign renal mesenchymoma. A case necessitating bilateral nephrectomy. Arch Intern Med *120*:78, 1967.
31. Viamonte M Jr, Ravel R, Politano V, et al: Angiographic findings in a patient with tuberous sclerosis. AJR 98:723, 1966.
32. Potter EL: Pathology of the Fetus and the Infant. 2nd Ed. Chicago, Year Book Medical Publishers, 1961, p 441.
33. Kidder LA: Congenital glycogenic tumors of the heart. Arch Pathol *49*:55, 1950.
34. Diamant S, Sharaz J, Holtzman M, et al: Echocardiographic diagnosis of cardiac tumors in symptomatic tuberous sclerosis patients. Clin Pediatr 22:297, 1983.
35. Fenoglio J, McAllister A, Ferrans J: Cardiac rhabdomyoma: A clinical and electron microscopic study. Am J Cardiol *38*:241, 1976.
36. Aughenbaugh GL: Thoracic manifestations of neurocutaneous diseases. Radiol Clin North Am 22:741, 1984.
37. Babcock TL, Snyder BA: Spontaneous pneumothorax associated with tuberous sclerosis. J Thorac Cardiovasc Surg 83:100, 1982.
38. Dwyer JM, Hickie JB, Gravan J: Pulmonary tuberous sclerosis: Report of three patients and a review of the literature. Q J Med *40*:115, 1971.
39. Malik SK, Pardee N, Martin CJ: Involvement of the lungs in tuberous sclerosis. Chest 58:538, 1970.
40. Sareen CK, Ruvalcaba RHA, Scotvold MJ, et al: Tuberous sclerosis. Am J Dis Child *123*:34, 1972.
41. Crowe FW, Schull WJ, Neel JV: A Clinical, Pathological and Genetic Study of Multiple Neurofibromatosis. Springfield, Ill, Charles C Thomas, 1956.
42. Steg NL, Wong AKC, Bogel MS, et al: The potential of computerized dermatoglyphia analyses as demonstrated through studies of patients with myelomeningoceles and neurofibromatosis. *In* D Bergsma, RB Lawrey (Eds): Numerical Taxonomy of Birth Defects and Polygenic Disorders. New York, Alan R Liss, 1977, p 158.
43. Ricciardi VM, Dobson CE, Chakraborty R, et al: The pathophysiology of neurofibromatosis. Am J Med Genet *18*:169, 1984.
44. Tiresius TWC: Historia Pathologica Singularis Cutis Turpitudinis. Leipzig, SL Crusius, 1793.
45. Smith RW: A Treatise on the Pathology, Diagnosis and Treatment of Neuroma. Dublin, Hodges & Smith, 1849.
46. Virchow R: Die krankhaften Geschwülste. Berlin, A Hirschwald, 1863. Vol 3, p 233.
47. Payne JF: Multiple neurofibromata in connection with molluscum fibrosum. Trans Pathol Soc Lond *38*:69, 1887.
48. von Recklinghausen K: Uber die multiplen Fibrome der Haut und ihre Beziehung zu den multiplen Neuromen. Berlin, A Hirschwald, 1882.
49. Fialkow PJ, Sagebeil RW, Gartler SM, et al: Multiple cell origin of hereditary neurofibromas. N Engl J Med *284*:298, 1971.
50. Hope DG, Mulvihill JJ: Malignancy in Neurofibromatosis. Adv Neurol 29:33, 1981.
51. Ricciardi VM: Von Recklinghausen neurofibromatosis. N Engl J Med *305*:1617, 1981.
52. Schenkein I, Bueker ED, Helson L, et al: Increased nerve-growth-stimulating activity in disseminated neurofibromatosis. N Engl J Med *290*:613, 1974.
53. Riopelle RJ, Ricciardi VM, Faulkner S, et al: Serum neuronal growth factor levels in von Recklinghausen's neurofibromatosis. Ann Neurol *16*:54, 1984.
54. Peltonen J, Foidart M, Aho HJ: Type IV and V collagens in von Recklinghausen's neurofibromas. Virchows Arch (Cell Pathol) *47*:291, 1984.
55. Norris JFB, Smith AG, Fletcher PJH, et al: Neurofibromatosis dermal hypoplasia: A clinical, pharmacological and ultrastructural study. Br J Dermatol *112*:435, 1985.
56. Perry H, Font R: Iris nodules in von Recklinghausen's neurofibromatosis. Arch Ophthalmol *100*:1635, 1982.
57. Burrows EH: Bone changes in orbital neurofibromatosis. Br J Radiol *36*:549, 1963.
58. Hunt JC, Pugh DG: Skeletal lesions in neurofibromatosis. Radiology *76*:1, 1961.
59. Seaman WB, Furlow LT: Anomalies of the bony orbit. AJR *71*:51, 1954.
60. Klatte EC, Franken EA, Smith JA: The radiographic spectrum in neurofibromatosis. Semin Roentgenol *11*:17, 1976.
61. Zatz LM: Atypical choroid plexus calcifications associated with neurofibromatosis. Radiology *91*:1135, 1968.
62. Leeds NE, Jacobson HG: Spinal neurofibromatosis. AJR *126*:617, 1976.
63. Levin B: Neurofibromatosis: Clinical and roentgen manifestations. Radiology *71*:48, 1958.
64. Meszaros WT, Guzzo F, Schorsch H: Neurofibromatosis. AJR *98*:557, 1966.
65. Crawford AH Jr, Bogamery N: Osseous manifestations of neurofibromatosis in childhood. J Pediatr Orthop *6*:72, 1986.
66. Benedict PH, Szabo G, Fitzpatrick TB, et al: Melanotic macules in Albright's syndrome and in neurofibromatosis. JAMA *205*:618, 1968.
67. Hsu LCS, Lee PC, Leong JCY: Dystrophic spinal deformities in neurofibromatosis. J Bone Joint Surg [Br] *66*:495, 1984.
68. Winter RB, Moe JH, Bradford DS, et al: Spine deformity in neurofibromatosis. J Bone Joint Surg [Am] *61*:677, 1979.
69. Gregg PJ, Price BA, Ellis HA, et al: Pseudoarthrosis of the radius associated with neurofibromatosis. Clin Orthop *171*:175, 1982.
70. Ostrowski DM, Eilert RE, Waldstein G: Congenital pseudoarthrosis of ulna: Cases and review of literature. J Pediatr Orthop *5*:463, 1985.
71. Morrissy RT: Congenital pseudarthrosis of the tibia. Clin Orthop *166*:14, 1982.
72. Angtuaco EJ, Binet EF, Flanigan S: Value of CT myelography in neurofibromatosis. Neurosurgery *13*:668, 1983.
73. Beggs I, Shaw DG, Brenton DP, et al: An unusual case of neurofibromatosis: Cystic bone lesions and coarctation of the aortic arch. Br J Radiol *54*:416, 1981.
74. Huson SM, Thrush DC: Central neurofibromatosis. Q J Med *218*:213, 1985.
75. Stern J, Jokahuc FA, Housepian EM: The architecture of optic nerve glioma with or without neurofibromatosis. Arch Ophthalmol 98:505, 1980.
76. Isu T, Miyasaka K, Abe H, et al: Atlantoaxial dislocation associated with neurofibromatosis. J Neurosurg *58*:451, 1983.
77. Patronas NJ, Zelkowitz M, Levin K: Ventricular dilatation in neurofibromatosis. J Comput Assist Tomogr *6*:598, 1982.
78. Treves F: Congenital deformity. Br Med J *2*:1140, 1884.
79. Weichert KA, Dine MS, Benton C, et al: Macrocranium and neurofibromatosis. Radiology *107*:163, 1973.
80. Holt JF, Kuhns LR: Macrocranium and macrencephaly in neurofibromatosis. Skel Radiol *1*:25, 1976.
81. Leone RG, Schatzki SC, Wolpow ER: Neurofibromatosis with extensive intracranial arterial occlusive disease. AJNR *3*:572, 1982.
82. Tomsick TA, Lukin RR, Chambers AA: Neurofibromatosis and intracranial arterial occlusive disease. Neuroradiology *11*:229, 1976.
83. Zochodne D: Von Recklinghausen's vasculopathy. AM J Med Sci *287*:64, 1984.

84. Paling MR: Plexiform neurofibroma of the pelvis in neurofibromatosis: CT findings. J Comput Assist Tomogr 8:476, 1984.
85. Clark RD, Hutter JJ Jr: Familial neurofibromatosis and juvenile chronic myelogenous leukemia. Hum Genet 60:230, 1982.
86. Weiner MA, Harris MB, Siegel RB, et al: Ganglioneuroma and acute lymphoblastic leukemia in association with neurofibromatosis. Am J Dis Child 136:1090, 1982.
87. D'Agostino AN, Soule EH, Miller RH: Sarcomas of the peripheral nerves and somatic soft tissues associated with multiple neurofibromatosis (von Recklinghausen's disease). Cancer 16:1015, 1963.
88. Sands MJ, McDonough MT, Cohen AM, et al: Fatal malignant degeneration in multiple neurofibromatosis. JAMA 233:1381, 1975.
89. Sack GH Jr: Malignant complications of neurofibromatosis. Clin Oncol 9:17, 1983.
90. Daneman A, Mancer K, Sonley M: CT appearance of thickened nerves in neurofibromatosis. AJR 141:899, 1983.
91. Coleman B, Arger PH, Dalinka MK, et al: CT of sarcomatous degeneration in neurofibromatosis. AJR 140:383, 1983.
92. Baker ND, Tchang FK, Greenspan A: Liposarcoma complicating neurofibromatosis. Report of 2 cases. Bull Hosp Joint Dis 42:172, 1982.
93. Dahlin DC: Bone Tumors: General Aspects. 3rd Ed. Springfield, Ill, Charles C Thomas, 1978.
94. Ducatman BS, Scheithauer BW, Dahlin DC: Malignant bone tumors associated with neurofibromatosis. Mayo Clin Proc 58:578, 1983.
95. Hammond JA, Driedger AA: Detection of malignant change in neurofibromatosis by gallium-67 scanning. J Can Med Assoc 119:352, 1978.
96. Fawcett KJ, Dahlin DC: Neurilemmoma of bone. Am J Clin Pathol 47:759, 1967.
97. Holt JF, Dickerson WW: The osseous lesions of tuberous sclerosis. Radiology 58:1, 1952.
98. Kullmann L, Wouters HW: Neurofibromatosis, gigantism, and subperiosteal haematoma. Report of two children with extensive subperiosteal bone formation. J Bone Joint Surg [Br] 54:130, 1972.
99. Pitt MJ, Mosher JF, Edeiken J: Abnormal periosteum and bone in neurofibromatosis. Radiology 103:143, 1972.
100. Yaghmai I, Tafazoli M: Massive subperiosteal hemorrhage in neurofibromatosis. Radiology 122:439, 1977.
101. Locht RC, Huebert HT, McFarland DF: Subperiosteal hemorrhage and cyst formation in neurofibromatosis. Clin Orthop 155:141, 1981.
102. Mandell GA, Dalinka MK, Coleman BG: Fibrous lesions in the lower extremities in neurofibromatosis. AJR 133:1135, 1979.
103. Jaffe HL: Tumors and Tumorous Conditions of the Bones and Joints. Philadelphia, Lea & Febiger, 1958, p 249.
104. Schwartz AM, Ramos RM: Neurofibromatosis and multiple non-ossifying fibromas. AJR 135:617, 1980.
105. Itzchak Y, Katznelson D, Boichis H, et al: Angiographic features of arterial lesions in neurofibromatosis. AJR 122:643, 1974.
106. Rowen M, Dorsey TJ, Kegel SM, et al: Thoracic coarctation associated with neurofibromatosis. Am J Dis Child 129:113, 1975.
107. Nieman HL, Mena E, Holt JF, et al: Neurofibromatosis and congenital heart disease. AJR 122:146, 1974.
108. Hilal SK, Solomon GE, Gold AP, et al: Primary cerebral arterial occlusive disease in children. II. Neurocutaneous syndromes. Radiology 99:87, 1971.
109. Halpern M, Currarino G: Vascular lesions causing hypertension in neurofibromatosis. N Engl J Med 273:248, 1965.
110. Elias DL, Ricketts RR, Smith RB III: Renovascular hypertension complicating neurofibromatosis. Am Surg 51:97, 1985.
111. Kalff V, Shapiro B, Lloyd R, et al: The spectrum of pheochromocytoma in hypertensive patients with neurofibromatosis. Arch Intern Med 142:2092, 1982.
112. Webb WR, Goodman PC: Fibrosing alveolitis in patient with neurofibromatosis. Radiology 122:289, 1977.
113. Daly D, Kaye M, Estrada RL: Neurofibromatosis and hyperparathyroidism—a new syndrome? J Can Med Assoc 103:258, 1970.
114. Hurwitz S: Sipple syndrome. Arch Dermatol 110:139, 1974.
115. Saxena KM: Endocrine manifestations of neurofibromatosis in children. Am J Dis Child 120:265, 1970.
116. Lichtenstein L, Jaffe HL: Fibrous dysplasia of bone: A condition affecting one, several or many bones, the graver cases of which may present abnormal pigmentation of skin, premature sexual development, hyperthyroidism or still other extraskeletal abnormalities. Arch Pathol 33:777, 1942.
117. Warrick CK: Polyostotic fibrous dysplasia—Albright's syndrome. A review of the literature and report of four male cases, two of which were associated with precocious puberty. J Bone Joint Surg [Br] 31:175, 1949.
118. Albright F, Butler AM, Hampton AO, et al: Syndrome characterized by osteitis fibrosa disseminata, areas of pigmentation and endocrine dysfunction with precocious puberty in females. N Engl J Med 216:727, 1937.
119. McCune DJ: Osteitis fibrosa cystica; the case of a 9-year-old girl who also exhibits precocious puberty, multiple pigmentation of the skin and hyperthyroidism. Transaction of the Society for Pediatric Research, Annual Meeting, May 5, 1936. Am J Dis Child 52:743, 1936.
120. Lichtenstein L: Polyostotic fibrous dysplasia. Arch Surg 36:874, 1938.
121. Thannhauser SJ: Neurofibromatosis (von Recklinghausen) and osteitis fibrosa cystica localisata et disseminata (von Recklinghausen). Medicine 23:105, 1944.
122. Warrick CK: Some aspects of polyostotic fibrous dysplasia: Possible hypothesis to account for the associated endocrinological changes. Clin Radiol 24:125, 1973.
123. Firat D, Stutzman L: Fibrous dysplasia of the bone. Review of 24 cases. Am J Med 44:421, 1968.
124. Grabias SL, Campbell CJ: Fibrous dysplasia. Orthop Clin North Am 8:771, 1977.
125. D'Armiento M, Reda G, Camagna A, et al: McCune-Albright syndrome: Evidence for autonomous multiendocrine hyperfunction. J Pediatr 102:584, 1983.
126. DiGeorge AM: Albright syndrome: Is it coming of age? J Pediatr 87:1018, 1975.
127. Rieth KG, Comite F, Shawker TH, et al: Pituitary and ovarian abnormalities demonstrated by CT and ultrasound in children with features of the McCune-Albright syndrome. Radiology 153:389, 1984.
128. Steendijk R: Metabolic bone disease in children. In LV Avioli, SM Krane (Eds): Metabolic Bone Disease. Vol 2, New York, Academic Press, 1978, p 633.
129. Gibson MJ, Middlemiss JH: Fibrous dysplasia of bone. Br J Radiol 44:1, 1971.
130. Harris WH, Dudy HR Jr, Barry RJ: The natural history of fibrous dysplasia. J Bone Joint Surg [Am] 44:207, 1962.
131. Leeds N, Seaman WB: Fibrous dysplasia of the skull and its differential diagnosis. A clinical and roentgenographic study of 46 cases. Radiology 78:570, 1962.
132. Daffner RH, Kirks DR, Gehweiler JA Jr, et al: Computed tomography of fibrous dysplasia. AJR 139:943, 1982.
133. Ito H, Waga S, Sakakura M: Fibrous dysplasia of the skull with increased vascularity in the angiogram. Surg Neurol 23:408, 1985.
134. Lin JP, Goodkins R, Chase NE, et al: The angiographic features of fibrous dysplasia of the skull. Radiology 92:1275, 1969.
135. Matson DD: Neurosurgery of Infancy and Childhood. 2nd Ed. Springfield, Ill, Charles C Thomas, 1969, p 617.
136. Nance FL, Fonseca RJ, Burkes EJ Jr: Technetium bone imaging as an adjunct in the management of fibrous dysplasia. Oral Surg 50:199, 1980.
137. Resnik CS, Liniger JR: Monostotic fibrous dysplasia of the cervical spine: Case report. Radiology 151:49, 1984.
138. King M, Payne WS, Olafsson S, et al: Surgical palliation of respiratory insufficiency secondary to massive exuberant polyostotic fibrous dysplasia of the ribs. Ann Thorac Surg 39:185, 1985.
139. Benedict PH: Endocrine features in Albright's syndrome (fibrous dysplasia of bone). Metabolism 11:30, 1962.
140. Riddell DH: Malignant change in fibrous dysplasia. J Bone Joint Surg [Br] 46:251, 1964.
141. DeSmet A, Travers H, Neff JR: Chondrosarcoma occurring in a patient with polyostotic fibrous dysplasia. Skel Radiol 7:197, 1981.
142. Huvos AG, Higinbotham NL, Miller TR: Bone sarcomas arising in fibrous dysplasia. J Bone Joint Surg [Am] 54:1047, 1972.
143. Sanerkin NG, Watt I: Enchondromata with annular calcification in association with fibrous dysplasia. Br J Radiol 54:1027, 1981.
144. Schwartz BT, Alpert M: The malignant transformation of fibrous dysplasia. Am J Med Sci 241:35, 1964.
145. Van Horn PE, Dahlin DC, Bickel WH: Fibrous dysplasia: Clinical pathologic study of orthopedic surgical cases. Proc Staff Meet Mayo Clin 38:175, 1963.
146. Drolshagen LF, Reynolds WA, Marcus NW: Fibrocartilaginous dysplasia of Bone. Radiology 156:32, 1985.
147. Pelzmann KS, Nagel DZ, Salyer WR: Case report 114. Skel Radiol 5:116, 1980.
148. Benedict PH: Sex precocity and polyostotic fibrous dysplasia. Report of a case in a boy with testicular biopsy. Am J Dis Child 111:426, 1966.
149. Foster CM, Ross JL, Shawker T, et al: Absence of pubertal gonadotropin secretion in girls with McCune-Albright syndrome. J Clin Endocrinol Metab 58:1161, 1984.
150. Foster CM, Comite F, Pescovitz OH, et al: Variable response to a long-acting agonist of luteinizing hormone-releasing hormone in girls with McCune-Albright syndrome. J Clin Endocrinol Metab 59:801, 1984.
151. Danon M, Crawford JD: Peripheral endocrinopathy causing sexual precocity in Albright's syndrome. Pediatr Res 8:368, 1974.
152. Husband P, Graeme JAI, Snodgrass AI: McCune-Albright syndrome with endocrinological investigations. Report of a case. Am J Dis Child 119:164, 1970.
153. Senior B, Robboy SH: Sexual precocity with polyostotic fibrous dysplasia. N Engl J Med 292:199, 1975.
154. Hall R, Warrick CK: Hypersecretion of hypothalamic releasing hormones. A possible explanation of the endocrine manifestations of polyostotic fibrous dysplasia (Albright's syndrome). Lancet 1:1313, 1972.
155. Hamilton CRJ, Maloof F: Unusual types of hyperthyroidism. Medicine 52:195, 1973.
156. Scurry MT, Bicknell JM, Fajans SS: Polyostotic fibrous dysplasia and acromegaly. Arch Intern Med 114:40, 1964.
157. Dent CE, Gertner JM: Hypophosphatemic osteomalacia in fibrous dysplasia. Q J Med 45:411, 1976.
158. McArthur RG, Hayles AB, Lambert PW: Albright's syndrome with rickets. Mayo Clin Proc 54:313, 1979.
159. Pont MS, Elster AD: Lesions of skin and brain: Modern imaging of the neurocutaneous syndromes. AJR 158:1193, 1992.
160. Smith MS, Smalley S, Cantor R, et al: Mapping of a gene determining tuberous sclerosis to human chromosome 11g14-11g23. Genomics 6:105, 1990.
161. Braffman BH, Bilaniuk LT, Naidich TP, et al: MR of tuberous sclerosis: Pathogenesis of this phakomatosis, use of gadopentetate dimeglumine, and literature review. Radiology 183:227, 1992.

162. Nixon JR, Houser OW, Gomez MR, et al: Cerebral tuberous sclerosis: MR imaging. Radiology *170*:869, 1989.
163. McMurdo SK, Moore SG, Brant-Zawadzki M, et al: MR imaging of intracranial tuberous sclerosis. AJR *148*:791, 1987.
164. Iwasaki S, Nakagawa H, Kichikawa K, et al: MR and CT of tuberous sclerosis. AJNR *11*:1029, 1990.
165. Wood B, Lieberman E, Landing B, et al: Tuberous sclerosis. AJR *158*:750, 1992.
166. Bernstein J, Robbins TO: Renal involvement in tuberous sclerosis. Ann NY Acad Sci *615*:36, 1991.
167. Narla LD, Slovis TL, Watts FB, et al: The renal lesions of tuberous sclerosis. Pediatr Radiol *18*:205, 1988.
168. National Institutes of Health Consensus Development Conference. Neurofibromatosis Conference Statement. Arch Neurol *45*:575, 1988.
169. McCann PD, Herbert J, Feldman F, et al: Neuropathic arthropathy associated with neurofibromatosis. J Bone Joint Surg [Am] *74*:1411, 1992.
170. Robinson SC, Sweeney JP: Cauda equina lipoma presenting as acute neuropathic arthropathy of the knee. A case report. Clin Orthop *178*:210, 1983.
171. Sartoris DJ, Jones H: Case report 343. Skel Radiol *15*:60, 1986.
172. Feldman F, Johnson AM, Walter JF: Acute axial neuroarthropathy. Radiology *111*:1, 1974.
173. Aoki S, Barkovich AJ, Nishimura K, et al: Neurofibromatosis types 1 and 2: Cranial MR, findings. Radiology *172*:527, 1989.
174. Rouleau GA, Wertelecki W, Haines JL, et al: Genetic linkage of bilateral acoustic neurofibromatosis 2 (bilateral acoustic neurofibromatosis) to a DNA marker on chromosome 22. Nature *329*:246, 1987.
175. Holman RE, Grimson BS, Drayer DP, et al: Magnetic resonance imaging of optic gliomas. Am J Ophthalmol *100*:596, 1985.
176. Hesselink JR, Press GA: MR contrast enhancement of intracranial lesions with Gd-DTPA. Radiol Clin North Am *26*:873, 1988.
177. Friedman D: Segmental neurofibromatosis (NF-5): A rare form of neurofibromatosis. AJR *12*:971, 1991.
178. Case Records of the Massachusetts General Hospital: N Engl J Med *328*:496, 1993.
179. Weinstein LS, Shenker A, Gejman PV, et al: Activating mutations of the stimulatory G protein in the McCune-Albright syndrome. N Engl J Med *325*:1688, 1991.
180. Schwindinger WF, Francomano CA, Levine MA: Identification of a mutation in the gene encoding the alpha subunit of the stimulatory G protein of adenylyl cyclase in McCune-Albright syndrome. Proc Natl Acad Sci USA *89*:5152, 1992.
181. Shenker A, Moran A, Pescovitz O, et al: Severe non-endocrine manifestations of the McCune-Albright syndrome (MAS) associated with activating G protein mutations. Presented at the 102nd Annual Meeting of the Society for Pediatric Research, Baltimore, May 4–7, 1992 (abstract).
182. Landis CA, Masters SB, Spada A, et al: GTPase inhibiting mutations activate the L chain of G5, and stimulate adenylyl cyclase in human pituitary tumours. Nature *340*:692, 1989.
183. Weinstein LS, Shenker A, Spiegel AM: Activating G protein mutations are present in the majority of patients with McCune-Albright syndrome (MAS). Presented at the 74th Annual Meeting of the Endocrine Society, San Antonio, TX, June 24–27, 1992 (abstract).

Enostosis, Hyperostosis, and Periostitis

Donald Resnick, M.D., and Gen Niwayama, M.D.

Single or multiple areas of increased radiodensity commonly are detected on skeletal roentgenograms. These may appear as discrete foci within the spongiosa (enostosis) or on the surface of the cortex (osteoma), or as more diffuse and widespread areas of cortical hyperostosis or periostitis. In some cases, the detection of such osseous alterations indicates the presence of a distant (and significant) extra-skeletal lesion or an underlying systemic disorder.

ENOSTOSIS (BONE ISLAND)

Since the initial report of bone islands by Stieda in 1905,[1] in which the name "kompakten Knochenkerne" was used, numerous terms have been applied to these lesions, including bone nucleus, compact island,[2] focal sclerosis,[3] calcified island in bone,[4] sclerotic bone island,[5] and enostosis.[6] The considerable attention devoted to a description of enostoses is not surprising in view of their common appearance on skeletal roentgenograms.[7, 8] Although the true frequency of these lesions is not known, Onitsuka,[9] in a review of radiographs of 189 subjects, noted that the prevalence of rib and pelvic bone islands was 0.43 and 1.08 per cent, respectively. There appears to be no significant sex preference in the rate of occurrence of these lesions, and they are encountered in all age groups, with perhaps a decreased frequency in pediatric patients.[7] Any osseous site can be affected, but the lesions have a predilection for the pelvis, proximal femur, and ribs.[7–9] Involvement of the skull is distinctly unusual. In the tubular bones, an epiphyseal location is common.

Enostoses or bone islands appear radiographically as single or multiple intraosseous sclerotic areas with discrete margins in asymptomatic persons. They may be ovoid, round, or oblong in shape, and they usually are aligned with the long axis of the trabecular architecture. Thorny, radiating bony spicules extend from the center of the lesion, intermingling with the surrounding trabeculae of the spongiosa (Fig. 93–1). The lesions do not protrude from the

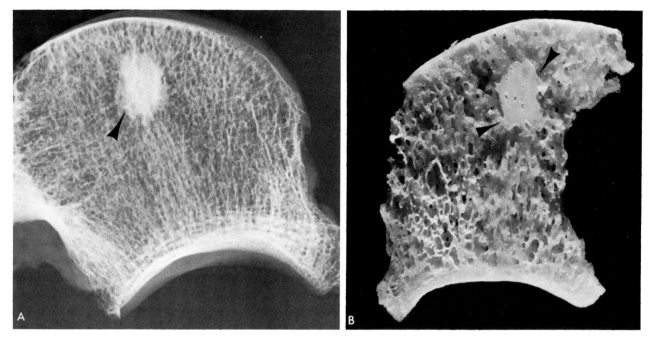

FIGURE 93–1. Enostosis: Talus. Observe the single osteosclerotic focus in the superior portion of the talus, possessing thorny radiating spicules that extend from the lesion into the surrounding spongiosa trabeculae (arrowheads).

cortical surface of the involved bone. Their size is variable; some are less than 1 × 1 mm, whereas others, especially in the pelvis, may reach proportions greater than 40 × 40 mm[10] (Fig. 93–2). Giant bone islands simulating osteoblastoma or low grade osteosarcoma on radiographic examination have been observed not only in the pelvis but also in the femur[442] and tibia.[443]

CT and MR imaging can be used effectively to further define the morphology and position of enostoses. Typically, with MR imaging the lesions are of low signal intensity on all pulse sequences. They may be located within the medullary cavity of the bone or abut the endosteal surface of the cortex. In the latter situation, the term endosteoma also may be applied to the lesion.

Initially, it generally was considered that bone islands were stable lesions representing no more than a radiographic curiosity, but there is evidence that the sclerotic areas may be more dynamic in nature.[7, 8, 11] They may increase or decrease in size (Fig. 93–2) or disappear completely. During periods of observation in adolescents, enostoses may appear for the first time and enlarge in proportion to bone growth.[9] Even in adult patients, such enlargement can be encountered, simulating the appearance of an osteoblastic skeletal metastasis. Ngan[12] has suggested that enostoses can be differentiated from metastatic foci by the absence of clinical findings. Furthermore, bone scintigraphy in cases of bone islands usually yields normal results, although a patient has been described with a large bone island of the ilium and a positive bone scan.[13] Other reports also have indicated positive bone scans in areas of enostoses.[288, 290, 291, 443–445] Such radionuclide uptake is encountered more commonly in cases of large bone islands and also appears to indicate an increased regional blood flow associated with new bone formation during the appearance and growth of the lesion.[445]

Nonetheless, the detection of one or more areas of in-

creased bone density in an elderly patient, especially in one suspected of having a prostatic carcinoma, can lead to difficulty in differential diagnosis. This is especially true when bone islands increase in size or appear in the axial skeleton. In the spine, enostoses may be apparent in 1 to 14 per cent of persons.[14, 315] At this location, they have been termed (sometimes inappropriately) endosteomas, and they create circular or triangular areas of increased density in the vertebral body that may reach 20 × 30 mm in size[6, 15, 16]; occasionally, they are seen in the posterior elements (Fig. 93–3). The lesions usually are homogeneous in density, with a well-defined margin and occasional radiating spicules (Fig. 93–4). They may border on the intervertebral discs or anterior or posterior surface of the vertebral body without expanding the vertebral contour. Radionuclide bone imaging of such lesions of the spine usually is normal,[6] serving to distinguish them from skeletal metastasis, infection, cartilaginous node formation, or intervertebral (osteo)-chondrosis. The absence of intervertebral disc space narrowing, of irregularity of the vertebral surface, and of radiolucent foci is a radiographic characteristic of spinal bone islands that aids in their differentiation from more significant processes.

Histologically, enostoses are composed of normal-appearing compact bone (Fig. 93–5). The haversian structure may be more remodeled than that of normal bone, but coarse fibrillar bone, cartilage remnants, and fibrous tissue usually are not apparent.[7, 11, 17, 316] The peripheral lamellar bone is connected to the thickened, spongy trabeculae, and their regular arrangement may be associated with slow bone formation not compensated for by bone resorption. The central core of the lesion can be irregular, suggesting the existence of a previous, more active site of bone remodeling.[17] These latter histologic observations suggest that active, albeit slight, remodeling capabilities exist in these lesions, explaining their occasional growth or disappear-

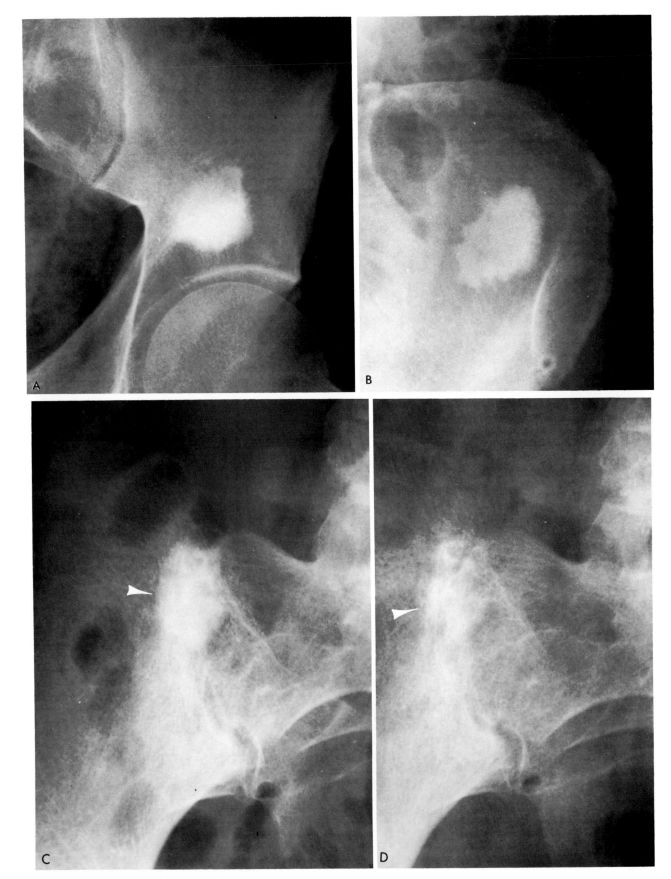

FIGURE 93–2. Enostosis: Pelvis.

   A, B Two examples of large enostoses of the pelvis. In this location, such lesions commonly are of this size. Note the homogeneous nature of the dense area and the radiating spicules extending into the adjacent bone.

   C, D Radiographs of the pelvis obtained several years apart reveal an enostosis of the ilium that has decreased in size (arrowheads).

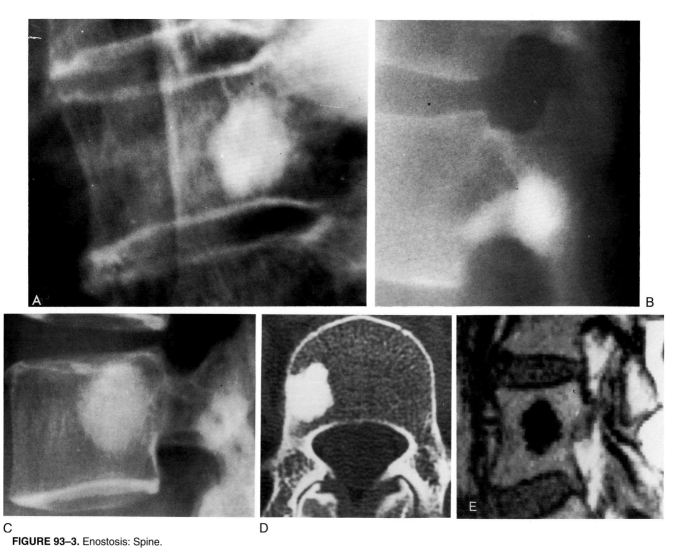

FIGURE 93–3. Enostosis: Spine.

A An example of an enostosis of the vertebral body is presented. It is relatively homogeneous and well defined.
(**A,** From Broderick TW, et al: Spine *3*:167, 1978.)

B This lesion extends from the pedicle and lamina into the posterior surface of the vertebral body. There is no expansion of osseous contour.

C, D A large enostosis in the posterolateral aspect of a lumbar vertebral body is shown by routine radiography and transaxial CT.

E A sagittal T1-weighted (TR/TE, 200/22) spin echo image shows the typical appearance and low signal intensity of an enostosis.

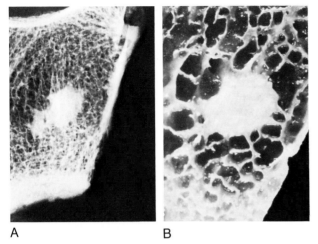

FIGURE 93–4. Enostosis: Spine. A 5 × 8 mm sclerotic lesion of the fifth lumbar vertebral body possesses thorny radiations. (From Resnick D, et al: Radiology *147*:373, 1983.)

ance, and their participation in any coexistent systemic disorder, such as hyperparathyroidism.[18]

The exact nature of enostoses is not clear. Their pathologic characteristics can be readily differentiated from those associated with bone infarction, infection, or neoplasms, such as osteoid osteoma or osteosarcoma. A traumatic cause appears unlikely. The lesions probably are developmental in nature, although a minimal ossification disorder also may be instrumental in their appearance.[9] Thus, a disturbance of the normal sequence of bone formation and resorption could lead to a localized excess of bone formation and the development of a bone island.[8] In the spine, the identification of cells resembling chondrocytes in some

bone islands suggests that cartilaginous nests or nodules may serve as a nidus on which lamellar bone is deposited (Fig. 93–6).[315]

In addition to skeletal metastases, the differential diagnosis of enostoses includes osteomas, osteoid osteomas, enchondromas, bone infarcts, fibrous dysplasia, and osteopoikilosis (Table 93–1). Osteomas protrude from the surface of the bone, a feature not present with enostoses. Osteoid osteomas, when located in the cortex, consist of lucent nidi, with or without calcification, and surrounding sclerosis. In a medullary location, a calcified nidus of an osteoid osteoma can create problems in differential diagnosis (Fig. 93–7). Enchondromas are characterized by lucent areas of variable size containing typical central calcification (Fig. 93–8), whereas bone infarcts are associated with sclerotic margins. In fibrous dysplasia, single or multiple lesions of variable density can be observed that have a predilection for the proximal femur. Osteopoikilosis leads to formation of multiple radiodense foci, each one of which resembles an enostosis radiographically and histologically.

OSTEOMA

An osteoma is a protruding mass composed of abnormally dense but otherwise normal bone that is formed in the periosteum.[19] Thus, the lesion represents no more than a localized exaggeration of intramembranous bone formation, and it is confined to areas of the bone that normally are produced by the periosteal membrane. Osteomas predominate in the skull and facial bones, although they occasionally may arise at other sites, including the pelvis and the tubular bones of the extremities. In the latter locations, osteochondromas containing cartilaginous caps are much more frequent and represent a different lesion.

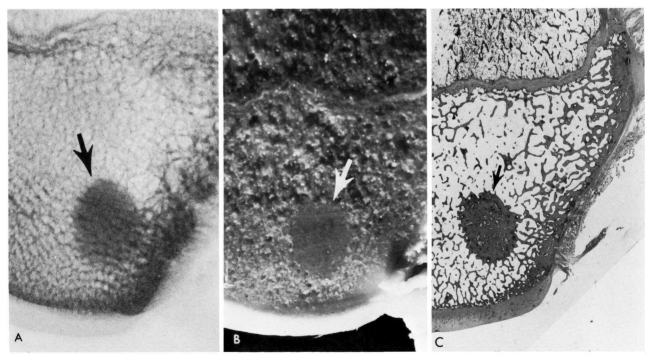

FIGURE 93–5. Enostosis: Pathologic abnormalities in extraspinal sites. Note the bone island within the epiphysis (arrows). It is connected to surrounding trabeculae by thorny excrescences. (From Lagier R, Nussle D: ROFO *128*:261, 1978. Courtesy of Georg Thieme Verlag, Stuttgart, Germany.)

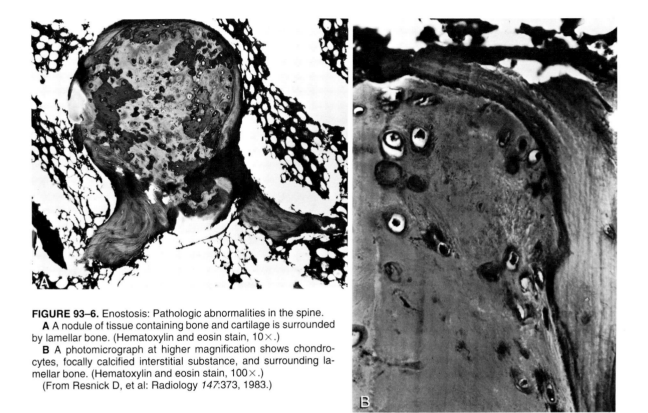

FIGURE 93–6. Enostosis: Pathologic abnormalities in the spine.

A A nodule of tissue containing bone and cartilage is surrounded by lamellar bone. (Hematoxylin and eosin stain, 10×.)

B A photomicrograph at higher magnification shows chondrocytes, focally calcified interstitial substance, and surrounding lamellar bone. (Hematoxylin and eosin stain, 100×.)

(From Resnick D, et al: Radiology *147*:373, 1983.)

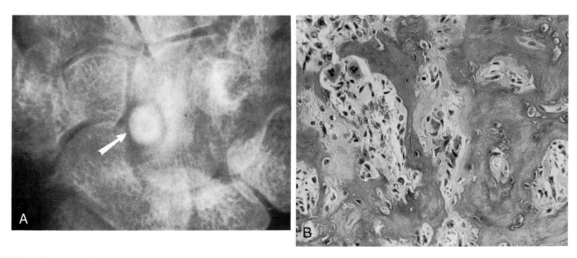

FIGURE 93–7. Osteoid osteoma.

A Observe the lesion of the capitate (arrow) with a partially calcified nidus and surrounding sclerosis. Soft tissue swelling and osteoporosis are evident.

B The center of the nidus of an osteoid osteoma contains irregular abnormal bone, cement lines, and vascular stroma (50×).

TABLE 93–1. Localized Radiodense Lesions

Lesion	Location	Appearance
Enostosis (bone island)	Medullary	Round or oblong, thorny radiating spicules
Osteoma	Cortical protrusion	Homogeneous, smooth or lobular, extend from osseous surface
Osteochondroma	Cortical and medullary protrusion	Cortical and spongiosa are continuous with parent bone, calcified cap
Enchondroma	Medullary	Lucent, well-circumscribed, central calcifications
Bone infarct	Medullary	Lucent, well or poorly circumscribed, peripheral shell of calcification
Osteoid osteoma	Cortical, medullary, or subperiosteal	Cortical: Lucent with or without calcification surrounded by sclerotic bone Medullary: Lucent or calcified, with little sclerosis Subperiosteal: Scalloped excavation with or without calcification and sclerosis

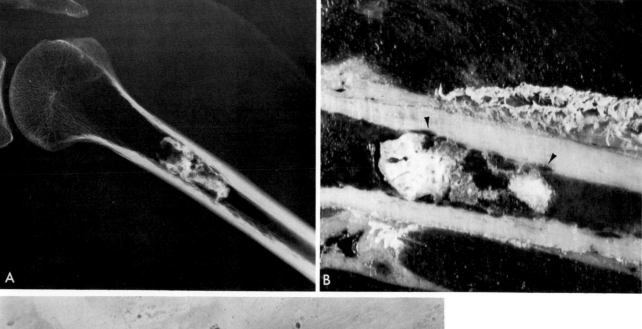

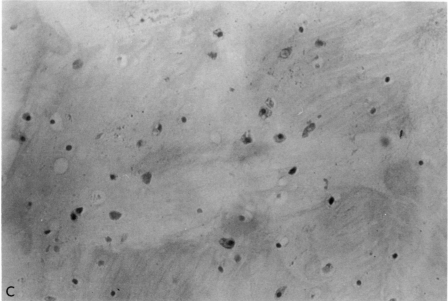

FIGURE 93–8. Enchondroma.

A, B A radiograph and photograph of a coronal section of the humerus reveal a calcified medullary lesion of the diaphysis of the bone. Note the "popcorn" appearance of the calcified deposits and the scalloping (arrowheads) of the endosteal margin of the cortex.

C The cartilage cells reveal only slight variation of the nuclei (430×).

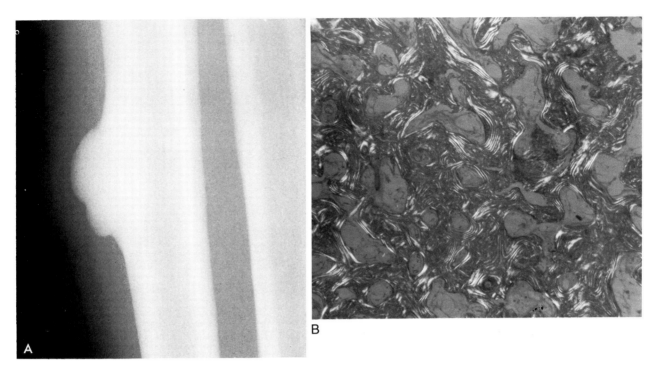

FIGURE 93–9. Osteoma: Tubular bones.
 A A protruding, homogeneously dense mass of the ulna is evident. It is of the same radiodensity and appearance as the underlying cortex. Note that there is no connection between the medullary bone of the ulna and the lesion.
 B A polarized photomicrograph (86×) reveals numerous osseous trabeculae with increased width and sparse intertrabecular space.

Osteomas are very frequent in the sinuses, especially the frontal sinus,[561] but they also are found in the ethmoid sinus and, rarely, in the sphenoid or maxillary sinuses.[20, 21, 317] Their frequency has been estimated to be 0.42 per cent in patients who have had sinus radiographs. Osteomas also arise from the inner and outer tables of the cranial vault,[318] the mandible, and the maxilla. Rarely, osteomas appear in the tubular bones of the extremities.[319] They have been detected in persons of all ages, although the lesions predominate in patients in the fourth and fifth decades of life. Men are affected more commonly. Osteomas generally are asymptomatic unless they protrude significantly into the sinus cavity (interfering with normal drainage and producing a mucocele), encroach on the orbital contents, extend into the cranial cavity, or prohibit normal dental formation or tongue movement.[446]

Osteomas are hard, nodular, or granular masses of bone that, on histologic examination, are found to consist of wide, irregularly arranged trabeculae of mature bone.[19] Prominent osteoid seams and osteoblasts may be evident. The intertrabecular tissue is sparse and may be highly vascular, with fibrous, fatty, and hematopoietic elements. The outer surface of the lesions is covered by a periosteal membrane, and a cartilaginous cap is not present.

On roentgenograms, the lesions appear as a single focus or as multiple radiodense foci that protrude into a sinus or extend from the surface of a parent bone (Figs. 93–9 and 93–10). Their outline is smooth or lobular, and they frequently are homogeneous in appearance. Rare instances of radiolucent osteomas, especially in the skull, have been described.[447] Once discovered, osteomas usually remain unchanged on serial studies. These radiographic characteristics differ from those of an enostosis, which is contained

within a bone, and an osteochondroma, which is continuous with the spongiosa and cortex of the underlying bone and may contain calcific foci.

Several descriptions exist of large, bulky osteomas arising from the cortical surface of the clavicle,[448] innominate bone,[449, 450] and tubular bones,[451] and in some of these descriptions the designation of parosteal osteoma has been used. The radiographic appearance of parosteal osteoma (Fig. 93–11) simulates that of parosteal osteosarcoma, ossifying parosteal lipoma, or post-traumatic heterotopic bone formation (myositis ossificans).

There are several opinions regarding the pathogenesis of osteomas. Jaffe[22] suggested that they are the sclerotized end-stage of fibrous dysplasia, whereas Aegerter and Kirkpatrick[23] considered osteomas to be hamartomas of bone.

Multiple osteomas of the mandible, calvarium, or tubular bones can accompany Gardner's syndrome[24–28] (Table 93–

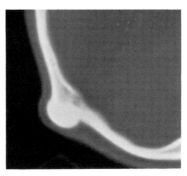

FIGURE 93–10. Osteoma: Cranial vault. CT reveals an osteoma arising from the external surface of the skull. (Courtesy of M. Taljanovic, M.D., Sarajevo, Bosnia.)

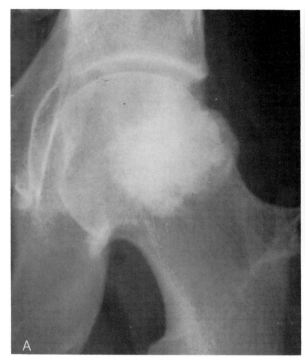

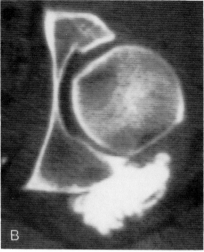

FIGURE 93–11. Parosteal osteoma: Innominate bone. Routine radiography (**A**) and transaxial CT (**B**) reveal a homogeneous, radiodense lesion arising about the hip with extension into the joint.

2). This is a familial autosomal dominant disease consisting of colonic polyposis, osteomatosis, and soft tissue tumors.[292, 293, 320–322, 452] The soft tissue tumors consist of epidermal or sebaceous cysts, subcutaneous fibromas and lipomas, and desmoid tumors.[322] Of these, the desmoid tumor occurs in 3 to 29 per cent of patients with Gardner's syndrome,[453] may arise prior to the clinical onset of polyposis, and following surgery, may occur in laparotomy scars in the anterior abdominal wall. Gallium scintigraphy has been used to localize these tumors (as well as sites of bone involvement).[454] Their MR imaging characteristics lack specificity (see Chapter 95).[453] The osseous lesions frequently precede the appearance of clinical and radiographic evidence of intestinal polyposis, so that their accurate recognition is important. Weary and colleagues[29] reported that 50 per cent of patients with Gardner's syndrome had osteomas, especially in the skull, sinuses, and mandible. The lesions also may be detected in the ribs and long bones; in the latter sites, however, the outgrowths may not be well defined but instead appear as localized, wavy cortical thickening, especially in the femur, tibia, and ulna (Fig. 93–12). In fact, any tubular bone, including those of the hands and feet, can reveal osseous protuberances or, more rarely, enostoses in this syndrome.[28] The vertebrae rarely are affected. Dental abnormalities include hypercementosis, supernumerary and unerupted teeth, odontomas, and dentigerous cysts.[311] The major differential diagnostic possibility is tuberous sclerosis, which can lead to similar bony excrescences, particularly in the metacarpals and metatarsals (Fig. 93–13).

OSTEOPOIKILOSIS

Osteopoikilosis (osteopathia condensans disseminata; spotted bones) is an asymptomatic osteosclerotic dysplasia initially described by Albers-Schönberg[30] and Ledoux-Lebard and associates[31] in the early twentieth century. Although the disorder is described as extremely rare,[32] the experience of many radiologists (including one of the authors) suggests that osteopoikilosis is more common than previous reports have indicated. The disorder is seen in both men and women and may become evident at any age, although its appearance below the age of 3 years is distinctly uncommon.[33] Inherited and sporadic cases of osteopoikilosis have both been reported. Studies of the familial occurrence indicate an autosomal dominant pattern of genetic transmission that may become more prominent in each succeeding generation.[34–37, 455]

Clinical manifestations usually are absent or mild. Cutaneous lesions may be evident in approximately 25 per cent of cases, consisting of closely situated, elevated, whitish fibrocollagenous infiltrations (dermatofibrosis lenticularis disseminata, or the Buschke-Ollendorff syndrome),[38–40, 323] a predisposition to keloid formation,[41, 42] and scleroderma-like lesions.[43, 44] Osteopoikilosis also has been associated with dwarfism,[40, 45] dystocia,[42] spinal stenosis,[325] and, in 15 to 20 per cent of patients, mild articular pain with or without joint effusion.[46]

Roentgenographic findings are diagnostic.[294] Numerous small, well-defined, homogeneous circular or ovoid foci of increased radiodensity are clustered in periarticular osseous regions. A symmetric distribution is observed,[456] with a predilection for the epiphyses and metaphyses of long tubular bones (Fig. 93–14), carpus, tarsus, pelvis, and scapu-

TABLE 93–2. Major Radiographic Abnormalities in Gardner's Syndrome

Colonic polyposis
Osteomas
Soft tissue tumors
Dental lesions

FIGURE 93–12. Gardner's syndrome: Bone abnormalities.

A Osteomas (arrows) of the outer table of the skull and mandible are evident.

B Observe wavy cortical thickening of the femur and lesions of the innominate bones that resemble enostoses.

(From Harned RK, et al: AJR *156*:481, 1991.)

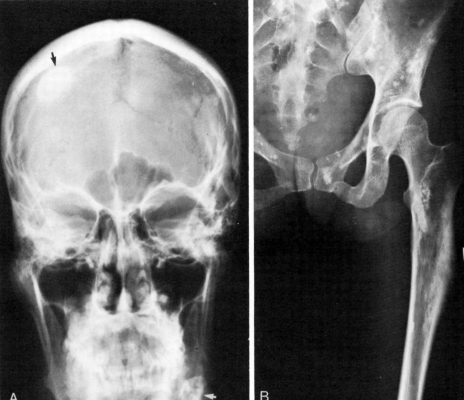

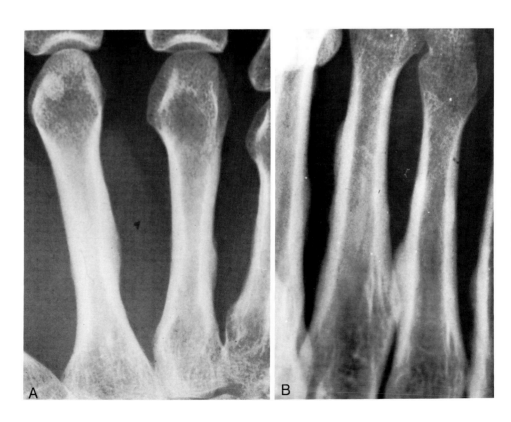

FIGURE 93–13. Tuberous sclerosis. Nodular osseous excrescences arise from the external cortex of the metacarpal and metatarsal bones. (Courtesy of V. Schiappacasse, M.D., Santiago, Chile.)

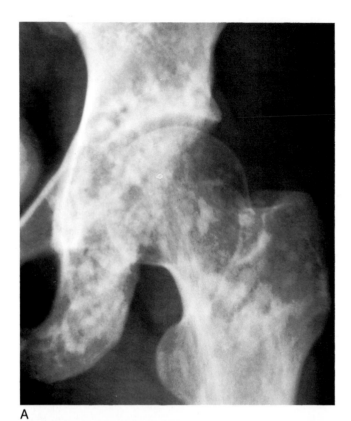

A

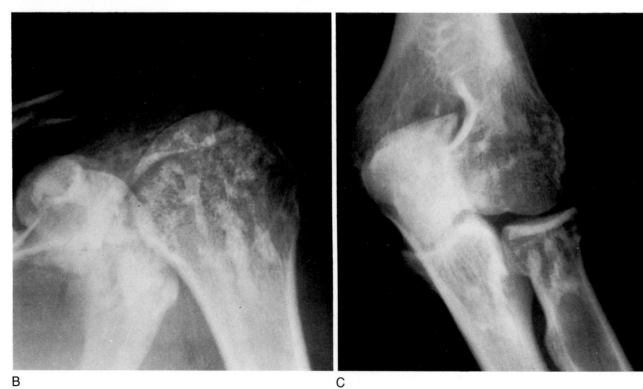

B   C

FIGURE 93–14. Osteopoikilosis: Typical sites of involvement.

A Hip. Note the circular or ovoid radiodense foci of the femur and pelvis without abnormality of the intervening joint space.

B, C Shoulder and elbow. The same radiographic characteristics are evident. Although epiphyses can be affected, metaphyseal foci commonly predominate.

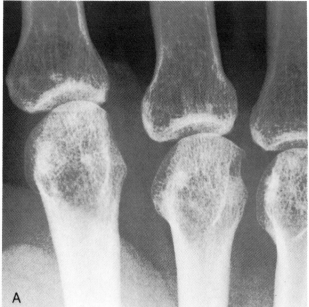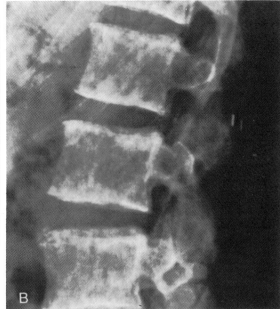

FIGURE 93–15. Osteopoikilosis: Less typical sites of involvement.
A Hand. Note several lesions in the metacarpal heads and proximal phalanges of the second, third, and fourth digits.
B Spine. Observe radiodense foci in the margins of the vertebral bodies and in the posterior osseous elements. This patient has had a laminectomy. (Courtesy of A. Brower, M.D., Norfolk, Virginia.)

lae; involvement of the ribs, clavicles, spine, and skull is rare and, when present, is less marked (Fig. 93–15). In some reports, involvement of the small tubular bones of the hands has been frequent (Fig. 93–15).[455] On serial roentgenograms, the radiopaque areas can increase or decrease in size and number or disappear.[37, 47] The dynamic nature of the lesions is more marked in children and adolescents than in adults, in whom the radiodense areas may change slowly or not at all.

Radionuclide examination with bone-seeking radiopharmaceutical agents usually reveals no evidence of increased activity about the skeletal lesions.[48, 49, 457]

Pathologically, the lesions of osteopoikilosis appear as oval or round foci of compact bone within the spongiosa.[50, 324] In the epiphyses of the tubular bones the foci rarely are in contact with the subchondral bone plate, whereas in the metaphyses they may be located eccentrically, abutting on the endosteal surface of the cortex. On histologic examination, the lesions are found to be composed of lamellar osseous tissue containing haversian systems (Fig. 93–16). Although osteoblasts, osteocytes, and even osteoclasts may be evident, residual calcified cartilage matrix is not seen, indicating that the foci probably are not formed through endochondral ossification of cartilage rests. The microscopic features of the lesion are identical to those encountered in bone islands.

The cause and pathogenesis of osteopoikilosis are not known. Some evidence suggests that a relationship exists between this condition and other osteosclerotic skeletal disorders, especially osteopathia striata and melorheostosis[50–52] (Table 93–3). Thus, round and linear areas of increased radiodensity can be encountered in multiple skeletal sites in the same patient, combined with flowing or undulating periosteal bone formation and even calvarial hyperostosis (hy-

perostosis frontalis interna). The resulting combination of abnormalities has been referred to as mixed sclerosing bone dystrophy (see later discussion). Osteopoikilosis (and these related disorders) may represent a hereditary failure to form normal trabeculae along lines of stress, in which small or large bony foci appear.[53, 324] As such, the lesions may arise as a consequence of altered osteogenesis. In this regard, a report of a patient with both osteopoikilosis and osteosarcoma is of interest[54] (Fig. 93–17). It has been suggested that this latter tumor may be related to active osteogenesis[55]; perhaps the chronic abnormal remodeling of bone that is evident in patients with osteopoikilosis can be associated with malignant transformation.[54] Cases of chondrosarcoma[458] and giant cell tumor[459] arising in patients with os-

TABLE 93–3. Diseases Associated with Various Hyperostotic Lesions

Lesion	Possible Associated Diseases
Osteoma	Gardner's syndrome
Osteopoikilosis	Osteopathia striata Melorheostosis Hyperostosis frontalis interna
Osteopathia striata	Osteopoikilosis Melorheostosis Osteopetrosis Cranial sclerosis Focal dermal hypoplasia
Melorheostosis	Linear scleroderma Osteopoikilosis Osteopathia striata Neurofibromatosis Tuberous sclerosis Hemangiomas

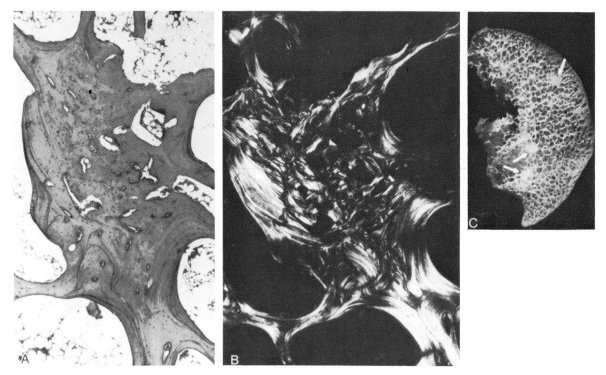

FIGURE 93–16. Osteopoikilosis.

A, B Within the deep region of a femoral head (which was excised following a subcapital fracture) in an elderly woman with osteopoikilosis, a focus of lamellar bone containing haversian systems is identified (**A** with ordinary light; **B** with polarized light). (Hematoxylin and eosin stain, 36×.)

C A photograph of the section of the femoral head reveals multiple areas of compact bone (arrows), each with the features of an enostosis. (From Lagier R, et al: Skel Radiol 11:161, 1984.)

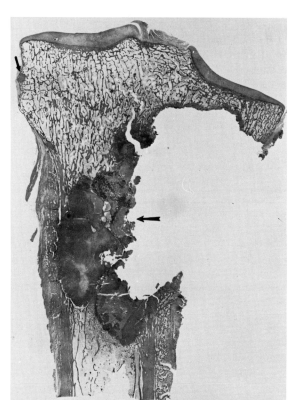

FIGURE 93–17. Osteopoikilosis and osteosarcoma. A histologic section of the proximal end of the tibia in a 48 year old man with both osteopoikilosis and osteosarcoma reveals a sarcomatous lesion containing a bone island (large arrow) and an additional subchondral bone island (small arrow). (From Mindell ER, et al: J Bone Joint Surg [Am] 60:406, 1978.)

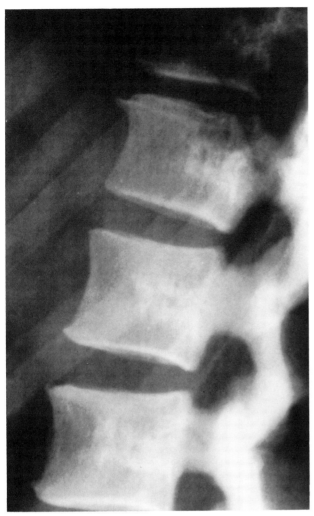

FIGURE 93–18. Osteomesopyknosis. Note small, centrally located sclerotic foci within the vertebral bodies.

teopoikilosis also have been described, but a definite association of such tumors and osteopoikilosis is not confirmed.

The major differential diagnostic considerations in cases of widespread focal round or oval radiodense lesions are osteopoikilosis, osteoblastic metastases, mastocytosis, and tuberous sclerosis. The symmetric distribution, the propensity for epiphyseal and metaphyseal involvement, and the uniform size of the foci are features that suggest osteopoikilosis, a diagnosis that is supported by a normal-appearing bone scan. Asymmetry, common involvement of the axial skeleton, including the spine, osseous destruction, variation in size, and positive scintigraphic findings characterize skeletal metastases. In both mastocytosis and tuberous sclerosis, symmetry, metaphyseal and epiphyseal preference, and uniform, well-defined foci are less striking than in osteopoikilosis.

A rare disorder, osteomesopyknosis resembles osteopoikilosis but leads to patchy osteosclerosis, principally in the axial skeleton (Fig. 93–18).[326, 327, 460, 461] It is an autosomal dominant condition that may be discovered as an incidental radiographic finding or on radiographs of the spine obtained in the investigation of chronic, mild thoracic and lumbar pain. Sclerosis of the endplates of the vertebral bodies resembles the rugger jersey appearance of renal os-

teodystrophy. A more focal or diffuse distribution of osteosclerosis also may be encountered in the vertebrae and innominate bones, and cystic lesions of the proximal portion of the femora occasionally occur. Generally discovered in adolescence or, less commonly, in childhood or adulthood, the radiographic alterations tend to be stable when observed on serial examinations.

OSTEOPATHIA STRIATA

Osteopathia striata (Voorhoeve's disease) was first described in 1924 by Voorhoeve[56] as a variant of osteopoikilosis. Subsequent reports of the disease have been few, verifying its very rare occurrence.[57–64, 296, 328] Men and women of any age can be affected, and a genetic transmission, probably an autosomal dominant one, has been suggested but is not definite. Clinical manifestations usually are absent, although joint discomfort has been encountered in some persons.[57] Facial deformity may be apparent.

Radiography reveals linear, regular bands of increased radiodensity that extend from the metaphyses of tubular bones for variable distances into the diaphyses, and that are interspersed with areas of rarefaction (Fig. 93–19). The length of the striations may be related to the growth rate of the involved bone; the longest lesions frequently are found in the femora.[59] In the flat bones, especially the ilium, a fan-like arrangement of radiodense striations radiates toward the iliac crests. Involvement of the small bones of the hands and feet, the skull and facial bones,[410] and the spine is unusual. Rarely, small exostoses are seen. The skeletal abnormalities usually are bilateral in distribution but may sometimes be unilateral.[60, 65]

Scintigraphy with bone-seeking radiopharmaceutical agents fails to reveal significant abnormalities.[49, 60]

Histologic findings rarely are recorded, although Willert and Zichner[61] noted abnormalities in biopsy specimens of two patients that suggested osteonecrosis.

Osteopathia striata may coexist with osteopoikilosis, melorheostosis, or osteopetrosis[50, 52, 63] (see Table 93–3). Metaphyseal flaring in some cases of osteopathia striata resembles the findings in Pyle's disease.[66] A relationship between osteopathia striata and focal dermal hypoplasia (Goltz's syndrome) has been noted.[58, 295, 329] This syndrome includes areas of skin atrophy and pigmentation, papillomas of mucous membranes, dystrophy of nails, digital abnormalities, scoliosis, tooth, eye, and ear anomalies, and mental retardation.[60, 67, 462] Radiographic features include syndactyly, adactyly, microcephaly, defects of segmentation of the vertebrae, and an association with multiple bone lesions resembling giant cell tumors.[462–464] In a group of 11 patients with focal dermal hypoplasia, nine demonstrated features of osteopathia striata.[58]

Osteopathia striata also has been associated with cranial sclerosis.[330–334] Although in some patients with this combination of findings, no other family members have similar changes,[331] the triad of osteopathia striata, cranial sclerosis, and macrocephaly has been separated as a rare and distinct syndrome demonstrating autosomal dominant hereditary characteristics.[334] Typically, macrocephaly appears first and may be detected prenatally by ultrasonography; osteopathia striata is present at birth or soon thereafter, and cranial sclerosis occurs gradually during childhood.[333] Additional

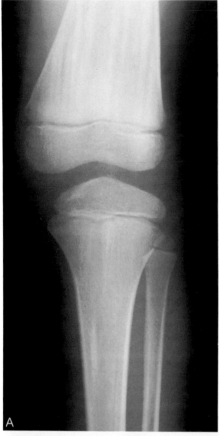

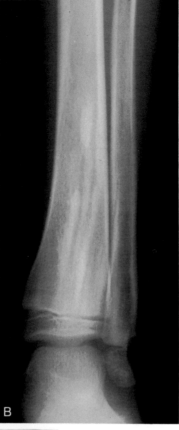

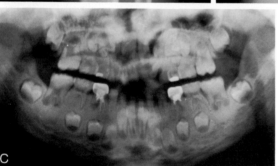

FIGURE 93–19. Osteopathia striata.
A, B In this 7 year old boy, note linear radio-dense areas principally in the metaphyses of the tibia and femur. (Courtesy of R. Tobin, M.D., San Diego, California.)
C In a different 7 year old boy, wavy sclerotic striations are evident in the mandible. (From Nakamura T, et al: Skel Radiol *14*:267, 1985.)

problems in this syndrome include cleft palate, cleft uvula, mental retardation, facial paralysis, and deafness.[335]

The cause and pathogenesis of osteopathia striata are not known. Its differential diagnosis includes prominent vertical trabecular formation that may be a normal variant[60]; the adult form of osteopetrosis, in which linear striations of long bones and pelvis may be encountered; enchondromatosis (Ollier's disease), in which oval-shaped lesions may produce metaphyseal bands of diminished density; and osteopoikilosis, in which oval or circular radiodense foci are seen.

MELORHEOSTOSIS

Melorheostosis is a rare bone disorder first described by Léri and Joanny in 1922.[68] It generally becomes manifest after early childhood, rarely in the first days of life,[68, 70] and in approximately 40 to 50 per cent of cases, the disease is evident by the age of 20 years.[71] Occasionally, patients in

the fourth and fifth decades of life may reveal evidence of melorheostosis.[69, 72] Men and women are affected equally, and no hereditary features have been established.

The clinical alterations of the disorder have been well documented[73–76] and are summarized in a comprehensive review of the subject.[77] Initial manifestations are variable. Intermittent swelling of joints can be evident. Pain and limitation of motion are more frequent in adults than in children,[299] and, with increasing muscle contractures, tendon and ligament shortening, and soft tissue involvement, these findings may become profound. Growth disturbances include increased circumference and angulation of affected limbs and an inequality of limb length.[336] Such disturbances can be severe and can lead to scoliosis, joint contracture and rigidity, and pes valgus, varus, or equinovarus. Soft tissue changes include tense, erythematous, and shiny skin, anomalous pigmentation, induration and edema of subcutaneous tissues, fibrosis, weakness and atrophy of muscles, and linear scleroderma (see discussion later in this chapter).

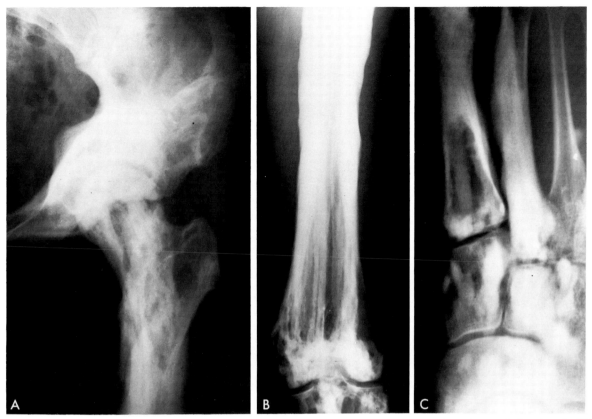

FIGURE 93–20. Melorheostosis. In this patient, characteristic radiographic abnormalities are evident throughout a single extremity. Note the hyperostosis of the left hemipelvis, para-acetabular region, and medial aspect of the proximal femur. In the distal femur, a peculiar linear radiodense pattern extends across the knee joint. Involvement of the medial rays of the foot also is seen. (Courtesy of R. Freiberger, M.D., New York, New York.)

These changes, which have been demonstrated with thermography,[72] may precede the osseous abnormalities for an extended period and may be evident at birth. The clinical manifestations may progress rapidly during childhood and more slowly during adult life.[465] Although life expectancy is not shortened, the disease can result in considerable deformity and disability and may require one or more orthopedic operations, including capsulotomy, fasciotomy, and even amputation.

Radiographic alterations are highly characteristic. Changes commonly are limited to a single limb, in which one or more bones may be affected. The lower extremity is involved more frequently than the upper extremity. Abnormalities also may be encountered in the skull and facial bones,[69, 466] ribs,[69, 73, 467] and vertebrae.[78, 337, 467] Changes in the scapulae, clavicles, and pelvis frequently are combined with alterations in the corresponding limb.

Peripherally located (cortical) hyperostosis is evident in one bone or a series of bones (Figs. 93–20 to 93–23). The appearance of the osseous excrescences extending along the length of the bone simulates that of candle wax flowing down the side of a lit candle. A wavy and sclerotic bony contour is produced that may involve one side of the tubular bones of the upper or lower extremity, reaching the carpus and tarsus as well as the metacarpals, metatarsals, or phalanges.[468] Endosteal hyperostosis is an associated feature that may partially or completely obliterate the medullary cavity (Figs. 93–24 and 93–25). In the carpal and tarsal

areas, more discrete round foci may resemble the findings of osteopoikilosis, whereas in the flat bones, such as those in the pelvis or the scapula, radiating or localized sclerotic patches are seen (Fig. 93–26). Bone masses may protrude into adjacent articulations, appearing as osteochondromas. Soft tissue calcification and ossification are not infrequent, having a predilection for para-articular regions, and may lead to complete ankylosis of the joint[297, 298, 469] (Figs. 93–27 to 93–29).

As opposed to the situation in osteopoikilosis and osteopathia striata, scintigraphy in cases of melorheostosis can reveal areas of increased skeletal accumulation of radionuclide,[49, 72, 79, 470] and the resulting scintigraphic image may simulate Paget's disease. This positivity, when compared with the negativity of scintigraphy in the former two disorders, may indicate the cortical location or greater size of the bony deposits or the presence of more metabolic activity. With MR imaging, bone and soft tissue lesions are of low signal intensity on all pulse sequences (Fig. 93–30).

On pathologic examination, thickened and enlarged bony trabeculae are found to contain normal-appearing haversian systems that may be irregularly arranged[71, 72] (Fig. 93–31). Within the marrow space, cellular fibrous tissue is apparent. Occasionally, cartilage islands revealing endochondral ossification and cellular fibrous tissue revealing intramembranous bone formation are encountered. Osteoblastic or osteoclastic activity usually is not prominent, however, and inflammatory lesions are lacking.[298]

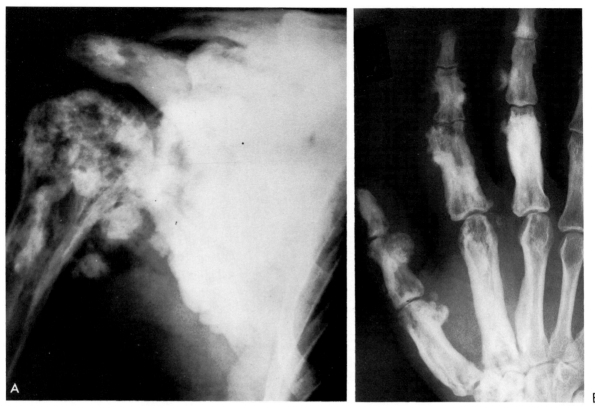

FIGURE 93–21. Melorheostosis. Observe the bizarre osseous overgrowth of the scapula, the hyperostosis of the proximal humerus, soft tissue ossification about the shoulder, and enlargement, deformity, and hyperostosis of the radial rays of the hand. The undulating irregular bony contours are typical of this condition. (Courtesy of J. Mink, M.D., and R. Gold, M.D., Los Angeles, California.)

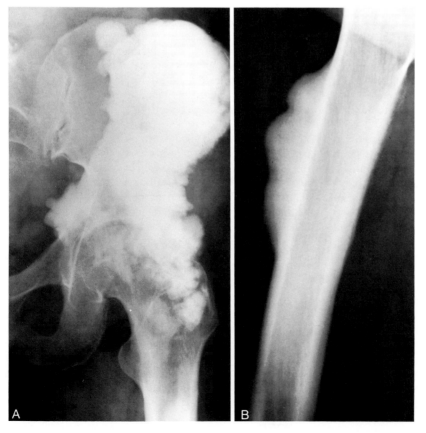

FIGURE 93–22. Melorheostosis. In a 71 year old woman, osseous excrescences are observed in the lateral portion of the ilium, acetabular region, and anterior surface of the femur, in combination with soft tissue ossification about the hip. (Courtesy of H. R. Fischer, M.D., Victoria, British Columbia, Canada.)

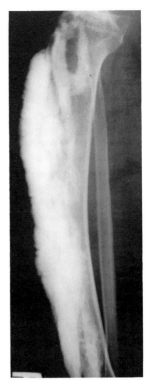

FIGURE 93-23. Melorheostosis. Observe bizarre excrescences, mainly involving the anterior aspect of the tibia. (Courtesy of R. Kerr, M.D., Los Angeles, California.)

Melorheostosis has been reported in association with other disorders[77] (see Table 93–3). Bandlike linear scleroderma overlying osseous excrescences has been noted.[73, 80–85] The histologic characteristics of the soft tissue involvement in these cases suggest that cutaneous abnormalities are secondary to the same proliferative disorder that produces the bony hyperostosis.[82] The association of melorheostosis with osteopoikilosis and osteopathia striata also has been reported[52, 86, 87]; in some cases of melorheostosis, the sclerotic foci in the carpus and tarsus that form part of the disease process itself may have been misinterpreted as evidence of osteopoikilosis.[77] Additional investigations have indicated possible associations between melorheostosis and neurofibromatosis,[88] tuberous sclerosis,[89] hypophosphatemic rickets,[471] and hemangiomas or other vascular lesions.[89, 90, 338] One report has described the occurrence of osteosarcoma of a femur involved with melorheostosis.[472] In the axial skeleton, melorheostosis has been accompanied by fibrolipomatous lesions in adjacent areas including the spinal canal and retroperitoneal tissues (Fig. 93–32).[337]

The cause and pathogenesis of melorheostosis are not known. Putti[91] postulated that vascular disturbances represented the primary cause of the disorder, and the role of vascular insufficiency has been emphasized by other investigators.[89, 90] An inflammatory process,[71] a degenerative disorder of connective tissue,[90, 92] an abnormality of innervation, and a defect in embryogenesis[73] have each been offered at one time or another as a possible etiologic factor.[77]

As one of the most striking characteristics of the disease is a peculiar pattern of distribution, clues to the pathogene-

sis of melorheostosis may be uncovered by analyzing this characteristic.[93] The segmental distribution of the lesions does not correspond to the anatomic course of blood vessels or mixed nerve roots of the limbs,[94] although it might result from a congenital disturbance initiated early in embryonic life prior to formation of the limb buds.[73, 95] Murray and McCredie[93] have emphasized the role of sclerotomes in the distribution of hyperostosis in melorheostosis. Sclerotomes represent zones of the skeleton supplied by individual spinal sensory nerves[96]; sclerotome maps can be constructed indicating patterns of skeletal innervation. In many cases of melorheostosis, skeletal alterations correspond to a single sclerotome or a part thereof, suggesting that the disease may represent the late result of a segmental sensory nerve lesion. The accompanying cutaneous lesions, including linear scleroderma, may be related to the same nerve segment, whereas para-articular ossification could result from involvement of the corresponding myotome.[93]

The radiographic abnormalities of melorheostosis are sufficiently characteristic to allow accurate diagnosis in most cases. Although hyperostosis can accompany tuberous sclerosis, neurofibromatosis, Gardner's syndrome, infantile cortical hyperostosis, and fibrous dysplasia, the distribution of bone deposition in these disorders does not reveal the unusual segmental features that appear in melorheostosis. In some patients with the latter disease, soft tissue calcification and ossification in para-articular regions may resemble the findings of idiopathic synovial (osteo)-chondromatosis, heterotopic ossification following burns or paralysis, osteomas, or soft tissue sarcomas.

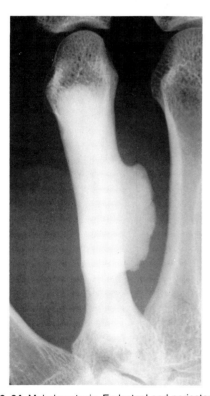

FIGURE 93-24. Melorheostosis. Endosteal and periosteal hyperostosis is evident in this 29 year old woman with a firm nontender mass that had been evident for 15 years. (Courtesy of G. Greenway, M.D., Dallas, Texas.)

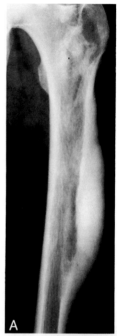

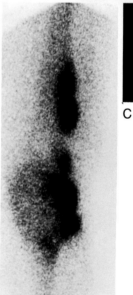

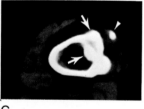

FIGURE 93–25. Melorheostosis. This 36 year old woman was evaluated for "bone tumors" in the left thigh. The lesions had been present for at least 8 years. Physical examination revealed an enlarged and tender thigh and hip.

A Observe nodular osseous densities on the lateral surface of and within the femur.

B A bone scan reveals abnormal uptake of the radiotracer in the femur and tibia.

C A transaxial CT scan of a portion of the femoral shaft shows osseous excrescences on the external and internal cortical surfaces (arrows) and soft tissue ossification (arrowhead).

(Courtesy of G. Greenway, M.D., Dallas, Texas.)

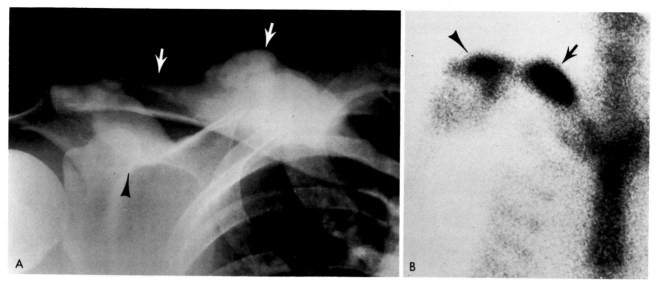

FIGURE 93–26. Melorheostosis. This 29 year old man had painful swelling of the right clavicle. A biopsy of the clavicle revealed findings of melorheostosis.

A Observe localized hyperostosis of the middle and distal portions of the clavicle (arrows) and the scapula (arrowhead). The process extended down the proximal aspect of the humerus.

B A technetium bone scan delineates increased activity in the clavicle (arrow) and scapula (arrowhead).

(Courtesy of W. Pogue, M.D., San Diego, California.)

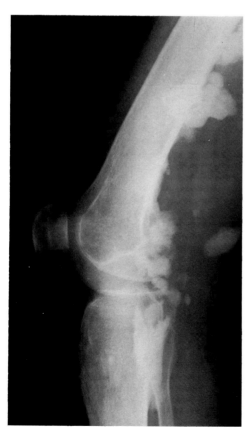

FIGURE 93–27. Melorheostosis. Prominent soft tissue calcification and ossification are noted along the posterior aspect of the thigh and the knee. Minor hyperostosis of the underlying cortex is evident.

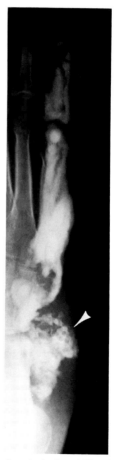

FIGURE 93–28. Melorheostosis. In addition to the typical osseous changes in the tarsus, metatarsal bone, and phalanges, observe prominent soft tissue ossification (arrowhead). (Courtesy of G. Greenway, M.D., Dallas, Texas.)

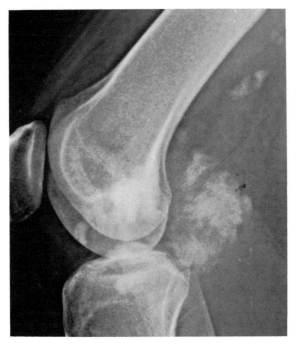

FIGURE 93–29. Melorheostosis. Observe extensive soft tissue ossification associated with radiodense foci in the femur and tibia. (Courtesy of R. Cone, M.D., San Antonio, Texas.)

MIXED SCLEROSING BONE DYSTROPHY

Although osteopoikilosis, osteopathia striata, and melorheostosis each possess characteristic radiologic abnormalities, some patients demonstrate findings of more than one of these disorders and, occasionally, of all three (Fig. 93–33). In 1964, Walker[70] termed this phenomenon mixed sclerosing bone dystrophy and, subsequently, others have described additional examples of this dystrophy.[52, 338–342, 432] As indicated by Whyte and collaborators,[341] some of these reports have contained cases inconsistent with those originally described by Walker,[70] including examples of osteopathia striata and cranial sclerosis (see previous discussion). Whyte and colleagues[341] identified four types of mixed sclerosing bone dystrophy: osteopathia striata, melorheostosis, osteopoikilosis, and focal osteosclerosis; osteopathia striata and cranial sclerosis with or without osteopoikilosis; osteopathia striata, generalized cortical hyperostosis, and metadiaphyseal widening with or without cranial sclerosis and osteopoikilosis of the ribs; and osteopoikilosis with diaphyseal periosteal proliferation. These types of mixed sclerosing bone dystrophy can be associated with a variety of vascular anomalies, including unilateral lymphangiectasia, capillary hemangiomas, and arteriovenous malformations,[338] and with Trevor's disease.[432]

OTHER SCLEROSING BONE DYSTROPHIES AND DYSPLASIAS

A number of other dysplastic and dystrophic disorders of bone are characterized by sclerosis, hyperostosis, and periostitis. Although these are addressed in Chapter 88, some additional comments are appropriate here owing to the clinical and radiographic characteristics that simulate or even overlap those observed in the sclerosing bone dystrophies.

Furthermore, because the causation and pathogenesis of many of these disorders are unknown and because two or more of them rarely may occur together, a uniformly accepted classification system does not exist. One system of nomenclature, adopted by the European Society of Pediatric Radiology, is presented in Chapter 88, but others continue to be introduced.

In one recent review, Greenspan[473] categorized the sclerosing bone dysplasias according to whether they involved endochondral bone formation, intramembranous bone formation, or both types. Disorders related to dysplasias of endochondral ossification were further divided into those affecting primary, or immature, bone (osteopetrosis and pyknodysostosis) and those affecting secondary, or mature, bone (enostosis, osteopoikilosis, and osteopathia striata). Dysplasias of intramembranous bone formation included diaphyseal dysplasia (Camurati-Engelmann disease), hereditary multiple diaphyseal sclerosis (Ribbing disease), and various types of endosteal hyperostosis (such as van Buchem's syndrome, Worth's syndrome, and sclerosteosis). Disorders affecting both endochondral and intramembranous ossification were subdivided into those affecting predominantly endochondral bone formation (dysosteosclerosis, metaphyseal dysplasia or Pyle's disease, and craniometaphyseal dysplasia); those affecting predominantly intramembranous bone formation (melorheostosis, craniodiaphyseal dysplasia, and progressive diaphyseal dysplasia with involvement of the base of the skull); and those in which two or more sclerosing bone dysplasias occurred together (various combinations of melorheostosis, osteopoikilosis, osteopathia striata, cranial sclerosis, osteopetrosis, progressive diaphyseal dysplasia, and generalized cortical hyperostosis).

As described in Chapter 20, the development of the human skeleton reflects an orderly process in which both endochondral ossification (the transformation of cartilage into bone) and intramembranous ossification (the transformation of mesenchymal cells through various phases of differentiation into bone without an intervening cartilaginous stage) occur simultaneously. Endochondral ossification is responsible for the formation of all tubular and flat bones, the vertebrae, the base of the skull, the ethmoids, and the medial and lateral ends of the clavicles; intramembranous ossification accounts for the formation of the frontal, parietal, and temporal bones and their squamae, the bones of the upper portion of the face, the tympanic parts of the temporal bone, the vomer, the medial pterygoid, and portions of the mandible and clavicle, as well as the periosteal and endosteal envelopes and the haversian envelope that are components of the cortex that surrounds the tubular and flat bones of the skeleton.[473] Therefore, a classification system based on alterations in endochondral ossification or intramembranous ossification, or both, emphasizes differences both in the specific osseous sites of involvement and in the portions of an individual bone (i.e., cortical or compact bone; trabecular or spongy bone) that are encountered in the various sclerosing bone dystrophies and dysplasias.

Certain dysplasias of intramembranous ossification lead to dramatic abnormalities of the tubular bones of the extremities affecting periosteal or endosteal surfaces of the diaphyseal cortex, or both types of surface, that simulate those occurring in other disorders addressed in this chapter. Although a family of diseases accompanied by endosteal

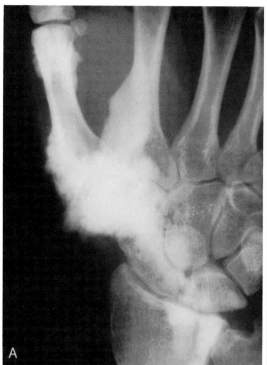
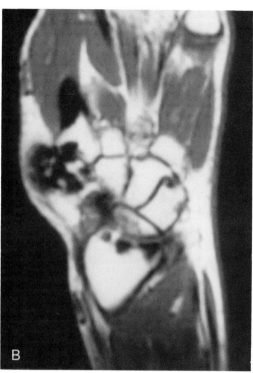
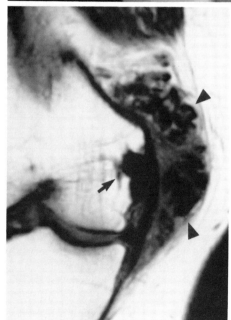

FIGURE 93–30. Melorheostosis: MR imaging.

A, B This 49 year old man had had an enlarging mass in the wrist for 34 years. The routine radiograph **(A)** reveals typical manifestations of melorheostosis. A coronal T1-weighted (TR/TE, 400/11) spin echo image **(B)** shows foci of low signal intensity in the distal radius, carpus, and second metacarpal bone. (Courtesy of G. Greenway, M.D., Dallas, Texas.)

C In a 32 year old man, a coronal T1-weighted (TR/TE, 550/20) spin echo MR image demonstrates bone (arrow) and soft tissue (arrowheads) lesions of low signal intensity involving the knee. (Courtesy of T. Broderick, M.D., Orange, California.)

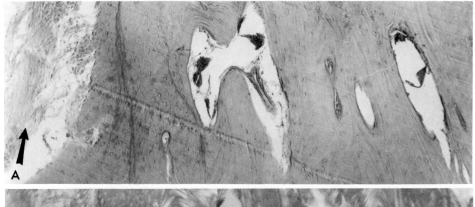

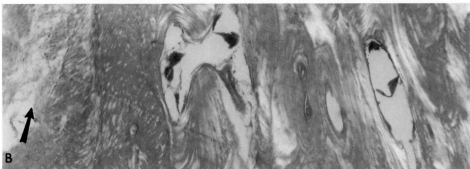

FIGURE 93–31. Melorheostosis. Nonpolarized (**A**) and polarized (**B**) photomicrographs reveal the hypertrophic bony trabeculae and periosteal fibrous tissue (arrows) (68×).

hyperostosis (Worth's syndrome, van Buchem's syndrome, sclerosteosis, and others) is included in this category (see Chapter 88), one disorder (diaphyseal dysplasia, or Camurati-Engelmann disease) and its variants (hereditary multiple diaphyseal sclerosis, or Ribbing's disease, and related conditions) deserve emphasis here.

A rare autosomal dominant disorder of the musculoskeletal system that was described initially by Camurati[474] in 1922 and then by Engelmann[475] in 1929 became known as *Camurati-Engelmann disease.* Owing to the diaphyseal location and progressive features of the skeletal abnormalities, Neuhauser and coworkers[476] in 1948 used the term *progressive diaphyseal dysplasia* to describe this disease. Subsequently, many articles have highlighted its major features.[477–482] This disease generally becomes manifest in the first decade of life, affecting boys more commonly than girls. Presenting clinical manifestations include muscle pain, weakness, and atrophy; a waddling and broad-based gait; bone pain; increased fatigability; and delayed puberty. The lower extremities are involved more frequently than the upper extremities. Laboratory parameters generally indicate normal values for urinary levels of hydroxyproline and serum levels of electrolytes; marrow and peripheral blood elements are normal as well.[473] Although somewhat variable in its clinical expression and course, the disorder usually is self-limited, resolving by the age of 30 to 35 years.[478, 482]

Radiographic findings include, foremost, fusiform thickening of the cortex in the diaphyseal portions of the tubular bones, involving (in order of decreasing frequency) the tibia, femur, fibula, humerus, ulna, and radius (Fig. 93–34).[473] Symmetric in distribution, the thickened cortex occurs as a result of both endosteal and periosteal bone formation. Narrowing of the medullary cavity is apparent.

Affected bone is sharply demarcated from normal bone, and the external contour of the bone usually is smooth.[473] Sparing of the epiphyses is a characteristic finding. Additional less constant sites of involvement include the bones of the hands and feet, the fibula, the innominate bone, the ribs, the spine, the clavicle, and the base of the skull. Scintigraphy, in combination with routine radiography, is effective in demonstrating the skeletal extent of the process,[482, 483] and CT has been used to further document the distribution of osseous involvement and the degree of endosteal and periosteal bone formation.[480]

Histopathologic findings of progressive diaphyseal dysplasia confirm the presence of cortical thickening owing to bone deposition on the endosteal and periosteal surfaces. Simultaneously occurring bone resorption and formation are characterized by intense osteoblastic and osteoclastic activity.

The cause of this disorder is unknown. Both familial and sporadic cases are described. Although reports of families with the disease are most consistent with an autosomal dominant mode of transmission, progressive diaphyseal dysplasia has variable penetrance, which has given rise to descriptions of lethal disease, of disabled patients, and of patients whose radiographic abnormalities almost were incidental findings.[481] Progressive diaphyseal dysplasia has been regarded as a disorder in which the genetic coding for haversian bone formation is either retarded or absent altogether,[481] and as one in which a deficient vascular supply to the periosteum and endosteum induces local hypoxia acting as a stimulus for bone formation.[473] Although reported inconsistencies in the clinical, histologic, and laboratory parameters of the disease contribute to the uncertainty of its causation and pathogenesis, the radiographic abnormalities of progressive diaphyseal dysplasia are remarkably constant

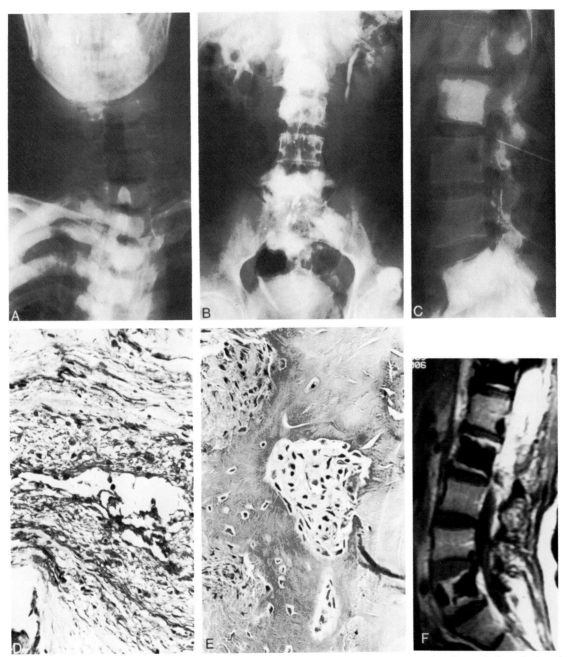

FIGURE 93–32. Melorheostosis. A 21 year old man developed quadriparesis due to a diffuse intramedullary lipoma in the spinal cord.

A–C Radiographs of the axial skeleton show hyperostosis and enostoses involving the upper ribs on the right, the thoracic and lumbar vertebrae, the sacrum, and the ilium. A previous laminectomy and myelogram had been performed.

D A histologic preparation of the intramedullary lipoma shows a vascular channel, probably a vein, within the fat with nonspecific subintimal fibrosis and associated luminal narrowing (100×).

E Histologic examination of the material derived from the second thoracic vertebral spinous process reveals increased woven bone (100×). (From Garver P, et al: Skel Radiol 9:41, 1982.)

F A sagittal T1-weighted (TR/TE, 600/20) spin echo image obtained 10 years later shows foci of low signal intensity within multiple thoracolumbar vertebral bodies and the high signal intensity of the intraspinal lipoma.

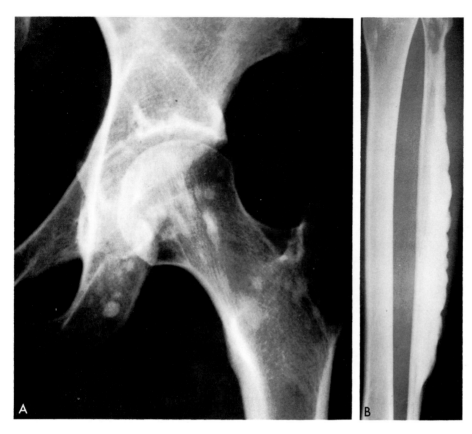

FIGURE 93–33. Mixed sclerosing bone dystrophy.

A The changes in the hip are diagnostic of osteopoikilosis, although some of the foci are elongated or linear in shape.

B Involvement of the fibula in the same patient consists of flowing, eccentrically located ossification, an appearance that is typical of melorheostosis.

(Courtesy of A. Brower, M.D., Norfolk, Virginia.)

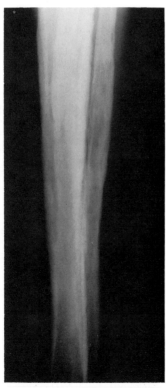

FIGURE 93–34. Diaphyseal dysplasia (Camurati-Engelmann disease). Note exuberant bone formation with thickening of the cortices in the diaphyses of the tibia and fibula. The opposite side was affected similarly. (Courtesy of S. Wootton, M.D., Denver, Colorado.)

and, although distinctive, create some diagnostic difficulty with regard to bone abnormalities accompanying primary and secondary hypertrophic osteoarthropathy.

A somewhat similar and perhaps related process with less extensive clinical and radiologic features has been designated *hereditary multiple diaphyseal sclerosis.* First described by Ribbing[484] in 1949 and sometimes referred to as Ribbing's disease, this disorder is entirely asymptomatic or leads to minor pain and tenderness in the affected extremity or extremities. As in progressive diaphyseal dysplasia, hereditary multiple diaphyseal sclerosis leads to osteosclerosis and hyperostosis of the diaphyses of tubular bones, especially the femur and tibia but also the fibula and radius (Fig. 93–35). The cortex is thickened, the medullary cavity is narrowed, and slight expansion of the bone may be evident.[473, 485] Skeletal involvement in Ribbing's disease, however, is much less widespread than that in progressive diaphyseal dysplasia, and asymmetry is the rule. Bone lesions may progress with time but eventually may become stationary.[477] Histopathologic abnormalities resemble those of Camurati-Engelmann disease, with evidence of periosteal bone formation and narrowing of haversian canals, except that bone resorption is not evident in hereditary multiple diaphyseal sclerosis.[484] Still, some regard the two disorders as related entities, differing only in the severity of the process.[473, 477]

In 1988, Abdul-Karim and associates[486] described five patients, ranging in age from 8 to 52 years, who presented with pain referred to the lower extremity. The pain was mild to moderate and increased with physical activity.

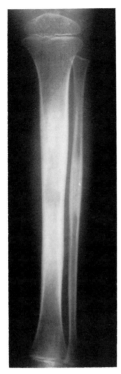

FIGURE 93–35. Hereditary multiple diaphyseal sclerosis (Ribbing's disease). Note the sclerotic regions in the diaphyses of the tibia and fibula. Radiolucent foci also are evident.

mary or secondary varieties, the syndrome may be incomplete, or additional features, such as thickening of skin on the face and scalp (pachydermia), may become prominent.

Primary hypertrophic osteoarthropathy also has been called pachydermoperiostosis, idiopathic hypertrophic osteoarthropathy, generalized hyperostosis with pachydermia, pachydermohyperostosis, idiopathic familial generalized osteophytosis, and Touraine-Solente-Golé syndrome. It was first described by Friedreich in 1868[97] and Marie in 1890.[98] In 1907, Unna[99] delineated the condition of cutis verticis gyrata, and in 1927 Grönberg[100] associated the latter condition with the one previously described by Friedreich.[101] Additional accounts of this entity followed,[102–111] including that of Touraine and associates[104] in 1935, which, when combined with more recent reports,[101, 112–119, 489–491] delineate in great detail the clinical and radiologic aspects of pachydermoperiostosis.

Clinical Abnormalities

Pachydermoperiostosis, a rare disease, demonstrates an autosomal dominant genetic transmission with marked variability of expression. More than one third of the reported patients have had a relative with a similar illness.[489] It predominates in men, is more severe in men than in women, and shows a predilection for blacks. An adolescent onset is typical, although cases appearing before puberty or in adult life have been recorded.[112, 113, 120] The clinical man-

There was no history of familial involvement, trauma, infection, or systemic illness. Intramedullary osteosclerosis was defined by routine radiography or CT, or both, and involved the midportion of the tibia, the distal portion of the tibia, the distal portion of the fibula, or the entire lower extremity. CT demonstrated the intramedullary location of the sclerosis and the absence of significant periosteal reaction. Bone scintigraphy was positive in all patients. Histopathologically, there was replacement of the normal spongiosa by marked sclerotic bone composed of an irregular arrangement of immature and mature trabeculae. These authors used the term *intramedullary osteosclerosis* to describe this disorder, and they referred to cases of similar but not identical findings that had been reported previously.[487, 488] Despite minor differences, the radiographic features of intramedullary osteosclerosis resemble those of Ribbing's disease (Fig. 93–36) and bear some resemblance also to stress-induced changes in the tubular bones of the lower extremities.

PRIMARY HYPERTROPHIC OSTEOARTHROPATHY (PACHYDERMOPERIOSTOSIS)

Hypertrophic osteoarthropathy represents a clinical syndrome consisting of clubbing of the digits of the hands and feet, enlargement of the extremities secondary to periarticular and osseous proliferation, and painful and swollen joints. The syndrome may be divided into two categories: primary (hereditary or idiopathic) hypertrophic osteoarthropathy and secondary hypertrophic osteoarthropathy.[562] The primary form represents approximately 3 to 5 per cent of all cases of hypertrophic osteoarthropathy. In either pri-

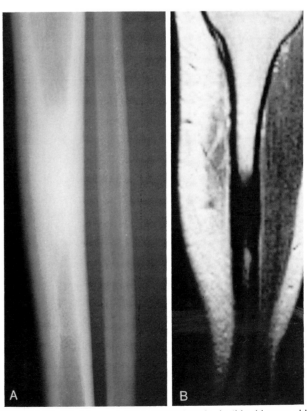

FIGURE 93–36. Intramedullary osteosclerosis. In this 44 year old woman with leg pain, routine radiography **(A)** shows mature endosteal and periosteal bone formation in the midshaft of the tibia. A coronal proton density weighted (TR/TE, 2000/40) spin echo MR image **(B)** reveals low signal intensity at the site of bone sclerosis. (Courtesy of A. Newberg, M.D., Boston, Massachussetts.)

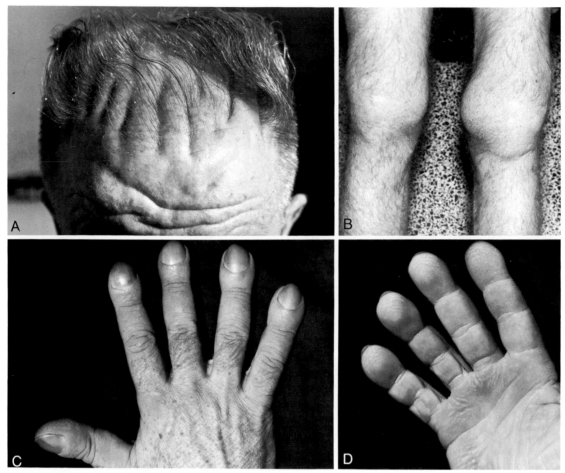

FIGURE 93–37. Primary hypertrophic osteoarthropathy (pachydermoperiostosis). Typical clinical features of this syndrome include furrowing and oiliness of the cutaneous tissue, enlargement of the hands with a paw-like appearance, digital clubbing, and swollen joints. (Courtesy of M. Dalinka, M.D., Philadelphia, Pennsylvania.)

ifestations are somewhat variable, depending on whether the patient demonstrates the complete syndrome (pachydermia, periostitis, cutis verticis gyrata), the incomplete form (sparing of the scalp), or the forme fruste (pachydermia with minimal or absent periostitis).[113, 116]

There is an insidious onset of enlargement of the hands and feet producing a paw-like appearance, clubbing of the distal ends of the fingers and toes, and convexity of the nails (Fig. 93–37). Coarsening of the skin of the face and scalp with ptosis, furrowing and oiliness of the cutaneous tissue, excessive sweating, enlargement and disruption of the normal contour of the extremities, fatigability, and vague pains in the bones and joints also are encountered. Pachydermoperiostosis generally progresses for approximately 10 years before arresting spontaneously. Chronic disabling complications may appear, however, with stiffness and restricted motion in the axial and appendicular skeleton, kyphosis, and neurologic manifestations due to osseous compression of the spinal cord or nerve roots as well as the cranial nerves (conductive and sensory hearing loss, vestibular dysfunction). Life expectancy is normal.

These clinical features are not constant in all persons with the disease. Pachydermia may be limited or absent,[120–125] or periostitis may not be apparent.[116] In some cases, the appearance resembles that of acromegaly, with thickened and coarsened cutaneous features,[126, 127] but macroglossia, mandibular and sellar enlargement, and visual defects are not evident.[50, 128] Furthermore, laboratory analysis fails to document the findings of acromegaly as growth hormone levels are normal.[116]

Of interest in some patients is the appearance of bone marrow failure and extramedullary hematopoiesis due to encroachment on the marrow space by the thickened cortex.[129, 130, 343] Hepatosplenomegaly and anemia in these persons may be associated with endocrine abnormalities,[129] although the latter findings also have been noted in patients with pachydermoperiostosis who do not have bone marrow failure.[131]

Radiographic Abnormalities

The predominant radiographic feature of pachydermoperiostosis is periostitis (Figs. 93–38 to 93–41). Widespread and symmetric findings occur, although osseous thickening is most pronounced in the tubular bones of the extremities, especially the tibia, fibula, radius, and ulna. Involvement of the carpus, tarsus, metacarpals, metatarsals, phalanges, and pelvis also is frequent. Thickening of the calvarium and base of the skull can be detected[111]; however, changes in the spine are unusual. In infants or young children, enlarge-

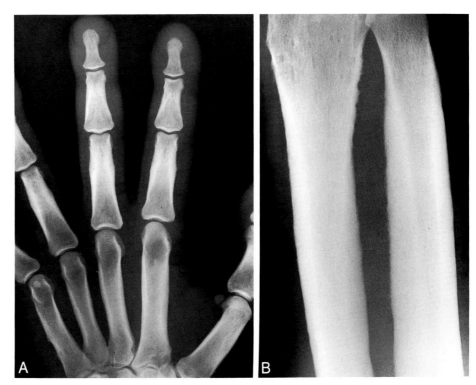

FIGURE 93–38. Primary hypertrophic osteoarthropathy (pachydermoperiostosis).

A In the hand, soft tissue prominence of the ends of the fingers and broad phalanges and metacarpal bones with thick cortices are observed.

B Note the shaggy or irregular periosteal bone formation with cortical thickening in the radius and ulna. The medullary canals are narrowed as a result of encroachment by the thick cortex.

(Courtesy of M. Dalinka, M.D., Philadelphia, Pennsylvania.)

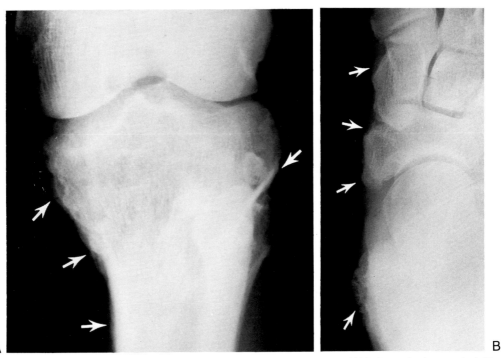

FIGURE 93–39. Primary hypertrophic osteoarthropathy (pachydermoperiostosis). A 55 year old black man had coarse facial features, clubbed digits, and painful but nontender bones; other family members had similar problems.

A Observe the periosteal proliferation in the proximal tibial epiphysis, metaphysis, and diaphysis (arrows).

B An irregular osseous surface on the medial malleolus and tarsus can be seen (arrows).

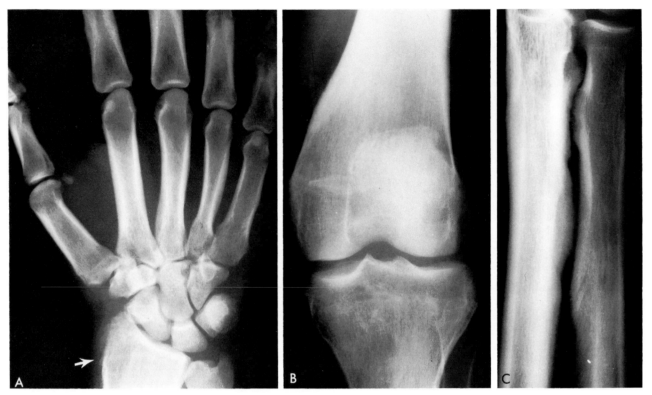

FIGURE 93–40. Primary hypertrophic osteoarthropathy (pachydermoperiostosis). A 26 year old man developed acromegalic features and cutaneous abnormalities.

    A In addition to periosteal proliferation of the distal radius (arrow), note the widened metacarpals and phalanges.

    B An expanded contour of the distal femur is associated with cortical thickening.

    C Exuberant osseous proliferation is evident along apposing surfaces of radius and ulna.

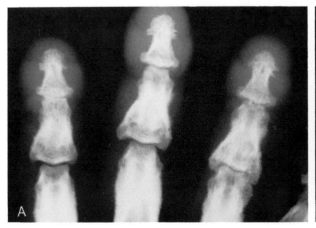

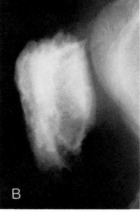

FIGURE 93–41. Primary hypertrophic osteoarthropathy (pachydermoperiostosis). Radiographic abnormalities in this patient include soft tissue clubbing and bone hypertrophy of the phalanges, including the tufts **(A)**, and patellar enthesophytes **(B)**. (Courtesy of C. Chen, M.D., Kaohsiung, Taiwan.)

TABLE 93–4. Some Causes of Diffuse Periostitis

Disease	Location	Characteristics
Primary hypertrophic osteoarthropathy (pachydermoperiostosis)	Tibia, fibula, radius, ulna (less commonly, carpus, tarsus, metacarpals, metatarsals, phalanges, pelvis, ribs, clavicle)	Diaphyseal, metaphyseal, and epiphyseal involvement Shaggy, irregular excrescences Diaphyseal expansion Clubbing Ligamentous ossification Cranial and facial changes
Secondary hypertrophic osteoarthropathy	Tibia, fibula, radius, ulna (less commonly, femur, humerus, metacarpals, metatarsals, phalanges)	Diaphyseal and metaphyseal involvement Single or laminated, regular or irregular proliferation Clubbing Periarticular osteoporosis, soft tissue swelling Underlying primary lesion
Thyroid acropachy	Metacarpals, metatarsals, phalanges (less commonly, other tubular bones)	Diaphyseal involvement Radial side predilection Dense, solid, and spiculated proliferation Clubbing Soft tissue swelling Thyroid gland abnormalities
Venous stasis	Tibia, fibula, femur, metatarsals, phalanges	Diaphyseal and metaphyseal involvement Undulating osseous contour Cortical thickening Soft tissue swelling, ulceration, ossification Phleboliths
Hypervitaminosis A	Ulna, metatarsals, clavicle, tibia, fibula	Diaphyseal involvement Undulating contour Epiphyseal deformities Soft tissue nodules Intracranial hypertension
Infantile cortical hyperostosis (Caffey's disease)	Mandible, clavicle, scapula, ribs, tubular bones	Periostitis and cortical hyperostosis May become extreme Cranial destruction Soft tissue nodules Deformities

ment and delayed closure of the cranial sutures have been observed in association with this disease.[344]

Superficially, the periosteal proliferation of the tubular bones resembles that typically seen in secondary hypertrophic osteoarthropathy, but such proliferation is not painful in pachydermoperiostosis,[490] and, further, careful radiographic analysis of periostitis in the primary and secondary forms reveals definite and significant differences (Table 93–4). Although the diaphyses and metaphyses can be affected in both conditions, periostitis commonly extends into the epiphyseal region in pachydermoperiostosis, producing shaggy excrescences about various articulations. In fact, ill-defined bony outgrowths are especially characteristic of this disease, differing from the linear deposits that most typically accompany secondary hypertrophic osteoarthropathy. These outgrowths also are encountered in the pelvis, particularly about the ischium, symphysis pubis, acetabulum, and iliac crest. It should be emphasized, however, that differences in the pattern and distribution of periosteal proliferation in primary and secondary hypertrophic osteoarthropathy are related, at least in part, to the earlier age of onset and longer duration of the former disorder, and that periostitis in secondary hypertrophic osteoarthropathy that begins early in life (as in patients with cyanotic congenital heart disease) more closely resembles the osseous proliferation that accompanies pachydermoperiostosis.[492]

In more advanced cases of pachydermoperiostosis, expansion of the diaphyses of the tubular bones and sclerosis of the spongiosa in both appendicular and axial skeletal sites are evident. The ribs and clavicles may be expanded diffusely, with coarsened trabeculae and prominent sclerotic islands. In addition to osseous thickening, the skull may reveal prominent sinuses, especially in the frontal and sphenoid regions, and moderate enlargement of the mandible (alveolar portions). Intervertebral disc space and foraminal narrowing, vertical or horizontal osseous ridges in the vertebral bodies, and ligamentous ossification are spinal manifestations of the disease. Soft tissue prominence of the distal digits may be associated with tuftal osteolysis (Fig. 93–42).[101, 345, 346] Osteolysis may occur after phalangeal hypertrophy, perhaps indicating that an orderly sequence consisting first of bone formation and then of bone destruction is typical of the tuftal abnormalities.[411, 412] The bony resorption produces tapering, pointing, truncation, or disappearance of terminal phalanges.

Ligamentous calcification and ossification may appear in portions of the appendicular skeleton, including the calcaneus, the ulnar olecranon, the patella, and the interosseous regions between radius and ulna and between tibia and fibula. Osseous bridges also may appear in the scapulae and sternum and may lead to bony ankylosis of articulations, particularly the joints of the hands and feet.

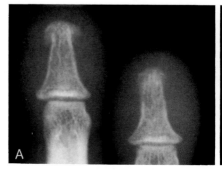 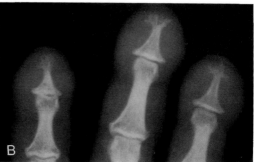

FIGURE 93–42. Primary hypertrophic osteoarthropathy (pachydermoperiostosis). Two examples are shown of soft tissue clubbing associated with mild **(A)** and severe **(B)** tuftal osteolysis. (A, Courtesy of R. Kerr, M.D., Los Angeles, California.)

Pathologic Abnormalities

Inspection of involved bones delineates a roughened surface due to periosteal deposition of bone.[50, 102, 112, 132] On cross section, the delineation between the original cortical bone and the periosteal new bone is less distinct in this condition than in secondary hypertrophic osteoarthropathy.[50] This difference may be related to the longer survival period encountered in patients with pachydermoperiostosis, allowing enough time for incomplete or complete incorporation of the periosteal deposits into the subjacent cortex.

Articular Abnormalities

Articular inflammation is less prominent in pachydermoperiostosis than in secondary hypertrophic osteoarthropathy. Pain and swelling are uncommon and, when present, are of only moderate severity and, perhaps, aggravated by alcohol abuse.[347] Joint effusions may be encountered.[114, 115] Aspiration of joint contents reveals noninflammatory synovial fluid, although in one patient calcium pyrophosphate dihydrate crystals were detected.[133] Histologic examination of the synovial membrane outlines mild cellular hyperplasia of the lining and thickening of the subsynovial blood vessels[134, 348, 349] (Fig. 93–43). With electron microscopy, multilayered basal laminae can be detected about small blood vessels in the subsynovial tissue.

In long-standing cases, increased rigidity and limitation of joint motion reflect mechanical interference due to periarticular osseous excrescences and intra-articular bony masses.[50] Carpal and tarsal ankylosis is particularly characteristic.

Etiology and Pathogenesis

A definite cause and pathogenesis of pachydermoperiostosis have not been unraveled. Although increased peripheral blood flow appears to be significant in the pathogenesis of secondary hypertrophic osteoarthropathy, measurements in patients with long-standing pachydermoperiostosis reveal diminished blood flow.[135] The cause and significance of this finding are not clear; it has been postulated that diminished peripheral blood flow may indicate secondary thickening of the arterial wall, as has been described in cases of secondary hypertrophic osteoarthropathy,[136] or massive connective tissue overgrowth, in the process of which small and medium-sized arteries are compressed or obliterated.[135] Whether or not a similar decrease in peripheral circulation

accompanies the early active phase of the disease is not known, although, in some investigations but not all,[491] an increase in blood flow in this active phase has been recorded.[348, 349] Perhaps, in early stages, an increase in peripheral blood flow through arteriovenous shunts bypasses the capillary beds, producing capillary stasis, local hypoxia, and connective tissue proliferation.[112] Pathologic studies documenting the occurrence of highly vascular periosteal new bone initially and avascular bone subsequently support the concept of changes in the peripheral circulation between the early and late stages of the disease.[349]

Differential Diagnosis

The irregular periosteal deposits that appear about metaphyses and epiphyses of tubular bones as well as axial skeletal sites in this condition are distinctive, and they usually are not encountered in secondary hypertrophic osteoarthropathy. This characteristic may indicate only that more irregular and extensive periostitis is seen in cases of hypertrophic osteoarthropathy of earlier onset or longer duration (as is typical of pachydermoperiostosis); some patients with congenital cyanotic heart disease and secondary hypertrophic osteoarthropathy have similar alterations.[492] The early age of onset, a family history of disease, and the absence of significant joint pain are clinical characteristics of pachydermoperiostosis that differ from those of secondary hypertrophic osteoarthropathy. In thyroid acropachy, fluffy, spiculated periosteal bone is encountered in the hands and feet. It rarely is observed elsewhere, a fact that, taken in combination with typical clinical characteristics such as exophthalmos and pretibial myxedema, ensures accurate diagnosis of thyroid acropachy. Some of the clinical and radiologic manifestations of acromegaly are observed in pachydermoperiostosis, but radiographic and laboratory signs of a pituitary tumor differentiate acromegaly from pachydermoperiostosis. In endosteal hyperostosis (van Buchem's disease), thickening of the cranial vault and cortices of the tubular bones are not combined with digital clubbing, skin changes, enlargement of paranasal sinuses, and irregular para-articular osseous excrescences. Similarly, in diaphyseal dysplasia (Camurati-Engelmann disease), endosteal and periosteal proliferation of the diaphyses of the tubular bones is characteristic. Macrodystrophia lipomatosa and the proteus syndrome are associated with bizarre bone proliferation and overgrowth, but additional clinical and radiologic manifestations allow their accurate diagnoses. Other disorders, such as Paget's disease, fibrous dysplasia,

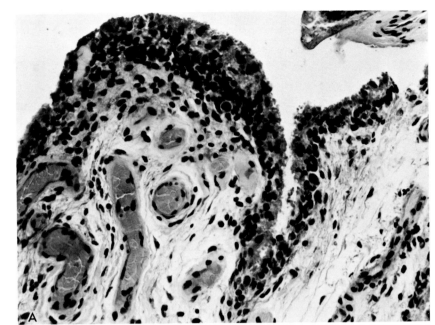

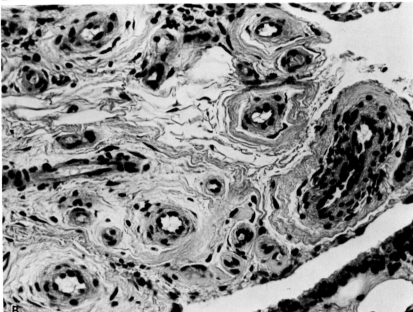

FIGURE 93–43. Primary hypertrophic osteoarthropathy (pachydermoperiostosis): Synovial abnormalities. A 40 year old man with pachydermoperiostosis and chronic articular symptoms underwent synovial biopsy of the right knee.

A Cellular hyperplasia of the synovial lining is evident (40×).

B Thickening of subsynovial blood vessels also is apparent (40×).

(From Lauter SA, et al: J Rheum *5*:85, 1978.)

and fluorosis, are easily differentiated from pachydermoperiostosis.

SECONDARY HYPERTROPHIC OSTEOARTHROPATHY

A description of clubbing of the digits was first provided by Hippocrates in the fifth century BC.[137] Following the descriptions of Bamberger in 1889[138] and Marie in 1890,[98] the entire syndrome of clubbing, arthritis, and periostitis became known. Currently, an extensive literature is available that describes the features of secondary hypertrophic osteoarthropathy.[139–144, 492] In many of the reports, the condition is termed hypertrophic pulmonary osteoarthropathy, emphasizing the fact that pulmonary problems represent a major cause of the periostitis. It has been estimated that

between 1 per cent[145, 146] and 12 per cent[147, 148] of patients with bronchogenic carcinoma develop hypertrophic osteoarthropathy, although estimates as high as 25 to 50 per cent have been recorded.[149] A 5 per cent incidence appears to be a typical approximation of the frequency of this complication in cases of bronchogenic carcinoma. Hypertrophic osteoarthropathy also is common in patients with pleural mesothelioma and may be apparent in as many as 50 per cent of these persons.[141, 150] Other intrathoracic diseases associated with this complication include pulmonary abscess, bronchiectasis, emphysema, Hodgkin's disease,[151–154] diaphragmatic tumors, and metastasis (sarcomas, carcinomas, and melanomas)[155–160, 312, 493–496] (Table 93–5). Hypertrophic osteoarthropathy rarely is encountered in cases of pulmonary tuberculosis[350] and sarcoidosis.[502, 503] Of all these potential intrathoracic causes, bronchogenic carcinoma is by

TABLE 93–5. Some Causes of Secondary Hypertrophic Osteoarthropathy

Pulmonary	Bronchogenic carcinoma
	Abscess
	Bronchiectasis
	Emphysema
	Hodgkin's disease
	Metastasis
	Cystic fibrosis
Pleural, diaphragmatic	Mesothelioma
Cardiac	Cyanotic congenital heart disease
Abdominal	Portal or biliary cirrhosis
	Ulcerative colitis
	Crohn's disease
	Dysentery
	Gastrointestinal polyposis
	Neoplasms
	Biliary atresia
Miscellaneous	Nasopharyngeal carcinoma
	Esophageal carcinoma
	Infected aortic or axillary artery grafts

far the most common underlying lesion. The frequency of hypertrophic osteoarthropathy is greater in those lung tumors that are peripherally situated, of squamous origin, and cavitary in nature. No relationship has been found between tumor size and the frequency and severity of hypertrophic osteoarthropathy.

Hypertrophic osteoarthropathy also has been associated with cyanotic congenital heart disease (tetralogy of Fallot, transposition of the great vessels, Eisenmenger's complex, patent ductus arteriosus with flow reversal, and other disorders),[161–166, 351, 425, 492, 497–499] and such extrathoracic conditions as portal and biliary cirrhosis,[167, 214, 413] cholestatic cirrhosis,[500] ulcerative colitis,[220, 352] Crohn's disease,[221, 222, 353] pseudomembranous enterocolitis,[354] gastrointestinal polyposis,[355, 356] nontropical sprue, and amebic and bacillary dysentery. In addition, nasopharyngeal,[166–171, 435] esophageal,[172, 350] gastric,[215] and pancreatic[173] neoplasms[216] can produce hypertrophic osteoarthropathy even in the absence of pulmonary metastasis. Hypertrophic osteoarthropathy confined to one or both lower or upper extremities is seen in patients with infected Dacron grafts of the aorta[303, 357, 504] or axillary artery.[433]

Hypertrophic osteoarthropathy is infrequent in childhood. In this age group, potential causes include pulmonary suppuration,[306, 434] cystic fibrosis,[301, 426, 427] congenital cyanotic heart disease, Hodgkin's disease, and metastasis,[174–179] as well as Crohn's disease, ulcerative colitis,[352] primary sclerosing cholangitis,[358] biliary atresia, or primary pulmonary neoplasms.

Clinical Abnormalities

Digital clubbing is a frequent but not invariable feature of hypertrophic osteoarthropathy[505]; however, its manifestation should not be equated with the full syndrome, as patients with diverse disorders can reveal clubbing without any associated findings of hypertrophic osteoarthropathy.[180] The initial alteration is thickening of the fibroelastic tissue at the base of the nail bed followed by increased fluctuance of the bed, and prominence, striations, shininess, and increased curvature of the nail itself.[506] Skin thickening and swelling of the limbs also can be evident.

Articular symptoms and signs are apparent at some time in approximately 30 to 40 per cent of patients and may be the presenting manifestation of hypertrophic osteoarthropathy. Typically, pain and tenderness appear about one or more articulations. The discomfort is aggravated by motion and is more pronounced at night. Neighboring subcutaneous tissues become swollen, and the overlying skin may appear warm and dusky red. The knees, ankles, wrists, elbows, and metacarpophalangeal articulations are involved most commonly,[359] occasionally in an asymmetric fashion.[181] When the small joints of the hands and wrists are affected, the findings resemble those of rheumatoid arthritis.[359] Synovial effusions are frequent, and the character of the fluid is noninflammatory.[181, 182, 507] The fluid is clear and viscous, mucin clot is good to fair, and low leukocyte counts and few neutrophils are seen.[182, 183] Elevated synovial fluid fibrinogen levels have been reported.[184]

These clinical manifestations are not uniform in all patients with hypertrophic osteoarthropathy and are dependent to some extent on the nature of the underlying lesion. Hypertrophic osteoarthropathy due to pulmonary neoplasm commonly is associated with an acute onset of digital clubbing, warmth and burning of the fingertips, and occasionally skin thickening and hyperhidrosis. Joint findings appear in approximately 30 to 35 per cent of cases, and may precede pulmonary symptoms and signs. Hypertrophic osteoarthropathy associated with other disorders may be characterized by an insidious onset of digital clubbing; arthritis, skin thickening, and hyperhidrosis may be mild or absent.

In cases of hypertrophic osteoarthropathy secondary to intrathoracic causes, thoracotomy frequently leads to prominent remission of the joint symptoms and signs within 24 hours, although radiographic findings may recede more slowly, requiring a period of months to years for complete resolution. Even patients with nonresectable tumors may benefit from thoracotomy. Other surgical procedures that can lead to a regression of the clinical manifestations include hilar neurectomy, vagotomy, and ipsilateral occlusion of the pulmonary artery.[217] Radiotherapy or chemotherapy[300] may be associated with similar improvement.[185, 289] Additionally, clinical relief has been recorded using intercostal nerve section, drugs that inhibit growth hormone, hypophysectomy, and even laparotomy.[186, 187, 218, 219, 360] Chemical vagotomy also may have beneficial results.[304, 305] Regrowth of the neoplasm commonly is associated with exacerbation of the clinical and radiographic findings.[148, 188] Hypertrophic osteoarthropathy related to chronic hepatic disease may benefit from liver transplantation,[500] although rejection of the transplanted liver has been associated with the initial appearance or recurrence of hypertrophic osteoarthropathy.[501]

Radiographic Abnormalities

Although, rarely, symptoms and signs of hypertrophic osteoarthropathy occur without obvious radiographic abnormality,[361] periostitis is the hallmark of the disease. Periosteal bone deposition initially appears in the proximal and distal diaphyses of the tibiae, fibulae, radii, ulnae, and (less frequently) the femora, humeri, metacarpals, metatarsals, and phalanges (with the exception of the terminal phalanges) (Fig. 93–44). With progression, periostitis becomes prominent in the metaphyseal regions as well as at musculotendinous insertions, but usually does not extend into the epiphyses. Epiphyseal extension of periostitis may be observed in patients with hypertrophic osteoarthropathy secondary to congenital cyanotic heart disease, however. Furthermore, in congenital cyanotic heart disease (Fig. 93–45), as well as in other disorders such as cystic fibrosis (Fig. 93–46) that lead to hypertrophic osteoarthropathy in the immature skeleton and that are of long duration, more

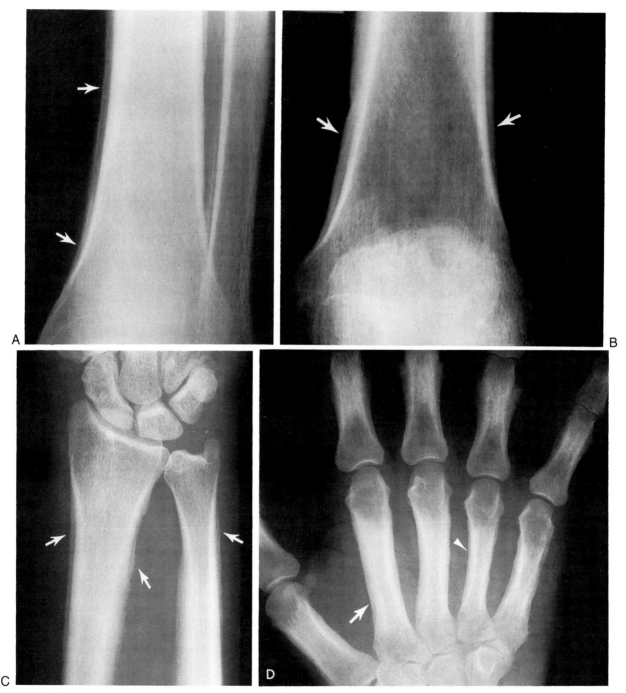

FIGURE 93–44. Secondary hypertrophic osteoarthropathy: Periostitis.
A Distal tibia and fibula. Elevation of the periosteal membrane in the diaphyses of these bones has resulted in linear deposition of new bone (arrows). Involvement ends at the metaphyses.
B Femur. Observe thick linear periosteal bone formation on the medial and lateral aspects of the femur (arrows). The endosteal surface of the cortex is not affected.
C Distal radius and ulna. In another classic location, observe linear periostitis of the diaphysis extending to the metaphysis of both bones (arrows).
D Metacarpal bones and phalanges. Linear periostitis of the metacarpal bones has produced bone that is either separated from (arrowhead) or firmly merged with (arrow) the underlying osseous tissue. Bony proliferation at muscular insertions of the phalanges also is seen. Note some degree of periarticular osteoporosis.

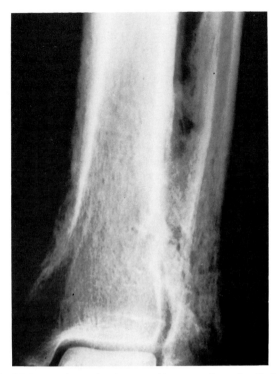

FIGURE 93–45. Secondary hypertrophic osteoarthropathy: Periostitis. Congenital cyanotic heart disease. Observe very irregular and prominent new bone formation in the tibia and fibula. (Courtesy of C. Pineda, M.D., Mexico City, Mexico.)

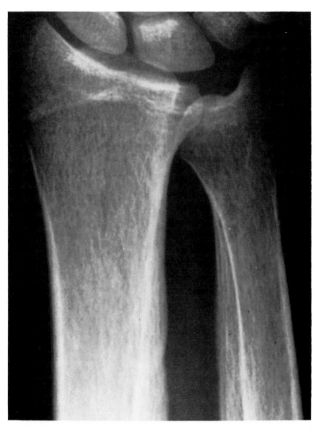

FIGURE 93–46. Secondary hypertrophic osteoarthropathy. Periostitis. Cystic fibrosis. The degree of bone formation in the distal portions of the radius and ulna is prominent. (Courtesy of M. Murphey, M.D., Washington, D.C.)

prominent periostitis may be seen. Rarely, in secondary hypertrophic osteoarthropathy, radiographic abnormalities may be detected in the scapulae, clavicles (Fig. 93–47), ribs, spine, and even the cranium and facial bones, although involvement at these latter sites is more obvious on scintigraphic examination (see discussion later in this chapter).

Various types of periostitis are seen: simple elevation of the periosteum with a radiolucent area between the periosteal bone and subjacent cortex; laminated or "onion-skin" appearance, with smooth layers of new bone formation; irregular areas of periosteal elevation; irregular, solid areas of periosteal cloaking with a wavy contour; and cortical thickening, with application of the periosteal bone to the outer surface of the cortex.[142] In fact, the appearance of the periostitis changes during the course of the process. Initially, it may appear as a single layer of new bone that is separate from the subjacent osseous structures. Subsequently, with exacerbations and remissions of the underlying disease, layered new bone formation can be evident, eventually merging with the cortical bone.

Digital clubbing leading to radiographically detectable soft tissue swelling also is evident. The finding is nonspecific, and may be associated with focal areas of tuftal hypertrophy or resorption (Fig. 93–48).[346]

Pathologic Abnormalities

Prior to the deposition of new bone by the periosteum, its outer or fibrous layer is the site of round cell infiltration.[50, 163, 189] Proliferation of the inner or cambium layer follows, leading to deposition of new bone on the original cortex (Fig. 93–49). Initially, the osseous deposits are separated from the cortex and are composed predominantly of

meshy trabeculae or coarse-fibered tissue.[50] As the deposits become more extensive, their deeper part becomes lamellar in character and the cortical bone may reveal focal areas of porosity. Eventually a clear demarcation between the periosteal and cortical bone is no longer identifiable. Endosteal deposition of bone is not prominent, a fact that is helpful in

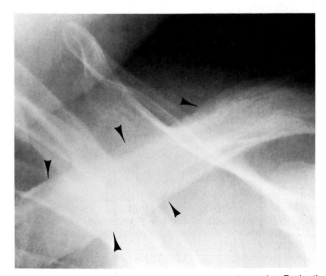

FIGURE 93–47. Secondary hypertrophic osteoarthropathy: Periostitis. Deposition of new bone (arrowheads) has resulted in diffuse enlargement of the clavicle.

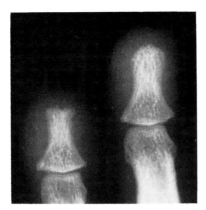

FIGURE 93–48. Secondary hypertrophic osteoarthropathy: Digital clubbing and osteolysis. In this patient with cyanotic congenital heart disease, soft tissue prominence and tuftal osteolysis are evident. (Courtesy of C. Pineda, M.D., Mexico City, Mexico.)

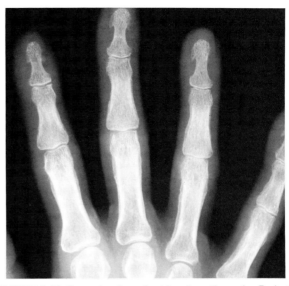

FIGURE 93–50. Secondary hypertrophic osteoarthropathy: Periarticular soft tissue swelling. Observe moderate periarticular swelling and prominent periostitis. The opposite hand showed similar abnormalities. Although the initial clinical diagnosis was rheumatoid arthritis, a chest radiograph revealed a poorly differentiated adenocarcinoma of the lung. (Courtesy of G. Greenway, M.D., Dallas, Texas.)

the accurate diagnosis of the radiographic and pathologic findings.

Holling and Brodey[144] have argued that descriptions of pathologic abnormalities in hypertrophic osteoarthropathy concentrate too heavily on the bone lesions. These investigators cite experimental studies in dogs in which exuberant new bone formation is preceded by an intense overgrowth of vascular connective tissue in portions of the affected limbs. This newly formed tissue surrounds tendons, bones, and even joints. Studies in humans reveal similar findings of newly formed vascular tissue investing osseous and periarticular structures; this tissue is composed of collagenous bundles supplied with many thick-walled blood vessels, often containing perivascular collections of lymphocytes.[136]

Articular Abnormalities

Pain and swelling about the knees, ankles, wrists, and even the fingers (Fig. 93–50) may be the presenting mani-

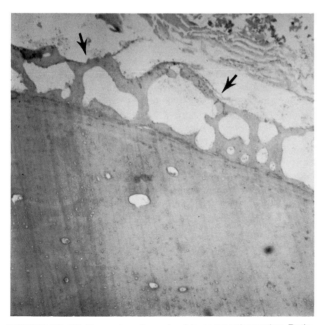

FIGURE 93–49. Secondary hypertrophic osteoarthropathy: Pathologic abnormalities. Note the lace-like deposition of bone (arrows) beneath the periosteum, which is uniting with the underlying cortex.

festation of hypertrophic osteoarthropathy,[182] simulating the clinical presentation of rheumatoid arthritis.[190, 191] This clinical dilemma is accentuated by the presence of soft tissue swelling, joint effusions, and periarticular osteoporosis on radiographic examination, and (rarely) by the simultaneous occurrence of true rheumatoid disease.[192] In hypertrophic osteoarthropathy, the predilection for large joint involvement with relative sparing of the interphalangeal articulations[193] as well as the absence of inflammatory synovial fluid on aspiration and an inflammatory synovial membrane on biopsy permits its differentiation from rheumatoid arthritis. Early reports of synovial membrane histology, however, cited evidence of chronic synovitis with fibrinoid degeneration, subsynovial congestion, cellular infiltration with lymphocytes, plasma cells, and histiocytes, and some degree of hyperplasia of synovial lining cells.[136] Even pannus formation and fibrous and bony ankylosis were noted in some specimens.[180] In hypertrophic osteoarthropathy secondary to congenital heart disease and cirrhosis, synovial biopsies also have demonstrated mild chronic inflammation[162] as well as synovial calcification.[194] Despite these reports, many investigators agree that considerable synovial inflammation is not a feature of hypertrophic osteoarthropathy, although increased inflammation could perhaps develop in disease of long duration[150, 182] (Fig. 93–51). Schumacher,[182] in an electron microscopic examination of the synovial membrane, detected electron-dense deposits in the vessel walls and prominent, fibrin-like material on the synovial surface, in the interstitium, and in some of the dense deposits. He speculated that the dense material arrived at the joint via the circulation, and that the prominent fibrin collections could have resulted from a microvascular injury to the synovial membrane allowing leakage of molecular weight proteins from the injured vessels.

In any case, it generally is regarded that the joint manifestations of hypertrophic osteoarthropathy are not specific, nor are they as inflammatory in nature as the changes in

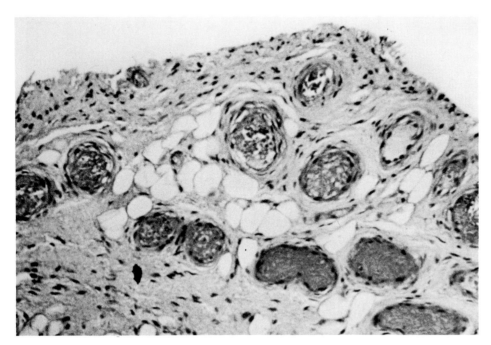

FIGURE 93–51. Secondary hypertrophic osteoarthropathy: Articular abnormalities. Marked congestion of small synovial vessels is unassociated with inflammatory cellular infiltration (180×).

(From Schumacher HR Jr: Arthritis Rheum *19*:629, 1976.)

rheumatoid arthritis. In experimental hypertrophic osteoarthropathy, specific articular findings also are not detectable.[195] Articular space narrowing, marginal and central erosions (as noted in patients with rheumatoid arthritis), and osseous excrescences and bony ankylosis (seen in patients with primary hypertrophic osteoarthropathy) are not found in persons with secondary hypertrophic osteoarthropathy.

Radionuclide Abnormalities

Radionuclide bone imaging represents a highly sensitive method of detecting abnormalities of primary or secondary hypertrophic osteoarthropathy.[196–203, 348, 349, 362, 363, 436] A diffuse, symmetric increased uptake in the diaphyses and metaphyses of tubular bones along their cortical margins creates a distinctive "double stripe" or "parallel track" sign (Fig. 93–52A). Associated synovitis can lead to increased radionuclide uptake in periarticular regions also. Unusual alterations include accumulation of radiopharmaceutical agents in the clavicles, scapulae, pelvis, and bones of the face, asymmetric uptake, and digital accumulation related to clubbing[199, 204, 302, 349] (Fig. 93–52B, C).

The scintigraphic abnormalities frequently appear before the roentgenographic findings, correspond well with clinical manifestations, and decrease following appropriate therapeutic regimens, such as surgery and radiation therapy. Occasionally, they may disappear without any treatment.[203] Recurrence of a tumor is followed by the return of an abnormal radionuclide pattern. Although an accumulation of radiopharmaceutical agents in the patient with malignant tumor also can represent evidence of skeletal metastasis, differentiation of the scintigraphic patterns in hypertrophic osteoarthropathy and in metastasis is not difficult (Fig. 93–53). Asymmetry, focal areas of increased activity, and prominent involvement of the axial skeleton and medullary spaces characterize the radionuclide abnormalities of metastatic disease involving the skeleton.[197, 198]

Pathogenesis

Since the early description of hypertrophic osteoarthropathy by Bamberger[138] and Marie,[98] numerous theories have been proposed to explain the pathogenesis of the condition, none of which is entirely adequate. Marie[98] believed that the primary disease elaborated a chemical irritant that, when absorbed, led to the osseous lesions. Other investigators also postulated the presence of a toxic substance that initiated a periosteal response.[205, 206] The humoral theory has been further developed through the years and has been encouraged by the detection of high urinary output of certain steroid metabolites in patients with hypertrophic osteoarthropathy.[211, 212] Some evidence, however, including the inability to produce hypertrophic osteoarthropathy in normal dogs following cross-circulation with affected dogs, has suggested that other factors are more important.[144]

A neurogenic mechanism in this condition has gained increasing support from the observation that prompt relief of symptoms and signs can follow surgical disruption of the vagus nerve.[187, 207] Vagal nerve interruption apparently reduces the increased blood flow that is present in cases of secondary hypertrophic osteoarthropathy.[208] It is postulated that neural impulses arise in the pulmonary or pleural lesion and pass as afferent impulses in the vagus nerve. Similar afferent pathways may exist when the causative lesion is located in certain additional viscera; in fact, many of the organs in which primary diseases lead to secondary hypertrophic osteoarthropathy are supplied by fibers from either the ninth or tenth cranial nerves.[213] The efferent pathways have not been delineated; denervation of affected limbs or high spinal anesthesia is without significant effect, either on clinical manifestations or limb blood flow. Sympathetic nerve activity appears to be unimportant, as sympathectomy produces little effect. Anticholinergic medication also has no effect, suggesting that vagal or other parasympathetic efferent nerves are not involved. If and when the efferent

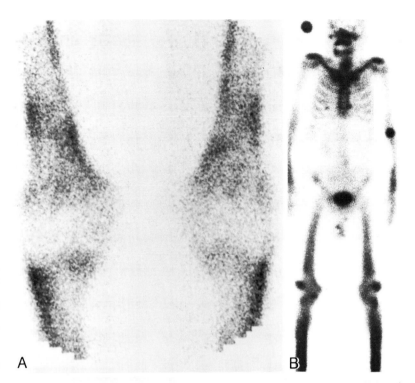

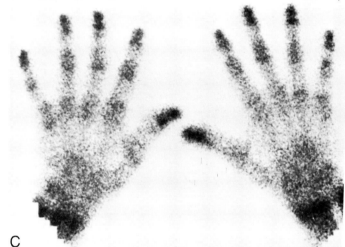

FIGURE 93–52. Secondary hypertrophic osteoarthropathy. Radionuclide abnormalities. Various patterns on bone scans.

A "Double stripe" or "parallel track" sign is present in the femora and tibiae.

B Diffuse uptake is observed in both the appendicular skeleton and the axial skeleton.

C Digital accumulation of radionuclide is evident.

(**B,** Courtesy of V. Vint, M.D., San Diego, California.)

limb of the arc can be fully delineated, the attractiveness of the neurogenic theory will increase dramatically.

The importance of increased blood flow in the pathogenesis of periostitis in hypertrophic osteoarthropathy has been emphasized. Pathologic studies of clubbed digits have outlined dilatation of vessels and dense neovascularity. The newly formed vascular channels envelop bones and joints, consisting of wide, thick-walled vessels, collagenous bundles, and cellular infiltration. Capillary flow studies that have used isotope washout rates have indicated increased vascular perfusion of affected areas in secondary hypertrophic osteoarthropathy.[209] Experimentally, periosteal changes can be produced in the dog by establishing a permanent fistula between the left auricle and pulmonary arteries; perhaps these changes are related to constantly excessive peripheral blood volume that increases periosteal nutrition and promotes bone proliferation.[210] A similar increase in blood flow could be expected in humans with cyanotic congenital heart disease and accounts for the clinical findings of warmth and burning that accompany hypertrophic osteoarthropathy. This type of flow consists of excessive blood that is poorly oxygenated and might produce local passive congestion and poor tissue oxygenation, with resulting stimulation of various connective tissues, including the periosteal membrane.[50] In most cases of hypertrophic osteoarthropathy, however, no evidence of arteriovenous shunting in the pulmonary circulation is demonstrated, and the appearance of periostitis in these situations may require the presence of some factor other than deoxygenated blood.

It is possible that several different mechanisms are responsible for secondary hypertrophic osteoarthropathy, considering the large number and diverse nature of the conditions that lead to it. A chemical substance, neurogenic

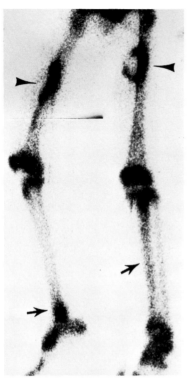

FIGURE 93–53. Secondary hypertrophic osteoarthropathy: Radionuclide abnormalities. This man had bilateral painful masses of the thigh and an abnormal chest radiograph. Biopsy of both the pulmonary and appendicular skeletal lesions confirmed the presence of bronchogenic carcinoma with metastasis. The radionuclide study using technetium indicates diffuse uptake in the diaphyses and metaphyses of the tubular bones, most marked about the ankles and in the tibiae (arrows). Focal accumulations are evident in both femora (arrowheads). A radiograph of the distal right leg (not shown) revealed periosteal proliferation indicative of hypertrophic osteoarthropathy. Metastatic lesions were found in both femora.

mechanism, or hypervascularity working alone or in combination may be responsible in a specific situation or disease. For example, hypertrophic osteoarthropathy in congenital cyanotic heart disease appears to be related to arterial oxygen unsaturation, increased systemic output, and severe right-to-left shunting, suggesting that the degree of lung bypass is a significant pathogenetic factor and that a chemical mediator in the visceral venous circulation that escapes inactivation or removal in the pulmonary capillary bed may be responsible.[351, 505] Hypertrophic osteoarthropathy complicating an infected aortic graft may correspond in distribution to the site of infection; unilateral or bilateral osseous changes in the lower extremities may indicate whether the sepsis spreads to one or both of the graft limbs.[357] This suggests that irritation of local nerves or septic emboli might account for the periosteal reaction, although other factors, including the patency of the graft, changes in regional blood flow, and a specific response of the Dacron material to infection, possibly are important.

Differential Diagnosis

Periostitis (and clubbing) also can be observed in primary hypertrophic osteoarthropathy (pachydermoperiostosis) and thyroid acropachy (see Table 93–4) (Fig. 93–54). In the former condition, the osseous excrescences are more irregular and extend into the epiphyses of the tubular bones. A family history of disease also is evident. In thyroid acropachy, periosteal proliferation has a predilection for the small bones of the hands and feet; significant or isolated abnormalities of the major tubular bones are distinctly unusual. Pretibial myxedema and a history of dysfunction of the thyroid gland are evident.

Chronic venous stasis can produce periostitis, usually confined to the lower extremities (see discussion later in this chapter). Cases of hypertrophic osteoarthropathy involving one or both lower extremities, without involving the upper extremity, have been reported but are very rare.[204, 223–225, 303] Furthermore, the nature of periosteal proliferation in the presence of venous insufficiency is unique.

Additional causes of diffuse periostitis or bone proliferation, such as hypervitaminosis A, infantile cortical hyperostosis, diffuse idiopathic skeletal hyperostosis, or fluorosis, usually are not confused with hypertrophic osteoarthropathy.

VASCULAR INSUFFICIENCY

Periosteal bone formation has been noted in association with chronic venous insufficiency.[226–230, 364] The lower extremities are affected almost exclusively, with involvement of the tibia, fibula, femur, metatarsals, and phalanges (see Table 93–4). The diaphyseal and metaphyseal segments are predominantly altered, and an undulating osseous contour is produced, with considerable new bone appearing on the outer aspect of the cortex (Figs. 93–55 and 93–56). Although initially separated from the underlying bone, the periosteal deposits soon merge with the cortex.

The frequency of periostitis increases with the severity and duration of the venous insufficiency, and the disorder may be detected in 10 to 60 per cent of patients with chronic disabling venous stasis.[227, 229, 231, 232] Although many patients also reveal soft tissue ulcerations, these cutaneous abnormalities are not always present in patients with venous periostitis, and the periostitis may be more severe in locations distant from the ulcerations. These observations indicate that infection is not fundamental to the appearance of periosteal proliferation. Similarly, although lymphatic insufficiency also may be noted in some patients with venous periostitis, it, too, does not appear to be a necessary component of the process. The pathogenesis of the periostitis may relate to hypoxia created by vascular stasis or hypertension, but a single mechanism has yet to be substantiated.

Soft tissue edema and ossification[365, 366] represent roentgenographic findings that commonly are associated with venous insufficiency and periostitis (Fig. 93–57). Single or multiple phleboliths may be apparent, and in some cases a diffuse reticular ossific pattern is evident. Metaplastic bone formation in the subcutaneous tissue is observed histologically.

Arterial insufficiency also has been associated with periosteal bone proliferation. This may occur in polyarteritis nodosa or other arteritides.[233, 508] Any bone can be affected, but most cases are confined to the lower extremity. Bilateral or unilateral changes are encountered.[509] The degree of bone formation usually is mild, but cases with exuberant periostitis have been reported (see Chapter 36).

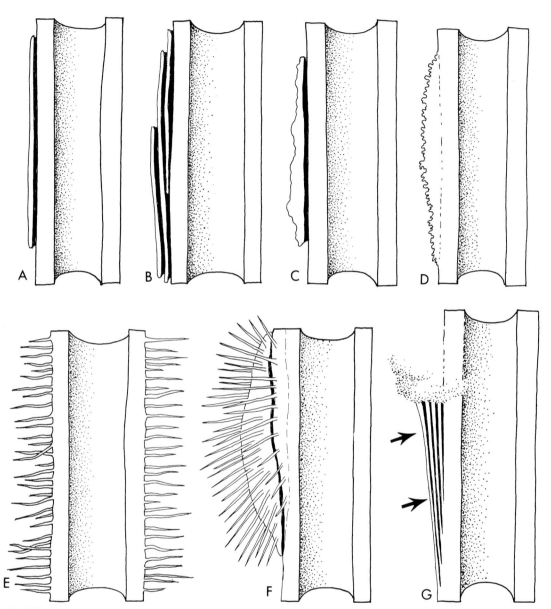

FIGURE 93–54. Differential diagnosis of periosteal new bone formation: Various types of periostitis are identified.

A Single layer of new bone, which may be observed in benign or malignant tumors, infection, and secondary hypertrophic osteoarthropathy.

B Multiple layers of new bone or "onion-skinning," which can be evident in infection, malignant tumors such as Ewing's sarcoma, hypertrophic osteoarthropathy, and other conditions.

C A thick linear osseous deposit, which can be separate from (as indicated here) or mixed with the underlying bone. This pattern is common in hypertrophic osteoarthropathy and venous stasis.

D An irregular osseous excrescence with spiculated contour that merges with the underlying cortex. This pattern can be observed in thyroid acropachy or primary hypertrophic osteoarthropathy (pachydermoperiostosis).

E Thin, linear osseous deposits that extend in a direction perpendicular to the underlying cortex, a pattern that is highly characteristic of Ewing's sarcoma.

F A sunburst pattern, in which linear deposits fan out from a single focus, an appearance that can be evident in osteosarcoma.

G A Codman's triangle, consisting of triangular elevation of the periosteum with one or more layers of new bone (arrows), a pattern that is suggestive but not diagnostic of malignancy.

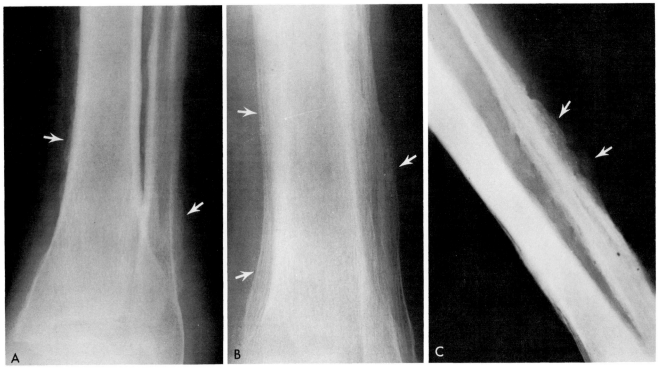

FIGURE 93–55. Chronic venous stasis: Periostitis.

A Observe undulating periosteal new bone in the diaphyses and metaphyses of the distal tibia and fibula (arrows). Soft tissue edema is present.

B In this patient, a laminated or solid coat of periosteal bone surrounds the distal tibia and fibula (arrows).

C A more nodular and irregular appearance of periosteal bone formation (arrows) characterizes the situation in this patient with chronic venous stasis and soft tissue infection.

INFANTILE CORTICAL HYPEROSTOSIS

Infantile cortical hyperostosis (Caffey's disease) is an uncommon disease, usually commencing in infancy, that affects predominantly the skeleton and adjacent fascial, muscular, and connective tissues.[234] It was first reported as a distinct entity in 1945 by Caffey and Silverman[235] and in 1946 by Smyth and coworkers.[236] Infantile cortical hyperostosis has a worldwide distribution, is evident in all racial strains, and affects boys and girls with approximately equal frequency.

Clinical Abnormalities

Almost without exception, the disease becomes evident in an infant less than 5 months of age; it may be apparent in the first days or weeks of life, and even has been recognized in utero.[237, 238] The average age of onset is 9 to 10 weeks. Familial instances (see later discussion) of the disease are recognized,[239–243, 367–370, 414] although most cases reported prior to 1960 were sporadic. Fever of abrupt onset, hyperirritability, and soft tissue swelling are typical. The swelling is especially prominent over the mandible but also can appear at other sites. On palpation, indurated, hard and tender soft tissue masses are noted, and these may be attached to the underlying bones. Such swelling reflects the soft tissue extension of periosteal reaction in the underlying bone, although it may antedate radiographic evidence of osseous abnormality. Discoloration and warmth are not evident. Subsidence of the soft tissue process is slow, and at

any time it may recur at the original site or at a new location.

Additional clinical features may include pallor, painful pseudoparalysis, and pleurisy.[234] Laboratory analysis may indicate an elevated erythrocyte sedimentation rate and an elevated serum level of alkaline phosphatase, a moderate leukocytosis, and anemia.

The clinical course is extremely variable. In many instances, clinical and radiographic features subside slowly over a period of a few months to a few years, but this self-limited quality is not uniform. Occasionally, active disease may persist, recurring intermittently for years, and leading to a marked delay in musculoskeletal development and crippling deformities.[234] Thus, residua of the disease may be evident even in the third and fourth decades of life.[234–248] In these instances, mandibular asymmetry,[235, 249] interosseous bony bridges,[247, 250, 251] and bowing of the limbs[239–240] can be observed.[242] Rarely, a severely affected infant will die, usually as a result of a secondary infection.[50, 252–254]

Radiographic Abnormalities

In any one patient, a single bone or many bones can be involved (see Table 93–4). Sequential involvement is typical, with one area being affected initially, followed in later stages of the disease by changes in other sites. The mandible, clavicles, and ribs are involved more often, and changes in these bones may be symmetric[255] (Fig. 93–58). Thoracic cage abnormalities can be combined with pleural

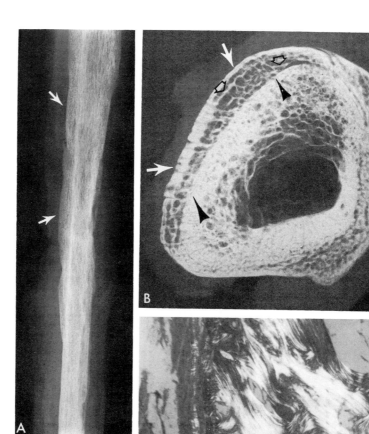

FIGURE 93–56. Chronic venous stasis: Periostitis.

A A radiograph of a removed fibula in a patient with venous insufficiency reveals the undulating nature of the periosteal bony deposition (arrows).

B A radiograph of a cross section through the upper fibular shaft outlines a ring of new bone (arrows) that has buried the original cortical surface (arrowheads). Note the laminated nature of the bony deposits (open arrows).

C On a polarized photomicrograph of the section (72×), note the periosteal fibrous tissue (arrow), periosteum with polarized collagen fibers (arrowhead), and hypertrophic polarized osseous trabeculae.

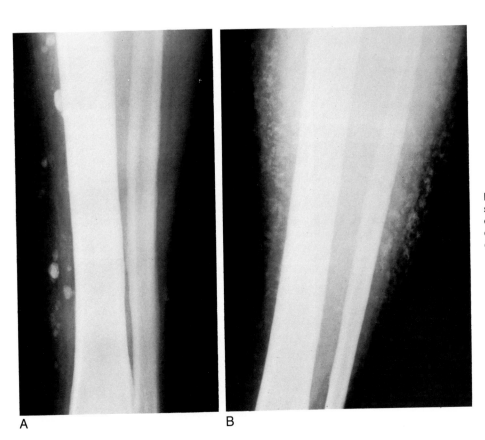

A   B

FIGURE 93–57. Chronic venous stasis: Soft tissue calcification and ossification. Examples of phlebolith calcification **(A)** and reticular ossification **(B)** are shown.

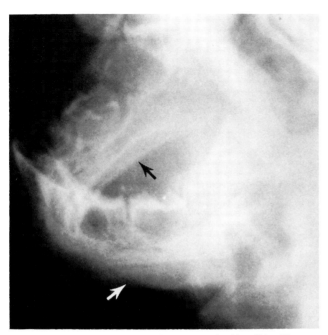

FIGURE 93–58. Infantile cortical hyperostosis: Mandible. Observe diffuse periosteal proliferation of the mandible (arrows).

effusions; such effusions occur ipsilateral to the side of costal hyperostosis. The scapulae are altered in approximately 10 per cent of cases, and involvement at this site may be monostotic or unilateral, exuberant, and associated with neurologic deficit and diaphragmatic elevation[256–258, 307, 371] (Fig. 93–59). Changes in the ilia, cranial vault (parietal and frontal regions), and tubular bones also are encountered.[259] In the tubular bones, asymmetry predominates, and the ulnae are involved most frequently, although changes in the tibiae, fibulae, humeri, femora, radii, metacarpals, and metatarsals may be seen[234, 260, 373] (Fig. 93–60). Alterations of the vertebrae, carpus, tarsus, and phalanges are unusual.

Cortical hyperostosis is the hallmark of the disease. New bone formation begins in the soft tissue swelling directly contiguous to the original cortex, becomes progressively more dense, and may reach profound proportions. Thus, the deposits of bone merge with the underlying osseous tissue, doubling or tripling the normal width of the parent bone. Predilection for the lateral arches of the ribs[372] and the diaphyses and metaphyses of tubular bones is evident. The epiphyseal ossification centers generally are spared. The endosteal surfaces also can undergo new bone formation, resulting in diminution of the medullary cavity.

Destructive lesions of the skull or, rarely, the tubular bones have been identified in some cases.[234, 262, 263, 415] These may be single or multiple, unilateral or bilateral; they may have a predilection for the frontal squamosa and may simulate histiocytosis or metastatic neuroblastoma. The lesions probably relate to focal resorption of peripheral layers of the cortex.

Radiographic improvement can occur in a period of weeks to months, to an extent that evidence of hyperostosis may be entirely lacking on follow-up examinations after 6 months to 1 year (Fig. 93–61). During healing, the cortical thickening may become lamellated with increased porosity, and the medullary canal can widen. Residual changes can

be encountered, such as diaphyseal expansion, longitudinal overgrowth and bowing deformities, osseous bridging between adjacent bones such as the radius and ulna, tibia and fibula, and ribs, exophthalmos, and facial asymmetry[261] (Fig. 93–62).

Although the radiographic abnormalities outlined earlier are virtually diagnostic of Caffey's disease, scintigraphy with bone-seeking radiotracers can be used to further document the extent of skeletal involvement (Fig. 93–63).[371, 373, 375]

Pathologic Abnormalities

Caffey[234] has reviewed in detail the pathologic data contained in previous descriptions of this disease[264] (Fig. 93–64). In the early stage, acute inflammatory changes appear in the periosteal membrane, consisting of edema and cellular infiltration with polymorphonuclear leukocytes. The thickened and inflamed membrane loses its peripheral limiting fibrous layer, blending with the adjacent fasciae, tendons, and muscles. Proliferation of connective tissue cells and of osteoblasts indicates considerable activity.[374, 416] Cortical resorption and porosity can be identified in this phase. In the subacute phase, inflammatory changes diminish. Beneath the periosteum, a layer of immature, coarse-fibered trabeculae of variable thickness becomes identifiable[50]; between trabeculae, vascularized connective tissue appears. In the late phases, the peripheral bone is removed, beginning in the interior and extending peripherally. Thus, dilatation of the medullary cavity is seen, with subsequent remodeling and shrinkage of the dilated, thin-walled bone shaft.

The involvement of adjacent soft tissue has been emphasized in these early reports. The presence of intimal prolif-

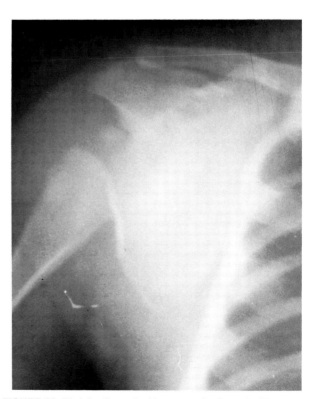

FIGURE 93–59. Infantile cortical hyperostosis: Scapula. Monostotic scapular disease has resulted in exuberant bone formation and considerable deformity and enlargement.

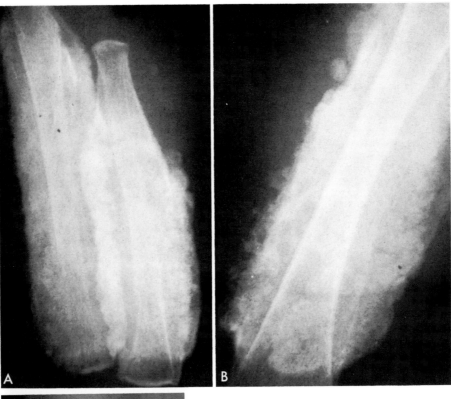

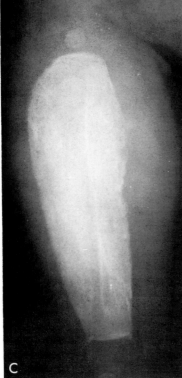

FIGURE 93–60. Infantile cortical hyperostosis: Tubular bones. Examples of radial and ulnar **(A),** femoral **(B),** and tibial **(C)** involvement are shown. The extent of new bone formation is remarkable. These deposits initially are evident in the soft tissues and later merge with the underlying bone.

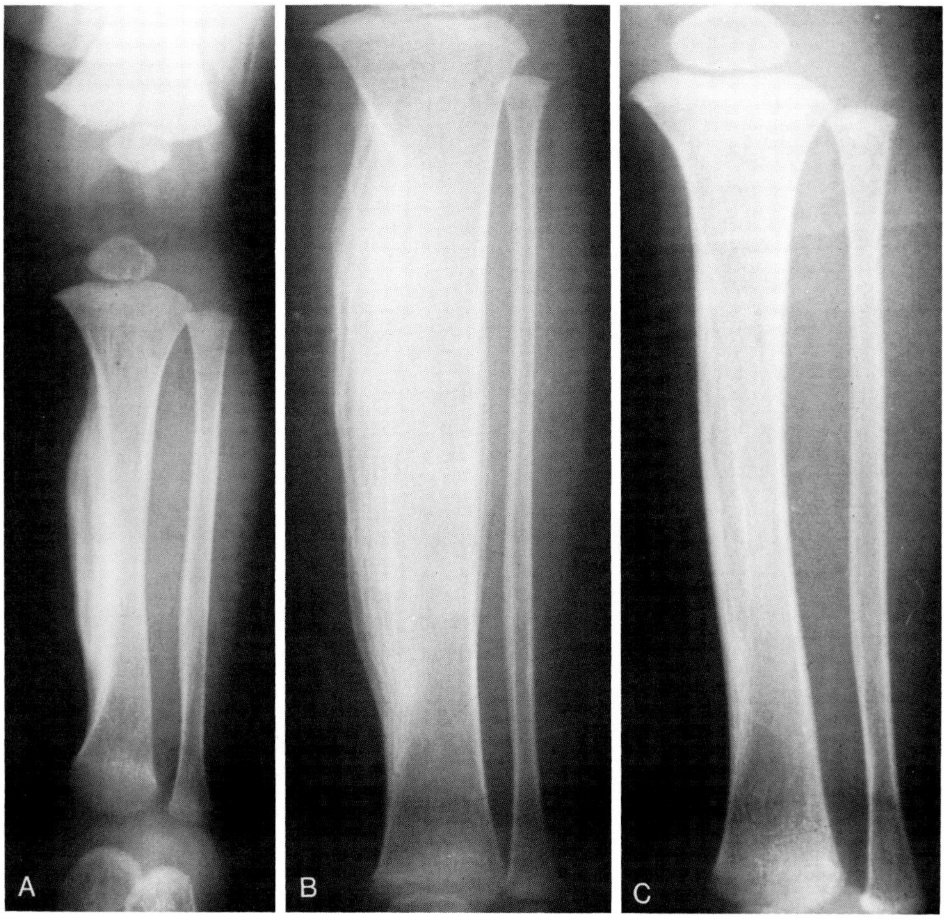

FIGURE 93–61. Infantile cortical hyperostosis: Improvement in skeletal lesions. Radiographs are shown of this child at the ages of 5 months **(A)**, 6 months **(B)**, and 10 months **(C)**. Note the marked improvement of the skeletal abnormalities in **C**. (Courtesy of H. S. Kang, M.D., Seoul, Korea.)

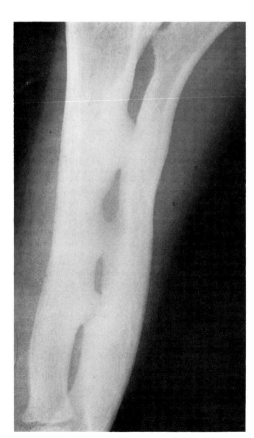

FIGURE 93–62. Infantile cortical hyperostosis: Residual changes. In this child, residual enlargement and deformity of the radius and ulna with interosseous bridging are apparent.

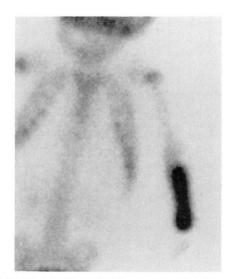

FIGURE 93–63. Infantile cortical hyperostosis: Scintigraphy. Bone scintigraphy in this 4 month old infant reveals intense uptake of the radionuclide in the left forearm, the site of radiographically evident hyperostosis of the radius and ulna.

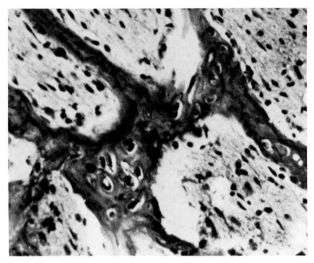

FIGURE 93–64. Infantile cortical hyperostosis: Pathologic abnormalities. A photomicrograph (270×) of a biopsy specimen from an involved bone indicates striking new bone formation and an inflammatory reaction characterized by acute and chronic cellular infiltration. (From Kaufmann HJ: Skel Radiol 2:109, 1977.)

eration of the small arteries in both the fascial and the osseous lesions has suggested to some investigators that hypoxia may be an initial event that stimulates soft tissue and bone proliferation.[253]

Etiology and Pathogenesis

Although there has been considerable speculation regarding the cause of infantile cortical hyperostosis, it remains unknown. There are many clinical and pathologic features suggesting that an infectious agent is responsible for the disease. The presence of severe and protracted fever, an elevated erythrocyte sedimentation rate, an occasional pleural exudate in association with thoracic cage lesions, and clustering of cases, both in time and in location, are clinical findings consistent with an infection.[265] The identification of acute inflammatory changes in the periosteum also raises the possibility of an infectious agent. The apparent immunity to recurrence after the initial course of the disease is not unlike that which is evident in certain viral diseases. A viral cause also is suggested by the demonstration of a virus in the hamster that has affinity for bones, including the mandible,[266] the lack of response to antibiotic therapy and sulfonamides, the alterations in serum proteins that resemble responses to known infections, and the elevation of gamma globulins that is consistent with an in-utero viral infection. No bacterial or viral agents have yet been identified in the disease, however, and serologic tests for such agents also have been unsuccessful.

Abnormalities of serum protein concentrations in infantile cortical hyperostosis also may indicate the importance of an altered immune status.[265] This possibility may explain the occurrence of the disease in patients with immunodeficient disorders,[267] although this association also could reflect the proclivity of such persons to develop infections. Further speculation exists that infantile cortical hyperostosis represents an allergic response to altered collagen tissue.[268] Hyperplasia and fibrinoid degeneration of collagen fibers may be prominent in this disorder and may promote altera-

tions in the surrounding osseous, muscular, soft tissue, and vascular tissues.

The appearance of infantile cortical hyperostosis in many members of a single family over one or more generations underscores the importance of genetic factors in the pathogenesis of the disease.[367–370] An autosomal dominant pattern of inheritance with incomplete penetrance and variable expressivity is seen. With a decrease in the number of sporadic cases that are encountered, familial infantile cortical hyperostosis may represent the major pattern of disease that is evident today.[368] Familial cases are characterized by an earlier age of onset (approximately 25 per cent have abnormalities at birth), less common mandibular involvement, and more common lower extremity involvement.[368] Changes in the ribs and scapulae are rare.[370]

Differential Diagnosis

Although periostitis and hyperostosis in an infant also can be observed in rickets and scurvy, the absence of epiphyseal or metaphyseal alterations and the resolution of clinical and roentgenographic features over a period of months in patients with infantile cortical hyperostosis allow its differentiation from these other disorders. Similarly, trauma, including that in the abused child, can lead to calcifying subperiosteal hematomas, but additional findings, such as microfractures and metaphyseal irregularity, are evident. In hypervitaminosis A, clinical and radiographic manifestations initially appear toward the end of the first year of life, metatarsal predilection is apparent, facial swelling and mandibular involvement are rare, and serologic testing indicates an elevation of vitamin A levels. The findings in osteomyelitis, leukemia, neuroblastoma, the kinky hair syndrome, and Camurati-Engelmann disease usually are not hard to differentiate from those of infantile cortical hyperostosis. The long-term administration of prostaglandin E_1 in infants with ductus-dependent cyanotic congenital heart disease is associated with periostitis and cortical hyperostosis, findings that are very similar to those of infantile cortical hyperostosis (see Chapter 74).[376–378]

HYPEROSTOSIS FRONTALIS INTERNA AND RELATED CONDITIONS

Hyperostosis frontalis interna is a descriptive term that is applied to hyperostosis involving predominantly the inner table of the frontal squama. Originally emphasized by Morgagni over 200 years ago,[50] this condition has been further delineated in numerous reports.[269, 270] It is of interest that Morgagni's original patient was an elderly woman with obesity and virilism, and these findings, combined with hyperostosis of the cranial vault, sometimes are referred to as "Morgagni's syndrome" or "metabolic craniopathy."[50] This association is neither constant nor frequent, however, as most persons with this cranial abnormality fail to reveal significant systemic manifestations.

Hyperostosis frontalis interna usually is observed in patients over the age of 40 years. Women predominate over men,[271] and many of the women are postmenopausal. In fact, Henschen[272] observed some degree of cranial hyperostosis in approximately 40 per cent of postmenopausal women. In these patients, rhizomelic obesity, facial hirsutism, hypertension, headache, depression, anxiety, and his-

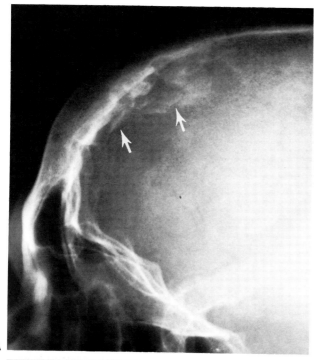

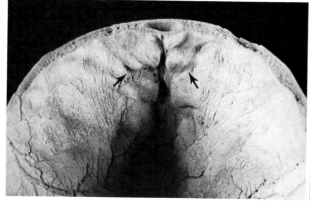

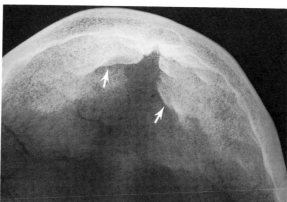

FIGURE 93–65. Hyperostosis frontalis interna.

A Note nodular hyperostosis of the inner table of the frontal bone (arrows).

B, C Nodular thickening of the inner table of the frontal bones in a symmetric distribution is seen (arrows).

torical evidence of menstrual irregularity are common but inconsistent findings.[50] Hyperostosis also has been considered a roentgenographic finding in insane patients[273] or an indication of brain loss.[274, 275]

Radiographically, the disorder leads to mild to moderate thickening of the inner table that is sessile or nodular in outline (Fig. 93–65). Single or multiple sclerotic patches can progress slowly over a period of many years. The outer cranial contour generally is not altered, and the position of the superficial veins and longitudinal sinus is not affected. In some cases, CT has indicated mild thickening of the outer table of the cranium.[379] Scintigraphically, increased uptake of the bone-seeking radionuclide is evident at an early stage of the process, and such uptake may be prominent at a time when radiographic abnormalities are mild.[510] These findings have led to speculation that hyperostosis frontalis interna initially is associated with high bone turnover and that with further development, the process becomes less active and finally quiescent.[510]

Pathologic examination frequently demonstrates excessive diploic bone, with thinning of either or both of the tables.[50] Bone deposition occurs on the inner table in asso-

ciation with spongy transformation (see Fig. 93–65). The roentgenographic findings are virtually diagnostic, although in some cases they may be misinterpreted as evidence of a meningioma,[380] Paget's disease, skeletal metastasis, or acromegaly. With regard to meningioma, conventional radiographs of the skull are positive in approximately 50 per cent of cases, demonstrating increased vascularity, tumor calcification, bone destruction, or hyperostosis alone or in any combination. Bone production is evident in about 30 per cent of cases. The patterns of cranial hyperostosis in meningioma are variable, and one or both tables may be affected (Fig. 93–66).[381] Deposition of new bone usually occurs in layers parallel to the cranial surface or as spicules arranged at right angles to the convexity of the skull.[380] A subdural layer of ossification along the hyperostotic bone, evident in the flat or en plaque form of meningioma, characteristically creates a lucent dural interface.[382] In some instances, cranial hyperostosis occurs at a distance from the tumor.[383] CT features of meningioma en plaque include periosteal deposition of bone, surface irregularity at the site of hyperostosis, and inward bulging of the cranial vault.[511]

Hyperostosis similar to that seen in the frontal region in

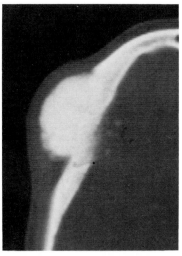

FIGURE 93–66. Meningioma: Cranial hyperostosis. In this example, destruction of the inner table and diploic portion of the skull is associated with an osteoma-like lesion extending from the outer table.

hyperostosis frontalis interna occurs in other areas of the cranial vault, especially the parietal region, and in a diffuse form[379] (Fig. 93–67). These patterns, which are less common than hyperostosis of the frontal bones, usually are symmetric in distribution and affect the inner and outer tables as well as the diploë. The occipital bone is uninvolved. The radiographic features of the diffuse variety of cranial hyperostosis, resemble those of Paget's disease, fibrous dysplasia (Fig. 93–68), acromegaly, hypoparathyroidism, and anemias.

OTHER DISORDERS

Numerous additional congenital disorders can lead to hyperostosis and increased skeletal density. These include osteopetrosis, pyknodysostosis, sclerosteosis, endosteal hyperostosis (van Buchem's disease, hyperostosis corticalis generalisata), hereditary hyperphosphatasia (juvenile Paget's disease), and idiopathic hypercalcemia (Williams' syndrome), some of which are discussed elsewhere in this book. Other causes of periostitis, such as hypervitaminosis A (Fig. 93–69A), prostaglandin medication (Fig. 93–69B), and a variety of tumors and infections also are discussed in other chapters.

Idiopathic Periosteal Hyperostosis with Dysproteinemia or Hyperphosphatemia

In 1966, Goldbloom and colleagues[276] reported two unrelated children who developed severe limb pain without

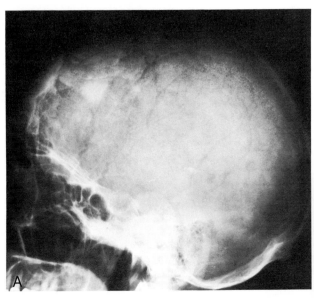

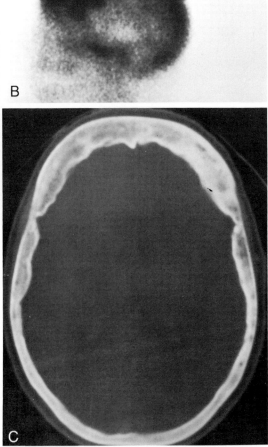

FIGURE 93–67. Generalized hyperostosis of the cranium.
  A Hyperostosis with thickening of the cranial vault predominates in the frontal regions but involves the parietal portions as well. The occiput is not affected.
  B Observe the diffusely increased accumulation of the bone-seeking radionuclide.
  C CT reveals irregular thickening of the diploic portion of the cranium in a diffuse fashion with relative sparing of the occiput.
  (Courtesy of J. Martin, M.D., San Diego, California.)

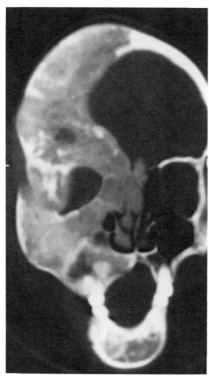

FIGURE 93–68. Fibrous dysplasia: Cranial and facial involvement. Note the classic features of bone enlargement and trabecular obliteration involving one side of the skull and face. Sinus obliteration, orbital deformity, and mandibular abnormalities are evident. (Courtesy of R. Stiles, M.D., Atlanta, Georgia.)

edema, clubbing, or joint symptoms following an upper respiratory tract infection and acute febrile illness. Neither patient had an intrathoracic lesion. Roentgenograms outlined marked periosteal bone formation involving the mandible, humeri, ulnae, metacarpals, femora, tibiae, fibulae, and metatarsals. A biopsy revealed subperiosteal bone deposition without inflammatory cells. Analysis of the serum from both patients showed decreased levels of albumin with an increase in the concentration of alpha-2 gamma globulin. With resolution of the fever over a period of weeks or months, the bone pain decreased and the radiographic findings improved. The cause of the changes remained unexplained, although an infectious agent, perhaps viral, is a significant possibility.[265]

The combination of periostitis and dysproteinemia subsequently has been observed in other patients[384] (Fig. 93–70), and similar patterns of periosteal new bone formation have been accompanied by elevated serum levels of alkaline phosphatase and hyperphosphatemia.[283, 385, 386, 512, 513] With regard to periostitis and hyperphosphatemia, male or female children usually are affected. Periosteal deposition typically is seen in the tubular bones, with predilection for the lower extremities (Fig. 93–71), although a more generalized skeletal distribution also is possible. In some instances, periods of clinical activity, consisting of pain and fever, are followed after a few weeks by those of remission in which initial periosteal deposits are incorporated into the cortex, leading to sclerosis and thickening; this feature has led to use of the term multifocal recurrent periostitis.[385, 417] Biopsy shows vascular connective tissue, periosteal bone formation, and cellular infiltration.[283] Although the cause of the syndrome is not clear, an infectious process is possible.

It is suggested that the hyperphosphatemia results from decreased renal excretion of phosphate.[386]

Hyperphosphatemia and periosteal bone formation have been identified in some children with tumoral calcinosis.[387] Except for the presence of soft tissue calcification, clinical and radiologic features in these cases are similar to those in the reported patients with periostitis and hyperphosphatemia, perhaps indicating a common cause and pathogenesis.

Plasma Cell Dyscrasia with Polyneuropathy, Organomegaly, Endocrinopathy, M Protein, and Skin Changes

In 1968, Shimpo[277] first described a unique syndrome characterized by severe progressive sensorimotor polyneuropathy that might be associated with a plasma cell dyscrasia, osteosclerotic bone lesions, production of M protein, hepatosplenomegaly, lymphadenopathy, endocrine dysfunction (diabetes mellitus, amenorrhea, gynecomastia, impotence, hypothyroidism), skin thickening and hyperpigmentation, papilledema, and episodes of anasarca. Additional reports of this syndrome soon appeared.[278–280] Although some of its radiographic features, including single or multiple solid or "bull's eye" osteosclerotic lesions, resemble findings in skeletal metastasis, plasma cell myeloma, cystic

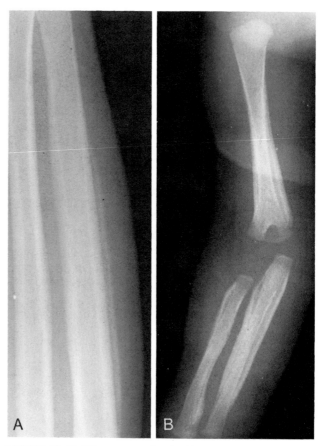

FIGURE 93–69. Other causes of periostitis.
A Hypervitaminosis A related to retinoid therapy. Observe linear periostitis of the ulna. (Courtesy of A. Newberg, M.D., Boston, Massachusetts.)
B Prostaglandin therapy. The humerus, radius, and ulna are involved. (Courtesy of M. Pathria, M.D., San Diego, California.)

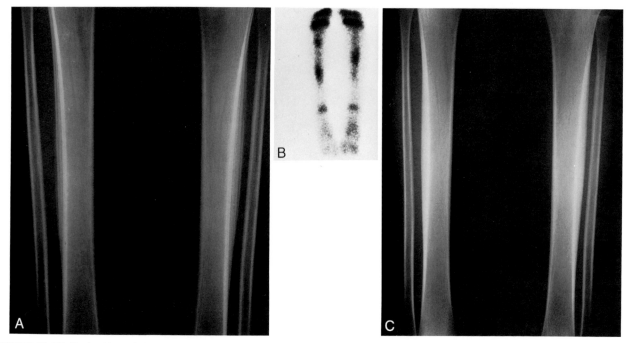

FIGURE 93–70. Periostitis and dysproteinemia. In this 6 year old Latin American girl, fever, headaches, and bilateral leg and forearm pain followed an upper respiratory tract infection. Elevated and abnormal levels of serum proteins were observed on laboratory examination. Clinical and radiologic alterations resolved over several months.

A An initial radiograph of the lower legs shows symmetric lamellated periosteal reaction in the lateral surface of the tibiae. The ulnae also were affected.

B A bone scan demonstrates patchy accumulation of the radionuclide in the tibiae.

C Eight months later, the periosteal bone has been incorporated into the cortex of the tibiae.

(From Grogan DP, Martinez R: Transient idiopathic periosteal reaction associated with dysproteinemia. J Pediatr Orthop *4*:491, 1984.)

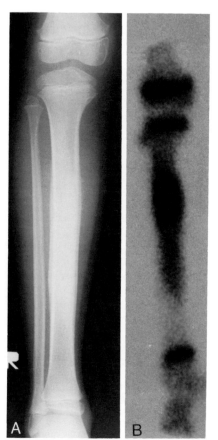

FIGURE 93–71. Periostitis and hyperphosphatemia. This 6 year old girl presented with pain and swelling of the right leg of a few weeks' duration. She had had similar symptoms in the same leg on three occasions during the previous 18 months. Hyperphosphatemia was evident on laboratory evaluation. A biopsy of the involved bone followed by histopathologic analysis revealed evidence of periosteal new bone without inflammation, and no microorganisms were recovered. The clinical and radiologic abnormalities resolved over a period of months, although 10 months later the opposite leg became involved.

A A radiograph shows periostitis and cortical thickening in the diaphysis of the right tibia.

B A bone scan demonstrates increased accumulation of the radionuclide in the affected region.

(From Talab YA, et al: J Pediatr Orthop *8*:338, 1988.)

angiomatosis, or tuberous sclerosis, a peculiar pattern of bone proliferation appears to be unique to this condition. It consists of fluffy, spiculated, hyperostotic areas that show a predilection for the sites of ligamentous attachment in the spine (apophyseal joints, transverse processes, laminae), as well as other axial and extra-axial locations[281, 388] (see Chapter 60). The genesis of the osteosclerotic lesions and bone proliferation is obscure. The abnormalities conceivably could result from the elaboration of an osteoblastic principle by the plasma cells or from osteoclast dysfunction. To facilitate recognition of the most constant and important features of the syndrome, the acronym POEMS has been suggested as appropriate[281]: polyneuropathy (P), organomegaly (O), endocrinopathy (E), M protein (M), and skin changes (S).

Periostitis Deformans

In 1952, Soriano[282] described a group of six patients, as young as 16 years of age, who developed a disorder characterized by outbreaks and remissions lasting for a period up to 20 years. Attacks were accompanied by toxic symptoms, pain, and anorexia lasting 2 to 12 months. Nodular subcutaneous tumors appeared rapidly. Osseous lesions developed, particularly in the forearms, hands, and legs, characterized by exuberant periosteal reaction. Histologic examination documented periosteal proliferation and osteoporosis. Spontaneous recovery occurred but residual bone deformities were encountered.

Fluorosis

Exuberant periosteal proliferation in the appendicular skeleton is encountered in patients with fluorosis, usually in combination with more well known axial skeletal alterations (Fig. 93–72) (see Chapter 74). These latter changes

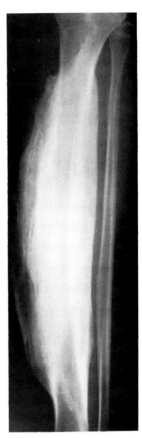

FIGURE 93–73. Neurofibromatosis. Exuberant subperiosteal bony deposition in the diaphysis of the tibia has resulted in an enlarged and bowed bone. (Courtesy of D. MacEwan, M.D., Winnipeg, Manitoba, Canada.)

include osteosclerosis, osteophytosis, and ligamentous calcification and ossification.

Neurofibromatosis

Massive subperiosteal proliferation is seen in patients with neurofibromatosis.[284–287] Involvement of the tubular bones of the lower extremity is characterized by bizarre, undulating periosteal deposits of varying size (Fig. 93–73). The pathogenesis of the changes is not clear; hypotheses include vascular abnormalities with subperiosteal hemorrhage, neurofibromatous infiltration of subperiosteal tissue, and an abnormally loose periosteum as a primary manifestation of the mesoderm dysplasia (see Chapter 92).

Diffuse Idiopathic Skeletal Hyperostosis

Hyperostosis is a common manifestation of this disorder (see Chapter 41). Such hyperostosis affects spinal and extraspinal sites, leading to diagnostic flowing ossification of the spine, bony excrescences at sites of tendinous and ligamentous attachment, para-articular osteophytes, and ligamentous calcification and ossification (Fig. 93–74).

Syndromes of Hyperostosis, Osteitis, and Skin Lesions (SAPHO Syndrome)

During the last two or three decades, extraordinary attention has been given to musculoskeletal problems associated

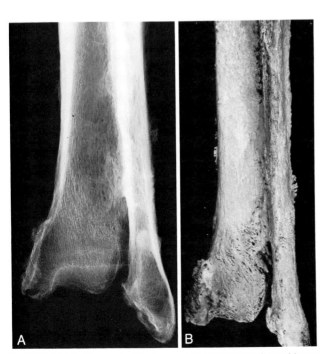

FIGURE 93–72. Fluorosis. Exuberant and irregular periosteal bone formation is evident on the surface of the tibia and fibula.

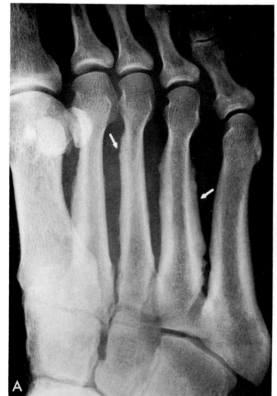

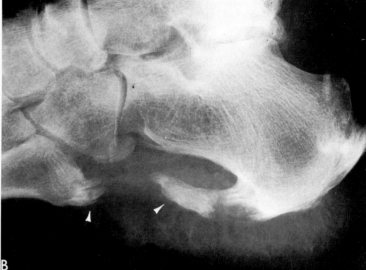

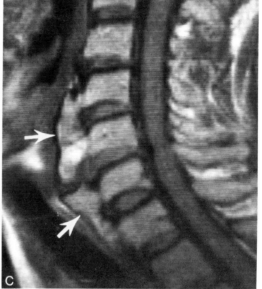

FIGURE 93–74. Diffuse idiopathic skeletal hyperostosis. In extraspinal sites, this disorder may be associated with periostitis (arrows) **(A)** and bony excrescences at tendinous attachments (arrowheads) **(B)**. In spinal sites, anterior ossification predominates. In a sagittal T1-weighted (TR/TE, 600/20) MR image **(C)**, note marrow with its high signal intensity (arrows) in the cervical osteophytes. **(C,** Courtesy of M. Solomon, M.D., San Jose, California.)

with a variety of cutaneous lesions, including acne conglobata, pustulosis palmaris et plantaris, and psoriasis (also see Chapter 29), and great difficulty has been encountered in the classification of such problems. Although a denominator common to many cutaneous syndromes is hyperostosis, osteitis, or periostitis, a number of reasons exist that make their classification difficult if not impossible. First, owing to similarities in some of the cutaneous abnormalities (e.g., pustular psoriasis and pustulosis palmaris et plantaris), accurate categorization of the skin disorder frequently is a diagnostic challenge, even for an experienced dermatologist. Second, although the morphology of the encountered skeletal alterations is remarkably constant, their distribution is not. Surely a predilection for involvement of the clavicle and anterior chest wall exists, but many instances have been recorded in which other sites, including the spine, innominate bone, and tubular bones, are affected with or without clavicular, rib, and sternal alterations. Another factor underscoring the difficulties in classification has been the appearance of similar skeletal abnormalities in the absence of skin

disease. In this situation it could be argued that the cutaneous involvement may have been overlooked or transitory or it may develop later in the course of the disease, but such speculation is not proved. Furthermore, the clinical characteristics as well as the histologic abnormalities are not uniform in these syndromes of bone and skin. Children and adults are affected, and the reported age of clinical onset of disease has spanned virtually every decade. Although agreement generally exists that biochemical parameters in patients with these syndromes are normal or mildly abnormal, the interpretation of the histopathologic findings derived from examination of samples provided by biopsy of affected skeletal sites has been inconsistent. Some regard the findings as indicative of nonspecific bone formation, whereas others have viewed them as indicative of osteomyelitis. Cultures of the recovered material usually have been nonrewarding, although *Propionibacterium acnes* has been implicated in some cases (see later discussion).

The list of names applied to these syndromes of bone and skin is long indeed and, as summarized by Kahn and

TABLE 93–6. SAPHO* Syndromes

Disorder	Typical Age of Onset	Pustulosis Palmaris et Plantaris	Anterior Chest Wall Involvement	Other Skeletal Sites of Involvement
Chronic recurrent multifocal osteomyelitis	First two decades of life	Evident in less than 40% of patients	+/−	+/−
Sternocostoclavicular hyperostosis	Fourth to sixth decades of life	Evident in 30 to 50% of patients	+†	+/−
Pustulotic arthro-osteitis	Adults	+†	−	+†

* *S* synovitis, *A* acne, *P* pustules, *H* hyperostosis, *O* osteitis.
† Must be present in order to establish the diagnosis.

Chamot,[514] includes acne-associated spondylarthropathy, arthro-osteitis with pustulosis palmoplantaris, chronic multifocal cleidometaphyseal osteomyelitis, chronic recurrent multifocal osteomyelitis, plasma cell osteomyelitis, intersternocostoclavicular ossification, juxtasternal arthritis and enthesitis, pustulotic arthro-osteitis, sternoclavicular hyperostosis, sternocostoclavicular hyperostosis, and tumorous osteomyelitis. The designations used in many publications have been based more on the location of the skeletal abnormalities or the interpretation of the skin lesions than on an understanding of the disease process.

In 1987, Chamot and coworkers[515] first employed the term SAPHO syndrome to designate collectively a group of disorders whose most common manifestation was osteitis of the anterior chest wall (Table 93–6). This acronym, representing the major findings of *s*ynovitis, *a*cne, *p*ustulosis, *h*yperostosis, and *o*steitis, subsequently has been used by other investigators as well.[514, 516–522] This term, although gaining support in Europe, has not yet been fully accepted. In support of the designation, Kahn and Chamot[514] emphasized that most previous reports of the different syndromes of bone and skin had related sternocostoclavicular hyperostosis, arthro-osteitis associated with pustulosis palmaris et plantaris, or arthro-osteitis associated with severe acne. In support of grouping these presentations into a single entity or syndrome, these investigators cited the following evidence: (1) Pustulosis and severe acne share the same basic histologic process (i.e., neutrophilic pseudoabscesses); (2) the bone involvement is radiologically and anatomically identical in cases with pustulosis, with acne, or without skin lesions; (3) preferential localization to the anterior chest wall is observed in all three conditions; (4) acute arthritis simulating infection may be observed with pustulosis, acne, and even psoriasis; and (5) sacroiliac joint involvement has been observed in each of the three conditions.[514]

One piece of evidence that supports a common pathophysiology in some of the syndromes of bone and skin has been the recovery of microorganisms of the species *Propionibacterium acnes* from affected areas. This microorganism is a common skin saprophyte that grows readily. *Propionibacterium acnes* has been found in the skin lesions of severe acne and in the bone and joint lesions of patients with pustulosis palmaris et plantaris.[514, 523, 524, 526] Furthermore, local injection of this microorganism may lead to joint lesions, including bone erosions.[525] Biopsies of involved articular and osseous sites in these syndromes, however, frequently have failed to demonstrate causative microorganisms, demonstrating only infiltrates of inflammatory cells, osteoclasts, and osteoblasts, with areas of Paget-like hyperostosis. The initial cellular reaction is composed primarily of polymorphonuclear leukocytes, but with disease chronicity, mononuclear cells, lymphocytes, plasma cells, and occasional multinucleated cells are encountered.[514] The early histologic features of inflammation when combined with later infiltration of plasma cells has led to one designation of the process: plasma cell osteomyelitis. Although therapy using antibiotics commonly has been employed in patients with these syndromes, the clinical results of such management have been ineffective or, at best, inconsistent.

Other evidence that supports a common pathogenesis in many of these syndromes is the localization and morphology of the skeletal lesions. Involvement of the sternum, clavicles, and anterior portions of the ribs is fundamental to the identification of adult patients with sternocostoclavicular hyperostosis (see later discussion) but also occurs in children with chronic recurrent multifocal osteomyelitis, and in both situations such involvement may be seen with or without pustulosis palmaris et plantaris. Similar localization is encountered in some patients with cutaneous evidence of psoriasis or acne conglobata. Elsewhere, subchondral lesions may be evident in many of these syndromes, particularly about cartilaginous joints (Fig. 93–75) such as the discovertebral junction and symphysis pubis but also about synovial articulations (Fig. 93–76) such as the sacroiliac joints. The distribution of lesions in tubular bones is more variable, although metaphyseal localization in chronic recurrent multifocal osteomyelitis is well known. Morphologically, bone sclerosis is a dominant radiographic abnormality.[563] Depending on its localization, such sclerosis may simulate that of osteitis condensans ilii or ankylosing spondylitis (sacroiliac joint), osteitis pubis (symphysis pubis), idiopathic hemispherical sclerosis of a vertebral body (discovertebral joint), or condensing osteitis of the clavicle (sternoclavicular joint). More diffuse sclerosis also is encountered, however, involving both sides of an articulation (simulating infection or the seronegative spondyloarthropathies), the entire clavicle (simulating Paget's disease or fibrous dysplasia), the innominate bone (simulating neoplasms such as lymphoma), and long segments of the tubular bones (simulating infection or neoplasm).

The precise cause of preferential involvement of the an-

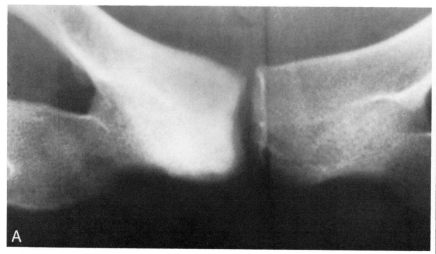

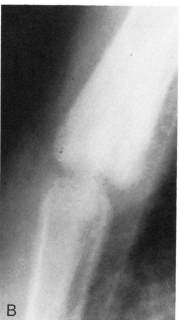

FIGURE 93–75. SAPHO syndrome: Involvement of cartilaginous joints.
A Symphysis pubis. Unilateral osteosclerosis is evident.
B Manubriosternal joint. The manubrium is sclerotic.
(Courtesy of J. Schils, M.D., Cleveland, Ohio.)

terior chest wall in patients with these various syndromes of bone and skin is unknown. Although radiographic abnormalities isolated to the manubriosternal joint without involvement of the spine or sacroiliac joints and without cutaneous abnormalities have been recorded in patients with or without inflammatory back pain,[527] such radiographic alterations of the anterior chest wall are associated more commonly with the seronegative spondyloarthropathies or pustulosis palmaris et plantaris. Jurik[528] reported radiographic abnormalities of the sternoclavicular joint in 17 per cent of patients with ankylosing spondylitis, 6 to 9 per cent of patients with reactive and psoriatic arthritis, and 48 per cent of patients with arthritis associated with pustulosis palmaris et plantaris. Jurik also reported that the manubriosternal joint was involved in 51 to 57 per cent of

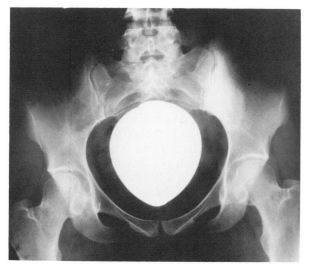

FIGURE 93–76. SAPHO syndrome: Involvement of synovial joints. Note ilial sclerosis adjacent to the left sacroiliac joint. The right side is normal. (From Wetzel R, et al: Intern Orthop (SICOT) 15:101, 1991.)

patients with ankylosing spondylitis or pustulosis palmaris et plantaris and in 18 to 24 per cent of patients with reactive or psoriatic arthritis.[528] Serial radiographs obtained over a period of years in patients with isolated involvement of the manubriosternal joint have revealed severe progressive involvement in those who later developed pustulosis palmaris et plantaris or acne vulgaris and progressive but less severe involvement in those who developed psoriasis or positivity for the HLA-B27 antigen.[529] The most pronounced abnormalities about the articulations of the anterior chest wall appear to correlate best with the presence of pustulosis palmaris et plantaris.[530, 531] The data underscoring a relationship between skin disease and such chest wall involvement are irrefutable, but the cause of this relationship remains elusive. Furthermore, cutaneous disorders including pustulosis palmaris et plantaris may be accompanied by changes in other skeletal sites without involvement of the anterior chest wall or with only minor abnormalities of the thoracic cage.[532–534] In fact, in children chronic recurrent multifocal osteomyelitis, which has an inconstant association with pustulosis palmaris et plantaris, may lead to prominent abnormalities of the tubular bones of the extremities in the absence of chest wall involvement (see later discussion and Chapter 64).

Is SAPHO an appropriate designation for these syndromes of bone and skin? This acronym certainly draws attention to the major clinical, radiologic, and pathologic components that are encountered. Synovitis (*S*), although not a consistent feature, is found in both the thoracic and extrathoracic sites of involvement (Fig. 93–77). Articular or periarticular inflammation and tenosynovitis are seen,[535] and peripheral polyarthritis or monoarthritis (simulating infection) may lead to joint space loss and marginal and central erosions of bone.[533, 534] Sacroiliac joint abnormalities, which are reported to be more often unilateral than bilateral,[514] are similar morphologically to the inflammatory changes of ankylosing spondylitis. Acne (*A*) and pustulosis (*P*) (Fig. 93–78) represent the types of skin involvement

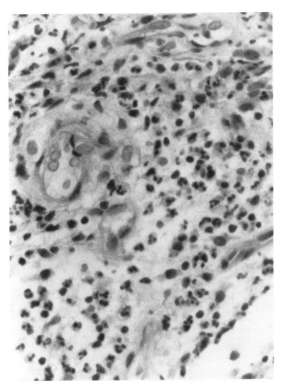

FIGURE 93–77. SAPHO syndrome: Synovitis. Synovial tissue derived from a symptomatic ankle joint reveals collections of monuclear cells and polymorphonuclear leukocytes (×140). (From Kawai K, et al: J Bone Joint Surg [Br] *70*:119, 1988.)

observed most commonly in these syndromes, although, as indicated previously, cutaneous abnormalities need not be present at the time of discovery of the skeletal lesions or, for that matter, at any time during the course of the disease. Pustular skin lesions are observed in pustulosis palmaris et plantaris, pustular psoriasis, and severe acne (conglobata or fulminans), and each of these cutaneous disorders may be accompanied by skeletal abnormalities. Hyperostosis (*H*), loosely defined as excessive osteogenesis, describes quite well the osteosclerosis that typifies these syndromes of bone and skin (Fig. 93–79*A*). Trabecular thickening of the spongiosa and cortical thickening related to both endosteal and periosteal bone proliferation are evident. The medullary cavity may be narrowed, and the external surface of the bone may be irregular. Osteitis (*O*), indicating inflammation of bone involving the haversian spaces, canals and their branches, and, generally, the medullary cavity,[536] is consistent with the histologic findings observed during examination of biopsy samples in some patients with these syndromes (Fig. 93–79*B*).

A potential criticism of the designation SAPHO syndrome relates not to the name itself but rather to the appropriateness of viewing these disorders of bone and skin as a single entity and, further, to the inclusion of the SAPHO syndrome in the same category as the seronegative spondyloarthropathies. For example, does chronic recurrent multifocal osteomyelitis, a disorder typically seen in the first two decades of life that generally is accompanied by lesions of the tubular bones and that may or may not be associated

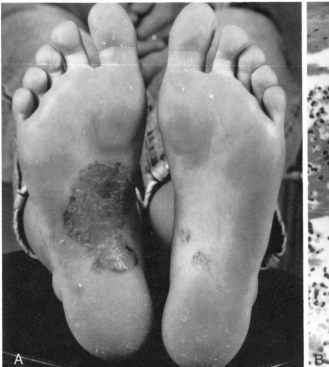
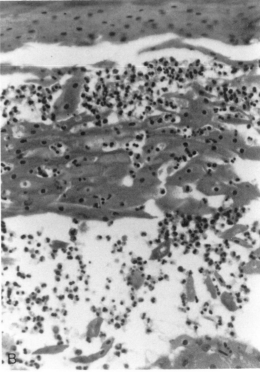

FIGURE 93–78. SAPHO syndrome: Pustulosis palmaris et plantaris.
  A A typical example is shown of the characteristic pustular lesions involving the soles of the feet. (From Wetzel R, et al: Intern Orthop (SICOT) *15*:101, 1991.)
  B Histopathologically, note the large number of polymorphonuclear leukocytes in a vesicle of the epidermis. There is infiltration of mononuclear cells in the transitional zone between dermis and epidermis (× 140). (From Kawai K, et al: J Bone Joint Surg [Br] *70*:117, 1988.)

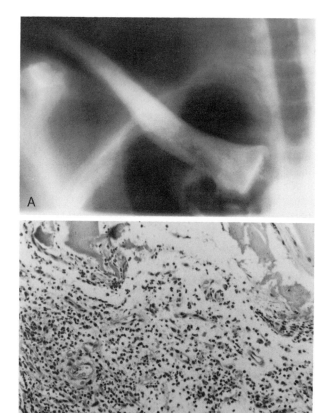

FIGURE 93–79. SAPHO syndrome: Hyperostosis and osteitis.

A Hyperostosis. There is sclerosis of the medial one half of the clavicle associated with radiolucent foci and erosions of the sterno-clavicular joint. (From Wetzel R, et al: Intern Orthop (SICOT) *15*:101, 1991.)

B Osteitis. A photomicrograph (×70) of a clavicular lesion shows inflammatory cells, mainly polymorphonuclear leukocytes and lymphocytes. (From Kawai K, et al: J Bone Joint Surg [Br] *70*:117, 1988.)

with clavicular changes and with pustular skin lesions, share causative and pathogenetic factors with the osteitis of severe acne, a disease usually seen in teenagers or young adults, or with sternocostoclavicular hyperostosis, a disorder classically seen in young and middle-aged adults that, by definition, involves the anterior chest wall? Is pustular psoriasis, when combined with sacroiliitis and spondylitis, a further manifestation of the SAPHO syndrome? Are instances of ankylosing spondylitis with exuberant bone sclerosis[521] or of enteropathic sacroiliitis with pustular skin lesions[520] sufficient evidence to confirm an association of these seronegative spondyloarthropathies with the SAPHO syndrome? The answers to these questions and others require further investigation and clarification.

At this time, it is most appropriate to consider that the SAPHO syndrome is composed of several disorders that share some clinical, radiologic, and pathologic characteristics. At one end of the spectrum of such disorders is chronic recurrent multifocal osteomyelitis and at the other end, sternocostoclavicular hyperostosis. In between is a less defined variety of musculoskeletal manifestations associated with pustulosis palmaris et plantaris and, perhaps, best described as pustulotic arthro-osteitis.

Chronic Recurrent Multifocal Osteomyelitis. This disorder, which is discussed more fully in Chapter 64 owing to the similarities of its manifestation to those of infection, also has been designated as plasma cell osteomyelitis, cleidometaphyseal osteomyelitis, and chronic symmetric osteomyelitis.[537–543.] As classically described, chronic recurrent multifocal osteomyelitis is a disease of unknown causation, affecting primarily children and adolescents and accompanied by local pain and swelling and, less commonly, systemic manifestations such as fever and weight loss. Although described most often in Scandinavia and Europe, it is being recognized with increased frequency throughout the world. The clinical course generally is marked by multiple remissions and exacerbations, and the eventual clinical outcome is one of permanent remission without significant sequelae. A significant relationship between this disorder and pustulosis palmaris et plantaris has been emphasized repeatedly in the literature, although fewer than 40 per cent of patients with chronic recurrent multifocal osteomyelitis reveal this skin lesion. Also, as classically described, chronic recurrent multifocal osteomyelitis affects a variety of tubular bones, especially the tibia and femur, with or without clavicular involvement (Fig. 93–80). In the tubular bones, a metaphyseal localization is frequent, and the radiographic abnormalities here and elsewhere (e.g., the clavicle) include, eventually, sclerosis and periostitis, with expansion and enlargement of the bone. These abnormalities are compatible with those of a chronic infection, although cultures of biopsy specimens are not rewarding.

Other, less typical, manifestations that have been described in patients whose disease has been labelled chronic recurrent multifocal osteomyelitis create difficulties in the classification of syndromes of bone and skin (see Chapter 64). Such manifestations include involvement of infants and middle-aged adults; localization in the flat and irregular bones, such as those of the pelvis, ribs, vertebrae, face,[564] and small bones of the hands and feet; findings of symmetric, asymmetric, or even unilateral or monostotic lesions; the presence of vertebral plana; the occurrence of exuberant alterations of the anterior chest wall resembling those of sternocostoclavicular hyperostosis; identification, albeit rare, of microorganisms on examination of biopsy material; and the presence of considerable residual deformity. Furthermore, as indicated previously, pustulosis palmaris et plantaris is an inconstant feature.

The diagnosis of chronic recurrent multifocal osteomyelitis can be applied most confidently to an illness of children and adolescents that demonstrates remissions and exacerbations, affects metaphyseal and subphyseal portions of tubular bones, produces clavicular sclerosis and enlargement, is accompanied histologically by findings of bone inflammation, is unassociated with recoverable microorganisms, and occurs in the clinical setting of pustular lesions of the hands and feet. In the absence of a significant number of these manifestations and dependent on the presence or absence of pustulosis palmaris et plantaris and anterior chest wall abnormalities, alternative (and possibly related) diagnoses, such as pustulotic arthro-osteitis, sternocostoclavicular hyperostosis, and nonspecific osteitis, should be considered.

Sternocostoclavicular Hyperostosis. In its classic form, sternocostoclavicular hyperostosis is characterized by dis-

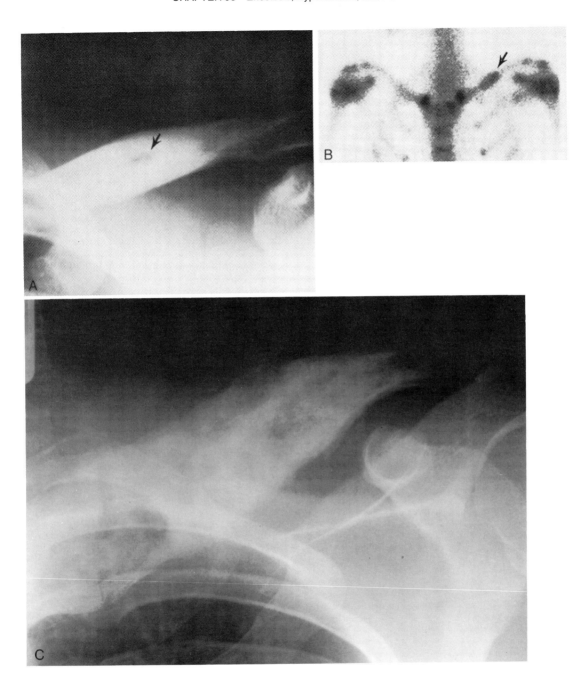

FIGURE 93–80. Chronic recurrent multifocal osteomyelitis.

A, B This 16 year old boy developed soft tissue swelling and pain, especially at night, which was relieved by aspirin. There was no fever or leukocytosis. The symptoms progressed over a 2 year period. The radiograph **(A)** reveals osteosclerosis in the midportion of the clavicle with fusiform enlargement of the bone. A radiolucent region (arrow) is evident within the sclerotic zone. A bone scan **(B)** shows increased accumulation (arrow) of the radionuclide in the clavicle. The lesion was excised. Fibrous tissue containing numerous plasma cells, lymphocytes, and mononuclear cells was evident. Organisms were not recovered from the tissue. The final pathologic diagnosis was chronic recurrent multifocal or plasma cell osteomyelitis.

(Courtesy of G. Greenway, M.D., Dallas, Texas.)

C In a different patient, a 19 year old man, observe bizarre bone proliferation and osteolytic foci in the clavicle.

tinctive bone overgrowth and soft tissue ossification of the clavicle, anterior portion of the upper ribs, and sternum.[308–310, 389–399, 418–422, 428–431, 523, 544–552] It is particularly frequent in Japan. Patients usually are in the fourth to sixth decades of life; men are affected more frequently than women. Bilateral alterations predominate. Clinical findings include pain, swelling, tenderness, and local heat in the anterior upper chest. Osseous overgrowth may lead to occlusion of the subclavian veins, producing considerable edema.[389, 549, 550]

A relationship of sternocostoclavicular hyperostosis and a cutaneous disorder of the hands and feet, pustulosis palmaris et plantaris, is recognized.[437] Approximately 30 to 50 per cent of patients with sternocostoclavicular hyperostosis reveal evidence of pustulosis palmaris et plantaris, typically occurring simultaneously with the lesions of the bones and joints but occasionally preceding or following such lesions. This skin disease is characterized by a protracted course with recurrent eruption of sterile pustules situated symmet-

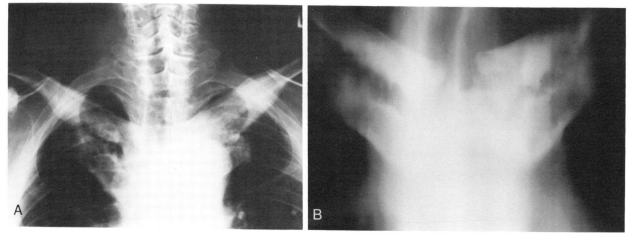

FIGURE 93–81. Sternocostoclavicular hyperostosis. Routine radiography **(A)** and conventional tomography **(B)** show hyperostosis of the sternum, clavicles, and anterior portions of the first ribs. (From Wetzel R, et al: Intern Orthop (SICOT) *15*:101, 1991.)

rically on the palms or soles, or on both.[390] Although rather distinctive in appearance, pustulosis palmaris et plantaris resembles pustular psoriasis,[400] and some investigators consider it a variant of psoriasis. This is of more than academic interest owing to the known association of psoriasis with osseous and articular manifestations, the features of which are similar in certain respects to those of sternocostoclavicular hyperostosis.[551, 553] The latter disorder is evident in approximately 10 to 20 per cent of patients with pustulosis palmaris et plantaris.[390] Findings resembling sternocostoclavicular hyperostosis also have been reported in association with other skin lesions, including severe acne and dissecting cellulitis of the scalp.[545, 553, 565]

The major radiographic abnormalities of sternocostoclavicular hyperostosis are seen in the anterior and upper portion of the chest wall.[313, 392] Ossification of varying degree involves the region of the costoclavicular ligament, inferior margin of the clavicle, and superior margin of the first rib (Fig. 93–81). Hyperostosis of the sternum, clavicle, and upper ribs is encountered and, in some cases, similar changes are evident at the manubriosternal junction (Fig. 93–82).[397, 398, 423, 424, 438] Additional changes occur in the vertebral column and include spinal outgrowths that resemble those of ankylosing spondylitis, diffuse idiopathic skeletal hyperostosis, or psoriatic spondylitis (Fig. 93–83). New bone formation in the cervical spine occasionally is exuber-

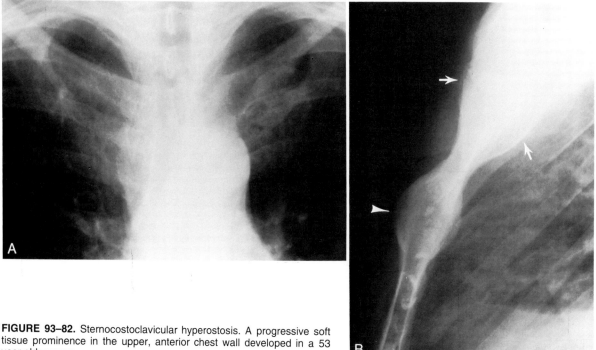

FIGURE 93–82. Sternocostoclavicular hyperostosis. A progressive soft tissue prominence in the upper, anterior chest wall developed in a 53 year old woman.

A An osseous mass is projected over the upper chest on both sides. There is obliteration of the inferior aspects of the clavicles, anterior margins of the first ribs, and sternoclavicular articulations.

B A lateral radiograph reveals the ossified mass (arrows) as well as ossification at the manubriosternal junction (arrowhead). (Courtesy of R. Kerr, M.D., Los Angeles, California.)

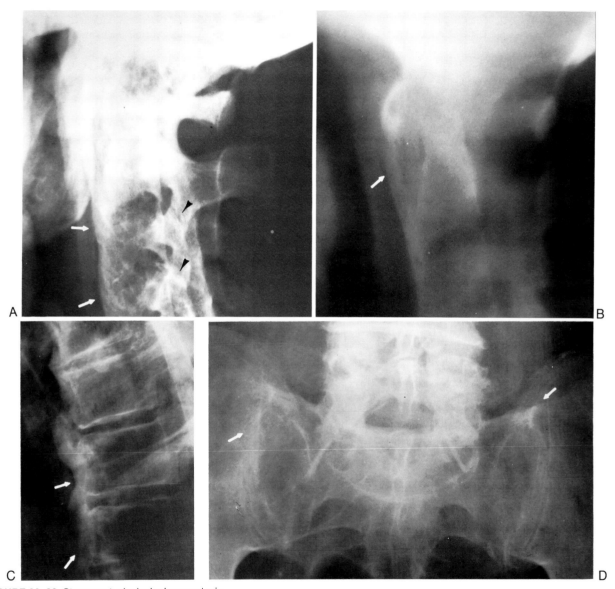

FIGURE 93–83. Sternocostoclavicular hyperostosis.

  A, B A lateral radiograph **(A)** and conventional tomogram **(B)** of the cervical spine indicate anterior ossification (arrows) and apophyseal joint ankylosis (arrowheads). Mild atlantoaxial subluxation is evident.

  C The flowing anterior ossification in the thoracic spine (arrows) is identical to that of diffuse idiopathic skeletal hyperostosis.

  D Ligamentous ossification (arrows) between sacrum and ilium is seen. There is no evidence of sacroiliitis.

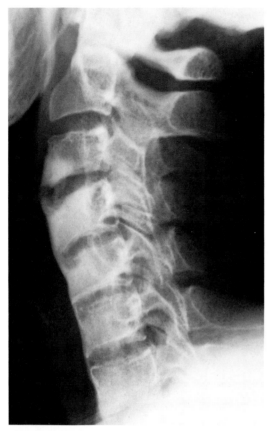

FIGURE 93–84. Sternocostoclavicular hyperostosis. Observe hyperostotic changes involving the anterior portion of the third to seventh cervical vertebral bodies and the development of syndesmophytes. (Courtesy of C. Resnik, M.D., Baltimore, Maryland.)

ant, predominating in the anterior aspect of the vertebral bodies and intervertebral discs and leading to obliteration of the anterior vertebral surface (Fig. 93–84). Discovertebral joint erosions simulating ankylosing spondylitis or infective spondylitis and ivory vertebral bodies simulating skeletal metastasis may be seen. Abnormalities of the sacroiliac articulation also are seen, consisting of either para-articular osseous bridging and ligamentous calcification simulating degenerative joint disease or intra-articular bone erosions, sclerosis, and fusion simulating ankylosing spondylitis (see Fig. 93–83).[391] Bilateral sacroiliac joint alterations occur, although a unilateral distribution of the disease is more frequent.[401, 553] Although clinical abnormalities, manifested as swelling, tenderness, and pain on motion, are detected in extra-axial articulations including, in order of decreasing frequency, the acromioclavicular joint, the metacarpophalangeal and proximal interphalangeal joints of the hand, the elbow, the knee, the hip, the ankle, and the wrist,[439] radiographic alterations generally are confined to soft tissue swelling, and bone erosions usually are not seen.[391] Periosteal proliferation and sclerosis, however, have been identified in some of the long tubular bones.[420, 421, 551, 553]

Laboratory examination reveals elevation of the erythrocyte sedimentation rate, mild leukocytosis, and, occasionally, increased serum levels of alkaline phosphatase. Serologic testing for rheumatoid factor and the histocompatibility antigen HLA-B27 usually yields negative results.

Histologic abnormalities detected on analysis of biopsy material from the ossified thoracic masses include considerable fibrosis and bone formation with mild accumulation of granulation tissue and round cell infiltration,[440] findings that resemble those of Paget's disease. With rare exceptions, microorganisms are not recovered from culture of this material. In one report, *Propionibacterium acnes* was cultured in tissue samples from seven of 15 patients who underwent biopsy of affected joints and para-articular bone.[523]

Sternocostoclavicular hyperostosis reveals a protracted course with periods of exacerbation and remission. A favorable clinical response to antibiotic therapy and prostaglandin inhibitors has been observed.[428] In some cases, patients do not seek medical attention until the degree of ossification and hyperostosis in the thoracic wall is profound, at which time findings on frontal chest roentgenograms are easily misinterpreted as evidence of neoplasm, such as lymphoma or bronchogenic carcinoma. CT or MR imaging is useful in delineating the osseous nature of the mass and its potential origin from the periosteum, perichondrium, and ligaments about the costal cartilage,[546, 548, 550, 552] and scintigraphy with bone-seeking radiopharmaceutical agents documents abnormal skeletal accumulation of the radiotracers[441, 547] (Figs. 93–85 and 93–86).

The cause and pathogenesis of the condition are not clear. Familial aggregation of cases rarely is evident. In some respects, sternocostoclavicular hyperostosis resembles chronic recurrent multifocal osteomyelitis (see Chapter 64): Both conditions are associated with pustulosis palmaris et plantaris and lead to hyperostosis of the clavicle.[402, 403] In other respects, it simulates Paget's disease, diffuse idiopathic skeletal hyperostosis, ankylosing spondylitis, and psoriatic spondylitis. The facts that pustulosis palmaris et plantaris and pustular psoriasis are nearly identical cutaneous lesions and that radiographic changes identical to those of sternocostoclavicular hyperostosis occur in some patients with biopsy-proven skin psoriasis[394] suggest a close relationship between the two disorders.

The diagnosis of sternocostoclavicular hyperostosis can be applied most confidently to an illness of adults in which bone hypertrophy and ligamentous ossification involves the structures of the anterior chest wall and in which other features, including pustular skin lesions, spinal and tubular bone involvement, and subclavian venous obstruction, may or may not be present. In the absence of such chest wall abnormalities, the diagnosis is not suitable. The presence of spinal or extraspinal alterations and pustulosis palmaris et plantaris in adult patients is best classified as pustulotic arthro-osteitis when the anterior chest wall is not affected.

Pustulotic Arthro-osteitis. Currently, this designation is best applied to adult patients with pustulosis palmaris et plantaris who reveal inflammatory changes of peripheral joints or sclerotic bone lesions in sites other than the anterior chest wall, or both findings. In a child or adolescent with similar findings, the diagnosis of chronic recurrent multifocal osteomyelitis is more appropriate. There are very few documented cases of adult patients who would meet these diagnostic criteria for pustulotic arthro-osteitis.[519, 533, 534, 566] Almost universally, reports of adult patients with pustulosis palmaris et plantaris and musculoskeletal involvement have indicated initial or subsequent involvement of the anterior chest wall. Such involvement almost always includes radiographic abnormalities although, rarely, clini-

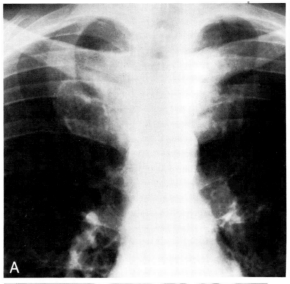

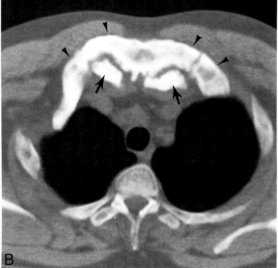

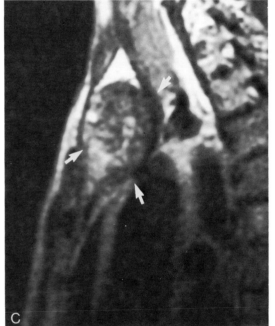

FIGURE 93–85. Sternocostoclavicular hyperostosis.

A, B The frontal radiograph of the chest **(A)** reveals the typical changes of this disease. CT **(B)** shows enlargement and irregularity of the medial ends of the clavicles (arrows) and ossification at the junction of the first rib and the sternum (arrowheads). Observe the increased radiodensity of the sternum, clavicles, and first ribs.
(Courtesy of J. Schreiman, M.D., Omaha, Nebraska.)

C In another patient, a sagittal T2-weighted (TR/TE, 2250/60) spin echo MR image reveals bone formation (arrows) about the sternum.
(Courtesy of D. Witte, M.D., Memphis, Tennessee.)

cal manifestations such as pain and tenderness about the sternoclavicular joints or sternum may occur in the absence of radiographic alterations. Furthermore, long-term observation of patients who initially meet the diagnostic criteria for pustulotic arthro-osteitis may indicate eventual involvement of the anterior chest wall.

Articular involvement in pustulotic arthro-osteitis generally is transient, although occasional descriptions exist in which persistent arthritis has led to rheumatoid arthritis-like abnormalities with joint space loss and bone erosions.[533, 534] In fact, the coexistence of pustulosis palmaris et plantaris and true rheumatoid arthritis has been reported.[554] Bone abnormalities in patients with pustulotic arthro-osteitis are seen in the spine, pelvis, and tubular bones and resemble those occurring in sternocostoclavicular hyperostosis with the exception that, by definition, the anterior chest wall is not involved.[524, 526, 555]

Almost all reported cases of the SAPHO syndrome, when analyzed according to these criteria, can be categorized as

examples of chronic recurrent multifocal osteomyelitis, sternocostoclavicular hyperostosis, or pustulotic arthro-osteitis. Theoretically, however, one could encounter a patient whose skeletal manifestations resemble those of pustulotic arthro-osteitis in whom pustular skin lesions are not evident.[567] In such instances, following the elimination of alternative diagnoses including a variety of tumors and infections, the manifestations should be regarded as evidence of nonspecific osteitis. If, with time, pustulosis palmaris et plantaris or anterior chest wall involvement occurs, or both become evident, a more specific diagnosis can be rendered.

Weismann-Netter-Stuhl Syndrome

This disorder, which also is termed toxopachyostéose diaphysaire tibiopéronière, was described in 1954 by Weismann-Netter and Stuhl.[404] Subsequently, additional reports appeared, many in the French literature.[314, 405–409, 556–559] The disorder affects both men and women of any age from infancy to the eighth or ninth decade of life. Short stature

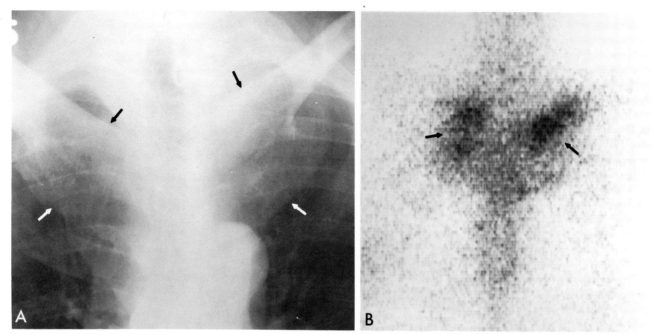

FIGURE 93–86. Sternocostoclavicular hyperostosis. This 72 year old man developed soft tissue swelling over the medial end of both clavicles. A radiograph **(A)** outlines considerable osseous overgrowth about the clavicles (arrows) with bony expansion and sclerosis. A bone scan **(B)** reveals bilateral accumulation of the radionuclide (arrows) in the areas of bony overgrowth.

and delayed ambulation are early features, and mental retardation sometimes is apparent. A family history of this syndrome is an inconsistent feature, although an autosomal dominant pattern of inheritance has been suggested.

The characteristic abnormality of the Weismann-Netter-Stuhl syndrome is bilateral bowing of the long tubular bones, principally the tibiae (Fig. 93–87). An anterior curvature of this bone is typical, with the apex of the curvature occurring at the junction of its middle and lower thirds. The posterior tibial cortex usually is thickened, and the adjacent fibula commonly is bowed and enlarged, with similar cortical thickening.[314] These fibular changes have been referred to as ''tibialization'' owing to the resulting similarity of the two bones. Additional sites of osseous bowing and deformity include, in order of decreasing frequency, the femur, the radius, the ulna, and the humerus.[314] A horizontal orientation of the sacrum, coxa vara deformity, flattening of the lower ribs, brachydactyly, patellar elongation, and squaring of the ilia sometimes are seen. A similar condition confined to the fibula has been designated pachydysostosis.[560]

The clinical and radiologic features of this syndrome resemble the saber shin of congenital or acquired syphilis (see Chapter 66), although in the latter disease, anterior cortical hyperostosis (rather than posterior hyperostosis) and absence of fibular involvement are typical.[314] Additional differential diagnostic considerations are Paget's disease, neurofibromatosis (Fig. 93–88), rickets, and osteogenesis imperfecta.

SUMMARY

Certain disorders are associated with localized or generalized cortical hyperostosis or periostitis. These include enostoses (bone islands), osteomas with or without associated Gardner's syndrome, osteopoikilosis, osteopathia striata,

melorheostosis, pachydermoperiostosis, secondary hypertrophic osteoarthropathy, vascular insufficiency, infantile cortical hyperostosis, hyperostosis frontalis interna, diffuse idiopathic skeletal hyperostosis, sternocostoclavicular hy-

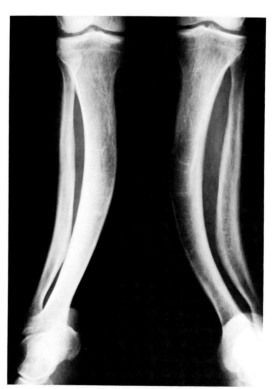

FIGURE 93–87. Weissmann-Netter-Stuhl syndrome. Observe bilateral bowing of the tibiae and fibulae. Anterior and medial bowing was documented on the basis of this and other radiographs (not shown), and the femora also were affected. The fibulae are markedly enlarged, resembling the tibiae. Cortical thickening is apparent. (Courtesy of A. Brower, M.D., Norfolk, Virginia.)

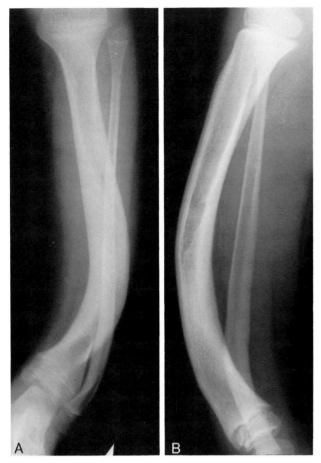

FIGURE 93–88. Neurofibromatosis. An appearance almost identical to the Weismann-Netter-Stuhl syndrome is evident.

perostosis, fluorosis, plasma cell dyscrasias, neurofibromatosis, and several rare or poorly defined syndromes. The changes must be distinguished from the periostitis that occurs as a response to an adjacent osseous process (neoplasm, infection, trauma) and from hyperostosis accompanying additional congenital disorders.

References

1. Stieda A: Ueber umschriebene Knochenverdichtungen im Bereich der Substantia spongiosa im Röntgenbilde. Bruns Beitr Klin Chir *45*:700, 1905.
2. Fischer H: Beitrag zur Kenntnis der Skelettvarietäten (überzählige Karpalia und Tarsalia, Sesambeine, Kompaktainseln). ROFO *19*:43, 1912.
3. Caffey J: Focal scleroses of the spongiosa (bone islands). *In* Pediatric X-ray Diagnosis. 6th Ed. Chicago, Year Book Publishers, 1972, Vol 2, p 961.
4. Steel HH: Calcified islands in medullary bone. J Bone Joint Surg [Am] *32*:405, 1950.
5. Meschan I: Roentgen Signs in Clinical Practice. Philadelphia, WB Saunders Co, 1966, Vol 1, p 372.
6. Broderick TW, Resnick D, Goergen TG, et al: Enostosis of the spine. Spine *3*:167, 1978.
7. Kim SK, Barry WF Jr: Bone island. AJR *92*:1301, 1964.
8. Kim SK, Barry WF Jr: Bone islands. Radiology *90*:77, 1968.
9. Onitsuka H: Roentgenologic aspects of bone islands. Radiology *123*:607, 1977.
10. Smith J: Giant bone islands. Radiology *107*:35, 1973.
11. Blank N, Lieber A: The significance of growing bone islands. Radiology *85*:508, 1965.
12. Ngan H: Growing bone islands. Clin Radiol *23*:199, 1972.
13. Sickles EA, Genant HK, Hoffer PB: Increased localization of ^{99m}Tc-pyrophosphate in a bone island: Case report. J Nucl Med *17*:113, 1976.
14. Schmorl G, Junghanns H: The Human Spine in Health and Disease. Translated by EF Besemann. 2nd Ed. New York, Grune & Stratton, 1971, p 327.
15. Ackermann W, Schwarz GS: Non-neoplastic sclerosis in vertebral bodies. Cancer *11*:703, 1958.
16. Epstein BS: The Spine. A Radiological Text and Atlas. 3rd Ed. Philadelphia, Lea & Febiger, 1969.
17. Lagier R, Nussle D: Anatomy and radiology of a bone island. ROFO *128*:261, 1978.
18. Hoffman RR Jr, Campbell RE: Roentgenologic bone-island instability in hyperparathyroidism. Case report. Radiology *103*:307, 1972.
19. Spjut HJ, Dorfman HD, Fechner RE, et al: Tumors of bone and cartilage. *In* Atlas of Tumor Pathology. Washington, DC, Armed Forces Institute of Pathology, 1971, Second Series, Fascicle 5, p 117.
20. Childrey JH: Osteoma of the sinuses, the frontal and the sphenoid bone. Report of fifteen cases. Arch Otolaryngol *30*:63, 1939.
21. Hallberg OE, Begley JW Jr: Origin and treatment of osteomas of the paranasal sinuses. Arch Otolaryngol *51*:750, 1950.
22. Jaffe HL: Tumors and Tumorous Conditions of the Bones and Joints. Philadelphia, Lea & Febiger, 1958, p 138.
23. Aegerter EE, Kirkpatrick JA Jr: Orthopedic Diseases: Physiology, Pathology, Radiology. 4th Ed. Philadelphia, WB Saunders Co, 1975, p 496.
24. Dolan KD, Seibert J, Seibert RW: Gardner's syndrome. A model for correlative radiology. AJR *119*:359, 1973.
25. Gardner EJ, Plenk HP: Hereditary pattern for multiple osteomas in a family group. Am J Hum Genet *4*:31, 1952.
26. Gardner EJ, Richards RC: Multiple cutaneous and subcutaneous lesions occurring simultaneously with hereditary polyposis and osteomatosis. Am J Hum Genet *5*:139, 1953.
27. Shiffman MA: Familial multiple polyposis associated with soft tissue and hard tissue tumors. JAMA *179*:514, 1962.
28. Chang CHJ, Piatt ED, Thomas KE, et al: Bone abnormalities in Gardner's syndrome. AJR *103*:645, 1968.
29. Weary PE, Linthicum A, Cawley EP, et al: Gardner's syndrome: A family group study and review. Arch Dermatol *90*:20, 1964.
30. Albers-Schönberg H: Eine seltene, bisher nicht bekannte Strukturanomalie des Skelettes. ROFO *23*:174, 1915–1916.
31. Ledoux-Lebard R, Chabaneix, Dessane: L'ostéopoecilie forme nouvelle d'ostéite condensante généralisée sans symptomes cliniques. J Radiol Electrol Med Nucl 2:133, 1916–1917.
32. Jonasch E: 12 Fälle von Osteopoikilie. ROFO *82*:344, 1955.
33. Busch KFB: Familial disseminated osteosclerosis. Acta Radiol *18*:693, 1937.
34. Szabo AD: Osteopoikilosis in a twin. Clin Orthop *79*:156, 1971.
35. Wilcox LF: Osteopoikilosis. AJR *30*:615, 1933.
36. Risseeuw J: Familiaire osteopoikilie. Ned Tijdschr Geneeskd *80*:3827, 1936.
37. Melnick JC: Osteopathia condensans disseminata (osteopoikilosis). Study of a family of 4 generations. AJR *82*:229, 1959.
38. Sutherland CG: Osteopoikilosis. Radiology *25*:470, 1935.
39. Windholz F: Über familiäre Osteopoikilie und Dermatofibrosis lenticularis disseminata. ROFO *45*:566, 1932.
40. Berlin R, Hedensiö B, Lilja B, et al: Osteopoikilosis—a clinical and genetic study. Acta Med Scand *181*:305, 1967.
41. Buschke A, Ollendorff H: Ein Fall von Dermatofibrosis lenticularis disseminata und Osteopathia condensans disseminata. Dermatol Wochenschr *86*:257, 1928.
42. Raskin MM: Osteopoikilosis. Possible association with dystocia and keloid. South Med J *68*:270, 1975.
43. Windholz F: Systemerkrankung des Skeleta (Osteopoikilie) kombiniert mit einer Affektion der Haut (Dermatofibrosis lenticularis disseminata). Wien Klin Wochnschr *44*:1611, 1931.
44. Weissmann G: Scleroderma associated with osteopoikilosis. Arch Intern Med *101*:108, 1958.
45. Pastinszky J, Csató Z: Uber Hautveränderungen bei Osteopoikilie (Buschke-Ollendorff Syndrom). Z. Hautkr *43*:313, 1968.
46. Bethge JFJ, Ridderbusch KE: Über Osteopoikilie und das neue Krankheitsbild Hyperostose bei Osteopoikilie. Ergeb Chir Orthop *49*:138, 1967.
47. Holly LE: Osteopoikilosis. Five year study. Am J Roentgenol *36*:512, 1936.
48. Grassberger A, Seyss R: Knochenszintigramm bei Osteopoikilosis familiaris. Radiol Clin North Am *44*:372, 1975.
49. Whyte MP, Murphy WA, Siegel BA: ^{99m}Tc-pyrophosphate bone imaging in osteopoikilosis, osteopathia striata, and melorheostosis. Radiology *127*:439, 1978.
50. Jaffe HL: Metabolic, Degenerative and Inflammatory Diseases of Bones and Joints. Philadelphia, Lea & Febiger, 1972.
51. Walker GF: Mixed sclerosing bone dystrophies. Two case reports. J Bone Joint Surg [Br] *46*:546, 1964.
52. Abrahamson MN: Disseminated asymptomatic osteosclerosis with features resembling melorheostosis, osteopoikilosis, and osteopathia striata. Case report. J Bone Joint Surg [Am] *50*:991, 1968.
53. Jancu J: Osteopoikilosis. A case report and a suggestion of its pathogenesis. Acta Orthop Belg *37*:284, 1971.
54. Mindell ER, Northup CS, Douglass HO Jr: Osteosarcoma associated with osteopoikilosis. Case report. J Bone Joint Surg [Am] *60*:406, 1978.
55. Dahlin DC: Pathology of osteosarcoma. Clin Orthop *111*:23, 1975.
56. Voorhoeve N: L'image radiologique non encore décrite d'une anomalie du squelette. Ses rapports avec la dyschondroplasie et l'osteopathia condensans disseminata. Acta Radiol *3*:407, 1924.
57. Fairbank HAT: Osteopathia striata. J Bone Joint Surg [Br] *32*:117, 1950.
58. Larrègue M, Maroteaux P, Michey Y, et al: L'osteopathie striée, symptome radiologique de l'hypoplasia dermique en aires. Ann Radiol *15*:287, 1972.
59. Gehweiler JA, Bland WR, Carden TS Jr, et al: Osteopathia striata—Voorhoeve's disease. Review of the roentgen manifestations. AJR *118*:450, 1973.

60. Carlson DH: Osteopathia striata revisited. J Can Assoc Radiol 28:190, 1977.

61. Willert HG, Zichner L: Osteopathia striata—juvenile metaphysäre Knochennekrosen. Z Orthop 111:836, 1973.

62. Bloor DU: A case of osteopathia striata. J Bone Joint Surg [Br] 36:261, 1954.

63. Hurt RL: Osteopathia striata—Voorhoeve's disease. Report of a case presenting the features of osteopathia striata and osteopetrosis. J Bone Joint Surg [Br] 35:89, 1953.

64. Fermin HEA: Osteorabdotose. Een voor het eerst door N. Voorhoeve beschreven bijzondere vorm van osteopathia condensans disseminata. Ned Tijdschr Geneeskd 106:1188, 1962.

65. Fairbank HAT: A case of unilateral affection of the skeleton of unknown origin. Br J Surg 12:594, 1925.

66. Culver GJ, Thumasathit C: Osseous changes of osteopathic striata and Pyle's disease occurring in a patient with an 11-year follow-up. A case report. AJR 116:640, 1972.

67. Ginsburg LD, Sedano HP, Gorlin RJ: Focal dermal hypoplasia syndrome. AJR 110:561, 1970.

68. Léri A, Joanny J: Une affection non décrite des os. Hyperostose "en coulée" sur toute la longueur d'un membre ou "melorhéostose." Bull Mem Soc Hop Paris 46:1141, 1922.

69. Widmann BP, Stecher WR: Rhizomonomelorheostosis. Radiology 24:651, 1935.

70. Walker GF: Mixed sclerosing bone dystrophies: Two case reports. J Bone Joint Surg [Br] 46:546, 1964.

71. Morris JM, Samilson RL, Corley CL: Melorheostosis: Review of the literature and report of an interesting case with a nineteen-year follow-up. J Bone Joint Surg [Am] 45:1191, 1963.

72. Bied JC, Malsh C, Meunier P: La mélorhéostose chez l'adulte. A propos de deux cas dont l'un traité par un diphosphonate. Rev Rhum Mal Osteoartic 43:193, 1976.

73. Campbell CJ, Papademetriou T, Bonfiglio M: Melorheostosis: A report of the clinical, roentgenographic, and pathological findings in fourteen cases. J Bone Joint Surg [Am] 50:1281, 1968.

74. Hove E, Sury B: Melorheostosis. Report on 5 cases with follow-up. Acta Orthop Scand 42:315, 1971.

75. Gold RH, Mirra JM: Case report 35. Skel Radiol 2:57, 1977.

76. Léri A, Lièvre JA: La mélorhéostose (hyperostose d'un membre en coulée). Presse Med 36:801, 1928.

77. Beauvais P, Fauré C, Montagne JP, et al: Leri's melorheostosis: Three pediatric cases and a review of the literature. Pediatr Radiol 6:153, 1977.

78. Masserini A: Sul morbo de Léri: Revisione della literatura e contributo casistico. Radiol Med Torino 31:183, 1944.

79. Janousek J, Preston DF, Martin NL, et al: Bone scan in melorheostosis. Letters to the editor. J Nucl Med 17:1106, 1976.

80. Dillehunt RB, Chuinard EG: Melorheostosis Léri: A case report. J Bone Joint Surg 18:991, 1936.

81. Gillespie JB, Siegling JA: Melorheostosis Léri. Am J Dis Child 55:1273, 1938.

82. Wagers LT, Young AW Jr, Ryan SF: Linear melorheostotic scleroderma. Br J Dermatol 86:297, 1972.

83. Muller SA, Henderson ED: Melorheostosis with linear scleroderma. Arch Dermatol 88:142, 1963.

84. Thompson NM, Allen CEL, Andrews GS, et al: Scleroderma and melorheostosis. Report of a case. J Bone Joint Surg [Br] 33:430, 1951.

85. Soffa DJ, Sire DJ, Dodson JH: Melorheostosis with linear sclerodermatous skin changes. Radiology 114:577, 1975.

86. Buchmann J: Osteopoikilie und Melorheostose. Beitr Orthop Traumatol 15:641, 1968.

87. Wellmitz G: Ein Beitrag zum Krankheitsbild der Melorheostose und Osteopoikilie. Beitr Orthop Traumatol 19:117, 1972.

88. McCarroll HR: Clinical manifestations of congenital neurofibromatosis. J Bone Joint Surg [Am] 32:601, 1950.

89. Hall GS: A contribution to the study of melorheostosis: Unusual bone changes associated with tuberous sclerosis. Q J Med 12:77, 1943.

90. Patrick JH: Melorheostosis associated with arteriovenous aneurysms of the left arm and trunk: Report of a case with long follow-up. J Bone Joint Surg [Br] 51:126, 1969.

91. Putti V: L'osteosi eburneizzante monomelica (una nuova sindrome osteopatica). Chir Organi Mov 11:335, 1927.

92. Valentin B: Über einen Fall von Melorheostose (Osteosclerosis, Osteosis eburnisans monomelica, Osteopathica hyperostotica). ROFO 37:884, 1924.

93. Murray RO, McCredie J: Melorheostosis and the sclerotomes: A radiological correlation. Skel Radiol 4:57, 1979.

94. Murray RO: Melorheostosis associated with congenital arteriovenous aneurysms. Proc R Soc Med 44:473, 1951.

95. Zimmer P: Über einen Fall einer eigenartigen seltenen Knochenerkrankung, Osteopathia hyperostotica—Melorheostose. Beitr Klin Chir 140:75, 1927.

96. Inman VT, Saunders JB: Referred pain from skeletal structures. J Nerv Ment Dis 99:660, 1944.

97. Friedreich N: Hyperostose des gesammten Skelettes. Virchows Arch Pathol Anat 43:83, 1868.

98. Marie P: De l'osteo-arthropathie hypertrophiante pneumique. Rev Med 10:1, 1890.

99. Unna PG: Cutis verticis gyrata. Monatsschr Praktische Dermatol 45:227, 1907.

100. Grönberg A: Is cutis verticis gyrata a symptom in an endocrine syndrome which has so far received little attention? Acta Med Scand 67:24, 1927.

101. Guyer PB, Brunton FJ, Wren MWG: Pachydermoperiostosis with acroosteolysis. A report of five cases. J Bone Joint Surg [Br] 60:219, 1978.

102. Uehlinger E: Hyperostosis generalisata mit Pachydermie. Virchows Arch Pathol Anat 308:396, 1941.

103. Vague J: La pachydermopériostose: pachydermie plicaturée avec pachypériostose des extrémités (syndrome de Touraine, Solente et Golé). Rev Rhum Mal Osteoartic 15:201, 1948.

104. Touraine A, Solente G, Golé L: Un syndrome osteó-dermopathique: La pachydermie plicaturée avec pachypériostose des extrémitiés. Presse Med 43:1820, 1935.

105. Langston HH: Bone dystrophy of unknown etiology (presented for diagnosis). Proc R Soc Med 43:299, 1950.

106. Angel JH: Pachydermo-periostosis (idiopathic osteo-arthropathy). Br Med J 2:789, 1957.

107. Brugsch HG: Acropachyderma with pachyperiostitis. Arch Intern Med 68:687, 1941.

108. Camp JD, Scanlan R: Chronic idiopathic hypertrophic osteoarthropathy. Radiology 50:581, 1948.

109. Sèze S de, Jurmand S-H: Pachydermopériostose. Bull Mem Soc Hop Paris 66:860, 1950.

110. Findlay GH, Oosthuizen WJ: Pachydermoperiostosis. The syndrome of Touraine, Solente and Golé. S Afr Med J 25:747, 1951.

111. Schönenberg H: Zum Krankheitsbild der Osteo-Arthropathie hypertrophiante (Pierre-Bamberger). Z Kinderheilkd 74:388, 1954.

112. Vogl A, Goldfischer S: Pachydermoperiostosis. Primary or idiopathic hypertrophic osteoarthropathy. Am J Med 33:166, 1962.

113. Ursing B: Pachydermoperiostosis. Acta Med Scand 188:157, 1970.

114. Herman MA, Massaro D, Katz S, et al: Pachydermoperiostosis: Clinical spectrum. Arch Intern Med 116:918, 1965.

115. Shawarby K, Ibrahim MS: Pachydermoperiostosis. A review of the literature and report on four cases. Br Med J 1:763, 1962.

116. Harbison JB, Nice CM Jr: Familial pachydermoperiostosis presenting as an acromegaly-like syndrome. AJR 112:532, 1971.

117. Fournier A-M, Mourou M: Pachydermopériostose. J Radiol Electrol Med Nucl 54:417, 1973.

118. Lazarus JH, Galloway JK: Pachydermoperiostosis. An unusual cause of finger clubbing. AJR 118:308, 1973.

119. Katoh T: Pachydermoperiostosis (syndrome of Touraine, Solente, and Golé). Jpn J Clin Dermatol 23:275, 1969.

120. Currarino G, Tierney RC, Giesel RG, et al: Familial idiopathic osteoarthropathy. AJR 85:633, 1961.

121. Keats TE, Bagnall WS: Chronic idiopathic osteoarthropathy. Radiology 62:841, 1954.

122. Berk M: Chronic idiopathic hypertrophic osteoarthropathy. Report of a case and review of the literature. N Engl J Med 247:123, 1952.

123. Cremin BJ: Familial idiopathic osteoarthropathy of children: A case report and progress. Br J Radiol 43:568, 1970.

124. Bartolozzi G, Bernini G, Maggini M: Hypertrophic osteoarthropathy without pachydermia. Idiopathic form. Am J Dis Child 129:849, 1975.

125. Bhate DV, Pizarro AJ, Greenfield GB: Idiopathic hypertrophic osteoarthropathy without pachyderma. Radiology 129:379, 1978.

126. Rimoin DL: Pachydermoperiostosis (idiopathic clubbing and periostosis): Genetic and physiologic considerations. N Engl J Med 272:923, 1965.

127. Bruwer A, Holman CB, Kierland RR: Roentgenologic recognition of cutis verticis gyrata. Mayo Clin Proc 28:63, 1953.

128. Roy JN: Hypertrophy of the palpebral tarsus, the facial integument and the extremities of the limbs associated with widespread osteo-periostitis: A new syndrome. Can Med Assoc J 34:615, 1936.

129. Metz EN, Dowell A: Bone marrow failure in hypertrophic osteoarthropathy. Arch Intern Med 116:759, 1965.

130. Neiman HL, Gompels BM, Martel W: Pachydermoperiostosis with bone marrow failure and gross extramedullary hematopoiesis. Report of a case. Radiology 110:553, 1974.

131. Chamberlain DS, Whitaker J, Silverman FN: Idiopathic osteoarthropathy and cranial defects in children (familial idiopathic osteoarthropathy). AJR 93:408, 1965.

132. Arnold J: Acromegalie, Pachyacrie oder Ostitis? Ein anatomischer Bericht über den Fall Hagner I. Beitr Pathol Anat 10:1, 1891.

133. Appelboom T, Busscher H, Famaey JP: Chondrocalcinosis as a possible cause of arthritis in pachydermoperiostosis? Letter to Editor. Arthritis Rheum 21:174, 1978.

134. Lauter SA, Vasey FB, Hüttner I, et al: Pachydermoperiostosis: Studies on the synovium. J Rheumatol 5:85, 1978.

135. Kerber RE, Vogl A: Pachydermoperiostosis. Peripheral circulatory studies. Arch Intern Med 132:245, 1973.

136. Gall E, Bennett GA, Bauer W: Generalized hypertrophic osteoarthropathy: Pathologic study of seven cases. Am J Pathol 27:349, 1951.

137. Hippocrates: The Book of Prognostics. In The Genuine Works of Hippocrates. Translated by F Adams. London, Sydenham Society, 1886.

138. Bamberger E: Protokoll der Kaisereiche und Koenigliche. Koenigliche Gesselschaft der Aertz in Wien. Sitzung vom 8 Marz, 1889. Wien Klin Wochenschr 2:225, 1889.

139. Vogl A, Blumenfeld S, Gutner LB: Diagnostic significance of pulmonary hypertrophic osteoarthropathy. Am J Med 18:51, 1955.

140. Berman B: Pulmonary hypertrophic osteoarthropathy. Arch Intern Med 112:947, 1963.

141. Temple HL, Jaspin G: Hypertrophic osteoarthropathy. AJR 60:232, 1948.

142. Greenfield GB, Schorsch HA, Shkolnik A: The various roentgen appearances of pulmonary hypertrophic osteoarthropathy. AJR *101*:927, 1967.

143. Holling HE, Brodey RS, Boland C: Pulmonary hypertrophic osteoarthropathy. Lancet 2:1269, 1961.

144. Holling HE, Brodey RS: Pulmonary hypertrophic osteoarthropathy. JAMA *178*:977, 1961.

145. Aufses AH: Primary carcinoma of the lung. 14 year survey. J Mt Sinai Hosp 20:212, 1953.

146. Jack GD: Bronchogenic carcinoma. Trans Med Chir Soc Edinb *132*:75, 1952–1953.

147. Hansen JL: Bronchial carcinoma presenting as arthralgia. Acta Med Scand Suppl 266:467, 1952.

148. Wierman WH, Clagett OT, McDonald JR: Articular manifestations in pulmonary diseases. An analysis of their occurrence in 1024 cases in which pulmonary resection was performed. JAMA *155*:1459, 1954.

149. Alvarez GH: Clinica del cáncer de pulmón. Rev Assoc Med Argent 62:690, 1948.

150. Berg R Jr: Arthralgia as a first symptom of pulmonary lesions. Dis Chest 16:483, 1949.

151. Peck B: Hypertrophic osteoarthropathy with Hodgkin's disease in the mediastinum. JAMA 238:1400, 1977.

152. Adler JJ, Sharma OP: Hypertrophic osteoarthropathy with intrathoracic Hodgkin's disease in the mediastinum. Am Rev Respir Dis *102*:83, 1970.

153. Kay CJ, Rosenberg MA, Burd R: Hypertrophic osteoarthropathy and childhood Hodgkin's disease. Radiology *112*:177, 1974.

154. Shapiro RF, Zvaifler NJ: Concurrent intrathoracic Hodgkin's disease and hypertrophic osteoarthropathy. Chest 63:912, 1973.

155. Aufses AH, Aufses BH: Hypertrophic osteoarthropathy in association with pulmonary metastases from extrathoracic malignancies. Dis Chest 38:399, 1960.

156. Gibbs DD, Schiller KF, Stovin PG: Lung metastases heralded by hypertrophic pulmonary osteoarthropathy. Lancet *1*:623, 1960.

157. Coury C: Hippocratic fingers and hypertrophic osteoarthropathy: Study of 350 cases. Br J Dis Chest 54:202, 1960.

158. Yacoub MH, Simon G, Ohnsorge J: Hypertrophic pulmonary osteoarthropathy in association with pulmonary metastases from extrathoracic tumors. Thorax 22:226, 1967.

159. Firooznia H, Seliger G, Genieser NB, et al: Hypertrophic pulmonary osteoarthropathy in pulmonary metastases. Radiology *115*:269, 1975.

160. Sethi SM, Saxton GD: Osteoarthropathy associated with solitary pulmonary metastases from melanoma. Can J Surg 17:221, 1974.

161. Fellows KE Jr, Rosenthal A: Extracardiac roentgenographic abnormalities in cyanotic congenital heart disease. AJR *114*:371, 1972.

162. McLaughlin GE, McCarty DJ Jr, Downing DF: Hypertrophic osteoarthropathy associated with cyanotic congenital heart disease. A report of two cases. Ann Intern Med 67:579, 1967.

163. Means MG, Brown NW: Secondary hypertrophic osteoarthropathy in congenital heart disease. Am Heart J 34:262, 1947.

164. Trevor RW: Hypertrophic osteoarthropathy in association with congenital cyanotic heart disease: Report of two cases. Ann Intern Med 48:660, 1958.

165. Shaw HB, Cooper RH: Pulmonary hypertrophic osteoarthropathy occurring in a case of congenital heart disease. Lancet *1*:880, 1907.

166. Shaffer HA Jr, Heckman JD: Hypertrophic osteoarthropathy associated with cyanotic congenital heart disease. J Can Assoc Radiol 24:265, 1973.

167. Han SY, Collins LC: Hypertrophic osteoarthropathy in cirrhosis of the liver. Report of two cases. Radiology 91:795, 1968.

168. Martin CL: Complications produced by malignant tumors of the nasopharynx. AJR *41*:377, 1939.

169. Diner WC: Hypertrophic osteoarthropathy. Relief of symptoms by vagotomy in a patient with pulmonary metastases from a lymphoepithelioma of the nasopharynx. JAMA *181*:555, 1962.

170. Papavasiliou CG: Pulmonary metastases from cancer of the nasopharynx associated with hypertrophic osteoarthropathy. Br J Radiol 36:680, 1963.

171. Zornoza J, Cangir A, Green B: Hypertrophic osteoarthropathy associated with nasopharyngeal carcinoma. AJR *128*:679, 1977.

172. Peirce TH, Weir DG: Hypertrophic osteoarthropathy associated with a non-metastasising carcinoma of the oesophagus. Ir Med J Assoc 66:160, 1973.

173. Heylen W, Baert AL: Hypertrophic osteoarthropathy secondary to malignant islet-cell tumor of the pancreas. J Belge Radiol 62:79, 1979.

174. Grossman H, Denning CR, Baker DH: Hypertrophic osteoarthropathy in cystic fibrosis. Am J Dis Child *107*:1, 1964.

175. Cavanaugh JJA, Holman GH: Hypertrophic osteo-arthropathy in childhood. J Pediatr 66:27, 1965.

176. Kay CJ, Rosenberg MA, Burd R: Hypertrophic osteoarthropathy and childhood Hodgkin's disease. Radiology *112*:177, 1974.

177. Petty RE, Cassidy JT, Heyn R, et al: Secondary hypertrophic osteoarthropathy. An unusual cause of arthritis in childhood. Arthritis Rheum *19*:902, 1976.

178. Ameri MR, Alebouyeh M, Donner MW: Hypertrophic osteoarthropathy in childhood malignancy. AJR *130*:992, 1978.

179. Howard CP, Telander RL, Hoffman AD, et al: Hypertrophic osteoarthropathy in association with pulmonary metastasis from osteogenic sarcoma. Mayo Clin Proc 53:538, 1978.

180. Mendlowitz M: Clubbing and hypertrophic osteoarthropathy. Medicine *21*:269, 1942.

181. Calabro JJ: Cancer and arthritis. Arthritis Rheum *10*:553, 1967.

182. Schumacher HR Jr: Articular manifestations of hypertrophic pulmonary osteoarthropathy in bronchogenic carcinoma. A clinical and pathological study. Arthritis Rheum *19*:629, 1976.

183. Ropes MW, Bauer W: Synovial Fluid Changes in Joint Disease. Cambridge, Mass, Harvard University Press, 1963, p 88.

184. Caughey D: Quoted by HR Schumacher. Arthritis Rheum *19*:629, 1976.

185. Steinfeld AD, Munzrider JE: The response of hypertrophic pulmonary osteoarthropathy to radiotherapy. Radiology *113*:709, 1974.

186. Greco FA, Kushner I: Loss of symptoms of pulmonary hypertrophic osteoarthropathy after laparotomy. Letter to Editor. Ann Intern Med *81*:555, 1974.

187. Holman CW: Osteoarthropathy in lung cancer: Disappearance after section of intercostal nerves. J Thorac Cardiovasc Surg 45:679, 1963.

188. Polley HF, Clagett OT, McDonald JR, et al: Articular reactions associated with localized fibrous mesothelioma of the pleura. Ann Rheum Dis *11*:314, 1952.

189. Crump C: Histologic der allgemeinen Osteophytose. (Ostéoarthropathie hypertrophiante pneumique.) Virchows Arch Pathol Anat *271*:467, 1929.

190. Ginsburg J: Hypertrophic pulmonary osteoarthropathy. Postgrad Med J *39*:639, 1963.

191. Mills JA: The connective tissue disease associated with malignant neoplastic disease. J Chronic Dis *16*:797, 1963.

192. Schechter SL, Bole GG: Hypertrophic osteoarthropathy and rheumatoid arthritis. Simultaneous occurrence in association with diffuse interstitial fibrosis. Arthritis Rheum *19*:639, 1976.

193. Hammarsten JF, O'Leary J: The features and significance of hypertrophic osteoarthropathy. Arch Intern Med 99:431, 1957.

194. Kieff ED, McCarty DJ Jr: Hypertrophic osteoarthropathy with arthritis and synovial calcification in a patient with alcoholic cirrhosis. Arthritis Rheum *12*:261, 1969.

195. Holmes JR, Price CH: Hypertrophic pulmonary osteoarthropathy with osteophytosis in a dog. Br J Radiol 31:412, 1958.

196. Rosenthal L, Kirsh J: Observations on the radionuclide imaging in hypertrophic pulmonary osteoarthropathy. Radiology *120*:359, 1976.

197. Terry DW Jr, Isitman AT, Holmes RA: Radionuclide bone images in hypertrophic pulmonary osteoarthropathy. AJR *124*:571, 1975.

198. Donnelly B, Johnson PM: Detection of hypertrophic pulmonary osteoarthropathy by skeletal imaging with ^{99m}Tc-labeled diphosphate. Radiology *114*:389, 1975.

199. Freeman MH, Tonkin AK: Manifestations of hypertrophic pulmonary osteoarthropathy in patients with carcinoma of the lung. Demonstration by ^{99m}Tc-pyrophosphate bone scans. Radiology *120*:363, 1976.

200. Kay CJ, Rosenberg MA: Positive ^{99m}Tc-polyphosphate bone scan in a case of secondary hypertrophic osteoarthropathy. J Nucl Med *15*:312, 1973.

201. Brower AC, Teates CD: Positive ^{99m}Tc-polyphosphate scan in case of metastatic osteogenic sarcoma and hypertrophic pulmonary osteoarthropathy. J Nucl Med *15*:53, 1974.

202. Costello P, Gramm HF, Likich J: Detection of hypertrophic pulmonary osteoarthropathy associated with pulmonary metastatic disease. Clin Nucl Med *2*:397, 1977.

203. Sagar VV, Meckelnburg RL, Piccone JM: Resolution of bone scan changes in hypertrophic pulmonary osteoarthropathy in untreated carcinoma of the lung. Clin Nucl Med *3*:472, 1978.

204. Rosenthall L, Hawkings D, Chuang S: Radionuclide demonstration of relative increased blood flow in uniappendicular secondary hypertrophic osteoarthropathy. Clin Nucl Med *3*:278, 1978.

205. Davis NJ Jr: Pulmonary hypertrophic osteoarthropathy. JAMA *24*:845, 1895.

206. Kessel L: Relation of hypertrophic osteoarthropathy to pulmonary tuberculosis. Arch Intern Med *19*:239, 1917.

207. Flavell G: Reversal of pulmonary hypertrophic osteoarthropathy by vagotomy. Lancet *1*:260, 1956.

208. Rutherford RB, Rhodes BA, Wagner HN: The distribution of extremity blood flow before and after vagectomy in a patient with hypertrophic pulmonary osteoarthropathy. Dis Chest 56:19, 1969.

209. Racoceanu SN, Mendlowitz M, Suck AF, et al: Digital capillary blood flow in clubbing: ^{85}Kr studies in hereditary and acquired cases. Ann Intern Med 75:933, 1971.

210. Mendlowitz M, Leslie A: Experimental simulation in the dog of cyanosis and hypertrophic osteoarthropathy which are associated with congenital heart disease. Am Heart J *24*:141, 1942.

211. Jao JY, Barlow JJ, Krant MJ: Pulmonary hypertrophic osteoarthropathy, spider angiomata, and estrogen hyperexcretion in neoplasia. Ann Intern Med 70:581, 1969.

212. Ginsburg J, Brown JB: Increased oestrogen excretion in hypertrophic pulmonary osteoarthropathy. Lancet 2:1274, 1961.

213. Carroll KB, Doyle L: A common factor in hypertrophic osteoarthropathy. Thorax 29:262, 1974.

214. Buchan DJ, Mitchell DM: Hypertrophic osteoarthropathy in portal cirrhosis. Ann Intern Med 66:130, 1967.

215. Singh A, Jolly SS, Bansal BB: Hypertrophic osteoarthropathy associated with carcinoma of the stomach. Br Med J 2:581, 1960.

216. Hollis WC: Hypertrophic osteoarthropathy secondary to upper gastrointestinal tract neoplasm. Case report and review. Ann Intern Med 66:125, 1967.

217. Wyburn-Mason R: Bronchial carcinoma presenting as polyneuritis. Lancet *1*:203, 1948.

218. Kourilsky R, Pieron R, Bonnet JL, et al: Bilateral vagotomy and hypophysectomy in a case of hypertrophic pulmonary osteoarthropathy caused by a secondary cancer of the lungs. Bull Mem Soc Med Hop Paris 77:113, 1961.

219. Holman CW: Osteoarthropathy in lung cancer: Disappearance after section of intercostal nerves. J Thorac Cardiovasc Surg 45:679, 1963.

220. Honska WL Jr, Strenge H, Hammarsten J: Hypertrophic osteoarthropathy and chronic ulcerative colitis. Gastroenterology 33:489, 1967.

221. Neale G, Kelsall AR, Doyle FH: Crohn's disease and diffuse symmetrical periostitis. Gut 9:383, 1968.

222. Pastershank SP, Tchang SPK: Regional enteritis and hypertrophic osteoarthropathy. J Can Assoc Radiol 23:35, 1972.

223. Dailey FH, Genovese PD, Behnke RH: Patent ductus arteriosus with reversal of flow in adults. Ann Intern Med 56:865, 1962.

224. King JO: Localized clubbing and hypertrophic osteoarthropathy due to infection in an aortic prosthesis. Br Med J 4:404, 1972.

225. Gibson T, Joye J, Schumacher HR, et al: Localized hypertrophic osteoarthropathy with abdominal aortic prosthesis and infection. Letter to Editor. Ann Intern Med 81:556, 1974.

226. Pearse HE Jr, Morton JJ: The stimulation of bone growth by venous stasis. J Bone Joint Surg 12:97, 1930.

227. Gally L, Arvay N: Les lésions osseuses dans les troubles circulatoires et trophiques des membres. J Radiol Electrol Med Nucl 31:690, 1950.

228. Horvath F, Hajos A: Altérations des os de la jambe dues aux troubles des circulations veineuse et lymphatique. J Radiol Electrol Med Nucl 40:257, 1959.

229. Fontaine R, Warter P, Weill F, et al: Les altérations morphologiques des os de la jambe déclenchées par les troubles circulatoires veineux des membres inférieurs. J Radiol Electrol Med Nucl 45:219, 1964.

230. Daumont A, Queneau P, Deplante JP, et al: Périostose hypertrophique et varices des membres inférieurs. Lyon Med 233:1261, 1975.

231. Melcore G, Chiarotte F: Quadro radiologico della gambe nell' insufficienza chronica venosa. Radiol Med (Torino) 58:867, 1972.

232. Graumann W, Braband H: Über periostveränderungen bei peripheren Durchblutungsstörungen. ROFO 92:337, 1960.

233. Lovell RRH, Scott GBD: Hypertrophic osteoarthropathy in polyarteritis. Ann Rheum Dis 15:46, 1956.

234. Caffey J: Pediatric X-ray Diagnosis. 7th Ed. Chicago, Year Book Medical Publishers, 1978, p 1430.

235. Caffey J, Silverman WA: Infantile cortical hyperostoses. Preliminary report on a new syndrome. AJR 54:1, 1945.

236. Smyth FS, Potter A, Silverman W: Periosteal reaction, fever and irritability in young infants. A new syndrome? Am J Dis Child 71:333, 1946.

237. Bennett HS, Nelson TR: Prenatal cortical hyperostosis. Br J Radiol 26:47, 1953.

238. Barba WP II, Freriks DJ: The familial occurrence of infantile cortical hyperostosis in utero. J Pediatr 42:141, 1953.

239. Van Buskirk FW, Tampas JP, Peterson OS Jr: Infantile cortical hyperostosis: Inquiry into its familial aspects. AJR 85:613, 1961.

240. Clemett AR, Williams JH: Familial occurrence of infantile cortical hyperostosis. Radiology 80:409, 1963.

241. Gerrard JW, Holman GH, Gorman AA, et al: Familial infantile cortical hyperostosis. J Pediatr 59:543, 1961.

242. Fráňa L, Sekanina M: Infantile cortical hyperostosis. Arch Dis Child 51:589, 1976.

243. Zeben W Van: Infantile cortical hyperostosis. Acta Paediatr 35:10, 1948.

244. Pajewski M, Vure E: Late manifestations of infantile cortical hyperostosis (Caffey's disease). Br J Radiol 40:90, 1967.

245. Taj-Eldin S, Al-Jawad J: Cortical hyperostosis. Infantile and juvenile manifestations in a boy. Arch Dis Child 46:565, 1971.

246. Swerdloff BA, Ozonoff MB, Gyepes MT: Late recurrence of infantile cortical hyperostosis (Caffey's disease). AJR 108:461, 1970.

247. Staheli LT, Church CC, Ward BH: Infantile cortical hyperostosis (Caffey's disease). Sixteen cases with a late follow-up of eight. JAMA 203:384, 1968.

248. Blank E: Recurrent Caffey's cortical hyperostosis and persistent deformity. Pediatrics 55:856, 1975.

249. Burbank PM, Lovestedt SA, Kennedy RLJ: The dental aspects of infantile cortical hyperostosis. Oral Surg 11:1126, 1958.

250. Caffey J: On some late skeletal changes in chronic infantile cortical hyperostosis. Radiology 59:651, 1952.

251. Scott EP: Infantile cortical hyperostosis. Report of an unusual complication. J Pediatr 62:782, 1963.

252. Holman GH: Infantile cortical hyperostosis. A review. Q Rev Pediatr 17:24, 1962.

253. Sherman MS, Hellyer DT: Infantile cortical hyperostosis. Review of the literature and report of five cases. AJR 63:212, 1950.

254. Matheson WJ, Markham M: Infantile cortical hyperostosis. Br Med J 1:742, 1952.

255. Kaufmann HJ, Mahboubi S, Mandell GA: Case report 39. Skel Radiol 2:109, 1977.

256. Holtzman D: Infantile cortical hyperostosis of the scapula presenting as an ipsilateral Erb's palsy. J Pediatr 81:785, 1972.

257. Padfield E, Hicken P: Cortical hyperostosis in infants: A radiological study of sixteen patients. Br J Radiol 43:231, 1970.

258. Marquis JR: Infantile cortical hyperostosis. A report of an unusual case. Radiology 89:282, 1967.

259. Jackson DR, Lyne ED: Infantile cortical hyperostosis. Case report. J Bone Joint Surg [Am] 61:770, 1979.

260. Harris VJ, Ramilo J: Caffey's disease: A case originating in the first metatarsal and review of a 12 year experience. AJR 130:335, 1978.

261. Minton LR, Elliott JH: Ocular manifestations of infantile cortical hyperostosis. Am J Ophthalmol 64:902, 1967.

262. Neuhauser EBD: Infantile cortical hyperostosis and skull defects. Postgrad Med 48:57, 1970.

263. Boyd RDH, Shaw DG, Thomas BM: Infantile cortical hyperostosis with lytic lesions in the skull. Arch Dis Child 47:471, 1972.

264. Eversole SL Jr, Holman GH, Robinson RA: Hitherto undescribed characteristics of the pathology of infantile cortical hyperostosis (Caffey's disease). Bull Johns Hopkins Hosp 101:80, 1957.

265. Silverman FN: Virus diseases of bone. Do they exist? AJR 126:677, 1976.

266. Dalldorf G: Viruses and human cancer. Bull NY Acad Med 36:795, 1960.

267. McEnery G, Nash FW: Wiskott-Aldrich syndrome associated with idiopathic infantile cortical hyperostosis (Caffey's disease). Arch Dis Child 48:818, 1973.

268. Sauterel L, Rabinowicz T: Contribution to the study of a new etiological aspect of infantile cortical hyperostosis. Ann Radiol 4:211, 1961.

269. Moore S: Hyperostosis Cranii. Springfield, Ill, Charles C Thomas, 1955.

270. Salmi A, Voutilainen A, Holsti LR, et al: Hyperostosis cranii in a normal population. AJR 87:1032, 1962.

271. Gershon-Cohen J, Schraer H, Blumberg N: Hyperostosis frontalis interna among the aged. AJR 73:396, 1955.

272. Henschen F: Über die verschiedenen Formen von Hyperostose des Schädeldachs. Acta Pathol Microbiol Scand Suppl 37:236, 1938.

273. Stewart RM: Localized cranial hyperostosis in the insane. J Neurol Psychopathol 8:321, 1928.

274. Dorst JP: Functional craniology: An aid in interpreting roentgenograms of the skull. Radiol Clin North Am 2:347, 1964.

275. Stewart RM: Hyperostosis frontalis interna: Its relationship to cerebral atrophy. J Ment Sci 87:600, 1941.

276. Goldbloom RB, Stein PB, Eisen A, et al: Idiopathic periosteal hyperostosis with dysproteinemia. A new clinical entity. N Engl J Med 274:873, 1966.

277. Shimpo S: Solitary myeloma causing polyneuritis and endocrine disorders. Nihon Rinsho (Jpn J Clin Med) 26:2444, 1968.

278. Meshkinpour H, Myung CG, Kramer LS: A unique multisystemic syndrome of unknown origin. Arch Intern Med 137:1719, 1977.

279. Trentham DE, Masi AT, Marker HW: Polyneuropathy and anasarca: Evidence in a new connective-tissue syndrome and vasculopathic condition. Ann Intern Med 84:271, 1976.

280. Waldenström JG, Adner A, Gydell K, et al: Osteosclerotic "plasmacytoma" with polyneuropathy, hypertrichosis and diabetes. Acta Med Scand 203:297, 1978.

281. Bardwick P, Zvaifler NJ, Gill G, et al: Plasma cell dyscrasia with polyneuropathy, organomegaly, endocrinopathy, M protein, and skin changes. The POEMS syndrome. Report of two cases and a review of the literature. Medicine 59:311, 1980.

282. Soriano M: Periostitis deformans. Ann Rheum Dis 11:154, 1952.

283. Melhem RE, Najjar SS, Knachadurian AK: Cortical hyperostosis with hyperphosphatemia: A new syndrome? J Pediatr 77:986, 1970.

284. Hooper G, McMaster MJ: Neurofibromatosis with tibial cysts caused by recurrent hemorrhage. A case report. J Bone Joint Surg [Am] 61:274, 1979.

285. Yaghmai I, Tafazoli M: Massive subperiosteal hemorrhage in neurofibromatosis. Radiology 122:439, 1977.

286. Kullmann L, Wouters HW: Neurofibromatosis, gigantism, and subperiosteal haematoma. Report of two children with extensive subperiosteal bone formation. J Bone Joint Surg [Br] 54:130, 1972.

287. Pitt MJ, Mosher JF, Edeiken J: Abnormal periosteum and bone in neurofibromatosis. Radiology 103:143, 1972.

288. Davies JAK, Hall FM, Goldberg RP, et al: Positive bone scan in a bone island. Case report. J Bone Joint Surg [Am] 61:943, 1979.

289. Rao GM, Guruprakash GH, Poulose KP, et al: Improvement in hypertrophic pulmonary osteoarthropathy after radiotherapy to metastasis. AJR 133:944, 1979.

290. Roback DL: Tc-99m-MDP bone scintigraphy and "growing" bone islands: A report of two cases. Clin Nucl Med 5:98, 1980.

291. Hall FM, Goldberg RP, Davies JAK, et al: Scintigraphic assessment of bone islands. Radiology 135:737, 1980.

292. Small IA, Shandler H, Husain M, et al: Gardner's syndrome with an unusual fibro-osseous lesion of the mandible. Oral Surg 49:477, 1980.

293. Rödl W: Das Gardner-syndrom—drei eigene Beobachtungen mit unterschiedlicher organmanifestation. ROFO 130:558, 1979.

294. Young LW: Radiological case of the month. Am J Dis Child 134:415, 1980.

295. Knockaert D, Dequecker J: Osteopathia striata and focal dermal hypoplasia. Skel Radiol 4:223, 1979.

296. Bass HN, Weiner JR, Goldman A, et al: Osteopathia striata syndrome. Clinical, genetic and radiologic considerations. Clin Pediatr 19:369, 1980.

297. Dissing I, Zafirovski G: Para-articular ossifications associated with melorheostosis Léri. Acta Orthop Scand 50:717, 1979.

298. Kinzinger H, Blaimont P, Wollast R: Un cas de mélorhéostose. Int Orthop (SICOT) 3:55, 1979.

299. Younge D, Drummond D, Herring J, et al: Melorheostosis in children. Clinical features and natural history. J Bone Joint Surg [Br] 61:415, 1979.

300. Evans WK: Reversal of hypertrophic osteoarthropathy after chemotherapy for bronchogenic carcinoma. J Rheumatol 7:93, 1980.

301. Nathanson I, Riddlesberger MM Jr: Pulmonary hypertrophic osteoarthropathy in cystic fibrosis. Radiology 135:649, 1980.

302. Ali A, Tetalman MR, Fordham EW, et al: Distribution of hypertrophic pulmonary osteoarthropathy. AJR *134*:771, 1980.

303. Sorin SB, Askari A, Rhodes RS: Hypertrophic osteoarthropathy of the lower extremities as a manifestation of arterial graft sepsis. Arthritis Rheum *23*:768, 1980.

304. López-Enriquez E, Morales AR, Robert F: Effect of atropine sulfate in pulmonary hypertrophic osteoarthropathy. Arthritis Rheum *23*:822, 1980.

305. d'Eshougues JR, Gille C, Smadja A: Interet du sulfate d'atropine dans les formes ''rheumatoides'' de la maladie de Pierre Marie: A propos du proiesverbal. Bull Soc Med Hôp Paris *113*:343, 1962.

306. Hamza M, Janier M, Moalla M, et al: Ostéo-arthropathie hypertrophiante de l'enfant. J Radiol *61*:369, 1980.

307. Finsterbush A, Husseini N: Infantile cortical hyperostosis with unusual clinical manifestations. Clin Orthop *144*:276, 1979.

308. Köhler H, Uehlinger E, Kutzner J, et al: Sternocostoclavicular hyperostosis: Painful swelling of the sternum, clavicles, and upper ribs. Ann Intern Med *87*:192, 1977.

309. Sonozaki H, Azuma A, Okai K, et al: Clinical features of 22 cases with ''intersterno-costo-clavicular ossification.'' Arch Orthop Trauma Surg *95*:13, 1979.

310. Camus JP, Prier A, Cassou B: L'hyperostose sterno-costo-claviculaire. Rev Rhum Mal Osteoartic *47*:361, 1980.

311. Scott RL, Pinstein ML, Sebes JI: Case report 129. Skel Radiol *5*:270, 1980.

312. Bhate DV, Chandraskhar H, Greenfield GB, et al: Case report 126. Skel Radiol *5*:258, 1980.

313. Resnick D: Sternocostoclavicular hyperostosis. AJR *135*:1278, 1980.

314. Amendola MA, Brower AC, Tisnado J: Weismann-Netter-Stuhl syndrome: Toxopachyostéose diaphysaire tibio-péronière. AJR *135*:1211, 1980.

315. Resnick D, Nemcek AA, Haghighi P: Spinal enostoses (bone islands). Radiology *147*:373, 1983.

316. Lagier R: L'ilot osseux benin solitare. Etude anatomo-radiologique d'un cas. Radiologie *3*:125, 1983.

317. Dolan KD, Babin RW, Smoker WRK: Case report 200. Skel Radiol *8*:233, 1982.

318. Von Babo H: Hyperostosen des Schadels. Nativ-aufnahme: Mikroradiographie. Radiologe *21*:12, 1981.

319. Stern PJ, Lim EVA, Krieg JK: Giant metacarpal osteoma. A case report. J Bone Joint Surg [Am] *67*:487, 1985.

320. Richards RC, Rogers SW, Gardner EJ: Spontaneous mesenteric fibromatosis in Gardner's syndrome. Cancer *47*:597, 1981.

321. Bessler W, Egloff B, Sulser H: Case report 253. Skel Radiol *11*:56, 1984.

322. Magid D, Fishman EK, Jones B, et al: Desmoid tumors in Gardner syndrome: Use of computed tomography. AJR *142*:1141, 1984.

323. Lippelt C, Petzel H: Dermatofibrosis lenticularis disseminata mit Osteopoikilie (Buschke-Ollendorff-Syndrom). Radiologe *22*:553, 1982.

324. Lagier R, Mbakop A, Bigler A: Osteopoikilosis: A radiological and pathological study. Skel Radiol *11*:161, 1984.

325. Weisz GM: Lumbar spinal canal stenosis in osteopoikilosis. Clin Orthop *166*:89, 1982.

326. Maroteaux P: L'osteomesopycnose. Une nouvelle affection condensante de transmission dominante autosomique. Arch Franc Pediatr *37*:153, 1980.

327. Proschek R, Labelle H, Bard C, et al: Osteomesopyknosis. J Bone Joint Surg [Am] *67*:652, 1985.

328. Clement A, Garrigues C, Coursault-Durand R, et al: Une affection osseuse rare, mais à ne pas méconnaître: L'ostéopathie striée. J Radiol *63*:673, 1982.

329. Barthels W, Boepple D, Petzel H: Die Osteopathia striata: Ein charakteristischer Röntgenbefund bei der fokalen dermalen Hypoplasi (Goltz-Gorlin-Syndrom). Radiologe *22*:562, 1982.

330. Cortina H, Vallcanera A, Vidal J: Familial osteopathia striata with cranial condensation. Pediatr Radiol *11*:87, 1981.

331. Paling MR, Hyde I, Dennis NR: Osteopathia striata with sclerosis and thickening of the skull. Br J Radiol *54*:344, 1981.

332. DeKeyser J, Bruyland M, DeGreve J, et al: Osteopathia striata with cranial sclerosis. Report of a case and review of the literature. Clin Neurol Neurosurg *85*:41, 1983.

333. Robinow M, Unger F: Syndrome of osteopathia striata, macrocephaly, and cranial sclerosis. Am J Dis Child *138*:821, 1984.

334. Horan FT, Beighton PH: Osteopathia striata with cranial sclerosis: An autosomal dominant entity. Clin Genet *13*:201, 1978.

335. Winter RM, Crawford MD, Meire HB, et al: Osteopathia striata with cranial sclerosis: Highly variable expression within a family including cleft palate in two neonatal cases. Clin Genet *18*:462, 1980.

336. Fryns JP, Pedersen JC, Vanfleteren L, et al: Melorheostosis in a 3-year-old girl. Acta Paediatr Belg *33*:185, 1980.

337. Garver P, Resnick D, Haghighi P, Guerra J: Melorheostosis of the axial skeleton with associated fibrolipomatous lesions. Skel Radiol *9*:41, 1982.

338. Kessler HB, Recht MP, Dalinka MK: Vascular anomalies in association with osteodystrophies—a spectrum. Skel Radiol *10*:95, 1983.

339. Kanis JA, Thomson JG: Mixed sclerosing bone dystrophy with regression of melorheostosis. Br J Radiol *48*:400, 1975.

340. Elkeles A: Mixed sclerosing bone dystrophy with regression of melorheostosis. Br J Radiol *49*:97, 1976.

341. Whyte MP, Murphy WA, Fallon MD, et al: Mixed-sclerosing-bone-dystrophy: Report of a case and review of the literature. Skel Radiol *6*:95, 1981.

342. Pascaud-Ged E, Rihouet J, Pascaud JL, et al: Mélorhéostose, ostéopoecilie et sclérodermie en bandes. Ann Radiol *24*:643, 1981.

343. Jeanmougin M, Civatte J, Pons A: Pachydermopériostose avec anémie par ostéosclérose. Ann Dermatol Venereol *109*:1067, 1982.

344. Reginato AJ, Schiapachasse V, Guerrero R: Familial idiopathic hypertrophic osteoarthropathy and cranial suture defects in children. Skel Radiol *8*:105, 1982.

345. Herbert DA, Fessel WJ: Idiopathic hypertrophic osteoarthropathy (pachydermoperiostosis). West J Med *134*:354, 1981.

346. Joseph B, Chacko V: Acro-osteolysis associated with hypertrophic pulmonary osteoarthropathy and pachydermoperiostosis. Radiology *154*:343, 1985.

347. Mueller MN, Trevarthen D: Pachydermoperiostosis: Arthropathy aggravated by episodic alcohol use. J Rheumatol *8*:862, 1981.

348. Jajic I, Pecina M, Krstulovic B, et al: Primary hypertrophic osteoarthropathy (PHO) and changes in the joints. Clinical, x-ray, scintigraphic, arteriographic and histologic examination of 19 patients. Scand J Rheumatol *9*:89, 1980.

349. Fam AG, Chin-Sang H, Ramsay CA: Pachydermoperiostosis: Scintigraphic, thermographic, plethysmographic, and capillaroscopic observations. Ann Rheum Dis *42*:98, 1983.

350. Barber PV, Lechler R: Hypertrophic osteoarthropathy: Two unusual causes. Postgrad Med J *59*:254, 1983.

351. Martinez-Lavin M, Bobadilla M, Casanova J, et al: Hypertrophic osteoarthropathy in cyanotic congenital heart disease. Its prevalence and relationship to bypass of the lung. Arthritis Rheum *25*:1186, 1982.

352. Oppenheimer DA, Jones HH: Hypertrophic osteoarthropathy of chronic inflammatory bowel disease. Skel Radiol *9*:109, 1982.

353. O'Neill S, Ryan M, Felding JF: Hypertrophic pulmonary osteoarthropathy and regional enteritis. Ir J Med Sci *150*:385, 1981.

354. Ueno Y, Cassell S, Barnett EV: Hypertrophic osteoarthropathy and pseudomembranous enterocolitis. J Rheumatol *8*:825, 1981.

355. Baert AL, Daele MC-V, Broeckx J, et al: Generalized juvenile polyposis with pulmonary arteriovenous malformations and hypertrophic osteoarthropathy. AJR *141*:661, 1983.

356. Simpson EL, Dalinka MK: Association of hypertrophic osteoarthropathy with gastrointestinal polyposis. AJR *144*:983, 1985.

357. Walter RD, Resnick D: Hypertrophic osteoarthropathy of a lower extremity in association with arterial graft sepsis. AJR *137*:1059, 1981.

358. Reginato AJ, Petrokubi R, Jasper CA: Juvenile hypertrophic osteoarthropathy associated with primary sclerosing cholangitis. Arthritis Rheum *23*:1391, 1980.

359. Segal AM, Mackenzie AH: Hypertrophic osteoarthropathy: A 10-year retrospective analysis. Semin Arthritis Rheum *12*:220, 1982.

360. Cerinic MM: Response of hypertrophic osteoarthropathy to drugs inhibiting growth hormone. J Rheumatol *11*:865, 1984.

361. Amin R: Hypertrophic osteoarthropathy without radiographic evidence of new bone formation. Postgrad Med J *59*:54, 1983.

362. Kroon HMJA, Pauwels EKJ: Bone scintigraphy for the detection and follow-up of hypertrophic osteoarthropathy. Diagn Imaging *51*:47, 1982.

363. Sty JR, Sheth K, Starshak RJ: Bone scintigraphy in childhood idiopathic hypertrophic osteoarthropathy. Clin Nucl Med *7*:421, 1982.

364. Dannels EG, Nashel DJ: Periostitis. A manifestation of venous disease and skeletal hyperostosis. J Am Podiatry Assoc *73*:461, 1983.

365. Lippmann HI, Goldin RR: Subcutaneous ossification of the legs in chronic venous insufficiency. Radiology *74*:279, 1960.

366. Mahoney PD, McGill JE, Bleicher JJ: Osteoma cutis: Computed tomography appearance. J Comput Tomogr *9*:61, 1985.

367. Newberg AH, Tampas JP: Familial infantile cortical hyperostosis: An update. AJR *137*:93, 1981.

368. Saul RA, Lee WH, Stevenson RE: Caffey's disease revisited. Further evidence for autosomal dominant inheritance with incomplete penetrance. Am J Dis Child *136*:56, 1982.

369. Emmery L, Timmermans J, Cristens J, et al: Familial infantile cortical hyperostosis. Eur J Pediatr *141*:56, 1983.

370. Maclachlan AK, Gerrard JW, Houston CS, et al: Familial infantile cortical hyperostosis in a large Canadian family. Can Med Assoc J *130*:1172, 1984.

371. Katz JM, Kirkpatrick JA, Papanicolaou N, et al: Case report 139. Skel Radiol *6*:77, 1981.

372. Gentry RR, Rust RS, Lohr JA, et al: Infantile cortical hyperostosis of the ribs (Caffey's disease) without mandibular involvement. Pediatr Radiol *13*:236, 1983.

373. Greer LW, Friedman AC, Madewell JE: Periosteal reaction of the femur in an infant with fever. JAMA *245*:1765, 1981.

374. Beluffi G, Chirico G, Colombo A, et al: Report of a new case of neonatal cortical hyperostosis. Histological and ultrastructural study. Ann Radiol *27*:79, 1984.

375. Taillefer R, Danais S, Marton D: Aspect scintigraphique de l'hyperostose corticale infantile (maladie de Caffey). J Can Assoc Radiol *34*:12, 1983.

376. Ueda K, Saito A, Nakano H, et al: Cortical hyperostosis following long-term administration of prostaglandin E_1 in infants with cyanotic congenital heart disease. J Pediatr *97*:834, 1980.

377. Benz-Bohm G, Emons D, Schickendantz S, et al: Kortikale hyperostosen unter langerfristiger prostaglandin E_2-therapie. Radiologe *24*:72, 1984.

378. Ringel RE, Brenner JI, Haney PJ, et al: Prostaglandin-induced periostitis: A complication of long-term PGE_1 infusion in an infant with congenital heart disease. Radiology *142*:657, 1982.

379. Dihlmann W: Computerized tomography in typical hyperostosis cranii (THC). Eur J Radiol *1*:2, 1981.

380. Huggins TJ, Ragsdale BD, Schnapf DO, et al: RPC from the AFIP. Radiology *141*:709, 1981.

381. Phemister DB: The nature of cranial hyperostosis overlying endothelioma of the meninges. Arch Surg 6:554, 1923.

382. Kim KS, Rogers LF, Lee C: The dural lucent line: Characteristic sign of hyperostosing meningioma en plaque. AJR 141:1217, 1983.

383. Rowbotham GF: The hyperostosis in relation with the meningioma. Br J Surg 26:593, 1939.

384. Grogan DP, Martinez R: Transient idiopathic periosteal reaction associated with dysproteinemia. J Pediatr Orthop 4:491, 1984.

385. Kozlowski K, Anderson R, Tink A: Multifocal recurrent periostitis. Report of two cases. ROFO 135:597, 1981.

386. Mikati MA, Melhem RE, Najjar S: The syndrome of hyperostosis and hyperphosphatemia. J Pediatr 99:900, 1981.

387. Clarke E, Swischuk LE, Hayden CK Jr: Tumoral calcinosis, diaphysitis, and hyperphosphatemia. Radiology 151:643, 1984.

388. Resnick D, Greenway G, Bardwick P, et al: Plasma cell dyscrasia with polyneuropathy, organomegaly, endocrinopathy, M-protein and skin changes. The POEMS syndrome. Distinctive radiographic abnormalities. Radiology 140:17, 1981.

389. Prost A, Dupas B, Rymer R, et al: Hypérostose sterno-costo-claviculaire. A propos de deux observations dont une forme partielle. J Radiol 61:807, 1980.

390. Sonozaki H, Kawashima M, Hongo O, et al: Incidence of arthro-osteitis in patients with pustulosis palmaris. Ann Rheum Dis 40:554, 1981.

391. Sonozaki H, Mitsui H, Miyanaga Y, et al: Clinical features of 53 cases with pustulosis arthro-osteitis. Ann Rheum Dis 40:547, 1981.

392. Resnick D, Vint V, Poteshman NL: Sternocostoclavicular hyperostosis. A report of three new cases. J Bone Joint Surg [Am] 63:1329, 1981.

393. Karasick S, Karasick D: Case report 188. Skel Radiol 8:74, 1982.

394. Fallet GH, Arroyo J, Vischer TL: Sternocostoclavicular hyperostosis: Case report with a 31-year follow-up. Arthritis Rheum 26:784, 1983.

395. Dohler R, Herrlinger JD: Hyperostosis der sternoklavikulargelenke—eine enthesopathie? Z Orthop 121:92, 1983.

396. Beraneck L, Crouzet J: Hyperostose sterno-costo-claviculaire. A propos d'un cas. Revue de la littérature. Sem Hop Paris 59:3443, 1983.

397. Manigand G, Faux N, Taillandier J, et al: Arthrites et ostéoarthrites inflammatoires au cours de pustulose palmo-plantaire. Une observation et revue de la literature. Sem Hop Paris 59:2257, 1983.

398. Nilson BE, Uden A: Skeletal lesions in palmar-plantar pustulosis. Acta Orthop Scand 55:366, 1984.

399. Pucar I, Durrigi TH, Skarica R: Pustulose arthroosteitis. Eine neue Entitat unter den rheumatischen Krankheiten? Z Rheumatol 43:148, 1984.

400. Ashurst PJC: Relapsing pustular eruptions of the hands and feet. Br J Dermatol 76:169, 1964.

401. Beraneck L, Kaplan G, Benoist M, et al: Hypérostose multiple avec sacro-iliite unilatérale. Une nouvelle spondyloarthropathie. Press Med 13:2001, 1984.

402. Appell RG, Oppermann HC, Becker W, et al: Condensing osteitis of the clavicle in childhood: A rare sclerotic bone lesion. Review of literature and report of seven patients. Pediatr Radiol 13:301, 1983.

403. Probst FP: Chronisch rekurrierende multifokale Osteomyelitis (CRMO). Radiologe 24:24, 1984.

404. Weismann-Netter R, Stuhl L: D'une ostéopathie congénitale éventuellement familiale. Presse Med 62:1618, 1954.

405. Weismann-Netter R, Rouaux Y: Toxopachyostéose diaphysaire tibiopéronière: Chez deux soeurs. Presse Med 64:799, 1956.

406. Larcan A, Cayotte JL, Gaucher A, et al: La toxopachyostéose de Weismann-Netter. Ann Med Nancy 2:1724, 1963.

407. Krewer B: Dysmorphie jambiere de Weismann-Netter: Chez deux vrais jumeaux. Presse Med 69:419, 1961.

408. Alavi SM, Keats TE: Toxopachyostéose diaphysaire tibiopéronière. Weismann-Netter syndrome. AJR 118:314, 1974.

409. Azimi F, Bryan PJ: Weismann-Netter-Stuhl syndrome (toxopachyostéose diaphysaire tibio-péronière). Br J Radiol 47:618, 1974.

410. Nakamura T, Yokomizo Y, Kanda S, et al: Osteopathia striata with cranial sclerosis affecting three family members. Skel Radiol 14:267, 1985.

411. Pineda CJ, Guerra J Jr, Weisman MH, et al: The skeletal manifestations of clubbing: A study in patients with cyanotic congenital heart disease and hypertrophic osteoarthropathy. Semin Arthritis Rheum 14:263, 1985.

412. Resnick D: Radiographic features of osteoarthropathy. Radiology 157:553, 1985.

413. Pignon JM, Moreau X, Chanudet X, et al: Osteo-arthropathie hypertrophiante et hepatopathies. Revue de la literature a propos d'un cas. Sem Hop Paris 61:1247, 1985.

414. Castel Y, Toudic L, Crenn P, et al: La maladie de Caffey (hyperostose corticale infantile). A propos d'une forme familiale. Ann Pediatr 32:143, 1985.

415. Leung VC, Lee KE: Infantile cortical hyperostosis with intramedullary lesions. J Pediatr Orthop 5:354, 1985.

416. Pazzaglia UE, Byers PD, Beluffi G, et al: Pathology of infantile cortical hyperostosis (Caffey's disease). Report of a case. J Bone Joint Surg [Am] 67:1417, 1985.

417. Festen JJM, Kuipers FC, Schaars AH: Multifocal recurrent periostitis responsive to colchicine. Scand J Rheumatol 14:8, 1985.

418. Goossens M, Vanderstraeten C, Claessens H: Sternocostoclavicular hyperostosis. A case report and review of the literature. Clin Orthop 194:164, 1985.

419. Sala RS, Gomez JM: Hiperostosis esternocostoclavicular: Presentacion de un caso y revision de la literatura. Med Clin (Barcelona) 84:483, 1985.

420. Gerster JC, Lagier R, Nicod L: Case report 311. Skel Radiol 14:53, 1985.

421. Patterson AC, Bentley-Corbett K: Pustulotic arthroosteitis. J Rheumatol 12:611, 1985.

422. Benhamou CL, Bardet M, Luthier F, et al: Arthrites chroniques des pustuloses palmo-plantaires. Bacterides d'Andrews. Rev Rhum Mal Osteoartic 52:487, 1985.

423. Jurik AG, Graudal H, deCarvalho A: Sclerotic changes of the manubrium sterni. Skel Radiol 13:195, 1985.

424. Jurik AG, Graudal H, de Carvalho A: Monarticular involvement of the manubriosternal joint. Skel Radiol 14:99, 1985.

425. Katariya S, Prasad PJ, Marwaha RK, et al: Hypertrophic osteoarthropathy in a young child with congenital cyanotic heart disease. Br J Radiol 59:75, 1986.

426. Crawford A-M, Rabin HR, Fritzler MJ: Hypertrophic pulmonary osteoarthropathy in cystic fibrosis. Rheumatol Int 5:283, 1986.

427. Rush PJ, Shore A, Coblentz C, et al: The musculoskeletal manifestations of cystic fibrosis. Semin Arthritis Rheum 15:213, 1986.

428. Chigira M, Maehara S, Nagase M, et al: Sternocostoclavicular hyperostosis. A report of nineteen cases with special reference to etiology and treatment. J Bone Joint Surg [Am] 68:103, 1986.

429. Sartoris DJ, Schreiman JS, Kerr R, et al: Sternocostoclavicular hyperostosis: A review and report of 11 cases. Radiology 158:125, 1986.

430. Resnick CS, Ammann AM: Cervical spine involvement in sternocostoclavicular hyperostosis. Spine 10:846, 1985.

431. Rosenthall L, Burke DL: A radionuclide and radiographic diagnosis of sternocostoclavicular hyperostosis. Clin Nucl Med 11:322, 1986.

432. Greenspan A, Steiner G, Sotelo D, et al: Mixed sclerosing bone dysplasia coexisting with dysplasia epiphysealis hemimelica (Trevor-Fairbank disease). Skel Radiol 15:452, 1986.

433. Ho A, Williams DM, Zelenock GB, et al: Unilateral hypertrophic osteoarthropathy in a patient with an infected axillary-axillary bypass graft. Radiology 162:573, 1987.

434. Drouat S, Khellaf M, Aissaout A, et al: À propos d'une maladie de Pierre-Marie-Bomberger chez un enfant. Ann Radiol 29:539, 1986.

435. Staalman CR: Hypertrophic osteoarthropathy in childhood malignancy. Diagn Imag Clin Med 55:233, 1986.

436. de Vries N, Datz FL, Manaster BJ: Case report 399. Skel Radiol 15:658, 1986.

437. Aberlé DR, Milos MJ, Aberlé AM, et al: Case report 407. Skel Radiol 16:70, 1987.

438. Jurik AG, Moller BN, Jensen MK, et al: Sclerosis and hyperostosis of the manubrium sterni. Rheumatol Int 6:171, 1986.

439. Chamot AM, Vion B, Gerster JC: Acute pseudoseptic arthritis and palmoplantar pustulosis. Clin Rheumatol 5:118, 1986.

440. Lagier R, Arroyo J, Fallet GH: Sternocostoclavicular hyperostosis. Radiological and pathological study of a specimen with ununited clavicular fracture. Pathol Res Pract 181:596, 1986.

441. Ueno K, Rikimaru S, Kawashima Y, et al: Bone imaging of sternocostoclavicular hyperostosis in palmoplantar pustulosis. Clin Nucl Med 11:420, 1986.

442. Ehara S, Kattapuram SV, Rosenberg AE: Giant bone island. Computed tomography findings. Clin Imag 13:231, 1989.

443. Gold RH, Mirra JM, Remotti F, et al: Case report 527. Skel Radiol 18:129, 1989.

444. Araki S, Otani T, Watanabe K, et al: Positive bone scan in a bone island. A histologically verified case in os capitatum. Acta Orthop Scand 60:369, 1989.

445. Greenspan A, Steiner G, Knutzon R: Bone island (enostosis): Clinical significance and radiologic and pathologic correlations. Skel Radiol 20:85, 1991.

446. Sadry F, Hessler C, Garcia J: The potential aggressiveness of sinus osteomas. A report of two cases. Skel Radiol 17:427, 1988.

447. Shibata Y, Yoshii Y, Tsukada A, et al: Radiolucent osteoma of the skull: Case report. Neurosurg 27:776, 1991.

448. Meltzer CC, Scott WW Jr, McCarthy EF: Case report 698. Skel Radiol 20:555, 1991.

449. Mirra JM, Gold RH, Pignatti G, et al: Case report 497. Skel Radiol 17:437, 1988.

450. Cervilla V, Haghighi P, Resnick D, et al: Case report 596. Skel Radiol 19:135, 1990.

451. Baum PA, Nelson MC, Lack EE, et al: Case report 560. Skel Radiol 18:406, 1989.

452. Harned RK, Buck JL, Olmstead WW, et al: Extracolonic manifestations of the familial adenomatous polyposis syndromes. AJR 156:481, 1991.

453. Casillas J, Sais GJ, Greve JL, et al: Imaging of intra- and extraabdominal desmoid tumors. RadioGraphics 11:959, 1991.

454. Hardoff R, Dov DB, Front A: Gallium 67 scintigraphy in the evaluation of Gardner's syndrome. Cancer 61:2353, 1988.

455. Benli IT, Akalin S, Boysan E, et al: Epidemiological, clinical and radiological aspects of osteopoikilosis. J Bone Joint Surg [Br] 74:504, 1992.

456. Chigira M, Kato K, Mashio K, et al: Symmetry of bone lesions in osteopoikilosis. Report of 4 cases. Acta Orthop Scand 62:495, 1991.

457. Tong ECK, Samii M, Tchang F: Bone imaging as an aid for the diagnosis of osteopoikilosis. Clin Nucl Med 13:816, 1988.

458. Grimer RJ, Davies AM, Starkie CM, et al: Chondrosarcome chez un patient porteur d'ostéopoïkilie. A propos d'un cas. Revue Chir Orthop 75:188, 1989.

459. Ayling RM, Evans PEL: Giant cell tumor in a patient with osteopoikilosis. Acta Orthop Scand 59:74, 1988.

460. Griffith TM, Fitzgerald E, Cochlin DL: Osteomesopyknosis: Benign axial osteosclerosis. Brit J Radiol 61:951, 1988.

461. Delcambre B, Flipo RM, Leroux JL, et al: Osteomesopyknosis. Report of two new cases. Skel Radiol 18:21, 1989.

462. Boothroyd AE, Hall CM: The radiological features of Goltz syndrome: Focal dermal hypoplasia. A report of two cases. Skel Radiol *17*:505, 1988.

463. Lynch RD, Leschrer RT, Nicholls PJ, et al: Focal dermal hypoplasia (Goltz syndrome) with an expansile iliac lesion. J Bone Joint Surg [Am] *63*:470, 1981.

464. Joannides T, Pringle JAS, Shaw DG, et al: Giant cell tumor of bone in focal dermal hypoplasia. Br J Radiol *56*:684, 1983.

465. Colavita N, Nicolais S, Orazi C, et al: Melorheostosis: Presentation of a case followed up for 24 years. Arch Orthop Trauma Surg *106*:123, 1987.

466. Williams JW, Monaghan D, Barrington NA: Cranio-facial melorheostosis: Case report and review of the literature. Br J Radiol *64*:60, 1991.

467. Raby N, Vivian G: Case report 478. Skel Radiol *17*:216, 1988.

468. Caudle RJ, Stern PJ: Melorheostosis of the hand. A case report with long-term follow-up. J Bone Joint Surg [Am] *69*:1229, 1987.

469. Khurana JS, Ehara S, Rosenberg AE, et al: Case report 510. Skel Radiol *17*:539, 1988.

470. Davis DC, Syklawer R, Cole RL: Melorheostosis on three-phase bone scintigraphy. Case report. Clin Nucl Med *17*:561, 1992.

471. Lee SH, Sanderson J: Case report: Hypophosphataemic rickets and melorheostosis. Clin Radiol *40*:209, 1989.

472. Böstman OM, Holmström T, Riska EB: Osteosarcoma arising in a melorheostotic femur. A case report. J Bone Joint Surg [Am] *69*:1232, 1987.

473. Greenspan A: Sclerosing bone dysplasias—a target-site approach. Skel Radiol *20*:561, 1991.

474. Camurati M: Di un raro caso di osteite simmetrica ereditaria degli arti inferiori. Chir Organi Mov *6*:662, 1922.

475. Engelmann G: Ein fall von osteopathia hyperostotica (sclerotisans) multiplex infantilis. ROFO *39*:1101, 1929.

476. Neuhauser EBD, Schwachmann H, Wittenborg M, et al: Progressive diaphyseal dysplasia. Radiology *51*:11, 1948.

477. Fallon MD, Whyte MP, Murphy WA: Progressive diaphyseal dysplasia (Engelmann's disease). Report of a sporadic case of the mild form. J Bone Joint Surg [Am] *62*:465, 1980.

478. Naveh Y, Kaftori JK, Alon U, et al: Progressive diaphyseal dysplasia: Genetics and clinical and radiologic manifestations. Pediatrics *74*:399, 1984.

479. Hundley JD, Wilson FC: Progressive diaphyseal dysplasia. Review of the literature and report of seven cases in one family. J Bone Joint Surg [Am] *55*:461, 1973.

480. Kaftori JK, Kleinhaus U, Naveh Y: Progressive diaphyseal dysplasia (Camurati-Engelmann): Radiographic follow-up and CT findings. Radiology *164*:777, 1987.

481. Wirth CR, Kay J, Bourke R: Diaphyseal dysplasia (Engelmann's syndrome). A case demonstrating a deficiency in cortical haversian system formation. Clin Orthop *171*:186, 1982.

482. Kumar B, Murphy WA, Whyte MP: Progressive diaphyseal dysplasia (Engelmann disease): Scintigraphic-radiographic-clinical correlations. Radiology *140*:87, 1981.

483. Lundy MM, Billingsley JL, Redwine MD, et al: Scintigraphic findings in progressive diaphyseal dysplasia. J Nucl Med *23*:324, 1982.

484. Ribbing S: Hereditary, multiple diaphyseal sclerosis. Acta Radiol *31*:522, 1949.

485. Paul LW: Hereditary multiple diaphyseal sclerosis (Ribbing disease). Radiology *60*:412, 1953.

486. Abdul-Karim FW, Carter JR, Makley JT, et al: Intramedullary osteosclerosis. Report of the clinicopathologic features of five cases. Orthopedics *11*:1667, 1988.

487. Horwitz T: Monomelic medullary osteosclerosis of unknown etiology. Radiology *36*:343, 1941.

488. Sotelo-Ortiz F: Monomelic medullary osteosclerosis. Case report. Bull Hosp J Dis *15*:95, 1954.

489. Martinez-Lavin M, Pineda C, Valdez T, et al: Primary hypertrophic osteoarthropathy. Semin Arthritis Rheum *17*:156, 1988.

490. Matucci-Cerinic M, Lotti T, Jajic I, et al: The clinical spectrum of pachydermoperiostosis (primary hypertrophic osteoarthropathy). Medicine *70*:208, 1991.

491. Matucci-Cerinic M, Cinti S, Morroni M, et al: Pachydermoperiostosis (primary hypertrophic osteoarthropathy): Report of a case with evidence of endothelial and connective tissue involvement. Ann Rheum Dis *48*:240, 1989.

492. Pineda CJ, Martinez-Lavin M, Goobar JE, et al: Periostitis in hypertrophic osteoarthropathy: Relationship to disease duration. AJR *148*:773, 1987.

493. Flueckiger F, Fotter R, Hausegger K, et al: Hypertrophic osteoarthropathy caused by lung metastasis of an osteosarcoma. Pediatr Radiol *20*:128, 1989.

494. Vico P, Delcorde A, Rahier I, et al: Hypertrophic osteoarthropathy and thyroid cancer. J Rheumatol *19*:1153, 1992.

495. Booth BW, Van Nostrand D, Graeber GM: Hypertrophic pulmonary osteoarthropathy and breast cancer. South Med J *80*:383, 1987.

496. Davies RA, Darby M, Richards MA: Hypertrophic pulmonary osteoarthropathy in pulmonary metastatic disease. A case report and review of the literature. Clin Radiol *43*:268, 1991.

497. Pineda C, Fonseca C, Martinez-Lavin M: The spectrum of soft tissue and skeletal abnormalities of hypertrophic osteoarthropathy. J Rheumatol *17*:626, 1990.

498. Pineda C: Diagnostic imaging in hypertrophic osteoarthropathy. Clin Exp Rheumatol *10*:27, 1992.

499. Martinez-Lavin M: Cardiogenic hypertrophic osteoarthropathy. Clin Exp Rheumatol *10*:19, 1992.

500. Huaux JP, Geubel A, Maldague B, et al: Hypertrophic osteoarthropathy related to end stage cholestatic cirrhosis: Reversal after liver transplantation. Ann Rheum Dis *46*:342, 1987.

501. Wolfe SM, Aelion JA, Gupta RC: Hypertrophic osteoarthropathy associated with a rejected liver transplant. J Rheumatol *14*:147, 1987.

502. Rahbar M, Sharma OP: Hypertrophic osteoarthropathy in sarcoidosis. Sarcoidosis *7*:125, 1990.

503. Alloway JA, Nashel DJ, Rohatgi PK: Sarcoidosis and hypertrophic osteoarthropathy. J Rheumatol *19*:180, 1992.

504. Stiles RG, Resnick D, Sartoris DJ, et al: Unilateral lower extremity hypertrophic osteoarthropathy associated with aortic graft infection. South Med J *81*:788, 1988.

505. Martinez-Lavin M: Digital clubbing and hypertrophic osteoarthropathy: A unifying hypothesis. J Rheumatol *14*:6, 1987.

506. Vázquez-Abad D, Pineda C, Martinez-Lavin M: Digital clubbing: A numerical assessment of the deformity. J Rheumatol *16*:518, 1989.

507. Schumacher HR Jr: Hypertrophic osteoarthropathy: Rheumatologic manifestations. Clin Exp Rheumatol *10*:35, 1992.

508. Sanders ME, Fischbein LC: Hypertrophic osteoarthropathy with Takayasu's arteritis. Clin Exp Rheumatol *5*:71, 1987.

509. Nash P, Fryer J, Webb J: Vasculitis presenting as chronic unilateral painful leg swelling. J Rheumatol *15*:1022, 1988.

510. Jacobsson H, Haverling M: Hyperostosis cranii. Radiography and scintigraphy compared. Acta Radiologica *29*:223, 1988.

511. Kim KS, Rogers LF, Goldblatt D: CT features of hyperostosing meningioma en plaque. AJR *149*:1017, 1987.

512. Cameron BJ, Laxer RM, Wilmot DM, et al: Idiopathic periosteal hyperostosis with dysproteinemia (Goldbloom's syndrome): Case report and review of the literature. Arthritis Rheum *30*:1307, 1987.

513. Talab YA, Mallouh A: Hyperostosis with hyperphosphatemia: A case report and review of the literature. J Pediatr Orthop *8*:338, 1988.

514. Kahn M-F, Chamot A-M: SAPHO syndrome. Rheum Dis Clin North Am *18*:225, 1992.

515. Chamot AM, Benhamou CL, Kahn MF, et al: Le syndrome acné pustulose hyperostose ostéite (SAPHO). Résultats d'une enquête nationale. 85 observations. Rev Rhum *54*:187, 1987.

516. Benhamou CL, Chamot AM, Kahn MF: Synovitis-acne-pustulosis hyperostosis-osteomyelitis syndrome (SAPHO). A new syndrome among the spondyloarthropathies? Clin Exp Rheumatol *6*:109, 1988.

517. Trotta F, Corte L, Bajocchi G, et al: Hyperostosis and multifocal osteitis: A purely rheumatological subset of the SAPHO syndrome. Clin Exp Rheumatol *8*:401, 1990.

518. Conrozier Th, Renevier JL, Tron AM, et al: Périostite ossifiante des péronés révélatrice d'un SAPHO. Rev Rhum *57*:225, 1990.

519. Kahn M-F, Bouvier M, Palazzo E, et al: Sternoclavicular pustulotic osteitis (SAPHO). 20-year interval between skin and bone lesions. J Rheumatol *18*:1104, 1991.

520. Kahn MF, Bouchon JP, Chamot AM, et al: Entérocolopathies chronique et syndrome SAPHO. 8 observations. Rev Rhum Mal Osteoartic *59*:91, 1992.

521. Olivieri I, Barbieri P, Padula A, et al: Ankylosing spondylitis with exuberant sclerosis or SAPHO syndrome. J Rheumatol *20*:202, 1993.

522. Kahn M-F: Reply. J Rheumatol *20*:203, 1993.

523. Edlund E, Johnsson U, Lidgren L, et al: Palmoplantar pustulosis and sternocostoclavicular arthro-osteitis. Ann Rheum Dis *47*:809, 1988.

524. Gerster JC, Lagier R, Livio JJ: Propionibacterium acnes in a spondylitis with palmoplantar pustulosis. Ann Rheum Dis *49*:337, 1990.

525. Trimble BS, Evers CJ, Ballaron SA, et al: Intraarticular injection of Propionibacterium acnes causes an erosive arthritis in rats. Agents Actions *21*:281, 1987.

526. Pillon P, Pajon A, Juvin R, et al: Hyperostose tibiale et Propionibacterium acnes. Rev Rhum Mal Osteoartic *59*:349, 1992.

527. The HSG, Cats A, van der Linden S: Isolated lesions of the manubriosternal joint in patients with inflammatory back pain and negative sacroiliac and spinal radiographs. Rheumatol Int *6*:245, 1986.

528. Jurik AG: Anterior chest wall involvement in seronegative arthritides. A study of frequency of changes at radiography. Rheumatol Int *12*:7, 1992.

529. Jurik AG, Graudal H: Monarthritis of the manubriosternal joint. A follow-up study. Rheumatol Int *7*:235, 1987.

530. Jurik AG: Seronegative arthritides of the anterior chest wall: A follow-up study. Skel Radiol *20*:517, 1991.

531. Jurik AG: Anterior chest wall involvement in patients with pustulosis palmoplantaris. Skel Radiol *19*:271, 1990.

532. Ralston SH, Scott PDR, Sturrock RD: An unusual case of pustulotic arthroosteitis affecting the leg, and erosive polyarthritis. Ann Rheum Dis *49*:643, 1990.

533. Takagi M, Oda J, Tsuzuki N, et al: Palmoplantar pustulotic arthro-osteitis of the peripheral joints with no sternocostoclavicular lesions. Ann Rheum Dis *51*:558, 1992.

534. Le Goff P, Baron D, Le Henaff C, et al: Arthrites destructrices périphériques au cours de la pustulose palmo-plantaire. A propos de trois observations. Rev Rhum Mal Osteoartic *59*:443, 1992.

535. Jurik AG, Helmig O, Graudal H: Skeletal disease, arthro-osteitis in adult patients with pustulosis palmoplantaris. Scand J Rheumatol *70*:3, 1988.

536. Dorland's Illustrated Medical Dictionary, Philadelphia, WB Saunders, 28th edition, 1994.

537. Laxer RM, Shore AD, Manson D, et al: Chronic recurrent multifocal osteomyelitis and psoriasis—a report of a new association and review of related disorders. Semin Arth Rheum *17*:260, 1988.

538. Brown T, Wilkinson RH: Chronic recurrent multifocal osteomyelitis. Radiology *166*:493, 1988.

539. Jurik AG, Møller BN: Chronic sclerosing osteomyelitis of the clavicle. A manifestation of chronic recurrent multifocal osteomyelitis. Arch Orthop Trauma Surg *106*:144, 1987.

540. Jurik AG, Helmig O, Ternowitz T, et al: Chronic recurrent multifocal osteomyelitis: A follow-up study. J Pediatr Orthop *8*:49, 1988.

541. Pelkonen P, Ryöppy S, Jaaskelainen J, et al: Chronic osteomyelitislike disease with negative bacterial cultures. Am J Dis Child *142*:1167, 1988.

542. Manson D, Wilmot DM, King S, et al: Physeal involvement in chronic recurrent multifocal osteomyelitis. Pediatr Radiol *20*:76, 1989.

543. Van Howe RS, Starshak RJ, Chusid MJ: Chronic recurrent multifocal osteomyelitis. Case report and review of the literature. Clin Pediatr *28*:54, 1989.

544. Wetzel R, Gondolph-Zink B, Puhl W: Pustular osteoarthropathy and its differential diagnosis. Intern Orthop (SICOT) *15*:101, 1991.

545. Ongchi DR, Fleming MG, Harris CA: Sternocostoclavicular hyperostosis: Two cases with differing dermatologic syndromes. J Rheumatol *17*:1415, 1990.

546. Chigira M, Shimizu T: Computed tomographic appearances of sternocostoclavicular hyperostosis. Skel Radiol *18*:347, 1989.

547. Prevo RL, Rasker JJ, Kruijsen MWM: Sternocostoclavicular hyperostosis or pustulotic arthroosteitis. J Rheumatol *16*:1602, 1989.

548. Farrés MT, Grabenwöger F: Die sternocostoclaviculäre Hyperostase: Raumforderung der oberen Thoraxapertur. Radiologe *28*:584, 1988.

549. van Holsbeeck M, Martel W, Dequeker J, et al: Soft tissue involvement, mediastinal pseudotumor, and venous thrombosis in pustulotic arthro-osteitis. Skel Radiol *18*:1, 1989.

550. Hallas J, Olesen KP: Sterno-costo-clavicular hyperostosis. A case report with a review of the literature. Acta Radiologica *29*:577, 1988.

551. Fallet GH, Lagier R, Gerster J-C, et al: Sternocostoclavicular hyperostosis (SCCHO) with palmoplantar pustulosis (PPP). Clin Exp Rheumatol *5*:135, 1987.

552. Dihlmann W, Hering L, Bargon GW: Das akquirierte Hyperostose-Syndrom (AHS). Synthese aus 13 eigenen Beobachtungen von sternokostoklavikulärer Hyperostose und über 300 Fällen aus der Literatur-Teil 1. Fortschr Rontgenstr *149*:386, 1988.

553. Dihlmann W, Hering L, Bargon GW: Das akquirierte Hyperostose-Syndrom. Teil 2. Fortschr Rontgenstr *149*:596, 1988.

554. Hoshino T, Minakami M: Rheumatoid arthritis associated with pustulosis palmoplantaris. Clin Orthop *216*:270, 1987.

555. Le Loet X, Bonnet B, Thomine E, et al: Manifestations ostéo-articulaires de la pustulose palmo-plantaire. Etude prospective de 15 cas. La Presse Medicale *20*:1307, 1991.

556. Durocher AM, Thévenon A, Dumolin E, et al: Toxopachyostéose de Weismann—Netter et Stuhl. Évolutive à l'âge adulte. Rev Rhum *57*:229, 1990.

557. Francis GL, Jelinek JJ, McHale K, et al: The Weismann-Netter syndrome: A cause of bowed legs in childhood. Pediatrics *88*:334, 1991.

558. Hary S, Houvenagel E, Vincent G, et al: La toxopachyostéose de Weismann-Netter et Stuhl. A propos de 30 observations. Rev Rhum Mal Ostéoartic *59*:65, 1992.

559. Hary S, Houvenagel E, Vincent G: Une observation de toxopachyostéose de Weismann-Netter et Stuhl avec localisations osseouse nouvelles. Rev Rhum Mal Ostéoartic *59*:73, 1992.

560. Maroteaux P, Freisinger P, Le Merrer M: Pachydysostosis of the fibula. J Bone Joint Surg [Br] *73*:842, 1991.

561. Earwaker J: Paranasal sinus osteomas: a review of 46 cases. Skel Radiol *22*:417, 1993.

562. Martínez-Lavin M, Matucci-Cerinic M, Jajic I, et al: Hypertrophic osteoarthropathy: Consensus on its definition, classification, assessment and diagnostic criteria. J Rheumatol *20*:1386, 1993.

563. Verbruggen LA, Shahabpour M, De Geeter F, et al: Femoral periosteal thickening in pustulotic arthroosteitis, including 3-year followup by magnetic resonance imaging. J Rheumatol *20*:1793, 1993.

564. Stewart A, Carneiro R, Pollock L, et al: Case report 834. Skeletal Radiol *23*:225, 1994.

565. Laasonen LS, Karvonen S-L, Reunala TL: Bone disease in adolescents with acne fulminans and severe cystic acne: Radiologic and scintigraphic findings. AJR *162*:1161, 1994.

566. Kasperczyk A, Freyschmidt J: Pustulotic arthroosteitis: Spectrum of bone lesions with palmoplantar pustulosis. Radiology *191*:207, 1994.

567. Dihlmann W, Schnabel A, Gross WL: The acquired hyperostosis syndrome: A little known skeletal disorder with distinctive radiological and clinical features. Clin Investig *72*:4, 1993.

94

Osteolysis and Chondrolysis

Donald Resnick, M.D., and Gen Niwayama, M.D.

Destruction of bone (osteolysis) or cartilage (chondrolysis) can become evident in innumerable neoplastic, infectious, metabolic, traumatic, vascular, congenital, and articular disorders. In fact, severe and progressive cartilaginous or osseous dissolution at multiple sites can lead to considerable clinical deformity in some of these disorders, such as rheumatoid arthritis, psoriatic arthritis, juvenile chronic arthritis, systemic lupus erythematosus, scleroderma, mixed connective tissue disease, multicentric reticulohistiocytosis, gout, calcium pyrophosphate dihydrate crystal deposition disease, neuropathic osteoarthropathy, osteonecrosis, hyperparathyroidism, renal osteodystrophy, plasma cell myeloma, skeletal metastasis, tuberculosis, fungal infections, and sarcoidosis; in addition, osteolysis may follow animal bites, irradiation, frostbite, and thermal and electrical burns.[1, 130, 141, 168, 174, 175] These conditions are discussed in detail elsewhere in this book. A group of heterogeneous conditions remains in which significant and severe osteolysis and chondrolysis may become manifest, and these disorders are described in this chapter.

OSTEOLYSIS

Occupational Acro-osteolysis

The 1950 report by Harnasch[2] focused attention on a new form of acro-osteolysis that appeared to represent an occupational hazard. This investigator noted shortened, thickened, and deformed fingers and widespread eczema in a blacksmith who had been handling oil and tar over a period of years. Subsequent reports by Suciu and coworkers[3] in 1963 and Cordier and colleagues[4] in 1966 implicated exposure to vinyl chloride monomer in the pathogenesis of acro-osteolysis, an observation that has been confirmed in numerous other investigations.[5-11] Routine radiographic surveys of persons in certain industrial plants have revealed that as many as 1 to 2 per cent of workers involved in the polymerization of vinyl chloride may develop acro-osteolysis.[10] Occasionally, exposure to vapors of other synthetic materials used in the manufacture of plastic products may produce similar abnormalities.[12] Initial clinical manifestations include fatigue, asthenia, nervousness, and insomnia.[10] A Raynaud's phenomenon-like disorder ensues, with digital pain, numbness, and tingling followed by the appearance of "drumstick" fingers and "watch-glass" nails. Some persons with this disorder may not develop radiographically evident changes, although arteriography can outline alterations in the palmar arches and digital arteries.[13, 137, 142] Additional clinical findings can include scleroderma-like plaques on the hands, wrists, and forearms, soft tissue nodules, hyperhidrosis and discoloration, and medial nerve compression in the carpal tunnel.[10] Further complications of vinyl chloride disease are hepatic fibrosis or tumor, splenomegaly, portal hypertension, thrombocytopenia, and pulmonary changes.[136]

The radiographic hallmark of the disorder is osteolysis that predominates in the terminal phalanges of the hands, although it also may affect other phalanges, the sacroiliac joints,[7, 8] the foot,[4, 7] and, rarely, additional skeletal structures,[10] including the mandible. Bandlike radiolucent areas across the waist of one or more terminal phalanges may be combined with tuftal resorption and beveling and osseous fragmentation (Fig. 94–1). The thumb is affected more commonly than the other digits. Similar changes may appear in the foot, and bone erosion and sclerosis about one or both sacroiliac joints resemble the changes of sacroiliitis found in association with the seronegative spondyloarthropathies. If the exposure to polyvinylchloride is halted, the patient may reveal slow improvement of the radiographic abnormalities. Consolidation and coalescence of phalangeal fragments can be evident, although some residua usually

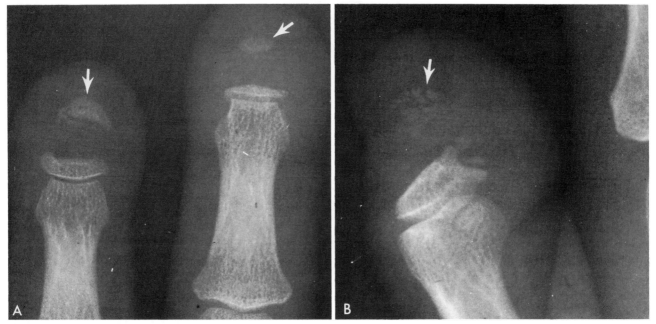

FIGURE 94–1. Occupational acro-osteolysis.

A Note bandlike resorption of the terminal phalanges of two digits, isolating small osseous fragments in the terminal tufts (arrows). Observe that the distal interphalangeal joints are intact.

B In the thumb, involvement is especially marked. The proximal portion of the terminal phalanx is tapered and small bony foci (arrow) are located distally.

persists, associated with shortening and clubbing of the digits. Elsewhere, roentgenographic improvement also may be recognized, and even the sacroiliac joint changes may regress. These improvements can be verified by scintigraphy, during which the accumulation of bone-seeking radiopharmaceutical agents in one or more skeletal sites can be seen to diminish after the elimination of contact with polyvinylchloride.[14]

The cause and pathogenesis of the condition are unclear. Wilson and associates[5] postulated that three factors were important, all of which were required for the development of the syndrome: a chemical insult, a physical insult, and a personal idiosyncrasy. The role of chemical or physical trauma would explain the predilection for involvement of the hand, the appearance of symmetric areas of osteopenia at skeletal sites of major muscle insertions, and the improvement in the clinical, radiographic, and scintigraphic alterations after cessation of the exposure to polyvinylchloride.[14] A disturbance in circulation, especially in the small peripheral arteries of the hands, may be attributable to a toxic chemical substance. The substance may act on the central or peripheral nervous system or directly on the walls of the arterioles and capillaries.[10] The lack of correlation between the duration of the exposure or the concentration of the toxic substances and the severity of the osteolysis, as well as the appearance of Raynaud's phenomenon without osteolysis in some persons, suggests that host factors also are important in the clinical expression of this disease. It is possible that exposure to polyvinylchloride initiates an immune complex disease in predisposed persons.[143]

The frequency of acro-osteolysis in workers involved in the polymerization of vinyl chloride has diminished in recent years.[10] This is due to an increase in the preventive measures currently being employed in this industry in view of the well-known skeletal and extraskeletal (angiosarcoma of the liver) complications of polyvinylchloride exposure.[15]

Bandlike resorption of the terminal phalanges in this condition differs from the usual pattern of osteolysis that may accompany vasculitis (Fig. 94–2), collagen vascular disorders (e.g., scleroderma) (Fig. 94–3), psoriasis (Fig. 94–4A), pityriasis rubra pilaris, gout, epidermolysis bullosa, frostbite, thermal and electrical burns, hypertrophic osteoarthropathy, septic shock, multicentric reticulohistiocytosis

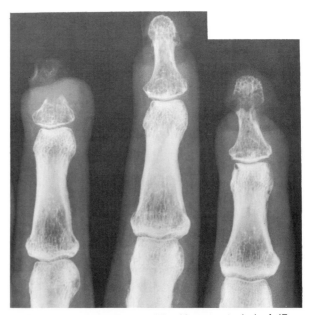

FIGURE 94–2. Rheumatoid vasculitis with acro-osteolysis. A 47 year old woman with classic rheumatoid arthritis and no evidence of another collagen vascular disorder developed digital gangrene, which eventually required distal phalangectomy. A radiograph of the left fingers reveals marked resorption and atrophy of distal soft tissues with self-amputation of the tufts of several digits. Note the absence of erosive arthritis. (From Rohlfing BM, et al: Br J Radiol 50:830, 1977.)

(Fig. 94–4*B*), and neuropathic osteoarthropathy.[141, 144, 145, 176] Similar bandlike resorption can be seen in hyperparathyroidism (in association with more characteristic alterations),[175] as a reaction to abnormal stress (Fig. 94–4*C*), after exposure to snake or scorpion venom,[168] and in certain familial conditions (see discussion later in this chapter).

Posttraumatic Osteolysis

Although some degree of bone loss is common after traumatic insult, particularly when complicated by fracture, in certain situations and sites the degree of posttraumatic osteolysis may appear excessive (Table 94–1). Knowledge of the existence and appearance of such osteolysis is important so that the resorption of bone that accompanies a traumatic insult is not mistaken for an inflammatory or neoplastic process.

Posttraumatic osteolysis can lead to progressive resorption of the outer end of the clavicle. According to Strauch,[16] this complication first was reported by Dupas in 1936. Numerous accounts of posttraumatic osteolysis of the clavicle now have appeared.[17–28, 146, 149, 195, 196] The process becomes apparent after single or repeated episodes of local trauma. Frequently, the traumatic insult is minor and unassociated with obvious fracture or dislocation; in fact, a similar process has been related to chronic stress (as in weight-lifters) without acute injury (see later discussion).[147, 177] The osteolytic process begins as early as 2 to 3 weeks and as late as several years after the injury. When untreated, it leads to lysis of 0.5 to 3 cm of bony substance from the distal end of the clavicle over a period of 12 to 18 months, which may be associated with erosion and cupping of the acromion, soft tissue swelling, and dystrophic calcification[22] (Fig. 94–5). Pain, diminished strength, local crepitation, and restricted mobility may be evident at this stage. After the lytic phase stabilizes, reparative changes occur

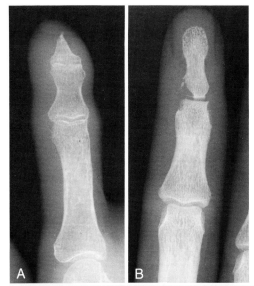
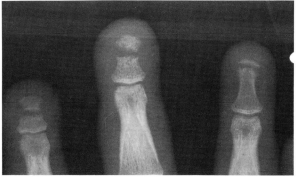

FIGURE 94–4. Other causes of acro-osteolysis.

A Psoriasis. In this 43 year old woman with psoriatic skin disease and stiffness in the hands, observe tapering of the terminal phalanx of the second finger with periarticular soft tissue prominence and deformity of the nail. Other fingers in both hands were affected similarly, and articular abnormalities were minimal. (Courtesy of G. Greenway, M.D., Dallas, Texas.)

B Multicentric reticulohistiocytosis. The extremely well marginated osseous erosions in the phalangeal portions of the distal interphalangeal joint are typical of this disease. (Courtesy of M. Dalinka, M.D., Philadelphia, Pennsylvania.)

C Stress changes. Unilateral abnormalities of the terminal phalanges occurred in this guitar player. The thumb was spared. The findings are consistent with stress fractures. (Courtesy of W. Murphy, M.D., Houston, Texas.)

over a period of 4 to 6 months, emphasizing the self-limited nature of the process. Eventually, the subchondral bone becomes reconstituted, although the acromioclavicular joint can remain permanently widened.[22]

Careful analysis of radiographs in the early posttraumatic period may allow identification of prominent soft tissues, osteoporosis, and small gaps in the subchondral bone plate of the clavicle that, when recognized and treated with immobilization, can shorten the course of the process.

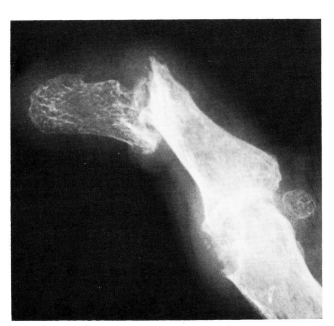

FIGURE 94–3. Scleroderma. Considerable destruction of the interphalangeal and metacarpophalangeal joints of the thumb is observed in this patient with scleroderma. This is an unusual manifestation of the disease. A similar pattern of joint destruction may accompany psoriatic arthritis and multicentric reticulohistiocytosis.

TABLE 94–1. Common Sites of Posttraumatic Osteolysis

Distal portion of the clavicle[16–28, 146, 149]	Distal portion of radius[21, 31]
Pubic and ischial rami[29, 150–153]	Carpus[21, 31]
Distal portion of ulna[21, 31]	Femoral neck[132]

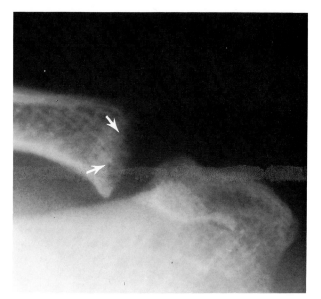

FIGURE 94–5. Posttraumatic osteolysis: Clavicle. In a 23 year old weight-lifter, irregular erosion of the distal portion of the clavicle (arrows) and, to a lesser extent, the acromion, with widening of the acromioclavicular joint, is seen. (Courtesy of P. Kaplan, M.D., Charlottesville, Virginia.)

The pathogenesis of posttraumatic osteolysis of the clavicle is not certain. Osteoclastic resorption, autonomic nervous system dysfunction, and catabolic hyperemia have been suggested as possible important factors.[17] Levine and coworkers[22] postulated that a slowly progressive, posttraumatic synovial reaction in the acromioclavicular joint could account for the osteolysis, citing such supporting evidence as acromial involvement, the presence of villous hyperplasia and marked vascular proliferation of the synovium after biopsy or resection (Fig. 94–6), and the osseous reconstitution after synovectomy.

Posttraumatic osteolysis of one or both clavicles also is observed in athletes, particularly weight-lifters, owing to chronic stress rather than acute injury.[147, 169, 177] A similar process can evolve in persons who lift heavy weights as part of their occupational activities. Clinical and radiologic abnormalities are virtually identical to those that occur after acute injury. Histologic inspection of resected clavicles in athletes has revealed intense osteoblastic activity consistent with a reparative response.[148] Microfractures may be evident in the subchondral bone, and the articular cartilage may contain fissures or other signs of degeneration.[148]

The differential diagnosis of osteolysis about the acromioclavicular joint includes, in addition to trauma, hyperparathyroidism, collagen vascular disorders, infection, rheumatoid arthritis, and other articular processes.

Posttraumatic osteolysis can become prominent at other skeletal sites as well. In the pubic or ischial rami, exaggerated resorption of bone about a fracture, with or without associated sclerosis, can simulate the appearance of a malignant process[29, 150–153, 170, 178] (Figs. 94–7 and 94–8). Furthermore, the pathologist may misinterpret the exuberant cartilage and disorderly membranous bone formation of a rapidly forming primary callus as evidence of a chondrosar-

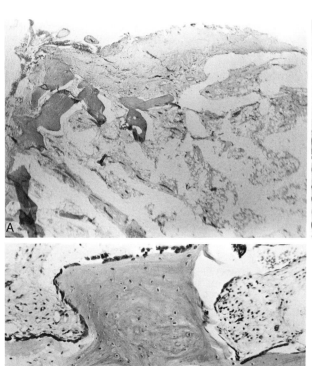

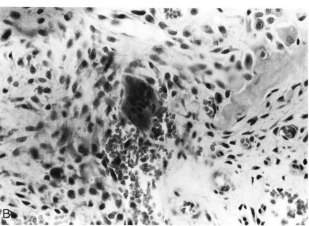

FIGURE 94–6. Posttraumatic osteolysis: Clavicle.

A Resection of the distal portion of the clavicle in a patient with posttraumatic osteolysis provided material for histologic analysis. In a low magnification photomicrograph, observe chronic inflammatory changes and fibrosis in the synovial membrane. (Hematoxylin and eosin stain, 4×.)

B At higher magnification of one area beneath the synovium, an osteoclast-type giant cell, fibrosis, and fibro-osseous metaplasia are seen. (Hematoxylin and eosin stain, 100×.)

C An area of reactive bone formation shows plump osteoblasts at the bone surfaces with fibrovascular, loose connective tissue in the intertrabecular spaces. (Hematoxylin and eosin stain, 40×.)

(Courtesy of T. Goergen, M.D., and P. Haghighi, M.D., San Diego, California.)

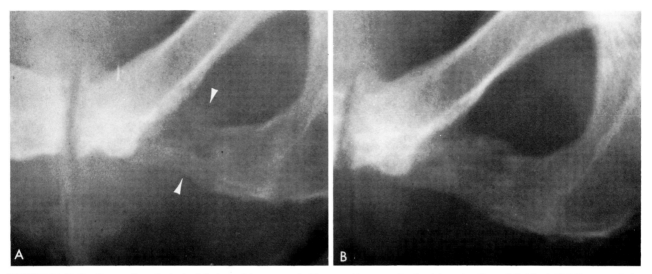

FIGURE 94–7. Posttraumatic osteolysis: Inferior pubic ramus. A 44 year old woman had pelvic pain after a fall. The initial film revealed an undisplaced fracture of the left inferior pubic ramus. The patient continued to experience pain.

A A radiograph obtained 4 weeks after the fracture reveals significant osteolysis about the fracture site (arrowheads). At this stage, the appearance resembles that of a pathologic fracture.

B Four weeks later, considerable healing at the fracture site is evident, indicating the true nature of the radiographic findings.

coma or other malignancy, thus compounding the diagnostic dilemma.[30] Such fractures occur as a result of either direct trauma or, frequently, chronic stress in an osteopenic skeleton (insufficiency fractures), sometimes in combination with similar fractures of the sacrum. The cause of osteolysis about these ramus fractures is not known, although instability, particularly in single ramus fractures,

should not be a factor. As there is no impaction of bone in these latter fractures, perhaps a lack of sound, direct bone contact is an explanation for the excessive osteolysis and delayed union.[29]

Prominent posttraumatic osteolysis also has been noted in the ulna, radius, and carpal bones.[21, 31] In the femoral neck, resorption and rotation at a fracture site can produce

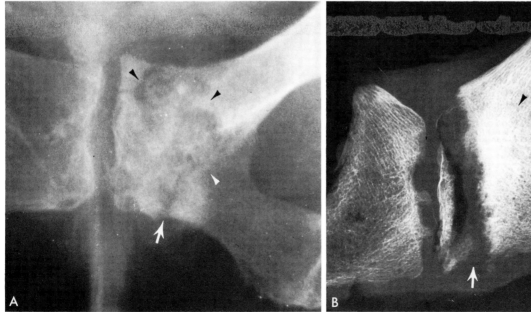

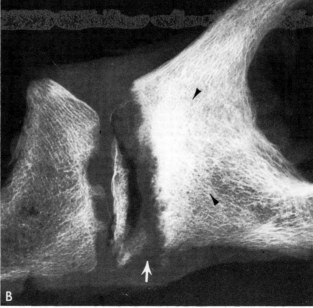

FIGURE 94–8. Posttraumatic osteolysis: Pubic bone. This 54 year old alcoholic woman complained of a dull left groin ache of 4 months duration and weight loss of 30 pounds. A history of trauma was denied. Because of the radiographic findings, which suggested a neoplastic process, an extensive search for other osseous or extraosseous lesions was undertaken and was unrewarding. A biopsy demonstrated areas of atypical cartilage, suggestive but not diagnostic of chondrosarcoma. A radical excision of the left pubic bone was performed. Histologic material was examined by five experienced bone pathologists, the diagnoses including chronic osteomyelitis, a benign cartilage tumor, and a reactive fibro-osseous proliferation most consistent with an ununited fracture. The patient later developed fractures of the sternum and ribs, although she continued to deny any significant trauma.

A A preoperative radiograph reveals a mixed lytic and sclerotic lesion of the left pubis (arrowheads) with a fracture (arrow).

B A radiograph of the removed bone indicates the probable benign nature of the lesion. The fracture line (arrow) is seen with surrounding bony eburnation (arrowheads).

a radiographic picture that may be misinterpreted as a malignant process[132, 139] (Fig. 94–9). Osteolysis after odontoid fracture[133] or atlantoaxial subluxation[134] can produce a separate bone at the tip of the dens, resembling or identical to the os odontoideum. Other sites of posttraumatic osteolysis are the skull,[179] sternum, and ribs.

Primary Osteolysis Syndromes

A diverse group of idiopathic disorders can lead to significant skeletal lysis. They differ in the presence or absence of genetic transmission, the associated clinical manifestations, and the major locations of osteolysis[32] (Table 94–2).

Acro-osteolysis Syndrome of Hajdu and Cheney. An unusual variety of cranioskeletal dysplasia was described by Hajdu and Kauntze in a sporadic case in 1948[33] and by Cheney in a family in 1965.[34] Further reports of this syndrome have appeared,[32, 35–45, 129, 135, 154, 172, 180, 181] allowing delineation of its clinical and radiologic manifestations. The disorder may be familial, with a dominant mode of inheritance, or sporadic and is manifested by short stature, low-set ears, recessed mandible, malocclusion and early loss of teeth, coarse hairs, pseudoclubbing of the digits, joint laxity, conductive hearing loss, and speech impairment. Radiographic features include osteolysis of distal phalanges of the hands and feet; a bizarre-shaped dolichocephalic skull with basilar impression, delayed closure of cranial sutures, multiple wormian bones, hypoplastic or absent frontal sinuses, prominent occipital ridge, and enlarged sella turcica; diminutive mandible and maxilla with poor dentition; generalized osteoporosis with vertebral compressions and deformities, and fractures of tubular bones; valgus deformities of the knees; and hypoplasia and subluxation of the proximal portion of the radius. Laboratory analysis usually is unremarkable, and renal function, which is altered in other osteolysis syndromes, is normal in this condition.

Osteolysis is especially characteristic (Figs. 94–10 and 94–11). Changes in the phalanges, which consist of resorption of tufts and bandlike areas of lucency, simulate ab-

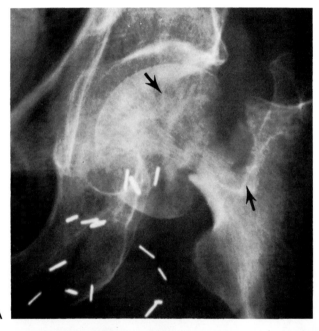

A

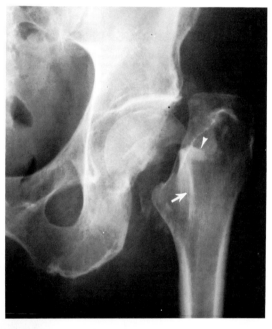

B

FIGURE 94–9. Posttraumatic osteolysis: Femoral neck.

A After a fracture of the femoral neck, resorption and rotation at the fracture site (arrows) can produce a radiographic picture resembling that of a malignant process.

B In another patient, a 61 year old man with a remote fracture of the femoral neck, observe the apparent disappearance of bone related both to true osteolysis and to rotation at the fracture site. A portion of the remaining femoral neck overlies the trochanteric region (arrow), and its superior margin can be identified (arrowhead).

C A transverse section of a cadaveric hip reveals a fracture of the femoral neck with rotation and anterior angulation at the fracture site. Such rotation, when exaggerated, simulates osteolysis on radiographic examination.

TABLE 94–2. Osteolysis Syndromes

Syndrome	Age of Onset	Major Site of Osteolysis	Patterns of Inheritance	Associated Features
Acro-osteolysis of Hajdu and Cheney[32–46]	Second decade	Distal phalanges; rarely tubular bones, mandible, acromioclavicular joints	Dominant or sporadic	Generalized bone dysplasia, fractures, osteoporosis
Massive osteolysis of Gorham[47–68]	Young adult	Variable; pelvic or shoulder girdles	Sporadic	Slowly progressive, extreme dissolution
Carpal-tarsal osteolysis: Multicentric osteolysis with nephropathy[77–84]	Infant, child	Carpal and tarsal areas, elbows	Sporadic; occasionally dominant	Osteoporosis, deformity, hypertension, renal failure, death
Hereditary multicentric osteolysis[85–90]	1–5 years	Carpal and tarsal areas, elbows, digitis	Dominant; occasionally recessive or sporadic	Progressive deformity
Neurogenic osteolysis[97, 98]	Childhood	Phalanges	Dominant or recessive	Sensory neuropathy, skin ulcerations
Acro-osteolysis of Joseph[101]	Childhood	Distal phalanges	Recessive	Otherwise healthy
Acro-osteolysis of Shinz[102]	Second decade	Phalanges	Dominant	Skin ulcerations, no neurologic defect
Farber's disease[95, 103]	Infancy	Elbows, wrists, knees, ankles	Sporadic	Subcutaneous nodules
Winchester's syndrome[104]	Infancy	Carpal and tarsal areas, elbows	Recessive	Osteoporosis, joint contractures, thick skin, corneal opacities
Osteolysis with detritic synovitis[105]	Adulthood	Widespread	Sporadic	Progressive

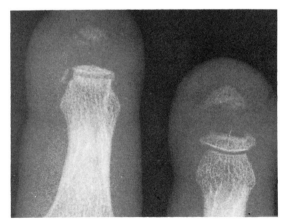
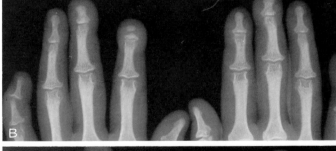
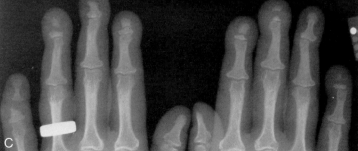

A

FIGURE 94–10. Acro-osteolysis of Hajdu and Cheney.
A The typical pattern of osteolysis of the digits is demonstrated. Note that resorption occurs in a band-like fashion across the waist of the terminal phalanges, isolating one or more phalangeal fragments. Soft tissue swelling also is evident. The appearance is identical to that in occupational acro-osteolysis. (Courtesy of M. Dalinka, M.D., Philadelphia, Pennsylvania.)
B, C In another patient, radiographs obtained at the ages of 18 years **(B)** and 29 years **(C)** show progressive acro-osteolysis. (Courtesy of H. Kroon, M.D., Leiden, The Netherlands.)

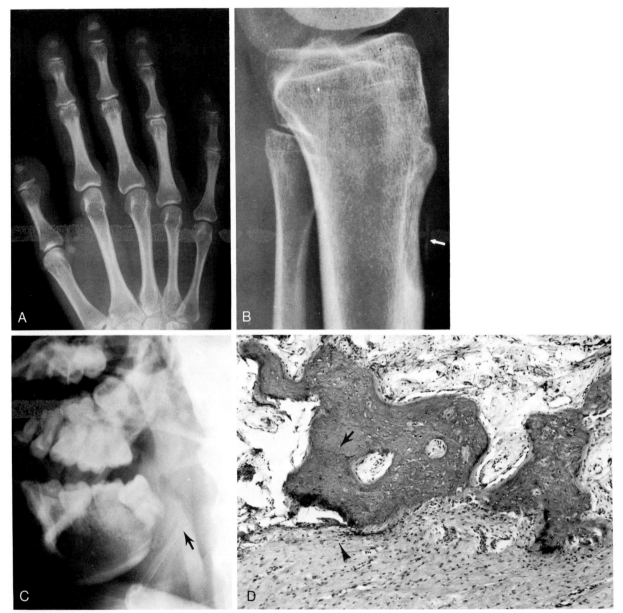

FIGURE 94–11. Acro-osteolysis of Hajdu and Cheney. A 20 year old woman developed progressive acro-osteolysis of the hands as well as of other skeletal sites. A family history of similar problems was not apparent.

A Note osteolysis of the terminal phalanges in all of the digits. The opposite hand was affected equally.

B A 5 cm long cortical defect containing a linear piece of bone (arrow) involves the anterior aspect of the proximal end of the tibia just inferior to the tibial tuberosity. The opposite knee also was affected.

C The right mandibular ramus is completely absent (arrow).

D A section of the lesion in the anterior proximal portion of the tibia shows erosion of bony trabeculae (arrow) that have a woven appearance. Osteoclasts are not seen. The periosteum (arrowhead) is labeled (90×).

(From Gilula CA, et al: Radiology *121*:63, 1976.)

normalities in occupation-induced (polyvinylchloride) acro-osteolysis, renal osteodystrophy, pyknodysostosis, Rothmund's syndrome, and collagen vascular disorders. Osteolysis also can be apparent in the tubular bones, mandibular rami, tarsal and metatarsal bones, and acromioclavicular joints.[46, 180] The radionuclide examination is characterized by abnormal accumulation of bone-seeking radiopharmaceutical agents at sites of osteolysis.[155] MR imaging can be used effectively to study the degree of involvement of the spinal cord in those patients who have basilar impression[182] as well as in those who in rare circumstances develop instability of the cervical spine.[183]

The pathogenesis of this syndrome is unknown. It may represent a manifestation of a generalized osseous dysplasia, as an abnormality of bone mineral and metabolism has not been documented. Bone and skin collagen appear normal on electron microscopy, although iliac crest biopsies demonstrate a decrease in skeletal mass.[44] The percentage of endosteal bone surfaces characteristic of bone formation may be diminished, and resorptive surfaces may be increased. Brown and colleagues[44] concluded, on the basis of their morphologic studies, that an abnormality of osteoblast function may be the cause of an alteration of structural protein. Their findings differed from those in hyperparathyroidism and hyperthyroidism. Elias and associates[32] obtained biopsy specimens of an area of active osteolysis in a phalanx and noted active replacement of central medullary bone by a fibrous and angiomatous process, characterized by the presence of small, thick-walled vessels and an unusual number of interspersed nerve fibers and mast cells. They suggested that a neurovascular dysfunction with local release of osteolytic mediators might be involved in the pathogenesis of the disorder.

Massive Osteolysis of Gorham. In 1954, Gorham and collaborators[47] reported two patients with a peculiar variety of massive osteolysis. One year later, Gorham and Stout,[48] in a more comprehensive report, detailed the previous descriptions of this entity in the literature,[49–55] and proposed the term hemangiomatosis for this condition. Subsequently, numerous other descriptions have appeared, some of which have introduced additional names, such as massive osteolysis, disappearing bone disease, vanishing bone disease, and Gorham disease.[56–68, 140, 171, 184–186]

The disease can become evident in men and women of all ages, although most cases are discovered before the age of 40 years. A family history is not apparent. The process may affect either the axial or the appendicular skeleton; numerous cases document the frequency of changes in the pelvic or shoulder regions. Clinical manifestations vary; some patients have a relatively abrupt onset of pain and swelling, whereas others describe an insidious onset of soft tissue atrophy and limitation of motion that is without pain unless an associated pathologic fracture develops. Of interest, some patients note the onset of the disorder after significant trauma. Laboratory analysis may show unremarkable results, with slight elevation of the serum alkaline phosphatase level.

The most dramatic aspect of massive osteolysis is its radiographic appearance (Fig. 94–12). Initially, radiolucent foci appear in the intramedullary or subcortical regions, which resemble findings in patchy osteoporosis. Slowly progressive atrophy, dissolution, fracture, fragmentation, and disappearance of a portion of the bone then occur, with tapering or "pointing" of the remaining osseous tissue and atrophy of soft tissue. The process subsequently extends to contiguous bones, the intervening joints affording no pro-

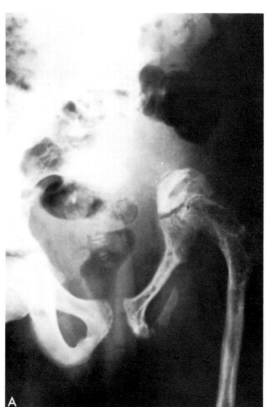
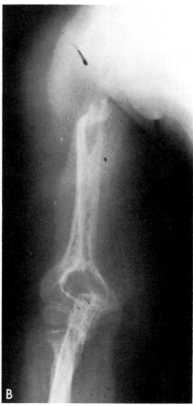

FIGURE 94–12. Massive osteolysis of Gorham.

A In this 14 year old boy, observe the dissolution of most of the left hemipelvis and the narrowed and tapered left femur. Radiolucent foci and a coarsened trabecular pattern are seen in the femur and pubic bone.

B In a 6 year old girl, resorption of the proximal half of the humerus is evident. The remaining bone is osteoporotic, with lucent lesions.

tection. Thus, osteolysis of the ilium may be associated with resorption of the proximal portion of the femur, whereas changes in the scapula may later be combined with osteolysis of the proximal end of the humerus, clavicle, and ribs. This pattern of regional destruction is dramatic and should suggest the correct diagnosis. Rarely, two or more anatomic regions are affected, separated by normal osseous structures. Apparently, any bone can be involved, including the small tubular bones of the hands and feet, the spine, the skull, and the mandible.[62, 64, 68, 69, 184] The degree of osseous destruction generally increases relentlessly over a period of years, although eventually it may stabilize. Occasional reports of massive osteolysis describe spontaneous recovery of some of the lost bone tissue[65] or clinical and radiologic improvement after radiotherapy.[166]

Arteriography may indicate stretching of vessels in the area of lysis.[59, 60] Prominent vascularity usually is not evident during this study, although direct injection of contrast medium into the lesion will result in opacification of the involved area.[66] As one main structural feature of the lesion is the presence of unusually wide capillary-like vessels (see discussion later in this chapter), it appears likely that the blood flow through these vessels is very slow. It has been suggested that the slow circulation produces local hypoxia and lowering of the pH, favoring the activity of various hydrolytic enzymes.[64]

Scintigraphy using bone-seeking radiopharmaceutical agents may demonstrate increased vascularity on initial images[156] and, subsequently, an area of decreased uptake corresponding to the site of diminished or absent bone tissue.[59]

In the early stages of the disorder, the pathologic features resemble those of skeletal hemangioma. In later stages, vascular fibrous tissue replaces the angiomatous tissue. Irregular wide spaces in cortical bone and enlarged marrow spaces in spongy bone contain numerous thin-walled, capillary-like vessels, most of them wider than normal capillaries and filled with blood cells.[64] Many of the abnormal vessels are situated in, and in direct contact with, osseous depressions. Inflammatory infiltrates generally are not evident.

The exact nature of the process is unknown. The resemblance of the pathologic characteristics to those of hemangiomas, coupled with the presence of soft tissue hemangiomatous or lymphangiomatous tissue and, occasionally, pleural effusions containing chyle, has suggested to some investigators, including Gorham and Stout,[48] that massive osteolysis represents a vascular derangement or a diffuse hemangiomatosis; this perhaps is due to a congenital condition in which hyperplastic vascular components form arteriovenous fistulae. Gorham and Stout[48] maintained that active hyperemia, changes in local pH, and mechanical forces promote bone resorption, that trauma might trigger the process by stimulating the production of vascular granulation tissue, and that osteoclastosis is not necessary. The virtual absence of multinucleated osteoclasts in areas of excessive bone resorption has been noted in other reports. Heyden and coworkers[64] observed strong activity of both acid phosphatase and leucine aminopeptidase in mononuclear perivascular cells that were in contact with remaining bone, perhaps indicating that these cells are important in the process of osseous resorption. As the perivascular cells may represent pericytes, the observation that pericytes may be precursors of mononuclear and multinuclear cells with osteolytic capacity is important.[64]

The possibility that massive osteolysis may represent a neoplastic proliferation of hemangiomatous (or lymphangiomatous) tissue also has been suggested in the past. It should be noted, however, that the process does not resemble closely ordinary hemangioma or lymphangioma of bone, or even cystic angiomatosis.[70–75]

Although the degree of osseous deformity in the disease may become severe, serious complications are not frequent. Paraplegia due to spinal cord involvement may occur in cases of vertebral osteolysis.[66] Death can result from thoracic cage, pulmonary, or pleural involvement that leads to compromise of respiratory function. Infection of bone and septic shock appear to be rare.[58]

Idiopathic Multicentric Osteolysis (Carpal-Tarsal Osteolysis). In 1976, Tyler and Rosenbaum[76] proposed the term idiopathic multicentric osteolysis for a rare disorder associated with extensive osteolysis, usually in the carpal or tarsal areas, that had previously been described under a variety of names; these included idiopathic osteolysis, essential osteolysis, progressive essential osteolysis, essential acro-osteolysis, familial osteolysis, hereditary osteolysis, carpal and tarsal agenesis, familial dysostosis carpi, and bilateral carpal necrosis. Idiopathic multicentric osteolysis was further classified into two basic types: multicentric osteolysis with nephropathy and hereditary multicentric osteolysis. Not all cases fit neatly into one of these two categories, so that a third designation, miscellaneous patterns, is required.

Multicentric Osteolysis with Nephropathy. This entity, which has been recognized in only a handful of cases, is characterized by an early age of onset (first few years of life) of osteolysis, associated with progressive renal failure that is commonly fatal by the third decade of life.[77–84, 173, 190] No family history of either osteolysis or renal disease is present. Presenting clinical manifestations include swollen, painful wrists with the presence or absence of foot deformities. Radiographs reveal progressive disappearance of the carpus and, less strikingly, the tarsus, with tapering of the adjacent tubular bones (Fig. 94–13). Osteolysis and subluxation about the elbow and congenital foot deformities also can be apparent. Rarely, other sites are affected. Renal alterations accompany the onset of osteolysis. Chronic glomerulonephritis results in hypertension, azotemia, and death in early adult life.

Hereditary Multicentric Osteolysis. This condition reveals a familial distribution, with most cases exhibiting a dominant mode of transmission, although the trait occasionally is recessive.[76, 85–90, 157, 158] In the dominant variety, the onset of disease usually occurs at the age of 3 to 4 years, with articular complaints involving the wrists and ankles. Subsequently, an asymptomatic period arises in adolescence in which a varying amount of carpal and tarsal osteolysis is associated with progressive deformity. In the recessive variety, the clinical course basically is similar.

Radiographs in both dominant and recessive forms outline dissolution of carpus and tarsus that, in most cases, is not associated with tapering of the adjacent tubular bones (Figs. 94–14 to 94–16). This latter characteristic, which differs from the ''penciling'' of tubular bones that is evident in multicentric osteolysis with nephropathy, is not

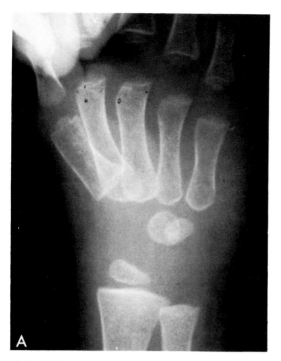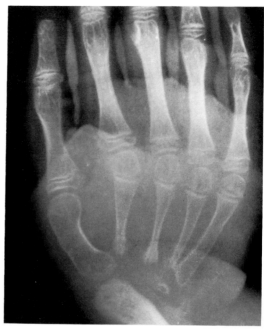

FIGURE 94–13. Multicentric osteolysis with nephropathy. A 14 year old boy developed progressive symmetric osteolysis involving hands, wrists, elbows, and feet, with associated renal failure and hypertension. Family history was not contributory.
  A Radiograph obtained in the second year of life fails to reveal osseous resorption.
  B At 14 years of age, osteolysis of the carpal bones, metacarpal bases, radius, and ulna is seen. The opposite side was affected similarly. (**B,** From MacPherson RI, et al: J Can Assoc Radiol 24:98, 1973.)

constant, and patients with hereditary multicentric osteolysis can reveal such tapering of metacarpals, distal end of the radius, and ulna. Rarely, osteolysis at additional sites can be encountered, including the elbows, shoulders, clavicles, hips, knees, ankles, feet, and ribs.[76, 158]

Miscellaneous Patterns. Some cases of idiopathic multicentric osteolysis may not fall precisely into one of these two groups. Thus, nonfamilial cases of carpal and tarsal osteolysis may be discovered that do not reveal renal disease.[85, 91, 92, 161] Similar sporadic cases with late age of onset[160] or involvement of osseous sites other than the carpal and tarsal areas[159, 187] have been described. Conversely, examples of carpal-tarsal osteolysis with evidence of renal involvement may demonstrate familial patterns (dominant mode of inheritance), although the nephropathy may differ in type and degree from that in the sporadic (nonfamilial) cases.[93, 94, 167] Erickson and colleagues[94] speculated that a child of a patient with a mild form of multicentric osteolysis with nephropathy conceivably could demonstrate features of the disease, revealing a dominant form of inheritance.

An extensive classification of the types of carpal and tarsal osteolysis has been proposed by Beals and Bird,[95] who addressed themselves to the difficulty of separating cases of such osteolysis on the basis of absence or presence of recognizable modes of inheritance and absence or presence of renal disease. It is apparent that dominant and recessive genetic patterns can be identified, that renal disease is not confined to nonhereditary cases, that the presence of so-called sporadic cases may not rule out a genetic transmission, and that other syndromes can reveal similar radiographic patterns.[162, 189]

Pathology and Pathogenesis. The involved tissues in idiopathic multicentric osteolysis usually reveal an increased content of fibrous elements and increased vascularity, with little evidence of inflammation.[95] Osteolysis is accompanied by osteoclastic activity. Bone formation appears normal, and reparative changes may be evidenced by the presence of woven bone formation.[85] Biopsies of involved joints may reveal no significant abnormalities of the synovial membrane and encroachment on cartilage by fibrocellular tissue.

The pathogenesis of the process is unknown. A primary defect may occur in the osseous and cartilaginous tissues, or these latter sites may be affected secondarily as a result of primary involvement and proliferation of articular fibrous tissue. Occasional reports of increased urinary hydroxyproline excretion[85] and elevated serum phosphatase levels may indicate the progressive destruction of bone or the presence of an underlying metabolic disorder characterized by increased bone turnover; however, the evidence of increased collagen turnover is inconsistent.[95]

Differential Diagnosis. The major radiographic characteristic of the various forms of idiopathic multicentric osteolysis is the striking resorption of bone that predominates in the carpal and tarsal areas (and occasionally in the elbows). This distribution differs from that typically associated with other varieties of osteolysis, such as occupational acro-osteolysis (phalanges), posttraumatic osteolysis (distal end of the clavicle, pubic and ischial rami, femoral neck, ulna, radius), acro-osteolysis syndrome of Hajdu and Cheney (phalanges), massive osteolysis of Gorham (variable distribution with predilection for pelvic and shoulder gir-

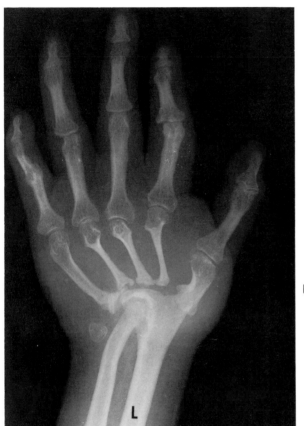

A

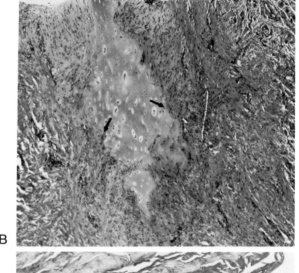

B

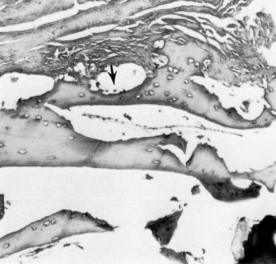

C

FIGURE 94–14. Hereditary multicentric osteolysis.

A This patient developed wrist symptoms and signs when he was an infant. A radiograph of the left wrist at age 40 years outlines absence of all but one of the carpal bones, hypoplasia of the metacarpal bones, and fusion of the fifth proximal interphalangeal joint. The right wrist was involved similarly.

B A biopsy of the left wrist of the 5 year old child of the patient in **A,** who had the same disease, delineates fibrocellular tissue encroaching on the cartilage (arrows) (120×).

C Two years later, biopsy of the same wrist demonstrates a thin rim of cortical bone beneath the periosteum with subperiosteal resorption (arrow) (120×).

(**A, C,** From Whyte MP, et al: Arthritis Rheum *21*:367, 1978.)

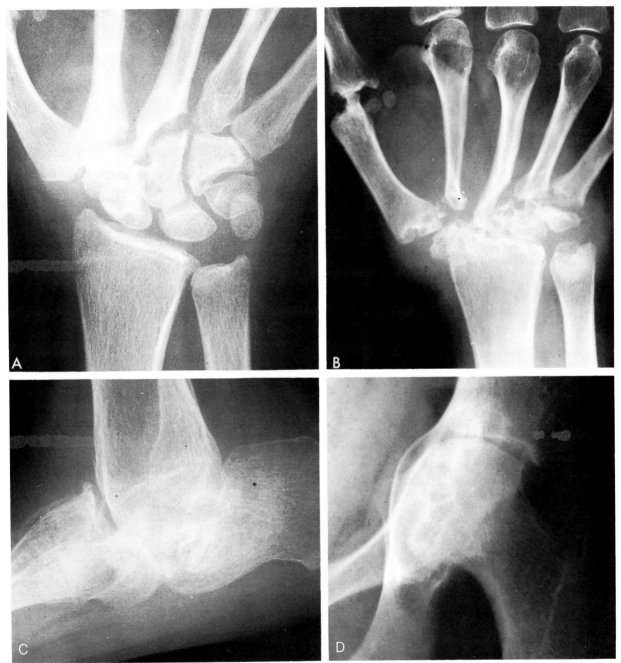

FIGURE 94–15. Hereditary multicentric osteolysis. This child developed progressive osteolysis at multiple skeletal sites without evidence of renal disease.

A, B Radiographs of the wrist obtained at the ages of 16 and 22 years reveal progressive resorption of the carpus and metacarpal bases, with soft tissue swelling. The tapered appearance of the proximal metacarpal bones and the osseous erosions at several metacarpophalangeal joints are readily apparent.

C A radiograph of the foot at age 16 years demonstrates the great degree of lysis of most of the tarsal bones. The tibia is articulating with the calcaneus.

D Unusual aspects of this case are the joint space narrowing, osseous erosion, and acetabular protrusion of the left hip.

(Courtesy of A. Brower, M.D., Norfolk, Virginia.)

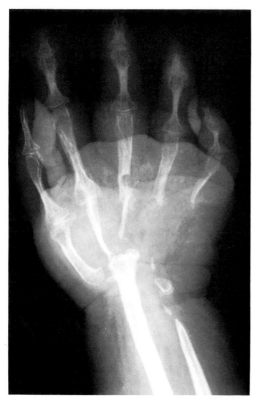

FIGURE 94–16. Hereditary multicentric osteolysis. The 48 year old woman had a childhood onset of the disease, a family history of similar abnormalities, and normal renal function. Disappearance of most of the carpal bones and the fourth and fifth metacarpals, tapering of the remaining metacarpals, phalanges, and ulna, and diminution of width of most of the bones are apparent; some of these changes were related to previous surgery. (Courtesy of S. Shaul, M.D., Yakima, Washington.)

dles), multicentric reticulohistiocytosis (hands, feet, wrists, ankles) (Fig. 94–17), acro-osteolysis syndrome of Joseph or of Shinz (phalanges), and neurogenic acro-osteolysis (phalanges). The changes may resemble those in juvenile

chronic arthritis (Fig. 94–18) (see Chapter 27). Winchester's syndrome, Farber's disease, and neuropathic osteoarthropathy in leprosy and diabetes mellitus (Fig. 94–19). Accurate diagnosis requires knowledge of the associated clinical manifestations, including the presence and mode of inheritance and the appearance of renal disease.

Other Osteolysis Syndromes

Neurogenic Acro-osteolysis. Both recessive and dominant forms of progressive peripheral bone destruction associated with sensory neuropathy have been described.[96] The disease becomes clinically apparent in childhood and is associated with skin ulcerations and progressive resorption of phalanges of the hands and feet.[97, 98] Vitamin B_{12} determinations in the spinal fluid of some patients have indicated abnormalities that suggest vitamin B_{12} hypovitaminosis as a possible direct cause of the disease.[99] A somewhat similar pattern of osteolysis, with more widespread bone destruction, has been noted in Vietnamese patients who revealed severe scarring of the skin, no neurologic alterations, and positive serologic tests for syphilis.[100] Some of these latter patients may have had the acro-osteolysis syndrome of Shinz (see next paragraph).

Acro-osteolysis of Joseph or of Shinz. Joseph and associates[101] described a single sibship with recessive inheritance of osteolysis of the distal phalanges in otherwise normal boys. Shinz[102] observed a form of peripheral osteolysis characterized by a dominant inheritance, onset in the second decade of life, destruction of phalanges of the hands and feet, and ulcerating skin lesions, without neurologic abnormalities. Acro-osteolysis syndromes similar to those of Joseph and of Shinz have been identified in adult patients without a family history of disease.[188]

Farber's Disease. Farber's disease is characterized by an onset in infancy of progressive, painful periarticular swelling, joint rigidity and contracture, osteolysis, and subcutaneous nodules.[95] It may represent a disorder of mucopolysaccharide metabolism of the fibroblast.[103]

Winchester's Syndrome. Winchester and associates[104]

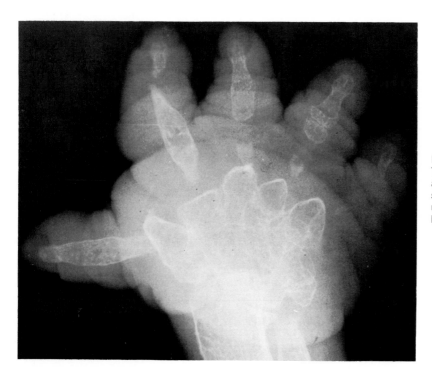

FIGURE 94–17. Multicentric reticulohistiocytosis. The degree of osteolysis of metacarpal bones and phalanges is striking. Carpal fusion and resorption of the distal portions of the radius and ulna are evident. (Courtesy of D. Chambers, M.D., Norfolk, Virginia.)

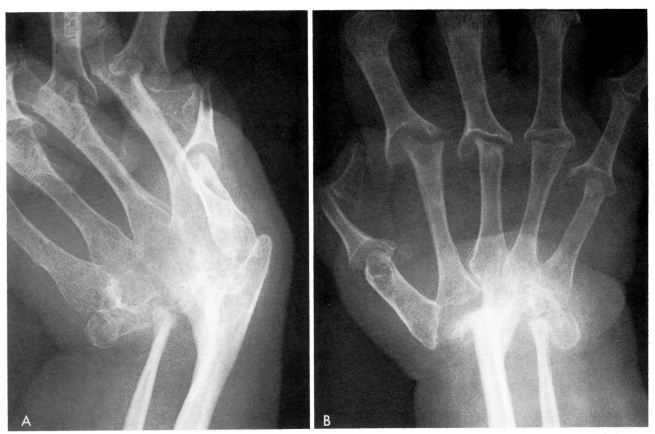

FIGURE 94–18. Still's disease. Observe the extreme destruction and resorption of carpus, radii, ulnae, metacarpal bones, and phalanges. The findings are not unlike those of carpal-tarsal osteolysis syndromes. (Courtesy of V. Vint, M.D., La Jolla, California.)

described a disorder with recessive inheritance manifested as extensive and progressive destruction of the carpus, tarsus, and elbows beginning in infancy and associated with increased acid mucopolysaccharides in cell cultures, but not in the urine.[95] Additional findings include dwarfism, coarsened facial features, peripheral corneal opacities, arthralgias and joint stiffening, progressive deformities of the trunk and limbs, and generalized and profound osteoporosis. Al-

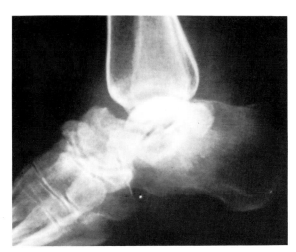

FIGURE 94–19. Neuropathic osteoarthropathy in diabetes mellitus. Osteolysis and bone fragmentation in the tarsus are observed in this condition. In this case, note the fracture of the midportion of the talus with ischemic necrosis of its proximal segment. (Courtesy of U.S. Naval Hospital, San Diego, California.)

though originally classified as a form of mucopolysaccharidosis, Winchester's syndrome may be regarded more accurately as a nonlysosomal connective tissue disease.[95]

Osteolysis with Detritic Synovitis. In 1978, Resnick and coworkers[105] described a new pattern of osteolysis in both the appendicular and the axial skeleton in a 71 year old woman without a family history of similar abnormalities. A severely destructive and mutilating arthropathy of the hands was associated with bone resorption of the phalanges, metacarpals, metatarsals, clavicles, tubular bones, and spine (Fig. 94–20). Pathologic examination documented the presence of superficial ulceration and necrosis of the synovium, fibrosis of deeper connective tissue, subsynovial fibrin deposition, focal areas of palisaded synovial cells, infrequent inflammatory cells, and numerous shards of necrotic bone embedded within fibrotic synovium and periarticular fibrous tissue. The radiographic characteristics resembled, in part, the findings of hyperparathyroidism; however, the absence of more classic features of subperiosteal and subchondral resorption, the presence of severe digital deformities, and the normal values for serum calcium, phosphorus, and parathyroid hormone levels made this latter diagnosis untenable.

Familial Expansile Osteolysis. In a series of articles, Wallace and coworkers[191–193] described an autosomal dominant bone disorder, beginning in childhood, adolescence, or early adulthood, that shared some clinical, radiologic, and histologic features with Paget's disease. Hearing loss represented an early clinical manifestation, sometimes becoming apparent before 5 years of age. Bone pain and dental

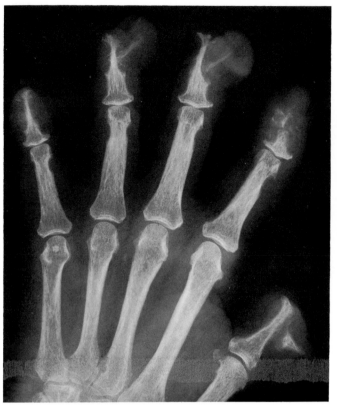

A

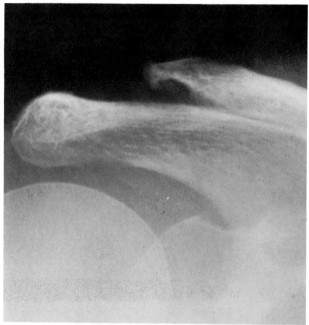

B

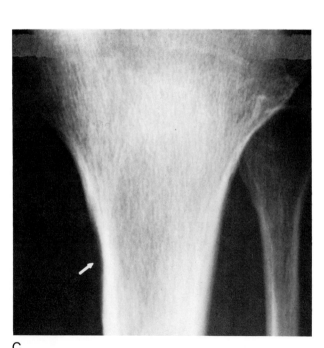

C

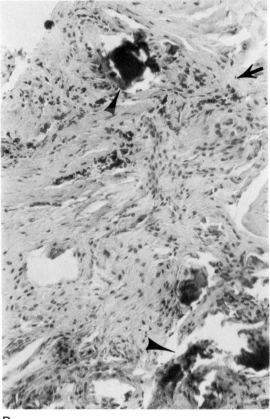

D

FIGURE 94–20. Osteolysis with detritic synovitis. A 71 year old woman developed a severely destructive and mutilating arthropathy of her hands. She had no pertinent family, occupational, or traumatic history.

A Note almost complete resorption of all terminal phalanges with proximal subluxation of the remaining bone, resorption along both radial and ulnar aspects of the phalanges and metacarpal bones, and articular spaces that appear unremarkable.

B Lysis of the distal end of the clavicle has produced a shortened and tapered osseous contour.

C Bony lysis of the medial aspect of the tibia (arrow) is identical to that which occurs in hyperparathyroidism.

D Biopsy specimen from an involved distal interphalangeal joint shows multiple bony fragments in the synovial and subsynovial tissue (arrowheads) and hemosiderin deposition (arrow) (160×).

(**A, B,** From Resnick D, et al: Arch Intern Med *138*:1003, 1978. Copyright 1978, American Medical Association.)

4482

manifestations, consisting of tooth mobility and fracture, also were observed. Radiographic abnormalities consisted of both generalized and focal changes. In the former category, disordered modeling and a coarsened trabecular pattern were evident, especially in the humerus, radius, ulna, and tibia. The trabecular changes included small radiolucent foci and were characterized as a "fishnet" appearance. Three grades of focal changes, all of which predominated in the appendicular skeleton, were identified: osteolytic lesions leading to cortical thinning and involving increasing portions of the bone, advancing with a flame-shaped osteolytic front; multiloculated and trabeculated osteolytic lesions producing bone expansion; and marked deformity and expansion of the bone with or without pathologic fractures. Histologic examination of bone biopsy specimens revealed a spectrum of findings, some resembling those of Paget's disease, including disorganized trabeculae, increased fibrous and vascular tissue, and, eventually, fatty replacement of medullary bone.

As these cases involved 42 members over five generations descended from a single North Ireland family, further reports are required to define this apparently new and disabling syndrome fully. Its radiographic features, although resembling fibrous dysplasia or Paget's disease, appear to be unique.

CHONDROLYSIS

Cartilage loss or destruction is an important complication of many articular disorders, including rheumatoid arthritis, seronegative spondyloarthropathies, septic arthritis, degenerative joint disease, and relapsing polychondritis (see Chapters 25 to 30, 32, and 39). In addition, cartilage atrophy can appear following disuse, immobilization, or paralysis, perhaps related to interruption of normal patterns of chondral nutrition (Fig. 94–21) (see Chapter 77). Finally, chondrolysis may appear as a complication of a slipped capital femoral epiphysis or on an idiopathic basis.

Chondrolysis Occurring After Slipped Capital Femoral Epiphysis

The association of chondrolysis with slipped capital femoral epiphysis was recognized first by Waldenström in 1930.[106] Subsequent reports are numerous,[107–115] and chondrolysis currently is recognized as a definite and important complication of slipping of the capital femoral epiphysis. Excellent reviews of the subject are provided in an article by Goldman and associates[116] and in one by Ingram and collaborators.[163]

The reported frequency of chondrolysis in association with slipped femoral capital epiphysis varies from approximately 1 per cent[110] to 40 per cent,[117] much of the variation being related to differences in patient selection and the clinical and radiographic criteria used for diagnosis. A high rate of occurrence is recorded in black, Hawaiian, and Hispanic patients.[108, 110, 113, 118] Both men and women are affected, and the frequency of chondrolysis in women is relatively high in view of the male predominance in cases of uncomplicated slipped epiphyses.[116] The age of the patient, the acuteness and extent of the epiphyseal separation, and the method of treatment probably are of minor importance in influencing the frequency of this complication, although chondrolysis may be more frequent in patients

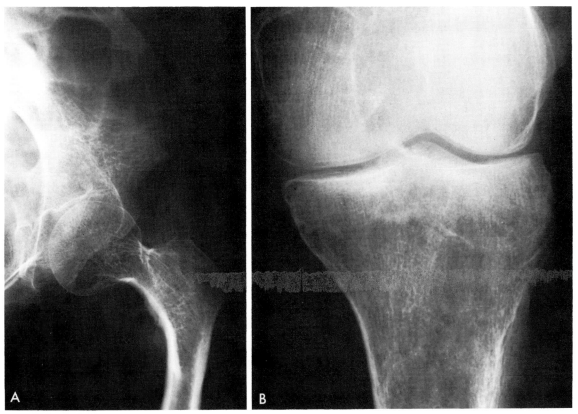

FIGURE 94–21. Cartilage atrophy. After paralysis **(A)** or disuse **(B),** cartilage atrophy can lead to diffuse loss of joint space.

treated by long-term immobilization or by surgical procedures other than in situ fixations. Ingram and associates[163]
described a decreased frequency of this complication in
mild or acute epiphyseal displacement.

Clinical manifestations of chondrolysis generally appear
within a year of the epiphyseal separation and, occasionally,
are observed simultaneously with the slipping itself. Pain,
tenderness, limitation of motion, and flexion contracture are
noted in the affected hip or, very rarely, in the hip that is
contralateral to that with the slipped capital femoral epiphysis. These findings may not allow precise or early diagnosis, as similar manifestations can accompany the slipping
process itself, the severity of the clinical abnormalities is
extremely variable, and additional complications of epiphyseal slipping may produce almost identical clinical alterations.[116] The diagnostic dilemma is accentuated further
by the absence of characteristic laboratory abnormalities.
Thus, correct interpretation of radiographic findings becomes important in establishing a specific diagnosis.

Goldman and coworkers[116] emphasized three radiographic features of chondrolysis (Fig. 94–22). Initially,
periarticular osteoporosis appears and may persist for variable amounts of time, probably reflecting the pathologically
evident increased vascularity of the subchondral osseous
tissue.[107, 109] The second finding is rapid narrowing of the
joint space that most typically affects the entire articulation
or is isolated to the superior aspect of the joint. Superior
joint space diminution is especially common when osteonecrosis also is present (7 to 25 per cent of cases)[109, 113] or
when osteotomies have been used in the treatment of the
epiphyseal slipping.[116] Third, thinning and disappearance of
the subchondral bone plate, osseous erosion, and flattening
can be seen, particularly at sites of chondral destruction,
about the fovea, and on both femoral and acetabular sur-

faces. Acetabular protrusion (which generally is mild), subchondral cysts (which usually are small or moderate in
size), and premature fusion of adjacent growth plates may
be apparent.

The radiographic findings appear in a relatively short
time and subsequently can stabilize, to be followed by
changes of cartilaginous and osseous repair characterized
by partial or complete "recovery" of the articular space,
bony eburnation or sclerosis, and osteophytosis. At other
times, especially in the presence of osteonecrosis, progressive deterioration of the joint is seen.

Pathologic alterations include thinning and pitting of the
articular cartilage of the acetabulum and femoral head, replacement of portions of the cartilaginous surface with fibrous tissue or fibrocartilage, and capsular thickening[108,
110, 119] (Fig. 94–23). The synovium initially undergoes proliferation with hypervascularity[116] and later is replaced by
fibrous tissue and a chronic inflammatory infiltrate.[107, 109, 163]

The cause and pathogenesis of chondrolysis in slipped
capital femoral epiphyses are not clear. The presence of
sparse synovial tissue has led to speculation that chondral
loss relates to poor cartilage nutrition from inadequate synovial fluid production,[106, 107] perhaps accentuated by prolonged immobilization that prevents appropriate diffusion
of nutrients into the cartilage. This theory is supported by
the similarity of the radiographic and pathologic findings to
those related to cartilage atrophy after extended periods of
inactivity and the occasional presence of chondrolysis of
both hips after bilateral immobilization for a unilateral
slipped capital epiphysis.[108, 120] Other investigators have emphasized the role of compromise of the subchondral vascular supply in the appearance of cartilage necrosis.[121–123] Evidence for this theory includes the occasional coexistence
of chondrolysis and osteonecrosis in the patient with a

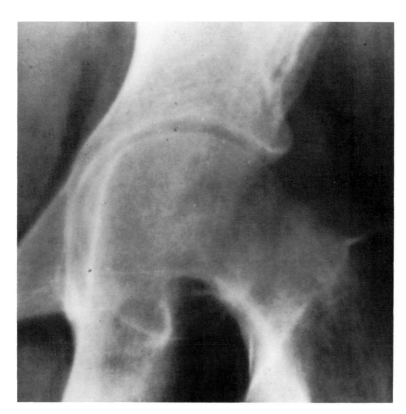

FIGURE 94–22. Chondrolysis after slipped femoral epiphysis: Radiographic abnormalities. Note osteoporosis, concentric joint space narrowing, protrusio
acetabuli deformity, and an abnormal alignment of the
femoral head and femoral neck.

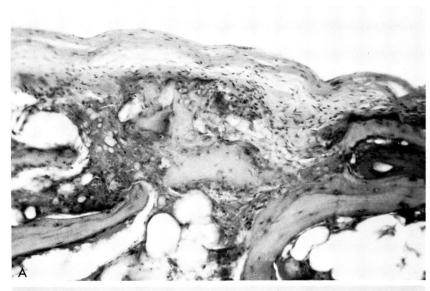

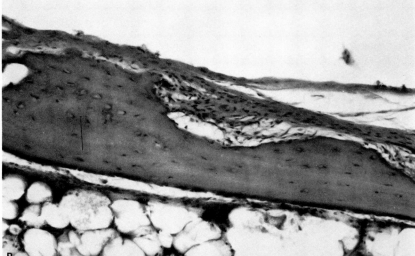

FIGURE 94–23. Chondrolysis after slipped capital femoral epiphysis: Pathologic abnormalities.

A Observe cartilage and subchondral bone erosions with an attempt at fibrous repair.

B In another photomicrograph, an attempt at fibrous repair in an area of cartilage erosion is seen.

(**A, B,** From Heppenstall RB, et al: Clin Orthop *103*:136, 1974.)

C, D A photograph and photomicrograph of a different femoral head indicate the severity of chondrolysis and subchondral bone erosion.

(**C, D,** Courtesy of R. B. Heppenstall, M.D., Philadelphia, Pennsylvania.)

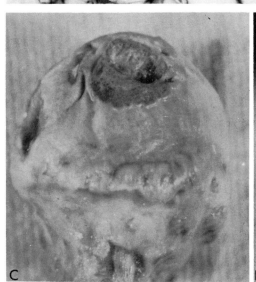

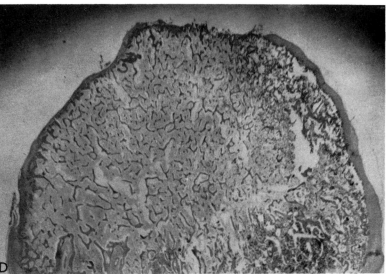

slipped capital femoral epiphysis and the appearance of similar cartilage loss accompanying osteonecrosis in patients without slipped capital femoral epiphyses.

Currently, it is believed that chondrolysis is a primary articular disorder distinct from osteonecrosis, although the basis for the cartilage loss has not been identified. In this regard, the study by Eisenstein and Rothschild is of interest.[115] These investigators noted biochemical abnormalities in patients with slipped capital femoral epiphyses, which included significant elevations in the serum levels of the immunoglobulins and C3 component of complement, the highest values being recorded for IgA, and with a greater elevation of the IgM fraction in those patients demonstrating chondrolysis. They suggested (1) that slipping of an epiphysis either produces an antigen that induces an autoimmune state or is a localized manifestation of a generalized process resembling a connective tissue disorder or inflammatory state; and (2) that a genetically determined subgroup of patients with slipped capital femoral epiphyses developed chondrolysis caused by the autoimmune-induced release of lysosomal enzymes and interference with synthetic processes of the articular cartilage.

The differential diagnosis of the radiographic features of chondrolysis accompanying slipped capital femoral epiphyses varies with the stage of the process.[116] Initially, the osteoporosis observed in chondrolysis is identical to that seen in various inflammatory synovial disorders, such as rheumatoid arthritis and infection, and in regional forms of osteoporosis, such as reflex sympathetic dystrophy, transient osteoporosis of the hip, and regional migratory osteoporosis. At this stage, aspiration of joint contents is mandatory to exclude the possibility of infection, and subsequent contrast opacification of the joint may be useful in confirming the presence of acute cartilage loss prior to diminution of the interosseous space. In the later stages of chondrolysis, loss of the articular space and subchondral osseous thinning and erosion simulate changes in infection, rheumatoid arthritis, and other inflammatory disorders but differ from the typical findings of reflex sympathetic dystrophy, regional migratory osteoporosis, and transient osteoporosis of the hip. The absence of systemic symptoms, of elevation of the erythrocyte sedimentation rate, and of leukocytosis in chondrolysis is a clinical clue that helps to exclude a septic process. In advanced stages of chondrolysis, differential diagnosis includes other disorders such as pigmented villonodular synovitis and idiopathic synovial (osteo)chondromatosis. At all stages, the history and clinical and radiographic manifestations of a slipped capital femoral epiphysis itself should serve as important indicators of the possible presence of chondrolysis to those physicians who are aware of this potential complication.

Idiopathic Chondrolysis of the Hip

The reports of Jones in 1971[124] and Moule and Golding in 1974[125] focused attention on the occurrence of chondrolysis of the hip joint in adolescent girls, particularly blacks, who did not have slipped capital femoral epiphyses. Sub-

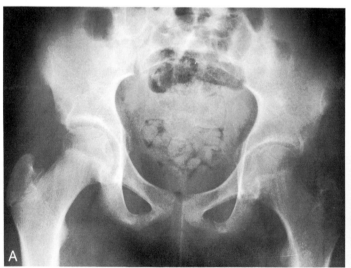
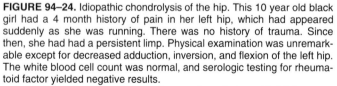
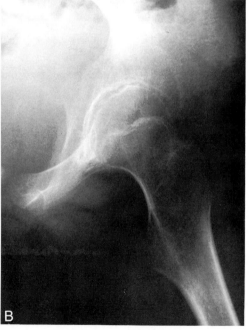

FIGURE 94–24. Idiopathic chondrolysis of the hip. This 10 year old black girl had a 4 month history of pain in her left hip, which had appeared suddenly as she was running. There was no history of trauma. Since then, she had had a persistent limp. Physical examination was unremarkable except for decreased adduction, inversion, and flexion of the left hip. The white blood cell count was normal, and serologic testing for rheumatoid factor yielded negative results.

A A radiograph demonstrates osteoporosis and symmetric joint space narrowing in the left hip. Conventional tomography confirmed the presence of these findings and revealed focal irregularity within the subchondral cortex of the capital femoral epiphysis. Aspiration arthrography demonstrated decreased thickness of the cartilage of both the acetabulum and the femoral head. Cultures of the joint fluid were sterile. The diagnosis at the time of this initial admission was synovitis of unknown cause. The patient was treated with restriction of weight-bearing and aspirin.

B Three months later, the patient was readmitted for evaluation of progressive loss of motion of the left hip. Radiograph at this time demonstrates a joint contracture with the hip held in external rotation. Progressive cartilage loss has occurred and diffuse osteoporosis persists. The findings are those of idiopathic chondrolysis of the hip.

(Courtesy of G. Greenway, M.D., Dallas, Texas.)

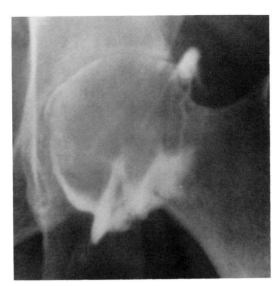

FIGURE 94–25. Idiopathic chondrolysis of the hip. In this teenage girl with clinical and radiographic manifestations of idiopathic chondrolysis, hip arthrography reveals diffuse loss of acetabular and femoral cartilage.

sequent investigators confirmed the presence of this entity, noting its occasional appearance not only in black female adolescents, but also in men, Hispanics, other whites, and Native Americans, and in persons over the age of 20 years.[126–128, 131, 138, 164, 165, 194] Monoarticular disease of the hip is typical, and clinical findings include pain, stiffness, restriction of motion, and the absence of a history of trauma. Radiographs outline periarticular osteoporosis, joint space narrowing that usually is diffuse or maximal on the weight-bearing surface, and irregularity and erosion of the subchondral bone (Fig. 94–24). In addition, slight enlargement and alteration in shape of the femoral head, an increase in width and periosteal bone formation of the femoral neck, narrowing of the growth plate, and mild protrusio acetabuli may be evident. The last-mentioned feature is reminiscent of that seen in primary protrusio acetabuli (Otto pelvis), and differentiating between the two conditions may be difficult.[165] Joint aspiration usually confirms the absence of an effusion or of organisms, and arthrography may demonstrate the irregularity and narrowing of the chondral surface (Fig. 94–25). Pathologic examination outlines changes in cartilage that are identical to those that occur in chondrolysis complicating slipped capital femoral epiphysis, including replacement of the deep layers of the articular cartilage, thinning of the superficial layers, and absence of widespread synovial inflammation. Some degree of villous formation, nodular lymphoid hyperplasia in the subsynovial areas, and perivascular infiltrates of lymphocytes, plasma cells, and monocytes may be noted. Fibrinoid necrosis and granulomas are not seen. The adjacent bone is osteoporotic, and cystic areas may be filled with synovium. Osteonecrosis also has been reported.[128]

Later stages of the process can be associated with obliteration of the articular space, cysts, osteophytes, and deformity.

Major alternatives in differential diagnosis include juvenile chronic arthritis and infection. Monoarticular involvement of the hip is somewhat unusual in juvenile chronic arthritis, although its clinical and radiologic features can

simulate those in idiopathic chondrolysis of the hip. Similarly, infection can lead to an identical radiographic picture, necessitating joint aspiration and culture of the fluid in all suspected cases of chondrolysis. Additional diagnostic considerations are transient osteoporosis of the hip, ischemic necrosis of the femoral head, primary protrusio acetabuli, and pigmented villonodular synovitis.

SUMMARY

A variety of disorders can lead to osteolysis and chondrolysis. In some, bone resorption is especially prominent in the phalanges of the hand and foot and may be related to occupational or inherited factors. Posttraumatic osteolysis can be evident at many sites, particularly the distal end of the clavicle, pubic and ischial rami, and femoral neck. Massive osteolysis of Gorham can lead to regional destruction and disappearance of bone. Idiopathic multicentric osteolysis shows a predilection for the carpal and tarsal areas and must be differentiated from juvenile chronic arthritis, Winchester's syndrome, and Farber's disease. Additional osteolysis syndromes include neurogenic acro-osteolysis, acro-osteolysis of Joseph or of Shinz, osteolysis with detritic synovitis, and familial expansile osteolysis. Chondrolysis of the hip can accompany a slipped capital femoral epiphysis or can appear on an idiopathic basis. It must be differentiated from juvenile chronic arthritis, infection, and regional osteoporosis.

References

1. Swezey RL, Bjarnason DM, Alexander SJ, et al: Resorptive arthropathy and the opera-glass hand syndrome. Semin Arthritis Rheum 2:1972–1973.
2. Harnasch H: Die Akroosteolysis ein neues Krankheitsbild. ROFO 72:352, 1950.
3. Suciu I, Drejman I, Valaskai M: Contributii la studiul imbolnavirilor produse de clorura de vinil. Med Interna 15:967, 1963.
4. Cordier JM, Fievez C, Lefevre MJ, et al: Acroosteolyse et lesides cutanées associées chez deux ouvriers affectes au nettoyage d'autodaves. Cah Med Travail 4:3, 1966.
5. Wilson RH, McCormick WE, Tatum CF, et al: Occupational acroosteolysis. Report of 31 cases. JAMA 201:577, 1967.
6. Markowitz SS, McDonald CJ, Fethiere W, et al: Occupational acroosteolysis. Arch Dermatol 106:219, 1972.
7. Dodson VN, Dinman BD, Whitehouse WM, et al: Occupational acroosteolysis. III. A clinical study. Arch Environ Health 22:83, 1971.
8. Harris DK, Adams WGF: Acro-osteolysis occurring in men engaged in the polymerization of vinyl chloride. Br Med J 3:712, 1967.
9. Stein G, Jühe S, Lange CE, et al: Bandförmige Osteolysen in den Endphalangen des Handskeletts. ROFO 118:60, 1973.
10. Gama C, Meira JBB: Occupational acro-osteolysis. J Bone Joint Surg [Am] 60:86, 1975.
11. Ross JA: An unusual occupational bone change. In AM Jelliffe, B Strickland (Eds): Symposium Ossium. Edinburgh, E & S Livingstone, 1970, p 321.
12. Kind R, Hornstein OP: Akroosteopathia ulcero-mutilans bei einem Kunststoffarbeiter. Dtsch Med Wochenschr 100:1001, 1975.
13. Bookstein JJ: Arteriography. In AK Poznanski (Ed): The Hand in Radiologic Diagnosis. Philadelphia, WB Saunders Co, 1974, p 75.
14. Murray IPC: Bone scanning in occupational acro-osteolysis. Skel Radiol 3:149, 1978.
15. Creech JL Jr, Johnson MN: Angiosarcoma of the liver in the manufacture of polyvinyl chloride. J Occup Med 16:150, 1974.
16. Strauch W: Posttraumatische Osteolysen des lateralen Klavikulaendes. Radiol Diagn 11:221, 1970.
17. Werder H: Posttraumatische Osteolyse des Schlüsselbeinendes. Schweiz Med Wochenschr 34:912, 1950.
18. Madsen B: Osteolysis of the acromial end of the clavicle following trauma. Br J Radiol 36:822, 1963.
19. Smart MJ: Traumatic osteolysis of the distal ends of the clavicles. J Can Assoc Radiol 23:264, 1972.
20. Jacobs P: Post-traumatic osteolysis of the outer end of the clavicle. J Bone Joint Surg [Br] 46:705, 1964.
21. Halaby FA, DiSalvo EI: Osteolysis: A complication of trauma. AJR 94:590, 1965.
22. Levine AH, Pais MJ, Schwartz EE: Posttraumatic osteolysis of the distal clavicle with emphasis on early radiologic changes. AJR 127:781, 1976.

23. Seymour EQ: Osteolysis of the clavicular tip associated with repeated minor trauma to the shoulder. Radiology 123:56, 1977.

24. Zsernaviczky J, Horst M: Kasuistischer Beitrag zur Osteolyse am distalen Klavikulaende. Arch Orthop Unfallchir 89:163, 1977.

25. Alnor P: Die posttraumatische Osteolyse des lateralen Claviculaendes. ROFO 75:364, 1951.

26. Hasselmann W: Die sog. posttraumatische Osteolyse des lateralen Claviculaendes. Monatsschr Unfallheilkd 58:242, 1955.

27. Ehricht HG: Die Osteolyse im lateralen Claviculaende nach Pressluftschaden. Arch Orthop Unfallchir 50:576, 1959.

28. Murphy OB, Bellamy R, Wheeler W, et al: Post-traumatic osteolysis of the distal clavicle. Clin Orthop 109:108, 1975.

29. Goergen TG, Resnick D, Riley RR: Post-traumatic abnormalities of the pubic bone simulating malignancy. Radiology 126:85, 1978.

30. Ackerman LV, Rosai J: Surgical Pathology. 5th Ed. St Louis, CV Mosby Co, 1974, p 1018.

31. Fischer E: Posttraumatische karpale Osteolysen nach isolierter Fraktur am distalen Radius. ROFO 112:541, 1970.

32. Elias AN, Pinals RS, Anderson HC, et al: Hereditary osteodysplasia with acroosteolysis (the Hajdu-Cheney syndrome). Am J Med 65:627, 1978.

33. Hajdu N, Kauntze R: Cranio-skeletal dysplasia. Br J Radiol 21:42, 1948.

34. Cheney WD: Acro-osteolysis. Am J Roentgenol 94:595, 1965.

35. Schulze R, Gulbin O: Beitrag zum Problem der Akroosteolyse (gleichzeitig ein Beitrag zur Kenntner der Patella profunda). ROFO 109:209, 1968.

36. Matisonn A, Ziady F: Familial acro-osteolysis. S Afr Med J 47:2060, 1973.

37. Harnasch H: Die Akroosteolysis, ein neues Krankheitsbild. ROFO 72:352, 1950.

38. Greenberg BE, Street DM: Idiopathic non-familial acro-osteolysis. Report of a case observed for five years. Radiology 69:259, 1957.

39. Papavasiliou CG, Gargano FP, Walls WL: Idiopathic nonfamilial acroosteolysis associated with other bone abnormalities. AJR 83:687, 1960.

40. Chawla S: Cranio-skeletal dysplasia with acro-osteolysis. Br J Radiol 37:702, 1964.

41. Dorst JP, McKusick VA: Acro-osteolysis (Cheney syndrome). Birth Defects 5(3):215, 1969.

42. Weleber RG, Beals RK: The Hajdu-Cheney syndrome. Report of two cases and review of the literature. J Pediatr 88:243, 1976.

43. Silverman FN, Dorst JP, Hajdu N: Acro-osteolysis (Hajdu-Cheney syndrome). Birth Defects 10:106, 1974.

44. Brown DM, Bradford DS, Gorlin RJ, et al: The acro-osteolysis syndrome: Morphologic and biochemical studies. J Pediatr 88:573, 1976.

45. Shaw DG: Acro-osteolysis and bone fragility. Br J Radiol 42:934, 1969.

46. Gilula LA, Bliznak J, Staple TW: Idiopathic nonfamilial acro-osteolysis with cortical defects and mandibular ramus osteolysis. Radiology 121:63, 1976.

47. Gorham LW, Wright AW, Shultz HH, et al: Disappearing bones: A rare form of massive osteolysis. Report of two cases, one with autopsy findings. Am J Med 17:674, 1954.

48. Gorham LW, Stout AP: Massive osteolysis (acute spontaneous absorption of bone, phantom bone, disappearing bone). J Bone Joint Surg [Am] 37:985, 1955.

49. Branch HE: Acute spontaneous absorption of bone. Report of a case involving a clavicle and a scapula. J Bone Joint Surg 27:706, 1945.

50. Dupas J, Baldelon P, Dayde G: Sur un cas d'ostéolyse progressive de la main gauche d'origine indéterminée. Rev Orthop 23:333, 1936.

51. Henderson MS: Acute atrophy of bone: Report of an unusual case involving the radius and ulna. Minn Med 19:214, 1936.

52. Simpson BS: An unusual case of post-traumatic decalcification of the bones of the foot. J Bone Joint Surg 19:223, 1937.

53. King DJ: A case resembling hemangiomatosis of the lower extremity. J Bone Joint Surg 28:623, 1946.

54. Leriche R: A propos des ostéolyses d'origine indéterminée. Mem Acad Chir 63:418, 1937.

55. Jackman WA: A case of spontaneous absorption of bone. Br J Surg 26:944, 1939.

56. Fornasier VL: Haemangiomatosis with massive osteolysis. J Bone Joint Surg [Br] 52:444, 1970.

57. Torg JS, Steel HH: Sequential roentgenographic changes occurring in massive osteolysis. J Bone Joint Surg [Am] 51:1649, 1969.

58. Kery L, Wouters HW: Massive osteolysis. Report of two cases. J Bone Joint Surg [Br] 52:452, 1970.

59. Thompson JS, Schuman DJ: Massive osteolysis. Case report and review of literature. Clin Orthop 103:206, 1974.

60. Imbert J-C, Picault C: Ostéolyse massive idiopathique ou maladie de Jackson-Gorham. Rev Chir Orthop 60:73, 1974.

61. Sage MR, Allen PW: Massive osteolysis. Report of a case. J Bone Joint Surg [Br] 56:130, 1974.

62. Iyer GV, Nayar A: Massive osteolysis of the skull. Case report. J Neurosurg 43:92, 1975.

63. Patrick JH: Massive osteolysis complicated by chylothorax successfully treated by pleurodesis. J Bone Joint Surg [Br] 58:347, 1976.

64. Heyden G, Kindblom L-G, Nielsen JM: Disappearing bone disease. A clinical and histological study. J Bone Joint Surg [Am] 59:57, 1977.

65. Campbell J, Almond HGA, Johnson R: Massive osteolysis of the humerus with spontaneous recovery. Report of a case. J Bone Joint Surg [Br] 57:238, 1975.

66. Halliday DR, Dahlin DC, Pugh DG, et al: Massive osteolysis and angiomatosis. Radiology 82:637, 1964.

67. Hambach R, Pujman J, Maly V: Massive osteolysis due to hemangiomatosis. Report of a case of Gorham's disease with autopsy. Radiology 71:43, 1958.

68. Heuck F: Case report 78. Skel Radiol 3:241, 1979.

69. Cadenat H, Combelles R, Fabert G, et al: Ostéolyse cryptogénétique de la mandibule. J Radiol Electrol Med Nucl 59:509, 1978.

70. Graham DY, Gonzales J, Kothari SM: Diffuse skeletal angiomatosis. Skel Radiol 2:131, 1978.

71. Schajowicz F, Aiello CL, Francone MV, et al: Cystic angiomatosis (hamartous haemolymphangiomatosis) of bone. A clinicopathological study of three cases. J Bone Joint Surg [Br] 60:100, 1978.

72. Rosenquist CJ, Wolfe DC: Lymphangioma of bone. J Bone Joint Surg [Am] 50:158, 1968.

73. Boyle WJ: Cystic angiomatosis of bone. A report of three cases and review of the literature. J Bone Joint Surg [Br] 54:626, 1972.

74. Singh R, Grewal DS, Bannerjee AK, et al: Haemangiomatosis of the skeleton. Report of a case. J Bone Joint Surg [Br] 56:136, 1974.

75. Brower AC, Culver JE Jr, Keats TE: Diffuse cystic angiomatosis of bone. Report of two cases. AJR 118:456, 1973.

76. Tyler T, Rosenbaum HD: Idiopathic multicentric osteolysis. AJR 126:23, 1976.

77. Derot M, Rathery M, Rosselin G, et al: Acroosteolyse du carpe, pied creus, scoliose et strabisme chez une jeune fille atteinte d'une insuffisance rénale. Bull Mem Soc Med Hôp Paris 77:223, 1961.

78. MacPherson RI, Walker RD, Kowall MH: Essential osteolysis with nephropathy. J Can Assoc Radiol 24:98, 1973.

79. Torg JS, Steel HH: Essential osteolysis with nephropathy. A review of the literature and case report of an unusual syndrome. J Bone Joint Surg [Am] 50:1629, 1968.

80. Mahoudeau D, Dubrisay J, Elissalde B, et al: Ostéolyse essentielle et néphrite. Bull Mem Soc Med Hop Paris 77:229, 1961.

81. Lagier R, Rutishauser E: Osteoarticular changes in a case of essential osteolysis. J Bone Joint Surg [Br] 47:339, 1965.

82. Marie J, Lévêque B, Lyon G, et al: Acro-ostéolyse essentielle compliquée d'insuffisance rénal d'évolution fatale. Presse Med 71:249, 1963.

83. Marie J, Salet J, Lévêque B: Polydystrophies sequelettiques avec ostéolyse progressive. Arch Fr Pediatr 8:752, 1951.

84. Marie J, Salet J, Lévêque B, et al: Syndrome ostéodystrophique de nature congénitale probable. Presse Med 64:2173, 1956.

85. Whyte MP, Murphy WA, Kleerekoper M, et al: Idiopathic multicentric osteolysis. Report of an affected father and son. Arthritis Rheum 21:367, 1978.

86. Thieffry S, Sorrel-Dejerine J: D'ostéolyse essentielle héréditaire et familiale. Presse Med 66:1858, 1958.

87. Kohler E, Babbit D, Huizenga B, et al: Hereditary osteolysis: A clinical, radiological and chemical study. Radiology 108:99, 1973.

88. Torg JS, DiGeorge AM, Kirkpatrick JA Jr, et al: Hereditary multicentric osteolysis with recessive transmission: A new syndrome. J Pediatr 75:243, 1969.

89. Coleman SS, Litton RJ, Christensen WR: Familial dysostosis carpi. J Bone Joint Surg [Am] 47:850, 1965.

90. Gluck J, Miller JJ: Familial osteolysis of the carpal and tarsal bones. J Pediatr 81:506, 1972.

91. Amin PH, Evans ANW: Essential osteolysis of carpal and tarsal bones. Br J Radiol 51:539, 1978.

92. Beals RK, Bird CB: Carpal and tarsal osteolysis. Birth Defects 11:107, 1973.

93. Shurtleff DB, Sparkes RS, Clawson DK, et al: Hereditary osteolysis with hypertension and nephropathy. JAMA 188:363, 1964.

94. Erickson CM, Hirschberger M, Stickler GB: Carpal-tarsal osteolysis. J Pediatr 93:779, 1978.

95. Beals RK, Bird CB: Carpal and tarsal osteolysis. A case report and review of the literature. J Bone Joint Surg [Am] 57:681, 1975.

96. McKusick VA: Mendelian Inheritance in Man, 3rd Ed. Baltimore, Johns Hopkins University Press, 1971.

97. Thévenard MA: L'acropathie ulcéro-mutilante familiale. Acta Neurol Psychiatr Belg 53:1, 1953.

98. Thévenard MA: L'acropathie ulcéro-multilante familiale. Rev Neurol 74:193, 1942.

99. Kozlowski K, Hanicka M, Garapich M: Neurogene ulcerierende Akropathie (Akroosteolyse-Syndrom). Monatsschr Kinderheilkd 119:169, 1971.

100. White AA III: Disappearing bone disease with arthropathy and severe scarring of the skin. A report of four cases seen in South Vietnam. J Bone Joint Surg [Br] 53:303, 1971.

101. Joseph R, Nézelof C, Guéraud L, et al: Acro-ostéolyse idiopathique familiale; renseignements fournis par la biopsie. Sem Hôp Paris 35:622, 1959.

102. Shinz HR: Roentgen-Diagnostics. New York, Grune & Stratton, 1951, Vol 1, p 734.

103. Bierman SM, Edgington T, Newcomer VD, et al: Farber's disease: A disorder of mucopolysaccharide metabolism with articular, respiratory, and neurologic manifestations. Arthritis Rheum 9:620, 1966.

104. Winchester P, Grossman H, Lim WN, et al: A new acid mucopolysaccharidosis with skeletal deformities simulating rheumatoid arthritis. AJR 106:121, 1969.

105. Resnick D, Weisman M, Goergen TG, et al: Osteolysis with detritic synovitis. A new syndrome. Arch Intern Med 138:1003, 1978.

106. Waldenström H: On necrosis of the joint cartilage by epiphyseolysis capitis femoris. Acta Chir Scand 67:936, 1930.

107. Cruess RL: The pathology of acute necrosis of cartilage in slipping of the capital femoral epiphysis. A report of two cases with pathological sections. J Bone Joint Surg [Am] 45:1013, 1963.

108. Lowe HG: Necrosis of the articular cartilage after slipping of the capital femoral epiphysis. Report of six cases with recovery. J Bone Joint Surg [Br] 52:108, 1970.

109. Heppenstall RM, Marvel JP Jr, Chung SMK, et al: Chondrolysis of the hip. Clin Orthop 103:136, 1974.

110. Tillema DA, Golding JSR: Chondrolysis following slipped capital femoral epiphysis in Jamaica. J Bone Joint Surg [Am] 53:1528, 1971.

111. El-Khoury GY, Mickelson MR: Chondrolysis following slipped capital femoral epiphysis. Radiology 123:327, 1977.

112. Ogden JA, Simon TR, Southwick WO: Cartilage space width in slipped capital femoral epiphysis: The relationship to cartilage necrosis. Yale J Biol Med 50:17, 1977.

113. Mauer RC, Larsen IJ: Acute necrosis of cartilage in slipped capital femoral epiphysis. J Bone Joint Surg [Am] 52:39, 1970.

114. Frymoyer JW: Chondrolysis of the hip following Southwick osteotomy for severe slipped capital femoral epiphysis. Clin Orthop 99:120, 1974.

115. Eisenstein A, Rothschild S: Biochemical abnormalities in patients with slipped capital femoral epiphysis and chondrolysis. J Bone Joint Surg [Am] 58:459, 1976.

116. Goldman AB, Schneider R, Martel W: Acute chondrolysis complicating slipped capital femoral epiphysis. AJR 130:945, 1978.

117. Wiberg G: Considerations on surgical treatment of slipped epiphysis with special reference to nail fixation. J Bone Joint Surg [Am] 41:253, 1959.

118. Orofino C, Innis JJ, Lowrey CW: Slipped capital femoral epiphysis in Negroes. A study of ninety-five cases. J Bone Joint Surg [Am] 42:1079, 1960.

119. Ponseti I, Barta CK: Evaluation of treatment of slipping of the capital femoral epiphysis. Surg Gynecol Obstet 86:87, 1948.

120. Jerre T: A study in slipped upper femoral epiphysis. With special reference to the late functional and roentgenological results and to the value of closed reduction. Acta Orthop Scand Suppl 6:1, 1950.

121. Hall JE: The results of treatment of slipped femoral epiphysis. J Bone Joint Surg [Br] 39:659, 1957.

122. Wilson PD: Discussion. Roentgenographic changes in nailed slipped epiphysis. J Bone Joint Surg [Am] 31:21, 1949.

123. Moore RD: Conservative management of adolescent slipping of the capital femoral epiphysis. Surg Gynecol Obstet 80:324, 1945.

124. Jones BS: Adolescent chondrolysis of the hip joint. S Afr Med J 45:196, 1971.

125. Moule NJ, Golding JSR: Idiopathic chondrolysis of the hip. Clin Radiol 25:247, 1974.

126. Wenger DR, Mickelson MR, Ponseti IV: Idiopathic chondrolysis of the hip. Report of two cases. J Bone Joint Surg [Am] 57:268, 1975.

127. Duncan JW, Schrantz JL, Nasca RJ: The bizarre stiff hip. Possible idiopathic chondrolysis. JAMA 231:382, 1975.

128. Sivanantham M, Kutty MK: Idiopathic chondrolysis of the hip: Case report with a review of the literature. Aust NZ J Surg 47:229, 1977.

129. Kozlowski K, Barylak A, Eftekhari F, et al: Acroosteolysis. Problems of diagnosis—report of four cases. Pediatr Radiol 8:79, 1979.

130. Bauer F, Lagier R, Wettstein P, et al: Anatomo-radiological study of a case of post-radiotherapeutic osteolysis of the hip. Strahlentherapie 155:396, 1979.

131. Duncan JW, Nasca R, Schrantz J: Idiopathic chondrolysis of the hip. J Bone Joint Surg [Am] 61:1024, 1979.

132. Roback DL: Posttraumatic osteolysis of the femoral neck. AJR 134:1243, 1980.

133. Fielding JW, Hensinger RN, Hawkins RJ: Os odontoideum. J Bone Joint Surg [Am] 62:376, 1980.

134. Hukuda S, Ota H, Okabe N, et al: Traumatic atlantoaxial dislocation causing os odontoideum in infants. Spine 5:207, 1980.

135. Iwaya T, Taniguchi K, Watanabe J, et al: Hajdu-Cheney syndrome. Arch Orthop Trauma Surg 95:293, 1979.

136. Binns CHB: Vinyl chloride: A review. J Soc Occup Med 29:134, 1979.

137. Koischwitz D, Marsteller HJ, Lackner K, et al: Veränderungen der Hand- und Fingerarterien bei der Vinylchloridkrankheit. ROFO 132:62, 1980.

138. Herman JH, Herzig EB, Crissman JD, et al: Idiopathic chondrolysis-an immunopathologic study. J Rheumatol 7:694, 1980.

139. Newberg AH, Howe JG: Posttraumatic osteolysis vs. fracture. AJR 135:1317, 1980.

140. Abrahams J, Ganick D, Gilbert E, et al: Massive osteolysis in an infant. AJR 135:1084, 1980.

141. Destouet JM, Murphy WA: Acquired acroosteolysis and acronecrosis. Arthritis Rheum 26:1150, 1983.

142. Falappa P, Magnavita N, Bergamaschi A, et al: Angiographic study of digital arteries in workers exposed to vinyl chloride. Br J Ind Med 39:169, 1982.

143. Grainger RG, Walker AE, Ward AM: Vinyl chloride monomer-induced disease: Clinical, radiological and immunological aspects. In L Preger, RE Steiner (Eds): Induced Disease: Drug, Irradiation, Occupation. New York, Grune & Stratton, 1980, p 191.

144. Joseph B, Chacko V: Acro-osteolysis associated with hypertrophic pulmonary osteoarthropathy and pachydermoperiostosis. Radiology 154:343, 1985.

145. Fernbach SK, Poznanski AK: Case report 231. Skel Radiol 10:43, 1983.

146. Quinn SF, Glass TA: Posttraumatic osteolysis of the clavicle. South Med J 76:307, 1983.

147. Cahill BR: Osteolysis of the distal part of the clavicle in male athletes. J Bone Joint Surg [Am] 64:1053, 1982.

148. Cahill BR: Correspondence. J Bone Joint Surg [Am] 65:421, 1983.

149. Bannwarth B, Asch L, Vogt JC, et al: Osteolyse post-traumatique de la clavicule. Rev Rhum Mal Osteoartic 49:643, 1982.

150. Hall FM, Goldberg RP, Kasdon EJ, et al: Post-traumatic osteolysis of the pubic bone simulating a malignant lesion. J Bone Joint Surg [Am] 66:121, 1984.

151. Hall FM: Post-traumatic pubic osteolysis simulating malignancy. J Bone Joint Surg [Am] 66:975, 1984.

152. McGuigan LE, Edmonds JP, Painter DM: Pubic osteolysis. J Bone Joint Surg [Am] 66:127, 1984.

153. Casey D, Mirra J, Staple TW: Parasymphyseal insufficiency fractures of the os pubis. AJR 142:581, 1984.

154. Cazalis P: Acro-osteolyse de la main. Ann Radiol 25:337, 1982.

155. Velchik MG: Acro-osteolysis in a patient with Hajdu-Cheney syndrome demonstrated by bone scintigraphy. Clin Nucl Med 9:659, 1984.

156. Lotz W, Ebert M, Fasske E: Die massive Osteolyse (Gorham-Stout-syndrom) mit lokaler Neurofibromatose. ROFO 137:55, 1982.

157. Hemingway AP, Leung A, Lavender JP: Familial vanishing limbs: Four generations of idiopathic multicentric osteolysis. Clin Radiol 34:585, 1983.

158. Sauvegrain J, Gaussin G, Blondet P, et al: Osteolyse multicentrique à transmission recessive. Quatre cas dans une nouvelle famille. Ann Radiol 24:638, 1981.

159. Tookman AG, Paice EW, White AG: Idiopathic multicentric osteolysis with acro-osteolysis. A case report. J Bone Joint Surg [Br] 67:86, 1985.

160. Renie WA, Pyeritz RE: Idiopathic multicentric osteolysis in a 78-year-old woman. Johns Hopkins Med J 148:165, 1971.

161. Lemaitre L, Remy J, Smith M, et al: Carpal and tarsal osteolysis. Pediatr Radiol 13:219, 1983.

162. Hardegger F, Simpson LA, Segmueller G: The syndrome of idiopathic osteolysis. Classification, review, and case report. J Bone Joint Surg [Br] 67:89, 1985.

163. Ingram AJ, Clarke MS, Clark CS Jr, et al: Chondrolysis complicating slipped capital femoral epiphysis. Clin Orthop 165:99, 1982.

164. Bleck EE: Idiopathic chondrolysis of the hip. J Bone Joint Surg [Am] 65:1266, 1983.

165. Hughes AW: Idiopathic chondrolysis of the hip: A case report and review of the literature. Ann Rheum Dis 44:268, 1985.

166. Hanly JG, Walsh NM, Breshihan B: Massive osteolysis in the hand and response to radiotherapy. J Rheumatol 12:580, 1985.

167. Tuncbilek E, Besim A, Bakkaloglu A, et al: Carpal-tarsal osteolysis. Pediatr Radiol 15:255, 1985.

168. Oteishat WA, Whitehouse GH, Hawass N-E-D: Acro-osteolysis following snake and scorpion envenomation. Br J Radiol 58:1035, 1985.

169. Kaplan PA, Resnick D: Stress-induced osteolysis of the clavicle. Radiology 158:139, 1986.

170. Jaffrès R, LeGoff P: Ostéolyse post-traumatique de l'os du pubis simulant une lesion maligne. Rev Rhum Mal Osteoartic 53:261, 1986.

171. Cannon SR: Massive osteolysis. A review of seven cases. J Bone Joint Surg [Br] 68:24, 1986.

172. Udell J, Schumacher HR Jr, Kaplan F, et al: Idiopathic familial acroosteolysis: Histomorphometric study of bone and literature review of the Hajdu-Cheney syndrome. Arthritis Rheum 29:1032, 1986.

173. Vichi GF, Falcini F, Pierattelli M, et al: Case report 401. Skel Radiol 15:665, 1986.

174. Rault R, Carpenter B: Pseudoclubbing in chronic renal failure. Q J Med 271:1063, 1989.

175. Wu AC, Gilula LA: Distal phalangeal brachydactyly secondary to healed renal osteodystrophy. Skel Radiol 16:312, 1987.

176. Duke RA, Barrett MR, Salazar JE, et al: Acro-osteolysis secondary to pityriasis rubra pilaris. AJR 149:1082, 1987.

177. Scavenius M, Iversen BF, Stürup J: Resection of the lateral end of the clavicle following osteolysis, with emphasis on non-traumatic osteolysis of the acromial end of the clavicle in athletes. Injury 18:261, 1987.

178. Ghezail M, Leroux JL, Chertok P, et al: Pubic post-fracture osteolysis simulating a malignancy. Clin Exp Rheumatol 9:635, 1991.

179. Hornig GW, Beatty RM: Osteolytic skull lesions secondary to trauma. Report of two cases. J Neurosurg 72:506, 1990.

180. Eyres KS, McCloskey EV, Fern ED, et al: Hajdu-Cheney syndrome: A report of two cases. J Orthop Rheumatol 5:163, 1992.

181. Kawamura J, Matsubayashi K, Ogawa M: Hajdu-Cheney syndrome. Report of a non-familial case. Neuroradiology 21:295, 1981.

182. Kawamura J, Miki Y, Yamazaki S, et al: Hajdu-Cheney syndrome: MR imaging. Neuroradiology 33:441, 1991.

183. Herscovici D Jr, Bowen JR, Scott CI Jr: Cervical instability as an unusual manifestation of Hajdu-Cheney syndrome of acroosteolysis. Clin Orthop 255:111, 1990.

184. Carneiro RDS, Steglich V: "Disappearing bone disease" in the hand. J Hand Surg [Am] 12:629, 1987.

185. Turra S, Gigante C, Scapinelli R: A 20-year follow-up study of a case of surgically treated massive osteolysis. Clin Orthop 250:297, 1990.

186. Friedman L, Horwitz T, Beck M, et al: Case report 672. Skel Radiol 20:307, 1991.

187. Pastakia B, Horvath K, Lack EF: Seventeen year follow-up and autopsy findings in a case of massive osteolysis. Skel Radiol 16:291, 1987.

188. Ikegawa S, Hoshikawa Y, Doi M: Idiopathic acro-osteolysis in an elderly woman. Arch Orthop Trauma Surg 111:181, 1992.

189. Kozlowski K, Bacha L, Brachimi L, et al: Multicentric/massive idiopathic osteolysis in a 17-year-old girl. Pediatr Radiol 21:48, 1990.

190. Warady BA, Haug SJ, Lindsley CB: Multicentric osteolysis: An infrequently recognized renal-rheumatologic syndrome. J Rheumatol 18:142, 1991.

191. Wallace RGH, Barr RJ, Osterberg PH, et al: Familial expansile osteolysis. Clin Orthop *248*:265, 1989.
192. Osterberg PH, Wallace RGH, Adams DA, et al: Familial expansile osteolysis. A new dysplasia. J Bone Joint Surg [Br] *70*:255, 1988.
193. Crone MD, Wallace RGH: The radiographic features of familial expansile osteolysis. Skel Radiol *19*:245, 1990.
194. van der Hoeven H, Keessen W, Kuis W: Idiopathic chondrolysis of the hip. A distinct clinical entity? Acta Orthop Scand *60*:661, 1989.
195. Jeandel P, Garbe L, Dischino M, et al: Ostéolyse post-traumatique de l'extremité distale de la clavicule. Etude anatomopathologique de deux observations. Rev Rhum Mal Osteoartic *59*:207, 1992.
196. Matthews LS, Simonson BG, Wolock BS: Osteolysis of the distal clavicle in a female body builder. A case report. Am J Sports Med *21*:150, 1993.

95

Soft Tissues

Donald Resnick, M.D., and Gen Niwayama, M.D.

Both localized and generalized processes can affect the soft tissues. In this chapter, a generalized radiographic approach to the differential diagnosis of such abnormalities is presented. Although note is made of changes accompanying some of the traumatic, infectious, and rheumatologic disorders that are discussed elsewhere in the book, the interested reader should refer to the appropriate sections for more detailed discussion. Instead, additional entities are included that are important to physicians engaged in the diagnosis and treatment of musculoskeletal diseases. By design, the analysis is direct and abbreviated, as a complete discussion of the multitude of soft tissue processes is beyond the scope of this textbook.

There is no uniformly accepted definition of soft tissue. A broad definition could include the epithelium, fibrous tissue, fat, and voluntary muscles with inclusion also of the vessels and nerves that supply these structures. Abnormalities of the skin are much more amenable to clinical than radiologic examination and are the subject of an entire medical subspecialty, dermatology. Conversely, processes of the subcutaneous and muscular tissues frequently are better evaluated by radiography and related techniques than by palpation, percussion, or auscultation. Routine radiographic manifestations of such processes may include mass formation, alteration in radiodensity, including exaggerated lucency, calcification and ossification, and resorption and contracture. In some instances, the constellation of findings is adequate for accurate diagnosis, although more typically supplementary methods such as CT and MR imaging are employed to further delineate the nature and extent of the process.

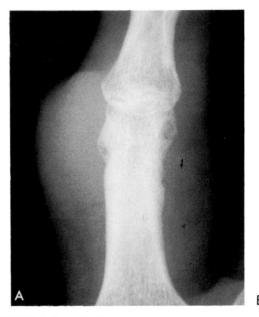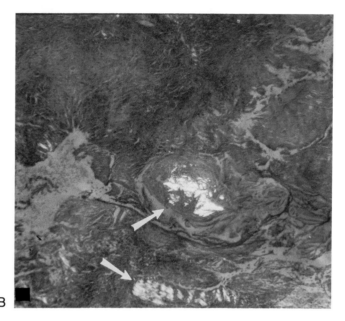

FIGURE 95–1. Gouty tophi.
   A A bulky mass about the proximal phalanx and proximal interphalangeal joint represents a tophus. Observe subjacent osseous erosion and flexion of the digit.
   B Polarized photomicrograph (250×) indicates urate crystal deposition (arrows) in a nodular fibrous lesion of the synovial tissue.

SOFT TISSUE MASSES

Available Diagnostic Techniques

The causes of soft tissue masses are diverse. Only a partial list would include the following: normal variations such as accessory muscles; primary and secondary neoplasms; articular diseases leading to tophi (gout) (Fig. 95– 1), nodules (rheumatoid arthritis), xanthomas (Fig. 95–2), and synovial cysts; collagen, metabolic, and endocrine disorders producing calcific collections (scleroderma, dermatomyositis, mixed connective tissue disease, hyperparathyroidism, renal osteodystrophy, hypervitaminosis D, milk-alkali syndrome); neurologic and traumatic conditions causing ossification (paralysis, immobilization, thermal burns); infections with abscess formation; hematomas;

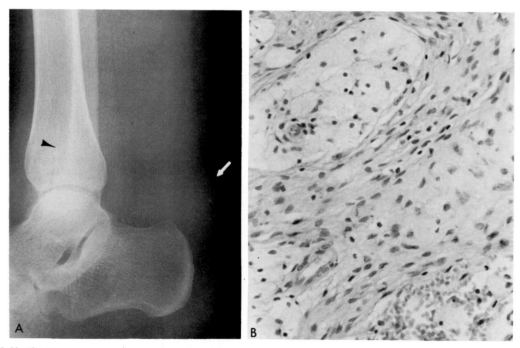

FIGURE 95–2. Xanthoma.
   A Observe xanthomatous infiltration in and around the Achilles tendon, producing lobulated soft tissue swelling (arrow). The anterior aspect of the distal fibula is eroded (arrowhead).
   B The photomicrograph (100×) demonstrates the typical appearance of a xanthoma.

aneurysms; foreign bodies; bursitis (Fig. 95–3) and tendinitis (Fig. 95–4); and hyperostotic processes of bone. In many instances, local or distant clinical findings provide important clues in the differential diagnosis of the various processes. In the discussion that follows, emphasis is given to some of the neoplasms and pseudoneoplastic processes of the soft tissues that can lead to a mass.

Routine Radiography and Related Techniques. The limitations of routine radiography in the assessment of soft tissue masses must be appreciated fully. Owing to its limited contrast resolution, this method is not ideally suited to sort out soft tissue processes. Although with proper technique, fat can be differentiated from muscle and other connective tissues, distinguishing among these soft tissues and between them and a soft tissue mass is poorly accomplished with conventional radiography. It frequently is necessary to alter the radiographic technique to maximize the information on the soft tissues that is obtained from the roentgenogram. Low kilovoltage (below 50 kVp), by exaggerating the differences in radiographic density of fat and muscle,[1] can be useful (see Chapter 5), although the adjacent osseous tissue is poorly evaluated with this technique. A fine-grain x-ray film is essential for anatomic detail,[2] and the use of a small focal spot x-ray tube allows radiographic magnification (see Chapter 4). These procedures increase local radiation exposure but may be justified in some cases because of the additional data supplied.

Considering the large number of soft tissue neoplasms that may be encountered, it is not surprising that the accurate preoperative radiographic diagnosis of the type of tu-

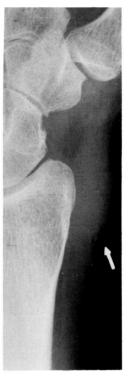

FIGURE 95–4. De Quervain's tenosynovitis. In this patient, localized soft tissue swelling adjacent to the radial styloid process (arrow) is a result of tenosynovitis. (Courtesy of J. Weston, M.D., Lower Hutt, New Zealand.)

mor frequently is difficult or impossible to accomplish. More feasible and more important, assessment of radiographic criteria may allow differentiation of a neoplastic from a non-neoplastic disorder, and a benign from a malignant process[2] (Table 95–1). This differentiation not always is possible, however, even using certain roentgenographic characteristics, and an accurate diagnosis must frequently await evaluation by the pathologist.

Tumor Size and Rate of Growth. The actual size of a mass provides little information about its nature. Although there is a tendency for malignant tumors to be larger than benign ones,[310, 331] benign processes may be large and malignant processes may be small. More significantly, serial or comparison films will allow assessment of the rate of growth. Very rapid enlargement of a mass can indicate hemorrhage, inflammation, or perhaps a malignant neoplasm but is not characteristic of a benign tumor. Conversely, absent or slow growth is typical of benign neoplasm.

Tumor Shape. As with tumor size, the amount of diagnostic information provided by the shape of the lesion is limited. Round masses more frequently are benign, whereas irregularly shaped masses are more commonly malignant.[310]

Tumor Location and Number. Some of the characteristic locations of certain tumors are indicated later in this chapter. Examples include the predilection of specific fibromatoses to involve the hands and the feet, of elastofibromas and desmoid tumors to appear about the shoulder, of xanthomatoses to affect tendons about the hands, elbows, and heels, and of synovial sarcomas to appear in the thighs or lower extremities. Non-neoplastic processes also have typical locations, such as the popliteal regions for synovial

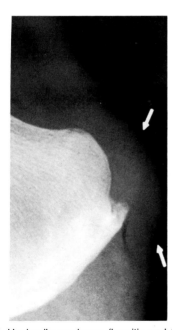

FIGURE 95–3. Haglund's syndrome (bursitis and tendonitis). Observe the soft tissue prominence (arrows) near the attachment of the Achilles tendon to the calcaneus, loss of the sharp interface between the Achilles tendon and the preachilles fat pad, and obscuration of the retrocalcaneal recess (the normal radiolucent area that exists between the Achilles tendon and the top of the calcaneus). This syndrome leads to pain in the posterior region of the heel and a "pump bump" and is characterized by retrocalcaneal bursitis. Achilles tendinitis, a superficial tendo Achilles bursitis, and a prominent bursal projection on the posterosuperior aspect of the calcaneus. (From Pavlov H. et al: Radiology *144*:83, 1982.)

TABLE 95–1. Radiographic Characteristics of Benign and Malignant Soft Tissue Tumors

	Benign Tumor	Malignant Tumor
Size	Variable	Variable
Rate of growth	Slow	Rapid*
Number	Single or multiple†	Single or multiple‡
Radiodensity	Vary from lucent (lipoma) to soft tissue density	Soft tissue density
Calcification or ossification	Possible§	Possible||
Tumor interface	Sharply demarcated	Poorly or sharply demarcated¶
Osseous involvement	Smooth pressure erosion with or without sclerosis	Smooth pressure erosion without sclerosis; cortical osteolysis due to hyperemia; cortical invasion

*Rapid growth can also indicate hemorrhage or infection.
†Examples of multiple lesions are lipomas, fibromas, hemangiomas, neurogenic tumors.
‡Examples of multiple lesions are metastases, Kaposi's sarcomas.
§Examples of calcifying tumors are hemangiomas, xanthomas, myxomas, lipomas, pilomatrixomas, chondromas.
\|\|Examples of calcifying or ossifying tumors are synovial sarcomas, rhabdomyosarcomas, malignant histiocytomas, chondrosarcomas, osteosarcomas.
¶Infection can also produce indistinctness of mass outline.

cysts. Deep masses more typically are malignant in nature.[331]

Certain masses frequently are multiple, including neurofibromas and other neurogenic tumors, Kaposi's sarcomas, lipomas, and even metastases.[2] Furthermore, multiple soft tissue masses appearing near a primary soft tissue neoplasm may indicate lymph node metastases, an obvious sign of tumor aggressiveness. Most soft tissue sarcomas disseminate via the hematogenous route, although metastasis to regional lymph nodes is not infrequent, especially in cases of alveolar rhabdomyosarcoma, clear cell sarcoma, epithelioid sarcoma, and angiosarcoma.[330]

Tumor Radiodensity. Lipomas produce radiolucent masses that frequently are well demarcated from the surrounding soft tissues (Fig. 95–5). Liposarcomas are less radiolucent and, when poorly differentiated, may contain few if any lucent zones. Most of the other soft tissue neoplasms are of approximately the same radiodensity as the adjacent tissue unless they contain zones of calcification or ossification. The precise density of any such neoplasm is better delineated with CT than with conventional radiography. Measurement of the attenuation values of a soft tissue tumor both before and after the intravenous administration of contrast material provides information regarding its homogeneity and vascularity, but, in most cases, a specific histologic diagnosis is not possible.

Tumor Calcification or Ossification. Calcification may appear in benign or malignant neoplasms as well as in nonneoplastic masses. Of the benign neoplasms, hemangiomas may reveal typical circular calcifications with lucent centers (phleboliths) (Fig. 95–6), whereas other tumors may be associated with sharply circumscribed peripheral calcific collections (e.g., myxoma, xanthoma, hamartoma, lipoma)[114] or with small or large foci of sandlike calcification (pilomatrixoma). Malignant neoplasms can lead to necrosis and hemorrhage, with secondary calcification that appears as irregular, faint amorphous zones of increased density on roentgenograms.[2] Such deposits are seen in synovial sarcomas,[101, 104] malignant histiocytomas,[115] and rhabdomyosarcomas. In addition, calcification can appear in pseudosarcomatous fasciitis.[51]

Extraskeletal chondrosarcomas or osteosarcomas may show irregular, poorly margined calcific and ossific deposits that differ from the other patterns of calcification.[2] The resulting deposits must be differentiated from small foci of metaplastic bone, which may appear in lipomas,[116]

liposarcomas, synovial sarcomas, epithelioid sarcomas, and malignant fibrous histiocytomas,[330] as well as from nonneoplastic ossifying processes of soft tissue, such as myositis ossificans traumatica.

Tumor Interface (Fig. 95–7). Benign neoplasms characteristically are sharply demarcated, and the surrounding tissue planes are displaced but not obliterated.[2] Malignant neoplasms can result in similar changes, however, although distortion and blurring of part of the interface between neoplasm and soft tissues can be seen in some cases. In inflammatory conditions, the entire interface may be obscured owing to fluid infiltration into the adjacent soft tissues.

Osseous Involvement (Figs. 95–8 and 95–9). Smooth resorption of cortical bone is more indicative of the proximity of a soft tissue process to subjacent bone than of its nature. Thus, benign and malignant neoplasms arising near

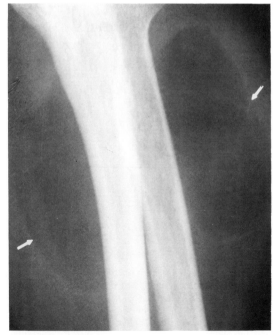

FIGURE 95–5. Soft tissue mass: Routine radiography—lipoma. In this 71 year old black woman, the radiograph reveals the typical characteristics of a lipoma (arrows). Observe the lucent and well-defined nature of this mass in the forearm. (Courtesy of G. Greenway, M.D., Dallas, Texas.)

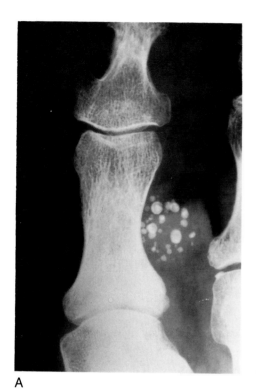

A

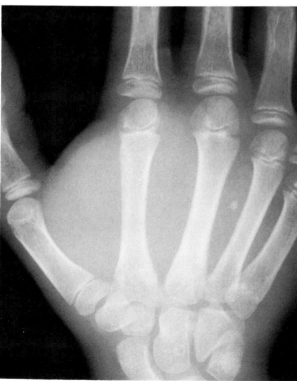

B

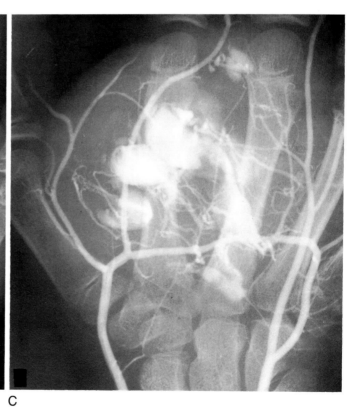

C

FIGURE 95–6. Soft tissue mass: Routine radiography—hemangioma.

A Circular calcifications, some of which contain lucent centers, within the mass of the great toe represent phleboliths.

B, C Cavernous hemangioma. An 11 year old black boy had a 1 year history of gradual swelling of the palm. The mass was soft and nontender. The radiograph **(B)** reveals soft tissue swelling of the thenar eminence as well as a phlebolith projected between the third and fourth metacarpal bones. Brachial arteriography **(C)** demonstrates large pools or lakes of contrast medium, which persisted late into the venous phase.

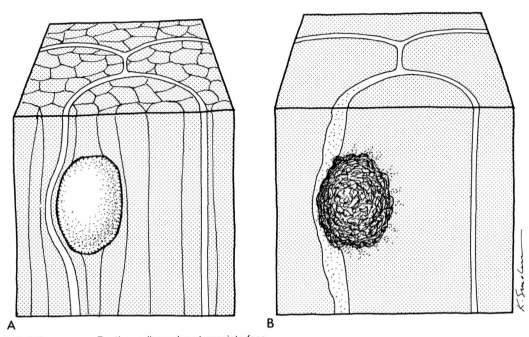

FIGURE 95–7. Soft tissue mass: Routine radiography—tumor interface.
  A Benign neoplasms may displace tissue planes, but the planes are not obliterated. The tumors frequently are well defined or marginated.
  B Malignant neoplasms can distort and obscure portions of the tissue planes. A poorly defined or irregular tumor outline can be seen.

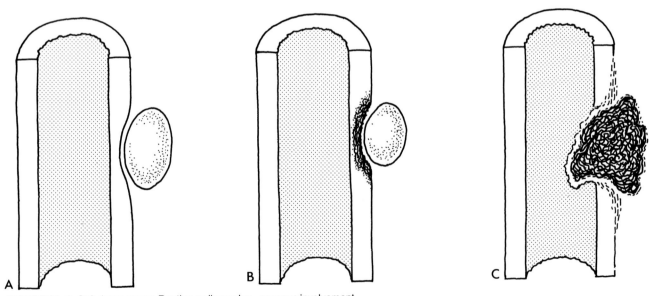

FIGURE 95–8. Soft tissue mass: Routine radiography—osseous involvement.
  A Smooth resorption of the cortical surface of a bone indicates the presence of an adjacent soft tissue mass but provides little information regarding its benign or malignant nature.
  B Cortical resorption associated with active sclerosis suggests a slowly evolving process and is more compatible with a benign neoplasm.
  C Irregular cortical destruction with medullary involvement and periostitis is strongly indicative of a malignancy or infection.

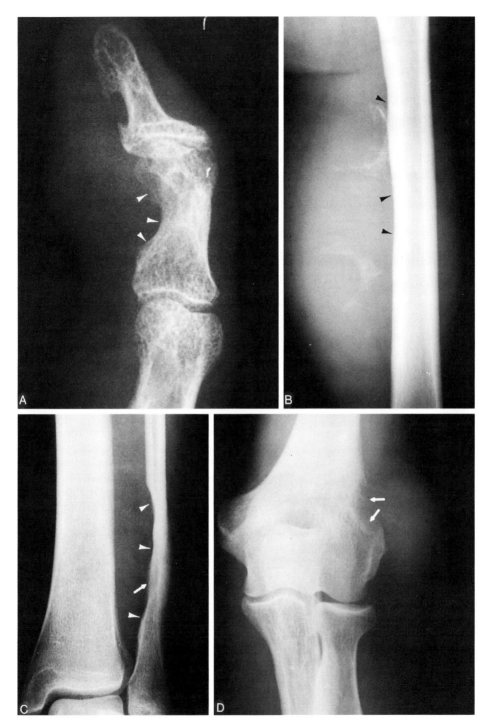

FIGURE 95–9. Soft tissue mass: Routine radiography—osseous involvement. Osseous involvement: Various patterns of bone erosion. Four cases demonstrate osseous changes that range from less aggressive **(A)** to more aggressive **(D).**

  A Pressure resorption of bone. The scalloped and smooth bone resorption (arrowheads) in the middle phalanx of a finger is indicative of pressure abnormalities without osseous invasion. (Giant cell tumor of a tendon sheath.)

  B Pressure resorption of bone. An undulating external cortical surface indicates pressure resorption (arrowheads) without bone invasion adjacent to a partially ossified soft tissue mass. (Undifferentiated sarcoma.) (Courtesy of G. Greenway, M.D., Dallas, Texas.)

  C Pressure resorption and possible bone invasion. Scalloped erosion of the medial portion of the fibula (arrowheads) and possible involvement of the medullary canal (arrow) are evident adjacent to a soft tissue mass containing faint calcification. Buttressing or thickening of the lateral fibular cortex also is seen. (Liposarcoma.) (Courtesy of M. Kelley, M.D., Charlotte, North Carolina.)

  D Bone invasion. Irregular osseous destruction (arrows) is indicative of a malignant soft tissue tumor. (Chondrosarcoma.) (Courtesy of G. Greenway, M.D., Dallas, Texas.)

bone can both produce pressure scalloping of the periosteal surface. Hyperemia due to vascularity of a neoplasm may contribute to cortical osteolysis.[2] The presence of sclerosis about the osseous defect suggests a slowly evolving process and is more typical of benign neoplasm; the absence of such bone formation is suggestive but not diagnostic of malignancy. The presence of irregular cortical destruction with or without medullary involvement is strongly indicative of a malignancy or infection.

Cortical hyperostosis subjacent to a soft tissue tumor usually implies a slow-growing process and should not be misinterpreted as bone invasion.[420] The finding, which may relate to traction periostitis, is most characteristic of lipomas but is observed in other neoplasms as well (Fig. 95–10). Furthermore, paraosseous soft tissue lesions such as ganglia may be accompanied by spiculated excrescences arising from the subjacent bone.

In the presence of a soft tissue mass and osseous abnormality, it may be difficult to differentiate a primary soft tissue tumor with osseous invasion from a bone tumor with soft tissue extension.[2] In general, the site of more extensive abnormality (bone versus soft tissue) represents the initial focus of the process. This rule is not without exception, however. Some osseous conditions, such as metastatic disease (thyroid, renal, bronchogenic, and prostatic carcinomas) and plasma cell myeloma, may produce extraordinary soft tissue components with minor bony destruction, whereas some soft tissue conditions, such as synovial sarcoma, may be present with a considerable amount of bony abnormality. The detection of a large soft tissue mass and resorption or destruction of more than one bone (e.g., metatarsals, metacarpals, radius and ulna, tibia and fibula) usually indicates the presence of a primary extraosseous neoplasm (Fig. 95–11).

Although not so frequent as lung metastasis, osseous metastasis can occur with virtually any of the malignant soft tissue tumors.[421, 422] In general, osteolysis predominates

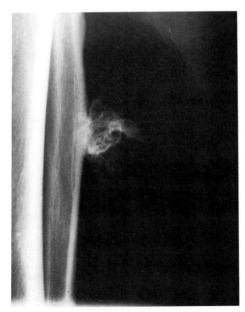

FIGURE 95–10. Soft tissue mass: Routine radiography—osseous involvement. Hypertosis in lipoma. As demonstrated here, lipomas arising close to bone may lead to bizarre hyperostosis. (Courtesy of J. Castello, M.D., Madrid, Spain.)

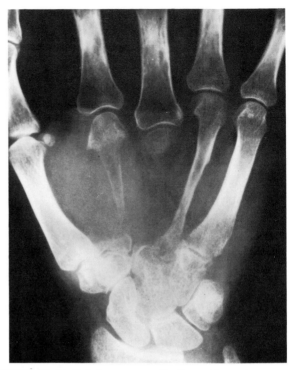

FIGURE 95–11. Soft tissue mass: Routine radiography—osseous involvement. The detection of resorption or invasion of more than one bone usually indicates the presence of a primary soft tissue process. In this case, erosion and destruction of multiple metacarpal bones have resulted from aggressive fibromatosis. (Courtesy of A. D'Abreu, M.D., Porto Alegre, Brazil.)

over osteosclerosis and involvement of the axial skeleton predominates over that of the appendicular skeleton.[422] Additional characteristics include motheaten bone destruction (although geographic destruction also is seen), cortical violation, soft tissue masses, and pathologic fracture.[422]

Conventional Tomography. With the increasing availability of CT and MR imaging, the role of conventional tomography in the evaluation of soft tissue masses has become limited. The interface between the process and the subjacent bone may be better visualized with this technique, and subtle changes in the osseous tissue may indicate the nature and aggressiveness of the soft tissue lesion. In general, however, the information supplied by conventional tomography in cases of soft tissue tumors is similar to that provided by routine radiography.

Xeroradiography. Xeroradiography with its edge contrast enhancement and great latitude is better suited for delineating soft tissue changes than is conventional radiography[3–5, 310] (see Chapter 6). This technique may define the characteristics of a tumor contour and the presence and extent of internal calcification or ossification. The expansile nature of a neoplasm occasionally can be differentiated from the retractile appearance of an organizing hematoma by xeroradiography.[5] Furthermore, both osseous and soft tissue structures can be evaluated on a single exposure, an advantage that cannot be obtained with conventional roentgenograms. Disadvantages of xeroradiography include the requirement for special equipment, limitation in field size, and high radiation exposure.

Ultrasonography. Ultrasonography has been used successfully to define the nature of certain soft tissue masses, particularly superficial ones, in both the axial and the appendicular skeleton,[322–324, 586–588] and it may be employed alone or in combination with other methods, such as CT. Most notably, synovial cysts and aneurysms are well delineated with ultrasonography, and this technique can be further applied to other masses as well (see Chapter 11). A subcutaneous or intramuscular abscess may possess echogenic properties similar to those of a tumor, although the concentration of weak echoes in a dependent portion of a lesion is more characteristic of necrotic debris within an abscess than of a neoplasm.[322] Ultrasonography can be used to delineate local recurrences of soft tissue sarcomas,[589, 590] and also to guide percutaneous needle aspiration of most lesions.[324]

Angiography. Angiography may be used to define the extent and vascular supply of a tumor and to differentiate a benign from a malignant neoplasm[11–14] (see Chapter 14). Differentiation of malignancy and hypervascular inflammatory masses may be more difficult,[2, 14] although evaluation of hemangiomas and vascular malformations can be accomplished with this technique.[15–17] Selective arterial injections, magnification and subtraction films, and administration of pharmacologic agents enhance the role of angiography.[277]

In general, there is a positive correlation between the extent of vascularity of a soft tissue tumor and the degree of malignancy.[591] Exceptions to this rule are encountered in cases of hemangioma, hemangiopericytoma, and hibernoma. It usually is not possible to distinguish between afferent and efferent vessels in malignant tumors; almost all vessels consist of simple vascular channels of varying caliber with capillary-like walls.[591] Vessels with smooth muscle tissue and elastin in their walls, often evident in benign tumors, rarely are seen in malignant tumors.

Scintigraphy. Scintigraphy with technetium (or other radiopharmaceutical agents) may delineate the presence and extent of soft tissue tumors[18, 19] (see Chapter 15). The mechanism of such uptake is incompletely understood, although increased blood flow, microcalcification, or a binding of the compounds by enzymes released in response to tissue damage may be important. Many of the tumors in which bone-seeking radioisotopes localize reveal radiographic or histologic evidence of calcification or ossification (Fig. 95–12), although this is not invariable. The vast majority of malignant soft tissue neoplasms will accumulate the radiotracer; however, as many as 50 per cent of benign tumors will do the same.[325] Because of the diverse nature of the processes that may produce accumulation of technetium (and other agents), the diagnostic capabilities of this technique are limited. Positive scans can accompany soft tissue neoplasm, infection, and diseases associated with local or widespread calcification. Although gallium initially was regarded as a tumor-localizing agent, it too may accumulate in inflamed or infarcted soft tissues.[29] Positive gallium scans are more characteristic of malignant soft tissue tumors than benign ones.[328] Gallium, however, may not accumulate in low grade malignant tumors or in some malignant tumors that do not possess necrotic or inflammatory portions. The results of studies using newer radiopharmaceutical agents, such as technetium 99m dimercaptosuccinic acid, for localization of soft tissue tumors have been promising,[959] although they are preliminary in nature.

Scintigraphy using bone-seeking radiotracers is capable of predicting osseous involvement with a high degree of accuracy in cases of soft tissue sarcomas[326, 327] and may be

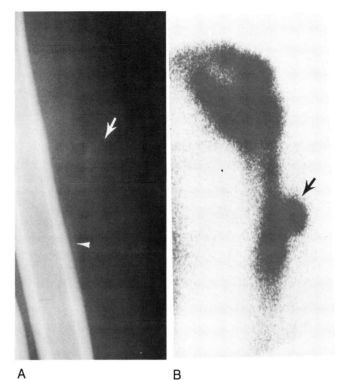

A   B

FIGURE 95–12. Soft tissue mass: Scintigraphy—myositis ossificans traumatica. This 13 year old girl collided with another skier in the mountains of New Zealand. Pain and a soft tissue mass developed over the following weeks.

A The radiograph shows faint soft tissue ossification (arrow) and periostitis (arrowhead) in the humerus.

B Intense uptake of the bone-seeking radionuclide (arrow) is apparent.

(Courtesy of M. Coel, M.D., Honolulu, Hawaii.)

more useful than CT in this respect.[327] Owing to this ability as well as the ability to detect regional or distant bone metastasis, bone scintigraphy (often combined with gallium scanning) is regarded as essential in the evaluation of patients suspected of having soft tissue sarcomas.[328, 592]

Computed Tomography. CT has been emphasized as a useful technique in evaluating soft tissue masses[6–10, 311–319] (see Chapter 8). The ability of this technique to define the exact dimensions of a lesion, the relationship of the tumor to nearby bone structures, and the density characteristics of the affected tissue is important both in correct diagnosis and in proper therapy.[302, 308] Certain limitations in the application of CT should be recognized. With the exception of a few types of masses, such as lipomas, the attenuation values do not allow a specific histologic diagnosis. Overestimation of tumor size on the basis of CT images is possible owing to adjacent soft tissue edema.[311] Similarly, if the soft tissue mass possesses attenuation characteristics identical to those of the adjacent tissues, defining the precise size of the lesion is not possible. The differentiation of actual invasion of neurovascular structures from simple distortion by the adjacent mass, even with the use of intravascular injection of contrast material, is difficult.[319]

Classification of a soft tissue tumor as benign or malignant solely on the basis of the CT findings also is difficult, although certain criteria have been emphasized in this distinction. CT features of a benign process include a smooth, well-defined border, lack of involvement of multiple muscle groups, and absence of blurring of surrounding fat (Fig. 95–13); features of a malignant process are poor margination, areas of diminished density, hazy blurring of adjacent fat, involvement of multiple muscle groups, and invasion of bone.[319] Locally aggressive but benign soft tissue neoplasms such as desmoid tumors can exhibit CT characteristics of a malignant process.[319]

In some instances, a careful analysis of all of the CT features of a soft tissue lesion (attenuation value, lesional border and position, calcification or ossification, change in appearance following administration of contrast material), especially when it appears to be benign in nature, will allow the formulation of a likely diagnosis. Examples of this situation include a synovial cyst (periarticular mass, well-defined border, attenuation value close to that of water) (Fig. 95–14), heterotopic ossification or myositis ossificans (dense rim or shell of ossification), and a peripheral aneurysm (well-defined, round inhomogeneous mass, partial opacification following the intravenous injection of contrast material, location in a neurovascular bundle) (Fig. 95–15).[317, 577] In these and other instances, the CT examination should be tailored to the specific situation; the decision regarding the need to administer intra-articular air or contrast material or to give a bolus intravenous injection of contrast material should be based on the evaluation of the initial CT scans.

CT can be used to monitor percutaneous needle biopsy of soft tissue masses[321] (see Chapter 16); however, the use of CT following complete or incomplete excisional biopsy of soft tissue sarcomas has met with varying success. Although this technique can identify new or residual abnormal tissue, differentiation among scar formation, hematoma, and tumor is difficult.[320]

Magnetic Resonance Imaging. Even the initial reports dealing with the assessment of soft tissue masses using MR

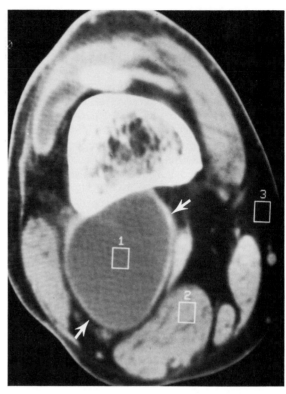

FIGURE 95–14. Soft tissue mass: CT—synovial (popliteal) cyst. In this 67 year old male physician who had had a meniscectomy 25 years earlier, pain and swelling developed behind the knee with a palpable (6 × 8 cm) mass in the popliteal fossa. Following the administration of intravenous contrast material, a transaxial CT scan at the level of the mass shows a well-circumscribed, lucent cystic lesion (24 Hounsfield units) with an enhanced wall (arrows), displacing the adjacent soft tissues and muscles (semimembranosus, biceps femoris). Clear, gelatinous fluid was aspirated from the mass. (Courtesy of G. Greenway, M.D., Dallas, Texas.)

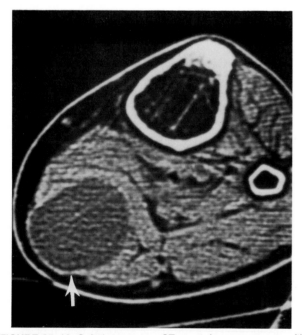

FIGURE 95–13. Soft tissue mass: CT—cyst. In a young man with an enlarging mass in the posterior aspect of the leg below the knee, a transaxial CT scan shows a well-defined lucent lesion (28 Hounsfield units) (arrow) in the gastrocnemius muscle. It did not communicate with the joint.

imaging were optimistic,[546–548, 578] indicating general superiority to CT in defining the extent of the process as well as the degree of osseous involvement. Subsequent investigations clearly have indicated that this early enthusiasm was well founded. The sensitivity of this technique when applied to the analysis of soft tissue disorders no longer is challenged, although other methods, particularly CT, provide similar and sometimes superior information in certain situations, such as the detection of calcification, ossification, and gas formation. It is the specificity of the MR imaging abnormalities that falls below some of the initial and unrealistic expectations.

With regard to the sensitivity of MR imaging in the evaluation of soft tissue tumors and tumorlike lesions, it was not unexpected that it would be tested by comparing it with that of CT scanning. Thus, in 1987 and 1988, several investigators generally concluded that MR imaging was superior to CT in the assessment of soft tissue tumors in the extremities.[593–595] In addition to the general disadvantages of CT (when compared with MR), which include some limitations in the choice of an initial imaging plane and the use of ionizing radiation, this method leads to some uncertainties in defining the margins of a soft tissue tumor. Although such tumors usually can be differentiated easily from subcutaneous fat, bone marrow, and cortex, their attenuation coefficients in many instances are similar to those of muscle. Thus, with CT, contrast differences between soft

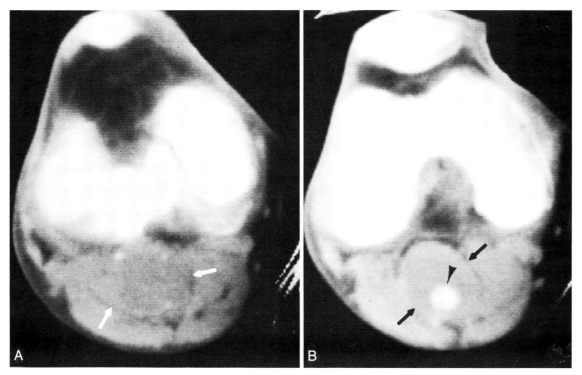

FIGURE 95–15. Soft tissue mass: CT—popliteal artery aneurysm.
   A A transaxial CT scan at the level of the knee, prior to the injection of contrast material, reveals a 3 cm inhomogeneous mass (arrows) with peripheral calcification in the popliteal fossa.
   B After an intravenous bolus injection of contrast material, a similar CT scan demonstrates the presence of an aneurysm (arrows) and its opacified lumen (arrowhead). The nonenhancing part of the mass represents atheroma or thrombus.
   (From Heikin JP, et al: Am J Roentgenol *142*:575, 1984. Copyright 1984, American Roentgen Ray Society.)

tissue tumors and adjacent musculature may be small.[593] By comparison, owing to the examiner's ability to modify the selected imaging parameters, MR imaging can define more accurately the relationship of the soft tissue tumor to surrounding muscles. Typically, this is accomplished through the use of both T1- and T2-weighted spin echo MR sequences. On T1-weighted MR images, most soft tissue tumors (the notable exception being lipomas) are of low signal intensity and easily are distinguished from fat with its high signal intensity; on T2-weighted MR images, most soft tissue tumors are of high signal intensity and can be differentiated from muscle. Some reports also have indicated that MR imaging is superior to CT in establishing the relationship of soft tissue tumors to vascular structures,[593] although the two methods provide similar information about tumor relationships with skeletal structures. With CT, administration of intravenous contrast material can be used to better define the extent of vascular tumors. Furthermore, in some investigations, the accuracy of MR and CT in allowing measurement of maximal soft tissue tumor diameter, detection of tumor depth, and delineation of tumor, neurovascular, osseous, and articular relationships has been equal, although MR imaging proved superior in defining involvement of anatomic compartments and individual muscles.[595] Establishment of the intracompartmental or extracompartmental location of a soft tissue tumor frequently requires multiplanar MR imaging, however.[596, 597] Diagnostic problems arise in accurate determination of the boundaries of a tumor by CT or MR imaging when it is accompanied by adjacent edema or hemorrhage, a situation that may be accentuated following biopsy.[595]

With regard to the specificity of MR imaging in cases of soft tissue tumors, it also was not unexpected that investigators, by modifying the parameters chosen for the examination, would seek to define imaging sequences that would provide data regarding the histologic nature of the process. Typically, on T1-weighted spin echo MR images, most soft tissue tumors, with the exception of those containing fat (Fig. 95–16) or vascular elements, or those with hemorrhage, have low signal intensity; usually, but not invariably, soft tissue tumors demonstrate high signal intensity on T2-weighted spin echo MR images (Fig. 95–17). In 1987, Sundaram and coworkers,[598] in an investigation of 48 soft tissue masses, noted seven tumors that, owing to short T2 values, had low signal intensity on T2-weighted spin echo MR images. These tumors, which were represented by aggressive fibromatosis, neurofibroma, cicatricial fibroma, and malignant fibrous histiocytoma, were characterized by relative acellularity and collagen composition, suggesting that these histologic features contributed to the low signal intensity. Although this MR finding, as well as others to be noted later, adds some specificity, the potential for tissue characterization by MR imaging remains limited. In this regard, Pettersson and colleagues[599] found no correlation between the T1 and T2 relaxation times and the histopathologic type of soft tissue (or bone) tumor. These values did differ from those of normal tissues, with the exception of the relaxation times of lipomas that were identical to those of normal fat, and there was no significant differences in these times between malignant and benign tumors. Moreover, without chemical shift imaging, different contributions to T1 and T2 from different populations of protons

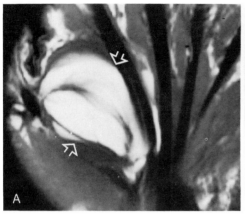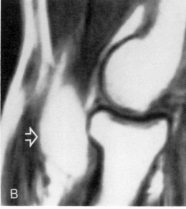

FIGURE 95–16. Soft tissue mass: MR imaging—lipoma.

A On a coronal T1-weighted (TR/TE, 500/11) spin echo MR image of the palmar region of the wrist, note the high signal intensity of the lipoma (arrows).

B This sagittal T1-weighted (TR/TE, 600/20) spin echo MR image shows a lipoma (arrow) with high signal intensity anterior to the elbow.

(e.g., water, lipid) cannot be determined.[599] Areas of necrosis and liquefaction, however, have considerably higher T2 values than those of tumors and surrounding normal tissue, and data derived from both the analysis of relaxation times and spectroscopy may prove useful for tissue characterization.[600, 960]

Of more practical importance the question regarding the specificity of MR imaging findings in allowing differentiation of benign and malignant tumors of soft tissues needs to be addressed. Kransdorf and associates,[601] in a review of MR images of 112 soft tissue masses of various causes, were able to provide a specific diagnosis in 24 per cent of cases. Such diagnosis was possible owing to the characteristic changes in signal intensity known to occur on T1- and T2-weighted spin echo MR images in instances of lipoma, hemangioma, hematoma, arteriovenous malformation, and pigmented villonodular synovitis. Despite previous data

suggesting that clearly defined margins and homogeneous signal intensity on T2-weighted images were indicative of benignancy, these investigators found that there were no reliable MR imaging criteria for differentiating benign from malignant soft tissue masses. They indicated that histologically high-grade malignant tumors may appear on MR images as well-defined, homogeneous soft tissue masses without surrounding edema or involvement of adjacent bone; and that histologically benign tumors may appear on MR images as poorly defined, inhomogeneous masses with surrounding edema and apparent involvement of adjacent bone.[601] Berquist and coworkers,[602] in a study of 95 consecutive soft tissue masses (50 benign and 45 malignant), examined the reliability of MR imaging findings to allow differentiation of benign and malignant tumors by interpreting the MR images twice: once without clinical history and the second time with clinical history. Knowledge of clinical data was most helpful to the "inexperienced" interpreter. Although there was overlap in the signal intensities, signal homogeneity, size, and margin outline in cases of benign and malignant tumors, the specificity and accuracy of diagnosis averaged 90 per cent for both types of tumor. No malignant soft tissue tumor was less than 3 cm in diameter; although 22 per cent of benign lesions were less than 3 cm in diameter, 50 per cent of such lesions were greater than 5 cm in diameter. Benign tumors tended to be well marginated, had homogeneous signal intensity, and did not encase neurovascular structures or invade bone; malignant tumors generally had irregular margins and inhomogeneous signal, and more often encased neurovascular structures and involved bone. Wetzel and Levine[604] performed a nonblinded study of 14 primary soft tissue tumors of the foot, nine benign and five malignant. Twelve tumors (86 per cent) were correctly characterized as benign or malignant. Criteria such as location relative to joints (for pigmented villonodular synovitis) or in the plantar fascia (for fibromatosis) proved more helpful than smooth margins or homogeneous signal intensity in the recognition of benign processes. Furthermore, distinctive features such as internal septation in hemangiomas, peritendinous distribution in ganglion cysts, peritendinous growth in synovial sarcomas, and persistent low signal intensity on T2-weighted MR images in pigmented villonodular synovitis improved diagnostic accuracy.

Crim and associates,[603] in a retrospective analysis of 83 soft tissue masses (49 benign and 34 malignant), found standard spin echo MR images to be unreliable in providing

FIGURE 95–17. Soft tissue mass: MR imaging—liposarcoma. These coronal proton density (TR/TE, 2500/25) **(A)** and T2-weighted (TR/TE, 2500/85) **(B)** spin echo MR images show that the tumor has higher signal intensity in **B.** Although well marginated, the soft tissue mass is inhomogeneous in appearance.

information that allowed differentiation of benign and malignant processes. The majority of both benign and malignant masses had inhomogeneous signal intensity and at least partially irregular borders; malignant tumors uncommonly had smooth borders and homogeneous signal intensity. These authors also indicated that the MR features of hematomas were similar to those of hemorrhagic tumors, that some but not all hemangiomas could be identified with MR imaging owing to the presence of serpentine vessels, and that lipomas and liposarcomas might have overlapping signal intensity characteristics. In a more recent review of the subject, Greenfield and colleagues[605] concluded that although a benign tumor in an adult more typically is small in size, well circumscribed, and of homogeneous signal intensity, and that a malignant tumor more typically is large, poorly marginated, and of inhomogeneous signal intensity, many neoplasms reveal indeterminate MR imaging features so that biopsy of the lesion is required. This opinion also is echoed by others.[606]

Most of the previously cited MR investigations of soft tissue masses have relied on standard spin echo MR imaging in one or more planes. The benefits of both T1- and T2-weighted sequences have been emphasized repeatedly. Although short tau (inversion time) inversion recovery (STIR) imaging also was employed in some of these studies,[596] the utility of STIR sequences in the evaluation of suspected extremity tumors first was reported in detail by Shuman and associates in 1991.[607] In 45 sequential patients with such tumors, these investigators noted increased lesion conspicuity on STIR images in 35 patients and on spin echo MR images in 10 patients. STIR imaging proved superior to spin echo MR imaging in delineation of peritumoral edema or peripheral microscopic tumor infiltration, and the authors concluded that STIR sequences, by allowing detection of a greater volume of abnormality than spin echo sequences, may have important implications for local staging of tumors and for surgical and radiation therapy planning. With regard to other modifications of MR imaging protocols in cases of soft tissue masses, some evidence suggests that spin echo MR images obtained following the intravenous administration of gadolinium improve the differentiation of necrotic and viable areas within soft tissue neoplasms, information useful in planning percutaneous biopsy procedures.[608] It also suggests that dynamic assessment of enhancement of signal intensity using fast scanning sequences following such administration shows potential for differentiating between tumor and edema and between scar and recurrent tumor.[608]

The value of MR imaging in guiding tissue sampling of soft tissue tumors has been the subject of investigation. Rubin and coworkers[609, 610] emphasized the inhomogeneity of signal intensity in many soft tissue tumors that complicated the selection of sites to be biopsied, particularly in large, histologically complex neoplasms. They concluded that a more precise biopsy technique could be accomplished when the MR features are used to guide the biopsy procedure, ensuring that more representative tissue is obtained. Such features also may aid in the planning of biopsies when recurrent tumor following surgical and radiation therapy is suspected. Correct interpretation of the MR imaging findings in the postoperative period, however, is difficult, owing to the presence of regions of high signal intensity on T2-weighted spin echo MR images that may reflect surgical

changes rather than recurrent tumor. In such cases, the value of textural patterns in skeletal muscle on MR images as an aid to differential diagnosis has been emphasized.[611] When T2-weighted spin echo MR images reveal diffuse areas of high signal intensity in the soft tissues at the operative site, the finding of textural features typical of skeletal muscle at these sites on T1-weighted spin echo MR images appears to be highly specific for the absence of recurrent tumor; the absence of such features may be indicative of tumor recurrence.

Vanel and coworkers[961] have emphasized an imaging protocol that appears effective in the postoperative assessment of aggressive soft tissue tumors. The results of an initial T2-weighted spin echo sequence serve as an indicator as to whether or not additional MR imaging sequences are required. If there is no high signal intensity in the soft tissues in the T2-weighted images, the study is considered negative and finished. If a mass of high signal intensity is apparent in these images, a T1-weighted sequence obtained after the intravenous administration of a gadolinium compound is performed. Recurrent tumor typically shows enhanced signal intensity in this situation, whereas hygromas do not. In difficult cases, fast injection, fast image acquisition, and subtraction technique provide data that generally allow differentiation of tumor and inflammatory changes.

Incidence of Tumors

Establishing the true frequency of soft tissue tumors is difficult. As the vast majority (over 95 per cent) of such neoplasms are benign and either go undetected or are not evaluated enough to allow accurate histologic diagnosis, reliable data regarding their frequency are not available. Conversely, soft tissue sarcomas (and other malignant tumors) usually require medical attention, and therefore data reflecting their rate of occurrence do exist. It is estimated that soft tissue sarcomas, which occur more often in men than women and with increasing frequency with advancing age, represent approximately 1 per cent of all malignant tumors. For purposes of comparison, these neoplasms occur in the United States with a frequency rate similar to that of plasma cell myeloma and with greater frequency (2 to 1) than sarcomas of bone. They are far less common than carcinomas of the lung, breast, and colon and lymphomas.

Many types of soft tissue sarcomas have a predilection for certain age groups: examples include the occurrence of rhabdomyosarcoma mainly in children; the appearance of clear cell sarcoma, epithelioid sarcoma, and synovial sarcoma in young adults; and an increased frequency of malignant fibrous histiocytoma in middle-aged and elderly persons.[591] The last of these tumors represents about 30 to 35 per cent of all soft tissue sarcomas.

Patterns of Growth of Tumors

The patterns of local growth as well as distant metastasis of soft tissue tumors, especially sarcomas, have been studied extensively by Enneking and colleagues[329] and are well summarized by Enzinger and Weiss,[330] whose textbook should be consulted by those seeking a detailed analysis of soft tissue neoplasms. As sarcomas grow, they flatten or compress the surrounding normal soft tissues, producing a compression zone of condensed and atrophic tissue.[329] A reactive zone, consisting of edematous and neovascularized tissue, exists about the compression zone.[329] Together, these two zones constitute a pseudocapsule, which, on gross pathologic inspection as well as by various imaging techniques, is easily misinterpreted as encapsulation, resulting in an underestimation of tumor aggressiveness. Histologically, such neoplasms are poorly confined, infiltrating along connective tissue septa and between muscle fibers initially as tiny irregular tumor extensions and subsequently as nodular satellite lesions.[330] The precise location of the sarcoma within the soft tissues influences the rate and pattern of local tumor spread; those arising in a muscle compartment (intracompartmental) usually extend within that compartment before violating fascial boundaries, whereas those originating in loose areolar tissue (extracompartmental) spread more rapidly.[329, 330] The adventitia of blood vessels and the tracts created by biopsy or surgical procedures provide access for more widespread tumor dissemination.[330]

Distant metastases arising from soft tissue sarcomas are related principally to hematogenous routes, although spread to regional lymph nodes occurs. Osseous involvement in such tumors reflects either local invasion or distant hematogenous dissemination, and the resulting lesions are generally osteolytic in nature.

Staging systems for soft tissue sarcomas have been developed to provide information regarding the choice of appropriate therapy and the likelihood for local recurrence or systemic metastasis. Although several different systems are employed, factors such as the size of the primary tumor (T), the presence or absence of lymph node (N) involvement, and the presence or absence of distant metastasis (M) usually are considered, forming the basis of the TNM staging system. To this may be added a histologic grade (G) of the malignant tumor, resulting in a TNMG staging system.[330, 591] Additional factors that influence the ultimate prognosis relate to the anatomic location of the tumor (i.e., superficial vs. deep, axial vs. extra-axial) and to whether the tumor is intracompartmental or extracompartmental. Owing to these many variables, some regard the staging of soft tissue sarcomas as an exercise with little practical value.[591] The clinical prognosis, therefore, is difficult to define in any one case, although unfavorable prognostic indicators appear to include a high histologic grade of malignancy, a deep-seated tumor, an older patient, nonadequate surgical removal, development of local recurrence, and short duration of time between surgery and the appearance of local recurrence.[591]

Types of Tumors

Tumors of soft tissues can arise from the epidermis and the ectodermal structures of the skin, from the lymph nodes, and from two additional primitive tissue sources: the mesoderm and the neuroectodermal tissues of the peripheral nervous system.[20] From the primitive mesenchyme are derived the supportive and reticuloendothelial tissues and their corresponding tumors; from the neuroectoderm are formed the Schwann sheath and possibly the endoneurium and perineurium and their corresponding tumors. The result is an overwhelming list of potential primary soft tissue neoplasms. Several additional factors complicate the characterization and recognition of histologic patterns of soft tissue tumors. The histology of a neoplasm may be altered through a process of differentiation or dedifferentiation of the primary cell type or as a result of proliferation of fibroblast cells due to local tissue injury. Admixtures and conglomerations of various types of neoplastic cells can result, typical examples of which are the malignant mesenchymoma, synovioma, and teratoma. Furthermore, although tumors of certain types generally arise at sites where corresponding varieties of tissue are found normally, this is not a constant rule.[20] Thus, not only are the types of neoplasm frequently difficult to classify, but in addition their locations are quite variable, and an endless list of tumor types and sites results. Certain characteristics of relative frequency and distribution allow probable preoperative diagnoses, however, and typical histologic patterns in certain neoplasms allow a specific pathologic appraisal.

In general, benign tumors or tumor-like processes are far more frequent than malignant processes. At Columbia University, the ratio of benign to malignant "tumors" detected on pathologic examination over a 45-year period was approximately 5.5 to 1.[20] Analysis of hospital populations may indicate a corresponding ratio of 100 to 1.[330] In many classification systems, benign and malignant subdivisions are entered under each histogenetic group, although transformation of a benign tumor to a malignant one, with the exception of a malignant schwannoma originating from a neurofibroma, is extremely rare.[330] Primary benign tumors can be classified as fibroblastic processes (fibroma, various forms of fibromatosis), myxomatoses, fibrous histiocytomas, lipomatoses, xanthomatoses, myomatoses, angiomatoses, lymphangiomatoses, and muscular types; primary malignant tumors can be regarded as fibrosarcomas, malignant (fibrous) histiocytomas, liposarcomas, lipomyosarcomas, rhabdomyosarcomas, angiosarcomatoses, lymphoid and reticuloendothelial tumors, extraskeletal osteosarcomas and chondrosarcomas, synovial sarcomas, malignant mesenchymomas, and miscellaneous types.[20] If to this list are added the neurogenic tumors, metastatic deposits, and non-neoplastic masses, the diverse nature of soft tissue masses readily is apparent.

Of the primary malignant soft tissue tumors, liposarcoma, fibrous histiocytoma, rhabdomyosarcoma, unclassified sarcomas, leiomyosarcoma, and synovial sarcoma are encountered most commonly. The two most common malignant soft tissue tumors are malignant fibrous histiocytoma and liposarcoma. The frequency of the specific types of malignant tumors varies with the age of the patient, however. Of the benign neoplasms, lipomas, fibrohistiocytic tumors, and hemangiomas are relatively common.[331]

Tumors of Fat

Liposarcoma is a frequent malignant neoplasm of soft tissues, representing approximately 20 per cent of all soft tissue sarcomas. It usually is encountered in middle-aged and elderly patients[10, 21, 22, 287, 332, 612, 613] (Fig. 95–18) and is rare in children. It is common in the thigh, gluteal region, retroperitoneum, and leg. Liposarcomas of the thigh predominate in the quadriceps muscle and the popliteal fossa and are somewhat smaller than those of the retroperitoneum.[330] Liposarcomas in the distal portions of the extremities are very infrequent. They rarely arise from a preexisting lipoma and are encountered infrequently in the subcutaneous tissue.

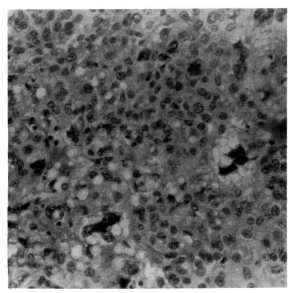

FIGURE 95–18. Liposarcoma. An 85 year old woman had a large mass in the left arm. Observe fat cells in various stages of differentiation. Bizarre giant nuclei and signet ring cells are seen (430×).

Four histologic categories of liposarcoma are recognized: well differentiated, myxoid, round cell, and pleomorphic.[612] Well-differentiated and pleomorphic liposarcomas are encountered most commonly in the retroperitoneum, and well-differentiated liposarcomas in this site (or in the mediastinum, the inguinal or testicular regions, or rarely the extremities) may reveal regions of malignant fibrous histiocytoma through a process of dedifferentiation.[612, 962, 963] Myxoid liposarcomas are the most common type of tumor, and round cell liposarcomas are poorly differentiated and associated with a poor prognosis; both of these types of liposarcomas predominate in the extremities and limb girdles.

On radiographs, an ill-defined mass of both water density and fat density may be observed. In general, more malignant lesions reveal increasing radiodensity, whereas less aggressive tumors have a greater fat content and increased lucency. Although uncommon, calcification or ossification is encountered in well-differentiated liposarcomas (Fig. 95–19). CT may reveal areas of low density in the mass (Fig. 95–20), but this finding is simulated by necrosis within a nonfatty tumor.[333] It must be emphasized that the CT appearance of liposarcomas, with the possible exception of well-differentiated liposarcomas, may not include areas of fat and, further, may resemble that of a benign process. The MR imaging features of liposarcomas are variable and dependent upon its composition.[614–617] Fat may or may not be present (Fig. 95–21), being most prominent in well-differentiated liposarcomas. Such well-differentiated tumors, however, also are characterized by septa, which reveal increased signal intensity on T2-weighted spin echo MR images, a feature not typical of ordinary lipomas.[617] Myxoid liposarcomas may be well defined and homogeneous in signal intensity, appearing as cystlike lesions on MR (and CT) examinations. Signal intensity inhomogeneity (Figs. 95–22 and 95–23) frequently is encountered in cases of pleomorphic and round cell liposarcomas.[617] Dedifferentiated liposarcomas are characterized by the presence of a well-defined nonlipomatous mass juxtaposed to a predomi-'nantly fatty tumor.[962]

One type of lipoma, the *infiltrating angiolipoma,* is composed of mature lipocytes with foci of angiomatous proliferation, is nonencapsulated, and is locally aggressive (Fig. 95–24). A distinctive radiographic appearance is evident, characterized by serpiginous densities intermixed with fat.[288] Phleboliths also may be seen.[549]

Lipomas are common lesions that typically are encountered in patients who are 30 to 50 years of age.[23, 24] Women are affected more frequently, and solitary lesions predominate. The tumors may be located throughout the body, although they show predilection for the subcutaneous tissues of the back, extremities, and thorax (Fig. 95–25). A well-defined radiolucent mass is detected on the roentgenogram. Ossification in the tumor occasionally is observed[334] (Fig. 95–26), and those lipomas located close to a bone may incite cortical thickening or hyperostosis[336] (see Fig. 95–10) or, rarely, bone erosion (Fig. 95–27). Elsewhere, soft tissue lipomas have been associated with congenital bone anomalies (including osseous overgrowth or malformation)[335, 538] and additional changes, such as melorheostosis (Chapter 93). CT and MR imaging reliably indicate the fatty nature of the tumor (Fig. 95–28). Histologically and chemically, the tumor tissue of a typical lipoma is similar to ordinary body fat. (Of interest, the fat of the lipoma is not available to the body in cases of starvation; in fact, as normal body fat undergoes wasting, the lipoma may actually increase in size[20]). Other mesenchymal elements, such as fibrous connective tissue, however, may be contained within a lipoma, leading to linear areas or septations with increased attenua-

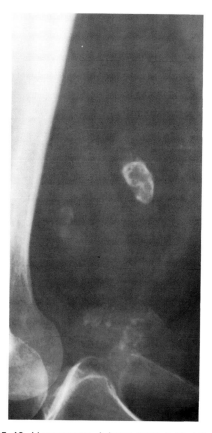

FIGURE 95–19. Liposarcoma. A large mass behind the femur is inhomogeneous in appearance with some areas of radiolucency and foci of ossification.

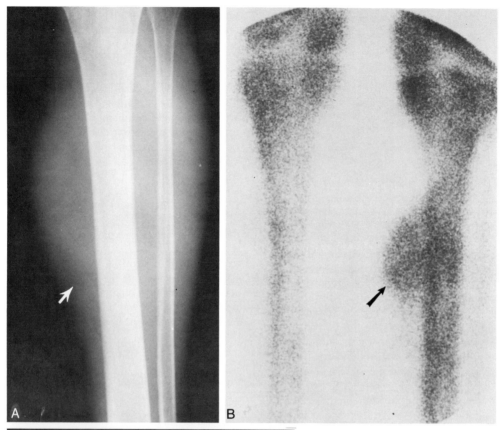

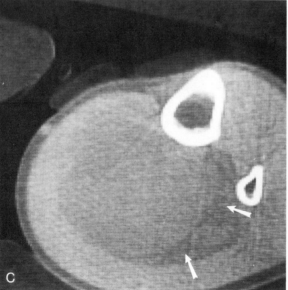

FIGURE 95–20. Liposarcoma. This 37 year old man had a 1 month history of calf pain and a mass with edema in the ipsilateral ankle.

A A soft tissue mass containing a small radiolucent area (arrow) is evident.

B The bone scan clearly indicates accumulation of the radiotracer in the mass (arrow). An ultrasound examination (not shown) revealed that the mass had mixed echogenicity.

C The transaxial CT scan shows an inhomogeneous lesion containing areas with low attenuation (arrows). It extends to the region of the interosseous membrane. Biopsy and subsequent amputation of the leg confirmed a myxoid and pleomorphic liposarcoma.

(Courtesy of G. Greenway, M.D., Dallas, Texas.)

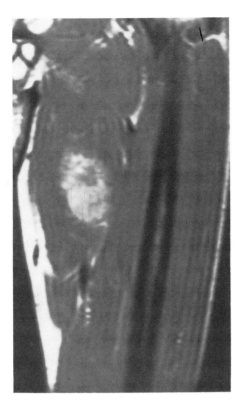

FIGURE 95–21. Liposarcoma. This intramuscular liposarcoma in the thigh is not well marginated and is inhomogeneous in signal intensity on a coronal proton density (TR/TE, 2500/20) spin echo MR image. In some regions, the signal intensity simulates that of fat; in others, it is identical to that of muscle.

tion on CT scans.[612] Soft tissue lipomas usually do not show enhancement on CT images following the intravenous administration of contrast material. MR images in cases of such lipomas reveal fat within the lesion, although linear areas of decreased signal intensity, representing septations, may be seen.[612]

One type of lipoma, designated an atypical, spindle cell or pleomorphic lipoma, is composed of a mixture of fat cells, pleomorphic giant cells, and interlacing bundles of dense, birefringent collagen.[618] Typically seen in men between the ages of 45 and 65 years and in the posterior neck or shoulder, atypical lipomas reveal areas of soft tissue density on CT (Fig. 95–29) and hyperintense regions on T2-weighted spin echo MR images.[612, 618] Rarely, bone erosion may be evident.[619]

Approximately 5 per cent of all patients with lipomas have multiple tumors,[330] an occurrence that is more frequent in men.[337] Additional varieties of fatty tumors are symmetric lipomatosis (in which diffuse and symmetric distribution of lipomas is recognized, with or without calcification[338] or severe peripheral and autonomic neuropathy[339, 550]), hibernoma and lipoblastoma (which are rare embryonal fatty tumors that occur in infancy, childhood, or adulthood) (Figs. 95–30 and 95–31),[25-27, 340, 551, 612, 620–622, 976] lipoma arborescens (in which fat collects beneath the synovial lining of the joint, especially the knee, producing swollen, villous projections),[28, 623–625] macrodystrophia lipomatosa (which can lead to grotesque enlargement of a digit) (Fig. 95–32),[626] congenital aggressive lipomatosis (in which a malformation of adipose tissue occurs early in life and is asso-

ciated with infiltration of adjacent tissues),[341] the Bannayan syndrome (which consists of lipomatosis, angiomatosis, and macroencephaly),[342] neural fibrolipoma (also designated fibrolipomatous hamartoma, which typically presents in early adulthood with a slowly enlarging mass in the volar aspect of the hand, wrist, or forearm),[612, 964, 965] and mesenchymoma (in which fatty, fibrous, vascular, smooth muscle, and osseous elements are evident). Furthermore, other soft tissue tumors such as hemangioma and elastofibroma may contain fatty tissue.[612]

Tumors of Fibrous Tissue

Fibrosarcomas occur in both adults (Fig. 95–33) and children, and they predominate in the external soft tissues rather than in the retroperitoneum, mediastinum, mesentery, or viscera.[20, 30, 31] The frequency of these soft tissue sarcomas has decreased dramatically since the recognition of malignant fibrous histiocytomas.[627] They are common in the region of the thigh and knee.[330] The neoplasms lack any specific radiographic characteristics. Calcification is seen but is much more frequent in synovial sarcomas.[330] *Infantile fibrosarcoma* is a rare but important tumor of children that, although histologically identical to fibrosarcoma in adults, carries a much better prognosis.[628] The peripheral soft tissues typically are affected, and local recurrence following excision is common.

The classification of benign fibrous tumors is complicated (Table 95–2). A *fibroma* represents a harmless pedunculated or filiform congenital malformation composed of the normal fibrous elements of the corium covered by epidermis.[20] Other varieties of benign fibrous proliferation are termed *fibromatoses*. In this latter group is a *desmoid tumor,* which arises in the abdominal and extra-abdominal musculature of men, women, and children and infiltrates the surrounding tissues in an insidious fashion, especially when located in extra-abdominal sites.[32–36, 278, 343–345, 552,]

Text continued on page 4512

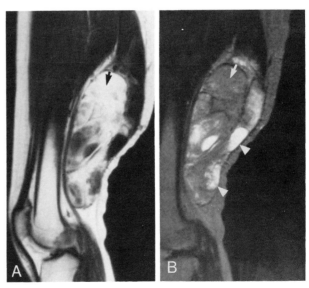

FIGURE 95–22. Liposarcoma. Sagittal T1-weighted (TR/TE, 500/16) **(A)** and T2-weighted (TR/TE, 2500/80) **(B)** spin echo MR images of a myxoid liposarcoma located behind the femur show inhomogeneity of signal intensity. Observe regions (arrows) of signal intensity identical to that of fat and others (arrowheads) with high signal intensity in **B.** (Courtesy of P. Ellenbogen, M.D., Dallas, Texas.)

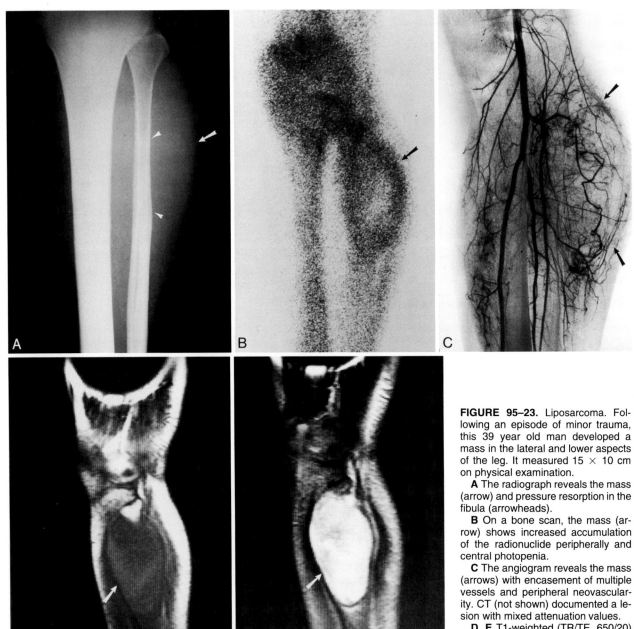

FIGURE 95–23. Liposarcoma. Following an episode of minor trauma, this 39 year old man developed a mass in the lateral and lower aspects of the leg. It measured 15 × 10 cm on physical examination.

A The radiograph reveals the mass (arrow) and pressure resorption in the fibula (arrowheads).

B On a bone scan, the mass (arrow) shows increased accumulation of the radionuclide peripherally and central photopenia.

C The angiogram reveals the mass (arrows) with encasement of multiple vessels and peripheral neovascularity. CT (not shown) documented a lesion with mixed attenuation values.

D, E T1-weighted (TR/TE, 650/20) **(D)** and T2-weighted (TR/TE, 2000/80) **(E)** sagittal MR images are shown. The mass (arrows) demonstrates inhomogeneous high signal intensity in **E.** Following intra-arterial doxorubicin hydrochloride (Adriamycin) infusion and radiotherapy, a myxoid liposarcoma was excised.

(Courtesy of G. Greenway, M.D., Dallas, Texas.)

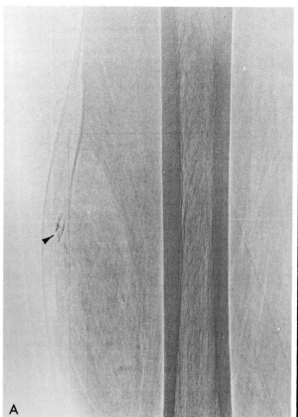
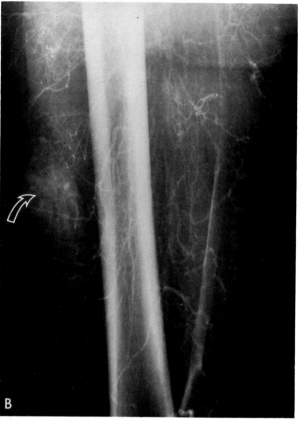
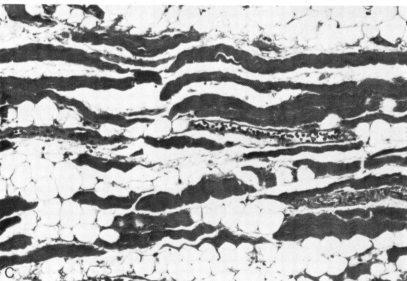

FIGURE 95–24. Infiltrating angiolipoma. A 35 year old woman had a soft, slightly tender mass in the anterolateral aspect of the thigh.

A Xeroradiography reveals small, sharply defined calcific dense areas in the periphery of the mass (arrowhead).

B The late arterial phase of a right femoral angiogram shows a tangle of irregular vessels and a tumor stain (arrow).

C Mature adipose tissue and longitudinally cut capillaries extend among darkly staining skeletal muscle fibers (150×).

(From Hunter JC, et al: Skel Radiol 4:79, 1979.)

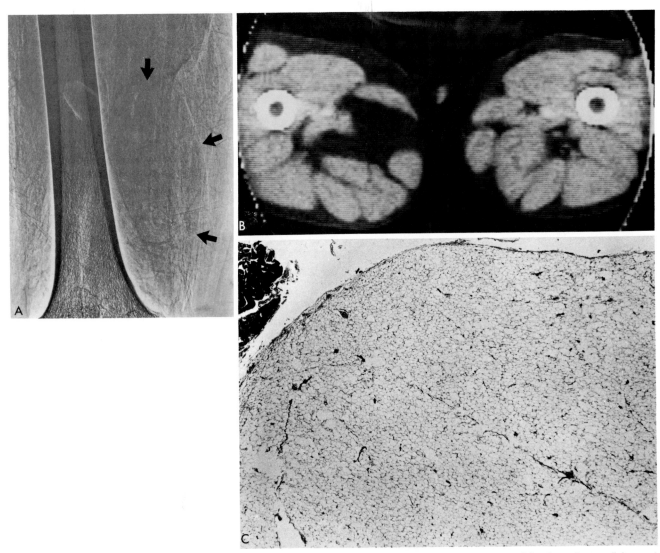

FIGURE 95–25. Lipoma. A 57 year old man had a 2 × 5 cm soft, nontender, movable but ill-defined mass overlying the anteromedial aspect of the thigh. Xeroradiography **(A)** demonstrates a poorly defined mass (arrows). CT **(B)** following administration of intravenous contrast material shows an area of low density medially, which extends from the subcutaneous fat to the area beneath the vastus medialis muscle. The CT number was −52 Hounsfield units (normal fat is −51 Hounsfield units). Photomicrograph **(C)** demonstrates adipose tissue containing a thin fibrous capsule (13.5×).

(From Hunter JC, et al: Skel Radiol *4:*79, 1979.)

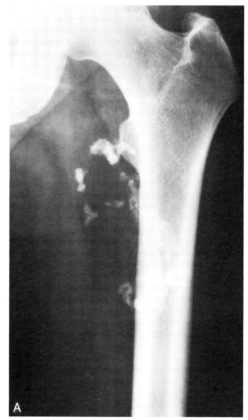

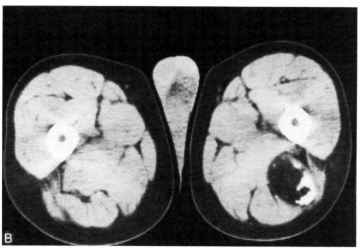

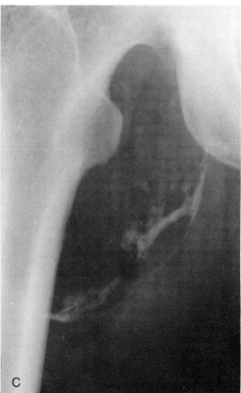

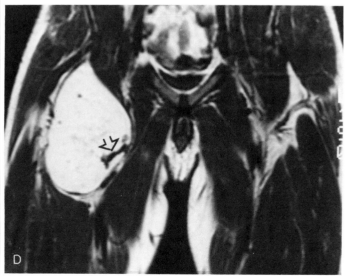

FIGURE 95–26. Lipoma: Soft tissue ossification.

A, B This 62 year old man developed a mass in the thigh measuring 3 × 3 cm. Conventional radiography and CT show irregular ossification in a radiolucent mass, which, at surgery, was found to be well encapsulated and on histologic examination contained areas of necrosis. (Courtesy of G. Greenway, M.D., Dallas, Texas.)

C, D A similar tumor is present in the right thigh of a 59 year old man. In **D,** a coronal T1-weighted (TR/TE, 966/17) spin echo image, areas of ossification (arrow) are of low signal intensity.

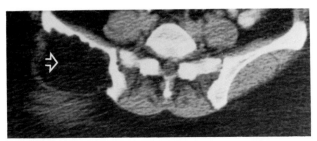

FIGURE 95–27. Lipoma: Bone erosion. In a 43 year old woman, an intramuscular lipoma (arrow) has led to erosion of the adjacent ilium. (Courtesy of G. Greenway, M.D., Dallas, Texas.)

[553, 629] Solitary lesions predominate but are not invariable[630] (Fig. 95–34). Recurrences are frequent.[344] The shoulder area is not an uncommon site of extra-abdominal desmoid tumors. Other frequent sites of involvement are the upper arm, thigh, neck, pelvis, forearm, and popliteal fossa, in order of descending frequency.[631] At any of these sites, pressure erosion of bone, cortical destruction, and a frond-like periosteal reaction may be evident.[345] At sonography, desmoid tumors have variable echogenecity, with smooth well-defined margins.[632] Hyperdensity is the predominant CT finding, and increased attenuation following the intravenous administration of contrast material is typical but not invariable.[632–634] With MR imaging, desmoids show inhomogeneous signal intensity, poor margination, and possible neurovascular and bone involvement, findings not unlike those of malignant tumors.[635] Persistent areas of low signal intensity, representing fibrous tissue or regions of increased collagen deposition, are evident in some cases, allowing more specific diagnosis (see later discussion). When desmoid tumors are located close to a joint, however, this MR imaging characteristic may be misinterpreted as evidence of pigmented villonodular synovitis.[966] Inhomogeneous enhancement of signal intensity within a desmoid tumor may follow intravenous administration of a gadolinium compound.[967]

Other types of fibromatoses are classified according to their location. *Recurring digital fibromas* (Fig. 95–35) of infancy represent a rare condition in which single or multiple fibromatous lesions arise from the fingers (and toes),

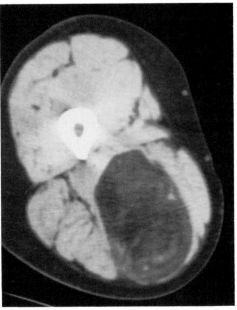

FIGURE 95–29. Atypical lipoma. An enlarging mass in the posterior portion of the thigh developed over a two-year period in this 34 year old man. A transaxial CT scan obtained following the intravenous administration of contrast material shows an inhomogeneous, enhancing intramuscular mass. Regions of higher attenuation are seen in the radiolucent lesion. Histologic analysis revealed a lipoma with fibrous septations and inflammatory cells. (Courtesy of G. Greenway, M.D., Dallas, Texas.)

affecting predominantly the dorsolateral aspect of the distal parts of adjacent digits.[37–39, 346–349, 579] They may reach considerable size but usually are painless. Their digital site of origin, their tendency to recur, and the presence of eosinophilic cytoplasmic inclusion bodies in some cases are characteristic features of this variety of fibromatosis. Furthermore, flexion contractures and hypoplastic or deformed metacarpals, metatarsals, or phalanges can be encountered. *Palmar* and *plantar fibromatoses*[330, 350] (Fig. 95–36) are terms applied to fibrous proliferations occurring in the palmar fascia (in association with Dupuytren's contracture) and plantar fascia. These lesions vary in size and commonly recur following local excision.

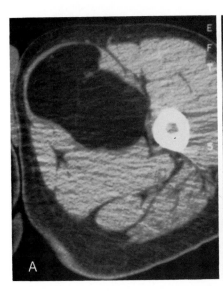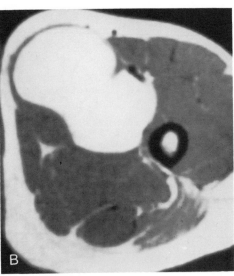

FIGURE 95–28. Lipoma. In a 19 year old man, a well encapsulated intramuscular lipoma shows a homogeneous appearance with features of fat with transaxial CT **(A)** and a transaxial T1-weighted (TR/TE, 600/15) spin echo MR image **(B).**

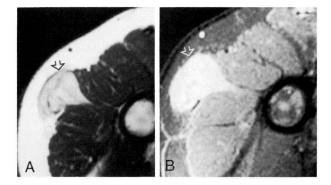

FIGURE 95–30. Hibernoma. In a 50 year old man, a mass extends from the deltoid muscle into the adjacent subcutaneous tissues. It is of intermediate to high signal intensity (arrow) on a transaxial T1-weighted (TR/TE, 400/15) spin echo MR image **(A)** and of high signal intensity (arrow) on a transaxial short tau inversion recovery (STIR) MR image (TR/TE, 2000/30; inversion time, 140 msec) **(B)**. (Courtesy of S. Eilenberg, M.D., San Diego, California.)

Juvenile aponeurotic fibroma is an aggressive variety of fibrous proliferation that arises in the aponeurotic tissues of the hands or feet of young children[40–42, 50] (Figs. 95–37 and 95–38). This lesion has a tendency to calcify, infiltrate adjacent tissues, and recur following incomplete excision. The aggressive histologic appearance and the recurrent nature of juvenile aponeurotic fibromatosis have raised the question of a low grade malignancy in some cases. Lichtenstein and Goldman[43] have postulated that this tumor is an atypical cartilaginous growth that may appear in many areas of the body in both children and adults. The designation of *musculoaponeurotic fibromatosis* sometimes is applied to desmoid-like lesions of muscles, fascia, or aponeurosis, most commonly observed in the limbs in persons of all ages.[636, 637] As in other forms of fibromatosis, signal heterogeneity characterizes the MR imaging appearance of musculoaponeurotic fibromatosis.[637]

Additional types of fibrous proliferation include *fibromatosis colli* (Fig. 95–39), which develops usually in the sternocleidomastoid muscle of infants and children and rarely may lead to osteolytic lesions of the clavicle;[351] *juvenile hyaline fibromatosis,* which is a rare hereditary disease (autosomal recessive) generally appearing in the first few years of life and resulting in multiple cutaneous tumors in the back, head, and extremities with inconstant dwarfism, flexion contractures of joints, mental retardation, and osteolytic lesions of the long and short tubular bones and skull[330, 352, 638–640]; *penile fibromatosis* (Peyronie's disease), which produces stiffening and deformity of the penis; *idiopathic retroperitoneal fibrosis,* in which fibrous proliferation of retroperitoneal tissues may lead to ureteral obstruction; *irradiation fibromatosis,* in which local superficial soft tissue fibrous proliferation relates to heavy irradiation; *progres-*

sive myositis fibrosa (hereditary polyfibromatosis), which represents an early stage of myositis ossificans before the development of bone formation; *elastofibroma,* in which unilateral or bilateral reactive lesions containing elastinophilic fibers develop in middle-aged and elderly persons, particularly those who are manual laborers or weight-lifters, especially between the scapula and chest wall (Fig. 95–40) and elsewhere about the shoulders[44–47, 641–646]; *pseudosarcomatous fasciitis,* related to fibroblastic proliferation in subcutaneous tissues, especially in the upper extremity, in children or men and women from infancy to old age[51] (Figs. 95–41 and 95–42); and *congenital generalized fibromatosis (infantile myofibromatosis)* affecting infants, in which fibrous proliferation occurs not only in the superficial soft tissues but also in viscera and bones[20, 353–355, 647–649, 951] (Fig. 95–43). The last-mentioned condition may be familial and the tumors may disappear spontaneously.[48, 49] The osseous lesions can arise in any site, are typically metaphyseal in location in the tubular bones, are variable in size, and may be associated with pathologic fractures.[353, 539] Furthermore, the bone lesions may be solitary or, more commonly, multiple; solitary lesions predominate in the craniofacial bones, and are accompanied by a benign clinical course, whereas multiple lesions may or may not be associated with visceral involvement which, when present, carries a poor prognosis.[648]

The fibromatoses, indeed, defy accurate classification owing to changing nomenclature, overlapping clinical, imaging, and pathologic manifestations, and in some cases the existence of intermediate forms that share features of more than one type of disorder.[650] Common to most of them are locally aggressive behavior, a tendency for recurrence following attempted surgical removal, and proliferation of be-

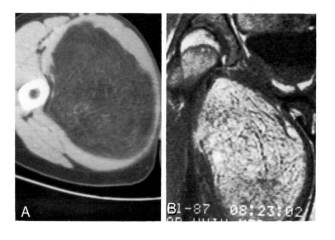

FIGURE 95–31. Lipoblastoma. This 12 year old girl developed a mass in the medial aspect of the right thigh over several years. It had increased significantly in size in the last few months and was painless. A transaxial contrast-enhanced CT image **(A)** shows a radiolucent mass in the adductor muscles, which is rather well defined. It contains linear regions of increased attenuation. A coronal T1-weighted (TR/TE, 528/25) spin echo MR image **(B)** shows that the mass has areas of signal intensity identical to that of fat, as well as linear regions of signal intensity close to that of muscle. (Courtesy of G. Greenway, M.D., Dallas, Texas.)

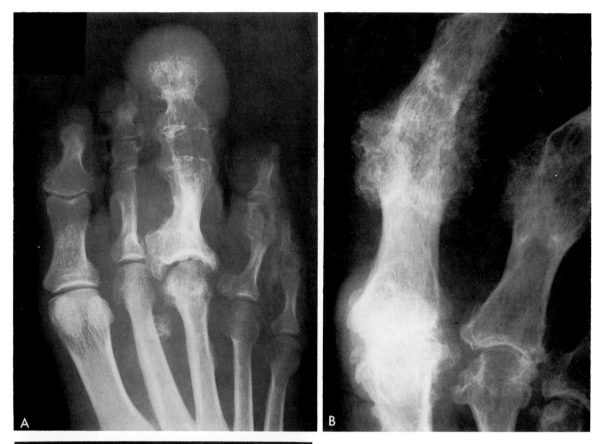

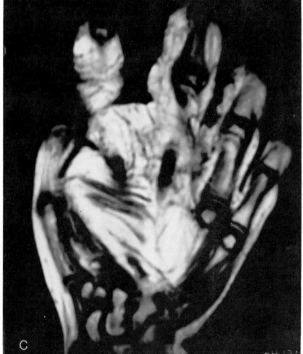

FIGURE 95–32. Macrodystrophia lipomatosa.

A, B Two examples reveal the massive enlargement of soft tissue and osseous tissue that can accompany this condition. Observe the degree of joint space narrowing, bony ankylosis, and proliferative alterations. (Courtesy of L. Ginsburg, M.D., Long Beach, California.)

C In a third case, a T1-weighted (TR/TE, 600/20) spin echo MR image shows fatty infiltration involving mainly the palm and second and third digits. (Courtesy of S. Wootton, M.D., Denver, Colorado.)

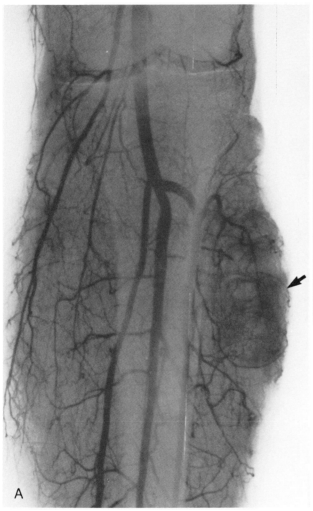

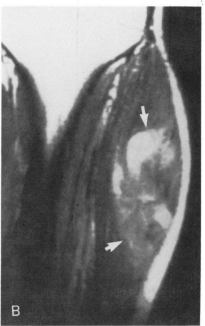

FIGURE 95–33. Fibrosarcoma. A 45 year old man developed a mass in the lateral aspect of the knee. Angiography **(A)** shows a hypervascular tumor (arrow) deriving its blood supply from the anterior tibial artery. A coronal T1-weighted (TR/TE, 750/40) spin echo MR image **(B)** shows inhomogenity of signal intensity (arrows). A grade II fibrosarcoma was diagnosed on histologic examination. (Courtesy of G. Greenway, M.D., Dallas, Texas.)

TABLE 95–2. Benign Fibrous Proliferations and Fibromatoses

Diagnosis	Typical Age of Presentation	Typical Location	Miscellaneous Data
Fibrous Proliferations of Infancy and Childhood			
Fibrous hamartoma	Infancy	Axillary, inguinal regions	Solitary, rarely recur
Congenital generalized fibromatosis (infantile myofibromatosis)	Infancy	Soft tissue, viscera, bone	Solitary or multiple, may regress, rarely recur
Infantile digital fibromatosis	Infancy	Fingers and toes	Solitary or multiple, may regress, commonly recur
Fibromatosis colli	Infancy	Sternocleidomastoid muscle	Solitary, rarely bilateral, may regress, rarely recur, associated torticollis
Juvenile aponeurotic fibroma	Infancy, childhood, or adolescence	Hands and feet	Solitary, may regress, commonly recur, may calcify
Juvenile hyaline fibromatosis	Childhood	Dermis and subcutis	Multiple, do not regress or recur
Infantile desmoid type fibromatosis	Infancy and childhood	Musculature	Solitary, commonly recur, no regression
Fibrous Proliferations of Adulthood			
Nodular fasciitis (pseudosarcomatous fasciitis)	Adulthood	Extremities	Solitary, may regress, rarely recur
Proliferative fasciitis	Adulthood	Extremities	Solitary
Proliferative myositis	Late adulthood	Trunk, shoulder girdle	Solitary
Elastofibroma	Late adulthood	Chest wall, scapula	Unilateral > bilateral
Keloid	Adolescence or adulthood	Face, shoulders, forearms, hands	Solitary or multiple, do not regress, common in blacks
Fibromatoses			
Palmar fibromatosis	Late adulthood	Hands	Unilateral or bilateral, associated Dupuytren's contracture
Plantar fibromatosis	Childhood or adulthood	Feet	Unilateral or bilateral, associated palmar fibromatosis
Peyronie's disease	Adulthood	Penis	May regress, associated palmar and plantar fibromatosis
Extra-abdominal fibromatosis (desmoid tumors)	Adulthood	Musculature	Rarely regress, commonly recur
Abdominal fibromatosis (desmoid tumors)	Early adulthood	Musculature	Commonly recur, occur during or after pregnancy
Intra-abdominal fibromatosis (pelvic fibromatosis, mesenteric fibromatosis, Gardner's syndrome)	Adulthood	Musculature, mesentery	May recur

Taken in part from Enzinger FM, Weiss SW: Soft Tissue Tumors, St. Louis, CV Mosby, 1983, p 71.

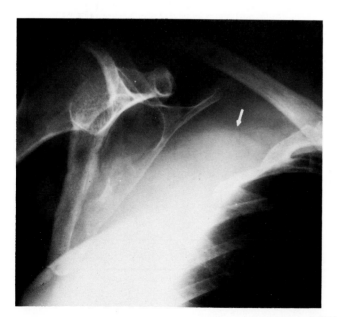

FIGURE 95–34. Extra-abdominal desmoid tumor. This 55 year old woman had a mass in the area of the right scapula. The radiograph outlines lateral displacement of the scapula by a large, poorly defined soft tissue mass (arrow). Equivocal osseous changes are apparent. At surgery, the mass, weighing 1240 gm, was found to have infiltrated the chest wall between the ribs. Histologic analysis confirmed the diagnosis of fibromatosis. (Courtesy of A. Bonakdarpour, M.D., Philadelphia, Pennsylvania.)

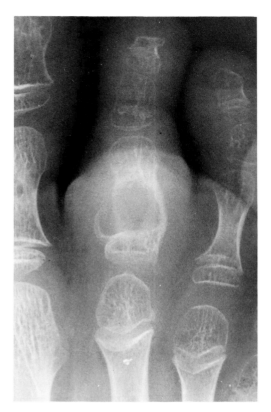

FIGURE 95–35. Recurring digital fibromas. In an 8 year old boy, a mass developed in the dorsal aspect of the foot, leading to soft tissue swelling and erosion of the proximal phalanx of the second toe. Although the original mass was removed surgically, the fibroma recurred.

nign fibrous tissue. Although the latter feature may be accompanied by persistent low signal intensity on both T1- and T2-weighted spin echo MR images (Fig. 95–44), signal intensity inhomogeneity is the rule which, when combined with locally aggressive characteristics, simulates the findings of malignant tumors.[635, 651–654] Thus, high signal intensity areas may be seen on T2-weighted images and, although well-defined margins may be apparent, poorly defined masses, especially those that have recurred, are encountered. Furthermore, when recurrent lesions are associated with relative acellularity, fibrosis, and persistent low signal intensity, the differentiation of a recurrent mass and postoperative fibrosis becomes difficult.[652] In one of the fibromatoses, elastofibroma, the detection of entrapped fat within a predominantly fibrous mass on MR images is reported to be characteristic[646] (Fig. 95–40).

Tumors of Muscle

Leiomyosarcomas (Fig. 95–45) are uncommon malignant neoplasms of soft tissues, primarily affecting adults.[52] They may arise in the retroperitoneum, the peripheral soft tissues, or the major blood vessels (medium-sized and large veins).[356, 655] Those occurring in the retroperitoneal region are most common and predominate in women. Soft tissue masses of variable size, hypervascularity, and bone invasion are encountered in cases of leiomyosarcoma.[357, 358] *Leiomyomas* (Fig. 95–46), the benign counterpart, can be found in the skin and subcutaneous or deep soft tissue.[53] They arise at variable sites, frequently from the smooth

muscle of small blood vessels, are single or multiple, and may calcify, usually in association with necrosis of part of the tumor.[290, 656–658]

Rhabdomyosarcoma (Figs. 95–47 to 95–50) can develop in a child or adult. It predominates in children between the ages of two and six years and in young adults between the ages of 14 and 18 years. It is rare after the age of 45 or 50 years. In the pediatric age group, the tumors (juvenile rhabdomyosarcoma, embryonal rhabdomyosarcoma) predominate in the head, neck, and urogenital tract, and affect both boys and girls.[20, 54–57, 279, 359, 659, 660] On radiographic examination, soft tissue masses, which rarely calcify or invade neighboring bone, are noted. Skeletal metastasis can resemble neuroblastoma[58] (Chapter 85). In adult rhabdomyosarcoma, many of the lesions are located in the deeper tissues of the extremities and torso, and few are found in the head and neck. Bone erosion is rare and is associated mainly with tumors of the hands and feet.[330]

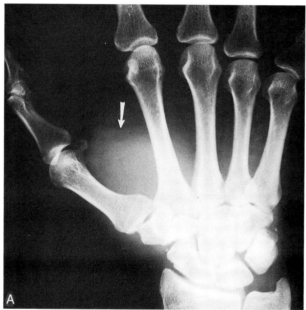

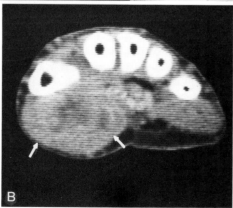

FIGURE 95–36. Palmar fibromatosis. A 47 year old man noticed a slowly enlarging mass beneath his thumb that interfered with his writing. The skin was red, and the lesion was firm and approximately 5 cm in diameter.

A Note the soft tissue mass (arrow).

B CT documents that the mass is inhomogeneous (arrows) and located in the adductor pollicis brevis and opponens pollicis muscles. Histologic examination of the excised mass revealed fibromatosis.

(Courtesy of G. Greenway, M.D., Dallas, Texas.)

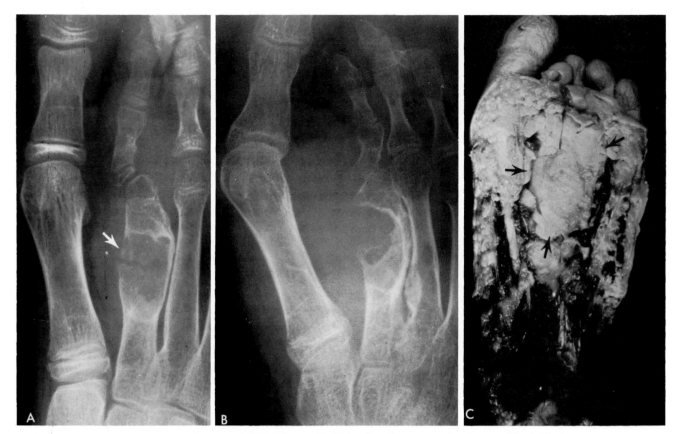

FIGURE 95–37. Juvenile aponeurotic fibromatosis. This 13 year old girl developed a mass on the dorsum of the left foot.

A An initial radiograph reveals a soft tissue mass with adjacent osseous involvement and a pathologic fracture through a well-circumscribed lesion in the second metatarsal (arrow). There is displacement and deformity of the proximal phalanx in the same digit. Excisional biopsy resulted in a diagnosis of either neurofibroma or desmoplastic fibroma.

B Approximately 3 years after **A,** a recurrent mass has produced further destruction and distortion of the neighboring bones.

C After amputation, the specimen shows the extent of the fibrous tumor invading the metatarsals (arrows). Atypical fibrous tissue was demonstrated on histologic examination.

(Courtesy of R. Freiberger, M.D., New York, New York, and J. Kaye, M.D., New York, New York.)

The *rhabdomyoma* is an extremely rare benign tumor composed of striated muscle cells that may occur in children or in adults.[20, 659] In most cases, it is observed in the face and neck, although a special variety occurs in the heart. The *myoblastoma* (granular cell tumor) is a growth of mesenchymal origin that can be benign or malignant, arising in striated muscle, skin, mucous membranes, alimentary tract, and many other places.[20, 59, 60]

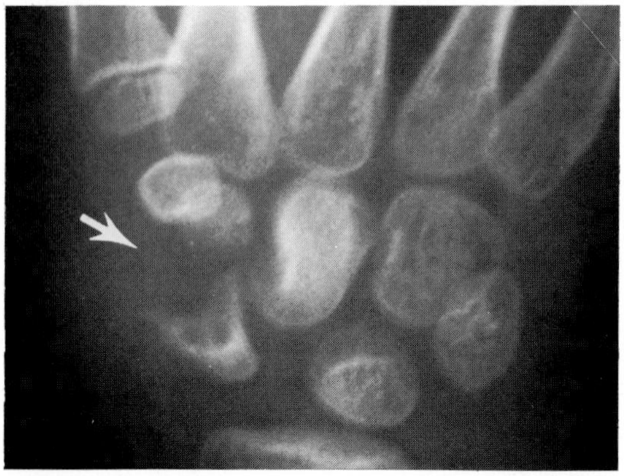

Myxomatoses

Many types of myxoid tumors and tumorlike lesions have been described, and inconstant nomenclature has led to problems in classification. Indeed, myxoid foci can be identified histologically in some liposarcomas, chondrosarcomas, and fibrous histiocytomas of soft tissue. Myxomatous lesions include ganglia, juxta-articular myxomas (also known as cystic myxomas, meniscal cysts, and ganglion cysts with myxoid lesion), and intramuscular myxoma. Although ganglion cysts have less developed myxoid components than juxta-articular myxomas,[661] these two lesions do share many features, including predilection for periarticular sites. They may lead to internal derangements of joints and, because of this, are discussed further in Chapter 70.

As classically described, the *ganglion* represents a cystic tumor-like lesion that usually is attached to a tendon sheath, particularly in the hands, wrists, and feet[20, 668, 669] (Figs. 95–51 and 95–52). It also arises from tendons, muscles, and semilunar cartilages. Unilocular or multilocular cystic swellings are observed, although their exact pathogenesis is not clear.[61] Synovial herniation and tissue degeneration are two suggested mechanisms for their development. Radio-

FIGURE 95–38. Juvenile aponeurotic fibromatosis. This 5 year old girl developed progressive pain and swelling of the wrist. Several of the carpal bones are invaded (arrow) by an adjacent soft tissue mass. Biopsy confirmed the diagnosis of juvenile aponeurotic fibromatosis. (Courtesy of H. Hricak, M.D., San Francisco, California.)

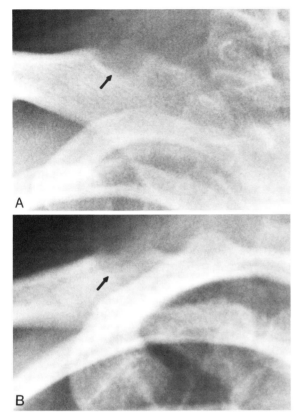

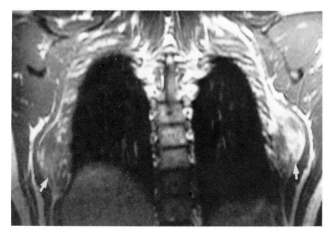

FIGURE 95–39. Fibromatosis colli. Examples of clavicular erosion (arrows) related to this condition are shown. (From Sartoris DJ, et al: Skel Radiol 10:34, 1983.)

FIGURE 95–40. Elastofibroma. In a 43 year old woman who was an avid weight-lifter, bilateral masses developed between the lower part of the scapula and the chest wall. This coronal T1-weighted (TR/TE, 500/20) spin echo MR image shows the two lesions (arrows), with inhomogeneous but mainly low signal intensity. Note areas of high signal intensity consistent with that of fat, however.

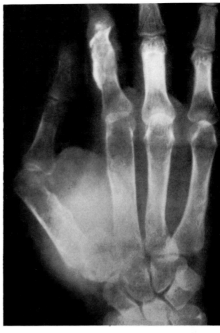

FIGURE 95–41. Nodular (pseudosarcomatous) fasciitis. This 35 year old woman had had long right index and middle fingers since birth. She developed swelling on the dorsum of the right hand over a 2 year period, which, following biopsy and amputation of the second digit, was diagnosed as nodular fasciitis. The mass recurred. A radiograph outlines amputation of the second digit, a soft tissue mass, bony erosion, and infiltration of the first and third metacarpals. (Courtesy of Naval Hospital, San Diego, California.)

graphic evaluation may reveal a soft tissue mass, surface bony resorption, and periosteal new bone formation, and arthrography or tenography may outline the communication of the mass with the underlying articular or tendinous structure. Ultrasonography also can be employed for accurate diagnosis.[972]

Ganglia arising about the proximal tibiofibular joint (Fig. 95–53) have been associated with compression of the common peroneal nerve.[360–362, 670] Those near the hip (and elsewhere) have been associated with chronic developmental dysplasia[683–685] (Fig. 95–54) and may communicate with subchondral cystic lesions,[363, 671] which frequently are interpreted as intraosseous ganglia (Chapter 39). The resulting imaging abnormalities may be diagnostic, revealing a radiolucent para-acetabular soft tissue mass with subjacent bone erosion[363, 364, 554] (Fig. 95–55). Cyst formation in the acetabular labrum, revealed by arthrography, CT, or MR imaging also has been described.[365, 555] In this location as well as in others, such as the glenohumeral joint (Fig. 95–56) and knee,[366, 556] intra-articular ganglia may lead to significant clinical manifestations. Examples of these include ganglia of the shoulder with entrapment of the suprascapular nerve,[672–674] ganglia arising from the cruciate ligaments,[675–680] and those at the insertion sites of the pes anserinus and popliteus tendons.[681, 682] Ganglionic degeneration of the periosteum may occur with or without a soft tissue or intraosseous component; cortical erosion and scalloping and distinctive, thick periosteal bone formation are observed[557, 558] (Fig. 95–57).

The *myxoma* is a rare connective tissue tumor that may appear at any age.[62, 367, 368, 540, 580] Intramuscular myxomas are most frequent in the fifth through seventh decades of life, predominating in women and in the thigh, shoulder, and, to a lesser extent, buttock and upper arm. Myxomas may demonstrate an invasive manner of growth, particularly within striated muscle, and can recur.[63] Solitary lesions of soft tissue outnumber multiple lesions. Rarely, they may calcify.[64, 367] Although myxomas arising in bone are rare, multiple soft tissue myxomas have been reported in associ-

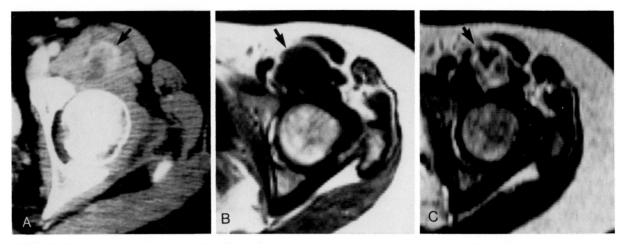

FIGURE 95–42. Nodular (pseudosarcomatous) fasciitis. A 44 year old woman developed pain and a mass in the left groin.

 A Transaxial CT following intravenous injection of contrast material shows a mass (arrow) in the left iliopsoas muscle with peripheral enhancement.

 B, C The mass (arrows) is of low signal intensity on a transaxial T1-weighted (TR/TE, 500/20) spin echo MR image **(B)** and is inhomogeneous in signal intensity on a transaxial T2-weighted (TR/TE, 2000/120) spin echo MR image **(C).** At the time of surgery, a mass embedded in the iliopsoas muscle was found that was adherent to the posterior surface of the fascia. A proliferative fasciitis was confirmed histologically.

 (Courtesy of G. Greenway, M.D., Dallas, Texas.)

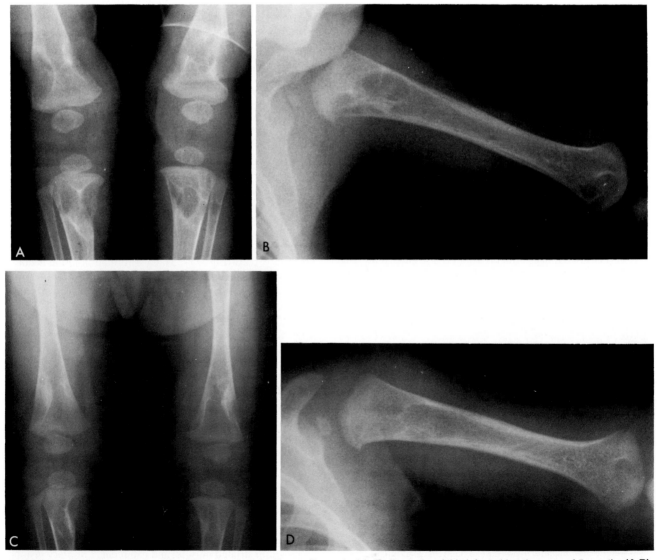

FIGURE 95–43. Congenital generalized fibromatosis (infantile myofibromatosis). Radiographs of this infant girl at the ages of 5 months **(A,B)** and 8 months **(C,D)** are shown. Multiple symmetrically distributed radiolucent foci, predominantly in the metaphyses of the tubular bones, represent sites of fibrous proliferation. Note the improvement of the abnormalities in the later films. (Courtesy of D. Weissberg, M.D., Orange County, California.)

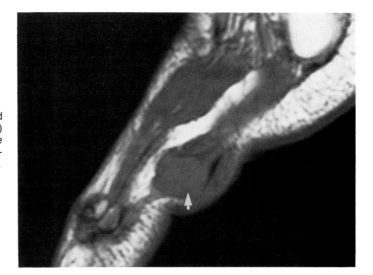

FIGURE 95–44. Plantar fibromatosis. A sagittal T1-weighted (TR/TE, 600/12) spin echo MR image reveals a mass (arrow) of low signal intensity in the plantar aspect of the foot. The mass remained of low signal intensity on T2-weighted MR images (not shown), and the opposite foot was affected similarly.

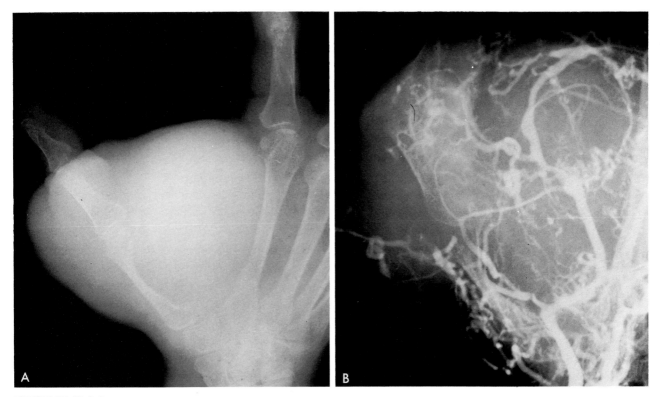

FIGURE 95–45. Leiomyosarcoma.

A 56 year old woman had a growing soft tissue mass in her hand and a pathologic fracture of the left femur. Observe the lobulated soft tissue mass in the thenar space, with pressure erosion of the first and second metacarpals and proximal phalanx of the thumb **(A)**. The angiogram **(B)** reveals irregular tumor vessels. (Courtesy of T. Staple, M.D., Long Beach, California.)

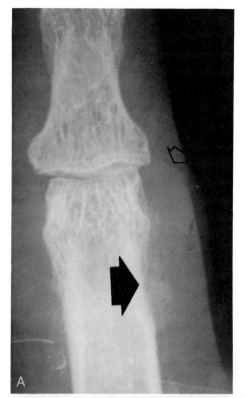

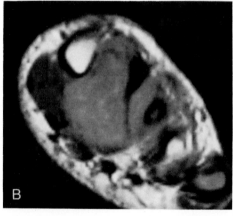

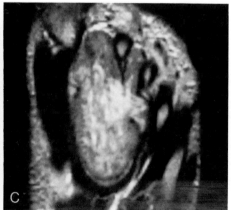

FIGURE 95–46. Leiomyoma.

A In this 62 year old man, a leiomyoma arising from a digital artery has led to a soft tissue mass (open arrow) with cortical erosion (arrow) of the adjacent proximal phalanx. (From Botte MJ, et al: Clin Orthop *260*:259, 1990.)

B, C An angioleiomyoma of the foot is seen as a tumor of low signal intensity on a coronal T1 weighted (TR/TE, 750/40) spin echo MR image **(B)** and of inhomogeneous signal intensity on a transverse T2 weighted (TR/TE, 2000/80) spin echo MR image **(C).** (Courtesy of A. Newberg, M.D., Boston, Massachusetts.)

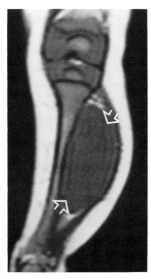

FIGURE 95–47. Rhabdomyosarcoma. This coronal T1-weighted (TR/TE, 500/20) spin echo MR image shows a mass (arrows) of low signal intensity producing pressure erosion of the tibia in a six month old girl. (Courtesy of T. Broderick, M.D., Orange, California.)

ation with fibrous dysplasia of the adjacent bone (Fig. 95–58).[65] This combination of findings sometimes is referred to as Mazabraud's syndrome.[968] The *myxosarcoma* is a rare malignant counterpart of the myxoma.

MR imaging has been used to study intramuscular myxomas as well as other myxoid containing tumors.[662, 663] Intra-

muscular myxomas typically are well circumscribed and are confined to the muscle. In T1-weighted spin echo MR images, their signal intensity is lower than that of skeletal muscle; increased signal intensity is evident in T2-weighted images (Fig. 95–59). The lesions usually are homogeneous in signal in both types of images. Following intravenous administration of gadolinium, enhancement of signal in the myxoma may[663] or may not[662] occur.

Tumors of Histiocytic Composition

Attention has recently been directed toward the soft tissue tumors dominated by the histiocyte[66–73, 292, 369–373, 377] and, specifically, toward a group of such tumors composed of cells that resemble fibroblasts and histiocytes. Although, in the past, it commonly had been assumed that the cellular origin of the fibrohistiocytic tumors was a histiocyte that could assume fibroblastic properties or a primitive mesenchymal element that could give rise to both fibroblasts and histiocytes, these concepts recently have been challenged, indicating that the precise nature of the progenitor cell is uncertain.[330] It is believed by some investigators that the histiocyte is derived from blood monocytes that originate in the bone marrow[374] and by others that the histiocyte represents an activated fibroblast.[375, 376] The application of more sophisticated investigative techniques, such as electron microscopy, while certainly providing a closer look at the cellular composition of the neoplasms, has done little to define their origin. The diversity of opinion regarding the derivation of cells that compose the fibrohistiocytic neoplasms has led to shifting nomenclature and complex clas-

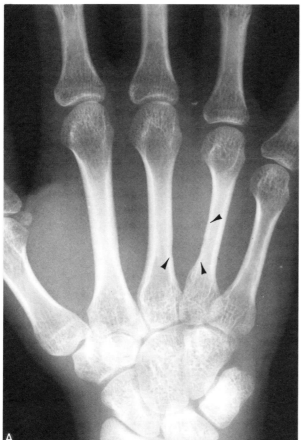

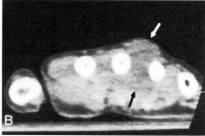

FIGURE 95–48. Rhabdomyosarcoma. A 15 year old girl developed a mass in the dorsum of the hand, which enlarged over the ensuing 3 months. It was firm and approximately 3 cm in diameter, palpable on both the dorsal and volar surfaces, and unattached to the skin, tendons, or bones.

A Observe erosion of both the third and the fourth metacarpals (arrowheads).

B The CT scan shows the location of the mass (arrows). There is no evidence of calcification. The final histologic diagnosis was an alveolar type of rhabdomyosarcoma. (Courtesy of G. Greenway, M.D., Dallas, Texas.)

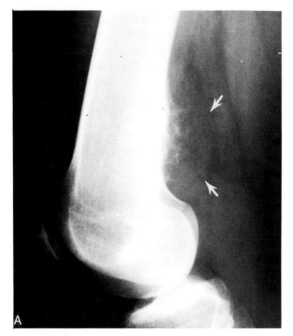
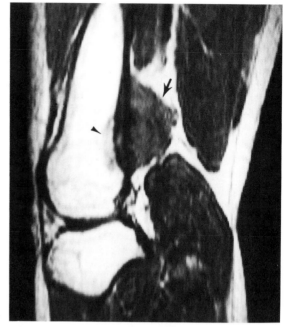

FIGURE 95–49. Rhabdomyosarcoma. A firm thigh mass and knee pain occurred in a 23 year old woman.

A A lateral radiograph shows the mass (arrows) with adjacent bone reaction in the femur. The posterior cortex of the bone is thickened.

B A sagittal T1-weighted (TR/TE, 600/20) spin echo MR image clearly demonstrates the tumor (arrow) and decreased signal intensity in the femur (arrowhead). This latter finding relates to marrow displacement by tumor or enlarged vessels. Note the similarity of the signal intensity of the tumor to that of the adjacent musculature. The final histologic diagnosis was alveolar rhabdomyosarcoma.

(Courtesy of G. Greenway, M.D., Dallas, Texas.)

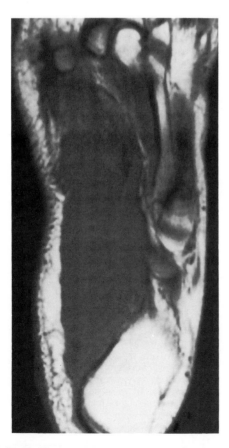

FIGURE 95–50. Rhabdomyosarcoma. In a 17 year old woman, a transverse T1-weighted (TR/TE, 618/18) spin echo MR image shows a large plantar mass of low signal intensity. It demonstrated high signal intensity on T2-weighted spin echo MR images (not shown). (Courtesy of R. Kerr, M.D., Los Angeles, California.)

sification systems and has cast doubt on the validity of data provided in older scientific publications dealing with these or similar tumors. Amid the chaos is the certainty that a number of both benign and malignant neoplasms of soft tissues (as well as of bone and supporting structures of various organs)[330] are characterized by a histologic pattern frequently dominated by spindle cells that exhibit, in some cases, a storiform pattern (resembling a woven mat) and, in others, a fascicular pattern and that may be admixed with myxoid, foam, giant, and inflammatory cells.

Atypical fibroxanthoma is a histologically malignant but clinically benign lesion that is apparent in the exposed skin on the face and neck of elderly persons and, less frequently, on the limbs and trunk of young persons.[330]

Malignant fibrous histiocytoma generally is evident in adult life, more frequently in men than in women, and in whites more often than in blacks or Asians; the lower extremity is the most common site of involvement (Figs. 95–60 and 95–61), followed by the upper extremity and retroperitoneum.[330] It typically involves deep fascia or skeletal muscle and only rarely is confined to the subcutis without fascial involvement.[370] It produces a mass of variable size with nonspecific radiologic features.[369] Infrequently, metaplastic bone and cartilage formation in the lesion is visible on conventional radiographs or CT; the resulting radiodense areas predominate at the periphery of the tumor, resembling the characteristics of myositis ossificans.[371, 559] In other instances, calcification is less organized and poorly defined.[369] Erosion of bone, periosteal reaction, and pathologic fractures can be observed. MR imaging features are not specific.[664, 665] Local recurrences and metastasis are encountered.[370, 581]

Histologically, five subtypes of malignant fibrous histiocytoma have been recognized: storiform-pleomorphic,

Text continued on page 4529

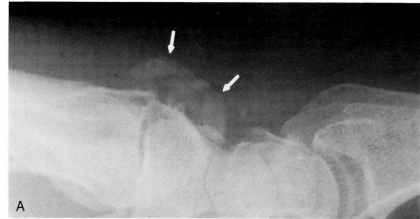

FIGURE 95–51. Ganglion.

A An unusual example of a calcified ganglion in the dorsum of the hand (arrows) is shown.

B A photomicrograph (80×) reveals the cystic wall of a ganglion, consisting of adipose and fibrous tissue. The surface layer is composed of flat lining cells.

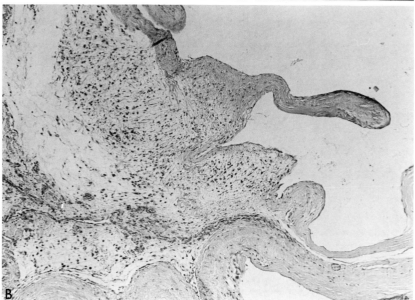

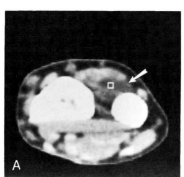

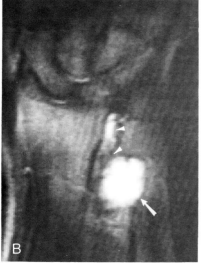

FIGURE 95–52. Ganglion. A 6 week history of a slightly painful mass in the extensor surface of the left forearm occurred in a 32 year old man. Ultrasonography (not shown) documented a cystic lesion, and a bone scan (not shown) was negative.

A On the transaxial CT scan, an ovoid lucent mass (arrow) dorsal to the distal portions of the radius and ulna is seen.

B The T2-weighted (TR/TE, 2000/80) coronal MR image shows high signal intensity (arrow) and communication with the inferior radioulnar joint (arrowheads). At surgery, a ganglion 2 cm in maximum dimension deep to the extensor muscles and abutting on the interosseous membrane communicated with the inferior radioulnar articulation.

(Courtesy of G. Greenway, M.D., Dallas, Texas.)

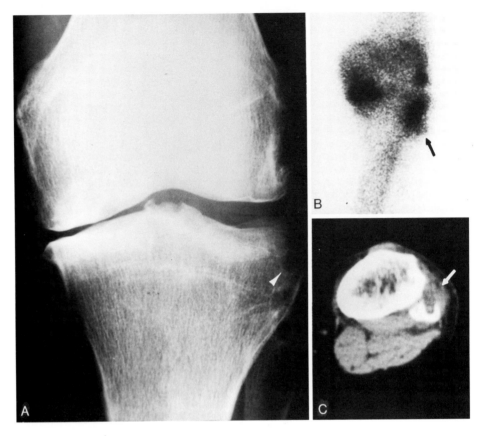

FIGURE 95–53. Ganglion. A 53 year old woman was referred for evaluation of a nonpainful mass in the lateral aspect of the knee with a preliminary diagnosis of soft tissue sarcoma.

A The initial radiograph shows osteoarthritis affecting mainly the medial femorotibial compartment and erosion of the tibia (arrowhead) and fibular head.

B A bone scan reveals abnormal accumulation of the radiotracer in the lesion (arrow) as well as in areas affected by osteoarthritis.

C A transaxial CT scan demonstrates the mass (arrow) and the osseous erosion. At surgery, a cystic lesion, filled with gelatinous yellow material, was found.

(Courtesy of G. Greenway, M.D., Dallas, Texas.)

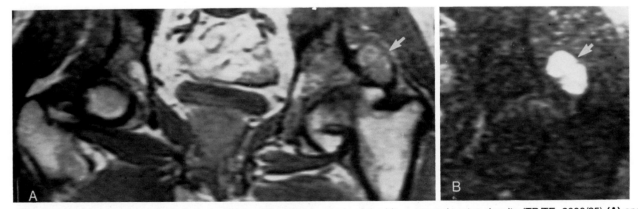

FIGURE 95–54. Ganglion. In this adult patient with developmental dysplasia of the hip, a coronal proton density (TR/TE, 2000/25) **(A)** and T2-weighted (TR/TE, 2000/50) **(B)** spin echo MR images reveal the para-acetabular ganglion (arrow), of high signal intensity in **B,** and the dysplastic hip. (Courtesy of A. Chevrot, M.D., Paris, France.)

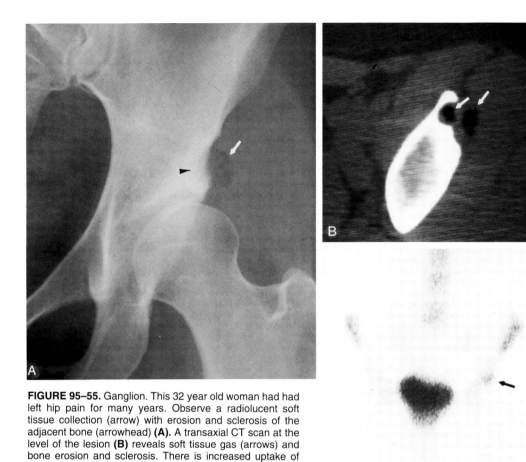

FIGURE 95–55. Ganglion. This 32 year old woman had had left hip pain for many years. Observe a radiolucent soft tissue collection (arrow) with erosion and sclerosis of the adjacent bone (arrowhead) **(A).** A transaxial CT scan at the level of the lesion **(B)** reveals soft tissue gas (arrows) and bone erosion and sclerosis. There is increased uptake of the bone-seeking radiopharmaceutical agent (arrow) **(C).** The imaging findings are virtually diagnostic of a ganglion, although this could not be proved as the patient refused surgery. (Courtesy of G. Greenway, M.D., Dallas, Texas.)

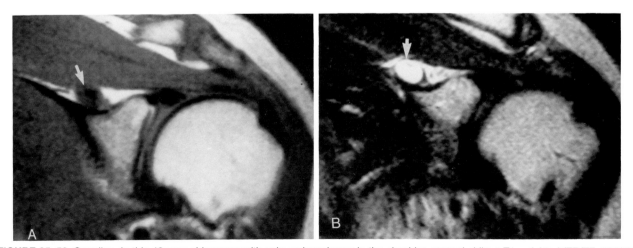

FIGURE 95–56. Ganglion. In this 43 year old woman with pain and weakness in the shoulder, coronal oblique T1-weighted (TR/TE, 560/20) **(A)** and T2-weighted (TR/TE, 1800/90) **(B)** spin echo MR images show a ganglion (arrows) in the suprascapular notch. Such ganglia are not rare, may be associated with tears of the glenoid labrum, and may produce an entrapment neuropathy involving portions of the suprascapular nerve (see Chapter 77).

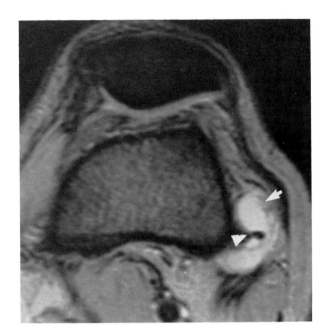

FIGURE 95–57. Ganglion. A periosteal ganglion adjacent to the lateral portion of the distal femur produced a local soft tissue mass in this 45 year old man. It is well shown on a transaxial multiplanar gradient recalled (MPGR) MR image (TR/TE, 267/15; flip angle, 25 degrees). Observe its high signal intensity (arrow) and subjacent bone proliferation (arrowhead).

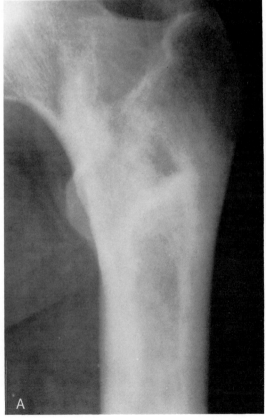

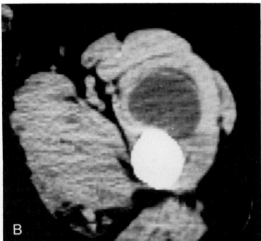

FIGURE 95–58. Myxoma and fibrous dysplasia. A 47 year old man with known polyostotic fibrous dysplasia developed a soft tissue mass in the anterior thigh. He had had a myxoma previously removed from the buttock.

A Routine radiography shows changes of fibrous dysplasia in the left femur.

B Transaxial CT reveals a well-defined intramuscular myxoma anterior to the involved portion of the femur. It has low attenuation. Note obliteration of the medullary cavity of the adjacent bone.

(Courtesy of M. Pathria, M.D., San Diego, California.)

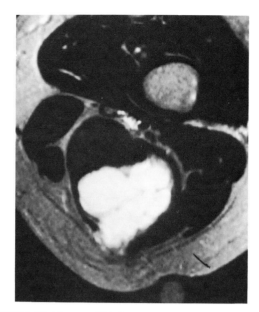

FIGURE 95–59. Myxoma. This intramuscular myxoma of the posterior thigh occurring in a 33 year old woman with fibrous dysplasia is well circumscribed and displays high signal intensity on a transaxial T2-weighted (TR/TE, 2200/90) spin echo MR image. (Courtesy of R. Stiles, M.D., Atlanta, Georgia.)

myxoid (myxofibrosarcoma), giant cell (malignant giant cell tumor of soft parts), inflammatory (xanthosarcoma, malignant xanthrogranuloma), and angiomatoid.[330] In general, they all possess similar clinical features with the following exceptions: the inflammatory malignant fibrous histiocytoma usually is located in the retroperitoneum and rarely in the extremities; and the angiomatoid malignant fibrous his-

tiocytoma frequently is seen in persons below the age of 20 years and is characterized by a less aggressive course (Fig. 95–62).[330, 378]

A more benign variety, the *fibrous histiocytoma,* occurs in adults and children and can lead to painful soft tissue masses (Fig. 95–63),[666] even in the fingers and toes[69, 70] (Fig. 95–64).

Xanthomatoses consist of a group of tumor-like proliferations characterized by the presence of a variable number of foam cells.[20] Some of the tumors are associated with metabolic and endocrine disorders, such as hypercholesterolemia and diabetes mellitus[74–77] (see Chapter 61). Many varieties are recognized (Fig. 95–65). *Tendinous xanthomas* are common about the fingers, heel, elbow, and knee, where they may erode subjacent bone. Calcification appears in 20 to 25 per cent of cases. CT[686] and MR imaging[687–689] have been used to study such xanthomas (Figs. 95–66 and 95–67); the latter method typically shows thickened tendons with heterogeneous signal intensity including regions of low signal intensity on T2-weighted spin echo MR images. A *fibrous xanthoma* (xanthofibroma) represents a small thickening of the corium covered by an intact epidermis (Fig. 95–68). Other types include *dermatofibrosarcoma protuberans,* located in the skin and deeper tissues, especially in the trunk and proximal portions of the extremities, which may grow to considerable size, recur, and rarely metastasize; *Bednar tumor,* which resembles dermatofibrosarcoma protuberans but possesses melanin pigment[330]; *sclerosing hemangioma,* which is a vascular lesion frequently found in the skin (Fig. 95–69); and *giant cell tumor of the tendon sheath,* which is detected in the hands and feet, attached to tendons, tendon sheaths, and fibrous capsules[291] (Figs. 95–70 to 95–72) (see later discussion in this chapter and Chapter 84). Rarely, *intraosseous xanthomas*

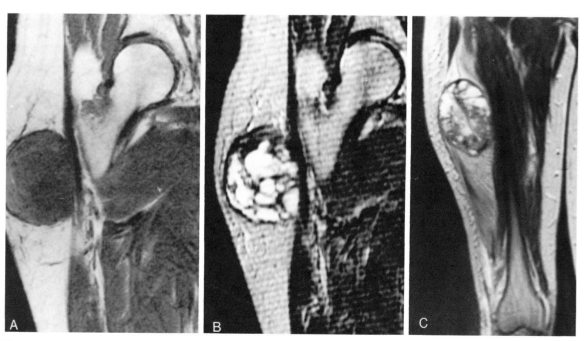

FIGURE 95–60. Malignant fibrous histiocytoma.

A, B In this 66 year old woman, a mass lateral to the proximal femur is located mainly in the subcutaneous tissue but also involves the fascia. It is well circumscribed and of low signal intensity on a coronal T1-weighted (TR/TE, 600/17) spin echo MR image **(A)** and of mixed signal intensity on a coronal T2-weighted (TR/TE, 2000/80) spin echo MR image **(B)**. In **B,** note linear foci of low signal intensity.

C In a 41 year old woman, a similar tumor is identified. Its signal intensity is inhomogeneous in a coronal T2-weighted (TR/TE, 3600/85) fast spin echo MR image. The appearance almost is identical to that in **B.** (**C,** Courtesy of M. Schweitzer, M.D., Philadelphia, Pennsylvania.)

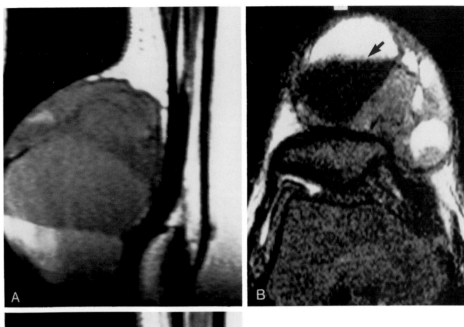

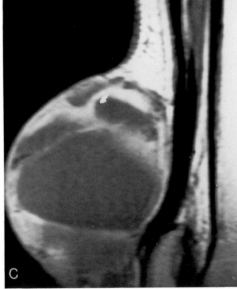

FIGURE 95–61. Malignant fibrous histiocytoma. A large soft tissue mass developed in the prepatellar region of a 57 year old man. On the sagittal T1-weighted (TR/TE, 886/15) spin echo MR image **(A)**, the mass reveals inhomogeneous signal intensity and lies in front of the quadriceps tendon and patella. A transaxial T2-weighted (TR/TE, 2700/80) spin echo MR image **(B)** again reveals signal inhomogeneity with a possible fluid level (arrow). Following the intravenous injection of gadolinium, a sagittal T1-weighted (TR/TE, 886/15) spin echo image **(C)** shows peripheral enhancement of signal intensity.

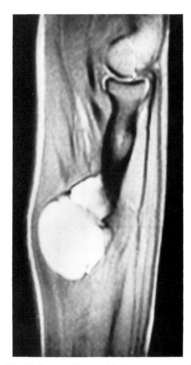

FIGURE 95–62. Malignant fibrous histiocytoma: Angiomatoid type. A 17 year old woman developed pain and swelling in the forearm of one month's duration. A sagittal T1-weighted (TR/TE, 450/11) spin echo MR image obtained with chemical presaturation (ChemSat) of fat reveals high signal intensity in the intramuscular tumor. At surgery, a blood-filled mass with a fibrous pseudocapsule was evident. (Courtesy of G. Greenway, M.D., Dallas, Texas.)

are recognized producing nonspecific, well-defined radiolucent lesions.

Angiomatoses

Angiomatoses are classified according to their tissue composition.[20] A *capillary hemangioma* is composed solely of capillaries. This tumor is common, usually appearing early in life in the skin or subcutaneous tissue. It sometimes is divided into three forms: juvenile hemangioma (strawberry nevus), verrucous hemangioma, and cherry angioma (senile angioma).[330] If the capillaries are widely dilated, the

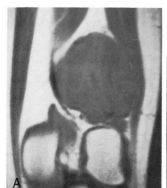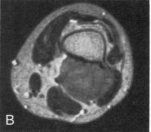

FIGURE 95–63. Fibrous histiocytoma. A 26 year old woman presented with a painful mass behind the knee. It is smooth and well marginated and shows predominantly low signal intensity on a coronal T1-weighted (TR/TE, 680/21) spin echo MR image **(A)** and a transaxial T2-weighted (TR/TE, 2000/85) spin echo MR image **(B).**

tumor is called a *cavernous hemangioma.* If a vascular tumor has thicker walls and contains smooth muscle cells, it is called a *venous hemangioma.* This tumor is less frequent than the capillary hemangioma, and it predominates in children in the upper portion of the body.[330] It may be large, may involve deep structures, and, unlike the capillary hemangioma, does not regress.[330] Capillary hemangiomas with prominent proliferation of the endothelial layer are called *benign hemangioendotheliomas,* whereas those with proliferation of pericytes are *benign hemangiopericytomas.*

The most recognized variety of benign hemangiopericytomas is the *glomus tumor.* This tumor is uncommon, occurs with equal frequency in men and women, and usually is detected in adults. It typically is located beneath the fingernail (subungual glomus tumor), leading to prominent symptoms that appear out of proportion to the size of the lesion (usually less than 1 cm)[330]; radiographs may reveal an eccentric intraosseous lucent lesion or cortical erosion in the terminal phalanx (Fig. 95–73). Ultrasonography reveals hypoechoic masses,[690] and MR images reveal nodules of low signal intensity on T1-weighted spin echo images and of high signal intensity on T2-weighted images[691] (Fig. 95–74). Less frequent sites of involvement include the palm, wrist, forearm, foot, eyelid, and chest wall as well as intraosseous locations, such as the metacarpal and phalangeal bones, ulna,[692] and patella.[330] Solitary tumors predominate but multiple lesions occasionally are encountered, especially in children. Recurrence of the tumor is rare, and malignant transformation is reportable.

Other benign types of angiomatoses are the *cirsoid aneurysm,* a vascular malformation consisting of arterial vessels; the *venous racemose aneurysm,* a malformation consisting of venous structures; *diffuse angiomatosis* due to capillary proliferation; a *lymphangioma,* a proliferation of lymphatic vessels; and *lymphangiopericytomas.* Syndromes associated with some of these vascular lesions include the *Kasabach-Merritt syndrome* (see Chapter 63), the *blue rubber bleb nevus syndrome* (blue cutaneous cavernous hemangiomas commonly associated with hemangiomas of the gastrointestinal tract),[379, 534, 667] *cystic hygroma* (hugely dilated lymphatic spaces occurring most typically in the neck with possible extension into the mediastinum and pleural spaces and in the axilla, in which osteolysis or bone hypertrophy may be present),[709, 710] and *Maffucci's syndrome* (multiple hemangiomas and enchondromas that may undergo malignant transformation).

Radiographs of hemangiomas and related lesions may reveal evidence of soft tissue masses containing circular calcified collections, termed phleboliths; in addition, osseous involvement, overgrowth, and articular abnormalities, especially in the knee, due to accompanying synovial lesions may be encountered[78–81, 693–696] (Figs. 95–75 and 95–76) (see Chapter 63). Arteriography may allow precise documentation of the pattern of vascular proliferation.

The evaluation of soft tissue, muscular, and synovial hemangiomas has been accomplished with MR imaging.[560, 612, 697–703] With regard to intramuscular hemangioma (Fig. 95–77), the lesion typically is poorly marginated and isointense relative to skeletal muscle on T1-weighted MR images; within the lesion on such images are delicate or coarse strands or bands that contain areas with signal intensity identical to that of fat.[612] On T2-weighted MR images, intramuscular hemangiomas are well marginated and hyper-

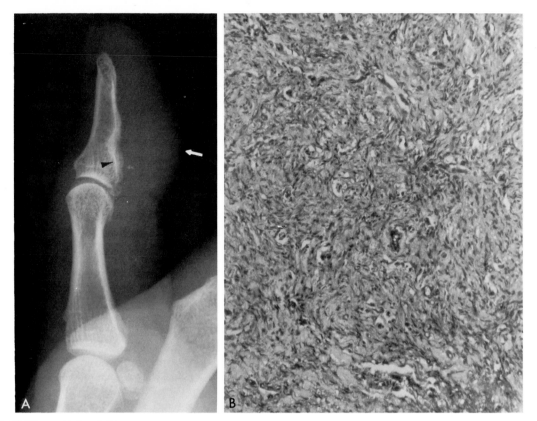

FIGURE 95–64. Fibrous histiocytoma.

A This 44 year old woman had developed a mass on her thumb over a 1 year period. Biopsy revealed a fibrous histiocytoma. Note the soft tissue mass on the volar surface of the thumb (arrow), with underlying periosteal bone formation (arrowhead).

B Histologic examination of a fibrous histiocytoma of the skin reveals bundles of collagen arranged in multiple directions with entrapped fat. The nuclei of the connective tissue cells are small and spindly, and the cells have relatively sparse cytoplasm (215×).

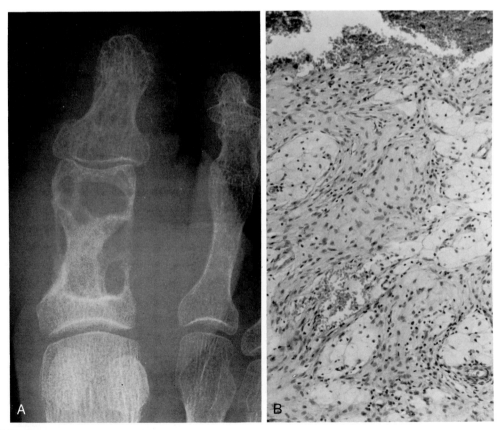

FIGURE 95–65. Xanthoma.

A In this patient with cerebrotendinous xanthomatosis, note the large soft tissue mass with invasion of the proximal phalanx of the great toe.

B Xanthomatous change, related to old hemorrhage, is revealed on this photomicrograph (200×).

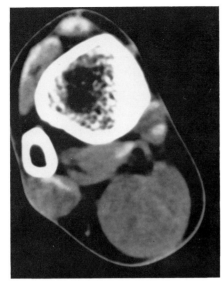

FIGURE 95–66. Xanthoma: Tendinous involvement. In this patient with cerebrotendinous xanthomatosis, multiple tendons including the peroneus and Achilles tendons are enlarged. Observe the smooth contour of the latter tendon, with inhomogeneous attenuation. (Courtesy of C. Chen, M.D., Kaohsiung, Taiwan.)

intense compared with subcutaneous fat and may contain segments that are isointense relative to fat or muscle. On either type of image, foci of low signal intensity representing phleboliths may be evident. Some types of intramuscu-

lar hemangiomas, particularly cavernous hemangiomas, contain large amounts of fatty tissue such that their MR imaging characteristics may be indistinguishable from those of a lipoma.[612] Serpentine areas within the hemangiomas can provide diagnostic aid[699] (Fig. 95–78). Masses of large tortuous vessels that are accompanied by rapidly flowing blood, which may be found in hemangiomas or arteriovenous malformations (Fig. 95–79), are characterized by regions of signal void.[697, 701, 711, 712] Deep and superficial extramuscular hemangiomas, as well as synovial hemangiomas, have similar MR imaging features.[701] Some variations in these features reflect modifications in the amounts of nonvascular tissue, which include fat, fibrous tissue, myxoid stroma, smooth muscle, hemosiderin, bone, and thrombus.[703] In some cases, fluid levels reflecting the presence of blood-filled cavities are seen on MR images (or CT scans),[969] although the finding is not specific, being evident in other soft tissue tumors as well.

On the malignant end of the spectrum, angiosarcomatoses are much less frequent. These lesions are classified according to the dominant cell pattern.[20] If endothelial cells predominate, a *malignant hemangioendothelioma* is present.[705] With pericytic proliferation, a *malignant hemangiopericytoma* is found.[704] A malignant tumor composed of lymphatic endothelioblasts frequently associated with lymphedema is termed a *lymphangiosarcoma* (see Fig. 95–166). This situation typically arises in women who have undergone radical mastectomies for carcinoma of the breast

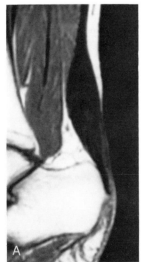

FIGURE 95–67. Xanthoma: Tendinous involvement. In a 45 year old woman, a sagittal T1-weighted (TR/TE, 600/12) spin echo MR image **(A)** shows fusiform enlargement of the Achilles tendon, which is of low signal intensity. A transaxial T2-weighted (TR/TE, 3600/102) fast spin echo MR image **(B)** reveals bilateral involvement of the Achilles tendon. The signal intensity of the involved tendons is low and homogeneous. A transaxial T1-weighted (TR/TE, 650/12) spin echo MR image obtained with chemical presaturation (ChemSat) of fat **(C)** shows inhomogeneity of signal intensity in both Achilles tendons. (Courtesy of M. Weisman, M.D., San Diego, California.)

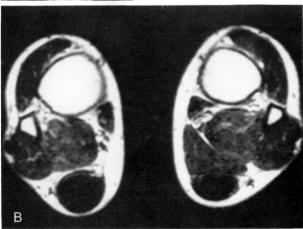

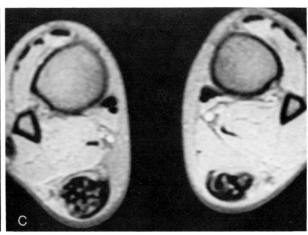

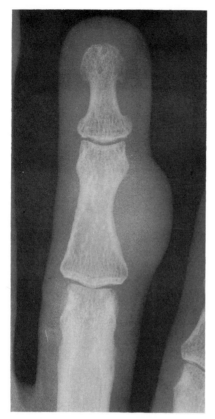

FIGURE 95–68. Fibrous xanthoma. A soft tissue mass adjacent to the middle phalanx has produced erosion of the adjacent bone. This pattern of bony resorption is indicative of pressure atrophy and is not a sign of malignancy.

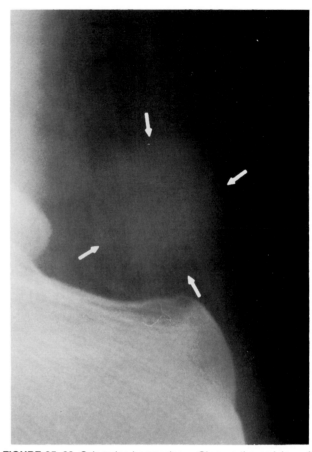

FIGURE 95–69. Sclerosing hemangioma. Observe the nodular soft tissue mass adjacent to the Achilles tendon (arrows).

and who develop chronic and severe lymphedema (Stewart-Treves syndrome).[380, 381, 706, 707] Lymphangiosarcomas (or angiosarcomas) less commonly complicate congenital, traumatic, or idiopathic lymphedema and are rare in cases of filarial lymphedema.[330, 708]

Kaposi's sarcoma is a complex vascular growth consisting of both capillaries and fibrosarcoma-like cells.[82–86, 382, 383] This lesion predominates in adult men and in persons with acquired immunodeficiency syndrome, and is especially common in blacks in certain parts of Africa. Cutaneous eruptions or nodules, frequently in the lower extremity, may lead to invasion of underlying bone (Fig. 95–80). Some patients also reveal evidence of malignant lymphoma, lymphatic leukemia, diabetes mellitus, and varicosities. The pathogenesis of Kaposi's sarcoma is not known.[307] Some investigators regard it as a neoplasm, whereas others suggest that it is a vascular or infectious process. The prognosis is guarded, especially in African patients; the survival time after diagnosis ranges from 5 to 20 years. Although individual lesions may heal, recurrences are the rule.

Cartilaginous and Osseous Tumors

Soft tissue *chondromas* are rare.[87, 561, 562, 952] The tumors occur predominantly in the third and fourth decades of life, especially in the hands and feet, although similar chondromas have been identified in the back,[713] mediastinum,[714] and other sites. They enlarge slowly and are well demarcated and lobulated. Radiographs reveal soft tissue masses frequently containing curvilinear, ringlike, or nodular calcifi-

cation (Fig. 95–81A). Subjacent cortical erosion and sclerosis may simulate the findings in a juxtacortical (periosteal) chondroma (Fig. 95–81B). Although local recurrences can be seen, metastasis is not evident, and the prognosis is good. Histologically, soft tissue chondromas show diver-

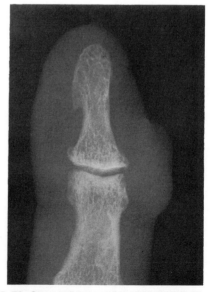

FIGURE 95–70. Giant cell tumor of tendon sheath. The soft tissue mass about the distal interphalangeal joint in this 50 year old man represents a giant cell tumor of the tendon sheath.

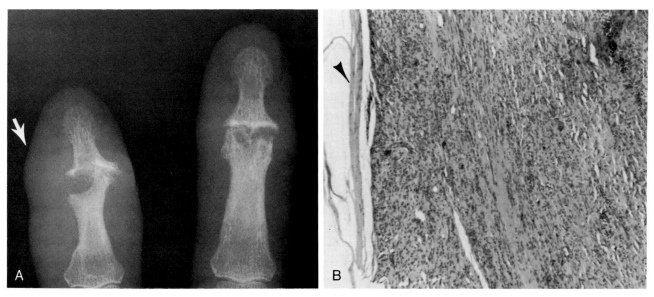

FIGURE 95–71. Giant cell tumor of tendon sheath.

A In a 55 year old woman with a 2 year history of pain and gradual swelling of the fingers, a soft tissue mass (arrow) can be identified about one distal interphalangeal joint. Underlying inflammatory osteoarthritis of the articulations is evident, and the combination of findings would suggest that the mass represents a mucous cyst. Biopsy of the affected joint demonstrated the findings of giant cell tumor of the tendon sheath. (From Crosby EB, et al: Radiology *122*:671, 1977.)

B A photomicrograph (86×) in a different case reveals a tendon capsule (arrowhead) with a tumor associated with moderately vascularized stroma, rather plump spindle-shaped or ovoid cells, and multinucleated giant cells.

FIGURE 95–72. Giant cell tumor of tendon sheath. The routine radiograph **(A)** reveals a soft tissue mass with involvement of the middle phalanx of the fourth toe. A T1-weighted (TR/TE, 400/15) transverse spin echo MR image **(B)** shows the lobulated soft tissue mass (arrows) of low signal intensity and bone involvement. (Courtesy of P. Ellenbogen, M.D., Dallas, Texas.)

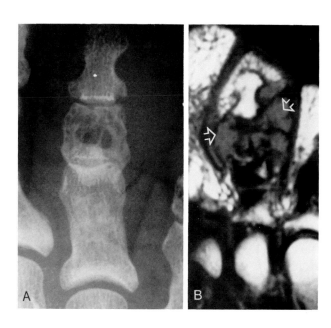

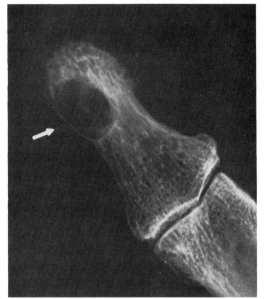

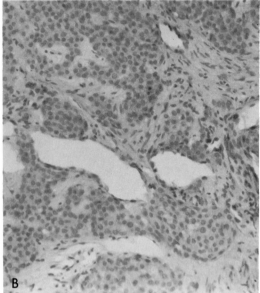

FIGURE 95–73. Glomus tumor.

A A well-defined cystic lesion of a terminal tuft is seen (arrow).

B A photomicrograph (215×) reveals multiple vascular channels surrounded by irregular extensions of cells with eosinophilic cytoplasm and bland, somewhat monotonous nuclei.

sity, containing areas of mature, lobulated hyaline cartilage that may be accompanied by fibrosis, myxoid change, calcification, or ossification. Occasionally, immature chondroblastic cells, resembling those of chondrosarcoma, are evident, and rarely lipoblast-like cells[715] or chondroblastoma-like cells[716] are noted.

An intracapsular chondroma (or osteochondroma) is a rare form of chondroma that most often arises in the knee, typically inferior to the patella[281, 563, 717] (Figs. 95–82 and 95–83). In this location, the lesion may attach to the meniscus, be located in the infrapatellar fat pad, and produce pain and locking of the joint.[293] The lesion may be a true tumor, although some of its histologic features are consistent with cartilaginous metaplasia of connective tissue in or around the joint capsule. Young adults usually are affected. Radiographs show a well circumscribed, partially or completely ossified mass that may erode the adjacent portions of patella and tibia. CT and MR imaging are useful in delineating the full extent of the process. Inhomogeneous signal intensity

characterizes the MR appearance of the intracapsular chondroma, and the patellar tendon may be displaced. This same lesion has been described as occurring in other sites; typically it is solitary, is often large, is partially or completely calcified, and may simulate a soft tissue chondrosarcoma

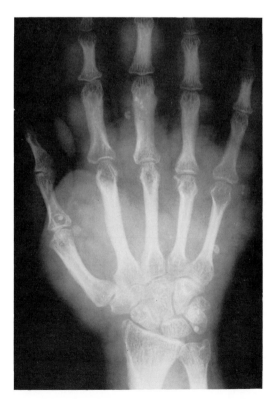

FIGURE 95–75. Hemangioma. Diffuse involvement of the hand is characterized by multiple soft tissue masses and phleboliths. This 28 year old man also had neurofibromatosis. An association of the latter condition and hemangiomatosis is recognized. (Courtesy of G. Greenway, M.D., Dallas, Texas.)

FIGURE 95–74. Glomus tumor. This subungual lesion (arrow) is of intense high signal on a transverse T2-weighted (TR/TE, 2000/80) spin echo MR image of the finger. (Courtesy of A. Deutsch, M.D., Los Angeles, California.)

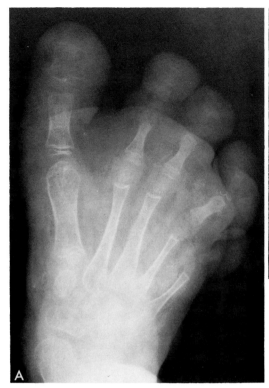

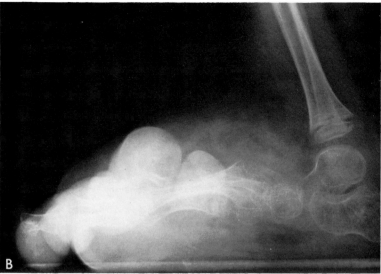

FIGURE 95–76. Lymphangioma. In this 4 year old boy, diffuse lymphangiomatosis of the tissues of the foot has produced nodular soft tissue enlargement. Osseous deformity also is present, but no phleboliths are apparent.

on radiographic examination. The designation of giant solitary synovial chondromatosis has been used.[971]

As extraskeletal chondromas commonly arise in close association with a tendon, tendon sheath, or joint capsule,[88, 89] the designation of *extra-articular synovial chondromatosis* or *tenosynovial chondromatosis* has been used to describe these lesions[384–387, 541, 718] (Fig. 95–84). Such chondromas should be differentiated from idiopathic (primary) synovial (osteo)chondromatosis (Fig. 95–85), in which metaplasia of the synovial lining in an articulation leads to numerous cartilaginous and osseous bodies (see later discussion and Chapter 84); idiopathic (primary) bursal (osteo)chondromatosis (Fig. 95–86), in which similar metaplasia occurs within a bursal sac that communicates with the joint; and secondary synovial (osteo)chondromatosis, in which an unrelated articular process is accompanied by disintegration of the joint surface, the production of one or more cartilaginous and osseous fragments, and irritation of the synovial membrane with its subsequent metaplasia. Tenosynovial chondromatosis usually is evident in the hand, wrist, foot, or, less frequently, knee. Synovial metaplasia arises in a tendon sheath, joint capsule, or extra-articular (noncommunicating) bursa, leading to cartilaginous nodules of variable size and number. A slowly enlarging smooth or lobulated mass (or, rarely, masses), containing multiple small calcified or ossified densities, develops either near a joint or at some distance from it. The resulting radiographic appearance is identical to that of a soft tissue chondroma; it is the histologic verification of a synovial origin that allows the differentiation of the two lesions. In some cases, both cartilage and fatty elements are present in the mass, suggesting the diagnosis of *tenosynovial lipochondromatosis*.[719] Furthermore, the occurrence of atypical and commonly bizarre chondrocytes in cases of tenosynovial chondromatosis can foster an incorrect diagnosis, such

as chondrosarcoma, unless the synovial site of initiation of the lesion is recognized. The facts that all evidence of the synovial origin may be obscured by the enlarging process in some cases of tenosynovial chondromatosis and that such masses may recur following surgery lead to further diagnostic difficulty.

Extraskeletal osteochondromas (see Fig. 95–81C) represent lesions that clinically and radiologically simulate soft tissue chondromas, tenosynovial chondromatosis, and soft tissue osteomas (see later discussion). Histologically, mature hyaline cartilage with extensive ossification is seen.[720] The typical presentation is that of an enlarging ossifying mass in the foot, hand, or wrist in an adult.[751] The existence of this lesion as a distinct entity is debated.

Idiopathic synovial (osteo)chondromatosis, discussed in Chapter 84, is an unusual condition involving joints with or without extension into nearby bursae. It results from metaplasia of subsynovial connective tissue into cartilage nodules that subsequently may calcify or ossify. The metaplastic or active stage of the disease may be self-limiting followed by an inactive stage in which the synovial membrane is quiescent. The cause of the condition is not clear. Familial cases have been reported but are rare.[721] Indeed, some investigators believe that the synovial metaplasia is a secondary phenomenon; the release of cartilage and chondrocytes into the synovial fluid of a joint may be followed by the uptake of such bodies by the synovial membrane and subsequent metaplasia.[722]

The clinical onset of idiopathic synovial (osteo)chondromatosis varies from childhood to the seventh or eighth decade of life, although most affected patients are young and middle-aged adults.[723, 724] The two most frequent sites of involvement are the knee and the hip, followed in descending order of frequency by the glenohumeral joint, elbow, and ankle. Any articulation may be involved, how-

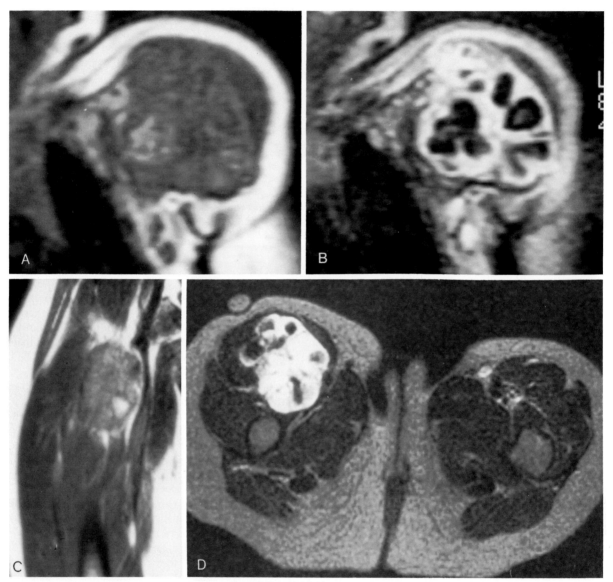

FIGURE 95–77. Hemangioma: Intramuscular type.

  A, B This hemangioma of the deltoid muscle in a 10 day old infant is characterized by inhomogeneous signal intensity on both the coronal proton density (TR/TE, 2000/30) **(A)** and T2-weighted (TR/TE, 2000/80) **(B)** spin echo MR images. In **B,** note lakelike foci of low signal intensity, perhaps representing areas of rapidly flowing blood. (Courtesy of T. Broderick, M.D., Orange, California.)

  C, D A hemangioma in the quadriceps femoris muscle in a three year old girl is inhomogeneous in signal intensity on the coronal T1-weighted (TR/TE, 800/20) **(C)** and the transaxial T2-weighted (TR/TE, 2000/80) **(D)** spin echo MR images. In **D,** foci of low signal intensity are consistent with areas of rapidly flowing blood. At surgery, a large vascular mass surrounded the femoral nerve. (Courtesy of G. Greenway, M.D., Dallas, Texas.)

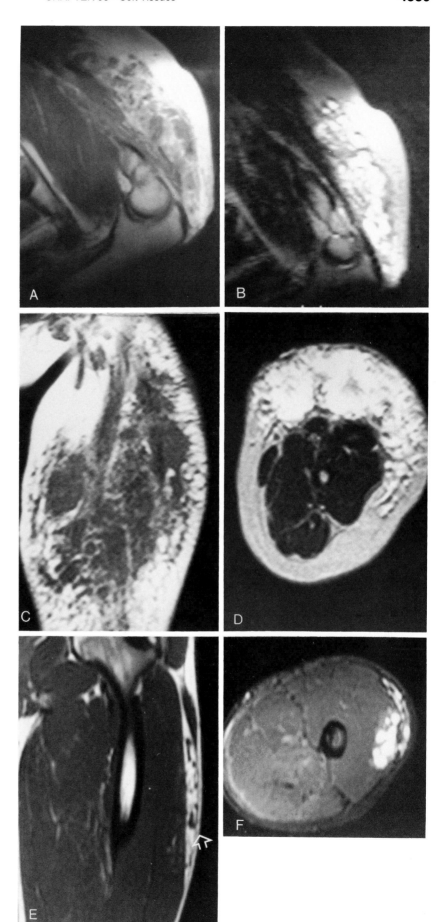

FIGURE 95–78. Hemangioma: Superficial type.

A, B In this 53 year old woman, a mass in the posterior aspect of the elbow had been present for several years. It was blue and nontender. A sagittal T1-weighted (TR/TE, 450/27) spin echo MR image **(A)** shows a nodular and serpentine mass of low signal intensity in the subcutaneous fat. On a sagittal T2-weighted (TR/TE, 2200/120) spin echo MR image **(B),** the lesion now is of high signal intensity. (Courtesy of G. Greenway, M.D., Dallas, Texas.)

C, D In this child, a superficial hemangioma in the thigh appears septated with nodular and linear regions. It is of low signal intensity on the coronal T1-weighted (TR/TE, 700/30) spin echo MR image **(C)** and of high signal intensity on the transaxial T2-weighted (TR/TE, 1800/100) spin echo MR image **(D).** (Courtesy of T. Mattsson, M.D., Riyadh, Saudi Arabia.)

E, F In a 19 year old man, a superficial hemangioma in the thigh is of low signal intensity (arrow) on the coronal T1-weighted (TR/TE, 500/20) spin echo MR image **(E)** and of high signal intensity on the short tau inversion recovery (STIR) transaxial image (TR/TE, 2000/40; inversion time, 140 msec).

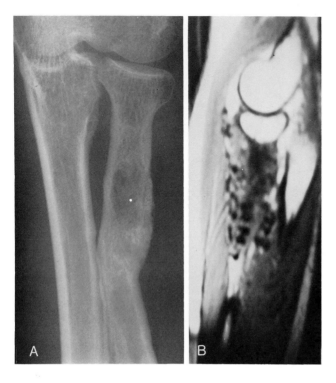

FIGURE 95–79. Arteriovenous malformation. An arteriovenous malformation developed after a radial fracture in a 31 year old woman. The routine radiograph **(A)** shows a deformed proximal radius with areas of osteolysis related to pressure erosion of bone. A sagittal T1-weighted (TR/TE, 600/20) spin echo MR image **(B)** shows tortuous vessels of low signal intensity.

ever, including the wrist, acromioclavicular and sternoclavicular joints, costovertebral joints, proximal tibiofibular articulation, small joints of the hand and feet, and temporomandibular joint.[725–731] Monoarticular disease is the rule but, rarely, more than one joint is affected. Extension of the process from the articulation to a nearby and often communicating bursa is recognized most frequently in the knee[732] and hip[733] but also may occur in the wrist, elbow, glenohumeral joint, and ankle. This phenomenon should be distinguished from involvement of the bursa alone (i.e., idiopathic bursal osteochondromatosis). Similarly, the process may extend from a joint to a surrounding tendon sheath. The clinical manifestations of idiopathic synovial (osteo)chondromatosis include pain, swelling, a mass, and restriction of joint motion. These findings may be profound, requiring operative or arthroscopic intervention designed to remove diseased synovium and any free intra-articular bodies.[734–736]

The radiographic features of this condition also are variable. Classically, idiopathic synovial (osteo)chondromatosis has been reported to produce multiple calcified or ossified bodies of approximately equal size scattered throughout the involved joint with little evidence of joint space narrowing, bone erosion, or osteoporosis (Fig. 95–85). Unfortunately, this classic appearance often is not encountered. First, in cases of synovial chondromatosis, there is no evidence of calcification or ossification, the purely cartilaginous bodies being undetectable by routine radiographic techniques. In such cases, conventional arthrography, computed arthrotomography, or MR imaging (see later discussion) is more diagnostic. In some instances of synovial (osteo)chondromatosis, the degree of calcification and ossification is limited, is not seen with routine radiography, and requires CT or computed arthrotomography for detection.[723, 737, 738] The calcification or ossification may appear as bodies in the joint lumen or as linear collections in the synovial membrane. Second, bone erosion is encountered,

especially in "tight" joints such as the hip[724] and wrist but also elsewhere. Typically, pressure defects at the articular margins are apparent, which can lead to pathologic fracture and are identical to those produced by pigmented villonodular synovitis. Typical sites for such erosion are the femoral neck, acetabular fossa, and humeral head and proximal metaphysis. Third, subchondral cysts also may be seen, again particularly about the hip.[739] Fourth, joint space loss occasionally is prominent. Usually, it is diffuse, resembling the changes in rheumatoid arthritis. Fifth, in cases of long duration and in which pain is prominent, periarticular osteoporosis is seen. In the hip, the resulting radiographic appearance resembles that of transient osteoporosis. Finally, subluxation of joints may be evident, presumably related to the synovial nodular proliferation, and it may lead to secondary osteoarthritis.[740]

MR imaging also has been used to investigate patients with idiopathic synovial (osteo)chondromatosis.[741–743, 970] The MR imaging abnormalities are dependent on the stage of the disease. In cases of synovial chondromatosis, in which intrasynovial cartilage nodules are uncalcified, the signal intensity of the process resembles that of fluid, being low on T1-weighted spin echo MR images and high on T2-weighted spin echo MR images (Fig. 95–87), and the condition may be misdiagnosed as a joint effusion. In cases of synovial (osteo)chondromatosis, foci of calcification appear as regions of low signal intensity on both T1- and T2-weighted images (Fig. 95–88), and with extensive calcification and ossification, ringlike structures with peripheral rims of low signal intensity and central regions of higher signal intensity identical to that of fat or cartilage are seen.

Synovial chondrosarcoma is extremely rare.[744–748, 973] The lesion may occur as a primary process or, more commonly, secondary to idiopathic synovial (osteo)chondromatosis. Adults are affected, and the knee and hip most commonly are involved. When synovial chondrosarcoma is superimposed on idiopathic synovial (osteo)chondromatosis, the

Text continued on page 4547

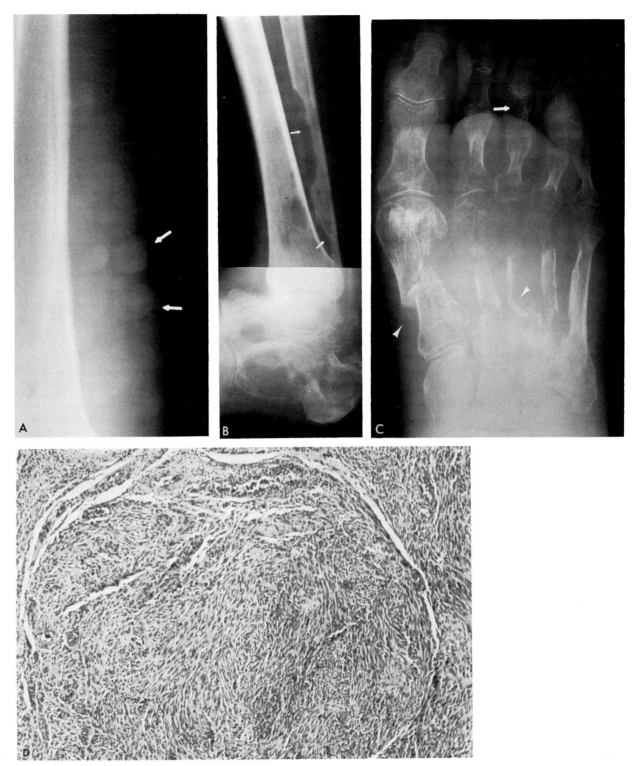

FIGURE 95–80. Kaposi's sarcoma.

A Nodular lesions of the soft tissues (arrows) are apparent.

B, C This 77 year old man with Kaposi's sarcoma reveals lytic destruction of the tibia, fibula, tarsals, metatarsals, and phalanges. Observe the eccentric location of many of the erosions (arrows) and pathologic fractures (arrowheads). (Courtesy of P. Ellenbogen, M.D., Dallas, Texas.)

D A photomicrograph (90×, 230×) demonstrates nodular masses composed of whorled spindle cells with occasional slits and vascular clefts. Cellular atypism and hemosiderin pigmentation are noted.

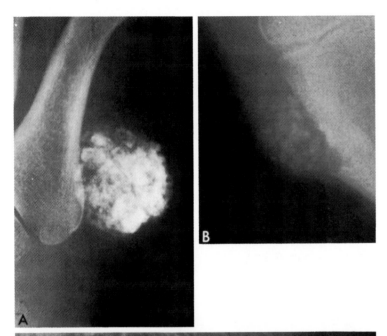

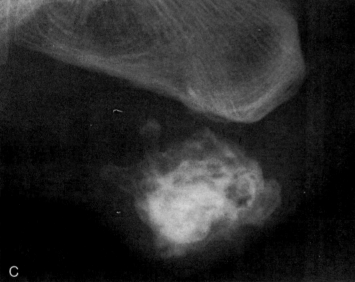

FIGURE 95–81. Chondroma and osteochondroma.

A Soft tissue chondroma. Observe the calcified soft tissue mass adjacent to the base of the fifth metatarsal bone.

B Juxtacortical (periosteal) chondroma. This 8 year old boy had a lump below the knee. A radiograph reveals a partially calcified and ossified soft tissue mass in the region of the anterior tibial tubercle. Minimal erosion of the cortex is seen. (From Kirchner SJ, et al: Am J Roentgenol *131*:1088, 1978. Copyright 1978, American Roentgen Ray Society.)

C Soft tissue osteochondroma. Note the irregularly calcified or ossified lesion beneath the calcaneus. (Courtesy of M. Dalinka, M.D., Philadelphia, Pennsylvania.)

FIGURE 95–82. Intracapsular chondroma. In this 55 year old man, a mass developed below the patella that interfered with his swinging of a golf club. The routine radiograph **(A)** reveals an ossified mass below the patella within the infrapatellar fat body. A sagital T1-weighted (TR/TE, 500/20) spin echo MR image **(B)** shows a mass of inhomogeneous but mainly low signal intensity displacing the patellar tendon. It had inhomogeneous high signal intensity on T2-weighted spin echo MR images (not shown). It was excised easily. (Courtesy of B. Sosnow, M.D., Phoenix, Arizona.)

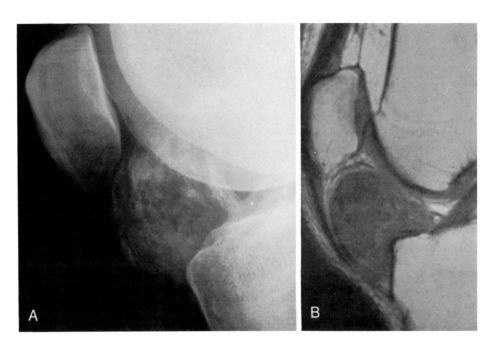

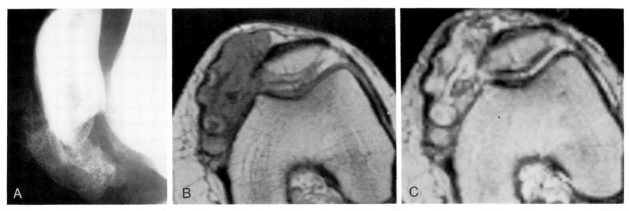

FIGURE 95–83. Intracapsular chondroma. A mass developed below the patella in a 40 year old woman. With routine radiography **(A),** the mass is seen to be ossified. Transaxial T1-weighted (TR/TE, 750/24) **(B)** and T2-weighted (TR/TE, 2000/80) **(C)** spin echo MR images show a lobulated soft tissue mass medial to the patella with distortion of the retinaculum. The mass is of inhomogeneous signal intensity, although its signal intensity is increased in **C.** Some of the signal intensity characteristics are those of fat, indicative of ossification with the presence of marrow. (Courtesy of A. Newberg, M.D., Boston, Massachusetts.)

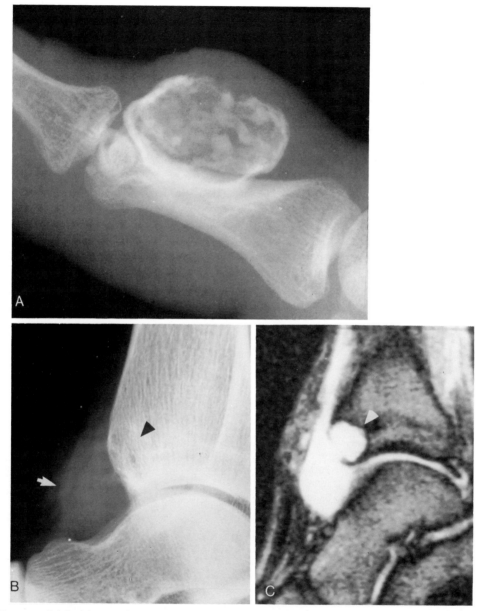

FIGURE 95–84. Tenosynovial chondromatosis.

A Note a partially ossified mass adjacent to the dorsal surface of the proximal phalanx of the thumb. Smooth erosion of the cortex of the phalanx is evident.

B, C In this 30 year old man, a mass in the anterior portion of the ankle limited dorsiflexion of the joint. Routine radiography **(B)** shows a soft tissue mass (arrow) with bone erosion (arrowhead) and spiculated bone reaction. A sagittal multiplanar gradient recalled (MPGR) MR image (TR/TE, 1000/30; flip angle, 28 degrees) **(C)** reveals high signal intensity in the mass and along the anterior surface of the tibia and bone erosion (arrowhead). Surgery confirmed that the lesion, composed of gelatinous material, was attached to the tibia and the anterior capsule of the ankle joint. (Courtesy of G. Greenway, M.D., Dallas, Texas.)

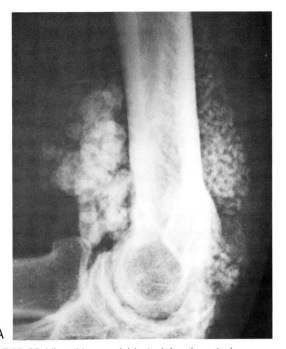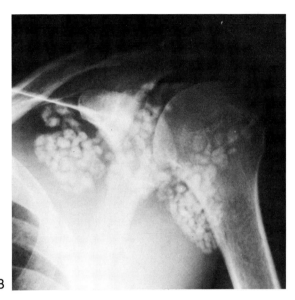

FIGURE 95–85. Idiopathic synovial (osteo)chondromatosis.
A, B Two examples are shown. Observe the uniform size of the radiodense collections, their confinement to the joint cavity, and the relative absence of additional articular abnormalities. (**B,** Courtesy of J. Slivka, M.D., San Diego, California.)

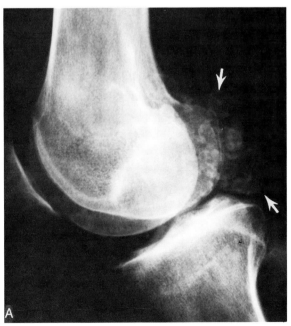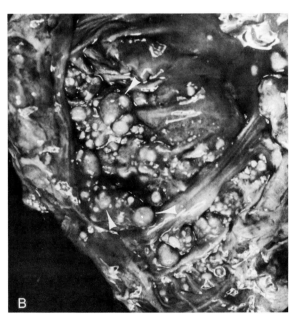

FIGURE 95–86. Idiopathic bursal (osteo)chondromatosis. On the radiograph **(A),** virtually all of the osseous bodies are confined to the area of a small popliteal cyst (arrows). Grossly **(B),** in such cases, osteocartilaginous nodules (arrowheads) are found in the synovial membrane and free in the bursal sac.

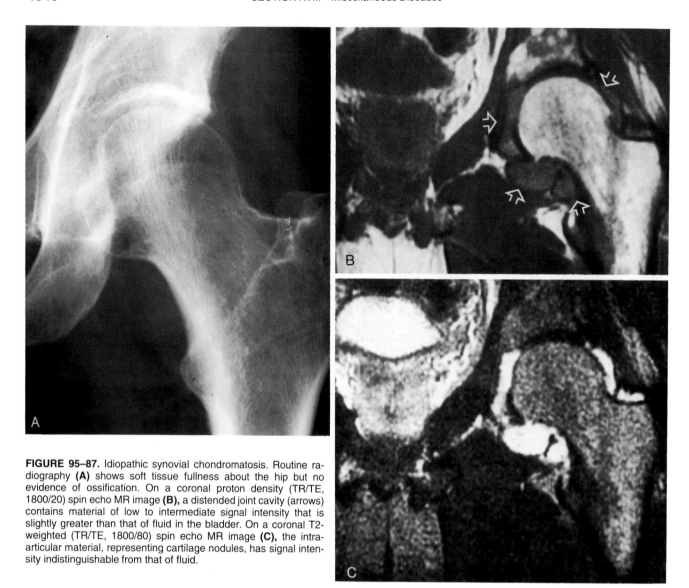

FIGURE 95–87. Idiopathic synovial chondromatosis. Routine radiography **(A)** shows soft tissue fullness about the hip but no evidence of ossification. On a coronal proton density (TR/TE, 1800/20) spin echo MR image **(B),** a distended joint cavity (arrows) contains material of low to intermediate signal intensity that is slightly greater than that of fluid in the bladder. On a coronal T2-weighted (TR/TE, 1800/80) spin echo MR image **(C),** the intra-articular material, representing cartilage nodules, has signal intensity indistinguishable from that of fluid.

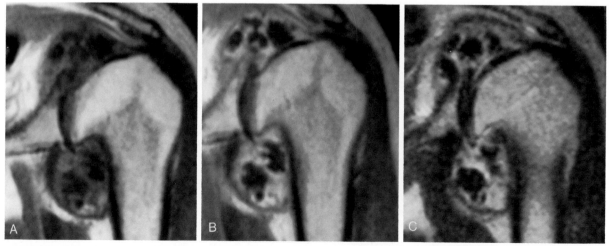

FIGURE 95–88. Idiopathic synovial (osteo)chondromatosis. Coronal oblique T1-weighted (TR/TE, 570/25) **(A),** intravenous gadolinium-enhanced T1-weighted (TR/TE, 570/25) **(B),** and T2-weighted (TR/TE, 1800/80) **(C)** spin echo MR images show a distended glenohumeral joint containing fluid of high signal intensity in **B** and **C** and calcified and ossified bodies of low signal intensity in all three images. (Courtesy of C. Ho, M.D., San Francisco, California.)

FIGURE 95–89. Synovial chondrosarcoma. This 65 year old man had had knee swelling for 15 years. A synovial chondrosarcoma had been documented at surgery more than 10 years previously, although the patient refused to undergo amputation of the limb at that time.

A A lateral radiograph of the knee shows an irregularly calcified soft tissue mass behind the knee.

B A sagittal T2-weighted (TR/TE, 2500/90) spin echo MR image reveals the extra-articular and intra-articular components of the tumor. Its signal intensity is inhomogeneous, although in places it is encapsulated. A resection of the mass confirmed the diagnosis of a low grade synovial chondrosarcoma.

(Courtesy of J. Hodler, M.D., Zurich, Switzerland.)

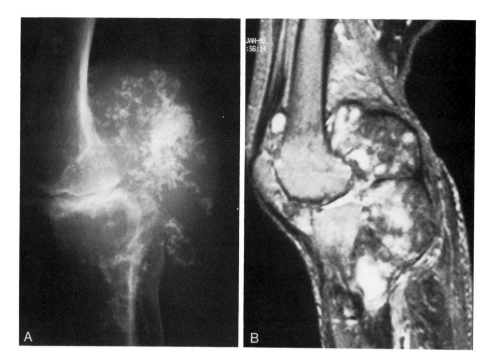

latter disorder generally has been present for many years. An intra-articular mass, often heavily calcified, is evident, and it may extend beyond the limits of the joint (Fig. 95–89). The pattern of calcification may be more irregular than that associated with idiopathic synovial (osteo)chondromatosis, and a poorly marginated mass with inhomogeneous signal intensity may be evident with MR imaging. Distant metastases, including pulmonary foci, may develop.

Extraskeletal soft tissue chondrosarcomas also are very uncommon.[90–93, 388, 582, 953, 954] These lesions are distinguished from those arising in a bone or in the periosteum and perichondrium. The soft tissues of the head and neck, extremities, shoulders, and buttocks typically are affected. Histologic features vary from well-differentiated cartilage proliferation to myxoid or mesenchymal elements.[306, 749, 750] The extraskeletal myxoid chondrosarcoma also is designated as a chordoid sarcoma, and it usually is observed in

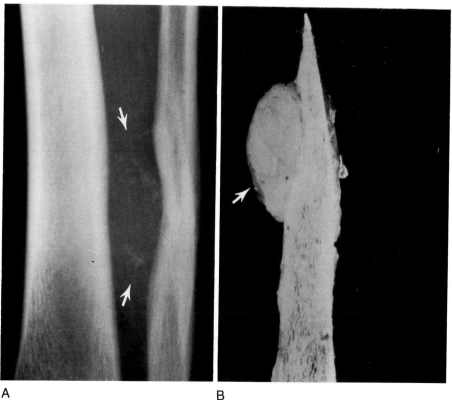

FIGURE 95–90. Chondrosarcoma. This 15 year old boy complained of swelling and pain. The radiograph **(A)** reveals a soft tissue mass with calcification (arrows) between the tibia and fibula, with erosion of both bones. Note buttressing or thickening of the outer aspect of the fibula. A photograph of a longitudinal section of the fibula **(B)** demonstrates the relationship of the mass to the bone (arrow). The final diagnosis was mesenchymal chondrosarcoma.

(Courtesy of R. Freiberger, M.D., New York, New York, and J. Kaye, M.D., New York, New York.)

middle-aged and elderly patients, especially in the thigh and popliteal fossa; the extraskeletal mesenchymal chondrosarcoma is more frequent in young adults, particularly women, and in the region of the head and neck, especially the cranial and spinal dura mater, the orbit, and the occipital portion of the neck.[330] It also may arise in an irradiated area. In either type of chondrosarcoma, a soft tissue mass with calcification and underlying osseous involvement can be detected radiographically (Fig. 95–90). Calcification is more typical of a mesenchymal than of a myxoid type of tumor.[749] CT can be used to further define the lesion and, in cases of mesenchymal chondrosarcoma, contrast-enhanced CT shows lobulation and peripheral tumoral enhancement, sometimes with central low attenuation areas.[750] In such cases, MR imaging reveals a soft tissue lesion of low signal intensity on T1-weighted spin echo MR images and high signal intensity on T2-weighted spin echo MR images and with regions of accentuated signal intensity following intravenous gadolinium administration[750] (Fig. 95–91). A similar MR imaging appearance is evident in cases of myxoid chondrosarcoma, although the signal intensity characteristics of this lesion appear to be more variable on the T1-weighted images.[974] The prognosis is variable; some lesions are highly aggressive, whereas others follow a more protracted course.

Osteomas arising in the skin are not rare, but, in most instances, this terminology is incorrect as the lesions represent bone metaplasia occurring in association with a variety of cutaneous processes, such as basal cell carcinoma, acne vulgaris, and surgical scars. True osteoma cutis is distinctly unusual, of unknown cause, and accompanied by soft tissue ossification of variable size.[389, 752] An association of this condition with pseudohypoparathyroidism, pseudopseudohypoparathyroidism, and clavicular dysgenesis has been noted. Disseminated cutaneous ossification in infants has also been described.[390] Osteomas of soft parts rarely are encountered. These lesions generally occur in the head, usually in the posterior portion of the tongue, but they also have been described in the thigh[753] (Fig. 95–92).

Soft tissue *osteosarcomas* likewise rarely are encountered.[94–97, 754–756, 955] These lesions are distinguished from medullary, periosteal, and parosteal osteosarcomas of bone, as well as from those arising from the surface of bone. They usually are evident in middle-aged and elderly patients, in the deeper tissues of the extremities, thighs, or shoulder region (Figs. 95–93 and 95–94). Patients may relate a history of prior irradiation or, more commonly, significant trauma, suggesting to some investigators that the neoplasms arise in foci of myositis ossificans. Radiographically, a soft tissue mass with calcification or ossification can be seen. On histologic examination, the osteosarcoma resembles the lesions that are encountered in bones.[294] Its areas of neoplastic osteoid and bone must be differentiated from small foci of metaplastic bone that may be observed in malignant fibrous histiocytoma, liposarcoma, epithelioid sarcoma, and synovial sarcoma.[330] The malignant potential of these tumors appears to be high. Indeed, widespread metastasis including that to bone may be seen.[756, 757]

Soft tissue neoplasms containing ossific and calcific foci must be distinguished from ''benign'' lesions such as myositis ossificans traumatica and pseudomalignant osseous tumors of soft tissue (see later discussion).

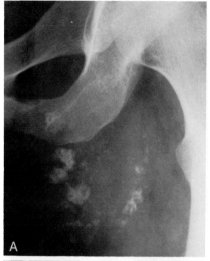
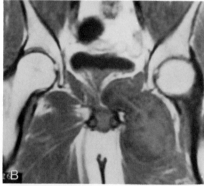
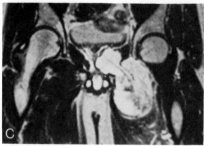

FIGURE 95–91. Chondrosarcoma. This 33 year old man developed a mass in the groin. Routine radiography **(A)** shows that the mass is calcified. On coronal T1-weighted (TR/TE, 500/20) **(B)** and T2-weighted (TR/TE, 2000/80) **(C)** spin echo MR images, the intramuscular tumor is inhomogeneous in signal intensity, with regions of low signal intensity in **C** related, in part, to calcific foci. It extends into the pelvis. (Courtesy of S. Fernandez, M.D., Mexico City, Mexico.)

Synovial Sarcomas

Synovial sarcomas are uncommon malignant neoplasms that can arise from within a joint but are more frequent in extra-articular locations.[98–103, 295, 391–399, 564] They are intimately related to tendons, tendon sheaths, bursal structures, and, less frequently, fasciae, ligaments, aponeuroses, and interosseous membranes.[330] A distinct predilection exists for involvement of the thigh and lower extremity. The single most common site is the region of the knee.[330] Involvement of the soft tissues in the axial skeleton is very rare.[759] Patients of all ages can be affected, including children,[758] although most are in the third and fourth decades of life.

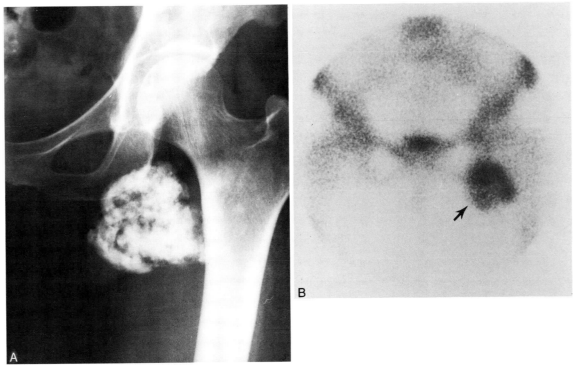

FIGURE 95–92. Osteoma. A 56 year old woman had a large mass in the thigh. A radiograph **(A)** and bone scan **(B)** document the lesion (arrow), which was interpreted histologically as an osteoma of soft parts. (Courtesy of G. Greenway, M.D., Dallas, Texas.)

Men are affected more frequently than women. On radiographs, a soft tissue mass is seen, which may reveal evidence of calcification in 20 to 30 per cent of cases and of osseous erosion or invasion in 5 to 20 per cent of cases[104]

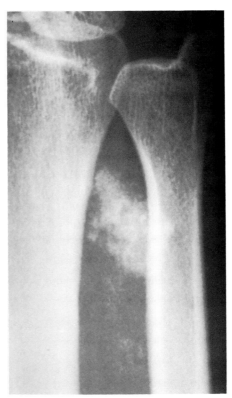

FIGURE 95–93. Osteosarcoma. An oblique radiograph of the forearm shows an irregularly ossified soft tissue mass in a 39 year old woman.

(Fig. 95–95). In some cases, extensive ossification of the mass leads to a radiographic appearance simulating that of a benign tumor.[763] Extensive bone destruction is rare, and reactive sclerosis is unusual. Angiography shows a fine network of tumor cells with an inhomogeneous capillary blush; neovascularity is greater in the monophasic (rather than biphasic) form of the tumor.[760] With MR imaging, synovial sarcomas usually reveal an inhomogeneous septated mass located close to a joint, tendon or bursa, possessing infiltrative margins, low signal intensity on T1-weighted spin echo images, and high signal intensity on T2-weighted spin echo MR images[761, 762] (Fig. 95–96). Fluid levels within the mass may be evident.[762, 956] MR imaging also may be used effectively to study the response of the tumor to chemotherapy.[761]

On histologic examination, synovioblastic and spindle-cell fibroblastic elements are seen (Fig. 95–97). The prognosis is poor. Those tumors that exhibit extensive calcification or ossification are associated with longer survival.[392] Recurrences are frequent and, in the majority of patients, sooner or later metastatic deposits appear, especially in the lungs, that on rare occasions may calcify.[105, 764] A benign variety of tumor, termed the *benign synovioma,* has been observed in the capsule of the knee.[20]

Tumors of Peripheral Nerves

The most important benign tumors of peripheral nerves are the *neurofibroma* and the *neurilemoma* (Fig. 95–98). Because of the similarity of the neoplastic cells of both of these tumors to the normal Schwann cell, some investigators regard them as closely related or identical neoplasms, whereas other authorities believe they should be classified separately, emphasizing their clinical and ultrastructural dif-

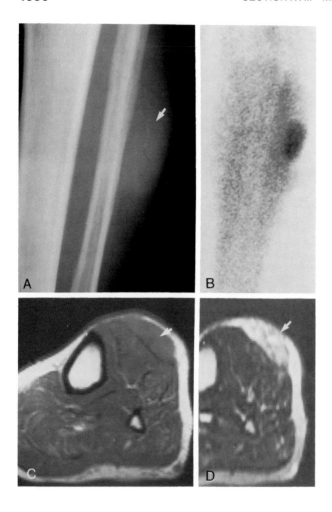

FIGURE 95–94. Osteosarcoma. A 65 year old man developed an enlarging mass in the lower leg over a three month period.

A Routine radiography shows a mass containing radiodense foci (arrow) lateral and anterior to the fibula.

B Increased uptake of the bone-seeking radionuclide is evident.

C, D Transaxial T1-weighted (TR/TE, 500/20) **(C)** and T2-weighted (TR/TE, 2100/120) **(D)** spin echo MR images show the location of the mass (arrows). It is subcutaneous, compressing the tibialis anterior, extensor hallucis longus, and extensor digitorum longus muscles. Its signal intensity is greater in **D** than in **C**.

(Courtesy of G. Greenway, M.D., Dallas, Texas.)

ferences.[330] The neurilemoma (benign schwannoma, neurinoma) is observed most commonly in adult men and women in the third to fifth decades of life.[400] This tumor typically arises from the spinal nerve roots and the cervical, sympathetic, vagus, peroneal, and ulnar nerves, appearing in the head, neck, and flexor surfaces of the upper and lower extremities.[330] The sciatic nerve also may be the source of a neurilemoma,[765] as can virtually any central or peripheral nerve.[767] It predominantly is a solitary, slowly growing lesion that, when large, leads to clinical manifestations that include pain, soft tissue prominence, and neurologic findings (Fig. 95–99). An association with neurofibromatosis (von Recklinghausen's disease) is recognized but uncommon. Neurilemomas are benign in their behavior; tumor recurrence is unusual, and malignant transformation is exceedingly rare.[401]

The neurofibroma may occur as a solitary lesion unassociated with neurofibromatosis, although a plexiform neurofibroma or multiple neurofibromas are characteristic of this latter disease. Although the discovery of a solitary neurofibroma should stimulate a thorough search for additional tumors as well as other manifestations of neurofibromatosis, its existence alone should not be regarded as synonymous with the diagnosis of von Recklinghausen's disease.[330] Solitary neurofibromas predominate in young adult men and women. They affect all areas of the body, appearing in the subcutis or dermis. They grow slowly, erode adjacent bone (such as the pedicle and lamina, leading to a widened neural foramin[768, 769]) and rarely undergo malignant degeneration.

The detection of localized neurofibromas or neurilemomas by conventional radiography (Fig. 95–100) is difficult unless they are large, are calcified, or affect adjacent structures, including the bones, leading to scalloped osseous erosions.[542] In this regard, the occurrence of a widened intervertebral foramen is a well-recognized manifestation of dumbbell-shaped lesions extending between the spinal canal and posterior mediastinum (Fig. 95–101), but it is a finding that can relate also to a tortuous or enlarged vertebral artery, congenital absence or hypoplasia of a pedicle, dermoids, teratomas, and hypertrophic interstitial polyneuritis (Dejerine-Sottas syndrome).[402–404] Although ultrasonography has been used as an imaging method for analysis of peripheral nerve tumors,[770] CT and MR imaging represent more effective means of delineating the lesions (Fig. 95–102), particularly those that are deep and nonpalpable, defining their position along the course of a nerve and their relationship to surrounding structures.[405–407, 543, 766, 771, 772] The tumors usually are well defined and smooth, with low attenuation values that may increase slightly following the administration of intravenous contrast material.[407–409, 566] A similar CT appearance may be evident in neurofibrosarcomas, although the presence of areas of low density, either round or linear, located centrally or peripherally, within a mass of higher density is more characteristic of malignancy.[409] It should be emphasized, however, that inhomogeneity of the lesion on the CT scans is not a finding specific for malignancy, being evident in benign tumors of nerves in which hypocellular and densely cellular areas

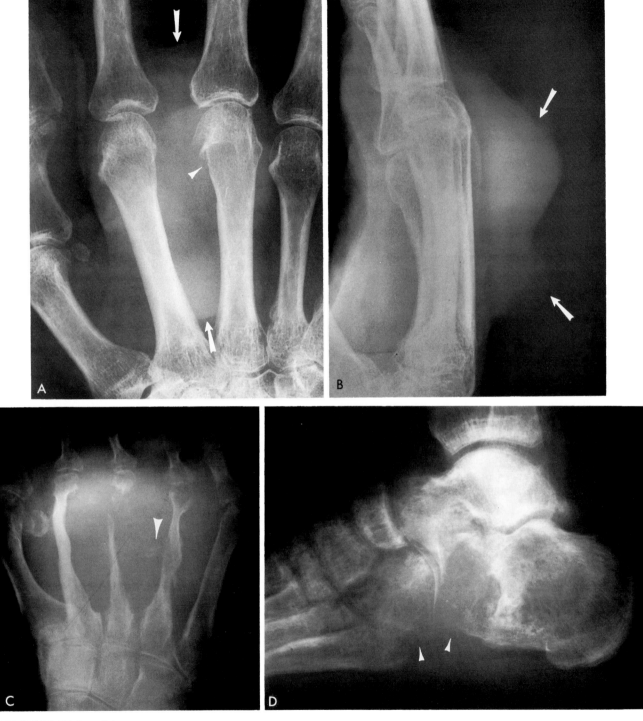

FIGURE 95–95. Synovial sarcoma.
   A, B The lobulated soft tissue mass (arrows) on the dorsum of the hand is eroding the second and third metacarpal bones (arrowhead).
   C This 25 year old woman developed an extensive mass on the left foot. Observe the pressure erosion of multiple metatarsal shafts with fracture and soft tissue calcification (arrowhead).
   D A 17 year old man had an enlarging mass of the foot. Destruction of the calcaneus and cuboid bones is seen (arrowheads). There is surrounding sclerosis, but the patient had previously received cobalt therapy. Osteoporosis also is evident.

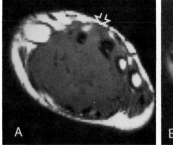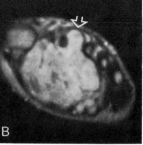

FIGURE 95–96. Synovial sarcoma. A calcified mass developed in the plantar aspect of the foot in a 14 year old girl. It is of low signal intensity on a coronal T1-weighted (TR/TE, 500/17) spin echo MR image **(A)** and of high signal intensity on a coronal T2-weighted (TR/TE, 2100/90) spin echo MR image **(B).** The intramuscular tumor is not homogeneous in signal intensity, however, and extends dorsally (arrows) between the second and third toes. The erosion and sclerosis of the second and third metatarsal bones were more obvious on routine radiographs (not shown). (Courtesy of M. Murphey, M.D., Washington, D.C.)

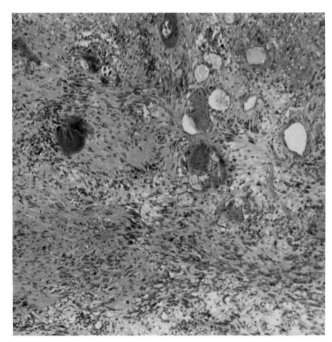

FIGURE 95–98. Neurilemoma. Neural bundles of spindle cells show a focal palisading configuration (90×).

coexist.[565] With regard to MR imaging,[773–777, 975] spinal, paraspinal or peripheral neurilemomas or neurofibromas can be evaluated. Most of the lesions reveal relatively low signal intensity on T1-weighted spin echo MR images and high signal intensity on T2-weighted images[773] (Fig. 95–103). On the latter images and on T1-weighted images following the intravenous administration of gadolinium, a target pattern may be identified, consisting of increased signal intensity at the periphery of the lesion and central low signal intensity.[777] This pattern, which may correspond to peripheral myxomatous tissue and central fibrous tissue, is absent in cystic, hemorrhagic, or necrotic lesions (which show hyperintensity and inhomogeneity on T2-weighted images) and in malignant schwannomas (which show similar hyperintensity and inhomogeneity).[777] MR imaging allows identification of the nerve trunk of origin and the relationship of the tumor to surrounding structures, although its size may be overestimated with this technique.[774]

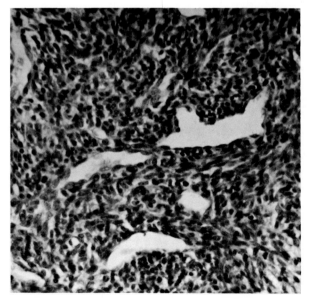

FIGURE 95–97. Synovial sarcoma. A photomicrograph (200×) demonstrates synovioblastic and spindle-cell fibroblastic elements with slit formation.

When MR imaging reveals a tumor in the vicinity of a large nerve trunk, a fusiform mass, and muscle atrophy along the longitudinal axis of surrounding or distally innervated musculature, a nerve sheath tumor is suggested[775] (Fig. 95–104).

Pseudotumorous benign lesions of peripheral nerves include the *nerve sheath ganglion* and *Morton's neuroma* (Fig. 95–105), a condition produced by degenerative changes in one or more intermetatarsal nerves that can lead to paroxysms of pain[106, 330, 778, 779] (see Chapter 77).

Fibrolipomatous hamartomas (also designated lipofibromatous hamartomas) are rare lesions related to the gradual infiltration of major nerves and their branches by fibrofatty tissue.[780–784] The hand usually is involved; most lesions affect the median nerve, although the radial and ulnar nerves also may be involved. The peroneal and digital nerves represent additional sites of involvement. Although the lesions are not malignant, clinical manifestations may become prominent. Fibrolipomatous hamartomas usually appear in children, adolescents, or young adults and can lead to an enlarging mass, macrodactyly, and a compression neuropathy. MR imaging reveals features of both fibrous and fatty tissue, and a serpentine-like appearance of the enlarged nerves is distinctive[781, 964, 965] (Fig. 95–106). On gross examination, a gray or yellow mass surrounding the involved nerve is seen which, histologically, relates to fibrofatty infiltration and epineural and perineural fibrosis.

Postamputation *stump neuromas* occurring at the severed ends of major nerves following limb amputations are well described.[785–787] Traumatic neuromas (Fig. 95–107) may be divided into two major categories reflecting the degree of damage sustained by the nerve: chronic friction or irritation to a nondisrupted, intact nerve trunk may give rise to internal, focal, fusiform swellings known as spindle neuromas; and severe trauma that partially avulses or totally transects a nerve (as in limb amputation) may lead to external

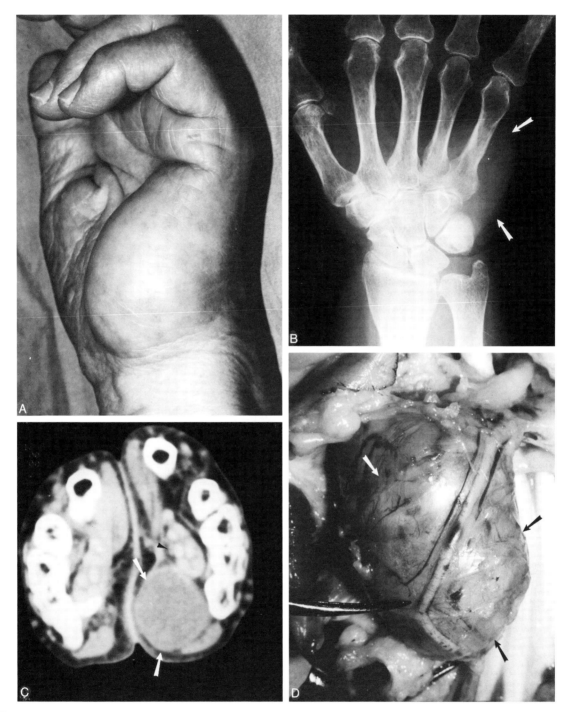

FIGURE 95–99. Neurilemoma. An 82 year old woman observed progressive pain, swelling, numbness, and weakness of the hand over an 18 month period. On physical examination, a firm soft tissue mass, atrophy of the ulnar intrinsic muscles, and local neurologic manifestations, including a carpal tunnel syndrome, were observed.

A The soft tissue mass is apparent.

B The radiograph reveals the mass (arrows) and the absence of bone involvement.

C A transaxial CT scan shows a soft tissue mass (arrows) near the hook of the hamate, compressing the structures within the carpal canal. The mass is not calcified, and its attenuation value was 27 Hounsfield units. Note the position of the median nerve (arrowhead).

D At surgery, a neurilemoma (arrows) was found to be located deep to the superficial arterial arch and nerves, and the sensory nerves to the ulnar side of the hand were stretched over the tumor. The motor branch of the ulnar nerve was pressed against the hook of the hamate, and the median nerve was compromised in the carpal tunnel. (Courtesy of G. Greenway, M.D., Dallas, Texas.)

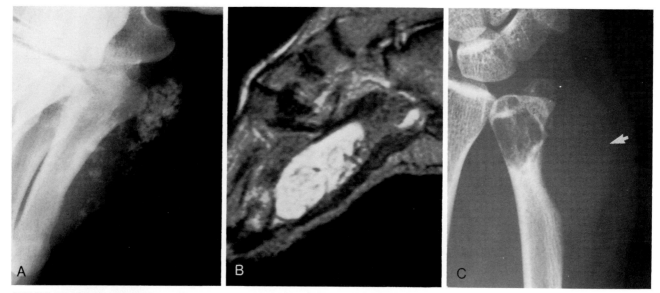

FIGURE 95–100. Neurilemoma.

A, B This tumor of the foot is calcified on routine radiography **(A)** and of inhomogeneous but mainly high signal intensity on a sagittal T2-weighted (TR/TE, 1000/80) spin echo MR image **(B)**.

C A neurilemoma of the ulnar nerve has produced a large soft tissue mass (arrow) with erosion of the ulna. **(C,** Courtesy of M. Mitchell, M.D., Halifax, Nova Scotia, Canada.)

growths such as lateral or terminal neuromas.[785] Traumatic neuromas represent the consequence of both the nerve injury itself and the abortive attempt at natural repair; in cases of limb amputation, the regenerating axon elongates and branches in various directions, and eventually a neuroma forms.[785] Postamputation neuromas become evident approximately one to 12 months after transection, are of variable size, have no malignant potential, and may be asymptomatic.[786] Pain and a mass may be evident, however. When assessing the cause of pain at the stump, other conditions such as soft tissue ulceration, heterotopic bone formation, bursitis and other inflammatory changes, retained foreign bodies, altered musculature, and scar formation also must be considered.[785]

CT analysis of stump neuromas reveals focal or generalized alteration in the caliber, size, or contour of the nerve trunk.[785] MR imaging findings (Fig. 95–108) include a fusiform mass with inhomogeneous signal intensity.[786, 787] Although most stump neuromas show regions of high signal intensity on T2-weighted images, strandlike regions of low signal intensity on such images may be seen.[787]

The *malignant schwannoma* is the major malignancy of the peripheral nerves. It may occur as an isolated phenomenon or, in less than 50 per cent of cases, with neurofibromatosis.[330, 567] Malignant schwannomas are seen in young and middle-aged men and women, appearing as enlarging masses, principally in the trunk and proximal portions of the extremities, in association with the sciatic nerve and brachial and sacral plexuses.[330] Pain and neurologic manifestations are variable in frequency and intensity.

As in cases of neurofibroma and neurilemoma, routine radiography (Fig. 95–109) provides little diagnostic information regarding malignant schwannomas. A mass is identified that in rare instances may calcify.[788] CT and MR imaging are better suited to identification of the lesion and its relationship to surrounding anatomic structures.[409] (Fig. 95–110). Thickening of the nerve in either a proximal or a

distal direction, or both, is compatible with neoplastic spread along the epineurium and perineurium.[330] A similar CT appearance of thickened nerves is encountered in patients with neurofibromatosis in whom malignancy is absent[406] (Fig. 95–111). MR imaging of malignant schwannomas (Fig. 95–112) shows an inhomogeneous mass, generally of low signal intensity on T1-weighted images and high signal intensity on T2-weighted images.[777, 789] A target pattern, seen in some benign nerve sheath tumors, is not present,[777] although differentiation of benign and malignant lesions may not be possible without histologic analysis. Malignant schwannomas, particularly those occurring in neurofibromatosis, carry a poor prognosis.

Additional malignant tumors of peripheral nerves include *neuroepitheliomas* (neuroblastomas), usually seen in the extremities or chest wall in children, adolescents, and young adults, and extraspinal (soft tissue) *ependymomas.*[330, 790, 791]

Other Tumors

Additional benign neoplasms include a *mixed tumor* arising in the sweat glands of the corium, especially in the face and head; a *mesenchymoma*, containing a mixture of fibrous and mesenchymal tissue[289]; and a *mesothelioma*, usually apparent in the pleura. These tumors may have their malignant counterparts, such as *malignant mesenchymoma, malignant ectomesenchymoma,*[792] and *malignant mesothelioma.*[20] Certain of these neoplasms, such as mesenchymomas, may contain areas of fat and calcification.[793]

Clear cell sarcomas, also known as aponeurotic clear cell sarcomas and malignant melanomas of soft parts (Fig. 95–113), are malignant neoplasms that arise in the vicinity of tendons and aponeuroses of the upper and lower extremities, especially in the region of the foot and ankle, followed in order of decreasing frequency by the knee, thigh, and hand.[107] Although the age range of affected persons is large, most patients are young adults, particularly women.[330, 410–

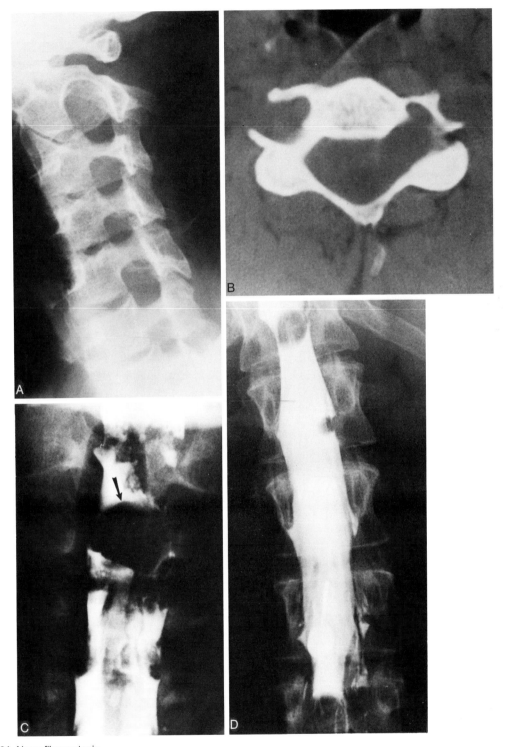

FIGURE 95–101. Neurofibromatosis.
  A, B Enlargement of the neural foramina in the cervical spine is well shown by both conventional radiography and transaxial CT.
  C, D Myelography documents the presence of multiple neurofibromas, appearing as eccentric filling defects in the spinal canal, the largest defect being evident in the cervical region (arrow).
  (Courtesy of V. Vint, M.D., San Diego, California.)

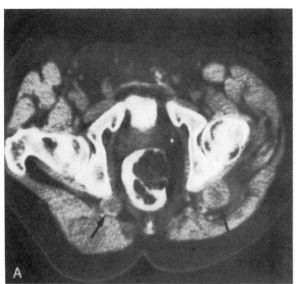

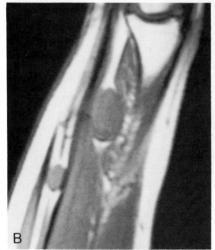

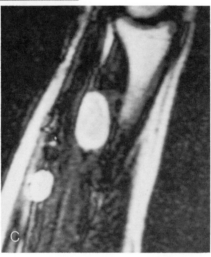

FIGURE 95–102. Neurofibroma.

A The transaxial CT scan reveals bilateral neurofibromas of the sciatic nerve (arrows). (From Lanziere CF, Hilal SK: Am J Roentgenol 143:165, 1984. Copyright 1984, American Roentgen Ray Society.)

B, C Two neurofibromas in the forearm are evident on sagittal T1-weighted (TR/TE, 549/13) **(B)** and T2-weighted (TR/TE, 2500/70) **(C)** spin echo MR images.

FIGURE 95–103. Neurilemoma.

A, B Common peroneal nerve. In this 40 year old man with a three week history of a mass in the popliteal fossa and paresthesias in the distribution of the common peroneal nerve, a coronal T1-weighted (TR/TE, 700/20) spin echo MR image **(A)** shows a fusiform mass (arrows) of low signal intensity. The distal portion of the nerve is evident inferiorly (arrowhead). A sagittal multiplanar gradient recalled (MPGR) MR image (TR/TE, 1000/20; flip angle, 45 degrees) shows high signal intensity in the lesion. (Courtesy of G. Greenway, M.D., Dallas, Texas.)

C–E Tibial nerve. Sagittal T1-weighted (TR/TE, 540/16) **(C)** and T2-weighted (TR/TE, 1800/80) **(D)** spin echo MR images and a sagittal T1-weighted (TR/TE, 540/18) spin echo MR image following the intravenous administration of gadolinium **(E)** show a well-defined mass posterior to the distal portion of the tibia. In **C,** the mass is of low signal intensity and the adjacent nerve (arrow) can be seen. Regions of high signal intensity in the mass are seen in **D** and **E.** (Courtesy of P. Kindynis, M.D., Geneva, Switzerland.)

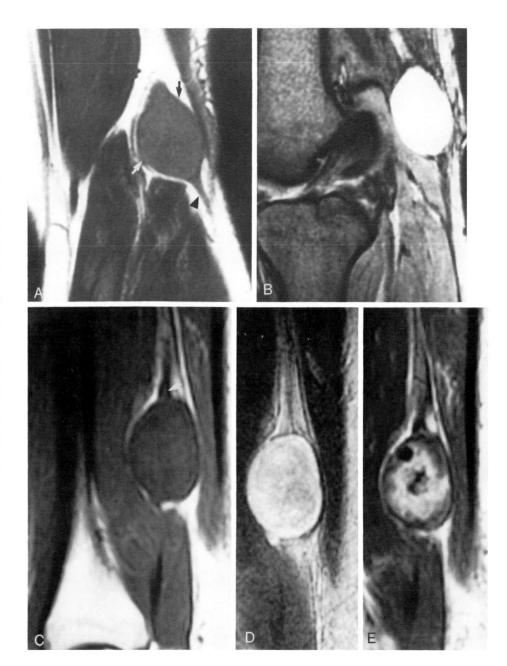

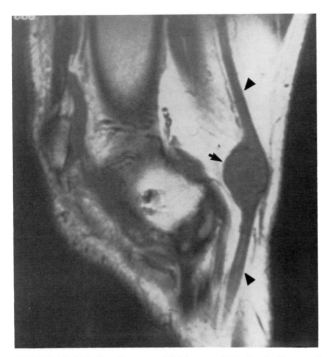

FIGURE 95–104. Neurilemoma. Tibial nerve. Note the fusiform soft tissue mass (arrow) of low signal intensity on a sagittal T1-weighted (TR/TE, 600/20) spin echo MR image. The adjacent portions of the nerve (arrowheads) are apparent. (Courtesy of R. Stiles, M.D., Atlanta, Georgia.)

[413, 794–796] A deep, slowly enlarging mass is typical. Rarely, multifocal lesions are encountered. Radiographs reveal the mass, the usual absence of calcification, and, rarely, the presence of bone erosion.[108, 795] Frequent tumor recurrences and distant metastasis underscore the poor prognosis of this tumor. The capacity of its constituent cells to produce melanin has suggested a relationship to malignant melanoma,[330] whereas other features are consistent with melanotic Schwann cell differentiation.[413]

An *alveolar soft part sarcoma* (malignant granular cell myoblastoma) usually is found in muscles but also may appear in the orbit, retroperitoneum, and elsewhere, in both children and young and middle-aged adults.[109–111, 414, 415] The thigh is a common site of involvement. The tumor grows slowly, may calcify (Fig. 95–114) or invade the underlying bone, and eventually may metastasize widely through the blood stream.[797, 798] Nonspecific MR (Fig. 95–115) and CT features are present,[957] and angiography (Fig. 95–114) re-

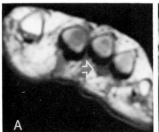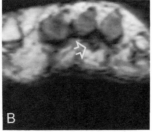

FIGURE 95–105. Morton's neuroma. Coronal T1-weighted (TR/TE, 450/14) **(A)** and T2-weighted (TR/TE, 4000/100) **(B)** spin echo MR images reveal a mass (arrows) of low signal intensity between the third and fourth metatarsal bones. Such low signal intensity is characteristic of this lesion.

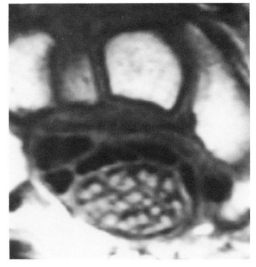

FIGURE 95–106. Fibrolipomatous hamartoma. Median nerve. In this 22 year old man with an enlarging mass in the palm, a T1-weighted (TR/TE, 550/15) transaxial spin echo MR image reveals tubular structures in the lesion of the median nerve. Some regions of the mass demonstrate signal intensity identical to that of fat, and others have low signal intensity.

veals the vascular nature of the tumor.[797] The histology resembles that of a paraganglioma, with subtle differences. The exact nature of the tumor remains uncertain.

An *epithelioid sarcoma* is a rare neoplasm arising principally in the fingers, hands, and forearms of young adults.[330, 416, 799] The lower extremities are involved less frequently than the upper extremities. Epithelioid sarcomas affect mainly the subcutaneous tissues, fascia, or tendon sheaths.[799] Solitary or multiple firm nodules in the subcutis and deeper tissues are evident. The cell of origin (i.e., a histiocyte, synovial cell, or some other type of cell) is not clear. On radiographs, a soft tissue mass may be observed. Calcification, ossification, hyperostosis, and cortical erosion

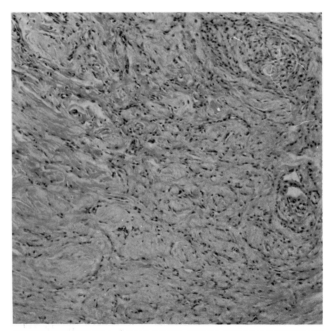

FIGURE 95–107. Traumatic neuroma. Dense dermal collagen tissue with entrapped pockets of neurofibrils is seen (90×).

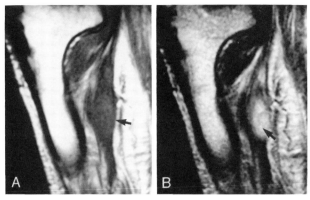

FIGURE 95–108. Stump neuroma. In a 20 year old man with a previous amputation of the leg below the level of the knee, sagittal T1-weighted (TR/TE, 700/20) **(A)** and T2-weighted (TR/TE, 2000/70) **(B)** spin echo MR images show a neuroma (arrows) of the tibial nerve with homogeneous, low signal intensity in **A** and inhomogeneous high signal intensity in **B**. (Courtesy of C. Sebrechts, M.D., San Diego, California.)

have been described[330, 417] (Fig. 95–116). MR imaging abnormalities are not specific (Fig. 95–117).

Malignant lymphoid and reticuloendothelial tumors such as *lymphoma, Ewing's sarcoma,* and *extraosseous plasma-*

cytoma rarely arise in the soft tissues.[20] *Primitive neuroectodermal tumor (PNET)* is discussed in Chapter 83.

Malignant melanoma (melanosarcoma) is a neoplasm of contested origin containing fibroblast-like cells, some of which contain melanin. It can arise from the skin and produce local and distant osseous destruction (see Chapter 85).

Squamous cell carcinoma of the skin (Fig. 95–118) can invade subjacent bone.[800, 958] This tumor can arise at various sites and is not uncommon in areas of chronic cutaneous irritation, such as about a draining sinus in association with osteomyelitis. *Subungual keratoacanthomas* are infiltrating, self-limiting, localized growths of squamous epithelium that can erode a terminal phalanx.[418, 419] *Pilomatrixomas* (calcifying epitheliomas) are benign soft tissue tumors occurring in the dermis or subjacent tissues, frequently in children.[112, 113] The lesions may be heavily calcified (Fig. 95–119). *Endometriosis,* occurring in women especially during their reproductive period, generally occurs in the pelvis or abdomen. Endometriosis appearing as a soft tissue mass in other locations is rare but is reported.[80]

Metastases

Single or multiple soft tissue or muscle[802] metastatic deposits can accompany a variety of primary malignant neoplasms (see Chapter 85). In general, a nonspecific soft tis-

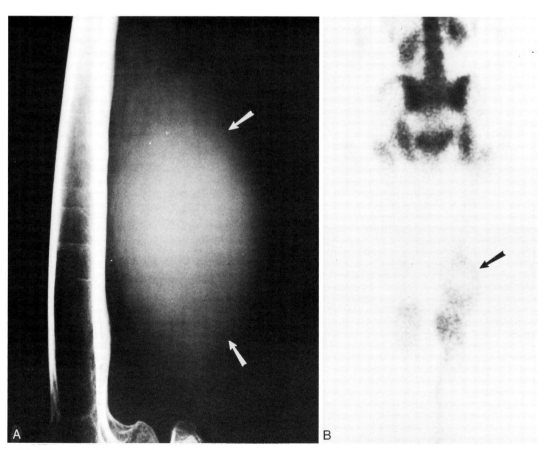

FIGURE 95–109. Malignant schwannoma. In a 25 year old woman with neurofibromatosis, a mass developed above the popliteal fossa and enlarged progressively over a 3 to 5 year period. On physical examination, it was movable, round, and 20 × 12 cm in size.

  A The radiograph reveals the mass (arrows).

  B On the bone scan, a rim of accentuated accumulation of the radionuclide is seen (arrow). Following an amputation, the diagnosis of a malignant schwannoma was firmly established.

(Courtesy of G. Greenway, M.D., Dallas, Texas.)

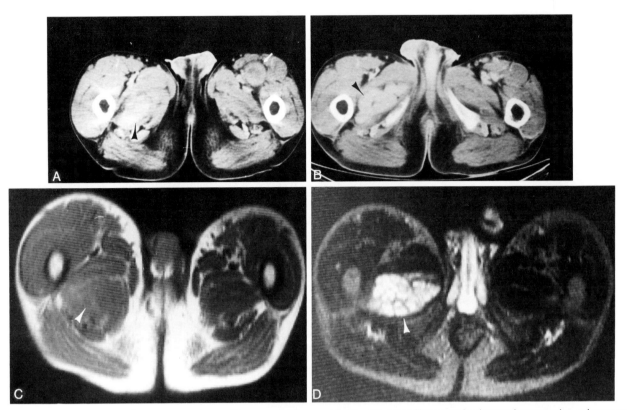

FIGURE 95–110. Malignant schwannoma and neurofibromas. A 26 year old man with neurofibromatosis observed progressive enlargement of the left thigh.

A The initial transaxial CT scan shows a mass (arrow) near the femoral nerve in the left thigh, and a larger mass (arrowhead) in close proximity to the vastus medialis in the right thigh. The tumor in the left leg was excised, allowing the diagnosis of a malignant schwannoma.

B A postoperative transaxial CT scan reveals the disappearance of the tumor in the left leg with the mass (arrowhead) in the right thigh still evident.

C, D T1-weighted (TR/TE, 800/20) **(C)** and T2-weighted (TR/TE, 2000/80) **(D)** transaxial MR images show the tumor in the right thigh (arrowheads), which demonstrates high signal intensity in **D** and which was considered to be a neurofibroma.

(Courtesy of G. Greenway, M.D., Dallas, Texas.)

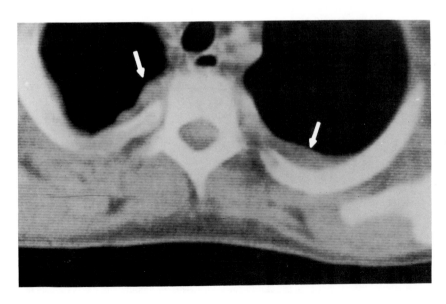

FIGURE 95–111. Neurofibromatosis. A transaxial CT scan shows bilateral thickened nerves (arrows) adjacent to the ribs. (Courtesy of A. Daneman, M.D., Toronto, Ontario, Canada.)

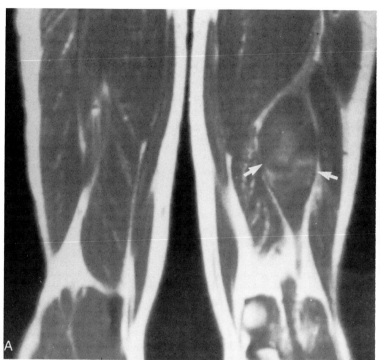

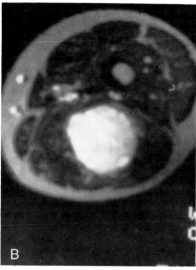

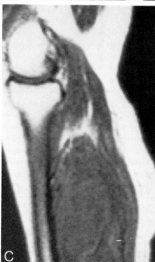

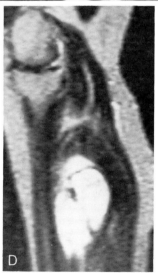

FIGURE 95–112. Malignant schwannoma.

A, B A 43 year old man complained of pain in the posterior thigh and tingling in the bottom of the foot. A firm mass was palpated. A coronal T1-weighted (TR/TE, 500/17) spin echo MR image **(A)** shows a mass (arrows) with slightly inhomogeneous but mainly low signal intensity, fusiform in shape, and situated in the vicinity of the sciatic nerve. A transaxial T2-weighted (TR/TE, 2500/90) spin echo MR image **(B)** reveals inhomogeneous high signal intensity in the mass. A radical excision of the tumor was performed.

C, D This 26 year old woman had pain and a tender mass near the gastrocnemius muscle. Sagittal T1-weighted (TR/TE, 555/26) **(C)** and T2-weighted (TR/TE, 2025/120) **(D)** spin echo MR images show a mass in the region of the posterior tibialis and soleus muscles. It is of low signal intensity in **C** and of high signal intensity in **D**. Note intralesional areas of low signal intensity in **D**.

(Courtesy of G. Greenway, M.D., Dallas, Texas.)

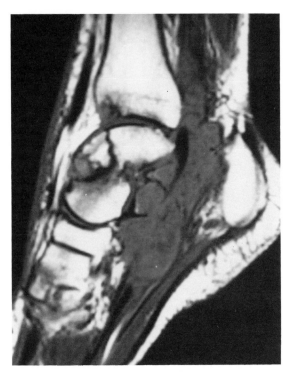

FIGURE 95–113. Clear cell sarcoma. On a sagittal T1-weighted (TR/TE, 700/20) spin echo MR image in a 57 year old woman, note the large tumor involving the plantar aspect of the foot, extending superiorly along the medial margin of the calcaneus and posteriorly, behind the tibia in the region of the flexor digitorum longus and flexor hallucis longus tendons. It is of low signal intensity. (Courtesy of C. Gundry, M.D., Minneapolis, Minnesota.)

sue mass is produced. The underlying bone can be eroded, and the osseous defects may resemble a ''cookie bite.'' In the authors' experience, bronchogenic carcinoma is the most frequent cause of metastases that lead to such a roentgenographic appearance (Fig. 95–120).

Synovial Disorders

A variety of synovial disorders can lead to intra-articular or periarticular masses. Such disorders include inflammatory joint diseases such as rheumatoid arthritis, the seronegative spondyloarthropathies, crystal deposition disorders, and septic arthritis, which are discussed elsewhere in this text. Three additional processes that may lead to prominent soft tissue enlargement are idiopathic synovial (osteo)chondromatosis, pigmented villonodular synovitis, and synovial cysts. The first of these is discussed in Chapter 84 and earlier in this chapter; the other two problems also are discussed in Chapter 84, but a few additional comments are appropriate here.

Pigmented Villonodular Synovitis. This synovial proliferative disorder typically occurs in adults in the third or fourth decade of life but also appears less frequently in older adults, adolescents, and even children. The knee is the most common site of involvement,[803] and additional frequently involved sites are the hip,[804] elbow, and ankle. Virtually any articulation can be affected, however, including such unusual locations as the joints of the vertebral column and the temporomandibular joint.[805] Monoarticular disease is the rule, with rare reports of bilateral or even

symmetrical involvement.[806, 807] A slight male predominance has been noted in some reports.[808] A history of trauma is evident in about 50 per cent of cases.

Clinical manifestations vary according to the type of disease present and its specific location (see later discussion). With diffuse involvement of a joint, slowly progressive pain and swelling, sometimes accompanied by warmth, tenderness, and stiffness, may be apparent, and a significant delay in diagnosis is common. With focal or localized involvement of a joint, symptoms and signs of an internal derangement may be apparent. Aspiration of joint contents classically reveals brown fluid consistent with chronic hemorrhage or fresh blood consistent with acute hemorrhage, or a combination of the two, although yellow fluid is recovered in some cases.

The difficulty encountered in providing a short summary of pigmented villonodular synovitis is related in part to inconsistencies in the methods used to classify the disorder. Indeed, a variety of names has been used to describe the condition, including (but not limited to) synovial endothelioma, synovial xanthoma, xanthomatous giant cell tumor, fibrohemosideric sarcoma, chronic hemorrhagic villous synovitis, and fibrous xanthoma of the synovial membrane.[809] In 1941, Jaffe and coworkers,[810] in a frequently quoted article on the subject, introduced the terms pigmented villonodular synovitis, pigmented villonodular bursitis, and pigmented villonodular tenosynovitis to describe the multiple manifestations of a histologic lesion characterized by a fibrous stroma, deposition of hemosiderin, histiocytic infiltration, and giant cells occurring in the synovial membrane of joints, bursae, and tendon sheaths.[809] In 1976, Granowitz and colleagues[811] further expanded this terminology by subdividing the disorder into a diffuse and a localized form, depending upon the extent of synovial involvement. Additional subclassifications of the process have emphasized its villous, nodular, or villonodular nature. Furthermore, in some varieties of this disorder, particularly its nodular and localized forms, hemosiderin deposition is minimal, leading to the designations of pigmented and nonpigmented types of involvement. When one considers all of these potential variations—articular, bursal, and tenosynovial localization; diffuse and localized forms; villous, nodular, and villonodular morphology; pigmented and nonpigmented forms—the complexity of the process and its accurate description become obvious. Finally, the use of the designation giant cell tumor of tendon sheath to describe a nodular lesion of the tendon sheaths in the hand and foot with histologic features similar to those of some forms of pigmented villonodular synovitis clouds the issue of nomenclature still further.[812, 813] Such nodular lesions are sometimes referred to as nodular tenosynovitis and can occur as localized processes in other locations, such as the foot, ankle, knee, and hip. Their relationship to the nodular form of pigmented villonodular synovitis as well as to fibromas of tendon sheath[814–817, 977] remains unclear and is better left to the attention of a pathologist than a radiologist.

The classic radiographic feature of diffuse, intra-articular pigmented villonodular synovitis includes soft tissue swelling or a joint effusion, preservation of joint space, the absence of osteoporosis, and the presence or absence of bone erosions and cysts.[803, 818–821] As in the case of idiopathic synovial (osteo)chondromatosis, however, modifications of these classic features must be recognized. Radio-

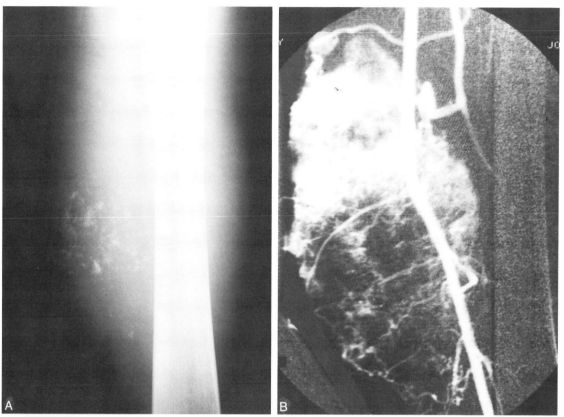

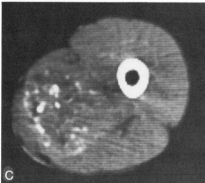

FIGURE 95–114. Alveolar soft part sarcoma. This 19 year old man developed an enlarging mass in the thigh.

A The radiograph shows a large soft tissue mass, medial to the femur, containing calcification.

B An angiogram documents increased vascularity in the mass. Arteriovenous shunting of blood also was found.

C The partially calcified mass in the adductor muscles contains areas of decreased attenuation on a transaxial CT scan.

(Courtesy of G. Greenway, M.D., Dallas, Texas.)

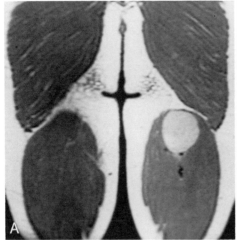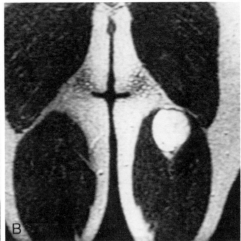

FIGURE 95–115. Alveolar soft part sarcoma. Coronal proton density (TR/TE, 2000/20) **(A)** and T2-weighted (TR/TE, 2000/80) **(B)** spin echo MR images in an 18 year old woman show a well-circumscribed mass in the semitendinosus muscle. The high signal intensity in **B** is typical of many benign and malignant tumors. (Courtesy of G. Greenway, M.D., Dallas, Texas.)

FIGURE 95–116. Epithelioid sarcoma. In a 52 year old woman with a wrist mass, routine radiography **(A)** shows subtle erosion of the triquetrum (arrow). A coronal T1-weighted (TR/TE, 550/20) spin echo MR image **(B)** demonstrates a mass (arrowhead) of low signal intensity eroding the triquetrum (arrow). (Courtesy of J. Kirkham, M.D., Minneapolis, Minnesota.)

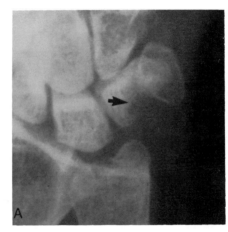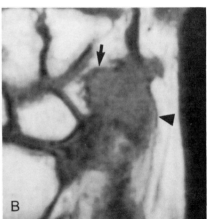

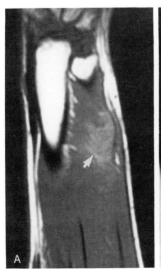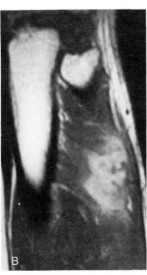

FIGURE 95–117. Epithelioid sarcoma. A forearm mass in a 22 year old man is well demonstrated with MR imaging. On a coronal T1-weighted (TR/TE, 650/20) spin echo image **(A),** the lesion (arrow) is located dorsal to the distal ulna. Its signal intensity is slightly higher than that of muscle. A coronal T1-weighted (TR/TE, 650/20) spin echo MR image following the intravenous administration of gadolinium **(B)** shows enhancement of the signal intensity of the tumor. The lesion is irregular in outline and not entirely homogeneous in appearance.

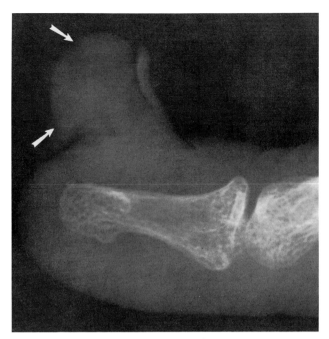

FIGURE 95–118. Squamous cell carcinoma of the nail bed. This 52 year old man developed an enlarging mass beneath the nail bed of the finger, which originally was believed to be a fungal infection. The large mass (arrows) required amputation of the digit.

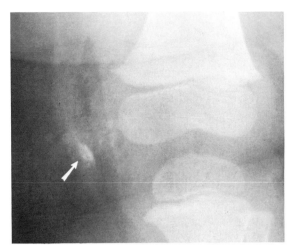

FIGURE 95–119. Pilomatrixoma (calcifying epithelioma). A calcified tumor (arrow) arose in the medial soft tissues of the knee in a 2 year old obese child.

graphs in such cases of pigmented villonodular synovitis may be entirely normal or may show minimal and nonspecific findings such as a joint effusion. Large effusions occasionally reveal a nodular outline or appear very radiodense, perhaps reflecting hemosiderin deposition. Minimal, moderate or, occasionally, dramatic loss of joint space may occur, especially in the hip.[822, 823] Bone erosions and sub-

chondral cysts, when present, can be prominent, particularly about "tight" joints such as the hip,[819] ankle, elbow and wrist; they also may be observed in joints with large capacity, such as the knee, where predilection for the patellofemoral region has been noted in some reports.[809] In the hip, bone lesions characteristically develop at the junction of the femoral head and femoral neck and in the acetabulum. The presence of osteoporosis does not eliminate the diagnosis of pigmented villonodular synovitis.

Many of the radiographic features of diffuse, intra-articular pigmented villonodular synovitis are identical to those seen in cases of idiopathic synovial chondromatosis in which calcification and ossification are absent. Despite the existence of occasional reports of pigmented villonodular

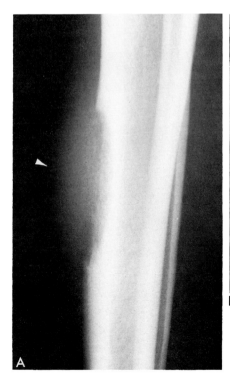

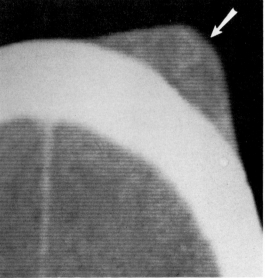

B **FIGURE 95–120.** Skeletal or soft tissue metastasis: Bronchogenic carcinoma.

A The "cookie bite" appearance of a tibial shaft is the result of a metastatic deposit from bronchogenic carcinoma. Note the soft tissue swelling (arrowhead).

B In a different patient, a soft tissue mass of the scalp (arrow) has resulted from metastasis due to bronchogenic carcinoma.

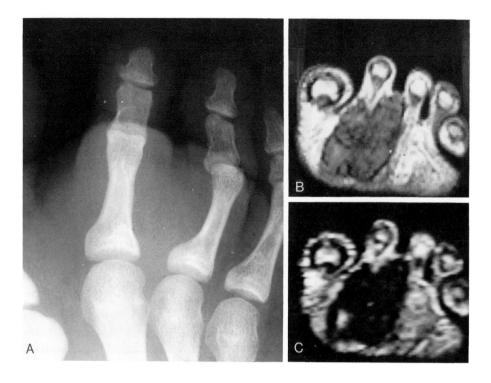

FIGURE 95–121. Giant cell tumor of tendon sheath. This 22 year old man had had foot pain for one year. A soft tissue mass was palpable in the plantar soft tissues between the second and third toes.

A Routine radiography confirms the presence of a soft tissue mass, leading to separation of the second and third digits. No bone erosion is evident.

B A transverse T1-weighted (TR/TE, 600/28) spin echo MR image reveals a mass of intermediate and low signal intensity.

C A transverse T2-weighted (TR/TE, 2100/120) spin echo MR image shows low signal intensity throughout the mass.

(Courtesy of G. Greenway, M.D., Dallas, Texas.)

synovitis that indicate radiographic[824] or histologic[825] evidence of calcification or metaplastic cartilage, the presence of such calcification generally eliminates the diagnosis of pigmented villonodular synovitis and, in the proper setting, favors the diagnosis of idiopathic synovial (osteo)-chondromatosis.

The radiographic features of pigmented villonodular synovitis also are modified in cases of bursal or tendon sheath involvement, including the nodular variety of tendon sheath disease known as giant cell tumor. In these instances, a diffuse or localized soft tissue mass (which calcifies only rarely[812]) is observed (Fig. 95–121). Subjacent erosion of bone may be encountered. The localized or nodular, intra-articular variety of pigmented villonodular synovitis usually is not detected with routine radiography (Fig. 95–122).

Additional imaging methods that can be used to study

the many forms of pigmented villonodular synovitis include arthrography (Chapter 13), arteriography, CT, and MR imaging. Arthrography reveals either a localized mass (localized or nodular form of the disease) or diffuse infiltration of the synovial membrane (diffuse form of the disease). Arteriography shows a richly vascular process with possible arteriovenous shunting, findings similar to those of a malignant tumor.[809] CT may reveal high attenuation values within the involved portions of the synovial membrane, consistent with an increased iron content.[826] Such elevated attenuation values are an inconstant feature, although CT with or without supplementary use of intravenous contrast material can be effective in defining the extent of the synovial process[827] and bone involvement.[828] With MR imaging, the deposition of hemosiderin in cases of pigmented villonodular synovitis leads to dramatic abnormalities characterized by regions of low signal intensity on both T1- and T2-weighted spin echo

FIGURE 95–122. Localized nodular synovitis. This 35 year old man developed recurrent effusions of the knee. He had had a history of a basketball injury with resulting ligamentous and meniscal tears.

A A coronal T2-weighted (TR/TE, 2350/80) spin echo MR image shows fluid of high signal intensity in the joint and subcutaneous tissues. A nodular mass (arrow) of low signal intensity is seen in the region of the infrapatellar fat body.

B A sagittal volumetric gradient recalled MR image (TR/TE, 18/4.6; flip angle, 30 degrees) reveals the mass (arrow) of low sig-

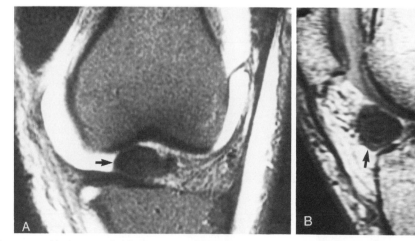

nal intensity. Histologic analysis of the resected lesion revealed findings compatible with the diagnosis of localized nodular synovitis or giant cell tumor of a tendon sheath.

(Courtesy of G. Greenway, M.D., Dallas, Texas.)

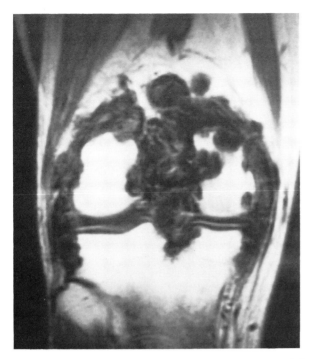

FIGURE 95–123. Diffuse (intra-articular) pigmented villonodular synovitis. A coronal T1-weighted (TR/TE, 650/28) spin echo MR image of the knee shows nodular soft tissue masses of low signal intensity, with joint distension and erosions of the femur and tibia.

MR images (Figs. 95–123 and 95–124) and, especially, on gradient echo MR images.[829–834] High signal intensity on T2-weighted spin echo MR images also is observed, indicative of joint fluid. The presence of hemosiderin deposition on MR images is a finding consistent with the diagnosis of pigmented villonodular synovitis, but it also is evident in some cases of hemophilia and other bleeding disorders, synovial hemangioma, neuropathic osteoarthropathy, and other processes associated with chronic hemarthrosis. MR imaging also may reveal the extent of bone involvement in diffuse pigmented villonodular synovitis and may allow the diagnosis of the localized or nodular form of the disease.[835, 836, 978]

The precise cause of pigmented villonodular synovitis is unknown.[809] The initial concept of it as a tumor largely has been abandoned. A metabolic, traumatic, or genetic basis for the disease has been considered, but the most widely held theory of pathogenesis is that of an inflammatory process with an unknown triggering mechanism.[809]

Synovial Cysts. Synovial cysts represent fluid-filled para-articular masses lined by a synovial membrane that may or may not communicate with the neighboring joint. Those that demonstrate such communication commonly distend with fluid when an effusion or synovial response, or both, appear in the adjacent joint, leading to elevation of intra-articular pressure. Typical processes accompanied by synovial cysts include rheumatoid arthritis (adult and, less

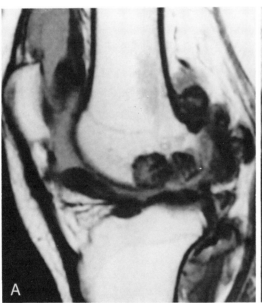
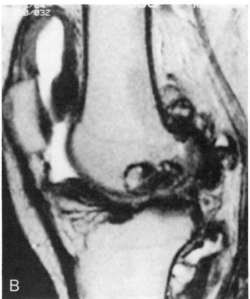
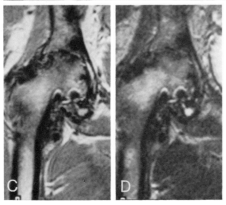

FIGURE 95–124. Diffuse (intra-articular) pigmented villonodular synovitis.

A, B Knee. Sagittal proton density (TR/TE, 2000/20) **(A)** and T2-weighted (TR/TE, 2000/80) **(B)** spin echo MR images show classic features of this disease. A joint effusion is of intermediate signal intensity in **A** and high signal intensity in **B**. Hemosiderin deposition accounts for the low signal intensity in the synovial nodules in **A** and **B**. Note the erosions of the distal femur. (Courtesy of T. Broderick, M.D., Orange, California.)

C, D Hip. Coronal proton density (TR/TE, 2216/28) **(C)** and T2-weighted (TR/TE, 2216/80) **(D)** spin echo MR images reveal regions of persistent low signal intensity in the right hip. Additional findings include erosions of the femoral neck and acetabulum, joint space loss, and a small amount of articular fluid appearing of high signal intensity in **D**. (Courtesy of P. Fenton, M.D., Toronto, Ontario, Canada.)

commonly, juvenile onset disease) (see Chapters 25, 26, and 27), the seronegative spondyloarthropathies (see Chapters 28, 29, and 30), osteoarthrosis (see Chapters 39 and 40), and crystal deposition diseases (see Chapters 43 and 44), although any monoarticular (e.g., septic arthritis, internal derangement) or polyarticular process associated with a large or recurrent joint effusion can lead to formation of a synovial cyst. Although synovial cysts can arise at many different periarticular locations, including those of the spine (see Chapter 40), they are encountered most commonly about the knee, hip, and to a lesser extent shoulder, elbow, wrist, foot, ankle, and hand. Indeed, synovial cysts can arise adjacent to sites of pseudarthrosis.[837] Large synovial cysts are most typical in cases of inflammatory arthritis, whereas small synovial cysts may indicate the presence of an internal derangement of the joint, such as a meniscal tear of the knee. In some locations, such as the semimembranosus-gastrocnemius region of the knee, a valvelike mechanism allows communication of the joint and cyst as a response to elevations in intra-articular pressure, serving as a mechanism for decompression of the joint. In other locations, the cyst and joint communicate freely without such a valve, or synovial cysts may be found that show no communication with the articulation. The differentiation of a noncommunicating synovial cyst and a ganglion cyst is best left to an experienced pathologist.

The most characteristic location of a synovial cyst is the posterior aspect of the knee related to distention of the gastrocnemius-semimembranosus bursa in response to a knee effusion. Such cysts become firm with full extension of the knee and soft when the joint is flexed, a phenomenon known as Foucher's sign.[838] These cysts, which are designated Baker's cysts, may dissect between the muscles of the leg (Fig. 95–125) or rupture with extravasation of fluid, producing clinical manifestations resembling those of thrombophlebitis. The diagnosis of a Baker's cyst can be accomplished with ultrasonography, radionuclide arthrography, standard arthrography, CT, computed arthrotomography, or MR imaging.[839–846] In addition to dissection or rupture, popliteal cysts may contain chondral or osteochondral bodies or rarely may calcify. Differential diagnostic considerations include meniscal and ganglion cysts of the knee,[847] anserine bursal distention,[848, 849] popliteal artery

aneurysm, entrapment or adventitial cystic disease,[850] and deep venous thrombosis or thrombophlebitis.

About the hip, fluid collections representing synovial cysts, distended iliopsoas bursae, or para-acetabular ganglia may be encountered.[851–857] They are most typical of rheumatoid arthritis (see Chapters 25 and 26) but also may be observed in osteoarthrosis (see Chapter 39) and other conditions. The iliopsoas bursa normally may communicate with the hip (see Chapter 22), so that its distension in cases of hip effusion is not unexpected. Complications of such distension include displacement of abdominal viscera and the bladder, venous obstruction, and entrapment of the femoral nerve.[852–854] CT and MR imaging[854, 855] are effective in accurate diagnosis. Chronic developmental dysplasia of the hip may be associated with tears of the acetabular labrum with intraosseous and para-acetabular ganglion cysts.[856] Such cysts in the soft tissues may be identified on plain films owing to the presence of gas.

Bursitis. Accumulation of fluid in bursal cavities may lead to soft tissue masses. Typical examples include iliopsoas bursitis,[854, 855] anserine bursitis,[848, 849] trochanteric bursitis,[858–860] cubital bursitis at the elbow,[861] prepatellar[862] and deep infrapatellar[863] bursitis, and bursitis about the Achilles tendon (Haglund's syndrome).[864] Bursal fluid may result from local irritation or trauma, or as a response to systemic rheumatologic conditions (e.g., rheumatoid arthritis, gout, seronegative spondyloarthropathies) or infection. Ultrasonography, CT, or MR imaging can be used for accurate diagnosis (Fig. 95–126). In some cases, the differentiation of bursitis and subcutaneous nodules, as in rheumatoid arthritis, with MR imaging may be difficult (Fig. 95–126).

SOFT TISSUE CALCIFICATION AND OSSIFICATION

The radiographic detection of calcification and ossification in the soft tissues provides an important clue to proper diagnosis. Although it certainly is helpful to distinguish between calcific and ossific radiodense lesions, this is not always possible, particularly if the collections are of small size. The documentation of ossification depends on the recognition of a trabecular pattern within the dense areas, a pattern that is identified more easily when large ossific

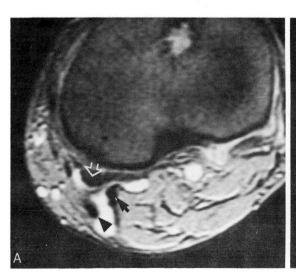
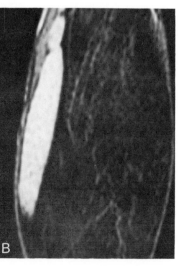

FIGURE 95–125. Synovial cyst: knee.

A A transaxial multiplanar gradient recalled (MPGR) MR image (TR/TE, 500/15; flip angle, 20 degrees) shows the site of origin of the synovial cyst. Note the fluid of high signal intensity passing posterior to the semimembranosus tendon (open arrow), medial to the tendon (closed arrow) of the medial head of the gastrocnemius muscle, and lateral to the semitendinosis tendon (arrowhead).

B A coronal T2-weighted (TR/TE, 2000/80) spin echo MR image in the same patient as in **A** shows the more distal extent of the synovial cyst, which is superficial to the medial head of the gastrocnemius muscle.

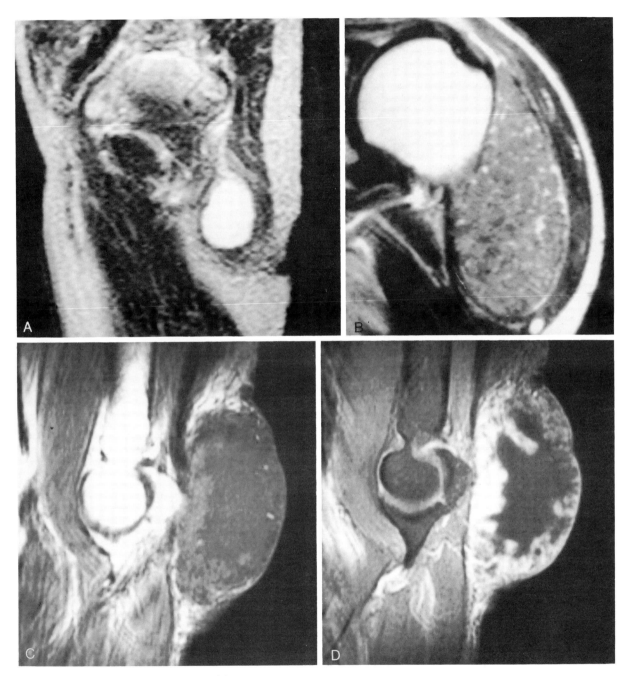

FIGURE 95–126. Bursitis and subcutaneous nodules.
 A Trochanteric bursitis. A sagittal T2-weighted (TR/TE, 1500/90) spin echo MR image reveals fluid of high signal intensity in the trochanteric bursa. (Courtesy of J. Dillard, M.D., San Diego, California.)
 B Subdeltoid bursitis. A coronal T2-weighted (TR/TE, 1800/90) spin echo MR image shows massive distention of the subdeltoid bursa. Areas of high signal intensity in the bursa represent fluid. Those of low signal intensity in the bursa are consistent with fibrous, or rice, bodies. (Courtesy of M. Tobias, M.D., Johannesburg, South Africa.)
 C, D Olecranon nodule in rheumatoid arthritis. This 76 year old man had multiple subcutaneous nodules. A sagittal T1-weighted (TR/TE, 700/14) spin echo MR image **(C)** shows a large soft tissue nodule posterior to the olecranon process. It is inhomogeneous but mainly of low signal intensity. Following the intravenous injection of a gadolinium compound, a sagittal T1-weighted (TR/TE, 600/14) fat-suppressed spin echo MR image **(D)** shows enhancement of the wall of this necrotic nodule. Additional diagnostic considerations include an infected subcutaneous nodule and septic olecranon bursitis.

masses are encountered. Calcification appears as irregular punctate, circular, linear, or plaque-like radiodense areas that do not possess trabecular or cortical structure. Diagnostic difficulty arises in the differentiation between calcification and ossification by radiographic methods, however, as calcification of ectopic bone initially will not reveal trabeculation, and ossifying neoplasms may produce poorly organized bone that does not possess a trabecular pattern.

Calcification

Greenfield[117] has classified the conditions that lead to deposition of calcium within soft tissues into three types: metastatic calcification related to a disturbance in calcium or phosphorus metabolism; calcinosis due to the deposition of calcium in skin and subcutaneous tissue in the presence of normal calcium metabolism; and dystrophic calcification related to calcium deposits in damaged or devitalized tissue in the absence of a generalized metabolic derangement. Causes of metastatic calcification include hyperparathyroidism, hypoparathyroidism, renal osteodystrophy (Fig. 95–127), hypervitaminosis D, milk-alkali syndrome, sarcoidosis, and processes associated with massive bony destruction, such as metastasis, plasma cell myeloma, and leukemia. In these disorders, collections of various sizes may appear in vis-

ceral and soft tissue locations; periarticular sites frequently are affected. The causes of generalized calcinosis include collagen vascular disorders, such as scleroderma and dermatomyositis, idiopathic tumoral calcinosis, and idiopathic calcinosis universalis (Fig. 95–128). The disorders leading to dystrophic calcification are many; neoplastic, inflammatory, and traumatic conditions are prime considerations, although tissue injury from any cause may produce lower carbon dioxide concentration, local alkalinity, and calcium deposition (Fig. 95–129).

The radiographic appearance in cases of soft tissue calcification usually does not allow a specific diagnosis. The terms calcinosis universalis, tumoral calcinosis, and calcinosis circumscripta should be regarded as descriptive designations for widespread, mass-like, or localized calcific deposits, respectively, and not as a single disease entity. Thus, "universal," "tumoral," or "circumscribed" deposits can accompany several collagen vascular or additional disorders or appear on an idiopathic basis.

In some conditions, the roentgenographic characteristics of the calcification are relatively diagnostic.[423] Circular or elliptical calcific collections with radiolucent centers may represent the phleboliths in hemangiomas or varicosities (Fig. 95–130), the calcified fatty deposits in panniculitis or Ehlers-Danlos syndrome (Fig. 95–131), or cysticercosis. A

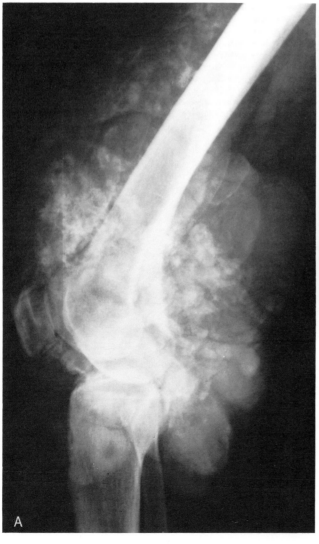

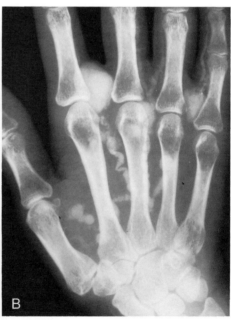

FIGURE 95–127. Metastatic soft tissue calcification. In renal osteodystrophy, periarticular, intra-articular, and vascular calcification may be evident. (**A,** Courtesy of J. Goobar, M.D., Ostersund, Sweden; **B,** Courtesy of M. Weisman, M.D., San Diego, California.)

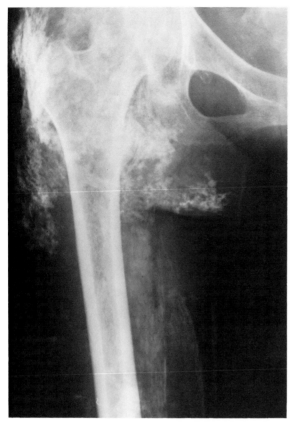

FIGURE 95–128. Generalized soft tissue calcinosis. A reticular pattern of soft tissue calcification is characteristic of dermatomyositis and collagen vascular overlap syndromes. (Courtesy of H.S. Kang, M.D., Seoul, Korea.)

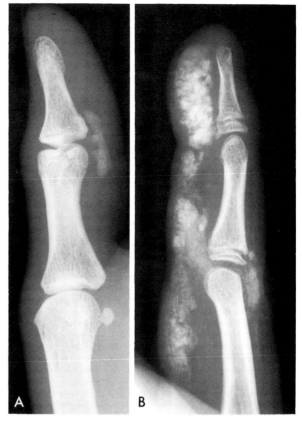

FIGURE 95–129. Dystrophic soft tissue calcification. Calcific deposits in the fingers of these two patients followed local injuries.

reticulated pattern of calcification is frequent in dermatomyositis.

The site of calcification also provides a clue to the correct diagnosis.[117–119] Examples include the periarticular deposits of hyperparathyroidism, renal osteodystrophy, milk-alkali syndrome, hypervitaminosis D, and collagen vascular disorders; the calcified joint capsules, tendons, or bursae of calcium hydroxyapatite or calcium pyrophosphate dihydrate crystal deposition disease; the lymph node collections that may appear in various granulomatous infections; the arterial calcifications of renal osteodystrophy, diabetes mellitus, and hypervitaminosis D; the calcified nerves of leprosy; chondrocalcinosis that appears in idiopathic calcium pyrophosphate dihydrate crystal deposition disease, hemochromatosis, hyperparathyroidism, and, rarely, other crystal deposition diseases; the calcified intervertebral discs that may accompany alkaptonuria, idiopathic calcium pyrophosphate dihydrate crystal deposition disease, hyperparathyroidism, immobilization, and trauma; the fingertip deposits that are seen in scleroderma and other collagen vascular disorders; the sheet-like collections of calcification in the lower leg indicating nerve and soft tissue injury in the compartment syndrome[424]; and calcification of the pinna of the ear, which may be evident in a variety of endocrine diseases, thermal or physical trauma, and perichondritis.

The uptake of ⁹⁹ᵐTc-labeled phosphate compounds by metastatic calcifications is a well recognized but nondiagnostic phenomenon.[303, 304] As the collections contain apatite, it has been suggested that such uptake is due to the same process of surface adsorption on the hydroxyapatite

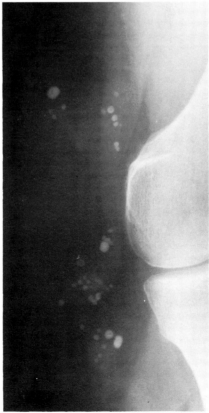

FIGURE 95–130. Hemangioma. Circular calcifications with lucent centers are typical of hemangiomas.

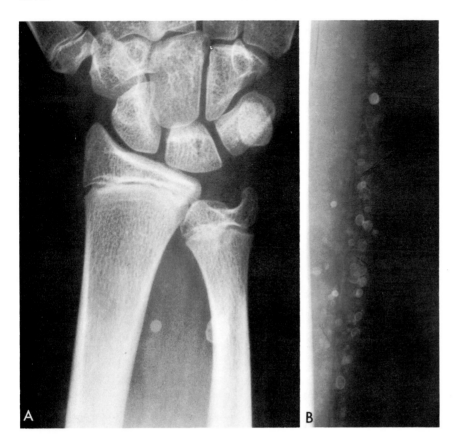

FIGURE 95–131. Ehlers-Danlos syndrome. Circular calcified fatty deposits with lucent centers can be seen in this syndrome. (Courtesy of M. Dalinka, M.D., Philadelphia, Pennsylvania.)

crystal that takes place in bone.[120] Alternative explanations suggest that the polyphosphate radical is metabolized in the same manner as ionic phosphate or that uptake is mediated by enzymatic receptors, such as the phosphatases. No matter what the cause, the abnormal scintigraphic pattern, although defining the location and extent of soft tissue calcification, provides little help in reaching a specific diagnosis.

Many of the disorders leading to calcific deposits in the soft tissue are described in other sections of the book. Two additional entities are noted here.

Idiopathic Calcinosis Universalis. This rare disorder of unknown cause affects infants and children.[121–123] The deposits initially appear in the subcutaneous fat of the extremities but subsequently involve other connective tissues, such as muscles, ligaments, and tendons, and other body regions. It appears that calcium phosphate and calcium carbonate are deposited about normal fat cells in the absence of infection, infarction, inflammation, or hemorrhage. A foreign body reaction occurs, leading to cellular infiltration, giant cell formation, and fibrosis. Calcareous nodules coalesce, becoming large masses that may violate the skin, producing sinus tracts. Internal organs are not affected. Serum calcium and phosphorus levels are normal.

Radiographs reveal discrete conglomerations of calcium that are arranged in longitudinal bands (Fig. 95–132). In the infant, the deposits usually are limited to the subcutaneous fat, whereas in the child, both fat and connective tissue are affected.[123]

The major differential diagnosis is dermatomyositis.[124] Other processes such as calcified subcutaneous fat necrosis,[125] extravasation of calcium gluconate injection solutions,[126, 296] and hyperparathyroidism also must be considered.

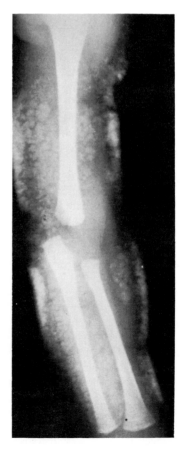

FIGURE 95–132. Calcinosis universalis (idiopathic). Longitudinal bands of calcification in the subcutaneous fat can be identified in this 3 month old male infant.

Idiopathic Tumoral Calcinosis. In 1943, Inclan and associates[127] first introduced the term tumoral calcinosis to describe the appearance of prominent periarticular calcified masses, especially about large joints such as the hip, the shoulder, and the elbow. Numerous descriptions of this entity now exist, although a variety of names have been used,[128] including lipocalcinogranulomatosis,[129] lipocalcinogranulomatous bursitis,[130] tumoral lipocalcinosis,[131, 132] calcifying collagenolysis,[133] and calcified bursae.[134] The designation of tumoral calcinosis is encountered most widely.[128, 135–141, 427–429]

Tumoral calcinosis usually becomes manifest in the second and third decades of life. Rarely, infants and young children are involved.[425, 426, 867, 873] Men are affected more commonly than women, and blacks especially are susceptible. A family history is apparent in 30 to 40 per cent of cases, and an autosomal dominant or recessive pattern of inheritance has been suggested. A previous episode of significant trauma is reported rarely. On clinical evaluation, firm, tumor-like, painless swellings are evident, especially about the hips and the shoulders as well as the elbows and ankles, and these may interfere with joint motion.[869] Solitary or, less commonly, multiple foci can be evident. The lesions usually involve the soft tissues or skeletal muscles but occasionally may be very superficial[870] or bursal[873] in location. The overlying skin usually is intact, although soft tissue ulcerations occasionally are apparent. Rare clinical manifestations include gingivitis and other lesions of the mucous membranes and an erythematous rash that may preceed the development of calcified soft tissue nodules.[871] The soft tissue lesions may recur following incomplete excision.

Laboratory analysis usually indicates normal or slightly elevated levels of serum calcium and normal levels of serum electrolytes, phosphorus, urea, uric acid, and alkaline phosphatase. The observation in some persons of (1) a slightly raised urinary level of hydroxyproline and hyperphosphatemia, (2) an increased intestinal absorption of dietary calcium coupled with radioactive studies with [47]Ca indicating rapid exchange of calcium between serum and masses, and (3) a family history of disease has suggested to some investigators that the disorder may be an inborn error of phosphorus metabolism.[143] More recent data have indicated that in patients with tumoral calcinosis and hyperphosphatemia, parathyroid hormone levels and renal responsiveness are normal and that parathyroid hormone-independent enhancement of phosphate reabsorption, possibly in the proximal tubule, may underlie the chronic hyperphosphatemia.[297] Dietary restriction of phosphorus or the use of aluminum-containing antacids that bind phosphorus in the gut have been reported to represent an effective therapeutic regimen.[428, 429, 869, 872]

Radiographs reveal circular or oval, well-demarcated masses of calcium about articulations (Figs. 95–133 and 95–134). A lobulated inhomogeneous appearance is characteristic. Radiolucent linear bands separate the calcific foci.[866] The individual lesions vary from 1 to 20 cm in diameter and may reveal fluid levels on erect, decubitus, or cross-table roentgenograms.[136, 137, 142] This finding, which also can be demonstrated with CT[430, 865] and MR imaging,[868] is not specific, being evident in other disorders associated with large soft tissue calcific collections (Fig. 95–134). Radionuclide studies with technetium compounds may out-

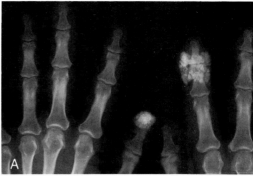
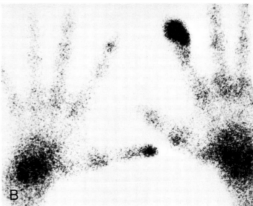

FIGURE 95–133. Tumoral calcinosis (idiopathic). A 51 year old white man had tumoral calcific deposits about multiple joints, including the shoulders, the hips, the feet, and the fingers. Soft tissue ulcerations had developed.
A A radiograph of the hands reveals dense nodular calcific deposits about a distal interphalangeal joint and the terminal tuft of the thumb.
B Bone scan with ^{99m}Tc-pyrophosphate delineates increased accumulation of radionuclide at sites of calcification.
(**A, B** From Brown ML, et al: Radiology *124*:757, 1977.)

line increased accumulation in areas of calcinosis.[140, 147, 305] Pathologic examination reveals a lobulated soft tissue mass containing fibrovascular fronds dividing it into several loculi. Yellowish-white in color, the masses exude a purulent calcified material or a pasty, chalky liquid. Analysis of this material documents accumulations of calcium phosphate, calcium carbonate, or a mixture of these. Although deposits are apatite in nature, they differ from normal bone mineral, being heavily mineralized and containing larger and more perfect hydroxyapatite crystals.[431] Histologic characteristics include active areas consisting of large numbers of mononuclear cells, probably histiocytes, and multinucleated giant cells, and vascular indolent areas consisting of foci of edematous and granulomatous or dense collagenous tissue with chronic inflammatory cells.[128]

The exact nature of idiopathic tumoral calcinosis is a mystery. The elevated serum phosphorus levels noted in some patients have been viewed as supporting the existence of an inborn error of metabolism,[143] perhaps related to an inherited reduction in renal tubular responsiveness to parathyroid hormone[144] or in renal handling of phosphate excretion.[432] Traumatic or infectious (parasitic) causes also have been suggested as factors that might stimulate the proliferation of primitive mesenchymal cells.[138, 145] Other investigators consider the disease a variant of calcinosis universalis, a reaction of surrounding soft tissue to ectopic

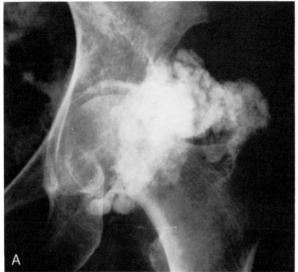

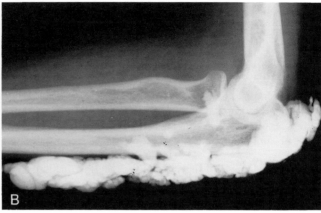

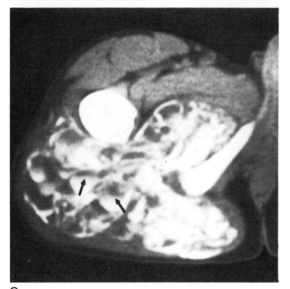

C

FIGURE 95–134. Tumoral calcinosis (idiopathic).

A, B In this 70 year old woman, prominent calcification is seen about the hip **(A)** and the elbow **(B)**. (Courtesy of H. Kroon, M.D., Leiden, the Netherlands.)

C In this patient, a transaxial CT scan at the level of the ischial tuberosities shows a large calcified periarticular mass with fluid levels (arrows). (Courtesy of A. Brower, M.D., Norfolk, Virginia.)

synovial membrane, or a degradation of periarticular collagen with dystrophic calcification. Calcification may indeed represent a secondary phenomenon related to a genetically determined defect in collagenous tissue.[128] Tumoral calcinosis has been described in association with massive osteolysis,[146] a pseudoxanthoma elasticum-like syndrome,[873] calcium pyrophosphate dihydrate crystal deposition disease,[873] dental abnormalities,[873] Engelmann's disease,[433] and Down's syndrome.[136] It also has been associated with recurrent pain and swelling in the legs and periostitis of tubular bones[434] (see Chapter 93). Some investigators suggest that the periosteal new bone formation occurring mainly in the diaphysis of tubular bones that may be seen in tumoral calcinosis is related to inflammatory changes in the bone marrow that occur as a response to hydroxyapatite crystal deposition and subsequent calcification.[873]

The diagnosis of idiopathic tumoral calcinosis is one of exclusion. Other processes, such as collagen vascular disorders, hyperparathyroidism, hypervitaminosis D, milk-alkali syndrome, and chronic renal disease, first must be eliminated by clinical, laboratory, and radiologic examinations. The periarticular localization of the calcifications in idiopathic tumoral calcinosis differs from the intra-articular

radiodense deposits of idiopathic synovial (osteo)chondromatosis and calcium pyrophosphate dihydrate crystal deposition disease, although these latter two disorders occasionally can affect extra-articular structures.[435]

Ossification

The disorders leading to ossification of soft tissues are more limited in number than those producing soft tissue calcification (Table 95–3). Heterotopic ossification appearing in association with neurologic disorders or problems

TABLE 95–3. Some Causes of Soft Tissue Ossification

Neurologic diseases
Physical and thermal injuries
Venous insufficiency
Neoplasms (e.g., parosteal osteosarcoma, extraskeletal osteosarcoma)
Pseudomalignant osseous tumor of soft tissue
Myositis (fibrodysplasia) ossificans progressiva
Melorheostosis
Surgical scars
Postoperative period

(see Chapter 77), thermal burns (see Chapter 72), and venous insufficiency (see Chapter 93) is discussed elsewhere in this book. In the first two situations, para-articular collections are frequent, which may lead to "ankylosis" of joints, whereas in the latter situation, small subcutaneous ossicles or a dense meshwork of osseous fibrils, usually in an edematous lower extremity, are observed.[436] Ossification appearing in scars also has been reported, creating plaque-like radiodense areas, especially on abdominal radiographs,[437, 438, 441, 442] but also on chest radiographs in women who have undergone a radical mastectomy.[439] Possible explanations for this phenomenon are detachment and stimulation of portions of the periosteum at the time of surgery and differentiation of immature connective tissue to osteoblasts as a reaction to injury. In the abdomen, ossification of scars is more frequent in men and is seen exclusively following vertical skin incisions.[438]

Ossification in soft tissues may occur as a result of intraosseous tumors, such as osteosarcoma, that extend into the adjacent soft tissues. In a similar fashion, some nontumorous conditions may extend from a bone, leading to apparent soft tissue ossification. A classic example is Paget's disease in which soft tissue masses containing osteoid tissue may appear. The resulting radiographic appearance may simulate that of a pagetic sarcoma (Fig. 95–135).

Osteosarcoma and other sarcomas of soft tissue represent additional causes of ossification (see earlier discussion). Foci of osteoid or new bone have appeared in association with melorheostosis (Fig. 95–136) and with proliferative myositis and ossifying fasciitis.[440] Metastases to soft tissues, including muscle, subsequently may ossify, and those to bone may induce nearby heterotopic ossification[443] (see Chapter 85).

In most of the situations mentioned previously, as well as those that are noted later in this chapter, radiographs may outline definite trabecular structure within the ossific collections, allowing differentiation of ossification from calcification. At certain times, serial roentgenograms will permit assessment of the maturity of the ossific deposit; initial cloud-like radiodense areas will mature into trabecular bone. Such an assessment is important, as removal of heterotopic bone prior to maturity in cases of burn or paraplegia may not afford long-term relief owing to rapid reaccumulation of the deposits. Unfortunately, roentgenographic changes and even serum alkaline phosphatase determinations do not adequately reflect the activity of the ossification process in many cases.[148, 149] Serial radionuclide studies using strontium[150] or technetium[151] compounds may be more accurate in this regard (see Chapter 15) and can be supplemented with bone marrow scans to assess the maturity of heterotopic ossification appearing in the paralyzed or burned patient or even in the person following local trauma, tetanus,[152, 157, 158, 444] or carbon monoxide poisoning.[153] CT and MR imaging also may be employed in the detection and serial monitoring of heterotopic ossification, particularly following trauma (see later discussion).

Ossification of Tendons and Ligaments. Although calcific tendinitis due to calcium hydroxyapatite or calcium pyrophosphate dihydrate crystal deposition is common and well recognized (see Chapters 44 and 45), ossification

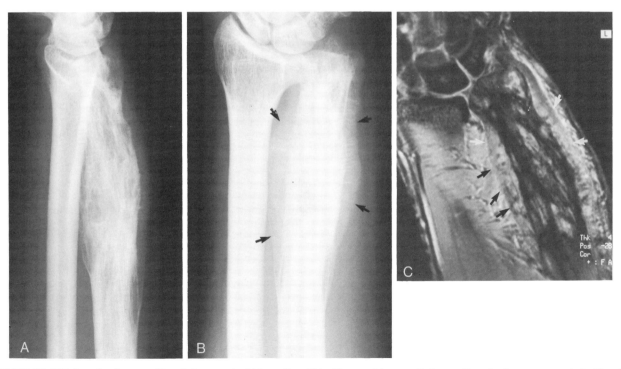

FIGURE 95–135. Paget's disease with soft tissue osteoid formation. This 44 year old man with known Paget's disease presented with pain and swelling of the forearm.

  A A radiograph obtained 6 years previously shows pagetic involvement of the distal portion of the ulna. Subtle spiculation of the surface of the bone is evident.

  B During his current evaluation, a radiograph reveals a periosseous mass (arrows) related to osteoid production.

  C A coronal multiplanar gradient recalled (MPGR) MR image (TR/TE, 578/18; flip angle, 30 degrees) shows the pagetic involvement of the ulna and surrounding osteoid (arrows). Biopsy confirmed the absence of a pagetic sarcoma.

  (Courtesy of P. Kaplan, M.D., Charlottesville, Virginia.)

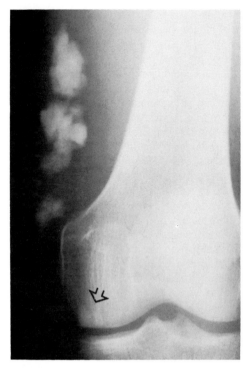

FIGURE 95–136. Melorheostosis. The beaded pattern of soft tissue ossification is characteristic of this disorder. Note the radiodense focus (arrow) within the distal femur.

within tendinous structures is relatively rare. Posttraumatic calcification and ossification of tendons or ligaments may be encountered at certain sites, such as the medial collateral ligament of the knee, where it is termed the Pellegrini-Stieda syndrome or disease, appearing as arcuate or curvilinear radiodense collections adjacent to the medial femoral condyle (Fig. 95–137). Ossification of the Achilles tendon also has been recognized,[154–156] although this appears to be an unusual finding (Fig. 95–138). The deposits may be unilateral or bilateral and originate in the body of the tendon or at its insertion into the calcaneus, producing a firm, nontender mass. A definite history of trauma or surgery is

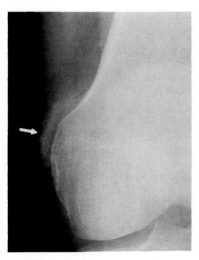

FIGURE 95–137. Pellegrini-Stieda syndrome. An example of post-traumatic ossification in the medial collateral ligament of the knee is shown (arrow).

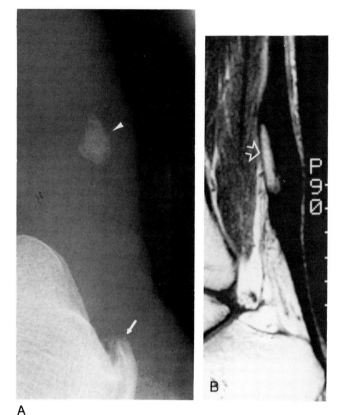

A

FIGURE 95–138. Ossification of the Achilles tendon.
  A Idiopathic ossification of this tendon (arrowhead) developed in this patient. Note the enlarged tendinous outline and the excrescence (arrow) at the site of tendinous attachment to the calcaneus. A history of trauma was not elicited.
  B In a different patient, a sagittal T1-weighted (TR/TE, 300/20) spin echo MR image shows Achilles tendon ossification (arrow) and thickening. (**B,** Courtesy of S. Moreland, M.D., San Diego, California.)

frequent but not invariable. Significant local symptoms and signs may indicate a fracture of the ossified deposit.[156, 569] MR imaging typically shows tendon thickening in the area of ossification (Fig. 95–138). A similar phenomenon of ossification occurs in the patellar tendon, usually as a response to repetitive trauma[874] or prior surgery,[875] and differs in appearance from patellar enthesophytes that occur at the osseous sites of attachment of the quadriceps and patellar tendons.

Calcification or ossification in the stylohyoid ligament is a frequent, incidental radiographic finding, although when excessive or when the styloid process itself is enlarged, or both, a specific syndrome (termed the Eagle syndrome) may occur.[445–450, 568] Dysphagia, abnormalities of taste, a ''lump'' in the throat, and pain are among the clinical manifestations of this syndrome and relate to the intimate association of the stylohyoid apparatus with such structures as the internal carotid artery, the internal jugular vein, the external carotid artery, and the accessory, hypoglossal, vagus, and glossopharyngeal nerves. In some cases, tonsillectomy scars contribute to the intensity of these manifestations. Radiographs reveal an elongated and ossified styloid process and ligament with either a smooth or irregular outline, which must be differentiated from normal variations in the length of this process and in the degree of ossification in the ligament

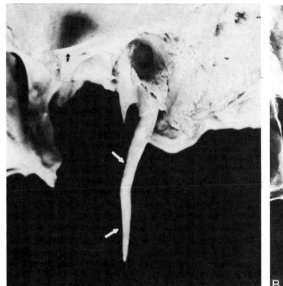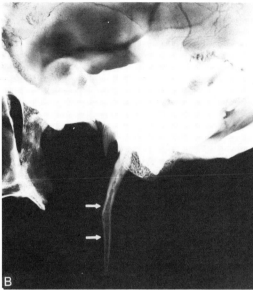

FIGURE 95–139. Ossification of the stylohyoid ligament (Eagle's syndrome). Observe the large ossified structure (arrows), which represents an elongated styloid process or ossified stylohyoid ligament, or both.

(Fig. 95–139). Of interest, ossified stylohyoid ligaments may fracture[451] and have been associated with mucopolysaccharidoses.[452] Such ossification also occurs in diffuse idiopathic skeletal hyperostosis.

Bony excrescences at sites of tendinous attachment should be differentiated from true tendinous ossification. These osseous outgrowths are frequent, especially in older patients, and may represent a manifestation of diffuse idiopathic skeletal hyperostosis (see Chapter 41). This disorder also can lead to true ossification in the substance of tendons and ligaments, a situation that additionally may be encountered in fluorosis (see Chapter 74).

Myositis Ossificans Traumatica. Sixty[159] to 75 per cent[160] of patients with localized soft tissue ossifications (myositis ossificans circumscripta) relate a clear history of trauma; the other patients either suffer from one of the systemic problems associated with soft tissue ossification, such as neurologic conditions, burns, and tetanus, or develop the lesions spontaneously.[161, 280] The spontaneous cases are termed myositis ossificans nontraumatica or pseudomalignant osseous tumor of soft tissue (see discussion later in this chapter). The radiographic and pathologic features of myositis ossificans traumatica and pseudomalignant osseous tumor of soft tissue virtually are identical.

The accuracy of the designation ''myositis ossificans'' for this lesion has been challenged on numerous occasions. Indeed, the absence of inflammation as well as muscular involvement in some cases would indicate the inappropriateness of this name.[162] It has been postulated that the soft tissue ossification results from damage to the interstitium, not to the muscle.[162, 163] The presence of osteoblastosis on histologic examination is irrefutable, but the source of the osteoblasts remains a mystery; they may originate from damaged periosteum or pleuripotent cells already present in the connective tissue.[161, 164, 165]

Myositis ossificans traumatica usually appears in adolescents or young adults; rarely, infants or children are affected.[169, 570] The sites of localization are areas susceptible to injury, such as the elbow, the thigh[309] (Fig. 95–140), the buttocks, and, less often, the shoulder and the calf.[159] The appearance of ossification following elbow injuries[166] (Fig. 95–141) or about the region of the quadriceps[167] is well recognized although virtually any site can be affected, including the hand,[170] the jaw,[453] and the spine.[454, 886] In general, the frequency of myositis ossificans traumatica is greater in the proximal than the distal portion of an extremity.[876] Post-traumatic ossification about the elbow occurs both medially and laterally, may encircle the collateral ligaments, and may injure the ulnar nerve.[877] When there has been a history of injury, specific radiographic features can be correlated with the time that has elapsed following trauma, although in some persons, the initiating injury may be of such minor nature as to be unrecognized or soon forgotten.[168] Post-traumatic ossification, however, appears to occur with a higher incidence when the initiating injury is severe.[876] Repetitive minor trauma induced by occupational or recreational activities is a well-known cause of such ossification, however.

Shortly after injury, a soft tissue mass or swelling becomes apparent, which may be associated with periosteal reaction in 7 to 10 days (Fig. 95–142). Flocculent dense lesions arise in the mass from 11 days to 6 weeks after the trauma.[161] The calcific dense areas gradually enlarge, and at 6 to 8 weeks a lacy pattern of new bone is sharply circumscribed about the periphery of the mass.[159] The soft tissue central core occasionally becomes encysted, and an enlarging central cavity combined with peripheral calcification and ossification resembles an eggshell. Maturity is reached in 5 to 6 months (Fig. 95–143), and the mass then shrinks. Complete or partial resorption of the ossified mass is reported to be more frequent in young persons.[876]

The recognition of a peripheral rim of calcification and ossification about a more lucent center cannot be overemphasized as an important radiographic manifestation of myositis ossificans (Figs. 95–144 and 95–145). Furthermore, a radiolucent band or zone between the lesion and the subjacent cortex also is a very important finding, reflecting the lack of intimacy between the ossified mass and neighboring

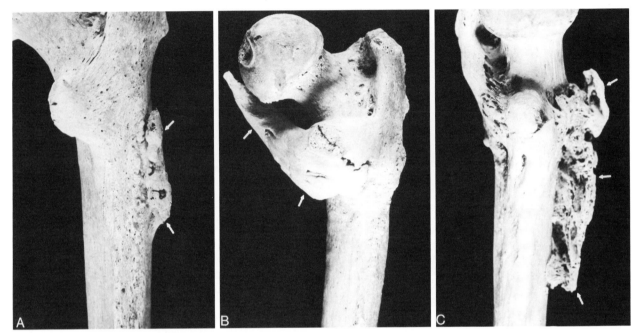

FIGURE 95–140. Myositis ossificans traumatica: Thigh. Three examples are shown (arrows).

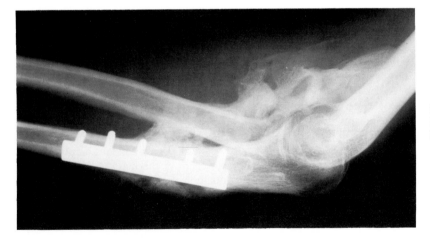

FIGURE 95–141. Myositis ossificans traumatica: Elbow. Heterotopic bone formation following elbow injuries is a well-recognized finding.

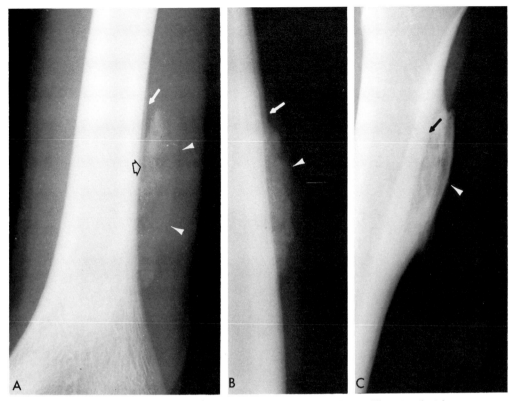

FIGURE 95–142. Myositis ossificans traumatica: Sequential radiographic abnormalities (three different patients).

A Shortly after injury, a soft tissue swelling appears that may be associated with periostitis (arrow). Ill-defined osseous dense areas (arrowheads) appear within 2 to 6 weeks following the traumatic insult. Note the lucent area (open arrow) between the ossifications and the underlying bone.

B Subsequently, a trabecular architecture can be seen in the mass (arrowhead) and the subjacent lucent area is obliterated. More mature periostitis (arrow) is seen.

C Eventually, the mass of mature bone (arrowhead) merges with the underlying cortex, producing a localized osseous expansion that resembles an osteochondroma. The original cortical line (arrow) can be recognized, however.

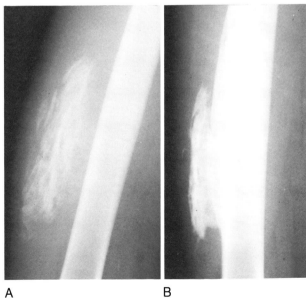

FIGURE 95–143. Myositis ossificans traumatica: Maturing ossification. In this 11 year old boy who fell from the stairs of a swimming pool, lateral radiographs of the femur 1 month **(A)** and 5 months **(B)** following the injury show maturation of the ossifying process. Initially separated from the bone, the process subsequently merges with the anterior femoral surface. (Courtesy of G. Greenway, M.D., Dallas, Texas.)

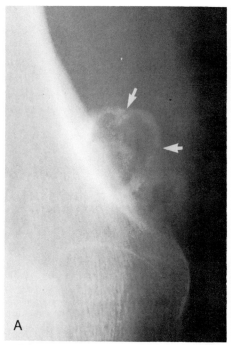

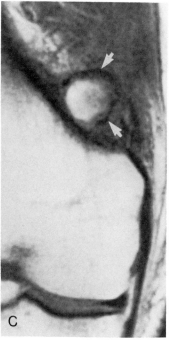

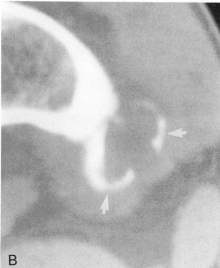

FIGURE 95–144. Myositis ossificans traumatica: Peripheral rim of calcification and ossification.

A A frontal radiograph shows a lesion applied to the medial cortex of the distal femur. Adjacent mature periosteal reaction is seen. Note the rimlike pattern of ossification (arrows).

B Transaxial CT confirms ossification (arrows) at the periphery of the mass and adjacent cortical thickening.

C A coronal T1-weighted (TR/TE, 600/20) spin echo MR image reveals low signal intensity at the margin of the lesion (arrows) and central higher signal intensity identical to that of fat or blood.

(Courtesy of M. Zlatkin, M.D., North Hollywood, Florida.)

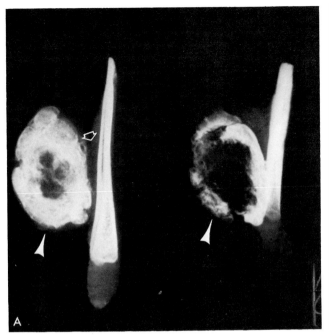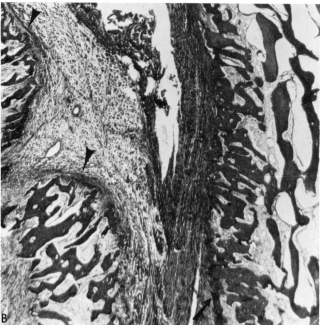

FIGURE 95–145. Myositis ossificans traumatica: Radiographic-pathologic correlation.

A Serial sections through a focus of myositis ossificans delineate a well-encapsulated lesion possessing a peripheral zone of ossification and a lucent center (arrowheads). Note the separation or clear zone (open arrow) between the lesion and the underlying bone.

B Fibrous tissue separates the maturing foci of myositis ossificans (arrowheads) from the periosteal new bone (arrow) and is the basis for the zone of radiolucency observed between the lesion and the parent bone.

(Courtesy of A. Norman, M.D., Valhalla, New York.)

bone, and allowing differentiation of myositis ossificans from parosteal osteosarcoma (see discussion later in this chapter). Topographic variations in the ossifying process can lead to radiographic alterations that may be more difficult to analyze, however[161] (Fig. 95–146). Direct damage to the cambium layer of the periosteum from the traumatic insult can lead to an ossifying subperiosteal hematoma[168] or

periosteoma, in which a sunburst periosteal reaction within the first 2 weeks easily may be misinterpreted as evidence of a malignant process. Second, a true hematoma of the muscle can create a soft tissue mass that is quite distant from the nearest bone and which may or may not ossify (ossifying hematoma) on subsequent examination.[171] In addition, a progressive variety of localized myositis ossifi-

FIGURE 95–146. Myositis ossificans traumatica: Atypical radiographic abnormalities. This one year old boy sustained an injury to the arm when he fell down the stairs.

A Although initial radiographs were normal, a radiograph obtained approximately two weeks after the injury shows extensive soft tissue swelling and periosteal new bone in the humerus and ulna.

B Eleven days later, increased periostitis and a mass containing irregular areas of ossification are evident.

C Six weeks after **B,** the ossification is more mature and organized. A blunt dissection with removal of as much of the mass as was possible provided material that on histologic analysis was typical of myositis ossificans.

(From Nuovo MA, et al: Skel Radiol *21:*87, 1992.)

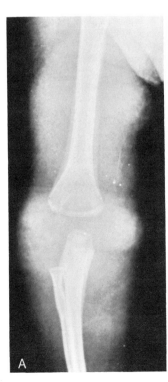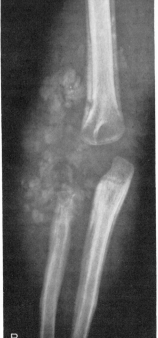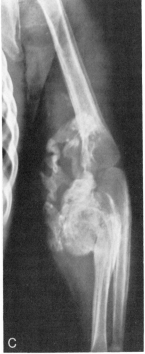

cans has been recorded that does not recur following surgery.[172, 173]

The microscopic changes of myositis ossificans have been well documented[161] (Fig. 95–147). Mesenchymal proliferation results in the accumulation of focal masses of collagen in which calcium salts are deposited. Heterotopic osteoblasts appear, produce matrix, and create a well-defined lesion possessing a fibrous capsule. The developing lesion demonstrates three distinct zones, a phenomenon that allows differentiation from sarcomatous processes.[162, 174] The center of the lesion contains rapidly proliferating fibroblasts with areas of hemorrhage and necrosis. A middle zone contains osteoblasts with islands of immature bone. Biopsy of cellular inner and middle layers alone may result in an erroneous diagnosis of a sarcoma. It is the outer zone of the lesion that reveals the true benign nature of the process. In this region, mature trabeculae are discovered that are clearly demarcated from the surrounding connective tissue. Thus, a peripheral shell of maturing bone exists about a soft cellular center, and maturation proceeds in a centripetal fashion with the center layer being the last to

ossify. Pathologic criteria that are helpful in differentiation of myositis ossificans from sarcoma are a zone phenomenon, the lack of invasion of adjacent tissues, and the inclusion of viable muscle fibers, which would be destroyed by an advancing tumor.[161]

Identification of myositis ossificans usually is possible on the basis of the clinical and radiologic findings (Fig. 95–148). Although other diagnostic techniques, such as arteriography,[175] ultrasonography,[176, 878, 879] scintigraphy,[455–457] and CT[458, 459, 880–882] (Fig. 95–144), occasionally may aid in the evaluation of this condition, they usually are not required for correct diagnosis but may be helpful in identifying the maturity of the lesion. MR imaging also has been employed to study myositis ossificans.[883–885] The MR imaging appearance of the ossifying lesions varies according to the stage of development and, in some cases, may simulate that of a soft tissue neoplasm. Less diagnostic difficulty is encountered in chronic lesions (Fig. 95–144), which tend to be well defined, possess a border of low signal intensity, and contain fat (with its characteristic signal intensity),[884] although occasional chronic lesions reveal regions of high

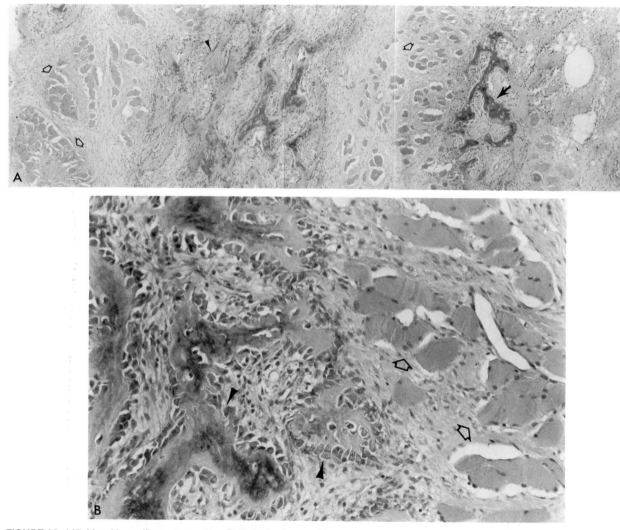

FIGURE 95–147. Myositis ossificans traumatica: Pathologic abnormalities.

A Muscular tissue can be identified (open arrows). In certain areas (intermediate zone), osteoid and immature bone formation in cellular fibrous tissue is seen (arrowhead); elsewhere (outer zone), maturation of ossification is evident (solid arrow) (68×).

B Observe muscle bundles (open arrows) and newly formed bone trabeculae with prominent osteoblasts (arrowheads) (170×).

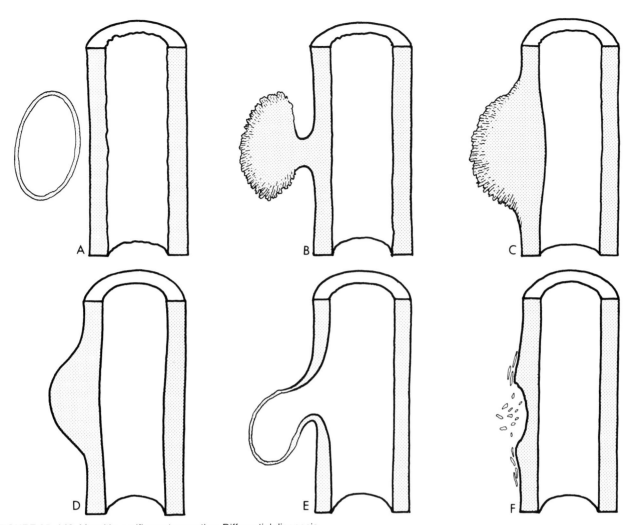

FIGURE 95–148. Myositis ossificans traumatica: Differential diagnosis.

A Myositis ossificans traumatica. The shell-like configuration of the ossification with a clear zone between it and the underlying bone is typical of this condition.

B Parosteal osteosarcoma. These lesions appear as central ossifying foci with irregular outlines and may be connected to the underlying bone by a stalk.

C Periosteal osteosarcoma. These tumors arise in the cortex of the diaphysis of a tubular bone and produce cortical thickening and spiculated osteoid matrix.

D Osteoma. Characteristic of this lesion is a localized excrescence that produces bulging of the cortical contour.

E Osteochondroma. An exostosis protrudes from the cortical surface. Its medullary and cortical bone is continuous with that of the underlying osseous structure.

F Juxtacortical (periosteal) chondroma. These periosteal lesions produce localized excavation of the cortex with periostitis. They may contain calcification.

signal intensity on T2-weighted images.[885] In acute or subacute stages of myositis ossificans, signal intensity inhomogeneity may be evident; high signal intensity on T2-weighted images may be seen (Figs. 95–149 and 95–150), particularly centrally in a proliferating core of fibroblasts and myofibroblasts.[884] When results of routine radiography or of other imaging methods are not diagnostic, histologic documentation may be necessary to establish a definite diagnosis; however, the pathologist must be wary of the ''pseudomalignant'' nature of the central portion of the lesion, which can complicate the evaluation. Furthermore, reports have been made of sarcomatous transformation in foci of myositis ossificans, usually taking the form of fibrosarcoma[178, 179] or osteosarcoma,[94, 177, 460, 461] an occurrence that could further complicate accurate histologic appraisal. Fortunately, the frequency of sarcomatous change in myositis ossificans appears to be very small.

Myositis ossificans must be differentiated from parosteal osteosarcoma, periosteal osteosarcoma, extraskeletal (soft tissue) osteosarcoma or chondrosarcoma, osteochondroma, osteoma, and juxtacortical chondroma (see Chapter 83). *Parosteal osteosarcomas*[180–182] arise in the metaphysis of tubular bones, especially along the posterior aspect of the distal femur (Fig. 95–151). Although a lucent zone may exist between the tumor and underlying bone, the zone usually is incomplete, as a pedicle extends from the neoplasm to the subjacent osseous tissue. Furthermore, a parosteal osteosarcoma is more heavily calcified in its central portion and base of attachment, the periphery is less dense and poorly circumscribed, and the tumor enlarges with time. *Periosteal osteosarcomas*[183, 184] arise in the cortex of the diaphysis of a tubular bone and lead to cortical thickening and spiculated osteoid matrix that is progressively denser from the periphery to the cortical base. *Extraskeletal*

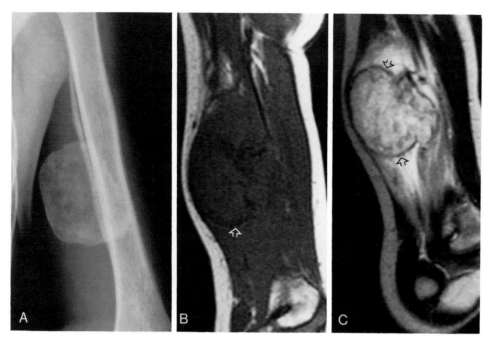

FIGURE 95–149. Myositis ossificans traumatica: MR abnormalities. This four year old boy fell on his arm.

A A radiograph obtained four weeks later shows classic features of myositis ossificans. Note the well-defined ossific mass and mature periosteal new bone formation in the humeral diaphysis.

B A sagittal oblique T1-weighted (TR/TE, 600/14) spin echo MR image shows a poorly defined intramuscular mass with signal intensity similar to that of muscle. Some foci of very low signal intensity are seen (arrow).

C A sagittal oblique T2-weighted (TR/TE, 3000/95) fast spin echo MR image reveals high signal intensity in the mass and surrounding tissues. Note the peripheral rim of low signal intensity (arrows), representing ossification.

(Courtesy of D. Witte, M.D., Memphis, Tennessee.)

osteosarcomas[94] are rare neoplasms that can cause difficulty in differential diagnosis. They grow slowly and affect older patients. An *osteochondroma* arises from and is connected to the subjacent bone; it possesses a cartilaginous cap (Fig. 95–152). Both the cortex and the spongiosa of the osteochondroma and parent bone are continuous. Occasionally, a mature focus of myositis ossificans may develop a cartilaginous cap and areas of cartilage,[162] whereas an osteo-

chondroma may give rise to a chondrosarcoma. In these cases, differential diagnosis may be more difficult. An *osteoma* is an osseous excrescence extending from the outer surface of the cortex (Fig. 95–153) that readily is differentiated from myositis ossificans (see Chapter 93), whereas a *juxtacortical (periosteal) chondroma* produces soft tissue calcification, an excavation of the cortex, and adjacent periosteal proliferation (Fig. 95–154).

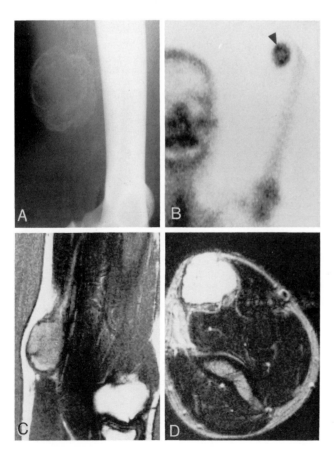

FIGURE 95–150. Myositis ossificans traumatica: MR abnormalities. This 22 year old man developed a mass in the arm following an injury.

A The mass is ossified and well defined. Note the shell-like pattern of ossification.

B A bone scan obtained with the arm held above the head shows accumulation of the radionuclide, particularly at the periphery of the lesion (arrowhead).

C A sagittal T1-weighted (TR/TE, 650/20) spin echo MR image shows a superficial anterolateral mass near the elbow, deforming the adjacent biceps, brachialis, and brachioradialis muscles. The interior of the mass is of intermediate signal intensity.

D A transaxial T2-weighted (TR/TE, 2400/90) spin echo MR image reveals the mass, of high signal intensity, the deformity of the adjacent musculature, and soft tissue edema.

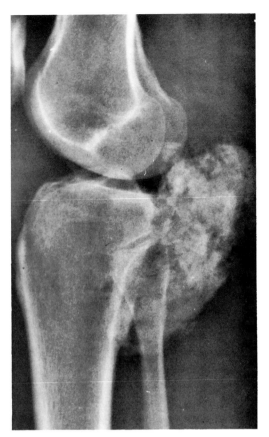

FIGURE 95–151. Parosteal osteosarcoma. An ossified rectangular mass arises from the posterior aspect of the proximal tibia. (Courtesy of J. Smith, M.D., New York, New York.)

Pseudomalignant Osseous Tumor of Soft Tissue. The presence of a nonmalignant tumor of soft tissue exhibiting sarcoma-like histologic features in its central portion and mature-appearing bone in its periphery was defined by Fine and Stout in 1956,[94] although previous reports can be found in the literature.[185–187] These lesions, which usually are termed pseudomalignant osseous tumors of soft tissue,[94, 160, 161, 188–191] appear in patients who do not relate a history of antecedent trauma. The lesions are well circumscribed, non-aggressive, and compatible with long-term survival. Men and women are affected, and most affected persons are in the second and third decades of life. Most tumors are located in the extremities or the gluteal regions,[462, 891] and they rarely are greater than 6 cm in diameter (Figs. 95–155 and 95–156). Those occurring in the hand and foot[887–889] resemble the findings of florid reactive periostitis (see later discussion). Soft tissue swelling with or without pain precedes the appearance of calcification and ossification by a short interval of approximately 2 to 3 weeks. Although previous trauma or infection is cited in some of the reports, this is an inconstant and infrequent feature. Radiographs reveal a well-circumscribed ossifying mass, with a dense periphery and lucent center. Periostitis may be identified and, in some instances, precedes soft tissue ossification. The course typically is benign, and, in some cases, the lesions have become smaller or disappeared.[890] Recurrence of the process after excision may be seen, and the recurrent lesions also may resorb spontaneously.[891]

The histologic characteristics include central connective tissue showing varying cell density with bundles of fibro-blasts, cellular pleomorphism with giant cells, and occasional mitotic figures; in addition, there is peripheral mature trabecular bone with spicules of osteoid tissue radiating toward the central areas of the lesion[189] (Fig. 95–157). These alterations resemble those in myositis ossificans traumatica, although muscle fibers, hematomas, and peripheral extension in the soft tissues are not found uniformly.

The major significance of pseudomalignant osseous tumor of soft tissue is the fact that it must be distinguished from malignant processes, especially osteosarcoma of soft tissue. The presence of the zone phenomenon, the peripheral location of the ossification, the limitation in size, and the absence of stromal cell atypism in pseudomalignant osseous tumor are helpful in this regard. The designation of this process as one distinct from myositis ossificans traumatica is based solely on the absence of a history of injury. Otherwise, the two processes are virtually indistinguishable. As both may resemble a malignant tumor on clinical, imaging, and pathologic examination, the term pseudomalignant osseous tumor of soft tissue may be applied appropriately to either. Furthermore, a third process (discussed subsequently), florid reactive periostitis, also shares many of these same features other than its predilection for the hands and feet. It, too, could be considered under the general "umbrella" term of pseudomalignant osseous tumor of soft tissue.

Florid Reactive Periostitis. In 1981, Spjut and Dorfman[463] described 12 children or adults who developed exuberant periosteal bone formation in the hands or, less commonly, the feet in association with local soft tissue swelling, pain, tenderness, or redness that was of weeks to

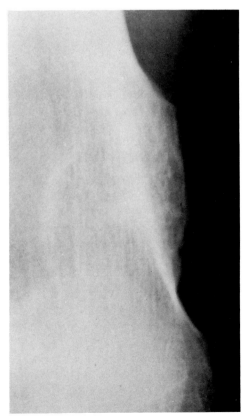

FIGURE 95–152. Osteochondroma. A broad-based osteochondroma of the distal femur is evident.

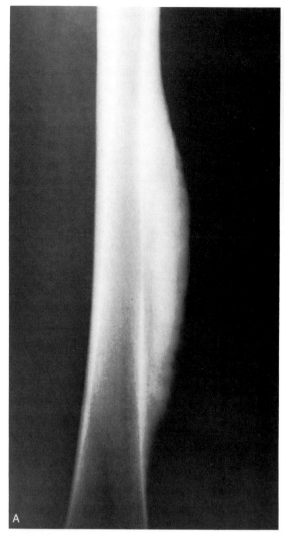

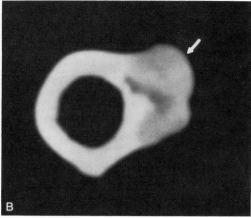

FIGURE 95–153. Osteoma. In a 32 year old man, a routine radiograph **(A)** reveals a long ossified lesion on the lateral surface of the femoral diaphysis. Transaxial CT **(B)** shows that the lesion (arrow) extends from the outer surface of the bone. It is slightly less dense than the adjacent cortex. An open biopsy led to the recovery of tissue that was interpreted as indicative of a parosteal osteoma. (Courtesy of G. Greenway, M.D., Dallas, Texas.)

years in duration. A history of trauma to the affected area was evident in only five of these patients. Radiographs revealed soft tissue prominence or mass formation, periostitis, or hyperostosis alone or in any combination. Histolog-

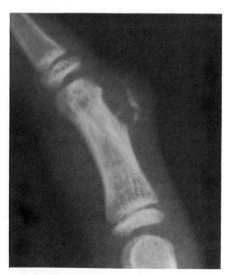

FIGURE 95–154. Juxtacortical (periosteal) chondroma. Typical findings are a soft tissue mass with or without calcification, with local excavation of the cortex and periostitis.

ically, the lesions were characterized by varying quantities of osteoid, bone, cartilage, and proliferating fibrous tissue and, in some instances, by a zoning phenomenon (osteoid centrally with mature bone at the periphery of the lesion) similar to that seen in myositis ossificans. These investigators referred to previous publications in which the same lesion was designated parosteal or nodular fasciitis,[464] tumor of soft parts containing bone and cartilage,[465] or fasciitis ossificans.[466]

Subsequent reports have documented further examples of florid periostitis, especially in the hands.[467–469, 895] Additional terms were applied to these lesions, including heterotopic chondro-ossification,[892] fibro-osseous pseudotumor of the digits,[893] pseudomalignant myositis ossificans of the hand,[894] pseudomalignant osseous tumor of soft tissue,[889] pseudomalignant, non-neoplastic osseous soft tissue tumor of the hand or foot,[887] and bizarre parosteal osteochondromatous proliferation.[897] Involvement of one of the proximal or middle phalanges predominates. A soft tissue mass containing calcification or ossification commonly dominates the radiographic findings and may occur prior to the development of osseous abnormality. The latter consists typically of periosteal reaction and, rarely, of cortical erosion or destruction (Fig. 95–158). These radiologic alterations are compatible with those of myositis ossificans or pseudomalignant osseous tumor of soft tissue, and it is certain that

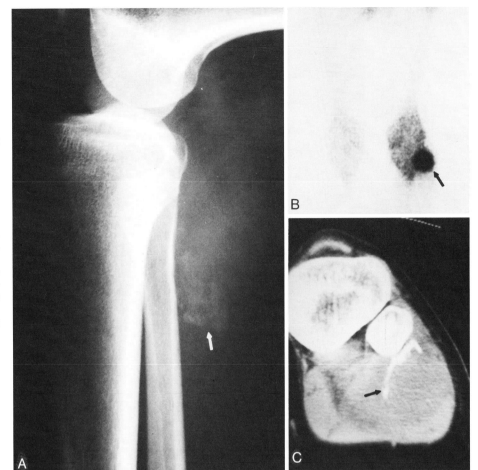

FIGURE 95-155. Pseudomalignant osseous tumor of soft tissue. An ossifying mass developed behind the knee in a 24 year old woman who repeatedly denied any injury to this region.

A Observe the mass containing peripheral ossification (arrow).

B Local accumulation of the bone-seeking radionuclide is evident (arrow).

C A relatively well-defined soft tissue mass with a partial rim of ossification (arrow) is seen posterior to the fibula in this transaxial CT image.

(Courtesy of V. Vint, M.D., San Diego, California.)

additional cases of this lesion have been interpreted as one or the other of these alternative diagnoses, depending on the presence or absence of a history of local trauma. Although simulating in some respects a malignant neoplasm, its histologic features lack cellular pleomorphism or atypical mitotic figures. Local excision generally is adequate, and the likelihood of lesional recurrence is small.

The differential diagnostic considerations in cases of florid reactive periostitis include mainly a number of other similar, if not identical, conditions related to periosteal proliferation of the phalanges of the hands and feet. As previously noted, many terms have been applied to these lesions. As indicated by Yuen and coworkers[896] common to all of these conditions is an initial stimulus, often related to trauma, that leads to hemorrhagic subperiosteal proliferation, which then matures. If the reaction remains contained within the periosteum, a localized fusiform periostitis develops that, with maturity, becomes incorporated into the cortex and, with remodeling, ultimately may resemble a broad-based cancellous protuberance.[896] This sequence fits the description of florid reactive periostitis. If the periosteum is breached, the reactive process then can extend into the loose areolar tissues around the fingers, producing a lobular rather than a fusiform lesion attached to the intact cortex. Owing to disruption of the periosteum, with its subperiosteal vascular plexus, a more limited blood supply results, which may lead to a failure of complete endochondral ossification. Cartilage foci remain, and the eventual appearance is that of bizarre parosteal osteochondromatous proliferation.[896] Local anatomic features, such as multiple septa on the volar aspect of the terminal phalanx, limit the extent of ossification. Clinical features such as pain, which is reported to be more prominent in florid reactive periostitis than in bizarre parosteal osteochondromatous proliferation, may relate to whether the periosteum is stretched, as in the former condition, or disrupted, as in the latter.[896] Therefore, it appears likely that all of these proliferative periosteal processes of the hands and feet are related, dif-

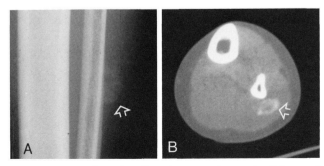

FIGURE 95-156. Pseudomalignant osseous tumor of soft tissue. A 40 year old woman noted a firm, tender, movable mass in the calf of three weeks' duration. There was no history of injury.

A Routine radiography shows a partially ossified soft tissue mass (arrow) adjacent to the fibula. The bone appears normal.

B Transaxial CT demonstrates a peripheral zone of ossification (arrow). The findings are typical of myositis ossificans.

(Courtesy of G. Greenway, M.D., Dallas, Texas.)

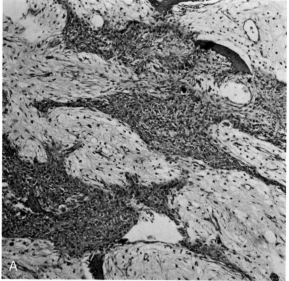

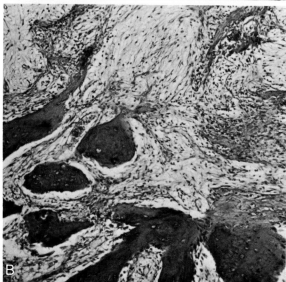

FIGURE 95–157. Pseudomalignant osseous tumor of soft tissue.

A In the central portion of the lesion, concentrated collections of spindle cells are observed, especially in pericystic locations. Loosely arranged spindle cells also are noted.

B In the peripheral portion of the lesion, regularly arranged mature spongy bone is seen separated by loosely arranged connective tissue.

(From Schulze K, et al: ROFO *129*:343, 1978. Courtesy of Georg Thieme Verlag, Stuttgart, Germany.)

fering only in the degree of pathologic and radiologic findings.

Myositis Ossificans Progressiva (Fibrodysplasia Ossificans Progressiva). Myositis ossificans progressiva is a rare disorder of mesodermal tissue in which inflammatory foci initially appear and proliferate in fibrous tissue.[192–202, 470–472, 544] It is discussed in depth in Chapter 87, and only a few comments will be included here. The hallmark of the disease is soft tissue ossification. Primary changes occur in the fibrous tissue, and the muscles are affected secondarily from the contiguous fascial coverings (Fig. 95–159). Histologic assessment of involved areas confirms the presence of ossified connective tissue and degenerating skeletal muscle. Early lesions are characterized by multifocal, intercon-

necting nodules composed of spindle-shaped fibroblast-like cells, in a distinctive connective tissue matrix, with centrally located osseous spicules; later lesions are composed of mature lamellar bone with adipose and hematopoietic tissue in the cancellous spaces, and a rim of fibroblast-like cells is lacking.[472] On roentgenograms, sheets of ossified tissue are encountered in the thoracic and abdominal walls and may bridge articulations, leading to contractures and "ankylosis"; osteophyte-like outgrowths of tubular bones also can be seen (Fig. 95–160). The findings can be striking, and in certain regions, such as the neck, a solid mass of bone may be found, associated with ossification of multiple intervertebral discs. Hypoplasia of vertebral bodies and intervertebral discs and bone ankylosis of apophyseal joints may be prominent, resembling findings in juvenile chronic arthritis or the Klippel-Feil syndrome.[470, 473] The natural history of the disease usually is one of ossification progressing from axial to appendicular locations and from cranial to caudal and proximal to distal anatomic sites.[898] A peculiar additional feature of the disease is the high rate of associated congenital anomalies of the thumb and big toe that are present at birth and that apparently are unrelated to the ossifying diathesis. Among others, these include microdactyly or adactyly, hallux valgus, ankylosis of interphalangeal and metatarsophalangeal joints, and clinodactyly of fingers. Additional abnormalities include cortical thickening in the medial and proximal portion of the tibia, a narrow lumbar spinal canal, and a decreased humeral-epicondylar angle.[471] Some of these congenital anomalies are consistent with defective induction of endochondral osteogenesis.[899]

The major differential diagnostic entity is idiopathic calcinosis universalis. This disease is associated with linear calcification appearing in the extremities, differing from the ossification of the axial skeleton that predominates in fibrodysplasia ossificans progressiva. In the latter disorder, para-articular osseous bridges may simulate the changes in neurologic illnesses or following burns, whereas the ossification about the spine can resemble the changes in ankylosing spondylitis or juvenile chronic arthritis. Accurate diagnosis generally is not difficult, especially when the anomalies of the toes and fingers are appreciated. Additional imaging methods are occasionally applied to the evaluation of patients with fibrodysplasia ossificans progressiva, although they generally are not required for diagnostic purposes. Bone scanning is useful in monitoring the extent of involvement,[571] and CT may provide information regarding early soft tissue abnormalities.[572] CT also can be used to define local pathologic findings of the disease, such as those in the gnathic bones.[900, 901] MR imaging has been applied to this condition in a limited fashion.[902]

Several reports exist of a developmental disorder of heterotopic ossification, recently designated *progressive osseous heteroplasia*, that appears to be distinct from myositis ossificans progressiva.[979, 980] Characteristic features include exclusive female involvement, noninflammatory osseous heteroplasia beginning in infancy, and progressive ossification of muscles, fascia, and deep connective tissue. This disorder, which also has been referred to as dysplastic cutaneous osteomatosis, familial ectopic ossification, and limited dermal ossification, is of unknown cause and pathogenesis. It may represent an inherited disease. The initial skin lesion has been described as a plaque or rash. Cutaneous ossification is a uniform feature, and extensive ossification

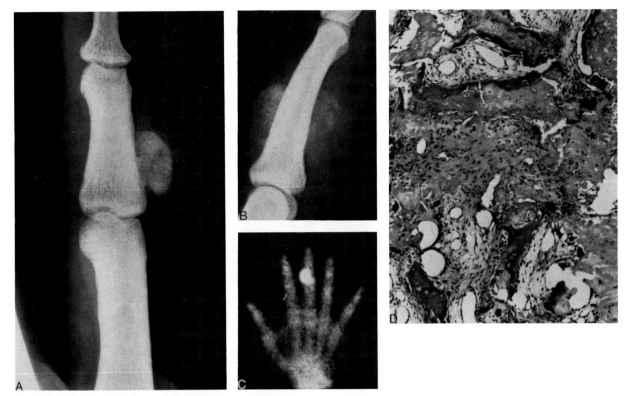

FIGURE 95–158. Florid reactive periostitis. Over a 4 month period, a 28 year old man developed an enlarging, nontender, slightly hyperemic, firm fixed mass in the dorsolateral aspect of the middle phalanx of the third finger. There was no history of local trauma.

A, B Posteroanterior and oblique radiographs reveal a soft tissue mass containing considerable ossification. It appears to be attached to the phalanx by a stalk.

C Intense uptake of the bone-seeking radionuclide is seen.

D The mass, which was found to be on a stalk and to have a fibrous soft tissue sheath, was excised. Islands of bone and cartilage separated by highly vascular fibrous connective tissue are apparent on histologic examination. Mitoses were rare. The lesion recurred 5 months later, and a third lesion developed in the opposite hand. Following excision of these last two masses (which yielded the same histologic diagnoses), two more digital lesions developed.

(From Porter AR, et al: AJR *144*:617, 1985. Copyright 1985, American Roentgen Ray Society.)

of subcutaneous and deep connective tissue appears in the limbs. Involvement of the axial skeleton is less constant. Laboratory findings may be unremarkable, although elevation of serum levels of alkaline phosphatase may be observed. Histologic assessment indicates the occurrence of intramembranous ossification in the soft tissues. Radiographically, sheets of ossification extend in a longitudinal fashion, paralleling the tubular bones and, eventually, merging with them. The disorder may progress relentlessly, leading to significant patient morbidity, or stabilize.[980]

SOFT TISSUE BANDS AND CONTRACTURES

Amniotic (or Streeter's) constriction bands have been recognized for over 150 years.[203–208] These soft tissue grooves or depressions can affect any portion of a limb, but most frequently they involve the fingers. They represent the most common cause of a terminal malformation of the limb.[903] Their cause is debated. Streeter[203] and Glessner[209] proposed that constriction rings could develop from defective germ plasm, perhaps related to an insult to the fetus at the time of differentiation of the limb buds.[203] Although the occurrence of such rings in identical twins[474] supports the germ-plasm-defect theory, anatomical differences in the sites of constriction in twins and the affliction of one twin with sparing of the other raise serious questions regarding

its validity. Torpin and coworkers,[210] Blanc and associates,[206] and Latta[211] postulated that premature rupture of the fetal amnion without injury to the chorion could produce raw surfaces and strings that attach to and mechanically entrap the limb, leading to rings and amputations. Abbe[212] proposed that the central nervous system could exert a deficient control on the developing tissue that could result in congenital bands. The role of intra-amniotic infection or trauma[213] also has been emphasized. With regard to trauma, the experimental production of limb malformations in rat fetuses by amniocentesis suggested that hemorrhages in the mesenchymal tissue of the limb produced by excessive uterine contractures during a critical period of limb development could be important in the pathogenesis of constriction bands.[213]

The frequency of such bands is recorded variously as 1 in 5000 to 1 in 45,000 births.[206, 209, 214, 215] It actually may be greater than these figures would suggest, as some bands may be associated with early fetal death, in which case careful histologic analysis of the placenta is required for accurate diagnosis.[475] The cases are sporadic, as no familial history has been noted. Many of the patients are products of first pregnancies and of young mothers with bleeding episodes in the third trimester of pregnancy,[216] and additional deformities of nails or other structures are frequent.[208] Common associated anomalies are clubbed feet and cleft

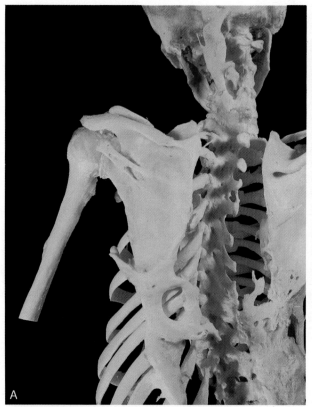

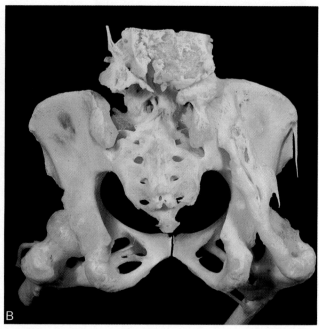

FIGURE 95–159. Myositis ossificans progressiva (fibrodysplasia ossificans progressiva). A 36 year old woman died from respiratory difficulties and pneumonia resulting from progressive soft tissue ossification that had begun at the age of 10 years. Painful masses, which were associated with heat and soft tissue edema, initially had developed around the shoulder girdles, thorax, hips, and knees and, over a period of years, had hardened to an osseous consistency. Involvement of the sternocleidomastoid muscles led to torticollis and neck rigidity, and she had become virtually confined to a wheelchair. Following the death of the patient, the entire skeleton was macerated, providing an extraordinary display of the gross pathologic findings of the disease.

These findings include a fixed position and tilting of the head, a large ossified band extending from the lower portion of the occiput and attaching to the seventh cervical vertebra, bone fusion of cervical laminae and spinous processes, and ossification of intervertebral discs. A rotary scoliosis in the thoracic spine, a bamboo vertebral column, and fusion of the scapulae to the underlying posterior portion of the ribs are also seen. Bands of scapular ossification extend in an inferior direction, merging with the ribs. Note the osseous bridging of the anterior portions of multiple ribs, bone ankylosis of the glenohumeral joints, and ossified masses on the posterior aspect of the right ilium merging with the greater trochanter of the femur. There also are complete bone ankylosis of the sacroiliac joints, flexion and immobility of the hips, new bone formation in the diaphysis of the left femur, and a large osseous ridge extending from the femur posteriorly across the knee with ankylosis of the adjacent proximal tibiofibular joint. (**A, B, D,** From Resnick D, et al: Skel Radiol *10*:131, 1983.)

Illustration continued on opposite page

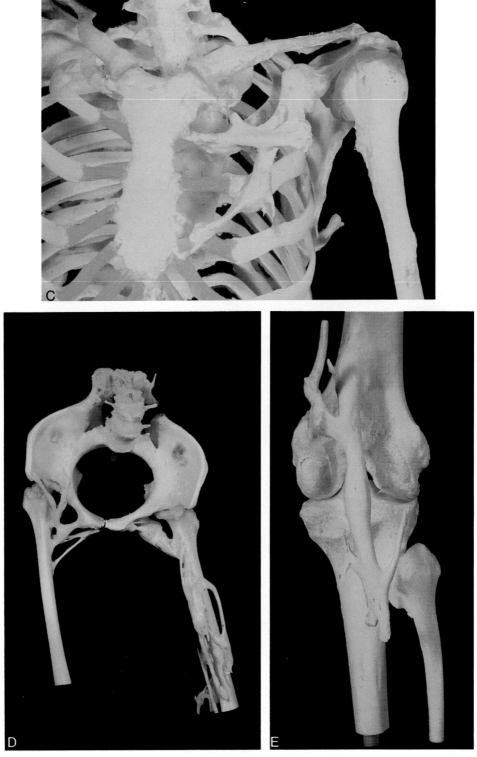

FIGURE 95–159 *Continued*

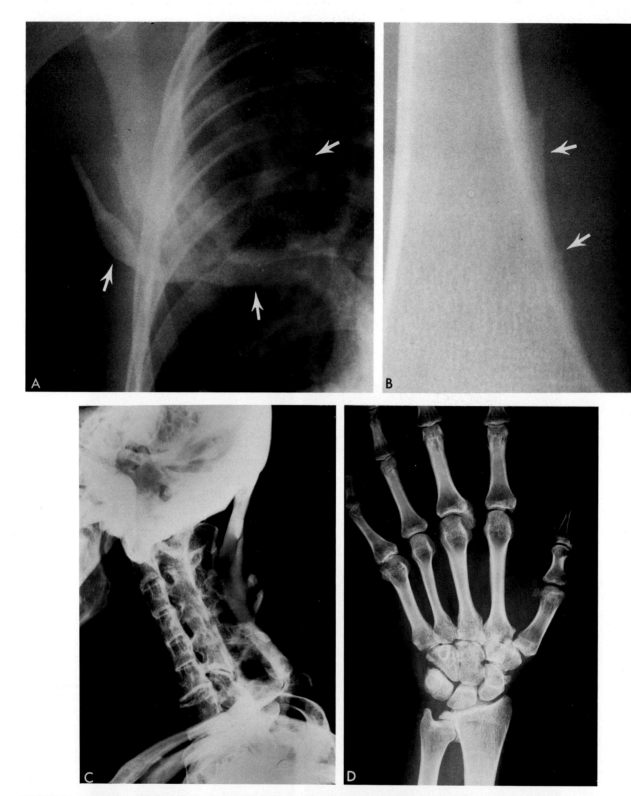

FIGURE 95–160. Myositis ossificans progressiva (fibrodysplasia ossificans progressiva).

A Sheet-like ossified bridges about the shoulder girdle are typical (arrows).

B Broad-based excrescences (arrows) can be seen in the tubular bones.

C In the cervical spine, hypoplastic vertebral bodies and intervertebral discs and bone ankylosis of apophyseal joints resemble the findings of juvenile chronic arthritis. A band of ossification extending from the occiput to the seventh cervical vertebra is evident. (Same patient as in Figure 95–159.)

D Note hypoplasia of the proximal phalanx of the thumb and peculiar excrescences arising from the bases of several proximal phalanges, particularly those of the second and third digits. (Same patient as in Figure 95–159.)

(**C, D,** From Resnick D, et al: Skel Radiol *10*:131, 1983.)

lip and palate. A compression neuropathy of the peroneal nerve caused by a constriction band below the knee is a recognized factor in the causation of the clubfoot deformity.[477] The midline facial anomalies also result from the constrictive and disruptive effects of adjacent abnormal strands of amniotic tissue.[478] On clinical examination, scarred rings are found to encircle a digit or limb, and temperature gradients and sensory deficits may be evident across the constricted areas.[217] Multiple and symmetrically distributed lesions are typical. In the hand, the central digits are affected most frequently, and the thumb commonly is spared.[477] Radiographs delineate the soft tissue constrictions that extend for a variable depth and may contact the subjacent bone.[474, 476] It is the visualization of soft tissue deficit that allows differentiation of this condition from congenital defects.[216] The underlying bones may be poorly developed or absent, and distal to the lesions, calcification,[545] lymphedema, or fatty accumulation may be encountered. Syndactyly or amputation also can be evident (Fig. 95–161).

Acquired rings also may occur, perhaps related to an encircling foreign object, such as a rubber band.[216] Ainhum (see Chapter 66) is a tropical disease in which a deep constricting band appears about the fifth toe or other digits on one or both feet.

Soft tissue contractures can accompany many congenital disorders, such as arthrogryposis multiplex congenita,[218] Leri's pleonosteosis,[219] and contractural arachnodactyly[220]; acquired conditions, such as Volkmann's ischemic contracture,[221] thermal burns, and neurologic injury; and various rheumatologic diseases, such as rheumatoid arthritis and systemic lupus erythematosus. Additional well-known examples in the hand are Dupuytren's contracture of the palmar fascia (Fig. 95–162); camptodactyly, in which a flexion contracture involves predominantly the proximal interphalangeal articulation of the fifth digit[222]; clinodactyly, in which a curvature of a finger occurs in a mediolateral plane[223]; and Kirner's deformity, in which palmar bending of the shaft of a terminal phalanx may be associated with epiphyseal separation.[224] In fact, many syndromes are associated with crooked fingers or crooked toes.[216] Furthermore, other skeletal sites can be affected, and the list of disorders associated with soft tissue contractures is extensive. One interesting example is the appearance of contracted and deformed soft tissues and bones associated with the former Chinese custom of binding women's feet[583] (Fig. 95–163). Another example is the popliteal pterygium syndrome, consisting of a popliteal web extending from the ischium to the heel, deformities of the foot and toes, toenail dysplasia, flexion contracture of the knee, and cleft palate.[573, 904, 905] Other findings of this autosomal dominant disorder include scoliosis, rib anomalies, and hypoplasia of the tibiae and patellae.[905] Although the pterygium varies in appearance and severity, a shortened sciatic nerve commonly is found in the web's posterior subcutaneous margin, making corrective surgery precarious.[905]

Of these soft tissue contractures, it is the one described by Dupuytren more than 150 years ago that has received the greatest attention: "Retraction of the fingers, gentlemen, and particularly that of the ring-finger has been observed for many years, but it is only very lately that the cause of this deformity has been investigated with success."[479, 480] Typically seen in middle-aged and elderly adults, more commonly in men, and infrequently in

Chinese, Indian, and black ethnic groups, Dupuytren's contracture involves the fingers in one or both hands, especially the third through fifth digits. This anatomic distribution may be influenced by the presence of an associated disease, such as diabetes mellitus, in which the third, fourth, and first digits are affected principally.[480] Although the pathologic alterations occur in the palm, the precise site of origin of the process is debated, with some investigators (including Dupuytren) favoring the palmar fascia and others implicating the subcutaneous tissue or the palmar aponeurosis. Well-oriented collagenous matrix increases in amount and is transformed into nodules, cords and laminated bands. The diseased tissue contains cells and collagen in varying proportions: The cells of the early or proliferative stage are fibroblasts; those of the active or involutional stage are myofibroblasts; and those of the advanced or residual stage are fibrocytes.[481] Gross contracture results from an active cellular process in which the digits are drawn closer together as the original tissue is being replaced.[482] Biomechanical forces contribute to the mechanism of contraction, in which the altered collagen exhibits abnormal patterns of stress during normal use of the hand that stimulate fibrous tissue deposition and progressive contracture.[481]

MR imaging has been used in a preliminary fashion to further define palmar involvement in Dupuytren's disease.[906] The signal intensity of the subcutaneous nodules and cords show some variation that appears to be dependent on their cellularity. The cords typically show low signal intensity similar to that of tendon on both T1- and T2-weighted spin echo MR images, consistent with the presence of dense collagen and few cells. The nodules usually reveal intermediate signal intensity similar to that of muscle on these spin echo MR images, consistent with more cellular tissue. As highly cellular lesions tend to have higher rates of recurrence after surgery than do hypocellular lesions, MR imaging may have some value in judging the prognosis of this condition.[906]

The cause of the disorder is not clear. In addition to diabetes mellitus, Dupuytren's disease has been associated with epilepsy and alcoholism. A strong genetic link has been documented, with an autosomal dominant mechanism of inheritance and almost total penetrance in men being found.[483] Accidental or occupational trauma, including vibration injury,[484] has been implicated in some cases, although this relationship is not constant and the dominant hand is not affected overwhelmingly.

SOFT TISSUE EDEMA

Traumatic or inflammatory processes can lead to localized soft tissue edema. In addition, venous or lymphatic obstruction from many diverse causes may produce edema that is recognized radiographically as enlargement of the soft tissue contour, obliteration of the fascial planes, and a fine or coarsened reticular pattern (Fig. 95–164). Soft tissue calcification or ossification may accompany the process (Fig. 95–165). Special studies, such as CT,[485, 486] phlebography, or lymphangiography, can accurately define the nature of the obstructive lesion. Lymphedema itself may result from various processes, including primary or congenital disorders,[225] trauma, infection (filariasis), irradiation, tumor, and surgery (e.g., following mastectomy). Lymphedema also may accompany thyroid acropachy, melorheostosis,

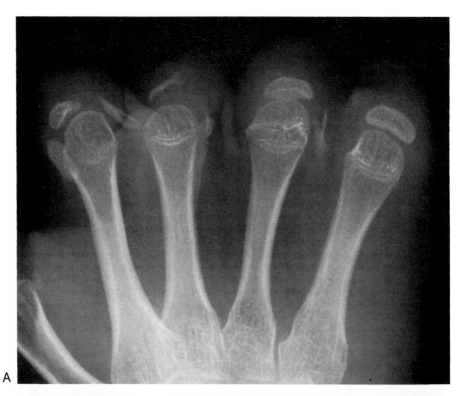

FIGURE 95–161. Amniotic (or Streeter's) constriction bands.

A Autoamputation of the fingers presumably is the result of amniotic bands, although the presence of small ossific foci about the metacarpal heads may indicate the occurrence of malformed phalanges and congenital defects of the hand.

B In this example, soft tissue constrictions can be seen (arrows), and there has been an amputation of a portion of the second digit. (Courtesy of J. Slivka, M.D., San Diego, California.)

C In this patient, soft tissue and osseous abnormalities involve the second, third, and fourth fingers, with autoamputation of portions of two fingers. (Courtesy of A. D'Abreu, M.D., Porto Alegre, Brazil.)

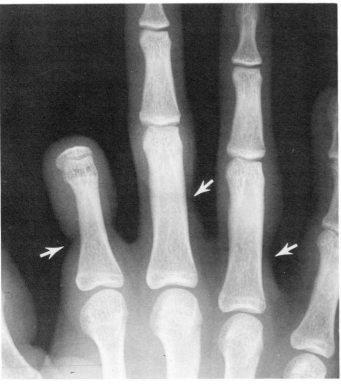

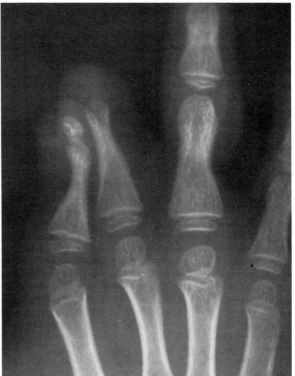

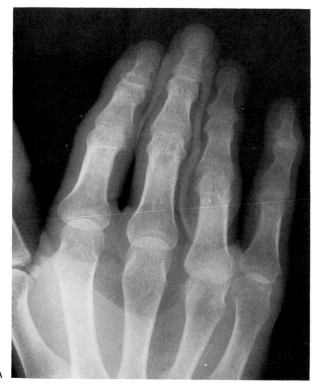 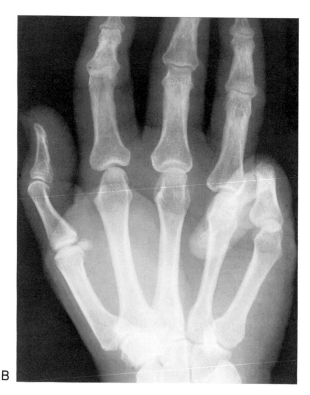

FIGURE 95–162. Dupuytren's contracture.
A Observe the flexion deformities about the metacarpophalangeal joints of the four ulnar digits.
B In this example, a severe flexion contracture is evident in the fifth finger with minor changes in the other digits.

infantile cortical hyperostosis, and acromegaly. The occurrence of lymphangiosarcomas in areas of long-term lymphedema has been discussed previously (Fig. 95–166).[380, 381, 907] Joint effusions in areas of lymphedema are described, related to an exudative arthropathy with extravasation of chyle in the joint space or chyle reflux.[487]

Common causes of diffuse swelling of an extremity include lymphedema, venous obstruction (phebedema), and lipedema. CT[908] and MR imaging[909–911] may be effective in differentiation among these conditions. In lymphedema, CT reveals fluid collections in the interstitial spaces of the soft tissue, which with chronicity are associated with fibrosis and a honeycomb pattern; in venous obstruction, CT shows an increase in the cross sectional area of the muscle compartment with a normal homogeneous layer of subcutaneous fat; in lipedema, typically seen in overweight women beyond the age of 20 years, CT demonstrates fat accumulation leading to an increase in size but a homogeneous appearance of subcutaneous fat.[908] With regard to MR imaging, lipedema (Fig. 95–167A) is associated with a homogeneously enlarged subcutaneous layer of fat that does not reveal enhancement of signal intensity after intravenous administration of gadolinium; phlebedema is accompanied by increased amounts of fluid within muscle and subcutaneous fat, with a moderate increase in signal intensity in muscle and a slight increase in signal intensity in subcutaneous tissue after gadolinium administration; and lymphedema (Fig. 95–167B) is associated with a honeycomb pat-

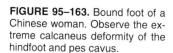

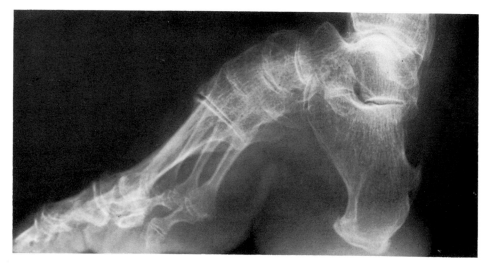

FIGURE 95–163. Bound foot of a Chinese woman. Observe the extreme calcaneus deformity of the hindfoot and pes cavus.

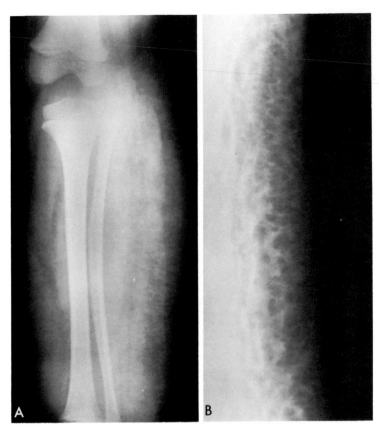

FIGURE 95–164. Lymphedema.

  A A 5 year old boy with congenital lymphedema reveals the typical striated pattern in the enlarged soft tissues.

  B A coned-down view in another patient delineates the reticular soft tissue pattern.

FIGURE 95–165. Edema: Soft tissue ossification.

  A Lymphedema has led to a fine reticular pattern of ossification. (Courtesy of A. Brower, M.D., Norfolk, Virginia.)

  B Venous insufficiency has produced a branching pattern of coarse ossification. (Courtesy of M. Nadel, M.D., Los Angeles, California.)

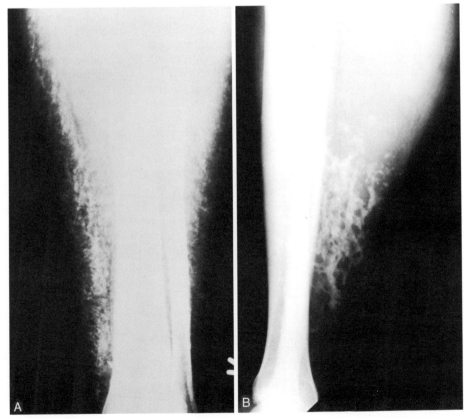

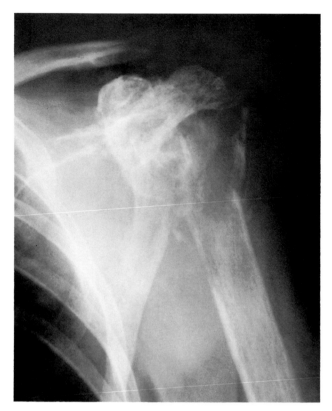

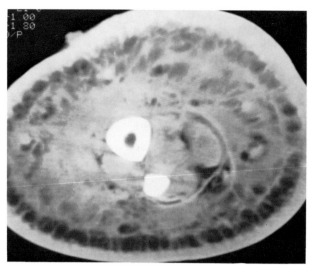

FIGURE 95–168. Lymphedema with lymphangiosarcoma. In this 26 year old woman with a 16-year history of idiopathic lymphedema in one lower extremity, a recent increase in the degree of swelling of the leg associated with mottled discoloration of the skin was noted. A transaxial contrast-enhanced CT scan of the involved lower leg shows increased attenuation of the subcutaneous fat, thickening of the fibrous septa, and a honeycomb pattern with lakes of encapsulated fluid, findings typical of lymphedema. In addition, however, extreme skin thickening, multiple cutaneous nodules, and fluid collections both within and surrounding muscle groups are observed. Following amputation of the leg, pathologic examination showed a diffusely infiltrating neoplasm that involved dermis, subcutis, and skeletal muscle.

(From Kazerooni E, et al: AJR *156*:543, 1991.)

FIGURE 95–166. Lymphedema with lymphangiosarcoma. In this patient with breast carcinoma, who had had a radical mastectomy and who had lymphedema of the arm, a lymphangiosarcoma developed, which led to osseous destruction of the proximal humerus. Irradiation effect also is evident. (Courtesy of D. McEwan, M.D., Winnipeg, Manitoba, Canada.)

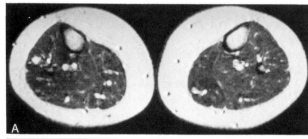

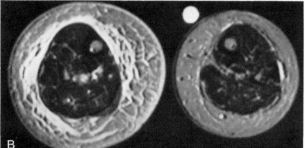

FIGURE 95–167. Lipedema and lymphedema.
A Lipedema. A transaxial T2-weighted (TR/TE, 2000/60) spin echo MR image shows homogeneous enlargement of the subcutaneous layer of fat in both legs.
B Lymphedema. A transaxial T2-weighted (TR/TE, 2000/60) spin echo image shows involvement of the right leg. A honeycomb pattern of increased signal intensity in the subcutaneous fat is evident.
(From Duewell S, et al: Radiology *184*:227, 1992.)

tern above the fascia between muscle and subcutaneous tissue, with a marked increase in signal intensity on T2-weighted images and a slight increase in signal intensity in the subcutaneous tissue after gadolinium administration.[909] CT (Fig. 95–168) and MR imaging also can be used to assess the occurrence of lymphangiosarcomas in regions of chronic lymphedema.

SOFT TISSUE EMPHYSEMA

Collections of gas, including air, in the soft tissues can be caused by several mechanisms. Air can be introduced iatrogenically into the soft tissues or joints during puncture for diagnostic or therapeutic purposes. Air also can penetrate the soft tissues in cases of communicating wounds or sinus tracts. Gas formation by bacteria such as Clostridium may lead to radiolucent streaks or bubbles in the subcutaneous or muscular tissues (see Chapters 64 and 66). This is not infrequent in diabetic patients (Fig. 95–169). Additional causes of gas or air in soft tissues include irrigation with hydrogen peroxide[489] and accidental injection of compressed air. In rare instances, soft tissue calcification may appear after subcutaneous emphysema.[490]

SOFT TISSUE FOREIGN BODIES

A variety of foreign bodies may become embedded or localize in the body's soft tissues owing to accidental or occupational trauma, surgical procedures (needles, sponges), acupuncture, or other causes.[923, 924] The identification of foreign bodies with conventional radiography or

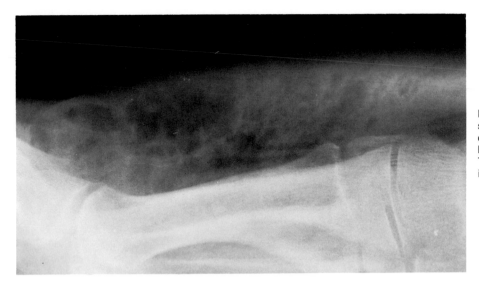

FIGURE 95–169. Soft tissue emphysema. Bubbly radiolucent soft tissue collections are not infrequent in diabetic patients with soft tissue infection. The causative microorganisms vary but in this case were *Escherichia coli.*

additional techniques is dependent on their composition, size, and anatomic location. Metallic fragments resulting from various missiles easily are detected on routine radiographs and, with gradual dissolution (especially in an intraarticular site), subsequently may lead to lead poisoning (see Chapter 76). Needles or metallic threads lodged in the soft tissues or bone also are readily apparent on conventional radiographs (Fig. 95–170). The identification of particles or fragments of glass or wood, two substances commonly associated with accidental injury, is more difficult and deserves special emphasis.

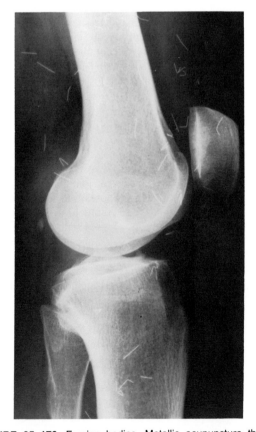

FIGURE 95–170. Foreign bodies. Metallic acupuncture threads. These threads, composed of gold, are seen easily with routine radiography. (Courtesy of H.S. Kang, M.D., Seoul, Korea.)

Glass and Wood

Although classically it has been taught that only leaded or pigmented glass is radiopaque, reports of some investigations have refuted this belief. Experimental studies in which all types of glass fragments have been placed in water or paraffin[491] or embedded in animal tissues[492–494] have indicated clearly the radiopaque nature of the glass. In clinical situations, the delineation of glass particles by conventional radiography depends on their size and orientation, their precise anatomic location (thick versus thin body parts), the nature of the surrounding tissue, and the specific radiographic technique (type of film, kilovoltage) that is employed (Fig. 95–171A). Furthermore, the radiopacity of some types of glass (beer and wine bottles) is greater than that of others (light bulbs).[494] Xeroradiography,[495] ultrasonography,[574, 575, 584] CT,[496, 912, 913] and MR imaging[914] can be helpful in defining small pieces of glass as well as plastic embedded in the soft tissues. With MR imaging, glass appears as a region of signal void that may be surrounded by a zone of inflammation.

The difficulties encountered in the delineation of foreign bodies composed of wood with standard radiography are well recognized.[497] Early detection is important, as sequelae of retained wood particles include granulomatous reactions,[585] osteitis,[915] and secondary infections (see Chapter 64); furthermore, although such particles initially have a density less than that of water, they soon absorb water and the differences in density become smaller.[496] Of the additional diagnostic techniques that are available, CT and ultrasonography (Fig. 95–172) have been most successful in detecting wood fragments.[498–500, 575, 912, 913, 916, 917] Wood appears as a region of signal void on MR images.[914]

Plant Thorns

An inflammatory reaction in the soft tissue, bone, or articular cavity is a potential complication of implantation of various types of foreign bodies, including surgical sponges,[501] glass particles,[502] Dacron threads,[503] and some of the materials used in arthroplasties (see Chapter 19). The reaction may appear soon after the introduction of the foreign material or years later. If, owing to its size or chemical nature, a foreign body cannot be eliminated during this

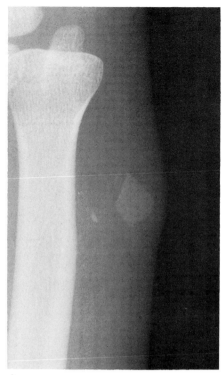

A

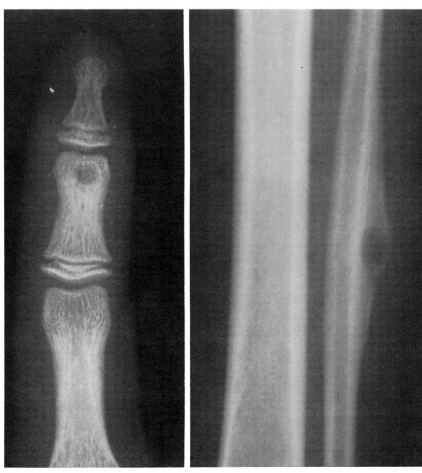

B   C

FIGURE 95–171. Foreign bodies.

A Glass shards. Several radiopaque areas in the distal forearm represent pieces of glass. Note soft tissue swelling.

B, C Plant thorns. Two examples of osteolytic lesions related to embedded plant thorns are shown. These lesions are well defined and, in **C,** there is associated periostitis. (**B,** Courtesy of G. Greenway, M.D., Dallas, Texas.)

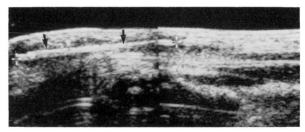

FIGURE 95–172. Foreign bodies. Wood splinter. This splinter (arrows) lodged in the volar surface of the wrist was not evident on routine radiography but is well shown on a sagittal scan with ultrasonography.

inflammatory reaction, encapsulation and granuloma formation may occur. Of particular importance is the granulomatous response present in the soft tissue, joint, or bone following the entry of certain types of plant thorns.

The organic foreign body reaction induced by plant thorns has been well summarized by Yousefzadeh and Jackson.[504] Date palm, sentinel palm, blackthorn, hawthorn, box thorn, bougainvillea, rose thorn, mesquite, and yucca are among the plants capable of eliciting such a reaction.[505-513] Although the clinical features vary somewhat according to the specific offending agent and its depth of penetration, the type of human tissue that is involved, and the presence or absence of associated bacterial infection, certain typical manifestations can be identified. Children are affected more frequently than adults, especially in cases of bone and joint involvement, although lesions of soft tissues are relatively common in adults. The extremities usually are affected, especially the hands and feet. Pain and soft tissue swelling are evident soon after the injury, and a puncture wound may be evident. Subsequently, a period of improvement in these manifestations is common, followed by the reappearance of symptoms and signs.[504] These biphasic clinical characteristics explain a delay in accurate diagnosis of the nature of the abnormality; the elapsed time between the injury and the surgical removal of the foreign body is commonly weeks or months and occasionally years. Operative and pathologic findings include a foreign body granuloma with giant cells or an abscess, or both.

The radiographic features vary according to the site of granuloma formation (Fig. 95–171B,C). Most frequently, an articulation, tendon sheath, or bursa is affected, although, rarely, the bone is the primary site of involvement. In the latter case, a well-circumscribed osteolytic lesion, termed a pseudotumor, with periostitis and soft tissue swelling is typical. Tenosynovitis or bursitis leads to soft tissue swelling and periosteal reaction, and arthritis (usually in a knee) is accompanied by an effusion.[918, 919, 921] The synovial fluid may be inflammatory in nature, and histologic inspection shows thickening of the synovial membrane with hyperemia and giant cell infiltration. Vegetable material may be identified in synovial tissues, particularly when special stains and polarized microscopy are employed.[922]

Granulomatous reactions following the introduction of plant thorns appear to relate to a component of the thorn itself or a surface contaminant. Surgical removal of the thorn is required for reversal of the process. Partial or total synovectomy may be necessary when the joint is involved.[919, 920]

Sea Urchin Spines

A similar granulomatous reaction of the soft tissues, synovial membrane, or bone has been observed following puncture wounds by the spines of a variety of sea urchins.[514-516, 922] The foot and heel are the typical sites of injury, which usually occurs while the patient is wading in shallow waters or scuba diving. Less commonly, a hand (Fig. 95–173), ankle, or knee is affected. The subsequent inflammatory response probably is related to the chemical composition of the spine; as the urchin spine is composed of calcium carbonate, a substance that should be immunologically inert, it may be that the surface, containing a thin layer of epithelium and various secretions, slime, and debris, is responsible for the foreign body reaction.[516] Systemic manifestations, including joint pain, swelling, malaise, and lymphadenopathy, are seen, perhaps indicating a slow but persistent release of antigenic material.[516]

SOFT TISSUE ATROPHY

Diffuse atrophy of soft tissue, including fat and muscle, is an accompaniment of chronic debilitating illnesses, lipoatrophic diabetes (Fig. 95–174), and malnutrition. Localized atrophy of soft tissue is evident in many different types of disorders, as indicated in other portions of this book, including collagen vascular diseases such as scleroderma, paralysis or prolonged disuse or immobilization of an extremity, thermal injury, and inflammatory or occlusive vascular processes. Causes of obstruction of peripheral arteries include arteriosclerosis obliterans (involvement of large and medium-sized arteries supplying the extremities, especially the legs, in older patients, men more commonly than women and diabetic persons more frequently than those without diabetes mellitus) and Buerger's disease or thromboangiitis obliterans (involvement of peripheral arteries and

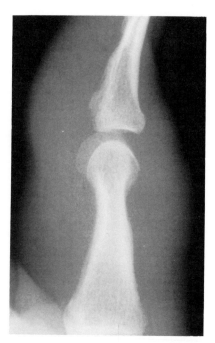

FIGURE 95–173. Foreign body. Sea urchin spine. Observe diffuse swelling of the thumb and erosion of the dorsal surface of the proximal phalanx.

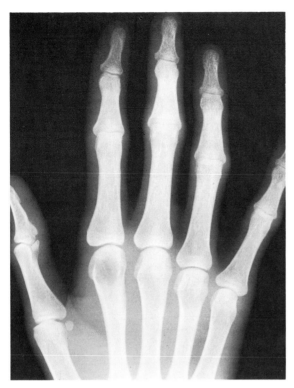

FIGURE 95–174. Soft tissue atrophy: Lipoatrophic diabetes. Note the loss of normal soft tissues throughout the hand in a 26 year old woman. (Courtesy of M. Dalinka, M.D., Philadelphia, Pennsylvania.)

veins in young adults, almost exclusively in men, especially Ashkenazic Jews, associated with cigarette smoking)[517] (Fig. 95–175).

Muscle atrophy (or rarely hypertrophy) occurs in certain neuromuscular disorders (see Chapter 77) and inflammatory conditions. CT and MR imaging are the techniques of choice in evaluating such atrophy.

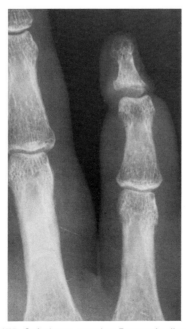

FIGURE 95–175. Soft tissue atrophy: Buerger's disease. Note the localized loss of soft tissue that may occur in this disease.

SOFT TISSUE HYPERTROPHY

Overgrowth of soft tissue alone or in combination with osseous enlargement may occur in a generalized or localized distribution. Generalized hypertrophy is a fundamental part of pituitary gigantism and acromegaly (see Chapter 55) but also is encountered in many other conditions, including cerebral gigantism, initially described by Sotos and collaborators in 1964.[518] This condition appears early in life and consists of excessively rapid growth, characteristic acromegalic-like facies, dilatation of the ventricles in the brain, and nonprogressive mental retardation.[519]

Hemihypertrophy, representing overgrowth of one half or one side of the body, usually involves muscular, vascular, skeletal, and nervous systems and may occur on an idiopathic basis or in association with neurocutaneous syndromes (neurofibromatosis, tuberous sclerosis, Sturge-Weber disease, Lindau-von Hippel disease), the Beckwith-Weidemann syndrome, or skin and vascular abnormalities (angiodysplasias, lymphatic abnormalities, lipomatosis).[520] Additional alterations associated with idiopathic congenital hemihypertrophy include a variety of tumors (especially Wilms' tumor, adrenocortical tumors, and hepatoblastoma) and renal abnormalities (nephromegaly and medullary sponge kidney).[520, 521]

Macrodactyly (Fig. 95–176) represents an increase in the size of all the structures (bones, tendons, nerves, vessels, subcutaneous fat, skin) in one or more digits of the hands and feet. It occurs on an idiopathic basis[522, 925] and in association with hemangiomas, lymphangiomas, and arteriovenous malformations. Similar enlargement is seen in neurofibromatosis, the epidermal nevus syndrome,[926] and macrodystrophia lipomatosa.[626]

In 1983, Wiedemann and coworkers[927] introduced the term *Proteus syndrome* to describe the altered pattern of growth seen in a congenital hamartomatous syndrome associated with partial gigantism of the hands and feet, hemihypertrophy, subcutaneous tumors, pigmented nevi, macrocephaly, and bone exostoses. Numerous reports followed,[928–935] and it became apparent that the Proteus syndrome was associated with diverse manifestations (Fig. 95–177). Clinical findings typically become apparent in the first few years of life. Regional gigantism and lymphangiomatous hamartomas are regarded as the two most essential features of the syndrome.[930]

Gigantism in the Proteus syndrome relates to excessive growth of a variety of tissues, including the epidermis, connective and adipose tissue, endothelium, and bone. Growth of the extremities is asymmetrical, and the tubular bones in one extremity become enlarged and elongated. Hyperplasia of subcutaneous tissues also is noted. In the palmar and plantar regions, this hyperplasia is manifested as cerebriform or gyriform lesions or, in the lower extremity, as moccasin feet.[930] Macrodactyly generally is present, with enlargement of some of the short tubular bones. Osteochondroma-like lesions arising from the short and long tubular bones are evident after the first few years of life.[933] Carpal and tarsal abnormalities are less constant.

The skull is affected in approximately 50 per cent of cases. Findings include macrocephaly in a symmetrical or asymmetrical distribution, cranial bossing (usually but not invariably involving the frontal region), and osteoma-like outgrowths of the cranium, external auditory canal, nasal

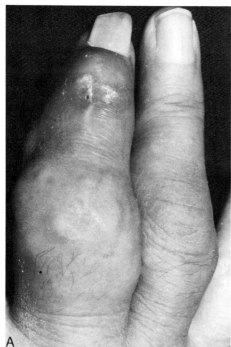

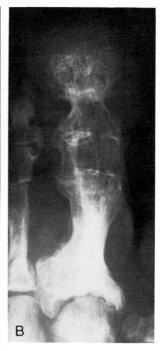

FIGURE 95–176. Macrodactyly: Various causes.

A, B Macrodystrophia lipomatosa. Shown are a clinical photograph of an enlarged and deformed finger in a 60 year old woman **(A)** and a radiograph of the toe in an adult patient revealing grotesque bone and soft tissue changes **(B).** (**A,** Courtesy of R. A. Frayha, M.D., Beirut, Lebanon; **B,** Courtesy of R. Sweet, M.D., Pomona, California.)

C, D Arteriovenous malformation. (Courtesy of M. Kelley, M.D., Orange County, California.)

E Neurofibromatosis.

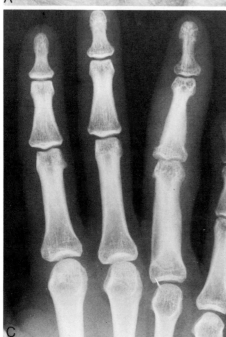

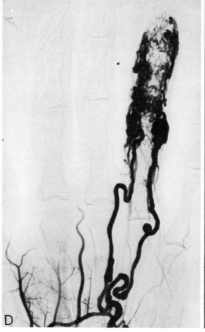

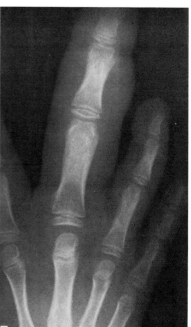

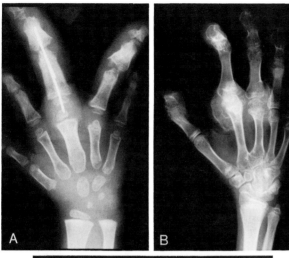

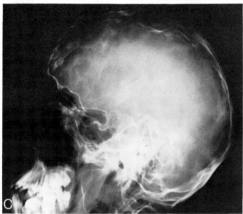

FIGURE 95–177. Proteus syndrome. The radiographic abnormalities of this syndrome are varied and, as shown in three affected patients, include macrodactyly with bone and soft tissue hypertrophy **(A)**, osteochondroma-like lesions of tubular bones **(B)**, and frontal bossing and a "copper-beaten" appearance of the cranial vault **(C)**. (From Nishimura G, et al: Australas Radiol 34:47, 1990.)

bridge, and alveolar ridges.[930] Spinal alterations include overgrowth of the vertebral bodies, irregularly shaped vertebrae, and dysplasia of pedicles and intervertebral discs.[930, 933]

The subcutaneous tumors in the Proteus syndrome vary in size but may be large. These tumors are not well encapsulated and histologically consist of large vascular channels with lipomatous and fibrous tissue; the histologic findings are best described as a lymphangiomatous hamartoma.[930] The overlying skin may demonstrate a deep purpura; the cutaneous changes may be confused with those accompanying a variety of other syndromes in which somatic overgrowth is a component, such as the café au lait spots of neurofibromatosis and the pigmented nevi of the Klippel-Trenaunay-Weber syndrome.[936] Lipomas, often distributed in the plantar and palmar regions, are an additional feature of the Proteus syndrome.[930]

Facial anomalies, occurring in about 30 per cent of cases, include malformed ears, high arched palate, malocclusion, depressed nasal bridge, and mandibular prognathism; ocular changes include strabismus, myopia, nystagmus, epibulbar tumor, cataracts, and ptosis.[930] Additional reported manifestations of the Proteus syndrome are mental retardation, seizures, pulmonary cystlike lesions, and pelvic lipomatosis.

The radiographic abnormalities of musculoskeletal involvement in this syndrome, which consist mainly of bone and soft tissue overgrowth and deformity, resemble those of neurofibromatosis, Ollier's disease, Maffucci's syndrome, macrodystrophia lipomatosa, the Klippel-Trenaunay-Weber syndrome, and the Bannayan-Zonana syndrome.[937, 938] Indeed, confusion among these syndromes is exemplified by the debate as to the cause of the deformities in Joseph Merrick, the "elephant man," who may have had the Proteus syndrome rather than neurofibromatosis.[939] Disorders such as the epidermal nevus syndrome and the linear sebaceous nevus syndrome share many features with the Proteus syndrome and may represent incomplete expressions of a similar entity.[930]

The ultimate prognosis of the Proteus syndrome appears favorable. Complications such as difficulty with ambulation, chronic dermatitis, bleeding within the subcutaneous masses, and joint instability or dislocation are seen, however.[930] Although cases of this syndrome are reported in which a malignant tumor developed, the precise frequency of this complication is not known but appears low.[930]

SPECIAL SYNDROMES OF SKIN AND SOFT TISSUE

Certain afflictions of the cutaneous and subcutaneous tissues can be associated with radiographic abnormalities. Some of the important afflictions are described here; however, others, such as ichthyosis, in which dry, scaly, thickened skin is observed, and fracture blisters, which occur after musculoskeletal injury, can produce soft tissue nodularity or irregularity (Fig. 95–178).

Epidermolysis Bullosa

This is a rare chronic skin disorder that results from poor adherence of the epidermis to the dermis, as a consequence of which vesicles, bullae, and ulcerations form either spontaneously or following minor traumatic insults.[226–230] The disorder is inherited in either a dominant or a recessive manner, and the latter form is more severe. Further division of the disease is made on the basis of specific clinical manifestations. Four types are recognized: the simple type, an autosomal dominant trait; the hyperplastic dystrophic type, also autosomal dominant; the dystrophic polydysplastic type, with recessive inheritance; and the lethal type, also with recessive inheritance.[230]

The simple variety is mild, becoming evident any time during the first year of life. Bullae appear in areas subjected to trauma, especially in the hands, feet, elbows, and knees, and they heal by epithelialization without scarring. Although new lesions may appear subsequently, the disease usually subsides after puberty. The hyperplastic dystrophic variety also is mild, becoming apparent before puberty. Bullae result from trauma, and the lesions heal with the development of hyperkeratosis and thin, atrophic scars. Fingernails and toenails may be lost, but the mucous membranes rarely are affected, and there is no interference with growth or development. The dystrophic polydysplastic type is severe. Bullae are noted at birth or shortly thereafter, developing after trauma or spontaneously. The mucous membranes of the eyes, nose, oropharynx, anus, and genital tract always are affected, and esophageal lesions may lead

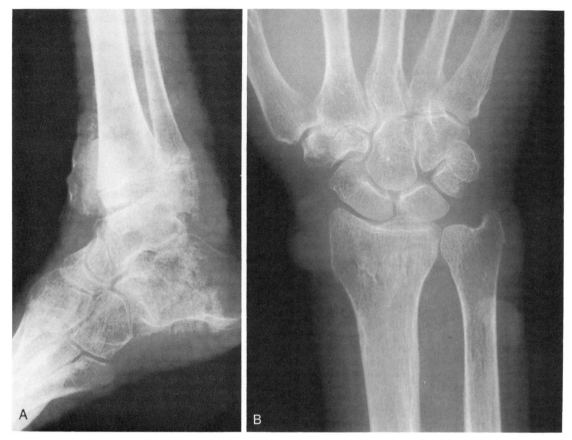

FIGURE 95–178. Soft tissue nodularity.
A Ichthyosis. Observe the soft tissue nodularity due to the presence of irregular skin thickening.
B Fracture blisters. In this elderly woman with a fracture of the distal radius, observe multiple fracture blisters about the wrist.

to dysphagia, spasm, scarring, and contractures. Malnourishment, retardation of physical development, thin, scarred atrophic skin, and hand deformities are encountered. The lethal type is rare, producing severe and widespread involvement with death in early infancy.

Radiographic findings are characteristic but not specific. They vary with the type of disease that is present. Flexion contractures of the metacarpophalangeal and interphalangeal articulations, webbing between the fingers, and distal trophic changes can be encountered (Fig. 95–179). The terminal phalanges of the hands (and, less frequently, the feet) are distorted, becoming pointed or wedged-shaped, resembling the findings in scleroderma. This resemblance may be accentuated by the rare appearance of soft tissue calcification in epidermolysis bullosa.[226] Such calcification is seen adjacent to the terminal tufts of the digits or, rarely, at other sites, typically in the superficial fascia.[940] The combination of flexion deformities of the fingers and toes and webbing is important in the diagnosis of this rare skin disease.[228] Additional changes in the hands and feet include subluxations, bone ankylosis of interphalangeal joints, resorption of metacarpal and metatarsal heads, shortened metatarsal bones, carpal and tarsal fusion or destruction, and cystic changes of the distal radius and ulna.[941] Osteoporosis, slender diaphyses of the tubular bones, perhaps due to chronic muscle atrophy, dental caries, periapical abscesses, loss of teeth, and esophageal strictures can be seen. The dental changes presumably are related to poor oral hygiene and extensive scarring in and around the mouth in

early life, although an intrinsic dysplasia also may be important.[229, 231] As a result of scarring in the face and the jaw, underdevelopment of the mandible and maxilla, and an increase in the mandibular angle with prognathism can be noted.[226, 227, 232] Further reported abnormalities are developmental dysplasia of the hip, scoliosis, and ankylosis of the knee.[941]

The pathologic findings have been well documented.[230] The bullae are tense, thin-walled structures filled with straw-colored fluid that occasionally is hemorrhagic or cloudy. The location of the bullae is variable. In the polydysplastic pattern, they are subepidermal; in other types, they are intraepidermal. Inflammation is not prominent. The characteristics of the healing stage also vary according to the pattern of disease. Scars are seen in those patients who do not have the simple variety of epidermolysis bullosa, and keloids, milia, and pigmentation can be evident.

A series of biochemical and histologic studies have been undertaken to define the cause and pathogenesis of the disease as well as to differentiate among the various clinical patterns. The mechanism of blister formation seems to be related to an abnormal synthesis of collagen or presence of an abnormal collagen produced in some other fashion.[233–238] A primary role for the proteolytic enzyme collagenase has been suggested; bioassays and radioimmunoassays have revealed increased levels of collagenase in both blistered and clinically normal skin in some patients with epidermolysis bullosa.[236] A structural defect at the basement membrane zone also may be important; deficient or absent anchoring

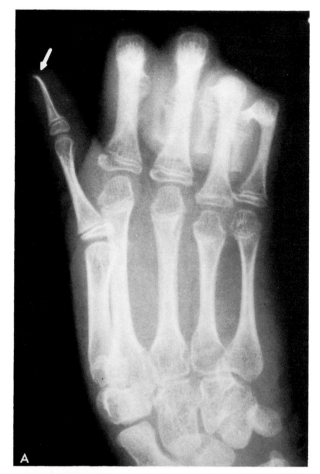

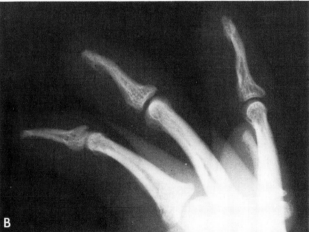

FIGURE 95–179. Epidermolysis bullosa.

A Observe contractures of the interphalangeal articulations, webbing between the digits, skin and bone atrophy, osteoporosis, epiphyseal deformity, and pointing of the terminal tufts of the phalanges, most evident in the thumb (arrow).

B In another patient, the tapered resorption of the terminal phalanges is well seen.

fibers have been reported in both blistered and clinically normal skin.[237] Such structural changes may produce an increased susceptibility of the basement membrane zone to proteolytic enzymes.[238] Other hypotheses regarding the cause of the disease include a hereditary vascular anomaly of the skin[239] and a congenital defect in the hyaluronidase-hyaluronic acid system.[240]

Occasionally patients with epidermolysis bullosa develop skin cancer[241, 242, 942] and a decreased tolerance to the effects of ionizing radiation.[243] With regard to the first complication, one or more squamous cell carcinomas may develop in various locations, including the extremities and oral, esophageal, and gastric mucosa; they are more frequent in patients with epidermolysis bullosa who are older than 30 years of age and who have the recessive types of the disease.[523] Metastases occur frequently, and prognosis is poor. An association of epidermolysis bullosa and bone sarcoma has been suggested[943] but is unproven.

Congenital Cutis Laxa (Generalized Elastolysis)

Congenital cutis laxa is an inherited disorder of connective tissue that becomes manifest at birth or, occasionally, in childhood or adulthood by a striking laxity of the skin, which hangs in pendulous folds over the entire body.[244–247] The cutaneous manifestations are associated with abnormalities of other organs and structures containing elastic tissue. Although the disorder may resemble Marfan's syndrome, Ehlers-Danlos syndrome, and pseudoxanthoma elasticum, it generally is regarded as a distinct entity. Autosomal dominant and recessive patterns exist in addition to an X-linked inherited pattern (see later discussion) and sporadic cases.[525] The congenital forms are characterized by a distinctive facies, with a long upper lip, short columella, and hook nose, resulting in a lugubrious, prematurely aged appearance.[525] Children with the dominant variety of the disease reveal cutaneous abnormalities, a normal life span, and few complications. Patients with the recessive forms are affected more severely and may die at an early age owing to pulmonary and cardiovascular involvement. The clinical manifestations, which include joint laxity and dislocation, large fontanelles with delayed sutural closure, and retardation of motor and intellectual development,[525] combined with biopsy studies that indicate sparse, fragmented, disrupted elastic fibers and an accumulation of material that resembles acid mucopolysaccharide, allow accurate diagnosis.

Radiographic manifestations (as well as clinical manifestations) vary according to the specific type of disease but may include hernias, diverticula of the gastrointestinal and genitourinary tracts, pulmonary emphysema, and diaphragmatic elevation. Numerous pronounced skin folds may be evident. Hypermobility and instability of joints, osteoporosis, and multiple fractures have been encountered.[526] Spontaneous rupture of patellar tendons and an association with plasma cell myeloma have been recorded.[248, 249] Arteriograms may reveal a tortuous, dilated aorta, peripheral pulmonary artery stenosis, and irregular and kinked peripheral vessels.

The cause is unknown. An abnormality of elastin, elastase, and elastase inhibitor biochemical complex has been suggested.[247, 250] A decreased activity of lysyl oxidase, an enzyme required for normal collagen and elastin cross-linking, has been observed in the skin and in cultures of dermal fibroblasts in patients with an X-linked form of cutis laxa,[524] a disease that actually may represent a type of Ehlers-Danlos syndrome.[525]

Eosinophilic Fasciitis (Shulman Syndrome)

Eosinophilic fasciitis, which is discussed in Chapter 34, consists of a scleroderma-like appearance, eosinophilia, hypergammaglobulinemia, and muscle fascia inflammation in the presence of normal skin.[251–253, 298–300] Men and women are affected and the age of onset varies from childhood to the seventh decade of life. Painful, swollen, indurated skin and subcutaneous tissues, especially in the distal portions of the forearms or legs, may lead to restricted motion in the hands and feet. Raynaud's phenomena and visceral manifestations of scleroderma are lacking. Biopsies outline sclerosis of the dermis and inflammation and fibrosis of the panniculus and deep fascia. Within 6 to 12 months, marked skin hardness can develop, and histologic changes may be very similar to those of scleroderma. Dramatic improvement following steroid medication has been noted. Although articular abnormalities are unusual, some reports of patients with eosinophilic fasciitis have stressed polyarticular manifestations with synovitis, mildly inflammatory synovial fluid, and the carpal tunnel syndrome.[300]

Erythema Nodosum

Erythema nodosum is a relatively uncommon inflammatory disorder leading to nodular cutaneous eruptions, which are red, tender, and warm but do not ulcerate. Located primarily on the lower legs, the lesions also can affect the hands, arms, face, and thighs. Microscopy outlines a nonspecific cutaneous vasculitis with subcutaneous infiltration of lymphocytes, granulocytes, histiocytes, and eosinophils.[254]

Erythema nodosum occurs as an idiopathic disorder (60 to 70 per cent of cases) or as a cutaneous manifestation of many systemic illnesses (30 to 40 per cent of cases), including infections (streptococcal, meningococcal, fungal, mycobacterial), sarcoidosis, Behçet's syndrome, ulcerative colitis, Crohn's disease, and leprosy, as well as following administration of certain drugs (oral contraceptives, sulfonamides).[254, 255] When it is idiopathic, the disease has a benign course, subsiding in a period of weeks or months.

Women are affected more often than men. Patients of all ages are involved, many being in the third and fourth decades of life. Clinical manifestations include fever, skin eruption, and joint abnormalities. The latter are observed in 50 to 75 per cent of cases and frequently precede the cutaneous alterations. Symmetric arthralgias and arthritis are noted in the knees and ankles and, less commonly, the wrists, elbows, shoulders, fingers, and hips. Affected articulations are swollen and tender, and a joint effusion may be detected on clinical and radiologic examination. Typically, no cartilaginous or osseous destruction is seen, and the articular abnormalities decrease and disappear in a few weeks to 6 months.[256] Recurrences of joint manifestations can appear simultaneously with the development of additional cutaneous lesions. An associated radiographic finding in either idiopathic or nonidiopathic cases is bilateral hilar adenopathy.

Laboratory analysis may indicate an elevated erythrocyte sedimentation rate and, possibly, hypergammaglobulinemia as well as positive sensitized sheep cell tests in low titer.

Erythema nodosum generally is considered to represent a hypersensitivity reaction to some agent or an allergic cutaneous vasculitis.[257]

Nevoid Basal Cell Carcinoma Syndrome (Gorlin's Syndrome)

Nevoid basal cell carcinoma syndrome is an inherited disorder that is characterized by multiple basal cell carcinomas, palmar pits, odontogenic keratocysts, rib and spine anomalies, brachydactyly, and various neurologic and ophthalmologic abnormalities.[258–265, 944] The disorder is inherited in an autosomal dominant pattern with variable expressivity[527, 528] and appears with equal frequency in both sexes.

Basal cell epitheliomas usually are seen near puberty, although they can be evident as early as 2 years of age. The lesions are slightly raised, translucent, and 1 to 10 mm in diameter and may reveal brown discoloration. Some are aggressive, with ulceration and local invasion. Typically affected sites are the face and trunk, although other regions can be involved. Less constant skin abnormalities include milia, comedones, sebaceous or epithelial cysts, and dyskeratosis.[260]

Dentigerous cysts of the mandible are common in this disorder but rarely produce clinical findings prior to the age of 6 to 7 years (Fig. 95–180). They may antedate the appearance of the skin lesions, and symptoms and signs related to these cysts may be the presenting manifestations of the disease. Swelling, pain, and spontaneous drainage are seen. Mandibular cysts can be single or multiple, vary in diameter from 1 or 2 mm to several centimeters, are located predominantly at the angle of the jaw, and appear as radiolucent lesions with ill-defined margins. Pathologic fractures and, rarely, ameloblastomas can develop from such lesions.[259, 266, 267] The cysts are follicular or dentigerous in type and are lined with epithelium that may be stratified squamous or abnormally keratinized. Their surgical removal may be followed by recurrence, perhaps related to activation of retained microcysts.

The common rib anomalies are splaying, synostosis, and bifid and cervical ribs[263] (Fig. 95–181). Unilateral or bilateral alterations in the first to fourth ribs are most typical. Shortening of the metacarpals, especially the fourth and fifth, also is a relatively common finding, similar to that which occurs in pseudohypoparathyroidism, multiple hereditary exostosis, and other conditions. In the spine, kyphoscoliosis, spina bifida occulta, block vertebrae, spondylolysis, spondylolisthesis,[529] and hemivertebrae can be seen. The list of additional skeletal manifestations in the basal cell nevus syndrome is impressive and includes shortened distal phalanges and notching of the inferior aspect of the scapula. In the skull, calcification of the falx cerebri (Fig. 95–181), dura, tentorium, and choroid, partial agenesis of the corpus callosum, hypertelorism, and anosmia[268] may occur. Mental retardation, congenital hydrocephalus, and changes in the eyes (dysgenesis oculi neuroblastica gliomatosa) have been noted. Several instances of medulloblastoma or meningioma in this syndrome have been recorded.[259, 262] Gonadal abnormalities include ovarian and uterine fibromas in the female and hypogonadism and cryptorchidism in the male.[260, 266]

Some reports have emphasized the occurrence of small, flame-shaped, cystic lucent areas in the phalanges and tubular bones of the arms[264, 265, 530–532] (Fig. 95–182). The lesions, which also may be observed in the metatarsals, femora, ribs, and, perhaps, any bone,[532] are multiple, elongated, and frequently eccentric in location. They may appear as enclosed medullary or cortical foci or as scalloped

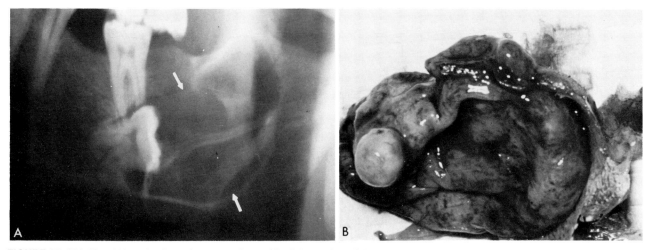

FIGURE 95–180. Nevoid basal cell carcinoma syndrome (Gorlin's syndrome): Mandibular abnormalities.
  A Dentigerous cysts (arrows) are common in this syndrome.
  B The size of the dentigerous cysts is variable, but they may reach several centimeters in diameter. (Courtesy of R. Smith, D.D.S., San Francisco, California.)

defects on the external surface of the bone and, in some cases,[531, 532] are combined with small sclerotic foci simulating osteopoikilosis (Fig. 95–183). The pathogenesis of these lucent areas is unknown, although they may relate to intraosseous epithelial cysts, lipomas, or fibromas, which do occur in other locations in this syndrome. The alterations may resemble those in sarcoidosis or tuberous sclerosis.

The presence of shortened metacarpals in as many as 50 per cent of patients with this syndrome, a finding that also is evident in pseudohypoparathyroidism and pseudopseudohypoparathyroidism, has raised the possibility of an as-

sociation among these disorders. This possibility is strengthened by the fact that soft tissue calcification occasionally is found in all of these diseases. Tissue response to parathyroid hormone has been reported to be less than normal in both the nevoid basal cell carcinoma syndrome and pseudohypoparathyroidism.[269] Other investigations have failed to document an abnormal parathyroid hormone response in patients with the nevoid basal cell carcinoma syndrome, however.[270, 271] In addition, serum calcium and phosphorus levels are normal in persons with this disease.[265] At this writing, the basic defect is not known.

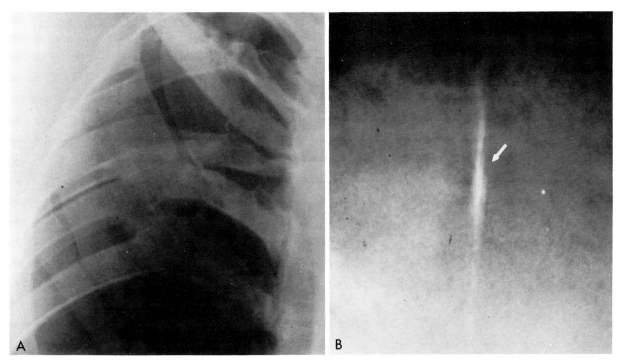

FIGURE 95–181. Nevoid basal cell carcinoma syndrome (Gorlin's syndrome): Other abnormalities.
  A Typical rib anomalies are demonstrated.
  B Calcification of the falx cerebri (arrow) is not unusual in this syndrome.

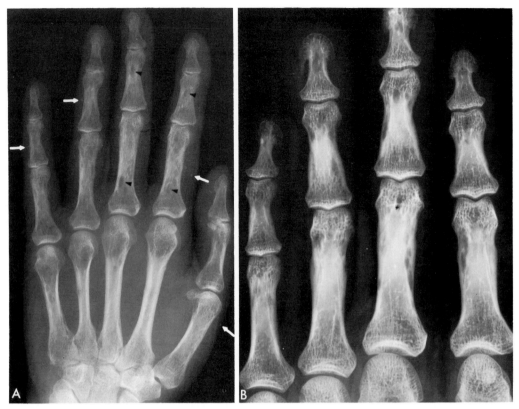

FIGURE 95–182. Nevoid basal cell carcinoma syndrome (Gorlin's syndrome): Cystic lesions of the hand.

A In this 65 year old woman, note multiple lucent lesions of the phalanges and the metacarpals (arrowheads), as well as small foci of soft tissue calcification (arrows).

B In a 25 year old man, note the flame-shaped configuration and eccentric location of many of the lucent lesions.

(From Dunnick NR, et al: Radiology *127*:331, 1978.)

Linear Nevus Sebaceus Syndrome

Linear nevus sebaceus syndrome is a recently recognized neurocutaneous syndrome characterized by an epidermal nevus, seizures, and mental retardation.[272–276] The syndrome may involve a variety of tissues of ectodermal and mesenchymal origin and, in this regard, resembles neurofibromatosis, tuberous sclerosis, the Proteus syndrome, the Sturge-Weber syndrome, and von Hippel-Lindau disease.[945] Malformations of the brain, viscera, and skeleton can lead to various radiographic alterations. These include asymmetry of the skull and facial bones, premature fusion of sutures, cerebral atrophy with ventricular dilatation, hydrocephalus, scoliosis, kyphoscoliosis, and deformities of the pelvis and long bones. The findings are not specific. The diagnosis should be considered when a variety of cranial, cerebral,

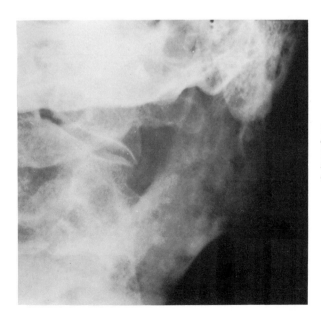

FIGURE 95–183. Nevoid basal cell carcinoma syndrome (Gorlin's syndrome): Sclerotic lesions of the mandible. Three members of a family (father, daughter, and son) had manifestations of the basal cell nevoid syndrome. A radiograph of the father, aged 50 years, is shown. Small oval osteosclerotic areas are seen.

(From Blinder G, et al: Skel Radiol *12*:196, 1984.)

and skeletal manifestations are detected in a mentally retarded child with seizures and typical skin lesions.

Rothmund-Thomson Syndrome

The Rothmund-Thomson syndrome, or congenital poikiloderma, is characterized by maculopapular and erythematous skin lesions with areas of hyperpigmentation. Additional manifestations include photosensitivity, cataracts, hypogonadism, and abnormalities of dentition.[946] Dwarfism, brachycephaly, and a birdlike facies may be seen.[947] Skeletal alterations include changes resembling osteopoikilosis (see Chapter 93), spinal anomalies or abnormal curvature, hypoplasia of the carpal bones, radius or ulna, tarsal fusion, foot deformities, tibial aplasia or hypoplasia, and patellar anomalies.[948] Cystic lesions of bone may be evident, and an association of this syndrome with osteogenic sarcoma is well known.[948, 949]

Panniculitis and Related Syndromes

Panniculitides represent inflammatory disorders of subcutaneous fat. Although several distinct forms of panniculitis have been recognized, clinical manifestations common to most forms include the presence of moderately tender nodules in the soft tissues, especially in the lower extremities, which may lead to discharge of liquefied fat and scarring.[533] These disorders are histologically classified into two patterns on the basis of the location of inflammation within the lobular arrangement of subcutaneous tissue: Inflammation around the central arterial system leads to changes affecting the entire lobule (lobular panniculitis); inflammation about the venous system produces septal changes (septal panniculitis).[282] Either pattern may occur with or without vasculitis. Erythema nodosum and subacute migratory panniculitis are examples of septal panniculitis; Weber-Christian disease, erythema induratum, and nodular vasculitis are examples of lobular panniculitis[282] (Table 95–4).

Weber-Christian disease is a contested entity. Some investigators believe it is a distinct pathologic condition, whereas others regard this disorder as a secondary manifestation of pancreatic disease.[283] Typically, a woman in the fourth or fifth decade of life is affected, with tender nodules in the trunk and buttocks as the presenting symptoms. Some of the lesions may ulcerate. Similar instances in children and infants have been described.[950] On histologic examination, the nodules initially are characterized by polymorphonuclear leukocytic infiltration in the fat and subsequently reveal fatty degeneration, macrophage accumulation, and lymphocyte and plasma cell infiltration.[282] Vascular changes and scar tissue may appear. Radiographic changes usually are absent.

Other varieties of lobular panniculitis are erythema induratum or nodular vasculitis (occurring in middle-aged women as bilaterally distributed painful nodules on the calves), pancreatic panniculitis (in which erythematous nodules and bone destruction accompany inflammatory or neoplastic diseases of the pancreas) (Fig. 95–184), and systemic vasculitis (in which subcutaneous nodules may appear during the course of systemic lupus erythematosus, periarteritis nodosa, Behçet's syndrome, and other vasculitic disorders).[282] Factitial panniculitis relates to inflammation and necrosis of fat produced by thermal, mechanical, or chemical trauma.[533]

Juxta-articular adiposis dolorosa or Dercum's disease also is a debated entity.[284, 576] In this disorder, generalized

TABLE 95–4. Characteristics of the Varying Panniculitides in Adults*

Condition	Clinical Features	Associated Conditions	Histopathologic Characteristics
Erythema nodosum	Tender erythematous nodules on lower extremities Fever Arthritis	Poststreptococcal sarcoidosis Inflammatory bowel disease	Septal panniculitis (no vasculitis)
Subacute nodular migratory panniculitis	Painless nodules on lower leg Yellow centers Sclerodermoid changes	None	Septal panniculitis
Weber-Christian disease	Chronic, recurrent, tender, erythematous nodules Systemic symptoms of foot necrosis	Pancreatic disease Infections Autoimmune disorders	Lobular panniculitis Foam cells Fibrosis in late stages (no vasculitis)
Nodular vasculitis	Tender nodules or plaques on posterior aspect of lower legs	None	Lobular panniculitis with vasculitis
Erythema induratum	Nodules on posterior aspect of legs	Tuberculosis	Lobular panniculitis with vasculitis and caseation necrosis
Lupus panniculitis	Nodules on face, buttocks, arms Overlying scars	Discoid lupus erythematosus Systemic lupus erythematosus	Septal and lobular panniculitis
Connective tissue panniculitis	Erythematous, tender plaques and nodules Resolution with atrophy	Unclassified connective tissue disease	Lymphohistiocytic invasion of fat lobules with caseation (no vasculitis)
Cytophagic panniculitis	Erythematous, tender nodules Fever Oral ulcers Serositis	Lymphadenopathy Organomegaly Pancytopenia	Lobular panniculitis with fat necrosis and hemorrhage
Pancreatic panniculitis	Erythematous nodules	Pancreatitis Pancreatic malignancy	Lobular panniculitis with necrosis of lipocytes and ghost cells

*From Thiers BH: Dermatol Clin North Am *1*:537, 1983.

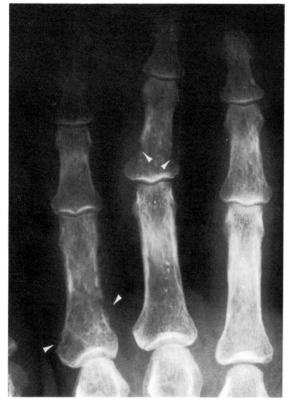

FIGURE 95–184. Pancreatic panniculitis. A 61 year old Mexican man had multiple painful and tender erythematous soft tissue nodules in both lower extremities and a 11.4 kg (25 lb) weight loss during the previous few months. He had a 2 month history of arthralgias. On physical examination, periarticular soft tissue swelling was evident in the hands, wrists, ankles, and knees. Aspiration of both knees yielded inflammatory cells and debris and, approximately 1 week later, thick cloudy fluid containing fat globules was removed from one knee. Serum levels of lipase and amylase were elevated. Anemia and an elevated erythrocyte sedimentation rate were additional laboratory findings. CT of the abdomen documented pancreatic enlargement, probably related to a tumor. Surgery was refused. The radiograph of one hand shows soft tissue swelling and osteolytic lesions with periostitis (arrowheads), consistent with fat necrosis. (Courtesy of R. Kerr, M.D., Los Angeles, California.)

obesity, weakness, fatigability, and emotional instability may be accompanied by painful, circumscribed or diffuse fatty deposits, frequently localized to the lower extremity. These may calcify or ossify (Fig. 95–185). Although some reports emphasize additional abnormalities of various endocrine glands, others doubt this association. In some patients, an autosomal dominant pattern of inheritance is evident.

Miscellaneous Syndromes and Conditions

Musculoskeletal manifestations associated with acne fulminans and acne conglobata are discussed in Chapter 29. Pyoderma gangrenosum, Sweet's syndrome, and papular mucinosis also are considered in Chapter 29. The Ehlers-Danlos syndrome is reviewed in Chapter 87, and tuberous sclerosis, neurofibromatosis, and fibrous dysplasia are discussed in Chapter 92. The blue rubber bleb nevus syndrome is noted earlier in this chapter.[379, 534] A discussion of the relationship of pustulosis palmaris et plantaris and sterno-costoclavicular hyperostosis is contained in Chapter 93. In the same chapter, the association of focal dermal hypoplasia (Goltz's syndrome)[535, 536] and osteopathia striata is described.

Keratodermia palmaris et plantaris is a rare autosomal inherited condition in which hyperkeratosis of the palms and soles develops in infancy or childhood. In occasional patients, clubbing and osteolysis or deformity of terminal phalanges have been noted.[285, 537]

Other varieties of hyperkeratosis have been associated with destructive changes of bone.[286, 301]

SUMMARY

The radiographic alterations in soft tissue disorders include masses, increased lucency, calcification or ossification, bands, contractures, foreign bodies, atrophy, hypertrophy, and edema. In most instances, the findings lack specificity, although at times, careful analysis may allow delineation of the benign or malignant nature of the process. Especially important is the differentiation of myositis ossificans traumatica from various malignant tumors and the recognition that widespread skeletal abnormalities may accompany certain cutaneous syndromes. Use of other diagnostic techniques, including xeroradiography, low KV radiography, ultrasonography, CT, MR imaging, angiography, and scintigraphy, may be required to supplement the radiographic evaluation and provide more accurate information regarding the extent of the soft tissue process and its relationship to adjacent structures.

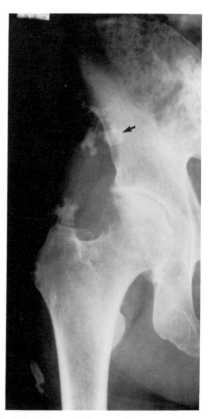

FIGURE 95–185. Adiposa dolorosa (Dercum's disease). Observe ossified nodules about the right hip. The shell-like appearance (arrow) is typical of fat necrosis. (Courtesy of L. Vaughn, M.D., San Diego, California.)

References

1. Frantzell A: Soft tissue radiography. Technical aspects and clinical applications in the examination of limbs. Acta Radiol (Suppl) *85:*1, 1951.
2. Martel W, Abell MR: Radiologic evaluation of soft tissue tumors. A retrospective study. Cancer *32:*352, 1973.
3. Friedmann G, Mödder U, Tismer R: Xeroradiographicsche Befunde bei osteosynthetische versorgten Frakturen. Röentgenblaetter *27:*586, 1974.
4. Wolfe JN: Xeroradiography of the bones, joints and soft tissues. Radiology *93:*583, 1969.
5. Otto RC, Pouliadis GP, Kumpe DA. The evaluation of pathologic alterations of juxtaosseous soft tissue by xeroradiography. Radiology *120:*297, 1976.
6. Hermann G, Rose JS: Computed tomography in bone and soft tissue pathology of the extremities. J Comput Assist Tomogr *3:*58, 1979.
7. Cohen WN, Seidelmann FE, Bryan PJ: Computed tomography of localized adipose deposits presenting as tumor masses. AJR *128:*1007, 1977.
8. Weinberger G, Levinsohn EM: Computed tomography in the evaluation of sarcomatous tumors of thigh. AJR *130:*115, 1978.
9. Wilson JS, Korobkin M, Genant HK, et al: Computed tomography of musculoskeletal disorders. AJR *131:*55, 1978.
10. Hunter JC, Johnston WH, Genant HK: Computed tomography evaluation of fatty tumors of the somatic soft tissues: Clinical utility and radiologic-pathologic correlation. Skel Radiol *4:*79, 1979.
11. Ney FG, Feist HH, Altemus LR, et al: The characteristic angiographic criteria of malignancy. Radiology *104:*567, 1972.
12. Levin DC, Watson RC, Baltaxe HA: Arteriography in diagnosis and management of acquired peripheral soft tissue masses. Radiology *104:*58, 1972.
13. Herzeberg DL, Schreiber MH: Angiography in mass lesions of the extremities. AJR *111:*541, 1971.
14. Cockshott WP, Evans KT: The place of soft tissue arteriography. Br J Radiol *37:*367, 1964.
15. Bliznak J, Staple TW: Radiology of angiodysplasias of the limb. Radiology *110:*35, 1974.
16. Bartley O, Wickbom I: Angiography in soft tissue hemangiomas. Acta Radiol *51:*81, 1959.
17. Levin DC, Gordon DH, McSweeney J: Arteriography of peripheral hemangiomas. Radiology *121:*625, 1976.
18. Richman LS, Gumerman LW, Levine G, et al: Localization of Tc⁹⁹ᵐ polyphosphate in soft tissue malignancies. AJR *124:*577, 1975.
19. Thrall JH, Ghaed N, Geslien GE, et al: Pitfalls in Tc⁹⁹ᵐ polyphosphate skeletal imaging. AJR *121:*739, 1974.
20. Stout AP, Lattes R: Tumors of the Soft Tissues. Atlas of Tumor Pathology, Series 2, Fascicle 1. Bethesda, Md, Armed Forces Institute of Pathology, 1967.
21. Edland RW: Liposarcoma. A retrospective study of fifteen cases, a review of the literature and a discussion of radiosensitivity. AJR *103:*778, 1968.
22. Pack GT, Pierson JC: Liposarcoma: A study of 105 cases. Surgery *36:*687, 1954.
23. Leffert RD: Lipomas of the upper extremity. J Bone Joint Surg [Am] *54:*1262, 1972.
24. Lin JJ, Lin F: Two entities in angiolipoma. A study of 459 cases of lipoma with review of literature on infiltrating angiolipoma. Cancer *34:*720, 1974.
25. Chung EB, Enzinger FM: Benign lipoblastomatosis. An analysis of 35 cases. Cancer *32:*482, 1973.
26. Brines OA, Johnson MH: Hibernoma, a special fatty tumor; report of a case. Am J Pathol *25:*467, 1949.
27. Vellios F, Baez J, Schumacker HB: Lipoblastomatosis: A tumor of fetal fat different from hibernoma. Report of a case with observations of the embryogenesis of human adipose tissue. Am J Pathol *34:*1149, 1958.
28. Weitzman G: Lipoma arborescens of the knee. Report of a case. J Bone Joint Surg [Am] *47:*1030, 1965.
29. Kaufman JH, Cedermark BJ, Parthasarathy KL, et al: The values of ⁶⁷Ga scintigraphy in soft-tissue sarcoma and chondrosarcoma. Radiology *123:*131, 1977.
30. Stout AP: Fibrosarcoma: The malignant tumor of fibroblasts. Cancer *1:*30, 1948.
31. Stout AP: Fibrosarcoma in infants and children. Cancer *15:*1028, 1962.
32. Bonakdarpour A, Pickering JE, Resnick EJ: Case report 49. Skel Radiol *2:*181, 1978.
33. Enzinger FM, Shiraki M: Musculo-aponeurotic fibromatosis of the shoulder girdle (extra-abdominal desmoid). Analysis of thirty cases followed up for ten or more years. Cancer *20:*1131, 1967.
34. Greenfield GB, Rubenstone AI, Lo M: Case report 31. Skel Radiol *2:*43, 1977.
35. Barber HM, Galasko CSB, Woods CG: Multicentric extra-abdominal desmoid tumours. Report of two cases. J Bone Joint Surg [Br] *55:*858, 1973.
36. Rosen RS, Kimball W: Extra-abdominal desmoid tumor. Radiology *86:*534, 1966.
37. Reye RDK: Recurring digital fibrous tumours of childhood. Arch Pathol *80:*228, 1965.
38. Bloem JJ, Vuzevski VD, Huffstadt AJC: Recurring digital fibroma of infancy. J Bone Joint Surg [Br] *56:*746, 1974.
39. Lakhanpal VP, Yadav SS, Sastry VRK, et al: Recurring digital fibromas of infancy. A case report. Acta Orthop Scand *49:*147, 1978.
40. Keasbey LE: Juvenile aponeurotic fibroma (calcifying fibroma): A distinctive tumor arising in the palms and soles of young children. Cancer *6:*338, 1953.
41. Vatopoulos PK, Garofalakis EE, Papathanassiou BT: Juvenile aponeurotic fibroma. Report of a case. Acta Orthop Scand *45:*158, 1974.
42. Keller RB, Baez-Giangreco A: Juvenile aponeurotic fibroma. Report of three cases and a review of the literature. Clin Orthop *106:*198, 1975.
43. Lichtenstein L, Goldman RL: The cartilage analogue of fibromatosis—a reinterpretation of the condition called juvenile aponeurotic fibroma. Cancer *17:*810, 1964.
44. Prete P, Thorne RP: Elastofibroma: A rare cause of periscapular pain. Arthritis Rheum *22:*792, 1979.
45. Renshaw TS, Simon MA: Elastofibroma. J Bone Joint Surg [Am] *55:*409, 1973.
46. Deutsch GP: Elastofibroma dorsalis treated by radiotherapy. Br J Radiol *47:*621, 1974.
47. Javors BR, Katz MC, Kwon CS: Case report 73. Skel Radiol *3:*183, 1978.
48. Schaffzin EA, Chung SMK, Kaye R: Congenital generalized fibromatosis with complete spontaneous regression. J Bone Joint Surg [Am] *54:*657, 1972.
49. Heiple KG, Perrin E, Aikawa M: Congenital generalized fibromatosis. A case limited to osseous lesions. J Bone Joint Surg [Am] *54:*663, 1972.
50. Karasick D, O'Hara AE: Juvenile aponeurotic fibroma. A review and report of a case with osseous involvement. Radiology *123:*725, 1977.
51. Broder MS, Leonidas JC, Mitty HA: Pseudosarcomatous fasciitis: An unusual cause of soft tissue calcification. Radiology *107:*173, 1973.
52. Stout AP, Hill WT: Leiomyosarcoma of the superficial soft tissues. Cancer *11:*844, 1958.
53. Bulmer JH: Smooth muscle tumours of the limbs. J Bone Joint Surg [Br] *49:*52, 1967.
54. Hornback NB, Shidnia H: Rhabdomyosarcoma in the pediatric age group. AJR *126:*542, 1976.
55. Moskowitz M, Rosenbaum HT, Sweet R, et al: Calcified embryonal rhabdomyosarcoma with local bone invasion. An unusual case. Radiology *91:*121, 1968.
56. McDowell CL, Cardea JA: Embryonal rhabdomyosarcoma of the hand. A case report. Clin Orthop *100:*238, 1974.
57. Bailey WC, Holaday WJ, Kontras SB, et al: Rhabdomyosarcomas in childhood: A review of 14 cases. Arch Surg *82:*943, 1961.
58. Simmons M, Tucker AK: The radiology of bone changes in rhabdomyosarcoma. Clin Radiol *29:*47, 1978.
59. Crane AR, Tremblay RG: Myoblastoma (granular cell myoblastoma or myoblastic myoma). Am J Pathol *21:*357, 1945.
60. Bielejeski TR: Granular-cell tumor (myoblastoma) of the hand. Report of a case. J Bone Joint Surg [Am] *55:*841, 1973.
61. Ghormley RK, Dockerty MB: Cystic myxomatous tumors about the knee: Their relation to cysts of the menisci. J Bone Joint Surg *25:*306, 1943.
62. Dutz W, Stout AP: The myxoma in childhood. Cancer *14:*629, 1961.
63. Stout AP: Myxoma; the tumor of primitive mesenchyme. Ann Surg *127:*706, 1948.
64. Milgram JW, Preininger RF: Calcifying myxoma. A case report. J Bone Joint Surg [Am] *55:*401, 1973.
65. Ireland DCR, Soule EH, Ivins JC: Myxoma of somatic soft tissues. A report of 58 patients, 3 with multiple tumors and fibrous dysplasia of bone. Mayo Clin Proc *48:*401, 1973.
66. Soule EH, Enriquez P: Atypical fibrous histiocytoma, malignant fibrous histiocytoma, malignant histiocytoma, and epithelioid sarcoma. A comparative study of 65 tumors. Cancer *30:*128, 1972.
67. Kyriakos M, Kempson RL: Inflammatory fibrous histiocytoma. An aggressive and lethal lesion. Cancer *37:*1584, 1976.
68. Solomon MP, Sutton AL: Malignant fibrous histiocytoma of the soft tissues of the mandible. Oral Surg *35:*653, 1973.
69. Spencer D, Wrighton JD: Histiocytoma presenting as swelling on the toe. Arch Dis Child *47:*828, 1972.
70. Helal B, Currey HLF, Vernon-Roberts B: Fibrous histiocytoma of the thumb. Br J Surg *61:*909, 1974.
71. Lo HH, Kalisher L, Faix JD: Epithelioid sarcoma: Radiologic and pathologic manifestations. AJR *128:*1017, 1977.
72. Bryan RS, Soule EH, Dobyns JH, et al: Primary epithelioid sarcoma of the hand and forearm. A review of thirteen cases. J Bone Joint Surg [Am] *56:*458, 1974.
73. DeLuca FN, Neviaser RJ: Epithelioid sarcoma involving bone. Clin Orthop *107:*168, 1975.
74. Hamilton WC, Ramsey PL, Hanson SM, et al: Osseous xanthoma and multiple hand tumors as a complication of hyperlipidemia. Report of a case. J Bone Joint Surg [Am] *57:*551, 1975.
75. Fahey JJ, Stark HH, Donovan WF, et al: Xanthoma of the Achilles tendon. Seven cases with familial hyperbetalipoproteinemia. J Bone Joint Surg [Am] *55:*1197, 1973.
76. Yaghmai I: Intra- and extraosseous xanthomata associated with hyperlipidemia. Radiology *128:*49, 1978.
77. Gattereau A, Davignon J, Langelier M, et al: An improved radiological method for the evaluation of Achilles tendon xanthomatosis. Can Med Assoc J [Br] *108:*39, 1973.
78. Neviaser RJ, Adams JP: Vascular lesions in the hand. Current management. Clin Orthop *100:*111, 1974.
79. McNeill TW, Ray RD: Hemangioma of the extremities. Review of 35 cases. Clin Orthop *101:*154, 1974.
80. Ayella RJ: Hemangiopericytoma. A case report with arteriographic findings. Radiology *97:*611, 1970.
81. Carroll RE, Berman AT: Glomus tumors of the hand. Review of the literature and report on twenty-eight cases. J Bone Joint Surg [Am] *54:*691, 1972.
82. Gorham LW: Kaposi's sarcoma involving bone: With particular attention to

angiomatous components of the tumor in relation to osteolysis. Arch Pathol 76:456, 1963.

83. Cox FH, Helwig EB: Kaposi's sarcoma. Cancer 12:289, 1959.

84. Bluefarb SM, Webster JR: Kaposi's sarcoma associated with lymphosarcoma. Arch Intern Med 91:97, 1953.

85. Aegerter EE, Peale AR: Kaposi's sarcoma. A critical survey. Arch Pathol 34:413, 1942.

86. Glatt OS: Kaposi's sarcoma. J Am Geriat Soc 21:469, 1973.

87. Chung EB, Enzinger FM: Chondroma of soft parts. Cancer 41:1414, 1978.

88. Murphy AF, Wilson JN: Tenosynovial osteochondroma in the hand. J Bone Joint Surg [Am] 40:1236, 1958.

89. Strong ML Jr: Chondromas of the tendon sheath of the hand. Report of a case and review of the literature. J Bone Joint Surg [Am] 57:1164, 1975.

90. Smith MT, Farinacci CJ, Carpenter HA, et al: Extraskeletal myxoid chondrosarcoma. A clinicopathological study. Cancer 37:821, 1976.

91. Guccion JG, Font RL, Enzinger FM, et al: Extraskeletal mesenchymal chondrosarcoma. Arch Pathol 95:336, 1973.

92. Angerval L, Enerbäck L, Knutston H: Chondrosarcoma of soft tissue origin. Cancer 32:507, 1973.

93. Hernandez R, Heidelberger KP, Poznanski AK: Case report 63. Skel Radiol 3:61, 1978.

94. Fine G, Stout AP: Osteogenic sarcoma of the extraskeletal soft tissues. Cancer 9:1027, 1956.

95. Kauffman SL, Stout AP: Extraskeletal osteogenic sarcomas and chondrosarcomas in children. Cancer 16:432, 1963.

96. Lorentzon R, Larsson SE, Boquist L: Extra-osseous osteosarcoma. A clinical and histopathological study of four cases. J Bone Joint Surg [Br] 61:205, 1979.

97. Adler CP: Case report 92. Skel Radiol 4:107, 1979.

98. Thompson DE, Frost HM, Hendrick JW, et al: Soft tissue sarcomas involving the extremities and the limb girdles. A review. South Med J 64:33, 1971.

99. Tillotson JF, McDonald JR, Janes JM: Synovial sarcomata. J Bone Joint Surg [Am] 33:459, 1973.

100. Pack GT, Ariel IM: Synovial sarcoma (malignant synvioma). A report of 60 cases. Surgery 28:1047, 1950.

101. Cadman NL, Soule EH, Kelly PJ: Synovial sarcoma. An analysis of 134 tumors. Cancer 18:613, 1965.

102. Cameron HU, Kostuik JP: A long-term follow-up of synovial sarcoma. J Bone Joint Surg [Br] 56:613, 1974.

103. Murray JA: Synovial sarcoma. Orthop Clin North Am 8:963, 1977.

104. Horowitz AL, Resnick D, Watson RC: The roentgen features of synovial sarcomas. Clin Radiol 24:481, 1973.

105. Desantos LA, Lindell MM Jr, Goldman AM, et al: Calcification within metastatic pulmonary nodules from synovial sarcoma. Orthopedics 1:141, 1978.

106. Reed RJ, Bliss BO: Morton's neuroma. Regressive and productive intermetatarsal elastofibrosis. Arch Pathol 95:123, 1973.

107. Enzinger FM: Clear-cell sarcoma of tendons and aponeuroses. An analysis of 21 cases. Cancer 18:1163, 1965.

108. Radstone DJ, Revell PA, Mantell BS: Clear cell sarcoma of tendons and aponeuroses treated with bleomycin and vincristine. Br J Radiol 52:238, 1979.

109. Smetana HF, Scott WF Jr: Malignant tumors of nonchromaffin paraganglia. Milit Surgeon 109:330, 1951.

110. Christopherson WM, Foote FW Jr, Stewart FW: Alveolar soft-part sarcomas. Structurally characteristic tumors of uncertain histogenesis. Cancer 5:100, 1952.

111. Dutt AK, Balasegaram M, Din OB: Alveolar soft-part sarcoma with invasion of bone. A case report. J Bone Joint Surg [Am] 51:765, 1969.

112. Forbis R Jr, Helwig EB: Pilomatrixoma (calcifying epithelioma). Arch Dermatol 83:606, 1961.

113. Haller JO, Kassner EG, Ostrowitz A, et al: Pilomatrixoma (calcifying epithelioma of Malherbe): Radiographic features. Radiology 123:151, 1977.

114. DuToit G Rang M: Congenital calcific hamartoma. A resolving lesion producing gastrocnemius contracture—report of a case. Clin Orthop 135:79, 1978.

115. Feldman F, Norman D: Intra- and extraosseous malignant histiocytoma (malignant fibrous xanthoma). Radiology 104:497, 1972.

116. Louis DS, Dick HM: Ossifying lipofibroma of the median nerve. J Bone Joint Surg [Am] 55:1082, 1973.

117. Greenfield GB: Radiology of Bone Diseases. 2nd Ed. Philadelphia, JB Lippincott Co, 1975, p 491.

118. Mathias K, Baumeister L: Röntgenologische Differentialdiagnose von Extremitäten-Verkalkungen. Radiologe 18:129, 1978.

119. Weber U, Pfeifer G: Beitrag zur Differentialdiagnose kalkdichter Weichteilverschattungen der Extremitäten. Z Orthop 115:256, 1977.

120. Epstein DA, Solar M, Levin EJ: Demonstration of long-standing metastatic soft tissue calcification by 99mTc diphosphonate. AJR 128:145, 1977.

121. Bauer W, Marble A, Bennett G: Further studies in a case of calcification of the subcutaneous tissue ("calcinosis universalis") in a child. Am J Med Sci 182:237, 1931.

122. Leistyna JA, Hassan HI: Interstitial calcinosis. Am J Dis Child 107:96, 1964

123. Caffey J: Pediatric X-ray Diagnosis, 7th Ed. Chicago, Year Book Medical Publishers, 1978, p 984.

124. Ozonoff MB, Flynn FJ Jr: Roentgenologic features of dermatomyositis of childhood. AJR 118:206, 1973.

125. Shackelford GD, Barton LL, McAlister WH: Calcified subcutaneous fat necrosis in infancy. J Can Assoc Radiol 26:203, 1975.

126. Harris V, Ramamurphy RS, Pildes RS: Late onset of subcutaneous calcifications after intravenous injections of calcium gluconate. AJR 123:845, 1975.

127. Inclan A, Leon P, Camejo MG: Tumoral calcinosis. JAMA 121:490, 1943.

128. Hacihanefioğlu U: Tumoral calcinosis. A clinical and pathological study of eleven unreported cases in Turkey. J Bone Joint Surg [Am] 60:1131, 1978.

129. Traca G, Hennebert P-N, Mazabraud A: Considérations sur un cas de lipocalcinogranulomatose. Presse Med 73:543, 1965.

130. Bancale A: Lipo-calcino-granulomatous bursitis (Teutschlaender's disease). Minerva Ortop 12:833, 1961.

131. Veress B, Malik MOA, El Hassan AM: Tumoural lipocalcinosis: A clinico-pathological study of 20 cases. J Pathol 119:113, 1976.

132. Hartofilakidas-Garofalidis G, Theodossiou A, Matsoukas J, et al: Tumoral lipocalcinosis. Acta Orthop Scand 41:387, 1950.

133. Thomson JG: Calcifying collagenolysis (tumoral calcinosis). Br J Radiol 39:526, 1966.

134. Ghormley RK: Multiple calcified bursae and calcified cysts in soft tissues. Trans West Surg Assoc 51:292, 1942.

135. Barton DL, Reeves RJ: Tumoral calcinosis. Report of three cases and review of the literature. AJR 86:351, 1961.

136. Sammarco GJ, Makley JT: Tumoral calcinosis and mongolism. A case report. Clin Orthop 91:164, 1973.

137. Kolawole TM, Bohrer SP: Tumoral calcinosis with "fluid levels" in the tumoral masses. AJR 120:461, 1974.

138. Slavin G, Klenerman L, Darby A, et al: Tumoral calcinosis in England. Br Med J 1:147, 1973.

139. Wilson AL, Chater EH: Tumoral calcinosis—an obscure disease. A report of four cases. J Irish Med Assoc 69:61, 1976.

140. Brown ML, Thrall JH, Cooper RA, et al: Radiography and scintigraphy in tumoral calcinosis. Radiology 124:757, 1977.

141. Currie H: Tumoral calcinosis. Br Med J 2:120, 1969.

142. Baldursson H, Evans EB, Dodge WF, et al: Tumoral calcinosis with hyperphosphatemia. A report of a family with incidence in four siblings. J Bone Joint Surg [Am] 51:913, 1969.

143. Lafferty FW, Reynolds ES, Pearson OH: Tumoral calcinosis. A metabolic disease of obscure etiology. Am J Med 38:105, 1965.

144. Wilber JF, Slatopolsky E: Hyperphosphatemia and tumoral calcinosis. Ann Intern Med 68:1044, 1968.

145. Harkess JW, Peters HJ: Tumoral calcinosis. A report of six cases. J Bone Joint Surg [Am] 49:721, 1967.

146. Frame B, Herrera LF, Mitchell DC, et al: Massive osteolysis and tumoral calcinosis. Am J Med 50:408, 1971.

147. Eugenidis N, Locher JT: Tumoral calcinosis imaged by bone scanning. Case report. J Nucl Med 18:34, 1977.

148. Bolger JT: Heterotopic bone formation and alkaline phosphatase. Arch Phys Med Rehabil 56:36, 1975.

149. Furman R, Nicholas JJ, Jivoff L: Elevation of the serum alkaline phosphatase coincident with ectopic-bone formation in paraplegic patients. J Bone Joint Surg [Am] 52:1131, 1970.

150. Muheim G, Donath A, Rossier AB: Serial scintigrams in the course of ectopic bone formation in paraplegic patients. AJR 118:865, 1973.

151. Tanaka T, Rossier AB, Hussey RW, et al: Quantitative assessment of para-osteo-arthropathy and its maturation on serial radionuclide bone images. Radiology 123:217 1977.

152. Gunn DR, Young WB: Myositis ossificans as a complication of tetanus. J Bone Joint Surg [Br] 41:535, 1959.

153. Bour H, Tutin M, Pasquier P, et al: Les paraostéoarthropathies au décours des comas oxycarbonés graves. Sem Hôp Paris 42:1912, 1966.

154. Ghormley JW: Ossification of the tendo Achillis. J Bone Joint Surg 20:153, 1938.

155. Marottoli OR: Osificaciones en el tendon de Aquiles. Rev Ortop Traumatol 11:53, 1941.

156. Lotke PA: Ossification of the Achilles tendon. Report of seven cases. J Bone Joint Surg [Am] 52:157, 1970.

157. Mitra M, Sen AK, Deb HK: Myositis ossificans traumatica: A complication of tetanus. Report of a case and review of the literature. J Bone Joint Surg [Am] 58:885, 1976.

158. Pitts NC: Myositis ossificans as a complication of tetanus. JAMA 189:237, 1964.

159. Norman A, Dorfman HD: Juxtacortical circumscribed myositis ossificans: Evolution and radiographic features. Radiology 96:301, 1970.

160. Paterson DC: Myositis ossificans circumscripta. Report of four cases without history of injury. J Bone Joint Surg [Br] 52:296, 1970.

161. Goldman AB: Myositis ossificans circumscripta: a benign lesion with a malignant differential diagnosis. Am J Roentgenol 126:32, 1976.

162. Ackerman LV: Extra-osseous localized non-neoplastic bone and cartilage formation (so-called myositis ossificans): Clinical and pathological confusion with malignant neoplasms. J Bone Joint Surg [Am] 40:279, 1958.

163. Adams RD, Denny-Brown D, Pearson CM: Diseases of Muscle: A Study in Pathology, 2nd Ed. New York, Harper & Row, 1962.

164. Mohan K: Myositis ossificans traumatica of the elbow. Int Surg 57:475, 1972.

165. Flynn JE, Graham JH: Myositis ossificans. Surg Gynecol Obstet 118:1001, 1964.

166. Thompson HC III, Garcia A: Myositis ossificans: Aftermath of elbow injuries. Clin Orthop 50:129, 1967.

167. Ellis M, Frank HG: Myositis ossificans traumatica with special reference to the quadriceps femoris muscle. J Trauma 6:724, 1967.

168. Gilmer WS Jr, Anderson LD: Reactions of soft somatic tissue which may progress to bone formation: Circumscribed (traumatic) myositis ossificans. South Med J 52:1432, 1959.

169. Dickerson RC: Myositis ossificans in early childhood. Report of an unusual case. Clin Orthop *79:*42, 1971.

170. Johnson MK, Lawrence JF: Metaplastic bone formation (myositis ossificans) in the soft tissue of the hand. Case report. J Bone Joint Surg [Am] *57:*999, 1975.

171. Zadek I: Ossifying hematoma in the thigh. A case report. J Bone Joint Surg [Am] *51:*386, 1969.

172. Maini PS, Singh M: Localized myositis ossificans progressiva. A case report. J Bone Joint Surg [Am] *49:*955, 1967.

173. Parkash S, Kumar K: Fibrodysplasia ossificans traumatica. A case report. J Bone Joint Surg [Am] *54:*1306, 1972.

174. Johnson LC: Histogenesis of myositis ossificans (Abstr). Am J Pathol *24:*681, 1948.

175. Yaghmai I: Myositis ossificans: Diagnostic value of arteriography. AJR *128:*811, 1977.

176. Kramer FL, Kurtz AB, Rubin C, Goldberg BB: Ultrasound appearance of myositis ossificans. Skel Radiol *4:*19, 1979.

177. Shanoff L, Spira M, Hardy SB: Myositis ossificans: Evolution to osteogenic sarcoma. Report of a histologically verified case. Am J Surg *113:*537, 1967.

178. Huvos AG, Higinbotham NL: Primary fibrosarcoma of bone: A clinicopathologic study of 130 patients. Cancer *35:*837, 1975.

179. Kagan AR, Steckel RJ: Heterotopic new bone formation: Myositis ossificans versus malignant tumor. AJR *130:*773, 1978.

180. Dwinnell LA, Dahlin DC, Ghormley RK: Parosteal (juxtacortical) osteogenic sarcoma. J Bone Joint Surg [Am] *36:*732, 1954.

181. Van der' Heul RO, von Ronnen JR: Juxtacortical osteosarcoma. Diagnoses, differential diagnoses, treatment, and an analysis of eighty cases. J Bone Joint Surg [Am] *49:*415, 1967.

182. Smith J, Ahuja SC, Huvos AG, et al: Parosteal (juxtacortical) osteogenic sarcoma. A roentgenological study of 30 patients. J Can Assoc Radiol *29:*167, 1978.

183. Unni KK, Dahlin DC, Beabout JW: Periosteal osteogenic sarcoma. Cancer *37:*2476, 1975.

184. deSantos LA, Murray JA, Finklestein JB, et al: The radiographic spectrum of periosteal osteosarcoma. Radiology *127:*123, 1978.

185. Mayer L, Friedman M: Extraskeletal bone-forming tumor of the fascia resembling osteogenic sarcoma. Bull Hosp Joint Dis *2:*187, 1941.

186. Mallory TB: A group of metaplastic and neoplastic bone- and cartilage-containing tumors of soft parts. Am J Pathol *8:*765, 1933.

187. Rhoads CP, Blumgart H: Two osteoblastomas not connected with bone, histologically identical with osteogenic sarcoma, and clinically benign. Am J Pathol *4:*363, 1928.

188. Schulze K, Treugut H, Schmitt WG: Die nicht traumatische Myositis ossificans circumscripta. ROFO *129:*343, 1976.

189. Chaplin DM, Harrison MHM: Pseudomalignant osseous tumour of soft tissue. Report of two cases. J Bone Joint Surg [Br] *54:*334, 1972.

190. Angervall L, Stener B, Stener I, et al: Pseudomalignant osseous tumour of soft tissue. A clinical, radiological, and pathological study of five cases. J Bone Joint Surg [Br] *51:*654, 1969.

191. Jeffreys TE, Stiles PJ: Pseudomalignant osseous tumour of soft tissue. J Bone Joint Surg [Br] *48:*488, 1966.

192. Lutwak L: Myositis ossificans progressiva. Mineral, metabolic and radioactive calcium studies of the effects of hormones. Am J Med *37:*269, 1964.

193. Letts RM: Myositis ossificans progressiva: A report of two cases with chromosome studies. Can Med Assoc J *99:*856, 1968.

194. Smith DM, Zeman W, Johnston CC Jr, et al: Myositis ossificans progressiva. Case report with metabolic and histochemical studies. Metabolism *15:*521, 1966.

195. Dixon TF, Mulligan L, Nassim R, et al: Myositis ossificans progressiva. Report of a case in which ACTH and cortisone failed to prevent ossification after excision of ectopic bone. J Bone Joint Surg [Br] *36:*445, 1954.

196. Smith R, Russell RGG, Woods CG: Myositis ossificans progressiva. Clinical features of eight patients and their response to treatment. J Bone Joint Surg [Br] *58:*48, 1976.

197. Holmsen H, Ljunghall S, Hierton T: Myositis ossificans progressiva. Clinical and metabolical observations in a case treated with a diphosphonate (EHDP) and surgical removal of ectopic bone. Acta Orthop Scand *50:*33, 1979.

198. Hentzer B, Jacobsen HH, Asboe-Hansen G: Fibrodysplasia (myositis) ossificans progressiva treated with disodium etidronate. Clin Radiol *29:*69, 1978.

199. Eaton WL, Conkling WS, Daeschner CW: Early myositis ossificans progressiva occurring in homozygotic twins. A clinical and pathological study. J Pediatr *50:*591, 1957.

200. Bassett CAL, Donath A, Macagno F, et al: Diphosphonates in the treatment of myositis ossificans progressiva. Letter to Editor. Lancet *2:*845, 1969.

201. Russell RGG, Smith R, Bishop MC, et al: Treatment of myositis ossificans progressiva with a diphosphonate. Lancet *1:*10, 1972.

202. Weiss IW, Fisher L, Phang JM: Diphosphonate therapy in a patient with myositis ossificans progressiva. Ann Intern Med *74:*933, 1971.

203. Streeter GL: Focal deficiencies in fetal tissues and their relation to intrauterine amputation. Contrib Embryol *22:*1, 1930.

204. Plotkin D: Congenital cicatrizing fibrous bands. Report of 2 cases. Arch Pediatr *68:*120, 1951.

205. Blackfield HM, Hause DP: Congenital constricting bands of the extremities. Plast Reconstr Surg *8:*101, 1951.

206. Blanc WA, Mattison DR, Kane R, et al: LSD, intrauterine amputations, and amniotic-band syndrome. Letter to Editor. Lancet *2:*158, 1971.

207. Field JH, Krag DO: Congenital constricting bands and congenital amputation of the fingers: Placental studies. J Bone Joint Surg [Am] *55:*1035, 1973.

208. Moses JM, Flatt AE, Cooper RR: Annular constricting bands. J Bone Joint Surg [Am] *61:*562, 1979.

209. Glessner JP Jr: Spontaneous intra-uterine amputation. J Bone Joint Surg [Am] *45:*351, 1963.

210. Torpin R, Goodman L, Gramling ZW: Amnion string swallowed by the fetus. Am J Obstet Gynecol *90:*829, 1964.

211. Latta JS: Spontaneous intrauterine amputations. Am J Obstet Gynecol *10:*640, 1925.

212. Abbe T: Report of a case of congenital amputation of fingers. Am J Obstet Dis Women *73:*1089, 1916.

213. Kino Y: Clinical and experimental studies of the congenital constriction band syndrome, with an emphasis on its etiology. J Bone Joint Surg [Am] *57:*636, 1975.

214. Chemke J, Graff G, Hurwitz N, et al: The amniotic band syndrome. Obstet Gynecol *41:*332, 1973.

215. Birch-Jensen A: Congenital Deformities of the Upper Extremities. Odense, Denmark, Andelsbogtrykkeriet, 1949.

216. Poznanski AK: The Hand in Radiologic Diagnosis. 2nd ed. Philadelphia, WB Saunders Co, 1984.

217. Barenberg LH, Greenberg B: Intra-uterine amputations and constriction bands. Report of a case with anesthesia below the constriction. Am J Dis Child *64:*87, 1942.

218. Friedlander HL, Westin GW, Wood WL Jr: Arthrogryposis multiplex congenita. A review of forty-five cases. J Bone Joint Surg [Am] *50:*89, 1968.

219. Rukavina JG, Falls HF, Holt JF, et al: Léri's pleonosteosis. A study of a family with a review of the literature. J Bone Joint Surg [Am] *41:*397, 1959.

220. Beals RK, Hecht F: Congenital contractural arachnodactyly. A heritable disorder of connective tissue. J Bone Joint Surg [Am] *53:*987, 1971.

221. Seddon JH: Volkmann's ischemia in the lower limb. J Bone Joint Surg [Br] *48:*627, 1966.

222. Currarino G, Waldman I: Camptodactyly. AJR *92:*1312, 1964.

223. Poznanski AK, Pratt GB, Manson G, et al: Clinodactyly, camptodactyly, Kirner's deformity and other crooked fingers. Radiology *93:*573, 1969.

224. Blank E, Girdany BR: Symmetric bowing of the terminal phalanges of the fifth fingers in a family (Kirner's deformity). AJR *93:*367, 1965.

225. Kinmonth JB, Taylor GW, Tracy GD, et al: Primary lymphedema. Clinical and lymphangiographic studies of a series of 107 patients in which the lower limbs were affected. Br J Surg *45:*1, 1957.

226. Hadley M, MacDonald AF: Epidermolysis bullosa. Br J Radiol *33:*646 1960.

227. Alpert M: Roentgen manifestations of epidermolysis bullosa. AJR *78:*66, 1957.

228. Becker MH, Swinyard CA: Epidermolysis bullosa dystrophica in children. Radiologic manifestations. Radiology *90:*124, 1968.

229. Brinn LB, Khilnani MT: Epidermolysis bullosa with characteristic hard deformities. Radiology *89:*272, 1967.

230. Horner RL, Wiedel JD, Bralliar F: Involvement of the hand in epidermolysis bullosa. J Bone Joint Surg [Am] *53:*1347, 1971.

231. Winstock D: Oral aspects of epidermolysis bullosa. Br J Dermatol *74:*431, 1962.

232. Moynahan EJ: Epidermolysis bullosa dystrophica with severe deformity of hands and pharyngeal stenosis, relieved by cortisone. Proc R Soc Med *54:*693, 1961.

233. Pearson RW, Spargo B: Electron microscope studies of dermal-epidermal separation in human skin. J Invest Dermatol *36:*213, 1961.

234. Pearson RW: Studies on the pathogenesis of epidermolysis bullosa. J Invest Dermatol *39:*551, 1962.

235. Sasai Y: A histochemical study on the mechanism of blister formation in epidermolysis bullosa group. Tohoku J Exp Med *85:*340, 1965.

236. Bauer EA, Gedde-Dahl T, Eisen AZ: The role of human skin collagenase in epidermolysis bullosa. J Invest Dermatol *69:*119, 1977.

237. Briggaman RA, Wheeler CE: Epidermolysis bullosa dystrophica-recessive: A possible role of anchoring fibrils in the pathogenesis. J Invest Dermatol *65:*203, 1975.

238. Mathias CGT, Daroczy J, Huttner I, Schopflocher P, Wilkinson R: Pityriasis rosea in a patient with epidermolysis bullosa dystrophica. J Cutan Pathol *6:*139, 1979.

239. Winer MN, Orman JM: Epidermolysis bullosa—a suggestion as to possible causation. Arch Dermatol *52:*317, 1945.

240. Lutowiecki J: Betrachtungen zur Klassifizierung und Differentzierung von bullösen Krankheiten. Hautarzt *15:*228, 1964.

241. Halpern LK: Development of squamous cell epithelioma in epidermolysis bullosa: report of a case. Arch Dermatol *56:*517, 1947.

242. Rasponi L: Il cancro sullepidermolisi bollosa distrofica. Arch Ital Dermatol Sif *23:*19, 1950.

243. Edland RW: Dystrophica epidermolysis bullosa. Tolerance of the bed and response of multifocal squamous cell carcinomas to ionizing radiation: Report of a case. AJR *105:*644, 1969.

244. Meine F, Grossman H, Forman W, et al: The radiographic findings in congenital cutis laxa. Radiology *113:*687, 1974.

245. Lally JF, Gohel VK, Dalinka MK, et al: The roentgenographic manifestations of cutis laxa (generalized elastolysis). Radiology *113:*605, 1974.

246. Merten DF, Rooney R: Progressive pulmonary emphysema associated with congenital generalized elastolysis (cutis laxa). Radiology *113:*691, 1974.

247. Harris RB, Heaphy MR, Perry HO: Generalized elastolysis (cutis laxa). Am J Med *65:*815, 1978.

248. Hashimoto K, Kanzaki T: Cutis laxa: Ultrastructural and biochemical studies. Arch Dermatol *111*:861, 1975.

249. Scott MA, Kauh YC, Luscombe HA: Acquired cutis laxa associated with multiple myeloma. Arch Dermatol *112*:853, 1976.

250. Goltz RW, Hult AM, Goldfarb M, et al: Cutis laxa. A manifestation of generalized elastolysis. Arch Dermatol *92*:373, 1965.

251. Shulman LE: Diffuse fasciitis hypergammaglobulinemia and eosinophilia: A new syndrome? J Rheumatol *1* (Suppl 1):46, 1974.

252. Caperton EM, Hathaway DE: Scleroderma with eosinophilia and hypergammaglobulinemia. The Shulman syndrome (Abstr). Arthritis Rheum *18*:391, 1975.

253. Rodnan GP, DiBartolomeo AG, Medsger TA Jr, et al: Eosinophilic fasciitis: Report of 7 cases of a newly recognized scleroderma-like syndrome (Abstr). Arthritis Rheum *18*:422, 1975.

254. Blomgren SE: Erythema nodosum. Semin Arthritis Rheum *3*:1, 1974.

255. Sams WM Jr, Winkelmann RK: The association of erythema nodosum with ulcerative colitis. South Med J *61*:676, 1968.

256. Truelove LH: Articular manifestations of erythema nodosum. Ann Rheum Dis *19*:174, 1960.

257. Fine RM, Meltzer HD: Erythema nodosum—a form of allergic cutaneous vasculitis. South Med J *61*:680, 1968.

258. Gorlin RJ, Goltz RW: Multiple nevoid basal-cell epithelioma, jaw cysts, and bifid rib. A syndrome. N Engl J Med *262*:908. 1960.

259. Gorlin RJ, Vickers RA, Kelln E, et al: The multiple basal-cell nevi syndrome. An analysis of a syndrome consisting of multiple nevoid basal-cell carcinoma, jaw cysts, skeletal anomalies, medulloblastoma, and hyporesponsiveness to parathormone. Cancer *18*:89, 1965.

260. Becker MH, Kopf AW, Lande A: Basal cell nevus syndrome: Its roentgenographic significance. Review of the literature and report of four cases. AJR *99*:817, 1967.

261. Kozlowski K, Baker P, Glasson M: Multiple nevoid basal cell carcinoma syndrome (report of five cases in a family). Pediatr Radiol *2*:185, 1974.

262. Stoelinga PJW, Peters JH, Van de Staak WJB, et al: Some new findings in the basal-cell nevus syndrome. Oral Surg *36*:686, 1973.

263. Lile HA, Rogers JF, Gerald B: The basal cell nevus syndrome. AJR *103*:214, 1968.

264. Novak D, Bloss W: Röntgenologische Aspekte des Basalzell-naevus-syndroms (Gorlin-Goltz-Syndrom). ROFO *124*:11, 1976.

265. Dunnick NR, Head GL, Peck GL, et al: Nevoid basal cell carcinoma syndrome: Radiographic manifestations including cystlike lesions of the phalanges. Radiology *127*:331, 1978.

266. Davidson F: Multiple naevoid basal cell carcinomata and associated congenital abnormalities. Br J Dermatol *74*:439, 1962.

267. Binkley GW, Johnson HH Jr: Epithelioma adenoides cysticum: Basal cell nevi, agenesis of corpus callosum and dental cysts. A clinical and autopsy study. Arch Dermatol *63*:73, 1951.

268. Wallace DC, Murphy KJ, Kelly L, et al: The basal cell naevus syndrome. Report of a family with anosmia and a case of hypogonadotrophic hypopituitarism. J Med Genet *10*:30, 1973.

269. Block JB, Clendenning WE: Parathyroid hormone hyporesponsiveness in patients with basal-cell nevi and bone defects. N Engl J Med *268*:1157, 1963.

270. Kaufman RL, Chase LR: Basal cell nevus syndrome: Normal responsiveness to parathyroid hormone. Birth Defects *7*:149, 1971.

271. Aurbach GD, Marcus R, Winickoff RN, et al: Urinary excretion of 3′,5′-AMP in syndromes considered refractory to parathyroid hormone. Metabolism *19*:799, 1970.

272. Marden PM, Venters HD Jr: A new neurocutaneous syndrome. Am J Dis Child *112*:79, 1966.

273. Solomon LM, Fretzin DF, Dewald RL: The epidermal nevus syndrome. Arch Dermatol *97*:273, 1968.

274. Bianchine JW: The nevus sebaceous syndrome of Jadassohn. A neurocutaneous syndrome and a potentially premalignant lesion. Am J Dis Child *120*:223, 1970.

275. Lovejoy FH Jr, Boyle WE Jr: Linear nevus sebaceous syndrome. Report of two cases and a review of the literature. Pediatrics *52*:382, 1973.

276. Leonidas JC, Wolpert SM, Feingold M, et al: Radiographic features of the linear nevus sebaceous syndrome. AJR *132*:277, 1979.

277. Kadir S, Athanasoulis CA, Waltman AC: Tolazoline-augmented arteriography in the evaluation of bone and soft-tissue tumors. Radiology *133*:792, 1979.

278. McDougall A, McGarrity G: Extra-abdominal desmoid tumors. J Bone Joint Surg [Br] *61*:373, 1979.

279. Bergiron C, Markovits P, Benjaafar M, et al: Lymphography in childhood rhabdomyosarcomas. Radiology *133*:627, 1979.

280. Jajic I, Rulnjevic J: Myositis ossificans localisata as a complication of tetanus. Acta Orthop Scand *50*:547, 1979.

281. Sarmiento A, Elkins RW: Giant intra-articular osteochondroma of the knee. J Bone Joint Surg [Am] *57*:560, 1975.

282. Morgan CJ Jr: Panniculitis and erythema nodosum. *In* WN Kelley, ED Harris Jr, S Ruddy, CB Sledge (Eds): Textbook of Rheumatology. Philadelphia, WB Saunders Co, 1981, p 1203.

283. Moore S: Relation of pancreatic disease to Weber-Christian disease. Can Med Assoc J *88*:1238, 1963.

284. Eisman J, Swezey RL: Juxta-articular adiposis dolorosa: What is it? Report of 2 cases. Ann Rheum Dis *38*:479, 1979.

285. Hedstrand H, Berglund G, Werner I: Keratodermia palmaris et plantaris with clubbing and skeletal deformity of the terminal phalanges of the hands and feet. Acta Dermatovenereol *52*:278, 1972.

286. Greenfield GB, Rosado W, Rothbart F: Benign proliferative skin lesions causing destructive and resorptive bone changes. AJR *97*:733, 1966.

287. Evans HL: Liposarcoma. Am J Surg Pathol *3*:507, 1979.

288. Chew FS, Hudson TM, Hawkins IF Jr: Radiology of infiltrating angiolipoma. AJR *135*:781, 1980.

289. Dorfman HD, Levin S, Robbins H: Cartilage-containing benign mesenchymomas of soft tissue. J Bone Joint Surg [Am] *62*:472, 1980.

290. Ledesma-Medina J, Oh KS, Girdany BR: Calcification in childhood leiomyoma. Radiology *135*:339, 1980.

291. Myers BW, Masi AT, Feigenbaum SL: Pigmented villonodular synovitis and tenosynovitis: A clinical epidemiologic study of 166 cases and literature review. Medicine *59*:223, 1980.

292. Zazzaro PF, Bosworth JE, Schneider V, et al: Gallium scanning in malignant fibrous histiocytoma. AJR *135*:775, 1980.

293. Milgram JW, Dunn EJ: Para-articular chondromas and osteochondromas. Clin Orthop *148*:147, 1980.

294. Wu KK, Guise ER: Extraosseous osteogenic sarcoma: A clinical analysis of ten cases. Orthopedics *3*:115, 1980.

295. Schiffman R: Epithelioid sarcoma and synovial sarcoma in the same knee. Cancer *44*:158, 1980.

296. Balsam D, Goldfarb R, Stringer B, et al: Bone scintigraphy for neonatal osteomyelitis; simulation by extravasation of intravenous calcium. Radiology *135*:185, 1980.

297. Mitnick PD, Goldfarb S, Slatopolsky E, et al: Calcium and phosphate metabolism in tumoral calcinosis. Ann Intern Med *92*:482, 1980.

298. Nassonova VA, Ivanova MM, Akhnazarova VD, et al: Eosinophilic fasciitis. Scand J Rheum *8*:225, 1979.

299. Moore TL, Zuckner J: Eosinophilic fasciitis. Semin Arthritis Rheum *9*:228, 1980.

300. Rosenthal J, Benson MD: Diffuse fasciitis and eosinophilia with symmetric polyarthritis. Ann Intern Med *92*:507, 1980.

301. Sekkat A, Benhayoune TS: A propos d'un cas de kératodermie Aïnhumoïde et mutilante. Ann Dermatol Venereol *107*:447, 1980.

302. Kan WC, Wiley AL Jr, Wirtanen GW, et al: High Z elements in human sarcomata: Assessment by multienergy CT and neutron activation analysis. AJR *135*:123, 1980.

303. Desai A, Eymontt M, Alavi A, et al: ⁹⁹ᵐTc-MDP uptake in nonosseous lesions. Radiology *135*:181, 1980.

304. Choy D, Murray IPC: Metastatic visceral calcification identified by bone scanning. Skel Radiol *5*:151, 1980.

305. Balachandran S, Abbud Y, Prince MJ, et al: Tumoral calcinosis: Scintigraphic studies of an affected family. Br J Radiol *53*:960, 1980.

306. Pringle J, Stoker DJ: Case report 127. Skel Radiol *5*:263, 1980.

307. Safai B, Good RA: Kaposi's sarcoma: A review and recent developments. Clin Bull *10*:62, 1980.

308. Stephenson TF: Computerized tomography of soft tissue abnormalities. Comput Tomogr *4*:181, 1980.

309. Jones BV, Ward MW: Myositis ossificans in the biceps femoris muscles causing sciatic nerve palsy. A case report. J Bone Joint Surg [Br] *62*:506, 1980.

310. Nessi R, Gattoni F, Mazzoni R, et al: Xeroradiography of soft tissue tumors. ROFO *134*:669, 1981.

311. Egund N, Ekelund L, Sako M, et al: CT of soft-tissue tumors. AJR *137*:725, 1981.

312. Soye I, Levine E, De Smet AA, et al: Computed tomography in the preoperative evaluation of masses arising in or near joints of the extremities. Radiology *143*:727, 1982.

313. Golding SJ, Husband JE: The role of computed tomography in the management of soft tissue sarcomas. Br J Radiol *55*:740, 1982.

314. Laursen K, Reiter S: Computed tomography in soft tissue disorders of the lower extremities. Acta Orthop Scand *51*:881, 1980.

315. Hermann G, Yeh H-C, Schwartz I: Computed tomography of soft-tissue lesions of the extremities, pelvic and shoulder girdles: Sonographic and pathological correlations. Clin Radiol *35*:193, 1984.

316. Bernardino ME, Jing B-S, Thomas JL, et al: The extremity soft-tissue lesion: A comparative study of ultrasound, computed tomography, and xeroradiography. Radiology *139*:53, 1981.

317. Heiken JP: CT of benign soft-tissue masses of the extremities. AJR *142*:575, 1984.

318. Apple JS, Gamba J, Martinez S: Diagnostic imaging of extremity soft tissue masses. Rev Interam Radiol *8*:45, 1983.

319. Weekes RG, McLeod RA, Reiman HM, et al: CT of soft-tissue neoplasms. AJR *144*:355, 1985.

320. Hudson TM, Schakel M, Springfield DS: Limitations of computed tomography following excisional biopsy of soft tissue sarcomas. Skel Radiol *13*:49, 1985.

321. Zornoza J, Bernardino ME, Ordonez NG, et al: Percutaneous needle biopsy of soft tissue tumors guided by ultrasound and computed tomography. Skel Radiol *9*:33, 1982.

322. Yeh H-C, Rabinowitz JG: Ultrasonography of the extremities and pelvic girdle and correlation with computed tomography. Radiology *143*:519, 1982.

323. Apple JS, Martinez S, Nelson PA, et al: Sonographic correlation in extremity soft-tissue masses. Noninvas Med Imaging *1*:75, 1984.

324. Braunstein EM, Silver TM, Martel W, et al: Ultrasonographic diagnosis of extremity masses. Skel Radiol *6*:157, 1981.

325. Chew FS, Hudson TM, Enneking WF: Radionuclide imaging of soft tissue neoplasms. Semin Nucl Med *11*:266, 1981.

326. Enneking WF, Chew FS, Springfield DS, et al: The role of radionuclide bone-

scanning in determining the resectability of soft-tissue sarcomas. J Bone Joint Surg [Am] 63:249, 1981.

327. Hudson TM, Schakel M II, Springfield DS, et al: The comparative value of bone scintigraphy and computed tomography in determining bone involvement by soft-tissue sarcomas. J Bone Joint Surg [Am] 66:1400, 1984.

328. Kirchner PT, Simon MA: The clinical value of bone and gallium scintigraphy for soft-tissue sarcomas of the extremities. J Bone Joint Surg [Am] 66:319, 1984.

329. Enneking WF, Spanier SS, Malawar MM: The effect of the anatomic setting on the results of surgical procedures for soft part sarcoma of the thigh. Cancer 47:1005, 1981.

330. Enzinger FM, Weiss SW: Soft Tissue Tumors. St Louis, CV Mosby Co, 1983.

331. Myhre-Jensen O: A consecutive 7-year series of 1331 benign soft tissue tumors. Clinicopathologic data. Comparison with sarcomas. Acta Orthop Scand 52:287, 1981.

332. Huebert HT: Liposarcoma: The Manitoba experience. Can J Surg 24:391, 1981.

333. De Santos LA, Ginaldi S, Wallace S: Computed tomography in liposarcoma. Cancer 47:46, 1981.

334. Tang TT, Chamoy L, Meyers A, et al: Congenital lipoma with ossification in the hand of a child. J Pediatr Surg 16:511, 1981.

335. Sauer JM, Ozonoff MB: Congenital bone anomalies associated with lipomas. Skel Radiol 13:276, 1985.

336. Demos TC, Bruno E, Armin A, et al: Parosteal lipoma with enlarging osteochondroma. AJR 143:365, 1984.

337. Rydholm A, Berg NO: Size, site and clinical incidence of lipoma. Factors in the differential diagnosis of lipoma and sarcoma. Acta Orthop Scand 54:929, 1983.

338. Enzi G, Biondetti PR, Fiore D, et al: Computed tomography of deep fat masses in multiple symmetrical lipomatosis. Radiology 144:121, 1982.

339. Enzi G: Multiple symmetric lipomatosis: An updated clinical report. Medicine 63:56, 1984.

340. Hertzanu Y, Mendelsohn DB, Louridas G: CT findings in hibernoma of the thigh. J Comput Assist Tomogr 7:1109, 1983.

341. Lachman RS, Finklestein J, Mehringer CM, et al: Congenital aggressive lipomatosis. Skel Radiol 9:248, 1983.

342. Bannayan GA: Lipomatosis, angiomatosis and macroencephalia. Arch Pathol Lab Med 92:1, 1971.

343. Kalifa G, Lalande G, Larde D, et al: Les fibromes desmoides chez l'enfant. Ann Radiol 25:25, 1982.

344. Rock MG, Pritchard DJ, Reiman HM, et al: Extra-abdominal desmoid tumors. J Bone Joint Surg [Am] 66:1369, 1984.

345. Abramowitz D, Zornoza J, Ayala AG, et al: Soft-tissue desmoid tumors: Radiographic bone changes. Radiology 146:11, 1983.

346. Iwasaki H, Kikuchi M, Mori R, et al: Infantile digital fibromatosis. Ultrastructural, histochemical, and tissue culture observations. Cancer 46:2238, 1980.

347. Nakayasu K, Maruo M, Ueda K, et al: Infantile digital fibromatosis. J Cutan Pathol 7:431, 1980.

348. Nakayasu K, Nishimura A, Maruo M, et al: Infantile digital fibromatosis. Arch Derm-Kyoto 75:167, 1980.

349. Mortimer G, Gibson AAM: Recurring digital fibroma. J Clin Pathol 35:849, 1982.

350. Kashuk KB, Pasternack WA: Aggressive infiltrating plantar fibromatosis. J Am Podiatry Assoc 71:491, 1981.

351. Sartoris DJ, Mochizuki RM, Parker BR: Lytic clavicular lesions in fibromatosis colli. Skel Radiol 10:34, 1983.

352. Stringer DA, Hall CM: Juvenile hyaline fibromatosis. Br J Radiol 54:473, 1981.

353. Brill PW, Yandow DR, Langer LO, et al: Congenital generalized fibromatosis. Case report and literature review. Pediatr Radiol 12:269, 1982.

354. Chung EB, Enzinger FM: Infantile myofibromatosis. Cancer 48:1807, 1981.

355. Jennings TA, Sabetta J, Duray PH, et al: Infantile myofibromatosis. Evidence for an autosomal-dominant disorder. Am J Surg Pathol 8:529, 1984.

356. Wile AG, Evans HL, Romsdahl MM: Leiomyosarcoma of soft tissue: A clinicopathologic study. Cancer 48:1022, 1981.

357. Ekelund L, Rydholm A: The value of angiography in soft tissue leiomyosarcomas of the extremities. Skel Radiol 9:201, 1983.

358. Kagan AR, Steckel RJ: Intramedullary extension of a soft-tissue neoplasm. AJR 139:807, 1982.

359. Ghavimi F: Rhabdomyosarcoma. Pediatr Ann 12:395, 1983.

360. Muckart RD: Compression of the common peroneal nerve by intramuscular ganglion from the superior tibio-fibular joint. J Bone Joint Surg [Br] 58:241, 1976.

361. Stack RE, Bianco AJ Jr, MacCarty CS: Compression of the common peroneal nerve by ganglion cysts. J Bone Joint Surg [Am] 47:773, 1965.

362. Firooznia H, Golimbu C, Rafii M, et al: Computerized tomography in diagnosis of compression of the common peroneal nerve by ganglion cysts. Comput Radiol 7:343, 1983.

363. McBeath AA, Niedhart DA: Acetabular cyst with communicating ganglion. A case report. J Bone Joint Surg [Am] 58:267, 1976.

364. Lagier R, Seigne JM, Mbakop A: Juxta-acetabular mucoid cyst in a patient with osteoarthritis of the hip secondary to dysplasia. Int Orthop (SICOT) 8:19, 1984.

365. Ueo T, Hamabuchi M: Hip pain caused by cystic deformation of the labrum acetabulare. Arthritis Rheum 27:947, 1984.

366. Muckle DS, Monahan P: Intraarticular ganglion of the knee. J Bone Joint Surg [Br] 54:520, 1972.

367. McCook TA, Martinez S, Korobkin M, et al: Intramuscular myxoma. Radio-

368. Ekelund L, Herrlin K, Rydholm A: Computed tomography of intramuscular myxoma. Skel Radiol 9:14, 1982.

369. Ros PR, Viamonte M Jr, Rywlin AM: Malignant fibrous histiocytoma: Mesenchymal tumor of ubiquitous origin. AJR 142:753, 1984.

370. Weiss SW, Enzinger FM: Malignant fibrous histiocytoma. An analysis of 200 cases. Cancer 41:2250, 1978.

371. Dorfman HD, Bhagavan BS: Malignant fibrous histiocytoma of soft tissue with metaplastic bone and cartilage formation: A new radiologic sign. Skel Radiol 8:145, 1982.

372. Fischer HJ, Lois JF, Gomes AS, et al: Radiology and pathology of malignant fibrous histiocytomas of the soft tissues: A report of ten cases. Skel Radiol 13:202, 1985.

373. Paling MR, Hyams DM: Computed tomography in malignant fibrous histiocytoma. J Comput Assist Tomogr 6:785, 1982.

374. Van Furth R: Origin and kinetics of monocytes and macrophages. Semin Hematol 17:125, 1970.

375. Groopman JE, Golde DW: The histiocytic disorders: A pathophysiologic analysis. Ann Intern Med 94:95, 1981.

376. Golde DW, Hocking WG, Quan SG, et al: Origin of human bone marrow fibroblasts. Br J Haematol 44:183, 1980.

377. Angervall L, Hagmar B, Kindblom L-G, et al: Malignant giant cell tumor of soft tissues: A clinicopathologic, cytologic, ultrastructural, angiographic, and microangiographic study. Cancer 47:736, 1981.

378. Kyriakos M, Kempson RL: Inflammatory fibrous histiocytoma. An aggressive and lethal lesion. Cancer 37:1584, 1976.

379. Hagood MF, Gathright JB: Hemangiomatosis of the skin and GI tract. Dis Colon Rectum 18:141, 1975.

380. McSwain B, Whitehead W, Bennett L: Angiosarcoma: Report of three cases of postmastectomy lymphangiosarcoma and one of hemangiosarcoma. South Med J 66:102, 1973.

381. Capo V, Ozzello L, Fenoglio CM, et al: Angiosarcomas arising in edematous extremities: Immunostaining for factor VII-related antigen and ultrastructural features. Hum Pathol 16:144, 1985.

382. Mann SG: Kaposi's sarcoma. Experience with ten cases. AJR 121:793, 1974.

383. Penn I: Kaposi's sarcoma in immunosuppressed patients. J Clin Lab Immunol 12:1, 1983.

384. Small R, Jaffe WL: Tenosynovial chondromatosis. Bull Hosp J Dis 41:37, 1981.

385. DeBenedetti MJ: Tenosynovial chondromatosis in the hand. J Bone Joint Surg [Am] 61:898, 1979.

386. Minsinger WE, Balogh K, Millender LH: Tenosynovial osteochondroma of the hand. A case report and brief review. Clin Orthop 196:248, 1985.

387. Karlin CA, De Smet AA, Neff J, et al: The variable manifestations of extraarticular synovial chondromatosis. Am J Roentgenol 137:731, 1981.

388. Luger AM, Ansbacher L, Farrell C, et al: Case report 158. Skel Radiol 6:291, 1981.

389. Karev A, Ben-Arieh Y: Osteoma cutis—a rare skin tumor in the finger. J Hand Surg 6:555, 1981.

390. Rotteleur G, Becquart P, Piette F, et al: L'ostéomatose cutanée diffuse du nourrisson. Arch Fr Pediatr 37:397, 1980.

391. Israels SJ, Chan HSL, Daneman A, et al: Synovial sarcoma in childhood. AJR 142:803, 1984.

392. Varela-Duran J, Enzinger FM: Calcifying synovial sarcoma. Cancer 50:345, 1982.

393. Ryan JR, Baker LH, Benjamin RS: The natural history of metastatic synovial sarcoma. Experience of the Southwest oncology group. Clin Orthop 164:257, 1982.

394. Wright PH, Sim FH, Soule EH, et al: Synovial sarcoma. J Bone Joint Surg [Am] 64:112, 1982.

395. Mayer DP, Clancy M, Bonakdarpour A, et al: Case report 152. Skel Radiol 6:221, 1981.

396. Buck P, Mickelson MR, Bonfiglio M: Synovial sarcoma. A review of 33 cases. Clin Orthop 156:211, 1981.

397. Azouz EM, Vickar DB, Brown KLB: Computed tomography of synovial sarcoma of the foot. J Can Assoc Radiol 35:85, 1984.

398. Potter GK, Walkes MH, Penny TR: Tendosynovial sarcoma. A clinicopathologic review of foot cases with a case report. J Am Podiatry Assoc 74:312, 1984.

399. Goodwin DRA, Salama R: Synovial sarcoma of the finger. Hand 14:198, 1982.

400. Geschickter CF: Tumors of the peripheral nerves. Am J Cancer 25:377, 1935.

401. Carstens H, Schrodt G: Malignant transformation of a benign encapsulated neurilemoma. Am J Clin Pathol 51:144, 1969.

402. Barratt JG: Enlargement of cervical intervertebral foramina by coiling of the vertebral artery. Australas Radiol 18:171, 1974.

403. Danziger J, Bloch S: The widened cervical intervertebral foramen. Radiology 116:671, 1975.

404. Patel DV, Ferguson RJL, Schey WL: Enlargement of the intervertebral foramina: An unusual cause. AJR 131:911, 1978.

405. Powers SK, Norman D, Edwards MSB: Computerized tomography of peripheral nerve lesions. J Neurosurg 59:131, 1983.

406. Daneman A, Mancer K, Sonley M: CT appearance of thickened nerves in neurofibromatosis. AJR 141:899, 1983.

407. Sutton D, Al-Kutoubi MA, DeSilva RDD, et al: Computed tomography in deep-seated peripheral neurofibromas. Clin Radiol 36:19, 1985.

408. Francis IR, Glazer GM: Peripheral neurofibromatosis. J Comput Assist Tomogr 7:374, 1983.
409. Coleman BG, Arger PH, Dalinka MK, et al: CT of sarcomatous degeneration in neurofibromatosis. AJR 140:383, 1983.
410. Pavlidis NA, Fisher C, Wiltshaw E: Clear-cell sarcoma of tendons and aponeuroses: A clinicopathologic study. Presentation of six additional cases with review of the literature. Cancer 54:1412, 1984.
411. Mukai M, Torikata C, Iri H, et al: Histogenesis of clear cell sarcoma of tendons and aponeuroses. Am J Pathol 114:264, 1984.
412. Eckardt JJ, Pritchard DJ, Soule EH: Clear cell sarcoma. A clinicopathologic study of 27 cases. Cancer 52:1482, 1983.
413. Azumi N, Turner RR: Clear cell sarcoma of tendons and aponeuroses; electron microscopic findings suggesting schwann cell differentiation. Hum Pathol 14:1084, 1983.
414. Brodsky AE, Dennis MD, Sassard WR: Alveolar soft-part sarcoma. A case report. J Bone Joint Surg [Am] 65:841, 1983.
415. Alexander C: Case report 270. Skel Radiol 11:229, 1984.
416. Sergiou SP, Reid DAC: Epithelioid sarcoma. Hand 12:304, 1980.
417. Prat J, Woodruff JM, Marcove RC: Epithelioid sarcoma: An analysis of 22 cases indicating the prognostic significance of vascular invasion and regional lymph node metastasis. Cancer 41:1472, 1978.
418. Levy DW, Bonakdarpour A, Putong PB, et al: Subungual keratoacanthoma. Skel Radiol 13:287, 1985.
419. Cramer SF: Subungual keratoacanthoma. A benign bone-eroding neoplasm of the distal phalanx. Am J Clin Pathol 75:425, 1981.
420. Rich PJ, King W III: Benign cortical hyperostosis underlying soft-tissue tumors of the thigh. AJR 138:419, 1982.
421. Kavanagh J, Yap B, Luna M, et al: Metastatic patterns of adult soft tissue sarcoma. Proc Am Assoc Cancer Res 21:480, 1980.
422. Wong WS, Kaiser LR, Gold RH, et al: Radiographic features of osseous metastases of soft-tissue sarcomas. Radiology 143:71, 1982.
423. Stewart VL, Herling P, Dalinka MK: Calcification in soft tissues. JAMA 250:78, 1983.
424. Viau MR, Pedersen HE, Salciccioli GG, et al: Ectopic calcification as a late sequela of compartment syndrome. Report of two cases. Clin Orthop 176:178, 1983.
425. Bostrom B: Tumoral calcinosis in an infant. Am J Dis Child 135:246, 1981.
426. Aprin H, Sinha A: Tumoral calcinosis. Report of a case in a one-year old child. Clin Orthop 185:83, 1984.
427. Bishop AF, Destouet JM, Murphy WA, et al: Tumoral calcinosis: Case report and review. Skel Radiol 8:269, 1982.
428. Kirk TS, Simon MA: Tumoral calcinosis. Report of a case with successful medical management. J Bone Joint Surg [Am] 63:1167, 1981.
429. Manaster J, Anderson TM Jr: Tumoral calcinosis: Serial images to monitor successful dietary therapy. Skel Radiol 8:123, 1982.
430. Gordon LF, Arger PH, Dalinka MK, et al: Computed tomography in soft tissue calcification layering. J Comput Assist Tomogr 8:71, 1984.
431. Boskey AL, Vigorita VJ, Sencer O, et al: Chemical, microscopic, and ultrastructural characterization of the mineral deposits in tumoral calcinosis. Clin Orthop 178:258, 1983.
432. Zerwekh JE, Sanders LA, Townsend J, et al: Tumoral calcinosis: Evidence for current defects in renal tubular phosphorus transport in 1,25 dihydroxy-cholecalciferol synthesis. Calcif Tissue Int 32:1, 1980.
433. Thurmon JF, Jackson J: Tumoral calcinosis and Engelmann disease. Birth Defects 12:321, 1976.
434. Clarke E, Swischuk LE, Hayden CK Jr: Tumoral calcinosis, diaphysitis, and hyperphosphatemia. Radiology 151:643, 1984.
435. Hensley CD, Lin JJ: Massive intrasynovial deposition of calcium pyrophosphate in the elbow. J Bone Joint Surg [Am] 66:133, 1984.
436. Kumar R, Roper PR, Guinto FC Jr: Subcutaneous ossification of the legs in chronic venous stasis. J Comput Assist Tomogr 7:377, 1983.
437. Odimba E, Stoppa R, Largueche S: Les ossifications hétérotopiques des cicatrices de laparotomie. Ann Chir 34:501, 1980.
438. Apostolidis NS, Legakis NCh, Gregoriadis GC, et al: Heterotopic bone formation in abdominal operation scars. Report of six cases with review of the literature. Am J Surg 142:555, 1981.
439. Fisher MS: Case report 186. Skel Radiol 7:277, 1982.
440. Daroca PJ Jr, Pulitzer DR, LoCicero J III: Ossifying fasciitis. Arch Pathol Lab Med 106:682, 1982.
441. Orda R, Baratz M, Wiznitzer T: Heterotopic bone formation in abdominal operation scars. Injury 15:334, 1984.
442. Lohela P, Orava S, Leinonen A: Heterotopic bone formation in abdominal midline scars. ROFO 139:412, 1983.
443. Rosenbaum LH, Nicholas JJ, Slasky BS, et al: Malignant myositis ossificans: Occult gastric carcinoma presenting as an acute rheumatic disorder. Ann Rheum Dis 43:95, 1984.
444. Ishikawa K, Izumi K, Kitagawa T: Heterotopic ossification of the hip as a complication of tetanus. Clin Orthop 166:249, 1982.
445. Eagle WW: Elongated styloid process: Further observations and a new syndrome. Arch Otolarngol 47:630, 1948.
446. O'Carroll MK: Calcification in the stylohyoid ligament. Oral Surg 58:617, 1984.
447. Mueller N, Hamilton S, Reid GD: Case report 248. Skel Radiol 10:273, 1983.
448. Lavallee M, Turcotte J-Y: Variations de la chaîne stylohyoïde et syndrome d'Eagle. Union Med Can 113:413, 1984.
449. Lorman JG, Biggs JR: The Eagle syndrome. AJR 140:881, 1983.

450. Messer EJ, Abramson AM: The stylohyoid syndrome. J Oral Surg 33:664, 1975.
451. McCorkell SJ: Fracture of an ossified stylohyoid ligament diagnosed by computed tomography. J Comput Assist Tomogr 8:544, 1984.
452. Oestreich AE: The stylohyoid ligament in Hurler syndrome and related conditions: Comparison with normal children. Radiology 154:665, 1985.
453. Arima R, Shiba R, Hayashi T: Traumatic myositis ossificans in the masseter muscle. J Oral Maxillofac Surg 42:512, 1984.
454. Mourad KA, Grant RW: Unusual post traumatic ossification within the intertransversarius muscle. Br J Radiol 56:55, 1983.
455. Drane WE: Myositis ossificans and the three-phase bone scan. AJR 142:179, 1984.
456. Orzel JA, Rudd TG: Heterotopic bone formation: Clinical, laboratory, and imaging correlation. J Nucl Med 26:125, 1985.
457. Moreno AJ, Yedinak MA, Spicer MJ, et al: Myositis ossificans with Ga-67 citrate positivity. Clin Nucl Med 10:40, 1985.
458. Amendola MA, Glazer GM, Agha FP, et al: Myositis ossificans circumscripta: Computed tomographic diagnosis. Radiology 149:775, 1983.
459. Zeanah WR, Hudson TM: Myositis ossificans. Radiologic evaluation of two cases with diagnostic computed tomograms. Clin Orthop 168:187, 1982.
460. Thyss A, Michiels JF, Caldani C, et al: Sarcome ostéogenique des tissus mous après myosite ossifiante posttraumatique. Presse Med 13:1333, 1984.
461. Eckardt JJ, Ivins JC, Perry HO, et al: Osteosarcoma arising in heterotopic ossification of dermatomyositis: Case report and review of the literature. Cancer 48:1256, 1981.
462. Oglivie-Harris DJ, Fornasier VL: Pseudomalignant myositis ossificans: Heterotopic new-bone formation without a history of trauma. J Bone Joint Surg [Am] 62:1274, 1980.
463. Spjut HJ, Dorfman HD: Florid reactive periostitis of the tubular bones of the hands and feet. A benign lesion which may simulate osteosarcoma. Am J Surg Pathol 5:423, 1981.
464. Hutter RVP, Foote FW, Francis KC, et al: Parosteal fasciitis. Am J Surg 104:800, 1962.
465. Mallory TB: A group of metaplastic and neoplastic bone and cartilage containing tumors of soft parts. Am J Pathol 9:765, 1933.
466. Kwittken J, Branche M: Fasciitis ossificans. Am J Clin Pathol 51:251, 1969.
467. De Smet L, Vercauteren M: Fast-growing pseudomalignant osseous tumour (myositis ossificans) of the finger. A case report. J Hand Surg [Br] 9:93, 1984.
468. Porter AR, Tristan TA, Rudy FR, et al: Florid reactive periostitis of the phalanges. AJR 144:617, 1985.
469. Jongeward RH Jr, Martel W, Louis DS, et al: Case report 304. Skel Radiol 13:169, 1985.
470. Resnick D, Sykes J, Collins W, et al: Case report 240. Skel Radiol 10:131, 1983.
471. Thickman D, Bonakdar-pour A, Clancy M, et al: Fibrodysplasia ossificans progressiva. AJR 139:935, 1982.
472. Cramer SF, Ruehl A, Mandel MA: Fibrodysplasia ossificans progressiva: A distinctive bone-forming lesion of the soft tissue. Cancer 48:1016, 1981.
473. Connor JM, Smith R: The cervical spine in fibrodysplasia ossificans progressiva. Br J Radiol 55:492, 1982.
474. Zionts LE, Osterkamp JA, Crawford TO, et al: Congenital annular bands in identical twins. A case report. J Bone Joint Surg [Am] 66:450, 1984.
475. Byrne J, Blanc WA, Baker D: Amniotic band syndrome in early fetal life. Birth Defects 18:43, 1982.
476. Zych GA, Ballard A: Congenital band causing pseudarthrosis and impending gangrene of the leg. A case report with successful treatment. J Bone Joint Surg [Am] 65:410, 1983.
477. Tada K, Yonenobu K, Swanson AB: Congenital constriction band syndrome. J Pediatr Orthop 4:726, 1984.
478. McCarthy S, Sarwar M, Virapongse C, et al: Craniofacial anomalies in the amniotic band disruption complex. Pediatr Radiol 14:44, 1984.
479. Dupuytren G: Permanent retraction of the fingers, produced by an affection of the palmar fascia. Lancet 2:222, 1834.
480. Noble J, Heathcote JG, Cohen H: Diabetes mellitus in the aetiology of Dupuytren's disease. J Bone Joint Surg [Br] 66:322, 1984.
481. McFarlane RM: The current status of Dupuytren's disease. J Hand Surg 8:703, 1983.
482. Brickley-Parsons D, Glimcher MJ, Smith RJ, et al: Biochemical changes in the collagen of the palmar fascia in patients with Dupuytren's disease. J Bone Joint Surg [Am] 63:787, 1981.
483. Ling RSH: The genetic factor in Dupuytren's disease. J Bone Joint Surg [Br] 45:709, 1963.
484. Roberts FP: A vibration injury: Dupuytren's contracture. J Soc Occup Med 31:148, 1981.
485. Hadjis NS, Carr DH, Banks L, et al: The role of CT in the diagnosis of primary lymphedema of the lower limb. AJR 144:361, 1985.
486. Gamba JL, Silverman PM, Ling D, et al: Primary lower extremity lymphedema: CT diagnosis. Radiology 149:218, 1983.
487. Das GC, Sen SB: Chylous arthritis. Br Med J 2:27, 1968.
488. Frayha RA, Mooradian A, Tabbara KF: Transudative knee effusions in Milroy's disease. J Rheumatol 8:670, 1981.
489. Friedman RJ, Gumley GJ: Crepitation simulating gas gangrene. J Bone Joint Surg [Am] 67:646, 1985.
490. Naidech HJ, Chawla HS: Soft-tissue calcification after subcutaneous emphysema in a neonate. AJR 139:374, 1982.

491. Felman AH, Fisher MS: The radiographic detection of glass in soft tissue. Radiology 92:1529, 1969.

492. Roberts WC: Radiographic characteristics of glass. Am J Roentgenol 115:636, 1972.

493. Tandberg D: Glass in the hand and foot. Will an x-ray film show it? JAMA 248:1872, 1982.

494. de Lacey G, Evans R, Sandin B: Penetrating injuries: How easy is it to see glass (and plastic) on radiographs? Br J Radiol 58:27, 1985.

495. Woesner ME, Saunders I: Xeroradiography: A significant modality in the detection of non-metallic foreign bodies in soft tissues. AJR 115:636, 1972.

496. Kuhns LR, Borlaza GS, Seigel RS, et al: In vitro comparison of computer tomography and radiography in the detection of soft tissue foreign bodies. Radiology 132:218, 1979.

497. Cracchiolo A: Wooden foreign bodies in the foot. Am J Surg 140:585, 1980.

498. Healy JF: Computed tomography of a cranial wooden body. J Comput Assist Tomogr 4:555, 1980.

499. Rhoades CE, Soye I, Levine E, et al: Detection of a wooden foreign body in the hand, using computed tomography—case report. J Hand Surg 7:306, 1982.

500. Bauer AR Jr, Yutani D: Computed tomographic localization of wooden foreign bodies in children's extremities. Arch Surg 118:1084, 1983.

501. Sexton CC, Lawson JP, Yesner R: Case report 174. Skel Radiol 7:211, 1981.

502. Cleland LG, Vernon-Roberts B, Smith K: Fibre glass induced synovitis. Ann Rheum Dis 43:530, 1984.

503. Vives P, de Lestang M, Dorde T, et al: Reaction ostéolytique tardive massive autour de fils trans-osseoux. Rev Chir Orthop 66:395, 1980.

504. Yousefzadeh DK, Jackson JH Jr: Organic foreign body reaction. Report of two cases of thorn-induced "granuloma" and review of literature. Skel Radiol 3:167, 1978.

505. Cahill N, King JD: Palm thorn synovitis. J Pediatr Orthop 4:175, 1984.

506. Balasubramaniam P, Prathap K: Pseudotumors due to oil palm thorn injury. Aust NZ J Surg 47:223, 1977.

507. Sugarman M, Stobie DG, Quismorio FP, et al: Plant thorn synovitis. Arthritis Rheum 20:1125, 1977.

508. Southgate GW, Murray RO: Case report 190. Skel Radiol 8:79, 1982.

509. Dickson RA, Kemp FH: Thorn-induced granulomata of bone. Hand 8:69, 1976.

510. Schenck JF, Strosberg JM: Use of thermography in the diagnosis of plant thorn synovitis. Arthritis Rheum 22:1037, 1979.

511. Kelly JJ: Blackthorn inflammation. J Bone Joint Surg [Br] 48:474, 1966.

512. Gerle RD: Thorn-induced pseudotumors of the bone. Br J Radiol 44:642, 1971.

513. Weston WJ: Thorn- and twig-induced pseudo-tumours of bone and soft tissues. Br J Radiol 36:323, 1963.

514. Strauss MD, MacDonald RI: Hand injuries from sea urchin spines. Clin Orthop 114:216, 1976.

515. Daupleix D, Dreyfus P, Amouroux J: Sea-urchin spine synovitis. One case associating synovitis due to sea-urchin spines and pasteurellosis. Rev Rhum Mal Osteoartic 49:219, 1982.

516. Cracchiolo A III, Goldberg L: Local and systemic reactions to puncture injuries by the sea urchin spine and the date palm thorn. Arthritis Rheum 20:1206, 1977.

517. Hagen B, Lohse S: Clinical and radiologic aspects of Buerger's disease. Cardiovasc Intervent Radiol 7:283, 1984.

518. Sotos JF, Dodge PR, Muirhead D, et al: Cerebral gigantism in childhood. A syndrome of excessively rapid growth with acromegalic features and a nonprogressive neurological disorder. N Engl J Med 271:109, 1964.

519. Poznanski AK, Stephenson JM: Radiographic findings in hypothalamic acceleration of growth associated with cerebral atrophy and mental retardation (cerebral gigantism). Radiology 88:446, 1967.

520. Kirks DR, Shackelford GD: Idiopathic congenital hemihypertrophy with associated ipsilateral benign nephromegaly. Radiology 115:145, 1975.

521. Miller RW, Fraumeni JF Jr, Manning MD: Association of Wilms' tumor with aniridia, hemihypertrophy and other congenital malformations. N Engl J Med 270:922, 1964.

522. Barsky AJ: Macrodactyly. J Bone Joint Surg [Am] 49:1255, 1967.

523. Schwartz RA, Birnkrant AP, Rubenstein DJ, et al: Squamous cell carcinoma in dominant type epidermolysis bullosa dystrophica. Cancer 47:615, 1981.

524. Byers PH, Siegel RC, Holbrook KA, et al: X-linked cutis laxa. Defective crosslink formation in collagen due to decreased lysyl oxidase activity. N Engl J Med 303:61, 1980.

525. Brown FR III, Holbrook KA, Byers PH, et al: Cutis laxa. Johns Hopkins Med J 150:148, 1982.

526. Sakati NO, Nyhan WL: Congenital cutis laxa and osteoporosis. Am J Dis Child 137:452, 1983.

527. Totten JR: The multiple nevoid basal cell carcinoma syndrome. Report of its occurrence in four generations of a family. Cancer 46:1456, 1980.

528. Fitzpatrick PJ, Thompson GA: Gorlin's syndrome or nevoid basal cell carcinoma syndrome. Can Med Assoc J 127:465, 1982.

529. Barnes DA, Borns P, Pizzutillo PD: Cervical spondylolisthesis associated with the multiple nevoid basal cell carcinoma syndrome. Clin Orthop 162:26, 1982.

530. Mabille JP, Legoux A, Lambert D: Les lacunes osseuses extramandibulaires de la naevomatose baso-cellulaire. Ann Radiol 23:679, 1980.

531. Hermann G, Som P: Case report 135. Skel Radiol 6:62, 1981.

532. Blinder G, Barki Y, Pezt M, et al: Widespread osteolytic lesions of the long bones in basal cell nevus syndrome. Skel Radiol 12:196, 1984.

533. Thiers BH: Panniculitis. Dermatol Clin North Am 1:537, 1983.

534. McCarthy JC, Goldberg MJ, Zimbler S: Orthopaedic dysfunction in the blue rubber-bleb nevus syndrome. J Bone Joint Surg [Am] 64:280, 1982.

535. Lynch RD, Leshner RT, Nicholls PJ, et al: Focal dermal hypoplasia (Goltz's syndrome) with an expansile iliac lesion. A case report. J Bone Joint Surg [Am] 63:470, 1981.

536. Hall EH, Terezhalmy GT: Focal dermal hypoplasia syndrome. Case report and literature review. J Am Acad Dermatol 9:443, 1983.

537. Schlansky R, Kucer KA, Deltoratius RJ, et al: Arthritis and distal tuft resorption associated with keratosis palmaris et plantaris. Arthritis Rheum 24:726, 1981.

538. Dimmock SA, Shaw DG, Pincott JR, et al: Case report 326. Skel Radiol 14:141, 1985.

539. Gold RH, Mirra JM: Case report 339. Skel Radiol 14:309, 1985.

540. Pettersson H, Hudson TM, Springfield DS, et al: Cystic intramuscular myxoma. Report of a case. Acta Radiol (Diagn) 26:425, 1985.

541. Patel MR, Desai SS: Tenosynovial osteochondromatosis of the extensor tendon of a digit: Case report and review of the literature. J Hand Surg [Am] 10:716, 1985.

542. Nichols J, Tehranzadeh J: Case report 325. Skel Radiol 14:136, 1985.

543. Owen RS, Fishman EK, Healy WL, et al: Case report 345. Skel Radiol 15:69, 1986.

544. Lindhout D, Golding RP, Tacts van Amerongen AHM: Fibrodysplasia ossificans progressiva: current concepts and the role of CT in acute changes. Pediatr Radiol 15:211, 1985.

545. Stoskopf CA, Poznanski AK, Gilbert A, et al: Calcification associated with terminal defects of the upper extremity. Radiology 152:689, 1984.

546. Petasnick JP, Turner DA, Charters JR, et al: Soft-tissue masses of the locomotor system: comparison of MR imaging with CT. Radiology 160:125, 1986.

547. Cory DA, Ellis JH, Bies JR, et al: Magnetic resonance imaging of extremity masses. Comput Radiol 10:99, 1986.

548. Totty WG, Murphy WA, Lee JKT: Soft-tissue tumors: MR imaging. Radiology 160:135, 1986.

549. DeOrchis D, Ozonoff MB: Infiltrating angiolipoma with phlebolith formation. Skel Radiol 15:464, 1986.

550. Enzi G, Angelini C, Negrin P, et al: Sensory, motor, and autonomic neuropathy in patients with multiple symmetric lipomatosis. Medicine 64:388, 1986.

551. Rigor VU, Goldstone SE, Jones J, et al: Hibernoma. A case report and discussion of a rare tumor. Cancer 57:2207, 1986.

552. Crisi G, Calo M, Mauri C: Case report 358. Skel Radiol 15:247, 1986.

553. Markhede G, Lundgren L, Bjurstam N, et al: Extra-abdominal desmoid tumors. Acta Orthop Scand 57:1, 1986.

554. Kay SP, Gold RH, Bassett LW: Meniscal pneumatocele. J Bone Joint Surg [Am] 67:1117, 1985.

555. Dorrell JH, Catterall A: The torn acetabular labrum. J Bone Joint Surg [Br] 68:400, 1986.

556. Present DA, Hudson TM, Enneking WF: Computed tomography of extraosseous ganglia. Clin Orthop 202:249, 1986.

557. McCarthy EF, Matz S, Steiner GC, et al: Periosteal ganglion: A cause of cortical bone erosion. Skel Radiol 10:243, 1983.

558. Grange WJ: Subperiosteal ganglion. A case report. J Bone Joint Surg [Br] 60:124, 1978.

559. Bhagavan BS, Dorfman HD: The significance of bone and cartilage formation in malignant fibrous histiocytoma of soft tissue. Cancer 49:480, 1982.

560. Cohen JM, Weinreb JC, Redman HC: Arteriovenous malformations of the extremities: MR imaging. Radiology 158:475, 1986.

561. Zlatkin MB, Lander PH, Begin LR, et al: Soft-tissue chondromas. AJR 144:1263, 1985.

562. Lagier R: Case report 354. Skel Radiol 15:179, 1986.

563. Böstman O, Karaharju E, Heikkonen L, et al: Extraskeletal ossifying chondroma in the knee. A case report. Acta Orthop Scand 56:87, 1985.

564. Treu EBWM, de Slegte RGM, Golding RP, et al: CT findings in paravertebral synovial sarcoma. J Comput Assist Tomogr 10:460, 1986.

565. Cohen LM, Schwartz AM, Rockoff SD: Benign Schwannomas: Pathologic basis for CT inhomogeneities. AJR 147:141, 1986.

566. Berlin Ö, Stener B, Lindahl S, et al: Vascularization of peripheral neurilemomas: Angiographic, computed tomographic, and histologic studies. Skel Radiol 15:275, 1986.

567. Ducatman BS, Scheithauer BW, Piepgras DG, et al: Malignant peripheral nerve sheath tumors. Cancer 57:2006, 1986.

568. Langlais R, Miles DA, Van Dis ML: Elongated and mineralized stylohyoid ligament complex: A proposed classification and report of a case of Eagle's syndrome. Oral Surg 61:527, 1986.

569. Fink RJ, Corn RC: Fracture of an ossified Achilles tendon. Clin Orthop 169:148, 1982.

570. Pazzaglia UE, Beluffi G, Columbo A, et al: Myositis ossificans in the newborn. A case report. J Bone Joint Surg [Am] 68:456, 1986.

571. Fang MA, Reinig JW, Hill SC, et al: Technetium-99m MDP demonstration of heterotopic ossification in fibrodysplasia ossificans progressiva. Clin Nucl Med 11:8, 1986.

572. Reinig JW, Hill SC, Fang M, et al: Fibrodysplasia ossificans progressiva: CT appearance. Radiology 159:153, 1986.

573. Herold HZ, Schmueli G, Baruchin AM: Popliteal pterygium syndrome. Clin Orthop 209:194, 1986.

574. Fornage BD, Schernberg FL: Sonographic diagnosis of foreign bodies of the distal extremities. AJR 147:567, 1986.

575. Little CM, Parker MG, Callowich MC, et al: The ultrasonic detection of soft tissue foreign bodies. Invest Radiol 21:275, 1986.

576. Bonatus TJ, Alexander AH: Dercum's disease (adiposis dolorosa). A case report and review of the literature. Clin Orthop 205:251, 1986.

577. Lee KR, Cox GG, Neff JR, et al: Cystic masses of the knee: Arthrographic and CT evaluation. AJR *148:*329, 1987.

578. Sundaram M, McGuire MH, Herbold DR, et al: High signal intensity soft tissue masses on T1 weighted pulsing sequences. Skel Radiol *16:*30, 1987.

579. Dabney KW, MacEwan GD, Davis NE: Recurring digital fibrous tumor of childhood: Case report with long-term follow-up and review of the literature. J Pediatr Orthop *6:*612, 1986.

580. Hashimoto H, Tsuneyoshi M, Daimaru Y, et al: Intramuscular myxoma. A clinicopathologic, immunohistochemical, and electron microscopic study. Cancer *58:*740, 1986.

581. Rydholm A, Syk I: Malignant fibrous histiocytoma of soft tissue. Correlation between clinical variables and histologic malignancy grade. Cancer *57:*2323, 1986.

582. Nakashima Y, Unni KK, Shives TC, et al: Mesenchymal chondrosarcoma of bone and soft tissue. A review of 111 cases. Cancer *57:*2444, 1986.

583. Blakeslee TJ, Chan RJ: Chinese bound foot. A literature review and case report. J Am Podiatr Assoc *76:*502, 1986.

584. Suramo I, Pamilo M: Ultrasound examination of foreign bodies. An in vitro investigation. Acta Radiol Diagn *27:*463, 1986.

585. Goldstein SA, Imbriglia JE: Erosion of the triquetrum and pisiform bones caused by a foreign body granuloma. J Hand Surg [Am] *11:*899, 1986.

586. Harcke HT, Grissom LE, Finkelstein MS: Evaluation of the musculoskeletal system with sonography. AJR *150:*1253, 1988.

587. Yamaguchi M, Takeuchi S, Matsuo S: Ultrasonic evaluation of pediatric superficial masses. JCU *15:*107, 1987.

588. Glasier CM, Seibert JJ, Williamson SL, et al: High resolution ultrasound characterization of soft tissue masses in children. Pediatr Radiol *17:*233, 1987.

589. Fornage BD, Lorigan JG: Sonographic detection and fine-needle aspiration biopsy of non-palpable recurrent or metastatic melanoma in subcutaneous tissues. J Ultrasound Med *8:*421, 1989.

590. Choi H, Varma DGK, Fornage BD, et al: Soft-tissue sarcoma: MR imaging vs. sonography for detection of local recurrence after surgery. AJR *157:*353, 1991.

591. Angervall L, Kindblom L-G, Rydholm A, et al: The diagnosis and prognosis of soft tissue tumors. Semin Diagn Pathol *3:*240, 1986.

592. Finn HA, Simon MA, Martin WB, et al: Scintigraphy with gallium-67 citrate in staging of soft-tissue sarcomas of the extremity. J Bone Joint Surg [Am] *69:*886, 1987.

593. Chang AE, Matory YL, Dwyer AJ, et al: Magnetic resonance imaging versus computed tomography in the evaluation of soft tissue tumors of the extremities. Ann Surg *205:*340, 1987.

594. Bland KI, McCoy M, Kinard RE, et al: Application of magnetic resonance imaging and computerized tomography as an adjunct to the surgical management of soft tissue sarcomas. Ann Surg *205:*473, 1987.

595. Demas BE, Heelan RT, Lane J, et al: Soft-tissue sarcomas of the extremities: Comparison of MR and CT in determining the extent of disease. AJR *150:*615, 1988.

596. Sundaram M, McGuire MH, Herbold DR: Magnetic resonance imaging of soft tissue masses: An evaluation of fifty-three histologically proven tumors. Magn Res Imag *6:*237, 1988.

597. Kalmar JA, Miller KD, Eick JJ, et al: A review of applications of MRI in soft tissue and bone tumors. Orthop *11:*417, 1988.

598. Sundaram M, McGuire MH, Schajowicz F: Soft-tissue masses: Histologic basis for decreased signal (short T2) on T2-weighted MR images. AJR *148:*1247, 1987.

599. Pettersson H, Stone RM, Spanier S, et al: Musculoskeletal tumors: T1 and T2 relaxation times. Radiology *167:*783, 1988.

600. Sostman HD, Charles HC, Rockwell S, et al: Soft-tissue sarcomas: Detection of metabolic heterogeneity with P-31 MR spectroscopy. Radiology *176:*837, 1990.

601. Kransdorf MJ, Jelinek JS, Moser RP Jr, et al: Soft-tissue masses: Diagnosis using MR imaging. AJR *153:*541, 1989.

602. Berquist TH, Ehman RL, King BF, et al: Value of MR imaging in differentiating benign from malignant soft-tissue masses: Study of 95 lesions. AJR *155:*1251, 1990.

603. Crim JR, Seeger LL, Yao L, et al: Diagnosis of soft-tissue masses with MR imaging: Can benign masses be differentiated from malignant ones? Radiology *185:*581, 1992.

604. Wetzel LH, Levine E: Soft-tissue tumors of the foot: Value of MR imaging for specific diagnosis. AJR *155:*1025, 1990.

605. Greenfield GB, Arrington JA, Kudryk BT: MRI of soft tissue tumors. Skel Radiol *22:*77, 1993.

606. Jelinek JS, Kransdorf MJ: MR imaging of soft-tissue masses. AJR *155:*423, 1990.

607. Shuman WP, Patten RM, Baron RL, et al: Comparison of STIR and spin-echo MR imaging at 1.5 T in 45 suspected extremity tumors: Lesion conspicuity and extent. Radiology *179:*247, 1991.

608. Seltzer S, Davis DO, Macht SD, et al: MRI of soft-tissue masses of the extremities. MRI Decisions, May/June 1990, p. 12.

609. Rubin SJ, Feldman F, Haber MM, et al: Magnetic resonance grid analysis of soft tissue lesions. Invest Radiol *26:*474, 1991.

610. Rubin SJ, Feldman F, Dick HM, et al: Heterogeneous in vivo MR images of soft tissue tumors: Guide to gross specimen sampling. Magn Res Imag *10:*351, 1992.

611. Biondetti PR, Ehman RL: Soft-tissue sarcomas: Use of textural patterns in skeletal muscle as a diagnostic feature in postoperative MR imaging. Radiology *183:*845, 1992.

612. Kransdorf MJ, Moser RP Jr, Meis JM, et al: Fat-containing soft-tissue masses of the extremities. RadioGraphics *11:*81, 1991.

613. Orson GG, Sim FH, Reiman HM, et al: Liposarcoma of the musculoskeletal system. Cancer *60:*1362, 1987.

614. London J, Kim EE, Wallace S, et al: MR imaging of liposarcomas: Correlation of MR features and histology. J Comput Assist Tomogr *13:*832, 1989.

615. Sundaram M, Baran G, Merenda G, et al: Myxoid liposarcoma: Magnetic resonance imaging appearances with clinical and histological correlation. Skel Radiol *19:*359, 1990.

616. Klein MH, Desai P: Case report 637. Skel Radiol *19:*545, 1990.

617. Jelinek JS, Kransdorf MJ, Shmookler BM, et al: Liposarcoma of the extremities: MR and CT findings in the histologic subtypes. Radiology *186:*455, 1993.

618. Bush CH, Spanier SS, Gillespie T III: Imaging of atypical lipomas of the extremities: Report of three cases. Skel Radiol *17:*472, 1988.

619. Braunschweig IJ, Stein IH, Dodwad MIM, et al: Case report 751. Skel Radiol *21:*414, 1992.

620. Nigrisoli M, Ruggieri P, Picci P, et al: Case report 489. Skel Radiol *17:*432, 1988.

621. Ehara S, Tokunaga S, Monma N, et al: Case report 675. Skel Radiol *20:*319, 1991.

622. Mahour GH, Bryan BJ, Isaacs H Jr: Lipoblastoma and lipoblastomatosis—A report of six cases. Surgery *104:*577, 1988.

623. Hubscher O, Costanza E, Elsner B: Chronic monoarthritis due to lipoma arborescens. J Rheumatol *17:*861, 1990.

624. Noel ER, Tebib JG, Dumontet Ch, et al: Synovial lipoma arborescens of the hip. Clin Rheumatol *6:*92, 1987.

625. Martinez D, Millner PA, Coral A, et al: Case report 745. Skel Radiol *21:*393, 1992.

626. Blacksin M, Barnes FJ, Lyons MM: MR diagnosis of macrodystrophia lipomatosa. AJR *158:*1295, 1992.

627. Scott SM, Reiman HM, Pritchard DJ, et al: Soft tissue fibrosarcoma. A clinicopathologic study of 132 cases. Cancer *64:*925, 1989.

628. Robinson W, Crawford AH: Infantile fibrosarcoma. Report of a case with long-follow-up. J Bone Joint Surg [Am] *72:*291, 1990.

629. Ayala AG, Ro JY, Goepfert H, et al: Desmoid fibromatosis: A clinicopathologic study of 25 children. Semin Diagn Pathol *3:*138, 1986.

630. Sundaram M, Duffrin H, McGuire MH, et al: Synchronous multicentric desmoid tumors (aggressive fibromatosis) of the extremities. Skel Radiol *17:*16, 1988.

631. Vizkelety T, Szendröi M: Desmoid tumors of the extremities. Intern Orthop (SICOT) *12:*249, 1988.

632. Casillas J, Sais GJ, Greve JL, et al: Imaging of intra- and extraabdominal desmoid tumors. RadioGraphics *11:*959, 1991.

633. Francis IR, Dorovini-Zis K, Glazer GM, et al: The fibromatoses: CT-pathologic correlation. AJR *147:*1063, 1986.

634. Rubenstein WA, Gray G, Auh YH, et al: CT of fibrous tissues and tumors with sonographic correlation. AJR *147:*1067, 1986.

635. Hartman TE, Berquist TH, Fetsch JF: MR imaging of extraabdominal desmoids: Differentiation from other neoplasms. AJR *158:*581, 1992.

636. Taylor LJ: Musculoaponeurotic fibromatosis. A report of 28 cases and review of the literature. Clin Orthop *224:*294, 1987.

637. Hawnaur JM, Isherwood I: Magnetic resonance imaging of musculoaponeurotic fibromatosis. Skel Radiol *19:*509, 1990.

638. O'Neill DB, Kasser JR: Juvenile hyaline fibromatosis. A case report and review of musculoskeletal manifestations. J Bone Joint Surg [Am] *71:*941, 1989.

639. Bedford CD, Sills JA, Sommelet-Olive D, et al: Juvenile hyaline fibromatosis: A report of two severe cases. J Pediatr *119:*404, 1991.

640. Suzuki S, Kasahara Y, Seto Y, et al: Juvenile hyaline fibromatosis. A case report. J Bone Joint Surg [Am] *74:*290, 1992.

641. Greenberg JA, Lockwood RC: Elastofibroma dorsi. A case report and review of the literature. Orthop Review *18:*329, 1989.

642. Marin ML, Austin JHM, Markowitz AM: Elastofibroma dorsi: CT demonstration. J Comput Assist Tomogr *11:*675, 1987.

643. Kapff PD, Hocken DB, Simpson RHW: Elastofibroma of the hand. J Bone Joint Surg [Br] *69:*468, 1987.

644. Ghiatas AA, Armstrong S, Tio FO: Case report 583. Skel Radiol *18:*619, 1989.

645. Massengill AD, Sundaram M, Kathol MH, et al: Elastofibroma dorsi: a radiological diagnosis. Skel Radiol *22:*121, 1993.

646. Kransdorf MJ, Meis JM, Montgomery E: Elastofibroma: MR and CT appearance with radiologic-pathologic correlation. AJR *159:*575, 1992.

647. Present DA, Abdelwahab IF, Zwass A, et al: Case report 575. Skel Radiol *18:*557, 1989.

648. Inwards CY, Unni KK, Beabout JW, et al: Solitary congenital fibromatosis (infantile myofibromatosis) of bone. Amer J Surg Path *15:*935, 1991.

649. Kozlowski K, Kan A, Marsden FW: Case report 684. Skel Radiol *20:*397, 1991.

650. Marty-Double C, Balmes P, Mary H, et al: Juvenile fibromatosis resembling aponeurotic fibroma and congenital multiple fibromatosis. One case with pleuropulmonary involvement. Cancer *61:*146, 1988.

651. Liu P, Thorner P: MRI of fibromatosis: with pathologic correlation. Pediatr Radiol *22:*587, 1992.

652. Feld R, Burk L Jr, McCue P, et al: MRI of aggressive fibromatosis: Frequent appearance of high signal intensity on T2-weighted images. Magn Res Imag *8:*583, 1990.

653. Quinn SF, Erickson SJ, Dee PM, et al: MR imaging in fibromatosis: Results in 26 patients with pathologic correlation. AJR *156:*539, 1991.

654. Kransdorf MJ, Jelinek JS, Moser RP Jr, et al: Magnetic resonance appearance of fibromatosis. A report of 14 cases and review of the literature. Skel Radiol 19:495, 1990.

655. Stallard D, Sundaram M, Johnson FE, et al: Case report 747. Skel Radiol 21:399, 1992.

656. Herrlin K, Willén H, Rydholm A: Deep-seated soft tissue leiomyomas. Skel Radiol 19:363, 1990.

657. Lubbers PR, Chandra R, Markle BM, et al: Case report 421. Skel Radiol 16:252, 1987.

658. Smith JW, Danon A, Padgett D, et al: Leiomyomas of the lower extremity. Orthop 14:594, 1991.

659. Agamanolis DP, Dasu S, Krill CE Jr: Tumors of skeletal muscle. Human Pathol 17:778, 1986.

660. Tantana S, Sotelo-Avila C, Pilla TJ, et al: Malignant rhabdoid tumor of the thoracic spine. Orthop 11:905, 1988.

661. Meis JM, Enzinger FM: Juxta-articular myxoma: A clinical and pathologic study of 65 cases. Human Pathol 23:639, 1992.

662. Abdelwahab AF, Kenan S, Hermann G, et al: Intramuscular myxoma: Magnetic resonance features. Brit J Radiol 65:485, 1992.

663. Peterson KK, Renfrew DL, Feddersen RM, et al: Magnetic resonance imaging of myxoid containing tumors. Skel Radiol 20:245, 1991.

664. Mahajan H, Kim EE, Wallace S, et al: Magnetic resonance imaging of malignant fibrous histiocytoma. Magn Res Imag 7:283, 1989.

665. Panicek DM, Casper ES, Brennan MF, et al: Hemorrhage simulating tumor growth in malignant fibrous histiocytoma at MR imaging. Radiology 181:398, 1991.

666. Fletcher CDM: Benign fibrous histiocytoma of subcutaneous and deep soft tissue: A clinicopathologic analysis of 21 cases. Amer J Surg Pathol 14:801, 1990.

667. Crosher RF, Blackburn CW, Dinsdale RCW: Blue rubber-bleb naevus syndrome. Brit J Oral Maxillofac Surg 26:160, 1988.

668. Watson HK, Rogers WD, Ashmead D IV: Reevaluation of the cause of the wrist ganglion. J Hand Surg [Am] 14:812, 1989.

669. Young L, Bartell T, Logan SE: Ganglions of the hand and wrist. South Med J 81:751, 1988.

670. Gambari PI, Giuliani G, Poppi M, et al: Ganglionic cysts of the peroneal nerve at the knee: CT and surgical correlation. J Comput Assist Tomogr 14:801, 1990.

671. Pope TL Jr, Fechner RE, Keats TE: Intra-osseous ganglion. Report of four cases and review of the literature. Skel Radiol 18:185, 1989.

672. Fritz RC, Helms CA, Steinbach LS, et al: Suprascapular nerve entrapment: Evaluation with MR imaging. Radiology 182:437, 1992.

673. Ogino T, Minami A, Kato H, et al: Entrapment neuropathy of the suprascapular nerve by a ganglion. J Bone Joint Surg [Am] 73:141, 1991.

674. Takagishi K, Maeda K, Ikeda T, et al: Ganglion causing paralysis of the suprascapular nerve. Diagnosis by MRI and ultrasonography. Acta Orthop Scand 62:391, 1991.

675. Garcia A, Hodler J, Vaughn L, et al: Case report 677. Skel Radiol 20:373, 1991.

676. Yasuda K, Majima T: Intra-articular ganglion blocking extension of the knee: Brief report. J Bone Joint Surg [Br] 70:837, 1988.

677. Kaempfee F, D'Amato C: An unusual intra-articular ganglion of the knee with interosseous extension. A case report. J Bone Joint Surg [Am] 71:773, 1989.

678. Chang W, Rose DJ: Ganglion cysts of the anterior cruciate ligament. A case report. Bull Hosp J Dis 48:182, 1988.

679. Brown MF, Dandy DJ: Intra-articular ganglia in the knee. J Arthros Rel Surg 6:322, 1990.

680. McLaren DB, Buckwalter KA, Vahey TN: The prevalence and significance of cyst-like changes at the cruciate ligament attachments of the knee. Skel Radiol 21:365, 1992.

681. Matsumoto K, Hukuda S, Ogata M: Juxta-articular bone cysts at the insertion of the pes anserinus. Report of two cases. J Bone Joint Surg [Am] 72:286, 1990.

682. Scapinelli R: A synovial ganglion of the popliteus tendon simulating a parameniscal cyst. Two case reports. J Bone Joint Surg [Am] 70:1085, 1988.

683. Dorrell JH, Catterall A: The torn acetabular labrum. J Bone Joint Surg [Br] 68:400, 1986.

684. Haller J, Resnick D, Greenway G, et al: Juxtaacetabular ganglionic (or synovial) cysts: CT and MR features. J Comput Assist Tomogr 13:976, 1989.

685. Klaue K, Durnin CW, Ganz R: The acetabular rim syndrome. A clinical presentation of dysplasia of the hip. J Bone Joint Surg [Br] 73:423, 1991.

686. Hertzanu Y, Berginer J, Berginer VM: Computed tomography of tendinous xanthomata in cerebrotendinous xanthomatosis. Skel Radiol 20:99, 1991.

687. Burnstein M, Buckwalter KA, Martel W, et al: Case report 427. Skel Radiol 16:346, 1987.

688. Liem MSL, Leuven G, Bloem JL, et al: Magnetic resonance imaging of Achilles tendon xanthomas in familial hypercholesterolemia. Skel Radiol 21:453, 1992.

689. Kenan S, Abdelwahab IF, Klein MJ, et al: Case report 754. Skel Radiol 21:471, 1992.

690. Fornage BD: Glomus tumors in the fingers: Diagnosis with US. Radiology 167:183, 1988.

691. Kneeland JB, Middleton WD, Matloub HS, et al: High resolution MR imaging of glomus tumor. J Comput Assist Tomogr 11:351, 1992.

692. Rozmaryn LM, Sadler AH, Dorfman HD: Intraosseous glomus tumor in the ulna. A case report. Clin Orthop 220:126, 1987.

693. Aalberg JR: Synovial hemangioma of the knee. A case report. Acta Orthop Scand 61:88, 1990.

694. Lenchik L, Poznanski AK, Donaldson JS, et al: Case report 681. Skel Radiol 20:387, 1991.

695. Wirth T, Rauch G, Rüschoff J, et al: Synovial haemangioma of the knee joint. Intern Orthop (SICOT) 16:130, 1992.

696. Visuri T: Recurrent spontaneous haemarthrosis of the knee associated with a synovial and juxta-articular haemangiohamartoma. Ann Rheum Dis 49:554, 1990.

697. Kaplan PA, Williams SM: Mucocutaneous and peripheral soft-tissue hemangiomas: MR imaging. Radiology 163:163, 1987.

698. Cohen EK, Kressel HY, Perosio T, et al: MR imaging of soft-tissue hemangiomas: Correlation with pathologic findings. AJR 150:1079, 1988.

699. Yuh WTC, Kathol MH, Sein MA, et al: Hemangiomas of skeletal muscle: MR findings in five patients. AJR 149:765, 1987.

700. Buetow PC, Kransdorf MJ, Moser RP Jr, et al: Radiologic appearance of intramuscular hemangioma with emphasis on MR imaging. AJR 154:563, 1987.

701. Hawnaur JM, Whitehouse RW, Jenkins JPR, et al: Musculoskeletal haemangiomas: comparison of MRI and CT. Skel Radiol 19:251, 1990.

702. Nelson MC, Stull MA, Teitelbaum GP, et al: Magnetic resonance imaging of peripheral soft tissue hemangiomas. Skel Radiol 19:477, 1990.

703. Greenspan A, McGahan JP, Vogelsang P, et al: Imaging strategies in the evaluation of soft-tissue hemangiomas of the extremities: correlation of the findings on plain films, angiography, CT, MRI, and ultrasonography in 12 histologically proven cases. Skel Radiol 21:11, 1992.

704. Lorigan JG, David CL, Evans HL, et al: The clinical and radiologic manifestations of hemangiopericytoma. AJR 153:345, 1989.

705. Ono CM, Mitsunaga MM, Lockett LJ: Intragluteal spindle cell hemangioendothelioma. Clin Orthop 281:224, 1992.

706. Sanchez RB, Quinn SF, Walling A, et al: Case report 569. Skel Radiol 18:485, 1989.

707. Kaufmann T, Chu F, Kaufman R: Post-mastectomy lymphangiosarcoma (Stewert-Treves syndrome: report of two long-term survivals. Brit J Radiol 64:857, 1991.

708. Muller R, Hajdu SI, Brennan MF: Lymphangiosarcoma associated with chronic filarial lymphedema. Cancer 59:179, 1987.

709. Zadvinskis DP, Benson MT, Kerr HH, et al: Congenital malformations of the cervicothoracic lymphatic system: Embryology and pathogenesis. Radio-Graphics 12:1175, 1992.

710. Law PJ, Hall CM: Clavicular overgrowth in association with cystic hygroma. Skel Radiol 20:597, 1991.

711. Rak KM, Yakes WF, Ray RL, et al: MR imaging of symptomatic peripheral vascular malformations. AJR 159:107, 1992.

712. Kransdorf MJ, McFarland DR, Moser RP Jr, et al: Case report 649. Skel Radiol 20:63, 1991.

713. Miki T, Yamamuro T, Shikata J, et al: Congenital soft-part chondroma. A case report. Clin Orthop 244:244, 1989.

714. Widdowson DJ, Lewis-Jones HG: Case report: A large soft-tissue chondroma arising from the posterior mediastinum. Clin Radiol 39:333, 1988.

715. Chan JKC, Lee KC, Saw D: Extraskeletal chondroma with lipoblast-like cells. Human Pathol 17:1285, 1986.

716. Isayama T, Iwasaki H, Kikuchi M: Chondroblastomalike extraskeletal chondroma. Clin Orthop 268:214, 1991.

717. Hayward I, Yaru N, Grafe M, et al: Knee pain and swelling in a 38-year-old woman. Inv Radiol 22:516, 1987.

718. Lipskeir E, Sagi A, Lifschitz-Mercer B: Extraarticular chondromatosis of the hand. A case report. Acta Orthop Scand 59:728, 1988.

719. Hayden JW, Abellera RM: Tenosynovial lipochondromatosis of the flexor hallucis, common toe flexor, and posterior tibial tendons. Clin Orthop 245:220, 1985.

720. Sowa DT, Moore JR, Weiland AJ: Extraskeletal osteochondromas of the wrist. J Hand Surg [Am] 12:212, 1987.

721. Steinberg GG, Desai SS, Malhotra R, et al: Familial synovial chondromatosis. J Bone Joint Surg [Br] 71:144, 1989.

722. Kay PR, Freemont AJ, Davies DRH: The aetiology of multiple loose bodies, Snow storm knee. J Bone Joint Surg [Br] 71:501, 1989.

723. Maurice H, Crone M, Watt I: Synovial chondromatosis. J Bone Joint Surg [Br] 70:807, 1988.

724. Norman A, Steiner GC: Bone erosion in synovial chondromatosis. Radiology 161:749, 1986.

725. Milchgrub S, Mulhollan T, Vuitch MF, et al: Case report 692. Skel Radiol 21:45, 1992.

726. Demeulemeester LJMJ, Bossuyt M, Casselman J, et al: Synovial chondromatosis of the temporomandibular joint. J Oral Maxillofac Surg 17:181, 1988.

727. DeBont LGM, Liem RB, Boering G: Synovial chondromatosis of the temporomandibular joint: A light and electron microscopic study. Oral Surg Med Pathol 66:593, 1988.

728. Pattee GA, Snyder SJ: Synovial chondromatosis of the acromioclavicular joint. A case report. Clin Orthop 233:205, 1988.

729. Nokes SR, King PS, Garcia R Jr, et al: Temporomandibular joint chondromatosis with intracranial extension: MR and CT contributions. AJR 148:1173, 1987.

730. Manco LG, DeLuke DM: CT diagnosis of synovial chondromatosis of the temporomandibular joint. AJR 148:574, 1987.

731. Pope TL Jr, Keats TE, de Lange EE, et al: Idiopathic synovial chondromatosis in two unusual sites: inferior radioulnar joint and ischial bursa. Skel Radiol 16:205, 1987.

732. Osburn AW, Bassett LW, Seeger LL, et al: Case report 609. Skel Radiol 19:237, 1990.

733. Ginai AZ: Case report 607. Skel Radiol 19:227, 1990.

734. Friedman B, Caspi I, Nerubay J, et al: Synovial chondromatosis of the hip joint. Orthop Review 17:994, 1988.

735. Coolican MR, Dandy DJ: Arthroscopic management of synovial chondromatosis of the knee. Findings and results in 18 cases. J Bone Joint Surg [Br] 71:498, 1989.

736. Okada Y, Awaya G, Ikeda T, et al: Arthroscopic surgery for synovial chondromatosis of the hip. J Bone Joint Surg [Br] 71:198, 1989.

737. Lagier R: Case report 451. Skel Radiol 16:660, 1987.

738. Blacksin MF, Ghelman B, Freiberger RH, et al: Synovial chondromatosis of the hip. Evaluation with air computed arthrotomography. Clin Imag 14:315, 1990.

739. Friedman B, Nerubay J, Blankstein A, et al: Case report 439. Skel Radiol 16:504, 1987.

740. Hardacker J, Mindell ER: Synovial chondromatosis with secondary subluxation of the hip. J Bone Joint Surg [Am] 73:1405, 1991.

741. Blandino A, Salvi L, Chirico G, et al: Synovial osteochondromatosis of the ankle: MR findings. Clin Imag 16:34, 1992.

742. Tuckman G, Wirth CZ: Synovial osteochondromatosis of the shoulder: MR findings. J Comput Assist Tomogr 13:360, 1989.

743. Burnstein MI, Fisher DR, Yandow DR, et al: Case report 502. Skel Radiol 17:458, 1988.

744. Bertoni F, Unni KK, Beabout JW, et al: Chondrosarcomas of the synovium. Cancer 67:155, 1991.

745. Manivel JC, Dehner LP, Thompson R: Case report 460. Skel Radiol 17:66, 1988.

746. Perry BE, McQueen DA, Lin JJ: Synovial chondromatosis with malignant degeneration to chondrosarcoma. Report of a case. J Bone Joint Surg [Am] 70:1259, 1988.

747. Hamilton A, Davis RI, Nixon JR: Synovial chondrosarcoma complicating synovial chondromatosis. Report of a case and review of the literature. J Bone Joint Surg [Am] 69:1084, 1987.

748. Hamilton A, Davis RI, Hayes D, et al: Chondrosarcoma developing in synovial chondromatosis. A case report. J Bone Joint Surg [Br] 69:137, 1987.

749. Casadei R, Ricci M, Ruggieri P, et al: Chondrosarcoma of the soft tissues. Two different sub-groups. J Bone Joint Surg [Br] 73:162, 1991.

750. Shapeero LG, Vanel D, Couanet D, et al: Extraskeletal mesenchymal chondrosarcoma. Radiology 186:819, 1993.

751. Li C, Arger PH, Dalinka MK: Soft tissue osteochondroma. A report of three cases. Skel Radiol 18:435, 1989.

752. Matsumoto K, Matsuda T, Hukuda S: Osteoma cutis associated with disordered ossification of the clavicle. A case report. Clin Orthop 246:106, 1989.

753. Schweitzer ME, Greenway G, Resnick D, et al: Osteoma of soft parts. Skel Radiol 21:177, 1992.

754. Greenspan A, Steiner G, Norman A, et al: Case report 436. Skel Radiol 16:489, 1987.

755. Present D, Bertoni F, Laus M, et al: Case report 565. Skel Radiol 18:471, 1989.

756. Doud TM, Moser RP Jr, Giudici MAI, et al: Case report 704. Skel Radiol 20:628, 1991.

757. Chung EB, Enzinger FM: Extraskeletal osteosarcoma. Cancer 60:1132, 1987.

758. Schmidt D, Thum P, Harms D, et al: Synovial sarcoma in children and adolescents. Cancer 67:1667, 1991.

759. Signorini GC, Pinna G, Freschini A, et al: Synovial sarcoma of the thoracic spine. A case report. Spine 11:629, 1986.

760. Lois JF, Fischer HJ, Mirra JM, et al: Angiography of histopathologic variants of synovial sarcoma. Acta Radiologic Diagn 27:449, 1986.

761. Mahajan H, Lorigan JG, Shirkhoda A: Synovial sarcoma: MR imaging. Magn Res Imag 7:211, 1989.

762. Morton MJ, Berquist TH, McLeod RA: MR imaging of synovial sarcoma. AJR 156:337, 1991.

763. Milchgrub S, Ghandur-Mnaymneh L, Dorfman HD, et al: Synovial sarcoma with extensive osteoid and bone formation. Amer J Surg Pathol 17:357, 1993.

764. Meyer CA, Kransdorf MJ, Moser RP Jr, et al: Case report 716. Skel Radiol 21:128, 1992.

765. Kelso TB, Ferrari CJ, Frassica FJ: Sciatica caused by a neurilemoma of the intrapelvic portion of the sciatic nerve. A case report. J Bone Joint Surg [Am] 75:603, 1993.

766. Barnowsky L, Dalal R: Extradural schwannoma manifested as an expansile vertebral lesion. AJR 159:1352, 1992.

767. Zuckerman JD, Powers B, Miller JW, et al: Benign solitary schwannoma of the foot. A case report and review of the literature. Clin Orthop 228:278, 1988.

768. Barboriak DP, Rivitz SM, Chew FS: Sacral neurofibroma. AJR 159:600, 1992.

769. Sanguinetti C, Specchia N, Gigante A, et al: Clinical and pathological aspects of solitary spinal neurofibroma. J Bone Joint Surg [Br] 75:141, 1993.

770. Fornage BD: Peripheral nerves of the extremities: Imaging with US. Radiology 167:179, 1988.

771. Matsumoto S, Hasuo K, Uchino A, et al: MRI of intradural-extramedullary spinal neuromas and meningiomas. Clin Imag 17:46, 1993.

772. Smith W, Amis JA: Neurilemoma of the tibial nerve. A case report. J Bone Joint Surg [Am] 74:443, 1992.

773. Burk DL Jr, Brunberg JA, Kanal E, et al: Spinal and paraspinal neurofibromatosis: Surface coil MR imaging at 1.5 T. Radiology 162:797, 1987.

774. Mann FA, Murphy WA, Totty WG, et al: Magnetic resonance imaging of peripheral nerve sheath tumors. Assessment by numerical visual fuzzy cluster analysis. Invest Radiol 25:1238, 1990.

775. Stull MA, Moser RP Jr, Kransdorf MJ, et al: Magnetic resonance appearance of peripheral nerve sheath tumors. Skel Radiol 20:9, 1991.

776. Suh J-S, Abenoza P, Galloway HR, et al: Peripheral (extracranial) nerve tumors: Correlation of MR imaging and histologic findings. Radiology 183:341, 1992.

777. Varma DGK, Moulopoulos A, Sara AS, et al: MR imaging of extracranial nerve sheath tumors. J Comput Assist Tomogr 16:448, 1992.

778. Redd RA, Peters VJ, Emery SF, et al: Morton neuroma: Sonographic evaluation. Radiology 171:415, 1989.

779. Alexander IJ, Johnson KA, Parr JW: Morton's neuroma: A review of recent concepts. Orthop 10:103, 1987.

780. Steentoft J, Sollerman C: Lipofibromatous hamartoma of a digital nerve. A case report. Acta Orthop Scand 61:181, 1990.

781. Walker CW, Adams BD, Barnes CL, et al: Case report 667. Skel Radiol 20:237, 1991.

782. Jacob RH, Buchino JJ: Lipofibroma of the superficial branch of the radial nerve. J Hand Surg [Am] 14:704, 1989.

783. Houpt P, van Leeuwen JBS, van der Bergen HA: Intraneural lipofibroma of the median nerve. J Hand Surg [Am] 14:706, 1989.

784. Silverman TA, Enzinger FM: Fibrolipomatous hamartoma of nerve. A clinico-pathologic analysis of 26 cases. Amer J Surg Pathol 9:7, 1985.

785. Singson RD, Feldman F, Slipman CW, et al: Postamputation neuromas and other symptomatic stump abnormalities: Detection with CT. Radiology 162:743, 1987.

786. Donnal JF, Blinder RA, Coblentz CL, et al: MR imaging of stump neuroma. J Comput Assist Tomogr 14:656, 1990.

787. Singson RD, Feldman F, Staron R, et al: MRI of postamputation neuromas. Skel Radiol 19:259, 1990.

788. Abdelwahab IF, Lewis MM, Klein MJ: Case report 441. Skel Radiol 16:573, 1987.

789. Levine E, Huntrakoon M, Wetzel LH: Malignant nerve-sheath neoplasms in neurofibromatosis: Distinction from benign tumors by using imaging techniques. AJR 149:1059, 1987.

790. Buckley SL, Burkus JK, Blasier RB: Malignant neuroepithelioma (peripheral neuroblastoma). A case report. Clin Orthop 243:220, 1989.

791. Varma DGK, Moulopoulos A, Sara AS, et al: Case report 682. Skel Radiol 20:391, 1991.

792. Kawamoto EH, Weidner N, Agostini RM Jr, et al: Malignant ectomesenchymoma of soft tissue. Cancer 59:1791, 1987.

793. Hertzanu Y, Hirsch M, Mozes M, et al: Case report 499. Skel Radiol 17:447, 1988.

794. Lucas DR, Nascimento AG, Sim FH: Clear cell sarcoma of soft tissues. Mayo Clinic experience with 35 cases. Am J Surg Pathol 16:1197, 1992.

795. Morishita S, Onomura T, Yamamoto S, et al: Clear cell sarcoma of tendons and aponeuroses (malignant melanoma of soft parts) with unusual roentgenologic findings. Case report. Clin Orthop 216:276, 1987.

796. Sartoris DJ, Haghighi P, Resnick D: Case report 423. Skel Radiol 16:325, 1987.

797. Lorigan JG, O'Keeffe FN, Evans HL, et al: The radiologic manifestations of alveolar soft-part sarcoma. AJR 153:335, 1989.

798. Munk PL, Connell DG, Müller NL, et al: Case report 501. Skel Radiol 17:454, 1988.

799. Bos GD, Pritchard DJ, Reiman HM, et al: Epithelioid sarcoma. An analysis of fifty-one cases. J Bone Joint Surg [Am] 70:862, 1988.

800. Bonfiglio M, Landas S: Case report 640. Skel Radiol 19:599, 1990.

801. Botha AJ, Halliday AEG, Flanagan JP: Endometriosis in gluteus muscle with surgical implantation. A case report. Acta Orthop Scand 62:497, 1991.

802. Sridhar KS, Rao RK, Kunhardt B: Skeletal muscle metastases from lung cancer. Cancer 59:1530, 1987.

803. Flandry F, McCann SB, Hughston JC, et al: Roentgenographic findings in pigmented villonodular synovitis of the knee. Clin Orthop 247:208, 1989.

804. Schwartz HS, Unni KK, Pritchard DJ: Pigmented villonodular synovitis. A retrospective review of affected large joints. Clin Orthop 247:243, 1989.

805. Khoury GM, Shimkin PM, Kleinman GM, et al: Computed tomography and magnetic resonance imaging findings of pigmented villonodular synovitis of the spine. Spine 16:1236, 1991.

806. Crosby EB, Inglis A, Bullough PG: Multiple joint involvement with pigmented villonodular synovitis. Radiology 122:671, 1977.

807. Gehweiler JA, Wilson JW: Diffuse biarticular pigmented villonodular synovitis. Radiology 93:845, 1969.

808. Myers BW, Masi AT, Feigenbaum SL: Pigmented villonodular synovitis and tenosynovitis. A clinical epidemiologic study of 166 cases and literature review. Medicine 59:223, 1980.

809. Flandry F, Hughston JC: Pigmented villonodular synovitis. J Bone Joint Surg [Am] 69:942, 1987.

810. Jaffe HL, Lichtenstein L, Sutro CJ: Pigmented villonodular synovitis, bursitis, and tenosynovitis. A discussion of the synovial and bursal equivalents of the tenosynovial lesion commonly denoted as xanthoma, xanthogranuloma, giant cell tumor or myeloplaxoma of the tendon sheath and some consideration of this tendon sheath lesion itself. Arch Pathol 31:731, 1941.

811. Granowitz SP, D'Antonio J, Mankin HL: The pathogenesis and long-term end results of pigmented villonodular synovitis. Clin Orthop 114:335, 1976.

812. Karasick D, Karasick S: Giant cell tumor of tendon sheath: spectrum of radiologic findings. Skel Radiol 21:219, 1992.

813. Covelli M, LaPadula G, Martino F, et al: Multiple giant cell tumour of tendon sheath (nodular tenosynovitis): a case report with a review of the literature. J Orthop Rheumatol 2:175, 1989.

814. Chung EB, Enzinger FM: Fibroma of tendon sheath. Cancer 44:1945, 1979.

815. Ogata K, Ushijima M: Tenosynovial fibroma arising from the posterior cruciate ligament. Clin Orthop 215:153, 1987.

816. Lourie JA, Lwin KY, Woods CG: Case report 734. Skel Radiol 21:273, 1992.

817. Pulitzer DR, Martin PC, Reed RJ: Fibroma of tendon sheath. A clinicopathologic study of 32 cases. Amer J Surg Pathol 13:472, 1989.

818. Breimer CW, Freiberger RH: Bone lesions associated with villonodular synovitis. AJR 79:618, 1958.

819. Rydholm U: Pigmented villonodular synovitis of the hip joint. Intern Orthop (SICOT) 11:307, 1987.

820. Smith JH, Pugh DG: Roentgenographic aspects of articular pigmented villonodular synovitis. AJR 87:1146, 1962.

821. Wright CJE: Benign giant-cell synovioma. An investigation of 85 cases. Brit J Surg 38:257, 1951.

822. Danzig LA, Gershuni DH, Resnick D: Diagnosis and treatment of diffuse villonodular synovitis of the hip. Clin Orthop 168:42, 1982.

823. Abrahams TG, Pavlov H, Bansal M, et al: Concentric joint space narrowing of the hip associated with hemosiderotic synovitis (HS) including pigmented villonodular synovitis (PVNS). Skel Radiol 17:37, 1988.

824. Baker ND, Klein JD, Weidner N, et al: Pigmented villonodular synovitis containing coarse calcifications. AJR 153:1228, 1989.

825. Janssens X, Veys EM, Cavelier C: Pigmented villonodular synovitis of the hip—association with osteochondromatosis. Clin Exp Rheumatol 5:329, 1987.

826. Rosenthal DI, Aronow S, Murray WT: Iron content of pigmented villonodular synovitis detected by computed tomography. Radiology 133:409, 1979.

827. Butt WP, Hardy G, Ostlere SJ: Pigmented villonodular synovitis of the knee: computed tomographic appearances. Skel Radiol 19:191, 1990.

828. Keenan WG: Computed tomography in pigmented villonodular synovitis of the hip. J Rheumatol 14:1181, 1987.

829. Spritzer CE, Dalinka MK, Kressel HY: Magnetic resonance imaging of pigmented villonodular synovitis: a report of two cases. Skel Radiol 16:316, 1987.

830. Kottal RA, Vogler JB III, Matamoros A, et al: Pigmented villonodular synovitis: A report of MR imaging in two cases. Radiology 163:551, 1987.

831. Weisz GM, Gal A, Kitchener PN: Magnetic resonance imaging in the diagnosis of aggressive villonodular synovitis. Clin Orthop 236:303, 1988.

832. Jelinek JS, Kransdorf MJ, Utz JA, et al: Imaging of pigmented villonodular synovitis with emphasis on MR imaging. AJR 152:337, 1989.

833. Sundaram M, Chalk D, Merenda J, et al: Case report 563. Skel Radiol 18:463, 1989.

834. Ugai K, Morimoto K: Magnetic resonance imaging of pigmented villonodular synovitis in subtalar joint. Report of a case. Clin Orthop 283:281, 1992.

835. Mandelbaum BR, Grant TT, Hartzman S, et al: The use of MRI to assist in diagnosis of pigmented villonodular synovitis of the knee joint. Clin Orthop 231:135, 1988.

836. Sherry CS, Harms SE: MR evaluation of giant cell tumors of the tendon sheath. Magn Res Imag 7:195, 1989.

837. Morris CS, Betran JL: Giant synovial cyst associated with a pseudarthrosis of a rib: MR appearance. AJR 155:337, 1990.

838. Canoso JJ, Goldsmith MR, Gerzof SG, et al: Foucher's sign of the Baker's cyst. Ann Rheum Dis 46:228, 1987.

839. Pathria MN, Zlatkin M, Sartoris DJ, et al: Ultrasonography of the popliteal fossa and lower extremities. Radiol Clin North Am 26:77, 1988.

840. Hall S, Littlejohn GO, Brand C, et al: The painful swollen calf. A comparative evaluation of four investigative techniques. Med J Austr 144:356, 1986.

841. Szer IS, Klein-Gitelman M, DeNardo BA, et al: Ultrasonography in the study of prevalence and clinical evolution of popliteal cysts in children with knee effusions. J Rheumatol 19:458, 1992.

842. Dungan DH, Seeger LL, Grant EG: Case report 707. Skel Radiol 21:52, 1992.

843. Lieberman JM, Yulish BS, Bryan PJ, et al: Magnetic resonance imaging of ruptured Baker's cyst. J Can Assoc Radiol 39:295, 1988.

844. Molpus WM, Shah HR, Nicholas RW, et al: Case report 731. Skel Radiol 21:266, 1992.

845. Wilson AJ, Ford LT, Gilula LA: Migrating mouse: A sign of dissecting popliteal cyst. AJR 150:867, 1988.

846. Fielding JR, Franklin PD, Kustan J: Popliteal cysts: a reassessment using magnetic resonance imaging. Skel Radiol 20:433, 1991.

847. Burk DL Jr, Dalinka MK, Kanal E, et al: Meniscal and ganglion cysts of the knee: MR evaluation. AJR 150:331, 1988.

848. Voorneveld C, Arenson AM, Fam AG: Anserine bursal distension: diagnosis by ultrasonography and computed tomography. Arthritis Rheum 32:1335, 1989.

849. Hall FM, Joffe N: CT imaging of the anserine bursa. AJR 150:1107, 1988.

850. Jasinski RW, Masselink BA, Partridge RW, et al: Adventitial cystic disease of the popliteal artery. Radiology 163:153, 1987.

851. Chalmers J, Chalmers N: Leg oedema due to a rheumatoid cyst in the pelvis. J Bone Joint Surg [Br] 74:390, 1992.

852. Van Mourik JBA, Josaputra HA, Axler A: Giant synovial cyst causing deep venous thrombosis: Brief report. J Bone Joint Surg [Br] 70:841, 1988.

853. Létourneau L, Dessureault M, Carette S: Rheumatoid iliopsoas bursitis presenting as unilateral femoral nerve palsy. J Rheumatol 18:462, 1991.

854. Toohey AK, La Salle TL, Martinez S, et al: Iliopsoas bursitis: Clinical features, radiographic findings, and disease associations. Semin Arthritis Rheum 20:41, 1990.

855. Varma DGK, Richli WR, Charnsangavej C, et al: MR appearance of the distended iliopsoas bursa. AJR 156:1025, 1991.

856. Haller J, Resnick D, Greenway G, et al: Juxtaacetabular ganglionic (or synovial) cysts: CT and MR features. J Comput Assist Tomogr 13:976, 1989.

857. Silver DAT, Cassar-Pullicino VN, Morrissey BM, et al: Gas-containing ganglia of the hip. Clin Radiol 46:257, 1992.

858. Varma DGK, Parihar A, Richli WR: CT appearance of the distended trochanteric bursa. J Comput Assist Tomogr 17:141, 1993.

859. Allwright SJ, Cooper RA, Nash P: Trochanteric bursitis: Bone scan appearance. Clin Nucl Med 13:561, 1988.

860. Traycoff RB: ''Pseudotrochanteric bursitis'': The differential diagnosis of lateral hip pain. J Rheumatol 18:1810, 1991.

861. Karanjia ND, Stiles PJ: Cubital bursitis. J Bone Joint Surg [Br] 70:832, 1988.

862. Bellon EM, Sacco DC, Steiger DA, et al: Magnetic resonance imaging in ''housemaid's knee'' (prepatellar bursitis). Magn Res Imag 5:175, 1987.

863. Taylor PW: Inflammation of the deep infrapatellar bursa of the knee. Arthritis Rheum 32:1312, 1989.

864. Chauveaux D, Liet P, Le Huec JC, et al: A new radiologic measurement for the diagnosis of Haglund's deformity. Surg Radiol Anat 13:39, 1991.

865. Chew FS, Crenshaw WB: Idiopathic tumoral calcinosis. AJR 158:330, 1992.

866. Resnik CS: Tumoral calcinosis. Arthritis Rheum 32:1484, 1989.

867. Rodriguez-Peralto JL, Lopez-Barea F, Torres A, et al: Tumoral calcinosis in two infants. Clin Orthop 242:272, 1989.

868. Zawin M, Katz LD, Lawson JP: Case report 500. Skel Radiol 17:450, 1988.

869. Gregosiewicz A, Warda E: Tumoral calcinosis: Successful medical treatment. A case report. J Bone Joint Surg [Am] 71:1244, 1989.

870. Croock AD, Silver RM: Tumoral calcinosis presenting as adhesive capsulitis: Case report and literature review. Arthritis Rheum 30:455, 1987.

871. Metzker A, Eisenstein B, Oren J, et al: Tumoral calcinosis revisited—common and uncommon features. Eur J Pediatr 147:128, 1988.

872. Davies MD, Clements MR, Mawer EB, et al: Tumoral calcinosis: Clinical and metabolic response to phosphorus deprivation. Quart J Med 242:493, 1987.

873. Martinez S, Vogler JB III, Harrelson JM, et al: Imaging of tumoral calcinosis: New observations. Radiology 174:215, 1990.

874. Lagier R, Gerster J-C: Disabling ossification of the patellar tendon. Ann Rheum Dis 50:338, 1991.

875. Kelly MA, Insall JN: Postpatellectomy extensive ossification of patellar tendon. A case report. Clin Orthop 215:148, 1987.

876. Puzas JE, Miller MD, Rosier RN: Pathologic bone formation. Clin Orthop 245:269, 1989.

877. Garland DE: A clinical perspective on common forms of acquired heterotopic ossification. Clin Orthop 263:13, 1991.

878. Kirkpatrick JS, Koman LA, Rovere GD: The role of ultrasound in the early diagnosis of myositis ossificans. A case report. Amer J Sports Med 15:179, 1987.

879. Peck RJ, Metreweli C: Early myositis ossificans: a new echographic sign. Clin Radiol 39:586, 1988.

880. Bressler EL, Marn CS, Gore RM, et al: Evaluation of ectopic bone by CT. AJR 148:931, 1987.

881. Laurin NR, Powe JE, Pavlosky WF, et al: Multimodality imaging of early heterotopic bone formation. J Canad Assoc Radiol 41:93, 1990.

882. Ackerman L, Ramamurthy S, Jablokow V, et al: Case report 488. Skel Radiol 17:310, 1988.

883. Ehara S, Nakasato T, Tamakawa Y, et al: MRI of myositis ossificans circumscripta. Clin Imag 15:130, 1991.

884. Kransdorf MJ, Meis JM, Jelinek JS: Myositis ossificans: MR appearance with radiologic-pathologic correlation. AJR 157:1243, 1991.

885. DeSmet AA, Norris MA, Fisher DR: Magnetic resonance imaging of myositis ossificans: analysis of seven cases. Skel Radiol 21:503, 1992.

886. Barea FL, Peralto JLR, López JG, et al: Case report 694. Skel Radiol 20:539, 1991.

887. Schütte HE, van der Heul RO: Pseudomalignant, nonneoplastic osseous soft-tissue tumors of the hand and foot. Radiology 176:149, 1990.

888. Nuovo MA, Norman A, Chumas A, et al: Myositis ossificans with atypical clinical, radiographic, or pathologic findings: A review of 23 cases. Skel Radiol 21:87, 1992.

889. Nash S, Rubenstein J, Morava-Protzner I: Case report 766. Skel Radiol 22:55, 1993.

890. Rööser B, Herrlin K, Rydholm A, et al: Pseudomalignant myositis ossificans. Clinical, radiologic, and cytologic diagnosis in 5 cases. Acta Orthop Scand 60:457, 1989.

891. Spencer JD, Missen GAK: Pseudomalignant heterotopic ossification (''myositis ossificans''). Recurrence after excision with subsequent resorption. J Bone Joint Surg [Br] 71:317, 1989.

892. Tatu WF, Phillips CD, Gurdak RG, et al: Heterotopic chondro-ossification: A case report. J Can Assoc Radiol 38:234, 1987.

893. Dupree WB, Enzinger FM: Fibro-osseous pseudotumor of the digits. Cancer 58:2103, 1986.

894. Kai Y, Masuda S, Ushijima M, et al: Pseudomalignant myositis ossificans occurring in the hand. J Hand Surg [Am] 12:634, 1987.

895. Holmes WS, Pope TL Jr, de Lange E, et al: Case report 413. Skel Radiol 16:163, 1987.

896. Yuen WF, Friedman L, Orr W, et al: Proliferative periosteal processes of phalanges: a unitary hypothesis. Skel Radiol 21:301, 1992.

897. Nora FE, Dahlin DC, Beabout JW: Bizarre parosteal osteochondromatous proliferation of the hands and feet. Am J Surg Pathol 7:245, 1983.

898. Cohen RB, Hahn GV, Tabas JA, et al: The natural history of heterotopic ossification in patients who have fibrodysplasia ossificans progressive. A study of forty-four patients. J Bone Joint Surg [Am] 75:215, 1993.

899. Kaplan FS, Tabas JA, Gannon FH, et al: The histopathology of fibrodysplasia ossificans progressiva. An endochondral process. J Bone Joint Surg [Am] 75:220, 1993.

900. Nunnelly JF, Yussen PS: Computed tomographic findings in patients with limited jaw movement due to myositis ossificans progressiva. J Oral Maxillofac Surg 44:818, 1986.

901. Kabala JE, Watt I, Hollingworth P, et al: Case report: Trismus and multifocal soft tissue ossification. A presentation of fibrodysplasia ossificans progressiva? Clin Radiol 40:523, 1989.

902. Caron KH, DiPietro MA, Aisen AM, et al: MR imaging of early fibrodysplasia ossificans progressiva. J Comput Assist Tomogr 14:318, 1990.

903. Greene WB: One-stage release of congenital circumferential constriction bands. J Bone Joint Surg [Am] 75:650, 1993.

904. Steinberg B, Saunders V: Popliteal pterygium syndrome. Oral Surg Med Pathol 63:17, 1987.

905. Oppenheim WL, Larson KR, McNabb MBB, et al: Popliteal pterygium syndrome: An orthopedic perspective. J Pediatr Orthop 10:58, 1990.

906. Yacoe ME, Bergman AG, Ladd AL, et al: Dupuytren's contracture: MR imaging findings and correlation between MR signal intensity and cellularity of lesions. AJR 160:813, 1993.

907. Kazerooni E, Hessler C: CT appearance of angiosarcoma associated with chronic lymphedema. AJR 156:543, 1991.

908. Vaughan BF: CT of swollen legs. Clin Radiol 41:24, 1990.

909. Duewell S, Hagspiel KD, Zuber J, et al: Swollen lower extremity: Role of MR imaging. Radiology 184:227, 1992.

910. Case TC, Witte CL, Witte MH, et al: Magnetic resonance imaging in human lymphedema: Comparison with lymphangioscintigraphy. Magn Res Imag 10:549, 1992.

911. Paajanen H, Brasch RC, Schmiedl U, et al: Magnetic resonance imaging of local soft tissue inflammation using gadolinium-DTPA. Acta Radiol Diagn 28:79, 1987.

912. Donaldson JS: Radiographic imaging of foreign bodies in the hand. Hand Clin 7:125, 1991.

913. Torfing KF, Teisen HG, Skjødt T: Computed tomography, ultrasonography and plain radiography in the detection of foreign bodies in pork muscle tissue. Fortschr Rongenstr 149:60, 1988.

914. Bodne D, Quinn SF, Cochran CF: Imaging foreign glass and wooden bodies of the extremities with CT and MR. J Comput Assist Tomogr 12:608, 1988.

915. Peters V, Rubin L, Gloster ES, et al: Foreign-body osteitis of the metacarpal bone. Clin Orthop 278:69, 1992.

916. Kobs JK, Hansen AR, Keefe B: A retained wooded foreign body in the foot detected by ultrasonography. A case report. J Bone Joint Surg [Am] 74:296, 1992.

917. Hansson G, Beebe AC, Carroll NC, et al: A piece of wood in the hand diagnosed by ultrasonography. Acta Orthop Scand 59:459, 1988.

918. Ramanathan EBS, Luiz CPJ: Date palm thorn synovitis. J Bone Joint Surg [Br] 72:512, 1990.

919. Doig SG, Cole WG: Plant thorn synovitis. Resolution following total synovectomy. J Bone Joint Surg [Br] 72:514, 1990.

920. Goupille P, Fouquet B, Favard L, et al: Two cases of plant thorn synovitis. Difficulties in diagnosis and treatment. J Rheumatol 17:252, 1990.

921. Larbre F, Louis J-J, Berard J, et al: Les arthrites a piquants vegetaux de l'enfant. A propos de Ce observations personelles. Pediatrie 41:601, 1986.

922. Reginato AJ, Ferreiro JL, O'Connor CR, et al: Clinical and pathologic studies of twenty-six patients with penetrating foreign body injury to the joints, bursae, and tendon sheaths. Arthritis Rheum 33:1753, 1990.

923. Abdul-Karim FW, Benevenia J, Pathria MN, et al: Case report 736. Skel Radiol 21:466, 1992.

924. Galuten A, Austin JHM: Permanent subcutaneous acupuncture needles: Radiographic manifestations. J Can Assoc Radiol 39:54, 1988.

925. Kalen V, Burwell DS, Omer GE: Macrodactyly of the hands and feet. J Pediatr Orthop 8:311, 1988.

926. Greenberg BM, Pess GM, May JW Jr: Macrodactyly and the epidermal nevus syndrome. J Hand Surg [Am] 12:730, 1987.

927. Wiedemann HR, Burgio GR, Aldenhoff P, et al: The Proteus syndrome. Eur J Pediatr 140:5, 1983.

928. Burgio GR, Wiedemann HR: Further and new details on the Proteus syndrome. Eur J Pediatr 143:71, 1984.

929. Costa T, Fitch N, Azouz EM: Proteus syndrome: Report of two cases with pelvic lipomatosis. Pediatr 76:984, 1985.

930. Vaughn RY, Howell CG, Parrish RA, et al: Proteus syndrome: Diagnosis and surgical management. J Pediatr Surg 28:5, 1993.

931. Azouz EM, Costa T, Fitch N: Radiologic findings in the Proteus syndrome. Pediatr Radiol 17:481, 1987.

932. Guy GE, Dorfman GS, Saskin H, et al: Case report 514. Skel Radiol 17:603, 1989.

933. Nishimura G, Kozlowski K: Proteus syndrome (report of three cases). Australas Radiol 34:47, 1990.

934. Wiedemann HR, Burgio GR, Aldenhoff P, et al. The proteus syndrome. Eur J Pediatr 140:5, 1983.

935. Burnstein MI, Kottamasu SR, Weiss L, et al: Case report 509. Skel Radiol 17:536, 1988.

936. Viljoen DL, Saxe N, Temple-Camp C: Cutaneous manifestations of the Proteus syndrome. Pediatr Dermatol 5:14, 1988.

937. Bialer MG, Riedy MJ, Wilson WG: Proteus syndrome versus Bannayan-Zonona syndrome: A problem in differential diagnosis. Eur J Pediatr 148:92, 1988.

938. Okumura K, Sasaki Y, Ohyama M, et al: Bannayan syndrome: generalized lipomatosis associated with megalencephaly and macrodactyly. Acta Pathol Jpn 36:269, 1986.

939. Tibbles JAR, Cohen MM Jr: The Proteus syndrome: the Elephant Man diagnosed. Brit Med J 293:683, 1986.

940. Panicek DM, Leeson SH: Superficial fascial calcification in epidermolysis bullosa. AJR 148:577, 1987.

941. Wong WL, Pemberton J: The musculoskeletal manifestations of epidermolysis bullosa: an analysis of 19 cases with a review of the literature. Brit J Radiol 65:480, 1992.

942. Lentz SR, Raish RJ, Orlowski EP, et al: Squamous cell carcinoma in epidermolysis bullosa. Treatment with systemic chemotherapy. Cancer 66:1276, 1990.

943. Yamauchi Y, Takahashi K, Shiotsu H: Osteogenic sarcoma of the tibia in a patient with epidermolysis bullosa dystrophica. Clin Orthop 228:273, 1988.

944. Gorlin RJ: Nevoid basal-cell carcinoma syndrome. Medicine 66:98, 1987.

945. Crawford SC, Boyer RS, Harnsberger HR, et al: Disorders of histogenesis: The neurocutaneous syndromes. Semin Ultrasound CT MR 9:247, 1988.

946. Gellis SS, Feingold M: Rothmund Thomson syndrome. Am J Dis Child 132:619, 1978.

947. Hall JG, Pagon RA, Wilson KM: Rothmund Thomson syndrome with severe dwarfism. Am J Dis Child 134:165, 1980.

948. Baró PR, Bastart FM, Bartrina JR, et al: Case report 529. Skel Radiol 18:136, 1989.

949. Kozlowski K, Scougall JS, Oates RK: Osteosarcoma in a boy with Rothmund Thomson syndrome. Pediatr Radiol 10:42, 1980.

950. Conway SP, Smithells RW, Peters WM: Weber-Christian panniculitis. Ann Rheum Dis 46:339, 1987.

951. Jenkins EA, Cawley MID: Infantile myofibromatosis: A cause of severe bone pain in a neonate. Brit J Rheumatol 32:849, 1993.

952. Bansal M, Goldman AB, DiCarlo EF, et al: Soft tissue chondromas: diagnosis and differential diagnosis. Skel Radiol 22:309, 1993.

953. Sundaram M, Percelay S, McDonald DJ, et al: Case report 799. Skel Radiol 22:449, 1993.

954. Kransdorf MJ, Meis JM: Extraskeletal osseous and cartilaginous tumors of the extremities. RadioGraphics 13:853, 1993.

955. Varma DGK, Ayala AG, Guo S-Q, et al: MRI of extraskeletal osteosarcoma. J Comput Assist Tomogr 17:414, 1993.

956. Jones BC, Sundaram M, Kransdorf MJ: Synovial sarcoma: MR imaging findings in 34 patients. AJR 161:827, 1993.

957. Hermann G, Abdelwahab IF, Klein MJ, et al: Case report 796. Skel Radiol 22:386, 1993.

958. Hiller N, Fisher D, Gottschalk-Sabag S, et al: Case report 809. Skel Radiol 22:539, 1993.

959. Kobayashi H, Sakahara H, Hosono M, et al: Soft-tissue tumors: Diagnosis with Tc-99m (V) dimercaptosuccinic acid scintigraphy. Radiology 190:277, 1994.

960. Sostman HD, Prescott DM, Dewhirst MW, et al: MR imaging and spectroscopy for prognostic evaluation in soft-tissue sarcomas. Radiology 190:269, 1994.

961. Vanel D, Shapeero LG, DeBaere T, et al: MR imaging in the follow-up of malignant and aggressive soft-tissue tumors: Results of 511 examinations. Radiology 190:263, 1994.

962. Kransdorf MJ, Meis JM, Jelinek JS: Dedifferentiated liposarcoma of the extremities: Imaging findings in four patients. AJR 161:127, 1993.

963. Ippolito V, Brien EW, Menendez LR, et al: Case report 797. Skeletal Radiol 22:604, 1993.

964. Declercq H, Man RD, Van Herck G, et al: Case report 814. Skeletal Radiol 22:610, 1993.

965. Cavallaro MC, Taylor JAM, Gorman JD, et al: Imaging findings in a patient with fibrolipomatous hamartoma of the median nerve. AJR 161:837, 1993.

966. Yao L, Toranji S, Doberneck SA, et al: Case report 818. Skeletal Radiol 23:217, 1994.

967. van Kints MJ, Tham TA Vroegindeweij D, et al: Magnetic resonance imaging findings in aggressive fibromatosis. Eur J Radiol 16:230, 1993.

968. Gober GA, Nicholas RW: Case report 800. Skeletal Radiol 22:452, 1993.

969. Ehara S, Sone M, Tamakawa Y, et al: Fluid-fluid levels in cavernous hemangioma of soft tissue. Skeletal Radiol 23:107, 1994.

970. Kramer J, Recht M, Deely DM, et al: MR appearance of idiopathic synovial osteochondromatosis. J Comput Assist Tomogr 17:772, 1993.

971. Edeiken J, Edeiken BS, Ayala AG, et al: Giant solitary synovial chondromatosis. Skeletal Radiol 23:23, 1994.

972. Bianchi S, Abdelwahab IF, Zwass A, et al: Ultrasonographic evaluation of wrist ganglia. Skeletal Radiol 23:201, 1994.

973. Kenan S, Abdelwahab IF, Klein MJ, et al: Case report 817. Skeletal Radiol 22:623, 1993.

974. Whitten CG, El-Khoury GY, Benda JA, et al: Case report 829. Skeletal Radiol 23:153, 1994.

975. Sullivan TP, Seeger LL, Doberneck SA, et al: Case report 828. Skeletal Radiol 23:149, 1994.

976. Seynaeve P, Mortelmans L, Kockx M, et al: Case report 813. Skeletal Radiol 23:137, 1994.

977. Bronstein RD, Sebastianelli WJ, DeHaven KE: Localized pigmented villonodular synovitis presenting as a loose body in the knee. J Arthrosc Rel Surg 9:596, 1993.

978. Jelinek JS, Kransdorf MJ, Schmookler BM, et al: Giant cell tumor of the tendon sheath: MR findings in nine cases. AJR 162:919, 1994.

979. Gardner RJ, Yun K, Craw SM: Familial ectopic ossification. J Med Genet 25:113, 1988.

980. Kaplan FS, Craver R, MacEwen GD, et al: Progressive osseous heteroplasia: A distinct developmental disorder of heterotopic ossification. J Bone Joint Surg [Am] 76:425, 1994.

INDEX

Note: Page numbers in *italics* refer to illustrations;
page numbers followed by (t) refer to tables.